HEAD AND NECK IMAGING CASES

The McGraw-Hill Radiology Series

Series Editor: Robert J. Ward, MD

This innovative series offers indispensable workstation reference material for the practicing radiologist. Within this series is a full range of practical, clinically relevant works divided into three categories:

- **Patterns:** Organized by modality, these books provide a pattern-based approach to constructing practical differential diagnoses.
- **Variants:** Structured by modality as well as anatomy, these graphic volumes aid the radiologist in reducing false positive rates.
- **Cases:** Classic case presentations with an emphasis on differential diagnoses and clinical context.

HEAD AND NECK IMAGING CASES

Osamu Sakai, MD, PhD
Chief of Neuroradiology
Professor of Radiology
Boston Medical Center
Boston University School of Medicine
Boston, Massachusetts

McGraw Hill Medical

New York Chicago San Francisco Lisbon London Madrid Mexico City
Milan New Delhi San Juan Seoul Singapore Sydney Toronto

The McGraw-Hill Companies

Head and Neck Imaging Cases

1 2 3 4 5 6 7 8 9 0 CTP/CTP 15 14 13 12 11

ISBN 978-0-07-154372-9
MHID 0-07-154372-4

This book was set in TradeGothic by Glyph International.
The editors were Michael Weitz and Christine Diedrich.
The production supervisor was Catherine Saggese.
Project management was provided by Vastavikta Sharma, Glyph International.
China Translation & Printing Services, Ltd. was printer and binder.

Library of Congress Cataloging-in-Publication Data

Head and neck imaging cases / [edited by] Osamu Sakai.
p. ; cm.
Includes index.
ISBN-13: 978-0-07-154372-9 (hard cover : alk. paper)
ISBN-10: 0-07-154372-4 (hard cover : alk. paper)
1. Head—Imaging—Case studies. 2. Neck—Imaging—Case studies. I. Sakai, Osamu.
[DNLM: 1. Head—radiography—Case Reports. 2. Neck--radiography—Case Reports. 3. Diagnosis, Differential—Case Reports. 4. Diagnostic Imaging—methods—Case Reports. 5. Otorhinolaryngologic Diseases—diagnosis—Case Reports. 6. Stomatognathic Diseases—diagnosis—Case Reports. WE 705]
RC936.H429 2011
617.5′10754—dc22

2011004190

To my wife, Mariko, and our sons, Yu and Shun.
Thank you very much for your encouragement,
unconditional support, and patience.

Each Case Highlights Findings, Differential Diagnoses, and Comments

Icons are used to create a grading system

The innovative grading system indicates the degree to which the images are representative of a case's typical appearance. The scale ranges from "typical" (five circles) to "rare" (one circle). Similarly, the differential diagnoses images are graded "common" (five squares) to "unusual" (one square). The aim is to provide the reader with a sense of appropriateness regarding the practical use of differential diagnoses.

IMAGE KEY

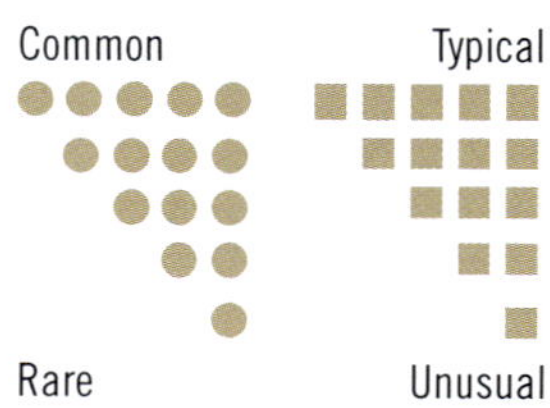

CONTENTS

Chapter 6: Suprahyoid Neck 537

Chapter 7: Salivary Gland 645

CONTRIBUTORS

Yoshinao Abe, MD, PhD
Professor and Chairman
Hirosaki University School of Medicine
Hirosaki, Japan

Ankit Agarwal
Research Scholar
Department of Radiology
Boston University School of Medicine
Boston, Massachusetts

Andrew Akman, MD, MBA
Clinical Instructor
Department of Radiology
Johns Hopkins Hospital
Baltimore, Maryland

Kurtis G. Birch
Student
Boston University School of Medicine
Boston, Massachusetts

Ilse Castro-Aragon, MD
Assistant Professor
Section Head Pediatric Radiology
Department of Radiology
Boston Medical Center
Boston University School of Medicine
Boston, Massachusetts

Margaret N. Chapman, MD
Resident
Department of Radiology
Boston Medical Center
Boston, Massachusetts

June F. Cheng, MD
Neuroradiology Fellow
Department of Radiology
Brigham and Women's Hospital
Boston, Massachusetts

Lawrence S. Chin, MD
Professor and Chair
Department of Neurosurgery
Boston University School of Medicine
Neurosurgeon-in-Chief
Boston Medical Center
Boston, Massachusetts

Francisco J. Contreras, MD, MS
Resident
Department of Radiology
Boston Medical Center
Boston, Massachusetts

Jessica Davison
Student
Boston University School of Medicine
Boston, Massachusetts

Brooke Devenney-Cakir, MD
Resident
Department of Radiology
Boston Medical Center
Boston, Massachusetts
Neuroradiology fellow
Department of Radiology
Hospital of the University of Pennsylvania
Philadelphia, Pennsylvania

Kevin P. Donahue, MD
Resident
Department of Radiology
Boston Medical Center
Boston, Massachusetts

Keith White Fleming, MDCM
Chief of Radiology
Radiology Specialists of Maine
Mid Coast Hospital and Parkview Adventist Medical Center
Brunswick, Maine

Dan C. Filitis, MA
Research Scholar
Department of Radiology
Boston University School of Medicine
Boston, Massachusetts

Elisa N. Flower, MD
Neuroradiology fellow
Department of Radiology
Boston Medical Center
Boston, Massachusetts

Akifumi Fujita, MD
Assistant Professor
Department of Radiology
Jichi Medical University School of Medicine
Shimotsuke, Tochigi, Japan

Anita Gohel, BDS, PhD
Associate Professor and Director
Oral Diagnosis and Radiology
Boston University
Henry M. Goldman School of Dental Medicine
Boston, Massachusetts

Carlos J. González, MD
Resident
Department of Radiology
Boston Medical Center
Boston, Massachusetts

Francois Guilbert, MD
Department of Radiology
Centre Hospitalier de'l Université de Montréal
Montreal, Canada

Rania Hito, MD
Resident
Department of Radiology
Boston Medical Center
Boston, Massachusetts

Hideki Hyodoh, MD, PhD
Assistant Professor
Department of Radiology
Sapporo Medical University School of Medicine
Sapporo, Japan
Visiting Professor
University of Belgrade
Belgrade, Serbia

Mayur Jayarao, MD, MSc
Department of Neurological Surgery
Boston Medical Center
Boston, Massachusetts

Junaid Kalia, MD
Department of Neurology
Medical College of Wisconsin and Froedtert Hospital
Milwaukee, Wisconsin

Takashi Kaneda, DDS, PhD
Professor and Chief
Department of Radiology
Nihon University School of Dentistry
Matsudo, Chiba, Japan

Hiroki Kato, MD
Assistant Professor
Department of Radiology
Gifu University School of Medicine
Gifu City, Japan

Shigeyoshi Kijima, MD
Resident
Department of Radiology
Jichi Medical University School of Medicine
Shimotsuke, Tochigi, Japan

John Kim, MD
Resident
Department of Radiology
Boston Medical Center
Boston, Massachusetts

Yukio Kimura, MD
Resident
Department of Radiology
Jichi Medical University School of Medicine
Shimotsuke, Tochigi, Japan

Takao Kodama, MD, PhD
Associate Professor
Department of Radiology
Faculty of Medicine
University of Miyazaki
Miyazaki, Japan

David Kozono, MD, PhD
Resident
Harvard Radiation Oncology Program
Boston, Massachusetts

Susan E. Langmore, PhD, CCC-SLP
Professor
Otolaryngology - Head and Neck Surgery
Boston Medical Center
Clinical Professor
Speech Language Hearing Sciences
Boston University
Boston, Massachusetts

Christina A. LeBedis, MSc, MD
Instructor
Department of Radiology
Boston Medical Center
Boston University School of Medicine
Boston, Massachusetts

Benjamin J. Ludwig, MD
Resident
Department of Radiology
Boston Medical Center
Boston, Massachusetts

Mostafa Mahmoud, MD
Assistant Professor
Department of Radiology
University of Ain Shams
Cairo, Egypt

Danielle Margalit, MD, MPH
Resident
Harvard Radiation Oncology Program
Boston, Massachusetts

Amol R. Mehta
Student
Department of Neuroscience
Boston University
Research Scholar
Department of Radiology
Boston University School of Medicine
Boston, Massachusetts

Asim Mian, MD
Assistant Professor
Department of Radiology
Boston Medical Center
Boston University School of Medicine
Boston, Massachusetts

Gabriel Monagas, MD
Resident
Department of Radiology
Boston Medical Center
Boston, Massachusetts

Akira M. Murakami, MD
Instructor
Department of Radiology
Boston Medical Center
Boston University School of Medicine
Boston, Massachusetts

Rohini Nadgir, MD
Assistant Professor
Department of Radiology
Boston Medical Center
Boston University School of Medicine
Boston, Massachusetts

Morio Nagahata, MD, PhD
Lecturer
Department of Radiology and Radiation Oncology
Hirosaki University Graduate School of Medicine
Instructor of the Neuroendovascular Therapy
Hirosaki University Hospital
Hirosaki, Aomori, Japan

Thanh Nguyen, MD, FRCPc
Assistant Professor
Department of Neurology, Neurosurgery, Radiology
Boston Medical Center
Boston University School of Medicine
Boston, Massachusetts

Alexander Norbash, MD, MHCM
Professor and Chair
Department of Radiology
Boston Medical Center
Boston University School of Medicine
Boston, Massachusetts

Jean Raymond, MD
Professor
Department of Radiology
Faculty of Medicine
Université de Montréal
Neuroradiologist
Department of Radiology
Centre hospitalier de l'Université de Montréal
Hôpital Notre-Dame
Montreal, Quebec, Canada

Susmitha Reddy, MBBS, MRCPCH, FRCR
Neuroradiology fellow
Department of Radiology
Boston Medical Center
Boston, Massachusetts

Paul B. Romesser, BA
Student
Boston University School of Medicine
Boston, Massachusetts

Daniel Roy, MD, FRCP
Professor
Department of Radiology
Radio Oncology and Nuclear Medicine
University of Montreal
Neuroradiologist
Montreal, Quebec, Canada

Timothy W. Ryan, MA
Research Scholar
Department of Radiology
Boston University School of Medicine
Boston, Massachusetts

Ari Sacks, MD
Intern
Carney Hospital
Dorchester, Massachusetts

Naoko Saito, MD, PhD
Assistant Professor
Department of Radiology
Saitama International Medical Center
Saitama Medical University
Saitama, Japan

Osamu Sakai, MD, PhD
Professor
Chief of Neuroradiology
Department of Radiology
Boston Medical Center
Boston University School of Medicine
Boston, Massachusetts

Atsuko Sakamoto, MD
Resident
Department of Radiology
Jichi Medical University School of Medicine
Shimotsuke, Tochigi, Japan

Yosuke Sato, MD
Resident
Department of Radiology
Jichi Medical University School of Medicine
Yakushiji, Shimotsuke, Tochigi, Japan

Bhavya Shah, MD
Resident
Department of Radiology
Boston Medical Center
Boston, Massachusetts

Cory Siegel, MD
Resident
Department of Radiology
Boston Medical Center
Boston, Massachusetts

Paramjit Singh, BS
Student
Boston University School of Medicine
Boston, Massachusetts

Rathan Subramaniam, MD, PhD, FRANZCR
Associate Professor
Department of Radiology
Boston Medical Center
Boston University School of Medicine
Boston, Massachusetts

Devaki Shilpa Sudha Surasi, MBBS
Research Fellow
Molecular Imaging and Nuclear Medicine
Department of Radiology
Boston Medical Center
Boston, Massachusetts

Misako Takeuchi, MD
Resident
Department of Radiology
Jichi Medical University School of Medicine
Shimotsuke, Tochigi, Japan

Minh Tam Truong, MD
Assistant Professor
Department of Radiology
Boston Medical Center
Boston University School of Medicine
Attending Radiation Oncologist
Department of Radiation Oncology
Boston Medical Center
Lecturer
Harvard Medical School
Assistant Radiation Oncologist
Massachusetts General Hospital
Boston, Massachusetts

Jimmy W. Wang, MD
Assistant Professor
Department of Radiology
Boston Medical Center
Boston University School of Medicine
Boston, Massachusetts

Memi Watanabe, MD
Research Scholar
Department of Radiology
Boston Medical Center
Boston University School of Medicine
Boston, Massachusetts

Alain Weill, MD, FRCPC
Professor of Radiology
Centre Hospitalier de l'Université de Montréal
Montreal, Canada

Daniel Weller, MD
Radiologist
Department of Radiology
St. Luke's Hospital Southcoast Hospital Group
New Bedford, Massachusetts

Osama O. Zaidat, MD, MS, FAHA, FAAN
Professor of Neurology
Neurosurgery and Radiology at Medical College of Wisconsin
Director
Neurointerventional Program Froedtert Hospital
Milwaukee, Wisconsin

FOREWORD

Head and neck imaging on interpretation combine an understanding of the anatomy with an accumulation of practical clinical experience. The only way to learn the anatomy is to sit down with a series of images and an anatomy book and follow various structures from slice to slice. Soon the anatomic relationships that allow a practical and, therefore, very helpful interpretation will become familiar and will help organize the approach to the task at hand. The more one studies these relationships, the more comfortable one becomes to give an effective challenge. Once there is a familiarity with the anatomy, the radiologist needs practical experience. Dr. Osamu Sakai's book provides a substantial experience that in most cases is very tightly connected to the anatomy. By the end of the book, the reader will be exposed to almost everything that he or she needs to know to practice head and neck radiology.

I have known Dr. Sakai for a long time. I had the pleasure of working with Osamu during his fellowship with us at the Massachusetts Eye and Ear Infirmary early in his career. Actually, it was not that early—Osamu had already done his training in Japan and came to us with a very good knowledge of the field. His natural abilities as a teacher were already evident. The most impressive thing about Osamu was his constant focus on the practical information hiding within an imaging study. He wanted to know the two or three things about each study that made a difference to the diagnosis or to the treatment plan. Of course he was curious about some of the more abstract aspects of a disease, but he always would come back to the single question, "What do we need to know?" His constant pursuit of that single question is the generative force that has evolved into this book.

This book follows very obviously from his direct practical approach. Each case focuses on a particular diagnosis and tells the reader the specific points that need to be considered to bring out the maximum amount of useful information. What is associated with the diagnosis? What are the most likely alternative diagnoses to be considered? The reader will certainly notice that the anatomy figures very prominently into the analysis of almost every case. If you can be precise about the anatomy, there are usually only a few potential diagnostic considerations. Move the location a centimeter or two, and the list of possibilities changes dramatically. Dr. Sakai's approach brings this concept into clear focus.

Each case in this book will bring the reader closer to the comfort zone for reading head and neck imaging. This book will be valuable to the student needing an initial exposure to head and neck. It will be valuable to the experienced radiologist seeking a bit more familiarity with this sometimes difficult field. The points made in the book are important information. They are what the radiologist needs to know.

I do think that the anatomy is important enough that any student should spend time just going through images, anatomy book in hand, identifying more and more structures. Then, to get the practical experience, read this book. If at the end you think that you need more experience to feel comfortable, read it again.

Hugh D. Curtin MD, FACR
Professor of Radiology
Harvard Medical School
Chief of Radiology
Massachusetts Eye and Ear Infirmary
Boston, Massachusetts

SERIES EDITOR'S FOREWORD

It is with great pleasure that I introduce our Head and Neck Imaging Cases volume. Osamu Sakai is a remarkably talented author who has labored to bring an outstanding breadth and depth of case material that encompasses the most essential head and neck imaging.

The text is organized systematcially for easy navigation and accessibility. Each case explores common presentations of the entity followed by typical imaging findings, differential diagnoses, a comments section, and useful pearls. The images are strategically formatted with the "index image" (the entity's most representative example) on the left and additional images on the right. A useful and practical differential diagnosis section follows.

The innovative grading system indicates the degree to which the images are representative of a case's typical appearance. The scale ranges from "typical" (five circles) to "rare" (one circle). Similarly, the differential diagnosis images are graded "common" (five squares) to "unusual" (one square). The aim is to provide a reader with a sense of appropriateness regarding the practical use of differential diagnoses.

Our ultimate aim for the series is to create a practical resource for radiologists at the workstation to reference on a regular basis. Please look forward to future Case editions as well as the corresponding Patterns and Variants volumes.

Congratulations to Dr. Sakai and his contributors. They have done an exemplary job in creating a practical and comprehensive work.

Robert J. Ward, MD, CCD
Series Executive Editor

Chief, Division of Musculoskeletal Radiology
Department of Radiology
Tufts Medical Center
Residency Associate Program Director
Director, Medical Student Education
Assistant Professor of Radiology and Orthopaedics
Tufts University School of Medicine
Boston, Massachusetts

Consultant
Sullivan's Island Imaging, LLC
Sullivan's Island, South Carolina

PREFACE

Many radiologists and physicians in other specialties may not be comfortable with head and neck imaging because of the complex head and neck anatomy and various pathologies. There are many structures in this small area, and understanding the fascia-defined spaces is challenging. Further, a few millimeter difference in disease extension may dramatically change the management. Radiology residents spend a great amount of time and energy learning head and neck imaging, and residents in surgical specialties struggle to integrate surgical and radiological anatomy. It is true that head and neck imaging is not easy for most radiologists, even for neuroradiologists.

This book *Head and Neck Imaging Cases* is written to pull head and neck imaging a few feet closer to you. You will become familiar with imaging findings of various head and neck diseases and conditions. This book covers common head and neck diseases and conditions we encounter in the daily practice, and also diseases, although rare, which have typical imaging findings to make a histological diagnosis. Further, normal variants and benign conditions which should not be mistaken as real abnormalities or malignancies are also included. Cases in this book are excellent materials to learn head and neck imaging easily, with visually attractive images and brief descriptions of the essences of the disease or condition. *Findings* gives you typical imaging findings of each case. *Differential Diagnoses* helps you consider other possibilities based on clinical presentation and imaging findings. *Comments* provide relevant background and essences of the disease or condition. *Pearls* are the core learning points of the case, which are exactly what I have been teaching to our residents and fellows in the daily practice. CT and MRI are the main modalities throughout this book, just like most practices. In addition, this book includes cases of fluoroscopy, PET-CT, conventional angiogram/interventional radiology, and radiotherapy in the head and neck. I believe familiarity with other modalities is helpful for radiologists to understand the real practice of head and neck imaging.

This book was intended to be a good resource for radiologists in practice initially. But I believe this reference will also be helpful for radiologists in training, as well as physicians and surgeons in other specialties, such as otolaryngology—head and neck surgery, ophthalmology, oral maxillofacial surgery, neurosurgery, neurology, and radiation oncology. It is impossible to master all aspects of head and neck imaging from a single book. But I hope this book will help you become more familiar with head and neck imaging, and more importantly will help you contribute to your patient's care through imaging.

ACKNOWLEDGMENTS

This book, *Head and Neck Imaging Cases*, would not have been possible without the inspiration and support from all of my mentors, former and current colleagues, and fellows and residents in and outside of radiology. I am especially thankful to Dr. Hideharu Sugimoto, Professor and Chairman of Radiology at Jichi Medical University, for mentoring me throughout my residency and instilling in me the importance of teaching others what I have learned. "We live on medicine," he said. "Experience and knowledge learned through practice should be shared with colleagues and given back to society." I am also very grateful to Dr. Hugh D. Curtin, Professor of Radiology at Harvard Medical School and Chief of Radiology at Massachusetts Eye and Ear Infirmary, for mentoring and teaching me the essentials of head and neck imaging. Dr. Curtin will forever be my teacher and is a true role model for all head and neck radiologists.

I thank Mr. Michael Weitz, Ms. Christine Diedrich, and all members of McGraw-Hill assigned to this book, as well as Dr. Robert Ward, Series Executive Editor, for their support and encouragement during the entire publishing process.

Last but not the least, I am indebted to the patients I have had the privilege of serving over the years. I have learned so much from them, and I sincerely thank them for all they have taught me.

Chapter 1

TEMPORAL BONES

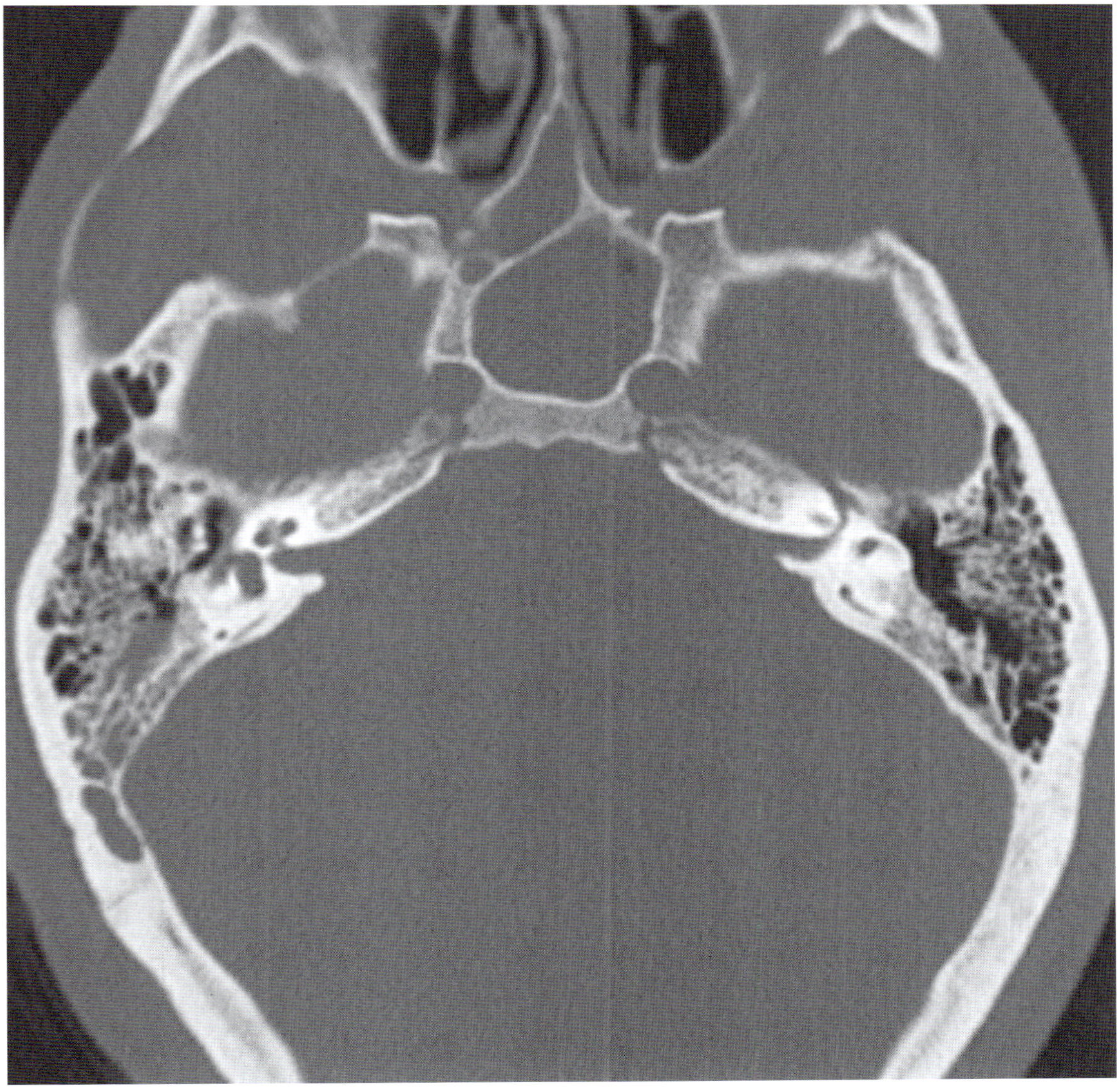

Case 1–1 Acute Otitis Media

Osamu Sakai, Keith Fleming

PRESENTATION

Acute onset of fever, ear pain, and middle ear effusion.

FINDINGS

Computed tomography (CT) demonstrates opacification of the tympanic cavity and mastoid air cells.

DIFFERENTIAL DIAGNOSIS

- Chronic otitis media: This condition demonstrates poor pneumatization of the petrous temporal bone and mastoid process, as well as sclerotic changes of the mastoid air cells.
- Langerhans cell histiocytosis: This is a rare condition generally seen in children. The clinical presentation may be similar to otitis media. Bone destruction and enhancing soft tissue are typical.
- Rhabdomyosarcoma: Clinically, this tumor can mimic otitis media. Patients often develop cranial nerve palsy and CT generally demonstrates aggressive bone destruction.

COMMENTS

This is a 10-year-old boy with ear pain and middle ear effusion.

Serous otitis media is a condition resulting in fluid accumulation in the tympanic cavity due to eustachian tube dysfunction. The eustachian tube is generally obstructed in the setting of viral or bacterial upper respiratory infection. This is the most common cause of hearing loss in children.

On CT, opacification of the tympanic cavity and pneumatized mastoid air cells is noted without erosion of the ossicles. There is no sclerosis or poor pneumatization of the mastoid air cells, findings which are commonly seen in chronic otitis media.

Suppurative mastoiditis is generally a bacterial infection. Pus is present in the middle ear. Bone destruction (coalescent mastoiditis) and extraosseous abscess formation are possible. Abscess along the sternocleidomastoid muscle (Bezold's abscess) can occur. Extension of infection to the petrous apex of the temporal bone may result in abducens nerve palsy and trigeminal neuralgia (Gradenigo syndrome).

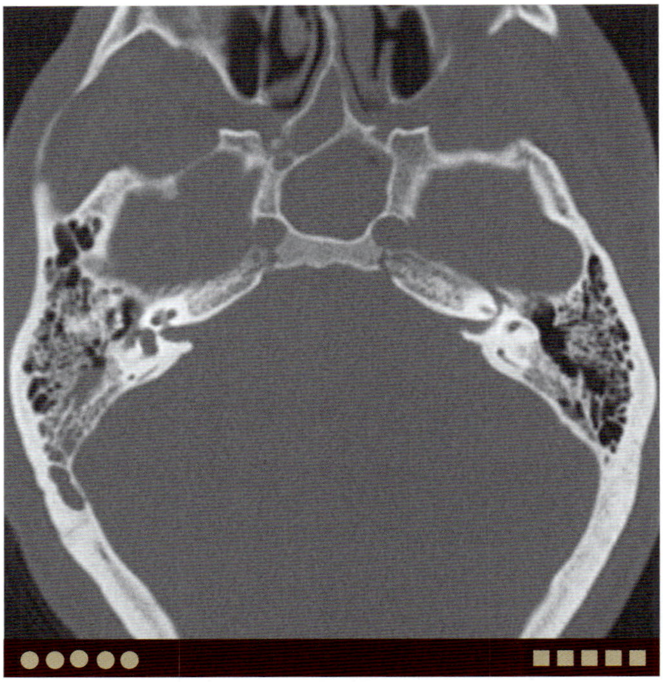

A. Serous otitis media. Axial CT demonstrates partial opacification of the right tympanic cavity and mastoid air cells without sclerosis or bone destruction.

It is important not to miss or ignore subtle changes in the mastoid air cells and trabeculation/bone marrow signal of the petrous bone. If petrous bone involvement is suspected clinically, MRI should be performed. Rhabdomyosarcoma and Langerhans cell histiocytosis demonstrate very similar clinical and radiological findings. These entities should always be considered in the differential diagnosis when diagnosing otitis media in children.

PEARLS

- **Serous otitis media is the most common cause of hearing loss in children. Opacification of the tympanic cavity and pneumatized mastoid air cells is seen without sclerosis or bone destruction.**
- **Bone destruction can be seen in coalescent mastoiditis.**
- **Rhabdomyosarcoma and Langerhans cell histiocytosis should be considered if aggressive bone destruction or cranial nerve impairment is noted.**

ADDITIONAL IMAGES (B-C)

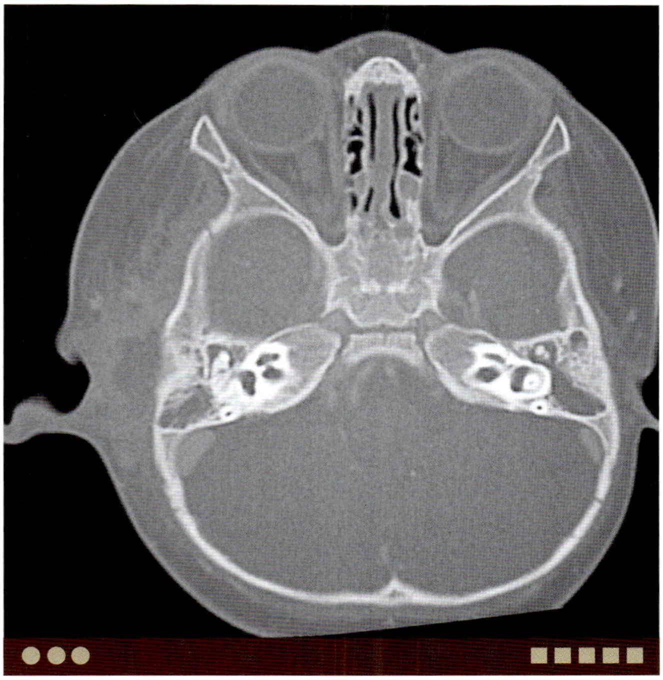

B. Complicated otomastoiditis in a 2-year-old boy. Axial CT demonstrates complete opacification of the mastoid air cells and tympanic cavities bilaterally. Note significant soft tissue swelling over the right mastoid.

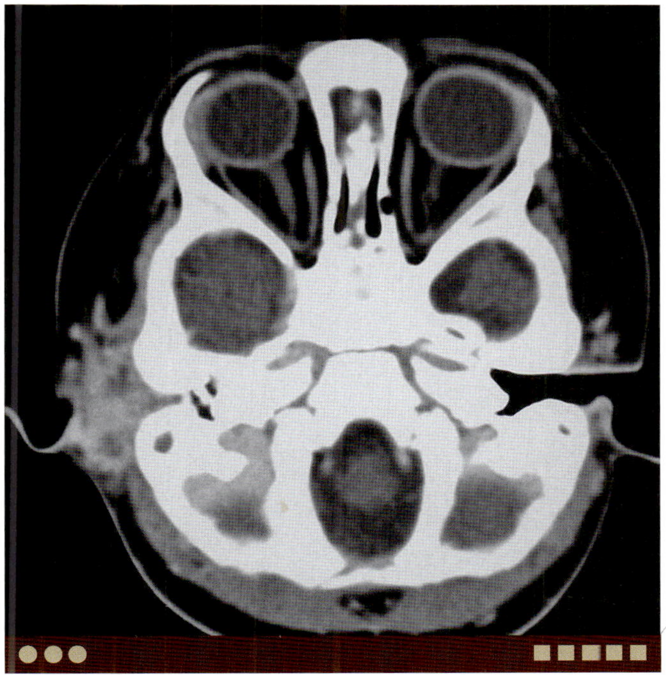

C. Complicated otomastoiditis, same patient as B. Axial postcontrast CT demonstrates heterogeneously enhancing soft tissue with low-density foci consistent with small abscesses.

DIFFERENTIAL DIAGNOSIS IMAGES (D-G)

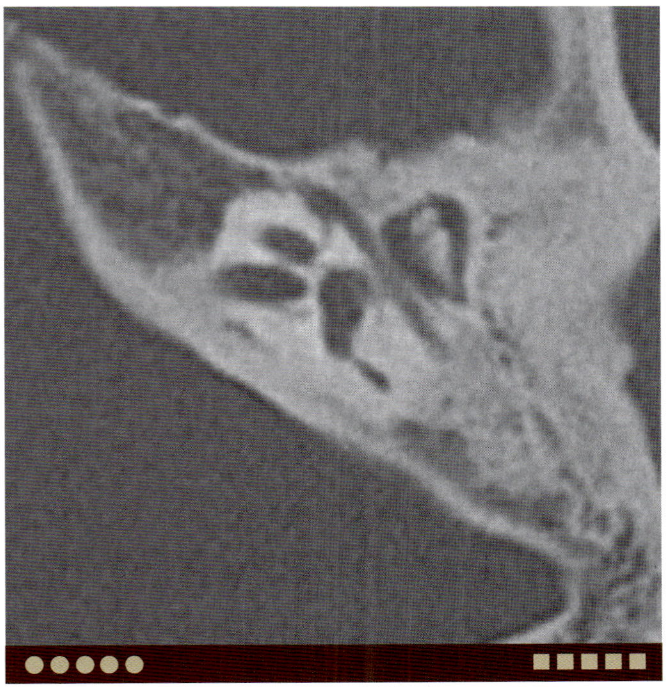

D. Chronic otitis media in a 25-year-old woman. Axial CT demonstrates opacification of the left epitympanum and mastoid air cells with diffuse sclerosis.

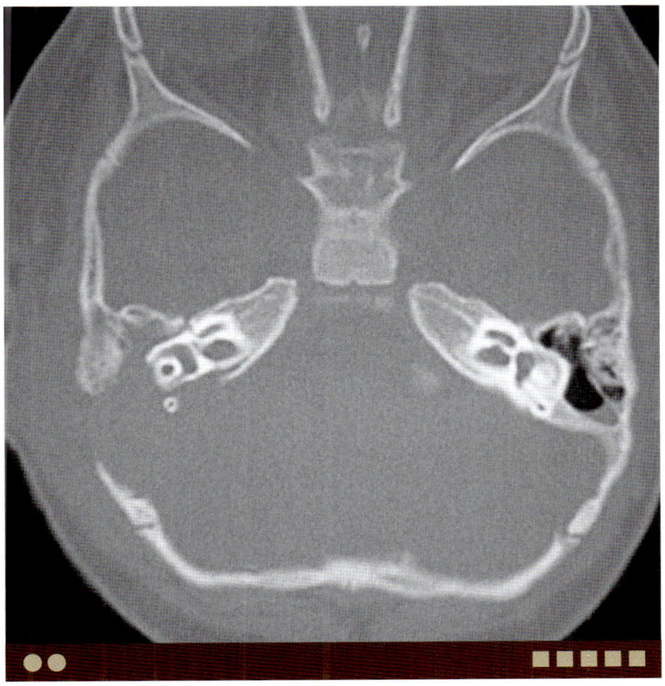

E. Langerhans cell histiocytosis in a 1-year-old infant. Axial CT demonstrates significant bone destruction of the right mastoid air cells. Note bone destruction is also seen in the otic capsule and petrous bone.

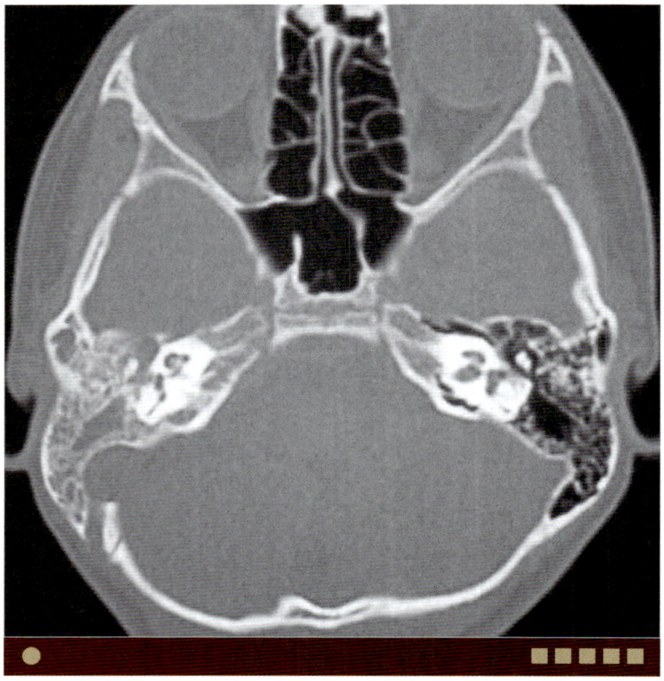

F. Rhabdomyosarcoma in a 10-year-old girl. Axial CT demonstrates opacification of the right mastoid air cells. Note bone destruction in the anterior mastoid.

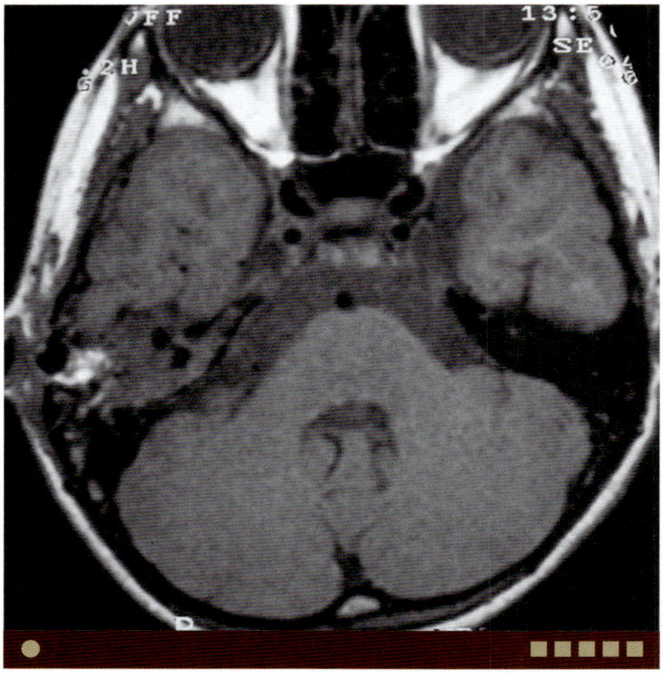

G. Rhabdomyosarcoma, same patient as F. Axial T1W magnetic resonance (MR) image demonstrates a soft tissue mass in the mastoid extending to the petrous portion as well as superficial soft tissue.

Case 1–2 Chronic Otitis Media

Osamu Sakai, Keith Fleming

PRESENTATION

Recurrent middle ear infection and ear discharge.

FINDINGS

Axial CT images demonstrate an opacified tympanic cavity and mastoid air cells with sclerotic changes of the bone surrounding these spaces.

DIFFERENTIAL DIAGNOSIS

- Acute otitis media: This condition demonstrates opacification of the mastoid air cells without sclerotic changes.
- Cholesteatoma: This is a common complication of chronic otitis media and results in bone erosion and destruction. Without bone erosion/destruction, it is difficult to differentiate cholesteatoma from uncomplicated chronic otitis media.
- Rhabdomyosarcoma: This clinically mimics otitis media. Imaging demonstrates aggressive bone destruction and enhancing soft tissue mass.
- Metastasis: Sclerotic metastases from prostate or breast cancer may demonstrate similar findings to chronic otitis media.
- Bone dysplasia: Diffuse sclerotic change can be seen in various bone dysplasias, such as osteopetrosis, fibrous dysplasia, and other benign fibroosseous lesions. Usually, aeration of the tympanic cavity is preserved.

COMMENTS

This is a 22-year-old man with recurrent middle ear infection and ear discharge.

Chronic otitis media is a chronic inflammatory and infectious condition resulting from various causes including acute otitis media, eustachian tube dysfunction, and trauma. The diagnosis of chronic otitis media is made clinically, and the main role of imaging is to identify complications.

On CT, poor pneumatization and sclerotic change of the mastoid air cells are present. Opacification of the pneumatized air cells is commonly seen. This is secondary to chronic inflammation and recurrent infections. Opacification of the tympanic cavity is seen in acute on chronic inflammatory and infectious conditions.

Generally, the presence of bone erosion and destruction suggests cholesteatoma. Therefore, careful evaluation of the ossicles, lateral wall of the epitympanum, scutum, lateral semicircular canal, and tegmen tympani should be performed to identify findings suggestive of cholesteatoma. However, erosive changes can also be seen in patients with long-standing infection.

Magnetic resonance imaging (MRI) is indicated to evaluate for intracranial complications and to rule out neoplastic processes when symptoms of meningitis or cranial nerve impairment are present.

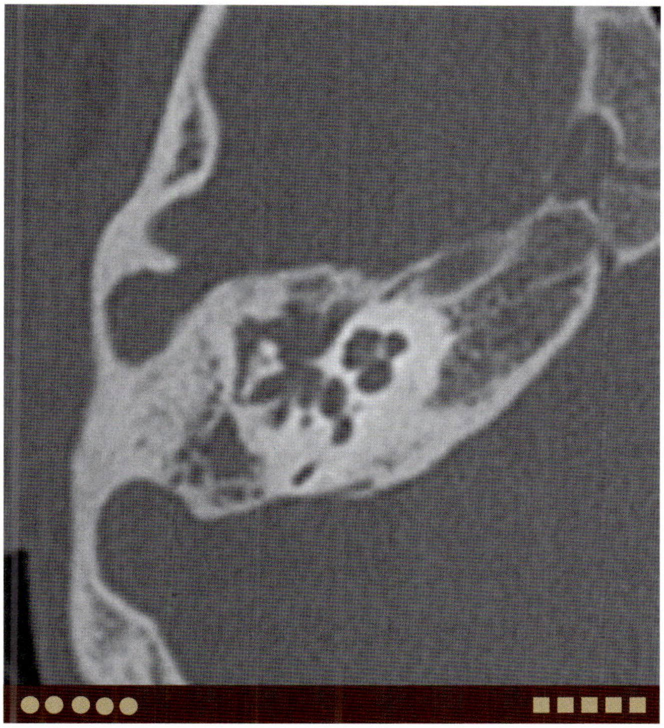

A. Chronic otitis media. Axial CT demonstrates completely opacified tympanic cavity and mastoid air cells with bone sclerosis. No bone destruction is noted.

PEARLS

- **Chronic otitis media is a chronic inflammatory and infectious condition resulting from various causes, such as acute otitis media, eustachian tube dysfunction, and trauma. The diagnosis is generally clinical, and the main role of imaging is to identify complications.**
- **The main imaging findings are tympanic cavity opacification, poor pneumatization and sclerotic change of the mastoid air cells, with opacification of the pneumatized air cells.**
- **The presence of bone erosion of the scutum, ossicles, lateral semicircular canal, and tegmen tympani suggests cholesteatoma.**

ADDITIONAL IMAGES (B-D)

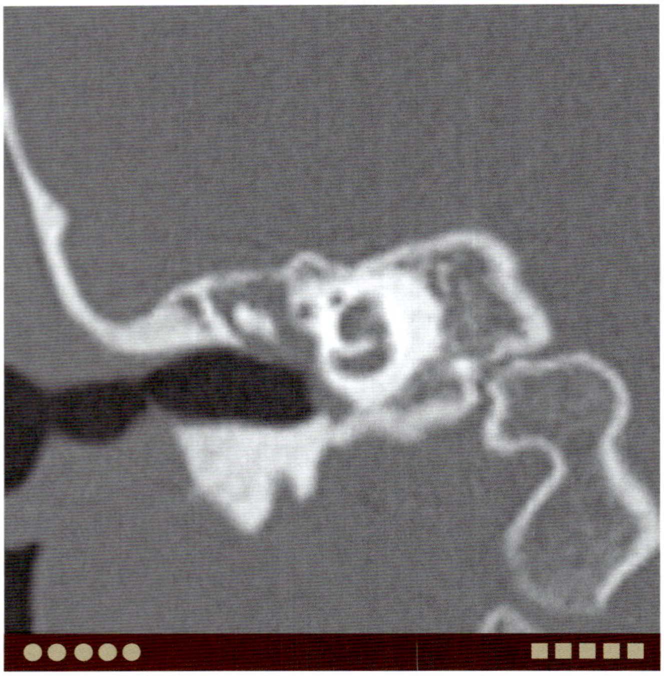

B. Chronic otitis media, same patient as A. Coronal CT demonstrates retracted tympanic membrane and opacified tympanic cavity. Sharp scutum is preserved. There is no bony destruction or erosion to suggest cholesteatoma.

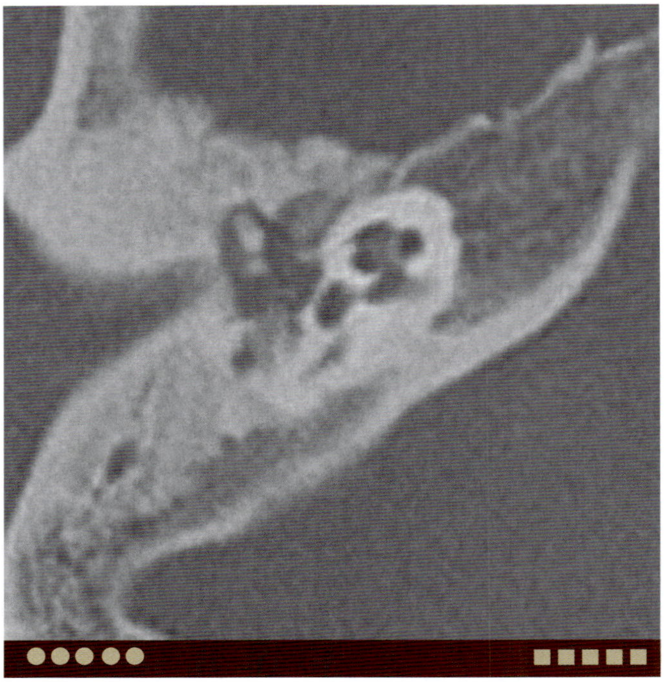

C. **Chronic otitis media** in a different patient. Axial CT demonstrates opacified tympanic cavity and sclerotic and poorly pneumatized mastoid air cells. No bone destruction is noted.

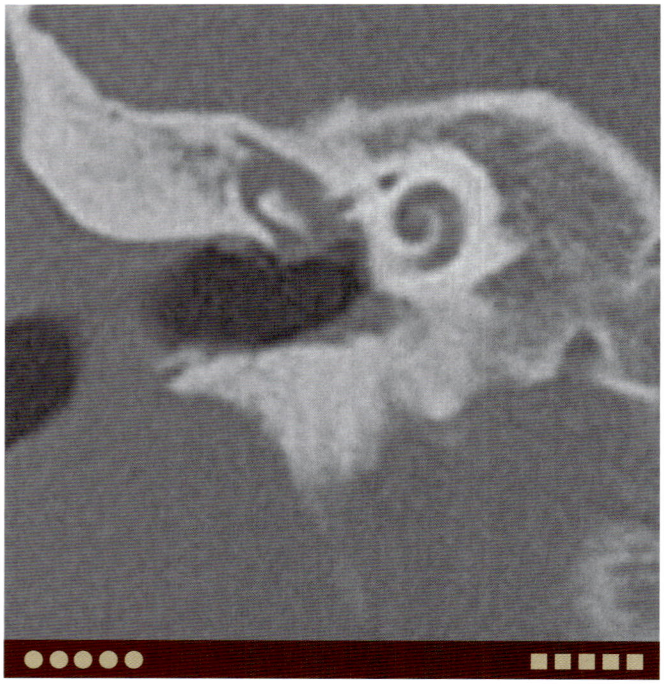

D. Chronic otitis media, same patient as C. Coronal CT demonstrates large tympanic membrane perforation and opacified tympanic cavity with intact scutum.

DIFFERENTIAL DIAGNOSIS IMAGES (E-G)

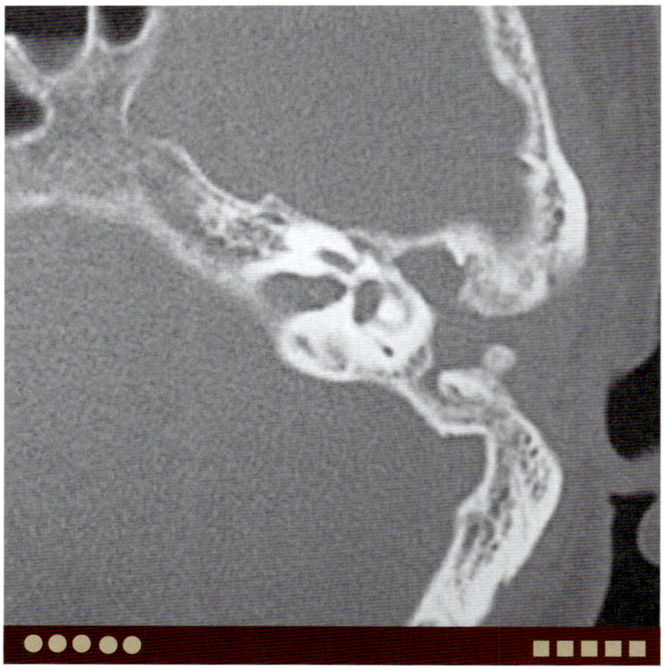

E. Cholesteatoma. Axial CT demonstrates opacified tympanic cavity with sclerotic changes in the mastoid air cells. Large bone defect from prior mastoidectomy is noted. Ossicles are completely eroded and not identified.

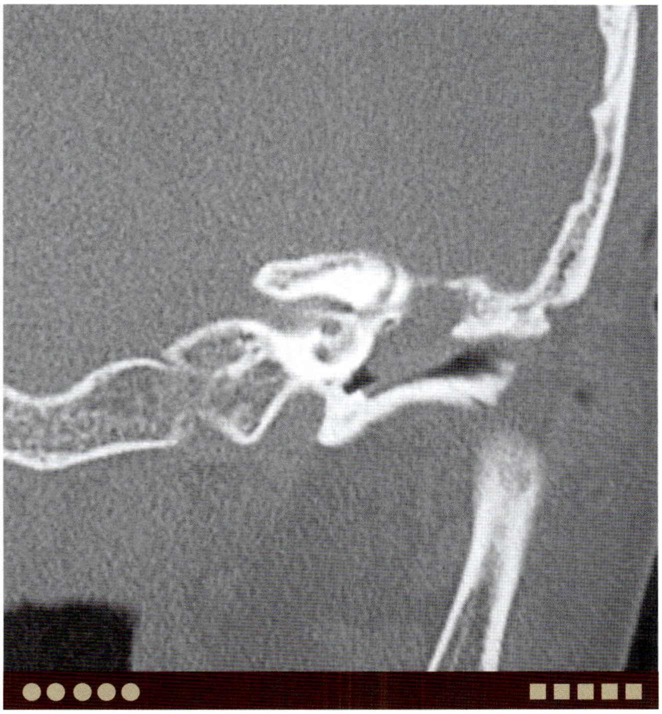

F. Cholesteatoma, same patient as E. Coronal CT demonstrates opacified tympanic cavity with eroded scutum and thinned tegmen tympani consistent with cholesteatoma. No ossicles are identified.

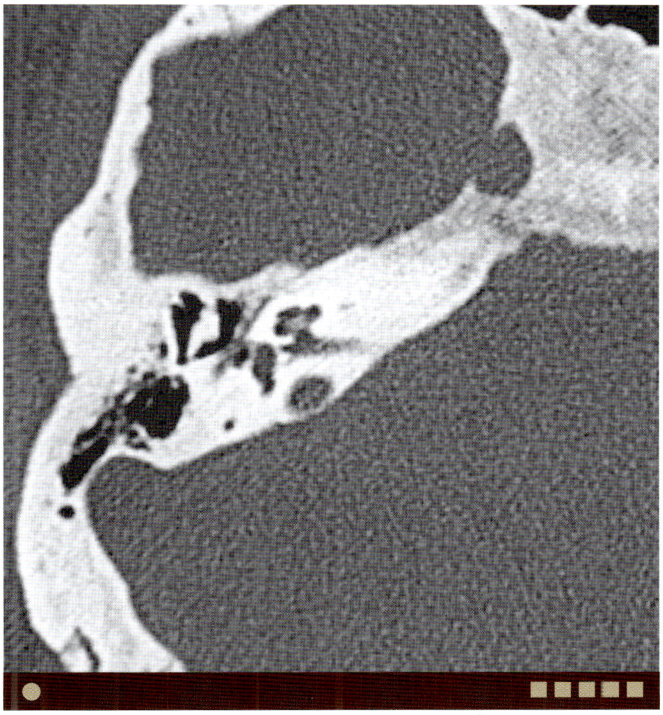

G. Osteopetrosis. Axial CT demonstrates diffuse sclerotic changes through the entire temporal bone. The aeration of the tympanic cavity is preserved, and the ossicles are intact.

Case 1–3 Cholesteatoma

Osamu Sakai, Keith Fleming

PRESENTATION

History of chronic otitis media and conductive hearing loss.

FINDINGS

CT demonstrates erosion of the scutum in addition to opacification of the tympanic cavity and mastoid air cells with sclerotic change due to chronic otitis media.

DIFFERENTIAL DIAGNOSIS

- Acute otitis media: Serous otitis media demonstrates opacification of the tympanic cavity and mastoid air cells without sclerotic changes. Coalescent mastoiditis can cause bone destruction but usually with typical clinical presentation of acute infection.
- Langerhans cell histiocytosis: This is a rare condition, commonly seen in children. Clinical presentation may be similar to otitis media. Bone destruction and enhancing soft tissue is generally seen.
- Rhabdomyosarcoma: This clinically mimics otitis media, commonly seen in children. Imaging demonstrates aggressive bone destruction and an enhancing soft tissue mass. Cranial nerve palsy is often noted.
- Metastasis: This demonstrates bone destruction and soft tissue mass with or without opacification and sclerotic changes of the mastoid air cells and tympanic cavity.

COMMENTS

This is a 74-year-old man with a history of chronic otitis media and conductive hearing loss, now with ear discharge.

Cholesteatoma is a middle ear mass resulting from accumulation of keratin due to migration of the squamous epithelium. In adults, most cholesteatomas are acquired sequela of chronic otitis media, resulting from a tear or retraction of the tympanic membrane. Histologically, cholesteatoma is identical to epidermoid.

Most acquired cholesteatomas occur in the pars flaccida of the tympanic membrane and form a mass in Prussak space, which is the space between the ossicles and the lateral wall of the epitympanum. Erosion of the scutum, lateral wall of the epitympanum, and ossicles is typical. Medial displacement of the ossicles can be an early sign of cholesteatoma. Occasionally, adhesion of the pars tensa of the tympanic membrane to the cochlear promontory results in cholesteatoma formation near the facial recess in the posterior tympanic cavity.

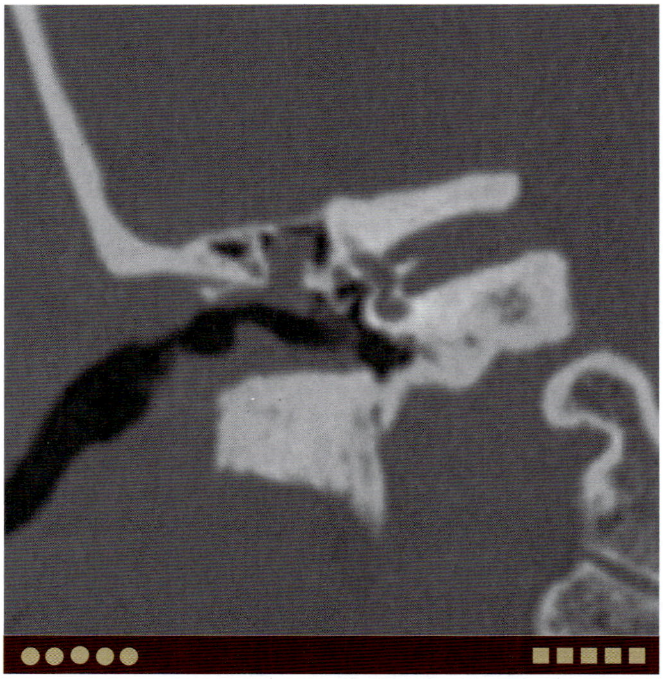

A. Cholesteatoma. Coronal CT of the right ear demonstrates a soft tissue mass eroding the scutum and displacing the ossicles medially.

CT demonstrates bone demineralization, erosion, and destruction in addition to findings of chronic otitis media. Erosion or destruction of the ossicles, scutum, lateral wall of the epitympanum, lateral semicircular canal, and tegmen tympani strongly suggests cholesteatoma. The ossicles can be displaced medially by pars flaccida cholesteatoma and laterally by pars tensa cholesteatoma. Without bone erosion or destruction, it is difficult to differentiate it from simple granulation tissue or fluid related to chronic otitis media.

PEARLS

- **Cholesteatoma is an accumulation of keratin by migrated squamous epithelium, and is histologically identical to an epidermoid.**
- **Erosion or destruction of the scutum, lateral wall of the epitympanum, ossicles, lateral semicircular canal, and tegmen tympani strongly suggests cholesteatoma.**
- **Automastoidectomy refers to spontaneous evacuation of cholesteatoma after extensive bone destruction, mimicking surgery.**

Imaging cannot rule out cholesteatoma. If a "pearly mass" is seen clinically, the diagnosis of cholesteatoma is made. The role of imaging is to define the extent of the lesion.

Bone erosion or destruction can be the only finding to suggest cholesteatoma. Occasionally, the contents of a cholesteatoma are completely drained by surgical intervention or drain spontaneously. The term, automastoidectomy (or natural mastoidectomy) refers to spontaneous evacuation/drainage of cholesteatoma after extensive bone destruction, mimicking surgery.

ADDITIONAL IMAGES (B-F)

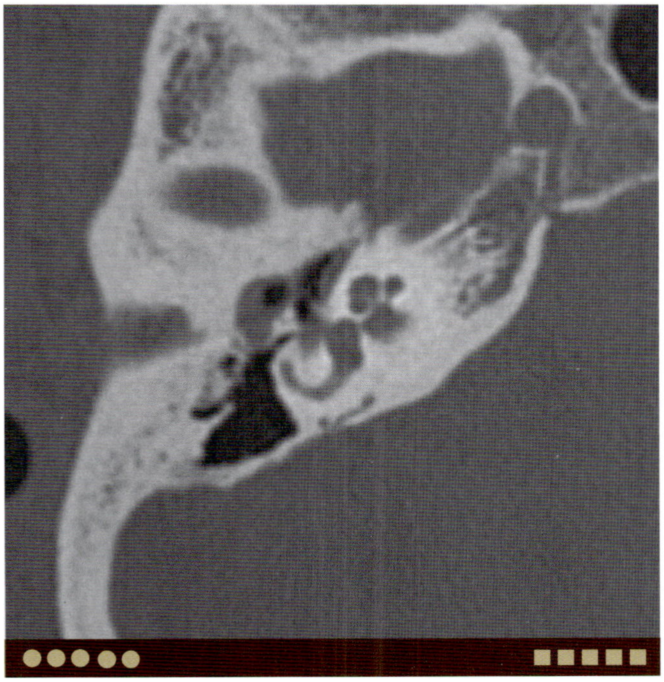

B. Cholesteatoma, same patient as A. Axial CT of the right ear demonstrates erosion of the lateral wall of the epitympanum and incus. Note sclerosis of the mastoid due to chronic inflammation.

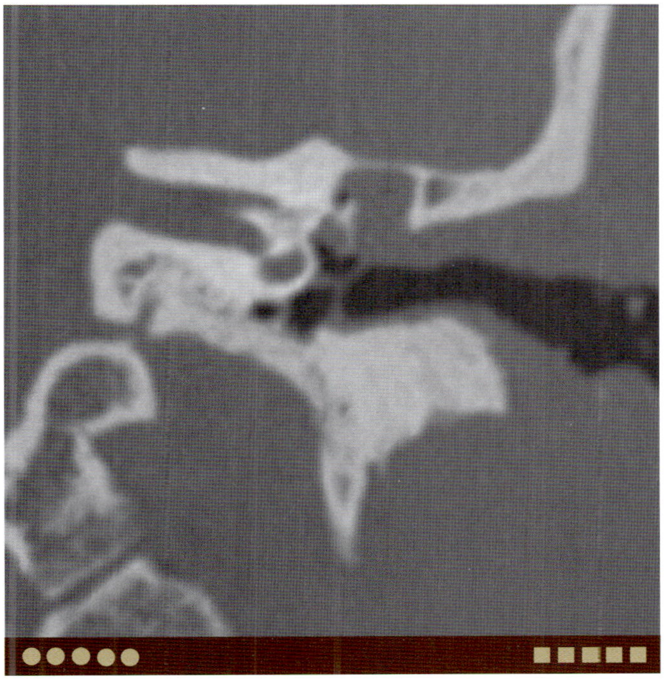

C. Cholesteatoma, same patient as A. Coronal CT of the left ear demonstrates a soft tissue mass eroding the scutum and ossicles.

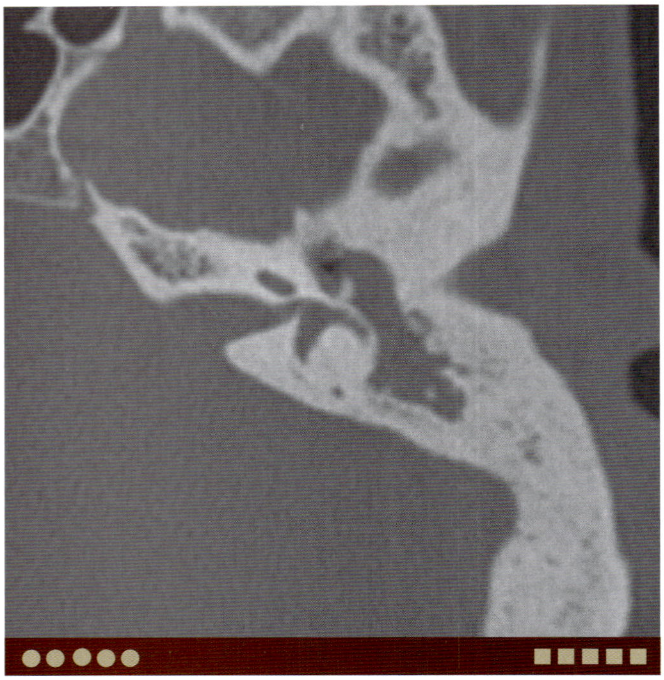

D. Cholesteatoma, same patient as A. Axial CT of the left ear demonstrates a soft tissue mass eroding the lateral wall of the epitympanum and ossicles.

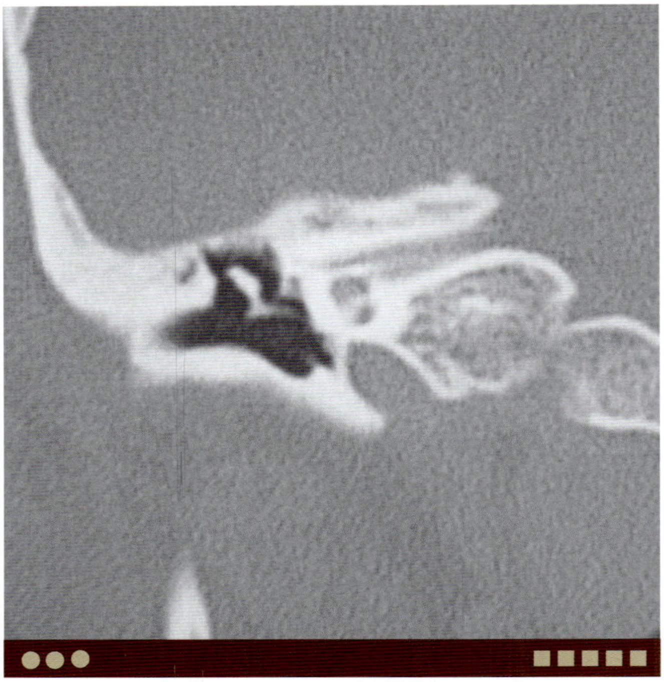

E. Cholesteatoma with spontaneous drainage in a 45-year-old man. Coronal CT demonstrates erosion of the scutum without opacification or soft tissue mass in the tympanic cavity after spontaneous drainage of cholesteatoma.

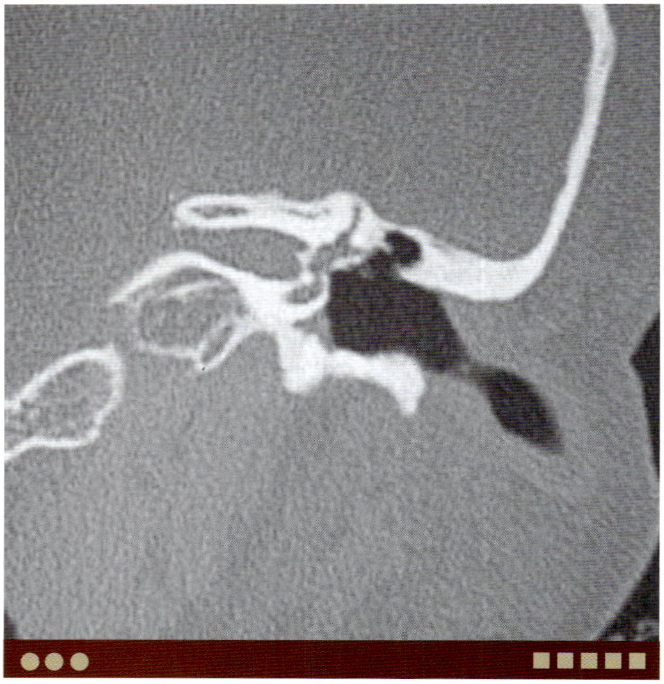

F. Cholesteatoma, automastoidectomy in a 55-year-old man. Coronal CT demonstrates erosion of the scutum and absence of the ossicles without history of prior surgery. Spontaneous evacuation of cholesteatoma after erosion of the scutum and ossicles.

DIFFERENTIAL DIAGNOSIS IMAGES (G-I)

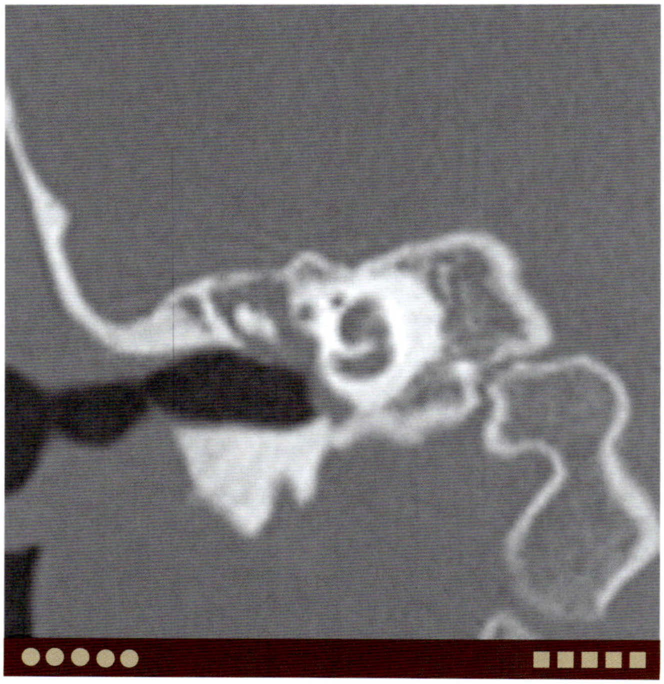

G. Chronic otitis media. Coronal CT demonstrates opacification of the right epitympanum without erosion of the scutum or ossicles.

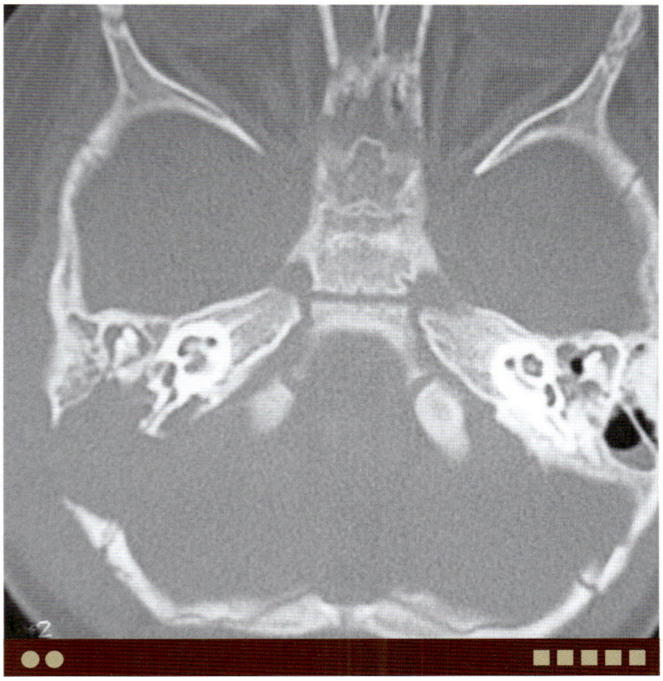

H. Langerhans cell histiocytosis. Axial CT demonstrates significant bone destruction of the right mastoid air cells. Note bone destruction is also seen in the otic capsule.

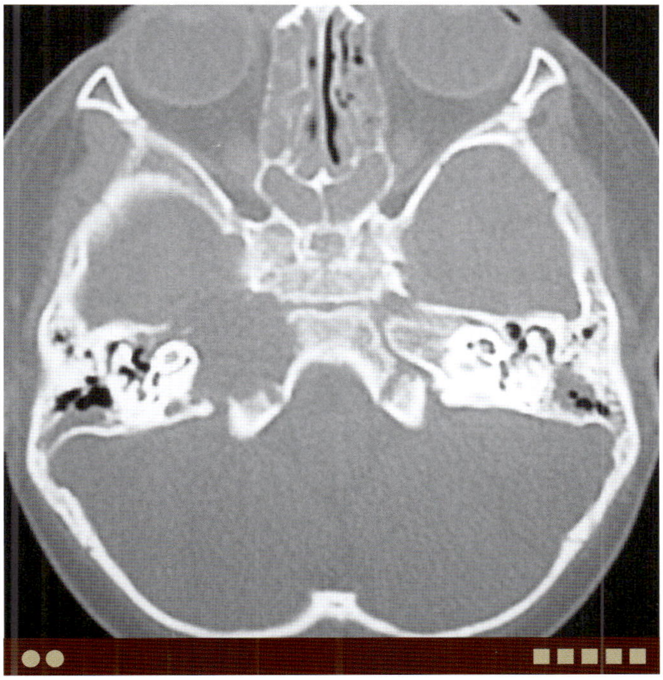

I. Rhabdomyosarcoma. Axial CT demonstrates opacification of the right mastoid air cells. Note bone destruction in the petrous bone and anterior mastoid.

Case 1–4 "Congenital" Cholesteatoma

Osamu Sakai, Keith Fleming

PRESENTATION

Conductive hearing loss.

FINDINGS

Axial CT demonstrates a soft tissue mass over the cochlear promontory without evidence of chronic otitis media.

DIFFERENTIAL DIAGNOSIS

- Acquired cholesteatoma: This condition usually demonstrates apparent evidence of underlying chronic otitis media.
- Glomus tympanicum: This is a hypervascular mass often seen around the cochlear promontory, which may cause pulsatile tinnitus.
- Facial schwannoma: This often arises from the genu and tympanic segment of the facial nerve with widening of the facial nerve canal.
- Persistent stapedial artery: This anomalous artery runs between the anterior and posterior crura and along the facial nerve in the tympanic cavity. The foramen spinosum is absent.

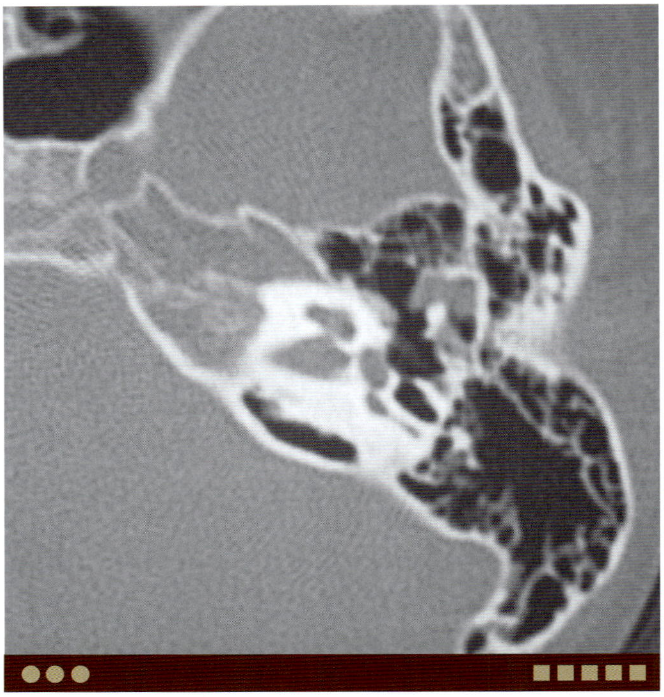

A. Congenital cholesteatoma. Axial CT demonstrates a focal mass anterolateral to the malleus without evidence of otitis media.

COMMENTS

This is an 8-year-old girl with history of conductive hearing loss.

Histologically, "congenital" cholesteatoma is identical to acquired cholesteatoma, a mass formed from accumulation of keratin by migrated squamous epithelium. It is often diagnosed in early childhood. There are various hypotheses regarding the mechanism of congenital cholesteatoma, which most likely occurs from aberrant migration of squamous epithelium before closure of the neural tube by 3 to 5 weeks of gestation.

On CT, a mass is seen without findings to suggest chronic otitis media. Congenital cholesteatoma is often seen in the anterior mesotympanum or in the peri-eustachian tube area. If the tympanic membrane is intact, and there is no history of recurrent otitis media, previous surgery or prior trauma, a congenital cholesteatoma should be suspected. If a congenital cholesteatoma obstructs the eustachian tube, chronic otitis media may occur.

A cholesteatoma arising in the petrous apex (epidermoid cyst) may show a similar appearance to a cholesterol cyst on CT. MRI is useful to differentiate these lesions. On MRI cholesteatoma usually demonstrates fluid signal, low on T1W and high on T2W images; while a cholesterol cyst typically shows high signal on both T1W and T2W images.

PEARLS

- **"Congenital" cholesteatoma can be seen without evidence of chronic otitis media. The etiology is unclear, and may be due to an epithelial migrational abnormality in utero.**
- **Congenital cholesteatoma is often seen in the anterior mesotympanum or in the peri-eustachian tube area, not in Prussak space (which is the typical location for acquired cholesteatoma).**
- **Petrous apex cholesteatoma may demonstrate a similar appearance to cholesterol cyst on CT. MRI is useful to differentiate these lesions.**

ADDITIONAL IMAGES (B-D)

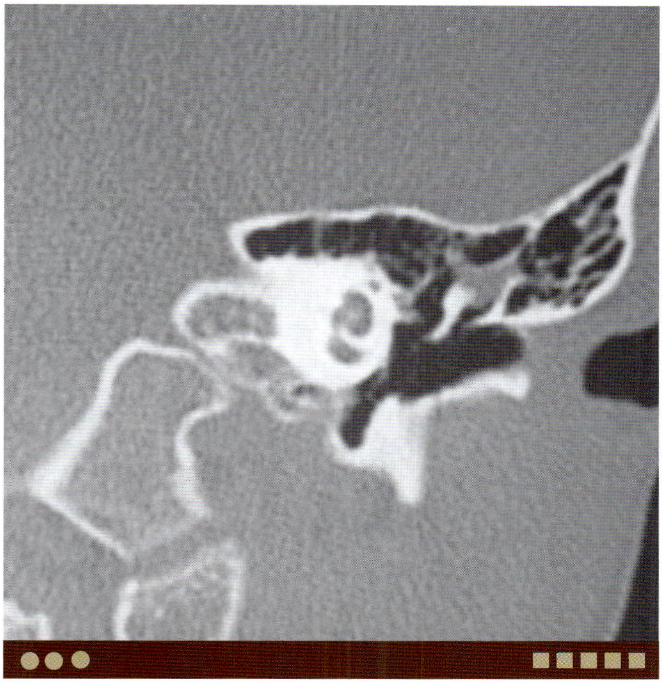

B. Congenital cholesteatoma, same patient as A. Coronal CT demonstrates a focal mass superolateral to the malleus without evidence of otitis media. Note sharp scutum and clear Prussak space.

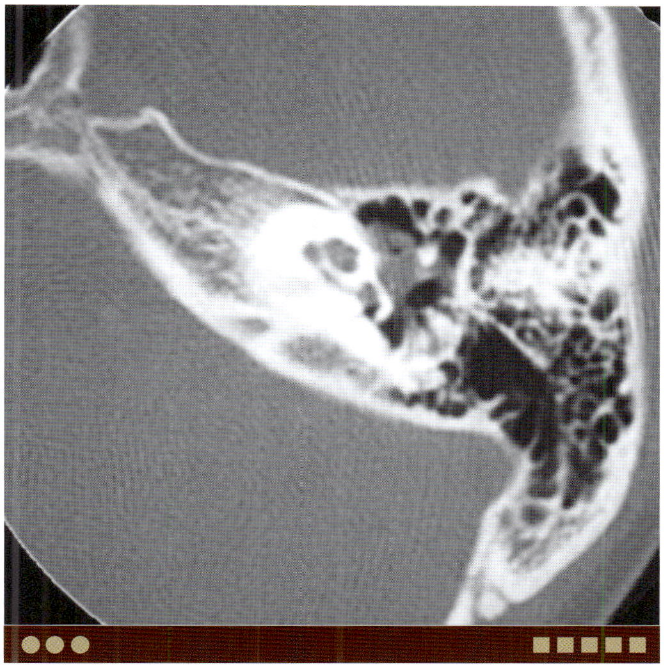

C. Congenital cholesteatoma in a 13-year-old adolescent. Axial CT demonstrates a soft tissue mass over the cochlear promontory, medial to the malleus and incus. There is no evidence of otitis media.

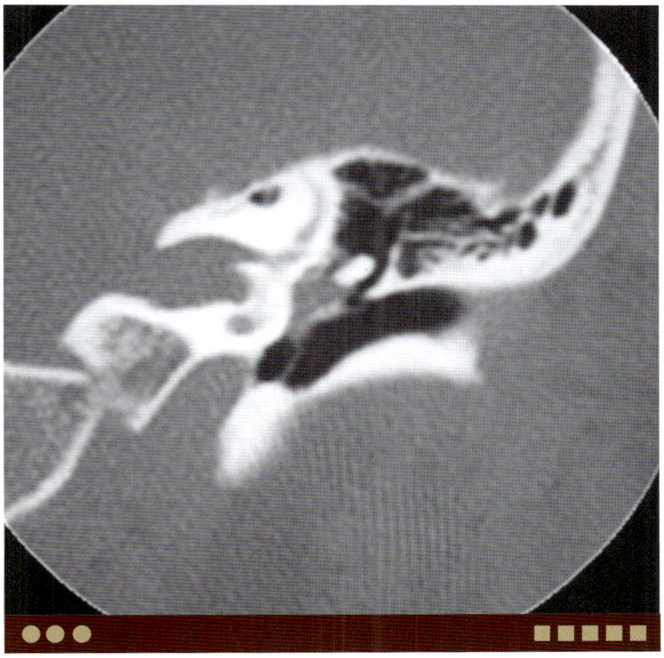

D. Congenital cholesteatoma, same patient as C. Coronal CT demonstrates a soft tissue mass over the oval window. Aeration of the rest of the tympanic cavity is well maintained.

DIFFERENTIAL DIAGNOSIS IMAGES (E-G)

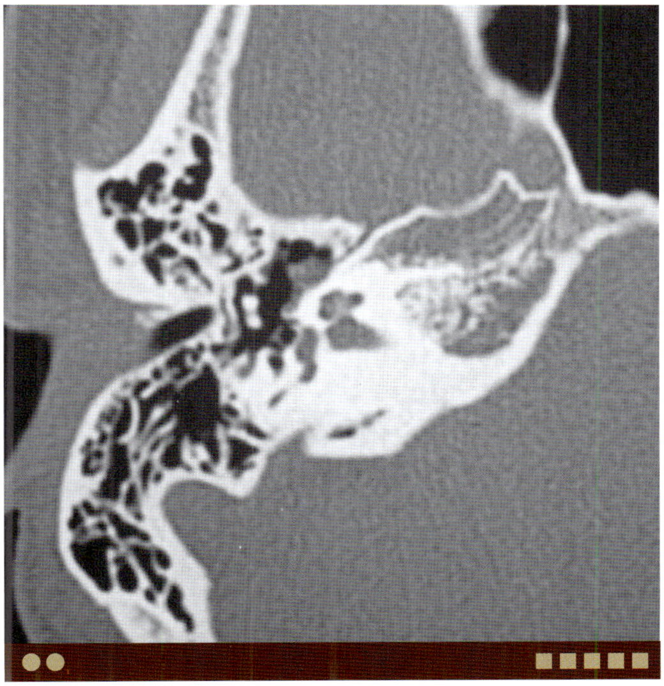

E. Facial nerve schwannoma. Axial CT demonstrates a soft tissue mass over the cochlear promontory.

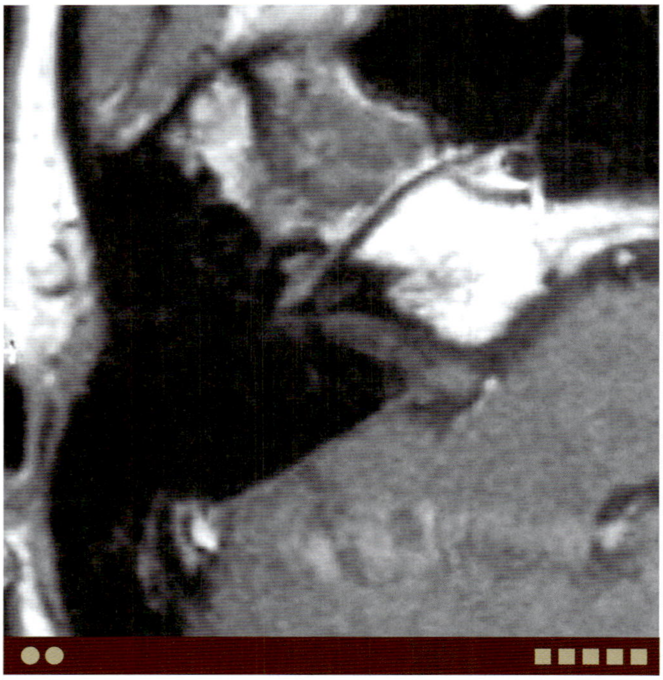

F. Facial nerve schwannoma, same patient as E. Axial postcontrast T1W MR image demonstrates enhancement of the mass.

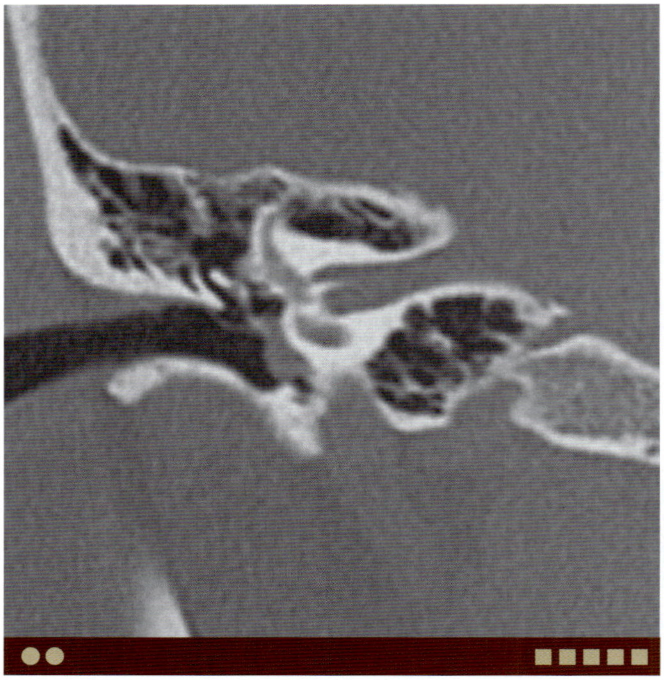

G. Glomus tympanicum. Coronal CT demonstrates a soft tissue mass over the cochlear promontory.

Case 1–5 Cholesteatoma: Labyrinthine Fistula

Osamu Sakai, Keith Fleming

PRESENTATION

History of chronic otitis media, now presents with new onset vertigo.

FINDINGS

CT demonstrates erosion of the wall of the lateral semicircular canal.

DIFFERENTIAL DIAGNOSIS

- Labyrinthitis: This occurs secondary to infection or inflammation with or without bone destruction of the otic capsule. Fistula formation is not necessary. Abnormal enhancement may be seen on MRI.
- Superior semicircular canal bone dehiscence: This is condition causes vertigo or other vestibular symptoms typically with loud noise (Tullio phenomenon).

COMMENTS

This is a 65-year-old man with history of chronic otitis media, now with vertigo.

Labyrinthine fistula is one complication of cholesteatoma. It has been reported to be found in 5% to 10% of patients with chronic otitis media and cholesteatomas. The lateral semicircular canal is most frequently involved, however, it can be seen in other locations, including the posterior and superior semicircular canal, as well as the vestibule. The patient often presents with vestibular symptoms, such as vertigo. The treatment involves either fibrin glue, autologous fascia, or perichondrium. The material is used to repair the fascia of the semicircular canal and cover the labyrinthine fistula defect.

CT can demonstrate fistula formation. Coronal images may over-diagnose labyrinth fistulae due to partial volume averaging effect, therefore, evaluation should be performed on both axial and coronal images. Pneumolabyrinth, air in the membranous labyrinth, can be seen with large fistulae.

MRI can demonstrate inflammatory changes in the membranous labyrinth secondary to the fistula formation. Loss of normal fluid signal on T2W images and abnormal enhancement on postcontrast T1W images in the membranous labyrinth may be seen.

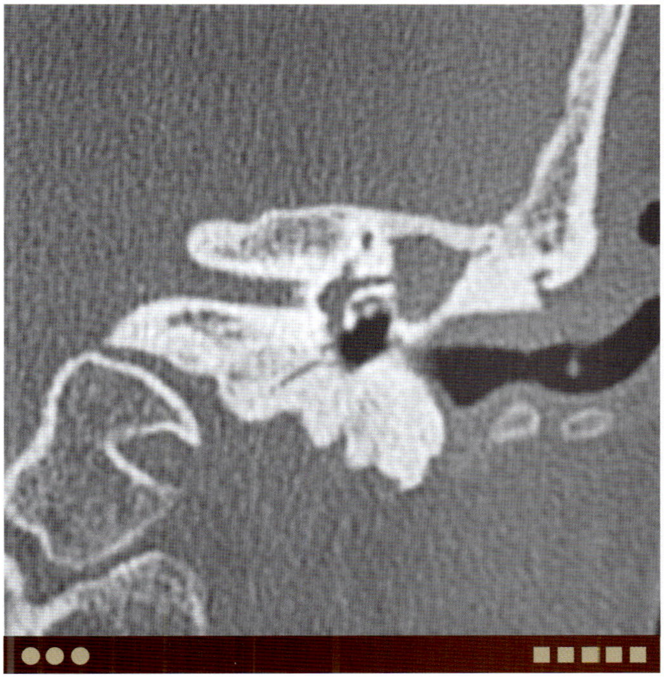

A. Labyrinthine fistula. Coronal CT demonstrates abnormal soft tissue eroding the lateral semicircular canal.

PEARLS

- **Labyrinthine fistula is a complication from cholesteatoma and most commonly seen involving the lateral semicircular canal.**
- **Evaluation should be performed on both axial and coronal images to avoid over diagnosis from partial volume averaging effect.**
- **MRI can demonstrate inflammatory changes in the membranous labyrinth secondary to the fistula formation.**

ADDITIONAL IMAGES (B-F)

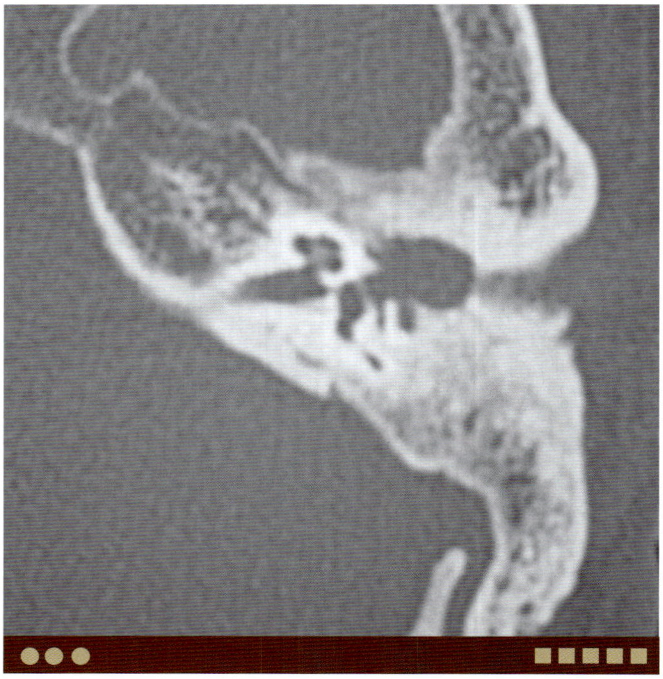

B. Labyrinthine fistula, same patient as A. Axial CT demonstrates abnormal soft tissue in the tympanic cavity, eroding the lateral semicircular canal as well as the lateral wall of the epitympanum.

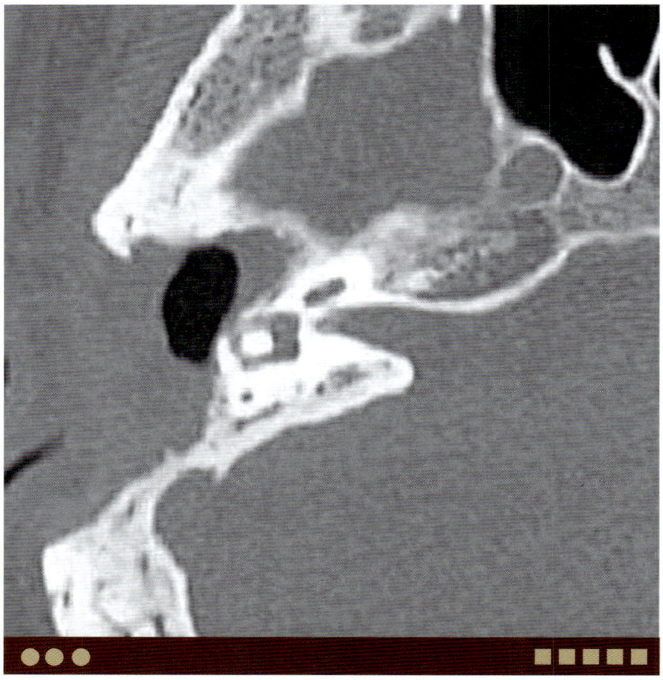

C. Labyrinthine fistula in a different patient. Recurrent cholesteatoma, status postradical mastoidectomy. Axial CT demonstrates a soft tissue mass occupying the tympanic cavity. Note bone defect in the anterolateral portion of the lateral semicircular canal.

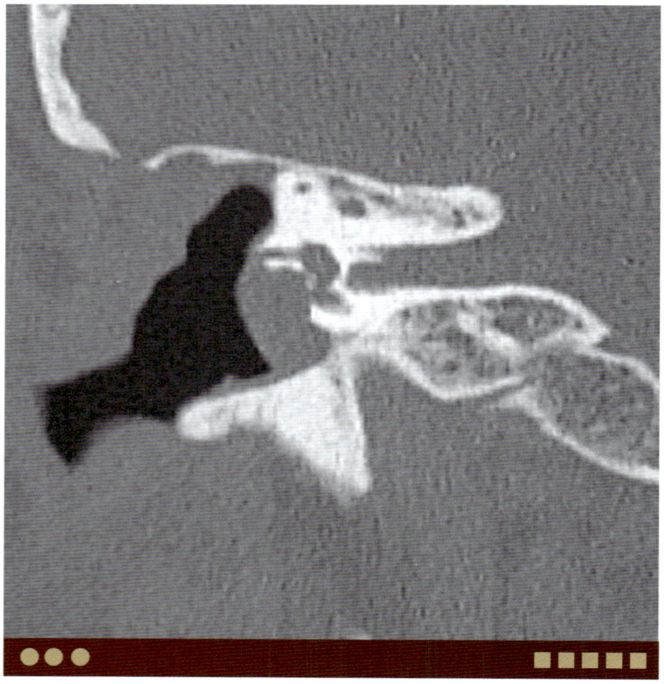

D. Labyrinthine fistula, same patient as C. Coronal CT demonstrates a soft tissue mass occupying the meso- and hypotympanum. Erosion of the lateral semicircular canal is again noted.

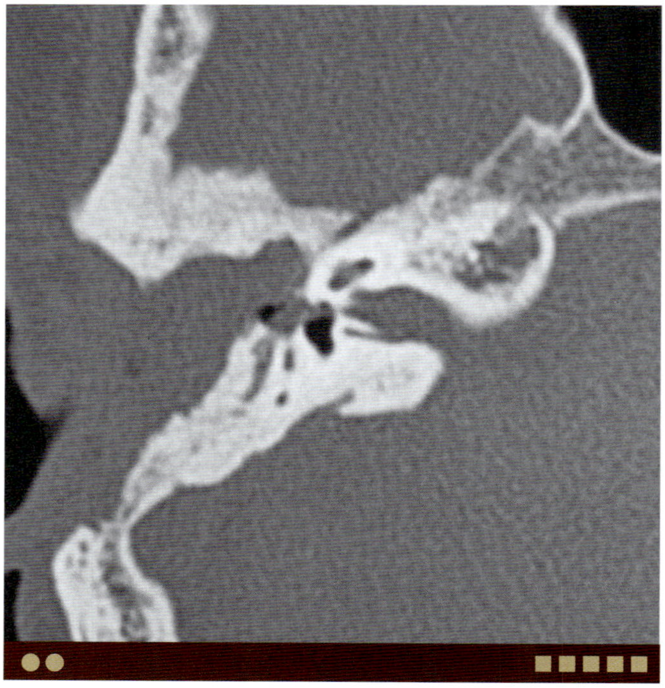

E. Labyrinthine fistula, pneumolabyrinth. Recurrent cholesteatoma, status postradical mastoidectomy. Axial CT demonstrates a soft tissue mass eroding into the lateral semicircular canal. Note the air density in the vestibule consistent with pneumolabyrinth.

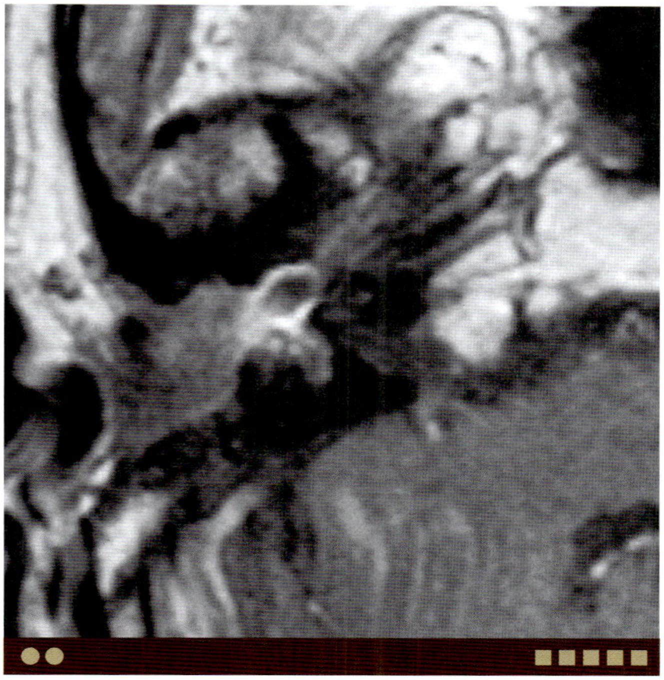

F. Labyrinthine fistula, same patient as E. Axial postcontrast T1W MR image demonstrates abnormal enhancement in the vestibule, consistent with labyrinthitis.

DIFFERENTIAL DIAGNOSIS IMAGES (G-H)

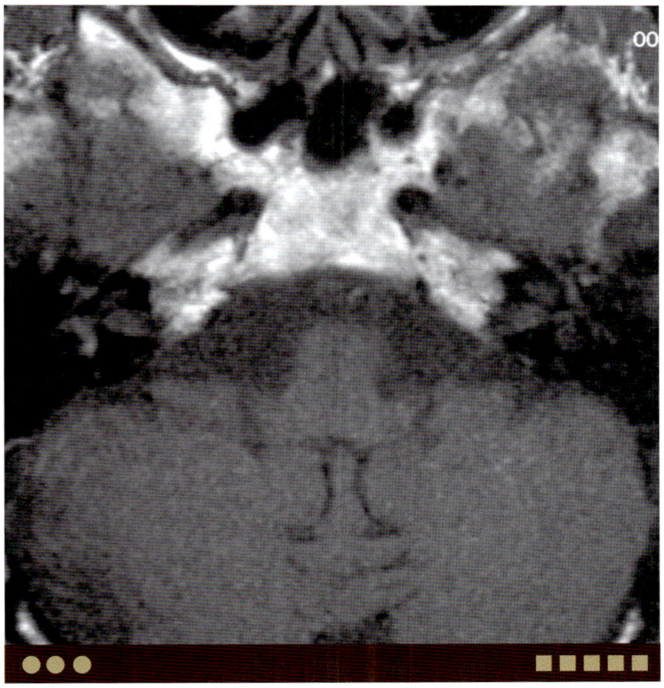

G. Labyrinthine hemorrhage. Axial T1W MR image demonstrates abnormal high signal in the right vestibule.

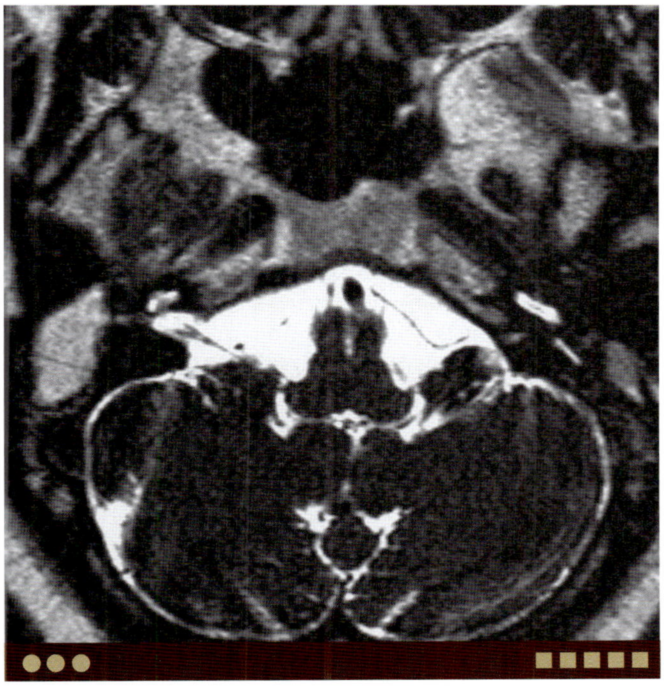

H. Labyrinthitis ossificans. Axial high-resolution T2W MR image demonstrates nonvisualization of the right vestibule and semicircular canals due to abnormal calcification/ossification. The patient is status postradial mastoidectomy.

Case 1–6 Cholesteatoma: Destruction of Tegmen Tympani

Osamu Sakai, Keith Fleming

PRESENTATION

Chronic otitis media and headache.

FINDINGS

Coronal CT demonstrates destruction of the tegmen tympani.

DIFFERENTIAL DIAGNOSIS

- Congenital/developmental bone dehiscence of the tegmen tympani: This is a congenital abnormality which may result in cephalocele and cerebrospinal fluid (CSF) leak without evidence of chronic otitis media.

COMMENTS

This is a 73-year-old man with history of chronic otitis media, who now presents with a new headache.

Destruction of the tegmen tympani by cholesteatoma may result in serious intracranial complications including meningitis, menigoencephalitis, abscess, cerebral herniation, and dural venous sinus thrombosis. On CT, evaluation of the intracranial structures is often limited. Careful evaluation of the soft tissue window images is important to avoid missing serious intracranial complications. Magnetic resonance imaging (MRI) is far superior to CT for evaluation of intracranial pathologies. MRI is indicated when intracranial complications are suspected.

On MRI, cholesteatoma is seen as a cystic lesion with slightly heterogeneous internal signal, generally demonstrating low signal on T1W and high signal on T2W images. Thin peripheral enhancement can be seen after contrast administration. It is important to evaluate the relationship between the tegmen tympani and temporal lobe on coronal images. A convex appearance of the inferior aspect of the temporal lobe raises the possibility of herniation. After contrast, careful evaluation for abnormal meningeal or parenchymal enhancement is important to rule out intracranial complications. Normal flow-voids and enhancement of the dural venous sinuses should always be confirmed to exclude the complication of dural sinus thrombosis.

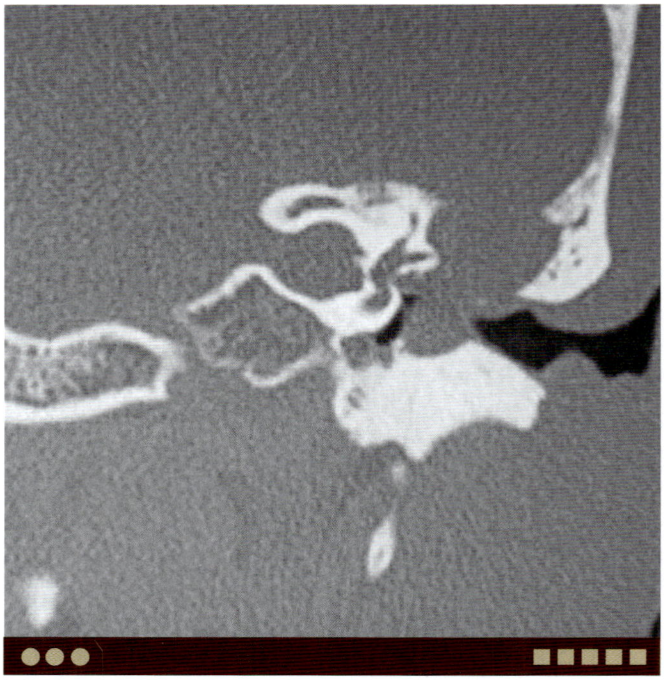

A. Cholesteatoma. Coronal CT demonstrates a soft tissue mass in the tympanic cavity with a large defect in the tegmen tympani.

MR venography can be performed to evaluate for dural venous sinus thrombosis, however, CT venography is easier to perform and interpret.

PEARLS

- **Destruction of the tegmen tympani by cholesteatoma may result in serious intracranial complications.**
- **A convex appearance of the inferior aspect of the temporal lobe suggests herniation.**
- **Contrast-enhanced MRI should be performed when intracranial complications are suspected.**

ADDITIONAL IMAGES (B-G)

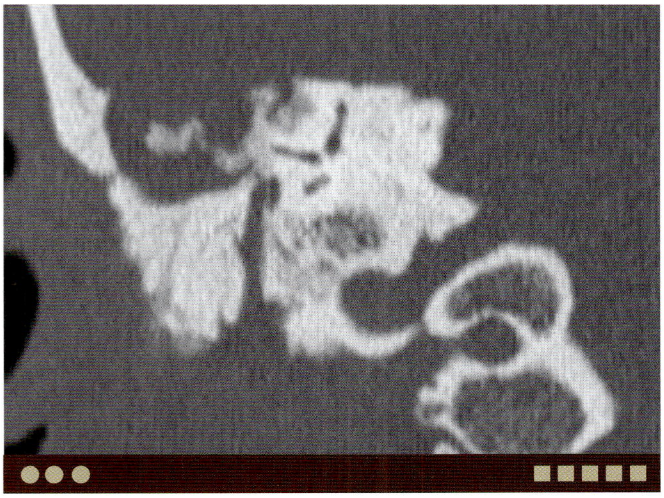

B. Cholesteatoma in a different patient. Coronal CT demonstrates a large-bone defect in the tegmen tympani. Note diffuse sclerotic change in the temporal bone due to chronic infection.

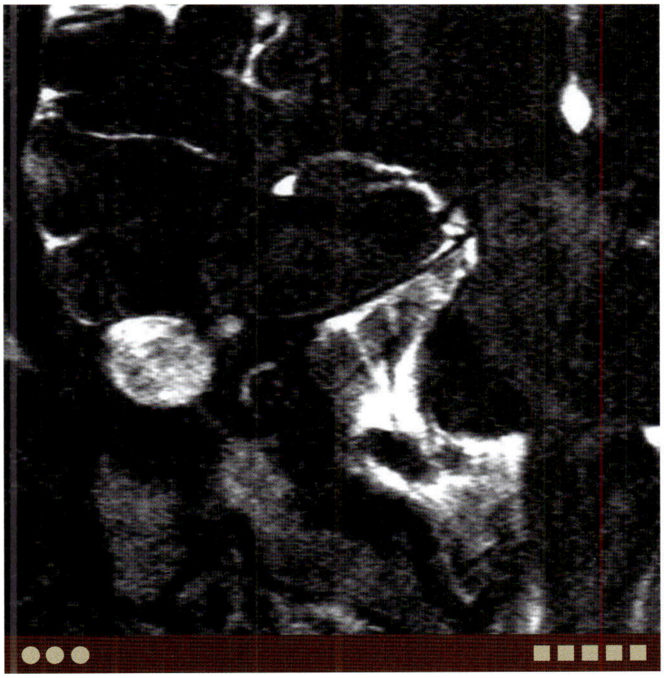

C. Cholesteatoma, same patient as B. Coronal T2W MR image demonstrates a hyperintense mass mildly compressing the inferior aspect of the temporal lobe.

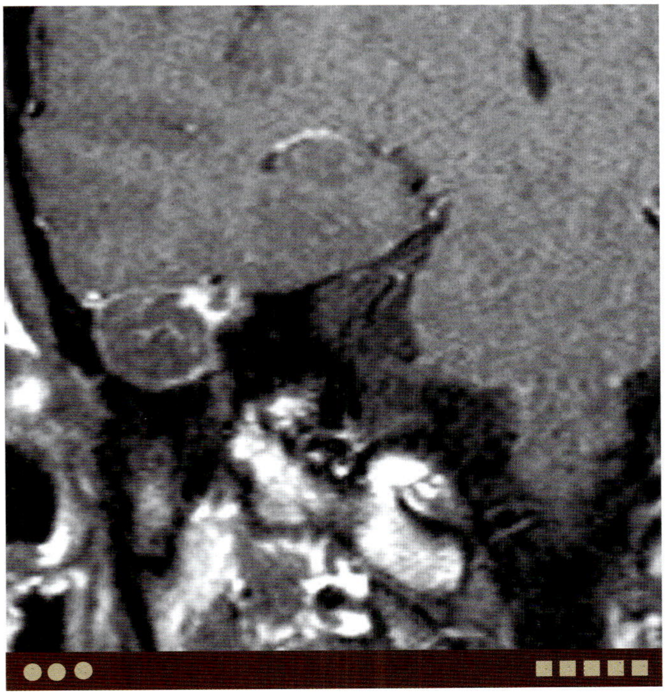

D. Cholesteatoma, same patient as B. Coronal postcontrast T1W MR image demonstrates peripheral enhancement of the lesion.

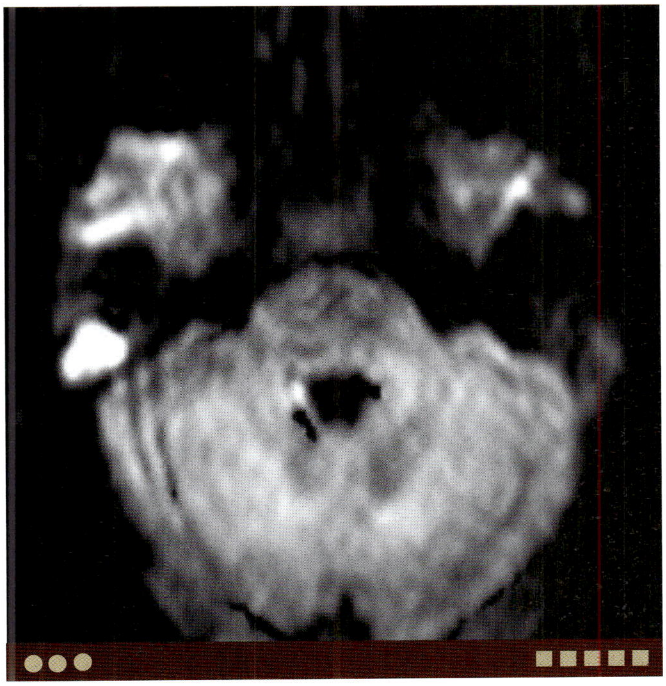

E. Cholesteatoma, same patient as B. Axial diffusion-weighted MR image (b = 1000) demonstrates high signal in the lesion.

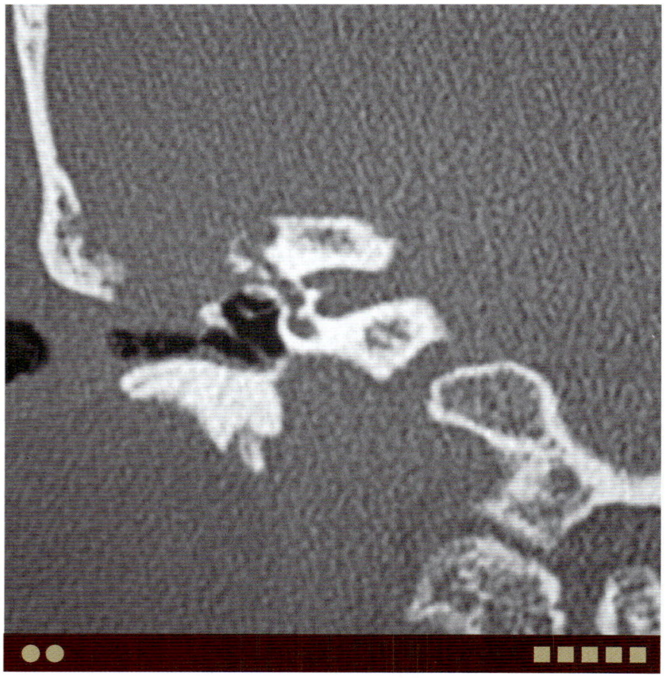

F. Cholesteatoma in a 57-year-old man. Coronal CT demonstrates a large tegmen tympani defect and abnormal soft tissue density in the epitympanum.

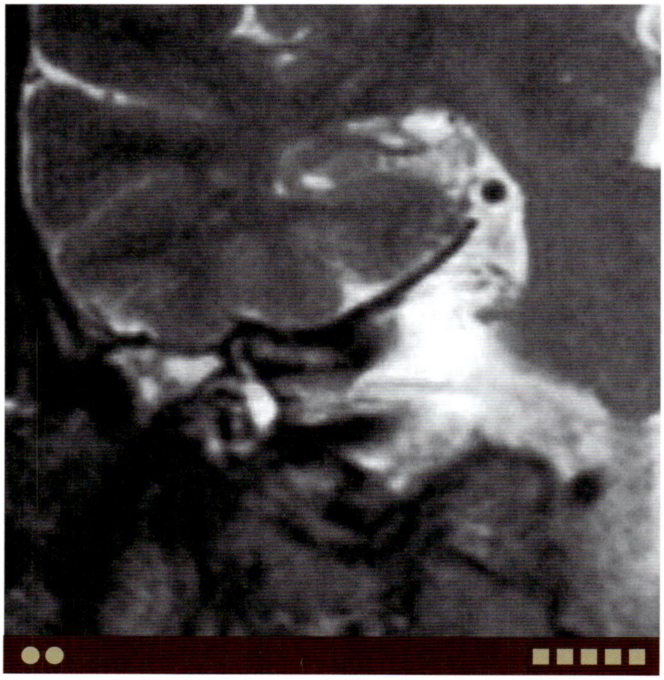

G. Cholesteatoma, same patient as F. Coronal T2W MR image demonstrates mild downward herniation of the temporal lobe through the bone defect.

DIFFERENTIAL DIAGNOSIS IMAGES (H-I)

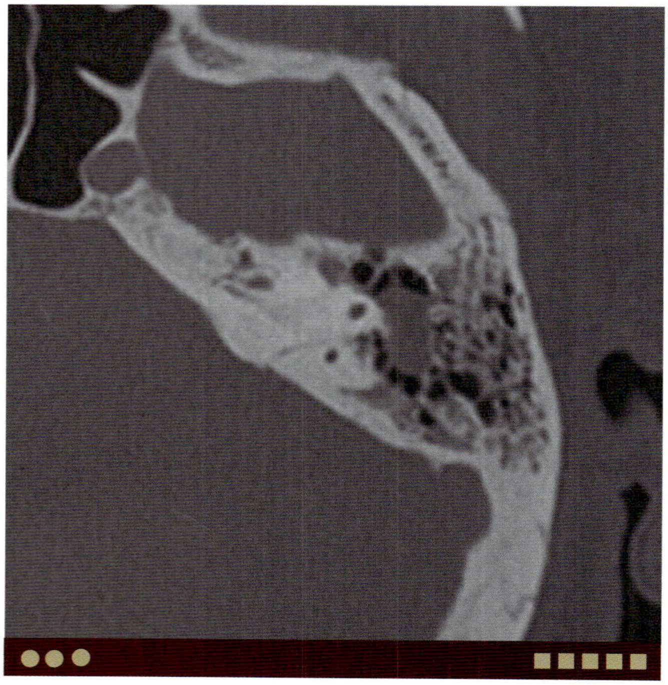

H. Cephalocele. Axial CT demonstrates a smooth soft tissue/water density mass in the mastoid.

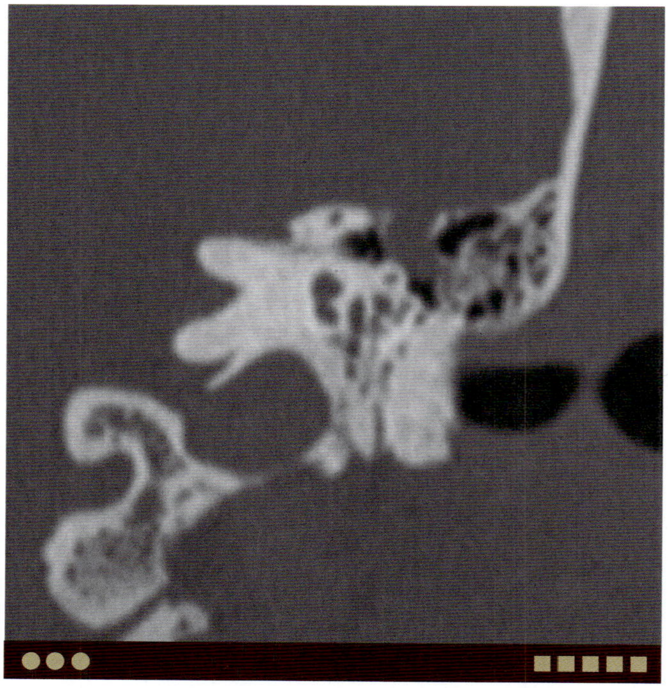

I. Cephalocele, same patient as H. Coronal CT demonstrates a soft tissue/water density mass extending inferiorly through the bone defect in the tegmen tympani.

Case 1–7 Tympanosclerosis

Osamu Sakai, Keith Fleming

PRESENTATION

Conductive hearing loss and chronic otitis media.

FINDINGS

CT demonstrates abnormal calcification in the opacified epitympanum.

DIFFERENTIAL DIAGNOSIS

- Chronic otitis media: This condition demonstrates opacification of the tympanic cavity and mastoid air cells with sclerotic changes of bone, but without calcification filling the tympanic cavity.
- Cholesteatoma: This demonstrates bone erosion or destruction rather than calcification or ossification.
- Otosclerosis: Also known as otospongiosis, otosclerosis begins as demineralization of the otic capsule, a totally different condition unrelated to tympanosclerosis.
- Labyrinthitis ossificans: This condition is calcification or ossification of the membranous labyrinth, not calcification in the tympanic cavity.

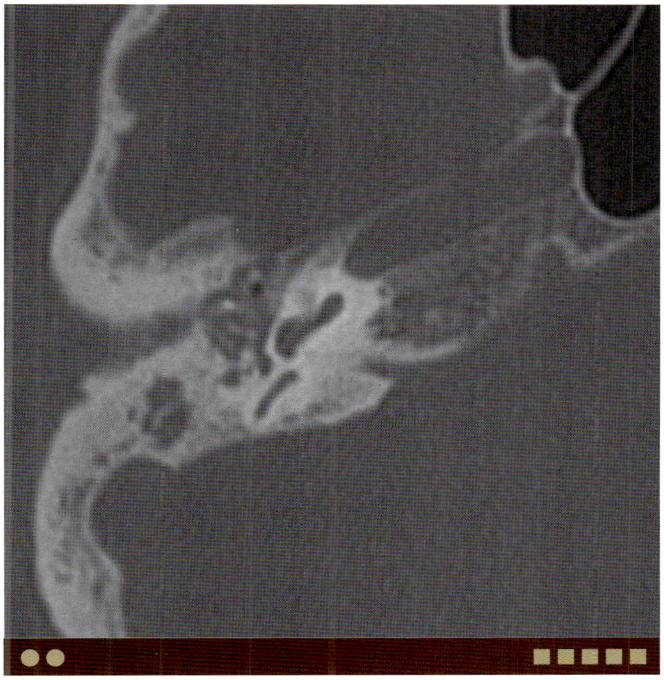

A. Tympanosclerosis. Axial CT demonstrates ill-defined calcifications in the opacified tympanic cavity. Note poorly pneumatized and diffusely sclerotic mastoid air cells due to chronic inflammation.

COMMENTS

This is a 72-year-old woman with conductive hearing loss.

Tympanosclerosis is a sclerosis of the tympanic cavity, usually due to chronic inflammation. This is a separate and unrelated condition from otosclerosis, which begins as demineralization of the otic capsule. Tympanosclerosis often occurs as a fibrous or hyaline deposit in the tympanic cavity, without apparent calcification or ossification. Tympanic membrane lesions are commonly seen, and the patient is often asymptomatic. Involvement of the annular ligament of the oval window results in fixation of the stapes and conductive hearing loss. Treatment of this complication requires stapedial surgery.

CT demonstrates calcification or ossification of the tympanic membrane or tympanic cavity in addition to the usual opacification and chronic inflammatory changes in the tympanic cavity and mastoid air cells seen with chronic otitis media. Ossification due to osteoblast migration is often seen in the epitympanum. Calcification or ossification may not be identified on CT; however, identification of calcification is helpful for preoperative evaluation as well as for prognosis. Calcification of the tympanic membrane is generally clinically apparent, however, it may be difficult to identify on CT.

PEARLS

- **Tympanosclerosis refers to sclerotic change narrowing or "filling in" the tympanic cavity, most commonly from chronic inflammation.**
- **CT demonstrates abnormal calcification or ossification in the tympanic membrane or tympanic cavity, most commonly seen in the epitympanum.**
- **Calcification of the tympanic membrane is easily seen clinically, however, it may be difficult to identify on CT.**

ADDITIONAL IMAGES (B-E)

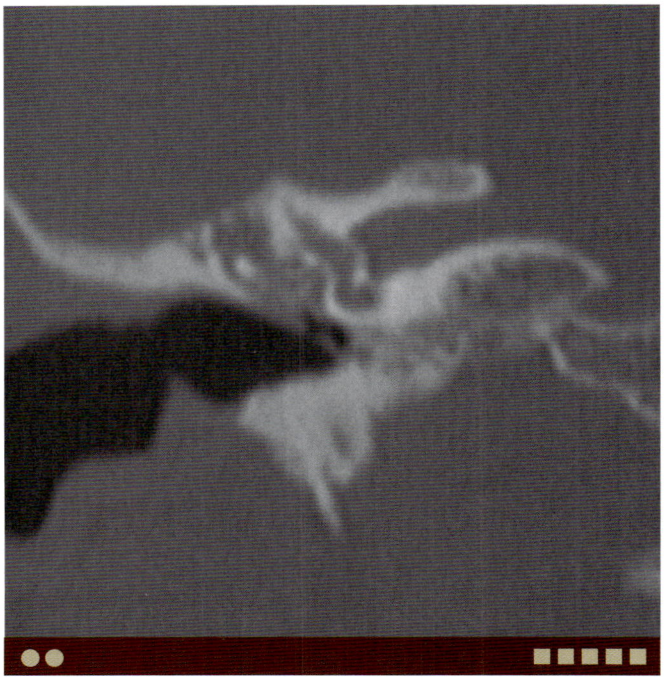

B. Tympanosclerosis, same patient as A. Coronal CT demonstrates ill-defined calcification in the opacified meso and epitympanum.

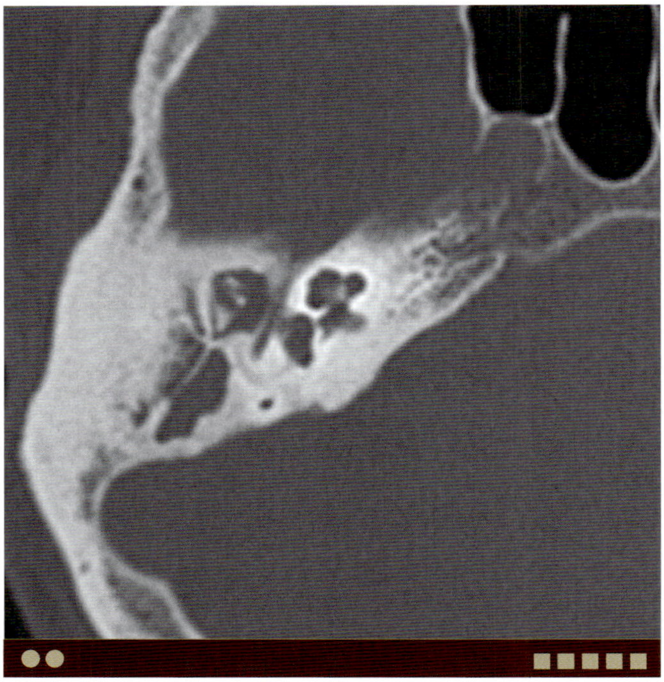

C. Tympanosclerosis in a 78-year-old woman. Axial CT demonstrates ill-defined punctate calcifications in the epitympanum. Note poorly pneumatized and opacified mastoid air cells and antrum due to chronic inflammation.

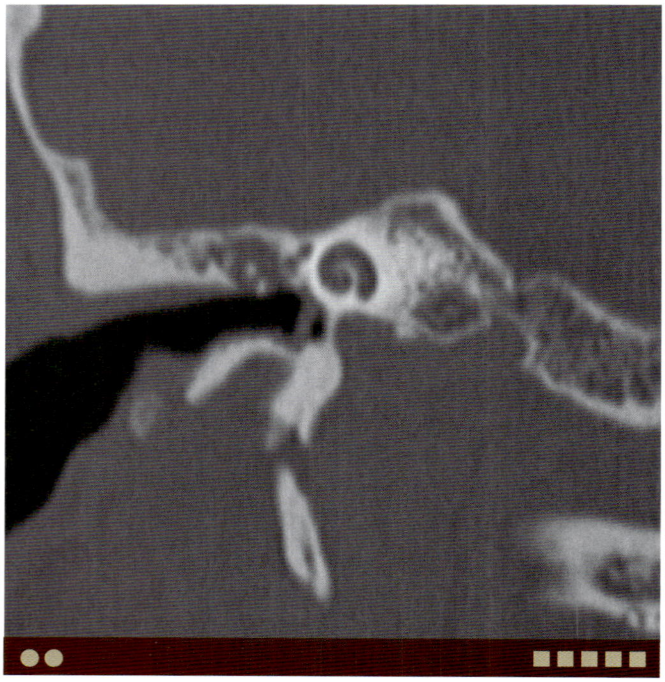

D. Tympanosclerosis, same patient as C. Coronal CT demonstrates ill-defined punctate calcifications in the epitympanum.

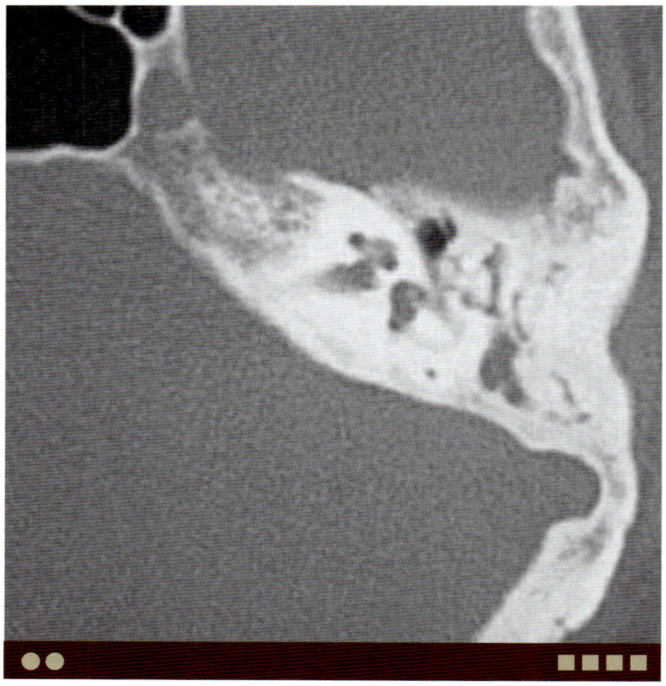

E. Tympanosclerosis in a 50-year-old woman. Axial CT demonstrates dense calcification around the malleus in the epitympanum.

DIFFERENTIAL DIAGNOSIS IMAGES (F-H)

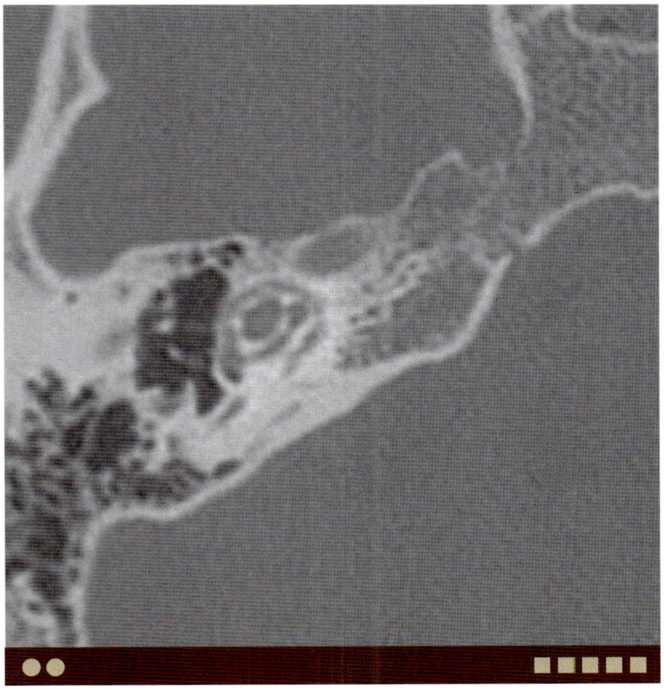

F. Otosclerosis, cochlear type. Axial CT demonstrates demineralization of the otic capsule. Pneumatization and aeration of the tympanic cavity and mastoid air cells are maintained.

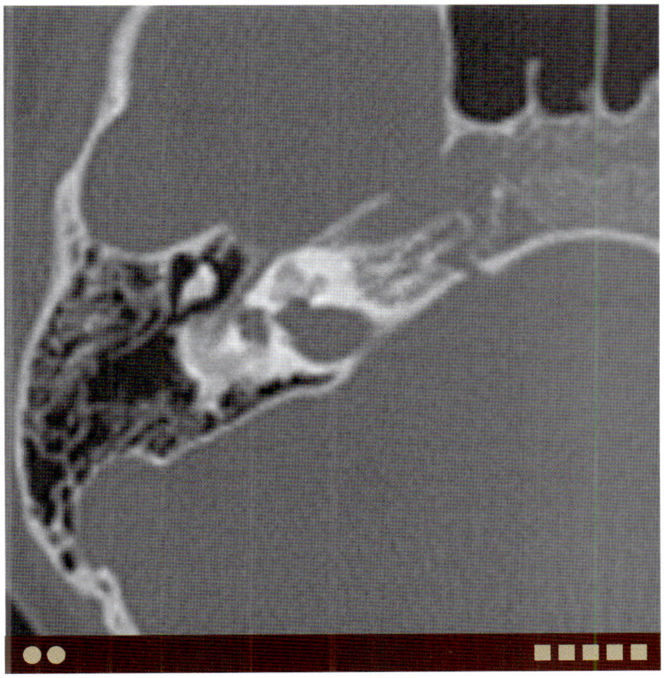

G. Labyrinthitis ossificans. Axial CT demonstrates ossification in the cochlea and lateral semicircular canal. Pneumatization and aeration of the tympanic cavity and mastoid air cells are maintained.

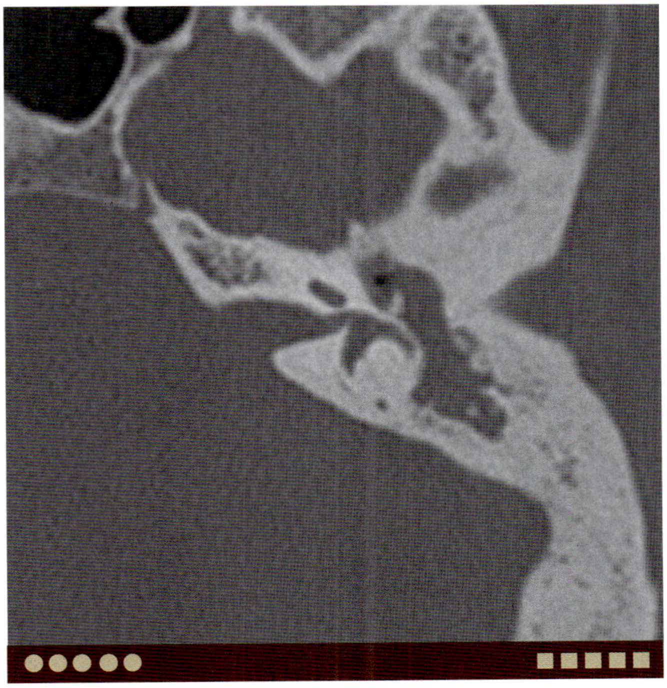

H. Cholesteatoma. Axial CT demonstrates a soft tissue mass eroding the lateral wall of the epitympanum and ossicles without calcification.

Case 1–8 Otosclerosis: Fenestral Type

Osamu Sakai, Keith Fleming

PRESENTATION

Progressive conductive hearing loss.

FINDINGS

CT demonstrates focal demineralization anteromedial to the oval window.

DIFFERENTIAL DIAGNOSIS

- Paget's disease: This often involves the entire skull. The otic capsule can be involved in late stage of Paget's disease, and may present findings similar to cochlear otosclerosis, rather than fenestral otosclerosis.
- Tympanosclerosis: The name sounds similar; however, this is a separate condition referring to calcification or ossification in the tympanic cavity from chronic infection/inflammation.
- Labyrinthitis ossificans: This is calcification or ossification in the membranous labyrinth, not an abnormality of the otic capsule.

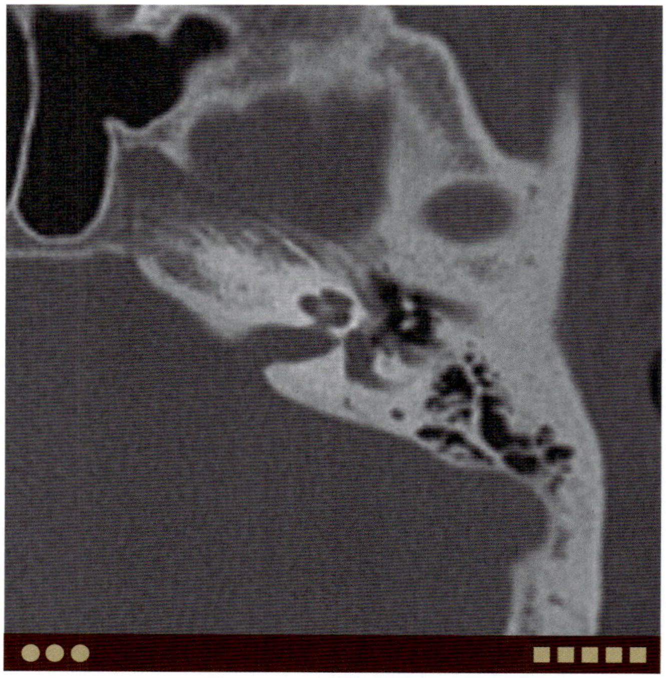

A. Fenestral otosclerosis. Axial CT demonstrates an area of decreased density with slight bone proliferation anteromedial to the oval window.

COMMENTS

This is a 38-year-old man with progressive conductive hearing loss.

Otosclerosis is rare condition characterized by demineralization of the otic capsule. Often called otospongiosis (a more accurate term), the lesion demonstrates demineralization of bone from increased vascularity, rather than sclerosis. Sclerotic change can be seen in the later stages of the disease. In the later sclerotic stage, it is difficult to diagnose on CT.

Otosclerosis can be divided into two types: fenestral type and retrofenestral or cochlear type. Fenestral type is a common type of otosclerosis in which the patient often presents with conductive hearing loss due to immobilization of the foot plate of the stapes. CT demonstrates focal demineralization in the *fissula ante fenestrum*, anteromedial to the oval window. The disease is often bilateral, therefore, careful evaluation of the contralateral side is essential. The patient often requires stapedial surgery, in which a metallic piston type of stapedial prosthesis is placed.

There is overlap with retrofenestral (cochlear) otosclerosis. Therefore, it is important to evaluate density of the entire otic capsule. Retrofenestral (cochlear) otosclerosis will be further discussed in the next section.

PEARLS

- **Otosclerosis is a condition resulting in demineralization of the otic capsule, not sclerosis. This condition is also known as otospongiosis.**
- **Fenestral otosclerosis is the common type, involving the *fissula ante fenestrum*, anteromedial to the oval window. This causes conductive hearing loss due to fixation of the foot plate of the stapes.**
- **Otosclerosis is often bilateral.**

ADDITIONAL IMAGES (B-E)

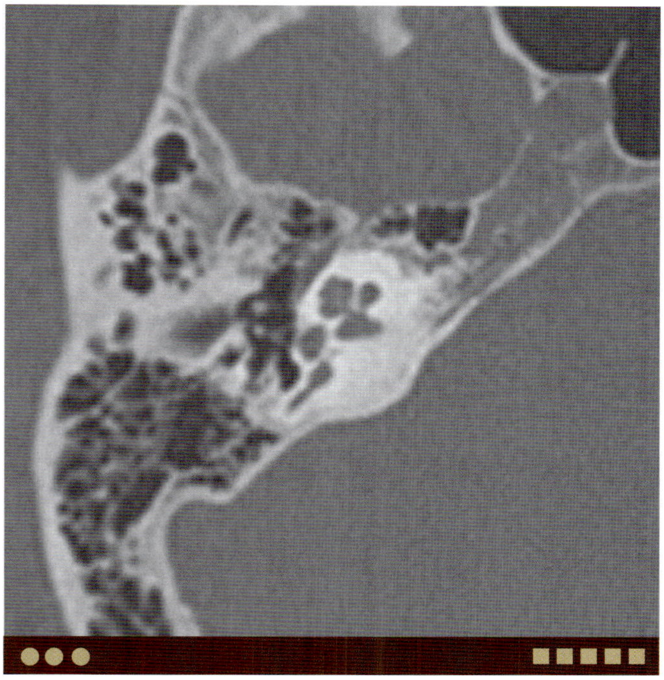

B. Fenestral otosclerosis in a 55-year-old man. Axial CT of the right ear demonstrates very subtle demineralization in the *fissula ante fenestrum*, anterior and medial to the oval window.

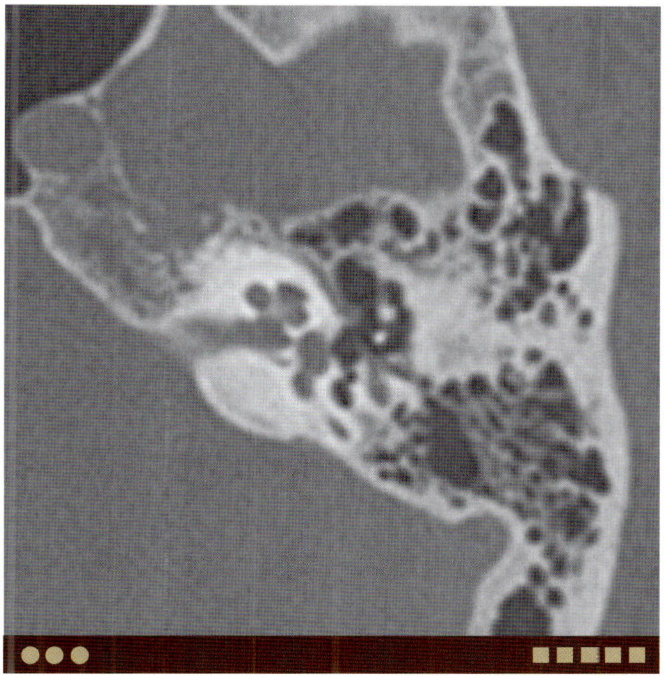

C. Fenestral otosclerosis, same patient as B. Axial CT of the left ear demonstrates an identical finding.

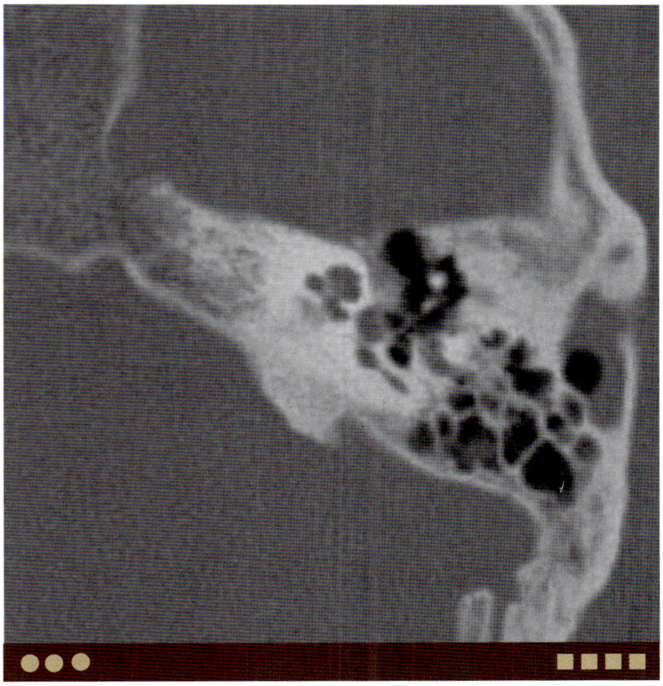

D. Fenestral otosclerosis in a 45-year-old woman. Axial CT demonstrates demineralization and prominent osseous proliferation in the *fissula ante fenestrum*, which contacts the stapes.

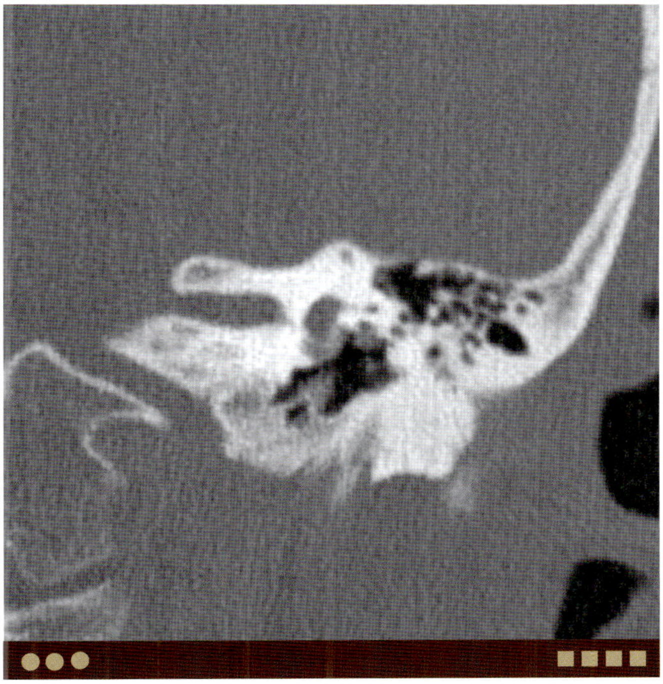

E. Fenestral otosclerosis, same patient as D. Coronal CT demonstrates prominent focal demineralization.

DIFFERENTIAL DIAGNOSIS IMAGES (F-G)

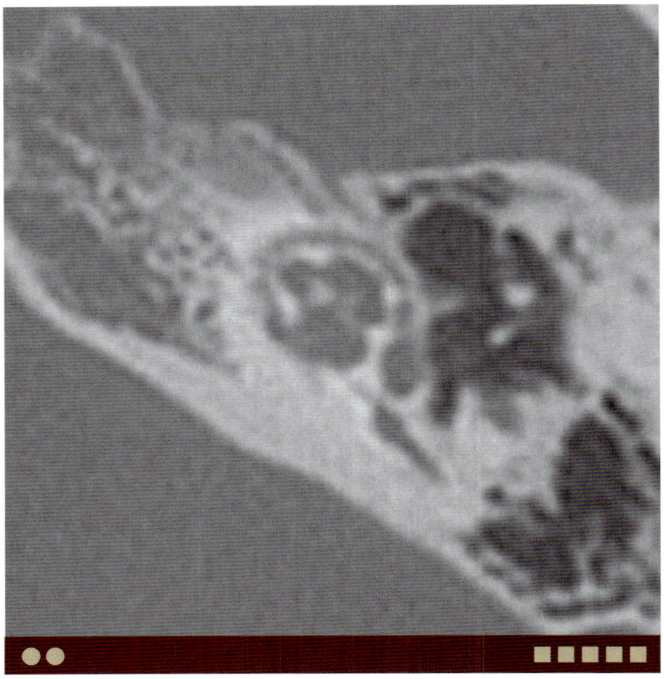

F. Cochlear otosclerosis. Axial CT demonstrates demineralization around the cochlea as well as in the *fissula ante fenestrum*.

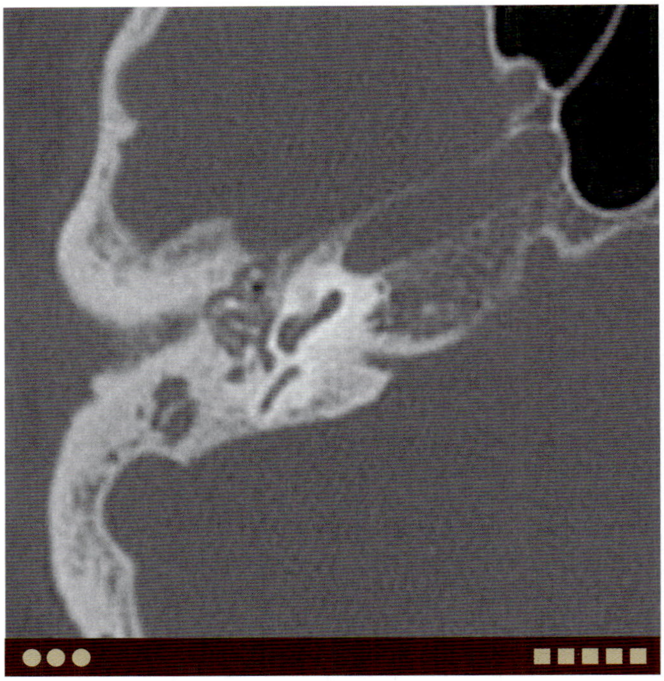

G. Tympanosclerosis. Axial CT demonstrates punctate calcification in the opacified epitympanum.

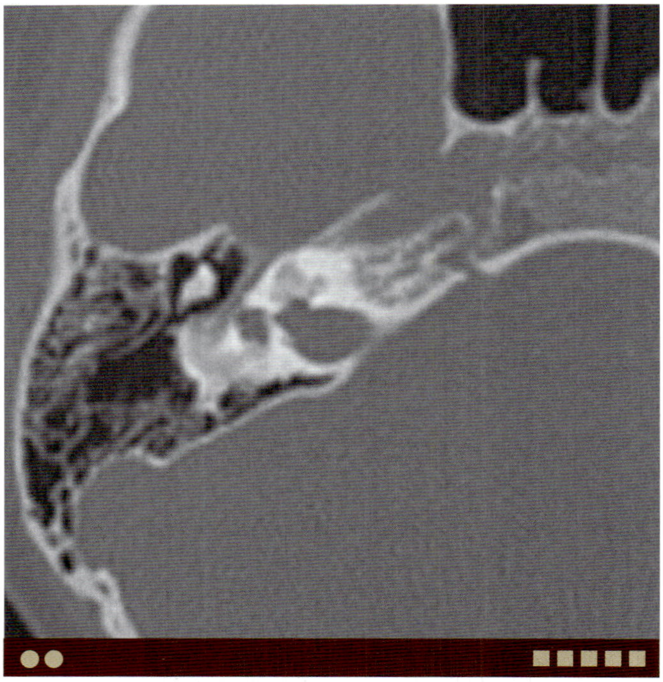

H. Labyrinthitis ossificans. Axial CT demonstrates ossification in the cochlea and lateral semicircular canal.

Case 1–9 Otosclerosis: Retrofenestral (Cochlear) Type

Osamu Sakai, Keith Fleming

PRESENTATION

Progressive mixed hearing loss.

FINDINGS

CT demonstrates demineralization of the otic capsule surrounding the cochlea.

DIFFERENTIAL DIAGNOSIS

- Osteogenesis imperfecta: This shows profound demineralization of the otic capsules bilaterally, very similar to cochlear otosclerosis.
- Paget's disease: This condition often involves the entire skull and skull base. The otic capsule may be involved in late stage of Paget's disease.
- Labyrinthitis ossificans: This is calcification or ossification in the membranous labyrinth, not an abnormality of the otic capsule.
- Tympanosclerosis: The name sounds similar, but this is a separate condition of calcification or ossification in the tympanic cavity from chronic infection/inflammation.

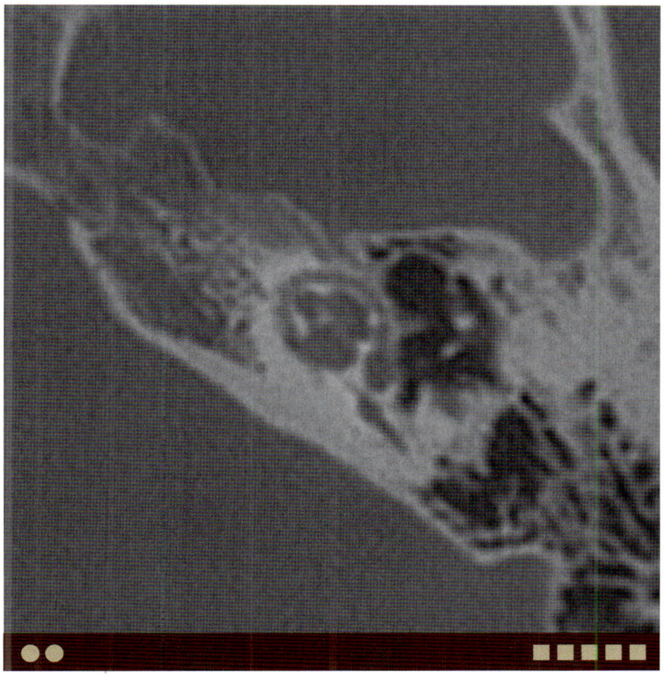

A. Cochlear otosclerosis. Axial CT demonstrates extensive demineralization of the otic capsule, forming an additional lucent zone outside of the basal turn of the cochlea, the "forth ring sign."

COMMENTS

This is a 19-year-old man with progressive bilateral mixed hearing loss.

Retrofenestral or cochlear type otosclerosis is a relatively rare form of otosclerosis, characterized by demineralization of the otic capsule around the cochlea. Patient presentation is usually a progressive mixed or sensorineural hearing loss. As discussed earlier, otosclerosis is a demineralization of the otic capsule, and more appropriately termed "otospongiosis" due to demineralization of increased vascularity, rather than sclerosis.

CT demonstrates demineralization of the otic capsule, which can be subtle. Extensive otic capsule demineralization is sometimes called the "forth ring sign." This is due to the demineralization resulting in an additional lucent ring surrounding the basal turn of the cochlea. The finding is often bilateral, although symptoms can be unilateral initially.

MRI demonstrates subtle, ill-defined intermediate signal in the otic capsule, with loss of the signal-void due to dense bone seen in normal patients. Abnormal enhancement is seen in the active phase of the disease, corresponding to increased vascularity and demineralization. MRI with contrast is useful to evaluate for activity of this condition. T2 high signal from the membranous labyrinth is usually preserved.

The main differential diagnosis is osteogenesis imperfecta, which demonstrates almost identical findings to retrofenestral or cochlear otosclerosis. Genetic consultation is required to establish the diagnosis.

PEARLS

- **Otosclerosis is a demineralization of the otic capsule, not sclerosis.**
- **Retrofenestral, or cochlear, otosclerosis is a relatively rare form of otosclerosis characterized by demineralization of the entire otic capsule. This usually presents with progressive mixed or sensorineural hearing loss.**
- **Retrofenestral (cochlear) otosclerosis is often bilateral and needs to be differentiated from osteogenesis imperfecta by clinical and genetic testing.**

ADDITIONAL IMAGES (B-F)

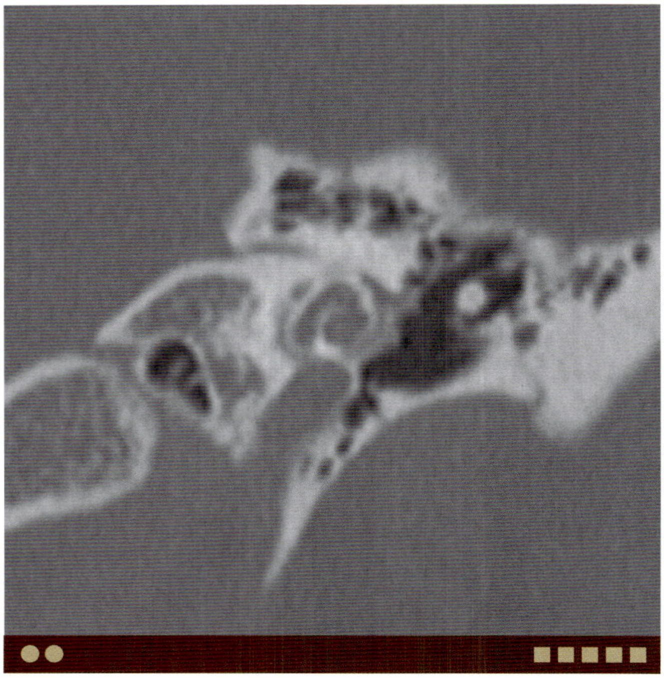

B. Cochlear otosclerosis, same patient as A. Coronal CT demonstrates demineralization around the cochlea.

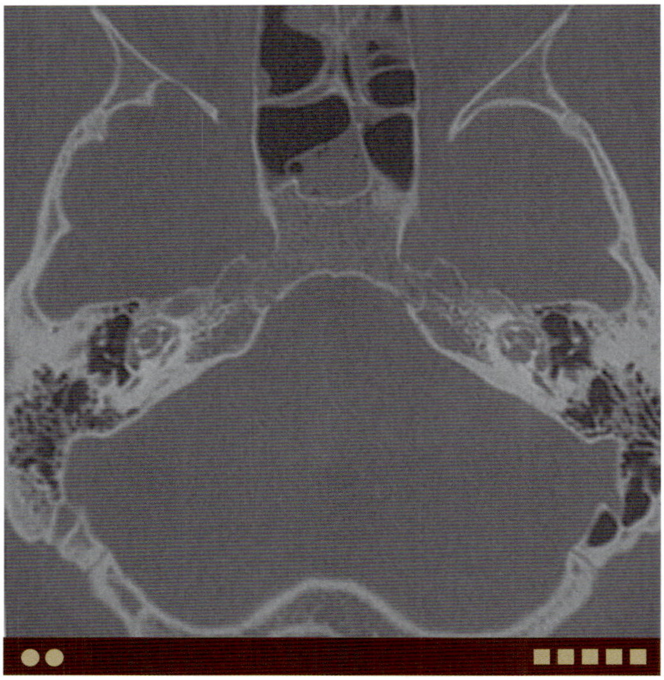

C. Cochlear otosclerosis in a different patient. Axial CT demonstrates demineralization of the otic capsule bilaterally.

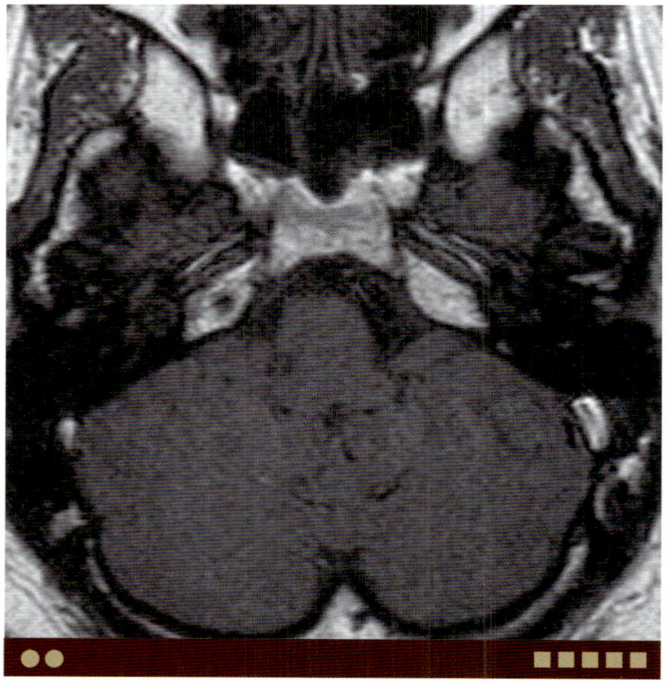

D. Cochlear otosclerosis, same patient as C. Axial T1W MR image demonstrates ill-defined intermediate signal in the otic capsule bilaterally.

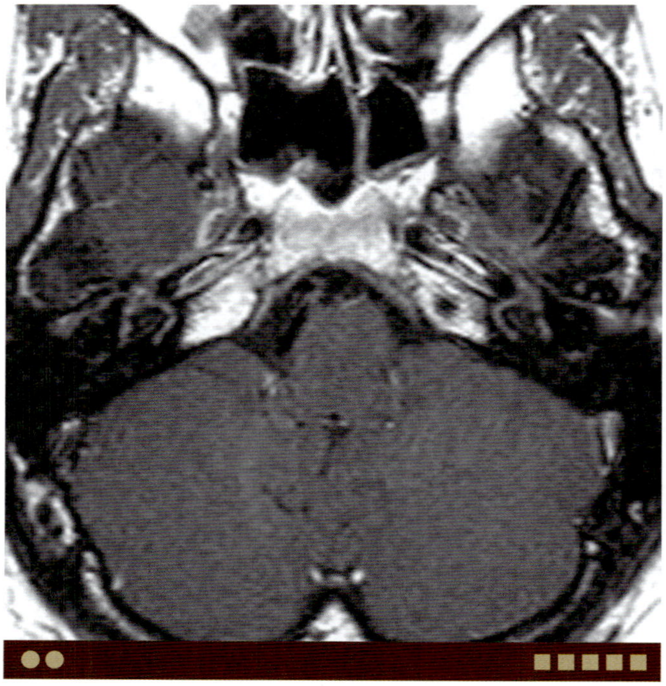

E. Cochlear otosclerosis, same patient as C. Axial postcontrast T1W MR image demonstrates abnormal enhancement of the otic capsule bilaterally.

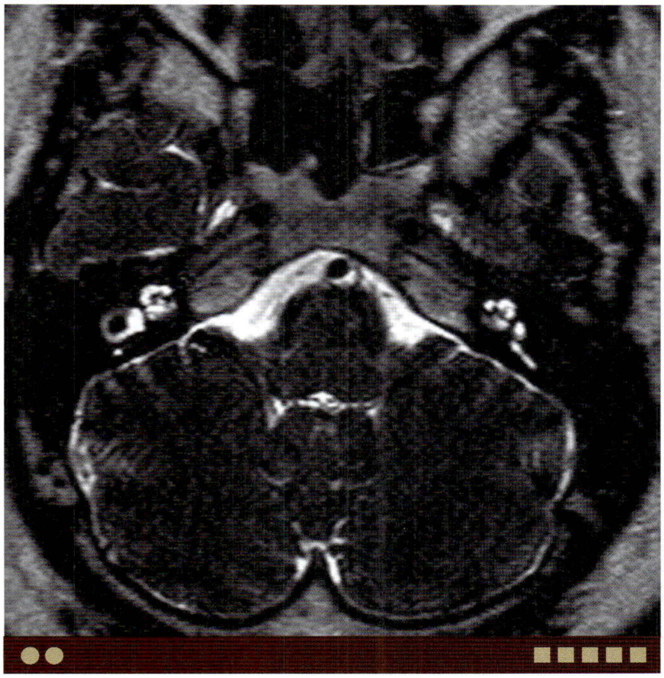

F. Cochlear otosclerosis, same patient as C. Axial T2W MR image demonstrates normal high signal in the membranous labyrinth bilaterally.

DIFFERENTIAL DIAGNOSIS IMAGES (G-I)

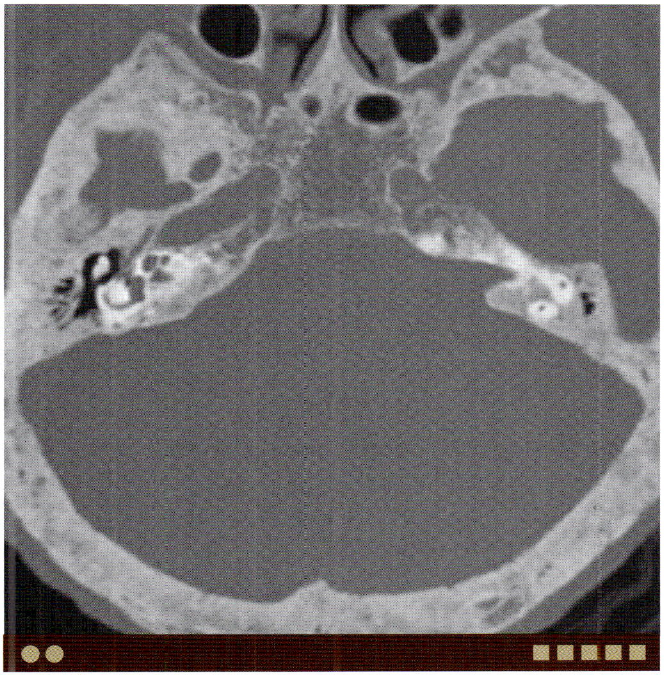

G. Paget's disease. Axial CT demonstrates heterogeneous demineralization and thickening of the entire skull base. Subtle demineralization is also seen in the otic capsule.

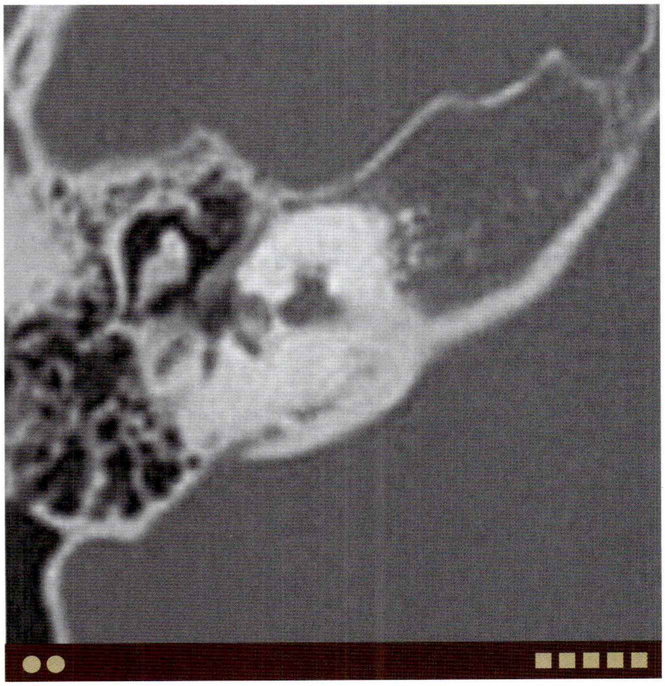

H. Labyrinthitis ossificans. Axial CT demonstrates ossification of the cochlea.

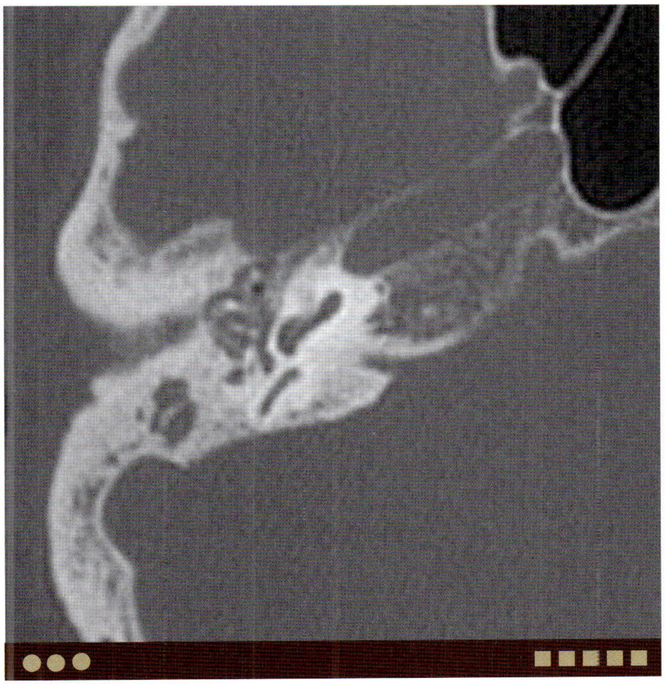

I. Tympanosclerosis. Axial CT demonstrates punctate calcification in the opacified epitympanum.

Case 1-10 Acoustic Neuroma (Vestibular Schwannoma)

Osamu Sakai, Keith Fleming

PRESENTATION

Sensorineural hearing loss.

FINDINGS

CT and MRI demonstrate an enhancing mass at the cerebellopontine angle (CPA).

DIFFERENTIAL DIAGNOSIS

- Meningioma: This is the second most common mass at the CPA after vestibular schwannoma. Typically, this is seen as a dural-based enhancing mass without extension into the internal auditory canal. A dural-tail sign is helpful, but may not be present.
- Epidermoid: This is the third most common mass at the CPA. Density and signal intensity are similar to CSF, and epidermoid may not be easily identified on CT or standard T1W and T2W images. However, epidermoids show significantly increased signal on diffusion-weighted images.
- Aneurysm: Pulsation and flow-artifact, as well as heterogeneous signal from blood products are helpful to make the diagnosis.
- Schwannomas from other cranial nerves: Schwannomas from other cranial nerves may extend into the CPA.

COMMENTS

This is a 55-year-old man with unilateral sensorineural hearing loss.

Acoustic neuroma is the most common CPA mass accounting for about 80% of masses in this region. Patients are often between 30 and 60 years old, with a slight female predominance. Although initial presentations are often cochlear nerve symptoms such as hearing loss and tinnitus, most acoustic neuromas arise from the vestibular nerve. Therefore, they should be referred to as vestibular schwannomas. Rarely, schwannomas arise from the cochlear nerve.

The cell of origin of a schwannoma is the Schwann cell, and the most common location of the lesion is at the orifice of the internal auditory canal (IAC), also known as the porus acousticus. The junction of the glial cells and Schwann cells is located at this point along the course of the cranial nerves.

On CT or MRI, widening of the bony canal is commonly seen. When the lesion grows further, it protrudes into the cistern and gives the "ice cream-on-cone" appearance. Schwannomas usually show homogeneous enhancement, however, cystic degeneration is often seen in larger tumors. With large tumors, peritumoral cysts can be seen in the adjacent brain parenchyma.

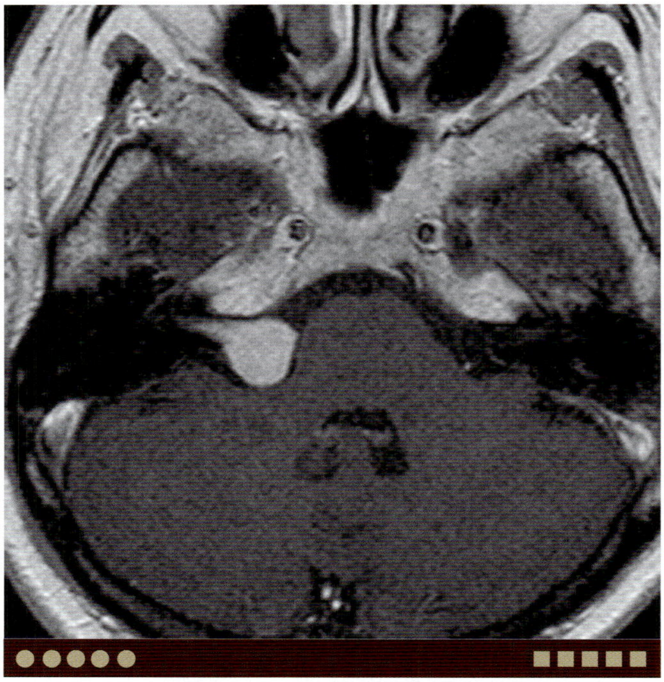

A. Vestibular schwannoma. Axial postcontrast T1W MR image demonstrates a homogeneously enhancing tumor centered at the orifice of the right IAC extending to the fundus, demonstrating the typical "ice cream-on-cone" appearance.

Although high-resolution T2W MR imaging depicts most schwannomas, postcontrast high-resolution T1W imaging is still the gold standard in diagnosing vestibular schwannomas. Adequate CSF contrast may not be obtained on T2W images in patients with small internal auditory canals. It is often difficult to diagnose schwannomas in the fundus of the IAC, cochlea, and vestibule without contrast. The membranous labyrinth should also be carefully evaluated, in addition to the entire IAC and the cisternal segments of the seventh and eighth cranial nerve complexes.

PEARLS

- **Acoustic neuroma is the most common CPA mass, accounting for approximately 80% of masses in this region. They usually arise from the vestibular nerve.**
- **Cystic degeneration is common, particularly in large tumors.**
- **Peritumoral cysts can be seen in brain parenchyma adjacent to large tumors.**
- **Bilateral vestibular schwannomas are pathognomonic for neurofibromatosis type II.**

Bilateral vestibular schwannomas are pathognomonic for neurofibromatosis type II. This is an abnormality of chromosome 22. These patients can have multiple schwannomas arising from other cranial nerves, as well as meningiomas and ependymomas.

ADDITIONAL IMAGES (B-H)

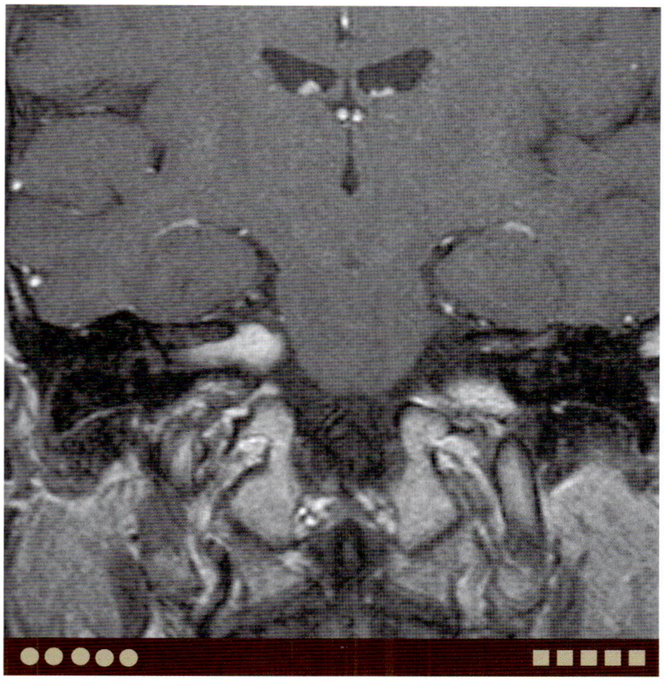

B. Vestibular schwannoma, same patient as A. Coronal postcontrast T1W MR image demonstrates a homogeneously enhancing tumor centered at the orifice of the right IAC extending to the fundus.

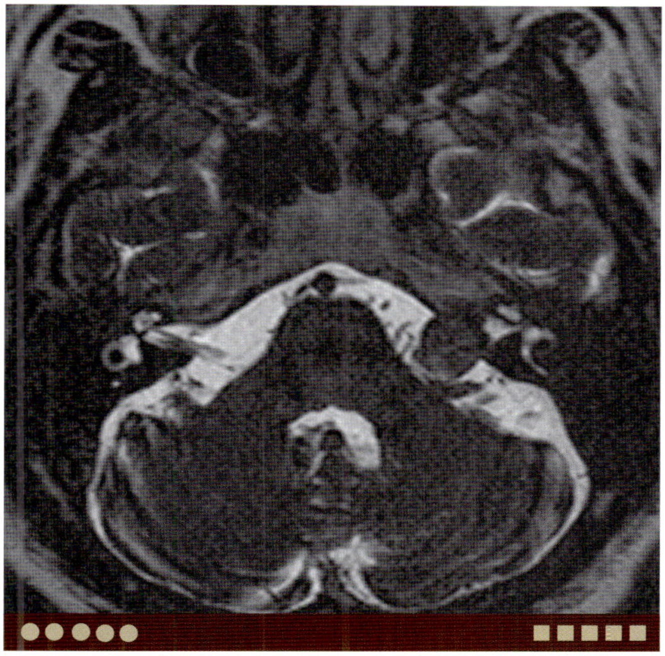

C. Vestibular schwannoma in a different patient. Axial high-resolution T2W MR image demonstrates a round mass slightly flaring the left IAC.

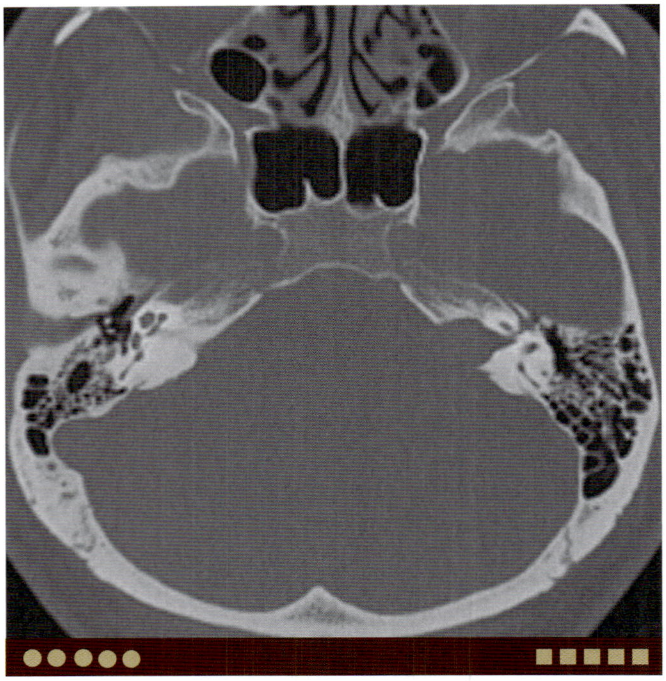

D. Vestibular schwannoma in a different patient. Axial CT demonstrates widened left IAC.

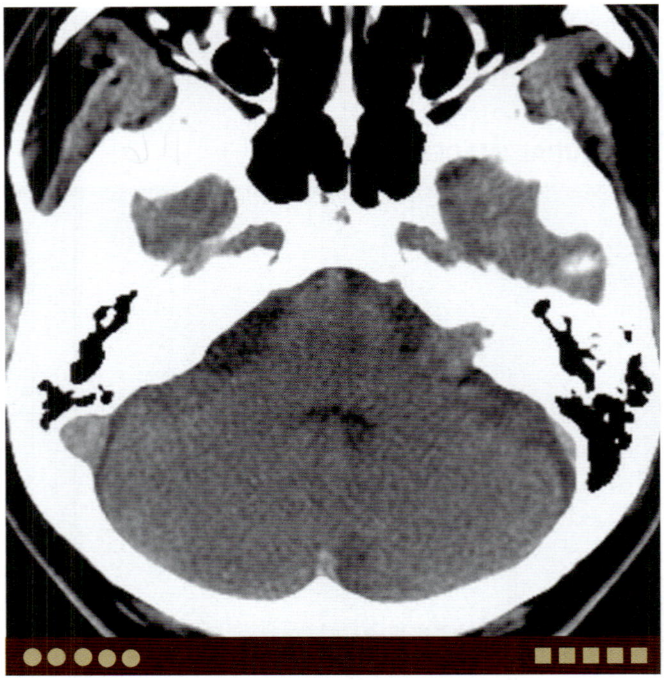

E. Vestibular schwannoma, same patient as D. Axial postcontrast CT demonstrates a mildly enhancing tumor at the orifice of the left IAC.

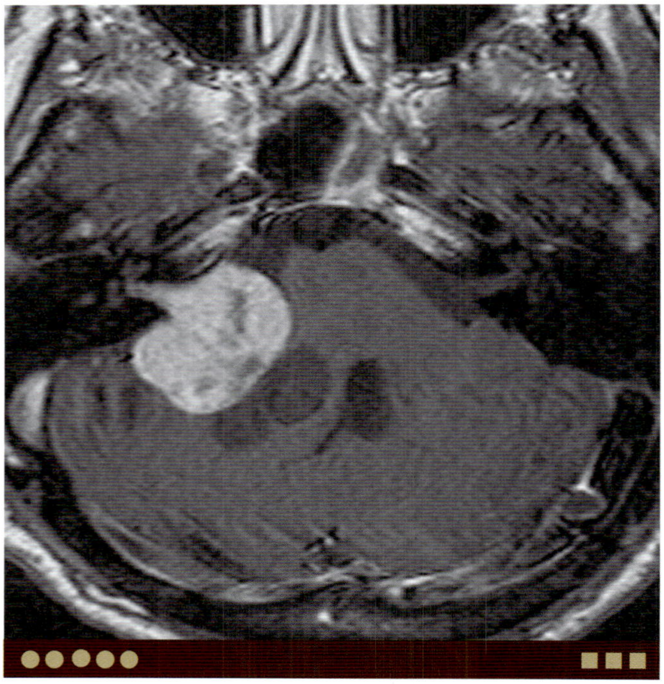

F. Vestibular schwannoma in a different patient. Axial postcontrast T1W MR image demonstrates a large tumor with a peritumoral cyst, posteromedial to the tumor in the right middle cerebellar peduncle.

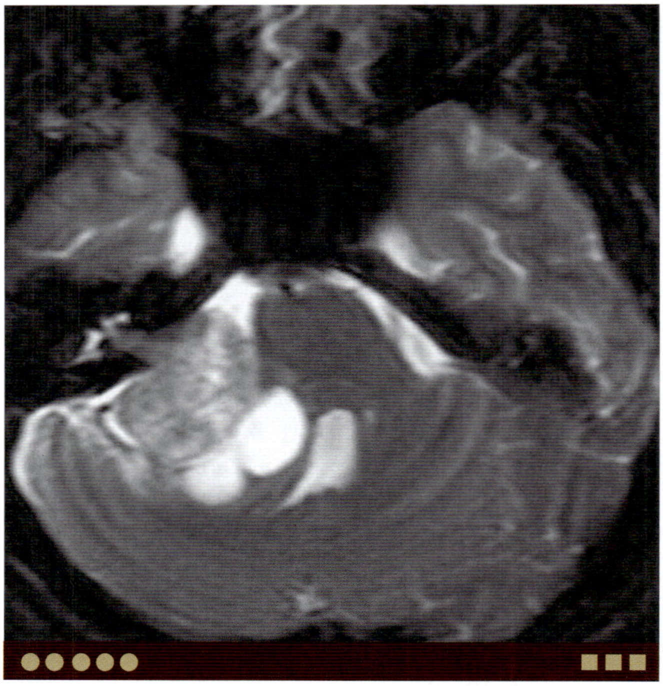

G. Vestibular schwannoma, same patient as F. Axial T2W MR image demonstrates a large, heterogeneous tumor with a peritumoral cyst in the right middle cerebellar peduncle.

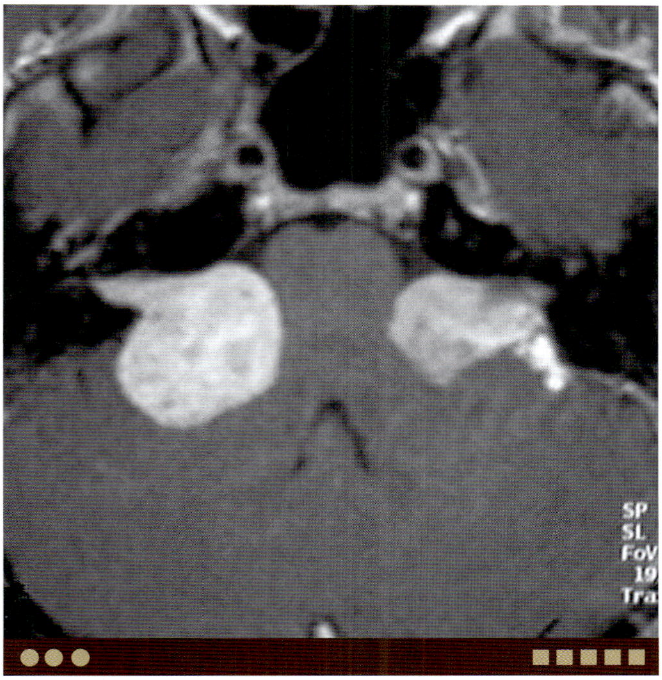

H. Bilateral vestibular schwannomas. Axial postcontrast T1W MR image demonstrates large bilateral vestibular schwannomas with mass-effect on the pons in a patient with neurofibromatosis, type II.

DIFFERENTIAL DIAGNOSIS IMAGES (I-J)

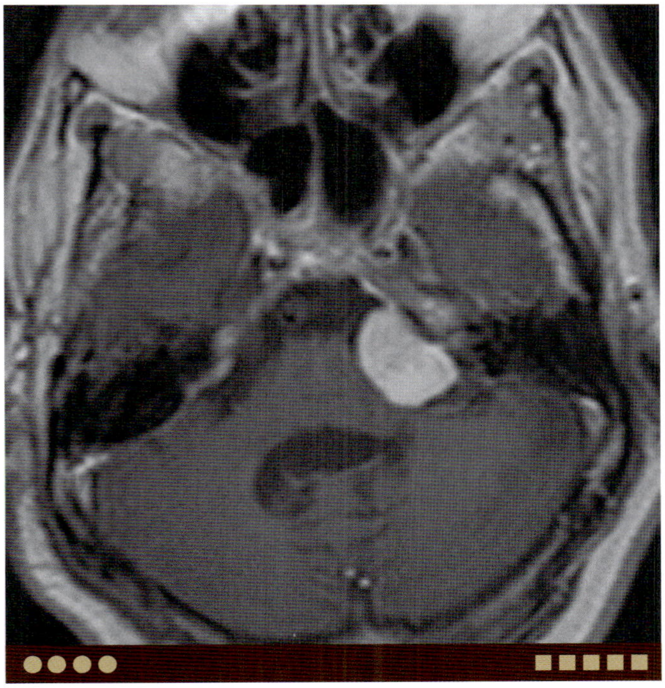

I. Meningioma. Axial postcontrast T1W image demonstrates a dural-based homogeneously enhancing tumor at the left CPA.

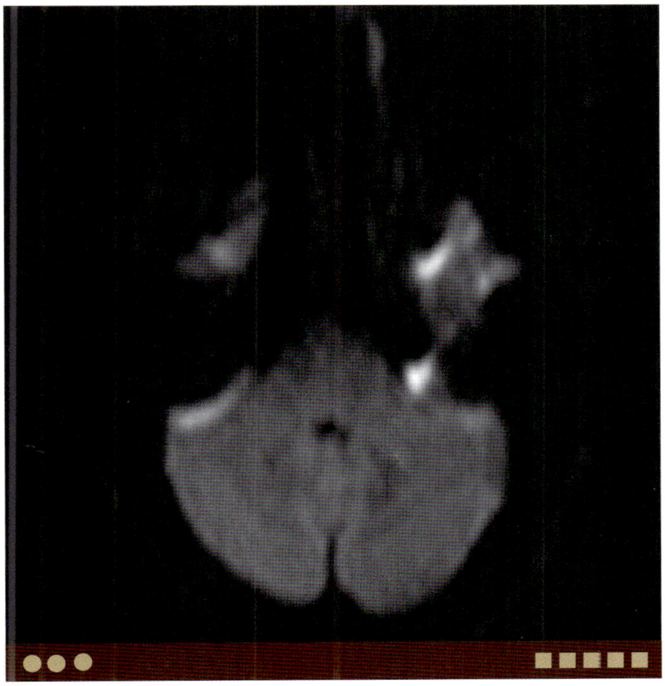

J. Epidermoid. Axial diffusion-weighted image demonstrates a high-signal lesion at the left CPA.

Case 1–11 Cochlear Schwannoma

Osamu Sakai, Rohini Nadgir

PRESENTATION

Sensorineural hearing loss.

FINDINGS

MR image shows an enhancing lesion in the cochlea and/or fundus of the internal auditory canal.

DIFFERENTIAL DIAGNOSIS

- Labyrinthitis: Abnormal enhancement after contrast, usually more diffuse and ill-defined distribution.
- Labyrinthine hemorrhage: This demonstrates increased signal on precontrast T1W images without enhancement.
- Lipoma: This demonstrates high signal on precontrast T1W images, decreased signal on fat-suppressed images and does not show enhancement.
- Schwannomas arising from the vestibular or facial nerves: These demonstrate identical signal patterns in different locations.

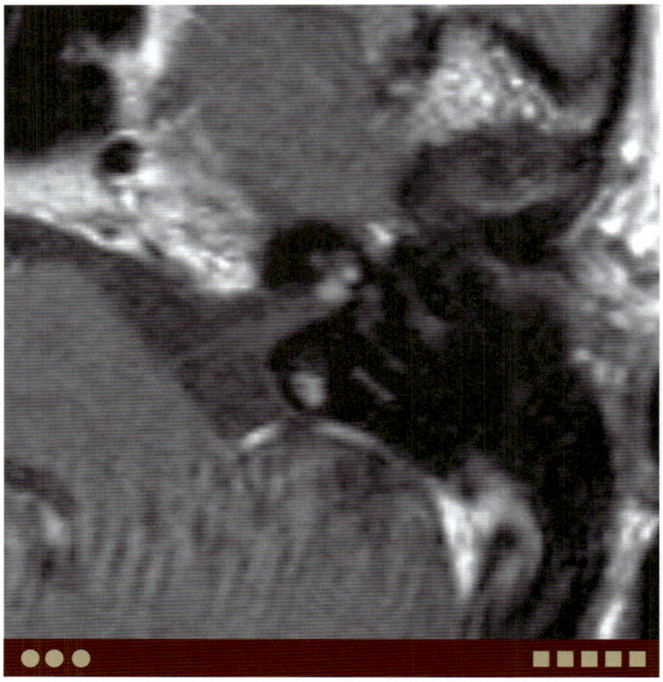

A. Cochlear schwannoma. Axial postcontrast T1W image demonstrates an enhancing lesion in the fundus of the IAC extending into the basal turn of the cochlea.

COMMENTS

This is a 41-year-old man with sensorineural hearing loss.

Schwannomas account for about 80% of cerebellopontine angle (CPA) masses and often arise at the orifice of the internal auditory canal (IAC), most commonly from the vestibular nerve. However, schwannoma can occur in the fundus of the IAC from the cochlear or vestibular nerves and also can be seen in the cochlea and vestibule. Therefore, it is important to investigate the membranous labyrinth and fundus of the IAC as well as the CPA carefully.

Cochlear schwannoma is rare. It has been reported that cochlear schwannoma accounts for 5% of CPA tumors. Clinically, a cochlear schwannoma mimics the clinical features of sudden deafness or Ménière's disease. Sudden or major hearing loss without associated vestibular symptoms or preoperative facial paralysis may be predictive of a cochlear schwannoma.

High-resolution T2W images are helpful to diagnose schwannoma without contrast. However, contrast-enhanced T1W imaging is often needed to confirm the diagnosis and define the extent of the lesion, particularly at the fundus of the IAC and in the membranous labyrinth.

PEARLS

- **Cochlear schwannoma is seen as an enhancing mass in the cochlea and/or fundus of the IAC.**
- **Careful evaluation of the membranous labyrinth is important in addition to evaluation of the CPA and IAC.**
- **Sudden or major hearing loss without associated vestibular symptoms or facial paralysis may suggest cochlear schwannoma.**

ADDITIONAL IMAGES (B-F)

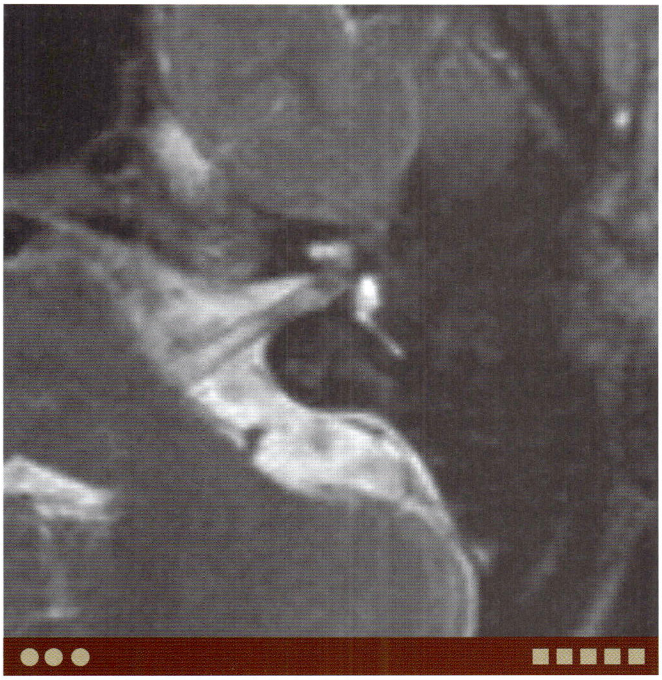

B. Cochlear schwannoma, same patient as A. Axial T2W image demonstrates loss of normal high signal from the cerebrospinal fluid in the fundus. The lesion in the basal turn of the cochlea is hardly appreciated.

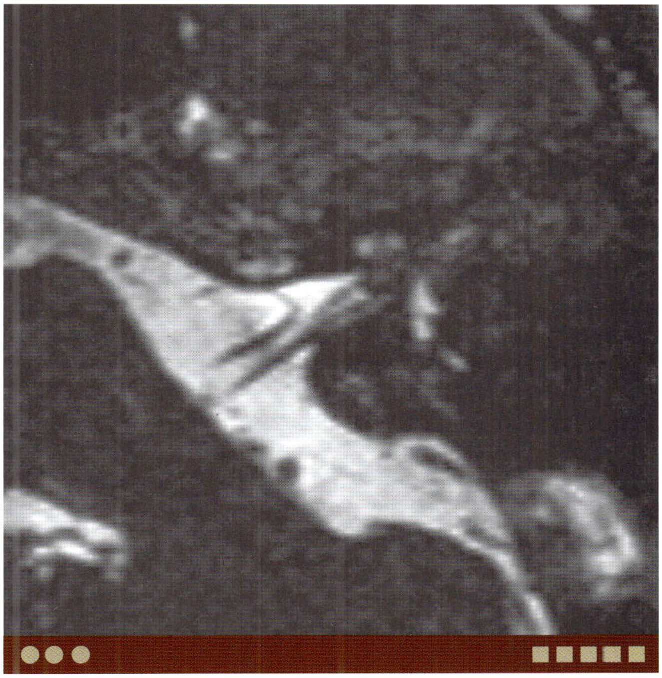

C. Cochlear schwannoma, same patient as A. Axial high-resolution T2W image demonstrates loss of normal high signal from fluid in the basal turn of the cochlea as well as in the fundus of the AC.

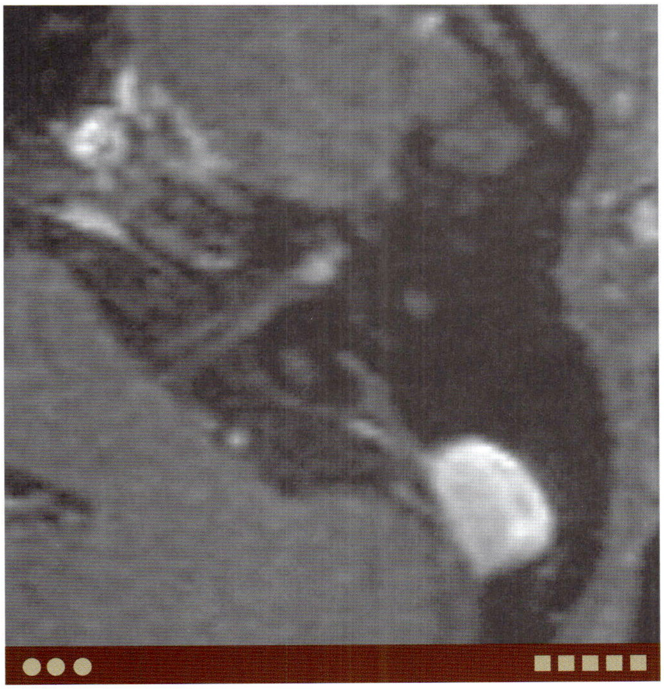

D. Cochlear schwannoma in the same patient as A. Axial postcontrast high-resolution T1W image demonstrates an enhancing lesion in the fundus extending into the basal turn of the cochlea.

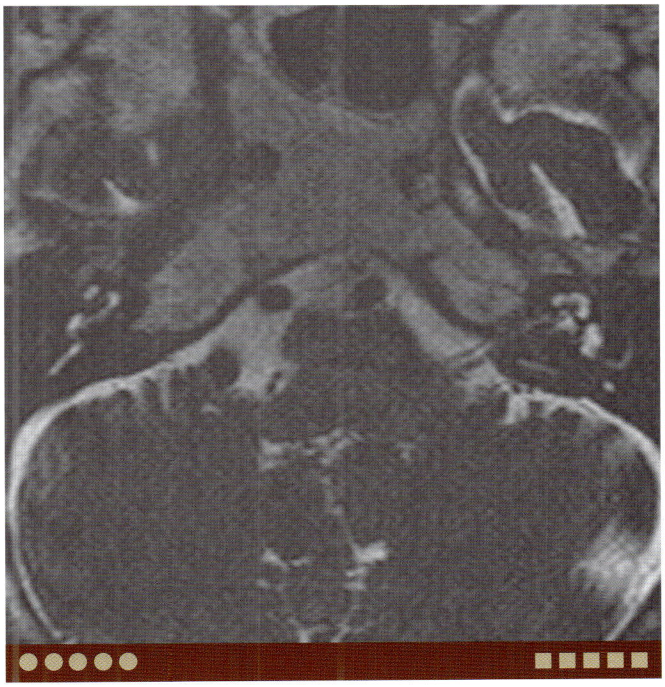

E. Cochlear schwannoma in a different patient. Axial high-resolution T2W image demonstrates loss of normal high signal from fluic in the middle turn of the right cochlea.

DIFFERENTIAL DIAGNOSIS IMAGES (E-H)

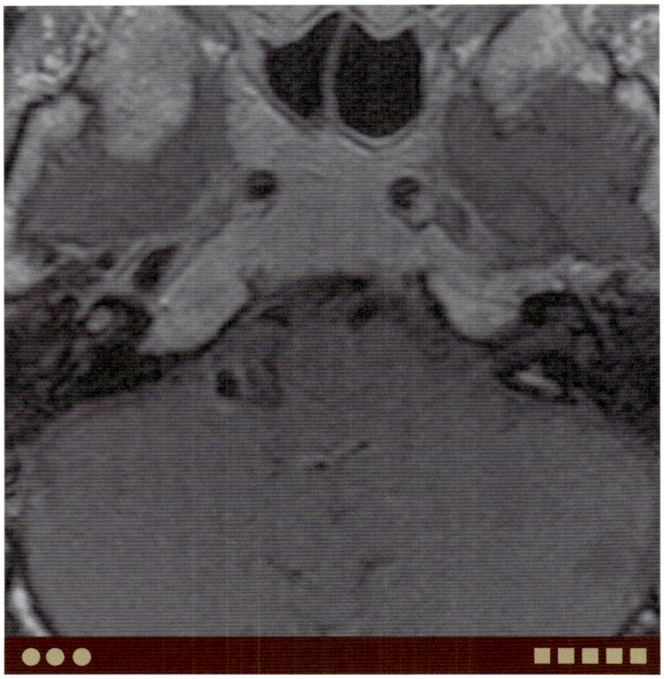

F. Cochlear schwannoma, same patient as E. Axial postcontrast high-resolution T1W image demonstrates enhancement of the lesion in the right cochlea.

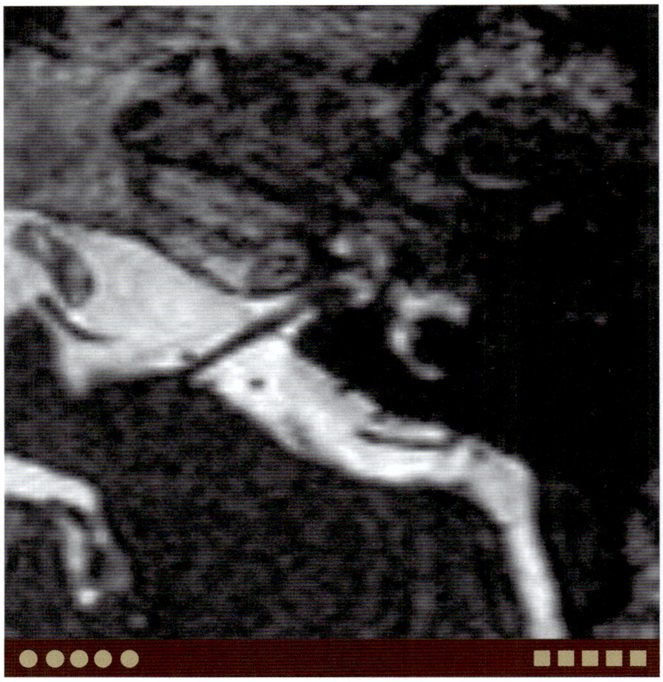

G. Vestibular schwannoma. Axial high-resolution T2W image demonstrates a small mass arising from the vestibular nerve in the posterior portion of the IAC.

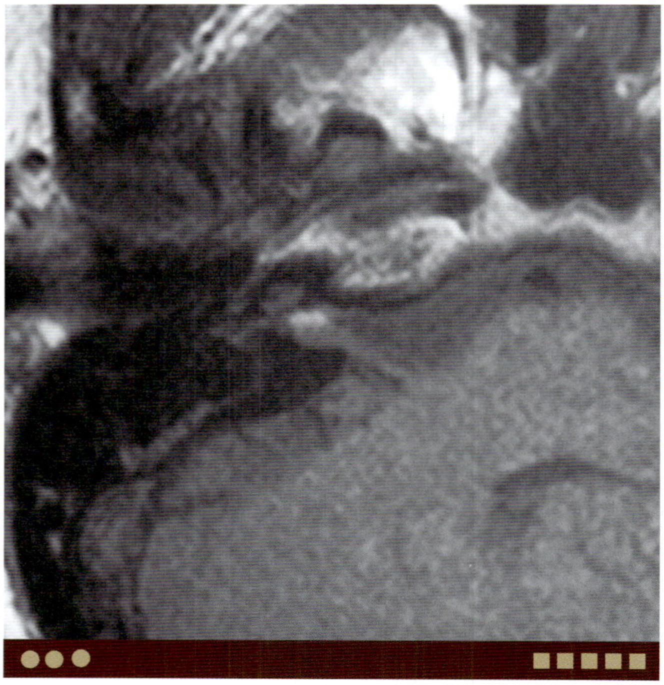

H. Lipoma. Axial noncontrast-enhanced T1W image demonstrates a small high-signal mass in the IAC.

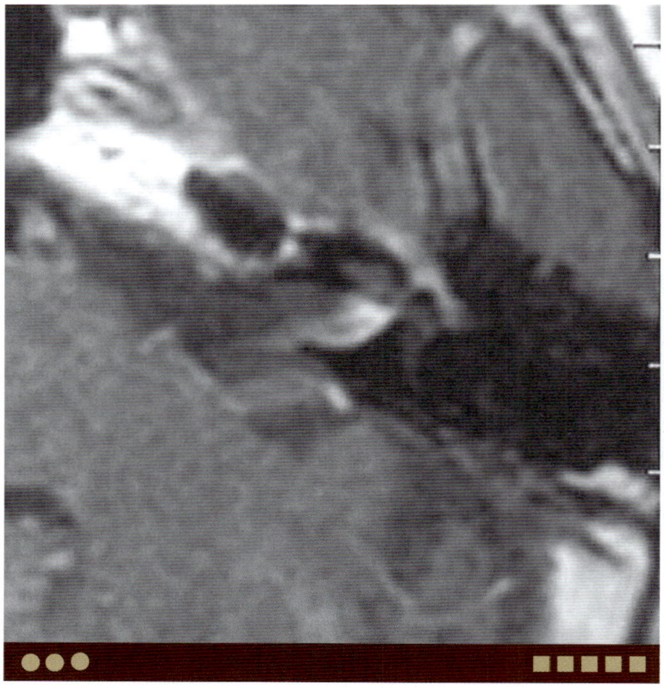

I. Bell's palsy. Axial postcontrast T1W image demonstrates abnormal enhancement in the intracanalicular segment of the facial nerve.

Case 1–12 Lipoma

Osamu Sakai, Rohini Nadgir

PRESENTATION

Sensorineural hearing loss.

FINDINGS

T1W MR image demonstrates a high-signal lesion in the internal auditory canal.

DIFFERENTIAL DIAGNOSIS

- Schwannoma: Postcontrast T1W demonstrates an enhancing lesion which is similar signal to lipoma. However, schwannoma demonstrates low signal on precontrast T1W images.
- Dermoid/epidermoid: Fat-containing dermoid or proteinaceous epidermoid can demonstrate similar findings.

COMMENTS

This is a 40-year-old woman with sensorineural hearing loss.

Lipoma in the internal auditory canal is rare. There is about 2:1 male-to-female predominance. Bilateral lesions have been reported. Hearing loss, dizziness, and tinnitus are the most common presenting symptoms.

Lipoma demonstrates fat density and is easily diagnosed on CT. On MRI, it shows high signal on T1W images and is readily diagnosed as well. However, if precontrast T1W imaging is skipped to minimize the scan time, lipoma may be misdiagnosed as schwannoma on postcontrast T1W and T2W images. Fat-containing lesions, such as dermoid and proteinaceous or hemorrhagic cystic lesions may demonstrate increased T1 signal. Fat-suppressed sequences are useful to confirm presence of fat in the lesion. Alternatively, CT can be performed to identify fat if it is not performed prior to MRI.

Conservative follow-up is the best treatment option for patients with lipomas. Surgery is indicated only when significant progressive or disabling symptoms are present because of the potential for significant morbidity with resection.

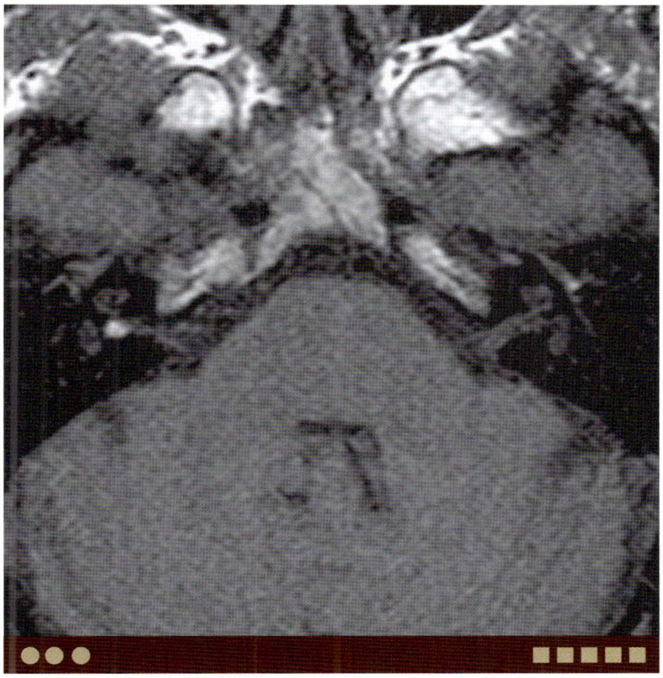

A. Lipoma. Axial T1W image demonstrates a small high-signal mass in the right internal auditory canal.

PEARLS

- **Lipoma demonstrates high signal on noncontrast T1W images.**
- **Lipoma demonstrates low density on CT.**
- **Lipoma is difficult to differentiate from schwannoma on postcontrast T1W and T2W images.**

ADDITIONAL IMAGES (B-G)

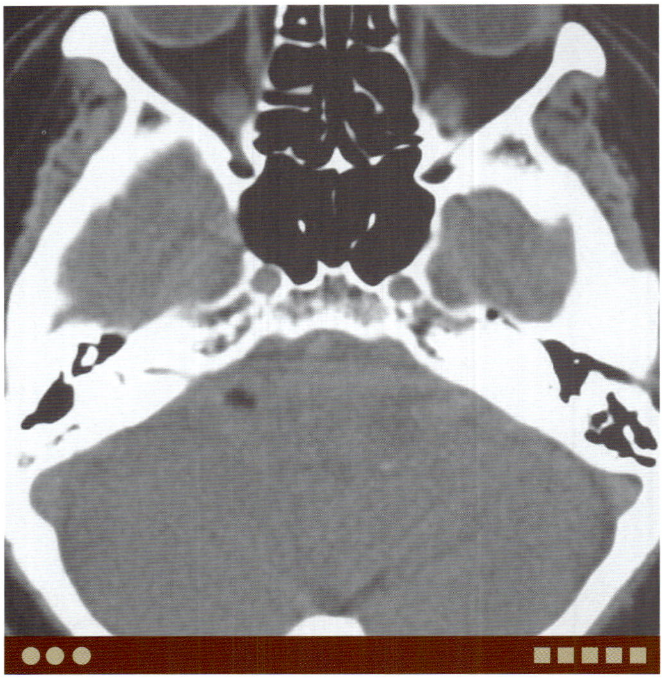

B. Lipoma in a different patient. Axial CT demonstrates a small low-density mass at the right CPA.

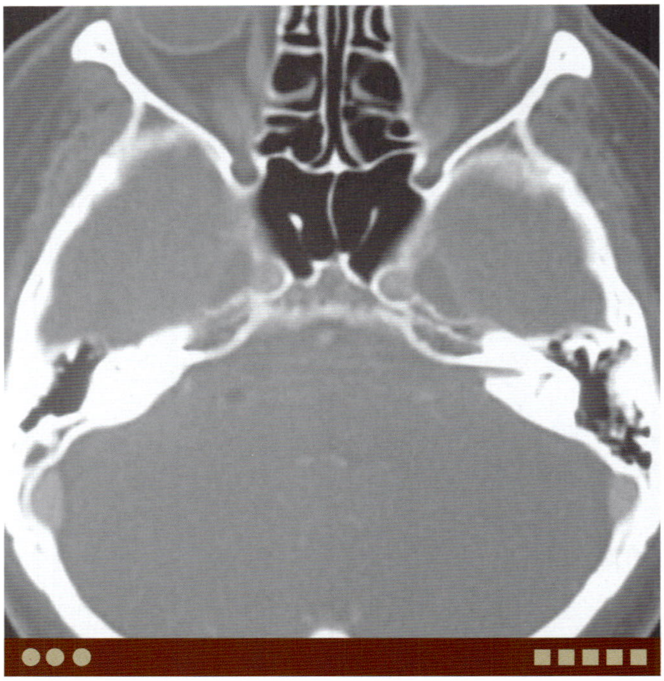

C. Lipoma, same patient as B. Axial CT with bone window confirms fat density, not air, of the lesion.

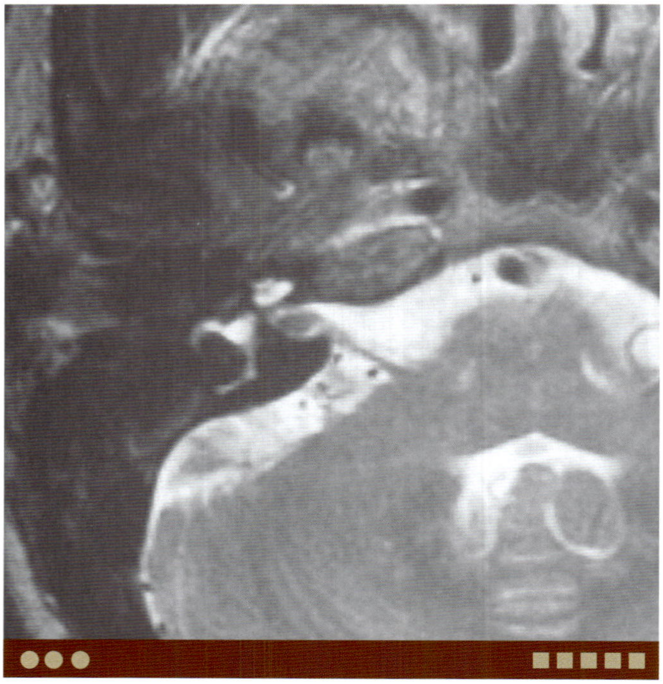

D. Lipoma in a different patient. Axial T2W image demonstrates a small mass demonstrating intermediate signal in the IAC.

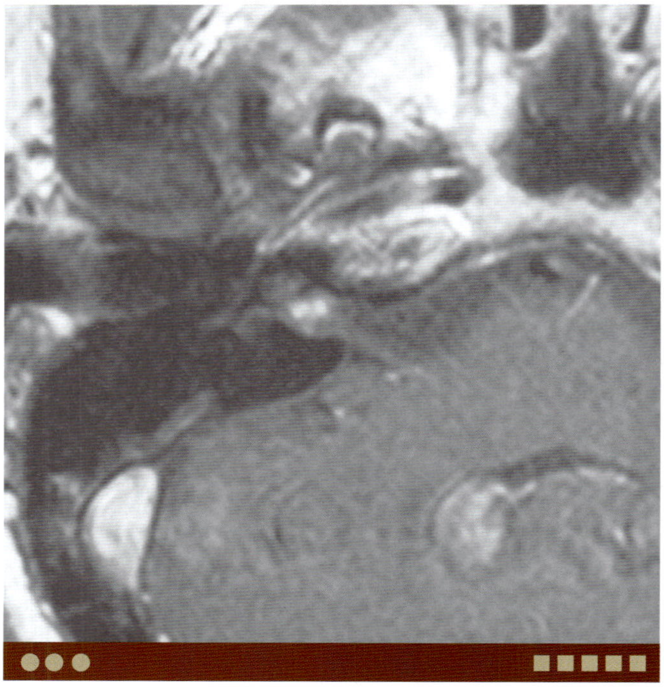

E. Lipoma, same patient as D. Axial contrast-enhanced T1W image demonstrates a small high-signal lesion in the IAC.

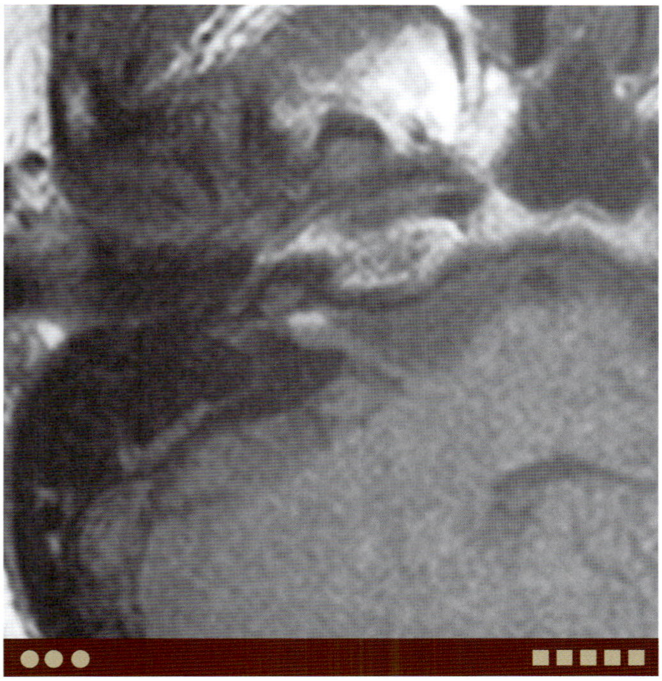

F. Lipoma, same patient as D. Axial noncontrast-enhanced T1W image demonstrates the lesion showing high signal without contrast.

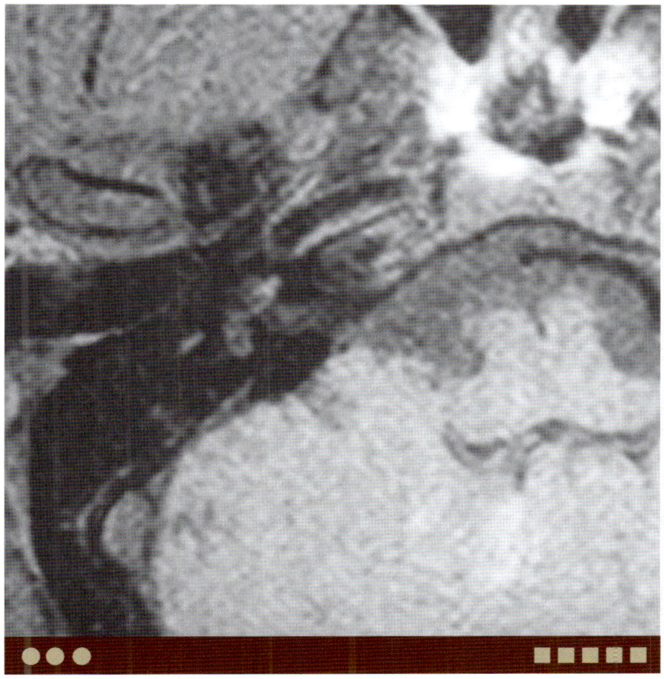

G. Lipoma, same patient as D. Axial noncontrast-enhanced fat-suppressed T1W image demonstrates suppressed signal of the lesion, which confirms fat.

DIFFERENTIAL DIAGNOSIS IMAGES (H-J)

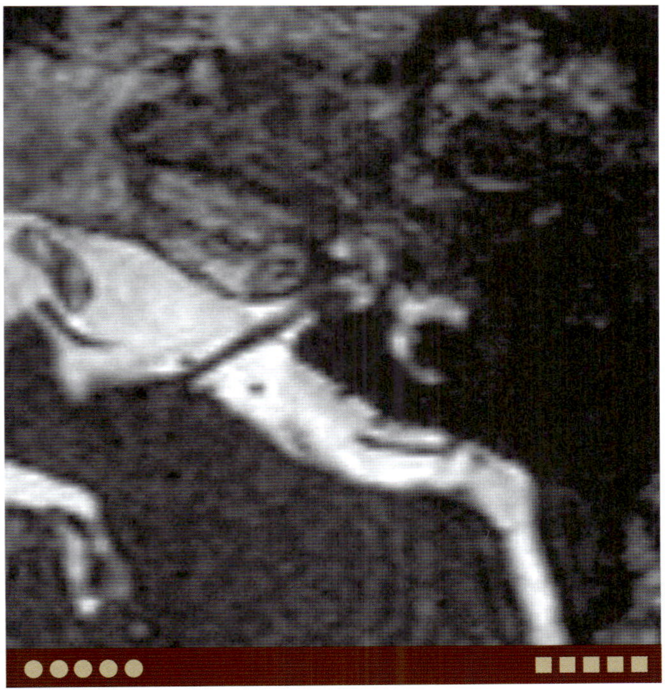

H. Vestibular schwannoma. Axial high-resolution T2W image demonstrates a small mass arising from the vestibular nerve in the posterior portion of the IAC.

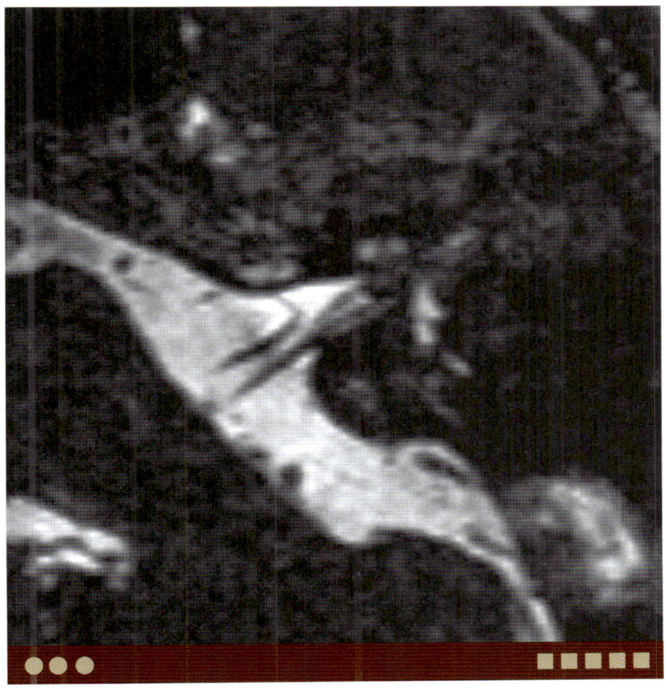

I. Cochlear schwannoma. Axial high-resolution T2W image demonstrates loss of normal high signal from fluid in the basal turn of the cochlea as well as in the fundus of the IAC.

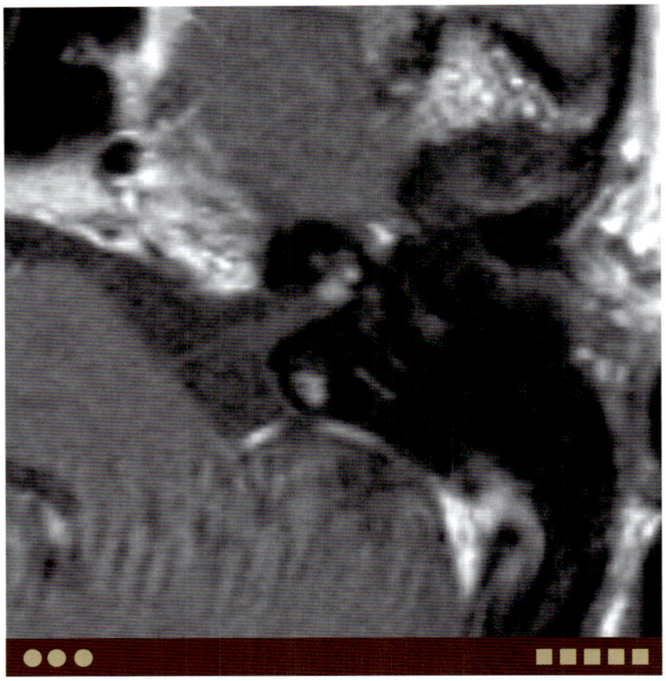

J. Cochlear schwannoma, same patient as I. Axial contrast-enhanced T1W image demonstrates an enhancing lesion in the fundus of the IAC extending into the basal turn of the cochlea.

Case 1–13 Labyrinthine Hemorrhage

Osamu Sakai, Rohini Nadgir

PRESENTATION

Sudden onset vertigo and hearing loss.

FINDINGS

T1W MR image shows abnormal high signal in the inner ear structures including cochlea and vestibule.

DIFFERENTIAL DIAGNOSIS

- Schwannoma: Enhancing tumors on postcontrast T1W images may show similar findings to labyrinthine hemorrhage, however, the high signal on precontrast T1W images can make the diagnosis of labyrinthine hemorrhage.
- Lipoma: Lipoma in the inner ear is a rare condition. Fat shows high signal on T1W MR images. Fat suppression MR sequence and CT can confirm the presence of fat.

COMMENTS

This is a 45-year-old woman with sudden onset of vertigo and hearing loss.

Labyrinthine hemorrhage is a rare condition and seen with trauma, coagulopathy, viral infection, and sickle cell anemia, however, the cause is often unknown. High-signal intensity on T1W images from methemoglobin in the inner structures, such as vestibule and cochlea, is characteristic, although it is very difficult to differentiate hemorrhage from proteinaceous exudate. The finding is usually subtle and high-resolution imaging and careful evaluation is necessary to make the diagnosis. Occasionally, increased signal can also be seen on T2W images.

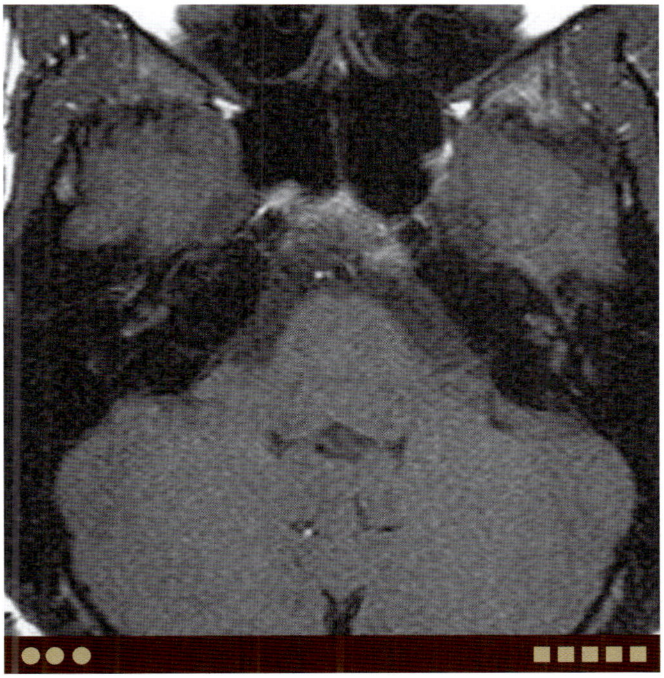

A. Labyrinthine hemorrhage. Axial T1W MR image demonstrates abnormal high signal in the cochlea and vestibule bilaterally.

PEARLS

- **High-signal intensity on T1W images from blood products, methemoglobin in the inner structures, such as vestibule and cochlea, is characteristic.**
- **Careful evaluation on high-resolution imaging is essential to make a diagnosis of labyrinthine hemorrhage.**
- **Sudden onset is a key clinical finding. Check underlying conditions such as trauma, coagulopathy, viral infection, and sickle cell anemia.**

ADDITIONAL IMAGES (B-D)

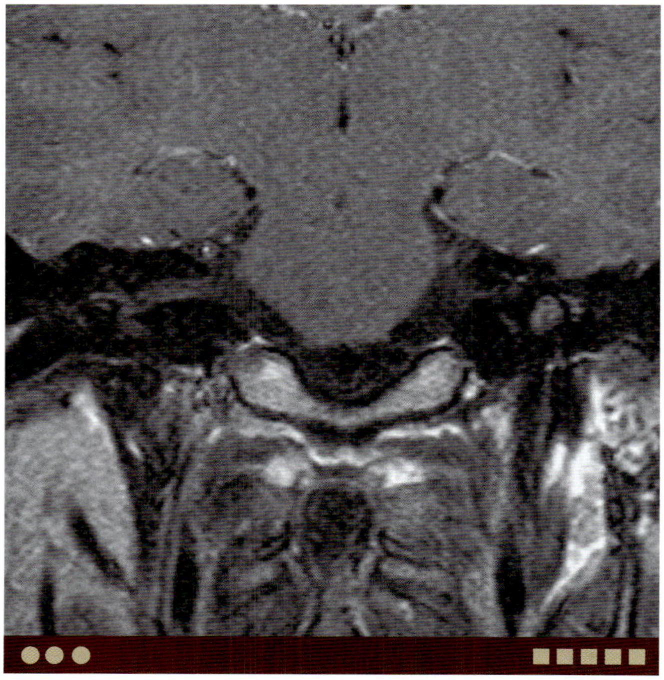

B. Labyrinthine hemorrhage, same patient as A. Coronal T1W image also demonstrates abnormal high signal in the membranous labyrinth, most prominent in the left cochlea.

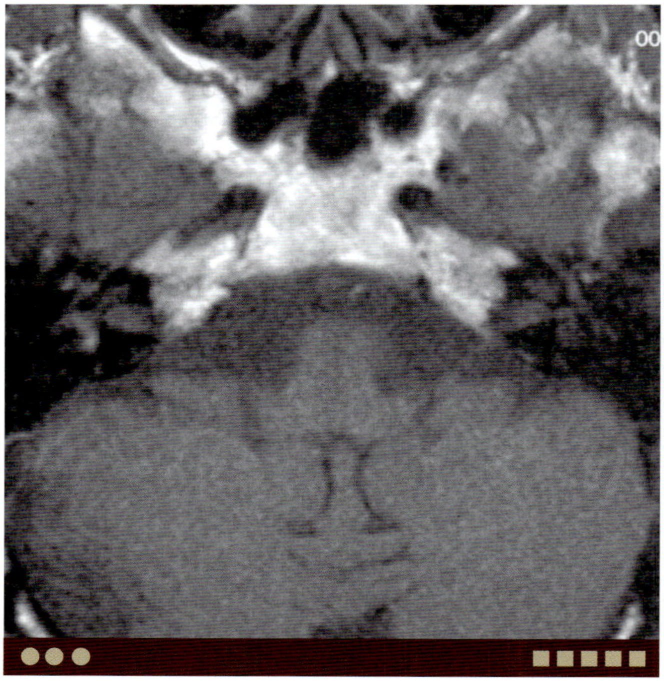

C. Vestibular hemorrhage in a 75-year-old man. Axial T1W MR image demonstrates abnormal high signal in the right vestibule.

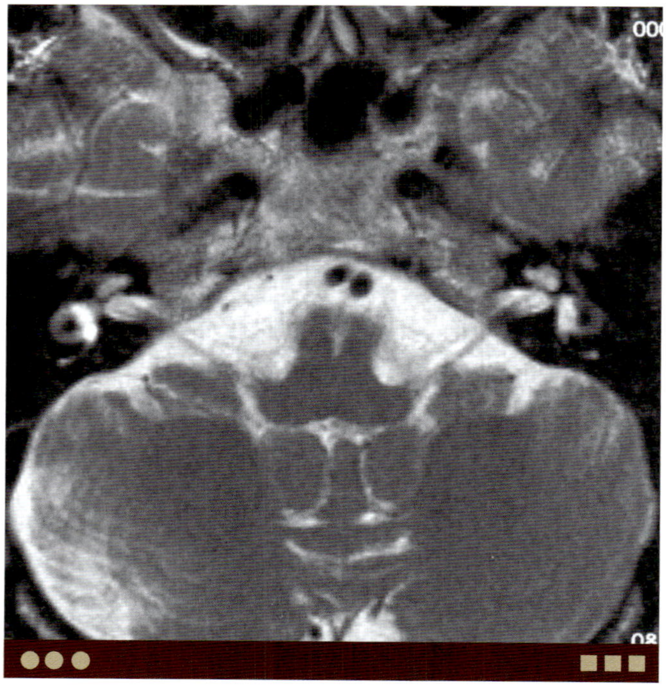

D. Vestibular hemorrhage, same patient as C. Axial T2W image also demonstrates abnormally increased signal in the right vestibule compared to the left.

DIFFERENTIAL DIAGNOSIS IMAGES (E-I)

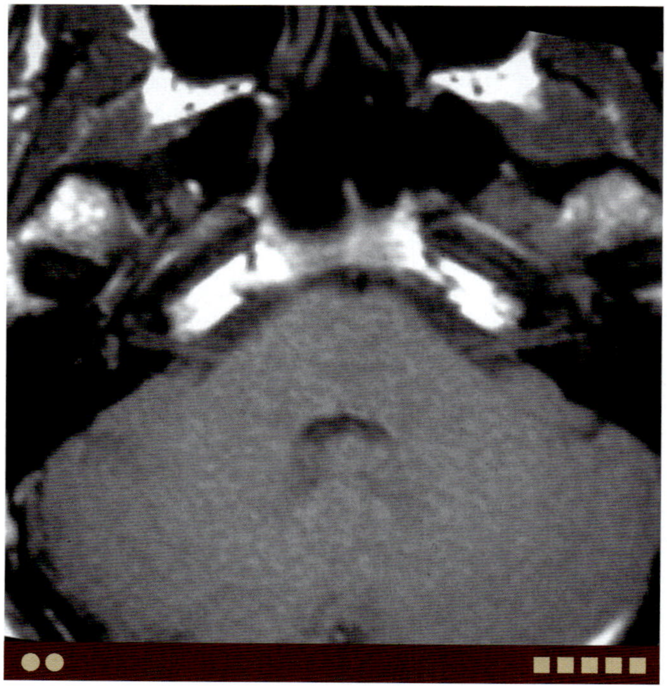

E. Vestibular schwannoma. Axial T1W MR image demonstrates intermediate signal in the right vestibule.

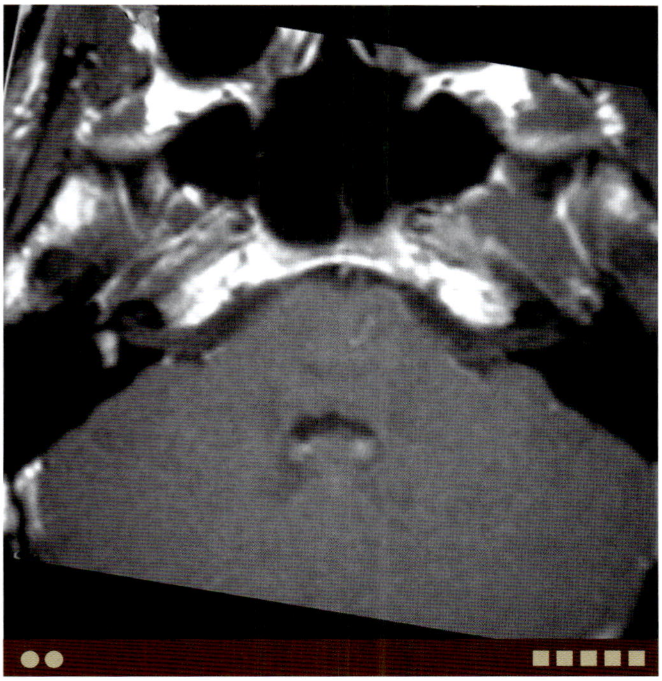

F. Vestibular schwannoma, same patient as E. Axial postcontrast T1W MR image demonstrates enhancement in the right vestibule.

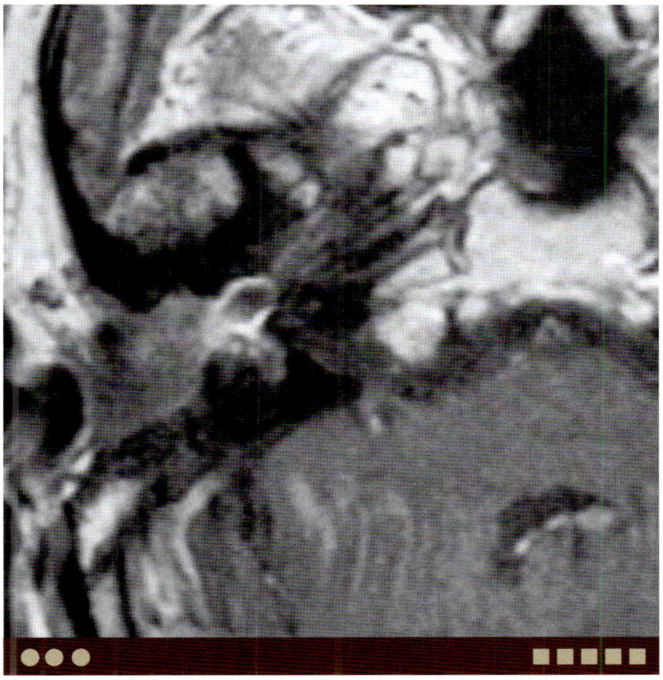

G. Labyrinthitis. Axial postcontrast T1W image demonstrates abnormal enhancement in the vestibule. The patient is status postradical mastoidectomy.

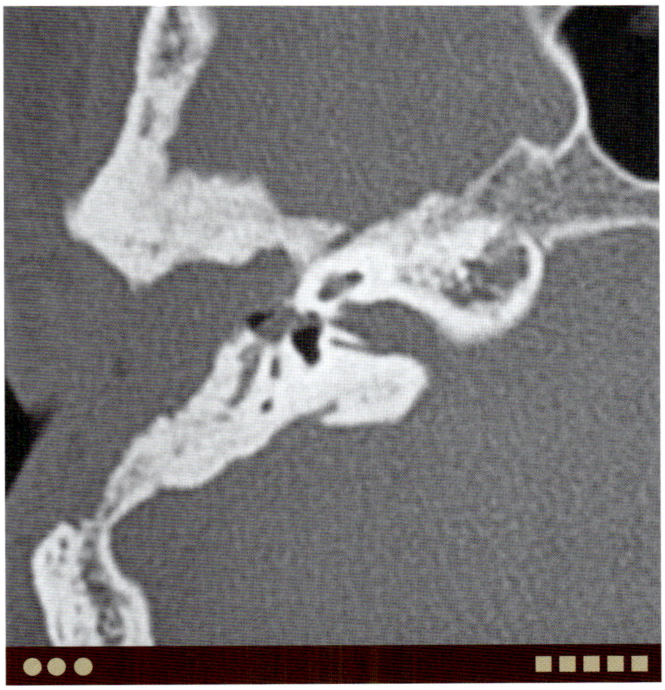

H. Labyrinthitis, same patient as G. Axial CT demonstrates destruction of the lateral semicircular canal and vestibule. Note air density in the vestibule, indicating pneumolabyrinth.

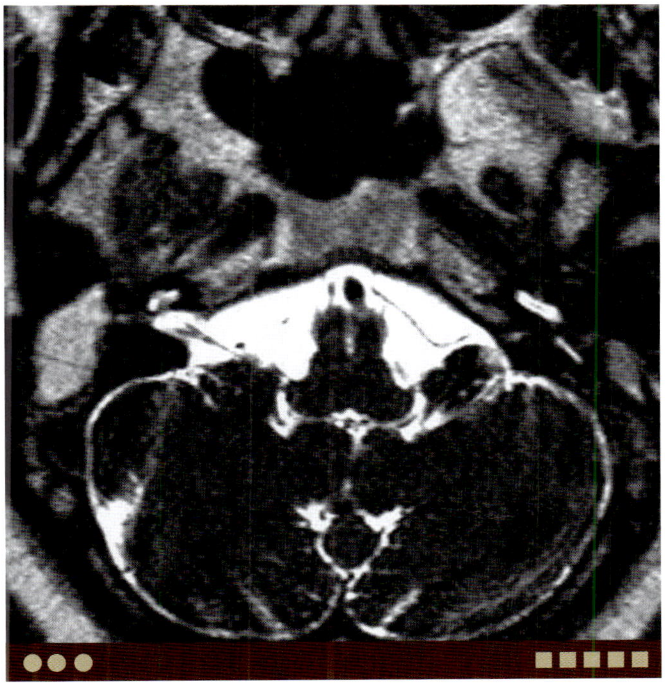

I. Labyrinthitis ossificans. Axial high-resolution T2W image demonstrates absence of normal high signal from the right vestibule and semicircular canals due to abnormal calcification/ossification. The patient is status postradical (please check the stylesheet) mastoidectomy.

Case 1–14 Labyrinthitis Ossificans

Osamu Sakai, Rohini Nadgir

PRESENTATION

Sensorineural hearing loss.

FINDINGS

CT demonstrates abnormal high density, ossification or calcification in the membranous labyrinth. T2W MR image demonstrates loss of normal high signal in the membranous labyrinth.

DIFFERENTIAL DIAGNOSIS

- Schwannoma: Schwannomas arising from the membranous labyrinth cause loss of T2 high signal. However, schwannomas show enhancement. CT does not demonstrate calcification or ossification.
- Otosclerosis: This condition causes demineralization of the otic capsule. The membranous labyrinth is usually preserved.
- Tympanosclerosis: This is a condition of sclerotic change, calcification, or ossification of the tympanic cavity, not the inner ear.

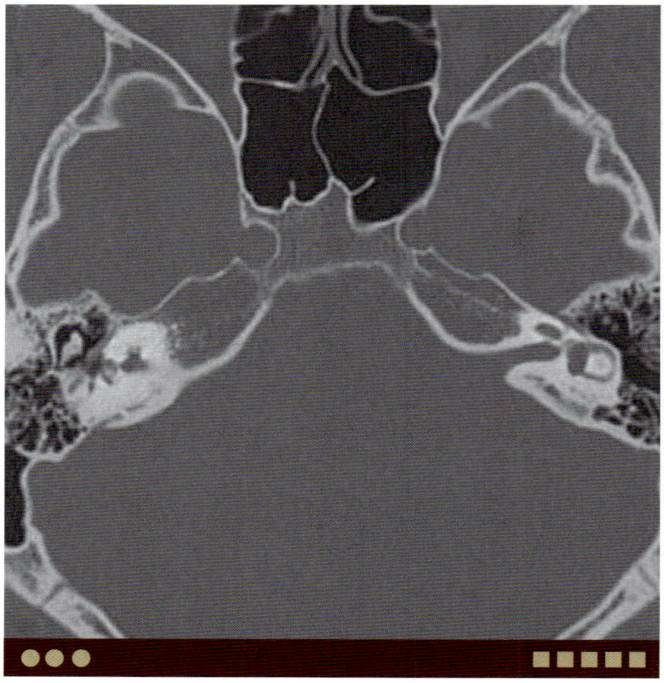

A. Labyrinthitis ossificans. Axial CT demonstrates ossification of the right cochlea.

COMMENTS

This is a 45-year-old man with sensorineural hearing loss.

Labyrinthitis ossificans is a condition characterized by pathologic calcification or ossification of the membranous labyrinth from various etiologies including trauma, inflammation and infection, and is associated with profound sensorineural hearing loss and impairment of vestibular function. This condition most commonly occurs as a sequela of inflammation/infection from trauma, otitis media, cholesteatoma, and surgery, or may be secondary to meningitis, particularly bacterial meningitis. Other etiologies include infarct, obstruction of the labyrinthine artery, autoimmune disease, leukemia, and otosclerosis.

On CT, abnormal high density is seen in the semicircular canals, vestibule, or cochlea. Bone destruction of the lateral semicircular canal may be seen in a patient with otitis media and cholesteatoma. Initially, increased density in the membranous labyrinth may not be apparent on CT, however, high-resolution T2W MR images demonstrate loss of normal water signal from the membranous labyrinth earlier, corresponding to fibrosis and subtle calcification/ossification. In a case with relatively fresh fibrosis or active inflammation, abnormal enhancement may be seen in the membranous labyrinth on contrast-enhanced MRI.

PEARLS

- **Labyrinthitis ossificans is a condition characterized by pathologic calcification or ossification of the membranous labyrinth.**
- **CT demonstrates abnormal high density in the semicircular canals, vestibule, or cochlea.**
- **High-resolution T2W MR images demonstrate loss of normal water signal from the membranous labyrinth corresponding to fibrosis or calcification/ossification.**

ADDITIONAL IMAGES (B-F)

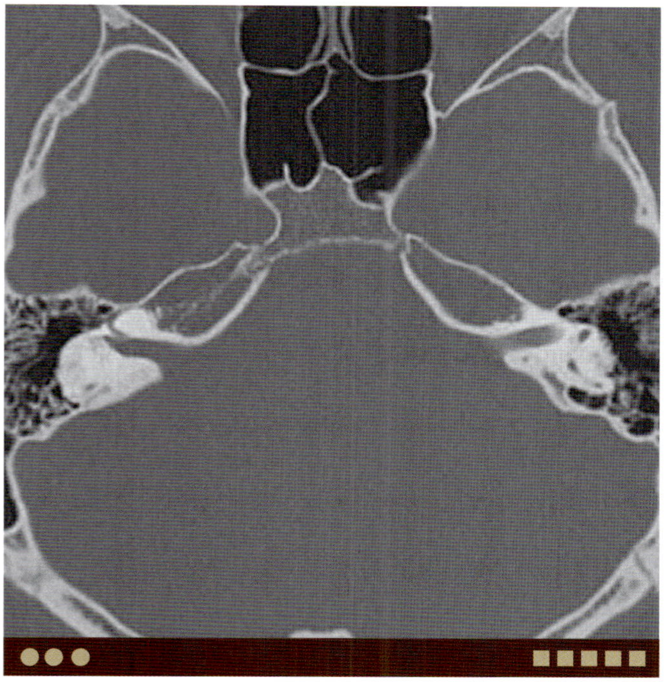

B. Labyrinthitis ossificans, same patient as A. Axial CT through a slightly higher level demonstrates ossification of the right semicircular canals and vestibule.

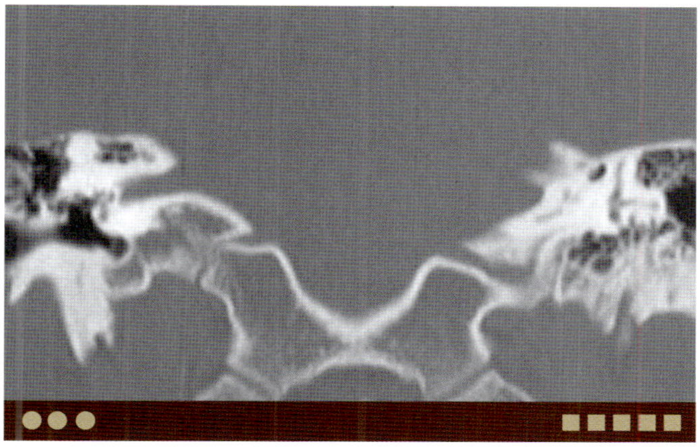

C. Labyrinthitis ossificans, same patient as A. Coronal CT also demonstrates ossification of the semicircular canals and vestibule on the right.

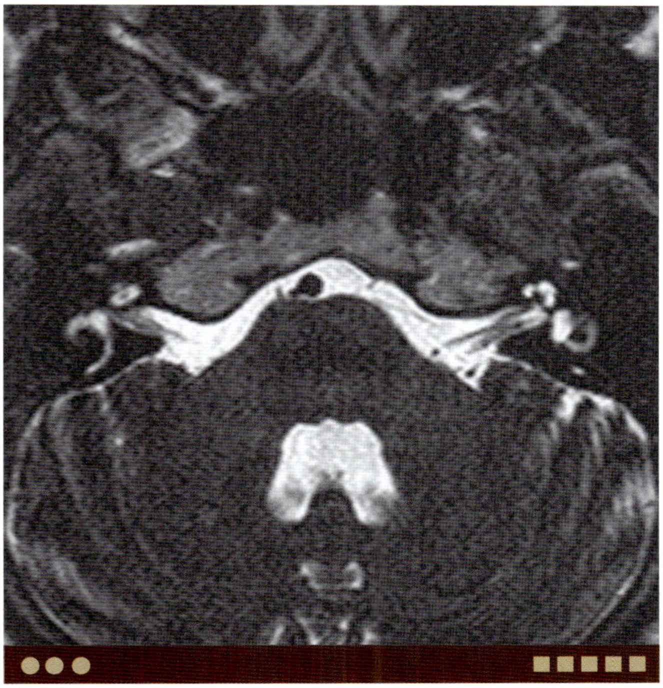

D. Labyrinthitis ossificans in a different patient. Axial high-resolution T2W image demonstrates loss of fluid signal in the posterolateral portion of the right lateral semicircular canal.

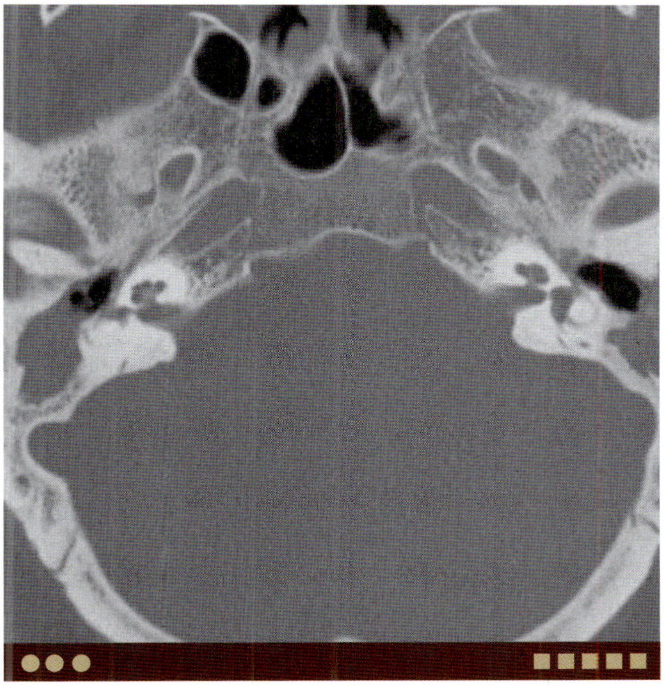

E. Labyrinthitis ossificans in a different patient. This patient is status post right radical mastoidectomy. Axial CT demonstrates abnormal ossification in the right lateral semicircular canal and vestibule.

DIFFERENTIAL DIAGNOSIS IMAGES (G-I)

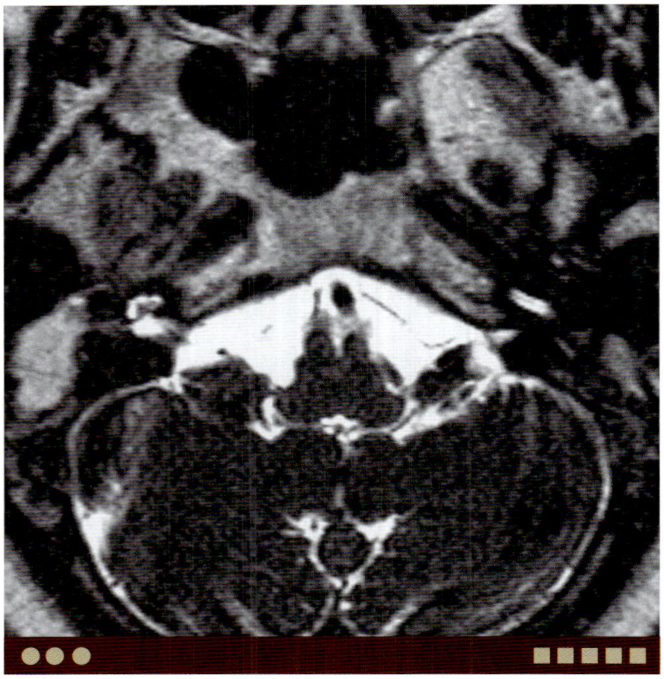

F. Labyrinthitis ossificans, same patient as E. Axial high-resolution T2W image demonstrates absence of fluid signal in the right lateral semicircular canal and vestibule.

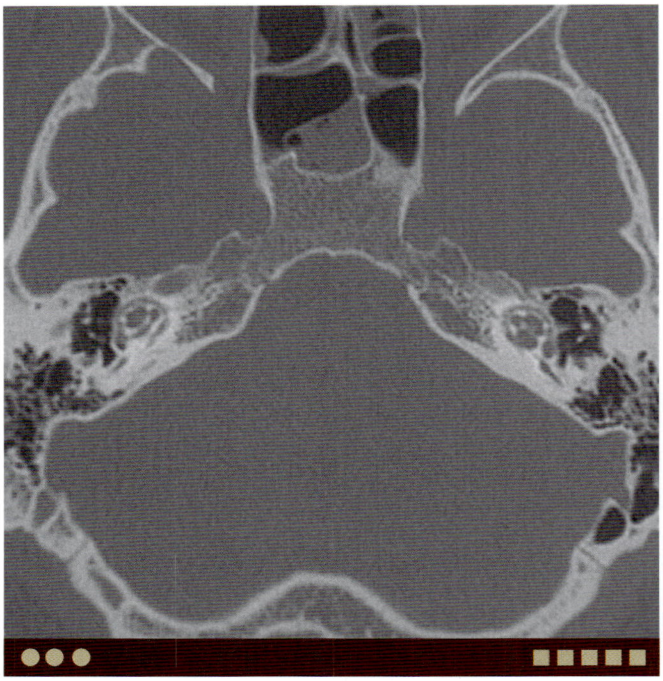

G. Cochlear otosclerosis. Axial CT demonstrates demineralization of the otic capsule bilaterally. Soft tissue/water density of the membranous labyrinth is preserved.

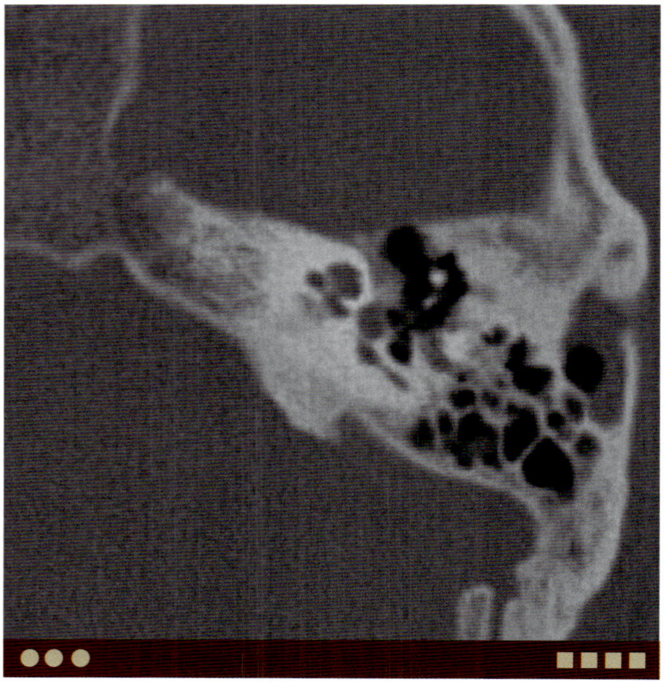

H. Fenestral otosclerosis. Axial CT demonstrates prominent osseous proliferation in the *fissula ante fenestrum*, anteromedial to the oval window.

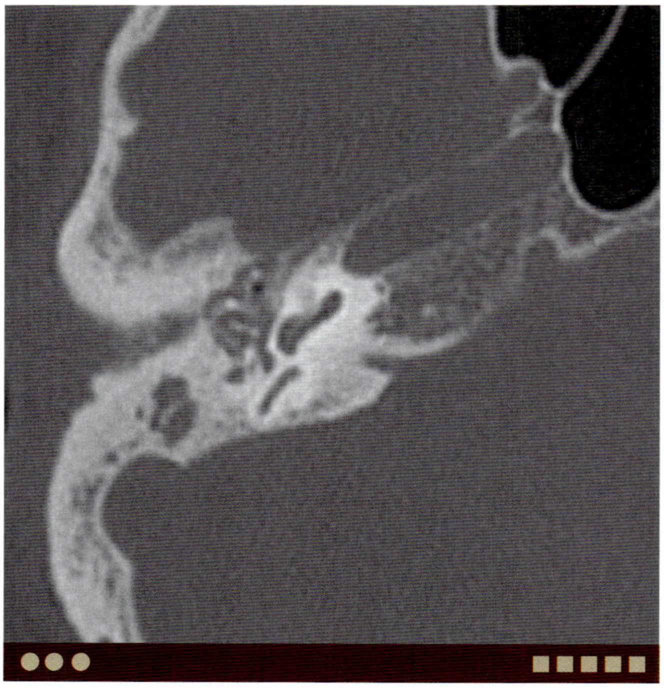

I. Tympanosclerosis. Axial CT demonstrates calcifications in the opacified epitympanum.

Case 1–15 Large Vestibular Aqueduct Syndrome

Osamu Sakai, Rohini Nadgir

PRESENTATION

Progressive sensorineural hearing loss.

FINDINGS

CT and MRI show enlarged vestibular aqueducts.

DIFFERENTIAL DIAGNOSIS

- Mondini deformity: This malformation consists of cochlear hypoplasia, enlarged vestibule, and enlarged vestibular aqueduct. Large vestibular aqueduct syndrome is in a spectrum of Mondini type anomaly.

COMMENTS

This is a 16-year-old girl with congenital and progressive sensorineural hearing loss.

Large vestibular aqueduct syndrome (LVAS) is a relatively common inner ear anomaly. LVAS is usually not an isolated anomaly and is closely associated with other inner ear anomalies, particularly cochlear anomalies including hypoplasia of the modiolus, and is considered as a part of Mondini type anomaly. The original description of Mondini deformity consisted of 1) a cochlea with one-and-one-half turns instead of the normal two-and-one-half turns, which demonstrates a normal basal turn and a cystic apex in place of the distal one-and-one-half turns; 2) an enlarged vestibule with normal semicircular canals; and 3) an enlarged vestibular aqueduct containing a dilated endolymphatic sac.

On CT, the diameter of the vestibular aqueduct is normally similar to that of the posterior semicircular canal or less than 1.5 mm in diameter. If it is larger than that, the diagnosis of large vestibular aqueduct syndrome should be considered and other anomalies in the inner ear structures, such as poor formation of cochlea and hypoplasia of the lateral semicircular canal, should be searched for. The lateral semicircular canal is formed at the late stage of inner ear development, therefore, almost all inner ear developmental anomalies carry some degree of lateral semicircular canal abnormality.

The normal vestibular aqueduct is usually not seen on MRI, even with high-resolution imaging. Therefore, visualization of vestibular aqueducts on MRI raises possibility of LVAS. Enlarged endolymphatic sac may demonstrate increased signal on T1W images due to proteinaceous contents. This can be seen as increased density on CT with soft tissue windows.

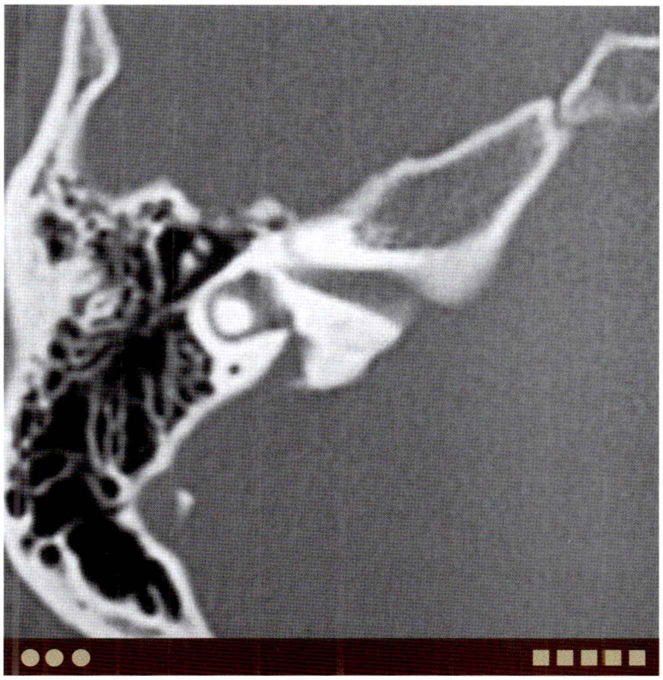

A. LVAS. Axial CT demonstrates enlarged vestibular aqueduct.

PEARLS

- **The diameter of the vestibular aqueduct is similar to that of the posterior semicircular canal or less than 1.5 mm.**
- **LVAS is often associated with other inner ear anomalies, particularly hypoplasia of the cochlea and lateral semicircular canals.**
- **Enlarged endolymphatic sac may demonstrate increased signal on T1W image or increased density on CT due to increased protein concentration.**

ADDITIONAL IMAGES (B-G)

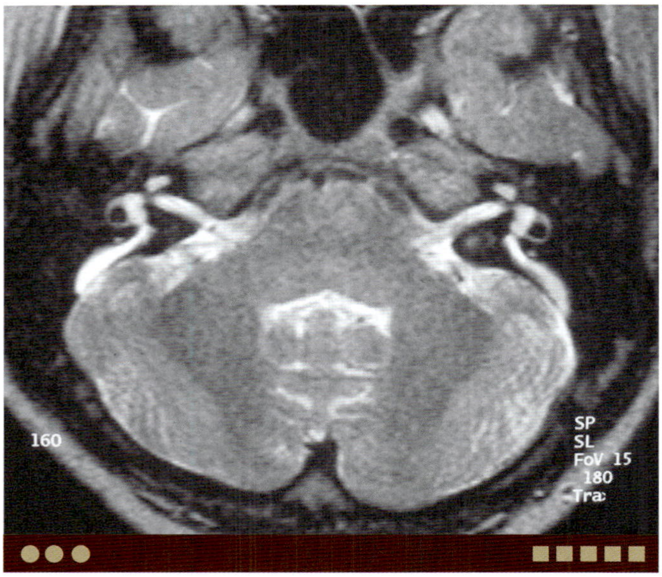

B. LVAS, same patient as A. Axial T2W image demonstrates enlarged endolymphatic sacs bilaterally.

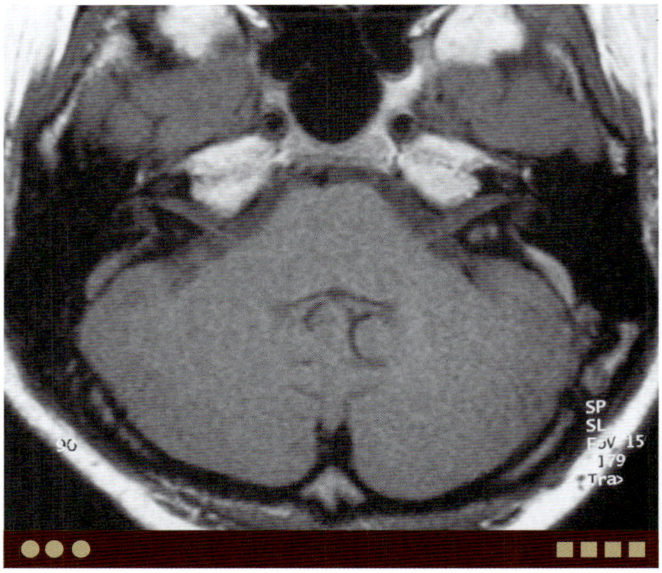

C. LVAS, same patient as A. Axial T1W image demonstrates increased signal in the enlarged endolymphatic sacs bilaterally, suggesting increased protein concentration within the sac.

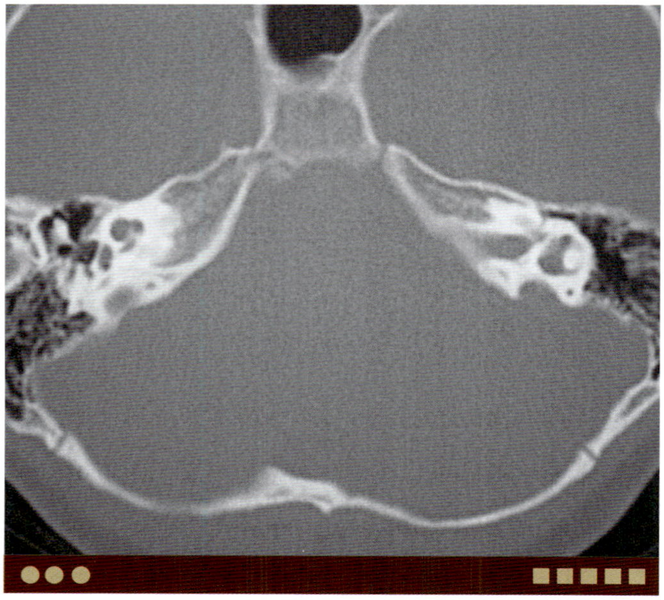

D. LVAS, 12-year-old girl. Axial CT demonstrates enlarged vestibular aqueducts bilaterally. Note globular appearance of the right cochlea, with poor separation of the apical and middle turns. Also, enlarged left vestibule is noted. These are common associated anomalies.

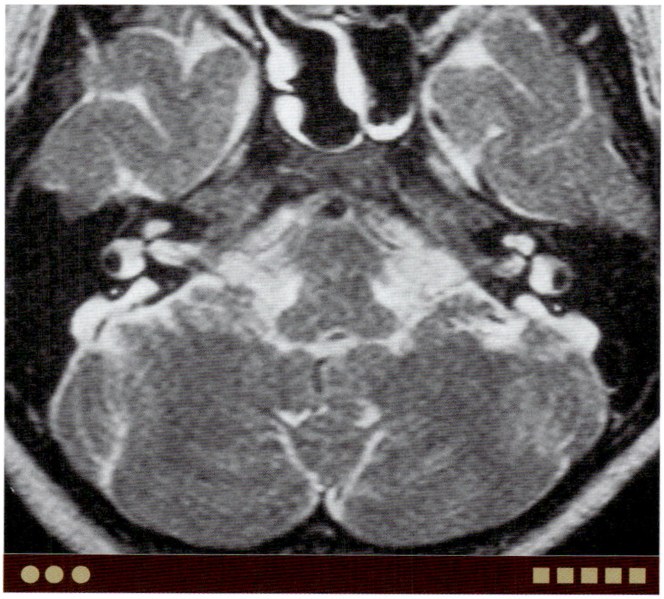

E. LVAS, same patient as D. Axial T2W image demonstrates enlarged endolymphatic sacs bilaterally as well as enlarged vestibules. Note hypoplasia of the bilateral lateral semicircular canals.

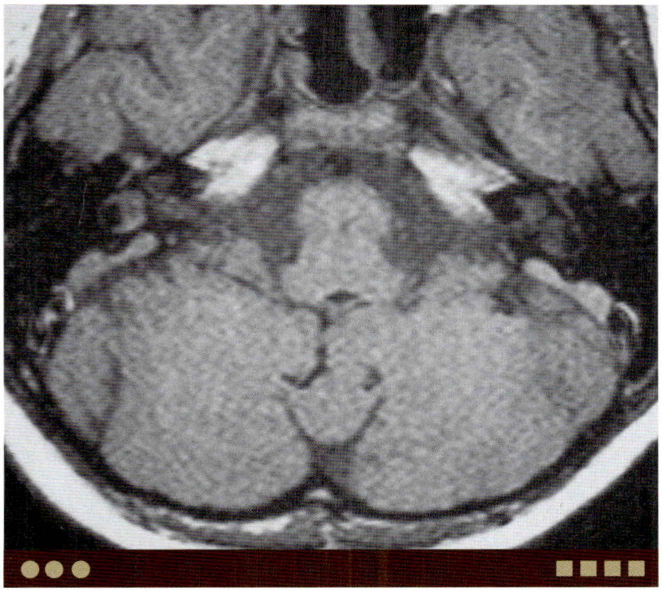

F. LVAS, same patient as D. Axial T1W image demonstrates increased signal in the enlarged endolymphatic sacs bilaterally, suggesting increased protein concentration within the sac.

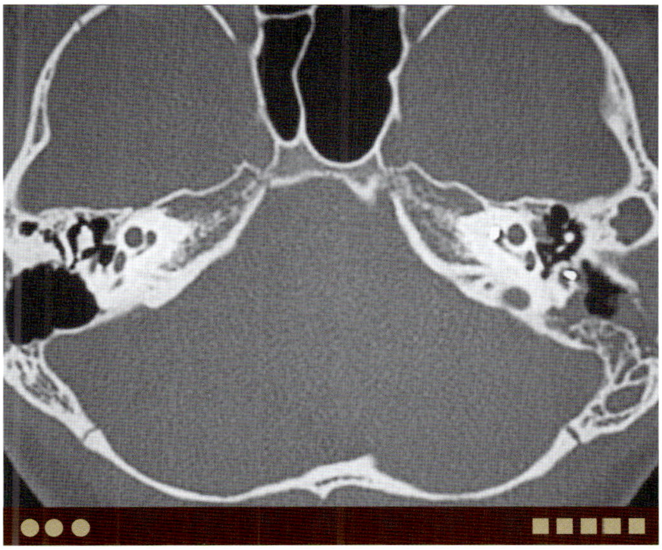

G. LVAS, same patient as D. Axial CT demonstrates a cochlear implant on the left. Globular appearance of the cochlea and poor separation of the apical and middle turns is noted bilaterally

DIFFERENTIAL DIAGNOSIS IMAGE

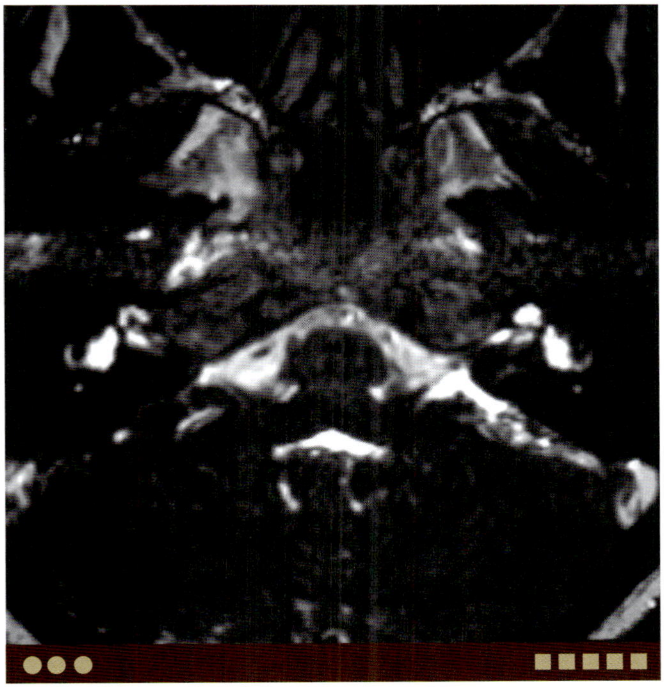

H. Modiolar hypoplasia. Axial T2W image demonstrates enlarged vestibules bilaterally. Note hypoplasia of the modiolus of the left cochlea.

Case 1–16 Hypoplasia of Modiolus

Osamu Sakai, Rohini Nadgir

PRESENTATION

Congenital sensorineural hearing loss.

FINDINGS

CT and MRI show small hypoplastic modiolus, the core of the cochlea, often associated with other anomalies of the inner ear.

DIFFERENTIAL DIAGNOSIS

- Mondini malformation: This condition consists of decreased number of turns of the cochlea, enlarged vestibule with normal semicircular canals, and enlarged vestibular aqueduct.

COMMENTS

This is a 9-year-old girl with congenital sensorineural hearing loss.

Recent advances in imaging enable evaluation of the modiolus, the core of the cochlea. On CT the modiolus is seen as a faint high density in the center of the basal turn of the cochlea, and on MRI it is seen as a low-signal structure in that location. This core of the "snail" should always be evaluated in patients with sensorineural hearing loss. Hypoplasia of the modiolus or cochlea is often associated with large vestibular aqueduct.

There is some debate regarding the first-line modality for congenital hearing loss; CT versus MRI. CT is quicker and easier to perform, has a higher success rate, and it is very useful to evaluate for integrity of bony structures. Radiation exposure is the disadvantage of CT. MRI is useful to evaluate for the membranous labyrinth, cochlear and vestibular nerves without ionizing radiation, however, MRI requires longer scan time, careful sedation in certain patients and dedicated high-resolution sequences. Many radiologists prefer CT as the first-line modality to evaluate for congenital inner ear anomalies.

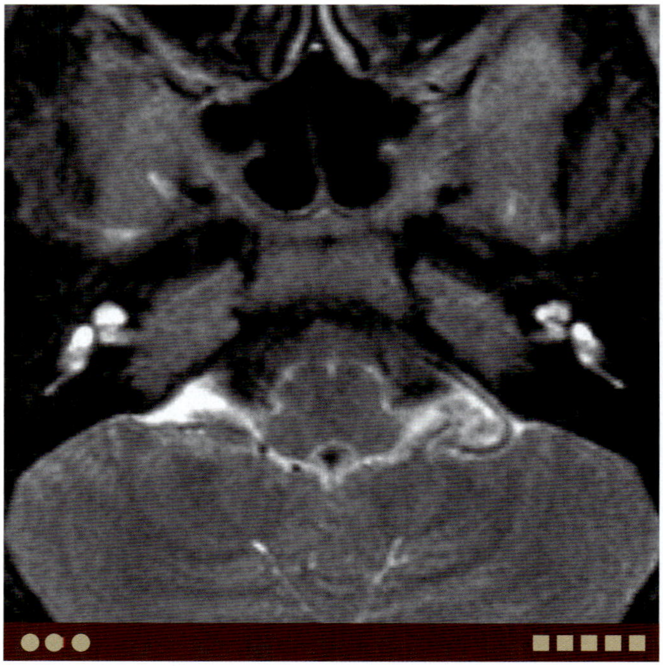

A. Modiolar hypoplasia. Axial T2W demonstrates globular appearance of the right cochlea without a low-signal core.

PEARLS

- **Small or absent core of the cochlea on T2W MR images.**
- **Absence of faint high density on CT in the center of the basal turn of the cochlea.**

ADDITIONAL IMAGES (B-C)

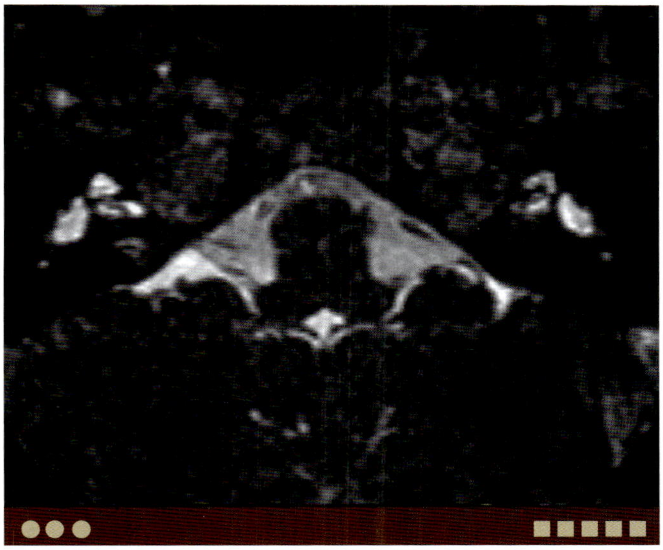

B. Modiolar hypoplasia, same patient as A. Axial high-resolution T2W image demonstrates absence of the modiolus on the right.

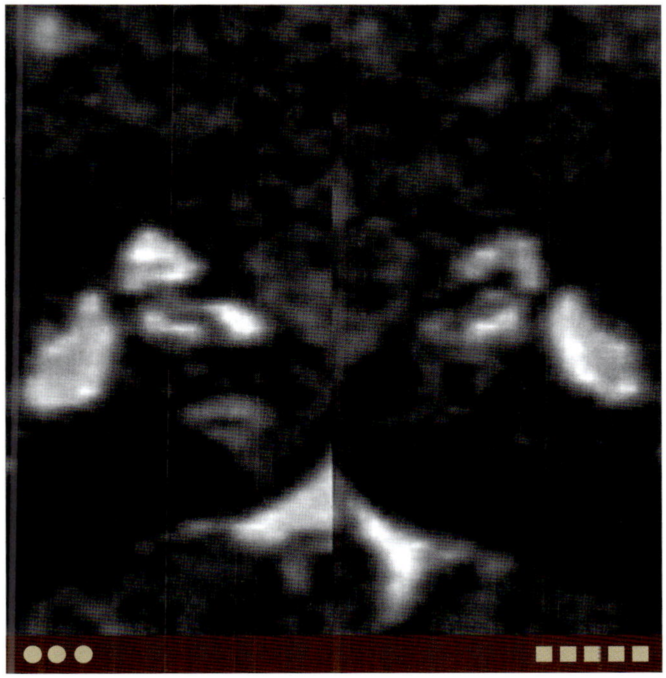

C. Modiolar hypoplasia, same patient as A. Magnified views of B demonstrates absence of the modiolus on the right.

DIFFERENTIAL DIAGNOSIS IMAGES (D-G)

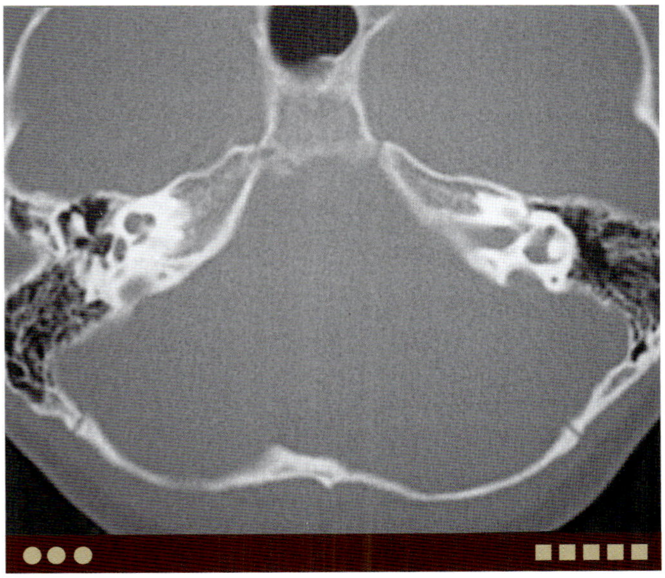

D. Large vestibular aqueduct syndrome. Axial CT demonstrates enlarged vestibular aqueducts bilaterally. Note globular appearance of the right cochlea, with poor separation of the apical and middle turns.

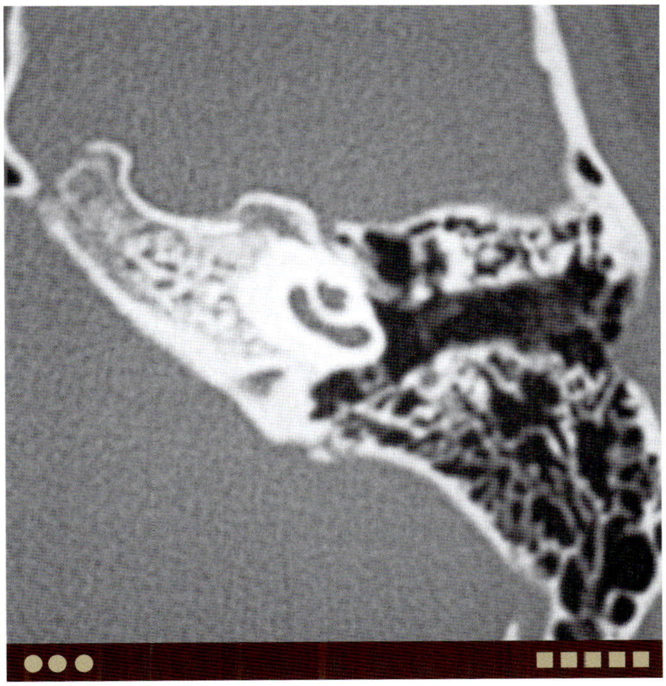

E. Cochlear dysplasia. Axial CT demonstrates flattening/deformity of the apical turn of the cochlea.

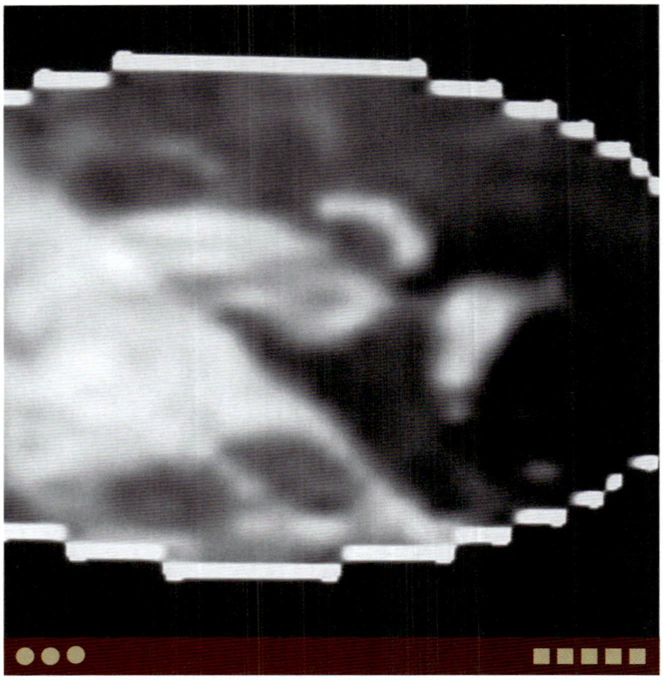

F. Cochlear dysplasia, same patient as E. Axial T2W image demonstrates flattening/deformity of the apical turn of the cochlea. The modiolus is identified.

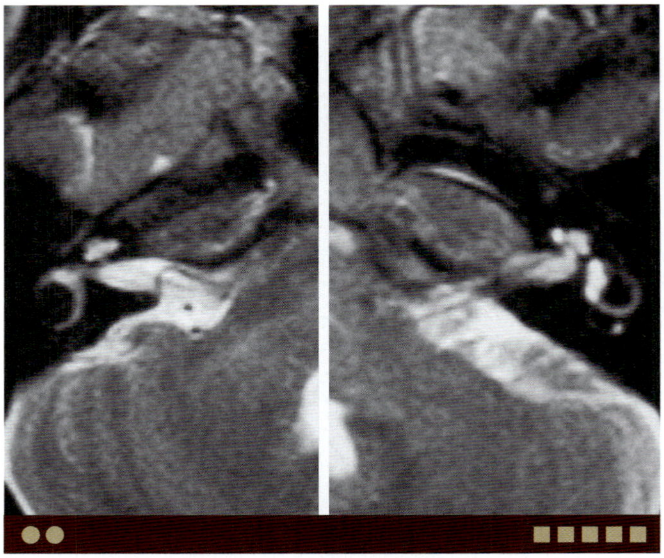

G. Hypoplastic cochlear nerve hole. Axial T2W image demonstrates a small cochlear nerve hole on the right. Note poor visualization of the right cochlear nerve compared with the left, suggesting hypoplasia.

Case 1–17 Glomus Tympanicum

Osamu Sakai, Rohini Nadgir

PRESENTATION

Pulsatile tinnitus.

FINDINGS

CT demonstrates a soft tissue density mass over the cochlear promontory without opacification of the tympanic cavity or mastoid air cells to suggest otitis media.

DIFFERENTIAL DIAGNOSIS

- Cholesteatoma: "Congenital" cholesteatoma can arise in the medial and inferior portion of the tympanic cavity without chronic otitis media.
- Schwannoma: This demonstrates similar findings to glomus tumors but often arises from the facial nerve. Therefore, expansion of the facial nerve canal is seen.
- Aberrant arteries: Aberrant internal carotid artery, fenestration of the internal carotid artery, and persistent stapedial artery are differential diagnoses for pulsatile tinnitus and "red drum." These should be differentiated by imaging.

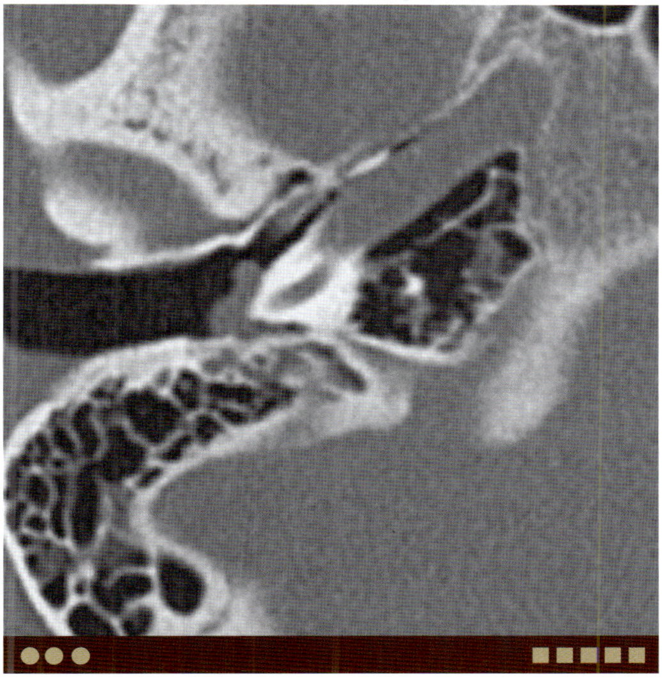

A. Glomus tympanicum. Axial CT demonstrates a soft tissue mass over the cochlea. Note clear tympanic cavity and mastoid air cells.

COMMENTS

This is a 53-year-old woman with pulsatile tinnitus. "Red drum" was noted in the otological examination.

Glomus tympanicum is a paraganglioma arising from the chemoreceptor. If it arises in the tympanic cavity, it is called glomus tympanicum. If it arises from the jugular foramen, it is called glomus jugulare. Large tumors often involve both the tympanic cavity and jugular foramen, and these are called glomus jugulotympanicum. Glomus tympanicum often arises from the nerve of Jacobson, a branch of the glossopharyngeus nerve, or the nerve of Arnold, a branch of the vagus nerve. It is often seen as a distinguished soft tissue density mass around the cochlear promontory.

Fisch classification is used for temporal bone paragangliomas, which is based on tumor extension and is closely related to mortality and morbidity: A—tumor limited to the middle ear cleft (glomus tympanicum), B—tumor limited to the tympanomastoid area with no infralabyrinthine compartment involvement, C—tumor involving the infralabyrinthine compartment of the temporal bone and extending to the petrous apex (C1; limited involvement of the vertical portion of the carotid canal, C2; invasion of the vertical portion of the carotid canal, C3; invasion of the horizontal portion of the carotid canal), and D—intracranial extension (D1; less than 2 cm in diameter, D2; greater than 2 cm in diameter).

Avid enhancement is seen on CT and MRI. "Salt-and-pepper appearance" from multiple abnormal vessels is well described in glomus tumors, however, it may not be seen in small tumors.

PEARLS

- **Glomus tympanicum is seen as an enhancing mass around the cochlear promontory without evidence of otitis media.**
- **"Salt-and-pepper appearance" may not be seen in small tumors.**
- **A large glomus tumor involving both the tympanic cavity and jugular foramen is called glomus jugulotympanicum.**

ADDITIONAL IMAGES (B-E)

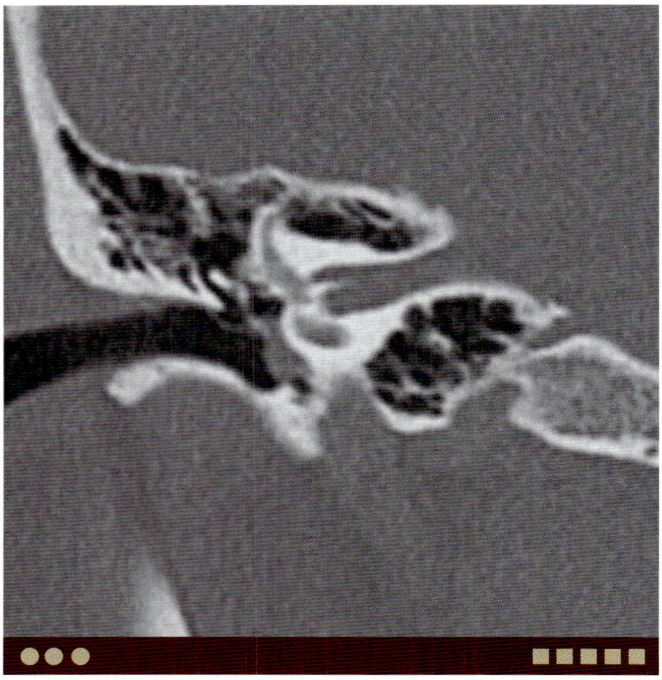

B. Glomus tympanicum, same patient as A. Coronal CT demonstrates a soft tissue mass over and inferior to the cochlear promontory.

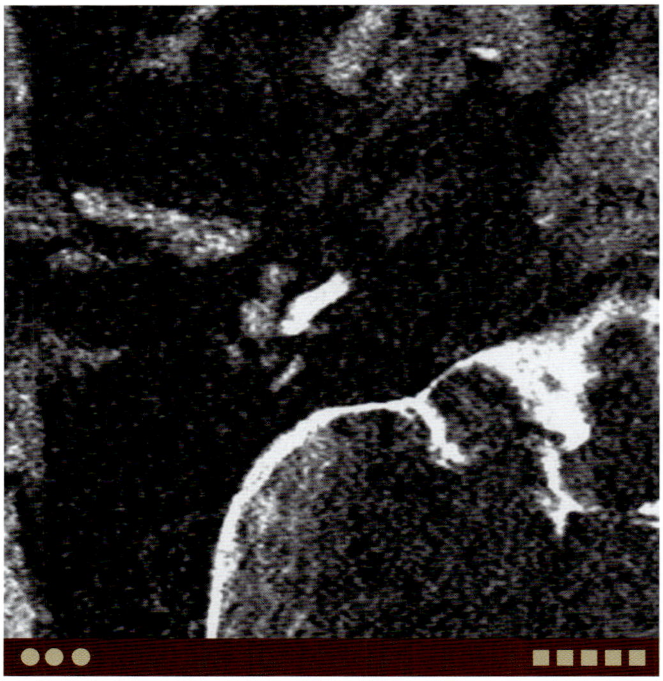

C. Glomus tympanicum, same patient as A. Axial T2W image demonstrates heterogeneously high signal within the lesion, lateral to the cochlea.

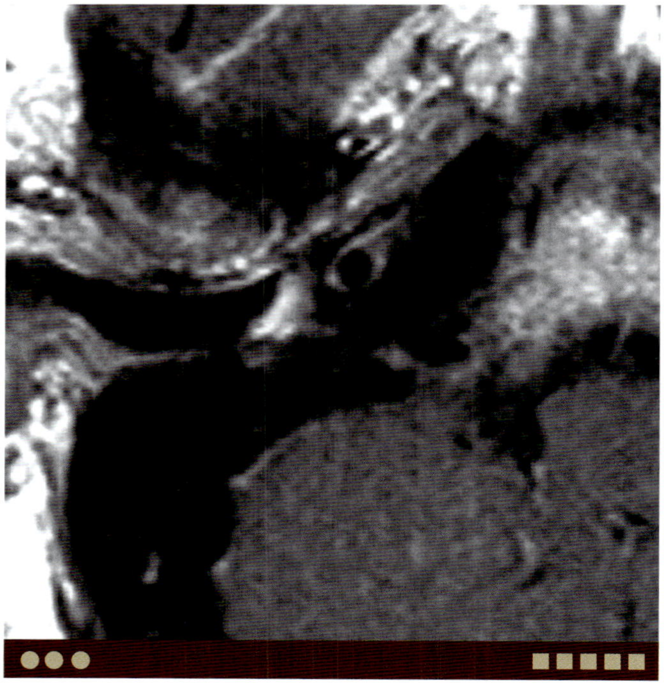

D. Glomus tympanicum, same patient as A. Axial postcontrast T1W image demonstrates enhancement of the lesion.

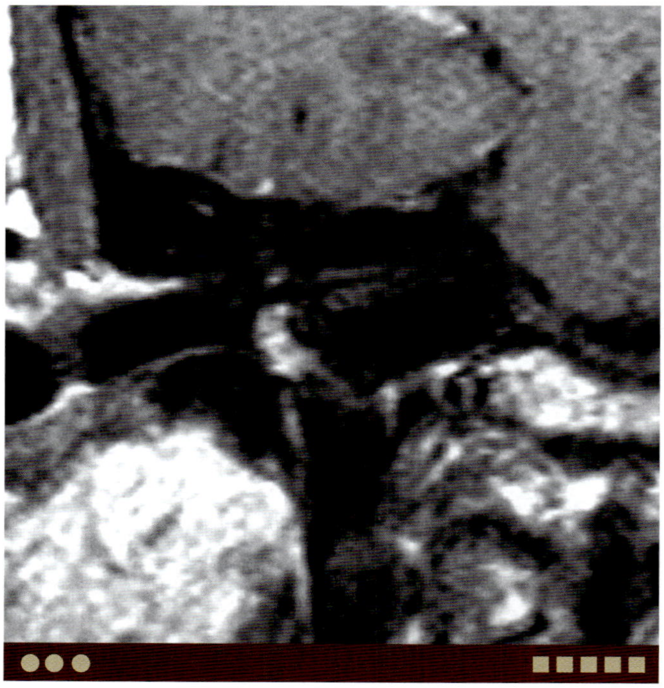

E. Glomus tympanicum, same patient as A. Coronal postcontrast T1W image demonstrates an enhancing tumor over the cochlea.

DIFFERENTIAL DIAGNOSIS IMAGES (F-H)

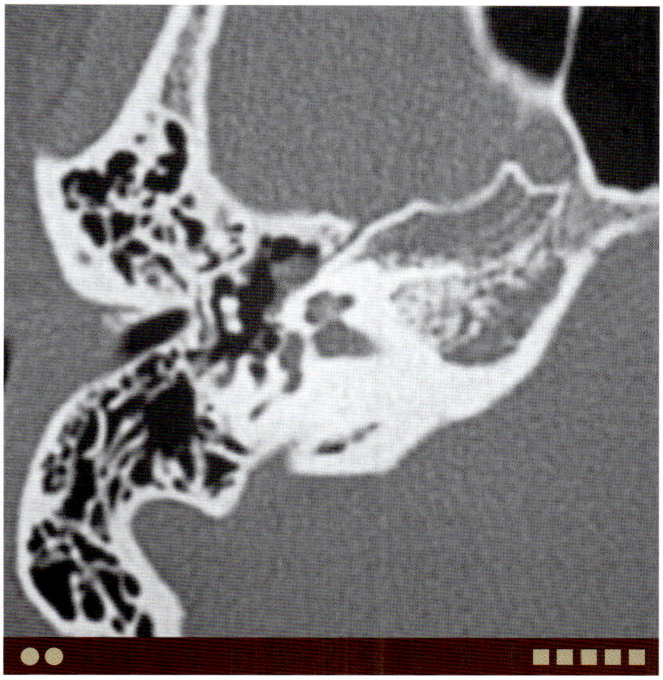

F. Facial nerve schwannoma. Axial CT demonstrates a soft tissue mass along the course of the facial nerve.

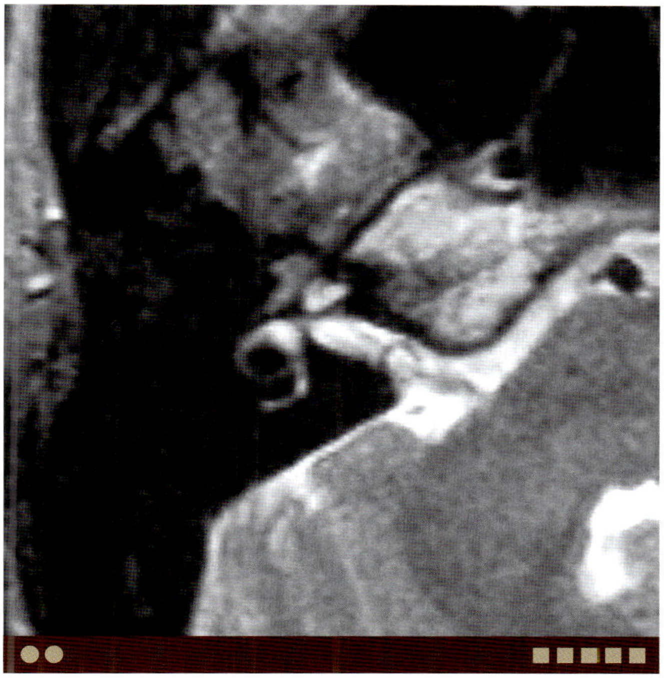

G. Facial nerve schwannoma, same patient as F. Axial T2W MR image demonstrates a mass in the genu extending to the tympanic segment of the facial nerve.

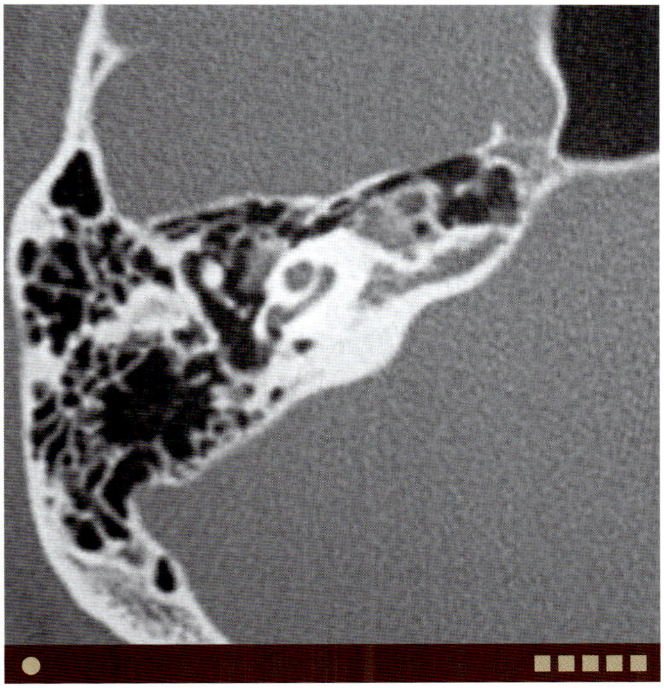

H. Facial nerve hemangioma. Axial CT demonstrates a soft tissue mass in the epitympanum.

Case 1–18 Glomus Jugulare

Osamu Sakai, Rohini Nadgir

PRESENTATION

Pulsatile tinnitus.

FINDINGS

CT demonstrates a soft tissue density mass in the jugular foramen with permeative changes in the adjacent osseous structures.

DIFFERENTIAL DIAGNOSIS

- Schwannoma: When this occurs in and around the jugular foramen, it usually shows smooth bone erosion or remodeling of the jugular foramen rather than permeative or infiltrative change. Schwannoma demonstrates homogeneous enhancement on MRI rather than "salt-and-pepper appearance," although cystic degeneration is often seen in large schwannomas.
- Meningioma: This usually demonstrates enhancement of the adjacent dura, "meningeal tail sign," in addition to mass formation. Hyperostosis is often seen rather than bone erosion or destruction.
- Metastasis: Metastases from thyroid, kidney, and liver cancers are very hypervascular and may demonstrate similar findings to paraganglioma. However, these are centered in the bone, not in the jugular foramen.

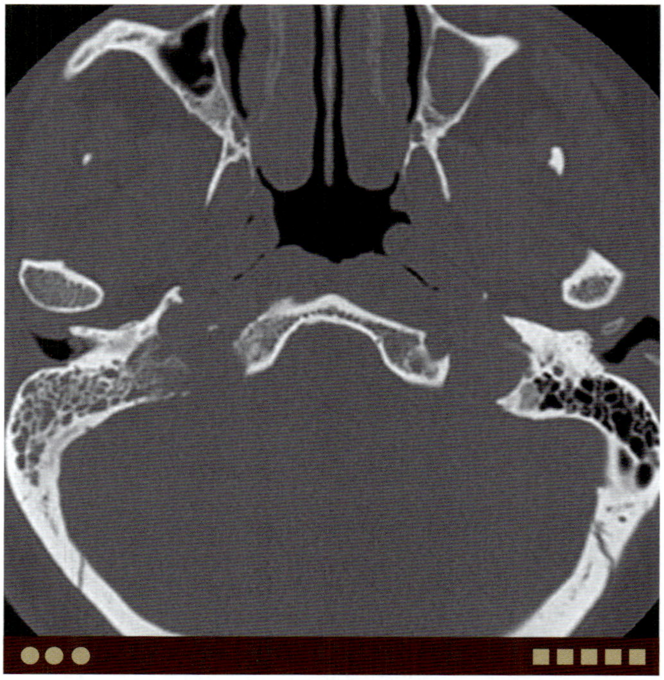

A. Glomus jugulare. Axial CT demonstrates extensive permeative bone destruction around the right jugular foramen.

COMMENTS

This is a 50-year-old man with pulsatile tinnitus.

Glomus jugulare is a paraganglioma arising at the level of the jugular foramen. At the time of diagnosis, it often involves the bone. Typically, glomus tumors demonstrate permeative or infiltrative changes in the adjacent osseous structures rather than bone erosion or hyperostosis. Therefore, CT is very useful to make the diagnosis. On MRI, "salt-and-pepper appearance" due to flow-voids from abundant tumor vessels is very typical; however, it may not be seen in small tumors.

After contrast, very rapid enhancement is seen on both CT and MRI, therefore, dynamic contrast-enhanced evaluation is helpful, particularly to differentiate the lesion from schwannoma and meningioma. In tumors with abundant tumor vessels and prominent flow-voids, degree of enhancement on conventional T1W images may be less compared with more solid lesions. Homogeneous strong enhancement on regular postcontrast T1W images may rather suggest schwannoma or meningioma than paraganglioma. Enhancement on MRI is different from that on CT, and also different from stains or vascularity demonstrated on catheter angiograms. Dynamic contrast-enhanced MRA is helpful to evaluate vascular anatomy as well as tumor vascularity, however, time-of-flight MRA is usually not very helpful except in very large tumors with prominent arteriovenous shunting.

PEARLS

- **Glomus jugulare is a paraganglioma arising at the level of the jugular foramen.**
- **CT demonstrates permeative or infiltrative changes in the adjacent osseous structures.**
- **"Salt-and-pepper appearance" is typically seen, however, may not be apparent in small tumors.**
- **A large tumor involving both the tympanic cavity and jugular foramen is called as glomus jugulotympanicum.**

ADDITIONAL IMAGES (B-F)

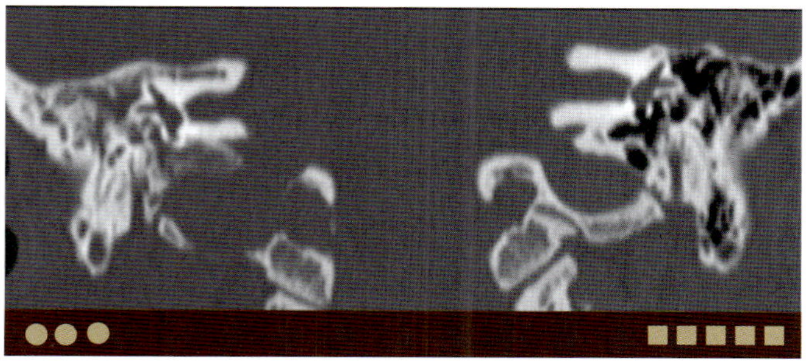

B. Glomus jugulare, same patient as A. Coronal CT demonstrates permeative osteolytic changes around the jugular foramen, inferomedial to the tympanic cavity.

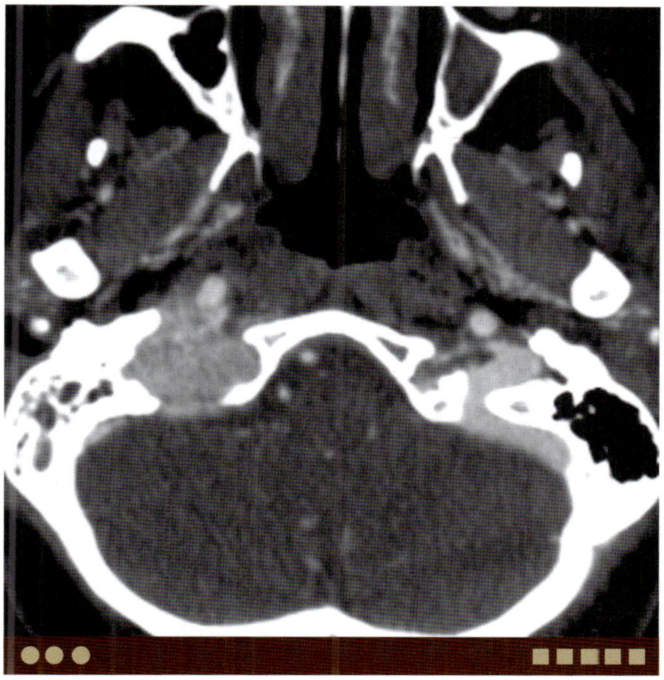

C. Glomus jugulare, same patient as A. Axial contrast-enhanced CT demonstrates an avidly enhancing lesion in the right jugular foramen.

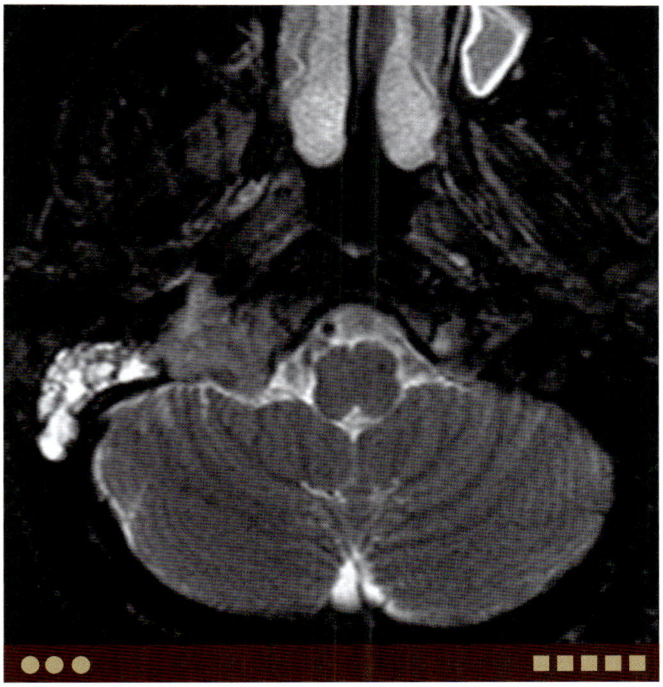

D. Glomus jugulare, same patient as A. Axial T2W image demonstrates a heterogeneous intermediate-signal lesion with internal flow-voids within the right jugular foramen.

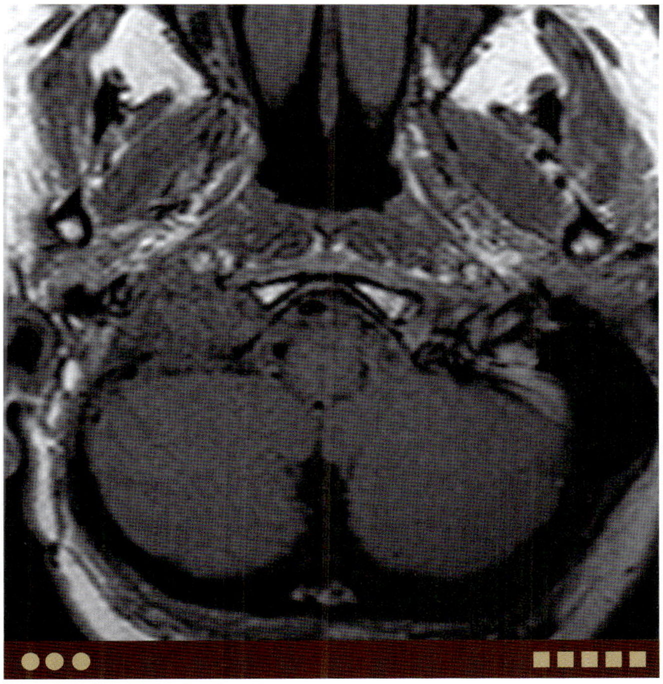

E. Glomus jugulare, same patient as A. Axial T1W image demonstrates a heterogeneous low-signal lesion within the right jugular foramen.

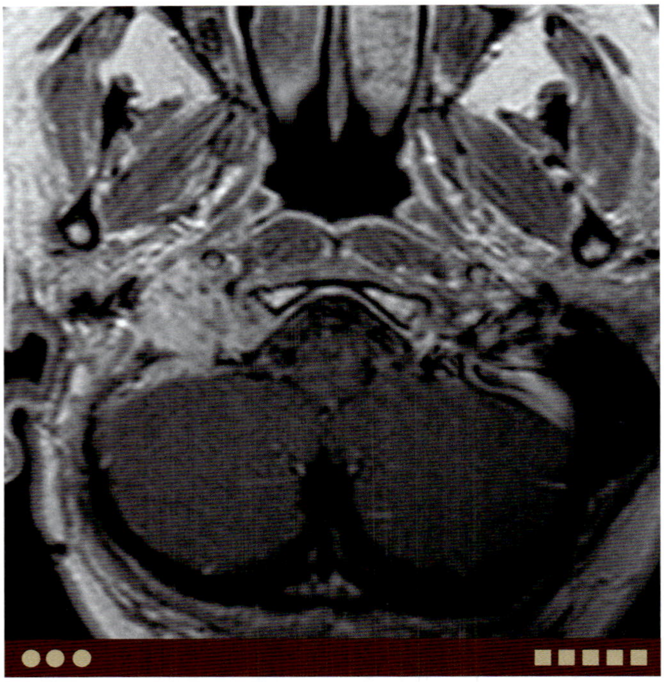

F. Glomus jugulare, same patient as A. Axial postcontrast T1W image demonstrates heterogeneous enhancement within the lesion.

DIFFERENTIAL DIAGNOSIS IMAGES (G-I)

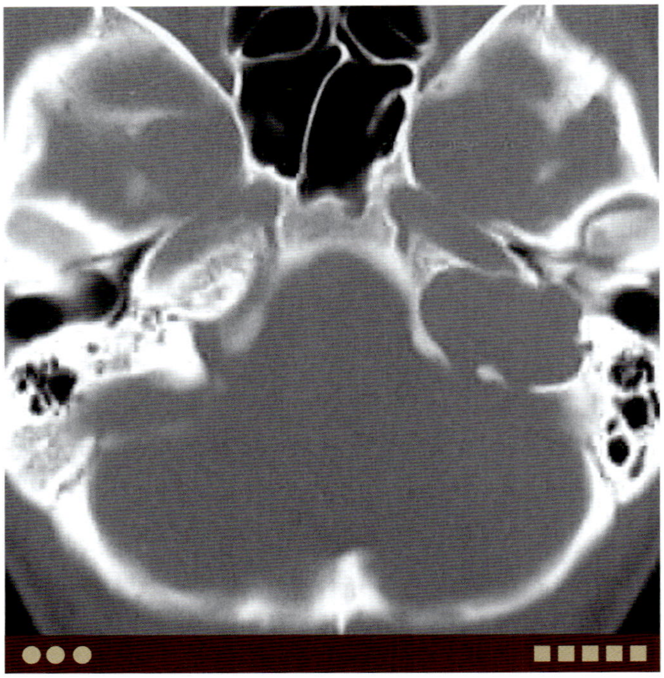

G. Schwannoma. Axial CT demonstrates smooth erosion, expansion of the left jugular foramen.

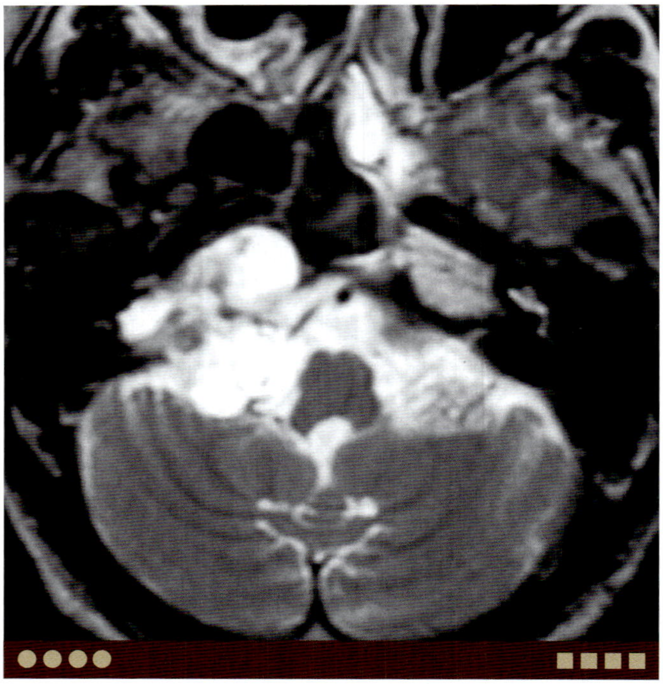

H. Schwannoma in a different patient. Axial T2W image demonstrates a lobulated heterogeneous high-signal tumor at the right jugular foramen without flow-voids.

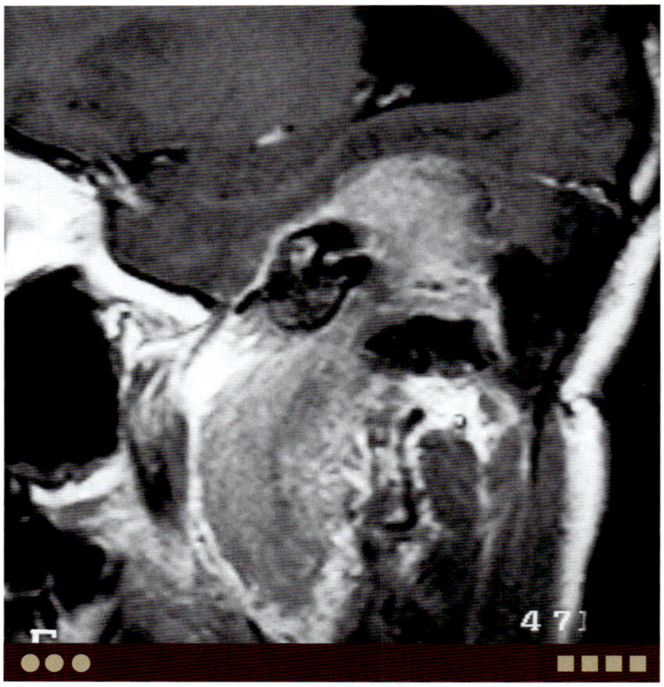

I. Meningioma. Sagittal postcontrast T1W image demonstrates extracranial extension of a heterogeneously enhancing tumor through the jugular foramen without flow-voids.

Case 1–19 Aberrant Internal Carotid Artery

Naoko Saito, Osamu Sakai

PRESENTATION

Pulsatile tinnitus.

FINDINGS

CT demonstrates an aberrant internal carotid artery running through the hypotympanum and entering the carotid canal through a dehiscence in the carotid plate.

DIFFERENTIAL DIAGNOSIS

- Glomus tympanicum: This is a paraganglioma in the tympanic cavity. CT shows a focal soft tissue density mass near the cochlear promontory. The mass avidly enhances on postcontrast CT and T1W MR images.
- High jugular bulb: This may extend into the hypotympanum with dehiscence of the bony covering. This occurs more commonly on the right side.
- Laterally displaced carotid artery (lateralized internal carotid artery): This runs into the tympanic cavity through a dehiscence of the bony carotid canal at petrous portion. Enlarged inferior tympanic canaliculus is not seen.

COMMENTS

This is a 41-year-old woman presented with pulsatile tinnitus. A red mass was noted in the lower tympanic cavity during otoscopy.

Aberrant internal carotid artery (ICA) is generally accepted to be a collateral pathway that occurs as a result of agenesis of the vertical segment of the ICA. The inferior tympanic artery arising from the ascending pharyngeal artery enters the temporal bone through the inferior tympanic canaliculus (Jacobson canal). It anastomoses with the caroticotympanic artery (the primitive hyoid artery) and establishes this aberrant collateral course.

An aberrant ICA can occur associated with other congenital vascular anomalies such as persistent stapedial artery and duplicated ICA, and also may be bilateral.

Four high-resolution CT findings of the aberrant ICA have been suggested: 1) absence of the vertical carotid canal, 2) enlargement of the inferior tympanic canaliculus, 3) an aberrant course of the artery through the hypotympanum, and 4) dehiscence of the carotid plate through which the artery enters the horizontal carotid canal. Contrast-enhanced CT and CT angiogram demonstrate aberrant course of the ICA and help to differentiate from tumors such as glomus tumor and cholesteatoma. MR angiogram is also useful to show a laterally positioned ICA.

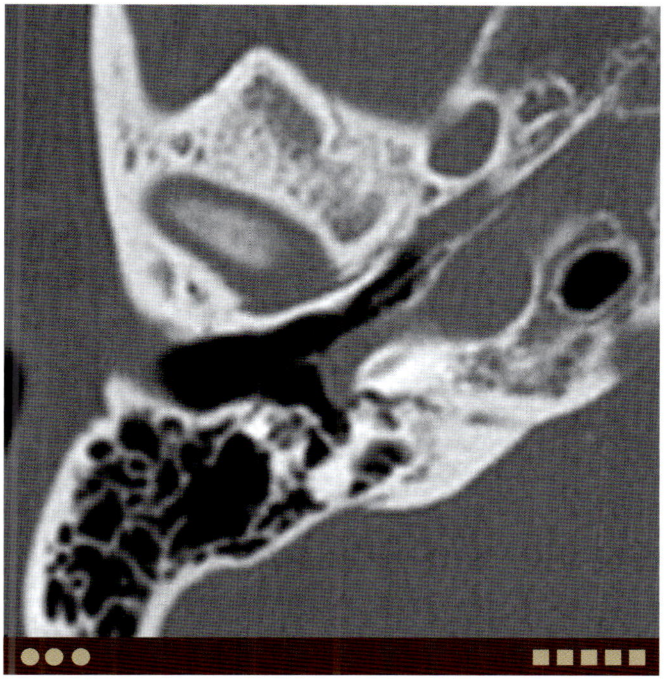

A. Aberrant internal carotid artery. Axial CT demonstrates soft tissue density mass running along the promontory and entering the carotid canal through a dehiscence in the carotid plate.

Clinical symptoms of aberrant ICA are tinnitus (with or without pulsation), hearing loss (mostly conductive), sensation of ear fullness, otalgia, and vertigo. Clinician often sees a red to bluish mass in the tympanic cavity during otoscopy. To avoid possible serious complications from surgery, it is important that an aberrant ICA should be considered and differentiated from the more commonly encountered lesions such as glomus tumor, cholesteatoma, and dehiscent jugular bulb. All these lesions may have similar clinical presentations.

PEARLS

- **1) Absence of the vertical carotid canal, 2) enlargement of the inferior tympanic canaliculus, 3) an aberrant course of the artery through the hypotympanum, and 4) dehiscence of the carotid plate through which the artery enters the horizontal carotid canal are the four major high-resolution CT findings.**
- **A persistent stapedial artery is often found in association with an aberrant ICA.**
- **Consideration of aberrant ICA in case of the retrotympanic mass is important to avoid serious complications from surgery.**

ADDITIONAL IMAGES (B-E)

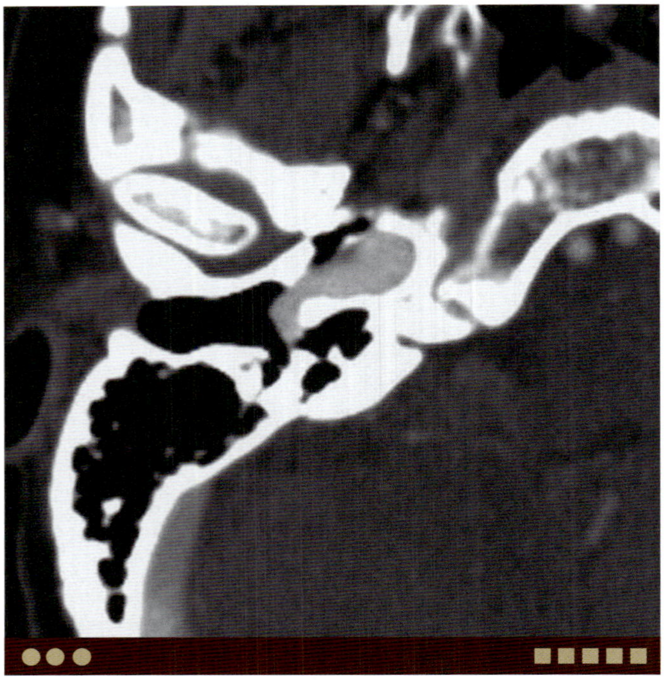

B. Aberrant internal carotid artery, same patient as A. Contrast-enhanced axial CT demonstrates the vascular structure running through the hypotympanum and joining the ICA.

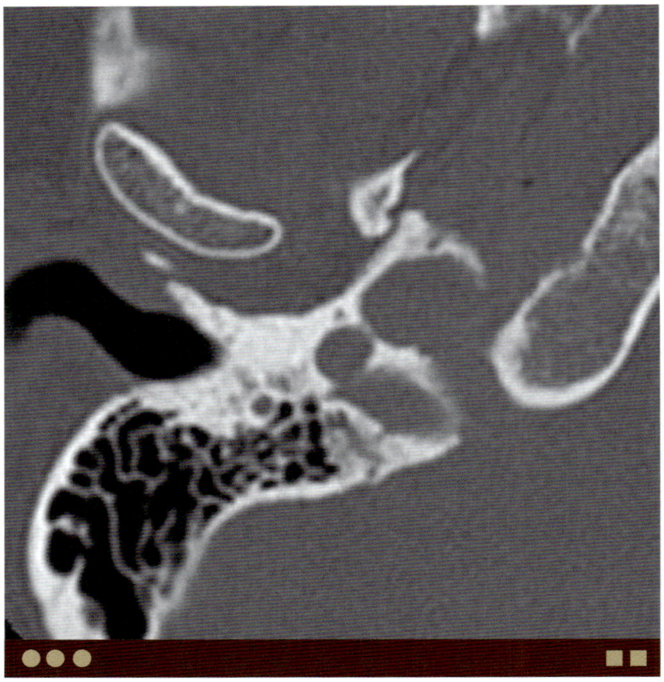

C. Aberrant internal carotid artery, same patient as A. Axial CT through the lower level demonstrates an enlarged inferior tympanic canaliculus. Vertical carotid canal is noted in this patient, representing a very rare anomaly, duplicated ICAs.

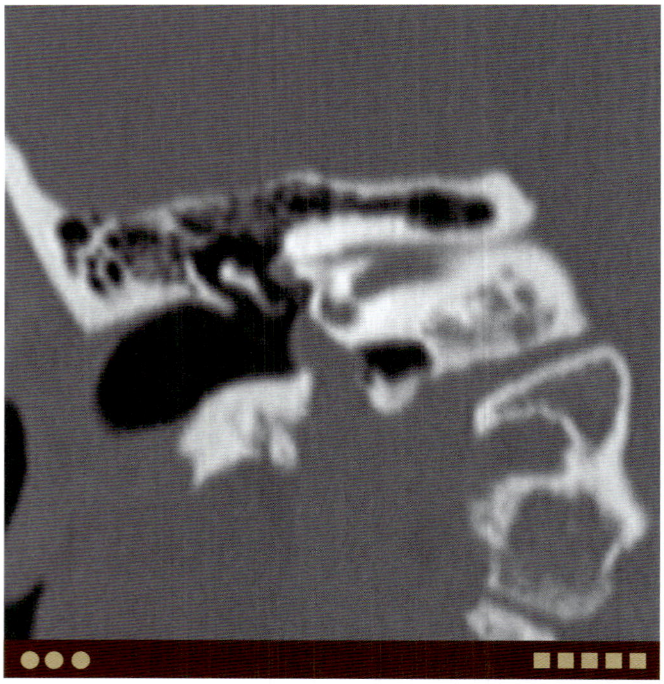

D. Aberrant internal carotid artery, same patient as A. Coronal CT demonstrates the aberrant ICA entering into hypotympanum through the inferior tympanic canaliculus.

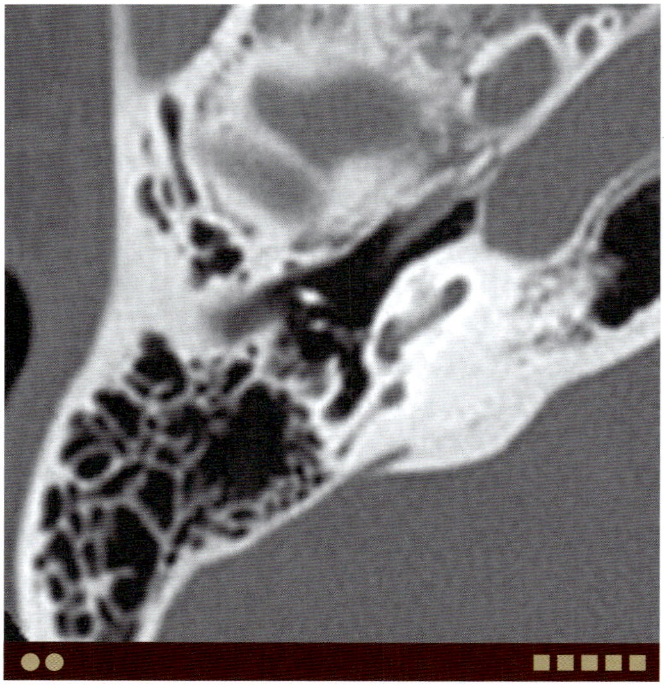

E. Aberrant internal carotid artery, same patient as A. Axial CT demonstrates a persistent stapedial artery arising from the aberrant ICA.

DIFFERENTIAL DIAGNOSIS IMAGES (F-H)

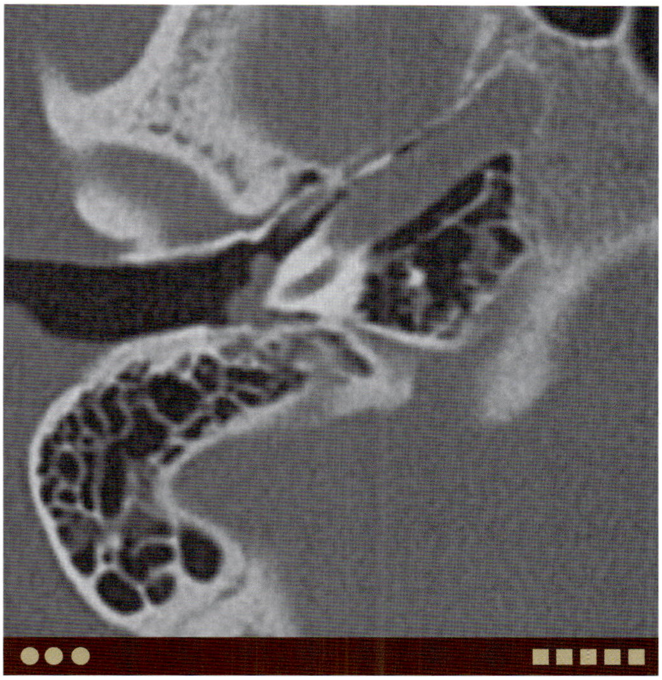

F. Glomus tympanicum. Axial CT demonstrates a focal soft tissue density mass over the cochlear promontory.

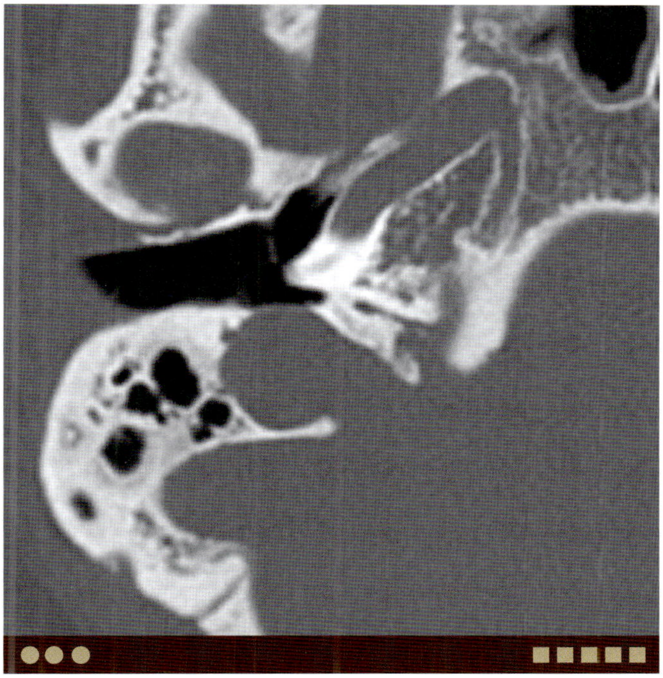

G. High jugular bulb. Axial CT demonstrates a high jugular bulb at the level of tympanic cavity. The bony covering is very thin.

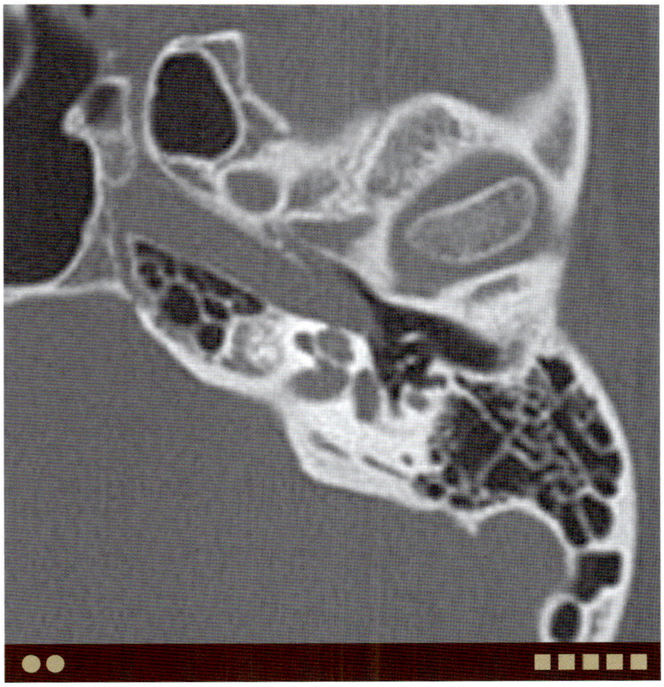

H. Laterally displaced carotid artery (lateralized ICA). Axial CT demonstrates a laterally displaced ICA running into the tympanic cavity through a dehiscence of the bony carotid canal in the petrous portion.

Case 1–20 External Auditory Canal Atresia

Osamu Sakai, Rohini Nadgir

PRESENTATION

Ear deformity, atresia of the external auditory canal (EAC).

FINDINGS

CT demonstrates atresia of the EAC.

DIFFERENTIAL DIAGNOSIS

- EAC exostosis: This condition is also known as surfer's ear. Osseous proliferation narrowing the EAC is noted, however, no anomaly is seen in the tympanic cavity.
- Goldenhar syndrome: This is first and second branchial arch anomaly and also known as hemifacial microsomia. In addition to anomalies in the temporal bone, incomplete development of the nose, soft palate, lip, and mandible is seen.

COMMENTS

This is a 10-year-old boy with right microtia.

Atresia of the EAC is more commonly seen in boys (M:F = 3:2), and about 30% of cases are bilateral and 15% are familial. Degree of atresia can be variable, from membranous soft tissue atresia to thick osseous atresia. Thicker atretic bony plate and smaller middle ear cavity suggest a more difficult reconstructive surgery and poorer outcome.

Anterior migration of the facial nerve is often seen with atresia of the EAC. Therefore, preoperative evaluation of the facial nerve course, particularly the tympanic and mastoid segments, is important to avoid intraoperative injury of the facial nerve. Sometimes, cholesteatoma occurs in association with EAC atresia and bone erosion and destruction can be seen secondary to cholesteatoma.

The EAC is derived from the first branchial arch. Therefore, malformation, fusion, and defects of the ossicles derived from the first branchial arch, such as malleus head, incus body, and short process are commonly seen. The malleus is often fused with the atretic bony plate. The second branchial arch forms the manubrium of malleus, long process of incus and stapes except a part of the footplate.

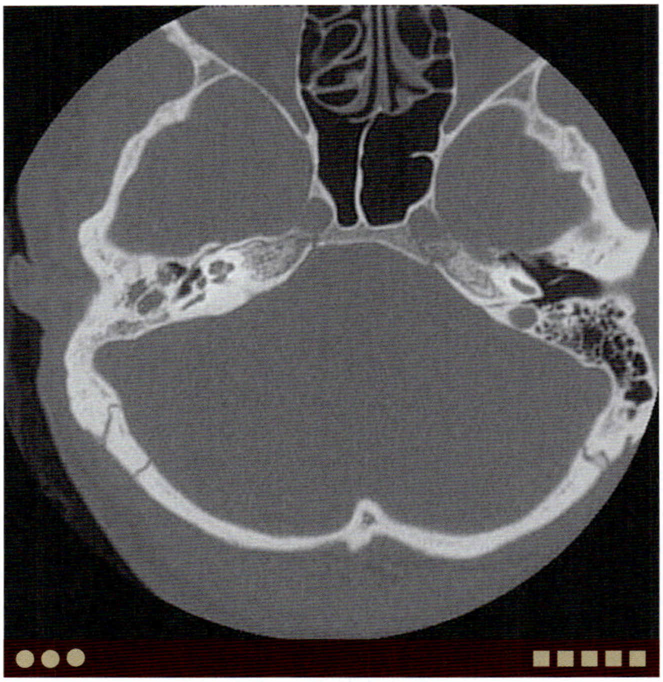

A. EAC atresia. Axial CT demonstrates atresia of the right EAC with decreased size and poor aeration of the tympanic cavity. Microtia is noted.

In general, external and middle ears are formed from the second branchial arch, while the inner ear is formed from the ectoderm (otocyst) earlier during gestation, therefore, malformations of these structures occur independently. However, malformation of both inner and middle ears can be seen in patients with trisomy 13, 18, and 21.

PEARLS

- **Degree of EAC atresia can be variable, from membranous soft tissue atresia to thick osseous atresia.**
- **Anterior migration of the facial nerve is often seen with EAC atresia.**
- **Cholesteatoma may occur in association with EAC atresia.**

ADDITIONAL IMAGES (B-E)

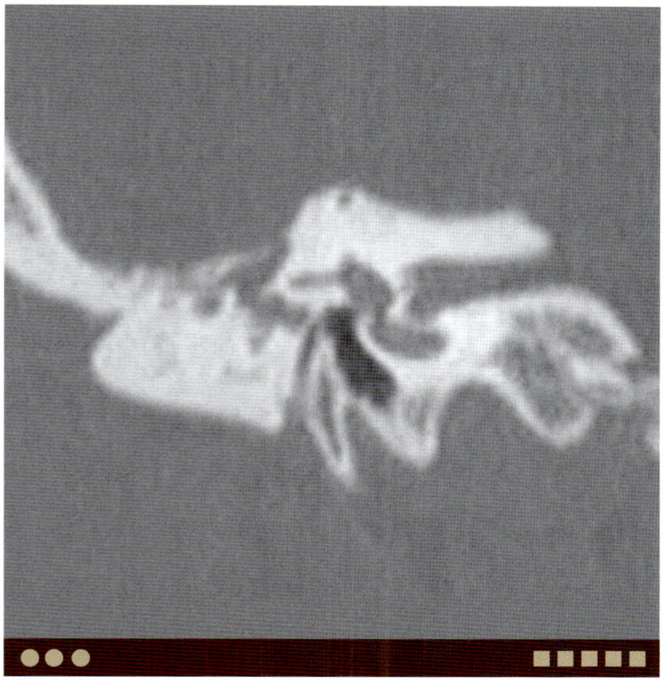

B. EAC atresia, same patient as A. Coronal CT demonstrates poorly formed tympanic cavity filled with soft tissue density and thick bony atresia. Note anomalous anterior course of the facial nerve.

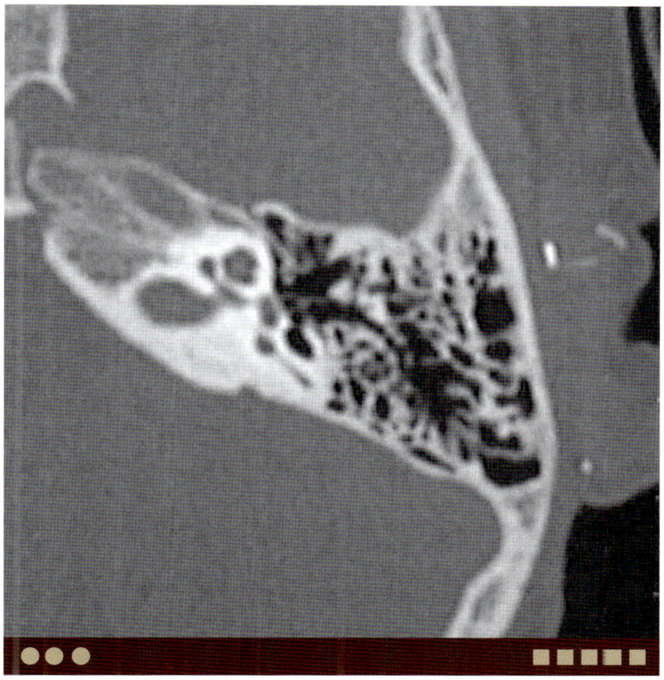

C. EAC atresia in a different patient. Axial CT demonstrates atresia of the EAC. However, aeration of the tympanic cavity and mastoid air cells is preserved. Note deformed malleus and incus.

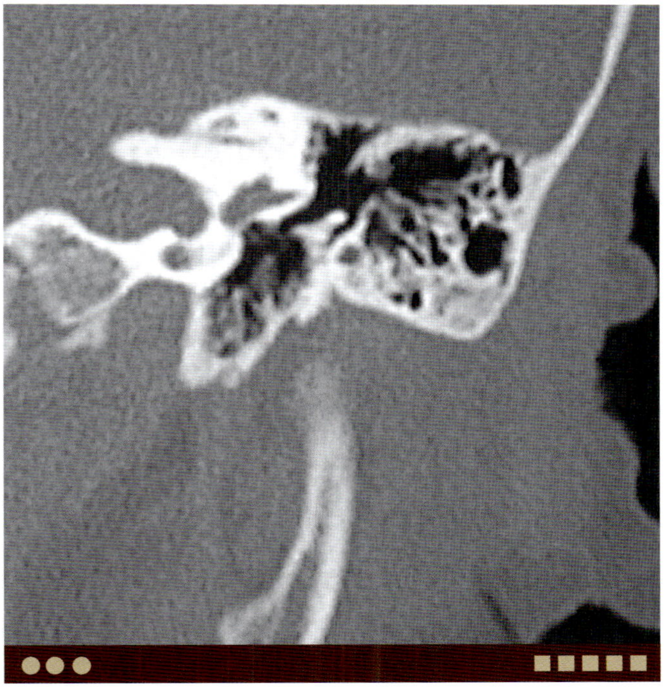

D. EAC atresia, same patient as C. Coronal CT demonstrates deformed malleus and incus fusing to the atretic bony plate. Aeration of the tympanic cavity and mastoid air cells is preserved. Microtia is noted.

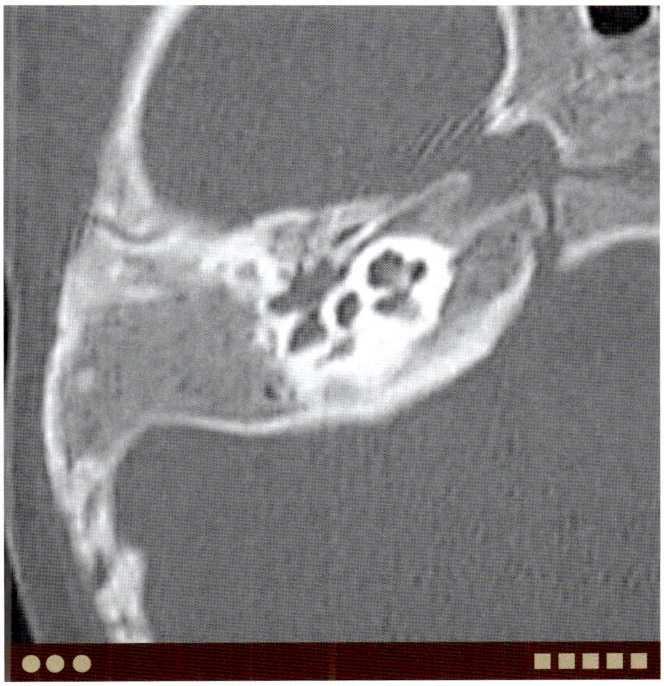

E. EAC atresia in a different patient. Axial CT demonstrates very thick atretic bony plate with poorly formed tympanic cavity filled with soft tissue density. No malleus or incus is identified.

DIFFERENTIAL DIAGNOSIS IMAGES (F-H)

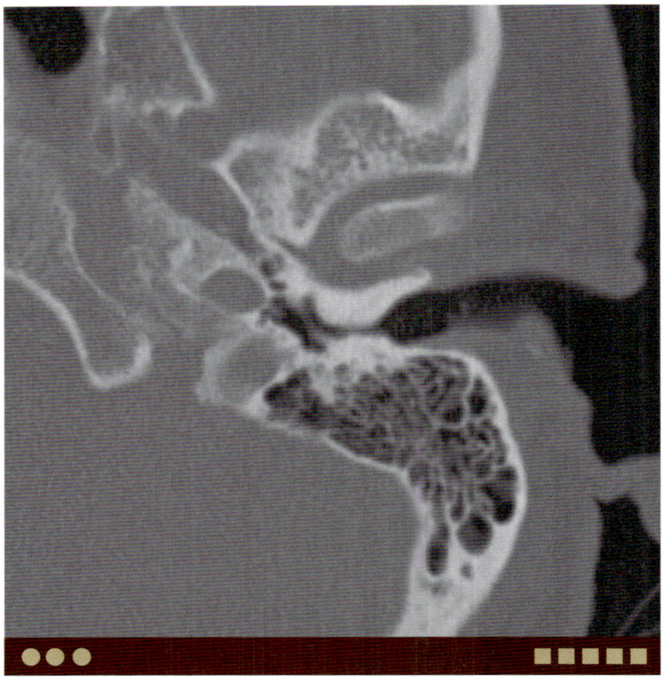

F. EAC exostosis. Axial CT demonstrates broad-based osseous proliferation narrowing the left EAC.

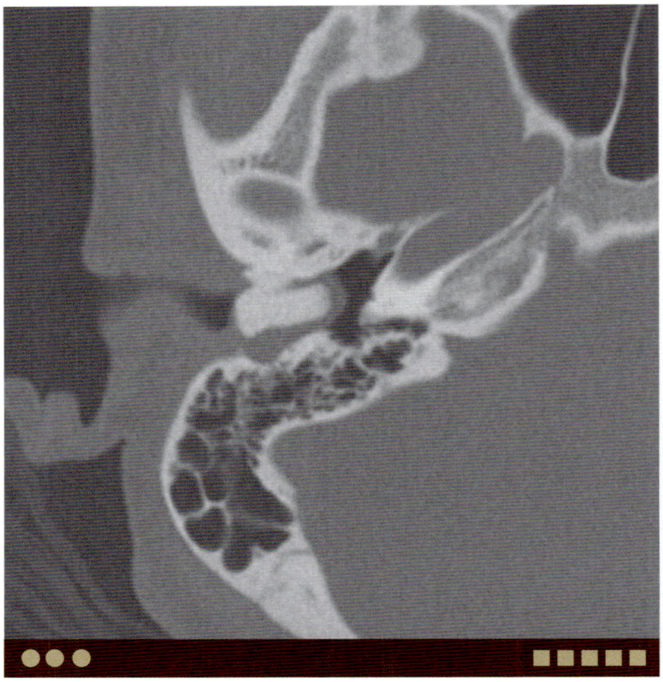

G. EAC osteoma. Axial CT demonstrates a pedunculated bony lesion in the right EAC.

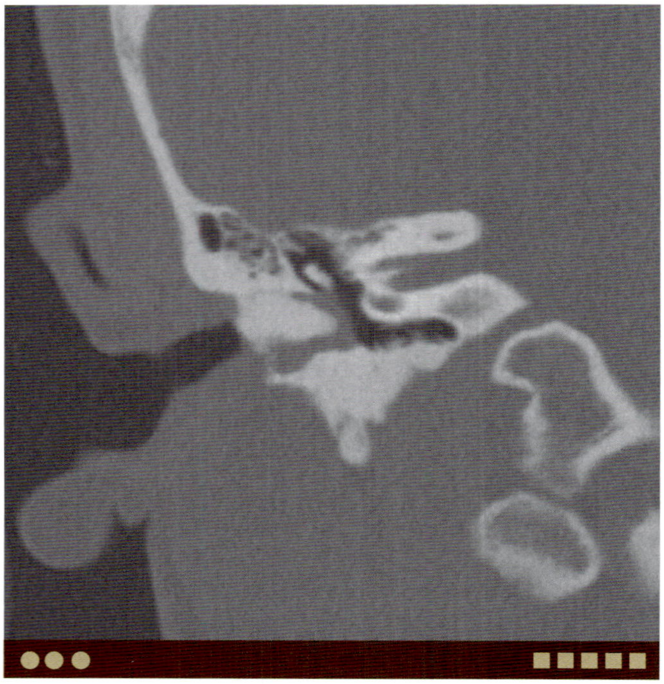

H. EAC osteoma, same patient as G. Coronal CT demonstrates a pedunculated bony lesion in the right EAC.

Case 1–21 Bell's Palsy

Osamu Sakai, Brooke Devenney-Cakir

PRESENTATION

Facial nerve palsy.

FINDINGS

Axial MRI demonstrates abnormal enhancement of the facial nerve.

DIFFERENTIAL DIAGNOSIS

- Schwannoma: This is the most common primary tumor arising from the facial nerve. Mass formation is noted in addition to abnormal enhancement, commonly seen in the genu and tympanic segment.
- Perineural tumor spread: This is commonly seen in patients with adenoid cystic carcinoma of the parotid gland. Obliteration of the fat in the stylomastoid foramen strongly suggests perineural tumor spread.
- Hemangioma: This is rare but the second most common tumor associated with the facial nerve. Bone remodeling or infiltrative change is seen around the facial canal.

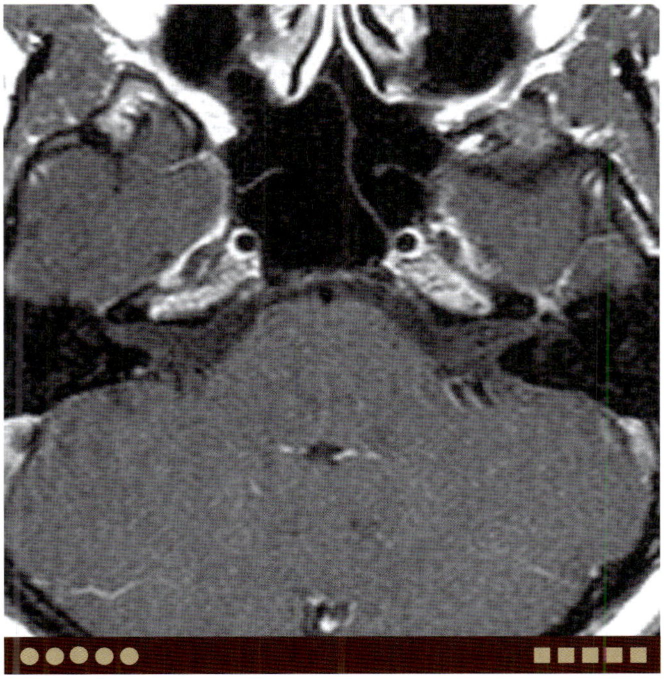

A. Facial nerve palsy. Axial postcontrast T1W image demonstrates abnormal enhancement of the genu of the left facial nerve compared with the right.

COMMENTS

This is a 28-year-old woman with Bell's palsy.

Bell's palsy is defined as an idiopathic facial nerve paralysis. By definition, it is idiopathic; however, most often associated with herpes simplex type 1 virus infection. It is usually self-limiting and imaging is not necessary. However, imaging is performed for prolonged paralysis which requires decompression surgery, and for recurrent or progressive facial nerve paralysis to rule out neoplastic processes such as schwannoma and hemangioma, as well as malignant tumors.

Ramsay Hunt syndrome is herpes zoster virus infection, causing sudden onset of hearing loss, ear pain, and facial nerve palsy. Occasionally, infection extends into the membranous labyrinth and C.N. VIII and causes vertigo and tinnitus.

Inflamed facial nerve demonstrates abnormal enhancement and slight enlargement on postcontrast T1W images. The facial nerve normally enhances in the genu to the mastoid segment, therefore, it is important to compare to the contralateral side. However, enhancement in the intracanalicular segment is always abnormal.

Evaluation of the intracranial structures is important to diagnosis intracranial pathologies causing facial nerve palsy, including infarct, demyelinating disease, tumors, granulomatous diseases, and infections.

PEARLS

- **Inflammation of the facial nerve demonstrates abnormal enhancement of the nerve.**
- **Normal enhancement can be seen in the genu and distal segments of the facial nerve. However, enhancement in the intracanalicular segment is abnormal.**
- **Evaluation of the intracranial structures is important to diagnose intracranial pathologies causing facial nerve palsy.**

ADDITIONAL IMAGES (B-G)

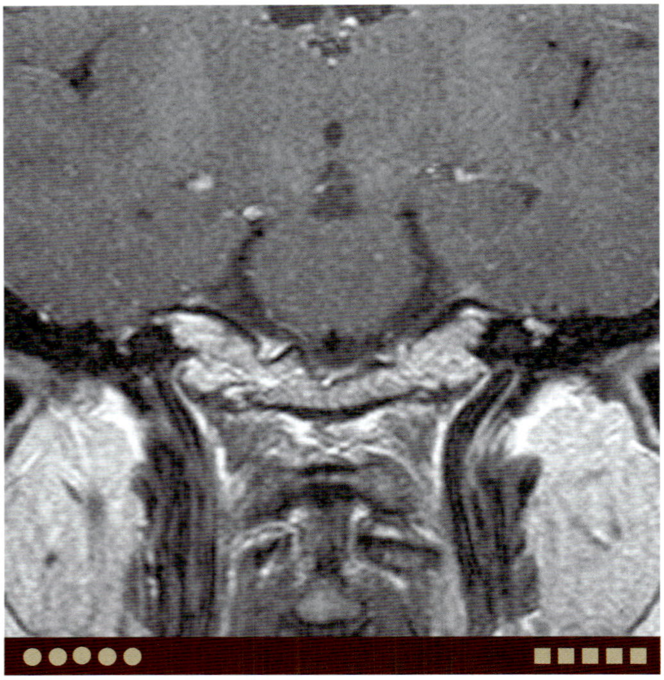

B. Facial nerve palsy, same patient as A. Coronal postcontrast T1W image demonstrates abnormal enhancement of the genu of the left facial nerve.

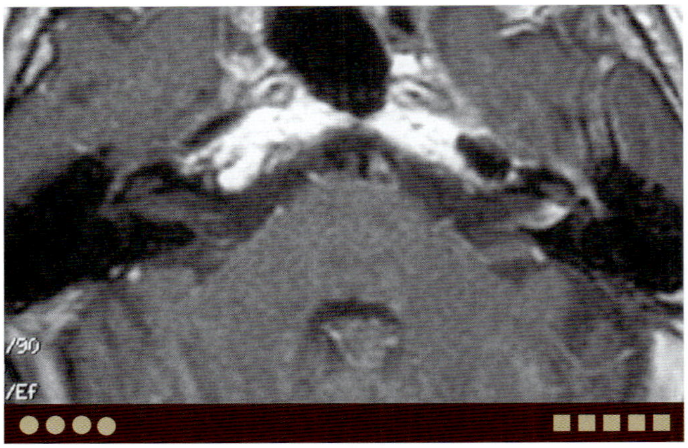

C. Facial nerve palsy, 76-year-old man with herpes zoster infection. Axial postcontrast T1W image demonstrates abnormal enhancement of the intracanalicular segment of the left facial nerve.

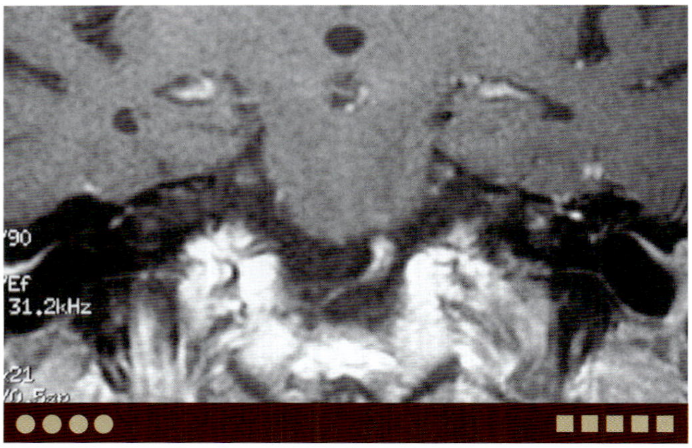

D. Facial nerve palsy, same patient as C. Coronal postcontrast T1W image demonstrates abnormal enhancement of the intracanalicular segment of the left facial nerve.

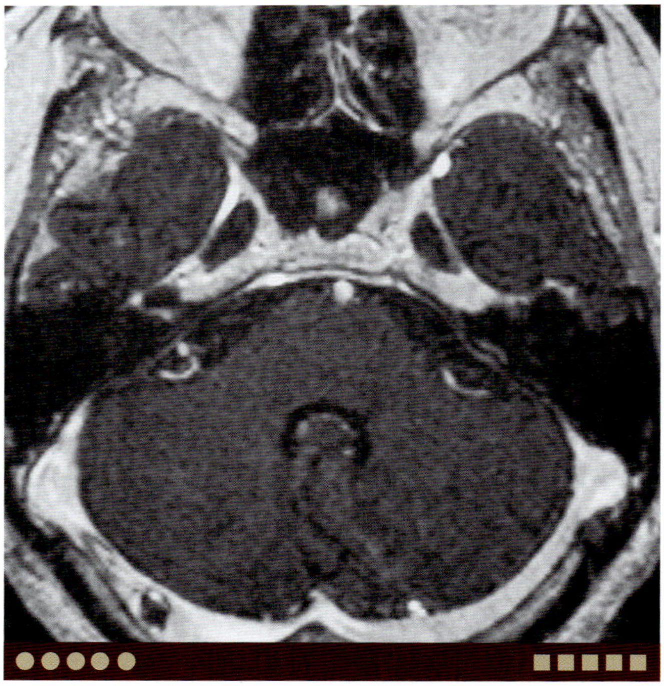

E. Facial nerve palsy in a different patient. Axial postcontrast T1W image demonstrates abnormal enhancement of the labyrinthine segment and genu of the right facial nerve.

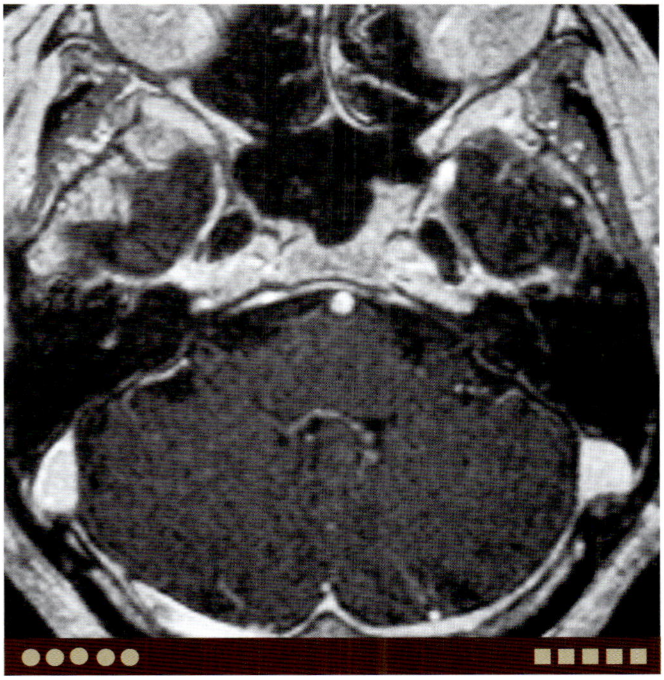

F. Facial nerve palsy, same patient as E. Axial postcontrast T1W image demonstrates abnormal enhancement of the mastoid segment of the right facial nerve.

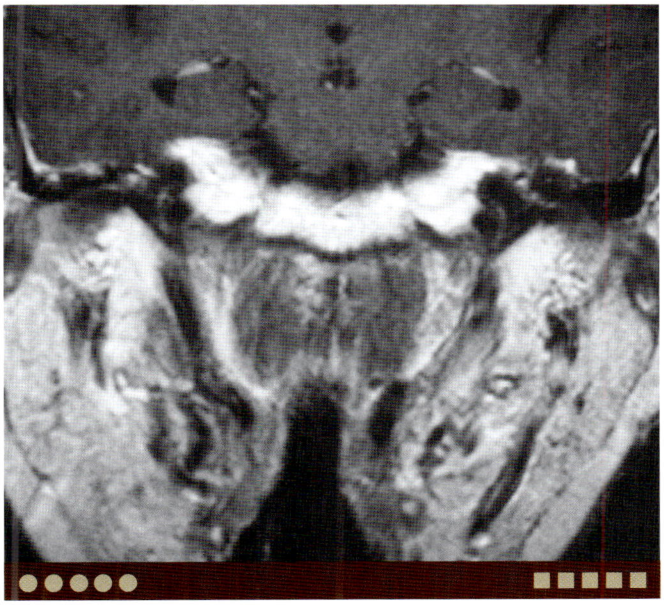

G. Facial nerve palsy, same patient as E. Coronal postcontrast T1W image demonstrates abnormal enhancement of the labyrinthine and tympanic segments of the right facial nerve.

DIFFERENTIAL DIAGNOSIS IMAGES (H-J)

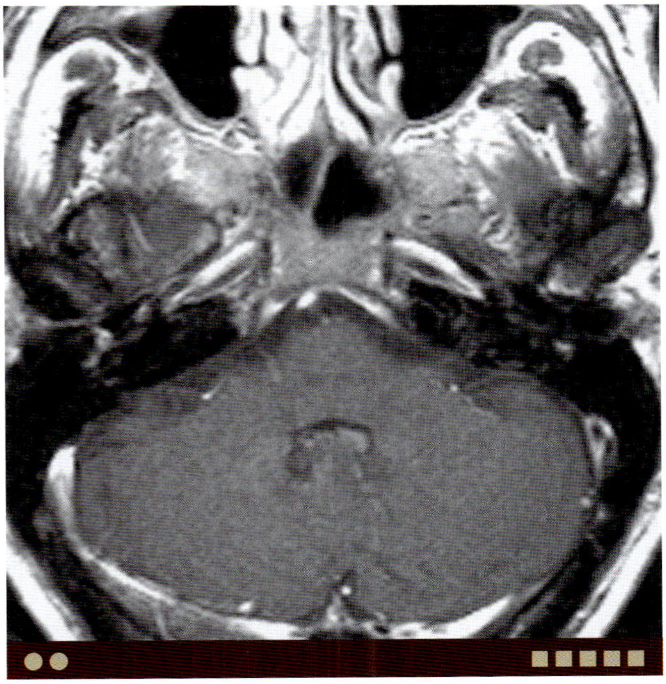

H. Schwannoma. Axial postcontrast T1W image demonstrates an enhancing globular lesion in the tympanic segment of the right facial nerve.

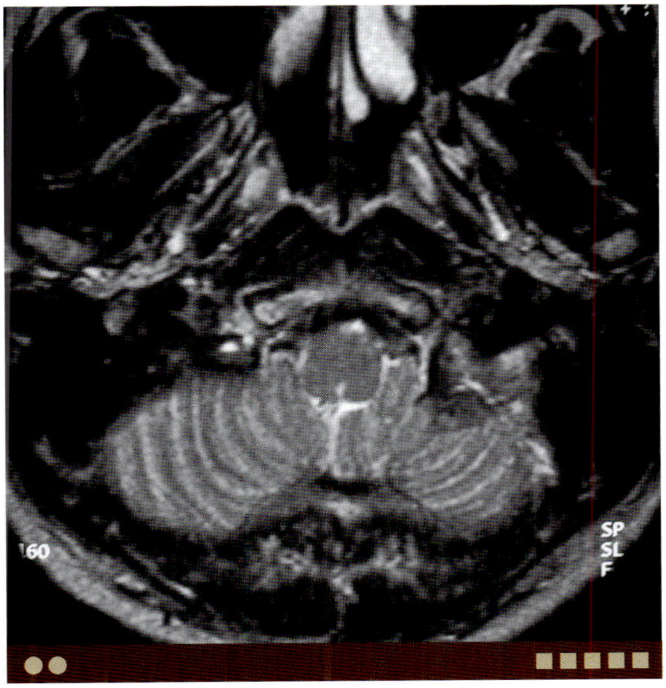

I. Hemangioma. Axial T2W image demonstrates a heterogeneous hyperintense lesion in the mastoid segment of the right facial nerve.

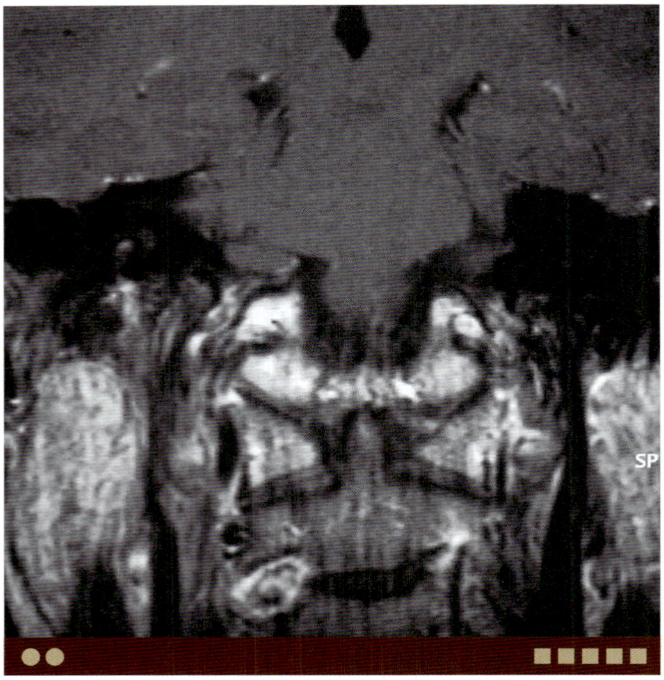

J. Hemangioma, same patient as I. Coronal postcontrast T1W image demonstrates a heterogeneously enhancing tubular lesion in the mastoid segment of the right facial nerve.

Case 1–22 Sarcoidosis: Heerfordt Syndrome

Osamu Sakai, Rohini Nadgir

PRESENTATION

Fever, parotid swelling, and facial weakness.

FINDINGS

Postcontrast T1W MR images show abnormal enhancement of the parotid glands and facial nerve.

DIFFERENTIAL DIAGNOSIS

- Bell's palsy: This is idiopathic facial nerve palsy. Abnormal enhancement of the facial nerve is seen without other abnormality.
- Schwannoma: This is the most common primary tumor arising from the facial nerve. Mass formation is noted in addition to abnormal enhancement, commonly seen in the genu and tympanic segments.
- Perineural tumor spread: This is commonly seen in patients with adenoid cystic carcinoma of the parotid gland. Obliteration of the fat in the stylomastoid foramen strongly suggests perineural tumor spread.
- Hemangioma: This is rare but the second most common tumor associated with the facial nerve. Bone remodeling or infiltrative change is seen around the facial canal.

COMMENTS

This is a 40-year-old woman with left facial nerve palsy.

Sarcoidosis can involve the facial nerve. Imaging findings are nonspecific and identical to that of Bell's palsy and Ramsay Hunt syndrome. Heerfordt syndrome, also known as uveo-parotid fever, is a subtype of sarcoidosis consisting of the triad of uveitis, parotid swelling, and facial nerve palsy, and is often accompanied with low-grade fever. Uveitis is seen in about 60% to 70% of patients with sarcoidosis and often is the first presenting symptom. Parotid swelling is seen in 6% of patients with sarcoidosis and is associated with tenderness; epithelioid granuloma is seen in biopsy specimen. Neurological abnormality is seen in about 5% of patients with sarcoidosis and 80% of those patients demonstrate peripheral nerve palsy. Facial nerve involvement is most common among cranial nerves involved. Heerfordt syndrome with complete symptoms is rare and is seen in only 0.3% to 0.7% of patients with sarcoidosis.

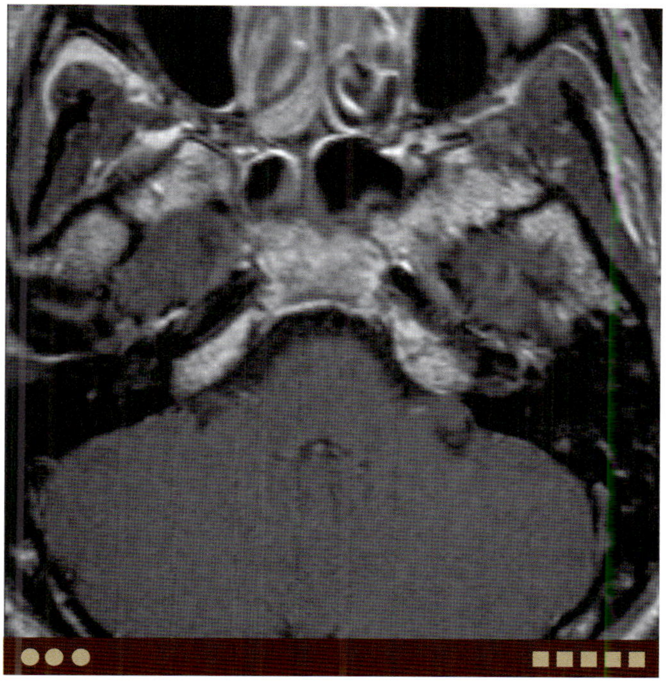

A. Sarcoidosis. Axial postcontrast T1W image demonstrates abnormal enhancement of the intracanalicular and labyrinthine segments and genu of the left facial nerve.

PEARLS

- **Sarcoidosis can involve the facial nerve.**
- **Heerfordt syndrome is a rare subtype of sarcoidosis consisting of the clincal triad of uveitis, parotid swelling, and facial nerve palsy and is often accompanied with low-grade fever.**

ADDITIONAL IMAGES (B-F)

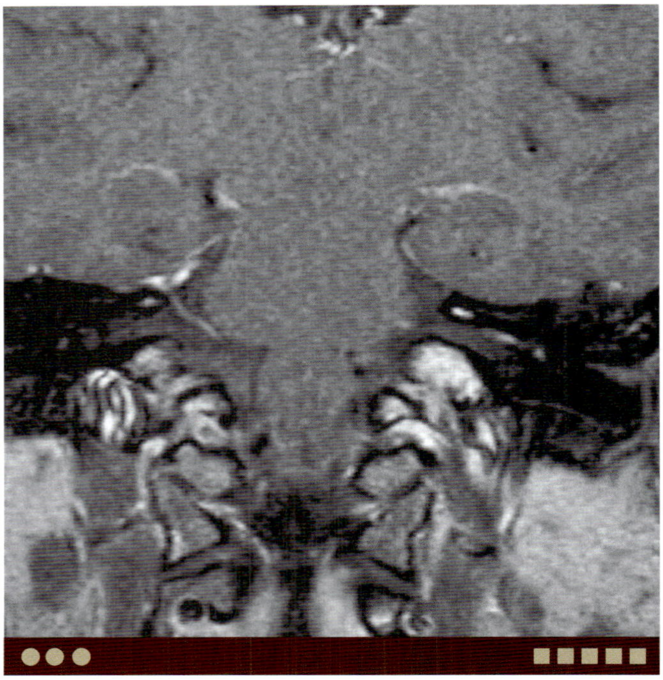

B. Sarcoidosis, same patient as A. Coronal postcontrast T1W image demonstrates abnormal enhancement of the intracanalicular segment of the left facial nerve.

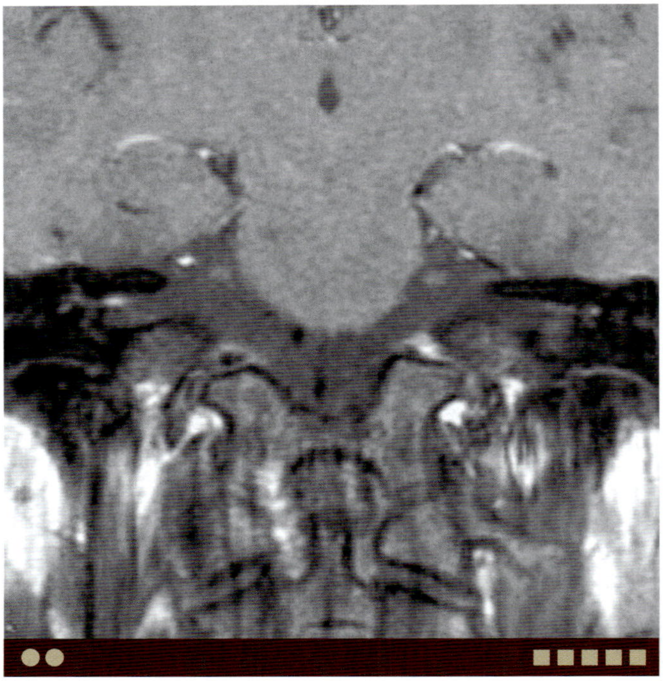

C. Heerfordt syndrome, 15-year-old adolescent with fever, bilateral parotid swelling, and right facial nerve palsy. Coronal postcontrast T1W image demonstrates abnormal enhancement of the intracanalicular segment of the right facial nerve.

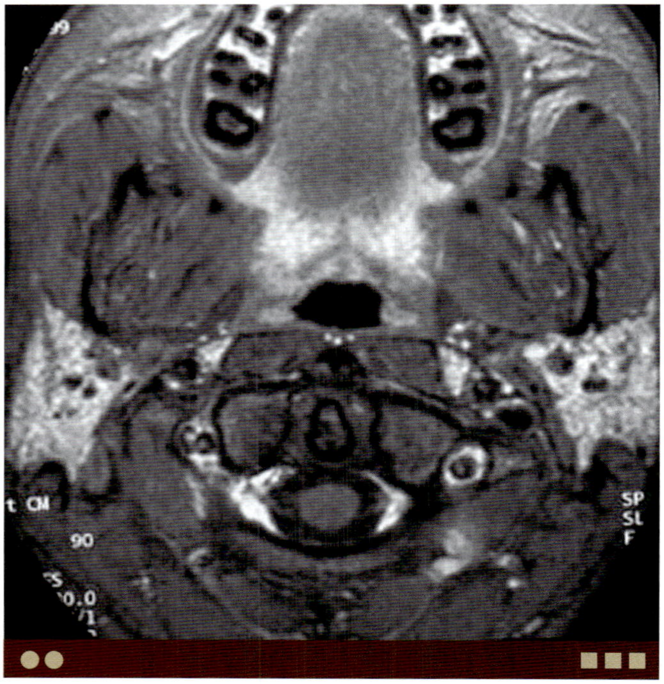

D. Heerfordt syndrome, same patient as C. Axial postcontrast fat-suppressed T1W image demonstrates abnormal enhancement of the bilateral parotid glands.

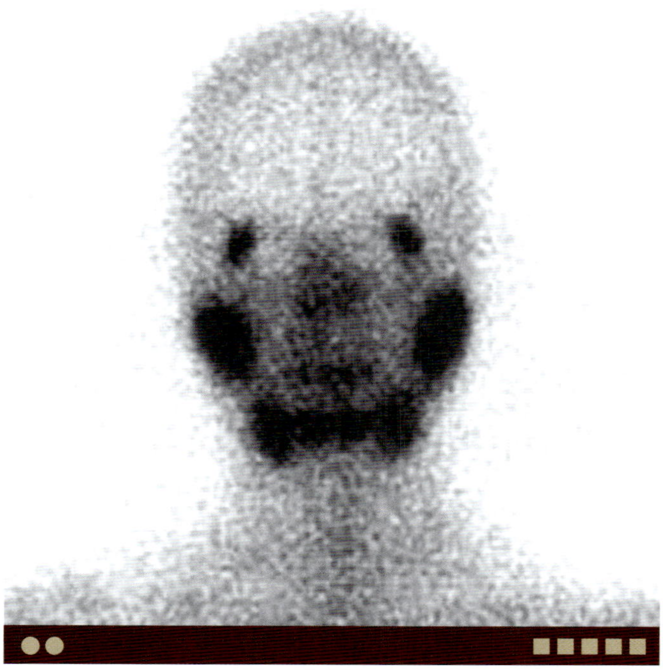

E. Heerfordt syndrome, same patient as C. Gallium-67 scan demonstrates "panda sign," increased accumulation of the radiotracer in the bilateral lacrimal and parotid glands as well as in the submandibular glands.

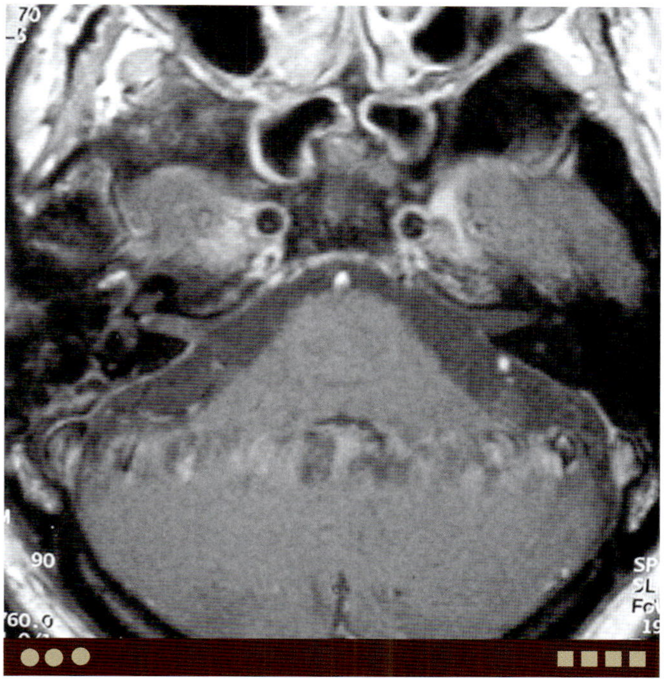

F. Sarcoidosis in a different patient. Axial T1W image demonstrates faint enhancement of the seventh and eighth nerve complex within the right internal auditory canal as well as abnormal dural enhancement.

DIFFERENTIAL DIAGNOSIS IMAGES (G-I)

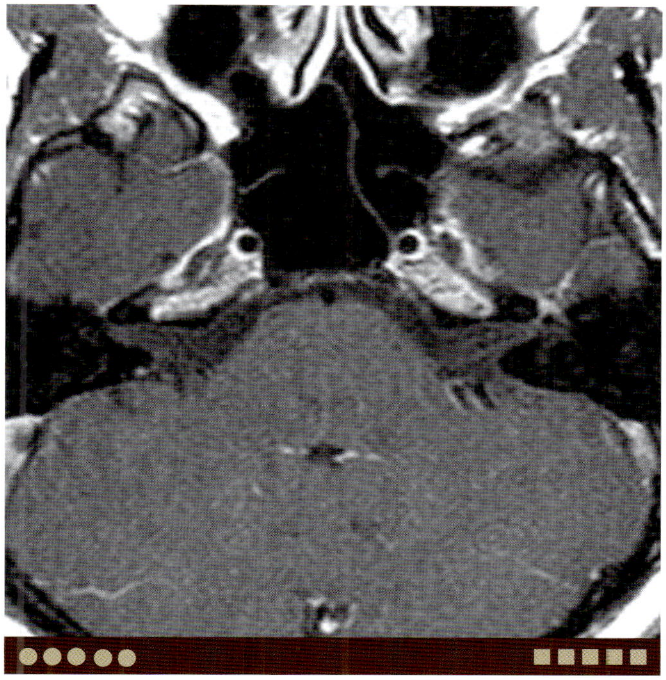

G. Bell's palsy. Axial postcontrast T1W image demonstrates abnormal enhancement of the genu and labrythine segments of the left facial nerve compared with the right.

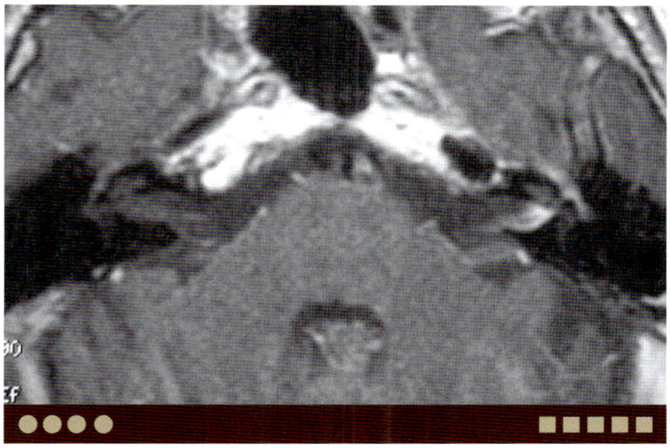

H. Herpes zoster infection. Axial postcontrast T1W image demonstrates abnormal enhancement of the intracanalicular segment of the left facial nerve.

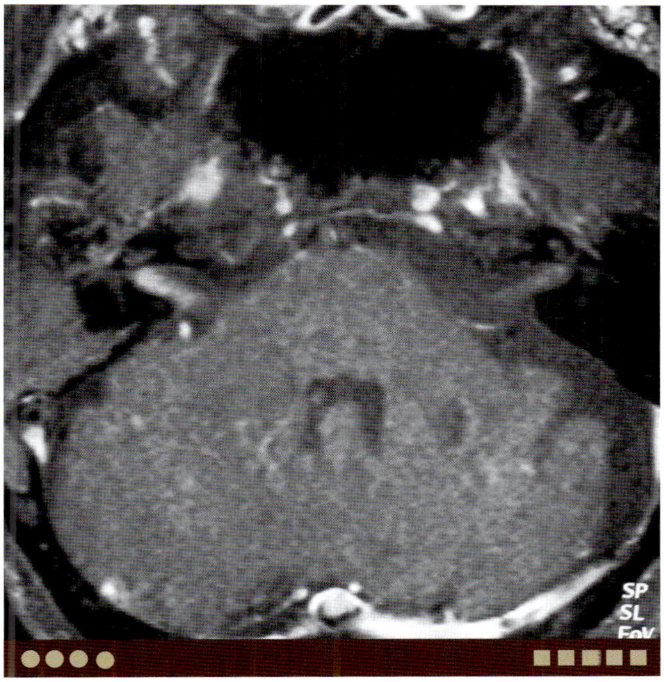

I. CSF tumor dissemination from breast cancer. Axial postcontrast T1W image shows abnormal enhancement along the seventh and eighth cranial nerve complex bilaterally, right more than left.

Case 1–23 Facial Nerve Schwannoma

Osamu Sakai, Rohini Nadgir

PRESENTATION

Slowly progressing facial nerve weakness.

FINDINGS

CT and MRI demonstrate an enhancing mass in the course of the facial nerve.

DIFFERENTIAL DIAGNOSIS

- Bell's palsy: This is defined as an idiopathic unilateral facial nerve paralysis. By definition, it is idiopathic; however, it is most often associated with herpes simplex type 1 virus infection. Abnormal enhancement of the facial nerve is noted without mass formation.
- Hemangioma: This is the second most common tumor associated with the facial nerve, although it is rare. This usually shows higher T2 signal than schwannoma.
- Perineural tumor spread: This is commonly seen with adenoid cystic carcinoma of the parotid gland. Obliteration of the fat in the stylomastoid foramen is often seen.

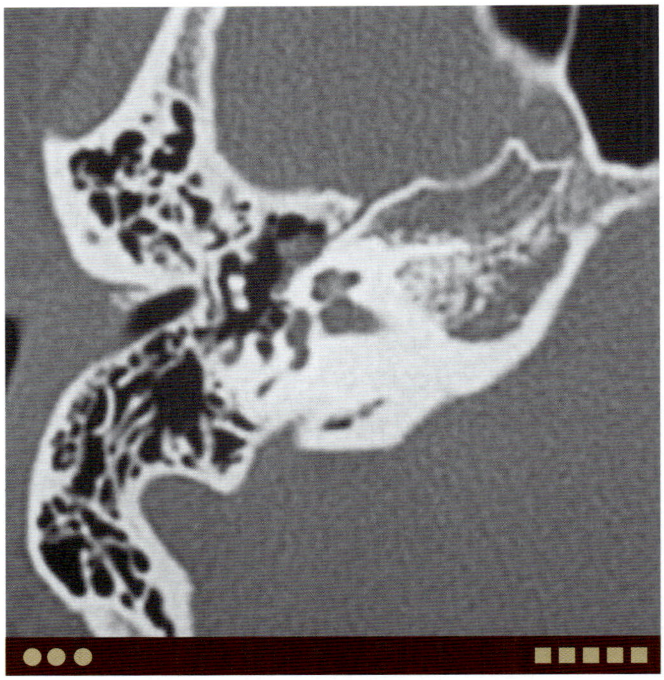

A. Schwannoma. Axial CT demonstrates a soft tissue mass over the cochlea.

COMMENTS

This is a 38-year-old woman with slowly progressive right-sided facial palsy.

Bell's palsy is the most common cause of facial nerve palsy. MRI is often performed in patients with prolonged or recurrent facial nerve palsy to rule out neoplastic processes such as schwannoma. Schwannoma is the most common tumor arising from the facial nerve, although it is not a very common location for schwannoma. The tympanic segment and genu are often involved and multiple schwannomas can be seen along the course of the facial nerve.

CT can demonstrate widening of the osseous canal in addition to soft tissue masses. Schwannomas show low signal on T1W, intermediate-to-high signal on T2W, and relatively homogeneous enhancement on MRI. Perineural tumor spread, commonly seen with adenoid cystic carcinoma, may demonstrate similar findings, however, typically perineural tumor spread shows lower signal on T2W and less enhancement compared with schwannoma.

PEARLS

- **Schwannoma is the most common tumor associated with the facial nerve, although it is not a very common location for schwannoma.**
- **Schwannoma most commonly involves the genu and tympanic segment of the facial nerve.**
- **Perineural tumor spread can be seen along the facial nerve.**

ADDITIONAL IMAGES (B-C)

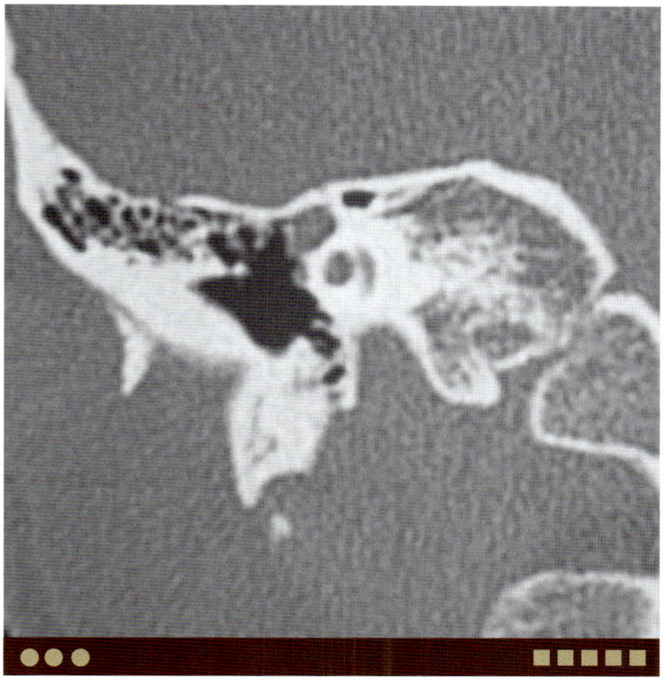

B. Schwannoma, same patient as A. Coronal CT demonstrates a soft tissue mass in the region of the genu of the facial nerve.

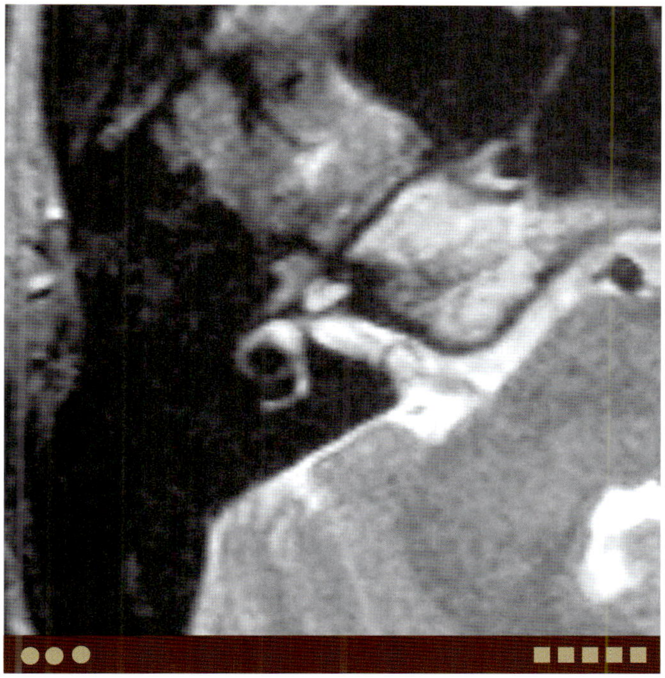

C. Schwannoma, same patient as A. Axial T2W MR image demonstrates an intermediate-signal mass in the genu extending to the tympanic segment of the facial nerve.

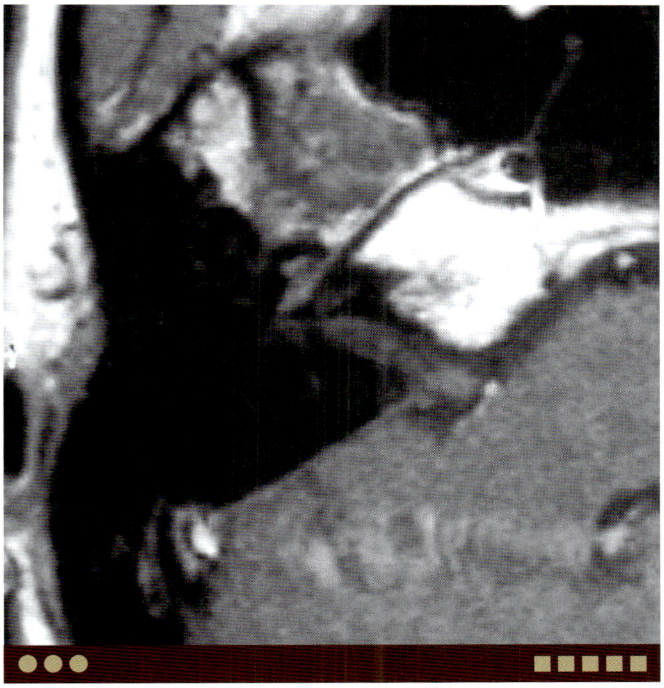

D. Schwannoma, same patient as A. Axial postcontrast fat-suppressed T1W image demonstrates enhancement of the lesion.

DIFFERENTIAL DIAGNOSIS IMAGES (E-H)

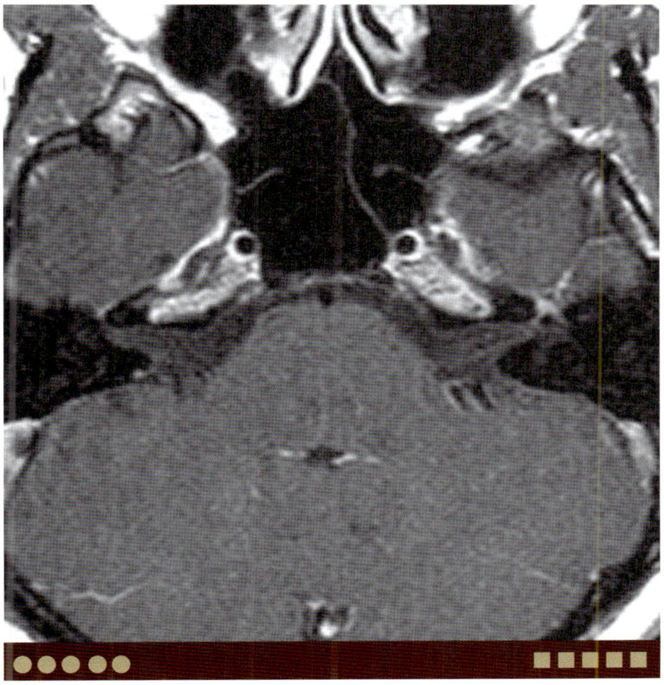

E. Bell's palsy. Axial postcontrast T1W image demonstrates abnormal enhancement of the genu of the left facial nerve compared with the right.

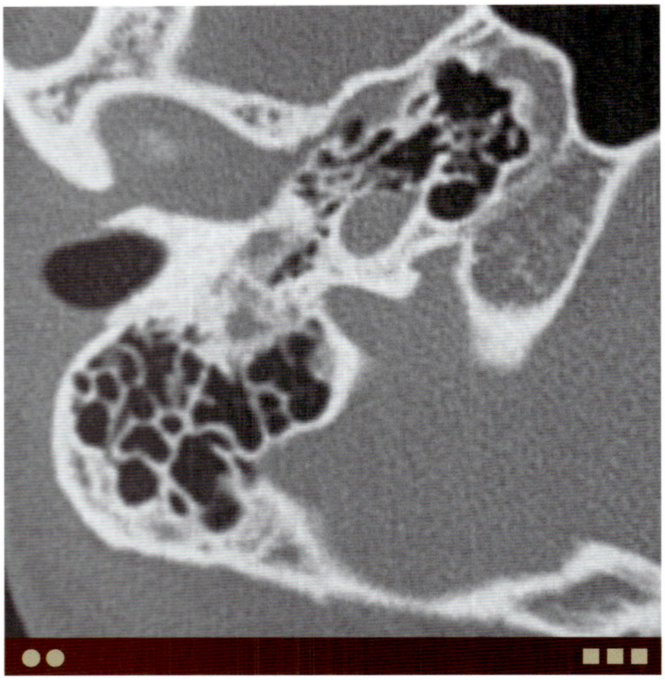

F. Facial nerve hemangioma. Axial CT demonstrates widening and infiltrative change of the mastoid segment of the facial nerve canal.

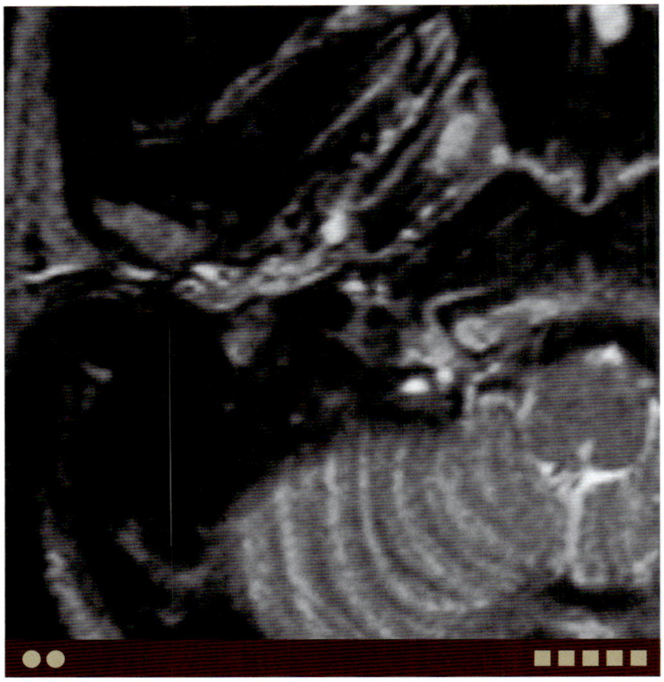

G. Facial nerve hemangioma, same patient as F. Axial T2W MR image demonstrates a slightly heterogeneous high-signal lesion involving mastoid segment of facial nerve.

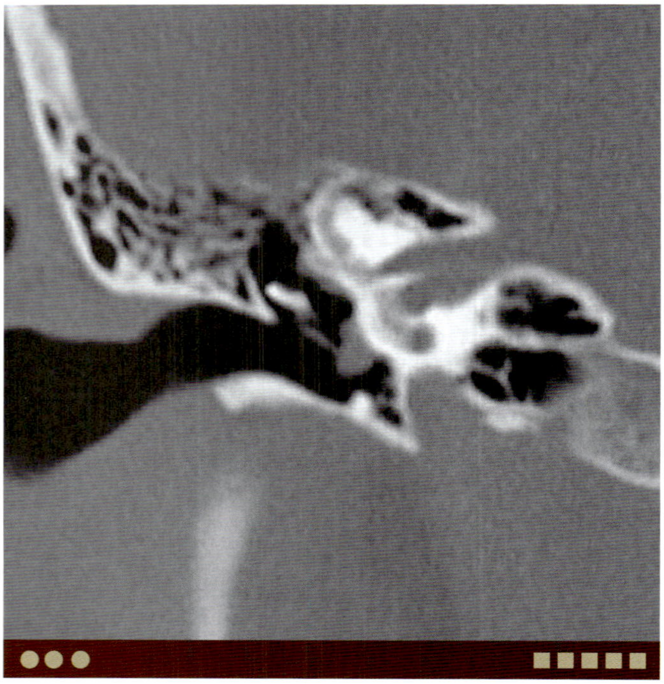

H. Glomus tympanicum. Coronal CT demonstrates a globular soft tissue mass over the coch ea.

Case 1–24 Semicircular Dysplasia

Osamu Sakai, Rohini Nadgir

PRESENTATION

Congenital sensorineural hearing loss.

FINDINGS

CT and MRI show large vestibule and hypoplastic lateral semicircular canal.

DIFFERENTIAL DIAGNOSIS

- Common cavity deformity: This is an anomaly of fusion of the cochlea and vestibule forming a single cavity. Semicircular canals may be normal.
- Large vestibular aqueduct syndrome: This show enlarged vestibular aqueduct wider than posterior semicircular canal or 1.5 mm in diameter on CT. Poor separation of the apical and middle turns of the cochlea is often noted.
- Labyrinthitis ossificans: With this condition, the semicircular canals are formed well, but ossified. Ossification of the membranous labyrinth may mimic dysplasia of the semicircular canal.

COMMENTS

This is a 25-year-old man with congenital sensorineural hearing loss.

The lateral semicircular canal is formed at the late stage of inner ear development, therefore, almost all inner ear developmental anomalies carry some degree of lateral semicircular canal abnormality. The most common appearance is a small and wide lateral semicircular canal with a small bony core of the lateral semicircular canal and a large vestibule. When more severely malformed, it forms single cavity with the vestibule without the bony core of the lateral semicircular canal. Other semicircular canals may or may not be affected. The cochlea may also be normal or hypoplastic.

On CT and MRI, a small bony core of the lateral semicircular canal is a clue to diagnosing mild semicircular dysplasia. This is one of the four check points to diagnose congenital inner ear anomalies: 1) hypoplastic lateral semicircular canal, 2) poor separation of the apical and middle turns of the cochlea, 3) enlarged vestibular aqueduct, and 4) small cochlear nerve hole (cochlear fossette).

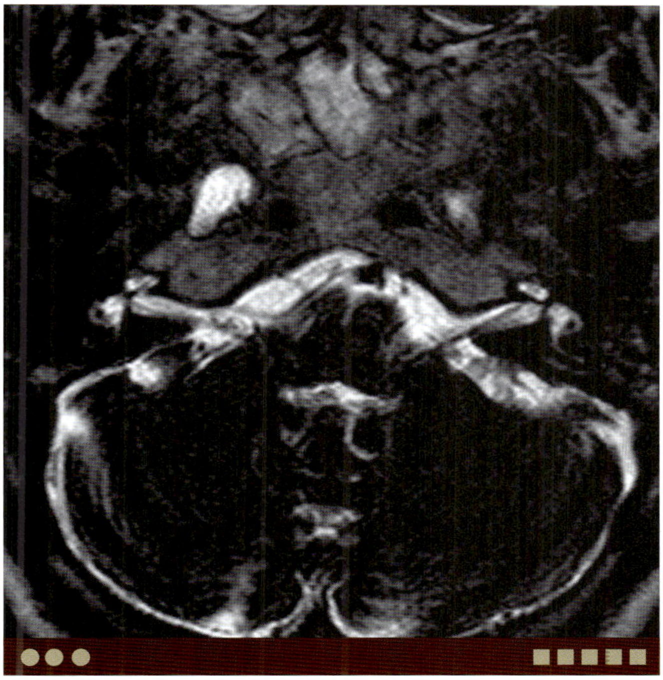

A. Lateral semicircular canal dysplasia. Axial high-resolution T2W MR image demonstrates small lateral semicircular canals with small bony core of the lateral semicircular canal and enlarged vestibule.

This condition may be seen associated with *CHARGE* syndrome. *CHARGE* syndrome is an autosomal dominant condition with genotypic heterogeneity manifesting *C*oloboma of the eye, *H*eart defects, *A*tresia of the nasal choanae, *R*etardation of growth and/or development, *G*enital and/or urinary abnormalities, and *E*ar abnormalities and deafness. Partial or complete semicircular canal hypoplasia is seen.

PEARLS

- **Lateral semicircular canal dysplasia is a relatively common inner anomaly. The mildest form demonstrates small and wide lateral semicircular canal with a small bony core.**
- **In more severely malformed cases, it forms single cavity with the vestibule without the bony core of the lateral semicircular canal.**

ADDITIONAL IMAGES (B-G)

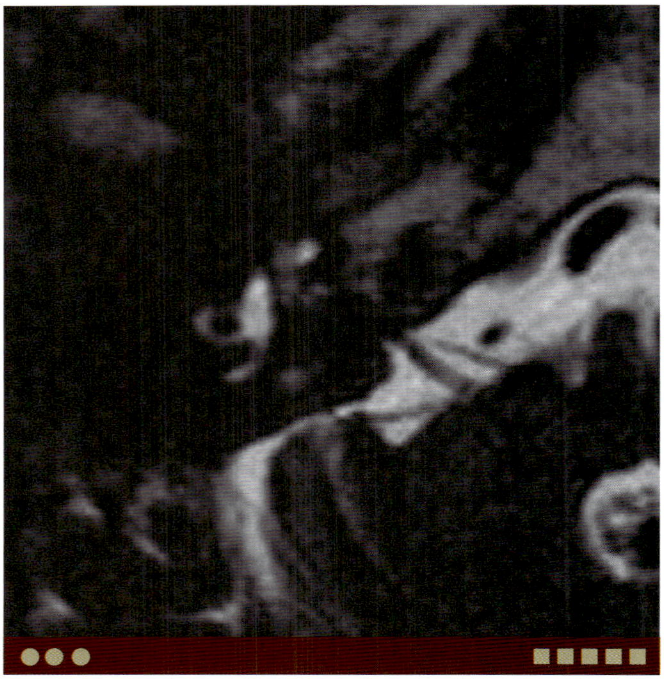

B. Lateral semicircular canal dysplasia in a different patient. Axial high-resolution T2W MR image demonstrates a small lateral semicircular canal and enlarged vestibule.

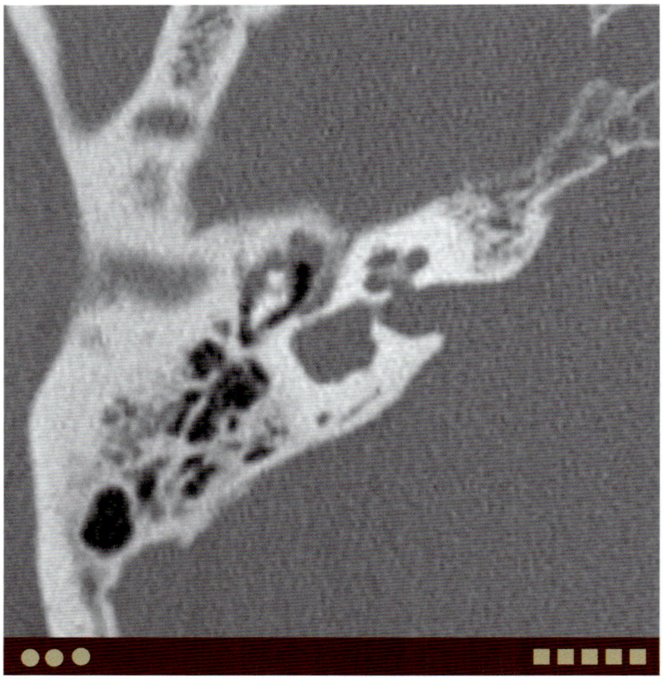

C. Lateral semicircular canal dysplasia in a different patient. Axial CT demonstrates single cavity of the lateral semicircular canal and vestibule.

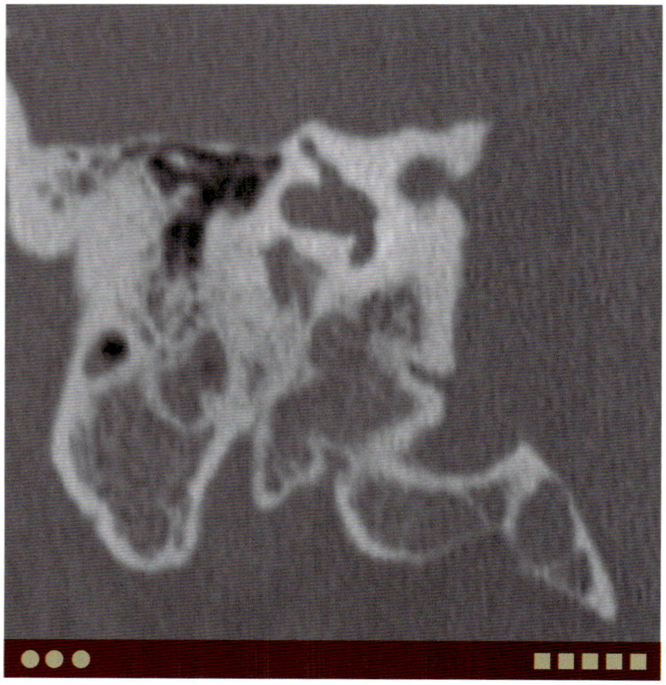

D. Lateral semicircular canal dysplasia, same patient as C. Coronal CT demonstrates widened lateral semicircular canal assimilated with the vestibule.

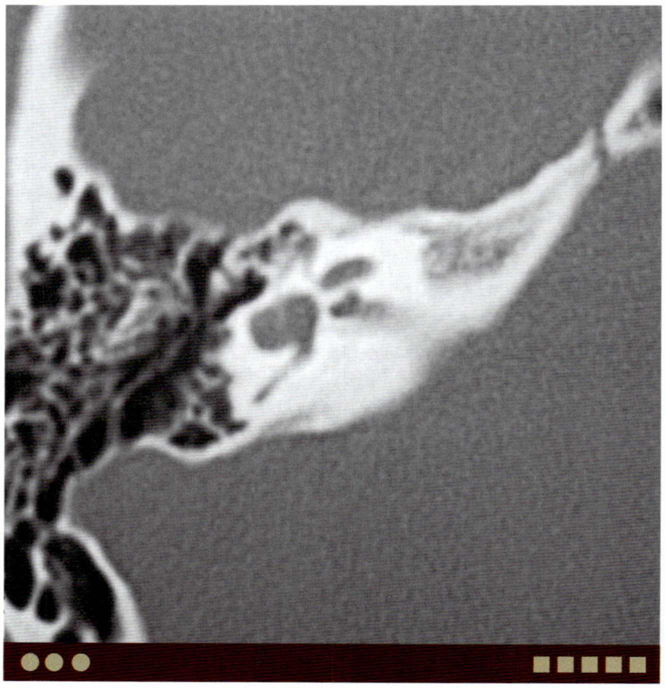

E. Lateral semicircular canal dysplasia in a different patient. Axial CT of the right ear demonstrates a single cavity of the lateral semicircular canal and vestibule.

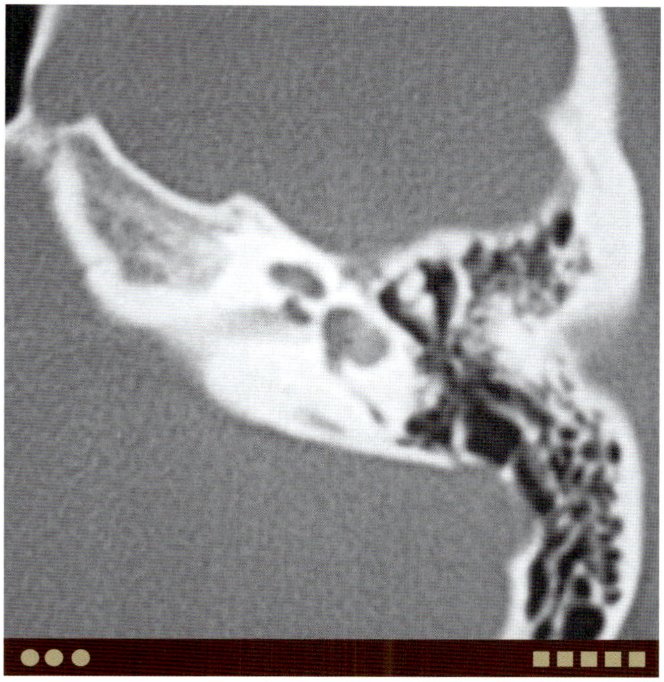

F. Lateral semicircular canal dysplasia, same patient as E. Axial CT of the left ear demonstrates the same finding.

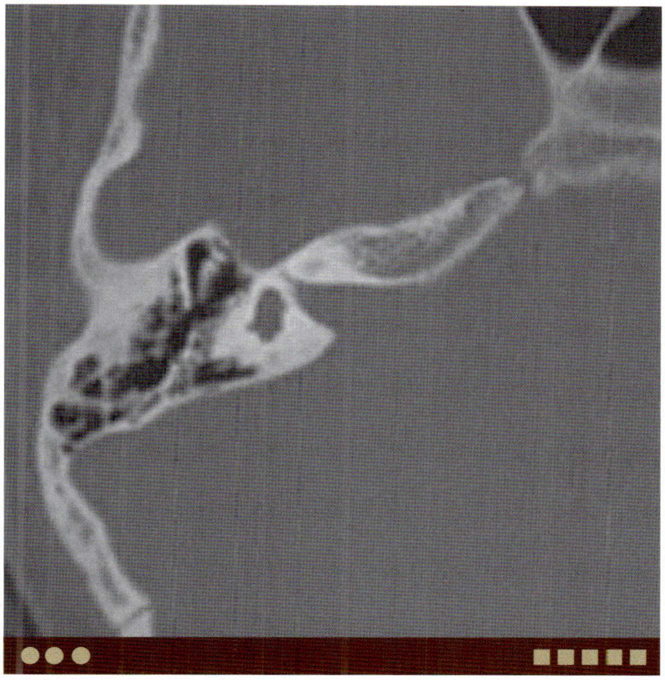

G. Lateral semicircular canal dysplasia in a different patient. Axial CT of the right ear demonstrates a poorly formed lateral semicircular canal.

DIFFERENTIAL DIAGNOSIS IMAGES (H-I)

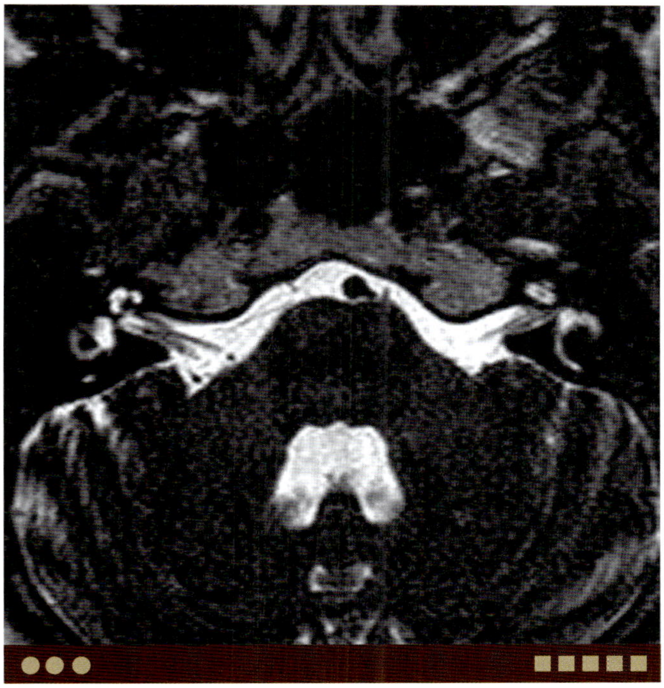

H. Labyrinthitis ossificans. Axial high-resolution T2W image demonstrates absence of normal high signal in the posterior portion of the left lateral semicircular canal.

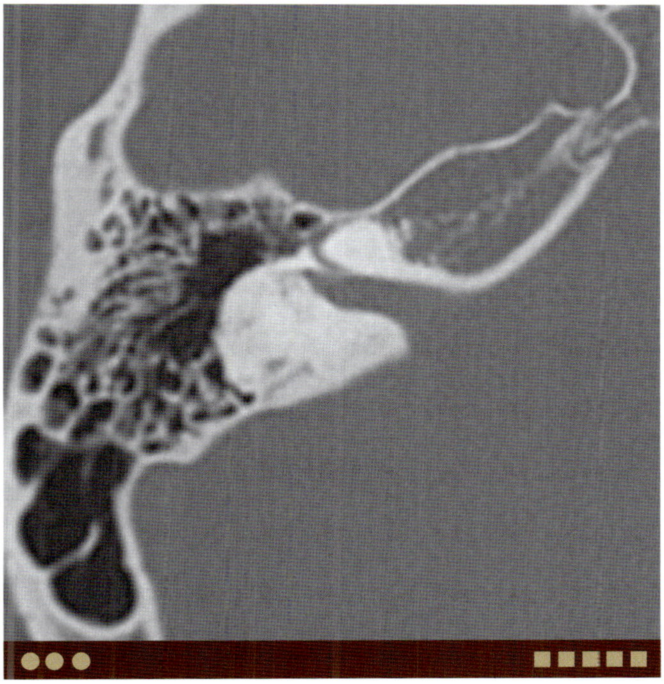

I. Labyrinthitis ossificans in a different patient. Axial CT demonstrates completely ossified lateral semicircular canal and vestibule.

Case 1–25 Temporal Bone Fracture: Longitudinal Versus Transverse

Naoko Saito, Osamu Sakai

PRESENTATION

Head trauma.

FINDINGS

CT demonstrates fractures of the temporal bone and opacified mastoid air cells and tympanic cavity.

DIFFERENTIAL DIAGNOSIS

- Pseudofractures: Normal structures such as cochlear aqueduct, subarcuate canal, and singular canal may be mistaken as a fracture.
- Congenital/developmental bone dehiscence of the tegmen tympani: Thin tegmen tympani is very common, often bilateral. However, opacification of the mastoid air cells raises the possibility of fracture with hemorrhage or CSF leak.

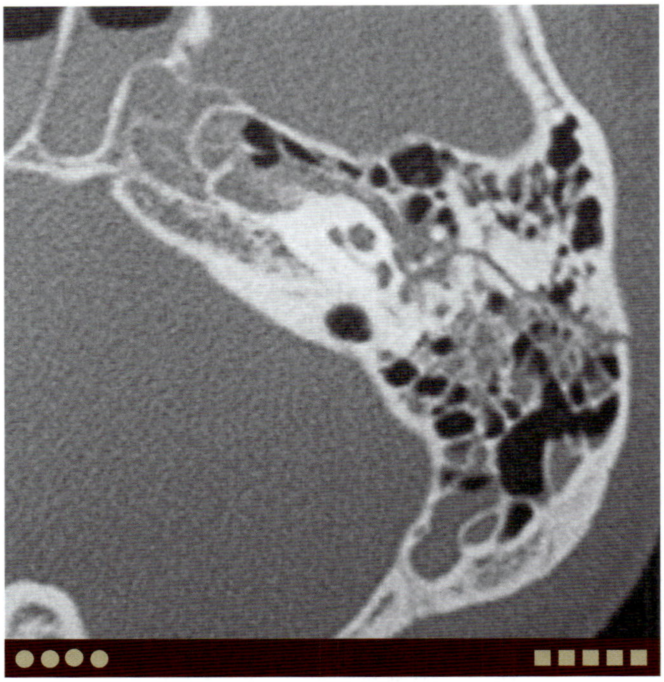

A. Longitudinal temporal bone fracture. Axial CT demonstrates a longitudinal temporal bone fracture disrupting the incudomalleolar joint and through the region of the genu of the facial nerve.

COMMENTS

This is a 55-year-old man with left-sided conductive hearing loss and facial nerve palsy after head trauma.

Temporal bone fractures are classically divided, with reference to the long axis of the petrous bone, into longitudinal (parallel to the axis) and transverse (perpendicular to the axis) fractures. However, most are oblique and often mixed, and clear classification is often difficult.

About 70% to 80% of fractures are longitudinal. Conductive hearing loss occurs in about 45% to 65% of longitudinal fractures because of the disruption of the ossicular chain, tympanic membrane perforation, and hemotympanum. Transverse fractures consist about 20% of temporal bone fractures and have higher risk for sensorineural hearing loss and facial nerve palsy. Sensorineural hearing loss occurs in about 25% to 50% of transverse fractures because of the cochlear nerve injury and disruption of the membranous labyrinth. Facial nerve injury occurs in about 35% to 50% and is most commonly seen in the labyrinthine portion. Facial nerve palsy can be seen immediately after the trauma due to direct injury or a few days later due to hemorrhage or edema.

On CT, careful evaluation of the otic capsule, entire course of the facial nerve, tegmen tympani, and ossicles is needed. Opacification of the mastoid air cells and tympanic cavity in the trauma setting is suspicious for fracture. Multiplanar reformation from thin slices should be performed to identify subtle fracture. Fluid density in the middle ear and paranasal sinuses may reflect hemorrhage or CSF leak. Fracture through the tegmen tympani without tympanic membrane perforation may not be noticed clinically since the CSF leakage drains through the eustachian tube into the nasopharynx.

Ossicular chain disruption may occur from either direct or indirect injury. Disruption between the incus and stapes is most common because when there is a significant acceleration force, displacement of the incus is likely to occur.

PEARLS

- **Temporal bone fractures are classically divided into longitudinal and transverse fractures.**
- **In longitudinal fractures, conductive hearing loss is often seen due to disruption of the ossicular chain.**
- **Transverse fractures have higher risk for sensorineural hearing loss and facial nerve injury.**

ADDITIONAL IMAGES (B-F)

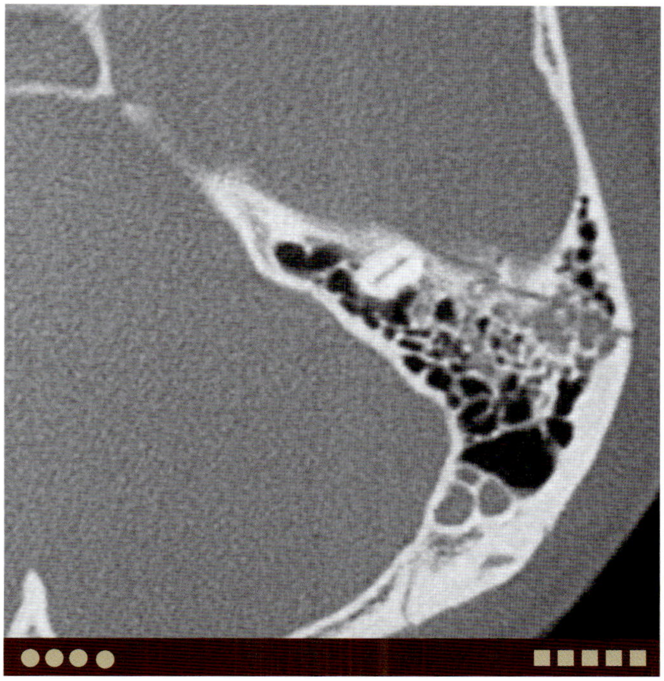

B. Longitudinal temporal bone fracture, same patient as A. Axial CT through higher level demonstrates a fracture involving the tegmen resulting in CSF leak and partial opacification of the mastoid air cells.

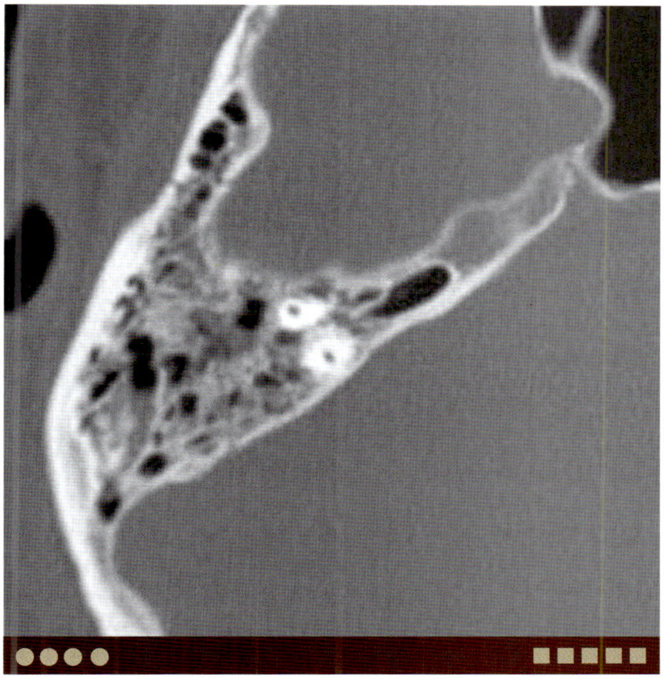

C. Transverse temporal bone fracture. Axial CT demonstrates a transverse temporal bone fracture crossing the mastoid portion.

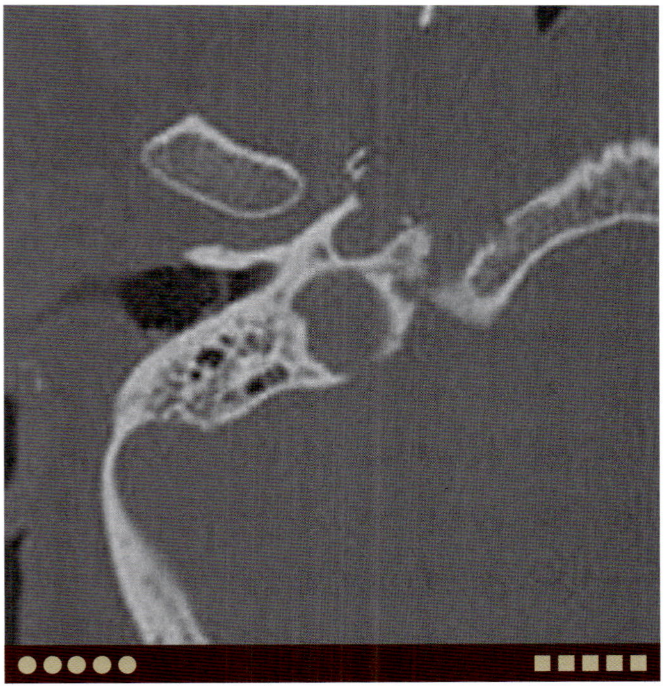

D. Temporal bone fracture in a different patient. Axial CT demonstrates very subtle lucency through the cortex of the mastoid with partial opacification of the air cells.

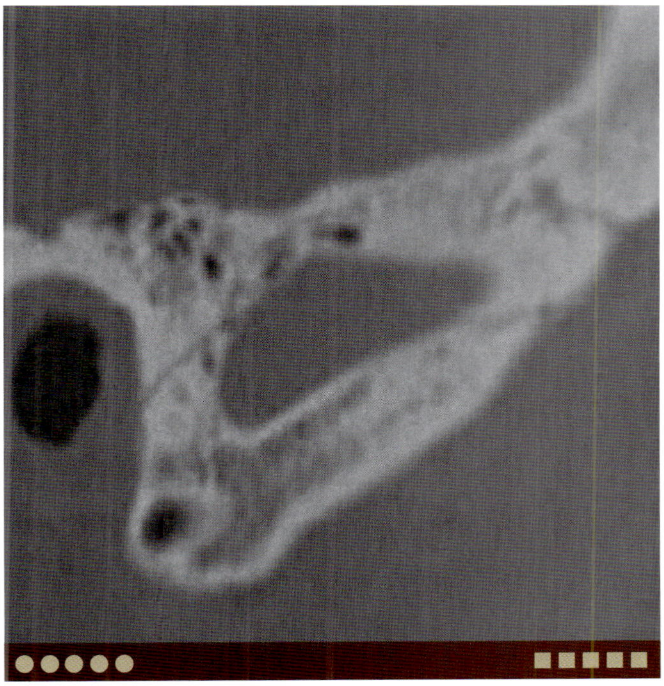

E. Temporal bone fracture, same patient as D. Sagittal reformatted CT image better demonstrates a fracture traversing the mastoid extending to the external auditory canal.

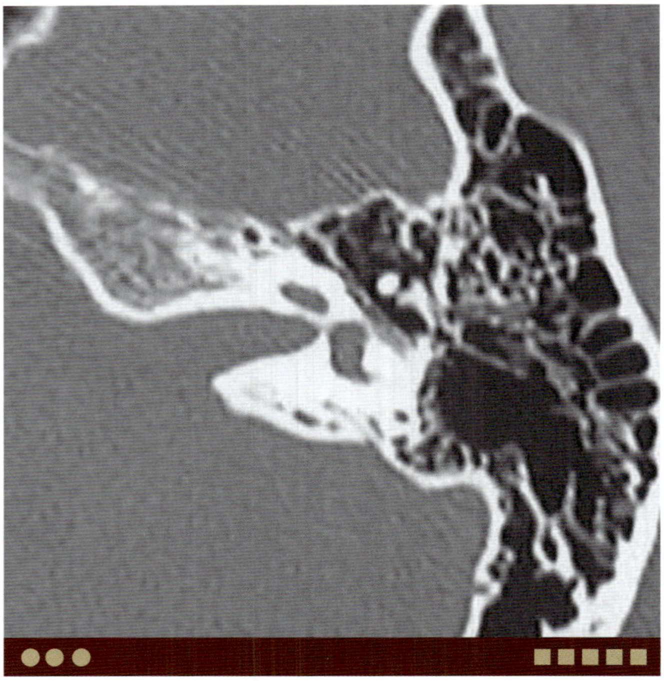

F. Incudomalleolar dislocation. Axial CT demonstrates separation of the malleus and incus.

DIFFERENTIAL DIAGNOSIS IMAGES (G-H)

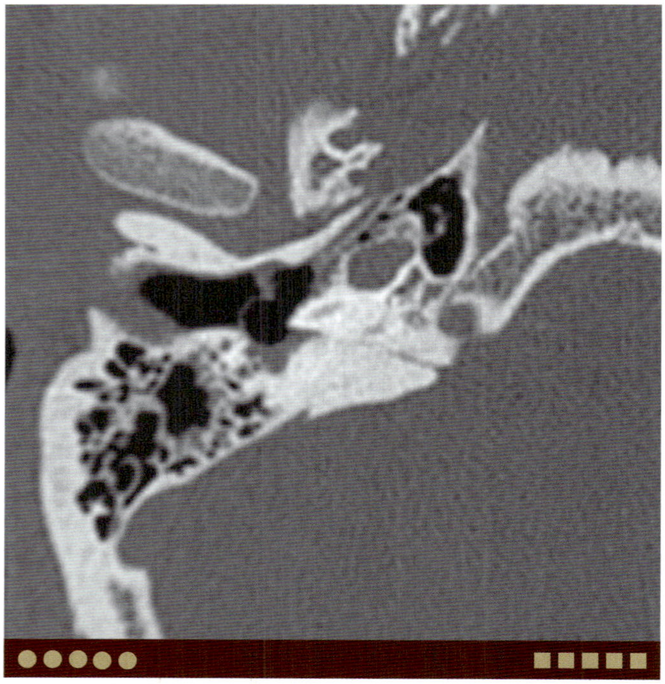

G. "Pseudofracture," cochlear aqueduct. Axial CT demonstrates a linear lucency inferoposterior to the cochlea. This is a normal structure.

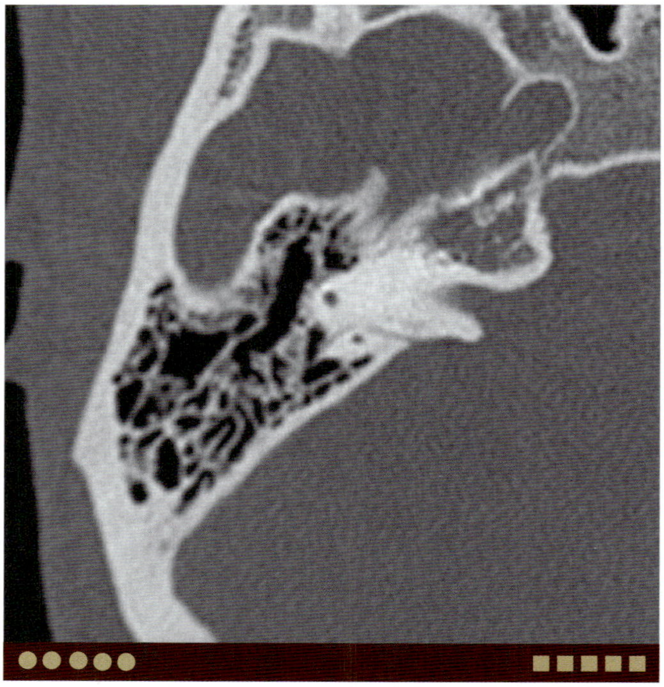

H. "Pseudofracture," subarcuate canal. Axial CT demonstrates a linear lucency through the superior semicircular canal. This is a normal structure and can be prominent in children.

Case 1–26 Temporal Bone Fracture: Recent Classifications

Naoko Saito, Osamu Sakai

PRESENTATION

Head trauma.

FINDINGS

CT demonstrates fractures of the temporal bone and opacified mastoid air cells and tympanic cavity.

DIFFERENTIAL DIAGNOSIS

- Pseudofractures: Normal structures such as singular canal and occipitomastoid suture may be mistaken as a fracture.

COMMENTS

This is a 36-year-old man after head trauma.

Additional classification systems of temporal bone fractures have been suggested, which demonstrate predictive ability for serious clinical outcomes associated with temporal bone fractures. One system categorizes fractures according to whether or not they involve the otic capsule. Another classifies them based on whether or not they extend into the petrous region of the temporal bone. The traditional classification of temporal bone fracture is based on fracture orientation in relation to the petrous ridge; longitudinal, transverse, and mixed fractures. This classification system is very well known, however, it has less correlation with clinical complications.

Otic capsule violating fractures, which have been described by Kelly and Tami in 1994, course through either the cochlea or the labyrinth. Otic capsule violating fractures consist of about 2.5% to 20% of temporal bone fractures. Dahiya et al. (1999) found that otic capsule violating fractures were two times more likely to have facial nerve injury, four times more likely to have cerebrospinal fluid (CSF) leak, and seven times more likely to have sensorineural hearing loss (SNHL) compared to otic capsule sparing fractures.

Petrous fractures, which have been described by Ishman and Friedland in 2004, are defined as the fractures extending to the petrous apex or the otic capsule, or both. Nonpetrous fractures are simply defined as fractures not involving them. Petrous fractures have better predictive ability for omplications than traditional classification system.

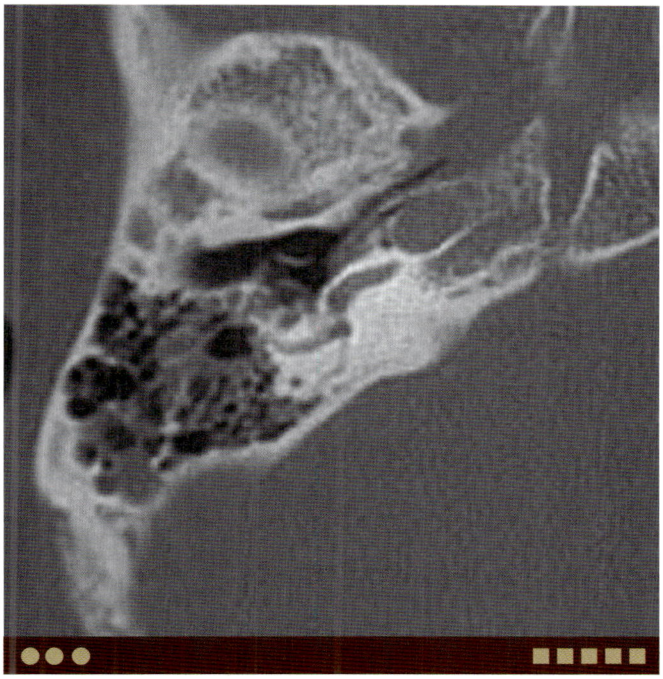

A. Otic capsule violating fracture. Axial CT demonstrates a fracture crossing the vestibular aqueduct, posterior semicircular canal, and vestibule.

Ishman et al. (2004) found that petrous fractures were 9.8 times more likely to have CSF leak, and also facial nerve injury and SNHL more strongly correlated with petrous fractures than nonpetrous fractures.

PEARLS

- **The main recent temporal bone fracture classifications are otic capsule violating/sparing fractures and petrous/nonpetrous fractures.**
- **These recent classification systems demonstrate predictive ability for serious clinical outcomes associated with temporal bone fractures.**
- **Otic capsule violating fractures have significantly higher risk for SNHL.**
- **Petrous fractures have higher risk for CSF leak.**

ADDITIONAL IMAGES (B-F)

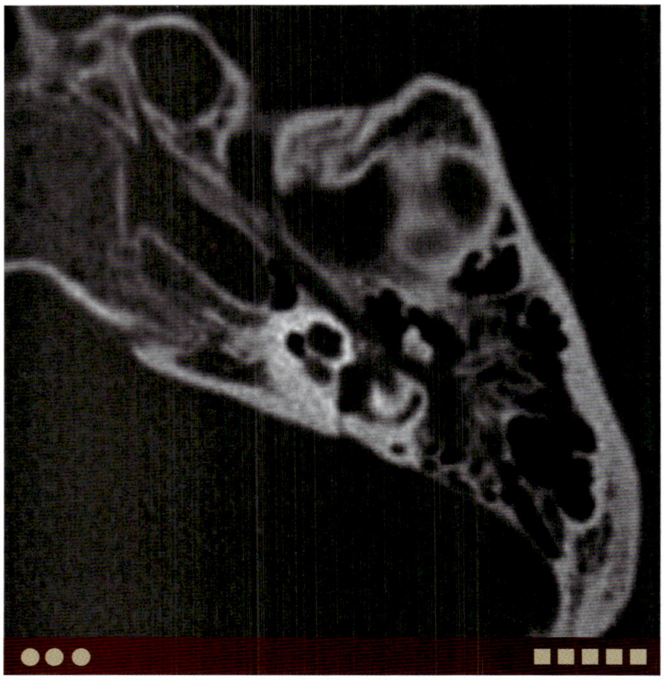

B. Otic capsule violating fracture in a different patient. Axial CT demonstrates a fracture crossing the vestibule. There is air in the vestibule and the basal turn of cochlea.

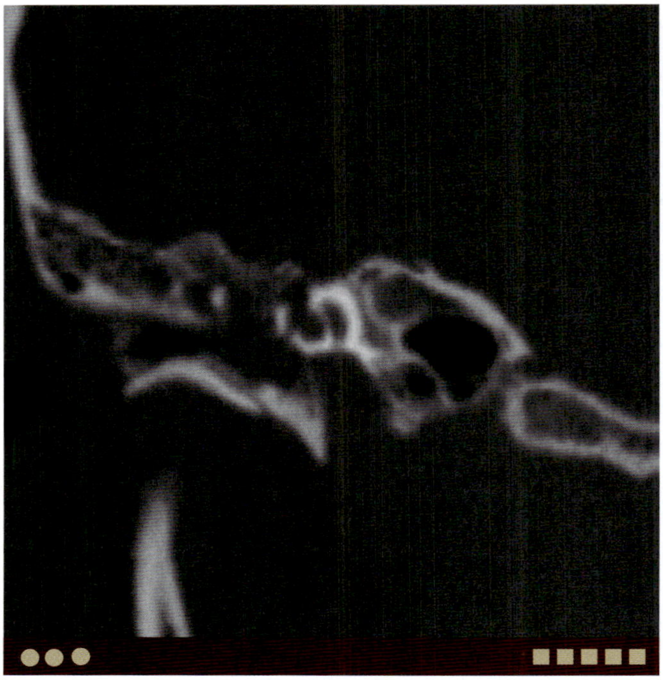

C. Otic capsule violating fracture in a different patient. Coronal CT demonstrates a fracture crossing the apical turn of the cochlea.

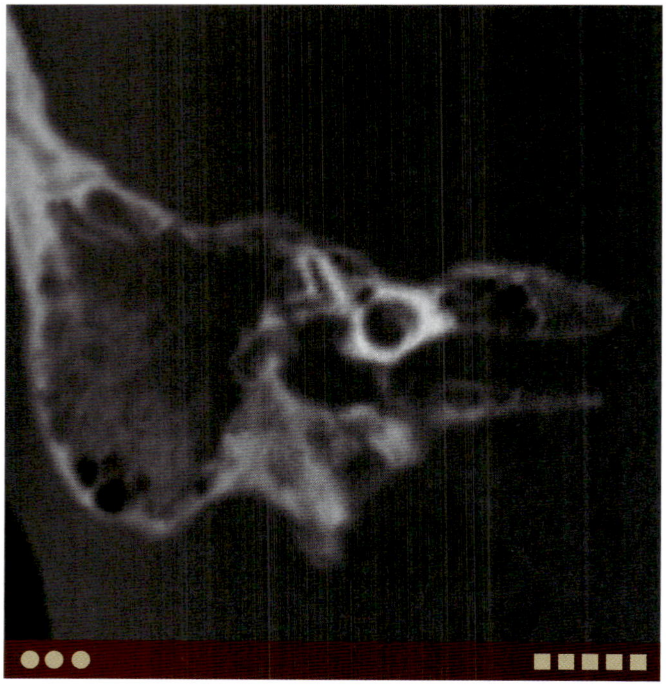

D. Otic capsule violating fracture, same patient as C. Oblique coronal CT demonstrates a fracture crossing the lateral semicircular canal.

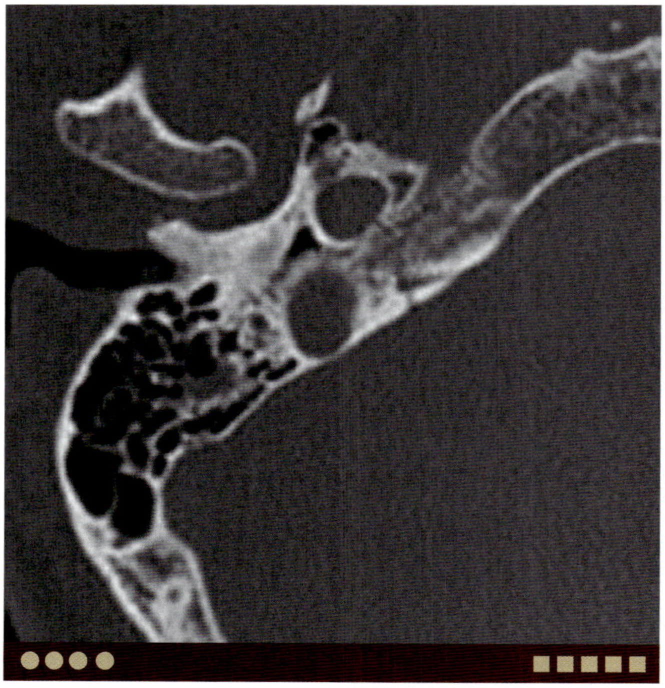

E. Petrous fracture in a different patient. Axial CT demonstrates a fracture involving the petrous apex. The fracture line crosses the carotid canal and the cochlear aqueduct.

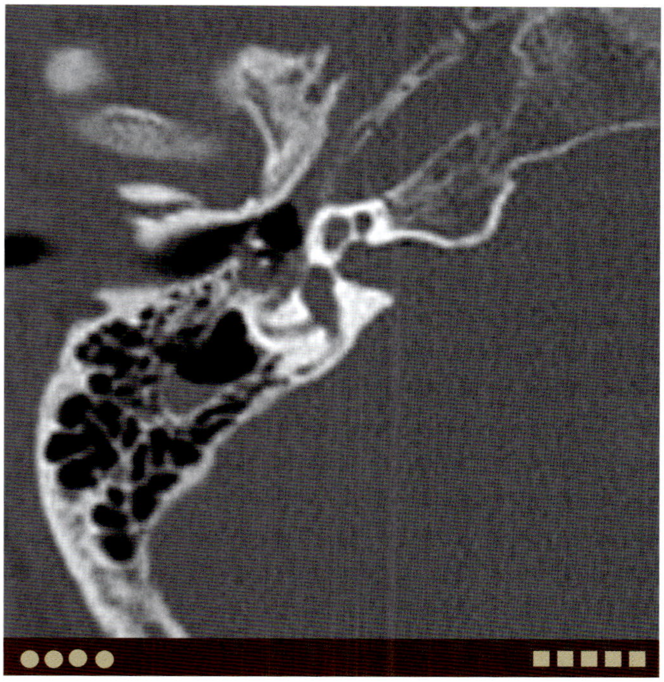

F. Petrous fracture, same patient as B. Axial CT through higher level demonstrates a fracture extending to the internal auditory canal.

DIFFERENTIAL DIAGNOSIS IMAGES (G-I)

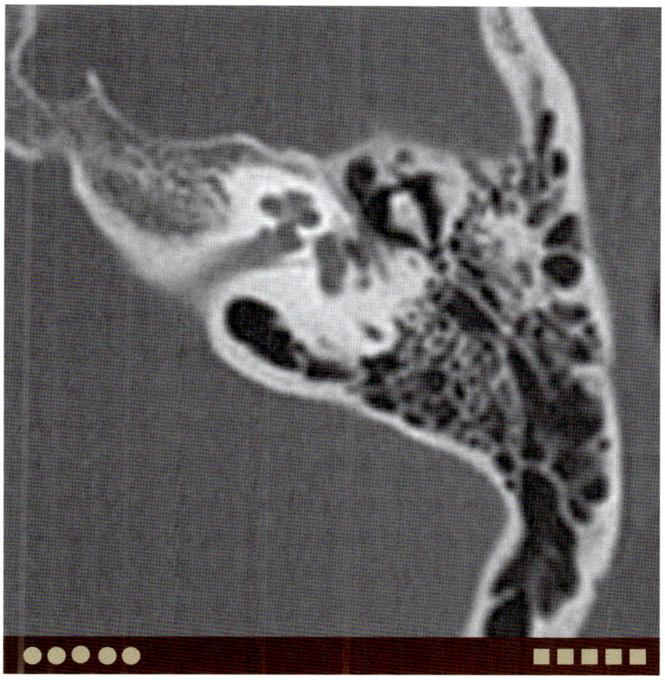

G. "Pseudofracture," singular canal. Axial CT demonstrates a linear lucency inferoposterior to the internal auditory canal reaching the labyrinth. This contains the singular nerve, a branch of the inferior vestibular nerve.

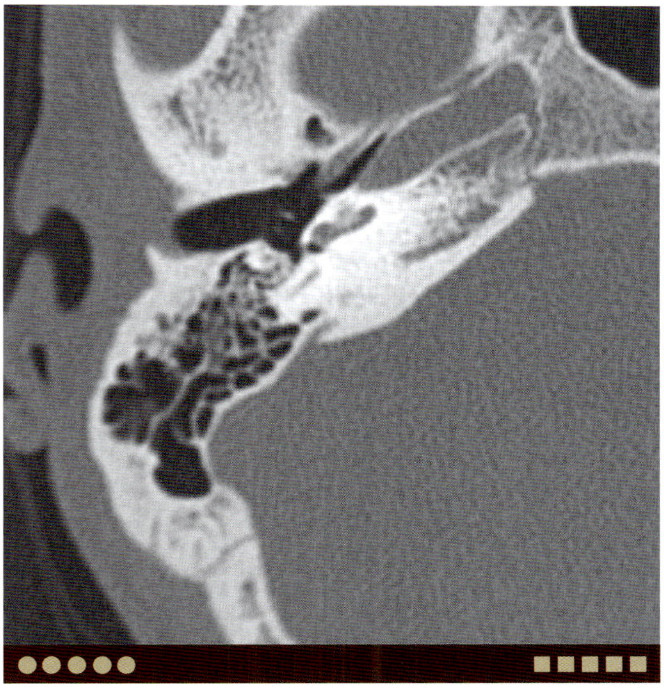

H. "Pseudofracture," petrooccipital fissure. Axial CT demonstrates a linear lucency between petrous apex and clivus. This is a normal structure.

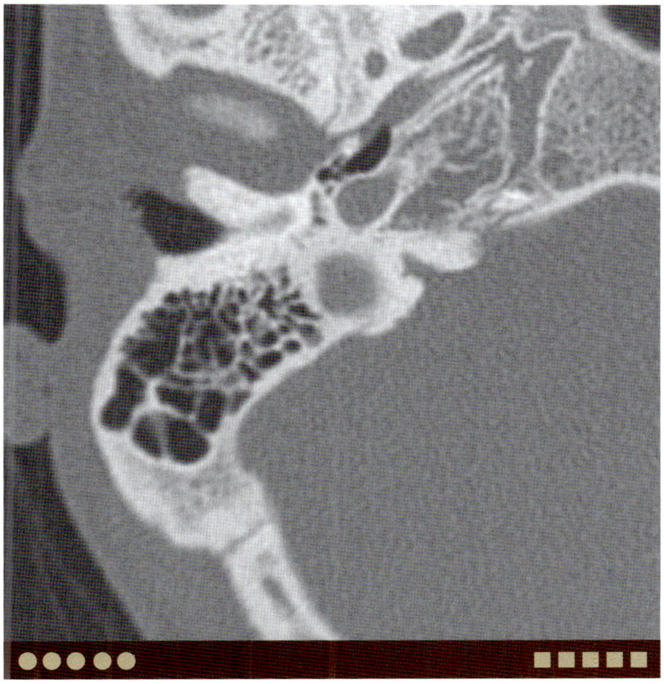

I. "Pseudofracture," occipitomastoid suture. Axial CT demonstrates a linear lucency between mastoid portion and occipital bone. This is a normal suture. Its appearance varies from smooth and well-corticated to irregular, coarse, and relatively wide.

Case 1–27 Temporal Bone Fracture: Vascular Involvement

Naoko Saito, Osamu Sakai

PRESENTATION

Head trauma.

FINDINGS

CT demonstrates fractures of the temporal bone crossing the vascular structures (carotid canal, jugular foramen, etc.). CT angiogram or venogram demonstrates vascular injury.

DIFFERENTIAL DIAGNOSIS

- Atherosclerosis: Stenosis and occlusion of the internal carotid artery (ICA) due to atherosclerosis is common. Calcified plaque is often seen at the site of stenosis or occlusion.
- Venous sinus thrombosis due to otomastoiditis: Venous sinus thrombosis can occur by direct extension of infection through defects in the inner mastoid cortex or via emissary veins. Epidural abscess and meningeal enhancement may also be observed.

COMMENTS

This is a 19-year-old man status post motor vehicle crash and head trauma.

Vascular injury may be present in patients with temporal bone fractures. About 10% to 50% of temporal bone fractures involve the carotid canal, however, they are not always associated with actual arterial injury. The most frequently fractured segment is the lacerum-cavernous junction, and the highest incidence of carotid artery injury occurs at the petrous segment of the carotid canal. Arterial vascular complications include pseudoaneurysm, spasm, dissection, occlusion, intimal injury, and carotid cavernous fistula. CT angiogram should be performed if there is a fracture crossing the carotid canal or there is air in the carotid canal. Further, even without direct evidence of carotid canal involvement, fractures through the petrous temporal bone and sphenoid bone near the carotid canal raise the possibility of vascular injury and further workup for vascular injury is appropriate.

Fractures through the sigmoid groove and jugular foramen are also observed. They are frequently associated with transverse fractures. Venous vascular complications include stenosis, thrombosis, external compression from an epidural hematoma, and venous extradural hematoma.

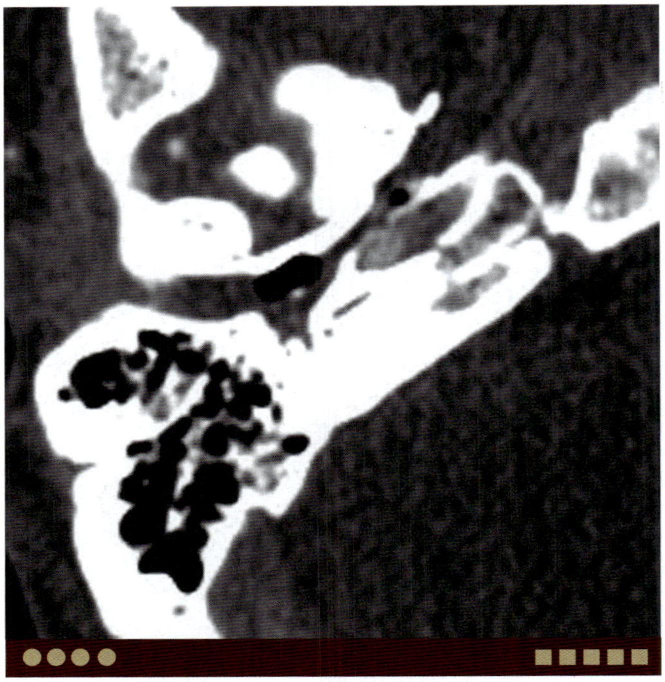

A. Segmental dissection of the ICA. CT angiogram demonstrates segmental stenosis of the ICA adjacent to the fracture, suggesting dissection of the ICA with intramural hematoma.

Clinical presentations of venous sinus occlusion are related to increased intracranial pressure: headache, nausea, altered mental status, and neurological deficit. CT venogram should be performed, if the fracture involves jugular foramen or sigmoid or transverse sinuses.

PEARLS

- **Vascular injury may be present in the patient with temporal bone fractures.**
- **CT angiogram should be performed if there is a fracture through or near the carotid canal in the petrous or sphenoid bones, or there is air in the carotid canal.**
- **CT venogram should be performed, if the fracture involves jugular foramen, or sigmoid or transverse sinuses.**

ADDITIONAL IMAGES (B-F)

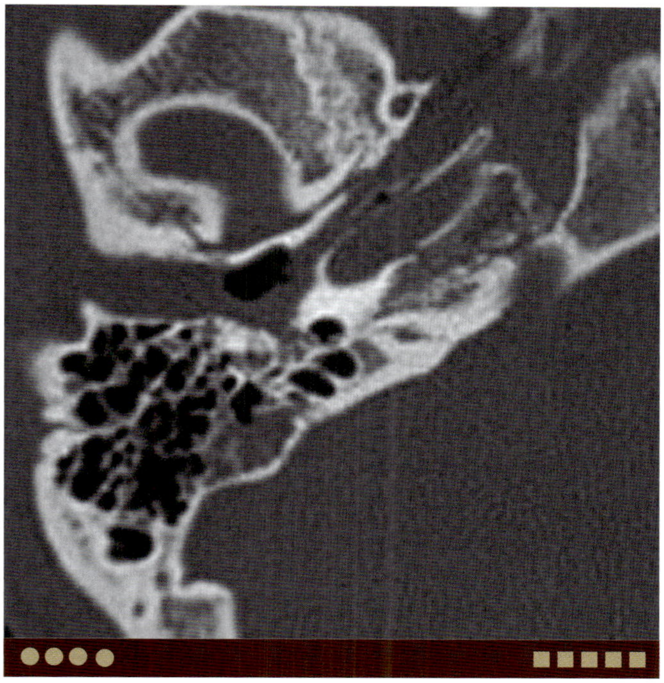

B. Segmental dissection of the ICA, same patient as A. Axial temporal bone CT demonstrates a transverse fracture crossing through the right carotid canal. Note hemotympanum.

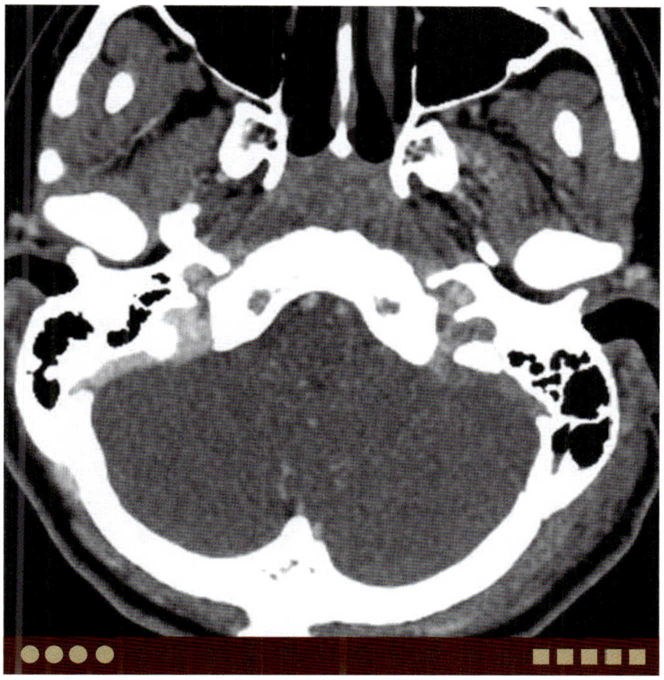

C. Venous thrombosis. CT venogram demonstrates a filling defect in the left jugular bulb and sigmoid sinus to suggest segmental thrombosis (4 days after head trauma).

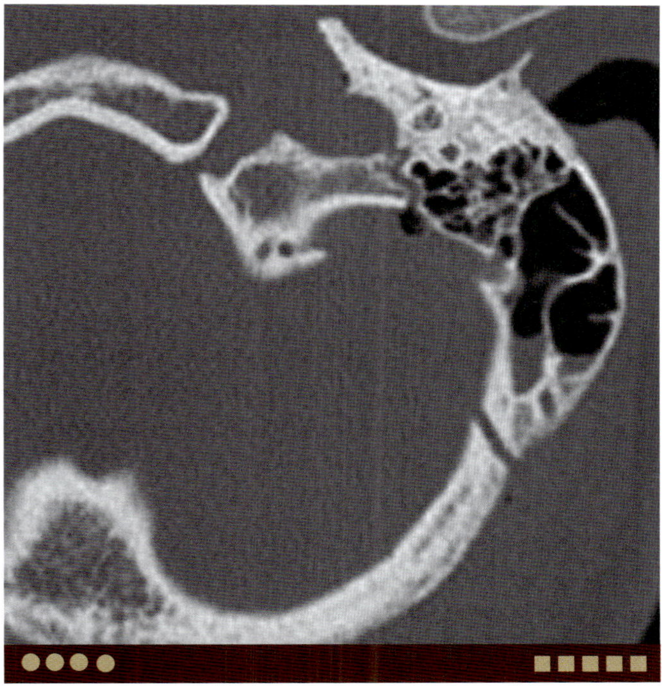

D. Venous thrombosis, same patient as C. Axial temporal bone CT demonstrates a transverse fracture with diastasis of the occipitomastoid suture. The fracture line passes through the sigmoid sinus and extends to the jugular foramen.

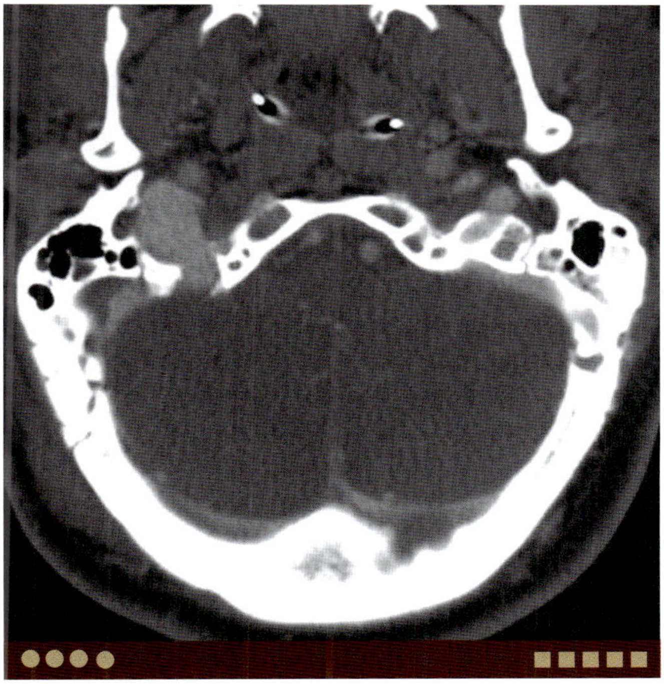

E. Sigmoid sinus narrowing due to hematoma. CT venogram demonstrates an extra-axial hematoma adjacent to the fractures, which displaces and narrows the right sigmoid sinus.

DIFFERENTIAL DIAGNOSIS IMAGES (G-H)

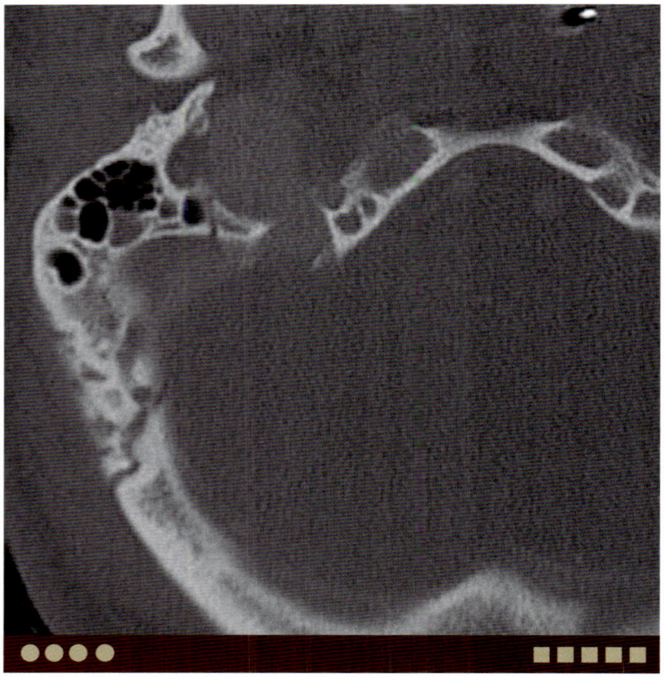

F. Sigmoid sinus narrowing due to hematoma, same patient as E. Axial temporal bone CT demonstrates a transverse fracture traversing the sigmoid sinus extending to the jugular foramen.

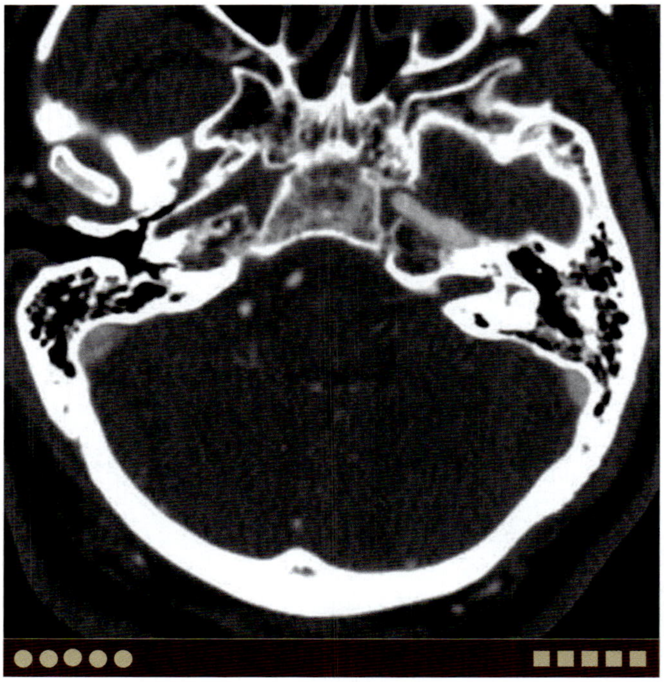

G. ICA occlusion due to atherosclerosis. CT angiogram demonstrates absence of contrast filling in the right ICA. CT angiogram of the neck revealed occlusion at the origin of ICA with a dense calcification (not shown).

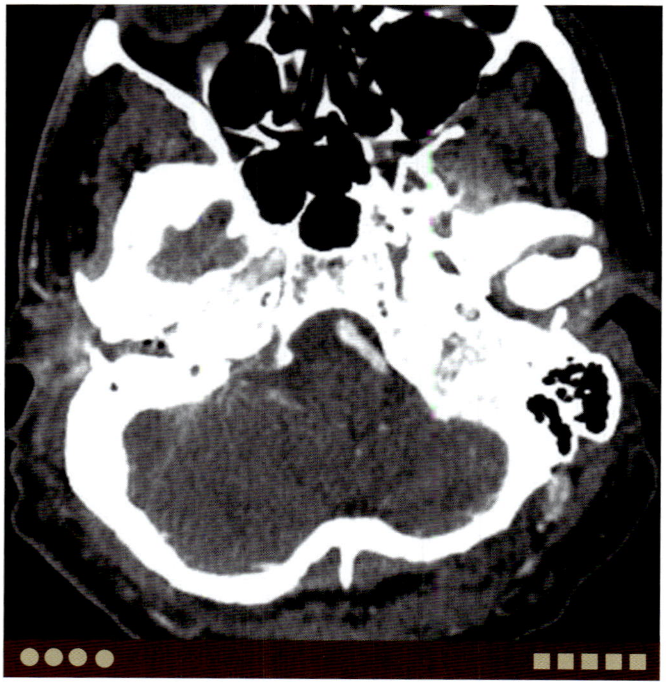

H. Venous sinus thrombosis due to otomastoiditis. CT venogram demonstrates a filling defect in the right sigmoid sinus and prominent dural enhancement. Note expansion of the thrombosed sinus.

Case 1–28 External Auditory Canal Squamous Cell Carcinoma

Akifumi Fujita, Osamu Sakai

PRESENTATION

Otorrhea and hearing loss.

FINDINGS

CT shows an external auditory canal (EAC) mass with bony destruction. MRI shows a heterogeneously enhancing EAC mass extending to adjacent soft tissues.

DIFFERENTIAL DIAGNOSIS

- Necrotizing external otitis (NEO): EAC mass with bony destruction and adjacent soft tissue involvement may mimic EAC SCCA, and it is difficult to differentiate it by imaging alone.
- EAC cholesteatoma: Cholesteatoma forms a soft tissue mass in the EAC and bone erosion, however, aggressive bone destruction or adjacent soft tissue involvement are not seen.
- Keratosis obturans: This condition does not cause bone erosion.

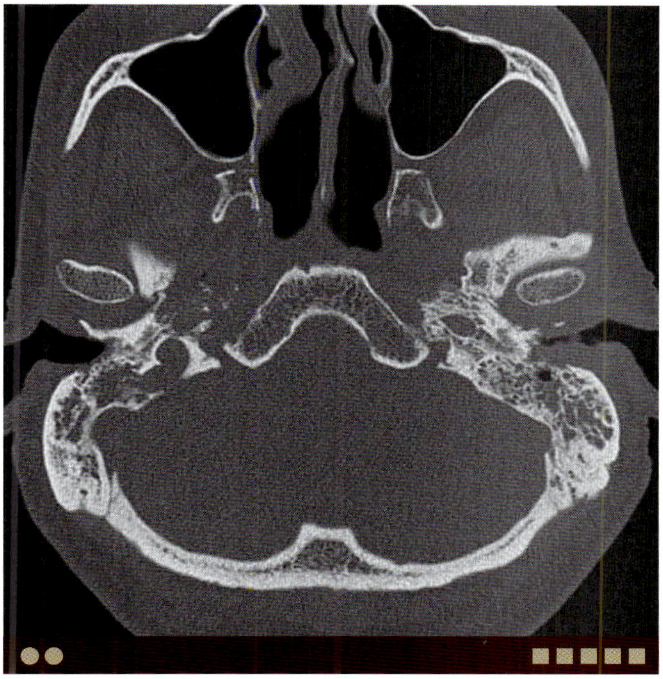

A. EAC SCCA. Axial CT demonstrates soft tissue swelling of the left EAC with bone destruction of the posterior wall.

COMMENTS

This is a 49-year-old man with persistent left otorrhea. He was initially diagnosed as chronic external otitis, however, the biopsy revealed SCCA.

Squamous cell carcinoma (SCCA) of the EAC often occurs in elderly woman centered within the wall of the EAC. Diagnosis is usually delayed because malignant tumor of the EAC is relatively rare, and the symptoms are similar to other benign otologic conditions such as chronic otitis media. Otorrhea, otalgia, and conductive hearing loss are common primary symptoms. Early stage disease with complete resection with free margins and radiotherapy has good prognosis. However, extensive disease, positive margins, dural involvement, facial nerve paralysis, lower cranial nerve involvement, and moderate-to-severe pain at presentation have been associated with poorer outcomes.

CT and MRI show nonspecific EAC soft tissue masses with heterogeneous enhancement. CT with bone algorithm is the best modality to depict the bone destructive changes that may lead to diagnosis of SCCA. MRI has advantage to demonstrate the extent of tumor to the surrounding soft tissues, skull base, and temporomandibular joint. Periauricular and peri/intraparotid nodes should be evaluated for nodal metastasis. Further, secondary involvement of the EAC from regional primary SCCA is much more common than primary EAC SCCA, therefore evaluation of the adjacent structures is crucial.

PEARLS

- **Diagnosis is usually delayed because malignant tumor of the EAC is relatively rare, and the symptoms are similar to other benign otologic conditions.**
- **Identifying bone destruction is a clue to make the diagnosis of EAC SCCA, however, presence of bony destruction means late stage disease which is associated with poor outcome.**
- **Dural invasion and cranial nerve involvement suggest poor outcome.**

ADDITIONAL IMAGES (B-G)

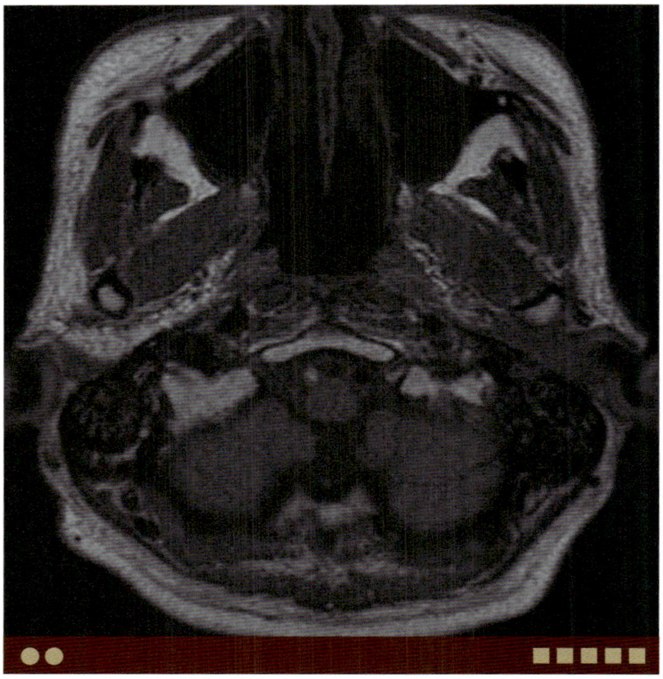

B. EAC SCCA, same patient as A. Axial T1W image demonstrates a low-signal tumor in the left EAC extending to the temporomandibular joint anteriorly and invading the mastoid posteriorly.

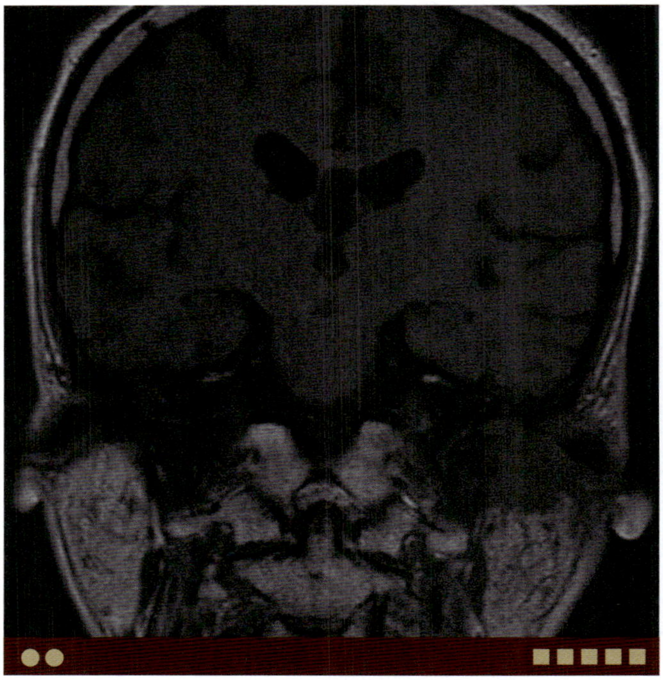

C. EAC SCCA, same patient as A. Coronal T1W image demonstrates invasion of the parotid gland.

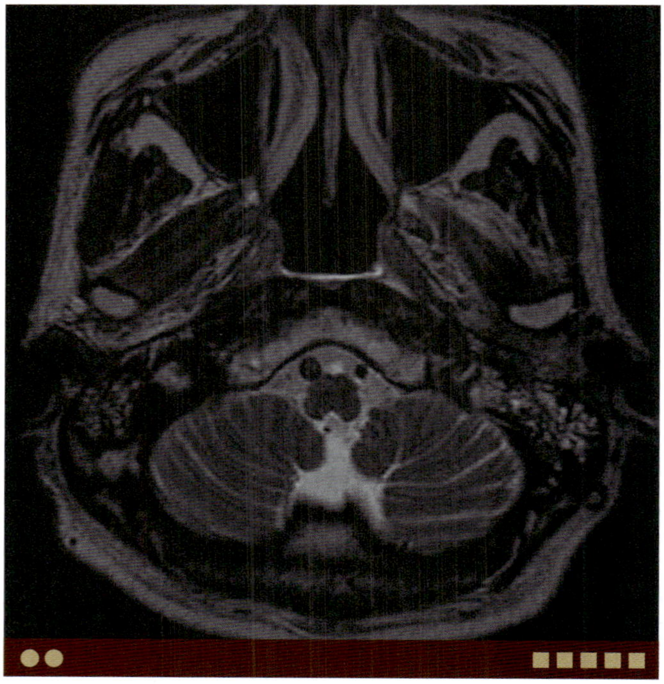

D. EAC SCCA, same patient as A. Axial T2W image demonstrates a heterogeneous signal tumor in the left EAC extending to the temporomandibular joint anteriorly and invading the mastoid posteriorly. Opacification is noted in the left mastoid air cells.

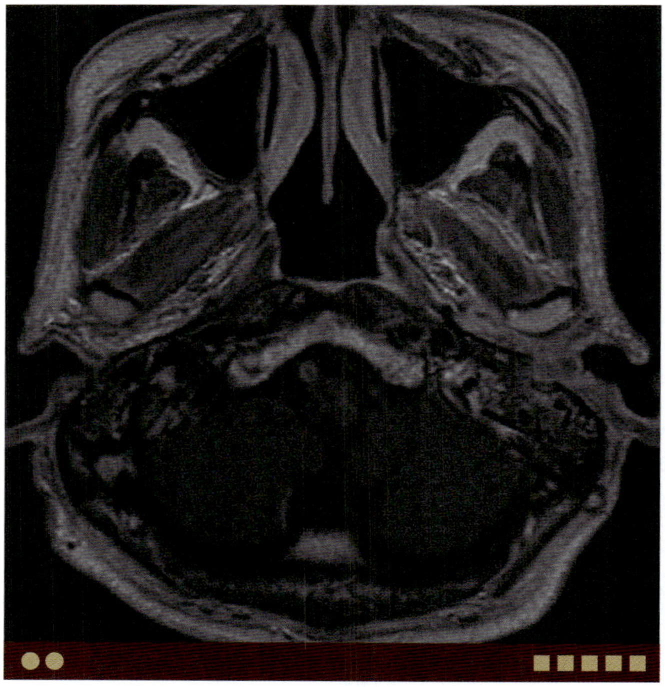

E. EAC SCCA, same patient as A. Axial postcontrast T1W image demonstrates heterogeneous enhancement of the tumor.

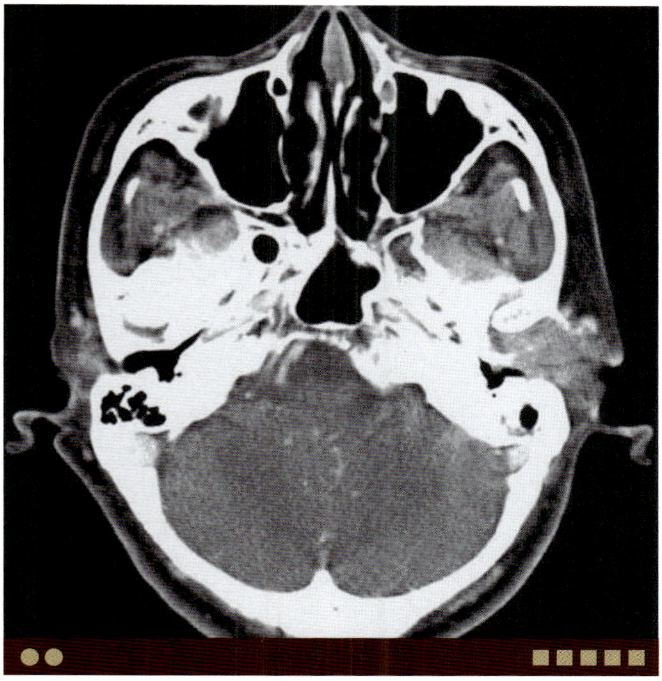

F. EAC SCCA in a different patient. Axial postcontrast CT demonstrates heterogeneously enhancing soft tissue tumor in the left EAC extending to the temporomandibular joint anteriorly.

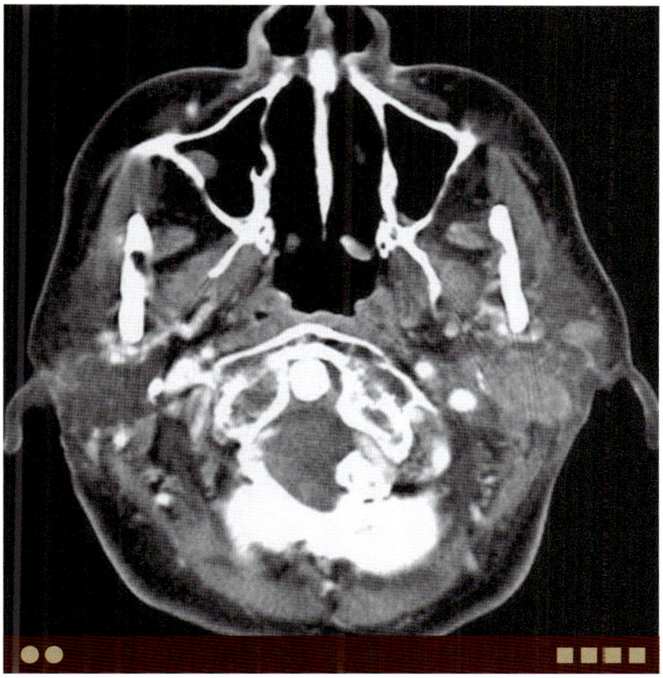

G. EAC SCCA, same patient as F. Axial postcontrast CT image demonstrates heterogeneously enhancing tumor invading the parotid gland. Intra-parotid nodal metastasis is also noted.

DIFFERENTIAL DIAGNOSIS IMAGES (H-I)

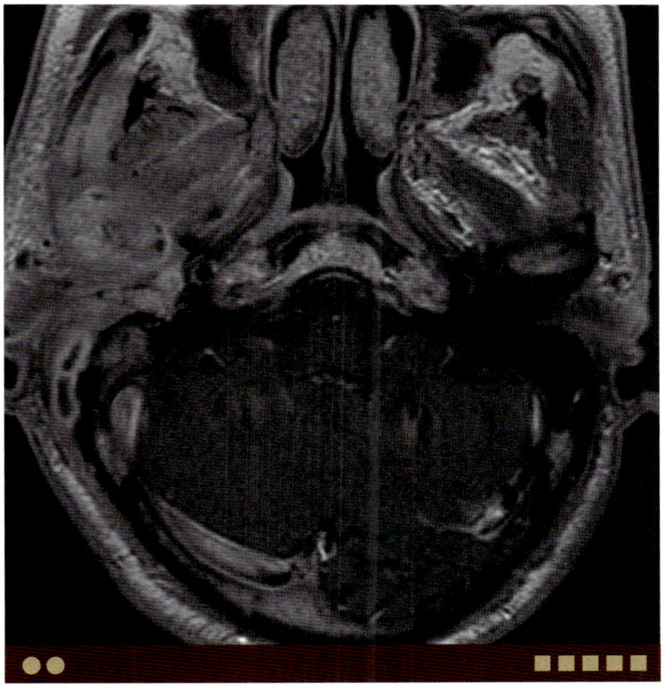

H. NEO. Axial postcontrast T1W image demonstrates diffuse swelling and heterogeneous enhancement of the right EAC, extending to the masticator space anteriorly. Subperiosteal abscess is noted posteriorly.

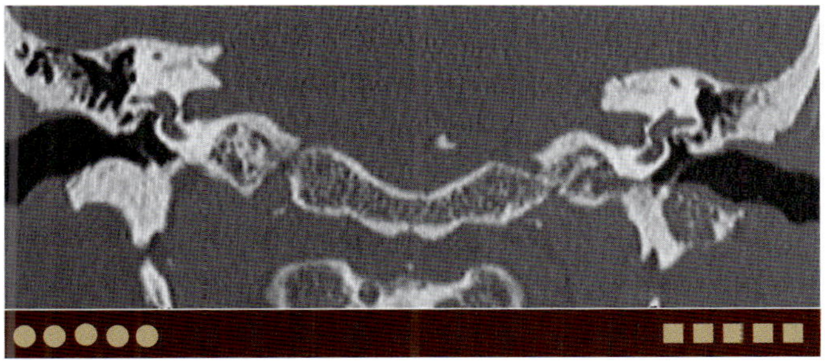

I. EAC cholesteatoma. Coronal CT shows a soft tissue mass eroding the inferior wall of the left EAC.

Case 1–29 Necrotizing External Otitis

Akifumi Fujita, Osamu Sakai

PRESENTATION

Otalgia and otorrhea.

FINDINGS

CT and MRI show diffuse soft tissue swelling and enhancement of the external auditory canal (EAC).

DIFFERENTIAL DIAGNOSIS

- EAC squamous cell carcinoma (SCCA): This usually demonstrates bone destruction in addition to mass formation. However, it is often difficult to differentiate it from NEO by imaging alone.
- EAC cholesteatoma: This condition typically forms a mass without adjacent soft tissue infection. Bone erosion/remodeling may be seen, however, aggressive bone destruction should not be present.
- Keratosis obturans: This condition may mimic cholesteatoma, however, bone erosion is not seen.
- Melanocytic nevus: This forms a flat or papillomatous lesion without bony erosion.

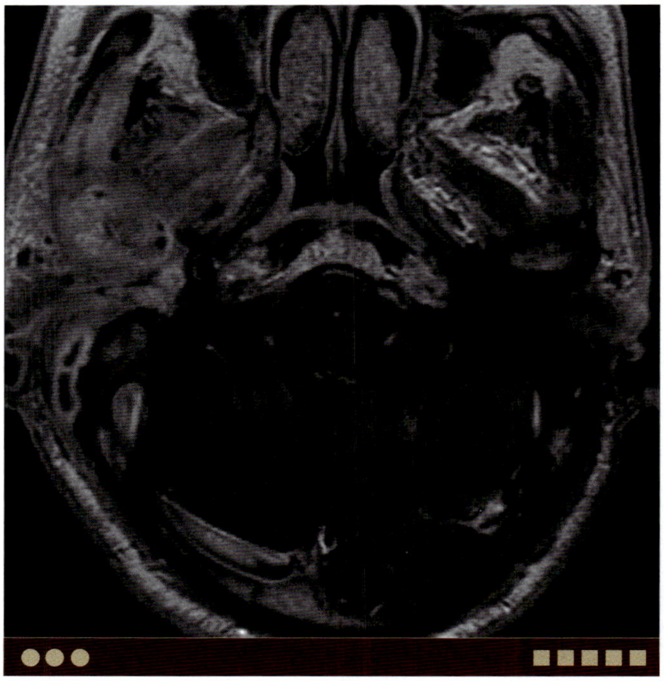

A. NEO. Axial postcontrast T1W image demonstrates diffuse swelling and enhancement of the right EAC, extending into the masticator space anteriorly. Posteriorly, periosteal abscess is also noted.

COMMENTS

This is a 67-year-old man with persistent right otalgia and otorrhea for 6 months. He is diabetic and *Psuedomonas aeruginosa* was cultured from the ear discharge.

Necrotizing external otitis (NEO) is a severe infection in the EAC. NEO mainly occurs in diabetic or immunocompromised patients, and most often the causative agent is *P. aeruginosa*. NEO begins in the EAC and involves the adjacent soft tissue structures. NEO typically extends via fissure of Santorini, and involves the retrocondylar fat, parapharyngeal fat, temporomandibular joint, and masticator muscles. Less common routes of spread include posteriorly into the mastoid process, and medially into the middle ear toward the petrous apex. Most common presenting symptom is persistent otalgia, but otorrhea, facial nerve palsy, and multiple lower cranial neuropathies may occur with disease progression.

CT can demonstrate swelling of the EAC soft tissue often with bony erosion and adjacent deep space cellulitis or abscesses. MRI is more helpful to show the extent of the infection, and has advantage of demonstrating bone marrow involvement and intracranial extension. The fat in and below the stylomastoid foramen should be carefully observed. Abnormal soft tissue density/signal and enhancement is often seen, particularly in patients with facial nerve palsy.

NEO can show similar imaging appearance to EAC SCCA, therefore, repeated biopsy may be necessary to exclude neoplastic process, particularly when the disease persists.

PEARLS

- **CT is preferred at the initial diagnosis to detect early cortical erosion of the EAC.**
- **MRI can demonstrate the adjacent soft tissue involvement better, and has advantage in early detection of osteomyelitis and intracranial extension compared with CT.**
- **Involvement of the facial nerve is often seen in and below the stylomastoid foramen. The fat pad should be carefully observed.**
- **NEO is often difficult to differentiate from EAC SCCA by imaging alone, therefore, repeated biopsy is often required.**

ADDITIONAL IMAGES (B-G)

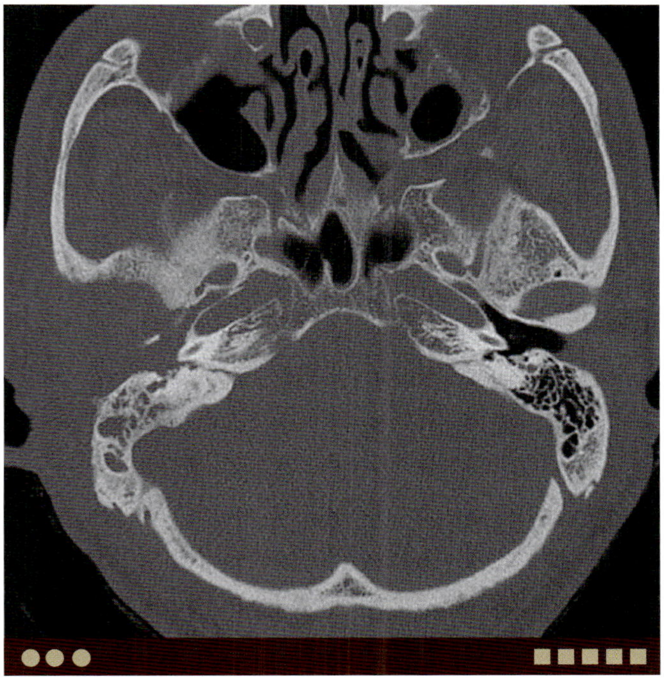

B. NEO, same patient as A. Axial bone algorithm CT demonstrates destruction of the anterior wall of the EAC and erosion is also noted in the posterior wall.

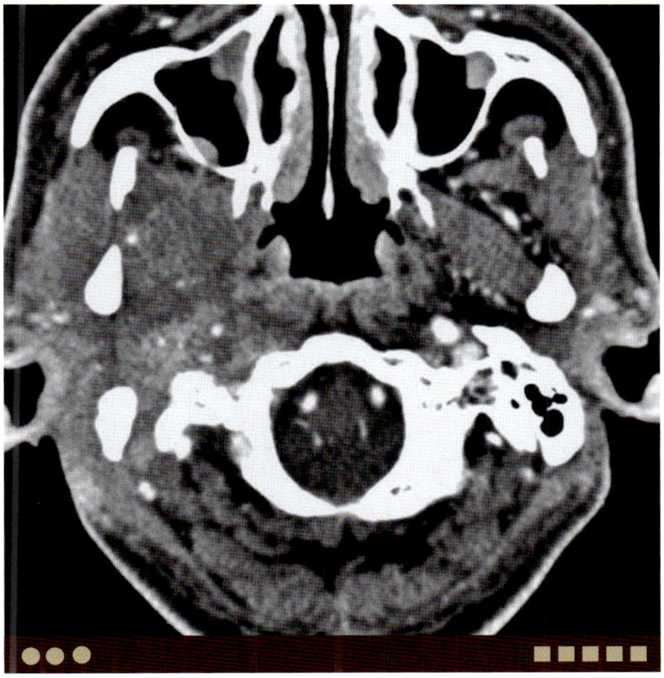

C. NEO, same patient as A. Axial soft tissue algorithm CT through the stylomastoid foramen demonstrates abnormal soft tissue density and enhancement, obliterating the stylomastoid fat pad.

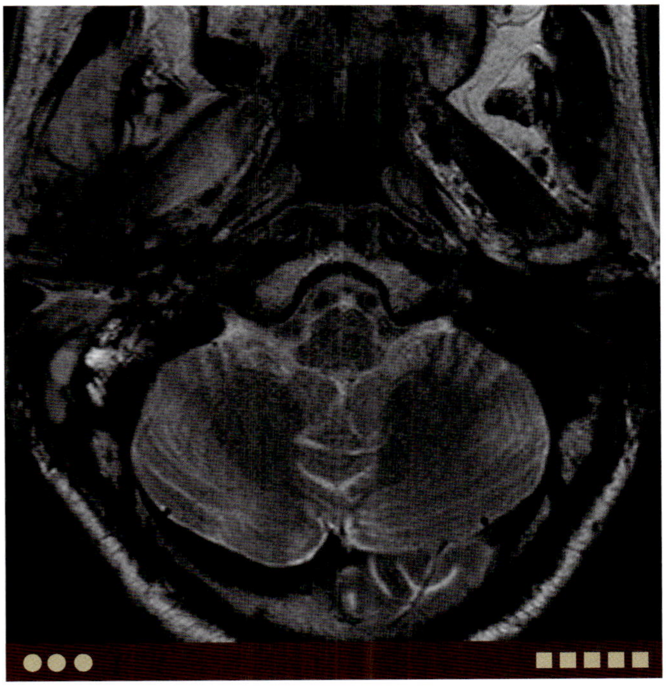

D. NEO, same patient as A. Axial T2W image demonstrates a heterogeneous signal lesion in the EAC and adjacent soft tissues, extending to the masticator space.

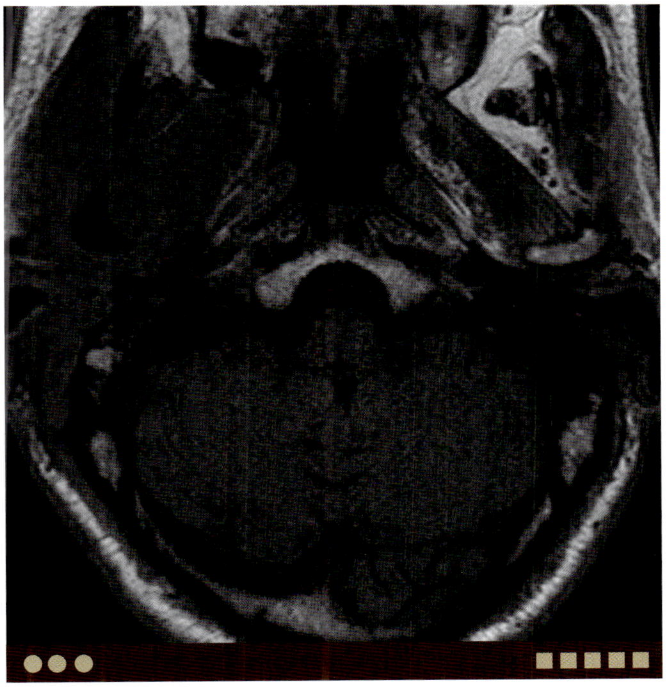

E. NEO, same patient as A. Axial T1W image demonstrates a low-signal lesion in the EAC and adjacent soft tissues, extending to the masticator space. Abnormal bone marrow signal is also noted in the right mandible.

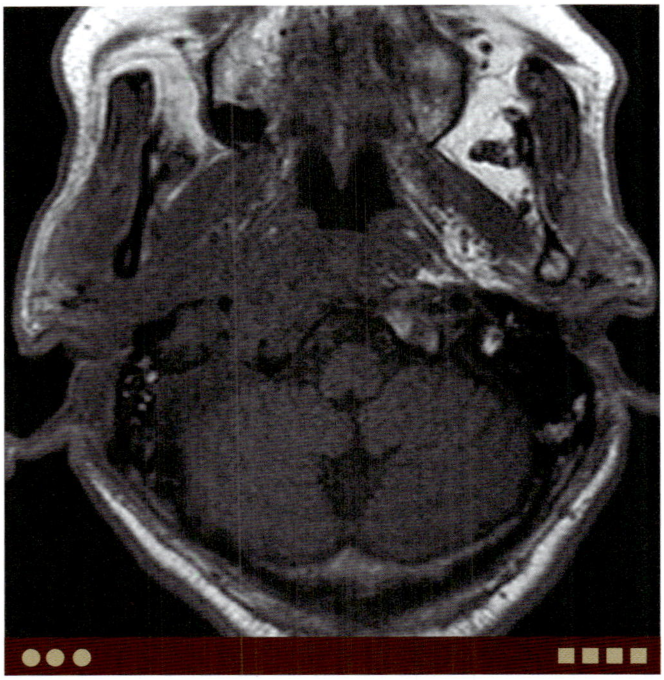

F. NEO, follow up MRI of the same patient as A. Axial T1W image shows interval improvement of the right EAC and masticator space soft tissue swelling, however, abnormal low signal persists in the petrous apex and jugular foramen.

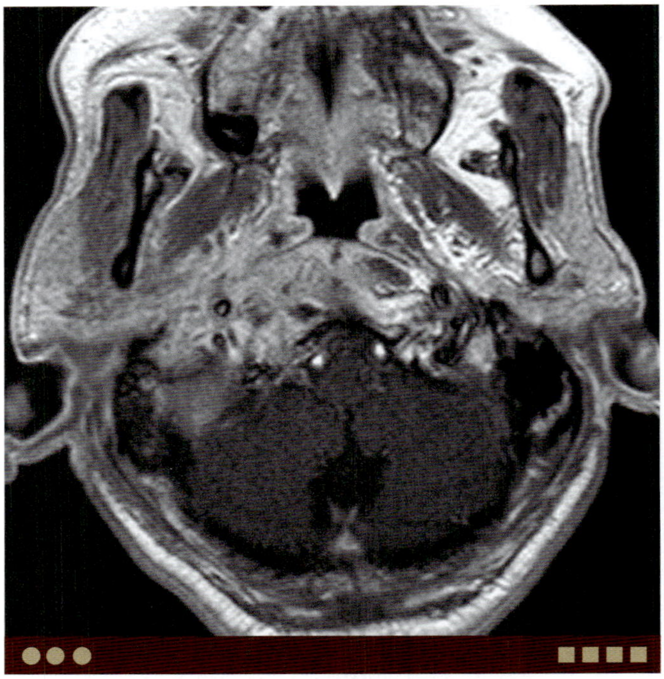

G. NEO, follow up MRI of the same patient as A. Axial postcontrast T1W image shows enhancement of the petrous apex and jugular foramen which suggests persistent active inflammation.

DIFFERENTIAL DIAGNOSIS IMAGES (H-I)

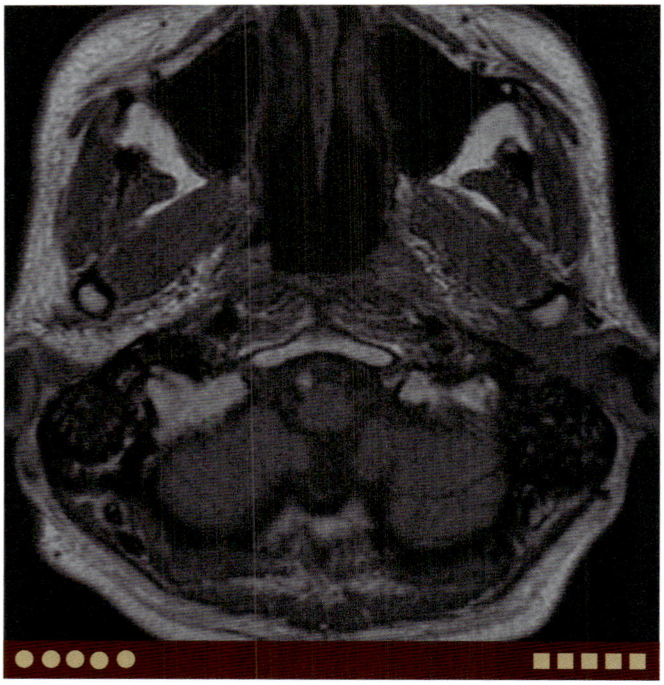

H. EAC SCCA. Axial T1W image demonstrates a large low-signal lesion involving the left EAC and extending anteriorly into the temporomandibular joint. It is difficult to differentiate from NEO by imaging alone.

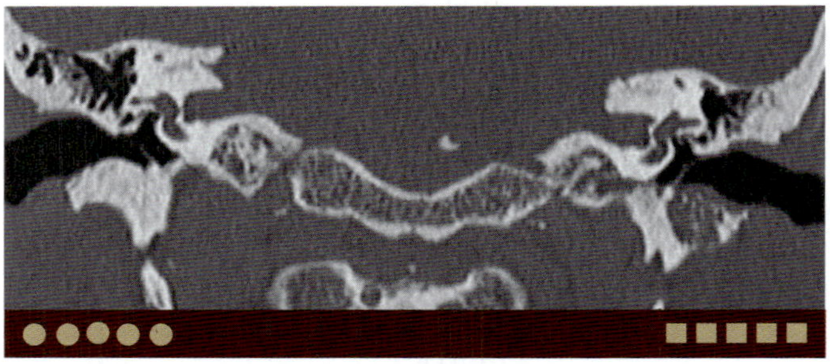

I. EAC cholesteatoma. Coronal bone algorithm CT shows a soft tissue mass with bone erosion in the inferior wall of the left EAC.

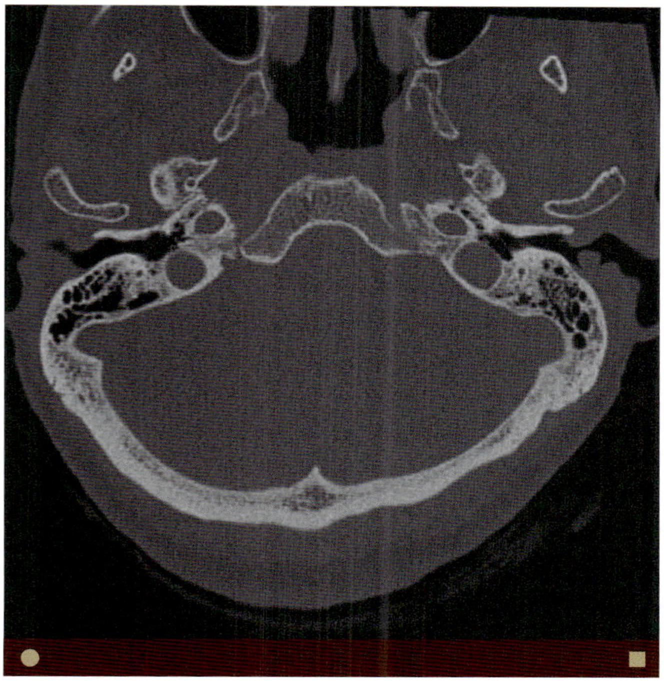

J. Melanocytic nevus. Axial bone algorithm CT shows a soft tissue mass protruding into the left EAC. Bone erosion is not noted.

Case 1–30 EAC Exostosis

Rania Hito, Osamu Sakai

PRESENTATION

Conductive hearing loss.

FINDINGS

CT shows osseous proliferation within the external auditory canal (EAC).

DIFFERENTIAL DIAGNOSIS

- Osteoma: This is a benign slow growing pedunculated bony lesion that often arises lateral to the isthmus of the EAC along the tympanosquamous suture.
- Osteochondroma: This is a benign cartilage-capped osseous growth arising from bone surface, which represents developmental abnormality rather than neoplastic process.
- EAC cholesteatoma: This condition typically forms a soft tissue density mass without adjacent soft tissue infection. Bone erosion/remodeling may be seen, not bone proliferation.
- Keratosis obturans: This condition may mimic cholesteatoma, however, bone erosion is not seen.

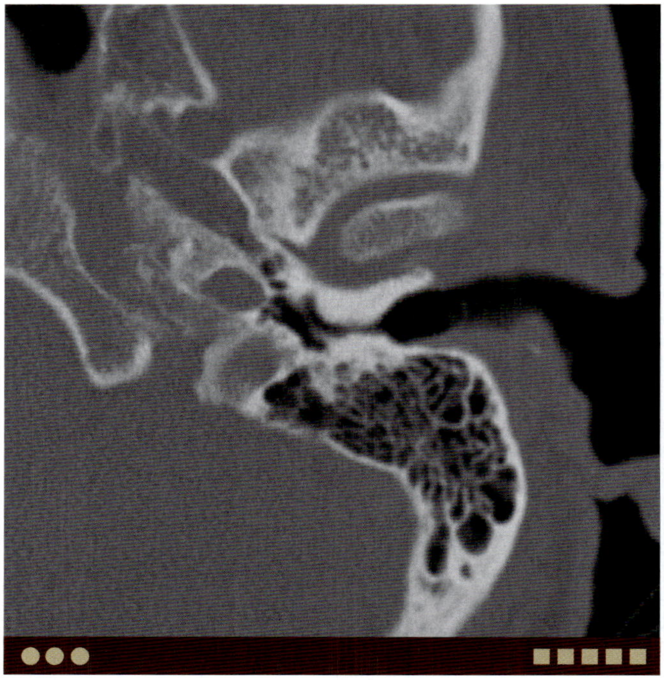

A. EAC exostosis. Axial CT demonstrates broad-based osseous proliferation narrowing the EAC.

COMMENTS

This is a 66-year-old man with conductive hearing loss.

Exostoses are benign osseous proliferations, usually broad-based, dense, composed of bone covered by periosteum and overlying squamous epithelium. They commonly arise medial to the tympanomastoid and tympanosquamous suture lines. Although presentation is usually marked by unilateral symptoms, often conductive hearing loss, these lesions are often bilateral. Repeated cold-water exposure and chronic otitis externa have been proposed as inciting agents for the formation of EAC exostoses, although etiologies are not clear. Several studies have found a high prevalence of exostoses in cold-water sports enthusiasts, leading to the name "surfer's ear."

Complications stem from obstructive lesions and include chronic otitis externa as well as postobstructive cholesteatoma. Treatment is surgical removal, reserved for cases where the lesions are obstructive and thus symptomatic.

Differential considerations for EAC exostosis include osteoma. Osteoma is a bony tumor that is often single, unilateral, pedunculated, and arises from the tympanosquamous or tympanomastoid suture. Although osteomas are often found in the fronto-ethmoid regions, they can occur in the maxillary and sphenoid sinuses as well as the mandible and temporal bone. Within the temporal bone, the EAC predominates as a location for osteomas. Differentiation between EAC exostoses and osteomas may not be crucial as treatment is essentially the same. Age of onset, presenting symptoms and complications are also similar. Histologically speaking, it has been argued that osteomas and exostoses are not different entities.

The role of CT in EAC exostoses is delineating the dimensions and complications, such as cholesteatoma developing medial to exostoses.

PEARLS

- **EAC exostoses are benign osseous proliferations, usually broad-based.**
- **Presenting symptoms are often unilateral, most commonly conductive hearing loss.**
- **Several studies have found a high prevalence of EAC exostoses in cold-water sports enthusiasts, leading to the name "surfer's ear."**

ADDITIONAL IMAGES (B-C)

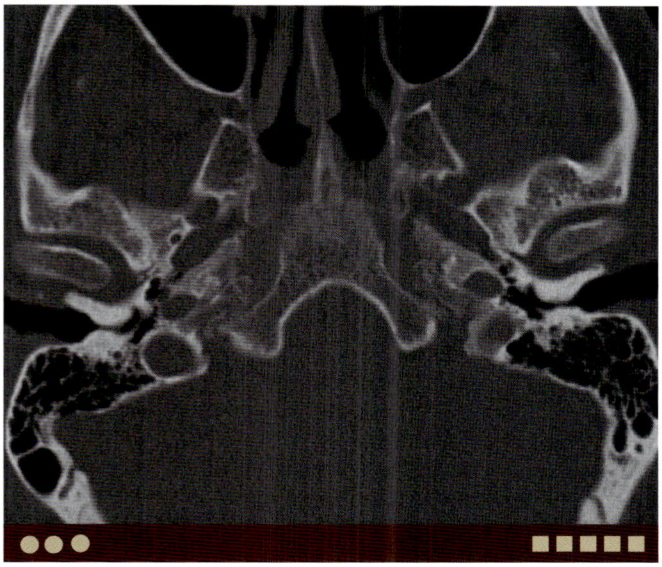

B. EAC exostosis, same patient as A. Axial CT demonstrates broad-based osseous proliferation narrowing the EAC bilaterally.

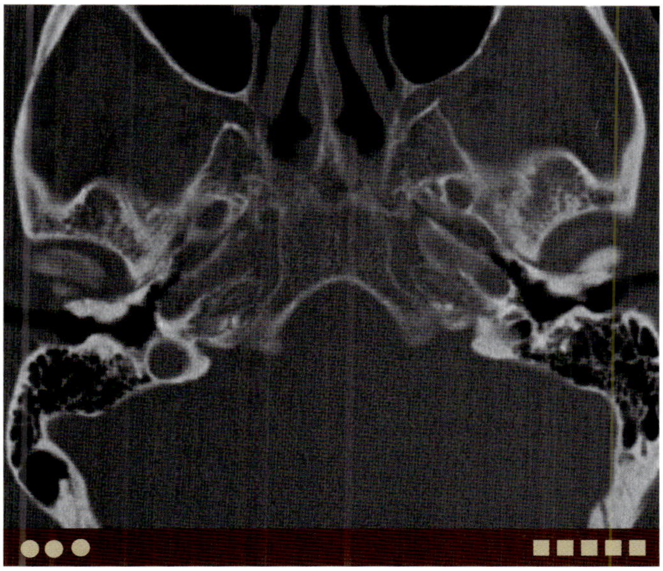

C. EAC exostosis, same patient as A. Axial CT demonstrates broad-based, slightly nodular, osseous proliferation narrowing the EAC bilaterally.

DIFFERENTIAL DIAGNOSIS IMAGES (D-F)

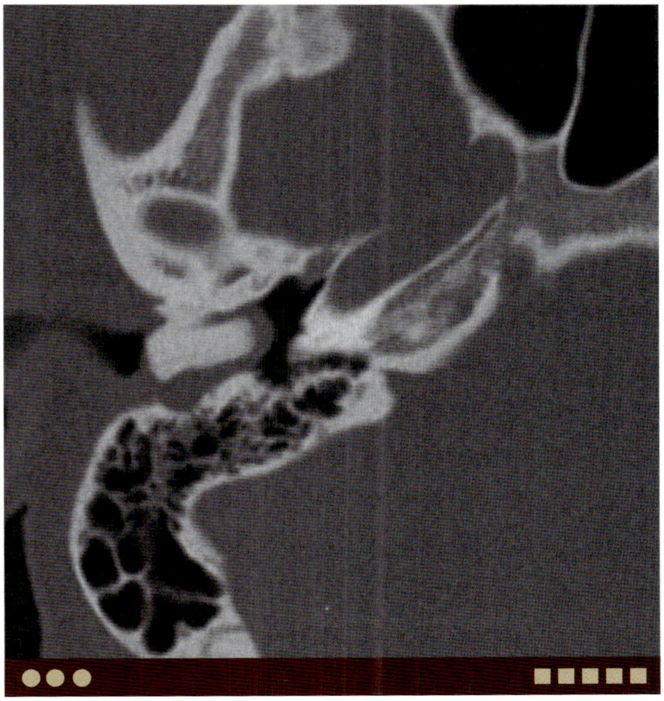

D. EAC osteoma. Axial CT demonstrates a pedunculated bony lesion with soft tissue density in the right EAC.

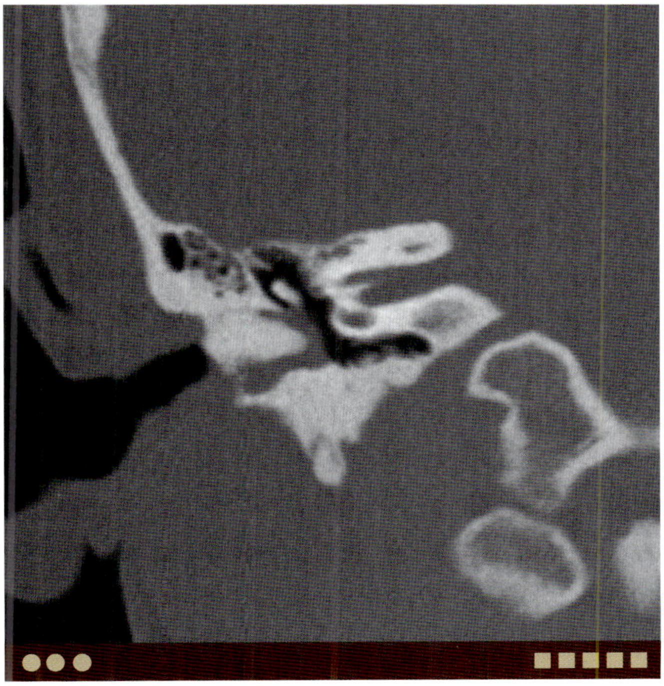

E. EAC osteoma same patient as D. Coronal CT demonstrates a pedunculated bony lesion in the right EAC with soft tissue density inferior and medial to the lesion.

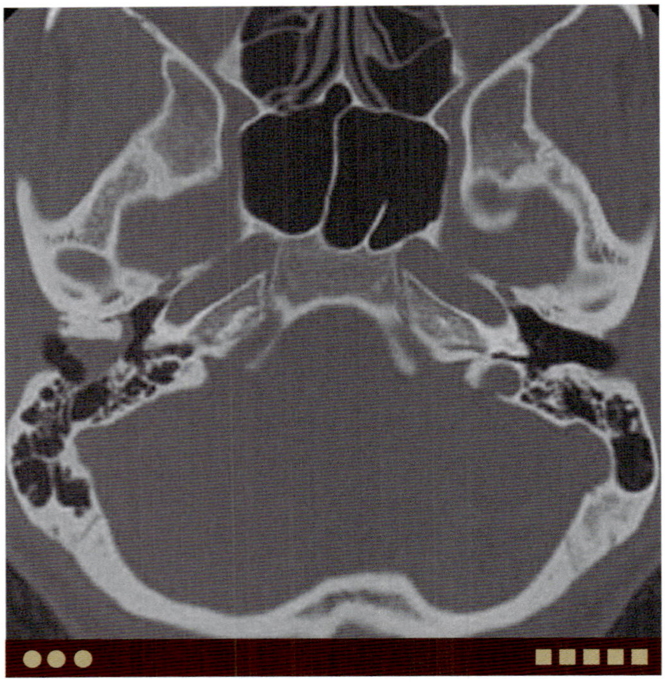

F. EAC osteoma, same patient as D. Axial CT demonstrates a pedunculated bony lesion in the right EAC with a large soft tissue density mass, which was revealed to be a cholesteatoma after surgery. Note intact left EAC.

Case 1–31 Persistent Stapedial Artery

Naoko Saito, Osamu Sakai

PRESENTATION

Pulsatile tinnitus.

FINDINGS

CT demonstrates a small vessel arising from the middle ear segment of the (aberrant) internal carotid artery runs through the crura of the stapes.

DIFFERENTIAL DIAGNOSIS

- Glomus tympanicum: This is a paraganglioma in the tympanic cavity. CT shows a focal soft tissue density mass over the cochlear promontory. Avid enhancement is seen on CT and MRI.
- Aberrant internal carotid artery: This anomaly causes pulsatile tinnitus, and may coexist with a persistent stapedial artery.
- Facial nerve schwannoma: CT and MRI demonstrate focal enlargement and enhancement of the facial nerve. Enlarged facial nerve canal with smooth margins is observed on CT.

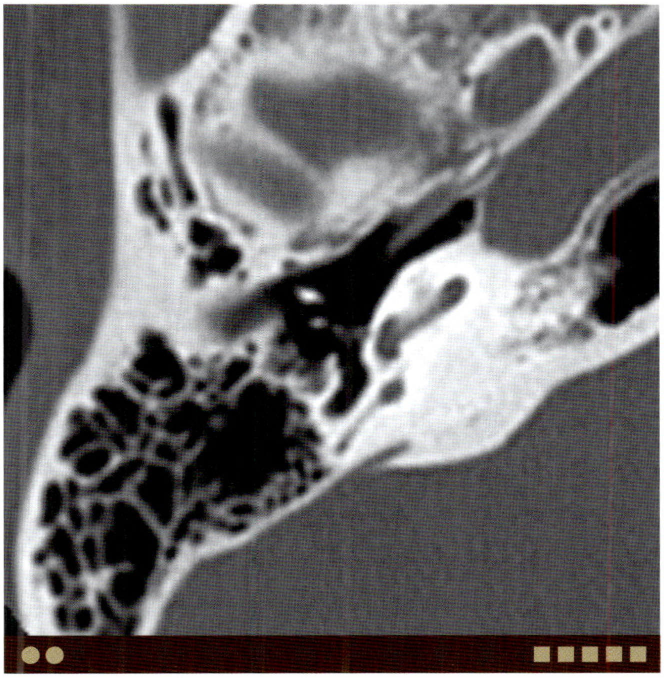

A. PSA. Axial CT demonstrates a small vessel running through the crura of the stapes, representing PSA.

COMMENTS

This is a 41-year-old woman presenting with pulsatile tinnitus. A red "mass" was noted in the tympanic cavity during otoscopy.

A persistent stapedial artery (PSA) is a rare congenital vascular anomaly, which can occur in isolation or in association with aberrant internal carotid artery (ICA). Rarely, PSA has been detected in patients with trisomy 13, 15, and 21, second branchial arch anomalies, Paget's disease, otosclerosis, neurofibromatosis, and thalidomide deformities.

PSA arises from the vertical petrous ICA or aberrant ICA and enters the tympanic cavity. It passes through the crura of the stapes and either enters the canal for the tympanic portion of the facial nerve or runs parallel to it in a separate canal. The PSA continues superiorly to supply the middle meningeal artery.

The imaging findings of a PSA are: 1) a small canaliculus leaving the carotid canal; 2) a linear structure crossing the tympanic cavity over the promontory; 3) an enlarged facial nerve canal or a separate canal parallel to the facial nerve; and 4) absence of the foramen spinosum through which the middle meningeal artery normally runs.

Clinical presentation of a PSA is conductive hearing loss, pulsatile tinnitus, or can be asymptomatic. Recognition of imaging findings is important to avoid possible serious complications from surgery.

PEARLS

- **PSA may occur in isolation or in association with aberrant ICA.**
- **PSA enters the tympanic cavity, passes through the crura of the stapes, and either enters the canal for the tympanic portion of the facial nerve or runs parallel to it in a separate canal.**
- **Absence of the foramen spinosum is an indirect sign of PSA.**

ADDITIONAL IMAGES (B-D)

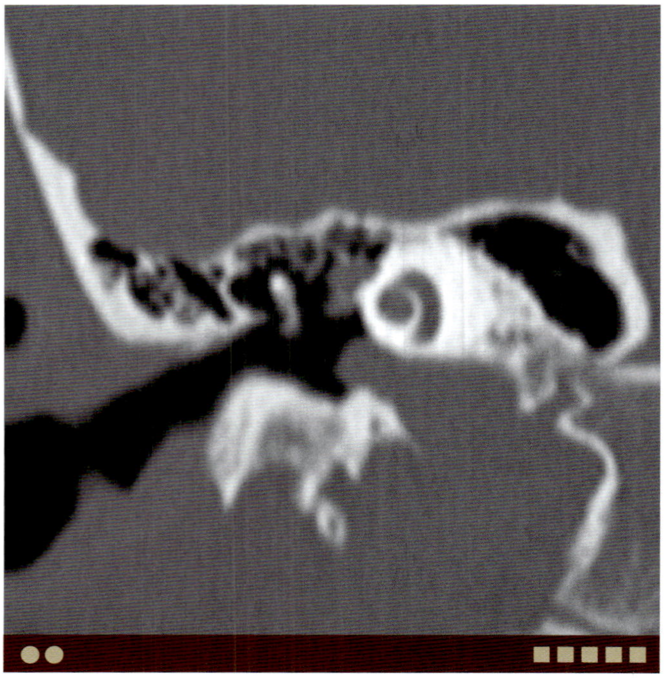

B. PSA, same patient as A. Coronal CT demonstrates the PSA coursing inferior to the anterior tympanic segment of the facial nerve. CT also shows an aberrant ICA entering into the tympanic cavity.

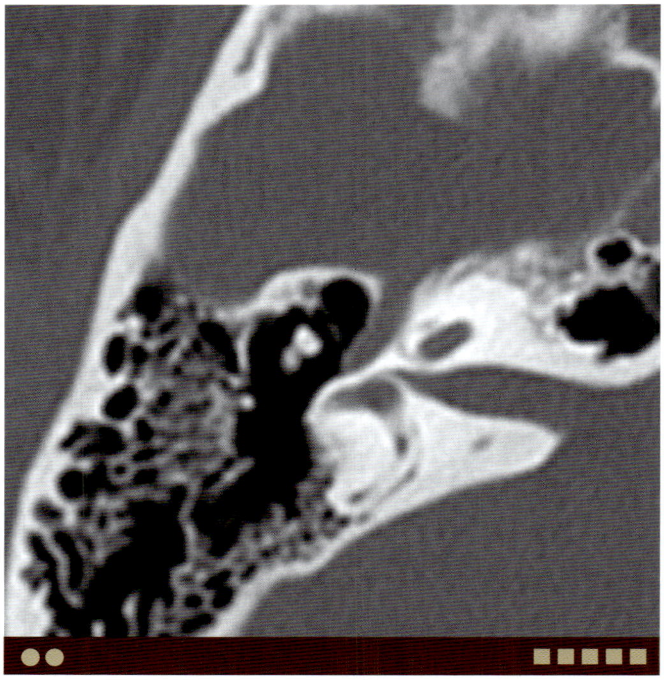

C. PSA, same patient as A. Axial CT through the upper level demonstrates the PSA entering a special opening located at the surface of the petrous bone superior to the geniculate ganglion.

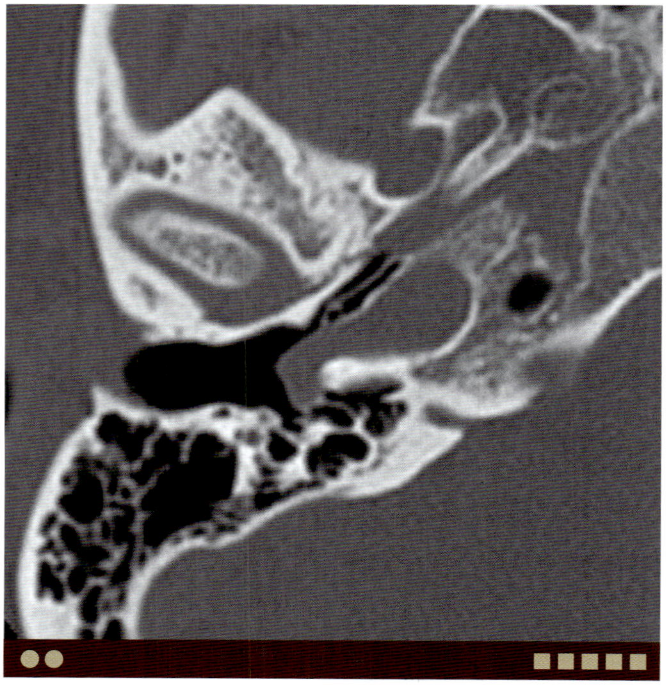

D. PSA, same patient as A. Axial CT through the lower level demonstrates absence of the foramen spinosum. CT also shows the aberrant ICA entering into the tympanic cavity.

DIFFERENTIAL DIAGNOSIS IMAGES (E-G)

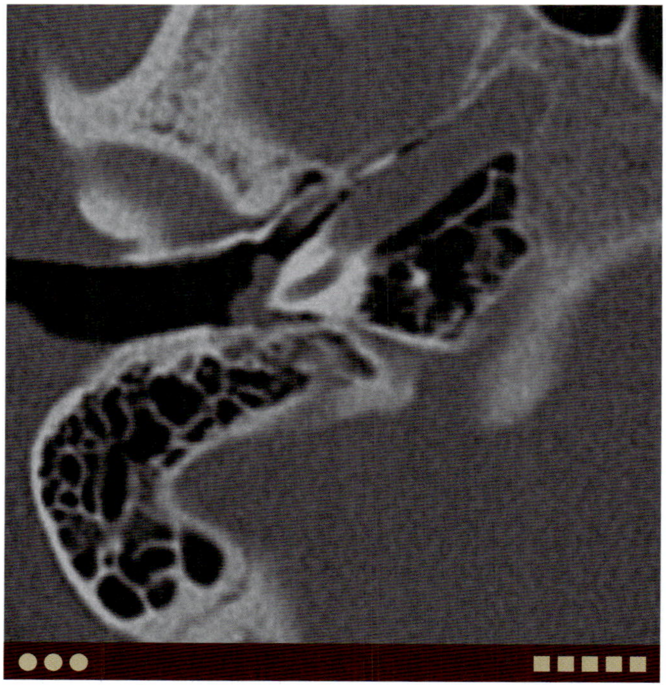

E. Glomus tympanicum. Axial CT demonstrates a focal soft tissue density mass over the cochlear promontory.

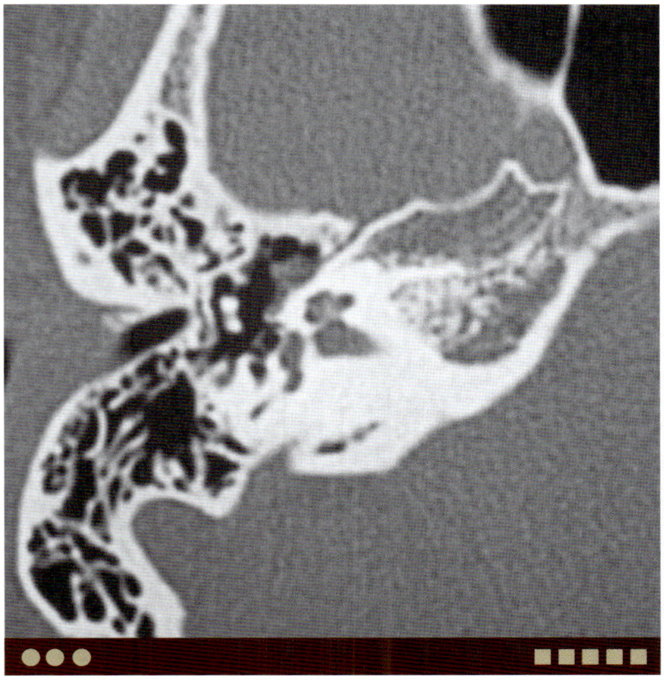

F. Facial nerve schwannoma. Axial CT demonstrates a soft tissue density mass over the cochlea.

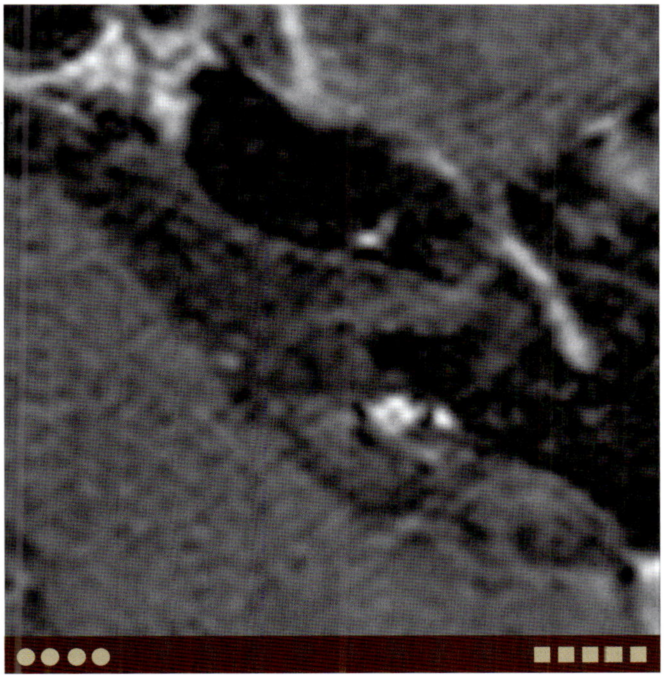

G. Bell's palsy. Axial postcontrast high-resolution T1W image demonstrates enhancement of the tympanic segment of the facial nerve.

Case 1–32 Neurofibromatosis Type 2: Bilateral Vestibular Schwannomas

Elisa Flower, Osamu Sakai

PRESENTATION

Bilateral hearing loss.

FINDINGS

MRI demonstrates enhancing tumors in the bilateral cerebellopontine angles (CPAs).

DIFFERENTIAL DIAGNOSIS

- Metastases: CSF dissemination of tumor cells demonstrates tumor implantations along the seventh and eighth cranial nerve complex, and are seen as enhancing masses at the CPAs.
- Sarcoidosis: Sarcoidosis and other granulomatous diseases may demonstrate abnormal enhancement along the seventh and eighth cranial nerve complex.
- Neurofibromatosis type 1 (NF1): NF1 is a distinct entity from NF2. Patients with NF1 may have optic pathway gliomas and parenchymal hamartomatous lesions intracranially.

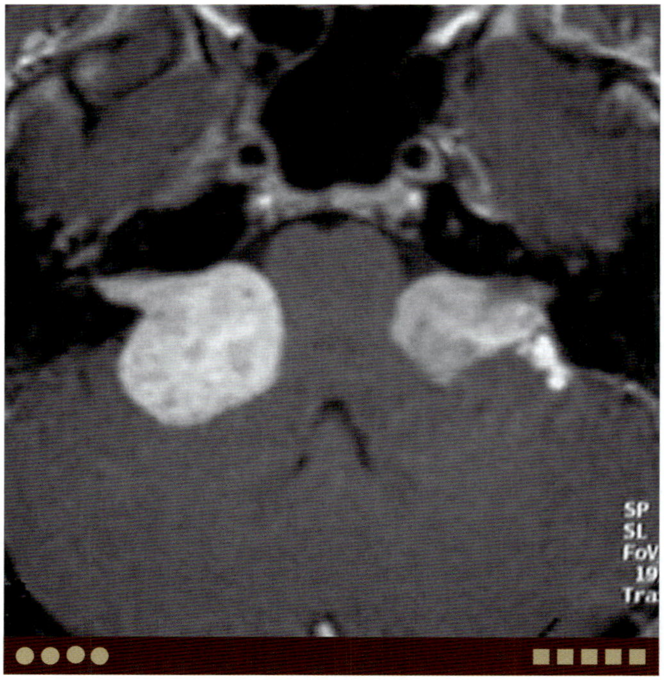

A. NF2, bilateral vestibular schwannomas. Axial postcontrast T1W MR image demonstrates enhancing tumors at the bilateral CPAs.

COMMENTS

This is an 11-year-old girl with bilateral sensorineural hearing loss.

Bilateral vestibular schwannomas are pathognomonic of neurofibromatosis type 2 (NF2). NF2 is an autosomal dominant condition transmitted on chromosome 22 characterized by *m*ultiple *i*nherited *s*chwannomas, *m*eningiomas, and *e*pendymomas (MISME). Half of cases develop secondary to sporadic mutation. It is a distinct entity from and much less common than neurofibromatosis type 1 (NF1).

Clinical diagnosis of NF2 can be made by either bilateral cranial nerve VIII schwannomas or first-degree relative with NF2 plus either unilateral cranial nerve (CN) VIII schwannoma or two of the following: schwannoma, neurofibroma, meningioma, or glioma. Posterior subcapsular lenticular opacity or juvenile cataract is also associated with NF2. Schwannomas are most frequently associated with the vestibular portion of the nerve. They may also involve peripheral nerves or other cranial nerves.

Patients typically present with sensorineural hearing loss. Vestibular schwannomas in patients with NF2 tend to arise early, in their third decade, as opposed to spontaneous lesions which usually occur later, in the fifth decade. Patients aged under 30 years diagnosed with unilateral acoustic schwannomas should be carefully evaluated for a contralateral lesion, other cranial nerve lesions, and have their spines screened for associated intramedullary spinal lesions.

Patients diagnosed with NF2 should be periodically screened for additional lesions. Genetic counseling and screening of family members should also be addressed.

PEARLS

- **Bilateral acoustic schwannomas are pathognomonic of NF2.**
- **Bilateral metastatic disease should be considered over NF2 in the older population.**
- **Patients aged under 30 years with unilateral acoustic schwannomas should be carefully evaluated for a contralateral lesion, other cranial nerve lesions, and have their spines screened for associated spinal lesions.**

ADDITIONAL IMAGES (B-F)

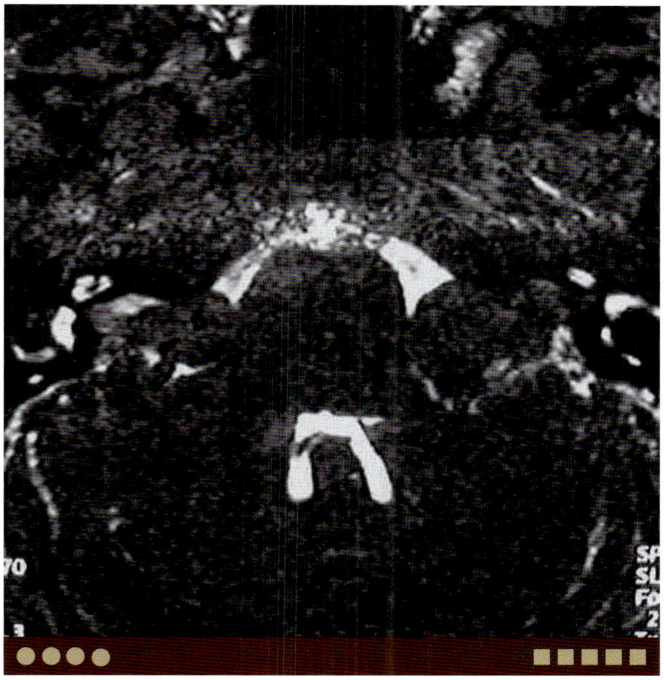

B. NF2, bilateral vestibular schwannomas, same patient as A. Axial high-resolution T2W MR image demonstrates round tumors at the orifice of the internal auditory canals bilaterally.

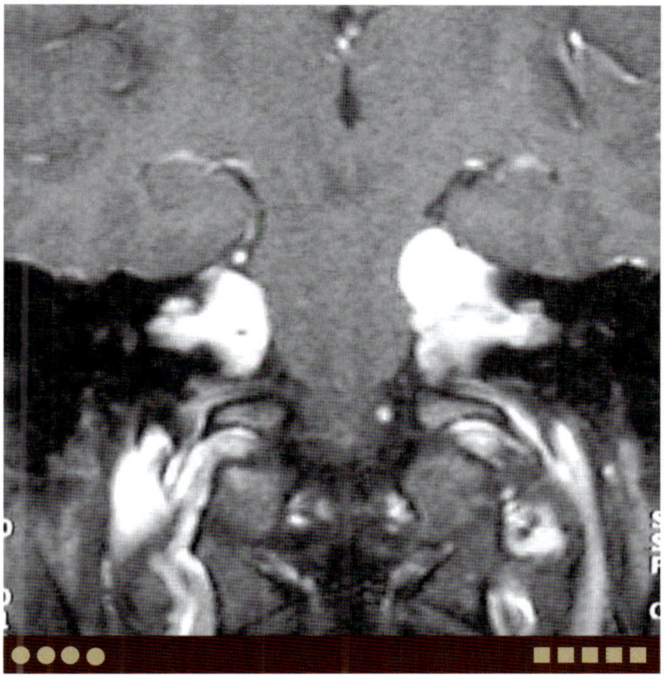

C. NF2, bilateral vestibular schwannomas, same patient as A Coronal postcontrast T1W MR image demonstrates enhancing tumors at the bilateral CPAs compressing the pons.

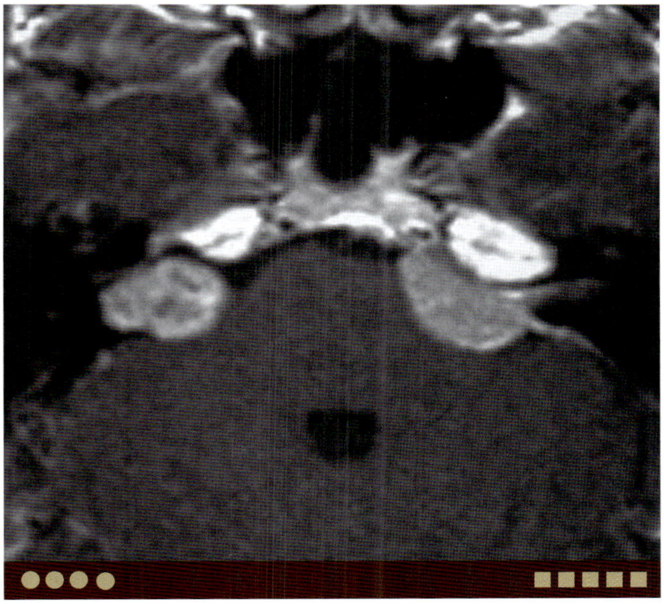

D. NF2, unilateral vestibular schwannoma and meningioma. Axial postcontrast T1W MR image demonstrates a vestibular schwannoma at the right CPA and a meningioma showing dural tail sign at the left CPA.

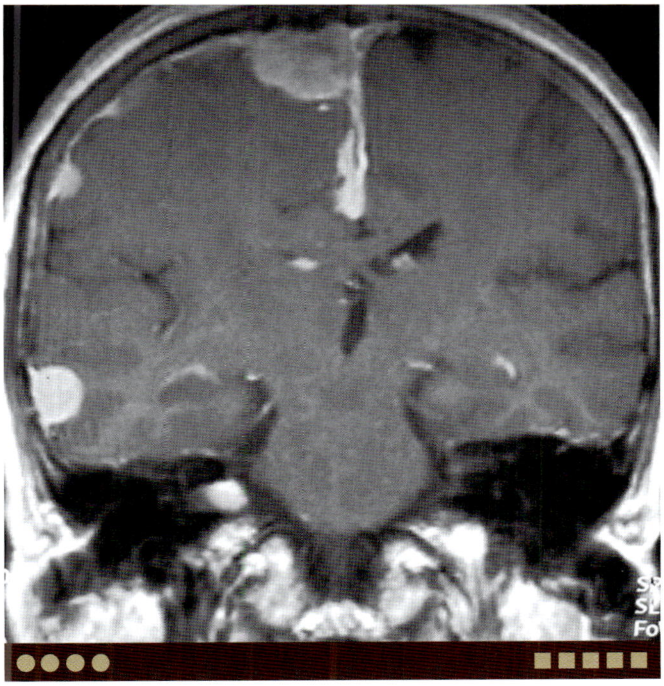

E. NF2, unilateral vestibular schwannoma and multiple meningiomas. Coronal postcontrast T1W MR image demonstrates a vestibular schwannoma at the right CPA and multiple meningiomas in the right cerebral hemisphere.

DIFFERENTIAL DIAGNOSIS IMAGES (G-J)

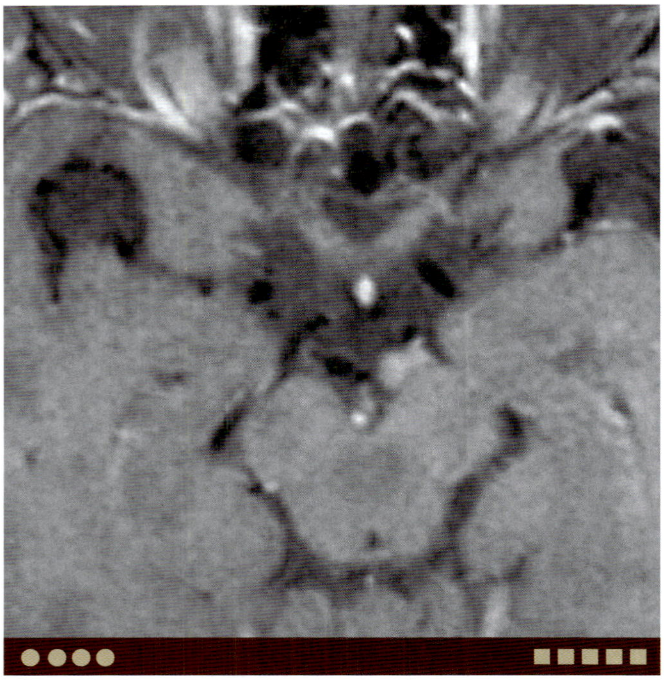

F. NF2, unilateral vestibular schwannoma and oculomotor nerve schwannoma. Axial postcontrast T1W MR image demonstrates an enhancing tumor at the origin of the left oculomotor nerve. This patient also had vestibular schwannoma (*not shown*).

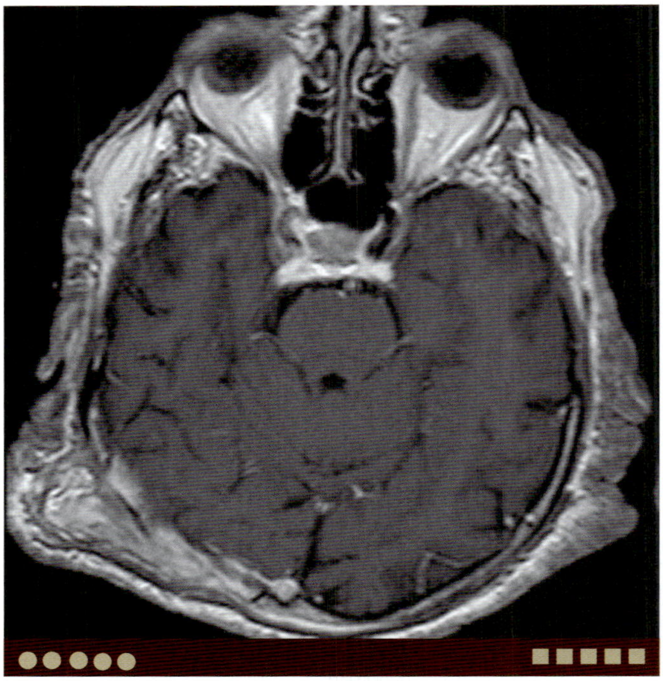

G. NF1. Axial postcontrast T1W image demonstrates numerous neurofibromas in the subcutaneous tissues.

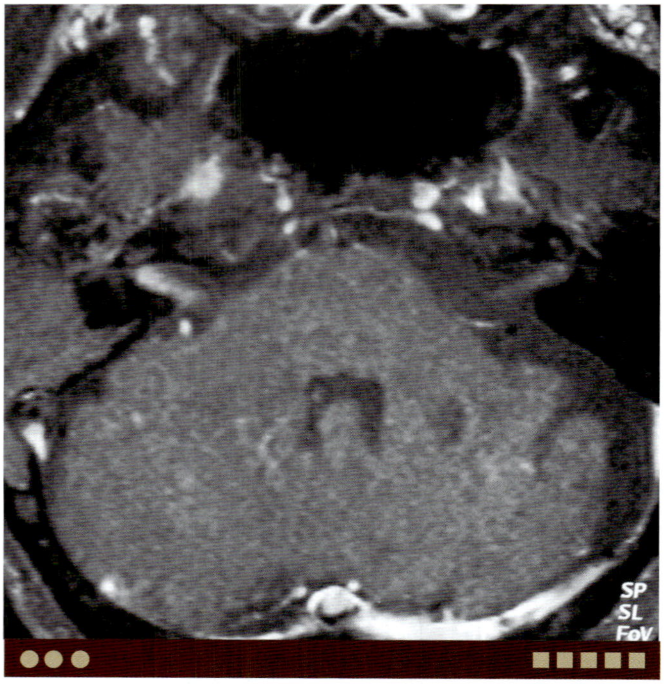

H. Metastasis, breast cancer. Axial postcontrast T1W image demonstrates enhancement of the bilateral CN VII/VIII complex, right more than left.

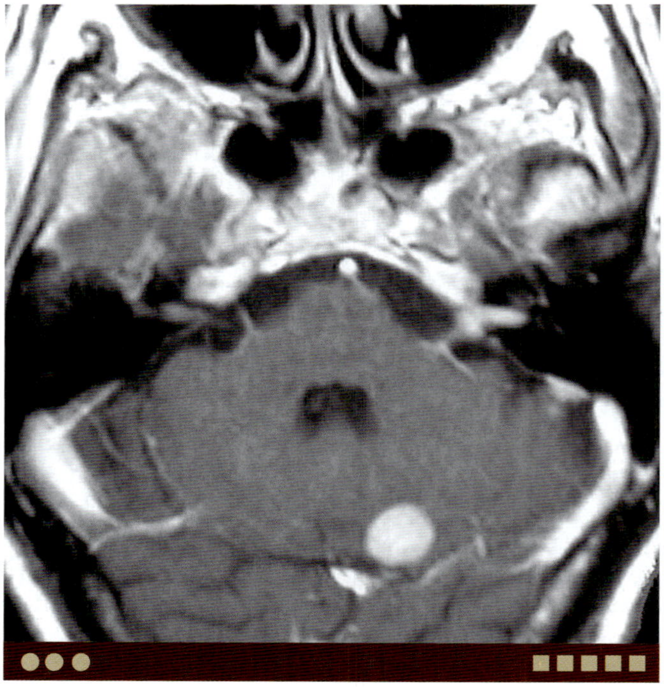

I. Metastasis, melanoma. Axial postcontrast T1W image demonstrates enhancement of the bilateral CN VII/VIII complex, left more than right. Further, a round enhancing metastatic lesion is seen along the left cerebellar tentorium.

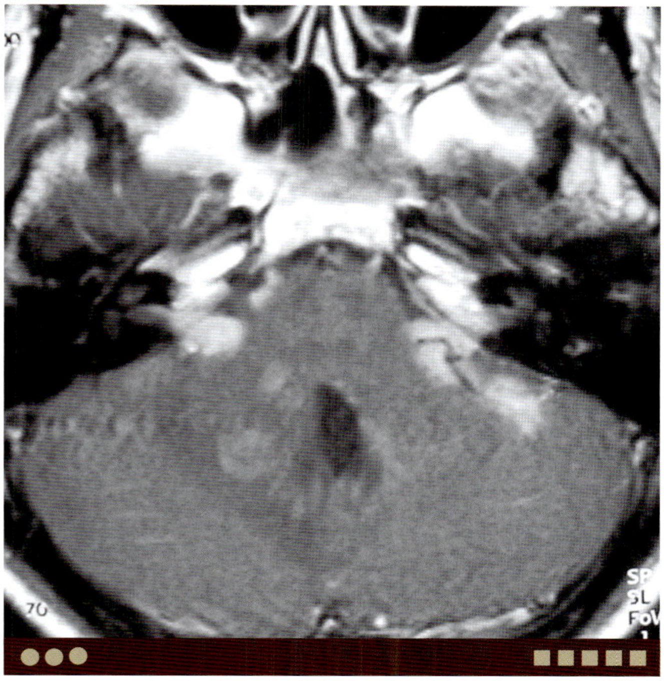

J. Metastasis, medulloblastoma. Axial postcontrast T1W MR image demonstrates enhancement of the bilateral CN VII/VIII complex, left more than right.

Case 1–33 Facial Nerve Hemangioma

Osamu Sakai, Rohini Nadgir

PRESENTATION

Slowly progressing facial nerve weakness.

FINDINGS

CT demonstrates demineralization of the facial nerve canal. MRI demonstrates an enhancing lesion along the facial nerve.

DIFFERENTIAL DIAGNOSIS

- Bell's palsy: This is the most common cause of facial nerve palsy. By definition, this is idiopathic, however, it is most often associated with herpes simplex type 1 virus infection. Abnormal enhancement of the facial nerve is noted without mass formation.
- Schwannoma: This is the most common primary tumor arising from the facial nerve. Mass formation is noted in addition to abnormal enhancement, commonly seen in the genu and tympanic segments.
- Meningioma: Meningioma rarely occurs in the area of the geniculate ganglion, but may show similar findings to hemangiomas and schwannomas.
- Perineural tumor spread: This is commonly seen with adenoid cystic carcinoma of the parotid gland. Obliteration of the fat in the stylomastoid foramen is an important finding to make a diagnosis. The T2 signal is usually lower than that of hemangioma.

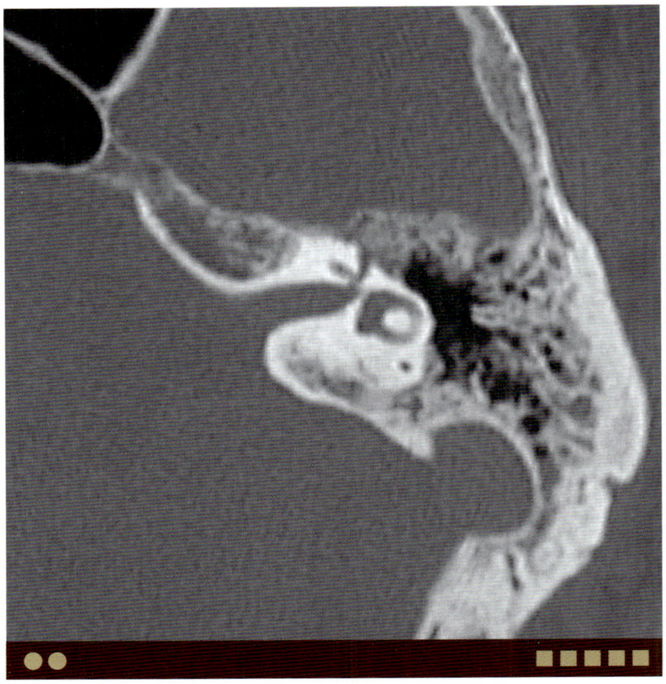

A. Hemangioma. Axial CT demonstrates demineralization at the level of the genu of the facial nerve.

COMMENTS

This is a 42-year-old woman with slowly progressive right-sided facial palsy.

Hemangioma of the facial nerve is a benign vascular tumor. This is the second most common tumor associated with the facial nerve after schwannoma, although it is rare. This is often seen in the area of the geniculate ganglion, although it can be seen anywhere along the course of the facial nerve. Hemangiomas grow very slowly and are most commonly found in middle-aged adults. Facial nerve dysfunction is the most common complaint, present in 60% of the cases, followed by hearing loss, which presents in 40% of cases.

CT demonstrates demineralization of the osseous canal in patients with hemangiomas, while erosion/remodeling is more commonly seen with schwannomas. On MRI, hemangioma demonstrates high signal on T2W images and enhancement. Perineural tumor spread, commonly seen with adenoid cystic carcinoma may demonstrate similar findings, however, typically perineural tumor spread shows lower T2 signal and less enhancement compared with hemangioma and schwannoma.

PEARLS

- **Hemangioma is the second most common tumor associated with the facial nerve.**
- **Hemangioma demonstrates demineralization of the facial nerve canal.**
- **Hemangioma demonstrates high T2 signal and enhancement.**

ADDITIONAL IMAGES (B-G)

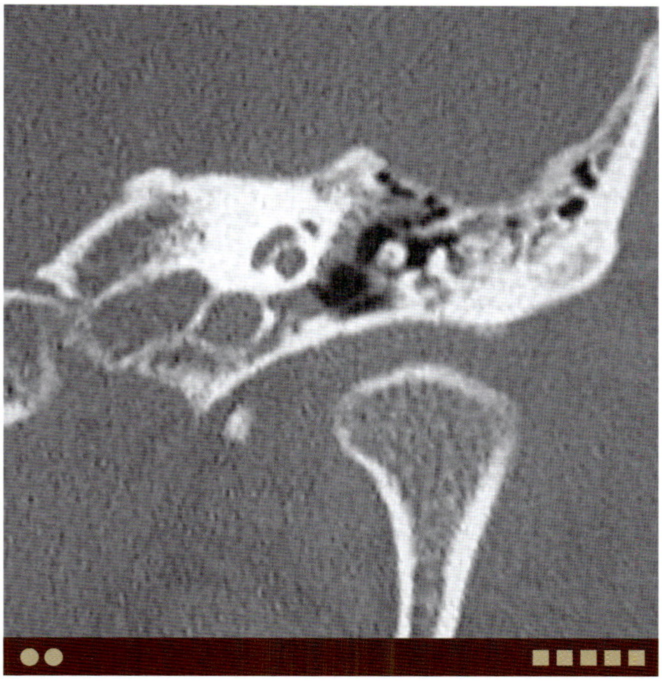

B. Hemangioma, same patient as A. Coronal CT demonstrates demineralization at the level of the genu of the facial nerve.

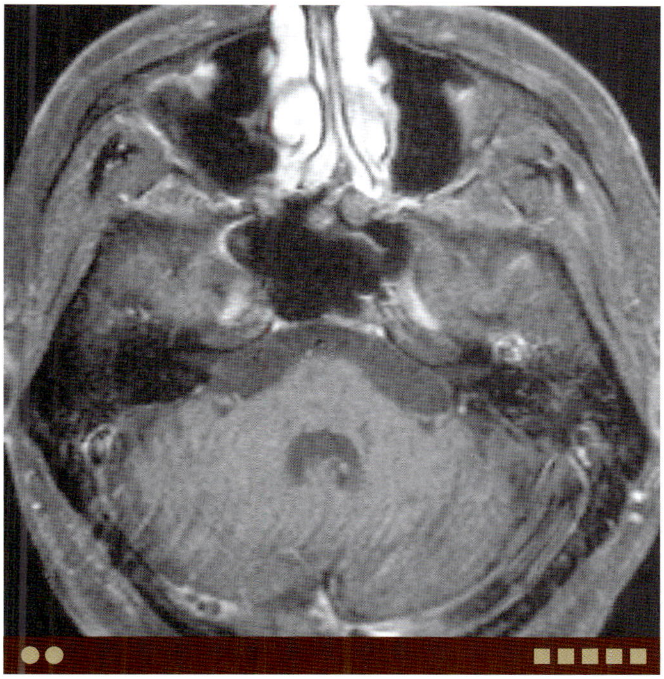

C. Hemangioma, same patient as A. Axial postcontrast fat-suppressed T1W image demonstrates enhancement of the lesion.

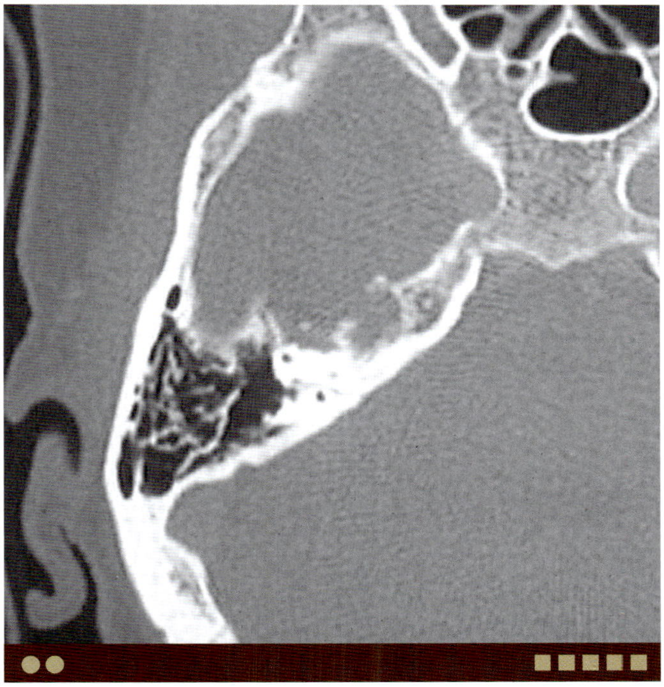

D. Hemangioma in a different patient. Axial CT demonstrates extensive demineralization of the petrous bone.

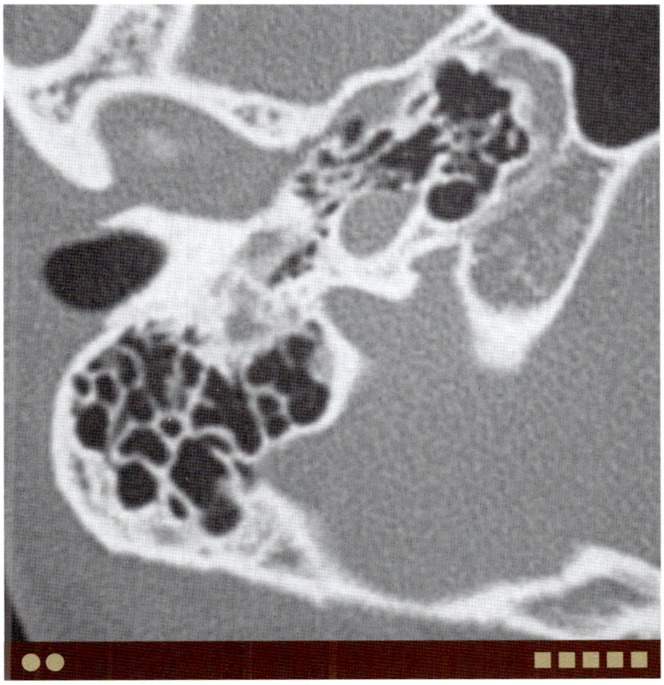

E. Hemangioma in a different patient. Axial CT demonstrates demineralization at the level of the mastoid segment of the facial nerve canal.

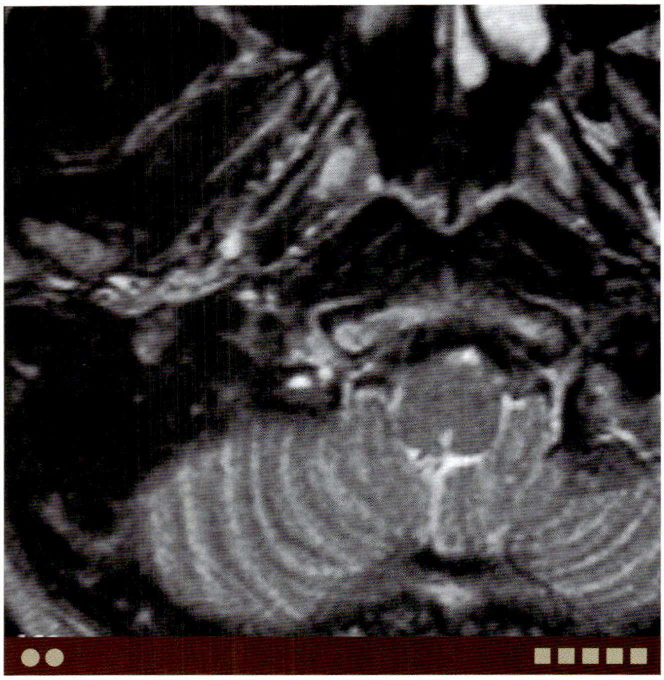

F. Hemangioma, same patient as E. Axial T2W MR image demonstrates heterogeneous high signal within the lesion.

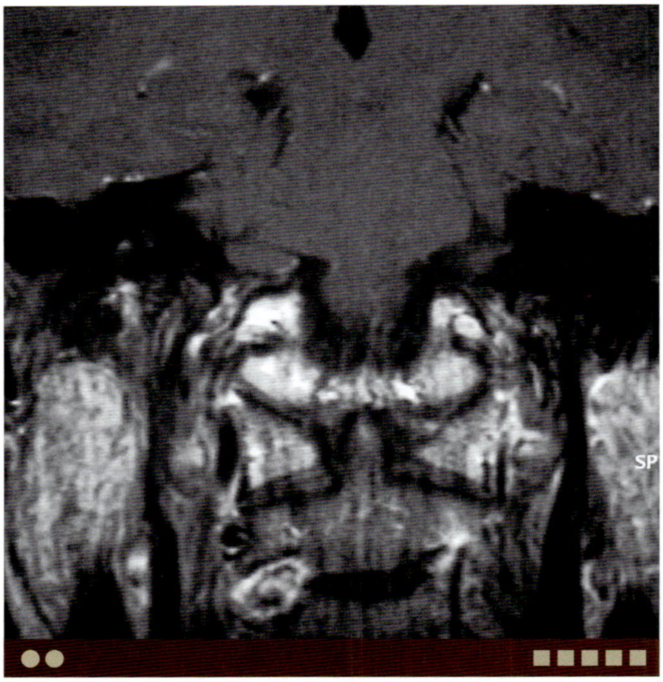

G. Hemangioma, same patient as E. Coronal postcontrast T1W image demonstrates enhancement of the lesion.

DIFFERENTIAL DIAGNOSIS IMAGES (H-J)

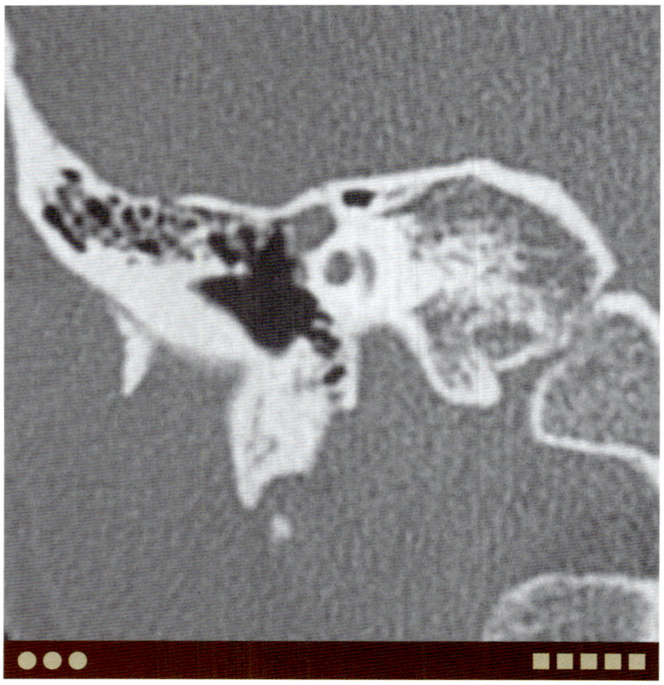

H. Schwannoma. Coronal CT demonstrates soft tissue mass and expansion at the level of the genu of the facial nerve.

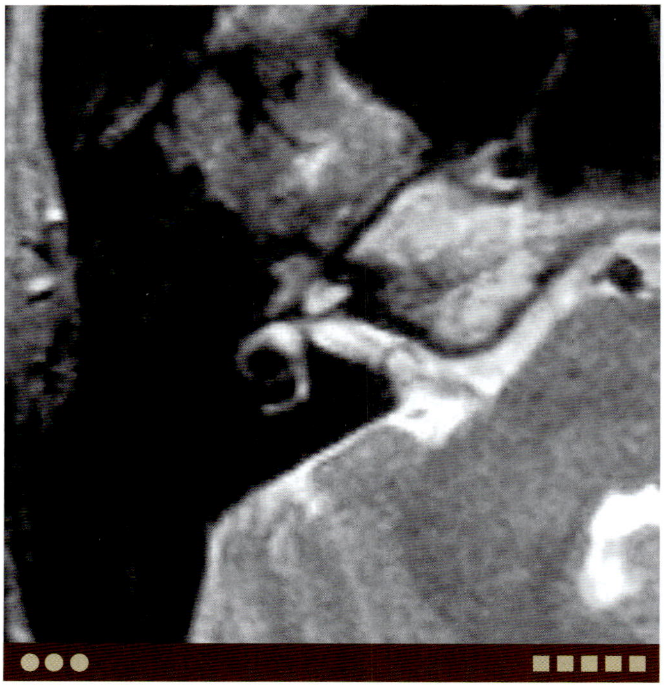

I. Schwannoma, same patient as H. Axial T2W MR image demonstrates slightly heterogeneous, intermediate-to-high signal in the tumor.

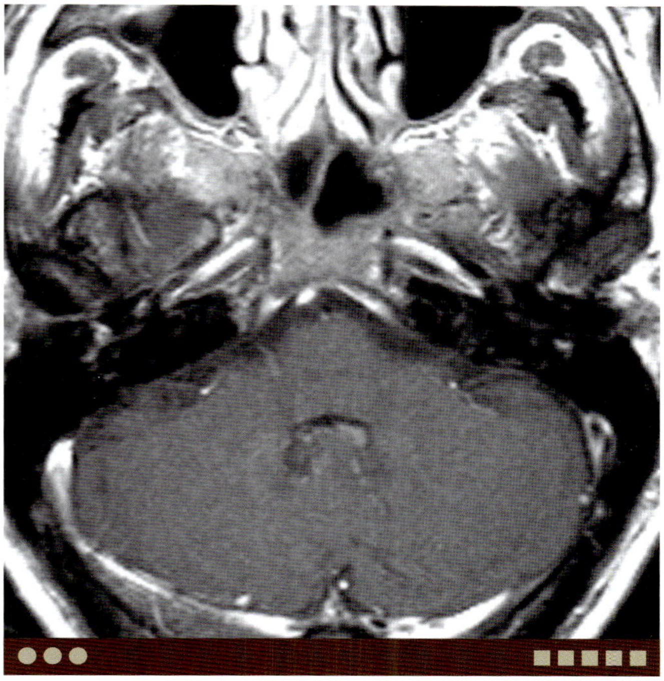

J. Schwannoma in a different patient. Axial postcontrast T1W MR image demonstrates an enhancing lesion in the genu and tympanic segment of the right facial nerve.

Case 1–34 Persistent Foramen Tympanicum

Hiroki Kato, Osamu Sakai

PRESENTATION

Temporomandibular joint pain.

FINDINGS

CT and MRI demonstrate a focal bone defect at the anteroinferior margin of the external auditory canal (EAC).

DIFFERENTIAL DIAGNOSIS

- Squamous cell carcinoma (SCCA) of the EAC: Although SCCA of the EAC is rare, SCCA is the most common malignancy of the EAC. Soft tissue lesion with bone destruction/erosion raises the possibility of SCCA.
- Cholesteatoma of the EAC: Cholesteatoma is occasionally seen in the EAC. Bone erosion rather than aggressive destruction is a common finding.
- Keratosis obturans: This is a keratin plug in the EAC without focal bony erosion or destruction, although diffuse EAC expansion may be present.
- EAC fracture: EAC fractures associated with temporal bone fractures are usually found in the posterosuperior quadrant near the tympanosquamous suture. EAC fractures secondary to blows to the mandible are located in the anterior wall (tympanic plate).

COMMENTS

This is a 35-year-old woman presented with a discomfort of the left ear during mastication.

Foramen tympanicum, also known as the foramen of Huschke, is a focal osseous defect of the EAC at its anteroinferior aspect, posteromedial to the temporomandibular joint (TMJ). This is a developmental anatomic variant in the tympanic portion of the temporal bone. At birth the entire temporal portion is not completely formed and the foramen tympanicum is present. It gradually regresses and completely seals before the age of 5 years in most children. Persistence of the defect after the age of 5 years is considered as an anatomic variant.

Foramen tympanicum may result in spontaneous herniation of soft tissue from the TMJ into the EAC, and cause TMJ pain and dysfunction. Soft tissue protrusion into the EAC can be apparent only when the patient closes the mouth, and it may completely resolve when the patient opens the mouth. Foramen tympanicum may incline individuals to TMJ pathology, and may be associated with salivary discharge into the EAC during mastication.

CT with multiplanar reformation is useful in detecting the foramen tympanicum, while MRI provides better information regarding the TMJ. On CT, anterior bone dehiscence of the EAC, along the posteromedial aspect of the glenoid fossa of the TMJ, is seen. Soft tissue protrusion from the TMJ into the EAC is sometimes seen when the mouth is closed.

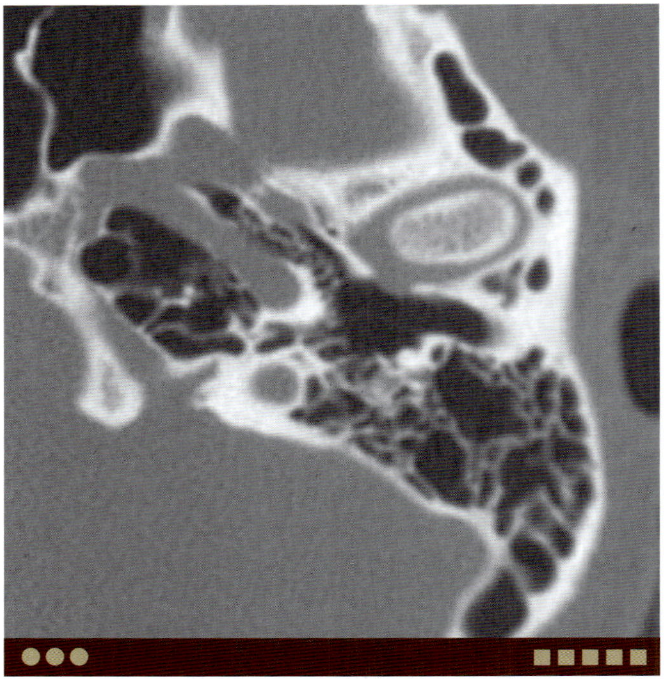

A. Persistent foramen tympanicum. Axial unenhanced CT demonstrates anterior bone dehiscence of the left EAC, posteromedial aspect of the glenoid fossa of the left TMJ.

PEARLS

- **Foramen tympanicum is a focal osseous defect of the EAC at its anteroinferior aspect, posteromedial to the TMJ.**
- **Soft tissue protrusion into the EAC can be apparent only when the mouth is closed, and it may completely resolve when the mouth is opened.**
- **Foramen tympanicum may cause TMJ pathology or salivary discharge into the EAC during mastication.**

ADDITIONAL IMAGE

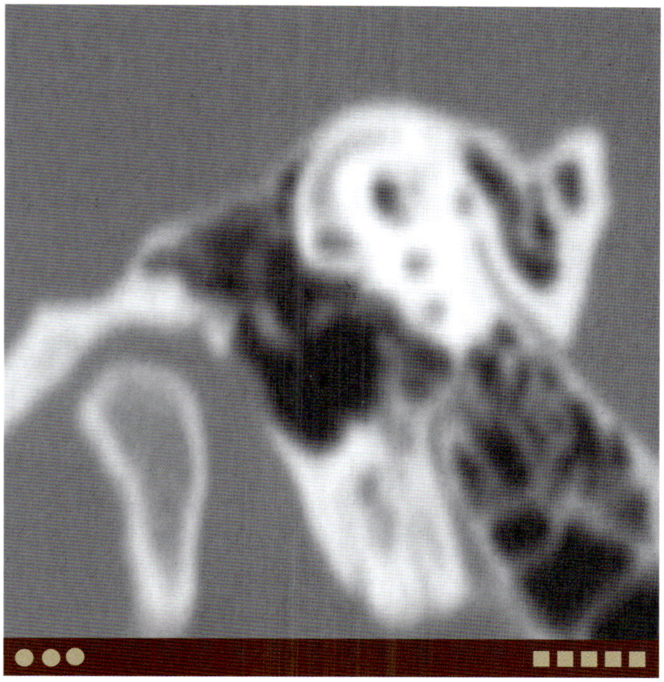

B. Persistent foramen tympanicum, same patient as A. Sagittal unenhanced CT demonstrates bone dehiscence in the posterosuperior aspect of the glenoid fossa.

DIFFERENTIAL DIAGNOSIS IMAGES (C-E)

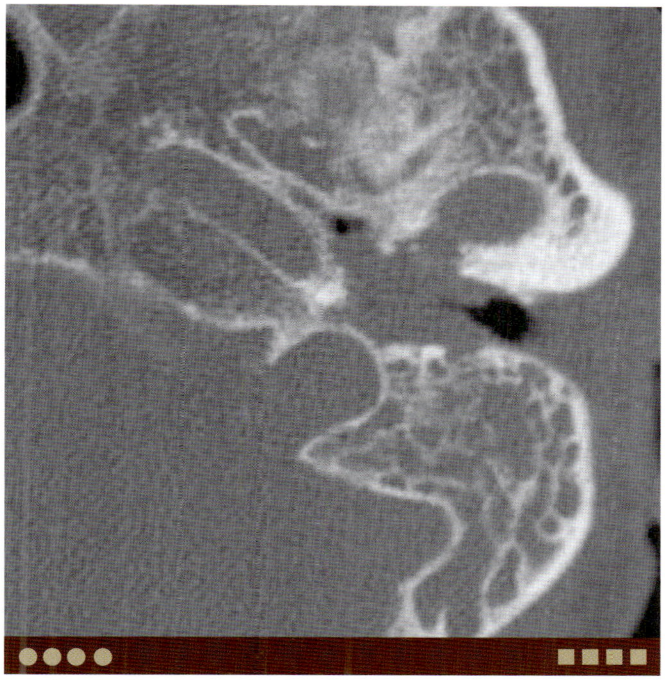

C. SCCA of the EAC. Axial unenhanced CT demonstrates a tumor within the left EAC destroying the anterior wall of the EAC.

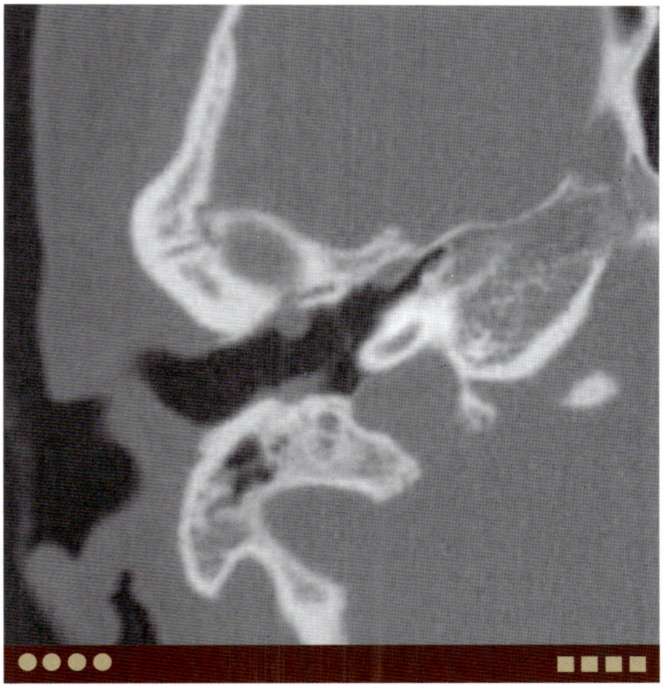

D. Cholesteatoma of the EAC. Axial unenhanced CT demonstrates a small soft tissue mass within the right EAC eroding the anterior wall of the EAC.

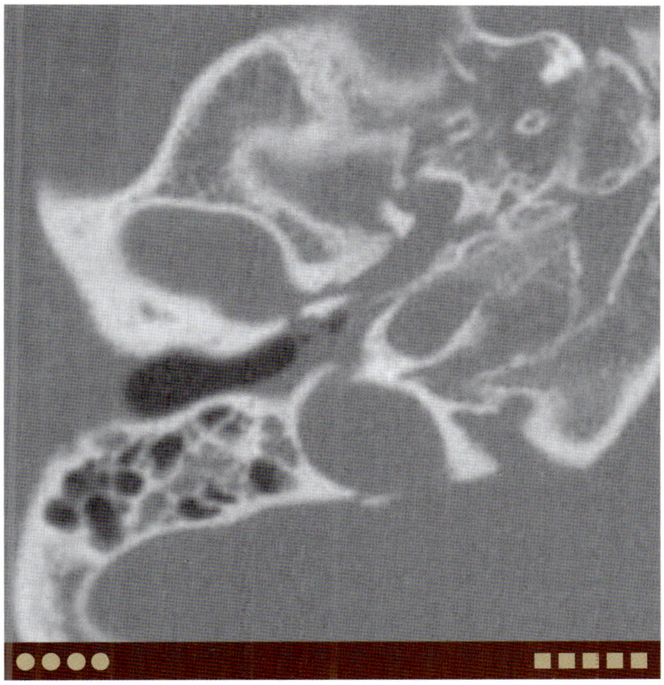

E. External auditory canal fracture. Axial unenhanced CT demonstrates a fracture through the anterior wall of the right EAC. Note another fracture through the jugular foramen.

Case 1–35 Dehiscent Jugular Bulb

Takao Kodama

PRESENTATION

Pulsatile tinnitus and vascular blue mass behind an intact tympanic membrane.

FINDINGS

CT shows focal bone dehiscence of the sigmoid (jugular) plate with protrusion of the jugular bulb (JB) into the tympanic cavity.

DIFFERENTIAL DIAGNOSIS

- JB diverticulum: CT shows a focal polypoid mass extending cephalad from the JB with intact sigmoid plate.
- Jugular foramen schwannoma: CT shows smoothly scalloped and enlarged jugular foramen. MRI reveals a dumbbell-shaped enhancing mass.
- Jugular foramen paraganglioma: Permeative-destructive bony change can be seen around the JB. MRI may show flow-voids suggesting a hypervascular tumor.
- Jugular foramen meningioma: JB margin may display permeative or hyperostotic changes. Postcontrast MRI may show "dural tail."

COMMENTS

This is a 12-year-old boy with left blue tympanic membrane.

The anatomy of the jugular venous system is highly variable. In addition to common variations such as unilateral large JB or high-riding JB, some rare variations such as dehiscence or diverticulum of the JB can be encountered.

Dehiscent or protruding JB is more common on the right side and is often associated with high-riding JB. Dehiscent JB was reported to be common in patients with Crouzon disease. Although many of the patients with dehiscent JB are usually asymptomatic, it can be a cause of pulsatile tinnitus. When a dehiscent JB protrudes into the middle ear, it is seen as a retrotympanic vascular mass and can be confused with a glomus tumor by otoscopy. Rarely, it can cause conductive hearing loss.

High-resolution CT is the best modality to evaluate variations of the JB. A soft tissue mass in the middle ear cavity contiguous with the JB and dehiscence of the sigmoid plate suggests dehiscent JB. The protruded JB may abut the ossicles. MRI is not needed to diagnose dehiscent JB.

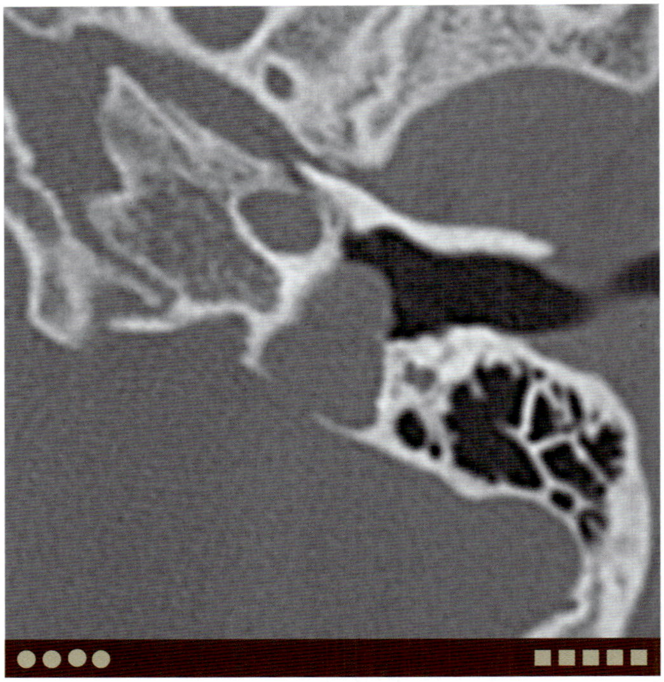

A. Dehiscent JB. Axial CT demonstrates a focal dehiscence of sigmoid plate with protrusion of the JB into the middle ear.

On T1W or T2W MR images, a JB may have heterogeneous signal intensity or flow-void and may not be distinguished from surrounding bony structures and air. Therefore, CT should be the first imaging modality to evaluate a patient with a retrotympanic vascular mass. Postcontrast study or MR venography may be useful to evaluate variations of the JB.

PEARLS

- **Dehiscent JB is one of the important differential diagnostic consideration in patients with pulsatile tinnitus or retrotympanic vascular mass.**
- **CT is the best modality to diagnose dehiscent JB. A soft tissue mass in the middle ear cavity contiguous with the JB and dehiscence of the sigmoid plate suggests dehiscent JB.**
- **T1W or T2W MR images are not useful to evaluate variations of the JB.**

ADDITIONAL IMAGES (B-F)

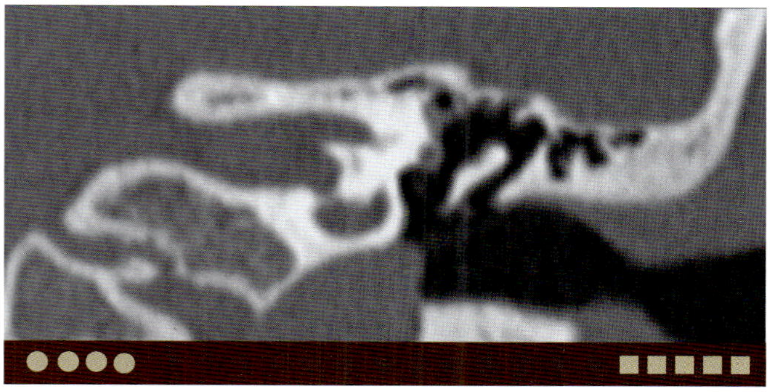

B. Dehiscent JB, same patient as A. Coronal CT demonstrates the upward protrusion of the JB.

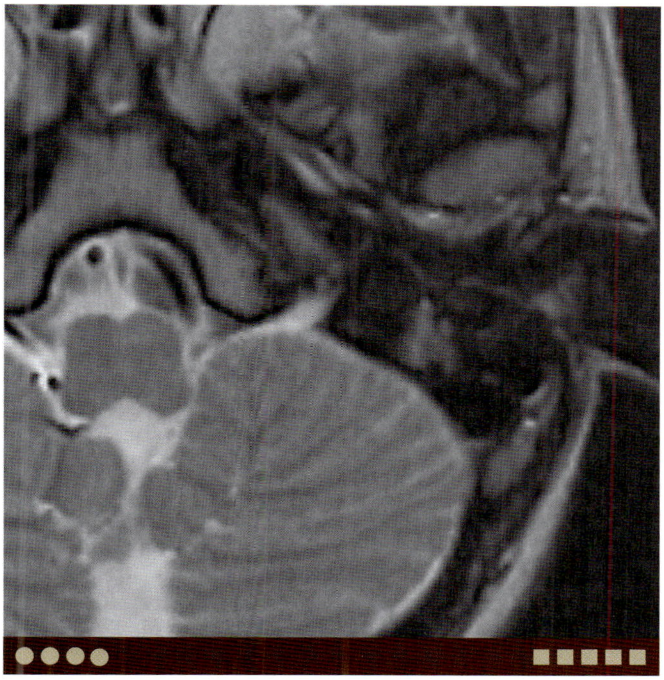

C. Dehiscent JB, same patient as A. Axial T2W image demonstrates flow-void of the JB. JB cannot be readily distinguished from surrounding bone and air.

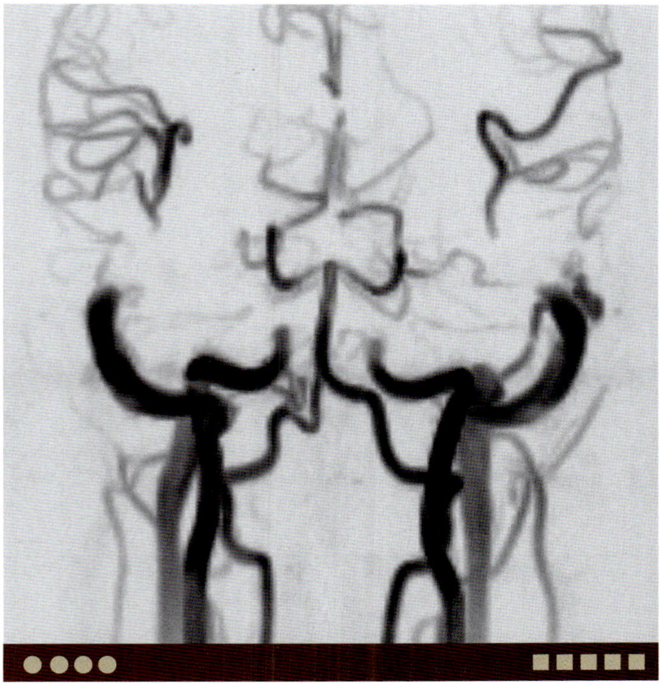

D. Dehiscent JB, same patient as A. Phase-contrast MRA reveals lateral protrusion of the left JB.

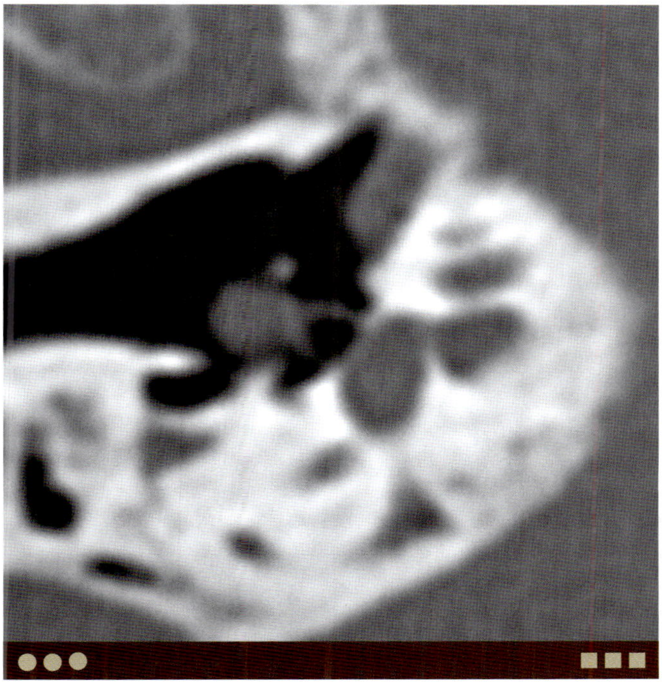

E. Dehiscent JB in a 12-year-old boy with right conductive hearing loss. Axial CT demonstrates soft tissue "mass" contacting with the stapes.

DIFFERENTIAL DIAGNOSIS IMAGES (G-J)

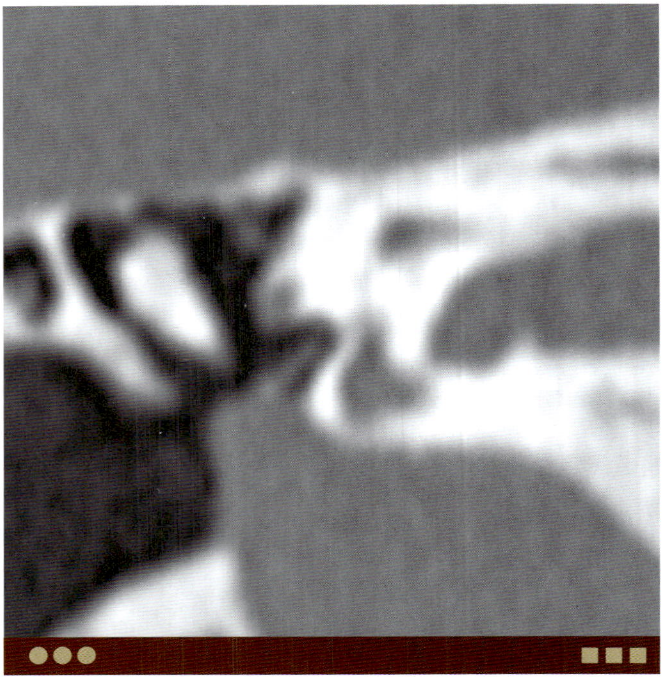

F. Dehiscent JB, same patient as E. Coronal CT demonstrates a dehiscent and protruding JB contacting with the stapes.

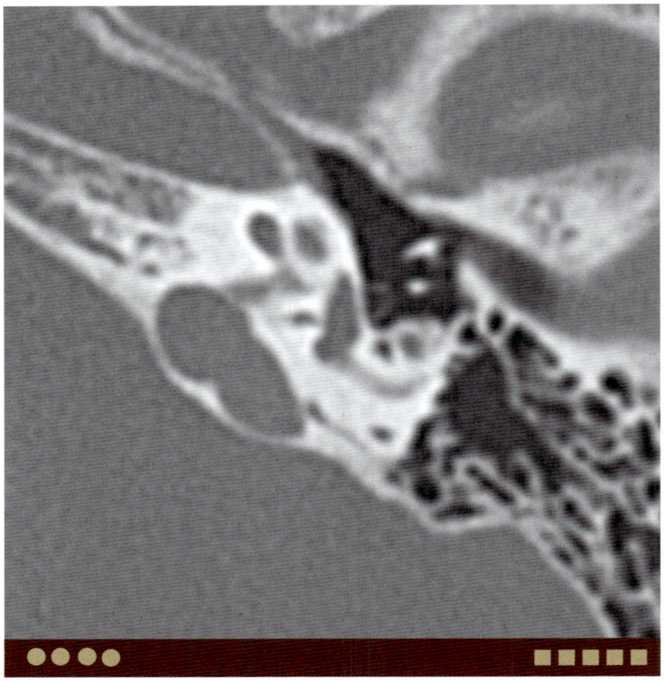

G. Diverticulum of the JB. Axial CT demonstrates left high-riding JB near the internal auditory canal.

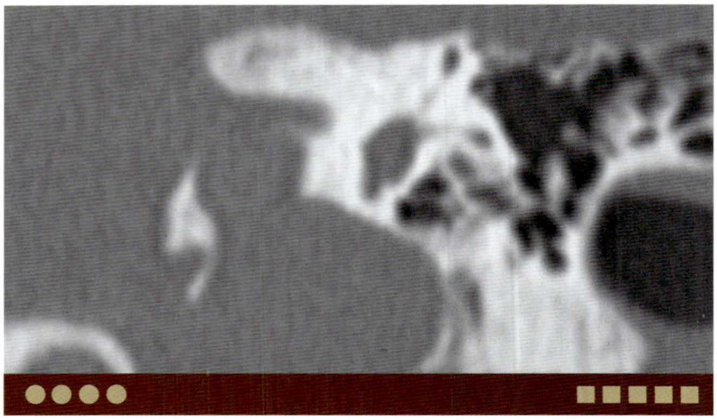

H. Diverticulum of the JB, same patient as G. Coronal CT reveals superomedial diverticular protrusion of the JB.

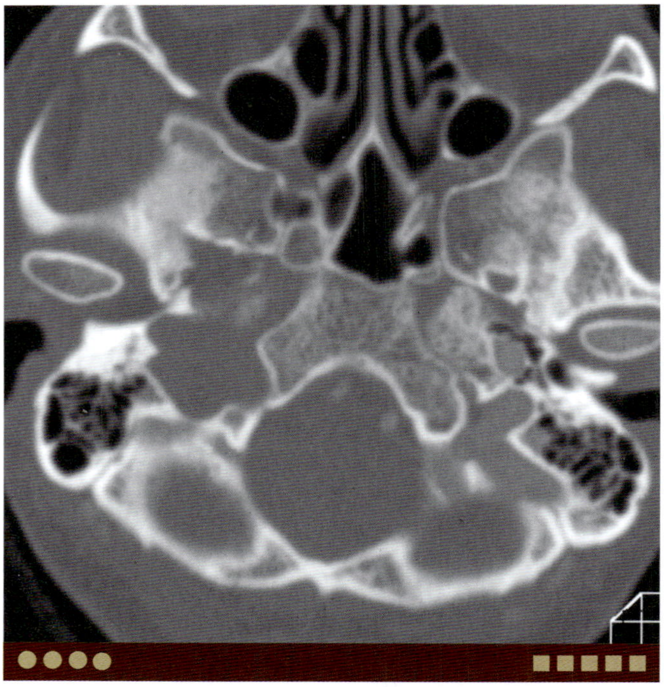

I. Jugular foramen schwannoma. Axial contrast-enhanced CT with bone window setting demonstrates smoothly scalloped and enlarged right jugular foramen. Enhancement of the right JB is not well seen.

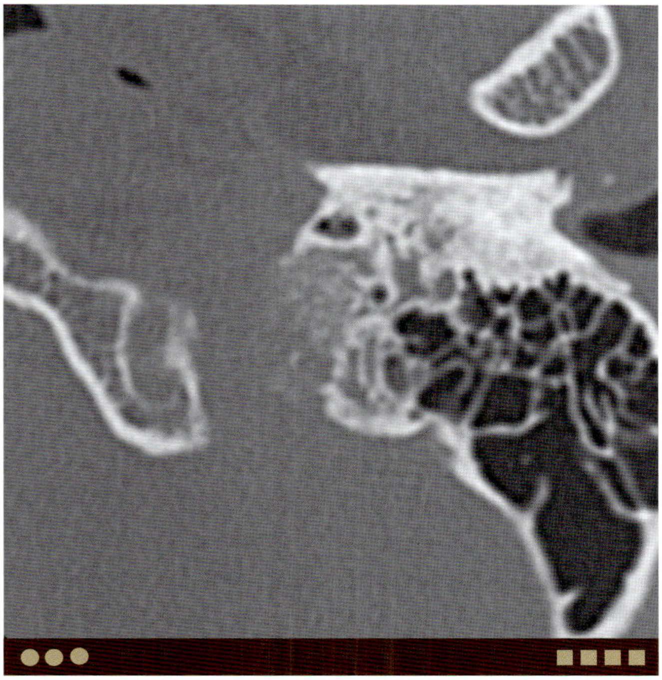

J. Jugular foramen meningioma. Axial high-resolution computed tomography demonstrates permeative change of the lateral wall of the jugular foramen.

Case 1–36 Endolymphatic Tumor

Takao Kodama

PRESENTATION

Hearing loss, tinnitus, vertigo, and facial nerve palsy.

FINDINGS

Temporal bone CT demonstrates permeative-destructive change of the posterior petrous ridge.

DIFFERENTIAL DIAGNOSIS

- Cholesterol cyst: MRI shows an expansile lesion with high signal on T1W and T2W images reflecting paramagnetic effect of methohemoglobin.
- Glomus jugulare paraganglioma: CT shows a mass in the jugular foramen with permeative-destructive change of the adjacent bone. MRI shows multiple flow-voids in the tumor to suggest vascular lesion.
- Meningioma or schwannoma of the jugular foramen: These tumors are centered in the jugular foramen.
- Primary and metastatic bone tumors: These tumors can occur anywhere in the temporal bone. Hypervascular tumors with destructive bony changes may show similar imaging findings to endolymphatic sac tumor.

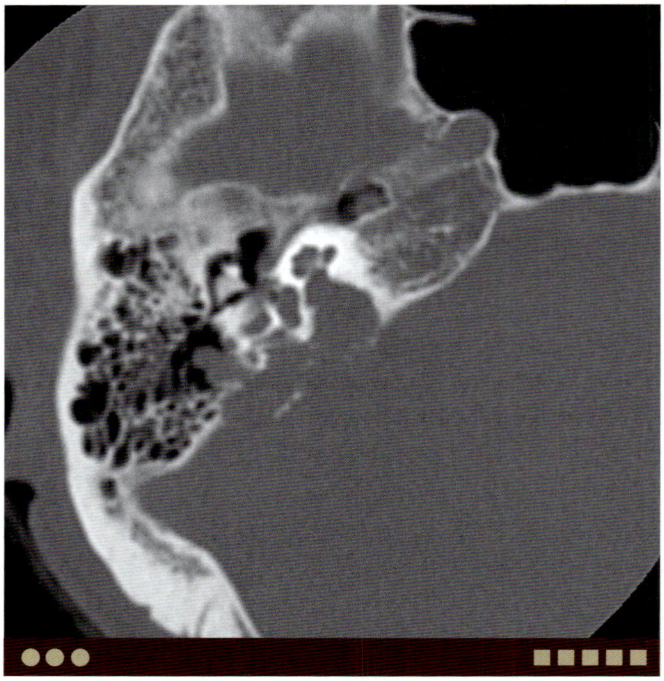

A. ELST. Axial temporal bone CT demonstrates permeative-destructive changes of the posterior wall of the temporal bone involving the vestibular aqueduct. Small calcifications are noted within the lesion. (A and B, courtesy of Dr. Mori, University of Tokyo, Japan)

COMMENTS

This is a 69-year-old woman with right hearing loss and tinnitus.

Endolymphatic sac tumor (ELST) was first established as a unique pathological entity by Heffner in 1989, with histological features of benign papillary-cystic neoplasm in the region of the posterior temporal bone. Although most ELSTs are sporadic, they are found in patients with von Hippel-Lindau (VHL) disease with an estimated incidence of 11% to 16%. Bilateral tumors may occur in as many as 15% to 30% of patients with VHL disease with ELSTs, and VHL is the only condition identified that is associated with bilateral ELSTs. ELSTs arise from the osseous portion (vestibular aqueduct) of the endolymphatic duct and sac system. Therefore, CT shows erosion of the posterior wall of the temporal bone involving the vestibular aqueduct. Posterior wall of the internal auditory canal may be destroyed and otic capsule invasion may be seen. The tumor may invade the inner and middle ear. Central spiculated calcification within the tumor and rim-like calcification are frequently seen. T1W MR images show hyperintense foci secondary to intratumoral hemorrhage. Flow-voids from high-flow tumor vessels can be seen in larger lesions. On postcontrast T1W images, heterogeneous intense enhancement is usually seen. Angiogram shows a hypervascular lesion with supply from branches of the external carotid artery (ECA). In large tumors, supply from branches of the internal carotid and vertebra-basilar artery is also seen.

PEARLS

- **ELST arises from the osseous portion of the endolymphatic duct and sac system centered at the vestibular aqueduct epicenter of the large tumors.**
- **Hyperintense foci on T1W image suggesting hemorrhage and intense enhancement are characteristic findings on MRI. Flow-voids can be seen in larger lesions.**
- **Angiography reveals a hypervascular tumor mainly supplied by branches of the EAC.**

ADDITIONAL IMAGES (B-F)

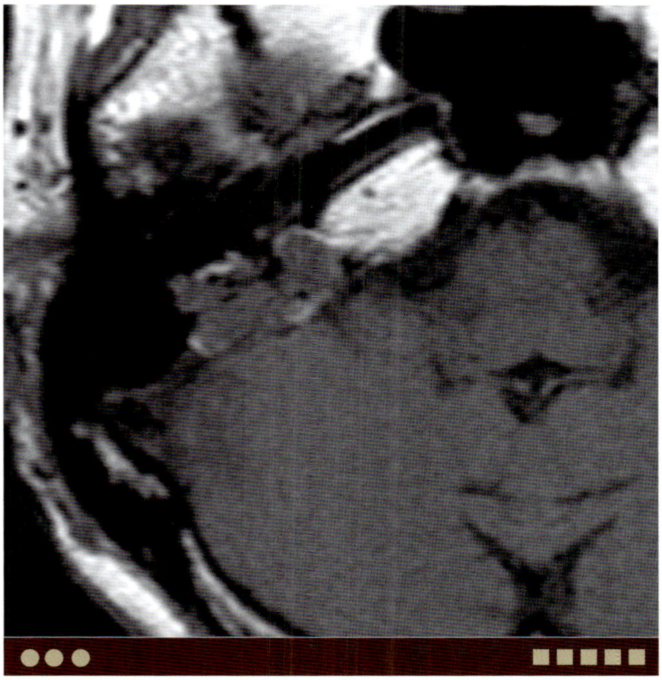

B. ELST, same patient as A. Axial T1W image demonstrates a low-signal soft tissue mass with hyperintense foci in the posterior petrous ridge.

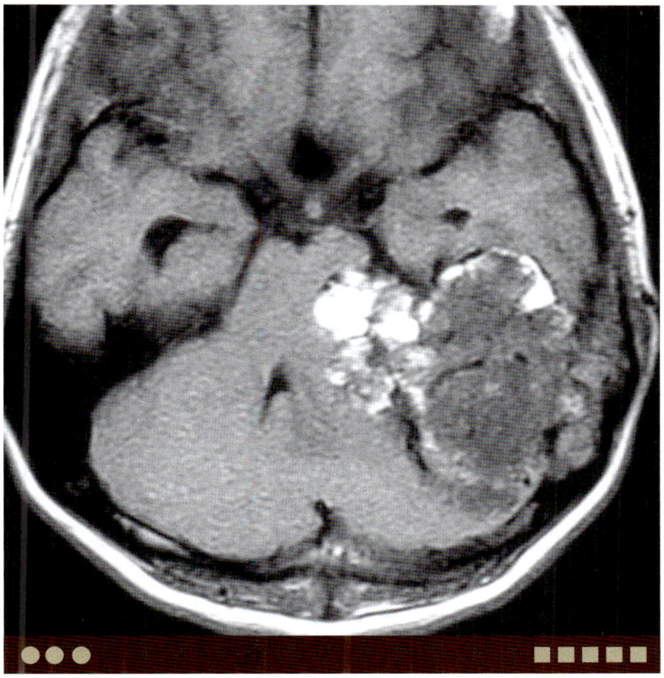

C. ELST in a different patient. Axial T1W image demonstrates a large tumor in the left temporal bone. Hyperintense foci suggesting hemorrhage and flow-voids are noted within the tumor (C-F, courtesy of Dr. Tomura, University of Akita, Japan).

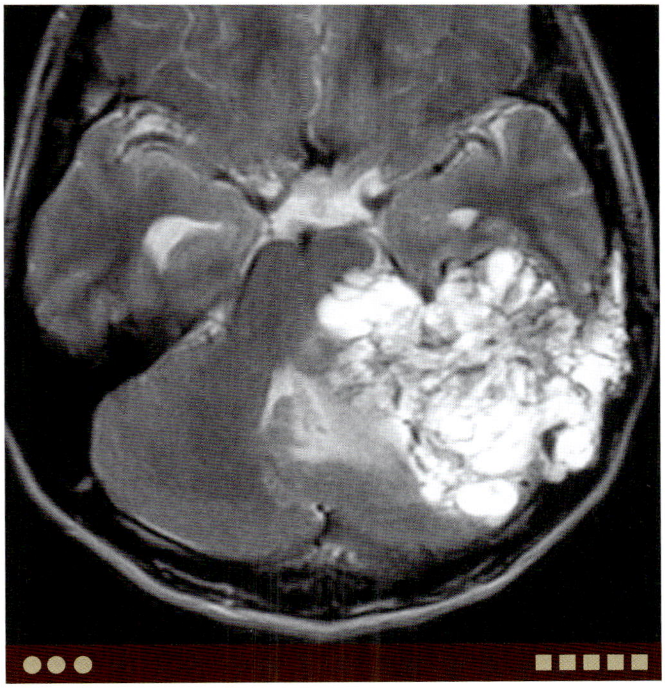

D. ELST, same patient as C. Axial T2W image demonstrates marked hyperintensity within the tumor.

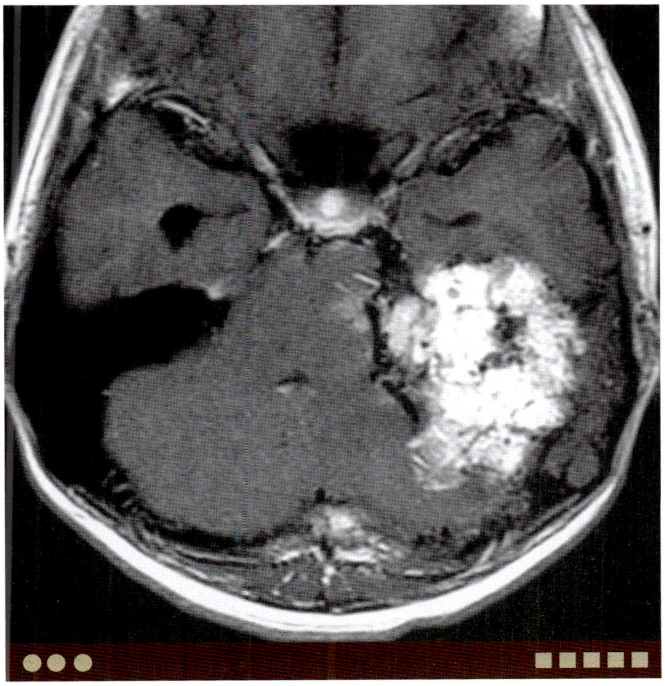

E. ELST, same patient as C. Axial postcontrast T1W image demonstrates marked enhancement of the tumor.

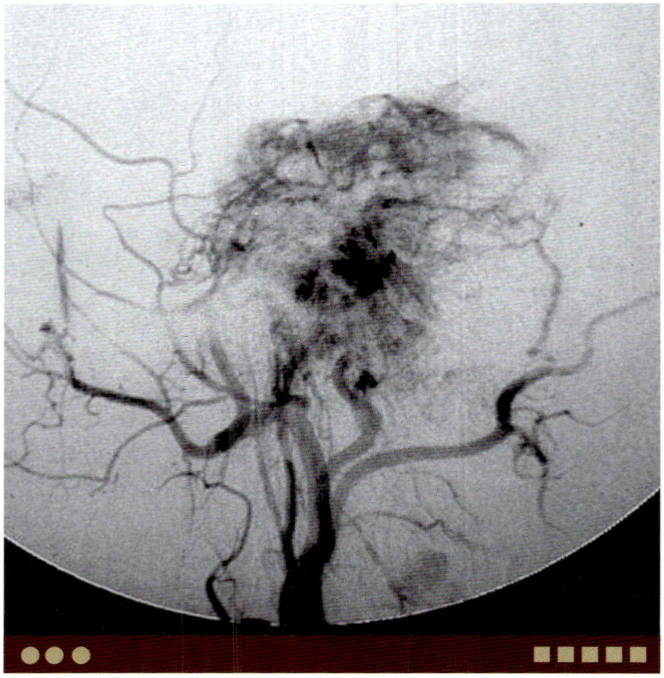

F. ELST, same patient as C. Left external carotid angiogram demonstrates heterogeneous tumor stain with supply from ECA branches.

DIFFERENTIAL DIAGNOSIS IMAGES (G-J)

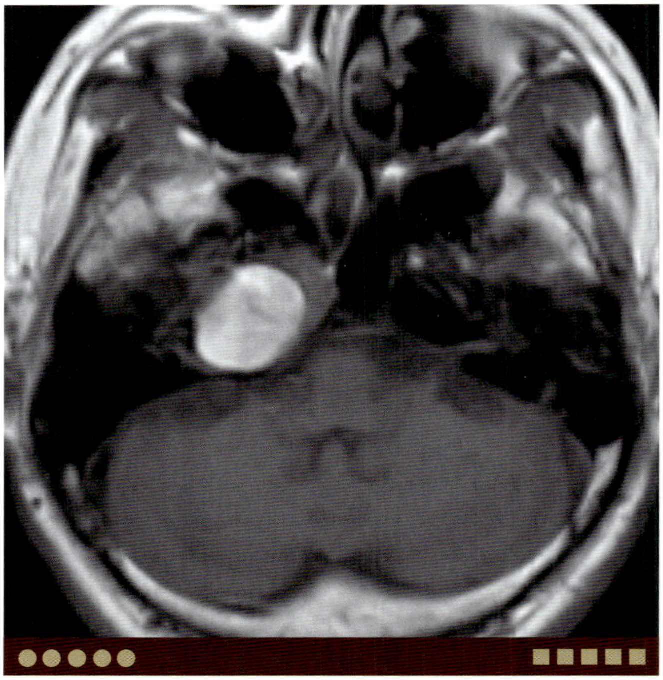

G. Cholesterol granuloma. Axial T1W image demonstrates a hyperintense expansile lesion in the right petrous apex.

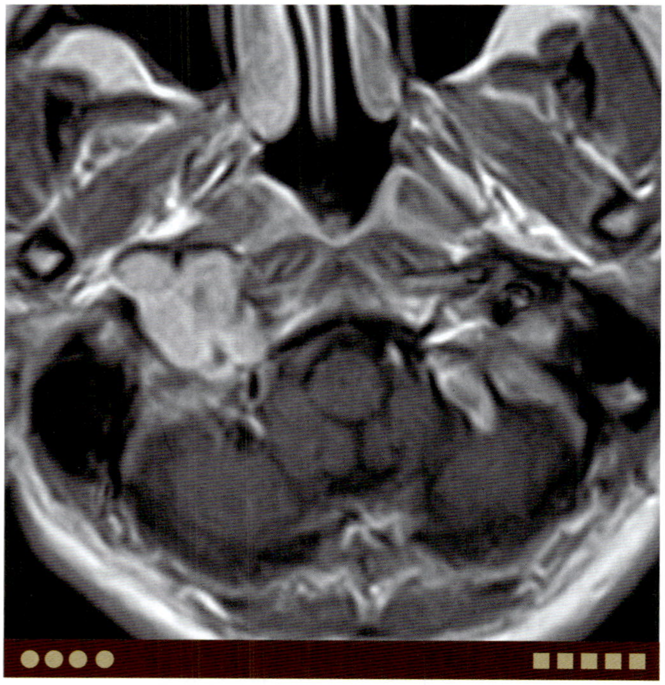

H. Jugular foramen schwannoma. Axial postcontrast T1W image demonstrates a well-demarcated enhancing lesion in the right jugular foramen.

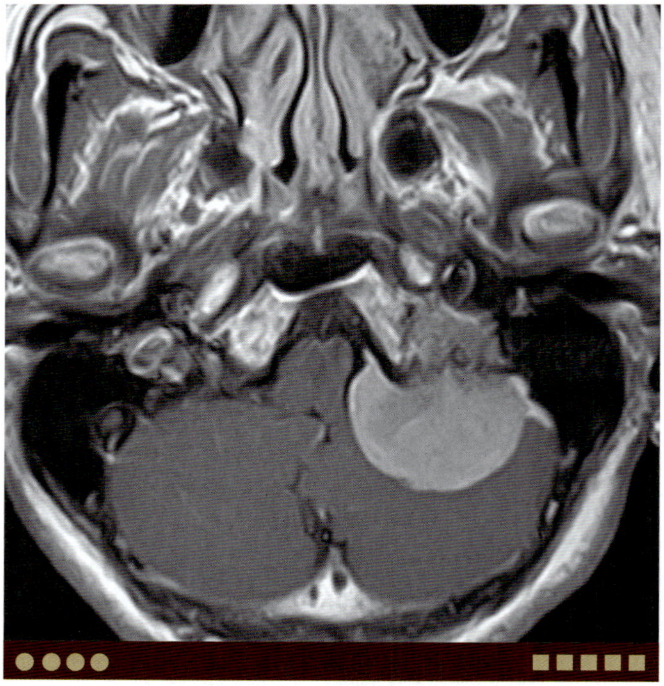

I. Jugular foramen meningioma. Axial postcontrast T1W image demonstrates an enhancing lesion with "dural tail."

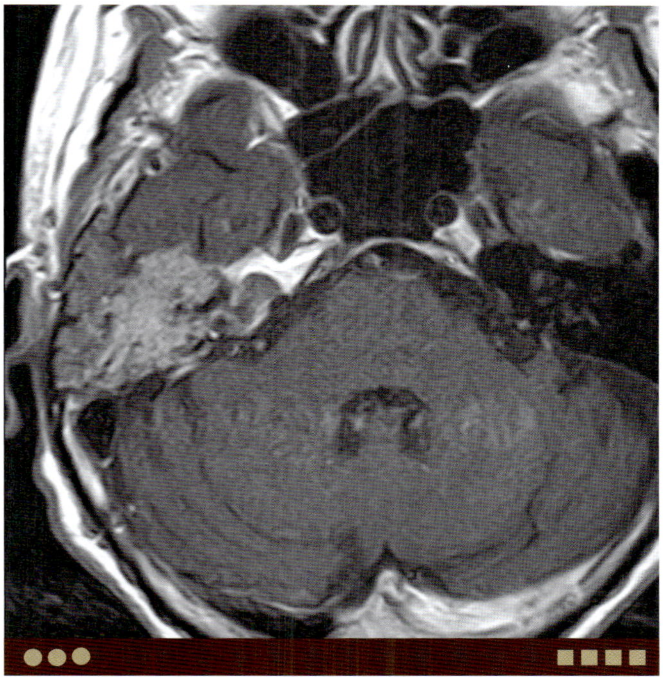

J. Metastatic hepatocellular carcinoma. Axial postcontrast T1W image shows an enhancing tumor with irregular margins in the right temporal bone. Flow-voids are noted within the tumor.

Case 1–37 Dural Arteriovenous Fistula

Takao Kodama

PRESENTATION

Pulsatile tinnitus.

FINDINGS

3D time-of-flight (TOF) MRA demonstrates abnormal visualization of venous structures.

DIFFERENTIAL DIAGNOSIS

- Normal visualization of dural sinus on 3D TOF MRA: Physiological reversed flow of the jugular vein can result in visualization of the sigmoid sinus on 3D TOF MRA, especially on the left side. Signal declines in the upper portion.
- Sigmoid sinus-jugular bulb pseudolesion: Increased signal or enhancement is seen in venous sinuses, particularly in the sigmoid sinus and jugular bulb depending on flow velocity and imaging parameters.
- Dural sinus thrombosis: Collateral or congested venous drainage can mimic dural arteriovenous fistula (AVF). Because the sinus thrombosis can be accompanied with dural AVF, angiography should be performed for diagnosis.
- Pial or mixed pial-dural arteriovenous malformation (AVM): AVM also shows abnormally dilated draining veins.

COMMENTS

This is a 46-year-old man with right pulsatile tinnitus.

Dural AVF is a heterogeneous group of lesions with common angioarchitecture of AV shunt in the dural sinus wall. It accounts for 10% to 15 % of all cerebrovascular malformations with AV shunting. Dural AVFs in adults are usually acquired. Although they may be idiopathic, they can occur as a result of trauma or venous occlusion. Dural AVFs can be associated with or secondary to dural venous sinus thrombosis. Venous drainage pattern including reflux to cortical veins is very important to speculate the risk and clinical outcome of dural AVFs (Cognard classification). In patients with pulsatile tinnitus and normal tympanic membrane, MRI and MRA should be initially performed. A thrombosed sinus may display isointensity on T1W and T2W images, and chronically thrombosed sinus usually enhances. Abnormal flow-voids can be seen in the dural sinus wall and retrograde drainage into cortical veins can be detected. Venous hypertension secondary to sinus occlusion can result in edema or hemorrhage in the brain parenchyma. Abnormal visualization of dural sinuses or cortical veins on 3D TOF MRA suggests AV shunting. Abnormal tiny vessels may be detected on MRA and careful investigation of source images is necessary. Time-resolved contrast augmented MRA may be useful for gross depiction of angioarchitecture and dynamics. In patients with "subjective" pulsatile tinnitus, catheter angiography should be performed even when MRI and MRA are negative. On catheter angiogram, multiple arterial feeders are typically seen, and dural branches of the external carotid artery are most common feeders.

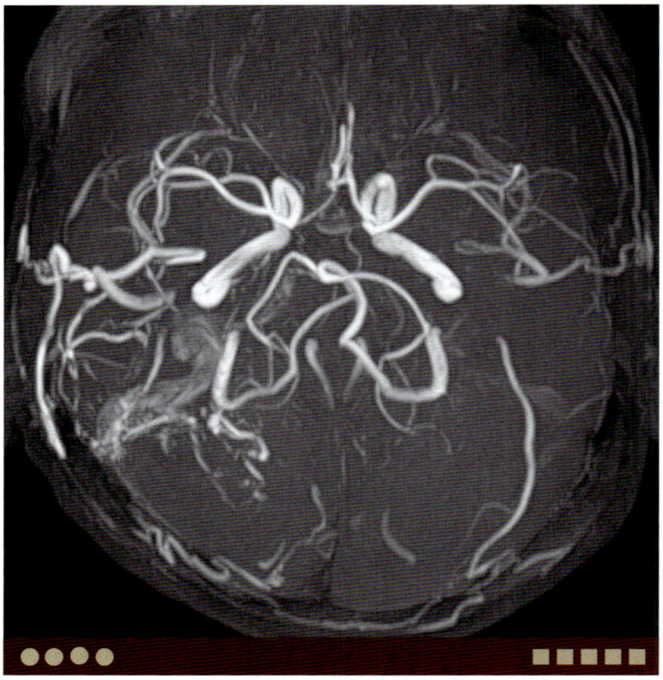

A. Dural AVF. 3D TOF MRA demonstrates abnormal visualization of the right sigmoid sinus with small "crack-like" vessels within the sinus wall.

PEARLS

- **Dural AVF is an important differential diagnostic consideration in patients with pulsatile tinnitus.**
- **Abnormal vessels in the wall of the dural sinus and AV shunting may be detected on MRI and MRA.**
- **MRI and MRA may be normal in patients with small dural AVF.**
- **If a patient has objective pulsatile tinnitus, catheter angiography is necessary to exclude dural AVF even with normal MRI and MRA.**

ADDITIONAL IMAGES (B-F)

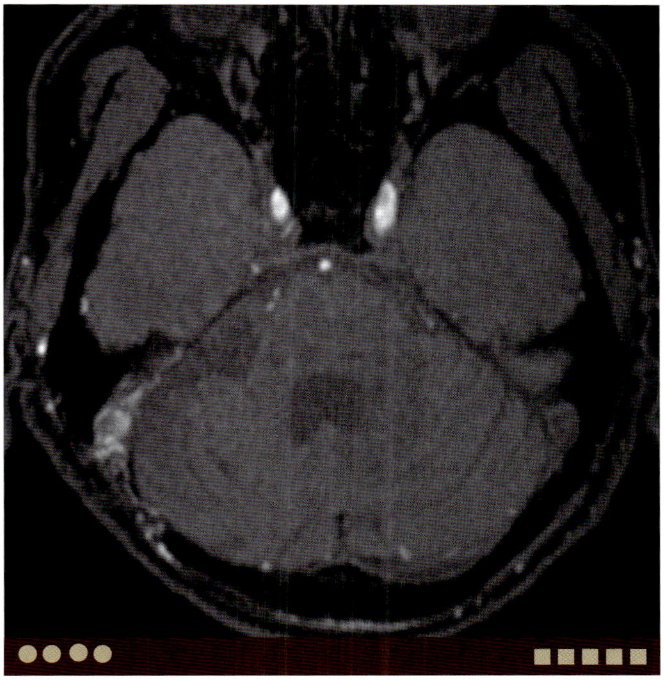

B. Dural AVF, same patient as A. Axial source image of 3D TOF MRA shows abnormal small vessels in and around the right sigmoid sinus more clearly.

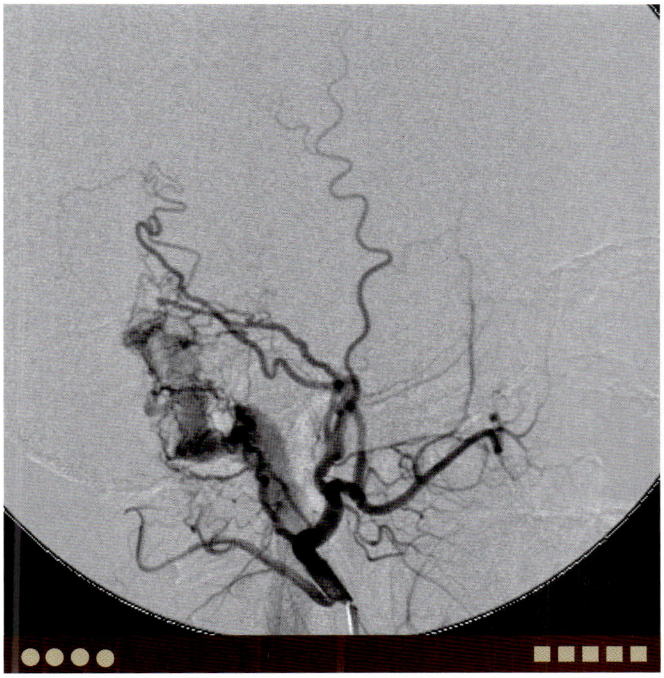

C. Dural AVF, same patient as A. Right external carotid angiogram demonstrates AV shunting in the wall of the patent sigmoid sinus (type I). Primary feeding arteries are the retroauricular artery, middle meningeal artery, and occipital artery.

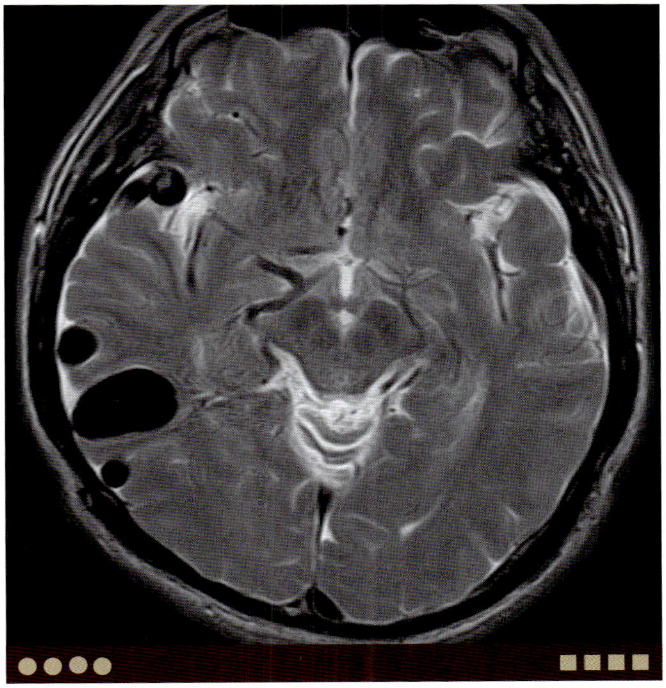

D. Dural AVF with sinus occlusion. Axial T2W image demonstrates significantly dilated cortical veins (flow-voids).

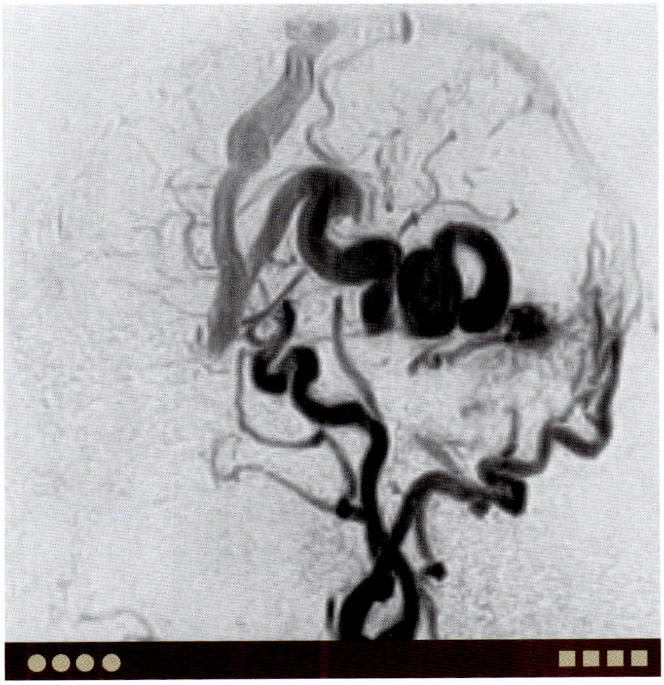

E. Dural AVF, same patient as D. Time-resolved contrast augmented MRA reveals dural AVF draining into a cortical vein with venous ectasia (type IV)

DIFFERENTIAL DIAGNOSIS IMAGES (G-J)

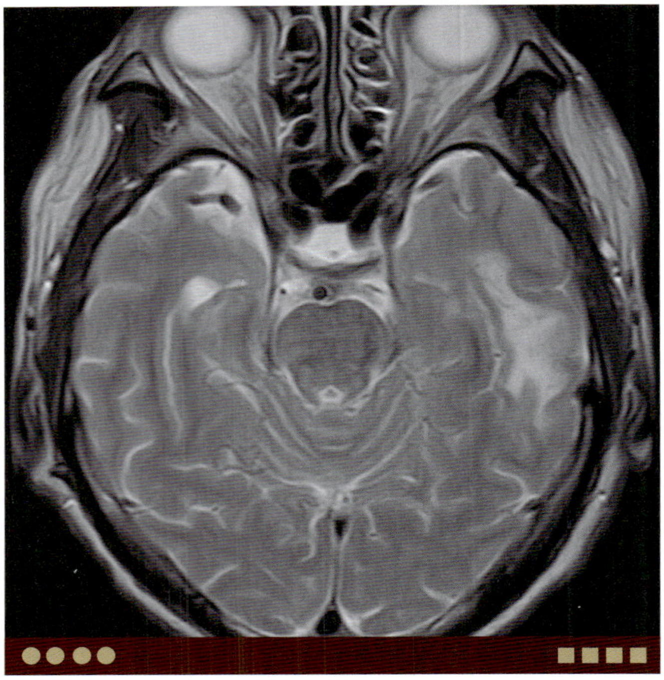

F. Dural AVF with sinus occlusion in a different patient. Axial T2W image demonstrates subcortical hyperintensity suggesting edema in the left temporal lobe.

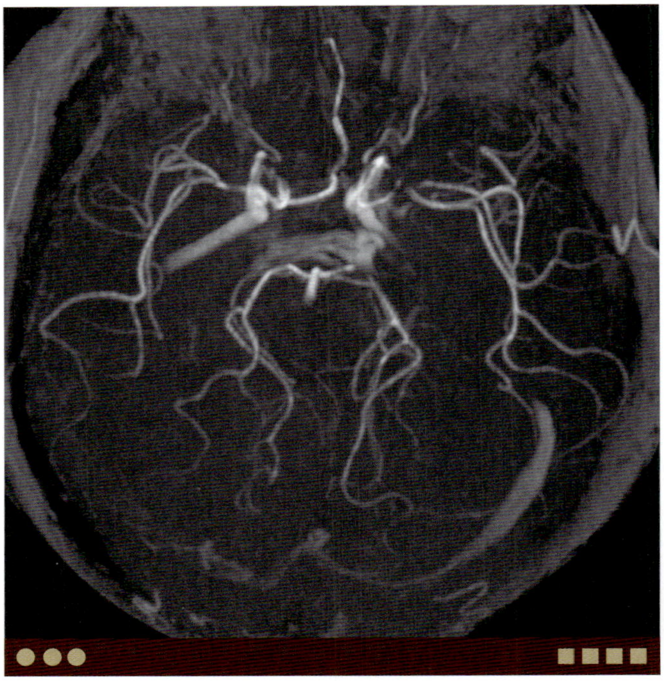

G. Normal visualization of the left transverse and sigmoid sinus on MRA. Retroclival venous plexus is also visualized.

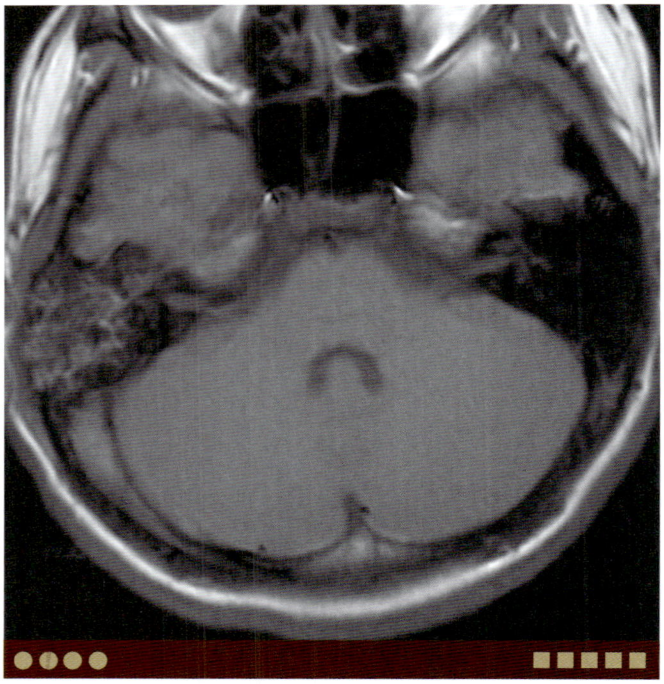

H. Transverse-sigmoid sinus thrombosis associated with temporal bone fracture. Right transverse sinus displays iso-to-slight hyperintensity on T1W MR image.

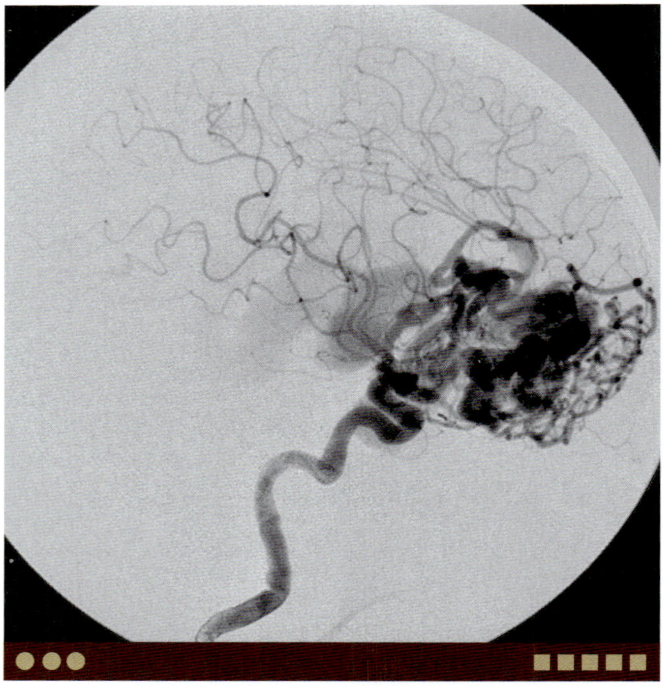

I. Mixed pial-dural AVM. Left internal carotid angiogram demonstrates AVM in the frontal base. Primary feeding arteries are branches of the middle cerebral artery.

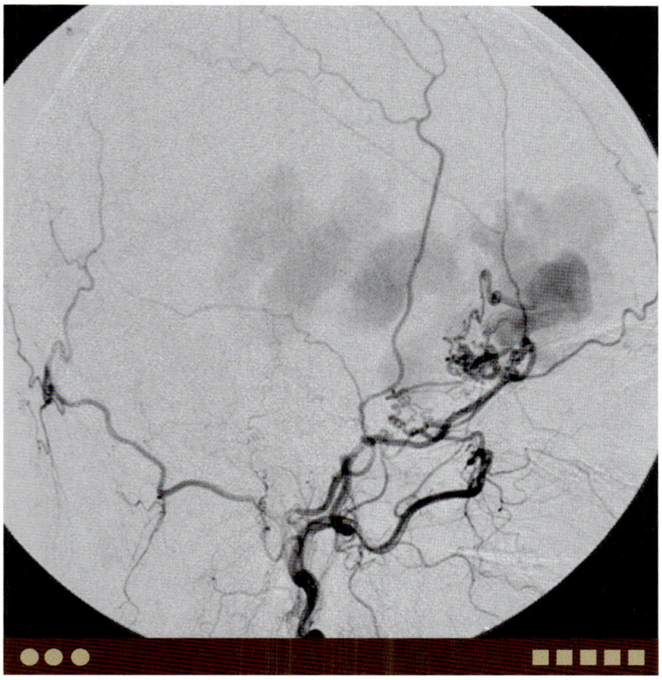

J. Mixed pial-dural AVM, same patient as I. Left external carotid angiogram demonstrates abnormal arteriovenous shunting via branches of the middle meningeal artery.

Case 1–38 Cystic Cochleovestibular Malformation, Incomplete Partition Type I

Takao Kodama

PRESENTATION

Congenital sensorineural hearing loss.

FINDINGS

The cochlea lacks the entire modiolus and cribriform area, resulting in a cystic appearance. There is an accompanying large cystic vestibule.

DIFFERENTIAL DIAGNOSIS

- Labyrinthine aplasia (Michel deformity): The entire labyrinth (cochlea vestibule, and semicircular canals) is absent.
- Cochlear aplasia: The cochlea is absent. Vestibule may be normal or hypoplastic.
- Common cavity deformity: The cochlea, vestibule, and semicircular canals form common cystic cavity.
- Incomplete partition type II (classic Mondini dysplasia): The cochlea consists of 1.5 turns in which the middle and apical turns coalesce to form a cystic apex. Large endolymphatic sac anomaly (large vestibular aqueduct syndrome) is frequently associated.
- Cochlear nerve hypoplasia with normal bony labyrinth: MRI with high-resolution heavily T2W image (MR cisternography) reveals defect of the cochlear nerve. The bony canal of the cochlear nerve may be stenotic.

COMMENTS

This is a 3-year-old boy with bilateral sensorineural hearing loss.

In most cases, imaging of a patient with congenital sensorineural hearing loss yields minimal findings, because most of these anomalies involve the membranous labyrinth. Jackler proposed a classification system of the inner ear anomalies based on the hypothesis that these anomalies result from a developmental arrest during different stages of embryogenesis. Incomplete partition including classic Mondini dysplasia results from late arrest of development and is the mildest form. Sennaroglu proposed two types of incomplete partition. Incomplete partition type I is characterized by a cystic appearance of the cochlea (cystic cochleovestibular malformation) and presumed to be caused by arrest of inner ear development at fifth week of embryogenesis. In type II, there is a cochlea comprised of normal basal turn and cystic apex accompanied by minimally dilated vestibule and enlarged vestibular aqueduct.

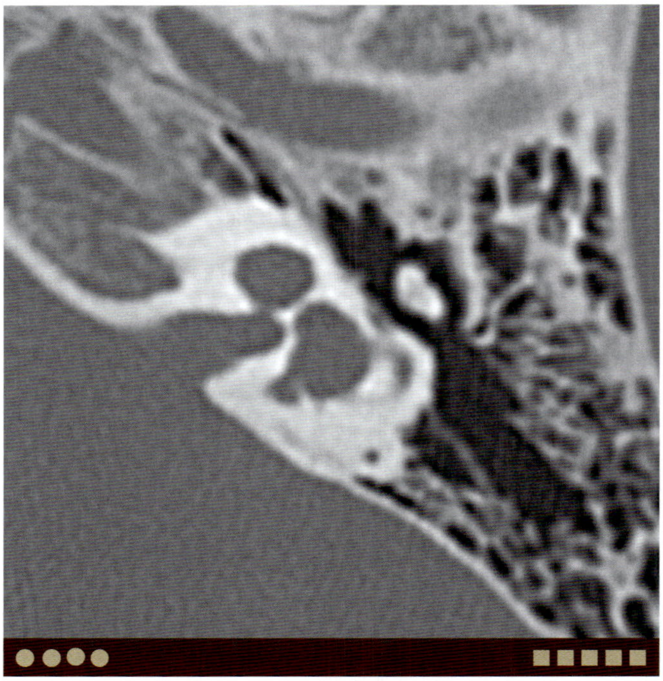

A. Cystic cochleovestibular malformation. Axial CT demonstrates cystic appearance of the cochlea with absent modiolus. The vestibule is mildly dilated.

Because no single classification is all-inclusive, most cochleovestibular malformations require precise description of specific anomalies pertaining to the cochlea, vestibule, semicircular canals, and aqueducts, not an eponym. Though bony labyrinth can be evaluated with CT, MRI with high-resolution T2W imaging is usually necessary to evaluate vestibulocochlear nerves.

PEARLS

- **Most cochleovestibular malformations require precise description of specific anomalies pertaining to the cochlea, vestibule, semicircular canals, and aqueducts.**
- **Anomalies of bony labyrinth can be evaluated by CT.**
- **MRI with MR cisternography is necessary to evaluate vestibulocochlear nerves.**

ADDITIONAL IMAGES (B-C)

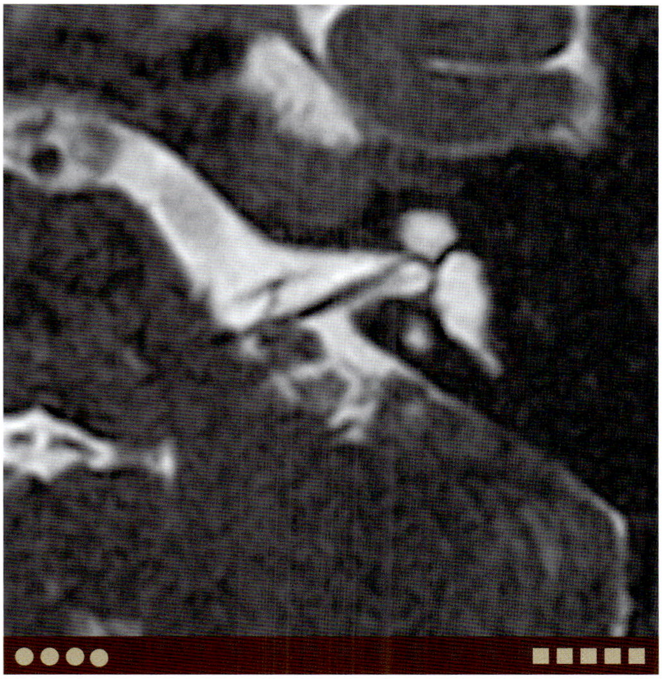

B. Cystic cochleovestibular malformation, same patient as A. Axial heavily T2W image reveals a normal vestibulocochlear nerve.

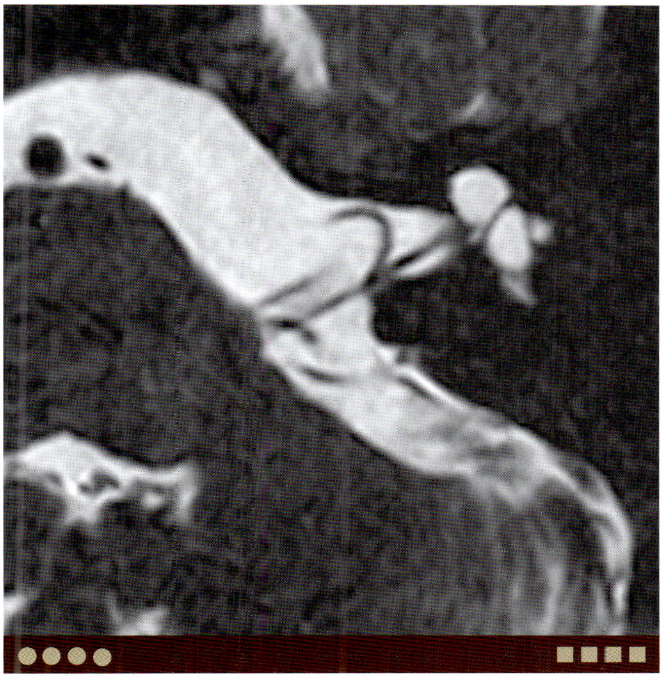

C. Cystic cochleovestibular malformation with cochlear nerve deficiency. Axial heavily T2W image reveals cochlear nerve deficiency with normal vestibular nerve.

DIFFERENTIAL DIAGNOSIS IMAGES (D-I)

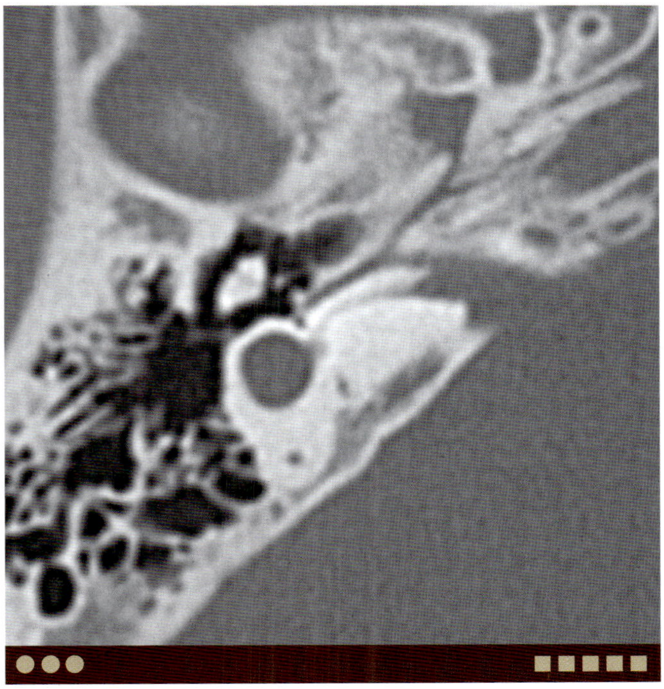

D. Cochlear aplasia. Axial CT shows absence of the cochlea with mildly dilated vestibule.

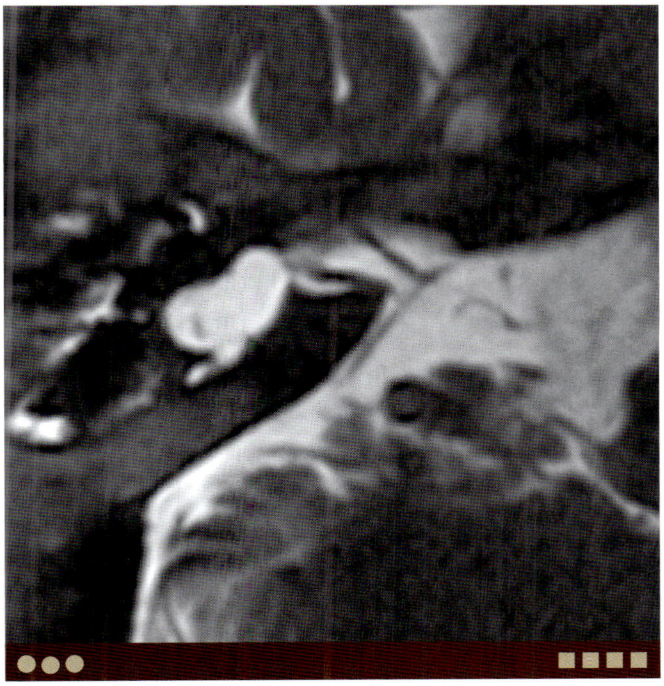

E. Common cavity deformity. Axial heavily T2W image demonstrates a common cystic cavity representing rudimentary cochlea and vestibule. Small posterior semicircular canal is present.

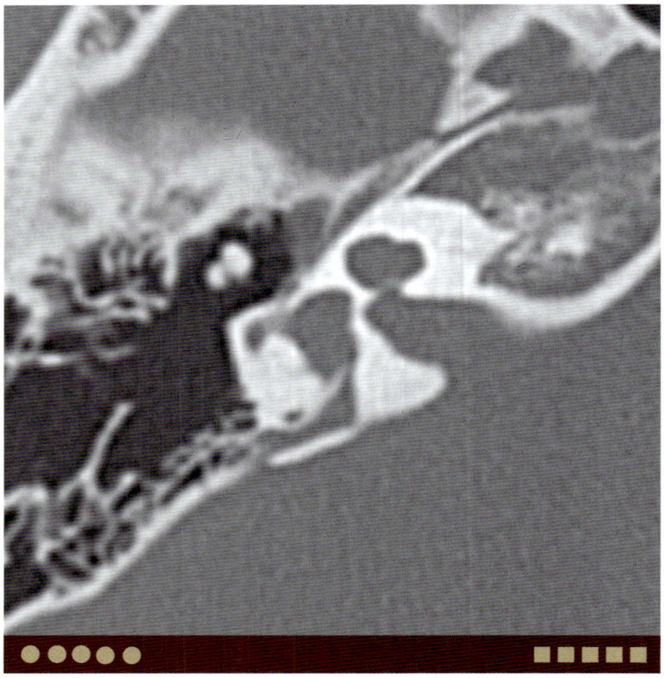

F. Large endolymphatic sac anomaly. Axial CT demonstrates modiolar deficiency and dilated vestibular aqueduct.

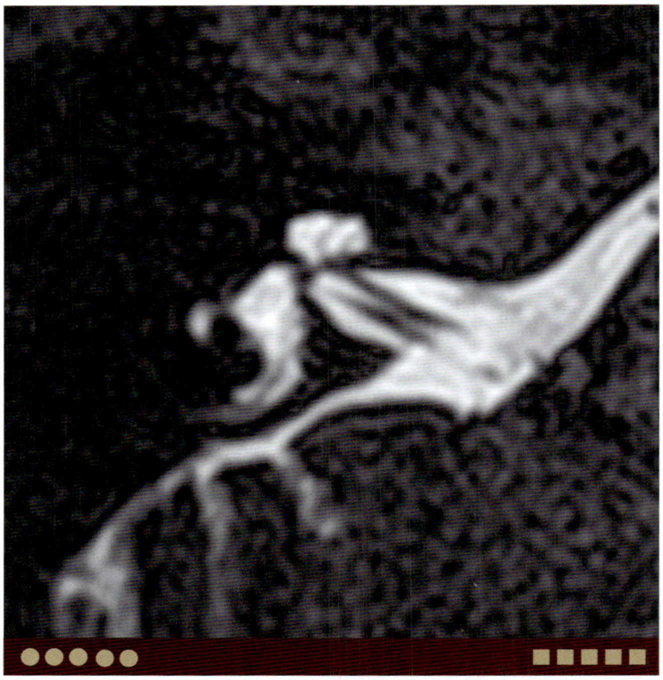

G. Large endolymphatic sac anomaly, same patient as F. Axial heavily T2W image shows dysplasia of the cochlea. The cochlear nerve is visualized normally.

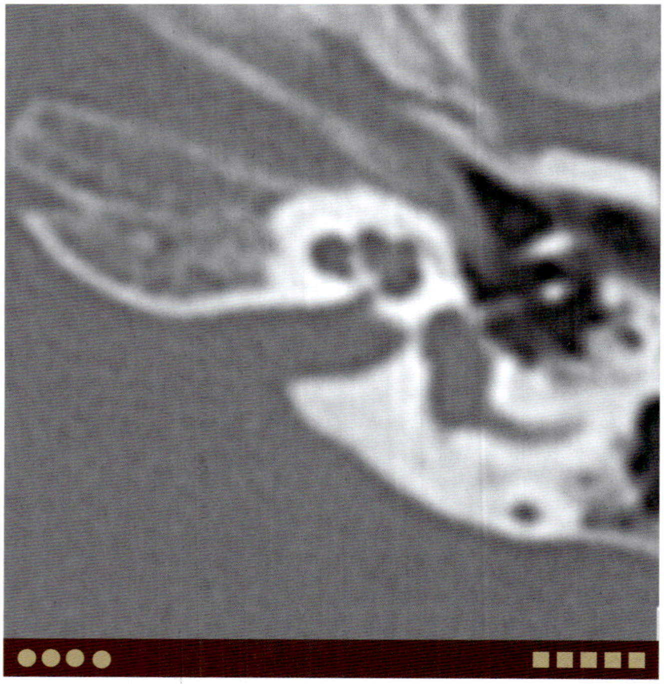

H. Cochlear nerve hypoplasia. Axial CT demonstrates normal cochlea, vestibule, and semicircular canals. The bony canal of cochlear nerve is stenotic.

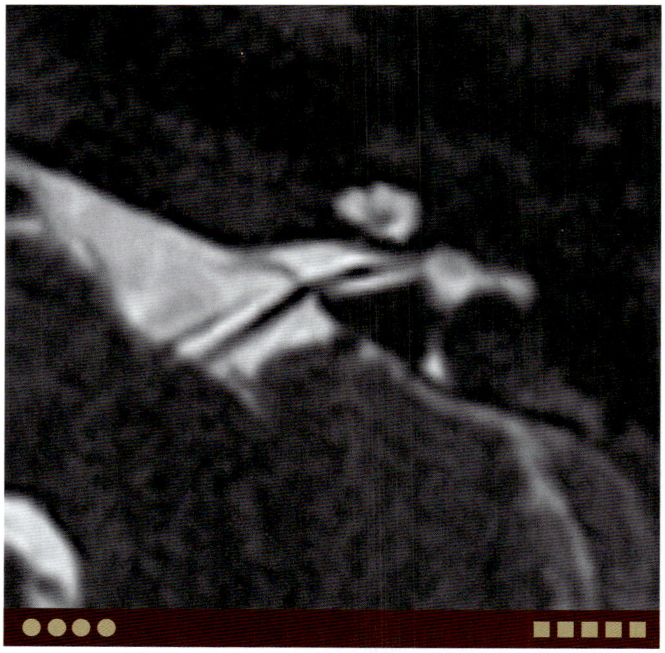

I. Cochlear nerve hypoplasia, same patient as H. Axial heavily T2W image reveals cochlear nerve deficiency and normal vestibular nerve.

Case 1–39 Semicircular Canal Bone Dehiscence

Rohini Nadgir, Osamu Sakai

PRESENTATION

Vertiginous symptoms and nystagmus in the setting of loud noises or pressure changes (Tullio phenomenon).

FINDINGS

Coronal CT demonstrates focal defect in the roof of the superior semicircular canal (SSC).

DIFFERENTIAL DIAGNOSIS

- Normal thinning of the superior or posterior semicircular canal walls: Normal thinning of bony coverage of the superior or posterior semicircular canals is often seen.
- Subarcuate venous malformation: This condition may cause bone defect in the SSC near the common crus.
- Erosion by cholesteatoma: The lateral semicircular canal is most susceptible to erosion by cholesteatoma, which results in labyrinthine fistula and vertiginous symptoms.
- Temporal bone fracture: Fractures through the temporal bone may involve the otic capsule and fracture planes could extend into the semicircular canals creating similar focal bony defect.

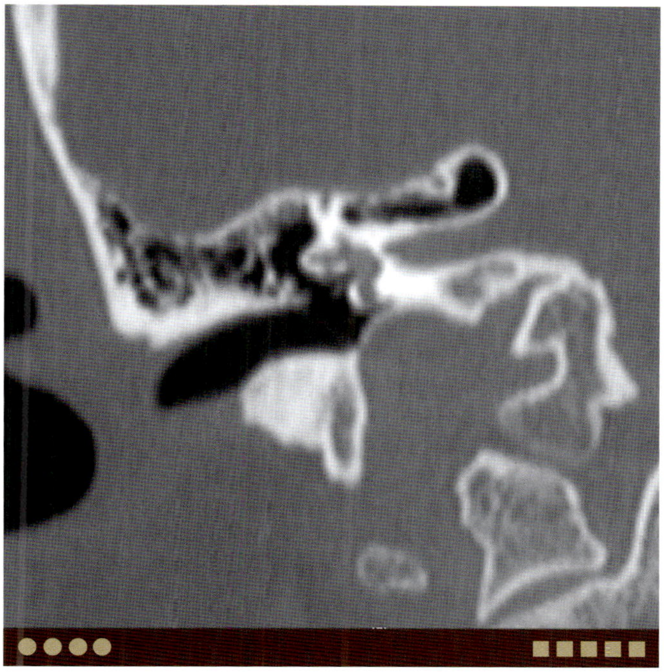

A. Superior semicircular canal bone dehiscence. Coronal CT demonstrates bone dehiscence of the roof of the superior semicircular canal.

COMMENTS

Focal dehiscence of the superior semicircular canal is seen more commonly on high-resolution CT temporal bone imaging than lateral or posterior canal dehiscence. Symptoms are attributed to the third "mobile" window, whereby the defect allows for pressure changes within the vestibule not normally experienced; this can allow for abnormal stimulation of hair cells within the vestibular apparatus, resulting in vertigo.

While the presentation of Tullio phenomenon is classically described, findings of canal dehiscence are often seen on imaging without the typical-associated clinical symptoms. It is nevertheless important to describe the finding, since truly symptomatic patients may benefit from surgical intervention, whereby the defect is packed via middle cranial fossa approach.

Thin section CT imaging of the temporal bones is required to make this diagnosis. Coronal reformations are a useful adjunct to interpretation. Some authors have suggested that additional reformations in the planes of Stenver and Poschl (perpendicular and parallel to the semicircular canal, respectively) can aid in the diagnosis.

Canal dehiscence is most often seen as an isolated finding, but can be seen as a consequence of some other destructive process that involves the arcuate eminence such as cholesteatoma, cholesterol cyst, aggressive infectious/inflammatory processes such as tuberculosis or syphillis, malignant neoplasms such as squamous cell carcinoma, and benign neoplasms such as facial nerve schwannomas and hemangiomas. Careful assessment for the integrity of other adjacent inner ear structures is important to exclude such associated processes.

PEARLS

- **Classically, patients present with vertiginous symptoms and nystagmus in the setting of loud noises or pressure changes (Tullio phenomenon).**
- **Thin section CT of the temporal bones is required to make this diagnosis. Multiplanar reformations can aid in the diagnosis.**
- **Canal dehiscence is most often seen as an isolated finding, but can be seen as a consequence of some other aggressive destructive inner ear process such as infection, inflammation, trauma, or benign and malignant neoplasms.**

ADDITIONAL IMAGES (B-G)

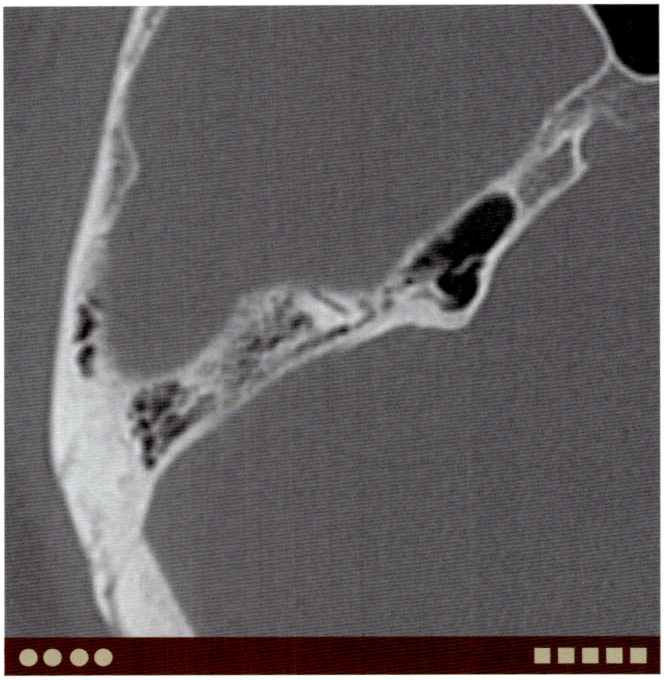

B. Superior semicircular canal bone dehiscence, same patient as A. Axial CT demonstrates bone dehiscence of the anterior portion of the SSC.

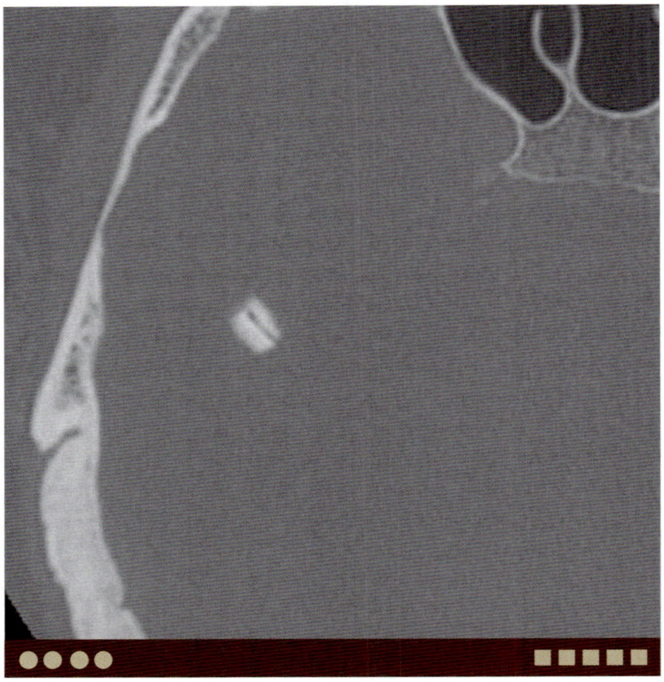

C. Superior semicircular canal bone dehiscence in a different patient. Axial CT demonstrates bone dehiscence of the posterior portion of the SSC.

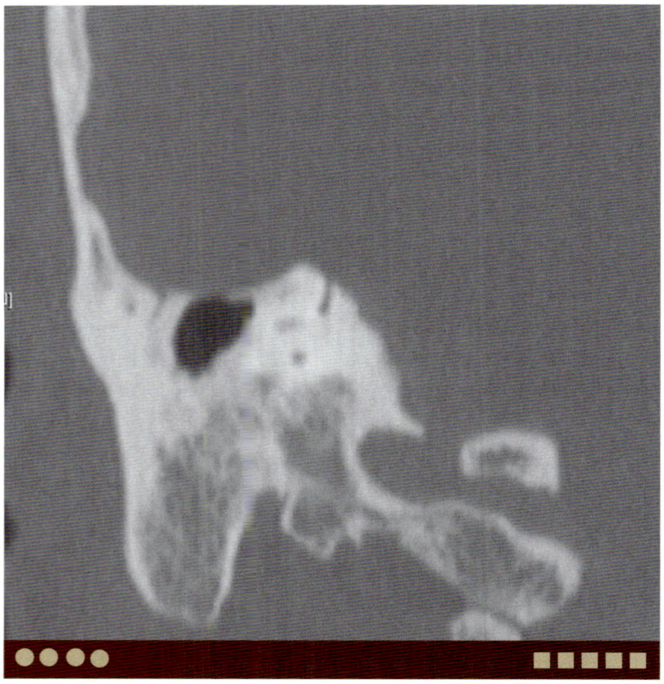

D. Superior semicircular canal bone dehiscence, same patient as C. Coronal CT demonstrates bone dehiscence of the roof of the SSC.

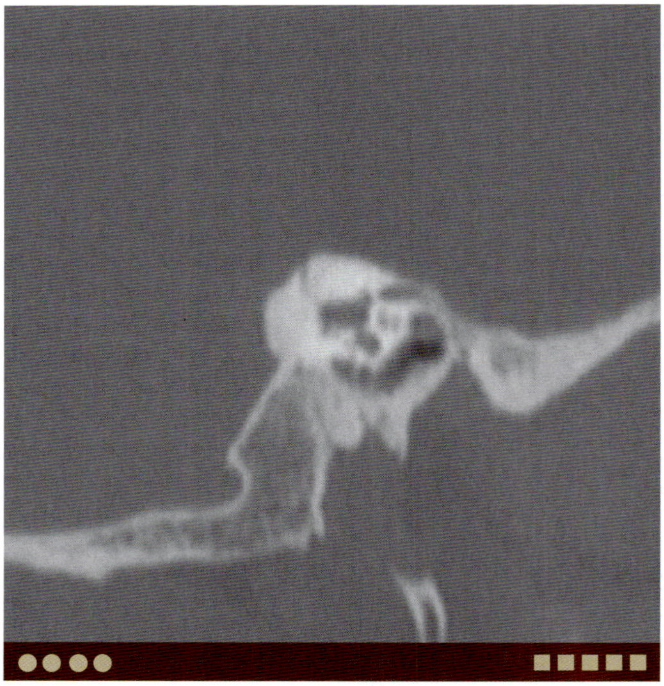

E. Superior semicircular canal bone dehiscence, same patient as C. Sagittal CT demonstrates bone dehiscence of the roof of the SSC.

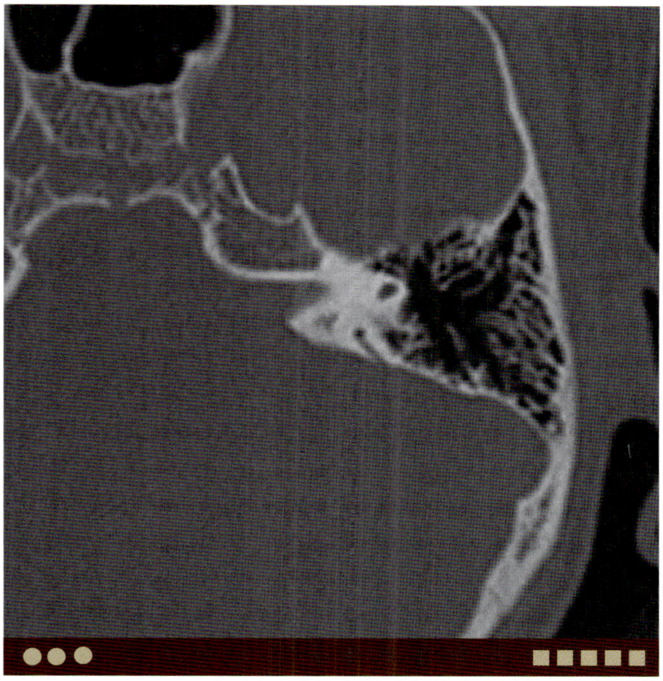

F. Posterior semicircular canal bone dehiscence. Axial CT demonstrates bone dehiscence of the posterior semicircular canal.

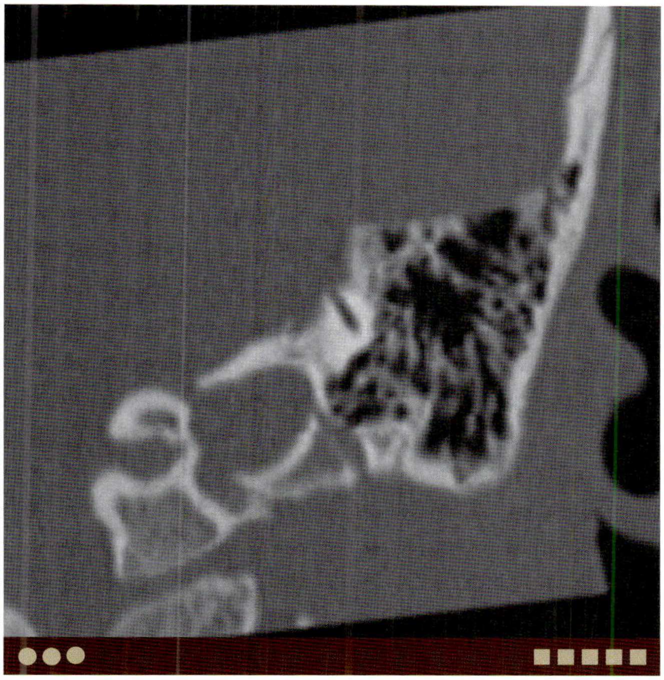

G. Posterior semicircular canal bone dehiscence, same patient as F. Coronal CT demonstrates bone dehiscence of the posterior semicircular canal.

DIFFERENTIAL DIAGNOSIS IMAGES (H-I)

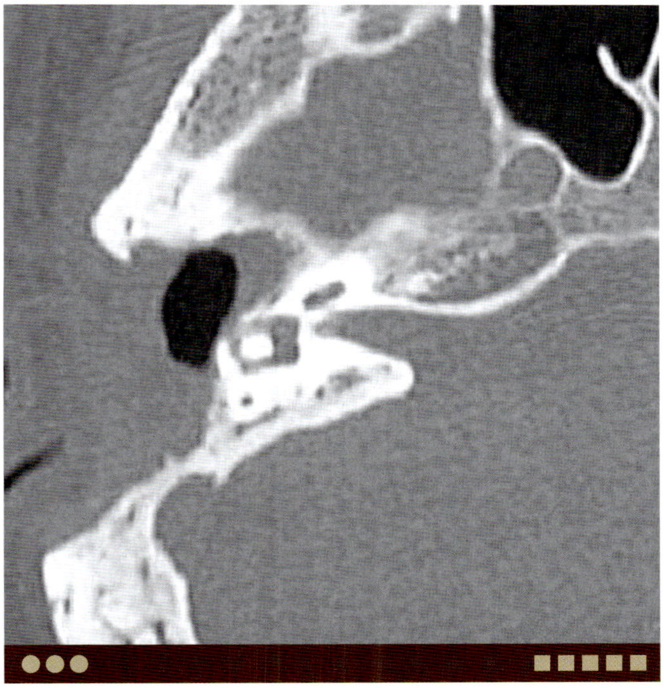

H. Labyrinthine fistula secondary to recurrent cholesteatoma, status postradical mastoidectomy. Axial CT demonstrates bone defect in the anterolateral portion of the lateral semicircular canal.

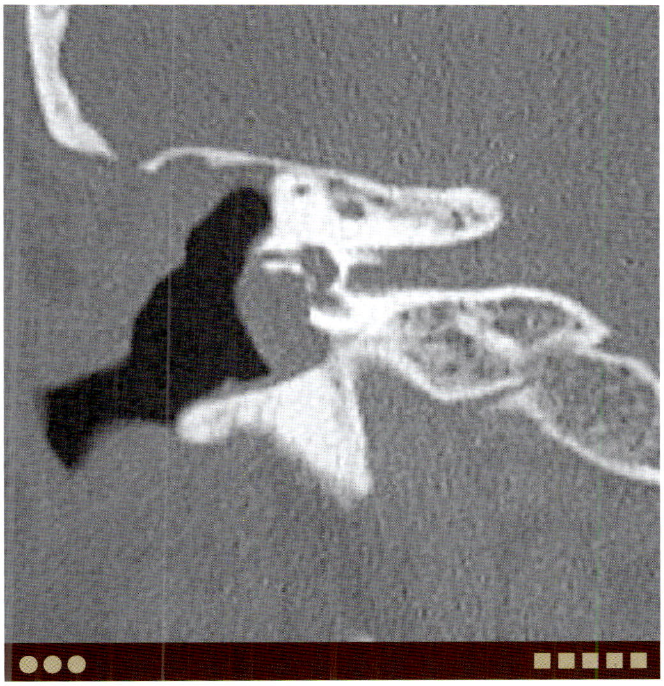

I. Labyrinthine fistula, same patient as H. Coronal CT demonstrates erosion of the lateral semicircular canal by the recurrent cholesteatoma.

Case 1-40 Cephalocele

Rohini Nadgir, Osamu Sakai

PRESENTATION

Typically asymptomatic, unless complicated by meningitis or CSF otorrhea.

FINDINGS

Smooth nonaggressive expansile defect in the mastoid or tympanic roof on CT. On high-resolution coronal MRI, herniation of meninges and CSF with or without brain tissue is seen through the defect.

DIFFERENTIAL DIAGNOSIS

- Arachnoid granulation: This is often seen in the dural venous sinuses as a "filling defect." This causes thinning of the skull and can be a cause of CSF leak, particularly when it occurs in the sphenoid bone.
- Cholesteatoma with tegmen dehiscence: Focal defects at the tegmen tympani can be resulted from bone erosion by cholesteatoma, which is often associated with other findings to suggest chronic otitis media and cholesteatoma, such as erosion of the scutum and ossicles.
- Erosive change from other middle or inner ear process: Any destructive process in the middle ear or skull base can be associated with bone defect that causes herniation of intracranial contents, including cholesterol cyst, aggressive infectious/inflammatory processes such as tuberculosis or syphillis, malignant neoplasms such as squamous cell carcinoma, and benign neoplasms such as facial nerve schwannomas and hemangiomas.

COMMENT

Cephalocele is a herniation of intracranial contents. This is most commonly an incidental finding on CT and MR imaging, unless the patient has complications of meningitis or CSF leak as a consequence. Cephaloceles can be congenital or acquired (posttraumatic or postsurgical). Regardless of cause, the defect should be surgically corrected in order to avoid serious complication of meningitis.

Coronal or sagittal thin slice CT can demonstrate the bone defect in the tegmen. Coronal or sagittal MRI is helpful to further evaluate the contents of herniated sac. If imaging demonstrates only CSF in the defect, the more appropriate term meningocele is used. If both brain and CSF are identified in the defect, it is called meningoencephalocele. However, more recently, the generalized term cephalocele is widely used for both conditions because differentiation is not always possible.

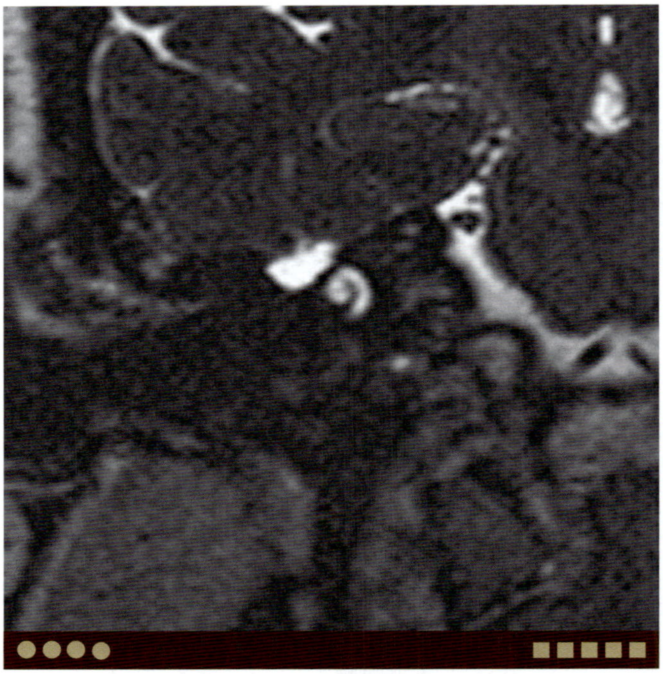

A. Cephalocele. Coronal T2W demonstrates a cystic lesion extending to the tympanic cavity through the tegmen.

In patients with associated meningeal signs, MRI is most useful to demonstrate possible secondary meningeal enhancement, subdural empyema, and brain abscess. In patients with CSF otorrhea, CT and MR imaging may not demonstrate very small defects; in these cases, Tc-99m or In-111-DTPA cisternography could be performed to confirm presence and general location of CSF leak.

PEARLS

- **Cephaloceles are typically asymptomatic, unless complicated by meningitis or CSF otorrhea.**
- **Thin section coronal or sagittal CT or MRI can detect bone defect and herniation of the intracranial contents through the defect.**
- **In patients with associated meningeal signs, MRI imaging is most useful to demonstrate possible secondary meningeal enhancement, subdural empyema, and brain abscess.**

ADDITIONAL IMAGES (B-F)

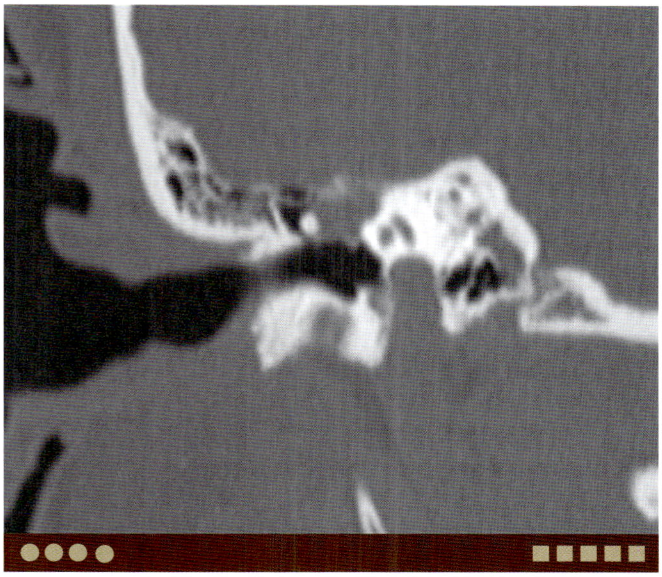

B. Cephalocele, same patient as A. Coronal CT demonstrates a cystic lesion extended through the ill-defined tegmen into the tympanic cavity, displacing the ossicles laterally.

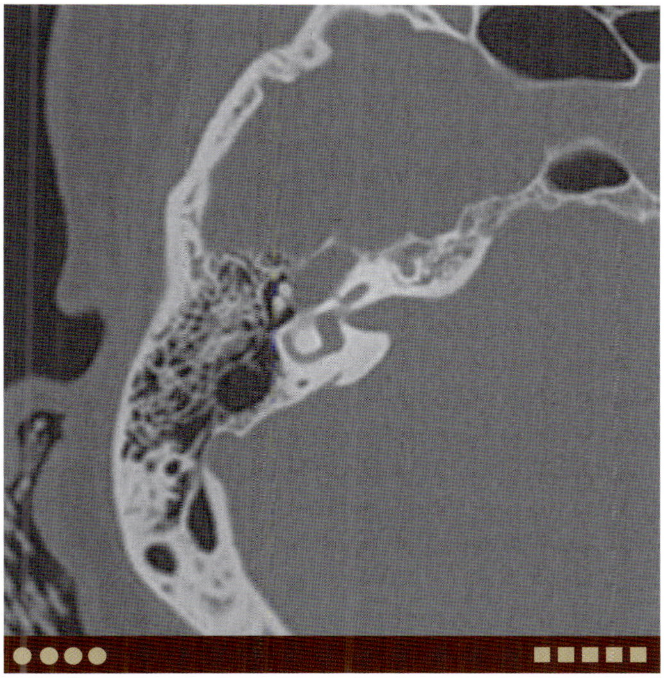

C. Cephalocele, same patient as A. Axial CT demonstrates a sharply marginated "mass" with bone remodeling in the tympanic cavity.

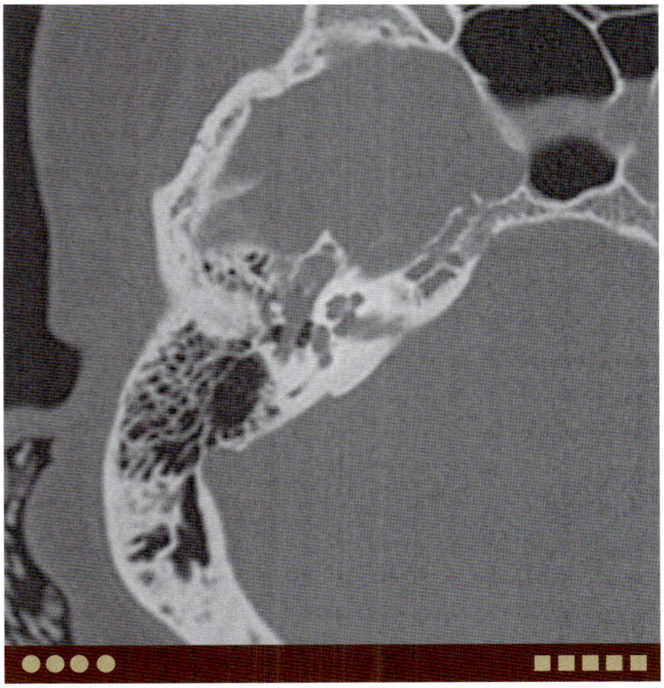

D. Cephalocele, same patient as A. Axial CT demonstrates the lesion extending along the tympanic segment of the facial nerve.

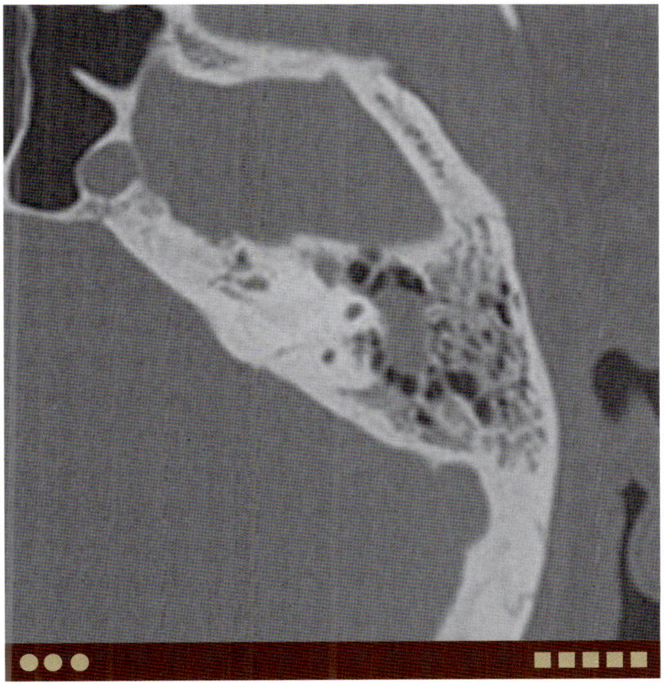

E. Cephalocele in a different patient. Axial CT demonstrates a smooth soft tissue/water density mass in the mastoid.

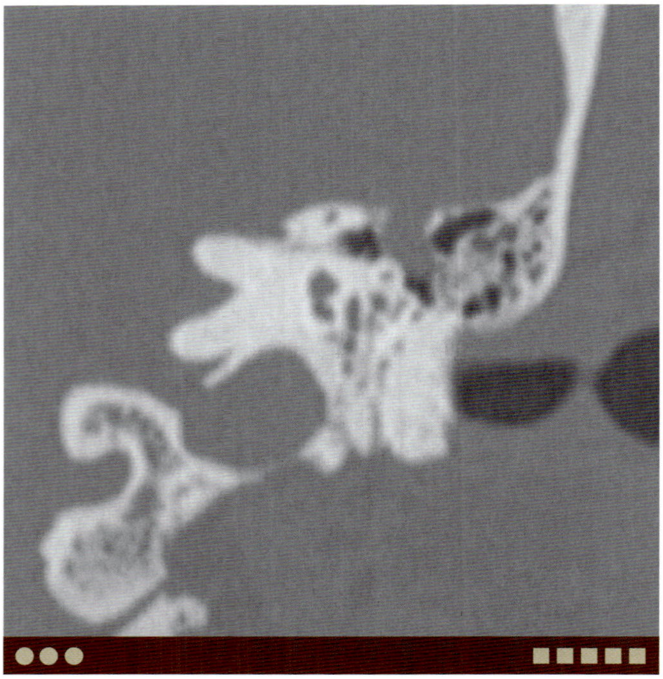

F. Cephalocele, same patient as E. Coronal CT demonstrates a soft tissue/water density mass extending inferiorly through the bone defect in the tegmen tympani.

DIFFERENTIAL DIAGNOSIS IMAGES (G-I)

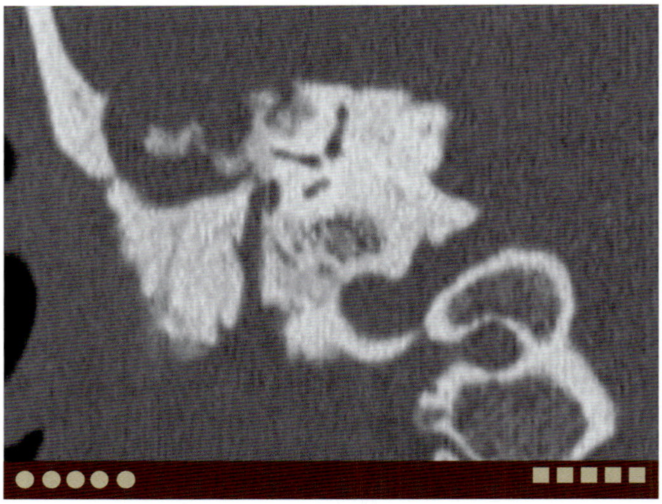

G. Cholesteatoma. Coronal CT demonstrates a large bone defect in the tegmen tympani. Note diffuse sclerotic change in the temporal bone due to chronic infection.

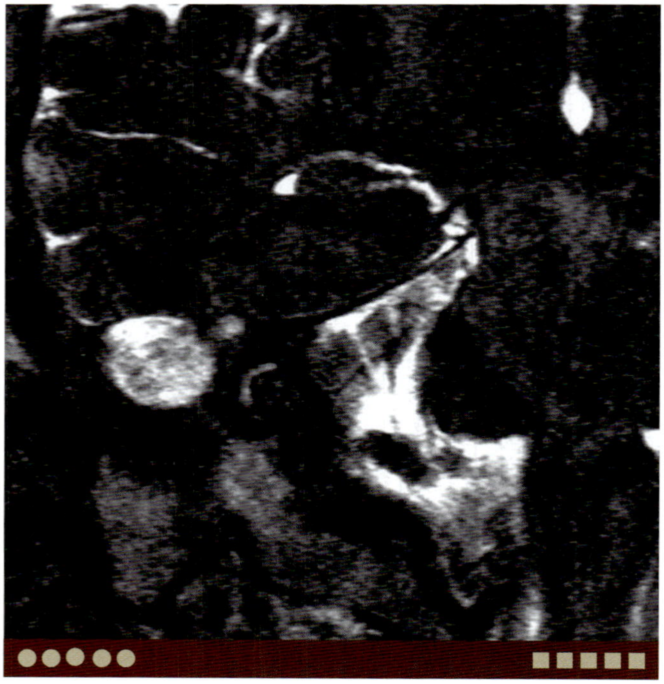

H. Cholesteatoma, same patient as G. Coronal T2W MR image demonstrates a cystic mass mildly compressing the inferior aspect of the temporal lobe.

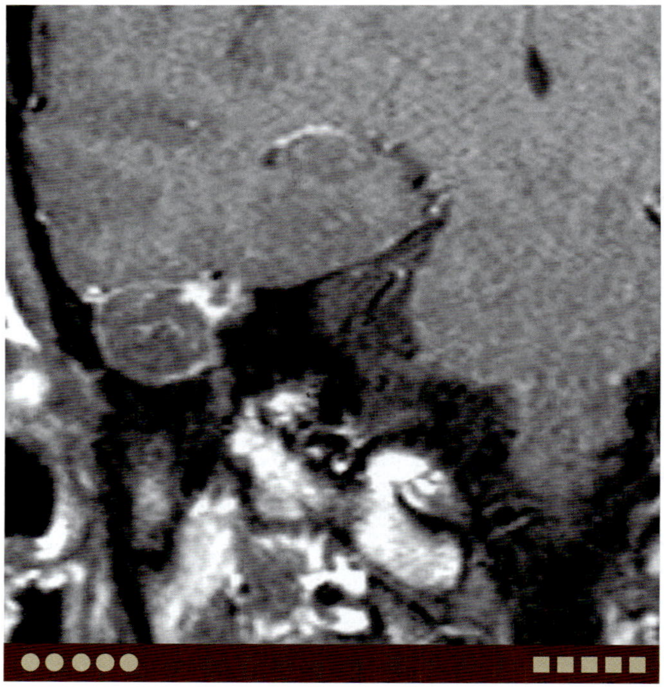

I. Cholesteatoma, same patient as G. Coronal postcontrast T1W MR image demonstrates peripheral enhancement of the lesion.

Case 1–41 Ossicular Anomaly

Takao Kodama

PRESENTATION

Congenital conductive hearing loss.

FINDINGS

Stapes superstructure and long process of the incus are not clearly identified.

DIFFERENTIAL DIAGNOSIS

- Erosion of ossicles associated with inflammatory middle ear disease: Long process of the incus can be eroded with chronic otitis media.
- Congenital cholesteatoma: Erosion of ossicles can be seen with a very small cholesteatoma.
- Luxation of the ossicular chain: Each ossicle is usually normal.

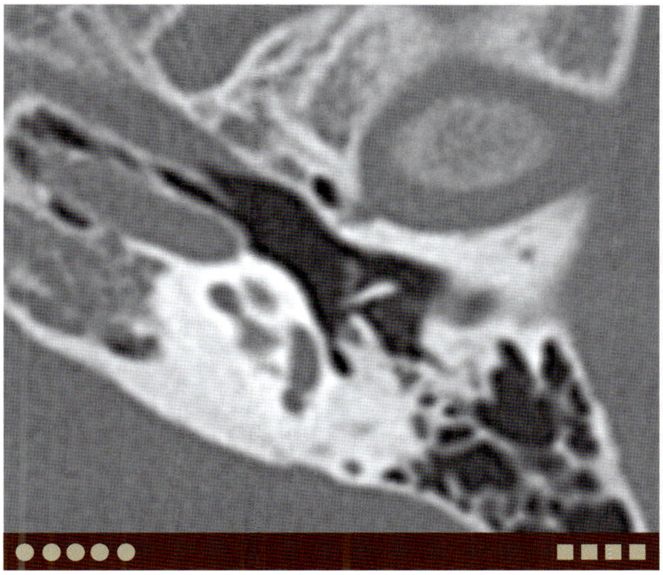

A. Ossicular anomaly. Axial CT demonstrates missing of the long process of the incus and stapes superstructure. The mastoid segment of the facial nerve course anteriorly.

COMMENTS

This is a 10-year-old boy with conductive hearing loss.

Congenital ossicular anomalies are commonly associated with dysplasia of the external auditory canal (EAC), and anomalies without external ear malformation are less common. Ossicular anomalies may be associated with some syndromes such as Klippel-Feil, Goldenhar, Treacher Collins, Pyle, and Apert syndromes.

Anomalies of the incudostapedial articulation are the most common isolated ossicular deformities when not associated with EAC dysplasia. The incudostapedial articulation develops between sixth and eighth weeks of gestation entirely from the second branchial arch. Anomalies (including absence) of the long process of the incus and the stapes superstructure are commonly seen. On axial CT, ossicular "parallel lines" in the mesotympanum is missed. The anomalies may be associated with oval window malformation. Stapes anomalies include aplasia, absence of the head and crura, hypoplasia, columnar-type deformity, and footplate fixation. CT diagnosis of congenital stapes fixation is only possible when the structures are thickened.

In cases with EAC dysplasia, the most commonly associated type of ossicular malformation is fusion of the malleus and incus resulting in absence of malleoincudal articulation. Patients with EAC dysplasia should be studied by CT, and the axial images are the most valuable for diagnosis of ossicular anomaly. Poor development of the middle ear cavity may be also seen.

The facial nerve course is often anomalous in the presence of ossicular anomalies as the nerve developed from the second branchial arch. The nerve is typically displaced inferiorly and medially, and may cross the oval window or lie inferior to it.

PEARLS

- **Congenital ossicular anomalies are commonly associated with EAC dysplasia.**
- **In cases with EAC dysplasia, the most commonly associated ossicular anomaly is fusion of the malleus and the incus.**
- **Anomalies of the incudostapedial articulation are the most common anomaly when not associated with EAC dysplasia.**
- **CT diagnosis of congenital stapes fixation is only possible when the involved structures are thickened.**

ADDITIONAL IMAGES (B-E)

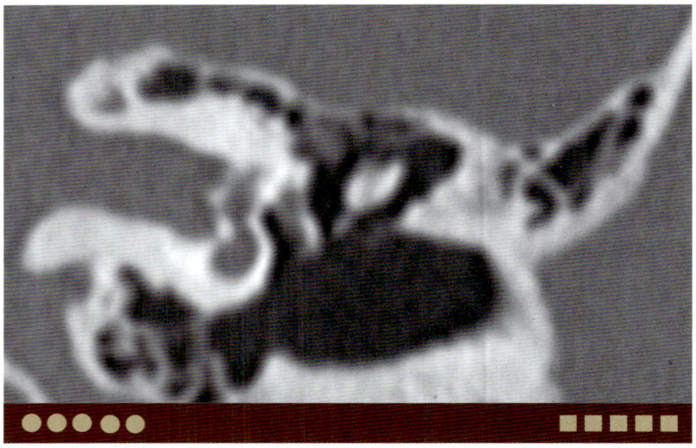

B. Ossicular anomaly, same patient as A. Coronal CT also reveals disconnections of the incudostapedial articulation. The facial nerve hangs over the oval window.

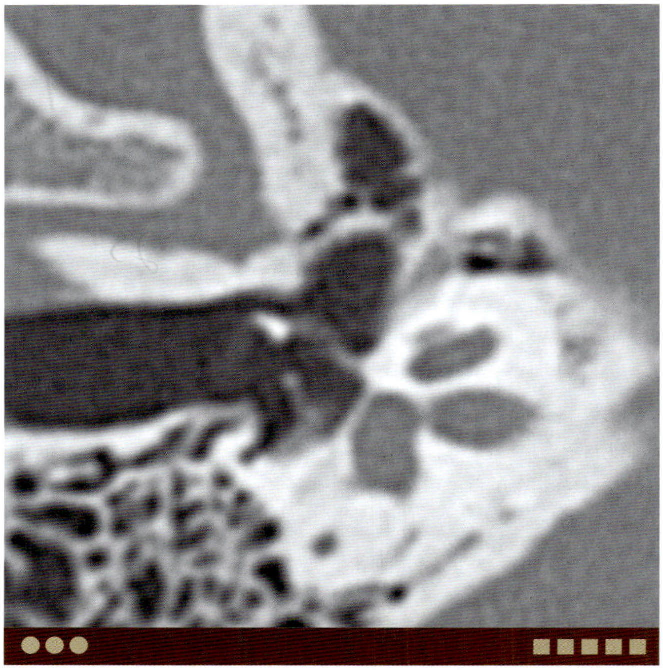

C. Congenital stapes anomaly ("monopod stapes"). On axial CT, the stapes superstructure consists of only a posterior crus.

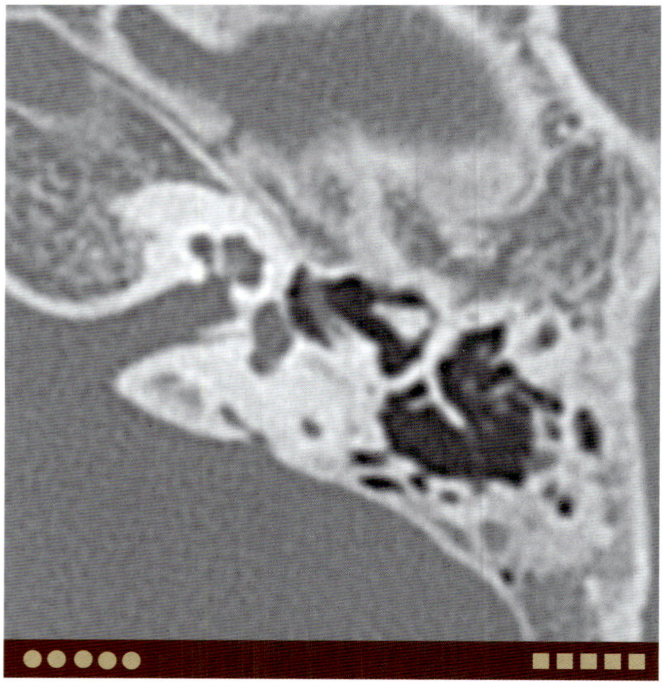

D. Atresia of EAC and microtia. On axial CT, the malleus and the incus are not clearly separated and only one anomalous ossicle is detected in the epitympanum.

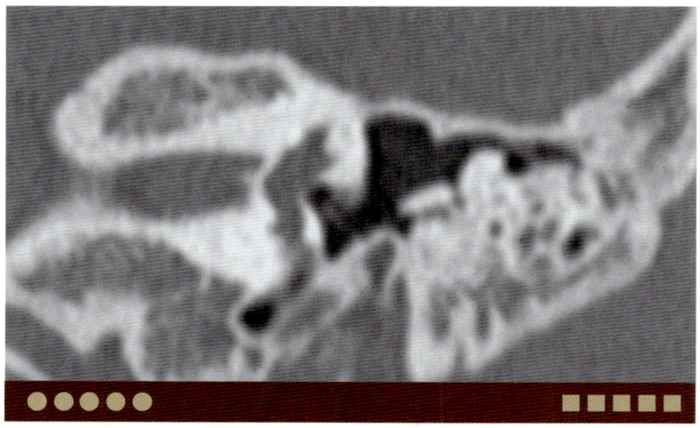

E. Atresia of EAC and microtia, same patient as D. Coronal CT demonstrates fusion of the anomalous ossicle to lateral wall of the epitympanum.

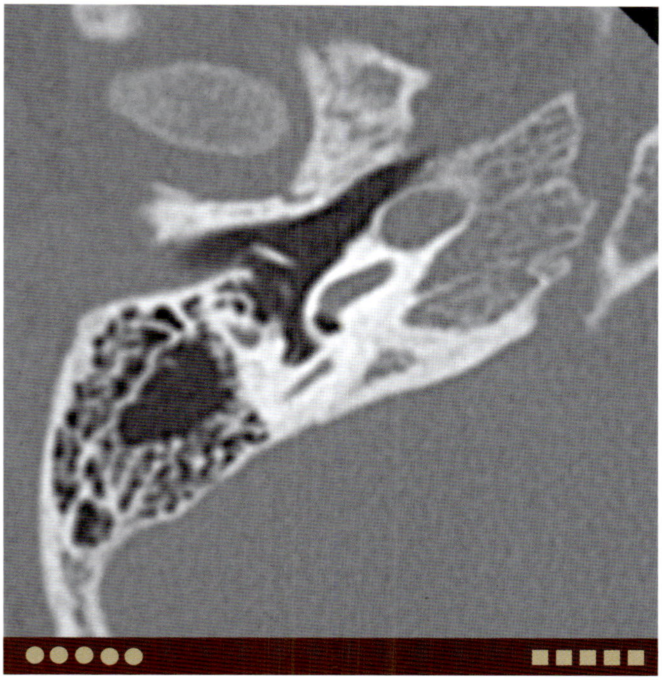

F. Inflammatory erosion of the long process of the incus. Axial CT reveals loss of the long process. Pathological findings suggested postinflammatory change.

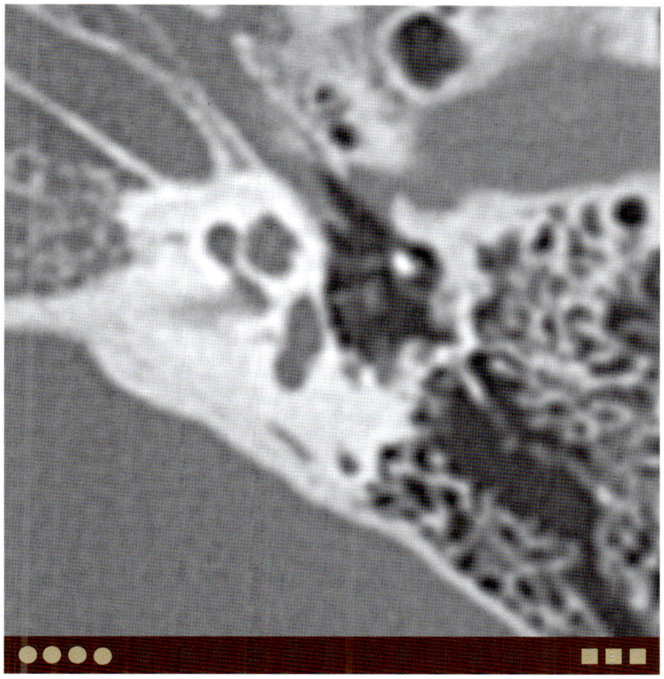

G. Congenital cholesteatoma. On axial CT, the long process of the incus cannot clearly be detected. Soft tissue suggesting a cholesteatoma is not apparent.

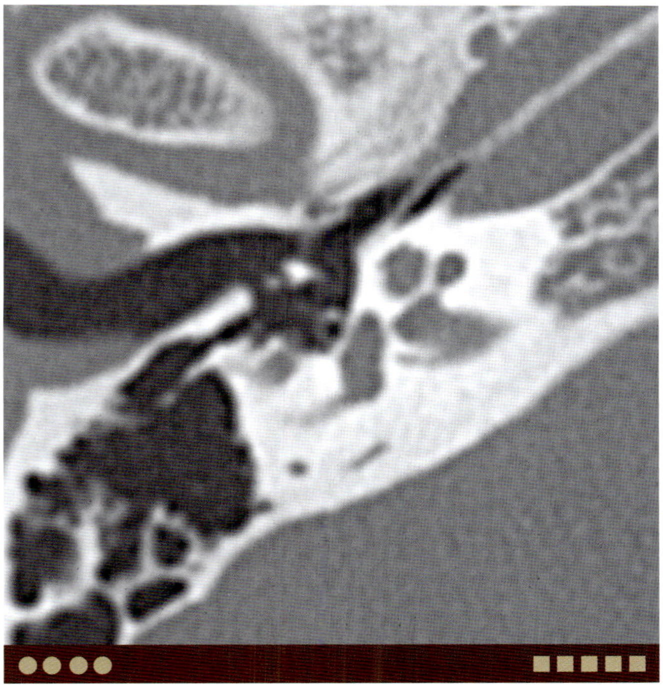

H. Ossicular luxation in a patient with a long history of conductive hearing loss. Axial CT demonstrates disconnection of the incudostapedial articulation.

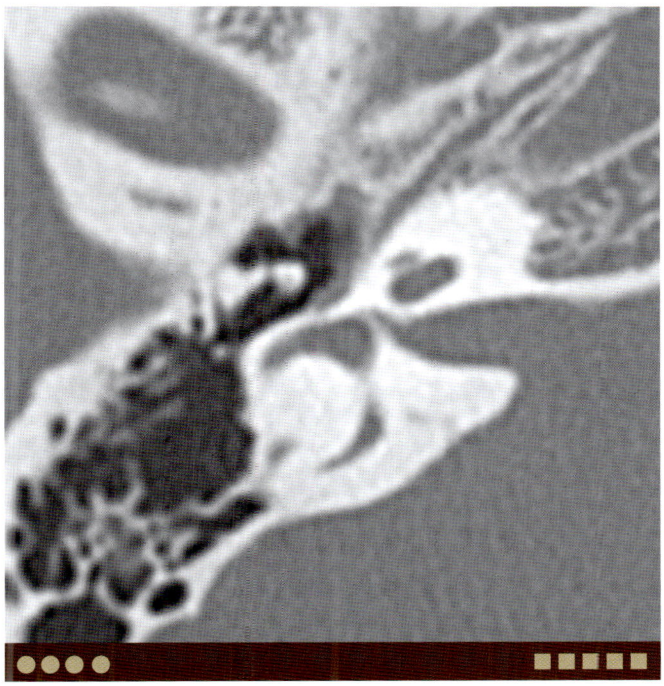

I. Ossicular luxation, same patient as H. Axial CT demonstrates luxation of the malleoincudal articulation.

Chapter 2

SKULL BASE

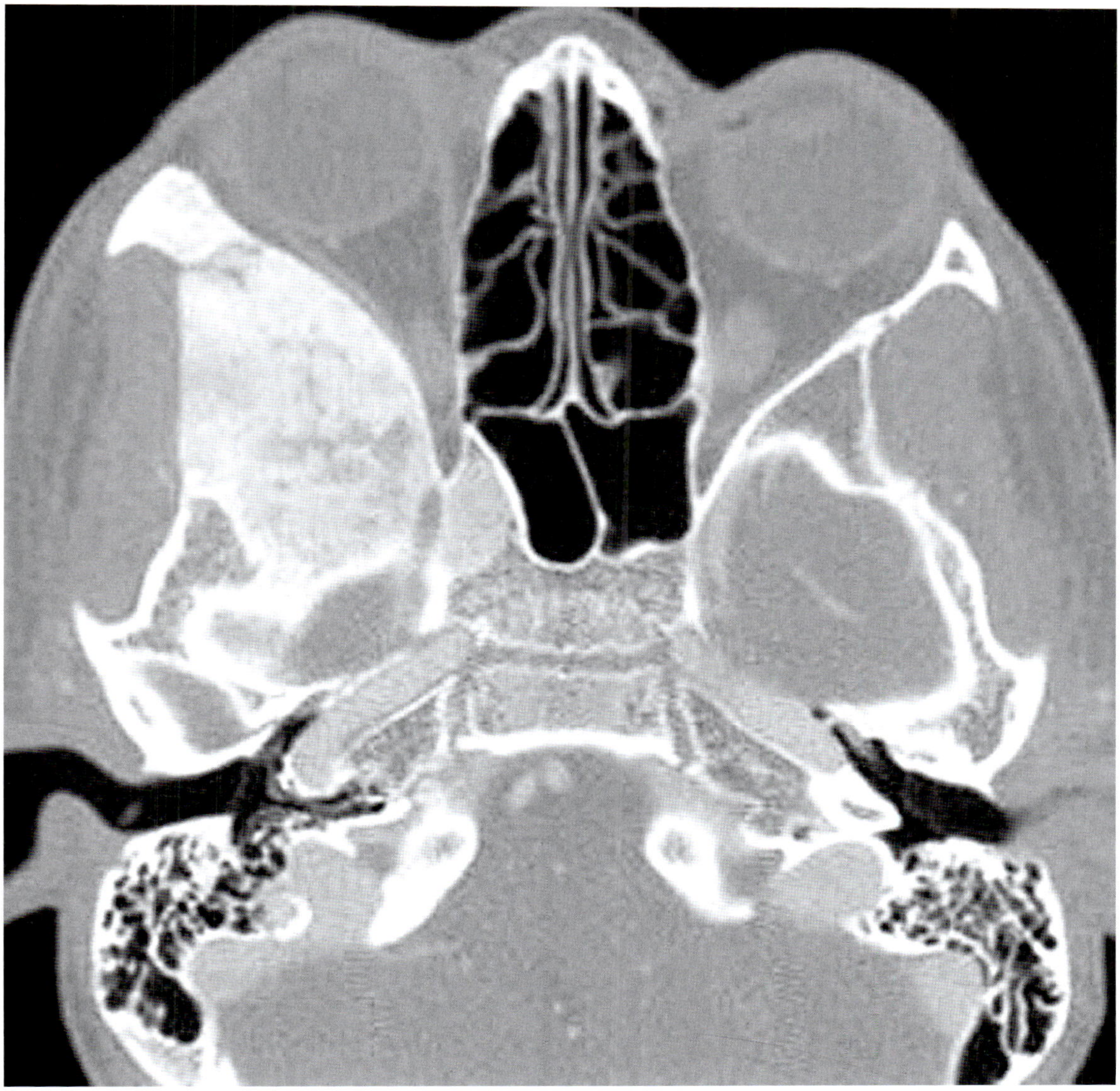

Case 2–1 Fibrous Dysplasia

Osamu Sakai, Rohini Nadgir

PRESENTATION

Facial asymmetry.

FINDINGS

CT demonstrates an expansile ground-grass density osseous lesion.

DIFFERENTIAL

- Ossifying fibroma This is a benign fibro-osseous lesion composed of lamellar bone with prominent osteoblastic rimming in dense fibrous stroma demonstrating nearly identical radiological findings to fibrous dysplasia.
- Paget's disease: This is a common disease of unknown etiology, usually seen in elderly people but unusual before age 40. Involvement of the skull and skull base is common, although any bone can be affected.

COMMENTS

This is a 16-year-old adolescent with facial asymmetry.

Fibrous dysplasia can occur anywhere in the body, however often seen in the face and skull base in the head and neck. This can be seen in any age group but often discovered before 20 years of age. It is subdivided into three types: monostotic, polyostotic, and Albright syndrome. Usually, it is unilateral, and in the head and neck, often involves contiguous bones on the same side. Skull and skull base lesions often cross midline, and maxillary and mandibular lesions on the same side, even discontinuous, are often encountered.

On CT, a ground-grass appearance is thought to be a typical finding; however, cystic change is also commonly seen. Radiologically, fibrous dysplasia may be difficult to differentiate from other benign fibro-osseous lesions. Narrowing of osseous canals and foramina is seen due to bone expansion and this occasionally results in cranial nerve impairment.

On MRI, fibrous dysplasia demonstrates low signal on T1W and variable signal on T2W images, depending on degree of fibrotic or osseous changes. "Fresh" fibrotic change demonstrates high signal on T2W images and strong enhancement after contrast.

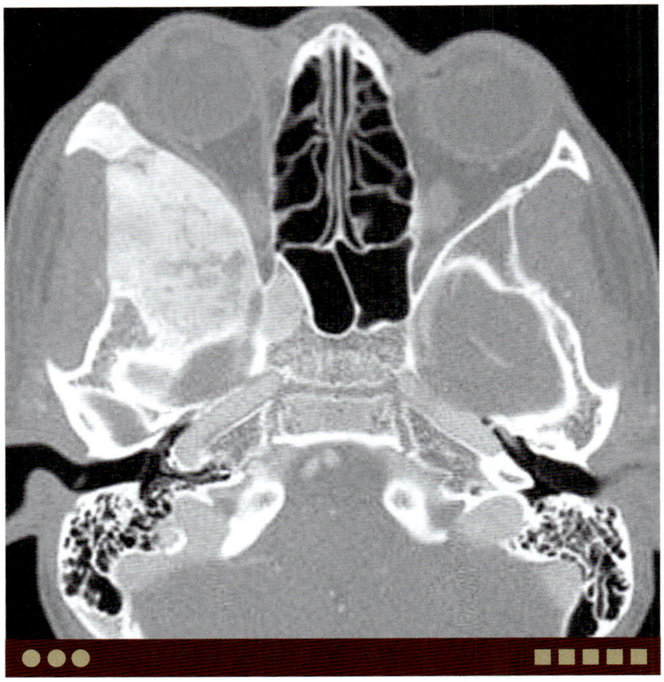

A. Fibrous dysplasia. Axial CT demonstrates a ground-grass appearance, slightly expansile lesion in the right sphenoid bone.

In Albright syndrome, skin lesions, precocious puberty and polyostotic fibrous dysplasia are seen. The patient is usually a young female.

PEARLS

- **Fibrous dysplasia is a common benign fibro-osseous lesion.**
- **It is usually unilateral and involves contiguous bones in the head and neck.**
- **A ground-grass appearance is a typical finding on CT; however, cystic change is also commonly seen.**
- **Fibrous dysplasia demonstrates low signal on T1W and variable signal on T2W images.**

ADDITIONAL IMAGES (B-E)

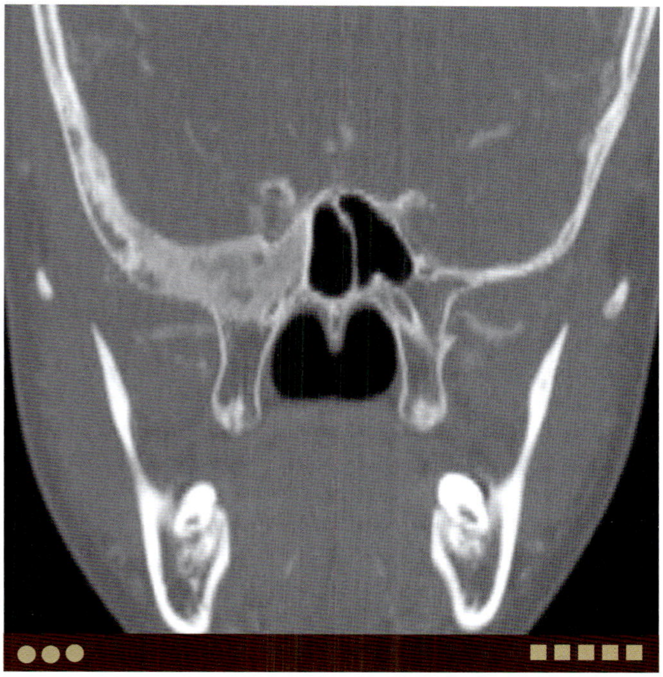

B. Fibrous dysplasia, same patient as A. Coronal CT demonstrates a ground-grass expansile lesion in the right sphenoid bone. Note the foramen rotundum and Vidian canal are involved and mildly narrowed.

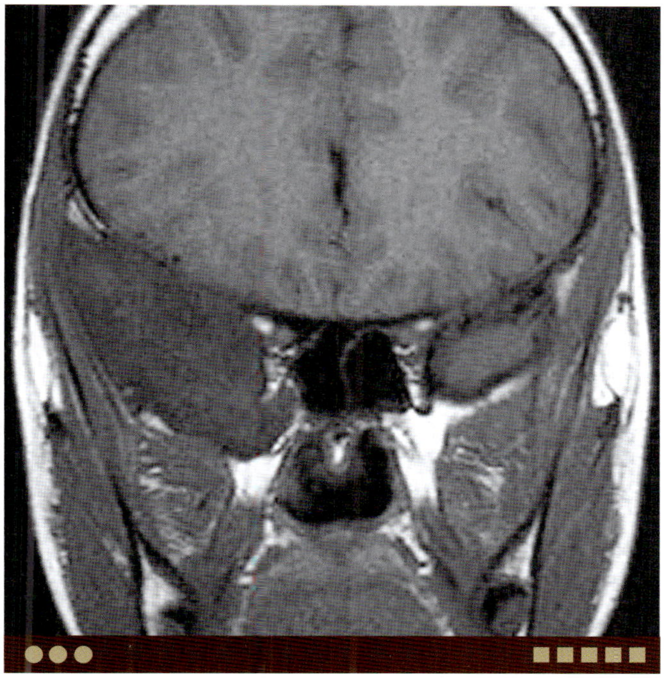

C. Fibrous dysplasia, same patient as A. Coronal T1W image shows an expansile lesion in the right sphenoid bone demonstrating slightly heterogeneous but predominantly low signal.

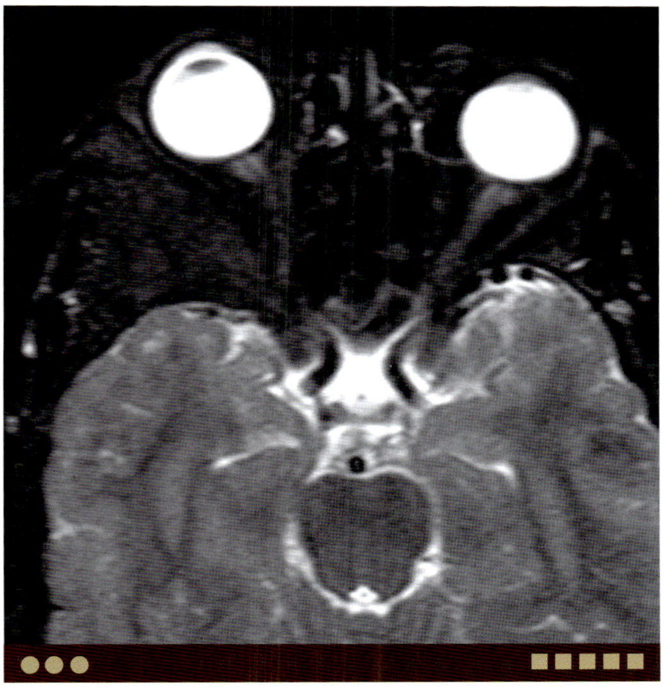

D. Fibrous dysplasia, same patient as A. Axial T2W image shows an expansile lesion in the right sphenoid bone demonstrating predominantly low signal. Note medial displacement of the right orbital contents.

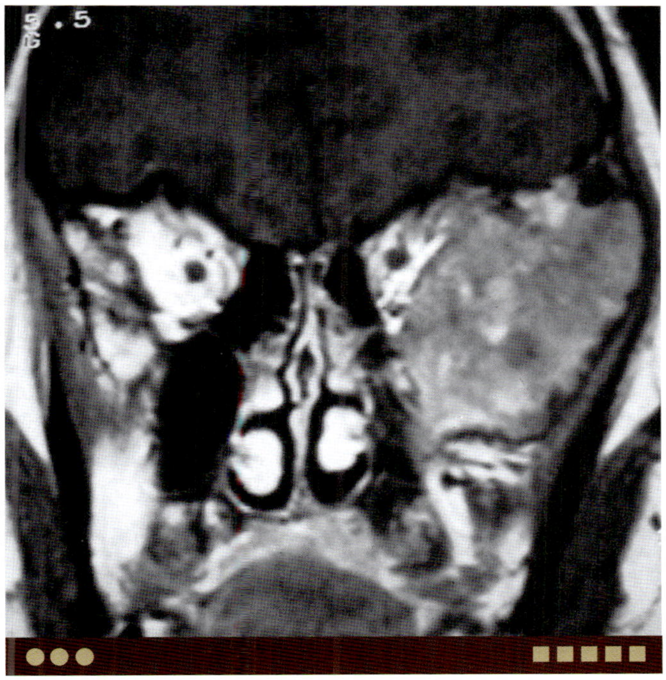

E. **Fibrous dysplasia** in a different patient. Coronal postcontrast T1W image shows heterogeneous avid enhancement in the left sphenoid lesion

DIFFERENTIAL DIAGNOSIS IMAGES (F-H)

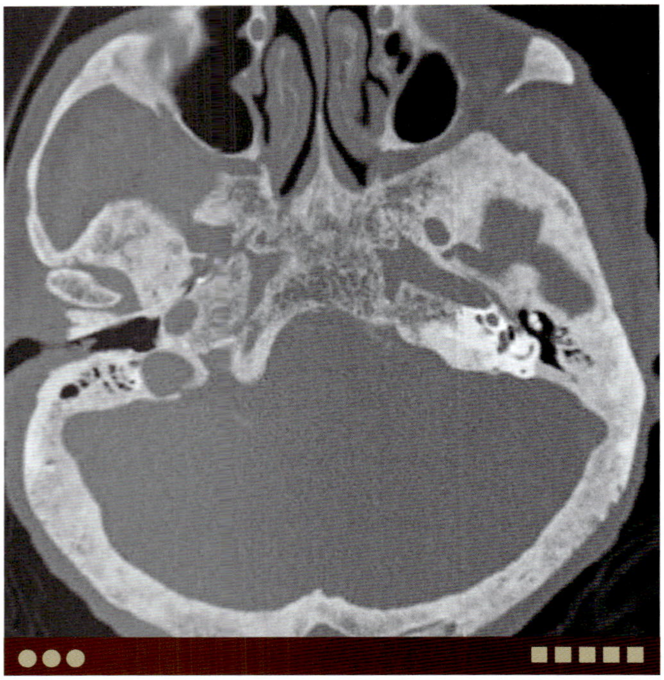

F. Paget's disease. Axial CT demonstrates coarse trabeculation and expansile change in the entire skull base and calvarium.

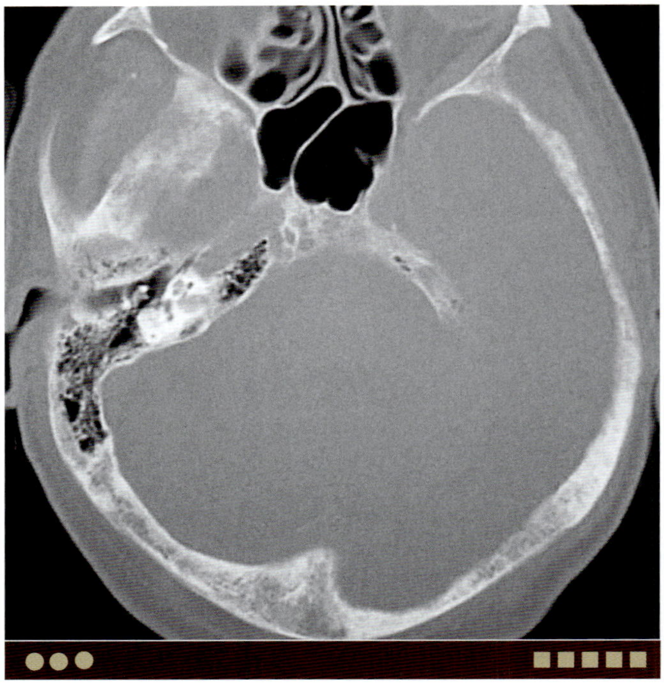

G. Metastasis from prostate cancer. Axial CT demonstrates diffuse permeative and sclerotic changes in the sphenoid, temporal, and occipital bones, right more than left.

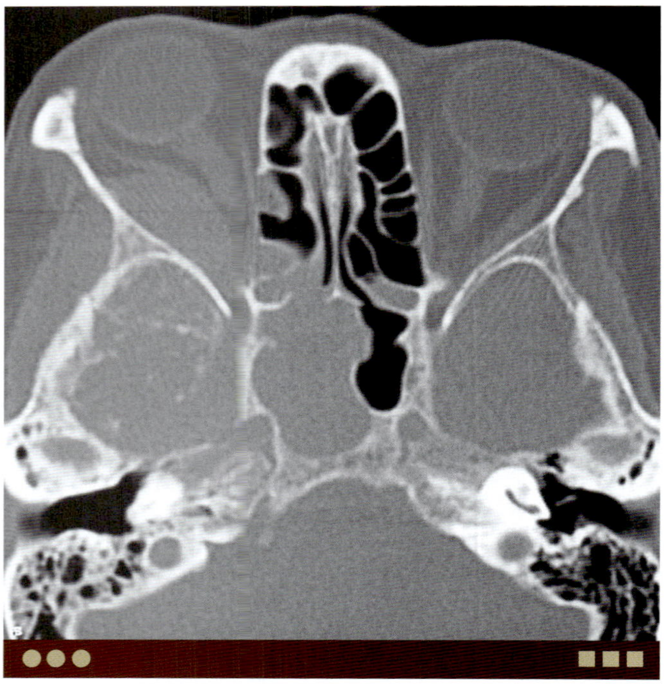

H. Metastasis from urethral cancer. Axial CT demonstrates a lesion centered in the right sphenoid triangle with a large soft tissue component extending into the orbit, sphenoid sinus, and middle cranial fossa.

Case 2–2 Jugular Foramen Schwannoma

Osamu Sakai, Rohini Nadgir

PRESENTATION

Hoarseness.

FINDINGS

CT demonstrates expansion of the jugular foramen.

DIFFERENTIAL

- Glomus jugulare: This lesion demonstrates permeative and infiltrative changes in the adjacent osseous structures rather than erosion or remodeling.
- Bone metastasis: These lesions are centered in the bone, not within the jugular foramen. Metastases from renal cell carcinoma, thyroid cancer, and hepatocellular carcinoma often demonstrate expansile osteolytic lesions.

COMMENTS

This is a 69-year-old woman with hoarseness.

Schwannoma is a benign tumor arising from the Schwann cell, commonly seen involving the cranial nerves and sympathetic nerves in the head and neck. Among the cranial nerves, this most often occurs in the vestibular nerve but also often seen in the trigeminal and facial nerves as well as in the lower cranial nerves.

Schwannomas show low signal on T1W and intermediate-to-high signal on T2W images. Homogeneous enhancement is commonly seen after contrast; however, with increase in size, cystic change is often seen. Schwannomas displace and compress the internal jugular vein but invasion or intravenous extension is very rare.

On CT, schwannomas shows similar density to the muscles and mild enhancement after contrast. Degree of enhancement is lower than meningioma or paraganglioma and is useful to differentiate from these lesions. Schwannoma tends to remodel or expand the jugular foramen, on the other hand sclerotic changes are seen with meningiomas and permeative/infiltrative changes are seen with paragangliomas.

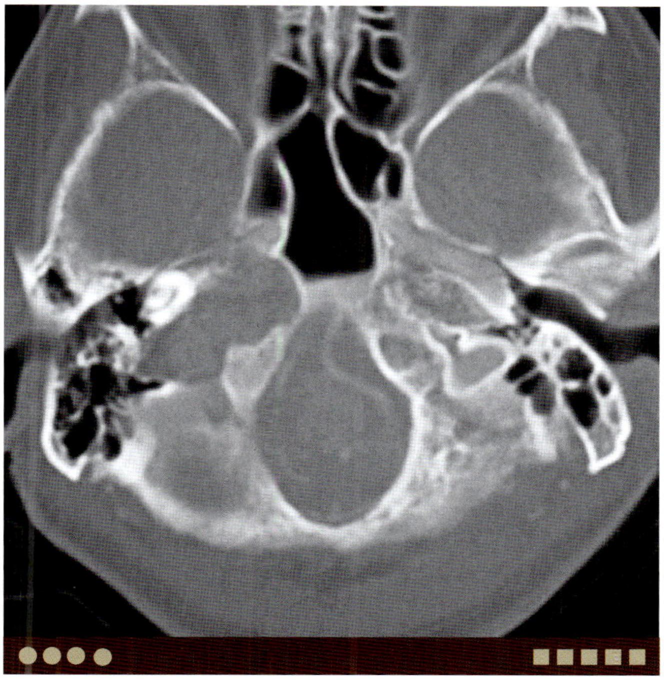

A. Vagus nerve schwannoma. Axial CT demonstrates expansion and erosion of the right jugular foramen.

Schwannomas arising from the lower cranial nerves displace the internal carotid artery anteromedially and internal jugular vein anterolaterally, while those from the sympathetic trunk displace the vessels laterally.

PEARLS

- **Schwannoma causes remodeling and expansion of the jugular foramen.**
- **Homogeneous enhancement is commonly seen after contrast on MRI.**
- **Schwannomas arising from the lower cranial nerves displace the internal carotid artery anteromedially and internal jugular vein anterolaterally.**

ADDITIONAL IMAGES (B-E)

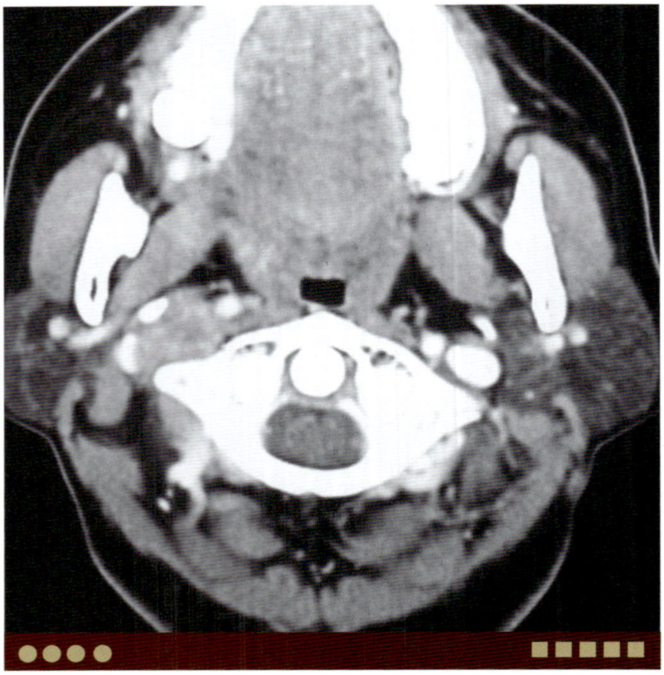

B. **Vagus nerve schwannoma** in a different patient. Axial postcontrast CT demonstrates a mildly enhancing tumor displacing the internal carotid artery anteromedially and internal jugular vein laterally.

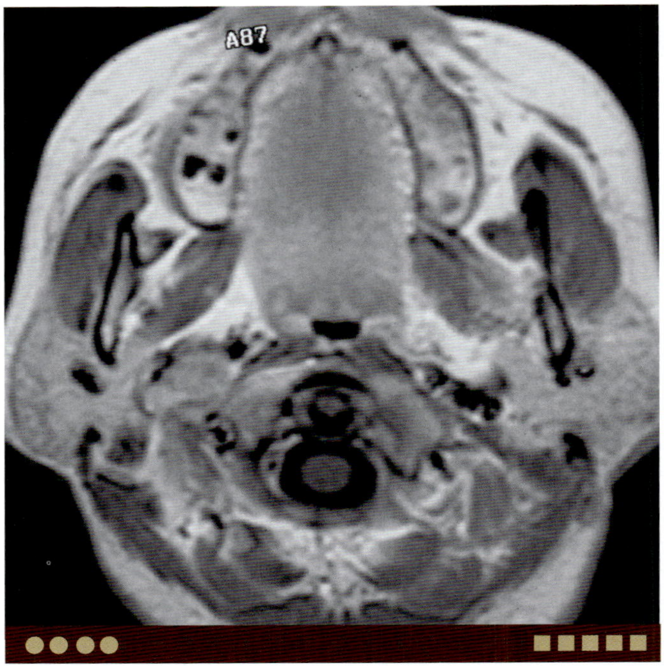

C. Vagus nerve schwannoma, same patient as B. Axial postcontrast T1W image demonstrates a mildly enhancing tumor.

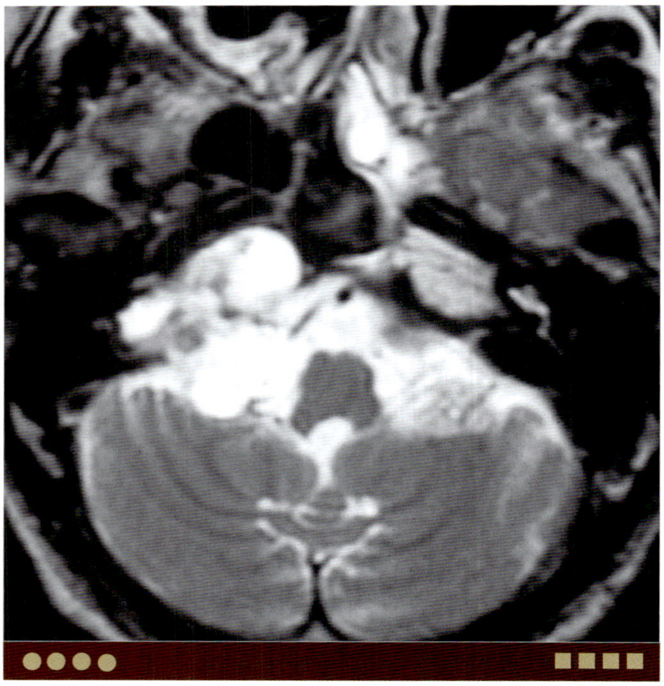

D. **Jugular foramen schwannoma** in a different patient. Axial T2W image demonstrates a lobulated heterogeneous tumor at the right jugular foramen.

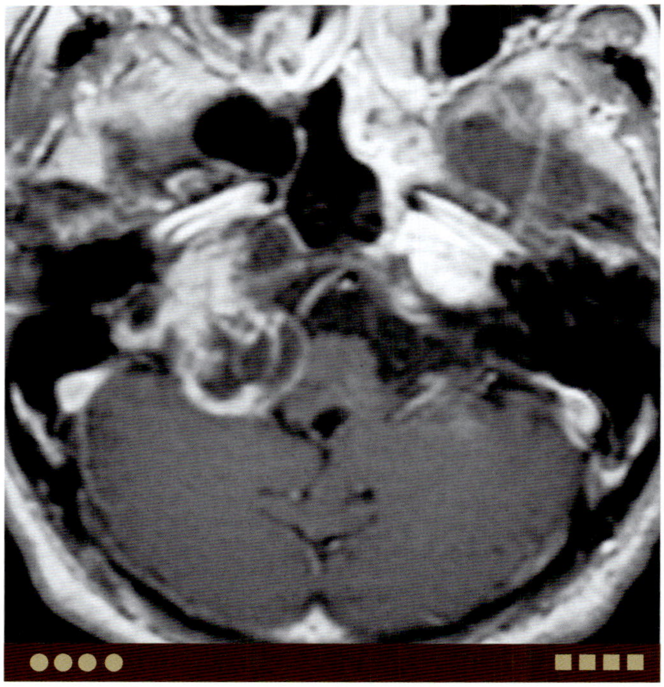

E. Jugular foramen schwannoma, same patient as D. Axial post-contrast T1W image demonstrates heterogeneous enhancement of the lesion with large areas of cystic degeneration.

DIFFERENTIAL DIAGNOSIS IMAGES (F-G)

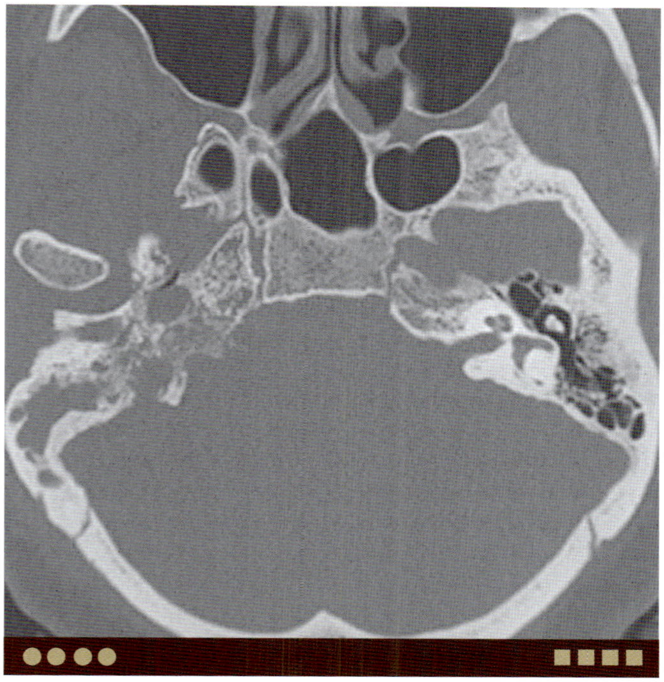

F. Paraganglioma. Axial CT demonstrates permeative/infiltrative osteolytic changes in the right temporal bone.

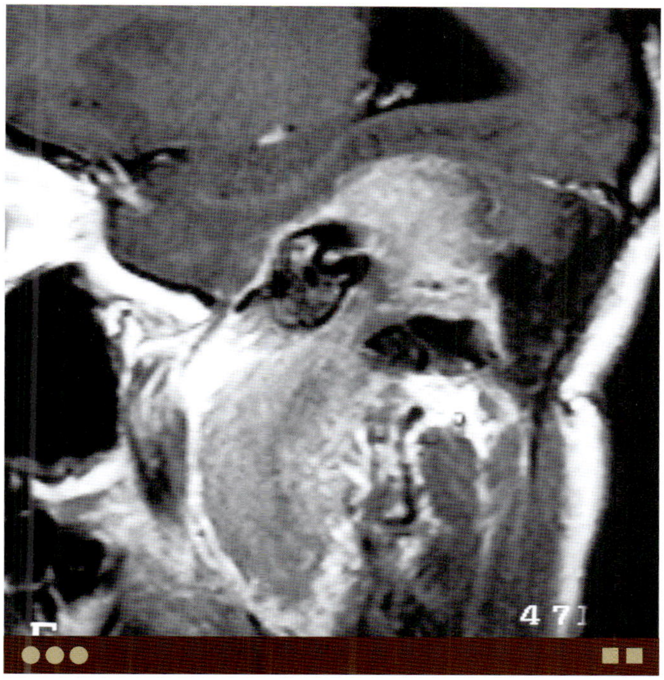

G. Meningioma. Sagittal postcontrast T1W image demonstrates extracranial extension of a heterogeneously enhancing tumor through the jugular foramen.

Case 2–3 Cholesterol Cyst

Osamu Sakai, Rohini Nadgir

PRESENTATION

Headache.

FINDINGS

An expansile lesion in the petrous apex demonstrates high signal on both T1W and T2W MR images.

DIFFERENTIAL

- Cholesteatoma/epidermoid cyst: This lesion demonstrates water signal; low on T1W and high on T2W images.
- Opacified petrous air cell/retention cyst: This demonstrates water signal; low on T1W and high on T2W images without expansile change.

COMMENTS

This is a 43-year-old man with headache.

Cholesterol cyst is a hemorrhagic mucocele which commonly occurs in the petrous apex. This condition occurs following chronic otitis media, however in the petrous apex, it often occurs without the history of otitis media. The etiology is unclear, however it is believed that the negative pressure in the air cells caused by obstruction results in edema of the mucosa, followed by hemorrhage. Then, foreign body reaction and formation of granulation tissue occur. Therefore, cholesterol cyst cannot occur without preexisting pneumatized petrous air cells.

On CT, an expansile cystic lesion with smooth margin is characteristic. The lesion demonstrates high signal on T1W MR images corresponding to proteinaceous and hemorrhagic contents. On T2W images, it usually demonstrates high signal, however decreased signal can be seen reflecting further increased protein concentration, hemosiderin deposition, and fibrosis.

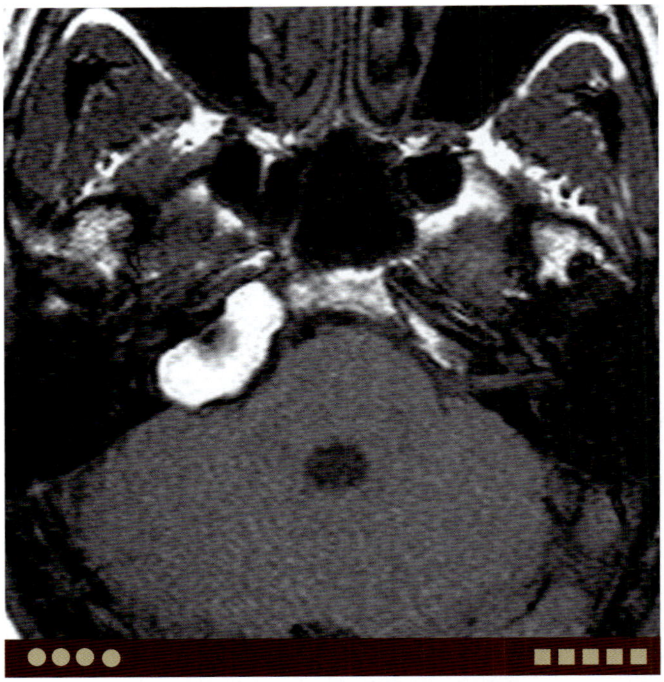

A. Cholesterol cyst. Axial T1W MR image demonstrates an expansile high-signal lesion in the right petrous apex.

PEARLS

- **Cholesterol cyst is seen in the petrous apex as an expansile cystic lesion.**
- **Cholesterol cyst typically demonstrates high signal on both T1W and T2W images. However, T2 signal may be decreased due to increased protein concentration, hemosiderin deposition, and fibrosis.**

ADDITIONAL IMAGES (B-F)

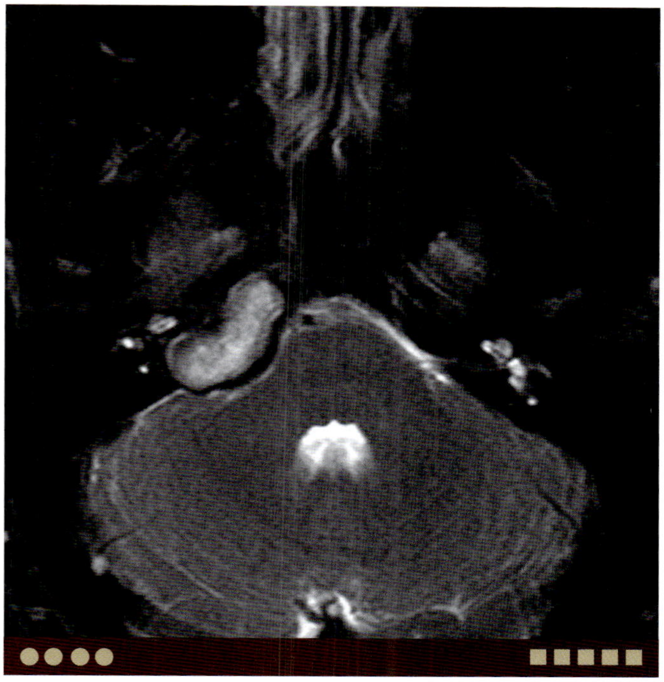

B. Cholesterol cyst, same patient as A. Axial T2W image demonstrates expansile, high-signal lesion in the right petrous apex.

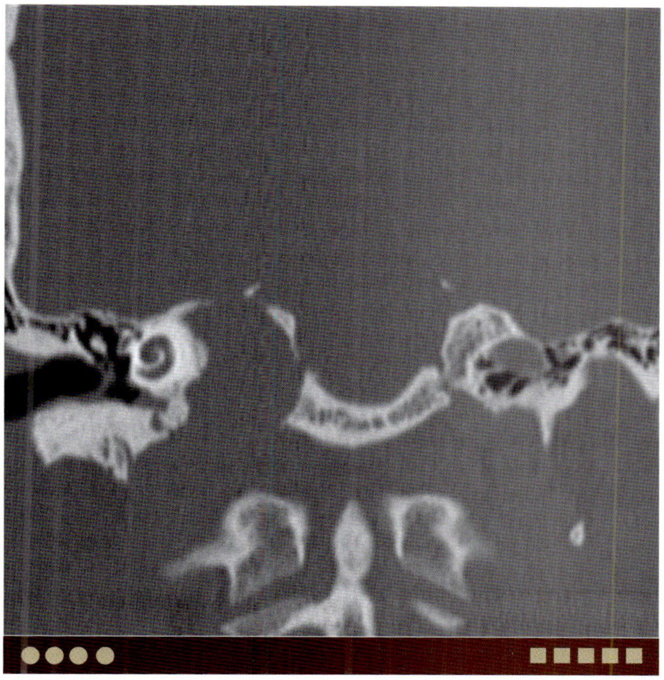

C. Cholesterol cyst, same patient as A. Coronal CT demonstrates an expansile lesion, medial to the cochlea in the right petrous apex eroding the bone.

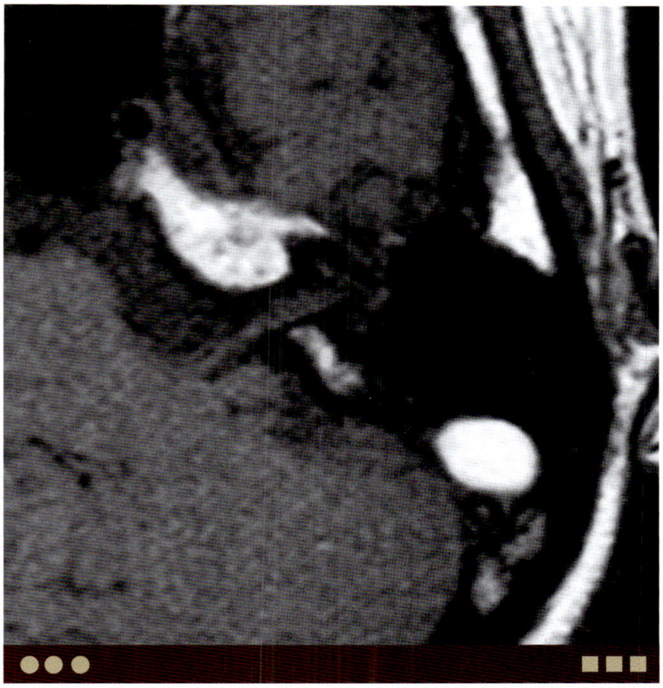

D. Cholesterol cyst in the mastoid. Axial T1W image demonstrates a high-signal cystic lesion in the mastoid air cell.

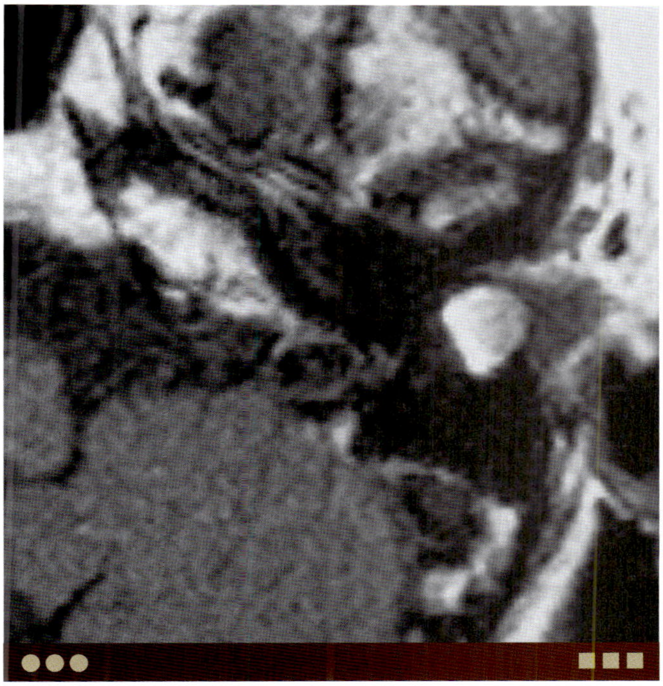

E. Cholesterol cyst in the mastoid in a different patient. Axial T1W image demonstrates a high-signal lesion in the mastoid extending into the external auditory canal.

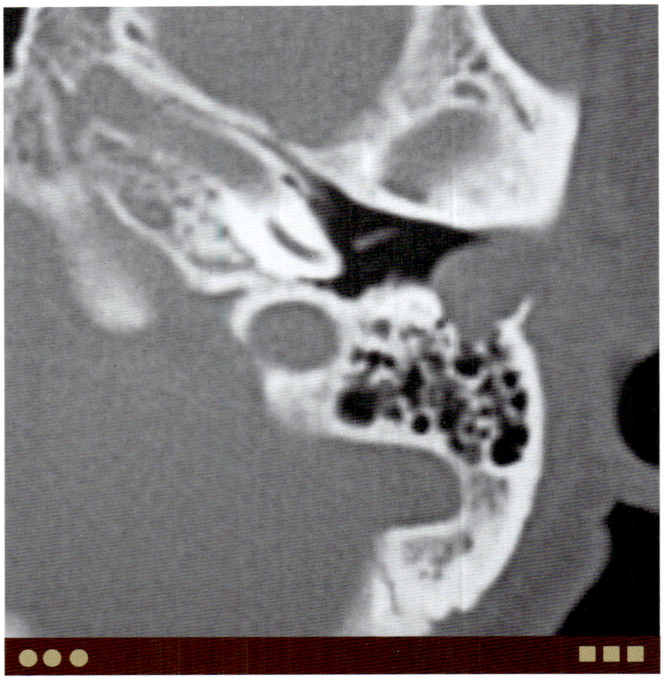

F. Cholesterol cyst in the mastoid, same patient as E. Axial CT demonstrates a lesion eroding the bone and protruding into the external auditory canal.

DIFFERENTIAL DIAGNOSIS IMAGE

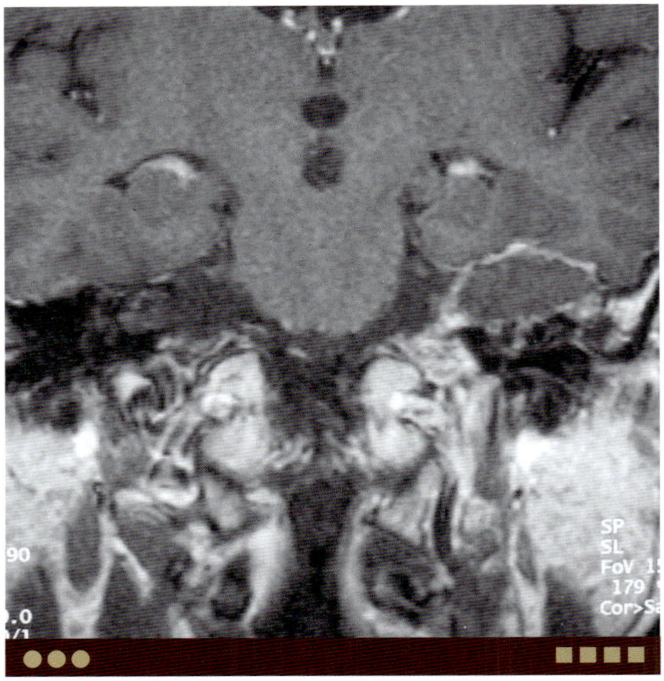

G. **Epidermoid**. Coronal postcontrast T1W image demonstrates a peripherally enhancing, expansile, low-signal lesion in the left petrous apex.

Case 2–4 Meningioma at the Cerebellopontine Angle

Osamu Sakai, Rohini Nadgir

PRESENTATION

Vertigo.

FINDINGS

Postcontrast MRI demonstrates an enhancing dural-based tumor at the cerebellopontine angle.

DIFFERENTIAL

- Vestibular schwannoma: This is the most common mass at the cerebellopontine angle, which often occurs at the porus acusticus and extends into the internal auditory canal.
- Aneurysm: This is seen as an avidly enhancing lesion on CT, however demonstrates heterogeneous signal due to flow on MRI. Bone erosion is occasionally seen.
- Metastasis: Dural metastasis may demonstrate similar findings to meningioma.

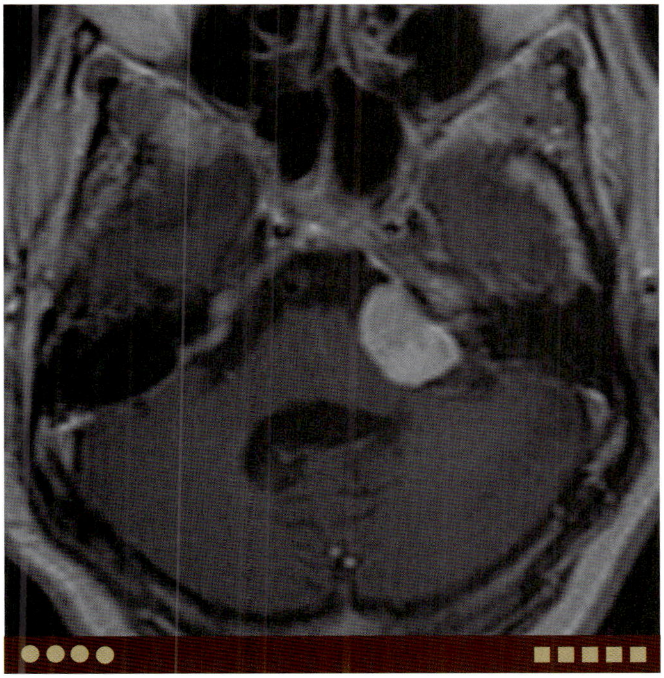

A. Meningioma. Axial postcontrast T1W image demonstrates an enhancing, dural-based, hemispheric mass centered outside the left internal auditory canal. Note dural tail sign anteromedial to the tumor.

COMMENTS

This is a 49-year-old woman with vertigo.

Meningioma is the second most common mass at the cerebellopontine angle (CPA) following the vestibular schwannoma, and accounts for 6% to 15% of all CPA tumors. Meningioma is often seen between 40 and 60 years of age with female predominance (M:F = 1:2). Clinical symptoms of vestibular schwannoma and CPA meningioma are very similar, including disequilibrium, headaches, facial numbness, and facial nerve paresis or palsy, although facial nerve symptoms are rare. Tinnitus and hearing loss are more common in vestibular schwannoma than in CPA meningioma.

Typically, meningioma is demonstrated as an avidly enhancing, hemispheric, dural-based mass centered outside of the internal auditory canal, although rarely it can be seen within the canal. Calcification within the lesion and hyperostosis of the adjacent osseous structure is common. This is a helpful finding to differentiate it from schwannoma, which often demonstrates bone erosion without calcification. On MRI, meningioma demonstrates similar signal intensity to the brain parenchyma on both T1W and T2W images, and avid enhancement after contrast. Linear enhancement of the adjacent dura, which is called the dural tail sign, is typically seen with meningioma. However, with a round meningioma at the cerebellopontine angle, dural tail sign may not be apparent.

PEARLS

- **Meningioma is the second most common mass at the cerebellopontine angle.**
- **Meningioma is typically demonstrated as a hemispheric dural-based mass centered outside the internal auditory canal.**
- **Meningioma typically demonstrates similar signal to the brain parenchyma on both T1W and T2W images, and avid enhancement.**
- **Calcification within the lesion and hyperostosis of the adjacent osseous structure are commonly seen.**

ADDITIONAL IMAGES (B-E)

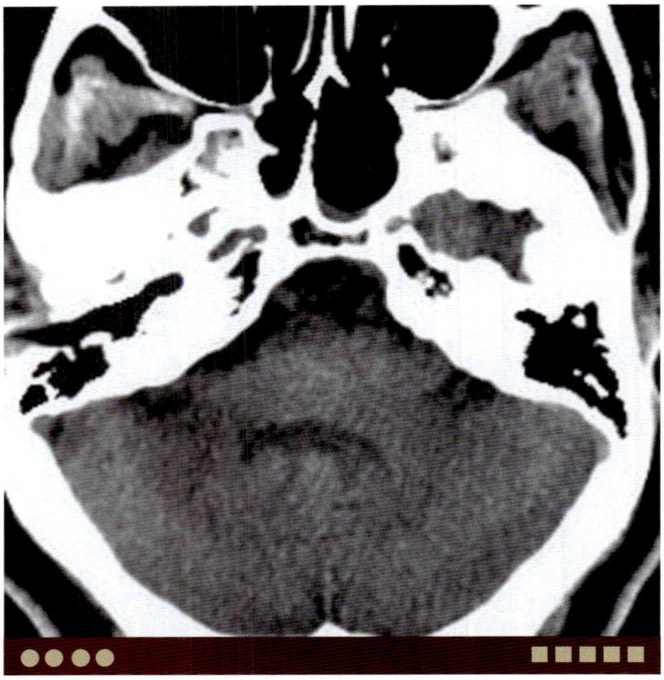

B. Meningioma, same patient as A. Axial CT shows the tumor demonstrating isodensity to the brain parenchyma.

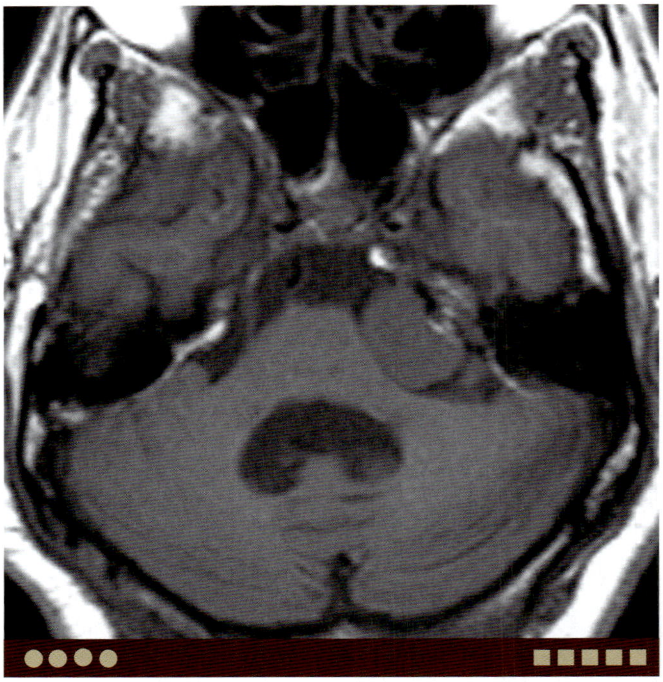

C. Meningioma, same patient as A. Axial precontrast T1W image shows the tumor demonstrating homogeneous low-to-isointense signal to the brain parenchyma.

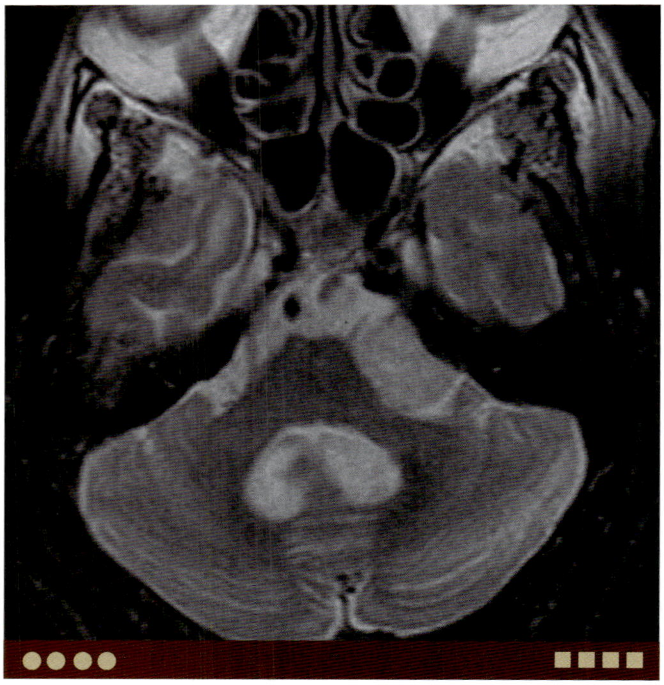

D. Meningioma, same patient as A. Axial T2W image shows the tumor demonstrating homogeneous high signal compared to the brain parenchyma.

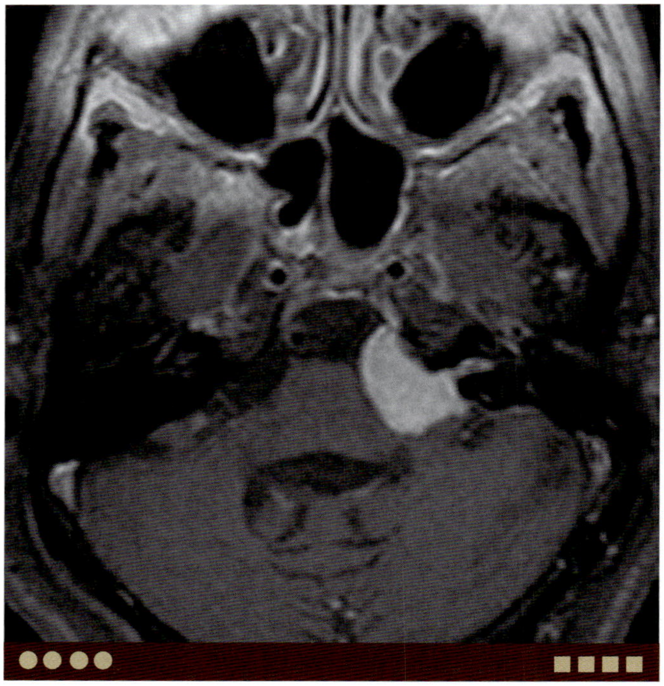

E. Meningioma in a different patient. Axial postcontrast fat-suppressed T1W image demonstrates tumor extension to the left internal auditory canal.

DIFFERENTIAL DIAGNOSIS IMAGES (F-G)

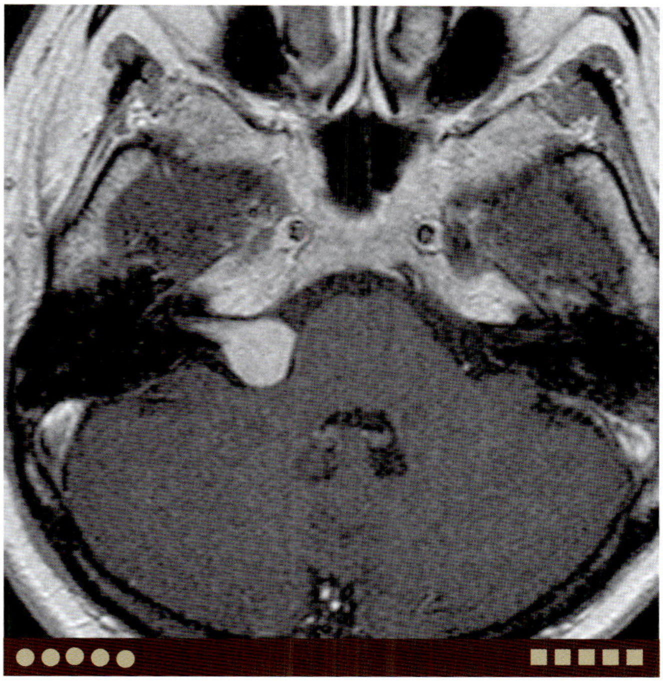

F. Vestibular schwannoma. Axial postcontrast T1W image demonstrates a homogeneously enhancing tumor extending from the right CPA into the internal auditory canal.

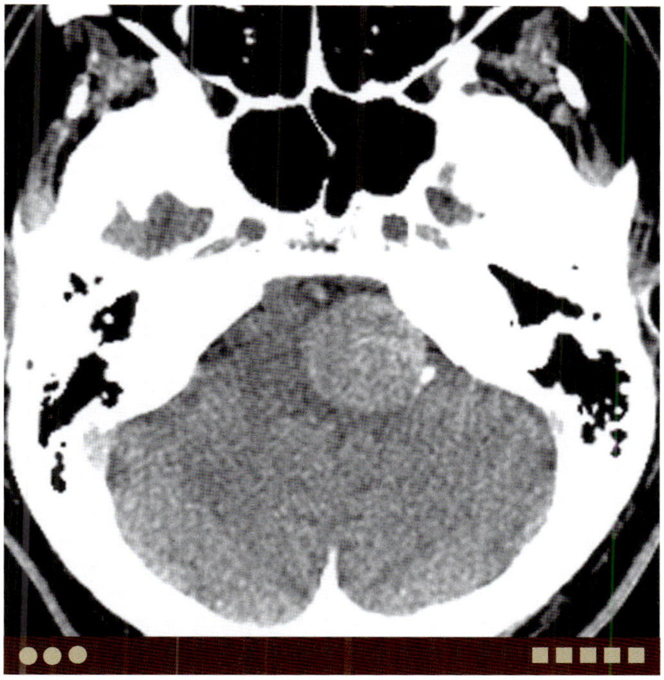

G. Aneurysm. Axial noncontrast CT demonstrates a slightly hyperdense round mass at the left CPA.

Case 2–5 Bone Marrow Abnormality Associated with Hematological Disorders

Osamu Sakai, Rohini Nadgir

PRESENTATION

History of lymphoma.

FINDINGS

T1W MR image demonstrates diffusely decreased bone marrow signal.

DIFFERENTIAL

- Hematological disorders: Diffuse marrow signal change is seen in patients with leukemia, lymphoma, myelodysplastic syndrome, sickle cell anemia, and other hematological disorders.
- Infection: Patients with human immunodeficiency virus (HIV) infection tend to demonstrate diffuse marrow signal abnormality.
- Paget's disease: Expanded marrow space with heterogeneous signal is usually seen.
- Osteopetrosis: Very dark signal with narrowed bone marrow space is noted.

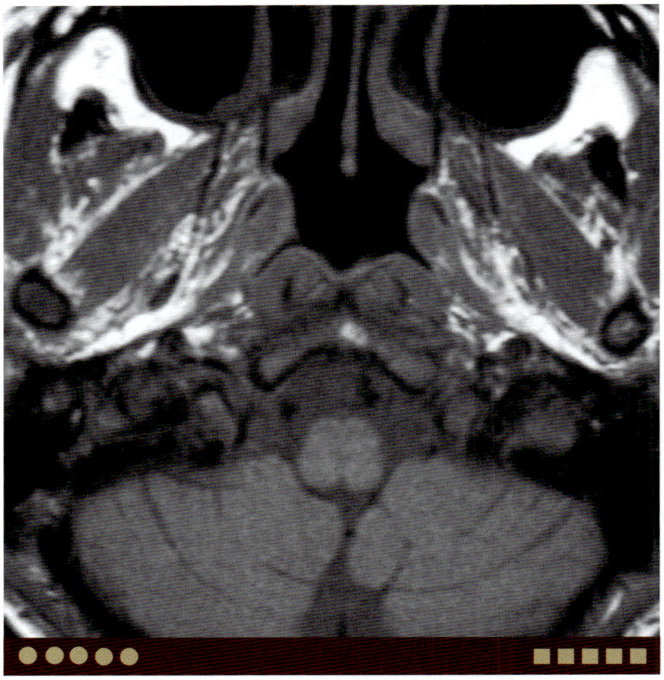

A. Lymphoma. Axial T1W MR image shows diffusely decreased marrow signal in the clivus as well as mandibular condyles.

COMMENTS

This is a 34-year-old man with lymphoma.

In adults, the bone marrow in the skull base and calvarium, including the clivus is usually fatty marrow and shows high signal on T1W MR images. High signal in the marrow on T1W images should be always identified when interpreting MRI, not only in patients with history of cancer or hematological disorders but also in patients without known malignancy. If there is decrease in signal in the marrow on T1W images, some type of infiltrative process must be suspected. This is a very nonspecific finding; however, it can be a clue to identify underlying serious conditions, such as leukemia, lymphoma, and HIV infection. Marrow signal abnormality is also often seen in patients receiving chemotherapy.

Diffuse expansion of the marrow space is often seen in patients with sickle cell anemia and thalassemia. Focal marrow space expansion can be seen in lymphoma, plasmacytoma, myeloma, and metastases.

The yellow marrow in the clivus may be variable among healthy individuals. Some investigators suggest marrow in the mandibular condyle is more reliable.

PEARLS

- **In adults, the bone marrow in the skull base and calvarium is usually fatty marrow and shows high signal on T1W images.**
- **Loss of normal high signal of the marrow on T1W images is seen in patients with various hematological disorders.**

ADDITIONAL IMAGES (B-F)

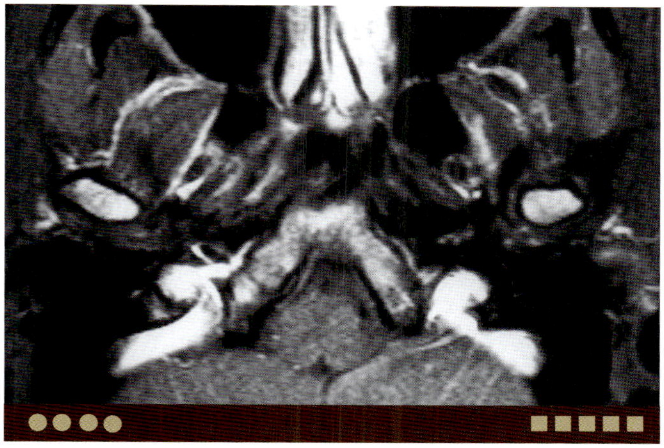

B. Acute myeloblastic leukemia. Axial postcontrast fat-suppressed T1W MR image demonstrates abnormal enhancement of the marrow in the clivus and mandibular condyles.

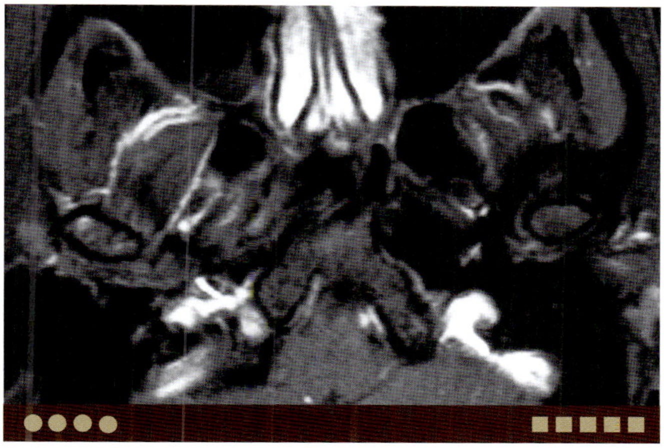

C. Acute myeloblastic leukemia, same patient as B, complete remission after chemotherapy. Axial postcontrast fat-suppressed T1W MR image demonstrates no abnormal enhancement of the marrow consistent with normal fatty marrow.

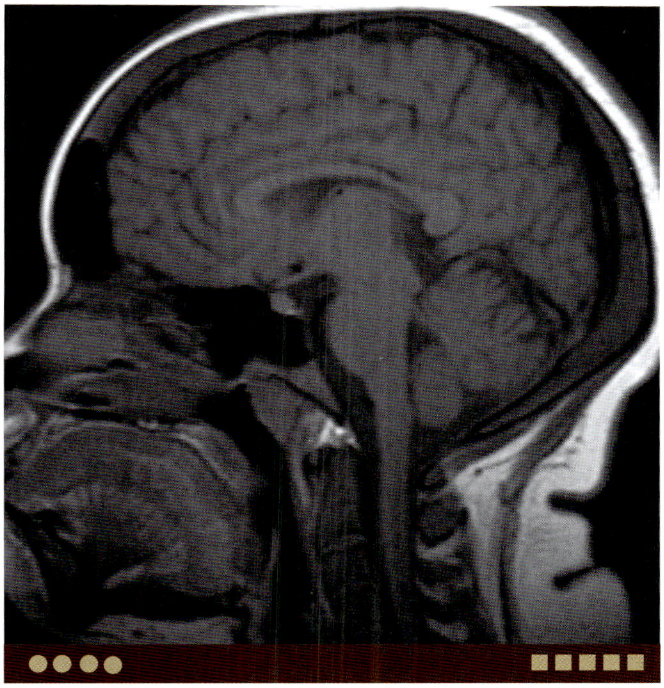

D. Sickle cell anemia. Sagittal T1W MR image demonstrates decreased bone marrow signal in the clivus and calvarium. Note slight expansion of the marrow space in the calvarium.

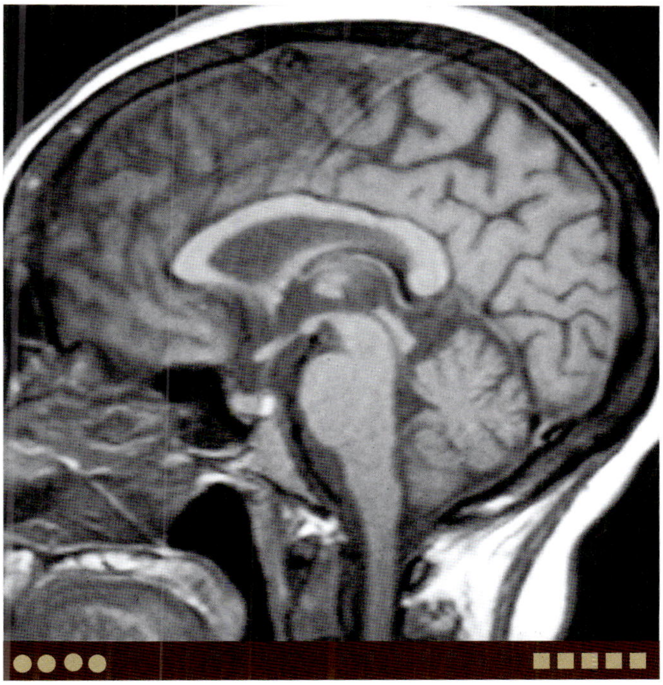

E. HIV infection. Sagittal T1W MR image demonstrates decreased bone marrow signal in the clivus and calvarium.

DIFFERENTIAL DIAGNOSIS IMAGE

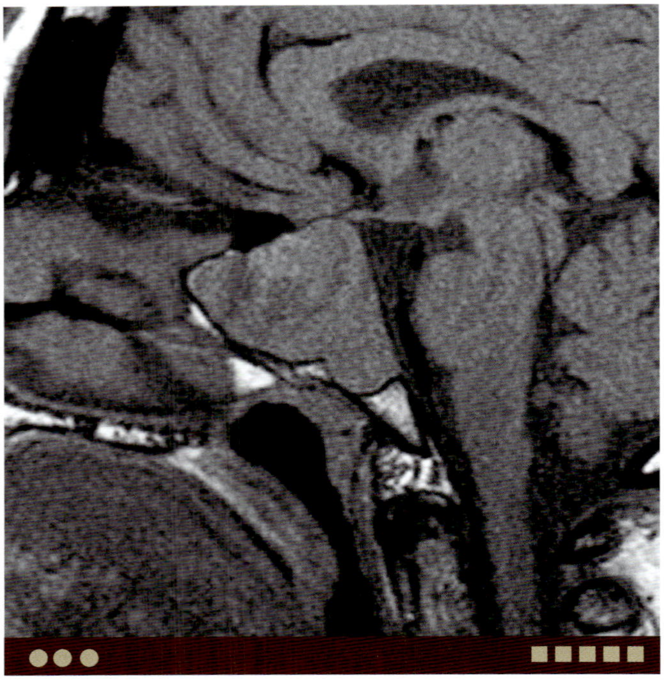

F. Lymphoma. Sagittal T1W MR image demonstrates an expansile low-signal lesion in the clivus occupying the sphenoid sinus.

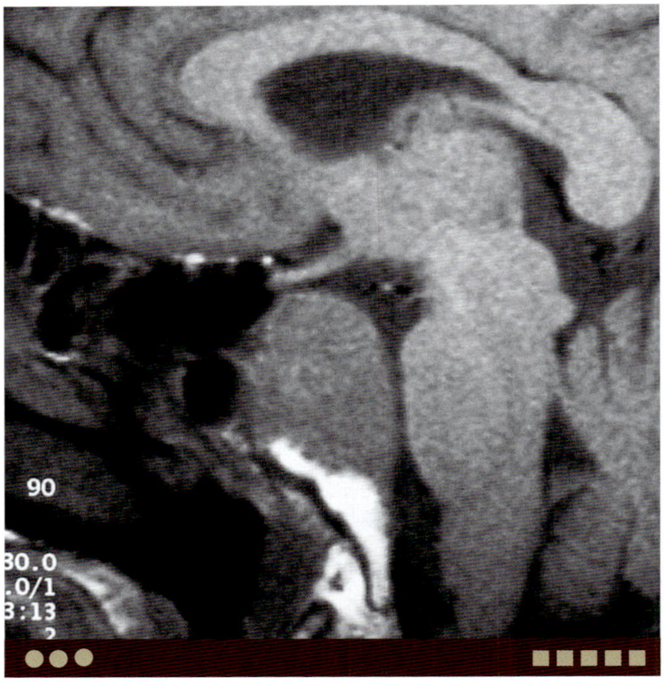

G. Metastasis from colon cancer. Sagittal postcontrast T1W MR image demonstrates an expansile mass in the clivus.

Case 2–6 Trigeminal Schwannoma

Osamu Sakai, Rohini Nadgir

PRESENTATION

Trigeminal neuralgia.

FINDINGS

MRI demonstrates a well-demarcated, spindle-shaped, enhancing lesion in the paracavernous region.

DIFFERENTIAL

- Meningioma: This is a dural-based mass demonstrating similar signal to the brain parenchyma on all sequences. Homogeneous avid enhancement with dural tail sign is a characteristic finding. Hyperostosis rather than erosion is commonly seen in the adjacent osseous structures.
- Neurofibroma: Similar appearing masses are often seen in patients with neurofibromatosis, although most neurofibromas are sporadic. Presence of central low signal on T2W images, "central core," sign is suggestive of neurofibroma rather than schwannoma, although this is not perfect to differentiate them.
- Perineural tumor spread: Adenoid cystic carcinoma is famous for this type of tumor spread; however, squamous cell carcinoma is the most common tumor causing this because it is the most common tumor in the head and neck.

COMMENTS

This is a 41-year-old woman with trigeminal neuralgia.

Trigeminal schwannoma is the second most common intracranial schwannoma following those arising from the seventh and eighth nerve complex. Intracranially, it often arises from the cisternal portion or in the Meckel's cave. If it extends inferiorly to the cerebellopontine angle, it may mimic schwannomas arising from the seventh and eighth nerve complex. Extension and expansion of the foramen rotundum or ovale is common.

On MRI, just as schwannomas arising from other nerves, trigeminal schwannoma usually is a spindle or dumbbell-shaped low signal on T1W and intermediate-to-high signal on T2W lesion which demonstrates homogeneous avid enhancement without meningeal tail sign after contrast. With increase in size, it tends to show cystic degeneration.

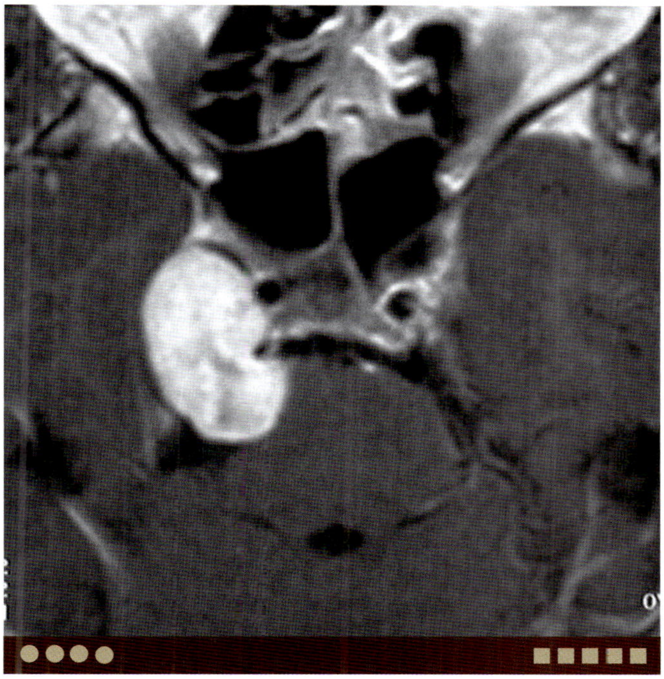

A. Trigeminal schwannoma. Axial postcontrast T1W image shows a dumbbell-shaped enhancing tumor in the right Meckel's cave and cisternal portion of the trigeminal nerve.

Trigeminal schwannomas tend to have a more cystic component than other schwannomas.

On CT, schwannoma enhances less than meningioma, although both demonstrates avid enhancement on MRI. Bone erosion is a common finding and helpful to differentiate it from meningioma, which often demonstrates hyperostosis.

PEARLS

- **Trigeminal schwannoma often arises in the Meckel's cave or the cisternal portion of the course of the trigeminal nerve.**
- **Trigeminal schwannoma usually demonstrates spindle or dumbbell-shape and low signal on T1W and intermediate-to-high signal on T2W images, and homogeneous enhancement without meningeal tail sign.**
- **Trigeminal schwannomas tend to have a more cystic component than other schwannomas.**

ADDITIONAL IMAGES (B-E)

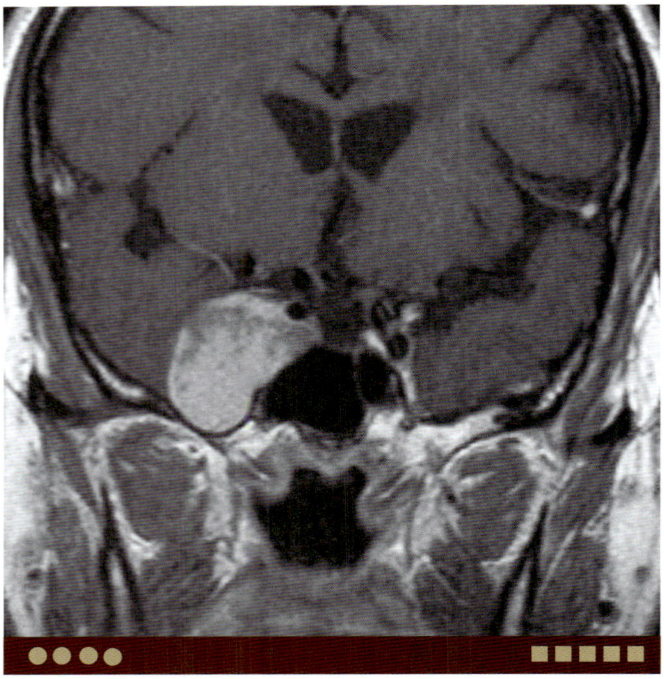

B. Trigeminal schwannoma in a different patient. Coronal postcontrast T1W image shows a well-demarcated enhancing tumor centered in the right Meckel's cave displacing the internal carotid artery medially. Note remodeling of the sphenoid bone inferior to the lesion.

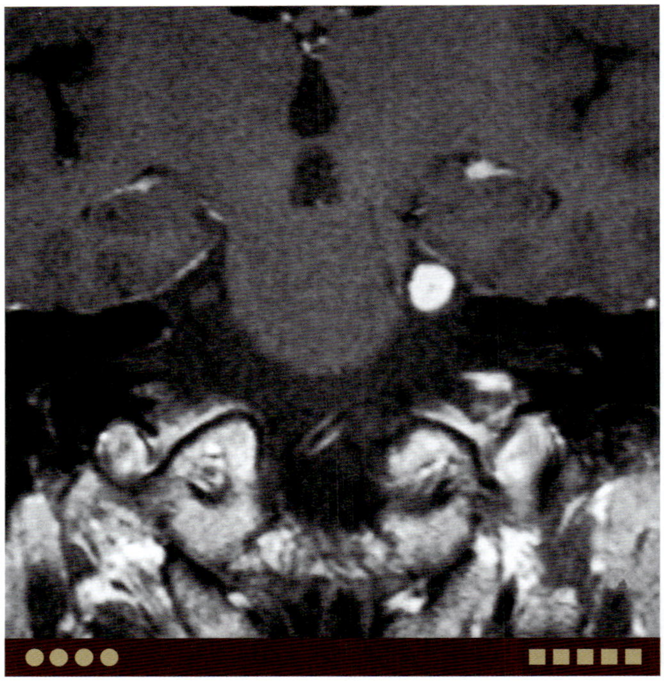

C. Trigeminal schwannoma in a different patient. Coronal postcontrast T1W image shows a round enhancing tumor arising from the cisternal portion of the left trigeminal nerve.

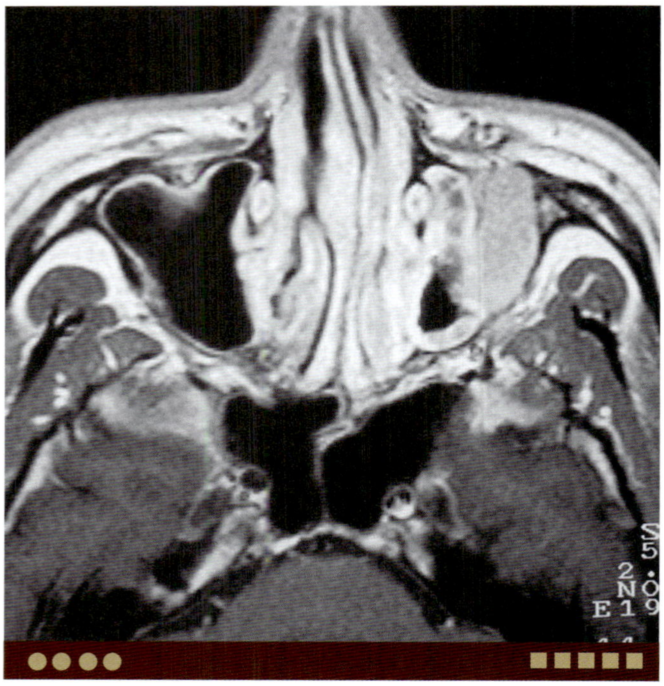

D. Trigeminal schwannoma in a different patient. Axial postcontrast T1W image shows an elongated homogeneously enhancing lesion along the course of the left infraorbital nerve.

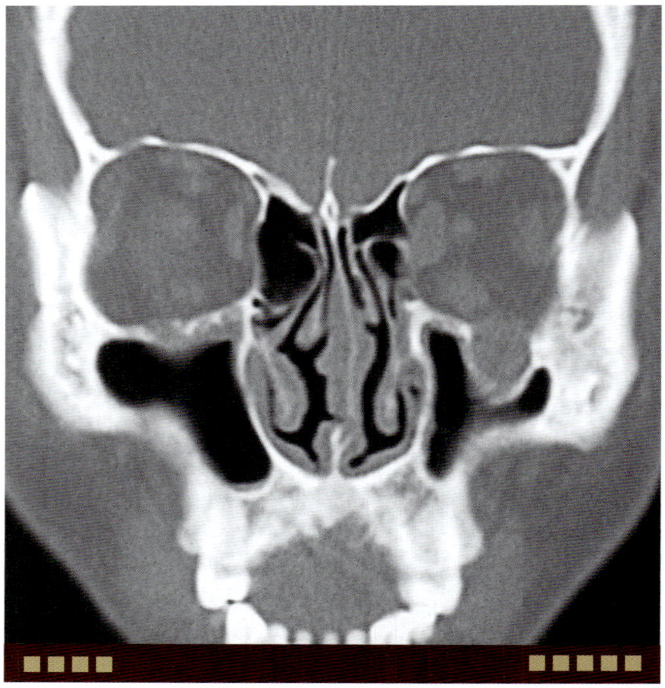

E. Trigeminal schwannoma, same patient as D. Coronal CT shows the tumor expanding the left infraorbital groove.

DIFFERENTIAL DIAGNOSIS IMAGES (F-I)

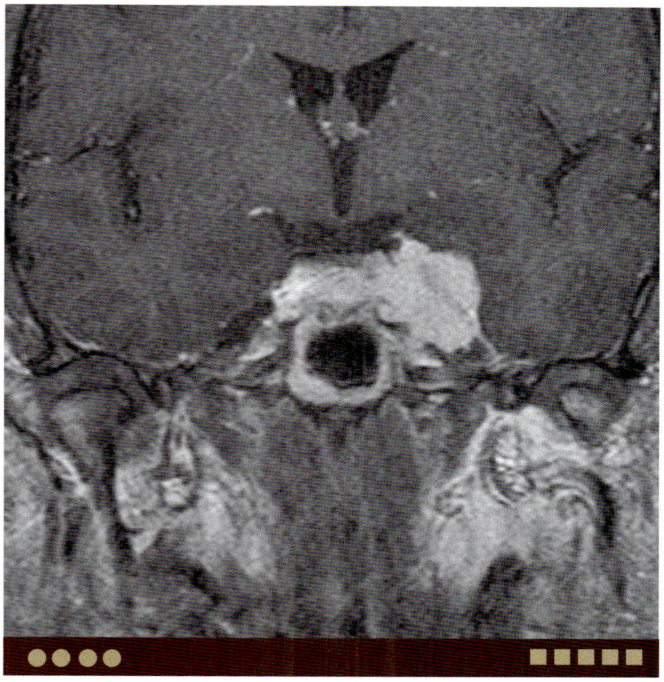

F. Meningioma. Coronal postcontrast T1W image demonstrates a slightly lobulated homogeneously enhancing lesion centered in the left paracavernous region.

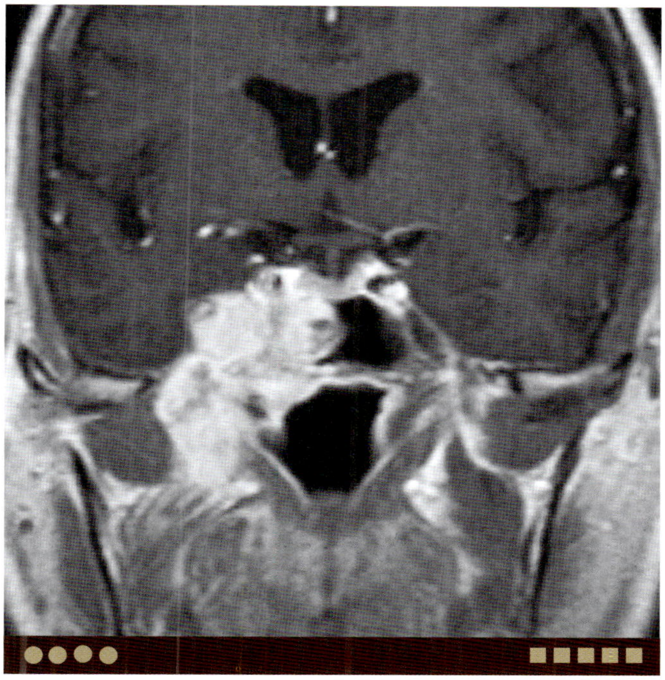

G. Perineural tumor spread, parotid adenoid cystic carcinoma. Coronal postcontrast T1W image demonstrates multilobulated heterogeneously enhancing tumor in and around the right Meckel's cave and foramen ovale, involving the trigeminal nerve.

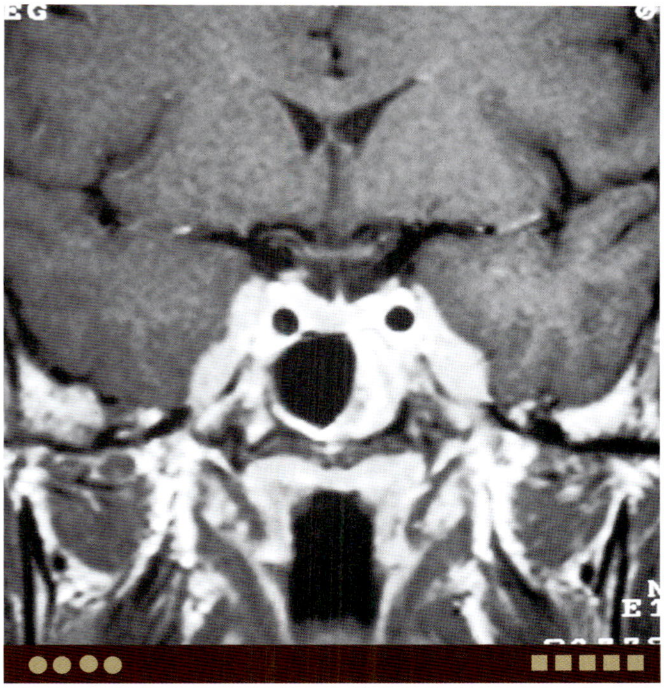

H. Perineural tumor spread, lymphoma. Coronal postcontrast T1W image demonstrates homogeneously enhancing tumors in the bilateral Meckel's caves involving the trigeminal nerves.

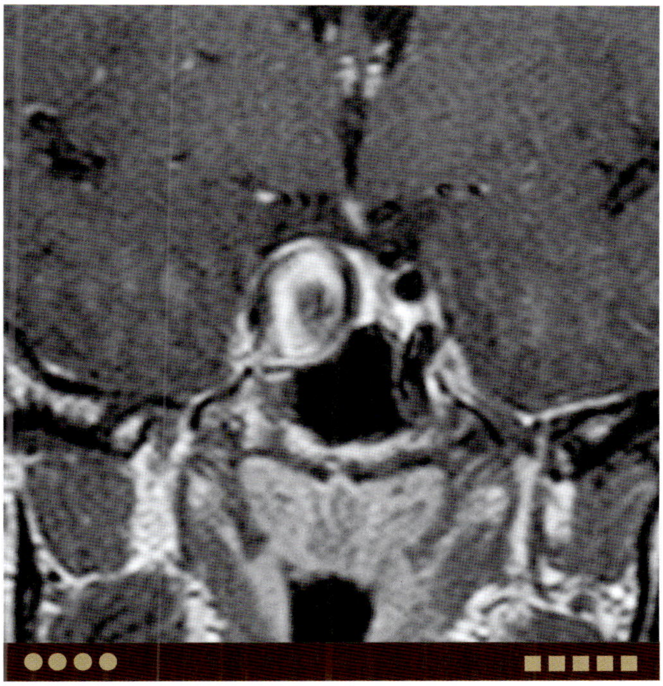

I. Internal carotid artery aneurysm. Coronal postcontrast T1W image demonstrates a heterogeneously enhancing lesion with internal signal voids from blood flow in the right paracavernous region.

Case 2–7 Chordoma

Osamu Sakai, Rohini Nadgir

PRESENTATION

Headache.

FINDINGS

CT demonstrates a soft tissue density mass with internal calcification involving the clivus. T2W MRI demonstrates heterogeneous high signal.

DIFFERENTIAL

- Chondrosarcoma: This demonstrates similar density on CT and signal pattern on MRI, however arises from the cartilage of the petroclival synchondrosis. Therefore, it locates off-midline.
- Nasopharyngeal carcinoma: This tumor can be almost completely submucosal and mimic bone tumors. However, signal on T2W images is lower than that of chordoma.
- Metastatic tumor: The clivus can have bone metastasis just as other osseous structures. Usually, signal on T2W images is lower than that of chordoma.

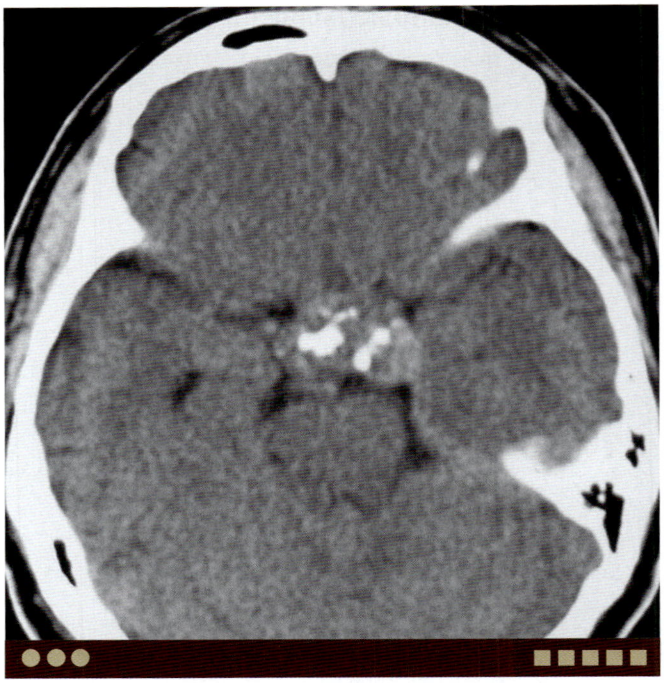

A. Chordoma. Axial CT shows a partially calcified mass in the suprasellar region.

COMMENTS

This is a 47-year-old man with chordoma.

Chordoma is a rare tumor arising from the notochord remnant, and often occurs in the clivus as well as in the sacrococcygeal region. This tumor can be seen at any age, however often occurs in men (male:female = 2:1) in the third to fifth decades. With increase in size, the tumor extends to the nasopharynx and shows similar appearance to submucosal extension of nasopharyngeal carcinoma.

Chordoma shows slightly increased density on CT, often with internal calcification, and heterogeneous, mild to intermediate enhancement. On MRI, it usually shows low-to-intermediate signal on T1W and very high signal with internal heterogeneity on T2W images, and heterogeneous, mild to intermediate enhancement. Similarly, very high signal on T2W images can be seen in chondrosarcoma, however chondrosarcoma arises from the petroclival synchondrosis and locates laterally and not in the midline. High signal on T2W images is useful to differentiate from nasopharyngeal carcinoma and lymphoma.

PEARLS

- **Chordoma is a rare tumor arising from the notochord remnant, and often occurs in the clivus.**
- **Chordoma arises in midline, while chondrosarcoma usually arises laterally, from the petroclival synchondrosis.**
- **Chordoma usually shows very high signal on T2W images, which is helpful to differentiate from nasopharyngeal carcinoma and lymphoma.**

ADDITIONAL IMAGES (B-D)

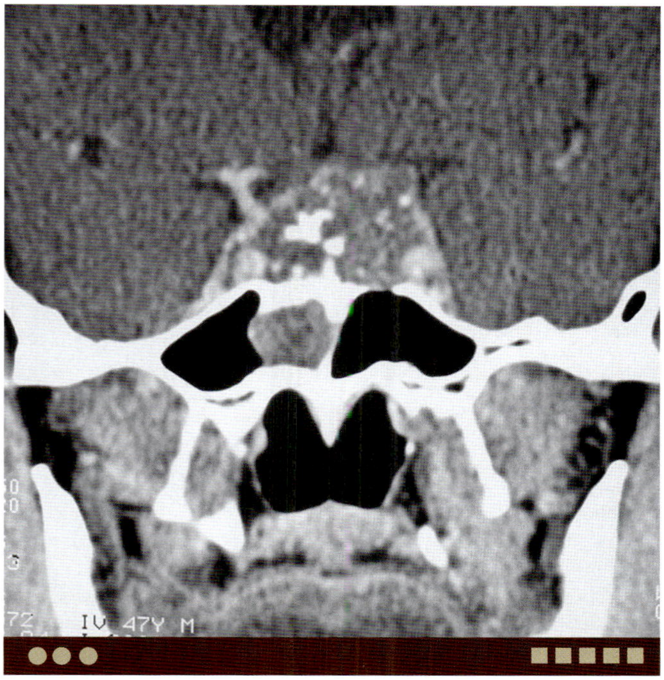

B. Chordoma, same patient as A. Coronal contrast-enhanced CT shows a mildly enhancing tumor involving the sella and sphenoid sinus.

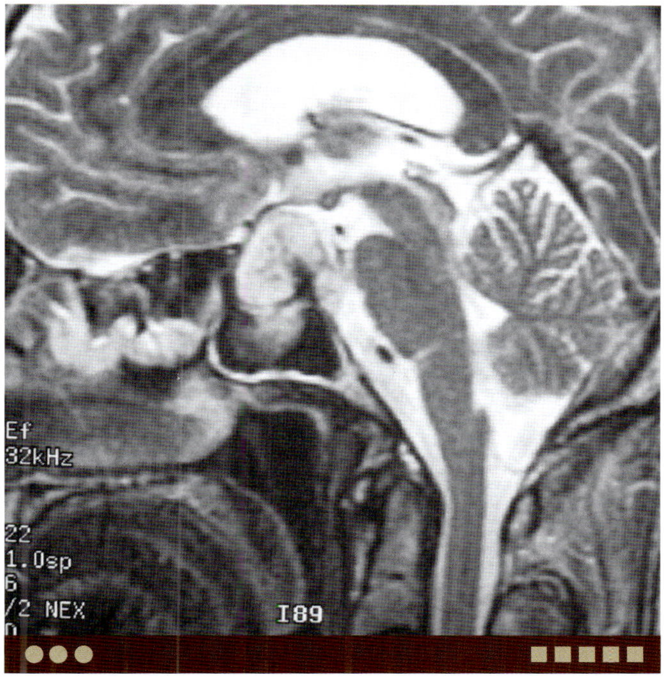

C. Chordoma, same patient as A. Sagittal T2W image shows a heterogeneous but predominantly high-signal mass involving the posterior clinoid and extending into the sphenoid sinus.

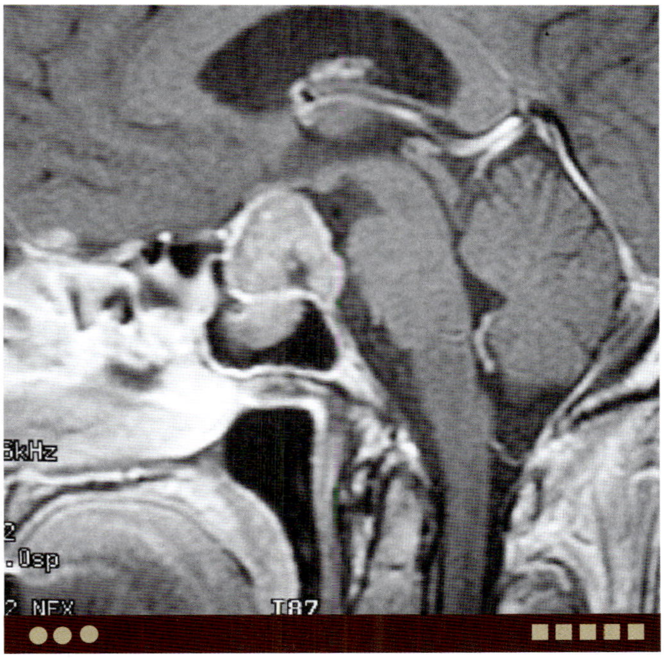

D. Chordoma, same patient as A. Sagittal postcontrast T1W image shows heterogeneous enhancement of the lesion.

DIFFERENTIAL DIAGNOSIS IMAGES (E-G)

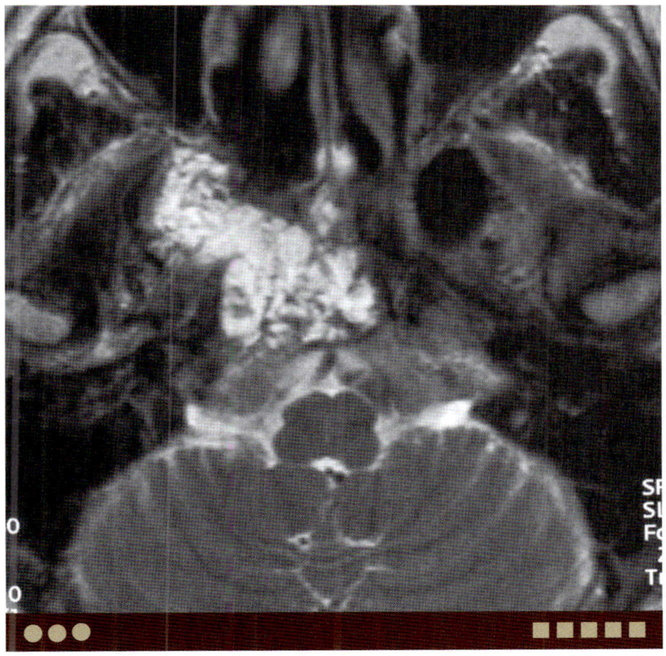

E. Chondrosarcoma. Axial T2W image demonstrates a predominantly high-signal lesion involving the body of the sphenoid and right pterygoid. Note very high T2 signal with multiple foci of dark signal and typical off-midline location to suggest chondroid origin.

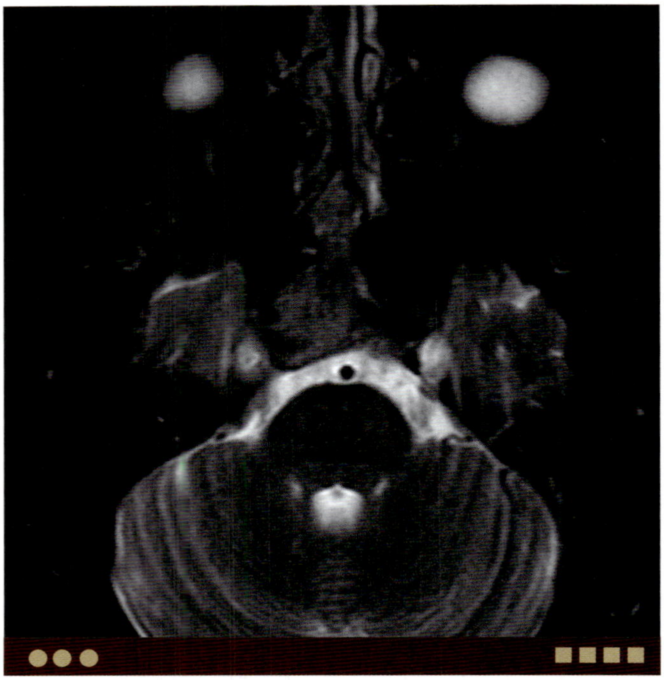

F. Lymphoma. Axial T2W image demonstrates a relatively homogeneous intermediate-signal lesion replacing the clivus.

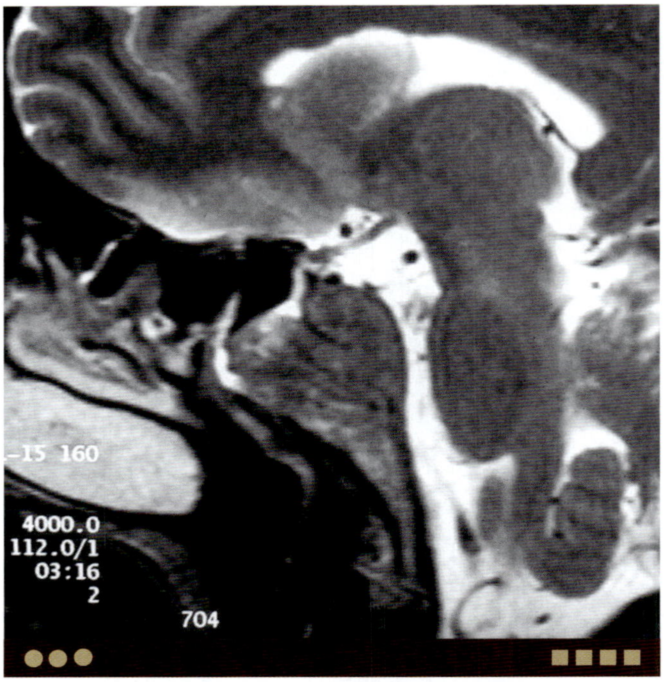

G. Metastasis from colon cancer. Sagittal T2W image demonstrates a slightly expansile intermediate-signal lesion occupying the clivus.

Case 2-8 Chondrosarcoma

Osamu Sakai, Rohini Nadgir

PRESENTATION

Headache.

FINDINGS

CT demonstrates a slightly lobulated, expansile lesion lateral to the clivus with internal heterogeneous calcification. T2W MR image demonstrates a heterogeneously high-signal mass lateral to the clivus.

DIFFERENTIAL

- Chordoma: This demonstrates similar signal pattern, however this arises from the notochord remnant and is located in midline.
- Nasopharyngeal carcinoma: This tumor can be almost completely submucosal and mimic bone tumors. However, signal on T2W images is lower than that of chondrosarcoma.
- Metastatic tumor: This involves the bone marrow rather than cartilage and therefore is more centrally located and demonstrates lower signal on T2W images compared with chondrosarcoma.

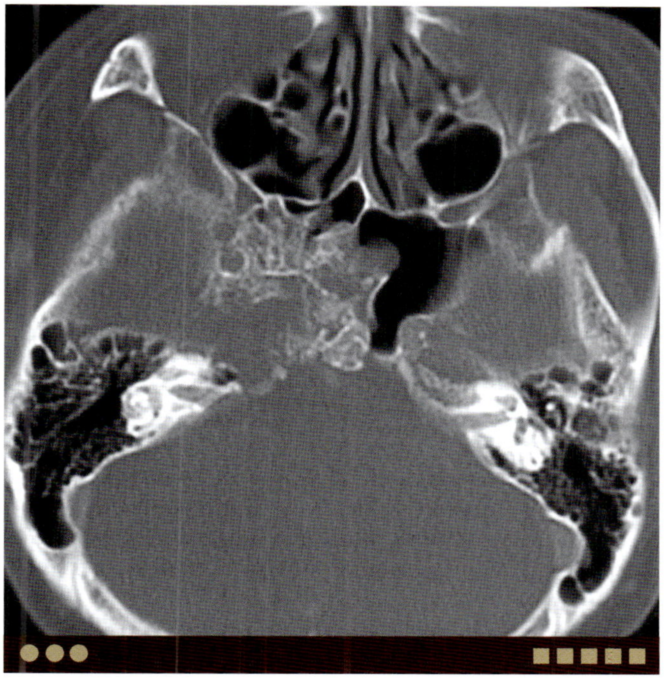

A. Chondrosarcoma. Axial CT shows a slightly lobulated, expansile lesion in the lateral aspect of the sphenoid bone on the right, with internal heterogeneous calcification.

COMMENTS

This is a 44-year-old man with headache.

In the central skull base, chondrosarcoma often arises from the petroclival synchondrosis, therefore it is located off-midline along the lateral aspect of the clivus. This is a key finding to differentiate it from chordoma, which arises from the notochord remnant and is located in the midline.

On CT, chondrosarcoma is seen as a soft tissue density mass, often slightly lobulated with internal calcification, often termed as "ring-and-arc" pattern. Low-to-intermediate enhancement is seen after contrast. On MRI, it usually shows low-to-intermediate T1 and very high T2 signal with internal heterogeneity due to presence of calcifications, and heterogeneous, mild to intermediate enhancement. Chondrosarcoma may show very similar signal pattern to chordoma on MRI; however, the location is different; chondrosarcoma locates off-midline and chordoma locates in midline. Very high signal on T2W images can be seen in both chondrosarcoma and chordoma, however this is helpful to differentiate from nasopharyngeal carcinoma, lymphoma, and metastasis.

Chondrosarcoma in the skull base can be seen as a part of Ollier disease and Maffucci syndrome.

PEARLS

- **Chondrosarcoma often arises from the petroclival synchondrosis in the central skull base and is located off-midline.**
- **"Ring-and-arc" pattern calcification is characteristic to suggest chondroid origin.**
- **Very high T2 signal is commonly seen and helpful to differentiate from nasopharyngeal carcinoma and lymphoma.**

ADDITIONAL IMAGES (B-E)

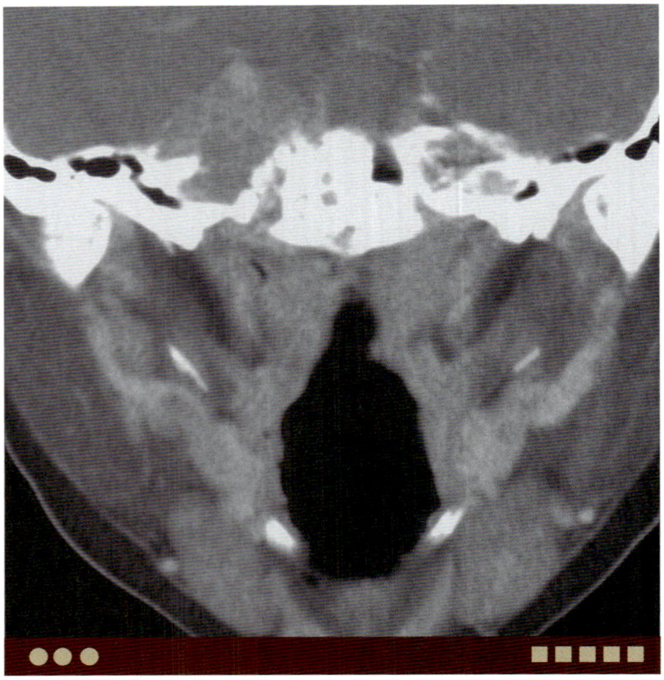

B. Chondrosarcoma, same patient as A. Coronal contrast-enhanced CT shows a slightly enhancing, expansile lesion arising from the junction of the clivus and petrous bone and extending superiorly and laterally.

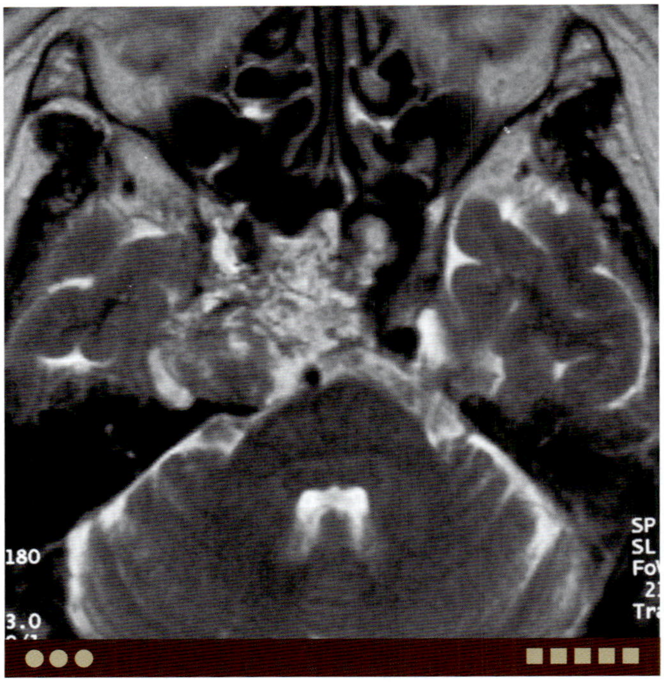

C. Chondrosarcoma, same patient as A. Axial T2W image demonstrates a lobulated, expansile lesion demonstrating predominantly high signal.

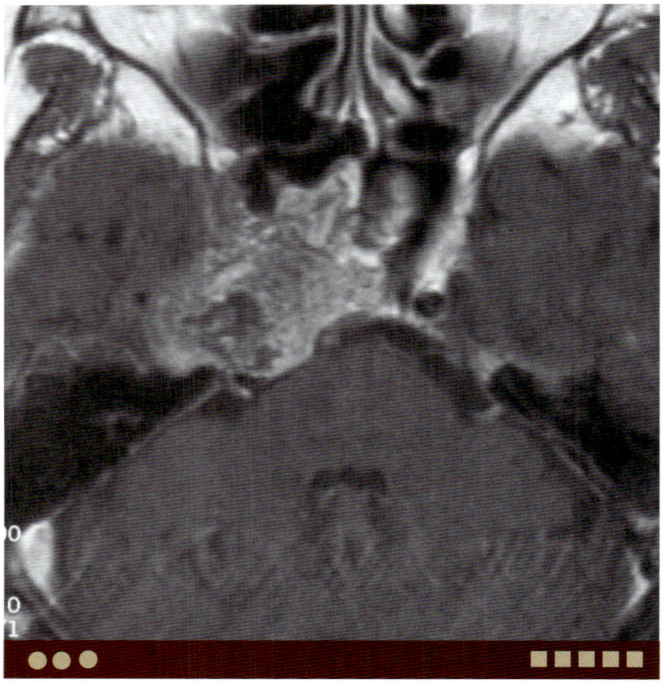

D. Chondrosarcoma, same patient as A. Axial postcontrast T1W image demonstrates a heterogeneous intermediate enhancement of the lesion.

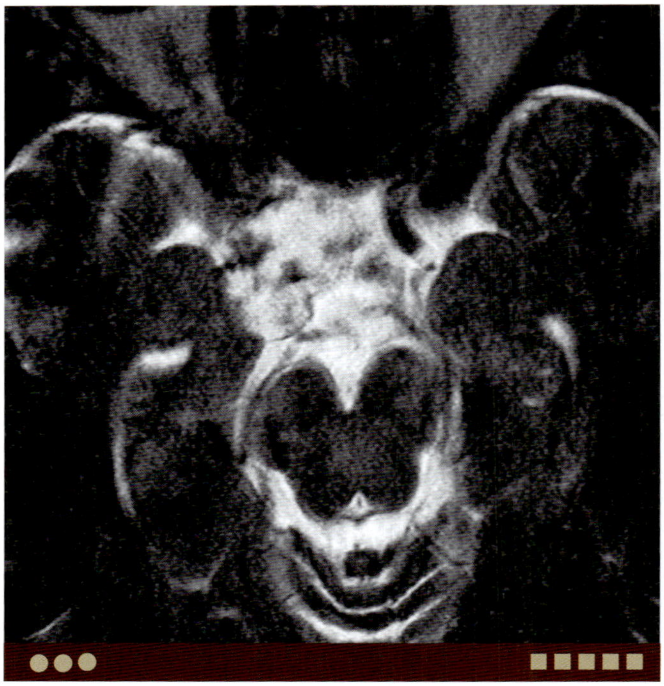

E. **Chondrosarcoma arising from the anterior clinoid**. Axial T2W image demonstrates a lobulated, high-signal lesion involving the right anterior clinoid.

DIFFERENTIAL DIAGNOSIS IMAGES (F-H)

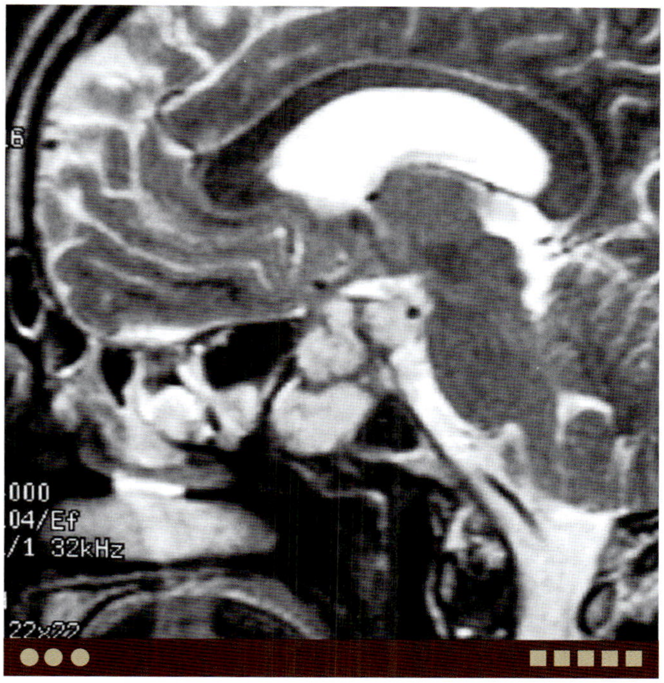

F. Chordoma. Sagittal T2W image demonstrates a lobulated, high-signal lesion involving the clivus and anterior clinoid in midline.

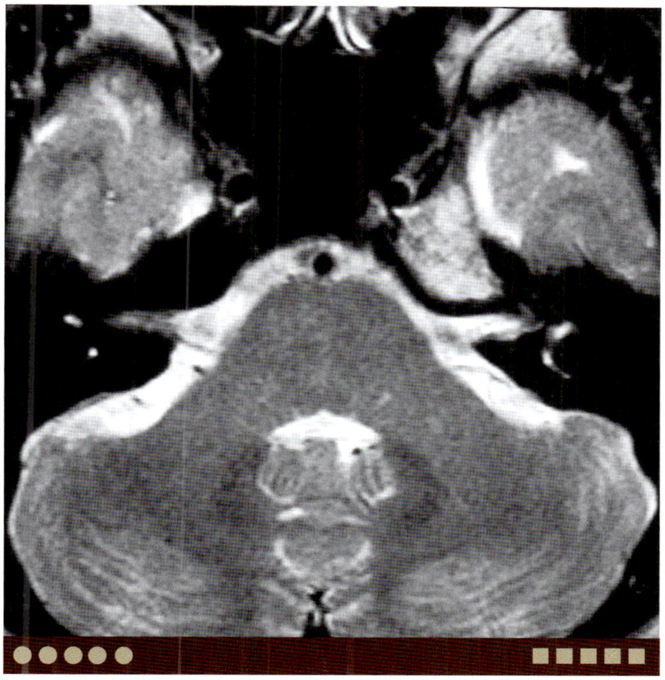

G. Nonpneumatized left petrous apex. Axial T2W image shows nonpneumatized left petrous apex demonstrating high signal from the normal fatty marrow without expansion or invasive findings.

Case 2-9 CSF Tumor Dissemination

Osamu Sakai, Rohini Nadgir

PRESENTATION

Headache.

FINDINGS

Postcontrast T1W images demonstrate abnormal enhancement along the cranial nerves and surface of the brain.

DIFFERENTIAL

- Sarcoidosis: This demonstrates similar findings to CSF tumor dissemination.
- Granulomatous infection: Tuberculosis and cryptococcosis demonstrate similar findings. Patients usually demonstrate clinical pictures for infection.

COMMENTS

This is a 77-year-old woman with breast cancer.

For diagnosis of meningeal carcinomatosis or CSF tumor dissemination, CSF analysis by lumbar puncture is essential to make the diagnosis. However, imaging is often performed to evaluate for conditions which may increase intracranial pressure prior to lumbar puncture, in order to avoid complications.

Noncontrast enhanced CT or MRI may demonstrate obliteration or poor definition of the sulci and cisterns and thickening of the cranial nerves. However, contrast-enhanced MRI is usually needed to demonstrate CSF tumor dissemination.

Postcontrast T1W images demonstrate leptomeningeal enhancement—abnormal enhancement along the surface of the brain and cranial nerves. When diagnosing metastatic brain tumors, it is very important to look for abnormal leptomeningeal or dural enhancement as well as bone metastasis. In patients with CSF tumor dissemination, cranial nerve palsy may be the initial presenting symptom. Thickening or swelling and enhancement of the affected nerve can be seen. Lesions along the seventh and eighth nerve complex may mimic acoustic tumors. Hydrocephalus is also occasionally seen.

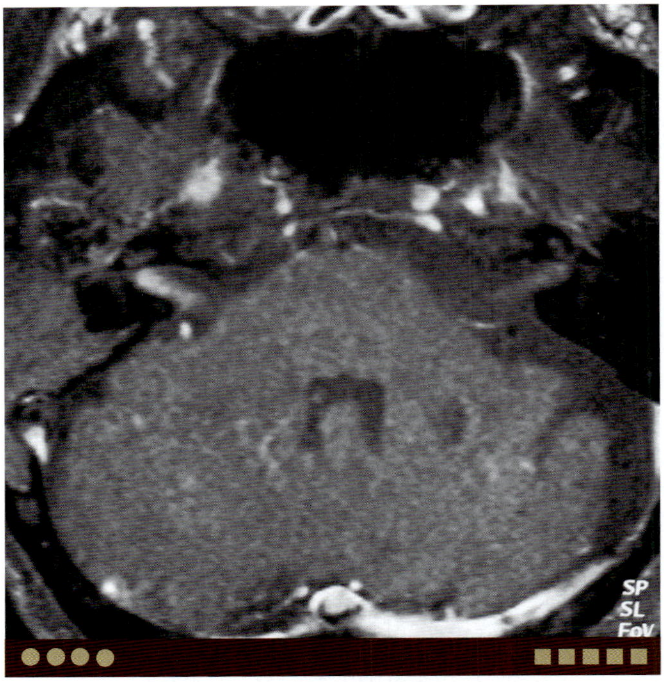

A. CSF tumor dissemination from breast cancer. Axial postcontrast T1W image shows abnormal enhancement along the seventh and eighth cranial nerve complex bilaterally, right more than left.

Sarcoidosis and other granulomatous diseases demonstrate similar findings to tumor dissemination. CSF analysis is needed to confirm the diagnosis. However, even in a patient with sarcoidosis, cerebral herniation related to lumbar puncture has been reported, and careful preprocedure evaluation of the patient is required.

PEARLS

- **Abnormal enhancement along the surface of the brain, sulci, and cranial nerves is a common finding for CSF tumor dissemination.**
- **Thickening/swelling and enhancement of the affected nerves can be seen.**
- **The findings are similar to that of sarcoidosis and other granulomatous diseases.**

ADDITIONAL IMAGES (B-E)

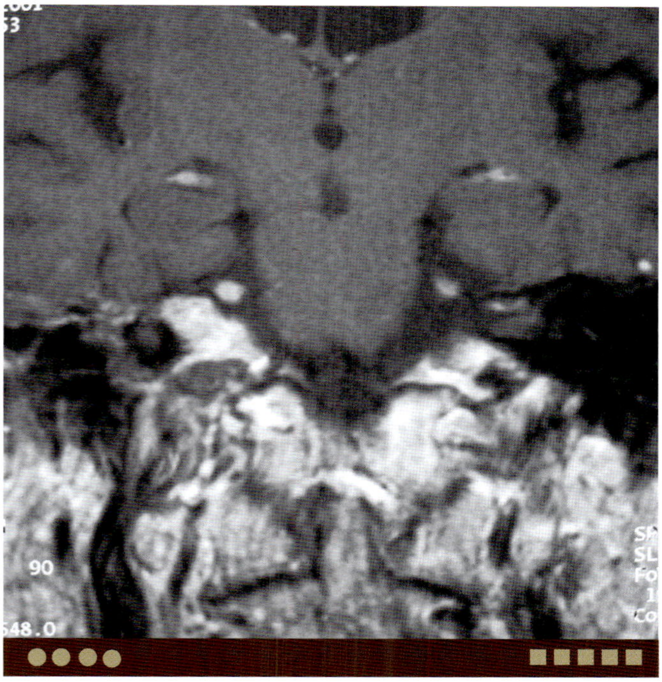

B. CSF tumor dissemination, same patient. Coronal postcontrast T1W image shows abnormal enhancement of the trigeminal nerves, right more than left.

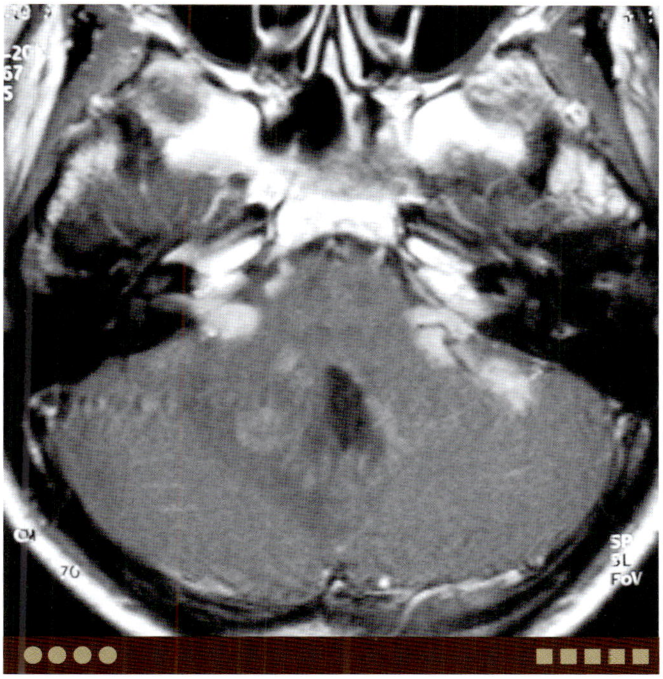

C. CSF tumor dissemination from medulloblastoma. Axial postcontrast T1W image shows abnormal enhancement along the seventh and eighth cranial nerve complex bilaterally as well as along the surface of the left cerebellar hemisphere.

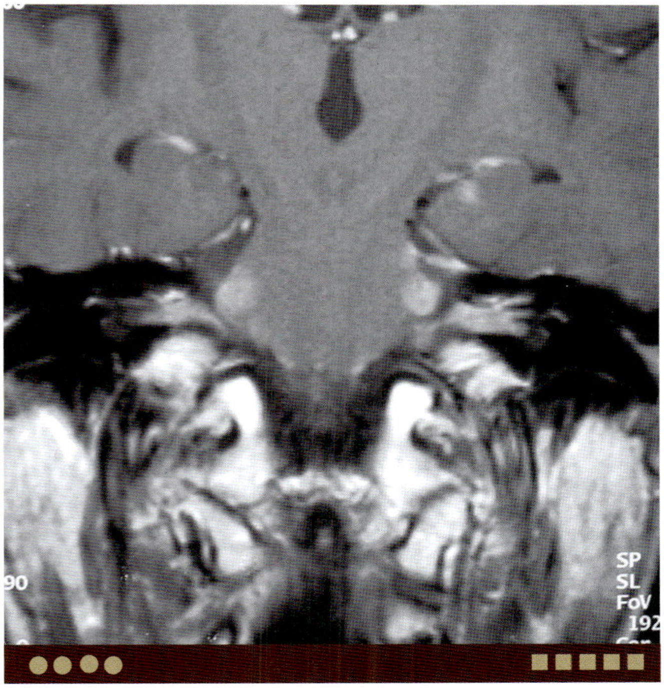

D. Same patient as C. Coronal postcontrast T1W image shows abnormal enhancement along the fifth cranial nerves and seventh and eighth cranial nerve complex bilaterally.

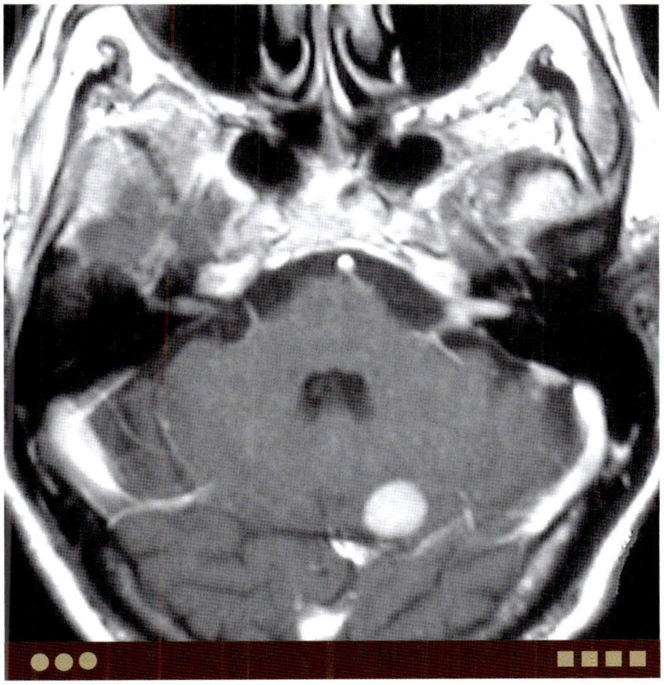

E. CSF tumor dissemination from melanoma. Axial postcontrast T1W image shows abnormal enhancement along the seventh and eighth cranial nerve complex bilaterally, left more than right. Note additional round lesion along the left cerebellar tentorium. The finding may mimic neurofibromatosis type 2.

DIFFERENTIAL DIAGNOSIS IMAGES (F-G)

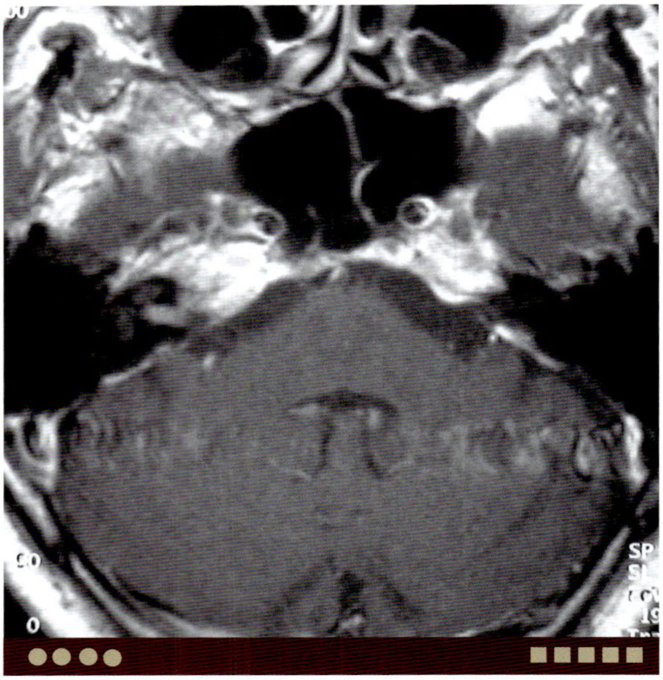

F. Vestibular schwannoma. Axial postcontrast T1W image shows abnormal enhancement in the right internal auditory canal.

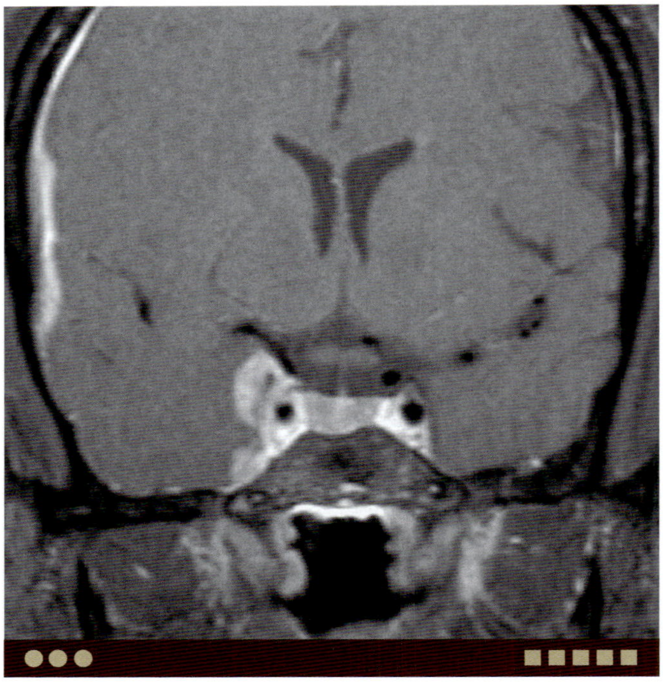

G. Sarcoidosis. Coronal postcontrast T1W image shows abnormal enhancement in the right paracavernous region. Additionally, abnormal dural enhancement is noted in the right frontotemporal region.

Case 2–10 Asymmetric Pneumatization of Petrous Apex

Osamu Sakai, Rohini Nadgir

PRESENTATION

Incidental finding.

FINDINGS

CT demonstrates pneumatized and nonpneumatized petrous apices.

DIFFERENTIAL

- Opacified pneumatized petrous air cells: This is a common condition, and demonstrates water density or signal in the pneumatized petrous air cells without bone remodeling or expansion.
- Cholesterol cyst: This demonstrates high signal both on T1W and T2W images due to proteinaceous or hemorrhagic contents with bone remodeling or expansion.
- Epidermoid cyst: This demonstrates bone remodeling or expansion similar to cholesterol cyst, however, signal pattern on MRI is different; high signal on T2W and low signal on T1W images.
- Chondrosarcoma: This occurs in the petroclival synchondrosis, the junction between the clivus and petrous bone, contains internal calcification, and usually demonstrates low signal on T1W images and high signal on T2W images to suggest chondroid tissue.

COMMENTS

This is a 25-year-old man scanned for headache.

Asymmetric pneumatization of petrous apex is a very common condition or normal variant. Air density in the pneumatized petrous apex and normal bone trabeculation in the nonpneumatized side are assuring findings for this benign condition on CT. However, this condition may be confusing on MRI, and occasionally this is misdiagnosed as cholesterol cyst, chondrosarcoma or metastatic tumor. Careful observation on multiple sequences is essential to make a diagnosis. Pneumatized petrous apex demonstrates no signal on all sequences, and nonpneumatized apex shows fatty marrow signal; high on T1W, intermediate-to-high on T2W, and low signal on fat-suppressed images. Bone remodeling, expansion, or destruction should not be seen.

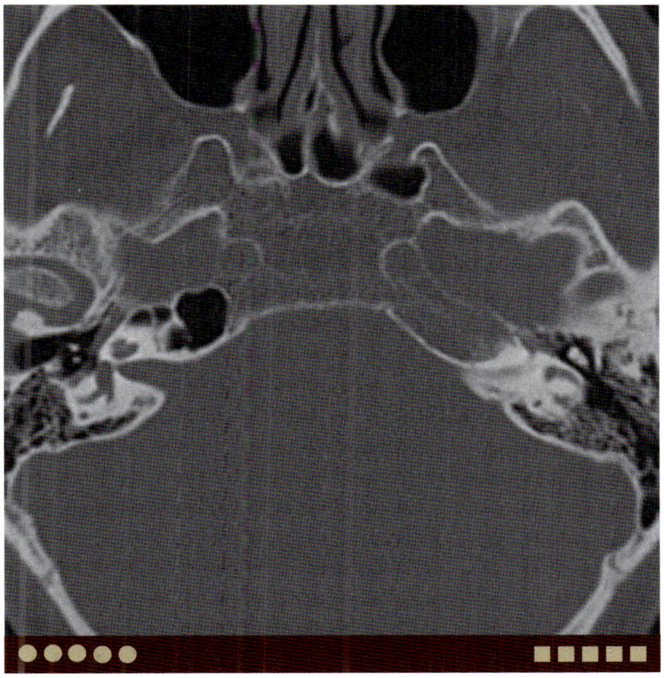

A. Asymmetric pneumatization of petrous apex. Axial CT shows pneumatized right and nonpneumatized left petrous apices.

PEARLS

- **Asymmetric pneumatization of the petrous apex is a normal variant.**
- **On MRI, pneumatized petrous apex demonstrates no signal and nonpneumatized apex shows fat signal; high on T1W, intermediate-to-high on T2W, and low signal on fat-suppressed images.**
- **On CT, pneumatized petrous apex demonstrates air density and nonpneumatized apex shows normal trabeculation and fat density.**

ADDITIONAL IMAGES (B-D)

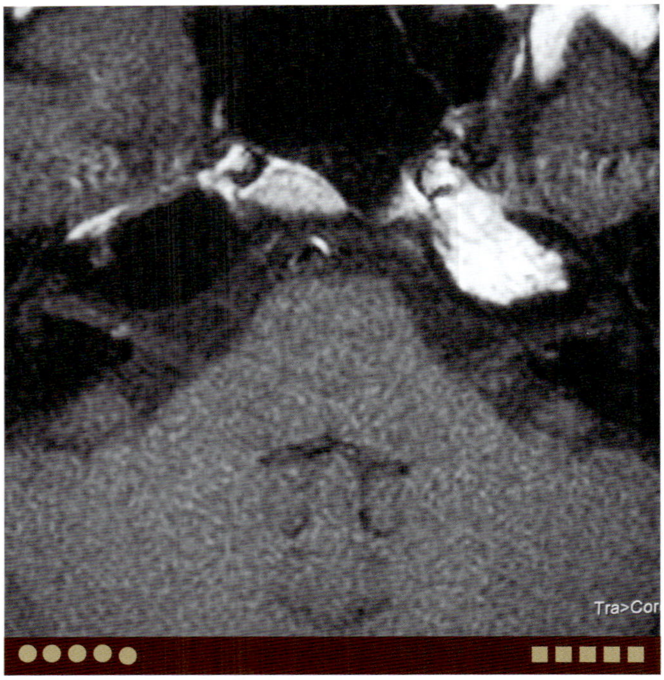

B. Asymmetric pneumatization of petrous apex in a different patient. Axial T1W MR image demonstrates high signal from the fatty marrow in the left petrous apex. Note normal trabeculation pattern in the marrow.

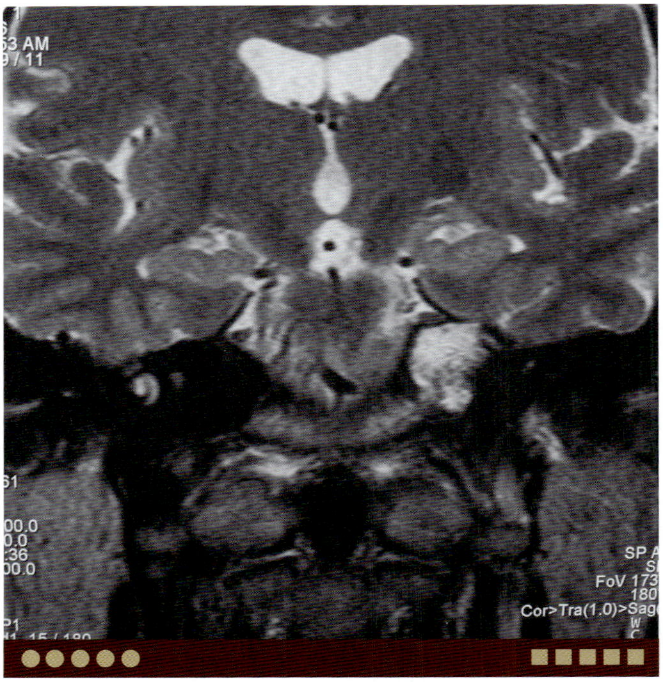

C. Asymmetric pneumatization of petrous apex, same patient as B. Coronal T2W MR image demonstrates high signal from the fatty marrow in the left petrous apex. Note normal trabeculation pattern in the marrow.

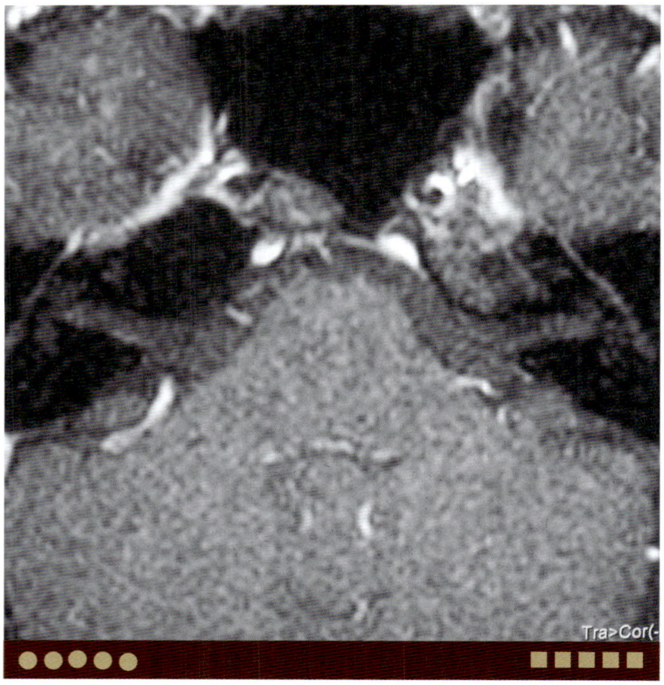

D. Asymmetric pneumatization of petrous apex, same patient as B. Axial postcontrast fat-suppressed T1W MR image demonstrates suppression of the signal in the left petrous apex confirming fatty marrow.

DIFFERENTIAL DIAGNOSIS IMAGES (E-G)

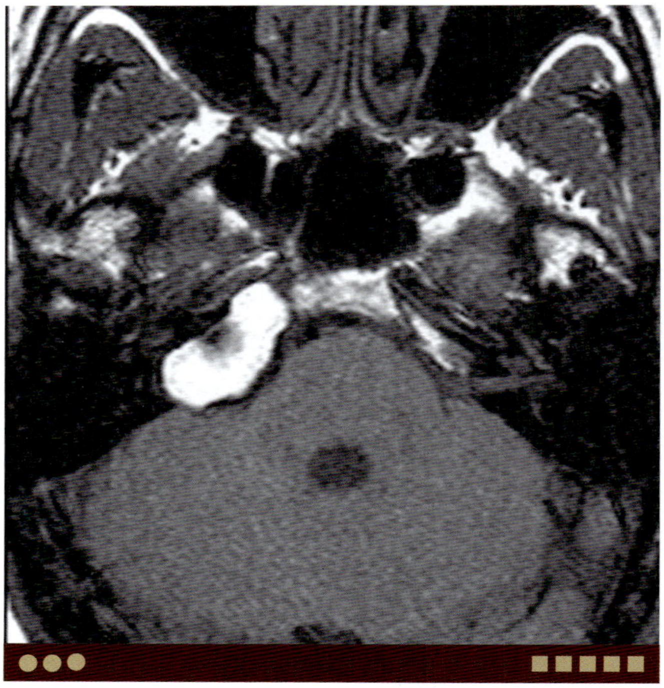

E. Cholesterol cyst. Axial T1W MR image demonstrates an expansile high-signal lesion in the right petrous apex.

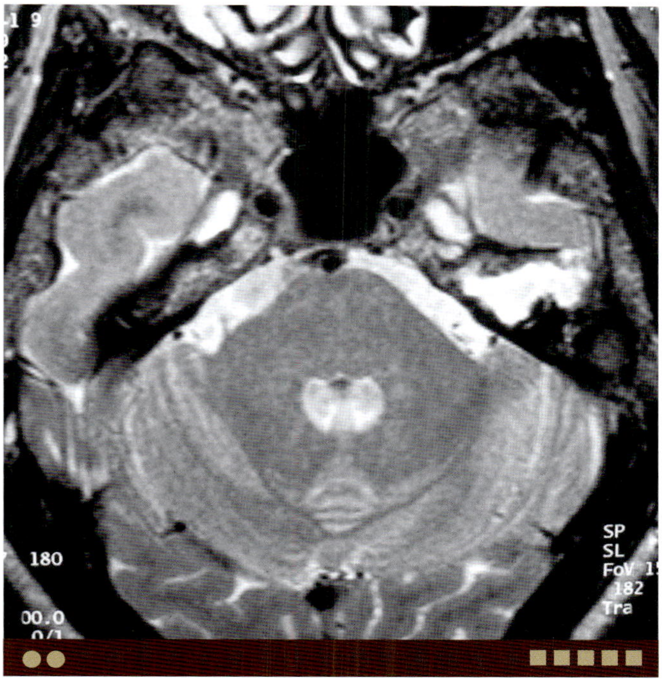

F. Epidermoid cyst. Axial T2W MR image demonstrates a slightly expansile high-signal lesion in the left petrous apex.

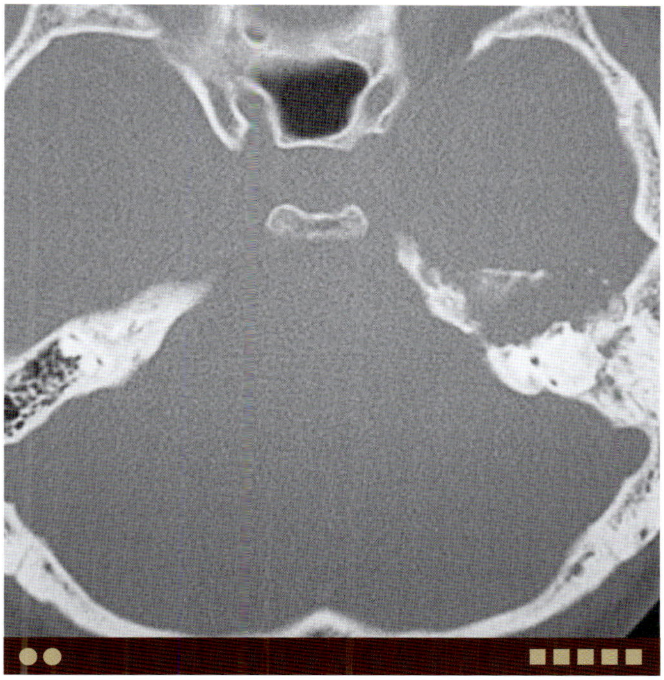

G. Epidermoid cyst, same patient as F. Axial CT demonstrates a slightly expansile lesion in the left petrous apex.

Case 2–11 Sarcoidosis

Osamu Sakai, Rohini Nadgir

PRESENTATION

Headache.

FINDINGS

Postcontrast T1W images demonstrate abnormal enhancement along the cranial nerves.

DIFFERENTIAL

- Carcinomatous meningitis/CSF tumor dissemination: This demonstrates leptomeningeal enhancement (abnormal enhancement of the surface of the brain and cranial nerves), similar to sarcoidosis. CSF analysis is needed to confirm the diagnosis.
- Granulomatous infection: Tuberculosis and cryptococcosis demonstrate similar findings. These patients usually demonstrate symptoms of infection.

COMMENTS

This is a 68-year-old woman with multiple cranial nerve palsies.

Sarcoidosis is a disease causing noncaseating epithelioid granulomas in multiple organs, such as lungs, lymphoid tissues, skin, orbits, etc. About 5% of patients with sarcoidosis show CNS involvement, and rarely the disease is limited in the CNS. Patients may initially present with cranial nerve palsy and diabetes insipidus. Most cases of sarcoidosis demonstrate similar findings to granulomatous meningitis or carcinomatous meningitis, most often prominently seen in the posterior cranial fossa and skull base, and it is almost impossible to differentiate sarcoidosis from these conditions by imaging alone. CSF analysis is essential to make a diagnosis. Secondary hydrocephalus can be also seen in these conditions. Serologically, increased angiotensin-converting enzyme (ACE) is common.

CSF analysis is needed to confirm the diagnosis as discussed. However, cerebral herniation related to lumbar puncture in a patient with sarcoidosis has been reported, and careful preprocedure evaluation of the patient is required.

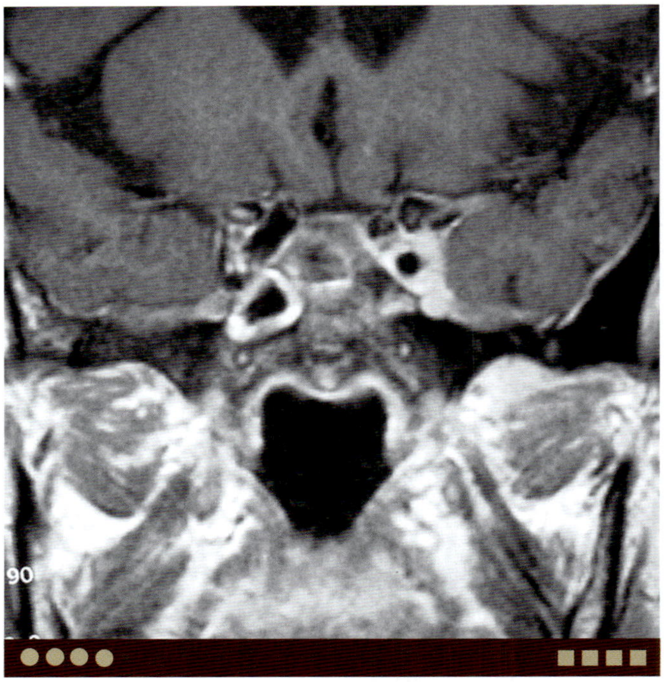

A. Sarcoidosis. Coronal postcontrast T1W image shows abnormal enhancement of the left Meckel's cave. Note swelling and abnomal enhancement of the second branch of the trigeminal nerve (V2).

PEARLS

- **Abnormal enhancement along the surface of the brain, sulci, and cranial nerves is a common finding in sarcoidosis.**
- **Thickening or swelling and enhancement of the affected nerve can be seen.**

ADDITIONAL IMAGES (B-D)

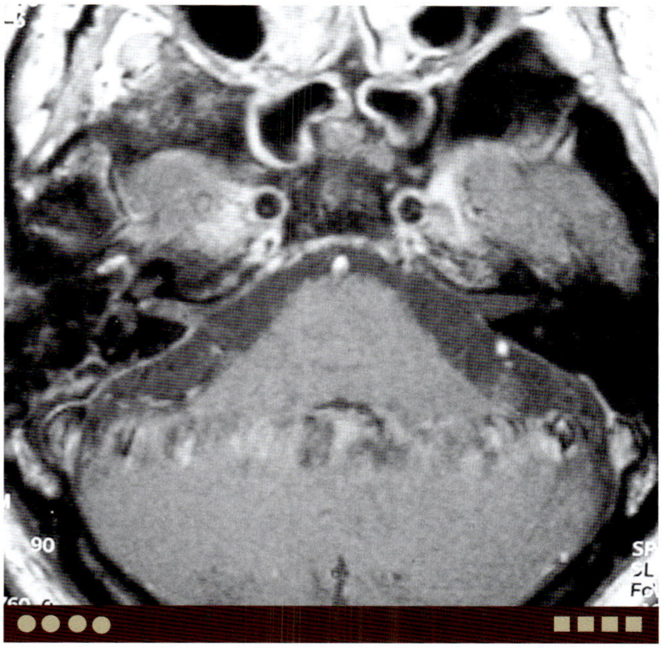

B. Sarcoidosis, same patient as A. Axial postcontrast T1W image shows abnormal meningeal enhancement in the middle cranial fossa, including in the right internal auditory canal. Note abnormal enhancement of the Meckel's cave, left more than right.

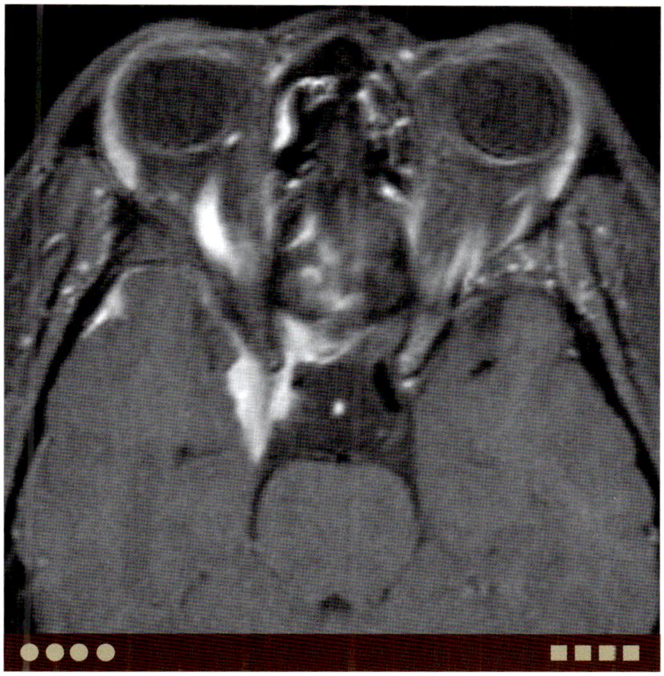

C. **Sarcoidosis** in a different patient. Axial postcontrast T1W image shows abnormal dural-based enhancement in the right paracavernous region. Note additional focal abnormal meningeal enhancement in the right temporal region.

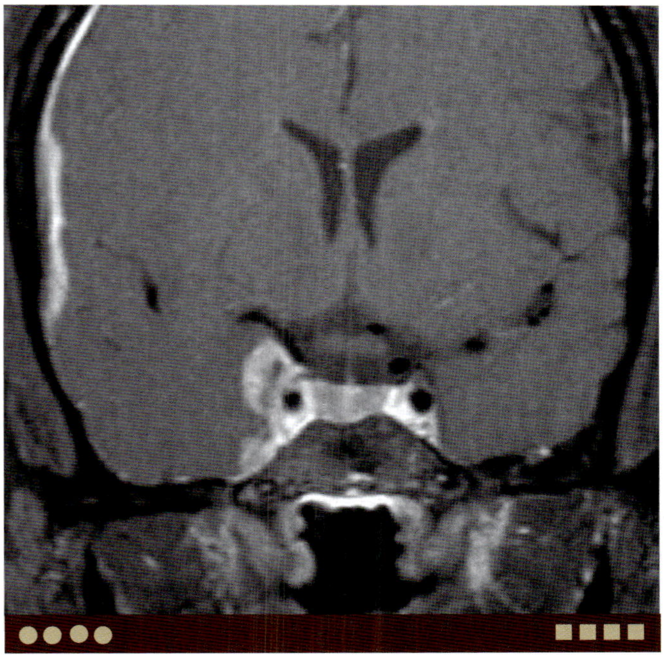

D. Sarcoidosis, same patient as C. Coronal postcontrast T1W image shows abnormal enhancement of the right paracavernous region. Abnormal dural-based enhancement is seen in the right frontotemporal region.

DIFFERENTIAL DIAGNOSIS IMAGES (E-G)

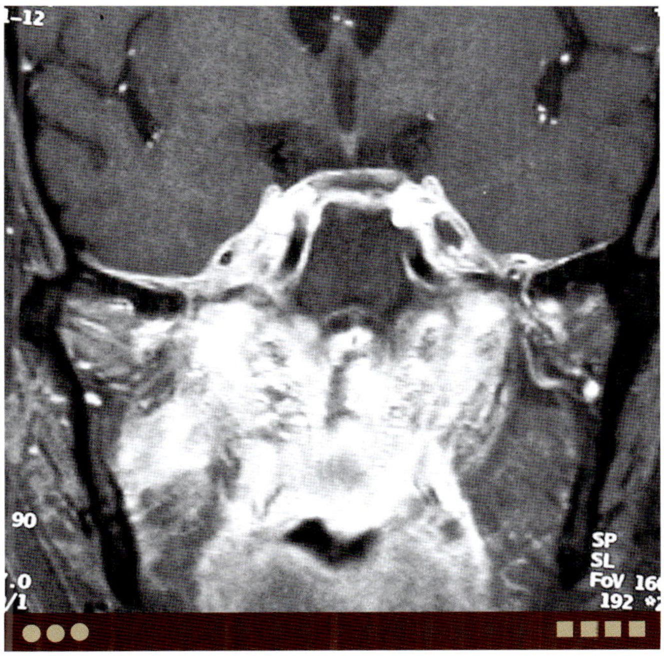

E. **Wegener's granulomatosis**. Coronal postcontrast T1W image demonstrates abnormal enhancement of the Meckel's cave and adjacent meninges bilaterally. Note diffuse abnormal enhancement of the pharyngeal mucosa with extension to the parapharyngeal and masticator spaces.

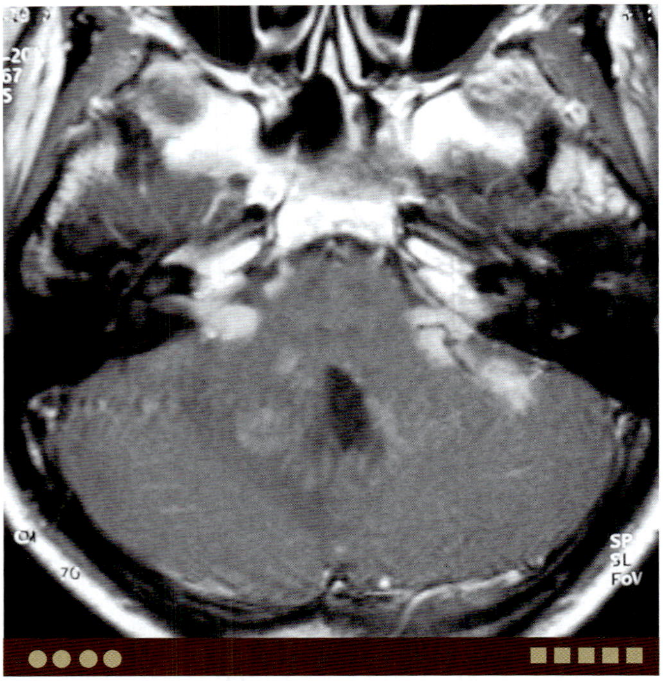

F. CSF tumor dissemination from medulloblastoma. Axial postcontrast T1W image shows abnormal enhancement along the seventh and eighth cranial nerve complex bilaterally as well as left cerebellar hemisphere.

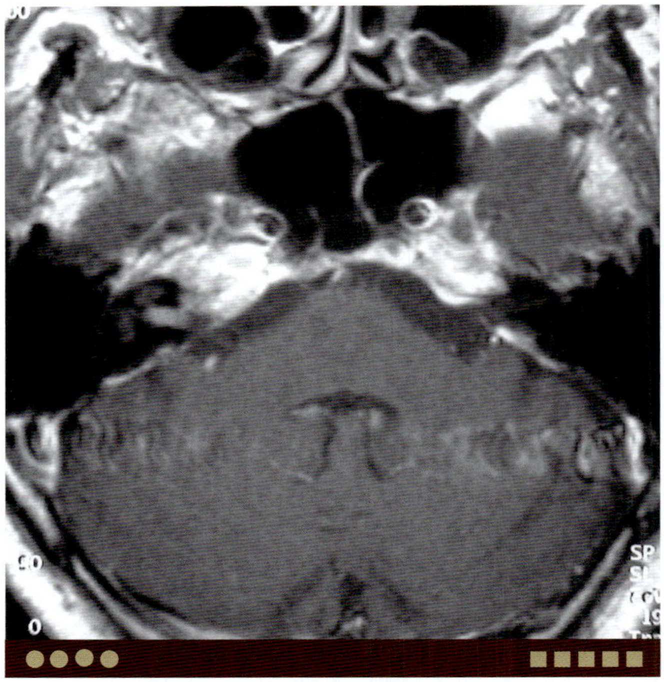

G. Vestibular schwannoma. Axial postcontrast T1W image shows abnormal enhancement in the right internal auditory canal.

Case 2–12 Pituitary Adenoma

Osamu Sakai, Rohini Nadgir

PRESENTATION

Visual field defect.

FINDINGS

Postcontrast T1W images demonstrate enlarged pituitary gland compressing the optic chiasm.

DIFFERENTIAL

- Craniopharyngioma: This often demonstrates calcification and cystic components which can be bright on T1W images due to proteinaceous contents.
- Rathke's cleft cyst: This is a congenital/developmental cystic lesion that often demonstrates increased signal on T1W images from proteinaceous contents.

COMMENTS

This is a 47-year-old woman with visual field defect.

Pituitary adenoma is the most common sellar or parasellar tumor and should be always included in the differential diagnosis of mass lesions in this location. Hyperfunctioning adenomas cause endocrinological abnormality, such as galactorrhea and amenorrhea and are found in relatively small sizes (< 1 cm, microadenoma). Nonhyperfunctioning adenomas are not clinically evident until they cause mass-effect upon the optic chiasm and visual field defects (typically bitemporal hemianopsia), and are therefore large at the time of diagnosis (> 1 cm, macroadenoma). Typically, pituitary adenoma grows superiorly and causes mass-effect on the optic chiasm, or laterally to involve the cavernous sinuses. However, occasionally it demonstrates significant inferior extension and is seen as a nasal mass on exam.

Typically, adenomas demonstrate similar signal to the brain parenchyma on all sequences, and relatively homogeneous enhancement. With increase in size, internal hemorrhage, necrosis, and cystic degeneration can occur and they can demonstrate more variable signal and heterogeneous enhancement.

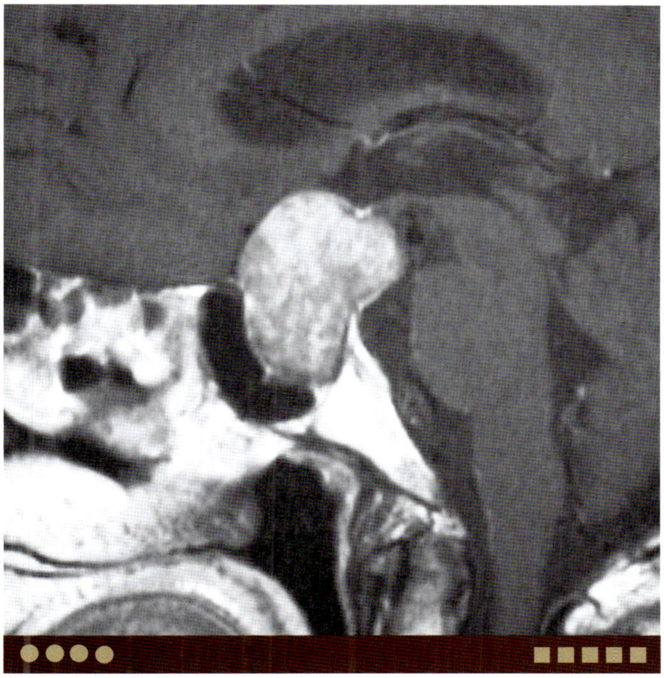

A. Pituitary adenoma. Sagittal postcontrast T1W MR image demonstrates a heterogeneously enhancing lesion centered in the sella.

PEARLS

- **Pituitary adenoma is the most common sellar or parasellar tumor.**
- **Hyperfunctioning adenomas are usually found due to endocrinological abnormality, while nonhyperfunctioning adenomas are often found on clinical presentation of visual field defect due to mass-effect on the optic chiasm.**
- **Pituitary adenomas can grow inferiorly and destroy the skull base.**

ADDITIONAL IMAGES (B-C)

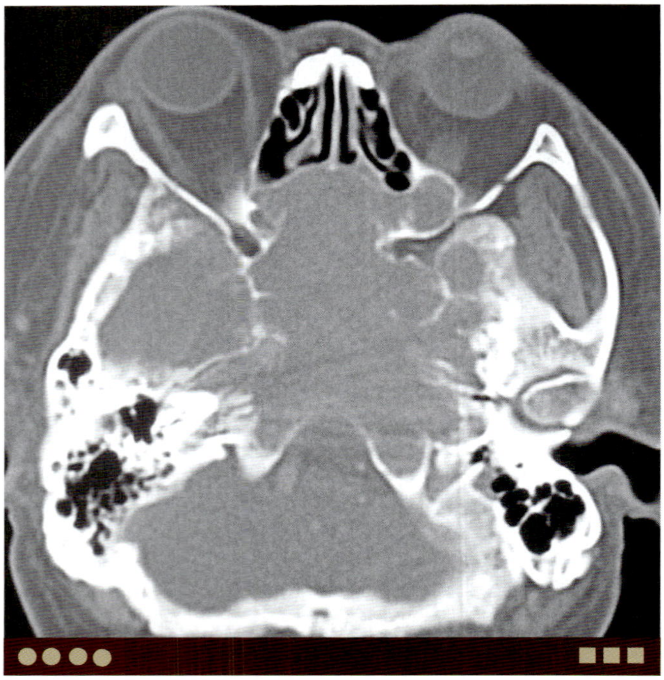

B. Pituitary adenoma in a different patient. Axial CT demonstrates a soft tissue mass destroying the skull base.

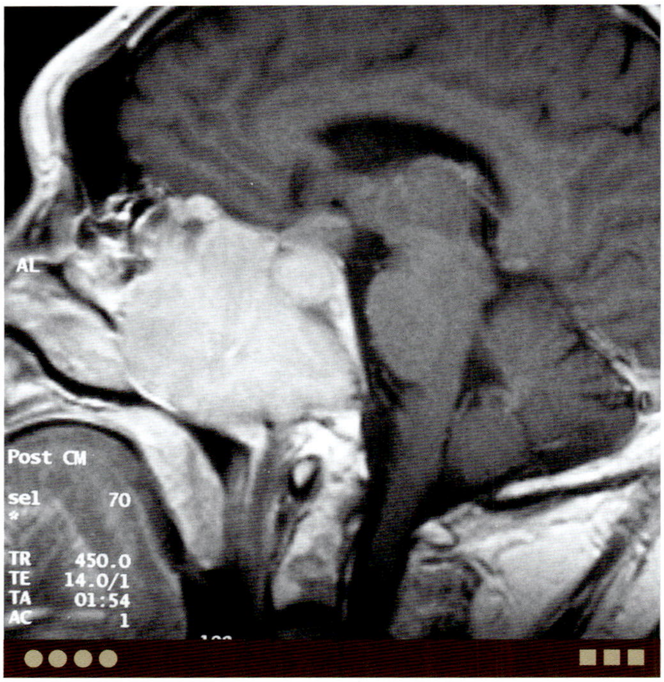

C. Pituitary adenoma, same patient as B. Sagittal postcontrast T1W MR image demonstrates a large homogeneously enhancing lesion invading the clivus, occupying the sphenoid and posterior ethmoid sinuses and extending to the nasal cavity.

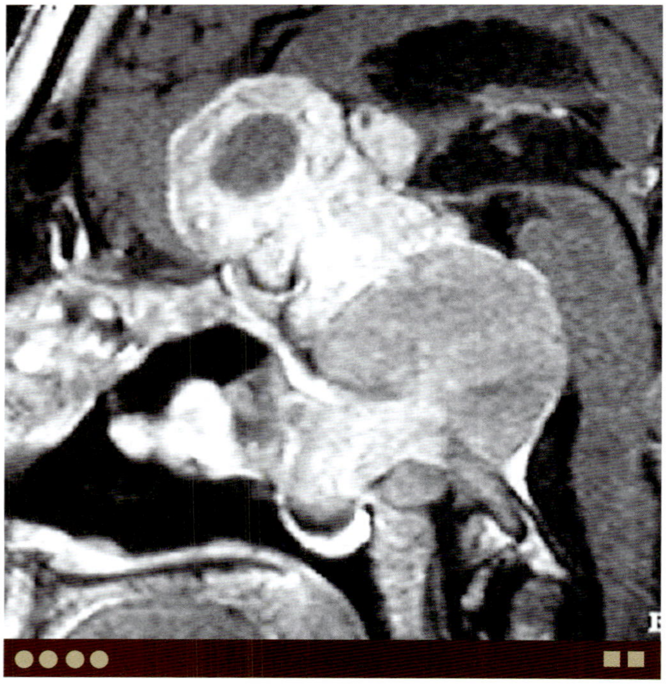

D. Pituitary adenoma in a different patient. Sagittal postcontrast T1W MR image demonstrates a large heterogeneously enhancing lesion invading the clivus and extending to the nasopharynx. Note significant superior and inferior extension of the tumor.

DIFFERENTIAL DIAGNOSIS IMAGES (E-G)

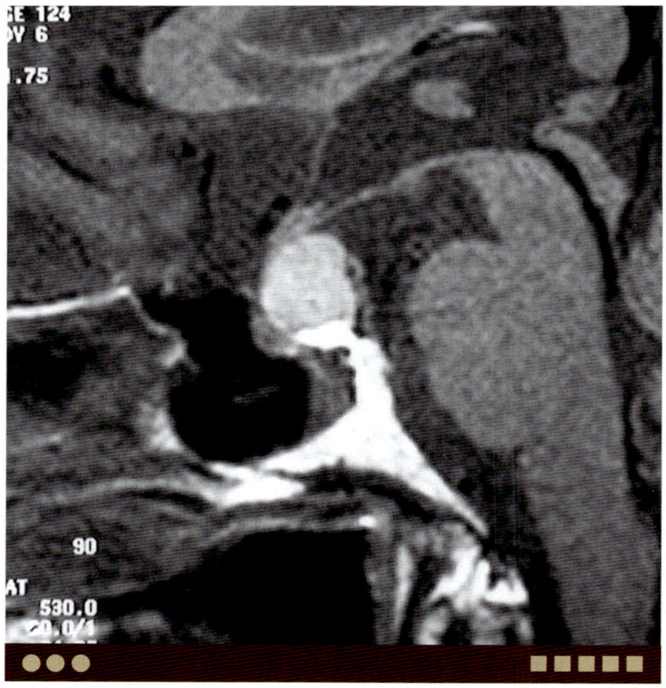

E. Rathke's cleft cyst. Sagittal T1W image demonstrates a large cystic lesion with high-signal contents in the sellar/suprasellar region without aggressive destructive findings.

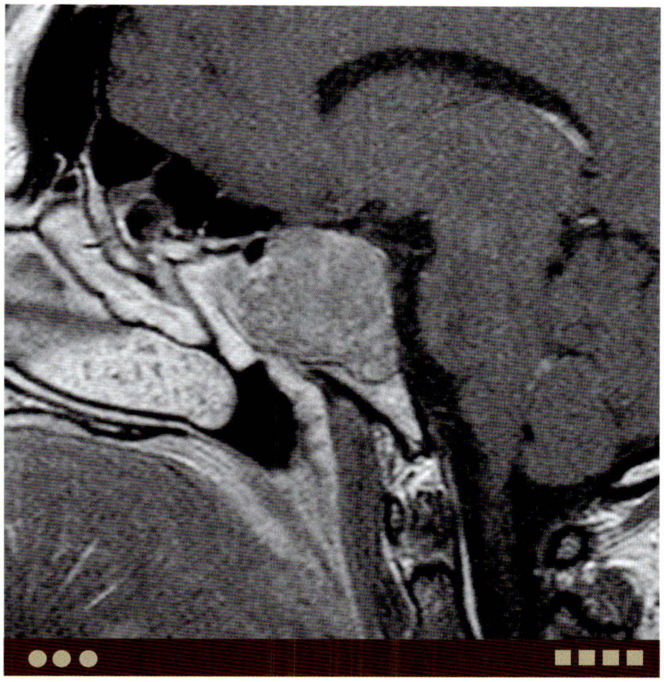

F. Lymphoma. Sagittal postcontrast T1W MR image demonstrates a mildly enhancing lesion invading the clivus and occupying the sphenoid sinus.

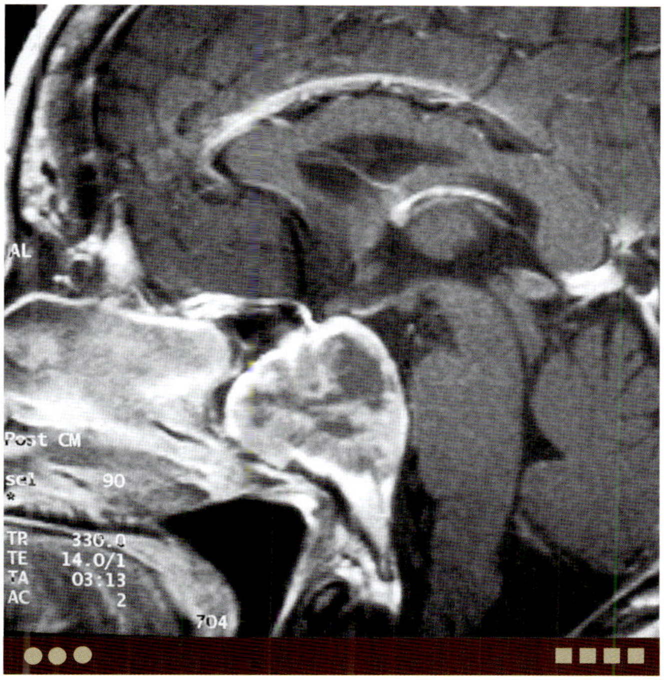

G. Metastasis from colon cancer. Sagittal postcontrast T1W MR image demonstrates a heterogeneously enhancing lesion invading the clivus and occupying the sphenoid sinus.

Case 2–13 Craniopharyngioma

Osamu Sakai, Rohini Nadgir

PRESENTATION

Visual field defect.

FINDINGS

CT demonstrates a partially cystic suprasellar mass with calcification.

DIFFERENTIAL

- Pituitary adenoma: This is the most common tumor in the sellar or suprasellar regions, and is occasionally cystic. However, calcification is rare.
- Rathke's cleft cyst: This is a congenital/developmental cystic lesion, often demonstrating increased T1 signal from proteinaceous contents, and should not have large solid portion.

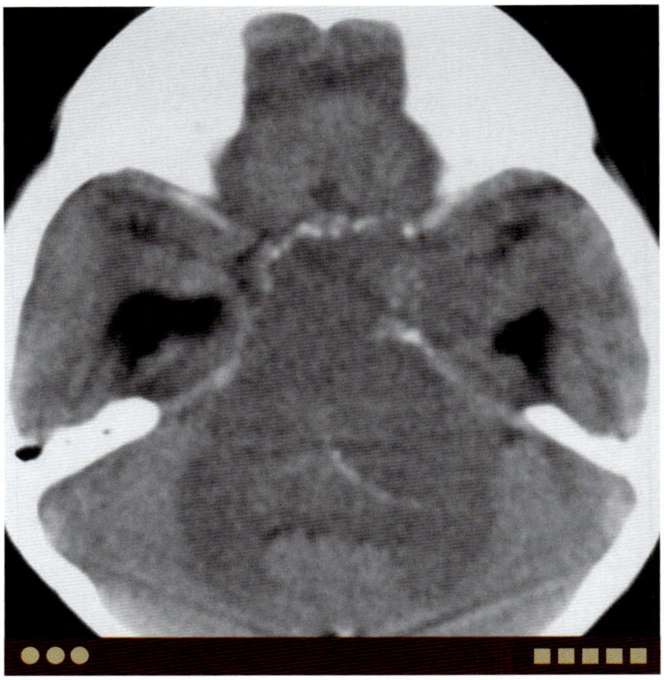

A. Craniopharyngioma. Axial CT shows a slightly lobulated cystic lesion with peripheral calcification. Note dilatation of the temporal horns of the lateral ventricles due to obstruction.

COMMENTS

This is a 3-year-old boy with headache and visual field defect.

Craniopharyngioma is a tumor arising from the squamous epithelium in the remnant of the pituitary-Rathke's pouch. This tumor is often seen in young children as well as adults in their fifties or sixties. It is histologically benign however locally aggressive and causes significant mass effect upon adjacent structures. Also, cases of malignant transformation into squamous cell carcinoma have been reported. Craniopharyngioma usually grows superiorly and causes mass effect upon the optic chiasm as well as frontal lobes. However, rarely it grows inferiorly and is noted as a nasal mass on exam.

On CT, it often demonstrates cystic portions and calcification. Presence of calcification is helpful to differentiate it from pituitary adenomas because calcification is rare in pituitary adenomas. On MRI, the cystic portion tends to demonstrate high signal on T1W images from "crankcase oil"—like proteinaceous contents. Craniopharyngioma tends to cause more mass effect compared to pituitary adenomas, and edema along the optic tract is more commonly seen, which can be a clue to differentiate it from pituitary adenomas.

PEARLS

- **Craniopharyngioma has two age peaks; young children and adults in their fifties and sixties.**
- **Cysts and calcification are commonly seen in craniopharyngiomas.**
- **Edema along the optic tract is more commonly seen with craniopharyngiomas compared with pituitary adenomas.**

ADDITIONAL IMAGES (B-E)

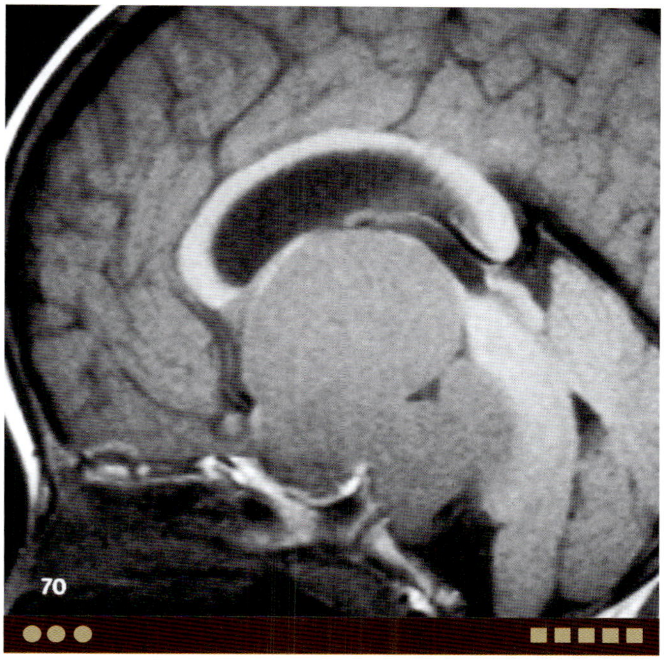

B. Craniopharyngioma, same patient as A. Sagittal T1W image demonstrates a large lobulated cystic lesion compressing the brainstem and remodeling the sella. Note slightly increased signal in the lesion compared with the cerebrospinal fluid suggesting increased protein concentration.

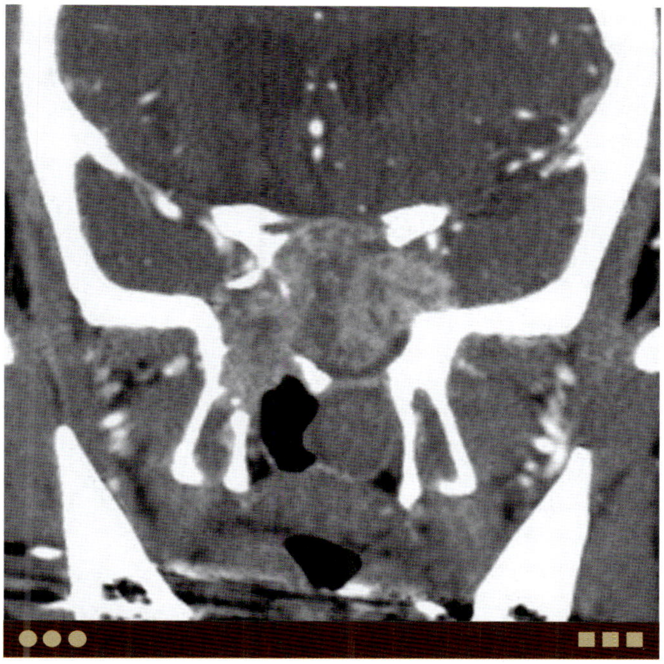

C. Craniopharyngioma in a different patient. Coronal postcontrast CT demonstrates a heterogeneously enhancing lesion destroying the skull base and extending into the sphenoid sinus and nasopharynx.

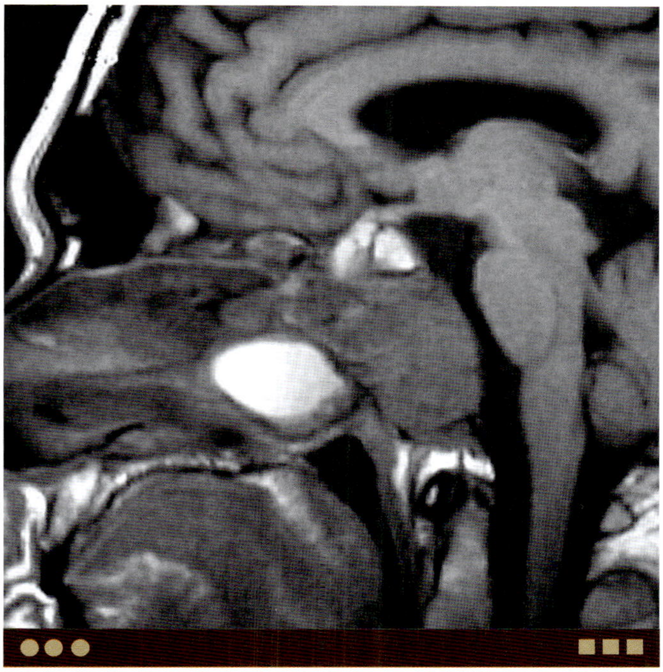

D. Craniopharyngioma in a different patient. Sagittal T1W image demonstrates a large multiloculated lesion destroying the clivus and extending into the sphenoid sinus and nasal cavity. Note significantly increased signal in some cystic components, a characteristic finding for craniopharyngioma.

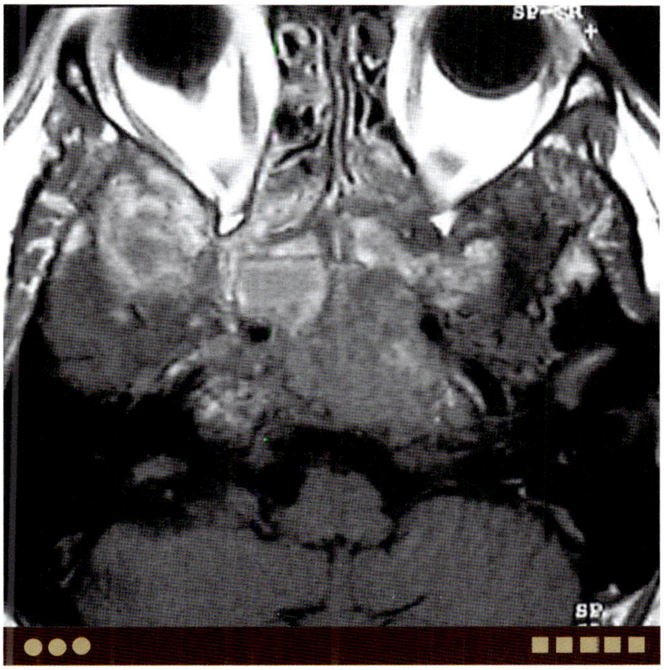

E. Craniopharyngioma in a different patient. Axial postcontrast T1W image demonstrates a large solid and cystic lesion destroying the clivus and causing mass effect upon the internal carotid arteries. The lesion demonstrates heterogeneous enhancement and cysts with increased T1 signal.

DIFFERENTIAL DIAGNOSIS IMAGES (F-G)

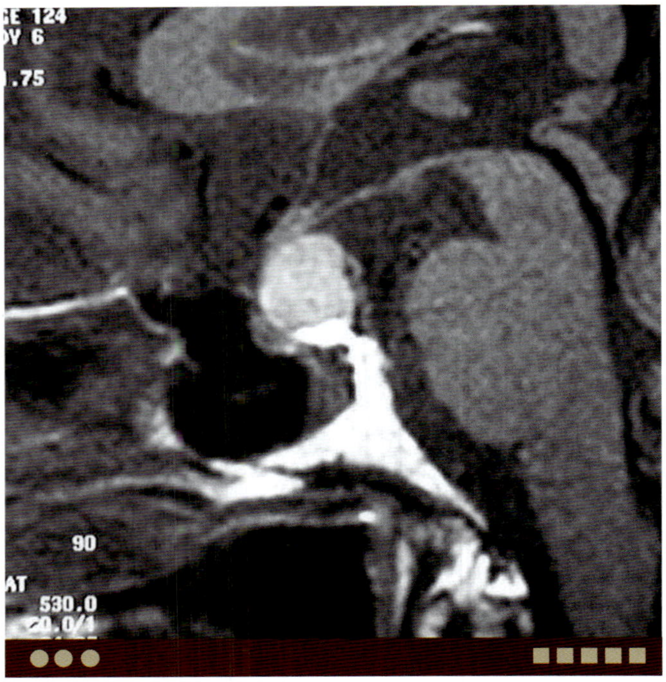

F. Rathke's cleft cyst. Sagittal T1W image demonstrates a large cystic lesion with high-signal contents in the sellar/suprasellar region without aggressive destructive findings.

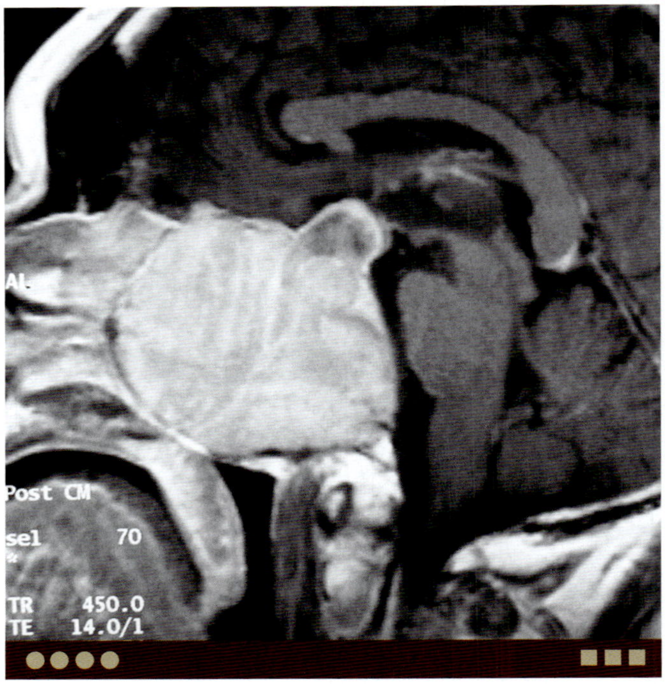

G. Pituitary adenoma. Sagittal postcontrast T1W image demonstrates a large enhancing lesion involving the clivus and extending into the posterior ethmoid air cells and nasal cavity. Note relatively homogeneous enhancement compared with craniopharyngioma.

Case 2–14 Petrous Apicitis

Osamu Sakai, Rohini Nadgir

PRESENTATION

Headache and fever.

FINDINGS

Postcontrast T1W MR images demonstrate abnormal enhancement in the petrous apex.

DIFFERENTIAL

- Opacified pneumatized petrous air cells: This is a very common condition, and demonstrates water density or signal in the pneumatized petrous air cells without bone remodeling.
- Rhabdomyosarcoma: This is an aggressive malignant tumor; however, clinical presentation may be similar to ordinary otitis media. MRI should be performed if clinical presentation involves cranial nerve palsy. MRI can demonstrate enhancing soft tissue tumor.
- Langerhans cell histiocytosis: Clinical presentation may be similar to ordinary otitis media. Osteolytic change and enhancing solid lesions are seen. Findings are often similar to that of rhabdomyosarcoma.
- Cholesterol cyst: This demonstrates high signal both on T1W and T2W images from proteinaceous and hemorrhagic contents with bone remodeling/expansion. No solid enhancement is seen.
- Epidermoid cyst: This demonstrates bone remodeling/expansion similar to cholesterol cyst, however signal pattern on MRI is different; high signal on T2W and low signal on T1W images is seen.

COMMENTS

This is a 6-year-old girl with otitis media.

Petrous apicitis is infection or inflammation in the petrous portion of the temporal bone, usually extending from otitis media or mastoiditis. This condition is relatively rare because of widespread use of antibiotics for middle ear infection. Influenza and pneumococcus are common pathogens.

Infection in this area can extend to the adjacent paracavernous region, which may result in cranial nerve involvement. Gradenigo triad includes mastoiditis, sixth nerve palsy, and pain in the fifth nerve distribution. However, it is rare to see all three symptoms due to current use of antibiotics. Delayed diagnosis and treatment increases risk of meningitis, sinus thrombosis, epidural abscess, and pseudoaneurysm, and early diagnosis is essential for favorable outcome.

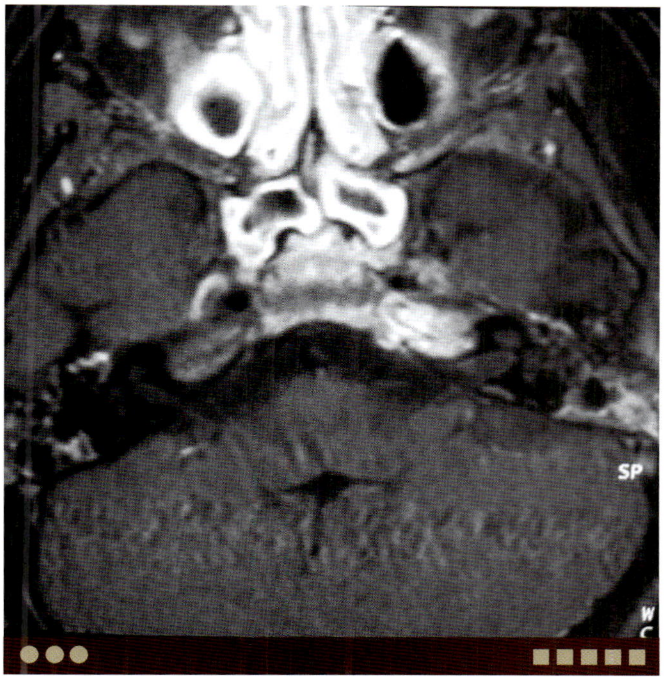

A. Petrous apicitis. Axial postcontrast fat-suppressed T1W image shows abnormal enhancement of the left petrous apex in addition to inflammatory change in the mastoid portion. Note narrowing of the left internal carotid artery compared with the right.

CT demonstrates opacification of the tympanic cavity and mastoid air cells as seen in ordinary otitis media. Extension of middle ear infection to the petrous apex may demonstrate abnormal soft tissue density with ill-defined osteolytic change in the late stage; however, it is difficult to identify this abnormality on CT in the early phase of this condition.

On MRI, loss of normal signal of the fatty marrow in the petrous apex and abnormal enhancement is easily seen. High-resolution images can demonstrate involvement of the cavernous sinus and cranial nerves. MRI is strongly recommended when petrous apicitis is clinically suspected, particularly in patients with cranial nerve impairment.

PEARLS

- **Petrous apicitis is infection/inflammation in the petrous portion of the temporal bone, usually extending from otitis media or mastoiditis.**
- **Gradenigo triad includes mastoiditis, sixth nerve palsy and pain in the fifth nerve distribution.**
- **Rhabdomyosarcoma shows similar clinical presentation to ordinary otitis media. MRI should be performed if cranial nerve palsy is noted.**

ADDITIONAL IMAGES (B-C)

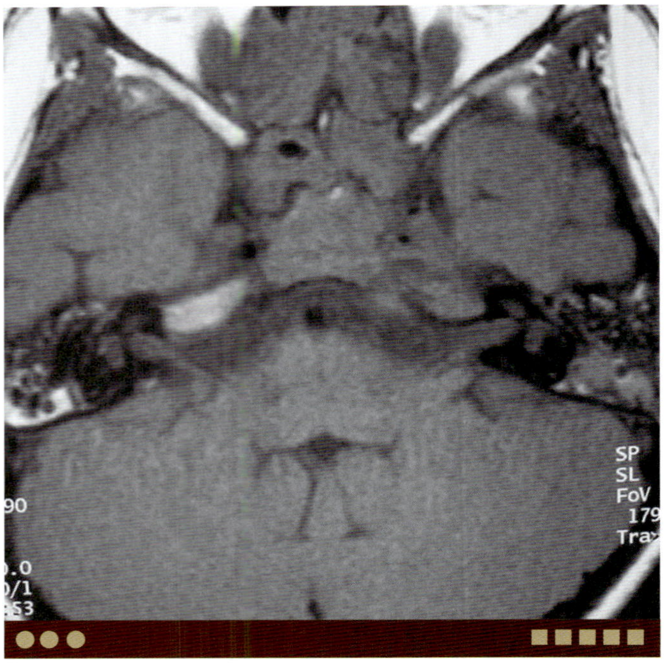

B. Petrous apicitis, same patient as A. Axial noncontrast-enhanced T1W image shows decreased signal in the left petrous apex consistent with inflammatory change. Narrowing of the left internal carotid artery is noted. Note normal fatty signal in the right petrous apex.

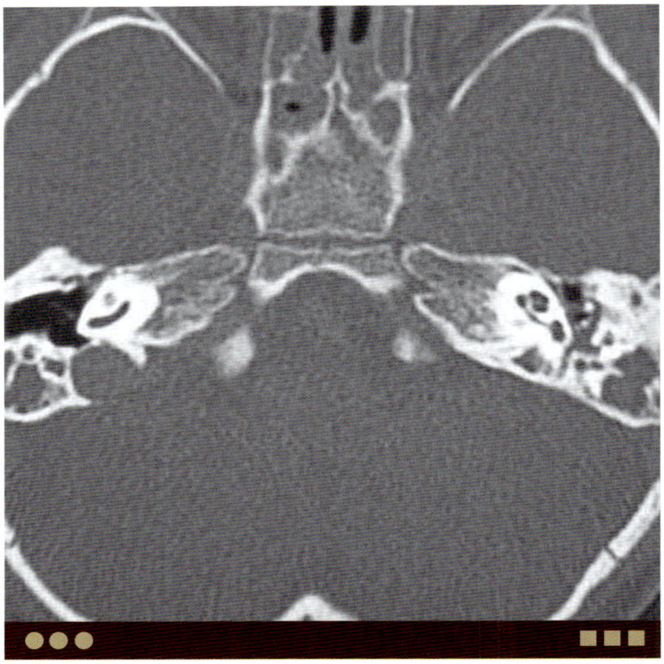

C. Petrous apicitis, same patient as A. Axial CT shows opacified left tympanic cavity and mastoid air cells. However, no apparent abnormality is noted in the left petrous apex.

DIFFERENTIAL DIAGNOSIS IMAGES (D-G)

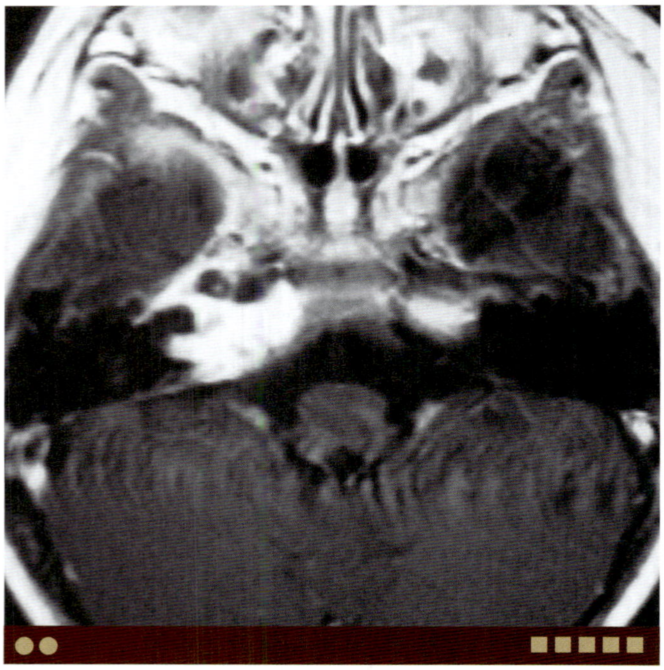

D. **Rhabdomyosarcoma**. Axial postcontrast T1W image shows abnormal enhancement of the right petrous apex extending to the right paracavernous region.

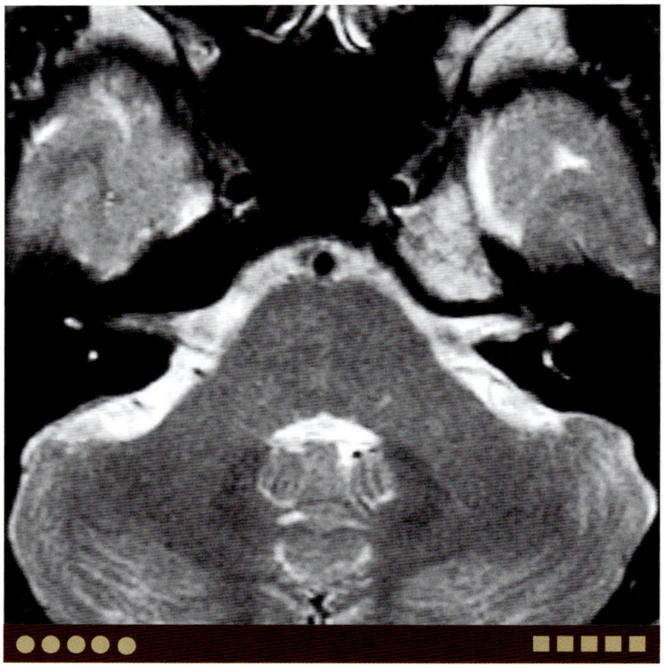

E. **Asymmetric pneumatization of the petrous air cells**. Axial T2W image shows intermediate-to-high signal from the fatty marrow in the left petrous apex. The right petrous apex is completely pneumatized and aerated, and demonstrates no signal.

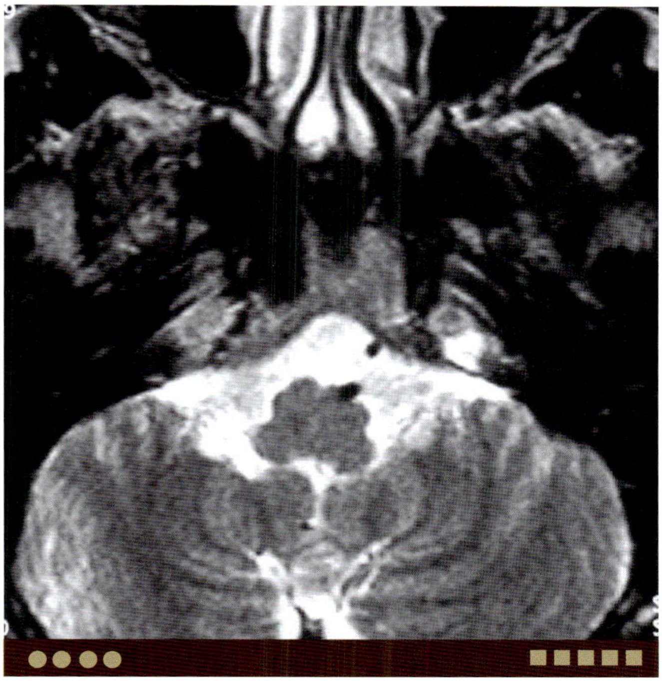

F. **Opacified petrous air cells**. Axial T2W image shows heterogeneous high signal in the left petrous apex. The right petrous apex demonstrates intermediate signal from the fatty marrow.

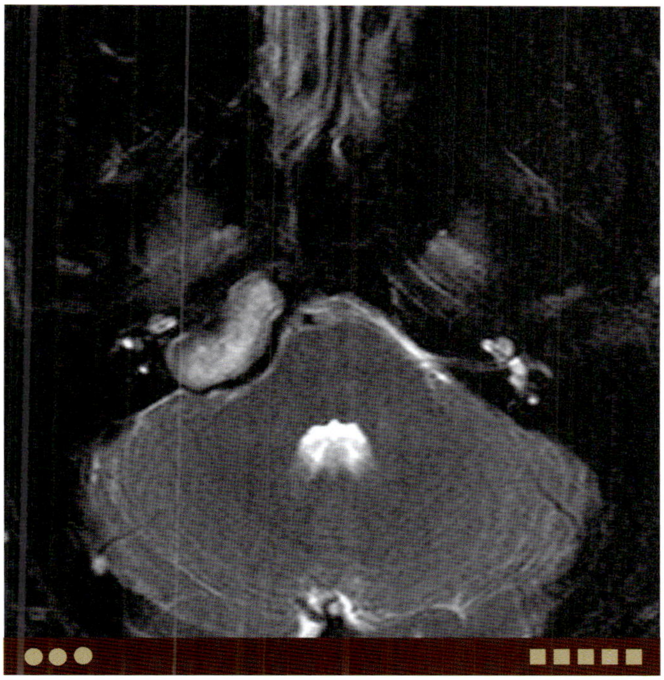

G. **Cholesterol cyst.** Axial fat-suppressed T2W image shows an expansile lesion demonstrating slightly heterogeneous but predominantly high signal in the right petrous apex.

Case 2-15 Epidermoid

Osamu Sakai, Rohini Nadgir

PRESENTATION

Vertigo and hearing loss.

FINDINGS

MRI demonstrates a cystic appearing lesion causing mass-effect upon adjacent structures in the cerebellopontine angle.

DIFFERENTIAL

- Arachnoid cyst: This lesion demonstrates water signal, low on T1W and high on T2W images without diffusion abnormality or associated enhancement.
- Schwannoma: Cystic degenerated schwannomas may be seen as a lobulated cystic lesion with slightly increased signal on T1W and slightly decreased signal on T2W images within the "cyst." Peripheral enhancement is seen after contrast.

COMMENTS

This is a 49-year-old woman with vertigo and hearing loss.

Epidermoid is proliferation of migrated ectoderm cells, which can be congenital/developmental or acquired from infection, trauma, or lumbar puncture. It often demonstrates lobulated or cauliflower-like appearance and the cyst wall is lined by squamous epithelium, containing cholesterol and keratin. It often occurs in the cerebellopontine angle cistern and middle cranial fossa.

On CT and MRI, epidermoid usually demonstrates similar density or signal to CSF, and subtle mass-effect to the adjacent structure may be the only imaging finding. Occasionally, it shows slightly increased density on CT and signal on T1W image due to proteinaceous content. Absence of signal loss from CSF pulsation on TSE T2W image in a focally widened extraaxial space can be a clue for presence of cystic lesions, although this can be seen with arachnoid cyst. Calcification can be seen in 10% to 25% of cases. Usually, almost no enhancement is noted. On high-resolution, heavily T2W images, it shows slightly decreased signal compared to the CSF, and relationship to the cranial nerves and vessels can be assessed. On diffusion weighted images, epidermoid shows very high signal and this is very helpful to differentiate it from arachnoid cyst.

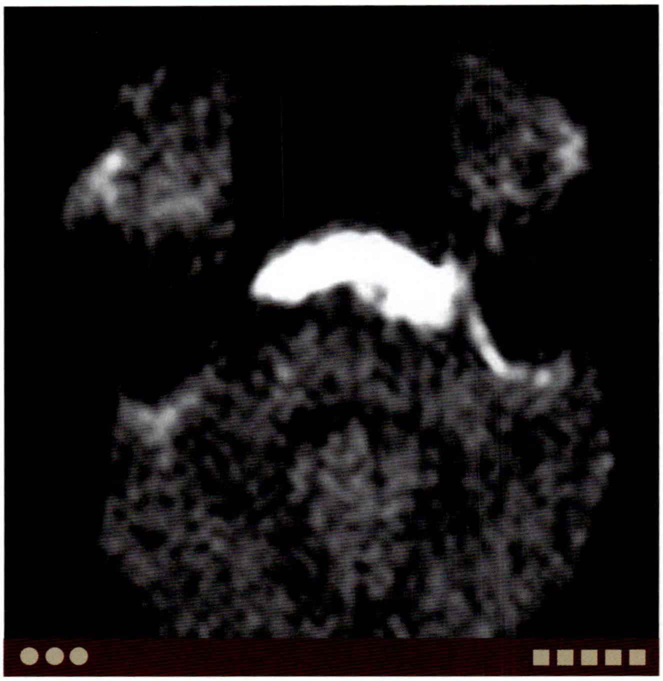

A. Epidermoid. Axial diffusion weighted image demonstrates a high-signal lesion in the prepontine cistern.

PEARLS

- **Epidermoid is seen as a lobulated or cauliflower-like shaped cystic lesion, and causes mass-effect upon adjacent structures.**
- **It shows similar density and signal to the CSF on CT and conventional MRI, but very high signal on diffusion weighted images.**

ADDITIONAL IMAGES (B-F)

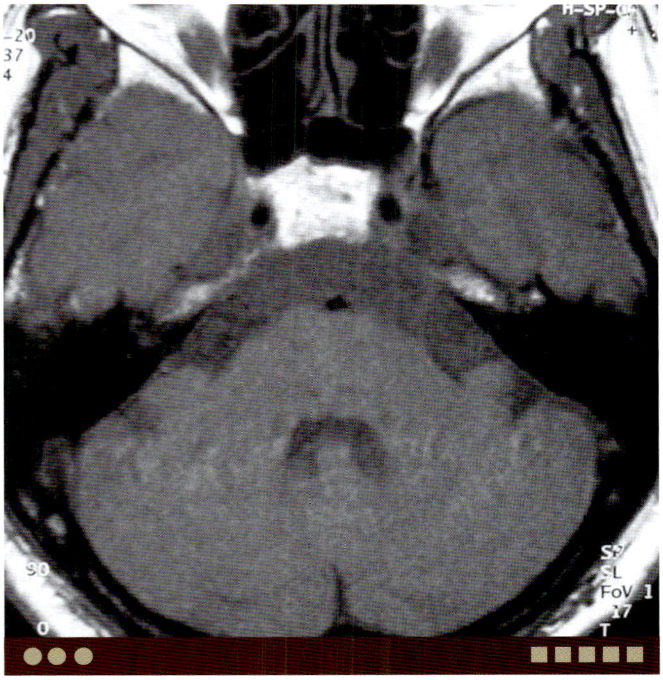

B. Epidermoid, same patient as A. Axial T1W image demonstrates widening of the prepontine cistern; however, the lesion is hardly appreciated.

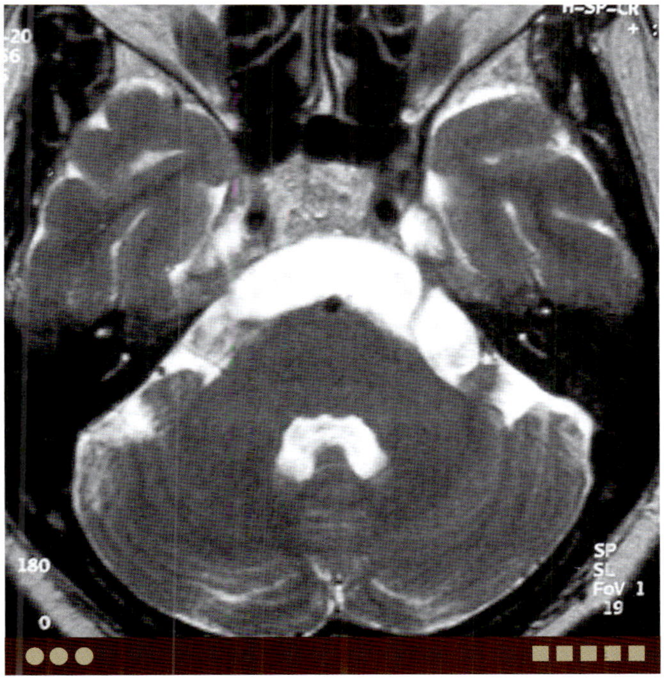

C. Epidermoid, same patient as A. Axial T2W image demonstrates widening of the prepontine cistern without CSF pulsation artifact. Note lateral displacement of the left trigeminal nerve.

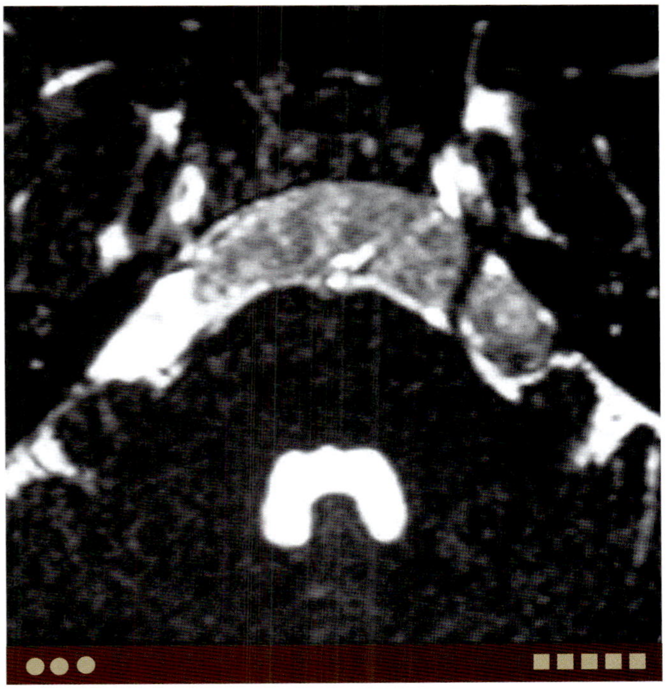

D. Epidermoid, same patient as A. Axial high-resolution T2W image shows the lesion demonstrating heterogeneously decreased signal.

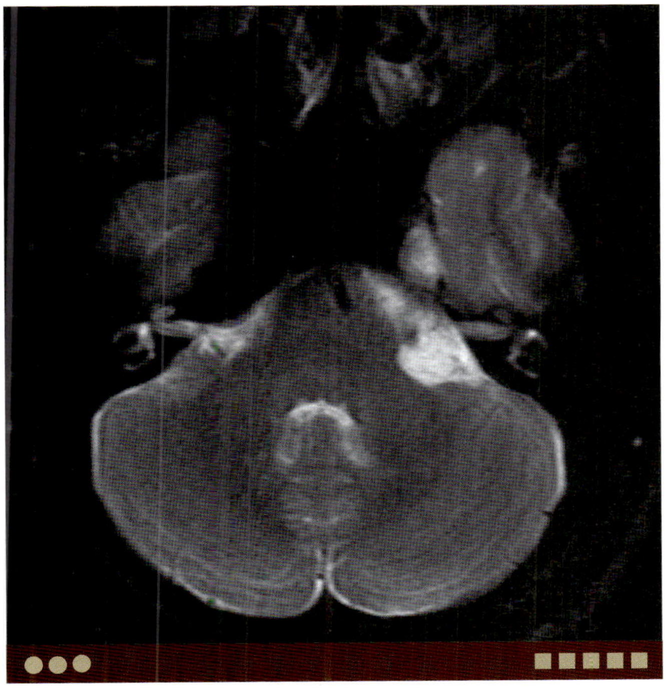

E. **Epidermoid** in a different patient. Axial T2W image demonstrates widening of the left CPA cistern.

DIFFERENTIAL DIAGNOSIS IMAGES (G-I)

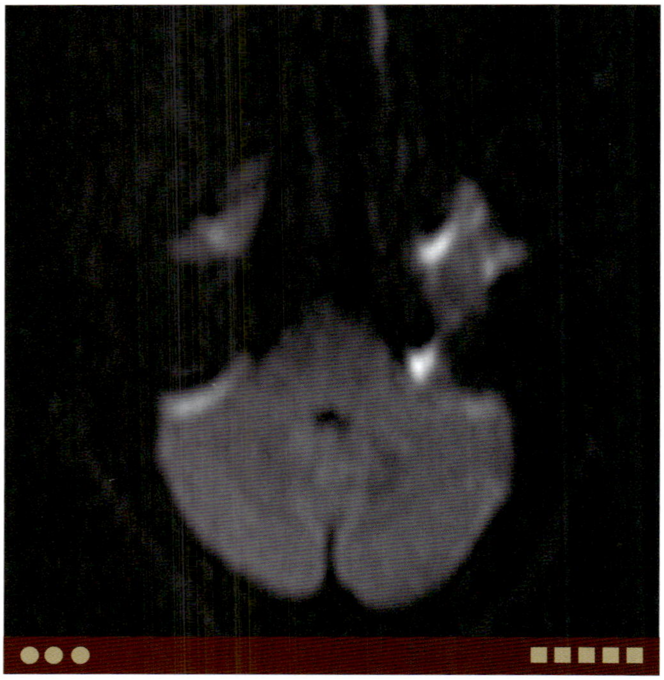

F. Epidermoid, same patient as E. Axial diffusion weighted image demonstrates a high signal in the left CPA lesion.

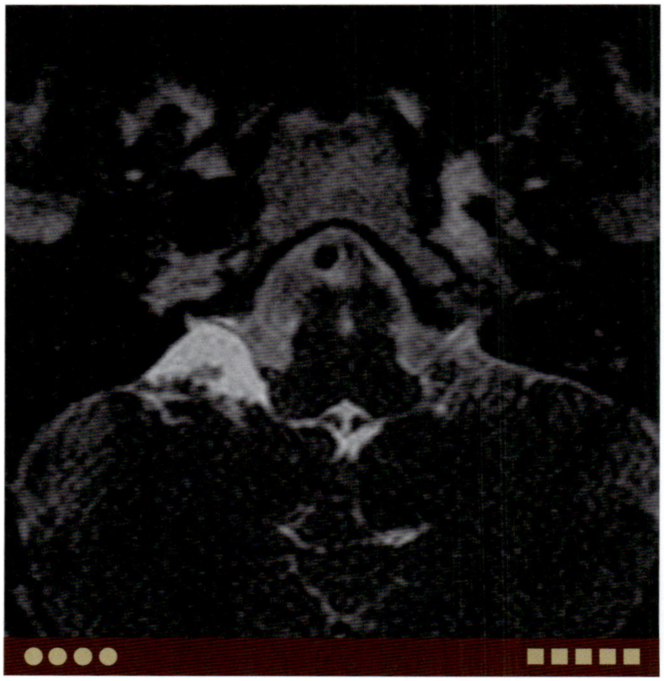

G. Arachnoid cyst. Axial high-resolution T2W image shows a high-signal lesion displacing the right lower cranial nerves.

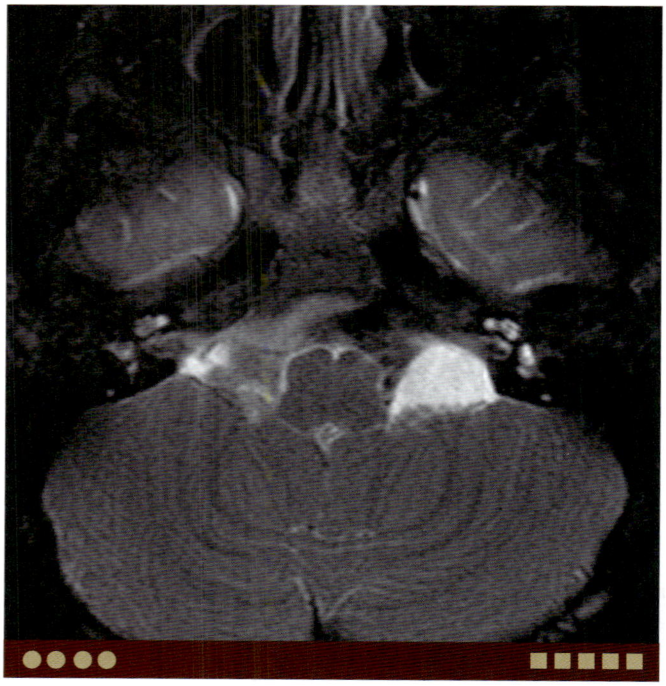

H. Arachnoid cyst in a different patient. Axial T2W image shows a cystic lesion in the left CPA causing mass-effect upon the adjacent cerebellar parenchyma.

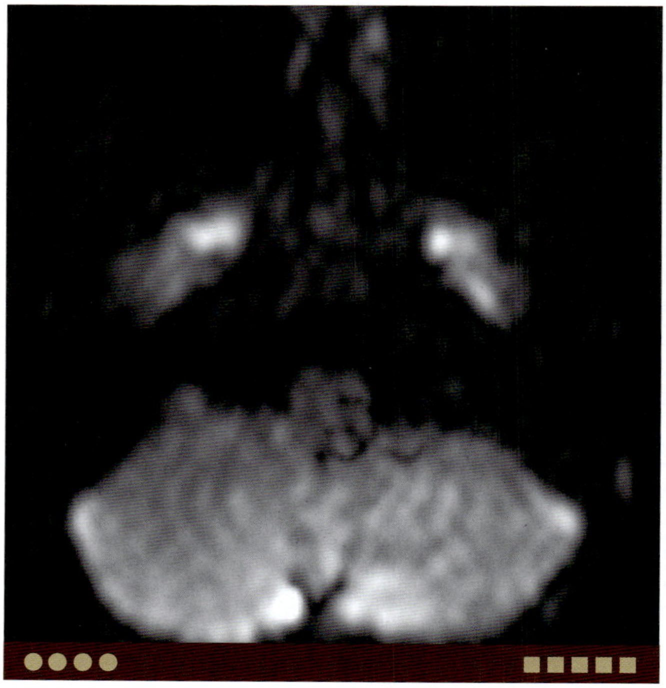

I. Arachnoid cyst, same patient as H. Axial diffusion weighted image shows low signal within the cystic lesion.

Case 2-16 Cephalocele (Meningocele and Encephalocele)

Osamu Sakai, Rohini Nadgir

PRESENTATION

Nasal mass.

FINDINGS

CT and MRI demonstrate a cystic appearing mass in the nasal cavity and bone defect in the roof of the ethmoid.

DIFFERENTIAL

- Nasal polyp: This is a solid lesion, but often demonstrates water density or signal. However, this should not have a bone defect at the skull base.
- Papilloma: This is a solid lesion and should not have a bone defect at the skull base.

COMMENTS

This is a 23-year-old woman with amenorrhea.

Cephalocele is defined as a herniation of cranial contents through a bone defect in the skull. Cephaloceles are classified according to their contents (meningocele: meninge and cerebrospinal fluid (CSF), meningoencephalocele: brain parenchyma in addition to meninges and CSF). These are congenital anomalies due to failure of closure of the neural tube. Despite many theories, the cause of cephalocele is not known. Cephalocele is commonly seen in the occipital region (occipital cephalocele) and these are diagnosed earlier, often at birth. On the other hand, trans-ethmoid and sphenoid cephaloceles are usually diagnosed later as a nasal obstruction, mass or CSF leak. Clinically, hypopituitarism and diabetes inspidus may be present. Unintentional injury to cephaloceles due to biopsy or resection can cause serious complications such as CSF leak, meningitis, and hemorrhage. Therefore, biopsy or resection of polypoid or cystic lesions in the nasal cavity or nasopharynx, particularly in young patients should not be performed without preoperative imaging evaluation. Cephalocele should be always in the differential diagnosis of nasal masses.

CT is used to evaluate for bone defect, and thin-slices with multiplanar reconstruction are needed. Smooth bone remodeling due to CSF pulsation can be seen at the skull base and paranasal sinuses in addition to bone defect. Cleft lip/palate and choanal atresia may be seen with cephaloceles. MRI is essential to evaluate contents of the protruded structures and other possible intracranial anomalies, such as agenesis/hypoplaisa of the corpus callosum, optic nerve/chiasmal anomalies, Chiari malformation, and hydrocephalus.

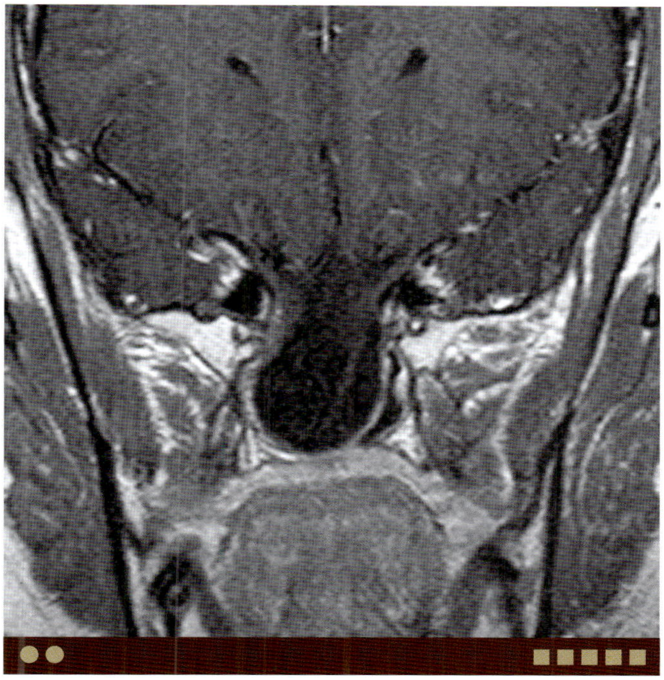

A. Cephalocele. Coronal postcontrast T1W MR image shows a cystic appearing lesion extending into the nasal cavity through a large defect in the roof of the ethmoid and contacting the palate.

PEARLS

- **Cephalocele is a failure of neural tube closure and herniation of the meninge and its contents (meningocele: meninges+CSF, meningo encephalocele: meninges+CSF+brain tissue).**
- **Trans-ethmoid and sphenoid cephaloceles can be present as a nasal mass later in life, while occipital cephaloceles are typically diagnosed at the birth.**
- **Cephalocele should always be included in the differential diagnosis of nasal masses, particularly in young patients.**

ADDITIONAL IMAGES (B-E)

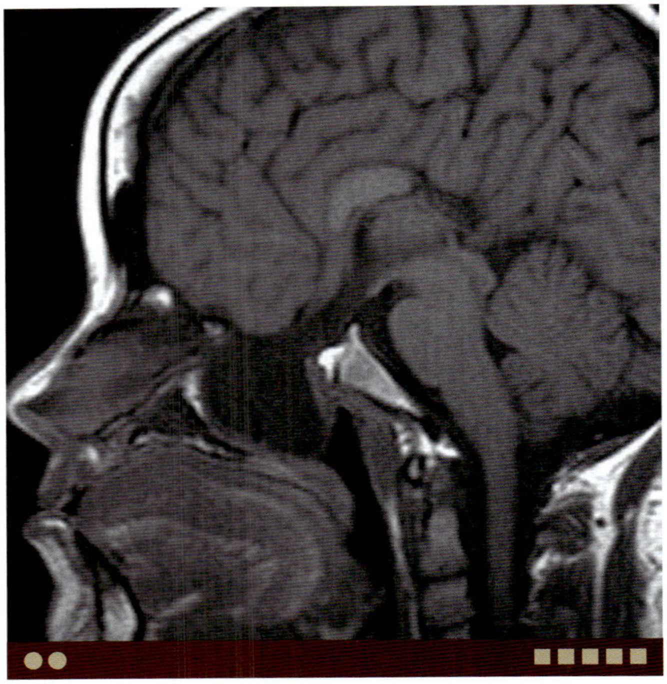

B. Cephalocele, same patient as A. Sagittal T1W MR image demonstrates communication between the cystic lesion and intracranial CSF through a large bone defect within the ethmoid and sphenoid roof. Note downward displacement of the frontal lobe and dysplastic corpus callosum.

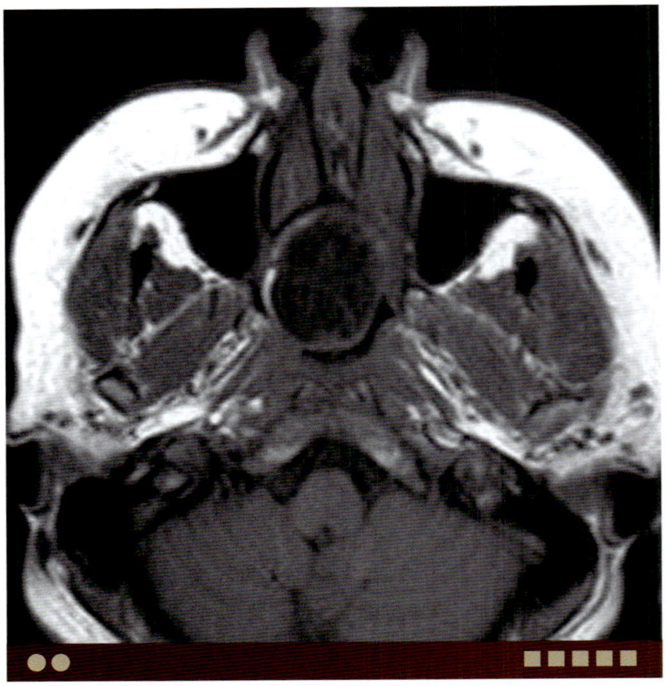

C. Cephalocele, same patient as A. Axial T1W MR image demonstrates a round low-signal lesion isointense to the CSF in the posterior nasal cavity extending to the nasopharynx.

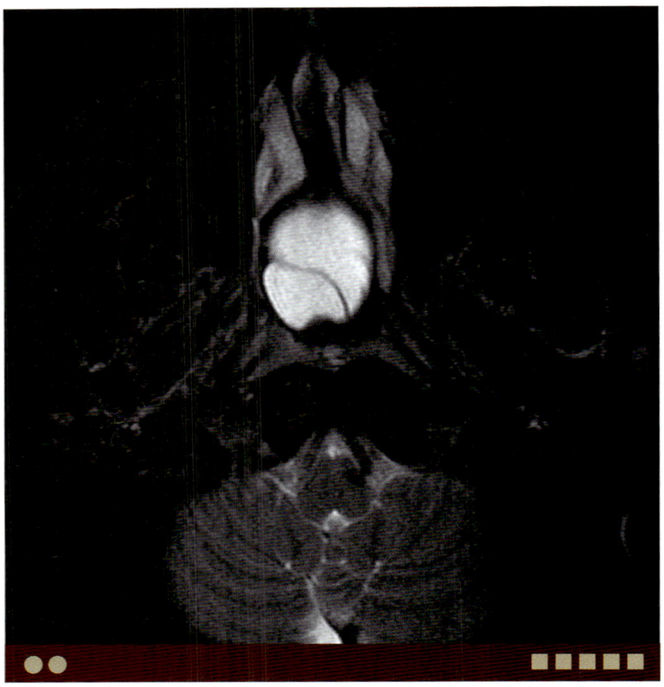

D. Cephalocele, same patient as A. Axial T2W MR image demonstrates a septated water signal lesion in the posterior nasal cavity extending to the nasopharynx.

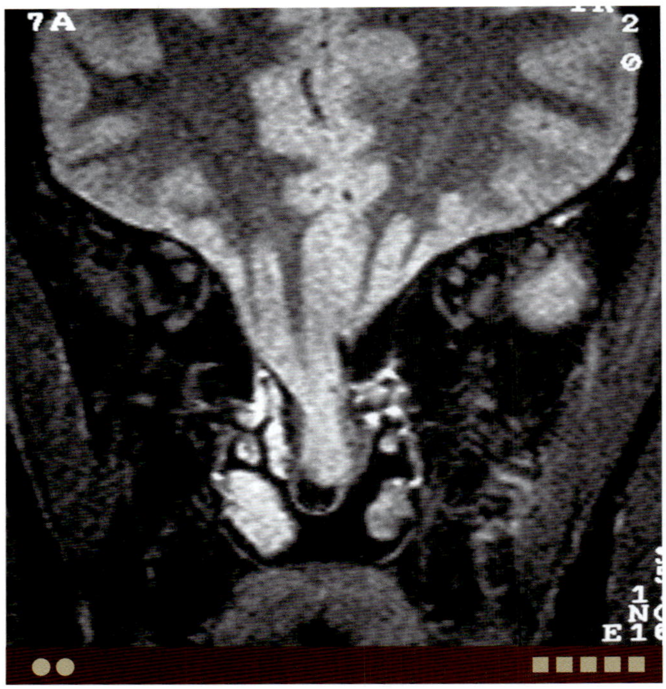

E. **Cephalocele** in a different patient. Coronal STIR MR image demonstrates herniation of the frontal lobes into the nasal cavity, right more than left.

DIFFERENTIAL DIAGNOSIS IMAGES (F-H)

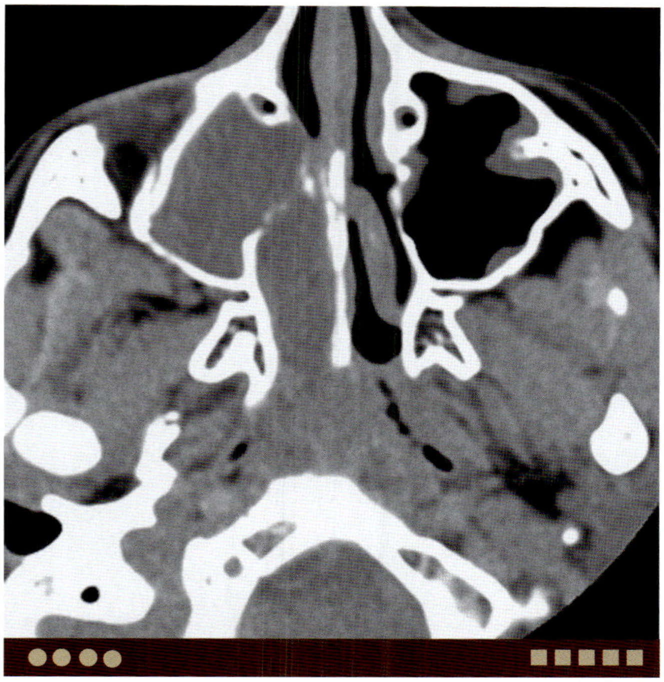

F. Antrochoanal polyp. Axial CT shows a large water density lesion occupying the posterior right nasal cavity as well as the right maxillary sinus.

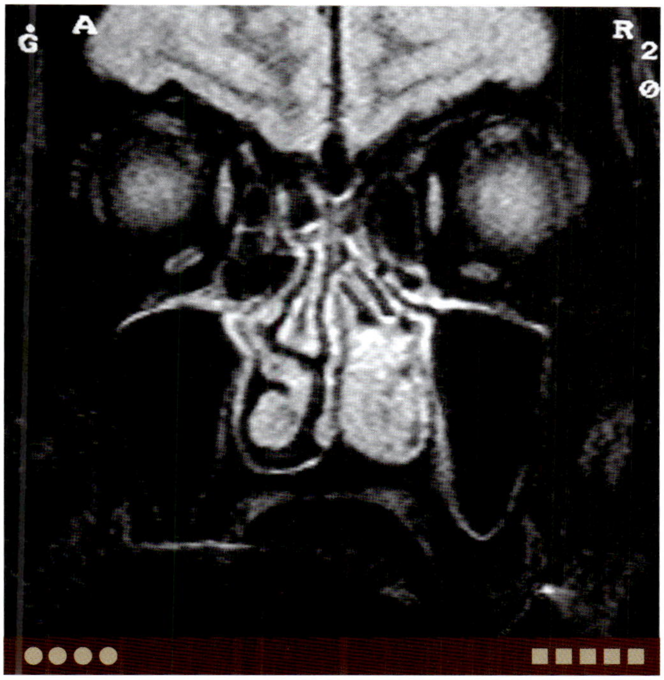

G. Nasal polyp. Coronal STIR MR image demonstrates a predominantly high-signal lesion occupying the left nasal cavity.

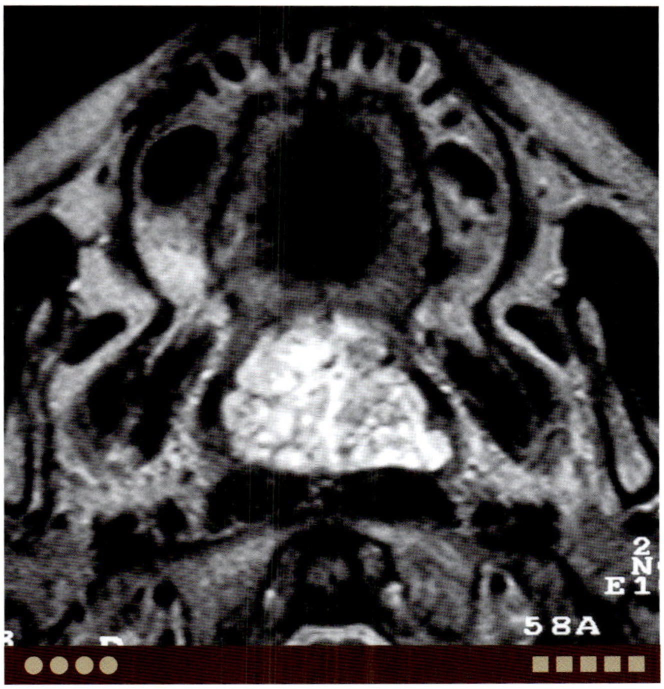

H. Nasal polyp, same patient as G. Axial T2W MR image demonstrates the lesion occupying the nasopharynx.

Case 2–17 Paget's Disease

Osamu Sakai, Rohini Nadgir

PRESENTATION

Increasing head size.

FINDINGS

CT demonstrates thickening and coarse trabeculation of the calvarium and skull base.

DIFFERENTIAL

- Fibrous dysplasia: The finding may be similar, however the lesion is more focal, and the patient is usually younger.
- Hyperparathyroidism: This condition is often clinically apparent and demonstrates diffuse ground-glass changes.
- Chronic osteomyelitis: The imaging finding may be similar, however, this can be usually differentiated by the history and clinical findings.
- Metastasis: Sclerotic metastases from prostate cancer may show similar findings.

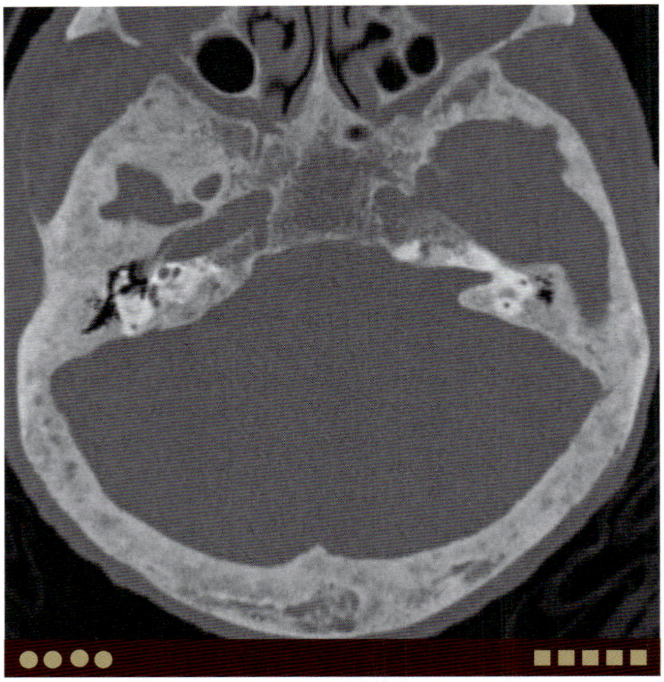

A. Paget's disease. Axial CT shows a coarse trabeculation and expansion of the marrow space in the skull base.

COMMENTS

This is a 71-year-old man with thickened skull.

Paget's disease is a fibro-osseous lesion of unknown etiology often seen in elderly people, involving any osseous structure. This condition is more common in Western countries involving about 10% of the population greater than 80 years of age. It is speculated that this may be caused by viral infection. Serous calcium and phosphate levels are within normal limits; however, significant increase of alkaline phosphatase is noted. The skull is involved in 30-50% of patients, particularly frontal and occipital bones. Due to intraosseous arteriovenous shunting, congestive hear failure may occur.

CT demonstrates thickening of the bone and coarse trabeculation with mixture of lytic and sclerotic changes, while fibrous dysplasia tends to show typical ground-glass appearance. When the skull base is involved, basilar impression can occur due to softening of the bone. Involvement of the temporal bone may result in narrowing of the internal auditory canal and demineralization of the otic capsule, usually preserving the cochlea until the very late stage. These may result in sensorineural hearing loss and tinnitus, which can be pulsatile.

On MRI, Paget's disease causes variable signal due to demineralization, hemorrhage, sclerosis and fatty change, and increased vascularity and blood flow. Strong heterogeneous enhancement is often seen after contrast. The local finding may be similar to other fibro-osseous lesions such as fibrous dysplasia, however, lesions of Paget's disease in the skull base and calvarium are usually more diffuse.

PEARLS

- **Paget's disease is often seen in elderly patients.**
- **Paget's disease often shows thickening of the bone and coarse trabeculation with mixture of lytic and sclerotic changes on CT and variable signal on MRI.**
- **Basilar impression may be present due to bone softening.**

ADDITIONAL IMAGES (B-D)

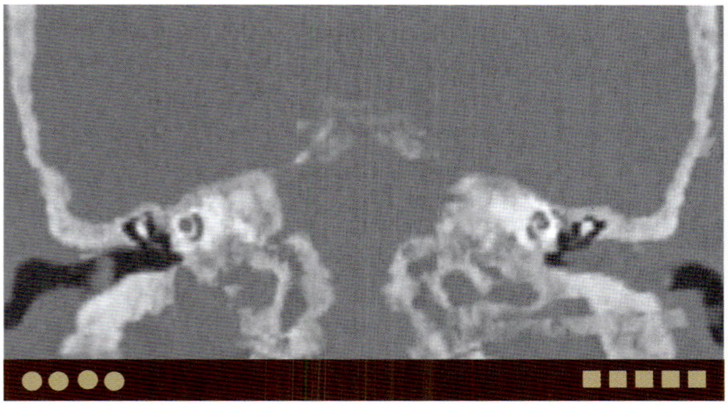

B. Paget's disease, same patient as A. Coronal CT shows a coarse trabeculation and expansion of the marrow space in the skull base.

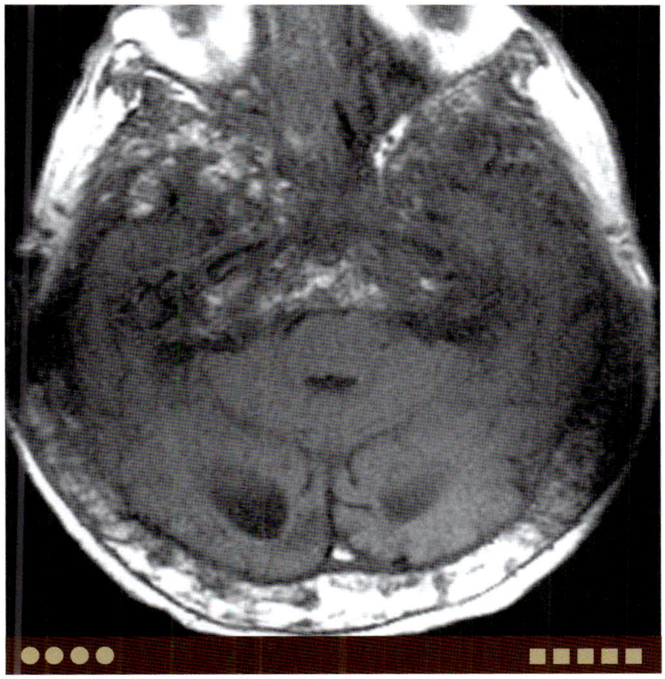

C. Paget's disease in a different patient. Axial T1W image shows diffuse, heterogeneous fatty changes and expansion of the marrow space in the entire skull base.

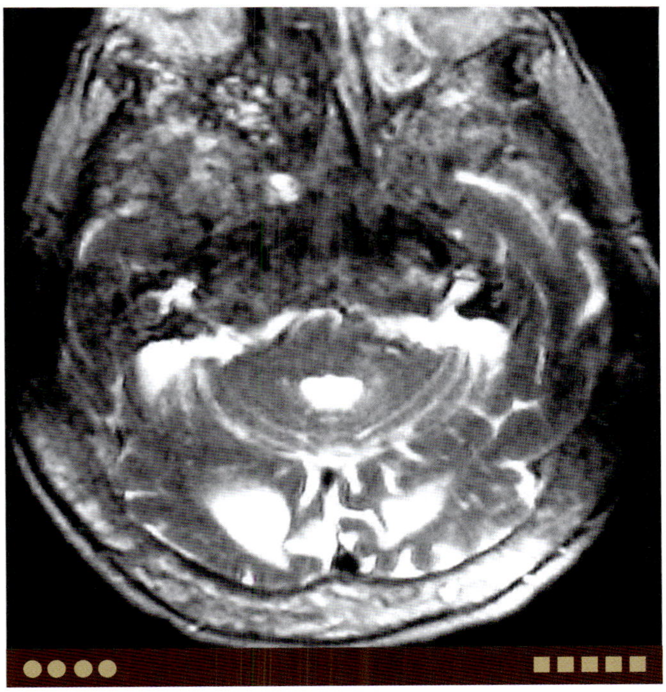

D. Paget's disease, same patient as C. Axial T2W image shows diffuse, heterogeneous high signal and expansion of the marrow space.

DIFFERENTIAL DIAGNOSIS IMAGES (E-H)

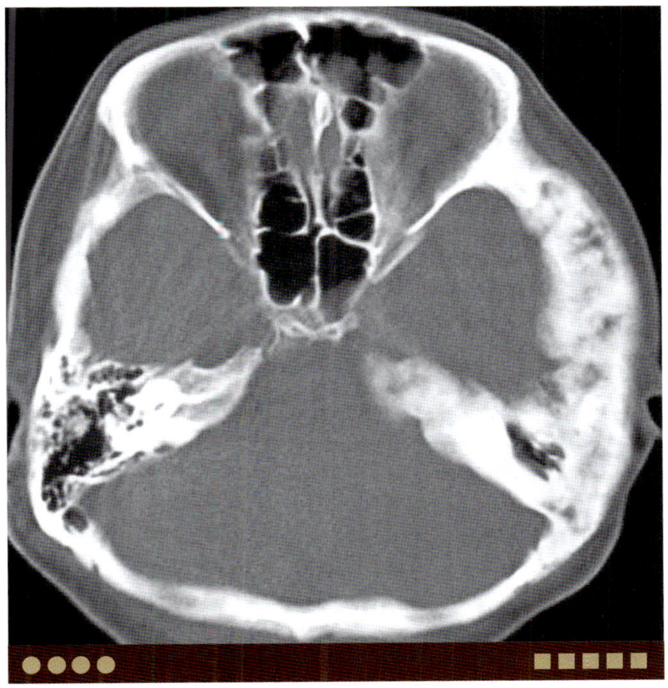

E. Fibrous dysplasia. Axial CT shows coarse trabeculation and expansion of the left temporal bone. Note more focal abnormality compared with Paget's disease.

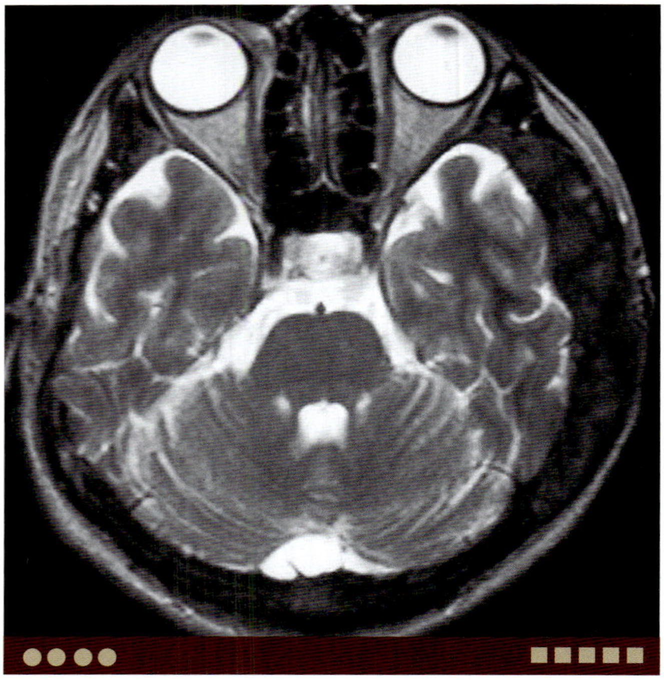

F. Fibrous dysplasia, same patient as E. Axial T2W image shows expansion of the left temporal bone demonstrating heterogeneous but predominantly low signal.

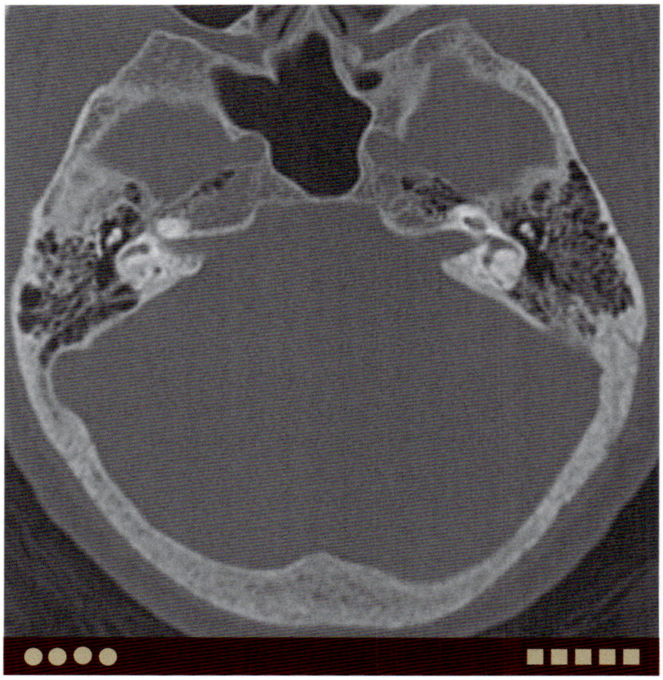

G. **Hyperparathyroidism**. Axial CT shows coarse trabeculation and diffuse demineralization in the entire skull base.

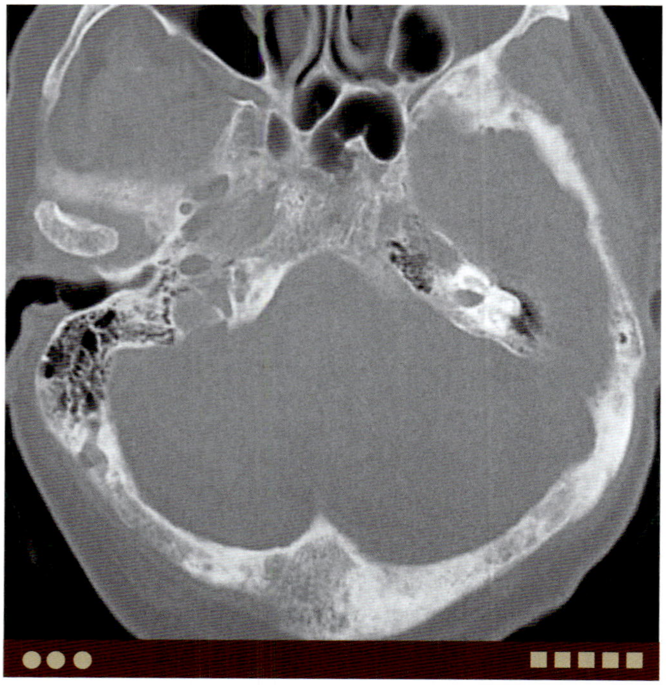

H. **Metastasis from prostate cancer**. Axial CT demonstrates diffuse permeative and sclerotic changes in the sphenoid, temporal, and occipital bones, right more than left.

Case 2–18 Perineural Tumor Spread

Osamu Sakai, Rohini Nadgir

PRESENTATION

Trigeminal neuralgia.

FINDINGS

CT and MRI demonstrate thickening of the cranial nerve, obliteration of the fat pad, and widening of the osseous canal/foramen.

DIFFERENTIAL

- Schwannoma: This occurs along the cranial nerve and demonstrates a spindle- or dumbbell-shaped lesion. Bone erosion rather than destruction is common with schwannoma.
- Neurofibroma: This is often seen in patients with neurofibromatosis, although most neurofibromas are sporadic. Thickened nerve is a common finding. Presence of central low signal on T2W images, central core sign is suggestive of neurofibroma rather than schwannoma.
- Aneurysm: Aneurysms from the cavernous portion of the internal carotid artery may be seen as a heterogeneously enhancing mass in the paracavernous region.

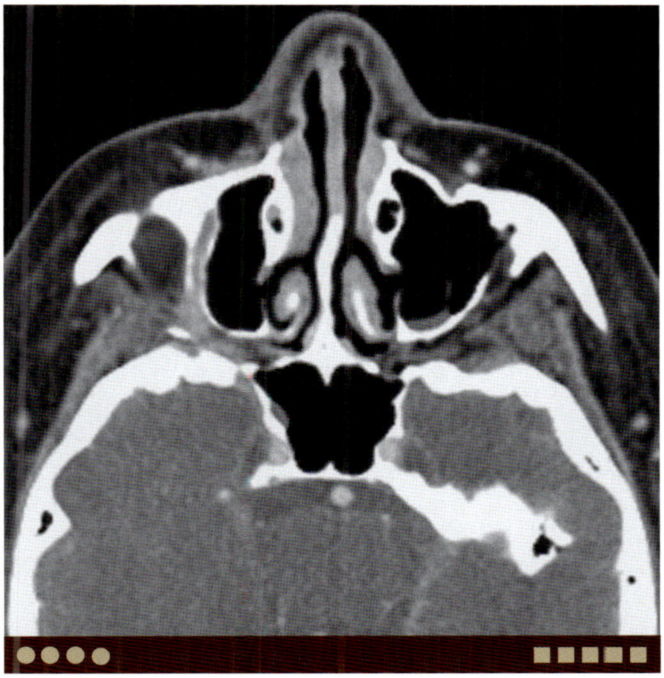

A. Perineural tumor spread, SCCA in the lip. Axial postcontrast CT shows a thickened, enhancing right infraorbital nerve. Note abnormal soft tissue density in the right pterygomaxillary fissure extending toward the pterygopalatine fossa.

COMMENTS

This is a 59-year-old man with trigeminal neuralgia.

Perineural tumor spread is often seen in patients with head and neck cancers. The tumor can extend intracranially through the foramina at the skull base; particularly along the facial nerve through the stylomandibular foramen, the second division of the trigeminal nerve (V2) through the foramen rotundum, the Vidian nerve through the Vidian canal, the hypoglossal nerve through the hypoglossal canal, and the third division of the trigeminal nerve (V3) through the foramen ovale. Adenoid cystic carcinoma and lymphoma are notorious for perineural tumor spread; however, squamous cell carcinoma (SCCA) is the most common tumor causing this because it is the most common tumor in the head and neck.

A failure in diagnosing this type of tumor extension may result in inadequate therapeutic planning. The patient's outcome or prognosis is seriously impaired by "recurrent" or "metastatic" disease, which was actually already present at the time of diagnosis and just continued to grow. A key concept for diagnosing perineural tumor spread just beneath the skull base is to observe the fat in or just inferior to the skull base foramina. Obliteration of the fat strongly suggests tumor spread, while the normal appearance of the fat reassures that tumor has not reached that point.

On CT, obliteration of the fat plane is the first finding. Later, erosion or destruction of the cortex of the canal or foramen can be seen. On MRI, enlargement and abnormal enhancement of the involved nerve is seen. Skip lesions may be present, therefore, careful evaluation of the entire course of the nerve is needed.

PEARLS

- **Perineural tumor spread is often seen in patients with head and neck cancers.**
- **Obliteration of the fat strongly suggests tumor spread, while the normal appearance of the fat is reassuring that tumor has not reached that point.**
- **Skip lesions may be present, therefore, careful evaluation of the entire course of the nerve is essential.**

ADDITIONAL IMAGES (B-G)

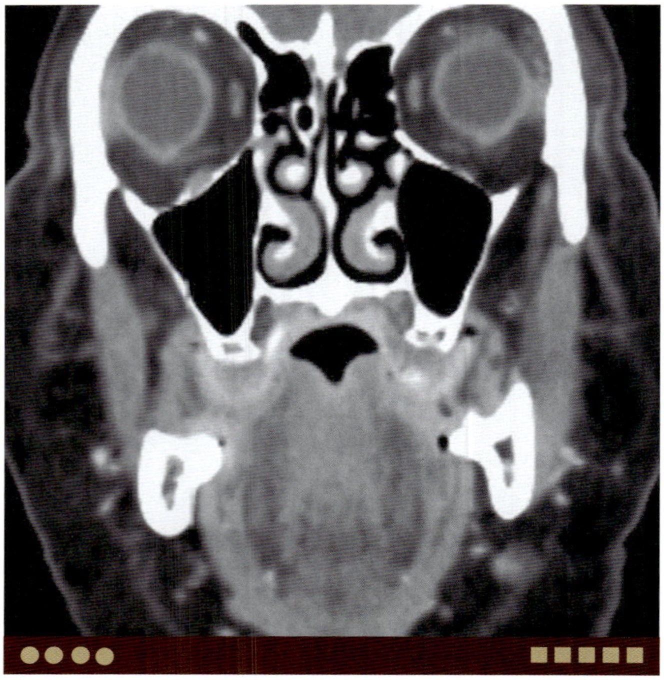

B. Perineural tumor spread, same patient as A. Coronal postcontrast CT shows a thickened, enhancing right infraorbital nerve.

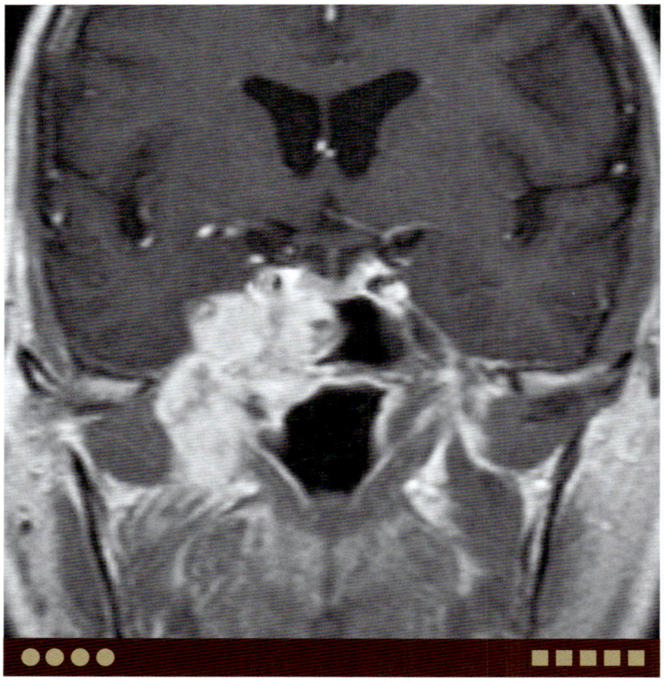

C. **Perineural tumor spread, adenoid cystic carcinoma of the parotid.** Coronal postcontrast T1W image shows a multilobulated heterogeneously enhancing tumor involving the right Meckel's cave and foramen ovale.

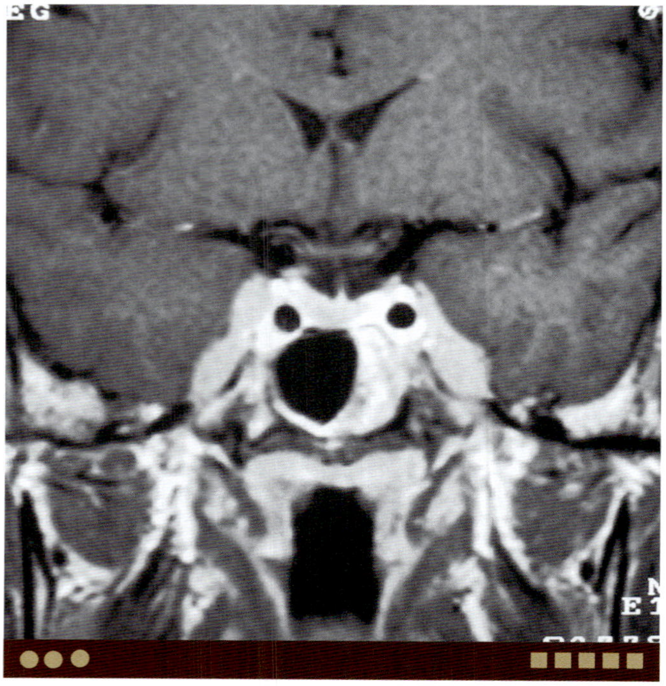

D. **Perineural tumor spread, lymphoma.** Coronal postcontrast T1W image shows enhancing tumors involving the Meckel's cave bilaterally and both trigeminal nerves.

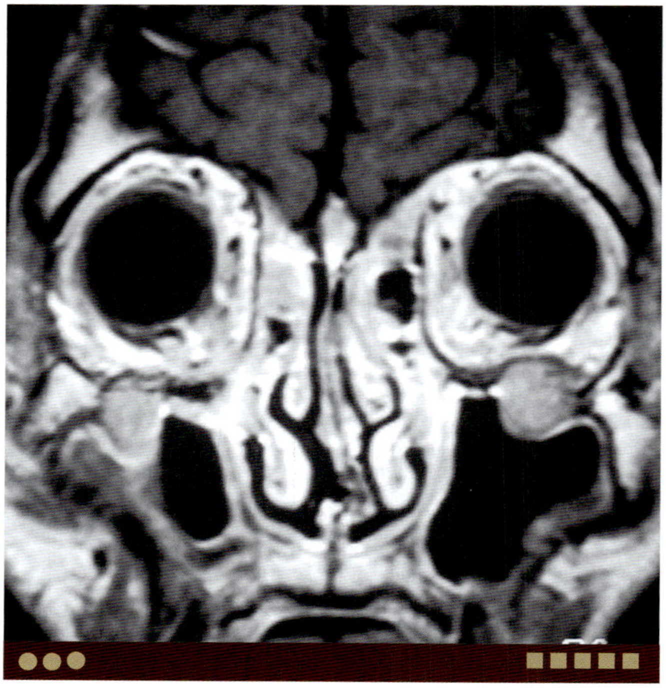

E. Perineural tumor spread, same patient as D. Coronal postcontrast T1W image shows enlargement and abnormal enhancement of the bilateral infraorbital nerves.

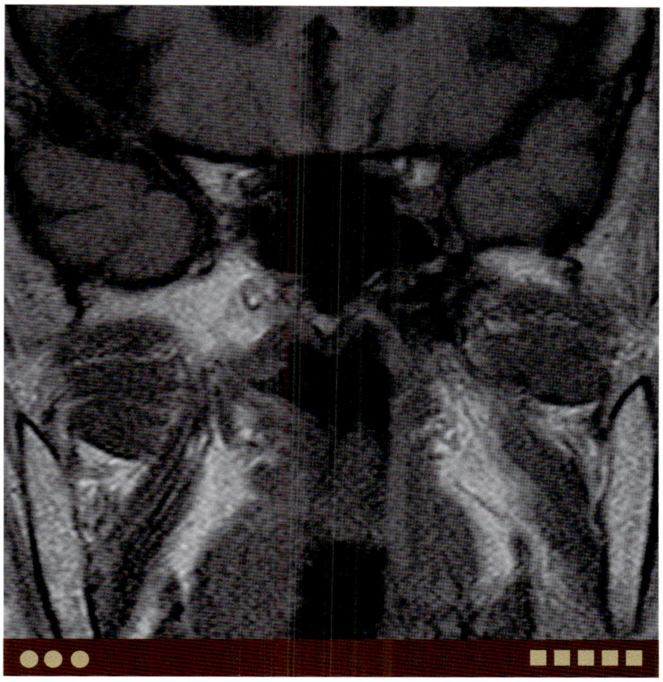

F. Perineural tumor spread, SCCA of the maxillary sinus. Coronal precontrast T1W image shows loss of fat signals in left foramen rotundum and Vidian canal. Note loss of high signal from the fatty marrow of the left pterygoid.

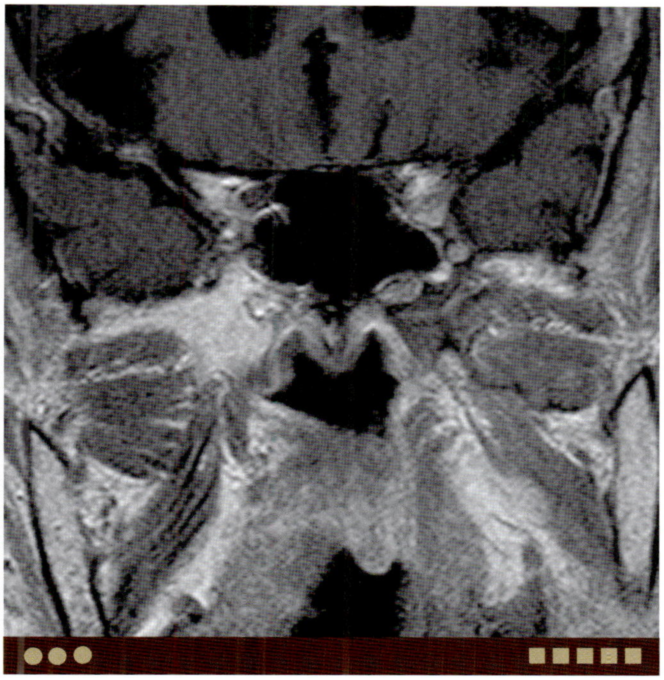

G. Perineural tumor spread, same patient as F. Coronal postcontrast T1W image shows swollen enhancing V2 and Vidian nerve consistent with perineural tumor spread.

DIFFERENTIAL DIAGNOSIS IMAGES (H-J)

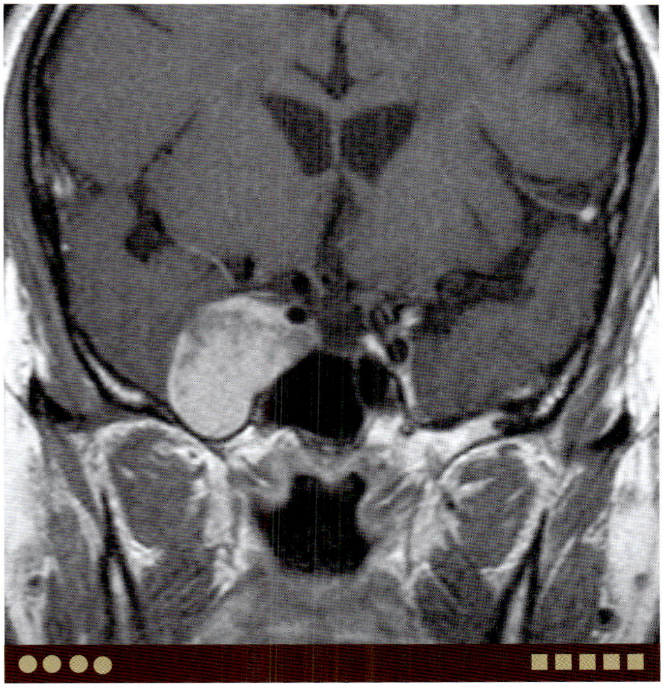

H. Trigeminal schwannoma. Coronal postcontrast T1W image shows a well-demarcated enhancing tumor centered in the right Meckel's cave.

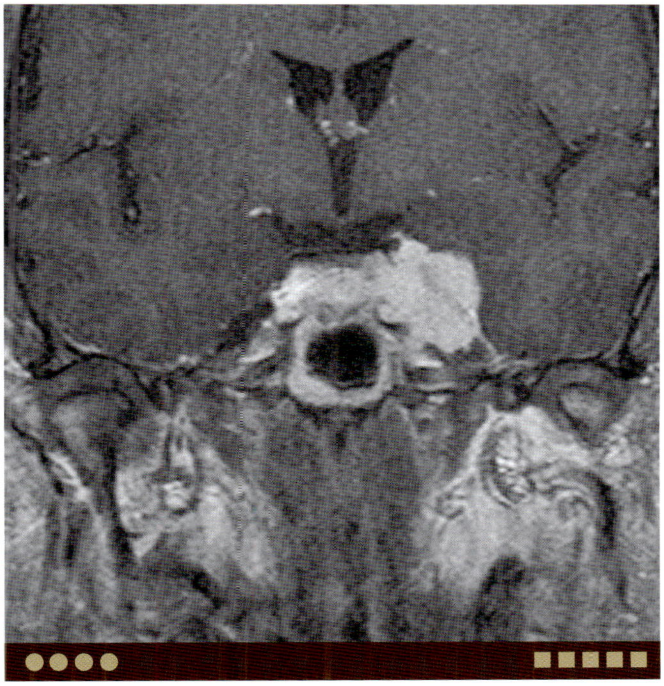

I. Meningioma. Coronal postcontrast T1W image demonstrates a slightly lobulated homogeneously enhancing lesion centered in the left paracavernous region.

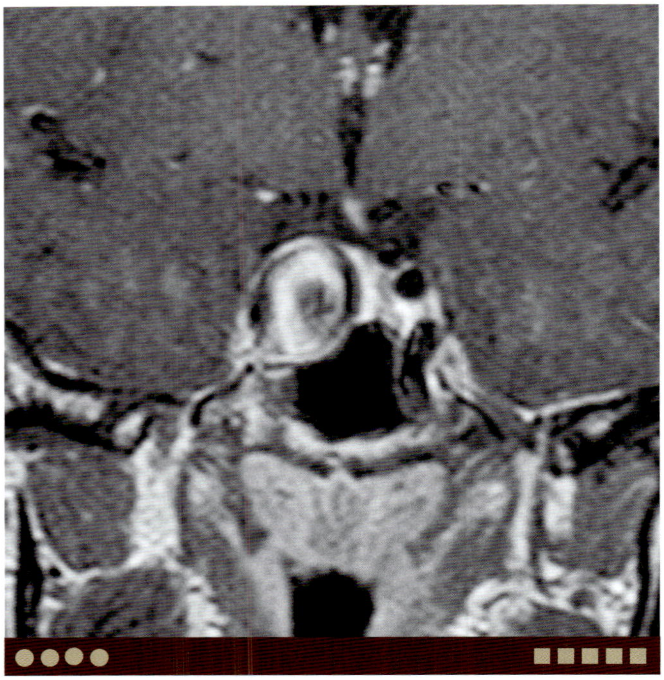

J. Internal carotid artery aneurysm. Coronal postcontrast T1W image shows a heterogeneously enhancing lesion with internal signal voids from blood flow in the right paracavernous region.

Case 2–19 Planum Sphenoidale Meningioma

Osamu Sakai, Rohini Nadgir

PRESENTATION

Anosmia.

FINDINGS

CT and MRI demonstrate an anterior skull base mass with hyperostosis.

DIFFERENTIAL

- Esthesioneuroblastoma: This is a mass arising from the upper nasal cavity, just below the cribriform plate, which often extends intracranially at the time of diagnosis. Avid enhancement is commonly seen.
- Neuroendocrine carcinoma: This is an epithelial tumor, which often arises in the nasal cavity as well as in the larynx. Imaging findings are similar to that of esthesioneuroblastoma.
- Squamous cell carcinoma: This is the most common tumor in the sinonasal cavity and occasionally invades the skull base.

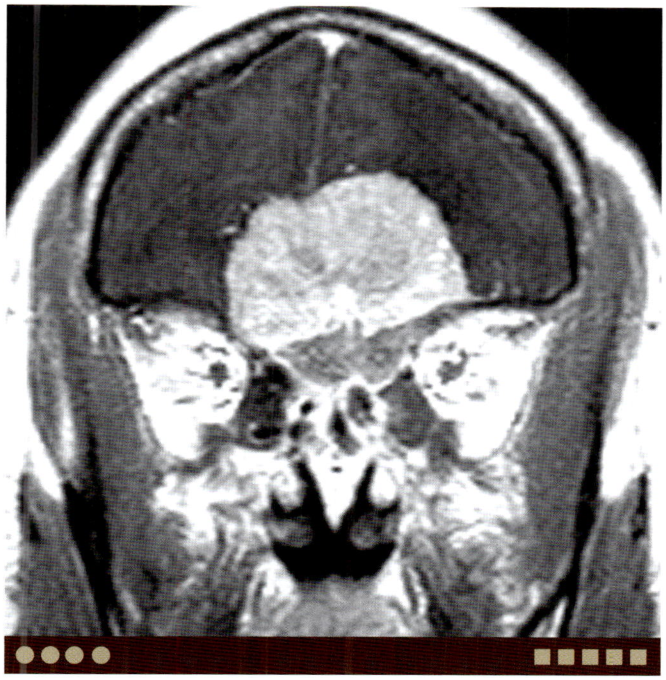

A. Planum sphenoidale meningioma. Coronal postcontrast T1W image shows a large avidly enhancing tumor with thickening of the anterior skull base. No extracranial extension is noted.

COMMENTS

This is a 45-year-old woman with anosmia.

Planum sphenoidale is one of the common sites for meningioma. It is located in midline posterior to the olfactory groove and anterior to the tuberculum sella. When large, planum sphenoidale meningiomas can cause mass-effect at the base of the frontal lobe.

Hyperostosis, "blistering" is more commonly seen with planum sphenoidale meningioma compared with meningiomas from other locations. CT, particularly with coronal or sagittal reconstructions nicely demonstrates hyperostosis in addition to an intracranial extra-axial dural-based mass.

On MRI, meningiomas often demonstrate isointense signal to the brain parenchyma on both T1W and T2W images, and avid enhancement with dural tail sign after intravenous contrast administration.

Extracranial extension of meningioma may occur, however it is rare. On the other hand, intracranial extension of esthesioneuroblastoma, which occurs in the upper nasal cavity, is common. Also, squamous cell carcinoma and sinonasal undifferentiated carcinoma often invades the skull base.

PEARLS

- **Planum sphenoidale is one of the common sites for meningioma, located in midline posterior to the olfactory groove and anterior to the tuberculum sella.**
- **Hyperostosis, "blistering" is commonly seen with planum sphenoidale meningioma.**
- **Extracranial extension of meningioma may occur, however intracranial extension of tumors originated from the sinonasal cavity is more common.**

ADDITIONAL IMAGES (B-D)

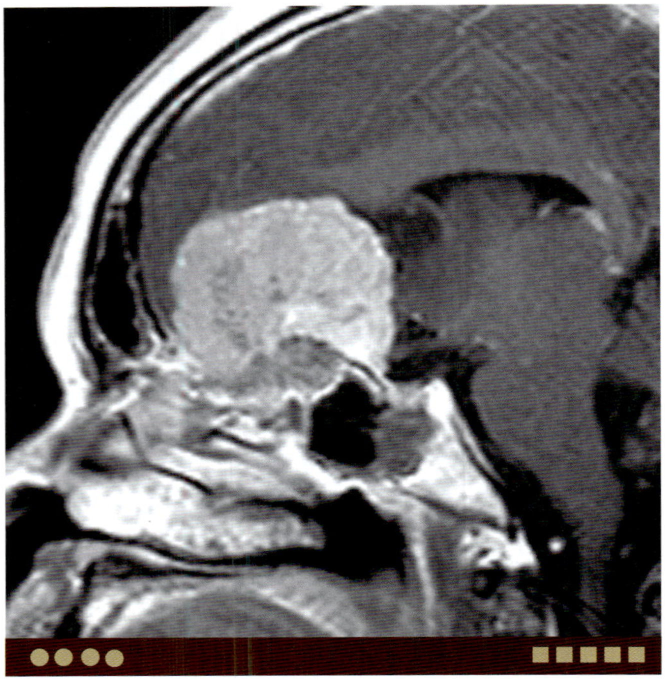

B. Meningioma, same patient as A. Sagittal postcontrast T1W image shows a large avidly enhancing dural-based tumor at the planum sphenoidale, anterior to the anterior clinoid. Note thickening of the anterior skull base.

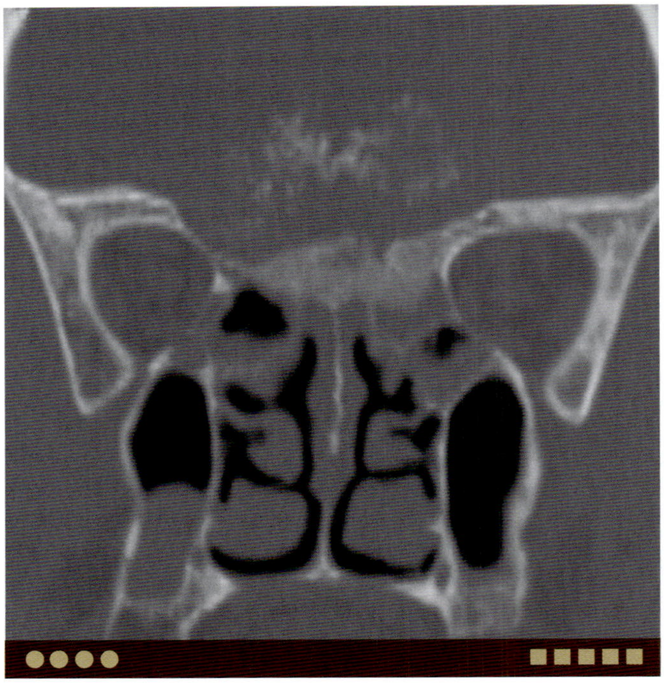

C. Meningioma, same patient as A. Coronal CT shows hyperostosis of the anterior skull base. Note heterogeneous calcification in the tumor.

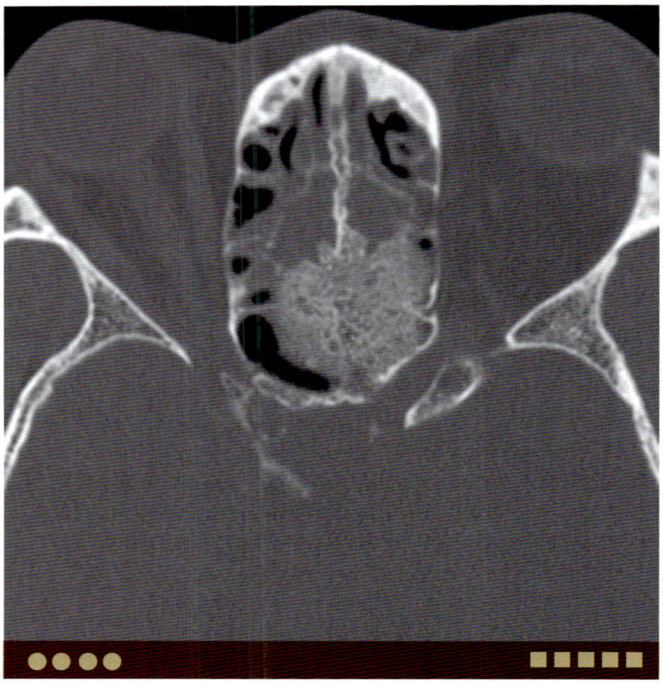

D. Meningioma, same patient as A. Axial CT shows focal hyperostosis in the posterior ethmoid air cells, left more than right.

DIFFERENTIAL DIAGNOSIS IMAGES (E-G)

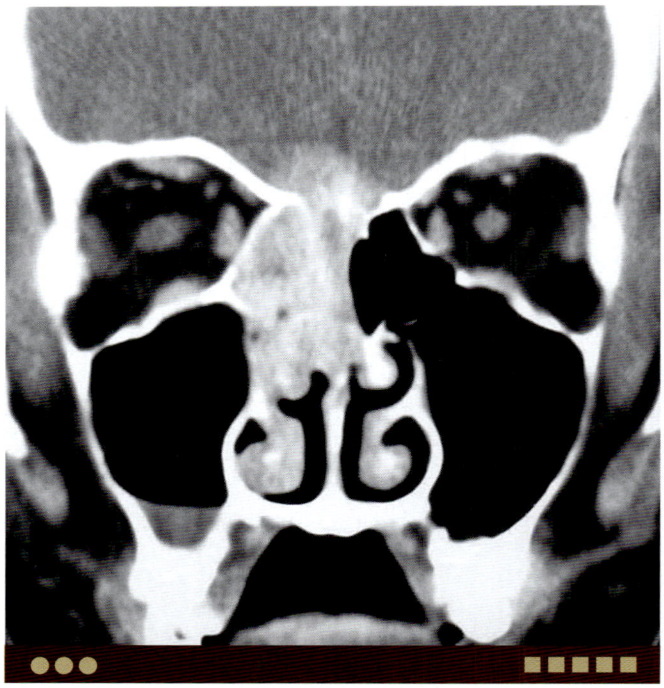

E. **Esthesioneuroblastoma**. Coronal postcontrast CT shows an enhancing tumor occupying the upper nasal cavity, invading the cribriform plate and extending intracranially.

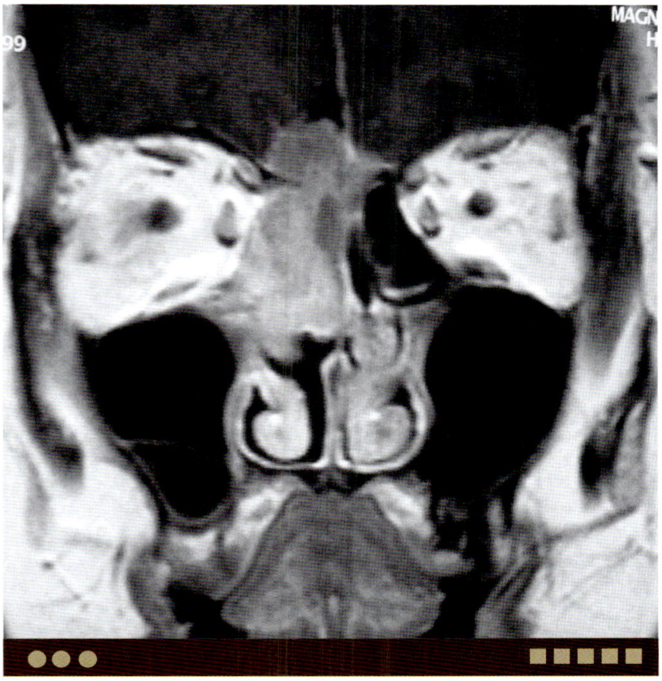

F. Esthesioneuroblastoma, same patient as E. Coronal postcontrast T1W image shows an enhancing upper nasal cavity tumor extending intracranially.

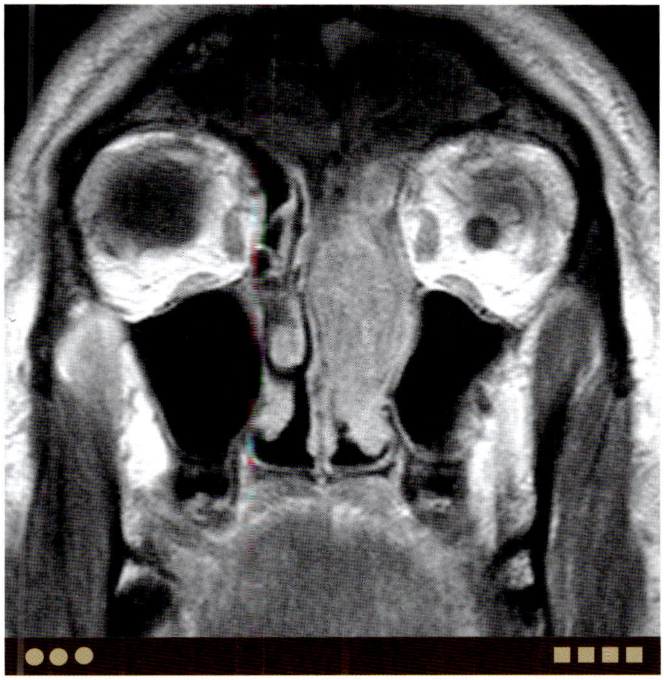

G. **Sinonasal undifferentiated carcinoma**. Coronal postcontrast T1W image shows a heterogeneously enhancing lesion occupying the left nasal cavity, anterior ethmoid and frontal sinuses without definite intracranial extension.

Case 2–20 Langerhans Cell Histiocytosis

Osamu Sakai, Rohini Nadgir

PRESENTATION

Swelling of the temporal region, clinically suspected acute mastoiditis.

FINDINGS

CT demonstrates opacified tympanic cavity and mastoid air cells with bone destruction.

DIFFERENTIAL

- Coalescent mastoiditis: This is bacterial infection and aggressive form of acute otitis media with bone destruction. Pus is seen in the middle ear. Bone destruction (mastoiditis) and abscess formation outside of the mastoid along the sternocleidomastoid muscle (Bezold's abscess) can occur.
- Rhabdomyosarcoma: This condition also clinically mimics otitis media. Patients often develop cranial nerve palsy and CT demonstrates aggressive bone destruction.

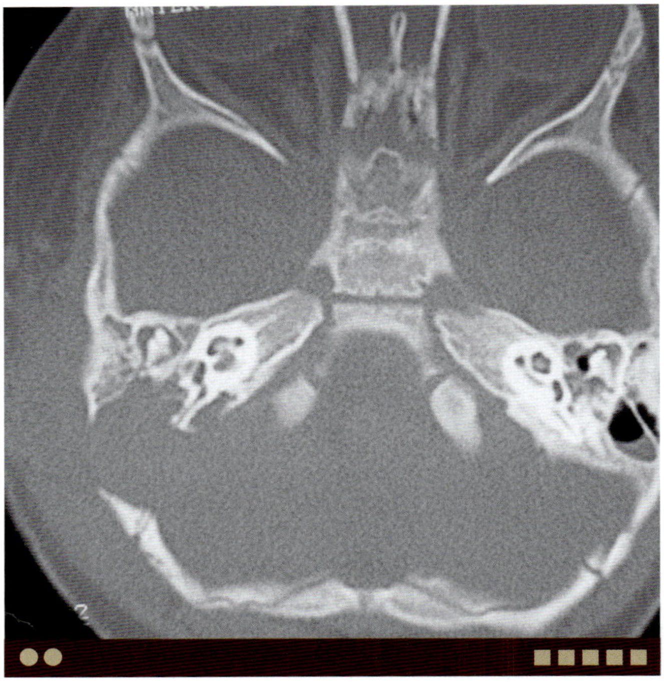

A. LCH. Axial CT demonstrates bone destruction in the posterior portion of the right mastoid.

COMMENTS

This is a 1-year-old boy with right temporal swelling. CT was performed to evaluate for acute mastoiditis.

Langerhans cell histiocytosis (LCH) is a rare condition which is characterized by the proliferation of specialized bone marrow–derived Langerhans cells and mature eosinophils. The term LCH is preferred to the older term, histiocytosis X. This condition can be divided into three forms: (1) Letterer-Siwe disease (acute fulminant, disseminated disease), (2) eosinophilic granulomas (solitary or few, indolent and chronic lesions of bone or other organs), and (3) Hand-Schüller-Christian disease (multifocal, chronic involvement, classically presented as the triad of diabetes insipidus, proptosis, and lytic bone lesions).

LCH occurs more in males (M:F = 2:1), from neonates to adults (Letterer-Siwe: younger than 2 years, Hand-Schüller-Christian syndrome: 2–10 years, eosinophilic granuloma: 5–15 years), and is more common among Caucasians.

LCH often presents similarly to acute otitis media, clinically and radiologically. Heterogeneous enhancement and bone destruction is commonly seen. More importantly, similar clinical and radiological findings are also seen with rhabdomyosarcoma which is a malignant tumor seen in children. Therefore, precise imaging evaluation, which can guide a biopsy is essential for management. LCH and rhabdomyosarcoma should be always in the differential diagnosis, when diagnosing otitis media in children, particularly with cranial nerve impairment.

CT demonstrates bone destruction with soft tissue mass with heterogeneous enhancement. MRI better demonstrates extent of the lesion, particularly in the bone marrow and soft tissue. Avid enhancement is often seen on MRI.

PEARLS

- **LCH is a rare condition, commonly seen in children.**
- **Bone destruction and enhancing soft tissue is seen on CT and MRI.**
- **LCH and rhabdomyosarcoma should be always in the differential diagnosis when diagnosing otitis media in children, particularly when aggressive bone destruction or cranial nerve impairment is noted.**

ADDITIONAL IMAGES (B-D)

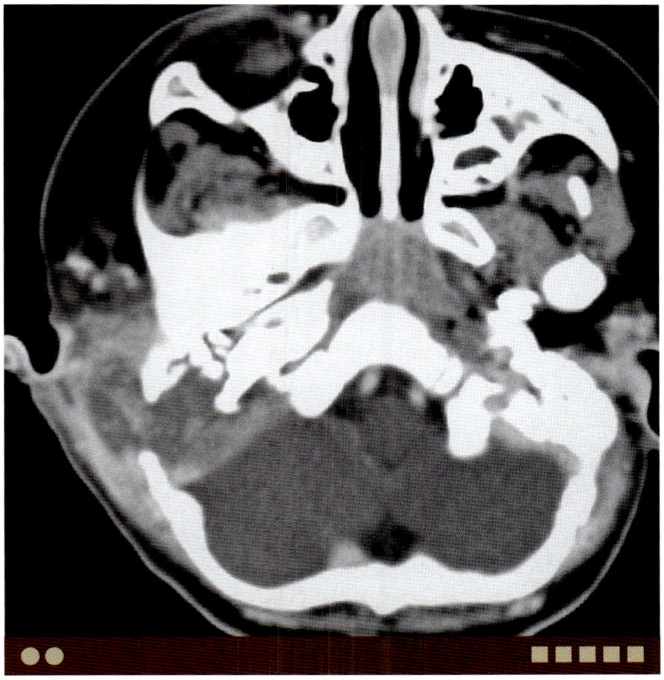

B. LCH, same patient as A. Axial postcontrast CT demonstrates a large heterogeneously enhancing lesion destroying the right temporal bone.

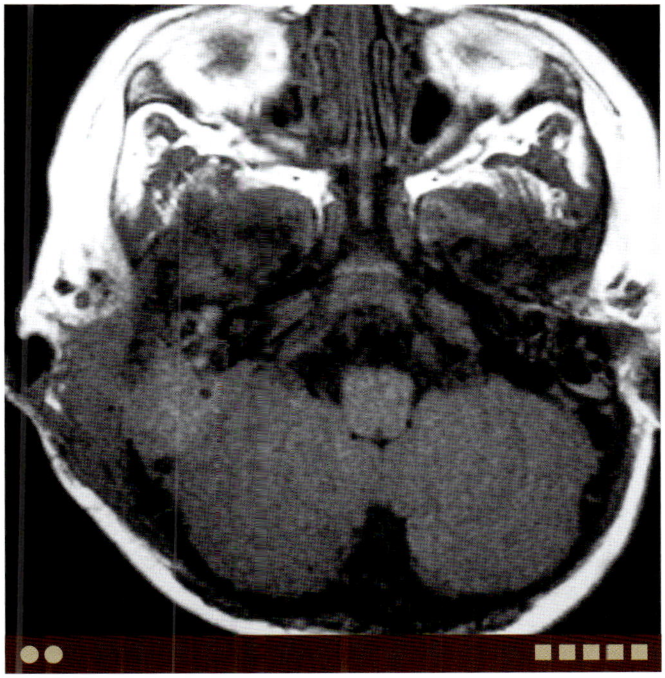

C. LCH, same patient as A. Axial T1W image shows the lesion demonstrating heterogeneous low signal with extraosseous extension.

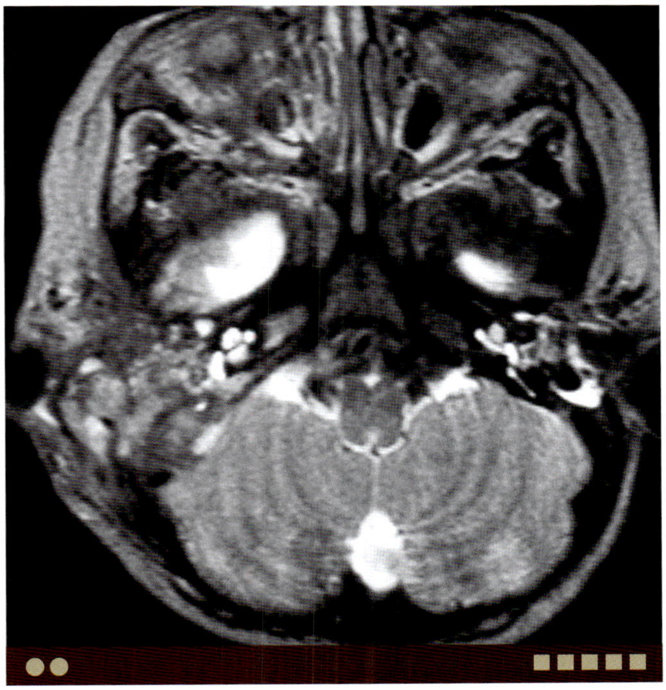

D. LCH, same patient as A. Axial T2W image shows the lesion demonstrating heterogeneous high signal.

DIFFERENTIAL DIAGNOSIS IMAGES (E-G)

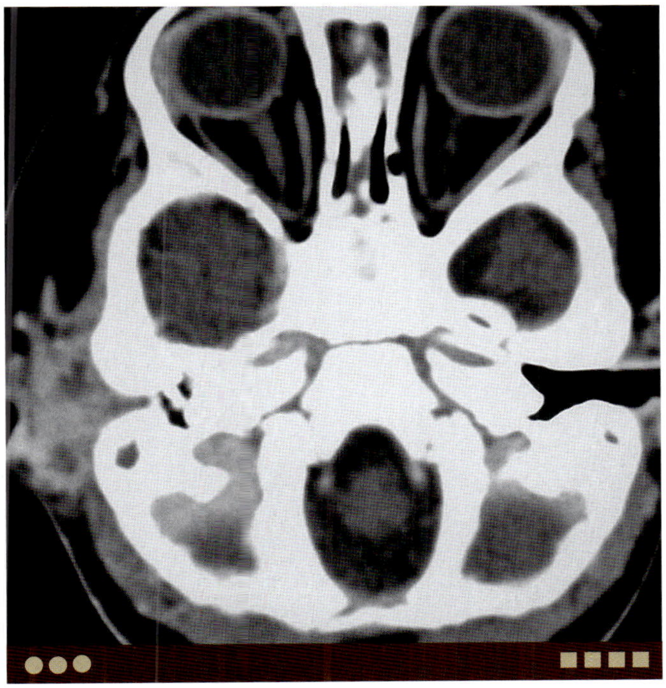

E. Acute mastoiditis. Axial postcontrast CT demonstrates a heterogeneously enhancing extraosseous lesion in the right temporal region.

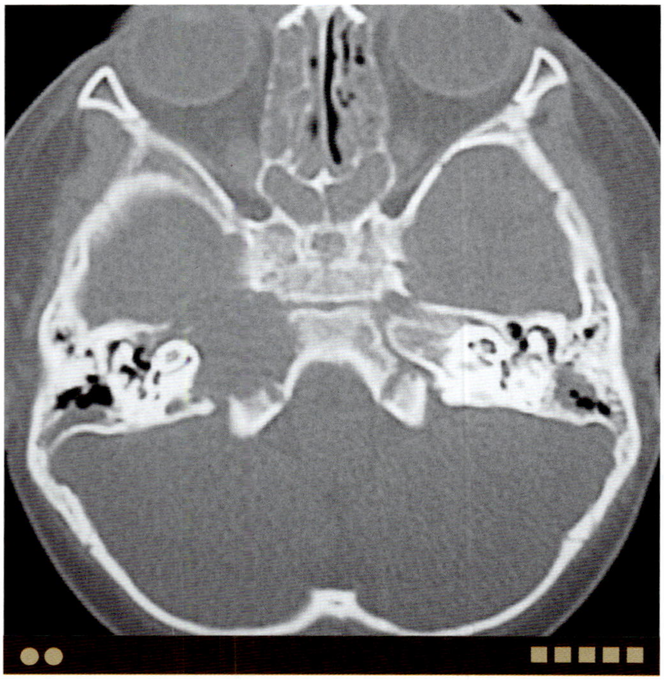

F. Rhabdomyosarcoma. Axial CT demonstrates an expansile osteolytic lesion in the right petrous apex. Partially opacified mastoid air cells are seen bilaterally.

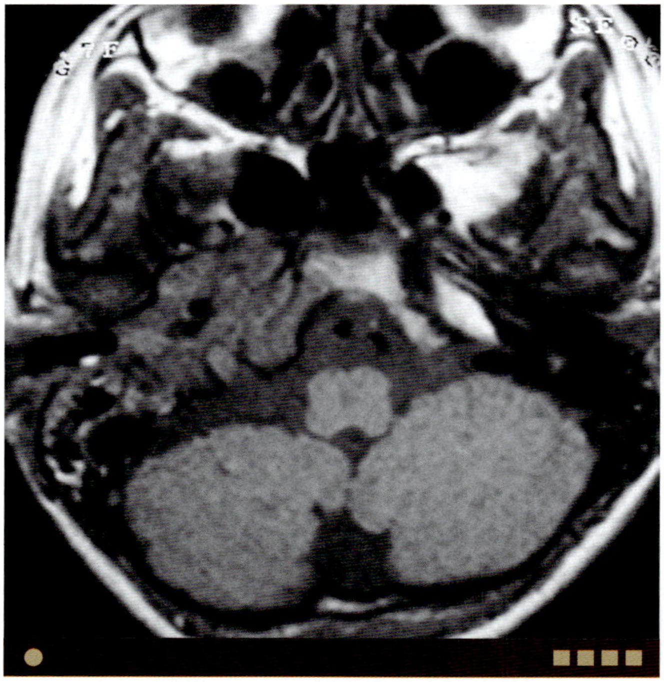

G. Rhabdomyosarcoma in a different patient. Axial T1W image demonstrates a slightly expansile heterogeneously low-signal lesion in the mastoid extending to the petrous portion. Note encasement of the right internal carotid artery.

Case 2–21 Rhabdomyosarcoma

Osamu Sakai, Rohini Nadgir

PRESENTATION

Evaluate for otitis media.

FINDINGS

CT demonstrates opacified tympanic cavity and mastoid air cells with bone destruction.

DIFFERENTIAL

- Coalescent mastoiditis: This is a bacterial infection and an aggressive form of acute otitis media with bone destruction. Pus is seen in the middle ear. Bone destruction (mastoiditis) and abscess formation outside of the mastoid along the sternocleidomastoid muscle (Bezold's abscess) can occur.
- Langerhans cell histiocytosis: This is a rare condition but commonly seen in children. Clinical presentation may be similar to otitis. Bone destruction and enhancing soft tissue is usually seen.

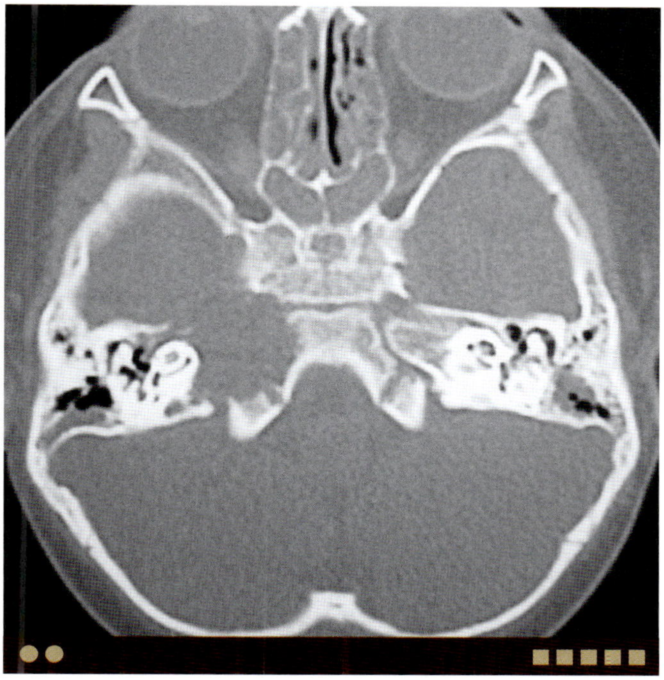

A. Rhabdomyosarcoma. Axial CT demonstrates partially opacified mastoid air cells bilaterally. Note bone the expansile osteolytic lesion in the right petrous apex.

COMMENTS

This is a 2-year-old boy with right temporal swelling with lower cranial nerve palsy. CT was performed to evaluate for otitis media.

Rhabdomyosarcoma is rare, however the most common soft tissue sarcoma in children, commonly seen in the head and neck (30–40%). Several distinct histologic types have been described, including embryonal (55%), botryoid (5%), alveolar (20%), and undifferentiated sarcoma (20%). Botryoid type arises in mucosal cavities, such as the nasopharynx and middle ear.

Rhabdomyosarcoma often presents with similar findings to acute otitis media clinically and radiologically. Therefore, this should always be in the differential diagnosis when diagnosing otitis media in children, particularly with cranial nerve impairment. Heterogeneously avid enhancement with bone destruction is commonly seen. Perineural tumor spread and intracranial extension is often seen in parameningeal tumors.

PEARLS

- **Rhabdomyosarcoma is rare, however the most common soft tissue sarcoma in children.**
- **Bone destruction and enhancing soft tissue is seen on CT and MRI.**
- **Rhabdomyosarcoma and Langerhans cell histiocytosis should be always in the differential diagnosis when diagnosing otitis media in children, particularly when aggressive bone destruction or cranial nerve impairment is noted.**

ADDITIONAL IMAGES (B-E)

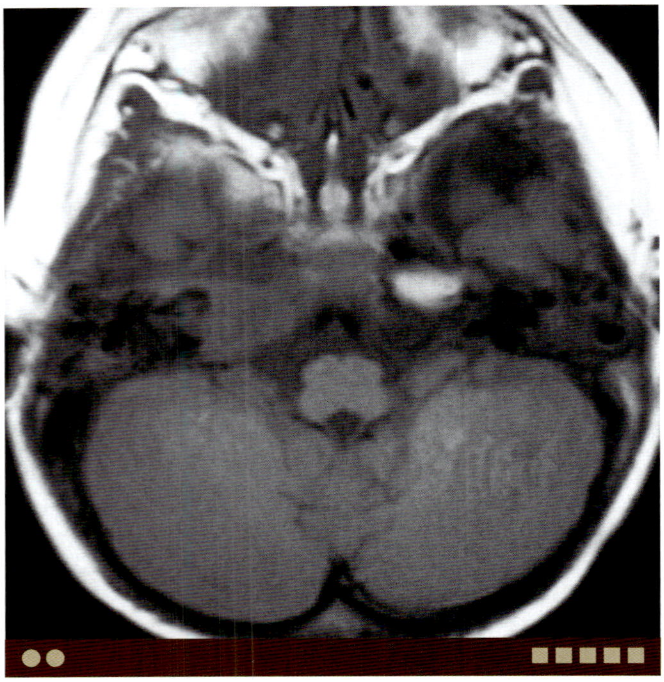

B. Rhabdomyosarcoma, same patient as A. Axial precontrast T1W image demonstrates a slightly expansile low-signal lesion in the right petrous apex, compared with preserved high signal from the normal fatty marrow in the left petrous apex.

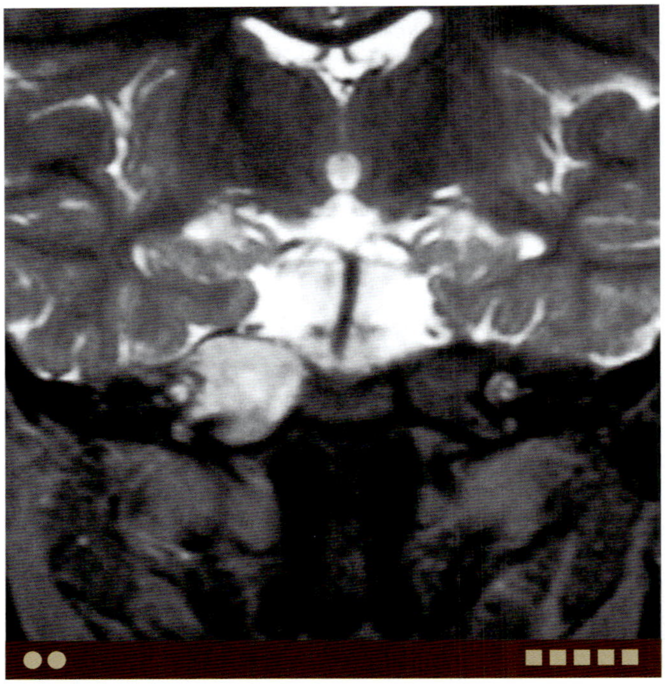

C. Rhabdomyosarcoma, same patient as A. Coronal T2W image shows the lesion demonstrating heterogeneous high signal.

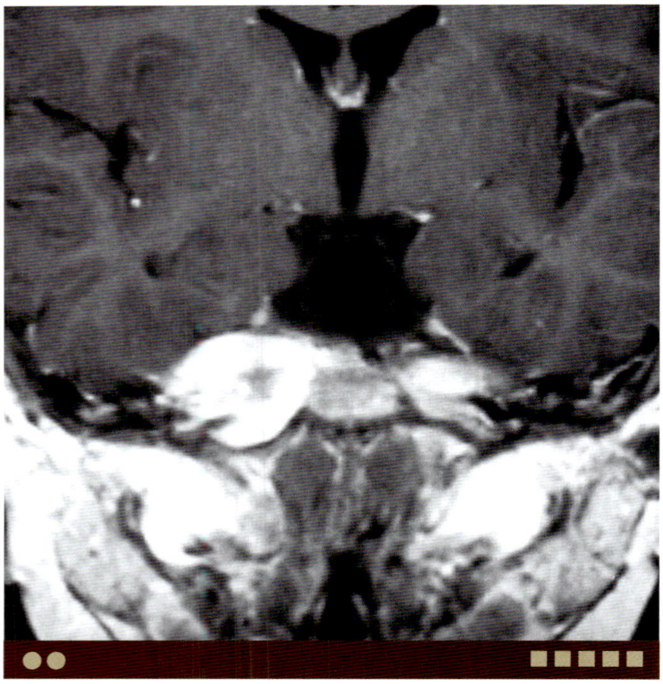

D. Rhabdomyosarcoma, same patient as A. Coronal postcontrast T1W image demonstrates avid enhancement of the lesion.

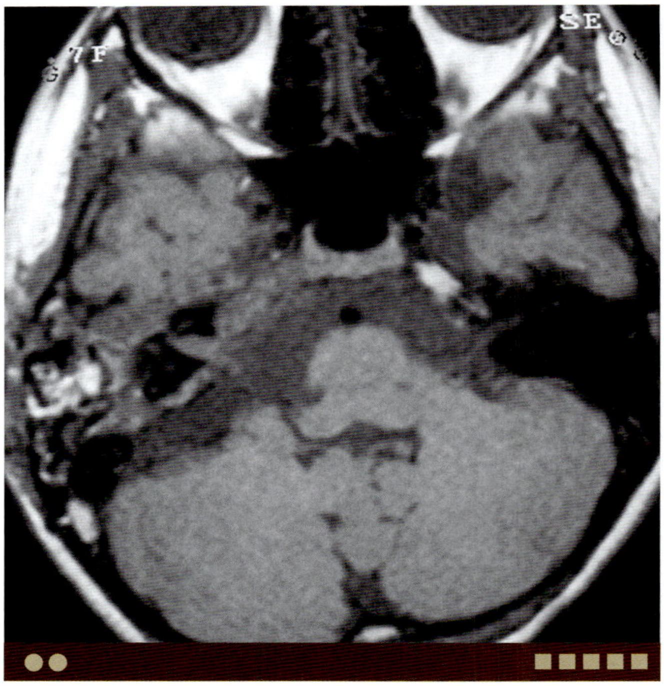

E. **Rhabdomyosarcoma** in a different patient. Axial T1W image demonstrates heterogeneous signal in the right mastoid air cells. The right petrous apex shows slight expansion and decreased signal. Note abnormal intermediate signals in the right internal auditory canal and along the posterior aspect of the petrous bone consistent with parameningeal tumor extension.

DIFFERENTIAL DIAGNOSIS IMAGES (F-G)

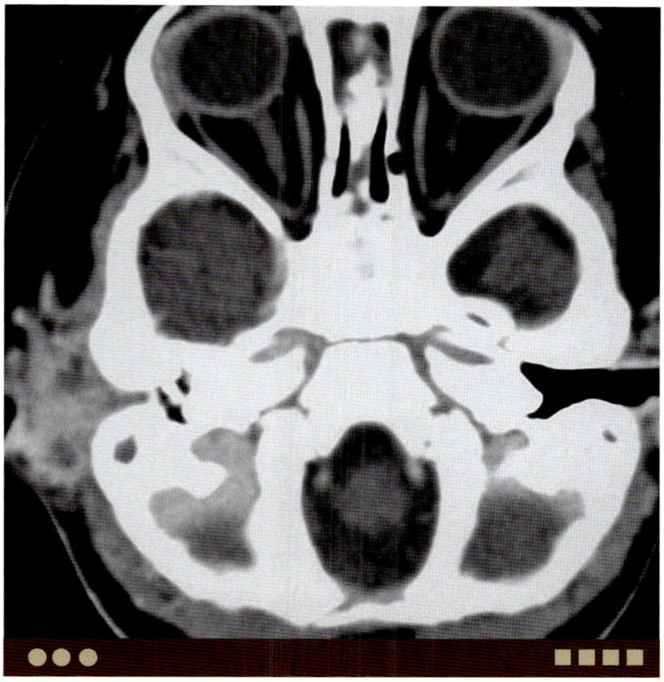

F. Complicated mastoiditis. Axial postcontrast CT demonstrates a heterogeneously enhancing extraosseous lesion in the right temporal region.

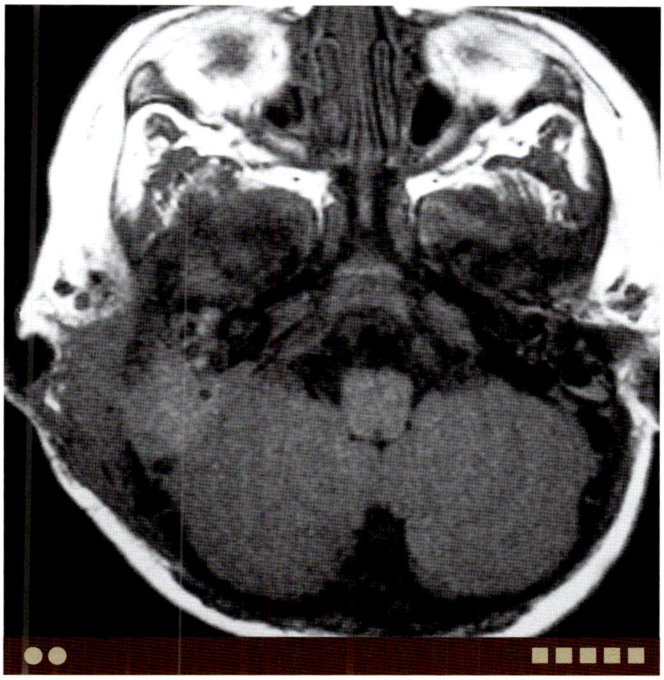

G. Langerhans cell histiocytosis. Axial T1W image demonstrates a heterogeneously low-signal lesion centered in the right mastoid extending into the superficial soft tissues.

Case 2–22 Lymphoma: Perineural Extension

Osamu Sakai, Rohini Nadgir

PRESENTATION

Trigeminal neuralgia.

FINDINGS

CT and MRI demonstrate thickening of the trigeminal nerve, obliteration of the fat pad below the foramen ovale, and masses in the paracavernous region.

DIFFERENTIAL

- Perineural tumor spread: Adenoid cystic carcinoma is well-known for perineural spread, however squamous cell carcinoma (SCCA) is the most common tumor causing this because SCCA is the most common malignancy in the head and neck.
- Schwannoma: This occurs along the cranial nerve and demonstrates a spindle- or dumbbell-shaped lesion. Bone erosion rather than destruction is common with schwannoma.
- Neurofibroma: This is often seen in patients with neurofibromatosis, although most neurofibromas are sporadic. Thickened nerve is a common finding.

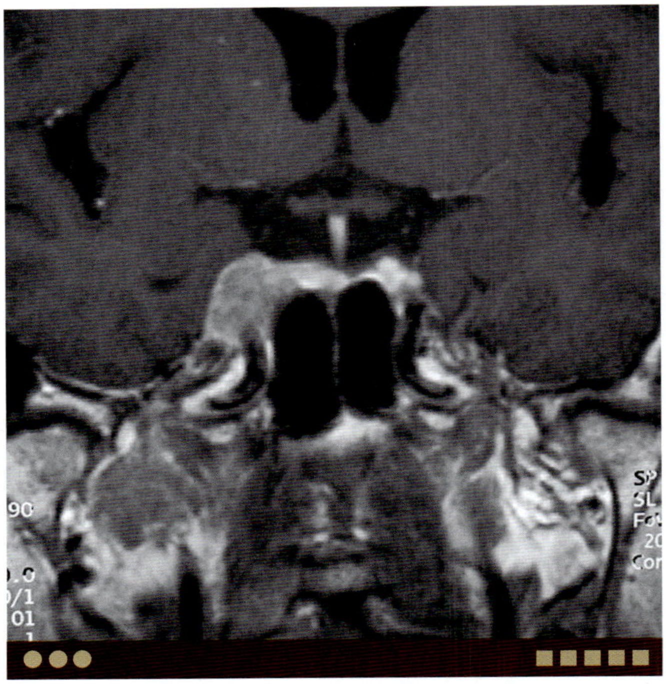

A. Lymphoma. Coronal postcontrast T1W image shows a mildly enhancing lesion involving the right paracavernous region. Note a larger region below the foramen ovale involving the V3.

COMMENTS

This is a 71-year-old man with trigeminal neuralgia.

Lymphoma in this region is usually B cell type non-Hodgkin lymphoma, like lymphomas in other areas of the head and neck. Lymphoma may be seen as a solid mass arising from the pharyngeal lymphoid tissue, mucosa or salivary glands, or may occur in the bone marrow. Lymphoma is a relatively soft tumor and invades and infiltrates into the adjacent organs preserving preexisting structures. Also, perineural extension is commonly seen.

On CT, lymphoma usually shows low-to-intermediate density similar to the muscle and mild enhancement. On MRI, it shows relatively low signal, slightly higher than the muscle on T1W images, and intermediate-to-high signal on T2W and STIR images. After contrast, it shows homogeneous mild-to-intermediate enhancement.

Perineural spread of lymphoma is often seen along the second division of the trigeminal nerve (V2) through the foramen rotundum, the Vidian nerve through the Vidian canal, the hypoglossal nerve through the hypoglossal canal, and the third division of the trigeminal nerve (V3) through the foramen ovale. Loss of normal fat pad in or below the canal/foramen is a key finding to make the diagnosis. This should be evaluated with precontrast T1W images because enhancing lesions may become less conspicuous after contrast. Fat-suppression may be useful; however, inhomogeneous suppression may be troublesome. Widening/expansion of the canal/foramen are often seen. Bone erosion may suggest a long-standing lesion, however, that does not imply benignity. Skip lesions may be present, therefore, it is important to evaluate the entire course of the nerve.

PEARLS

- **Perineural tumor spread is seen with lymphoma.**
- **Obliteration of the fat within or below canals/foramina strongly suggests tumor spread, while the normal appearance of the fat pad is reassuring.**
- **Skip lesions may be present, therefore, careful evaluation of the entire course of the nerve is essential.**

ADDITIONAL IMAGES (B-F)

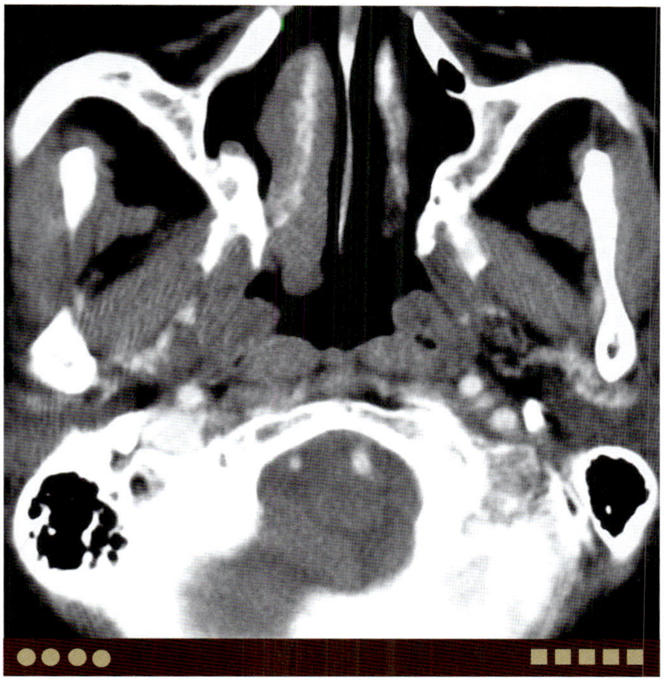

B. Lymphoma in a different patient. Axial postcontrast CT shows obliteration of the fat around the V3 on the right. The trigeminal fat pad is preserved on the left.

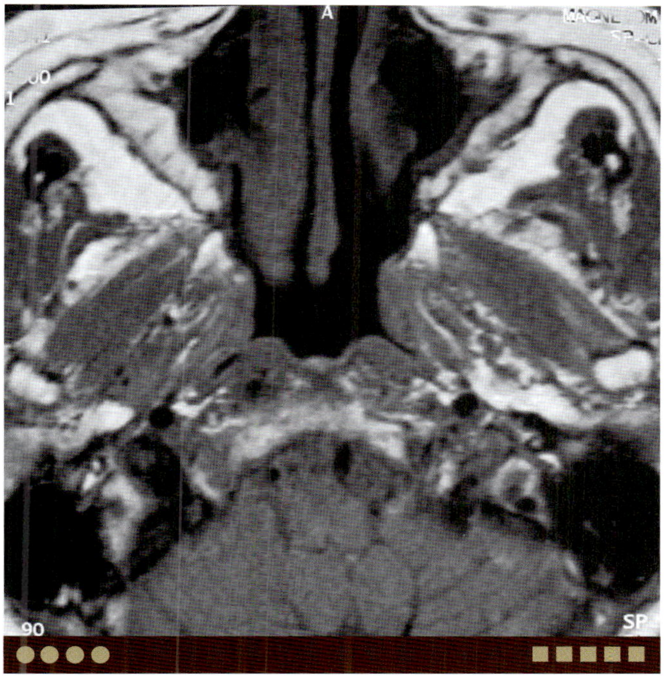

C. Lymphoma, same patient as B. Axial T1W image demonstrates obliteration of the fat around the V3 on the right. The fat is preserved on the left.

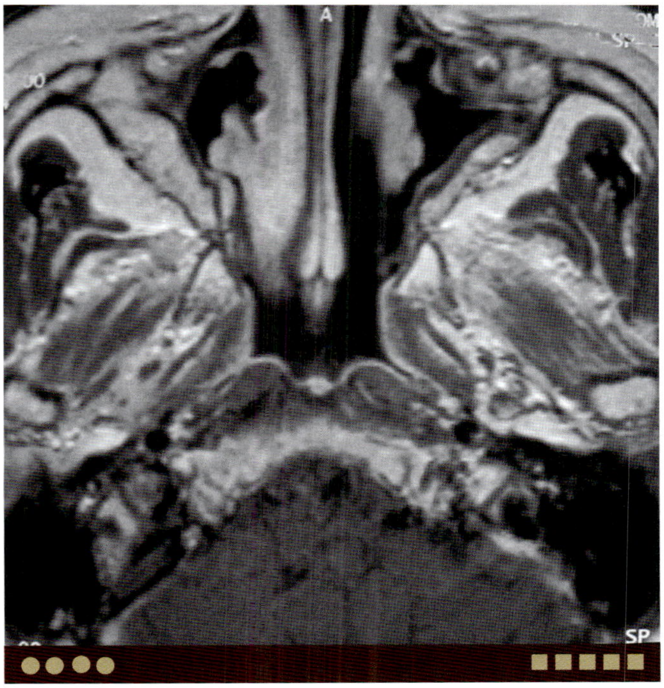

D. Lymphoma, same patient as B. Axial postcontrast T1W image demonstrates enhancement of the lesion. The lesion becomes less conspicuous after contrast.

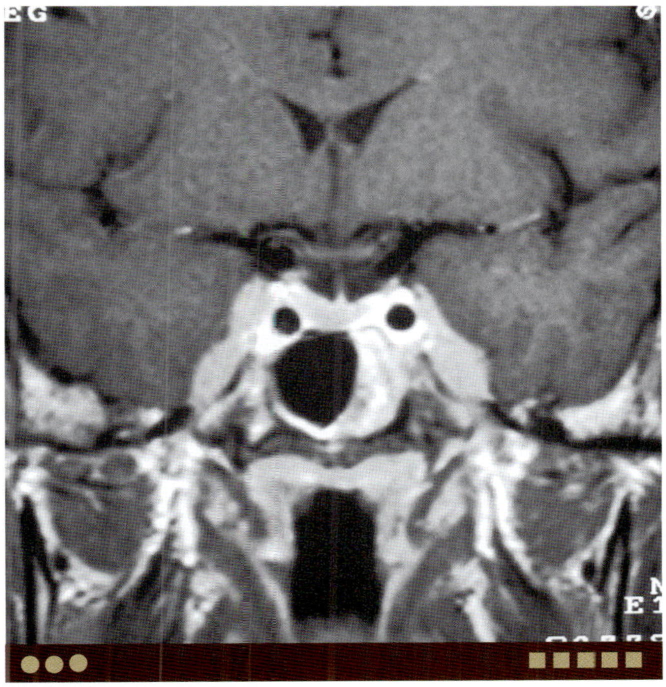

E. Lymphoma in a different patient. Coronal postcontrast T1W image shows enhancing lesions involving the Meckel's cave bilaterally and both trigeminal nerves.

DIFFERENTIAL DIAGNOSIS IMAGES (G-I)

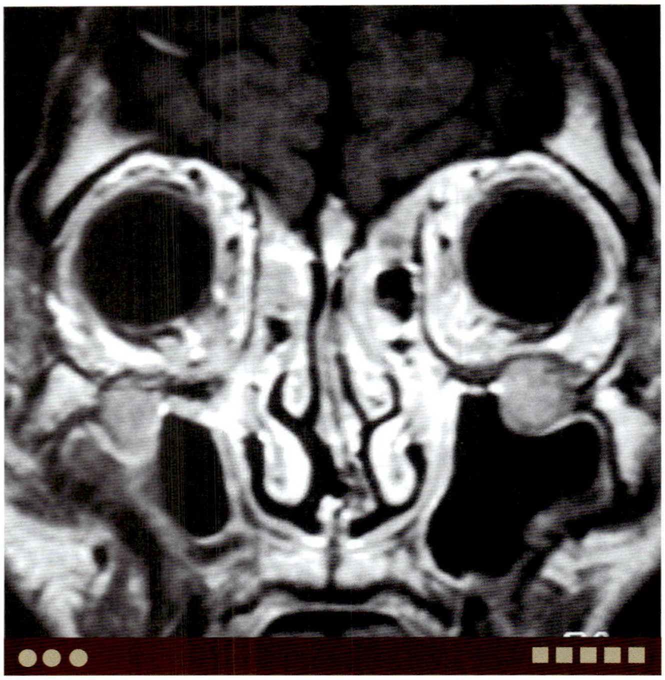

F. Lymphoma, same patient as E. Coronal postcontrast T1W image shows enlargement and abnormal enhancement of the bilateral infraorbital nerves.

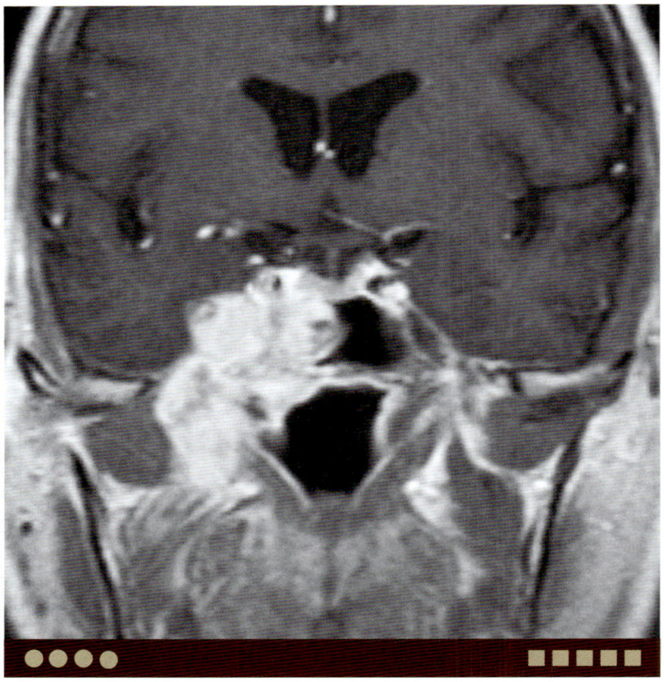

G. Perineural tumor spread, adenoid cystic carcinoma of the parotid. Coronal postcontrast T1W image shows a multilobulated heterogeneously enhancing tumor involving the right Meckel's cave and foramen ovale.

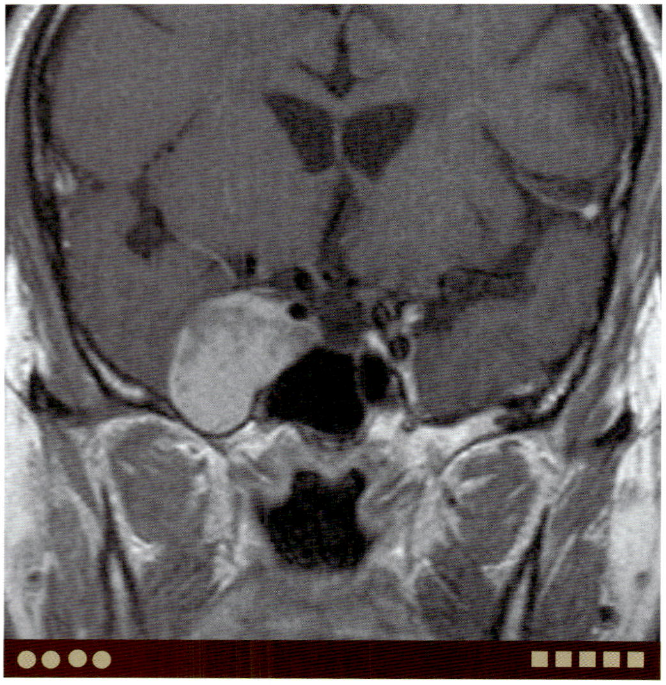

H. Trigeminal schwannoma. Coronal postcontrast T1W image shows a well-demarcated enhancing tumor centered in the right Meckel's cave displacing the internal carotid artery medially. Note remodeling of the sphenoid bone inferior to the lesion.

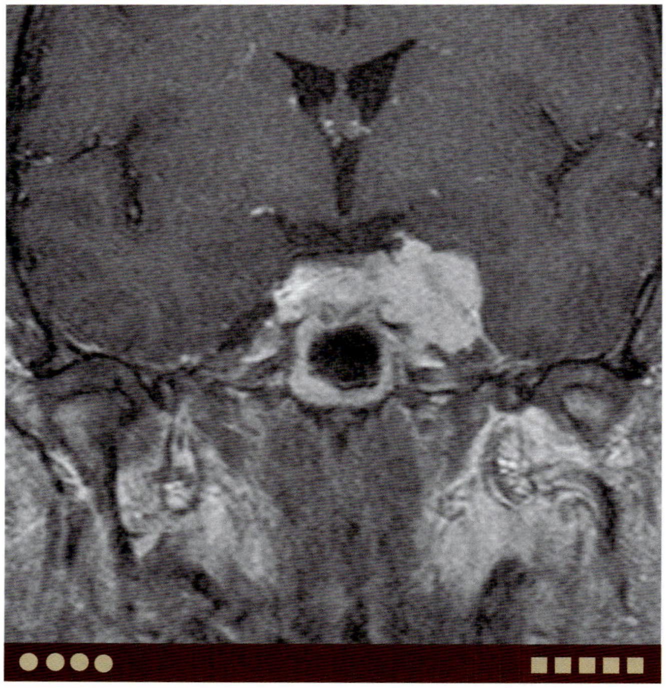

I. Meningioma. Coronal postcontrast T1W image demonstrates a slightly lobulated homogeneously enhancing lesion centered in the left paracavernous region.

Case 2–23 Sellar Dermoid

Rohini Nadgir, Osamu Sakai

PRESENTATION

Typically asymptomatic unless large enough to compress optic chiasm or cranial nerves within the cavernous sinus. Ruptured dermoids can present with severe headache and chemical meningitis.

FINDINGS

CT and MRI demonstrate a fat-containing lesion in the sella.

DIFFERENTIAL

- Internal carotid artery (ICA) aneurysm: On MRI, ICA aneurysms can be heterogeneous in signal due to flow and partial thrombosis. Gradient echo images can show susceptibility artifact. Pulsation artifact can be also seen.
- Rathke's cleft cyst: This is a congenital/developmental cystic lesion, often demonstrating increased T1 signal from proteinaceous contents, but should not contain fat; unchanged T1 hyperintensity on fat-suppressed images should confirm that no fat is present within this lesion.
- Craniopharyngioma: This tumor often demonstrates calcification and cystic components which can be T1 bright due to proteinaceous contents. T1 hyperintensity is typically not as bright as fat, but if there is a concern, unchanged T1 hyperintensity on fat suppressed images should confirm so that no fat is present within this lesion.
- Epidermoid: Cystic congenital lesion containing epithelial elements only. Fatty component should not be seen.
- Residual pantopaque: Pantopaque was used decades ago as a myelographic contrast agent. It has since been taken off the market due to complications of seizures and arachnoiditis. Occasionally, residual pantopaque can be seen intracranially or within the spinal canal on imaging, with imaging characteristics of fat due to its oil base.

COMMENTS

Dermoids are congenital cystic lesions that contain epithelial elements and dermal appendages. The epithelial elements account for the cystic component, whereas the dermal appendages account for the fatty components. If fatty component is identified on imaging, the diagnosis of dermoid is clear. However, occasionally the fatty component is microscopic and can only be identified histopathologically; in these cases, dermoids are not distinguishable from epidermoids on imaging.

Other T1 hyperintense lesions that occur in this location include Rathke's cleft cysts and cystic components within craniopharyngiomas. The T1 hyperintensity within these lesions is related to proteinaceous material, not fat. Typically, the cyst components are less T1 hyperintense than fat on MRI, but occasionally it may be difficult to tell the difference. Fat suppressed sequences are helpful in making the distinction, since the material within Rathke's cysts and craniopharyngiomas should maintain T1 hyperintensity on fat suppressed images, whereas signal will be suppressed in dermoid lesions.

Dermoids can be symptomatic in the sellar region if large enough to compress the optic chiasm or compress cranial nerves within the cavernous sinus. Dermoids can also rupture, resulting in clinically devastating chemical meningitis. On imaging, ruptured dermoid can be seen as numerous small droplets of fat within the subarachnoid spaces. For this reason, while these lesions are benign, surgical excision should be considered.

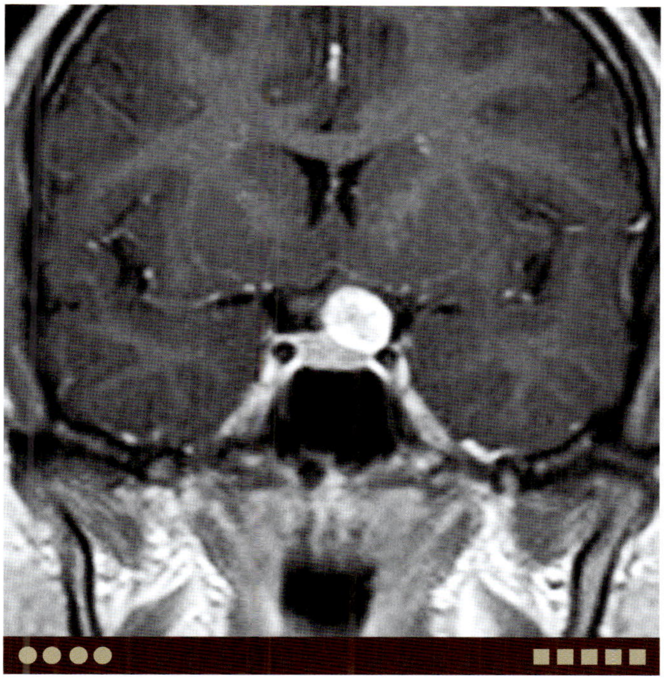

A. Dermoid. Coronal postcontrast T1W MR image demonstrates a round high-signal lesion in the left suprasellar region without pulsation artifact.

PEARLS

- **Dermoids are congenital cystic lesions that contain epithelial elements and dermal appendages, which account for fatty component that can be seen on CT and MR imaging.**
- **Intracranial dermoids can rupture, resulting in clinically devastating chemical meningitis.**

ADDITIONAL IMAGES (B-G)

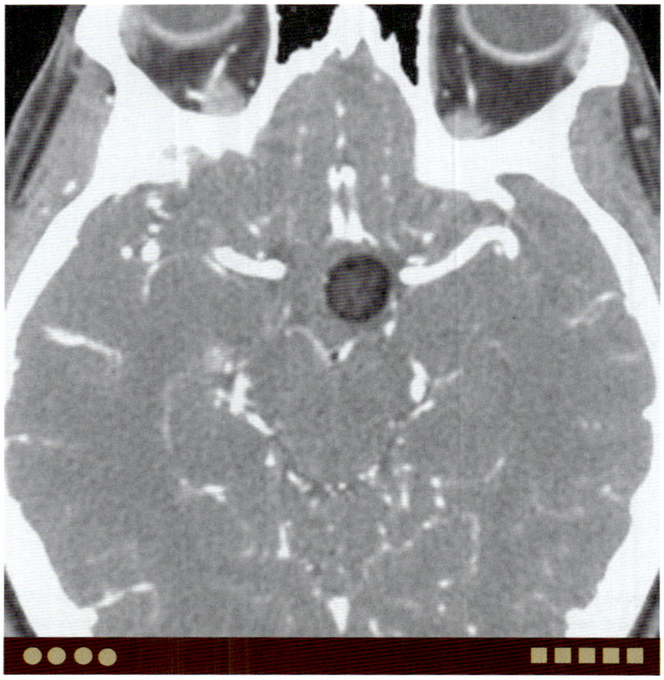

B. Dermoid, same patient as A. Axial CTA image demonstrates a round fat density lesion in the left suprasellar region.

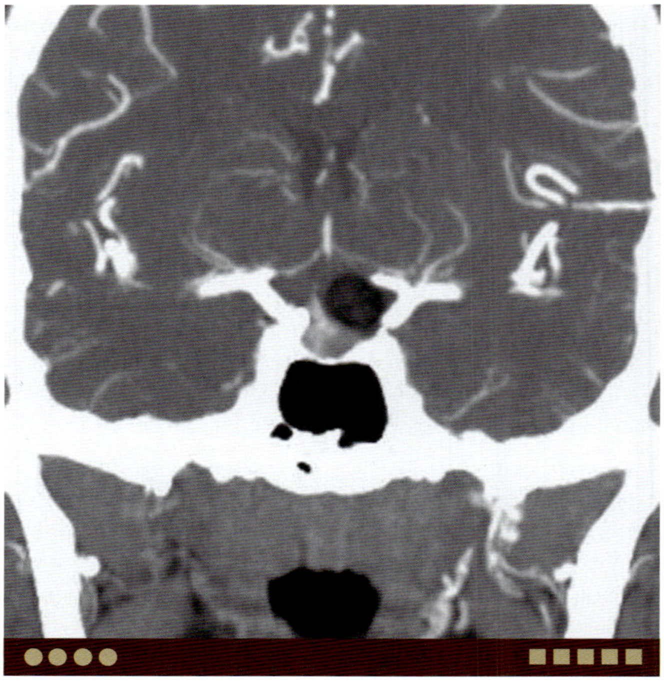

C. Dermoid, same patient as A. Coronal CTA MIP image demonstrates a round fat density suprasellar lesion.

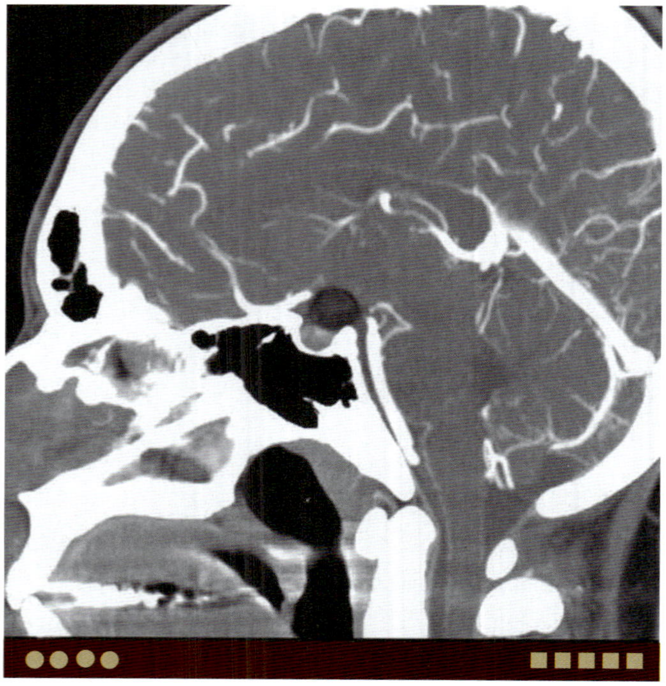

D. Dermoid, same patient as A. Sagittal CTA MIP image demonstrates a fat density suprasellar lesion.

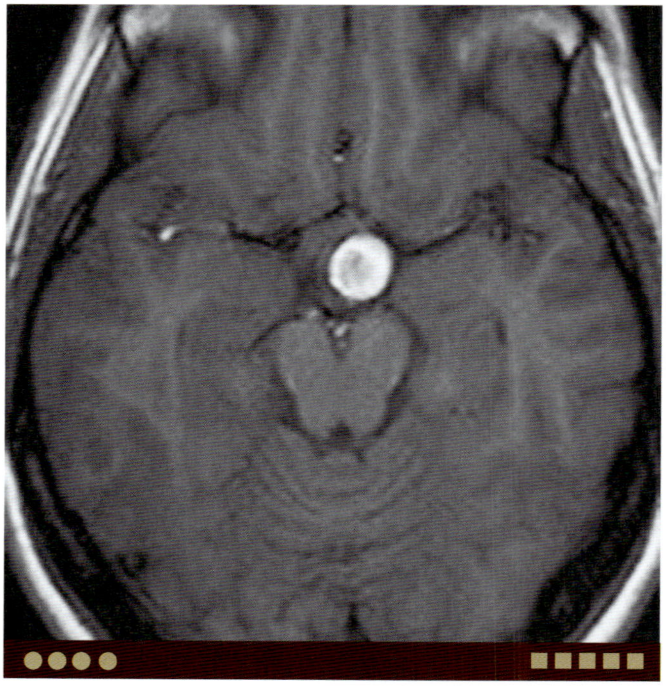

E. Dermoid, same patient as A. Axial T1W MR image demonstrates a round high-signal lesion in the left suprasellar region without pulsation artifact.

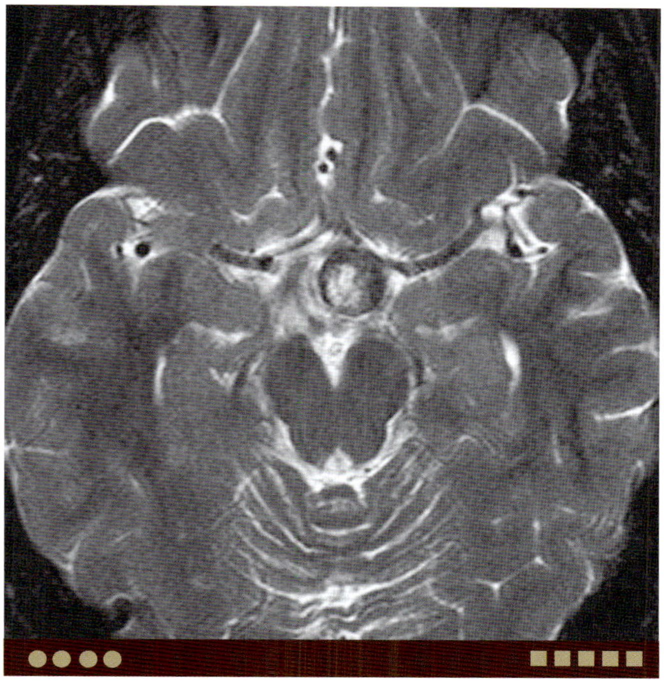

F. Dermoid, same patient as A. Axial fat-suppressed T2W MR image demonstrates a round heterogeneous signal lesion in the left suprasellar region without pulsation artifact. Note signal drop in the peripheral portion the lesion by fat-suppression.

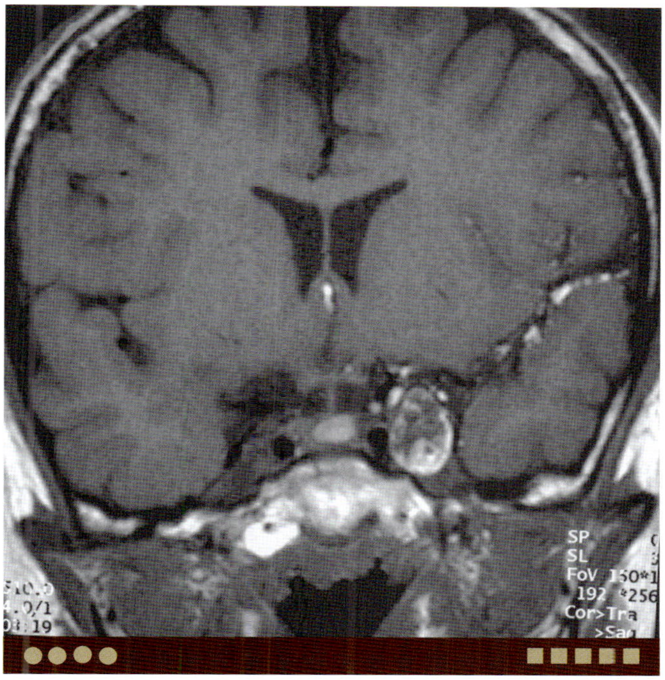

G. Ruptured dermoid in a different patient. Coronal T1W MR image demonstrates a paracavernous high-signal lesion and multiple high-signal droplets in the left Sylvian fissure.

DIFFERENTIAL DIAGNOSIS IMAGES (H-I)

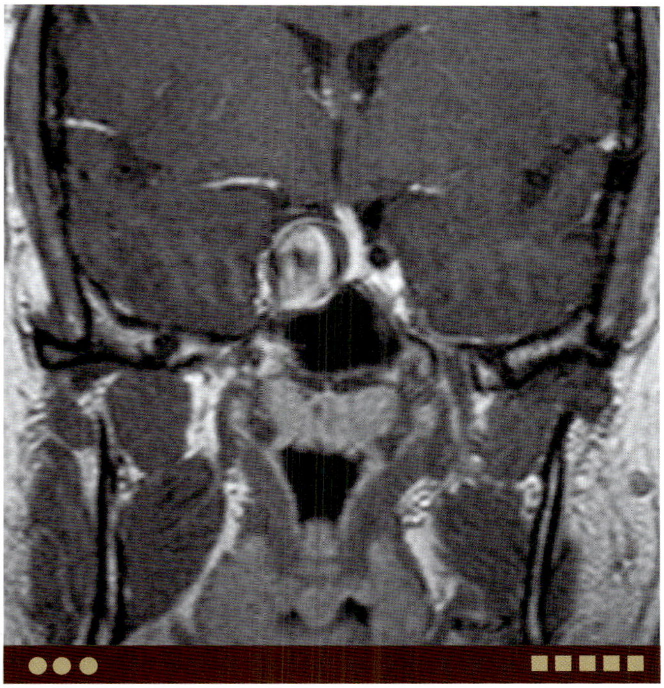

H. ICA aneurysm. Coronal postcontrast T1W MR image demonstrates a heterogeneously enhancing round lesion with pulsation artifacts in the right sellar/parasellar region. Normal right ICA flow void is not visualized.

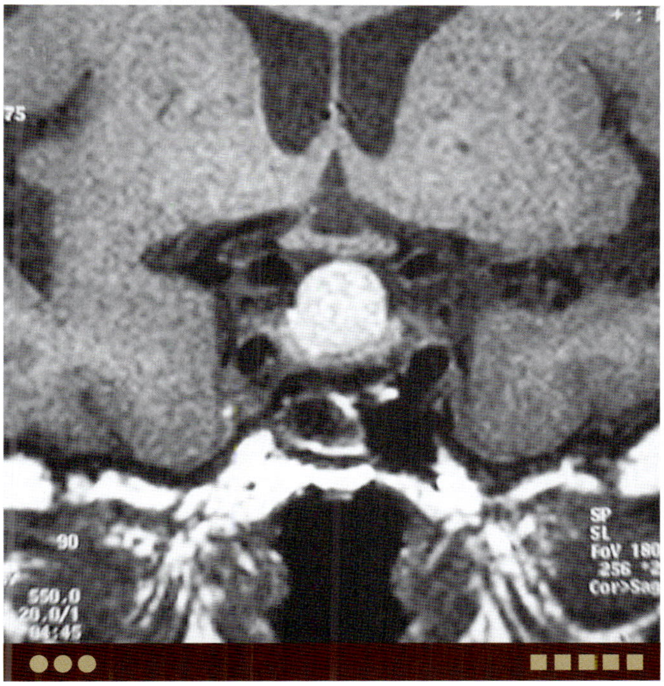

I. Rathke's cleft cyst. Coronal T1W image demonstrates a round high-signal lesion in the sellar/suprasellar region without pulsation artifact. Normal ICAs are seen bilaterally.

Case 2–24 Parasellar Internal Carotid Artery Aneurysm

Rohini Nadgir, Osamu Sakai

PRESENTATION

Pulsatile tinnitus, headache, or symptoms related to cranial nerve compression.

FINDINGS

MR images demonstrate a heterogeneously enhancing parasellar mass with pulsation artifact in the phase encoding direction. CT demonstrates smooth nonaggressive focal remodeling of the bony margin of the sella and avid enhancement.

DIFFERENTIAL

- Pituitary macroadenoma: These lesions are typically centered in the sella and can be seen arising from pituitary tissue. Macroadenomas can extend laterally into the cavernous sinus and/or superiorly to compress the optic chiasm. Pulsation artifact should not be seen.
- Craniopharyngioma: These tumors are typically complex with cystic and solid components and calcifications. They can become very large in size and invade the skull base and brain. There is a bimodal age distribution, with young children and older adults affected. Pulsation artifact should not be seen.
- Rathke's cleft cyst: These are sellar/suprasellar cystic lesions, often demonstrating T1 high signal from proteinaceous contents. Pulsation artifact should not be seen.
- Schwannoma: These lesions can occur in a parasellar location but are more typically homogeneously enhancing. Cystic degeneration can sometimes be seen. Pulsation artifact should not be seen.
- Meningioma: Like schwannomas, these lesions can occur in a parasellar location but are more typically homogeneously enhancing. Dural tail enhancement is most suggestive of meningioma. Pulsation artifact should not be seen.
- Metastases: When there is a clinical history of known primary tumor, metastastes should always be considered in the differential of sellar/parasellar mass. Pulsation artifact should not be seen.

COMMENTS

Parasellar ICA aneurysms are typically complex lesions associated with bony expansion but should also demonstrate flow related characteristics on imaging if not completely thrombosed at the time of diagnosis. Heterogeneous enhancement can be seen on contrast-enhanced CT if the aneurysm is partially thrombosed; internal flow within nonthrombosed components and intimate relationship with internal carotid artery can also be confirmed on CT angiogram or conventional catheter angiography.

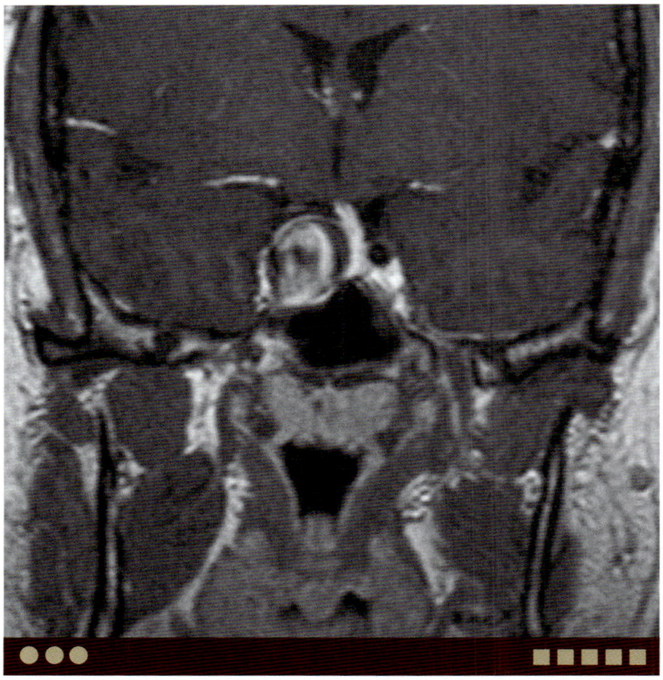

A. ICA aneurysm. Coronal postcontrast T1W MR image demonstrates a heterogeneously enhancing round lesion with pulsation artifacts in the right sellar/parasellar region. Normal right ICA flow void is not visualized.

On MRI, ICA aneurysms can be heterogeneous in signal on T1W and T2W images with heterogeneous enhancement due to complex flow dynamics and variable ages of clot material within the aneurysm. Gradient echo images can show susceptibility artifacts from blood products. Pulsation artifact in the phase-encoding direction can be seen if the aneurysm is not completely thrombosed.

The possibility of ICA aneurysm should always be considered within the differential of any sellar/parasellar mass. On MR imaging, if pulsation artifact is demonstrated through the lesion, ICA aneurysm becomes the primary diagnostic consideration. Biopsy should not be performed on any pulsatile lesions in this region, and conventional angiography should be considered for confirmation and treatment planning.

PEARLS

- **The possibility of ICA aneurysm should always be considered within the differential of any sellar/parasellar mass.**
- **On MR imaging, if pulsation artifact is demonstrated through the lesion, ICA aneurysm becomes the primary diagnostic consideration.**
- **Biopsy should not be performed and conventional angiography should be considered for confirmation and treatment planning.**

ADDITIONAL IMAGES (B-G)

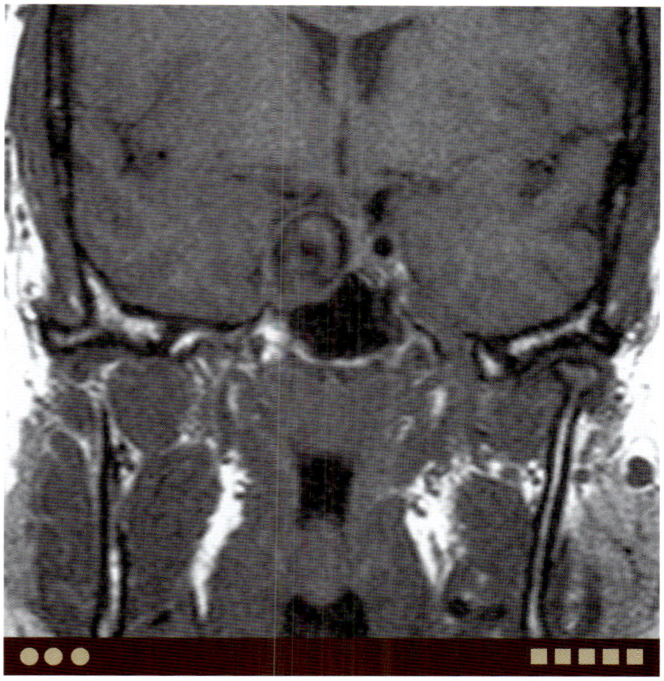

B. ICA aneurysm, same patient as A. Coronal T1W MR image demonstrates a round heterogeneous signal lesion with signal voids in the right sellar/parasellar region. Normal right ICA flow void is not visualized.

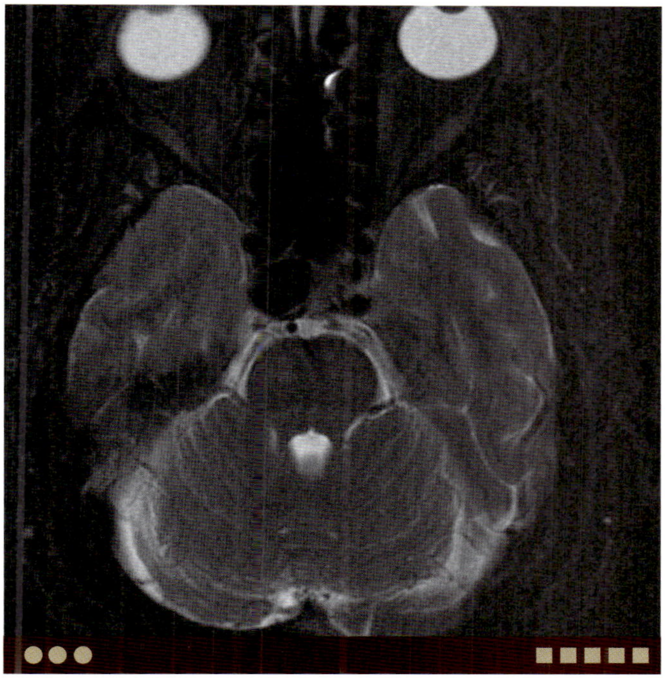

C. ICA aneurysm, same patient as A. Axial T2W MR image demonstrates a round signal void in the right parasellar/cavernous region.

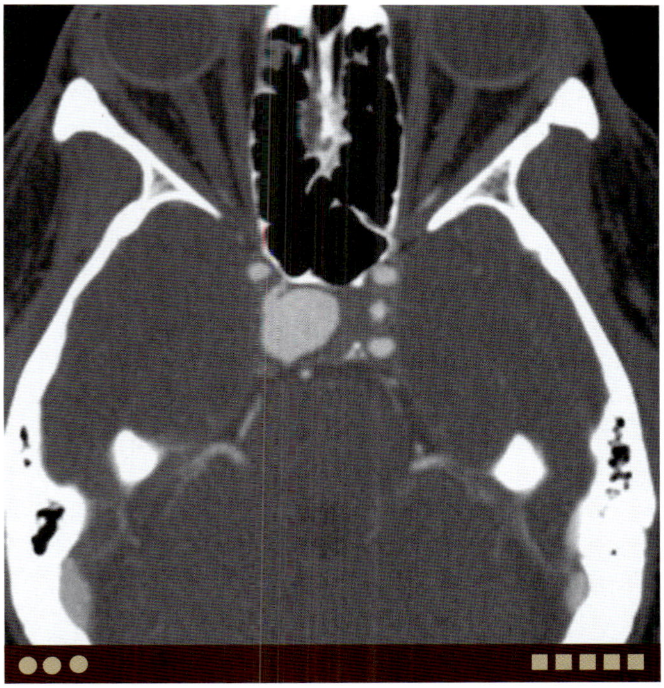

D. ICA aneurysm, same patient as A. Axial CTA image demonstrates a round homogeneously enhancing lesion in the right parasellar/cavernous region. Note erosion of the right posterior clinoid.

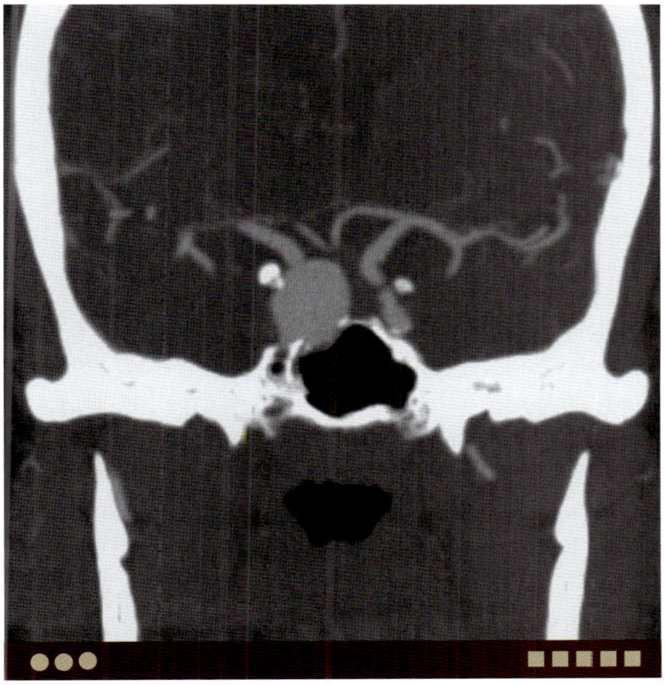

E. ICA aneurysm, same patient as A. Coronal CTA image demonstrates a round homogeneously enhancing lesion eroding the roof of the right sphenoid sinus.

ADDITIONAL IMAGES (B-C)

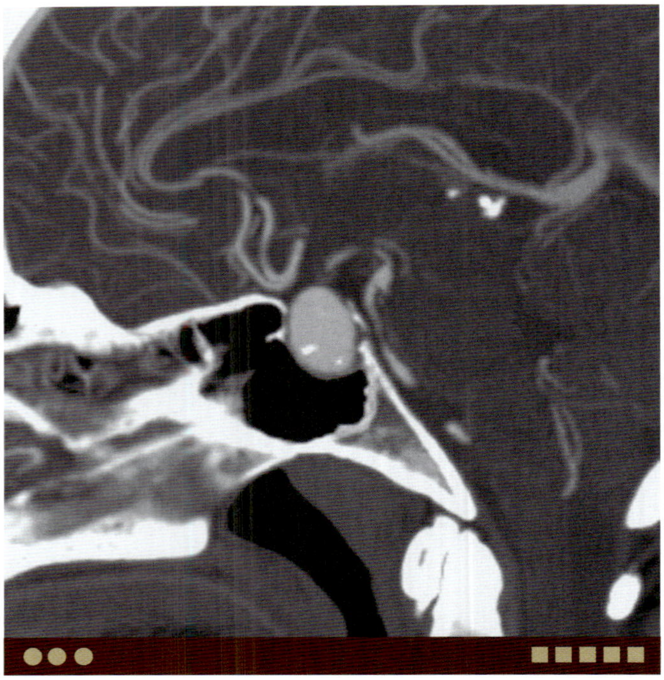

F. ICA aneurysm, same patient as A. Sagittal CTA image demonstrates a round homogeneously enhancing lesion eroding the floor of the sella.

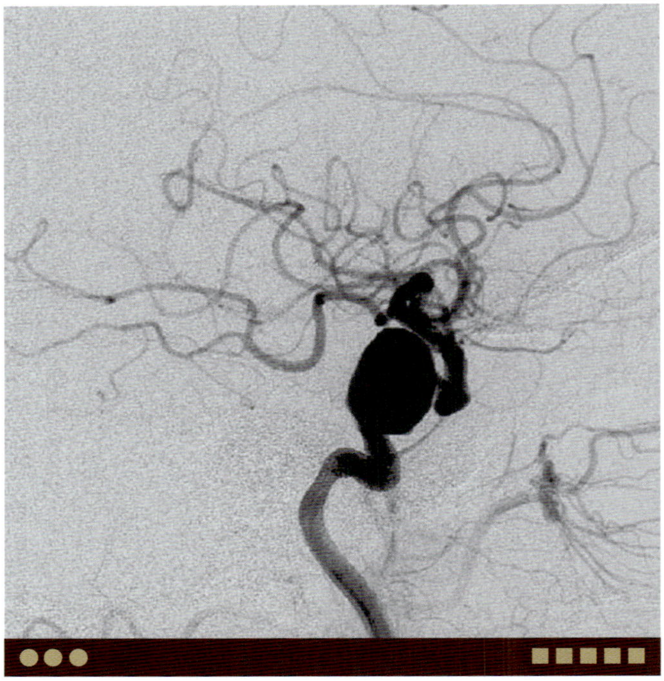

G. ICA aneurysm, same patient as A. Right ICA injection demonstrates a large aneurysm in the cavernous segment.

DIFFERENTIAL DIAGNOSIS IMAGES (H-J)

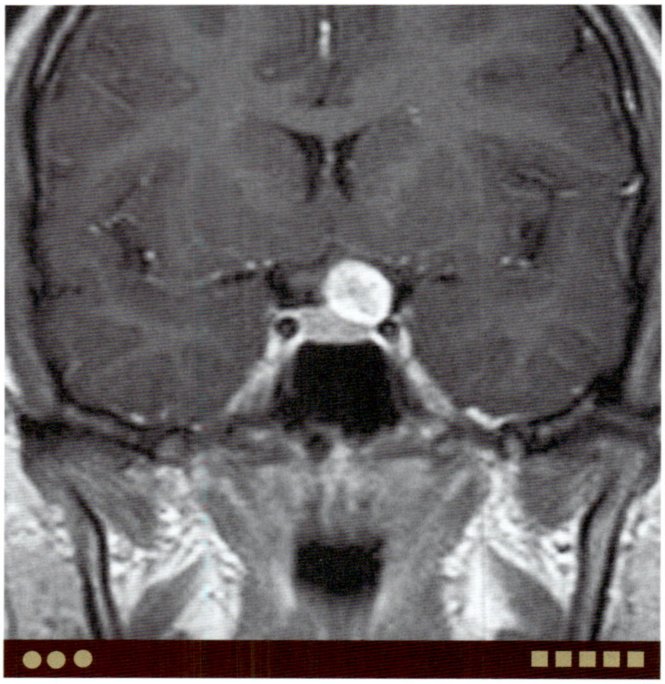

H. Dermoid. Coronal postcontrast T1W MR image demonstrates a slightly heterogeneous high signal, round lesion in the left suprasellar region. No pulsation artifact is seen.

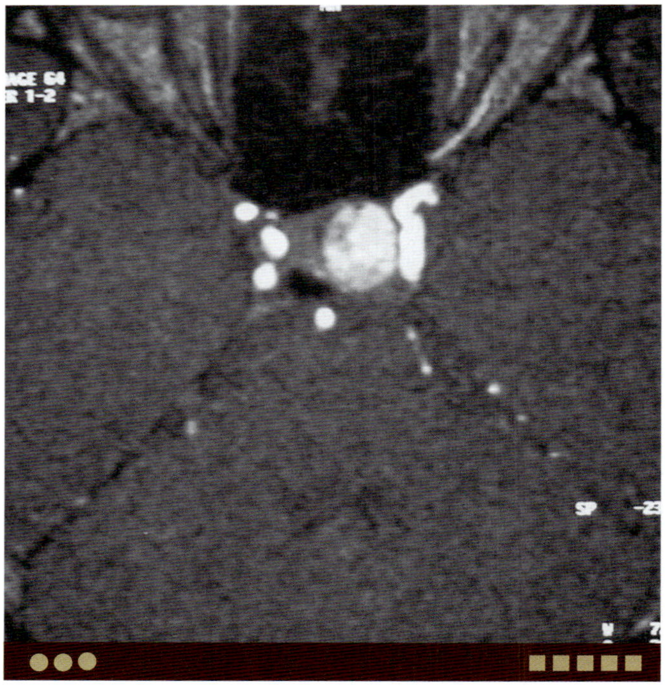

I. Rathke's cleft cyst. Axial time-of-flight MRA source image shows a round, high-signal lesion in the sella on the left.

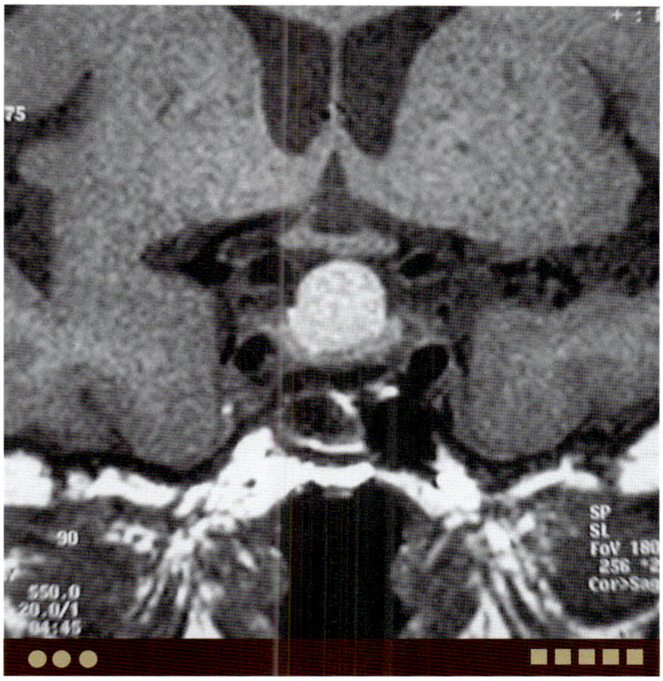

J. Rathke's cleft cyst, same patient as I. Coronal T1W image demonstrates a round high-signal lesion in the sellar/suprasellar region without pulsation artifact. Normal ICAs are seen bilaterally.

Case 2–25 Neurovascular Compression

Rohini Nadgir, Osamu Sakai

PRESENTATION

Tinnitus and/or neuralgia related to cranial nerve compression.

FINDINGS

Thin section T2W and time-of-flight MRA source images demonstrate a tortuous vertebral artery focally contacting and compressing the seventh and eighth nerve complex at the level of the root exit zone.

DIFFERENTIAL

- Normal anatomic relationship: Vertebral artery and major vertebrobasilar branches such as PICA and AICA can often be seen closely approximating cranial nerves within the cerebellopontine angle and internal auditory canal in asymptomatic patients.

COMMENTS

Neurovascular compression of cranial nerves at the skull base remains a relatively controversial diagnosis. Vessels related to the circle of Willis can often be seen approximating cranial nerves at the skull base in otherwise asymptomatic patients.

Occasionally, patients may truly have troublesome symptoms related to adjacent cranial nerves secondary to constant pulsation of the artery against the nerve. Such symptomatic patients may benefit from surgical intervention. MR imaging will demonstrate compression of the affected cranial nerve at the root exit zone, where the nerve arises from the brainstem. Elongation or stretching of the affected cranial nerve may be seen. Dural graft can be surgically placed between the vessel and affected nerve to alleviate symptoms.

Since tinnitus is a common reason for performing thin section T2W MR imaging through the skull base, if a close anatomic association is seen with respect to vessels and nerves, particularly at the nerve root exit zone, the finding should be reported.

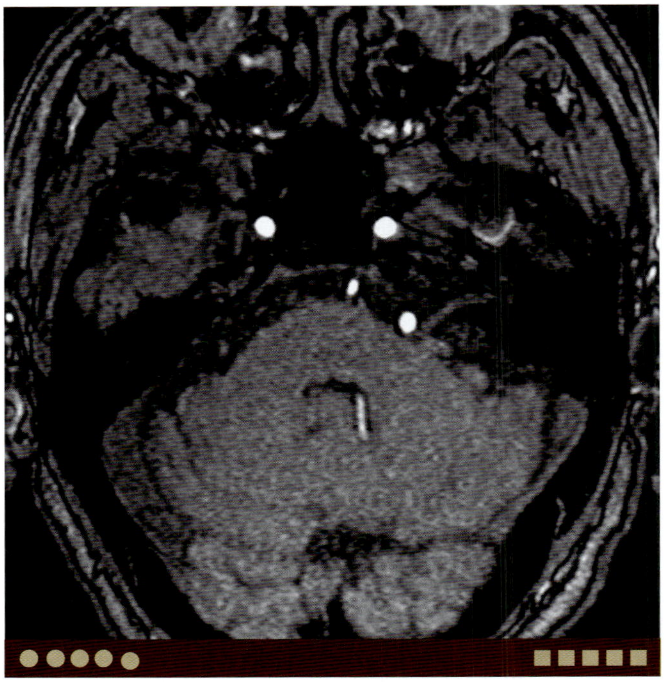

A. Neurovascular compression. Axial time-of-flight MRA source image shows the left vertebral artery compressing the seventh and eighth nerve complex at the level of the root exit zone.

PEARLS

- **Since tinnitus is a common reason for performing thin section T2W imaging through the skull base, if a close anatomic association is seen with respect to vessels and nerves, particularly at the root exit zone, the finding should be reported.**
- **Patients may truly have troublesome symptoms secondary to constant pulsation of artery against the adjacent nerve; such symptomatic patients may benefit from surgical intervention.**
- **Vessels related to the circle of Willis can often be seen approximating cranial nerves at the skull base in otherwise asymptomatic patients.**

ADDITIONAL IMAGES (B-D)

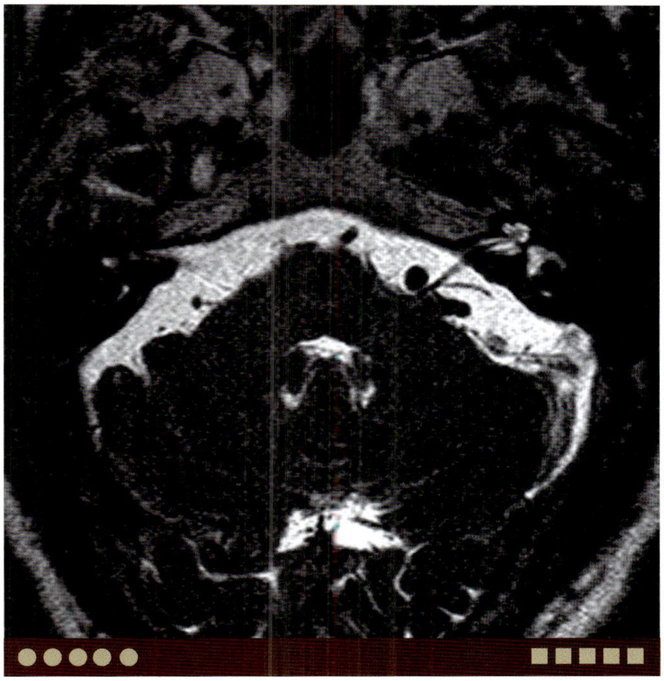

B. Neurovascular compression, same patient as A. Axial T2W DRIVE image shows the left vertebral artery compressing the seventh and eighth nerve complex at the level of the root exit zone.

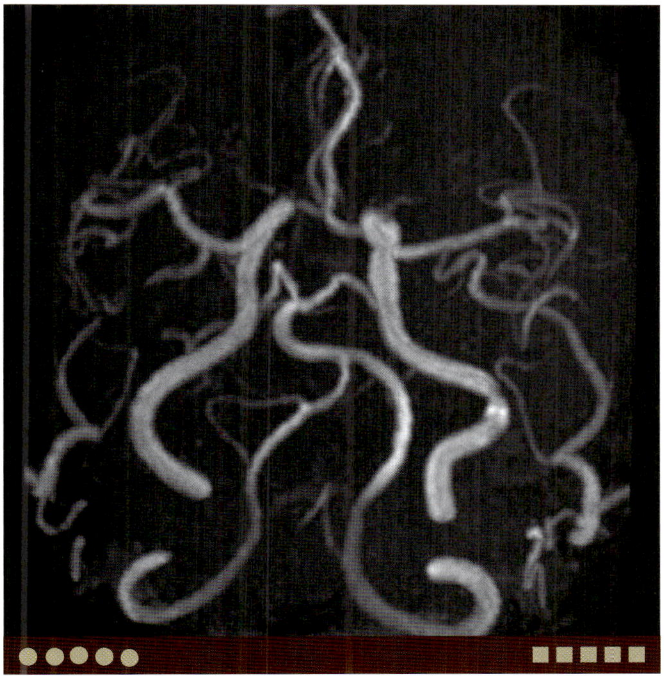

C. Neurovascular compression, same patient as A. MIP image of time-of-flight MRA shows elongated and somewhat tortuous left vertebral artery.

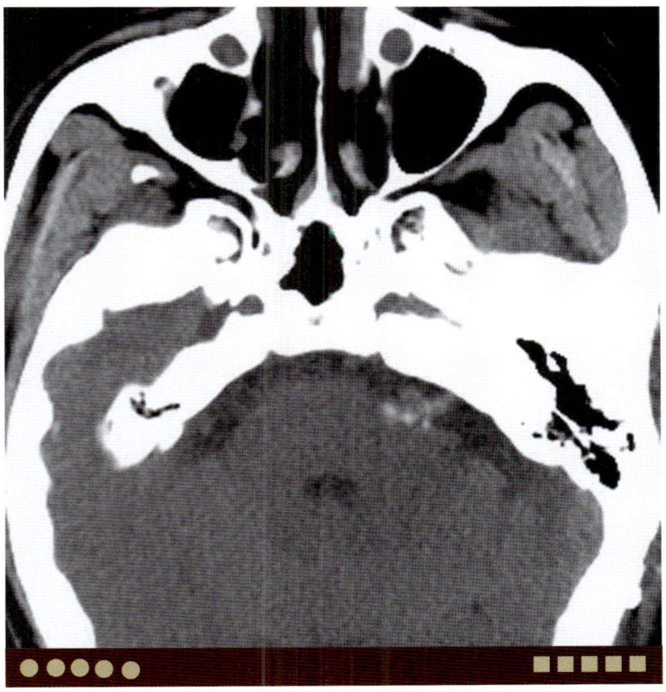

D. Neurovascular compression, same patient as A. CT after decompression surgery demonstrates high-density graft material at the left cerebellopontine angle.

DIFFERENTIAL DIAGNOSIS IMAGES (E-F)

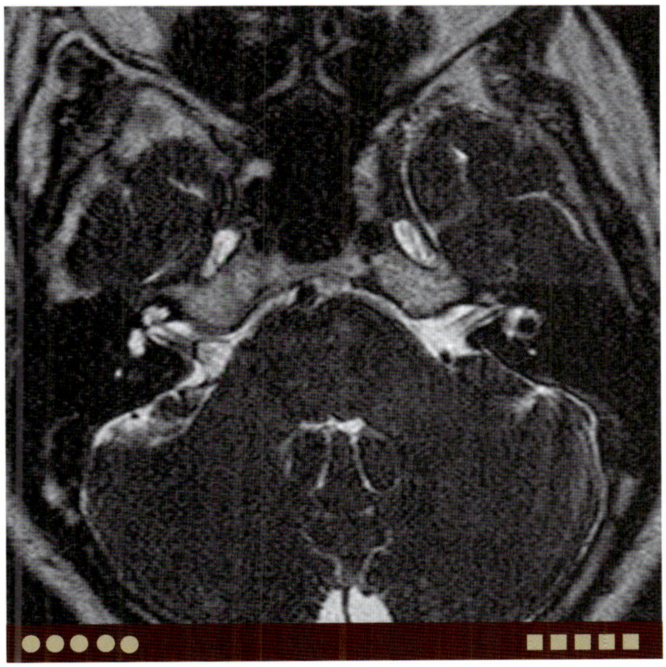

E. Normal AICA loop. Axial T2W DRIVE image shows normal AICA loop at the orifice of the right internal auditory canal.

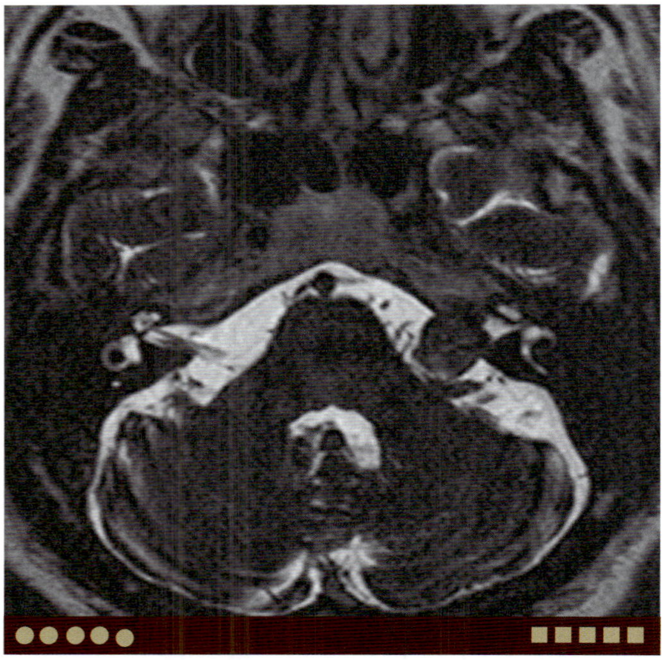

F. Vestibular schwannoma. Axial high-resolution T2W MR image demonstrates a round mass at the left cerebellopontine angle, slightly flaring the internal auditory canal.

Case 2–26 Rathke's Cleft Cyst

Osamu Sakai, Rohini Nadgir

PRESENTATION

Visual field defect, pituitary dysfunction, or asymptomatic, depending on size.

FINDINGS

MRI demonstrates a T1 high-signal cystic mass in the sellar/suprasellar region.

DIFFERENTIAL

- Pituitary adenoma: This is the most common tumor in the sellar or suprasellar regions, and is occasionally cystic. However, calcification is rare.
- Craniopharyngioma: Craniopharyngioma is a tumor arising from the squamous epithelium in the remnant of the Rathke's pouch. Presence of cystic components and calcification is characteristic.
- Internal carotid artery (ICA) aneurysm: On MRI, ICA aneurysms can be heterogeneous in signal due to flow and partial thrombosis. Gradient echo images can show susceptibility artifact. Pulsation artifact can be also seen.

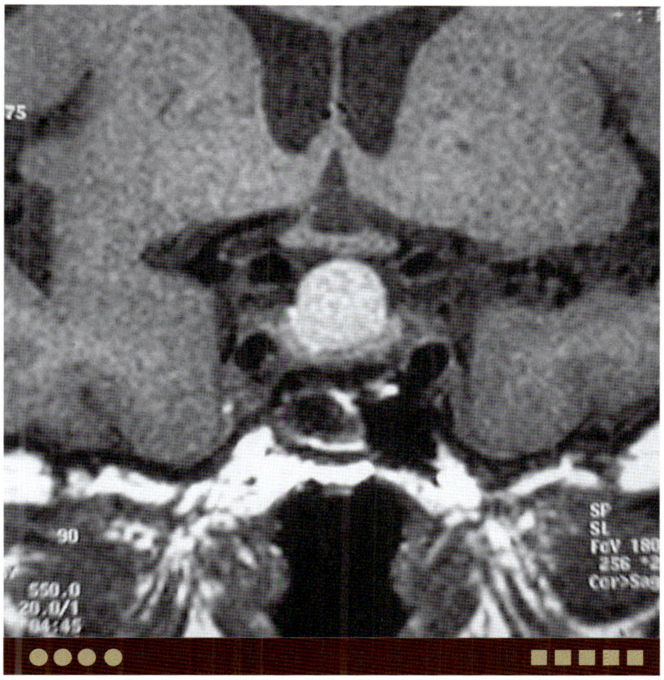

A. Rathke's cleft cyst. Coronal T1W image demonstrates a round high-signal lesion in the sellar/suprasellar region without pulsation artifact. Normal ICAs are seen bilaterally.

COMMENTS

This is a 70-year-old woman with headache and visual field defect.

Rathke's cleft cyst is a developmental anomaly arising from the Rathke's pouch, which is a normal component of development that eventually forms the anterior lobe, pars intermedia and pars tuberalis of the pituitary gland. The Rathke's pouch normally closes early in fetal development, however a remnant can persist as a cleft that lies within the pituitary gland.

Rathke's cleft cyst can be seen at any age. An intrasellar cyst is usually asymptomatic, while a larger cyst or suprasellar cyst may cause mass-effect on the pituitary gland and optic chiasm, and may result in pituitary dysfunction and visual field defect, respectively.

On CT, Rathke's cleft cyst is seen as a water density intrasellar/suprasellar cyst without calcification. On MRI, the cyst often shows high signal on T1W images secondary to proteinaceous contents. No solid component or enhancement should be seen.

PEARLS

- **Rathke's cleft cyst is a developmental anomaly arising from the Rathke's pouch, which is a normal structure that eventually forms the anterior lobe, pars intermedia and pars tuberalis of the pituitary gland.**
- **Rathke's cleft cyst is seen as a sellar/suprasellar cyst without calcification or enhancing solid component.**
- **Rathke's cleft cyst often shows high signal on T1W images secondary to proteinaceous contents.**

ADDITIONAL IMAGES (B-G)

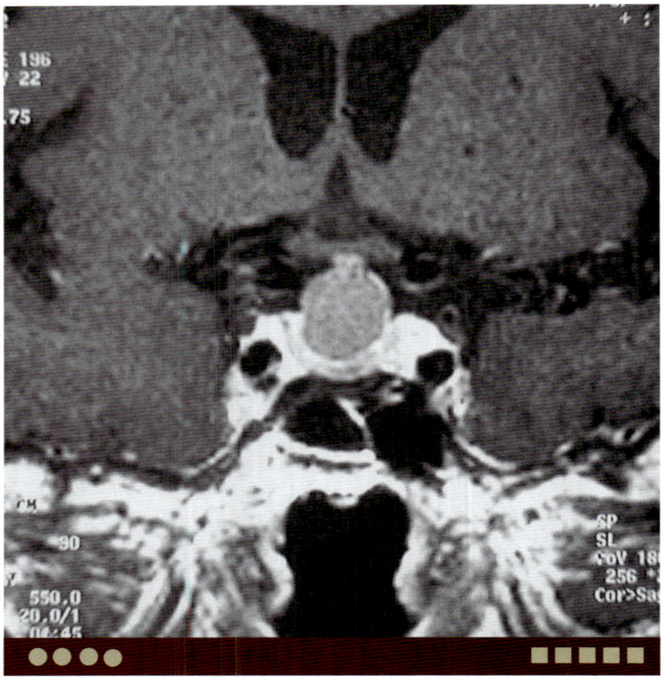

B. Rathke's cleft cyst, same patient as A. Coronal postcontrast T1W image demonstrates normal enhancement of the pituitary gland and cavernous sinuses. No enhancement is seen in the cyst.

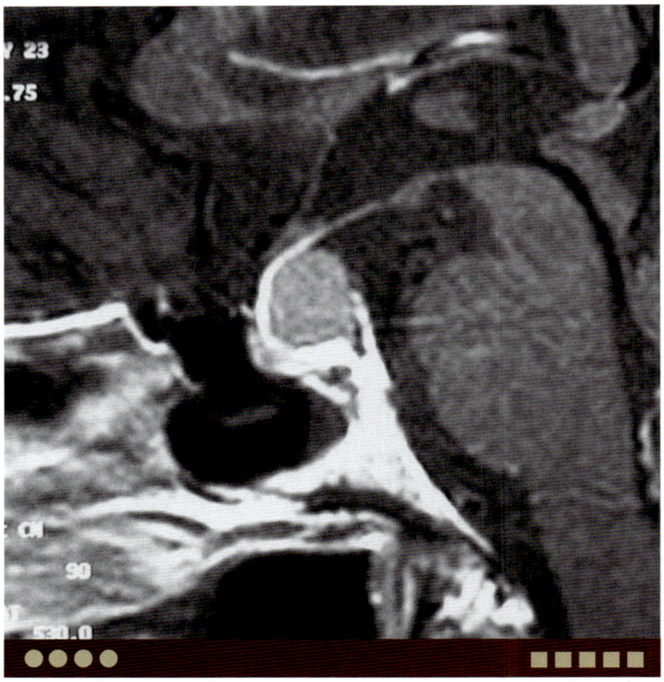

C. Rathke's cleft cyst, same patient as A. Sagittal postcontrast T1W image demonstrates the cyst stretching and displacing the pituitary stalk.

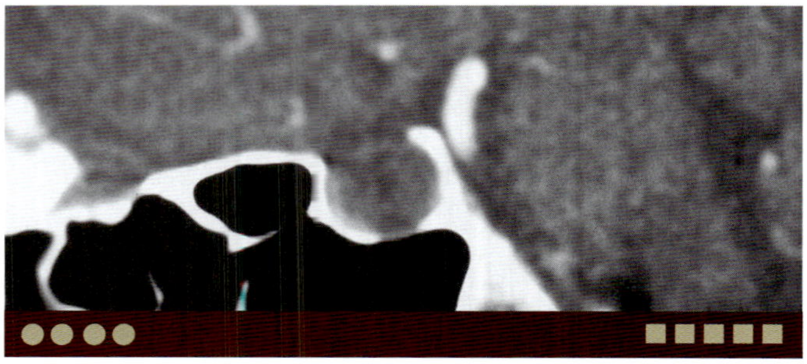

D. **Rathke's cleft cyst** in a different patient. Sagittal postcontrast CT demonstrates a slightly heterogeneous cystic lesion in the sella.

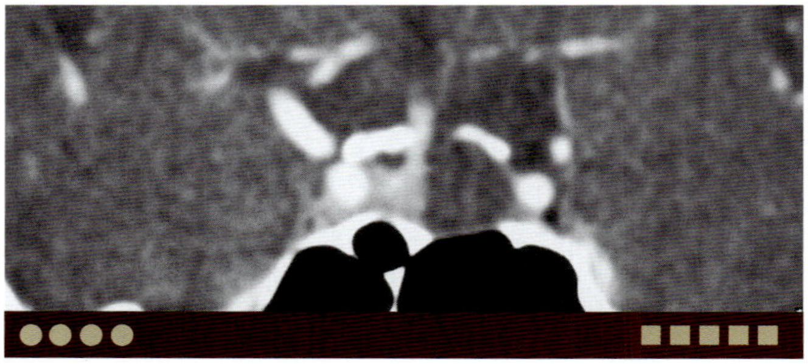

E. Rathke's cleft cyst, same patient as D. Coronal postcontrast CT demonstrates the cyst occupying the left half of the sella.

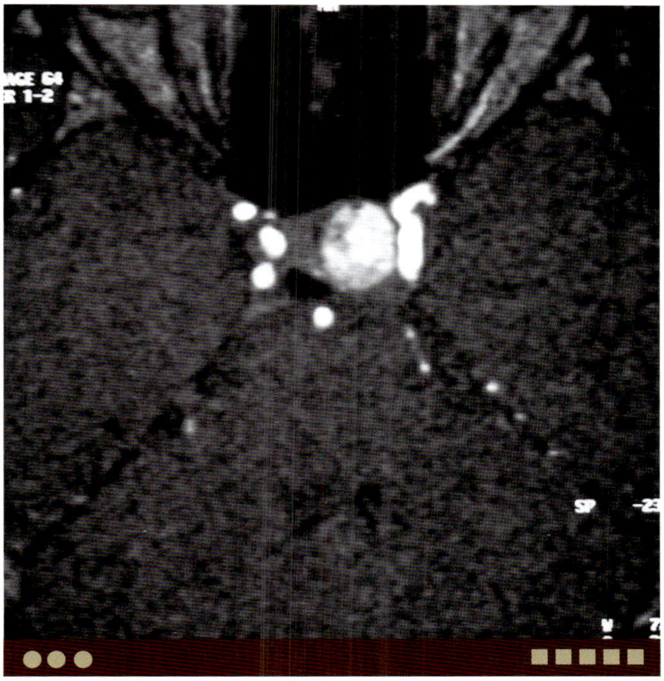

F. Rathke's cleft cyst, same patient as D. Axial time-of-flight MRA source image shows a round, high-signal lesion in the sella on the left.

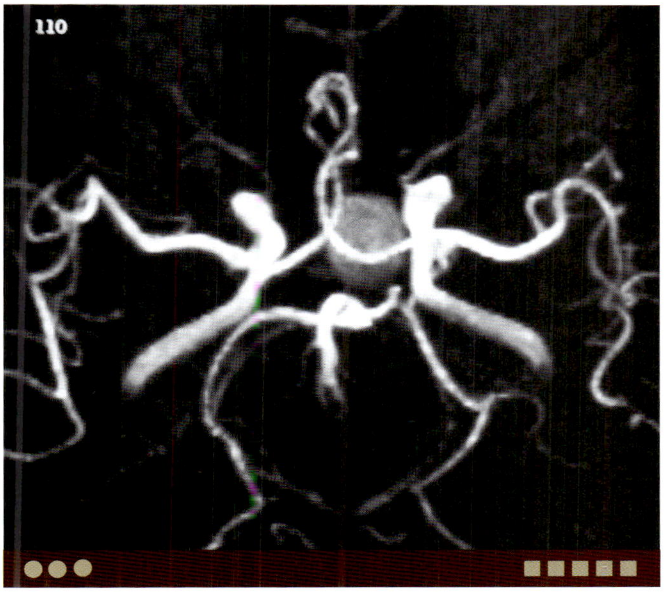

G. Rathke's cleft cyst, same patient as D. MIP image of MRA shows a round high-signal lesion mildly displacing the proximal portion of the left anterior cerebral artery.

DIFFERENTIAL DIAGNOSIS IMAGES (H-J)

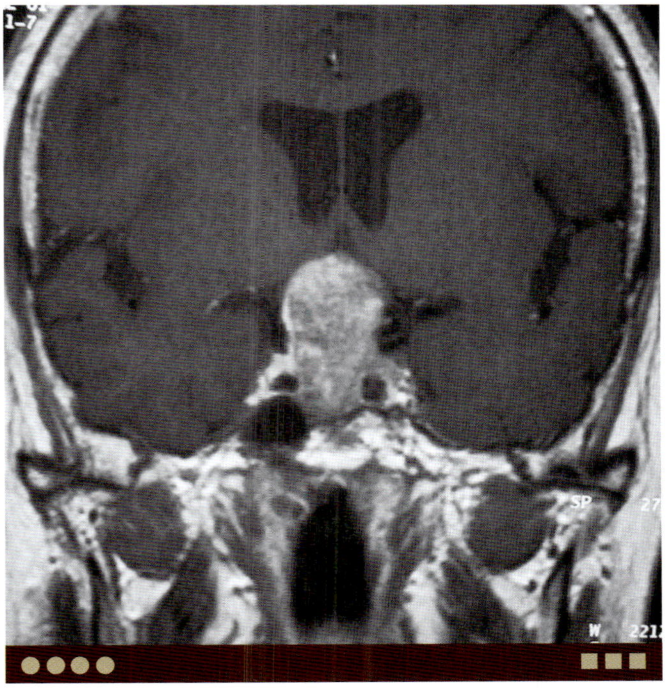

H. Pituitary adenoma. Coronal postcontrast T1W image demonstrates a large enhancing sellar/suprasellar lesion.

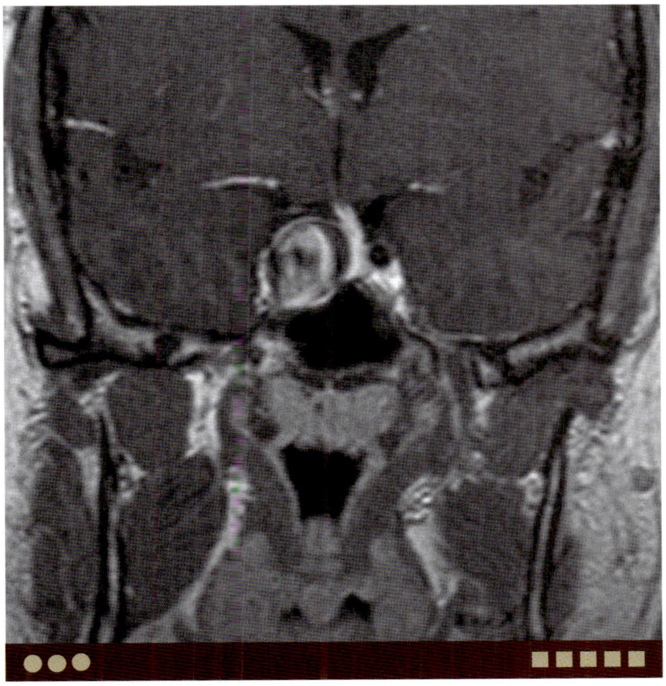

I. ICA aneurysm. Coronal postcontrast T1W image demonstrates a heterogeneously enhancing lesion in the right sellar/parasellar region. Note pulsation artifact.

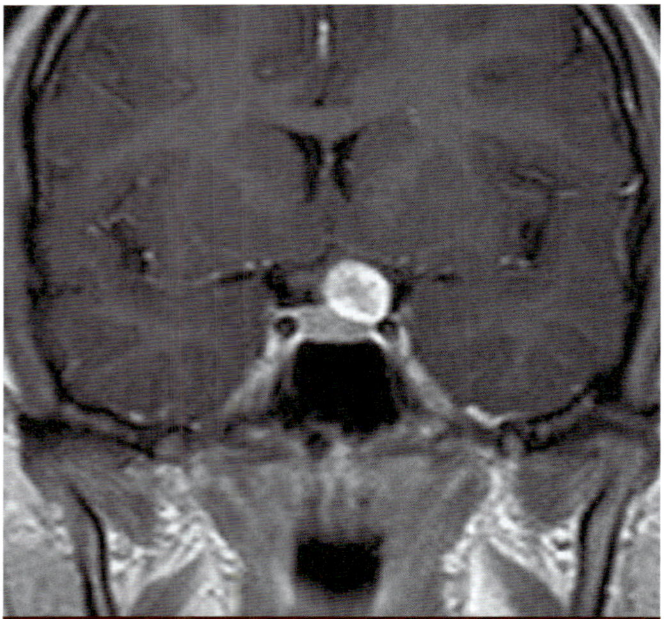

J. Dermoid. Coronal postcontrast T1W MR image demonstrates a slightly heterogeneous high-signal round lesion in the left suprasellar region without pulsation artifact.

Chapter 3

NASAL CAVITY AND PARANASAL SINUS

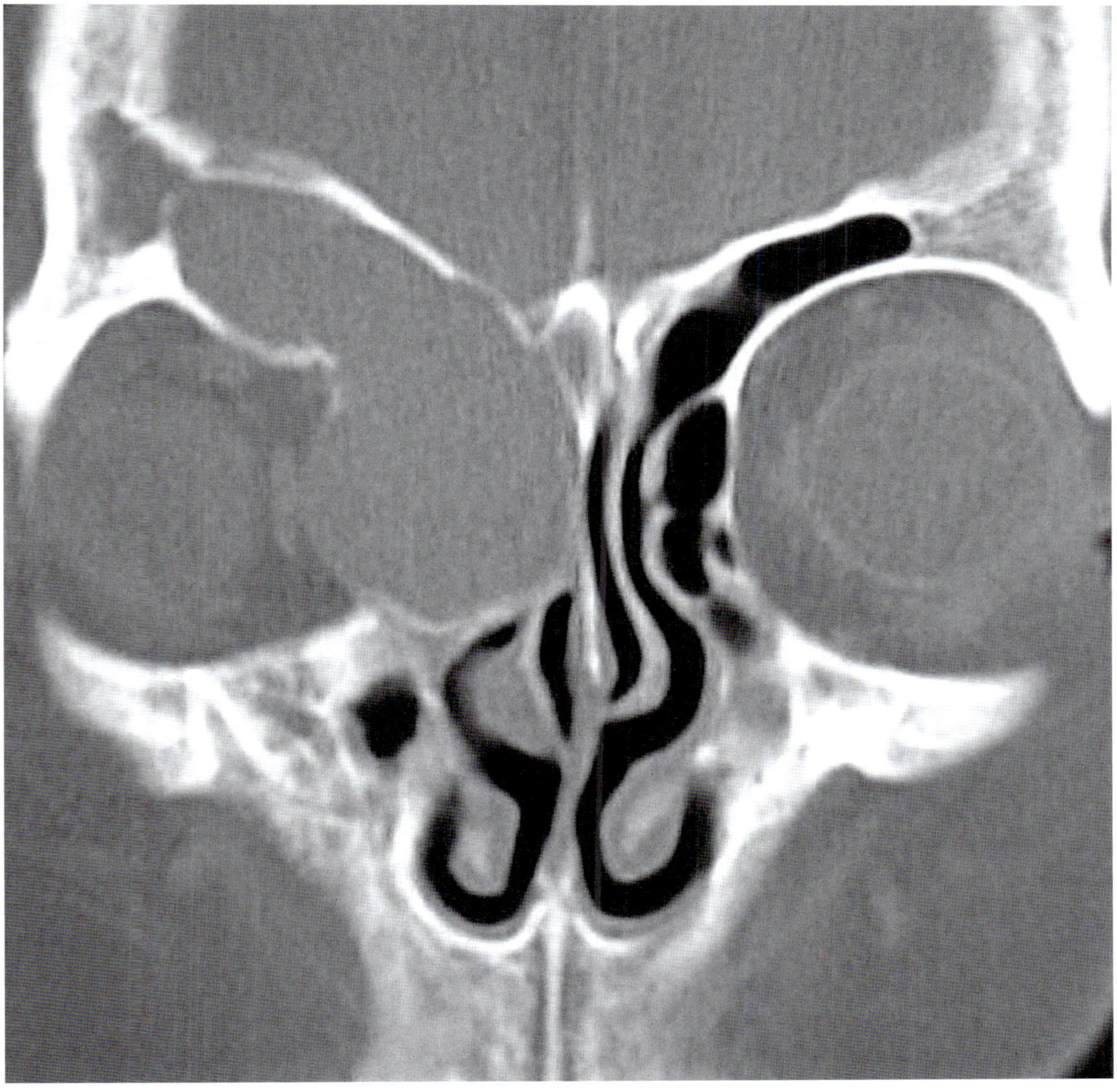

Case 3–1 Mucocele

Osamu Sakai, Susmitha Reddy

PRESENTATION

Unilateral proptosis.

FINDINGS

CT and MRI demonstrate an expansile cystic lesion in the paranasal sinuses.

DIFFERENTIAL DIAGNOSIS

- Retention cyst: This is secondary to mucous retention. It can be very proteinaceous and cause T1 and T2 shortening. If there is bone remodeling or erosion, it is called a mucocele.
- Fungus infection: This often demonstrates increased density on CT. Fungal sinus infection can be seen as allergic fungal sinusitis, mycetoma, or acute invasive sinusitis.
- Inverted papilloma: This can be seen anywhere in the sinonasal cavities but often arises from the lateral wall of the nasal cavity and extends into the maxillary sinus. Chronic expansion or remodeling of the ostiomeatal complex occurs. Increased density and calcification is often seen on CT.
- Hemorrhage: Hemorrhage causes high density on CT and variable T1 and T2 signal depending on the age of the blood products on MRI.
- Cephalocele: This is a failure of neural tube closure and herniation of the meninge and its contents (meningocele: meninges+CSF, meningoencephalocele: meninges+CSF+brain tissue).

COMMENTS

This is a 47-year-old woman with right exophthalmos due to fronto-ethmoidal mucocele.

Mucocele is a mucus collection obstructing a paranasal sinus or air cell resulting in bony remodeling or expansion. Without bony remodeling or expansion, the term obstructed sinus/air cell or retention cyst is used. Mucocele is often seen in the ethmoid and frontal sinuses. Although there is significant expansion and mass effect upon adjacent structures, the periosteum is usually preserved. Decompression and drainage is indicated when there is a significant mass-effect upon critical structures such as the orbit and brain parenchyma, or if the mucocele becomes infected or inflamed.

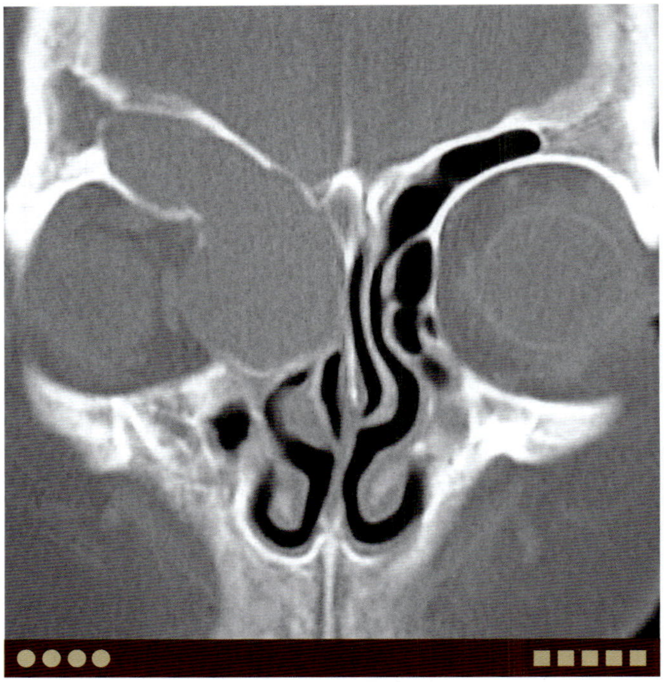

A. Mucocele. Coronal CT demonstrates a well-demarcated, expansile lesion centered at the right fronto-ethmoidal junction.

Mucocele initially shows density similar to water on CT. However, over time it may demonstrate increased density secondary to increased protein concentration. On MRI, mucocele can demonstrate variable signal depending on protein content. Increased signal on T1W and decreased signal on T2W images is commonly seen secondary to proteinaceous content. Very thick inspissated mucocele can demonstrate very low signal on both T1W and T2W images and may mimic air, such that the opacified sinus can be missed on MRI. T1 shortening effect from proteinaceous mucocele or retention cyst may demonstrate very high signal on time-of-flight MR angiography and mimic an aneurysm.

PEARLS

- **Mucocele occurs as a result of sinus or air cell obstruction with bone expansion or remodeling.**
- **It often occurs in the ethmoid and frontal sinuses.**
- **Variable densities and signals can be seen depending on protein concentration of the fluid. High density on CT and high signal on T1W MR images are seen with high protein content mucoceles.**

ADDITIONAL IMAGES (B-G)

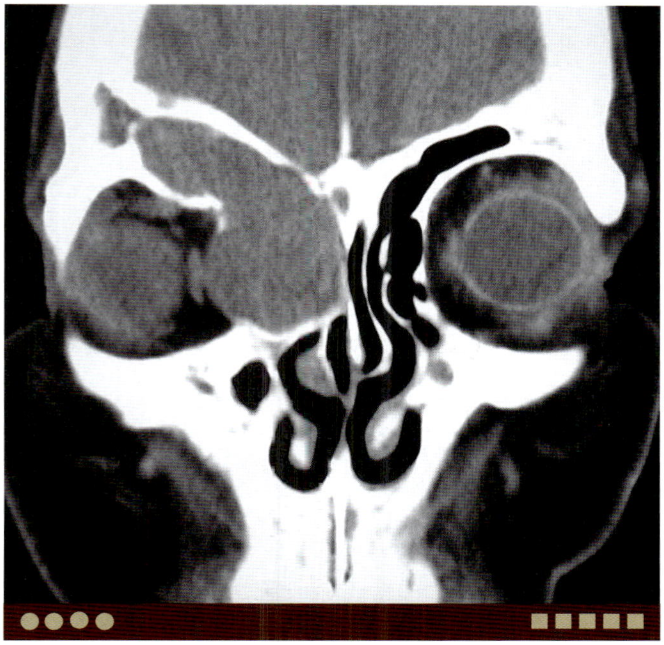

B. Mucocele, same patient as A. Coronal soft tissue windowed CT demonstrates homogeneous, increased density within the lesion compared with the left globe, suggesting increased protein concentration.

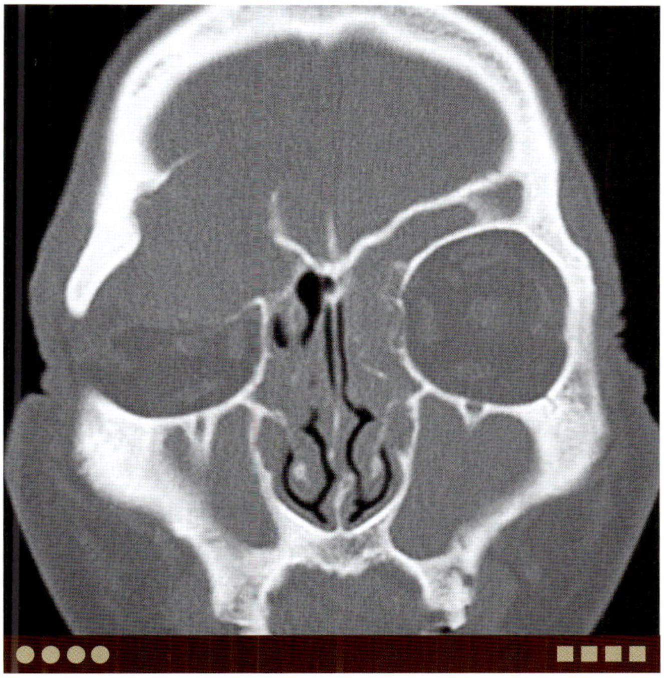

C. **Mucocele** in a different patient. Coronal CT demonstrates an expansile lesion in the right frontal sinus compressing the right orbital contents. Other visualized sinuses are nearly completely opacified. Note complete erosion of the superior and inferior walls of the right frontal sinus.

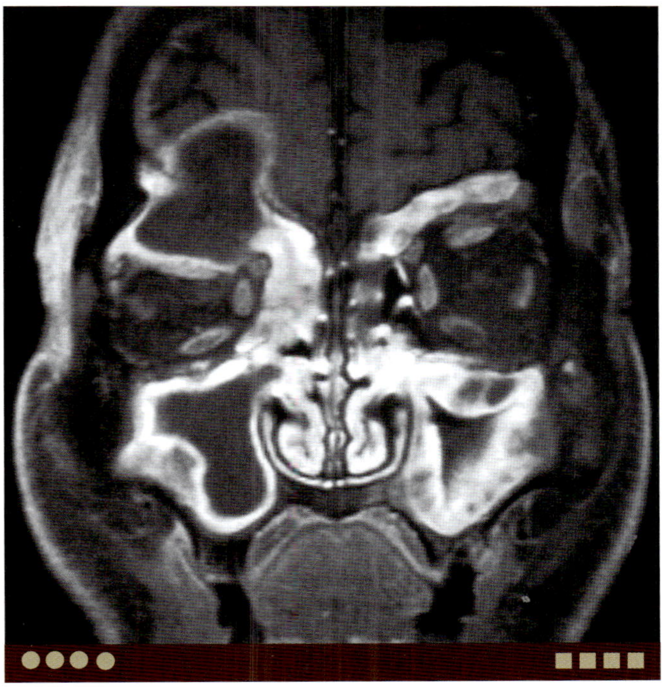

D. Mucocele, same patient as C. Coronal postcontrast fat-suppressed T1W image demonstrates enhancement of the wall of the mucocele as well as the rest of the paranasal sinuses secondary to inflammation.

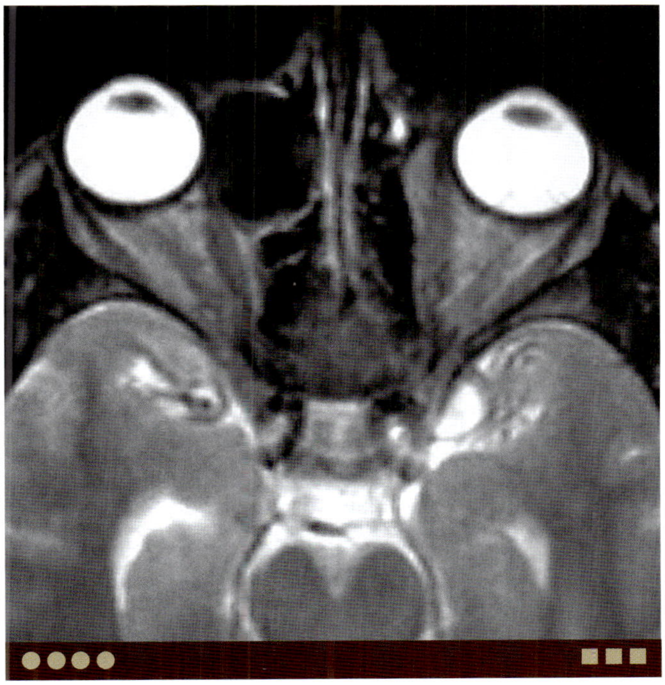

E. **Mucocele** in a different patient. Axial T2W image demonstrates a round expansile lesion with low signal similar to air in the right anterior ethmoid.

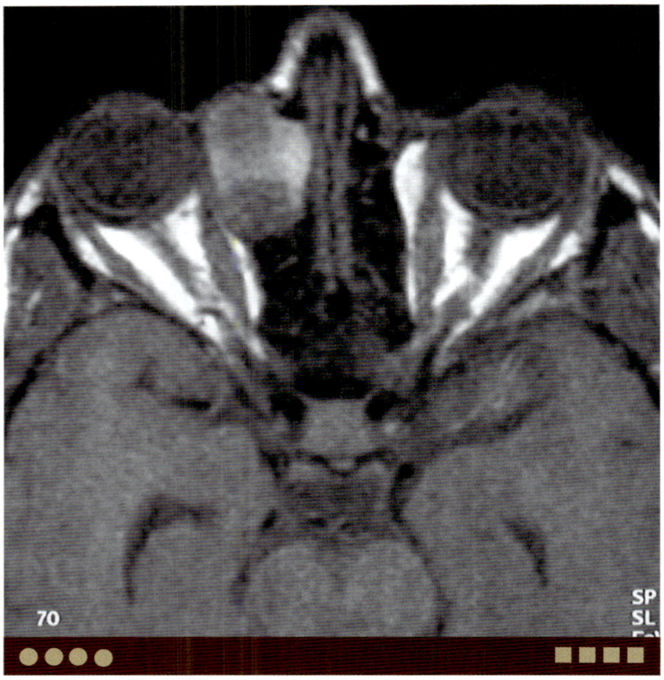

F. Ethmoid mucocele, same patient as E. Axial T1W image demonstrates some high signal in the lesion consistent with inspissated mucocele.

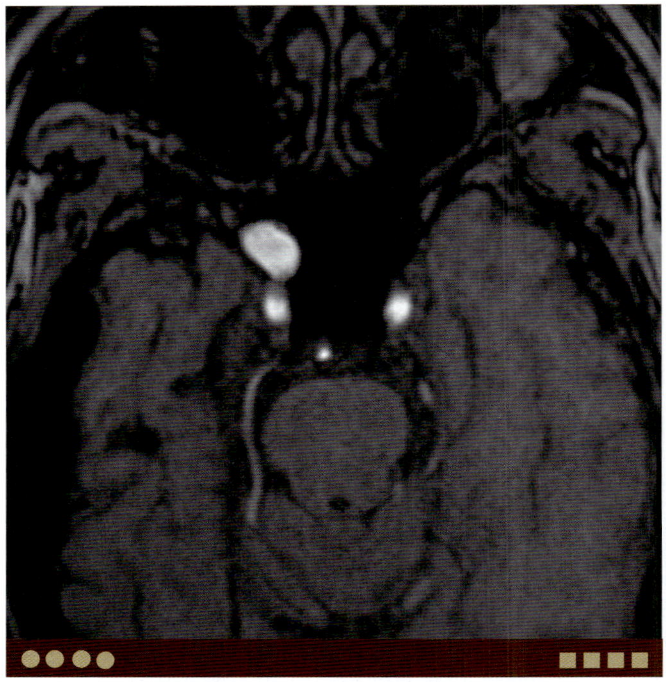

G. **Proteinaceous sphenoid retention cyst/mucocele**. Axial source image of 3D TOF MRA demonstrates a round high-signal lesion anterior to the right internal carotid artery (ICA), mimicking aneurysm.

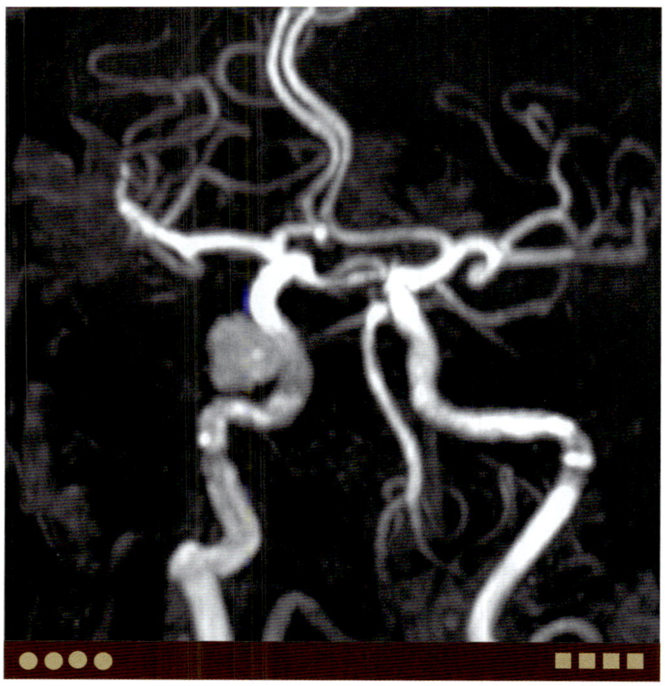

H. Proteinaceous sphenoid retention cyst/mucocele, same patient as G. Frontal projection of MIP reconstruction of 3D TOF MRA demonstrates a round lesion mimicking an aneurysm arising from the precavernous segment of the right ICA.

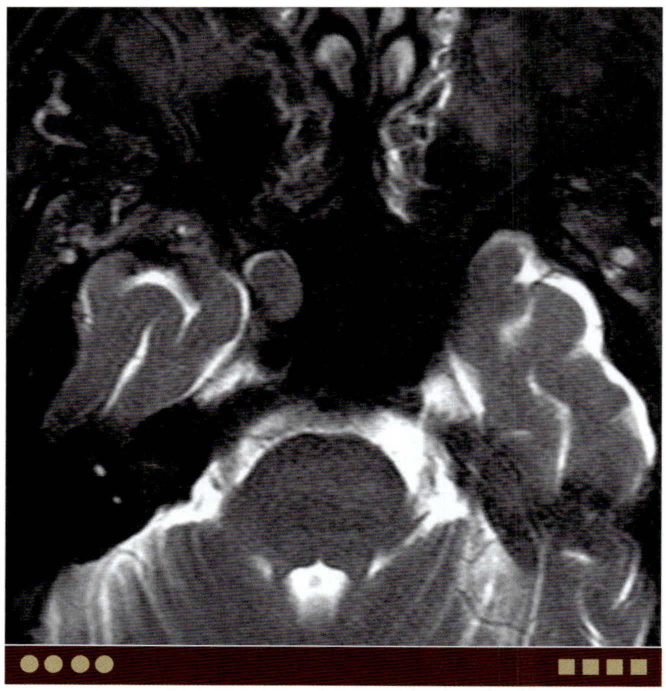

I. Proteinaceous sphenoid retention cyst/mucocele, same patient as G. Axial T2W MR image demonstrates an ovoid-shaped, intermediate-signal lesion consistent with a proteinaceous retention cyst/mucocele.

DIFFERENTIAL DIAGNOSIS IMAGE

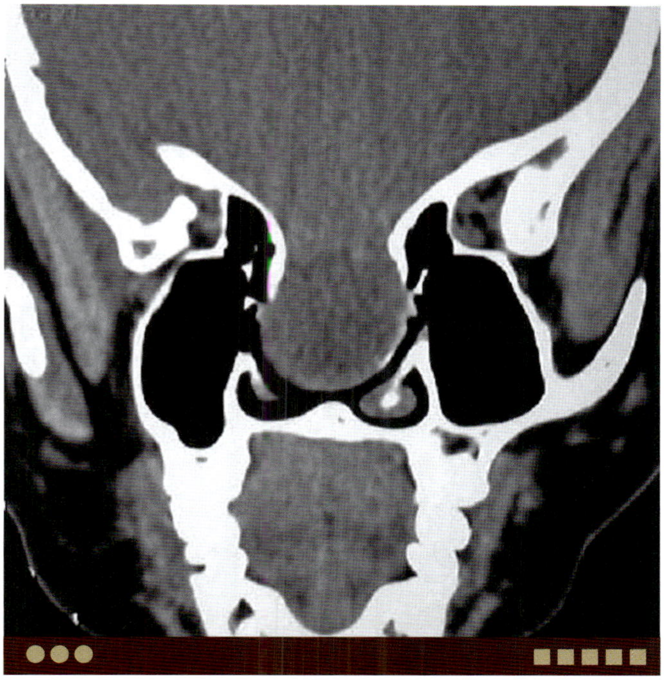

J. Cephalocele. Coronal CT demonstrates intracranial contents herniating through a large bony defect at the anterior skull base in the midline.

Case 3–2 Proteinaceous Mucus

Osamu Sakai, Susmitha Reddy

PRESENTATION

Chronic sinusitis.

FINDINGS

CT and T1W MR images demonstrate a lesion with high-density and high-signal intensity within the sinuses, respectively.

DIFFERENTIAL DIAGNOSIS

- Fungus infection: Allergic or invasive fungal infection demonstrates increased density and increased T1 signal due to T1 shortening effect by manganese produced by fungi as well as iron and calcium.
- Inverted papilloma This condition may demonstrate foci of calcification.
- Hemorrhage: Acute hemorrhage is seen as high density on CT. Density on CT and signal on MRI of the contents of the sinus depend on the age of the blood products.

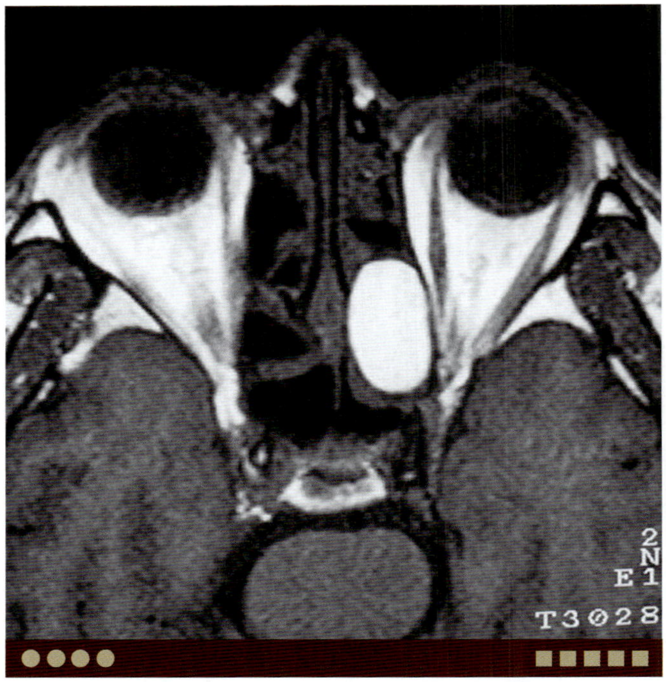

A. Proteinaceous mucocele. Axial T1W MR image demonstrates a slightly expansile ovoid lesion with homogeneous high signal in the left posterior ethmoid.

COMMENTS

This is a 61-year-old man with chronic sinusitis.

Retention cysts or mucoceles can be proteinaceous and demonstrate high density on CT or high signal on T1W MR images. Heterogeneous density on CT and variable signal on MRI images may be secondary to infection or hemorrhage. The difference between retention cyst and mucocele is whether bony remodeling is present or not. If there is bony remodeling or expansion, the lesion is called as mucocele.

Mucous retention initially demonstrates water density or signal; low on CT, low on T1W and high on T2W images. With increase in protein concentration, mucus shows increased density on CT, increased T1 and decreased T2 signal on MRI. Proteinaceous mucus may show very high signal on T1W images mimicking fat. Very thick, old inspissated proteinaceous mucus can demonstrate very low signal on both T1 and T2W images. This may mimic air and potentially an opacified sinus can be missed on MRI.

Inspissated proteinaceous secretion is the most common cause of "high density sinus," however, the differential diagnosis includes fungal infection (which can be allergic or invasive), hemorrhage, calcification or ossification, and inverted papilloma. Attention must be paid not to miss bony destruction to indicate a more aggressive process.

PEARLS

- **Mucus can demonstrate variable density on CT and signal on MRI depending on protein concentration.**
- **Proteinaceous mucus is the most common cause of high density or T1 high signal in the paranasal sinuses.**
- **Very thick, inspissated secretion may demonstrate dark signal on both T1 and T2W images, just like air, and complete opacification of the sinus can be missed on MRI.**

ADDITIONAL IMAGES (B-G)

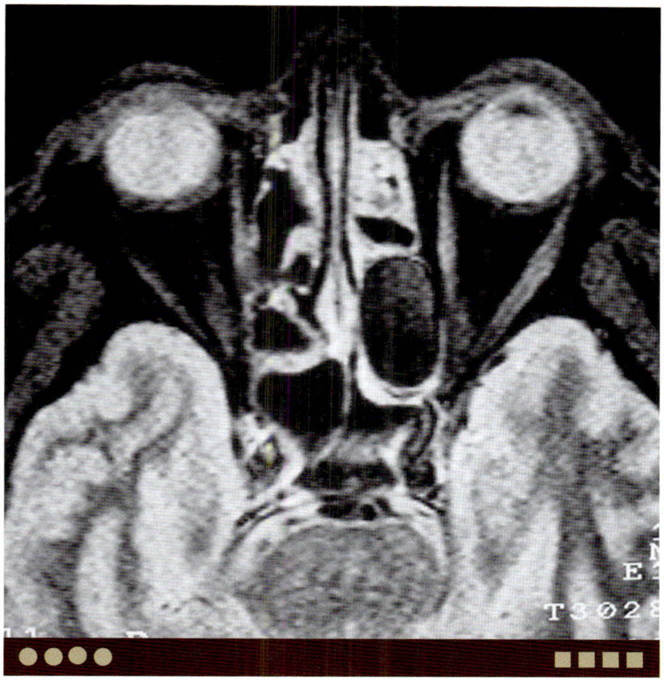

B. Proteinaceous mucocele, same patient as A. Axial STIR MR image shows signal drop with in the lesion, mimicking fat.

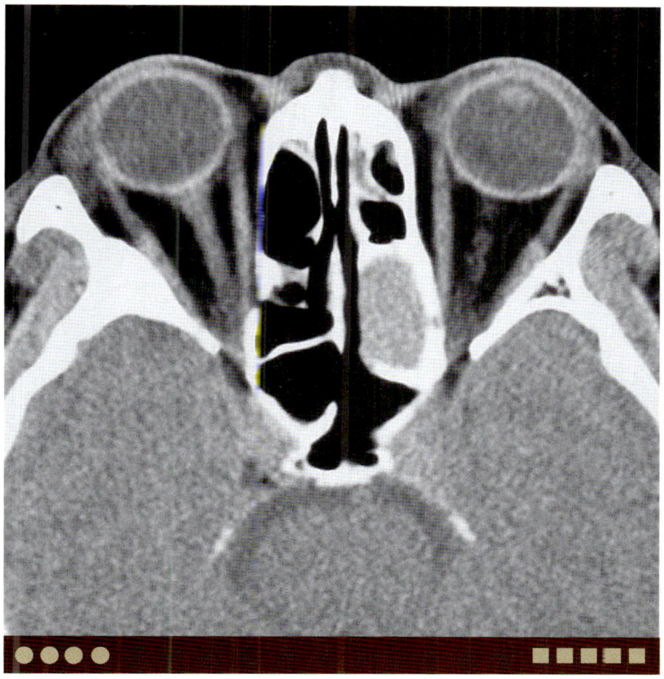

C. Proteinaceous mucocele, same patient as A. Axial noncontrast CT shows an ovoid high-density lesion consistent with thick, proteinaceous mucus retention.

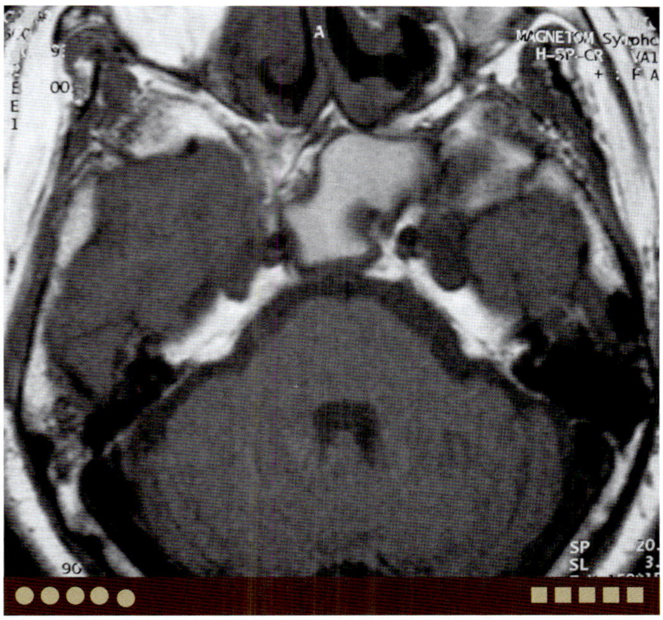

D. **Obstructed sphenoid sinus with proteinaceous mucus**. Axial T1W MR image demonstrates homogeneous high signal in the sphenoid sinus reflecting proteinaceous material with peripheral low signal representing thickened mucosa.

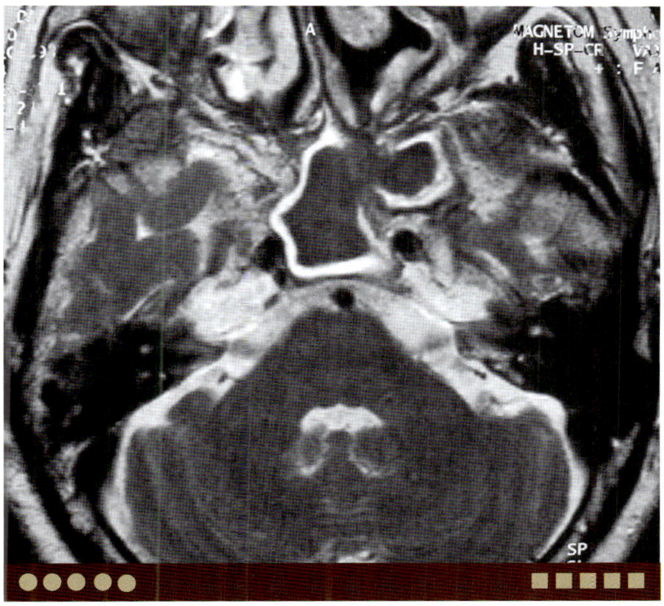

E. Obstructed sphenoid sinus with proteinaceous mucus, same patient as D. Axial T2W MR image demonstrates homogeneous low signal in the sphenoid sinus reflecting proteinaceous content with peripheral high signal from thickened inflamed mucosa.

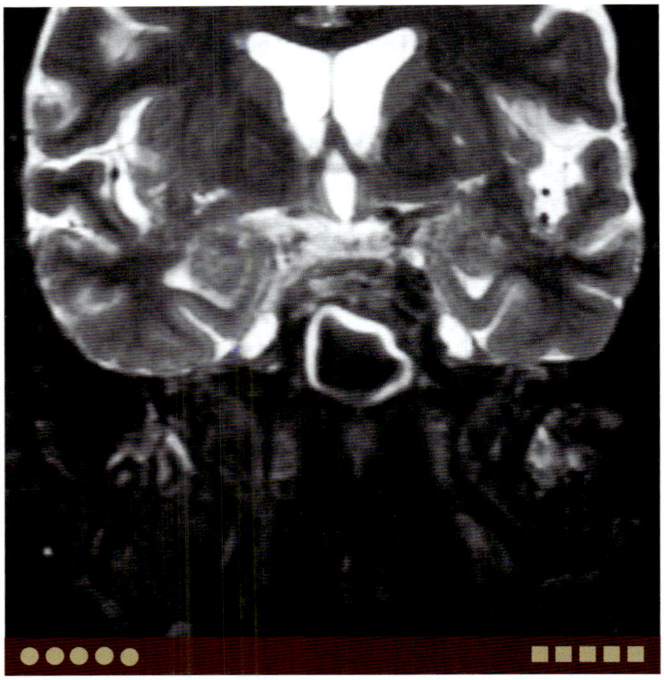

F. Obstructed sphenoid sinus with proteinaceous mucus, same patient as D. Coronal STIR MR image demonstrates complete signal loss within the sphenoid sinus except for the high signal within the thickened mucosa.

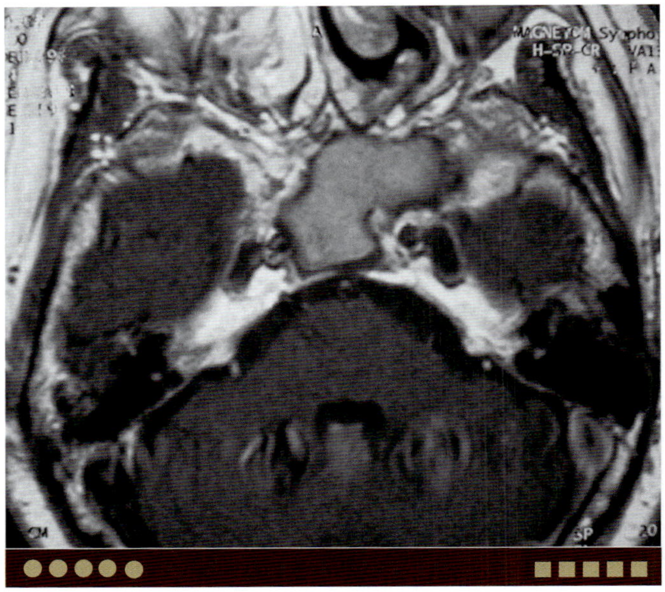

G. Obstructed sphenoid sinus with proteinaceous mucus, same patient as D. Axial postcontrast T1W MR image demonstrates no apparent abnormal enhancement.

DIFFERENTIAL DIAGNOSIS IMAGES (H-J)

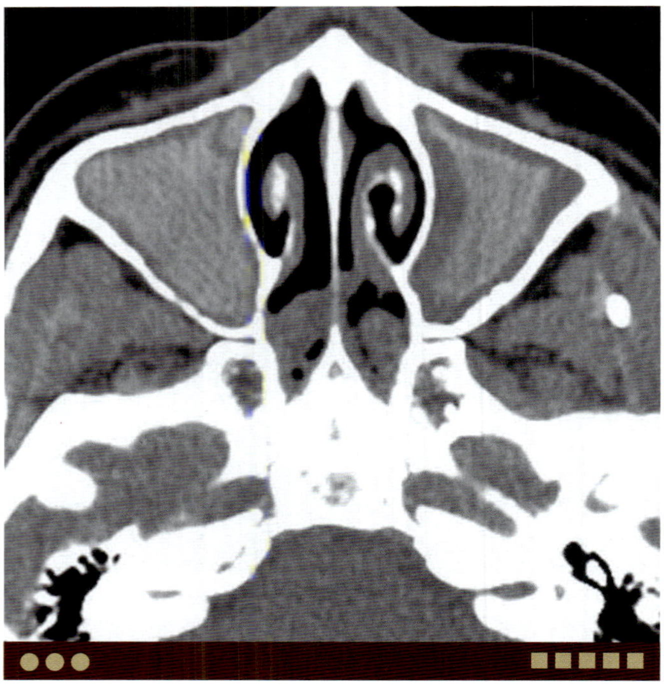

H. Allergic aspergillosis. Axial CT demonstrates complete opacification of bilateral maxillary sinuses with high-density material.

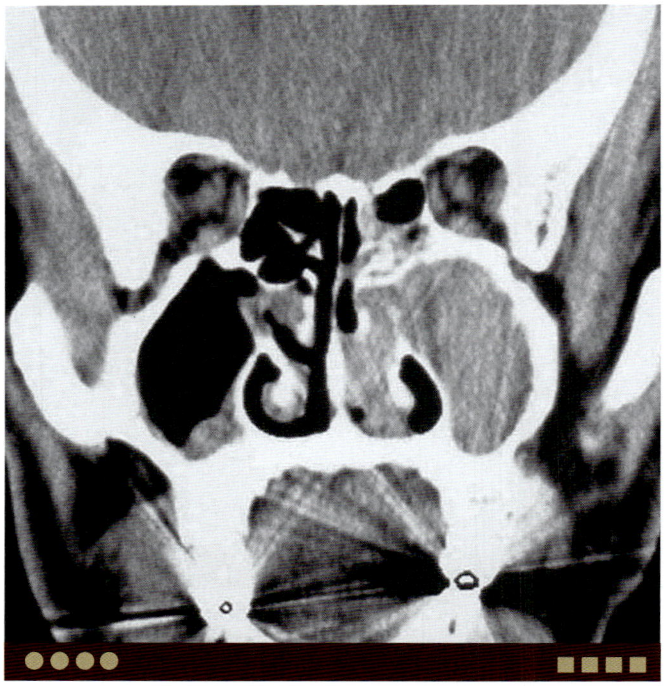

I. Inverted papilloma. Coronal CT demonstrates complete opacification of left maxillary sinus with high-density contents.

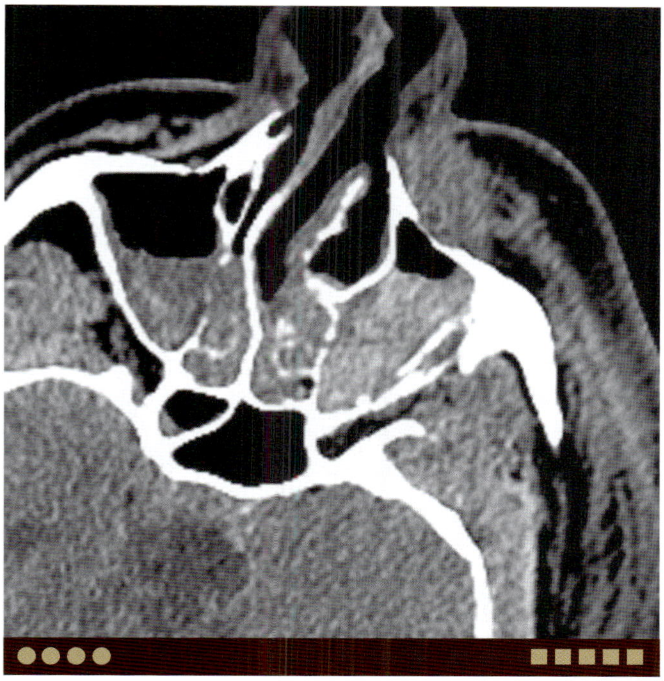

J. Maxillary sinus fracture with hemorrhage. Axial soft tissue window CT shows high-density material forming air-fluid level in the left maxillary sinus. Note fracture of the posterolateral wall.

Case 3–3 Postoperative or Posttraumatic Mucocele

Osamu Sakai, Susmitha Reddy

PRESENTATION

Cheek swelling, history of sinus surgery 20 years ago.

FINDINGS

CT demonstrates expansile cystic lesions in the maxillary sinuses causing exophthalmos.

DIFFERENTIAL DIAGNOSIS

- Nontraumatic mucocele: This is a mucocele without the history of surgery or trauma. Mucocele occurs secondary to obstruction of the air cell or sinus with expansion and bone remodeling/erosion.
- Retention cyst: This is mucous retention without bone remodeling or erosion.

COMMENTS

This is a 57-year-old man with history of sinus surgery 20 years ago, now presenting with right cheek swelling and right exophthalmos.

Postoperative mucocele is a mucocele formation after Caldwell-Luc surgery, usually more than 10 years after surgery. This is also called as postoperative maxillary cyst (POMC). Similar findings can be seen after maxillofacial fractures without the history of Caldwell-Luc surgery (posttraumatic mucocele). Recently, most sinus surgeries are endoscopically performed [functional endoscopic sinus surgery (FESS)] and Caldwell-Luc surgery is not the first line procedure for chronic sinusitis. However, postoperative mucocele is still encountered on rare occasions as it takes several years to become symptomatic. Usually, even with significant mass-effect such as exophthalmos, the periosteum is preserved.

Posttraumatic mucoceles can have multiple compartments. Preoperative CT has an important role in diagnosing exact location of the lesion and multiplicity of compartments to plan the endoscopic surgical repair.

Coronal bone window CT is the most important to assess the extent of the lesion, however soft tissue window images must be evaluated because occasionally expanded marrow space can be mistaken for fluid filled cyst on bone window images. MRI is usually not necessary for diagnosis, however, it can provide detailed information regarding its content, such as protein concentration, hemorrhage, and is helpful to rule out tumors.

Precise history taking is important to make the diagnosis; rarely tumors can show similar findings to postoperative mucocele.

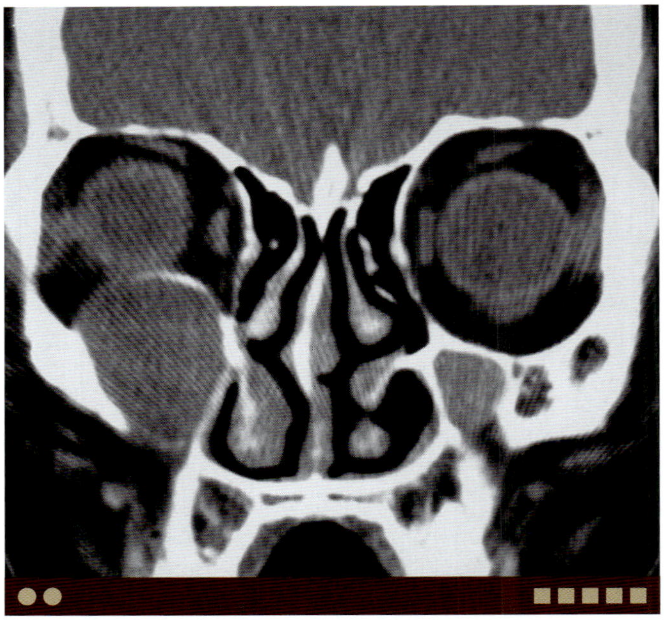

A. Postoperative mucocele. Coronal noncontrast CT demonstrates an expansile cystic lesion in the right maxillary sinus protruding into the right orbit. A small cystic lesion is also seen on the left.

PEARLS

- **Postoperative mucocele develops many years after sinus surgery, typically in the maxillary sinus in a patient with prior Caldwell-Luc surgery.**
- **Postoperative mucocele can have multiple compartments and evaluation with bone and soft tissue window images is crucial to plan the surgical procedure.**
- **MRI is not necessary to make a diagnosis, however it can provide detailed information regarding cyst contents and exclude neoplasm.**

ADDITIONAL IMAGES (B-G)

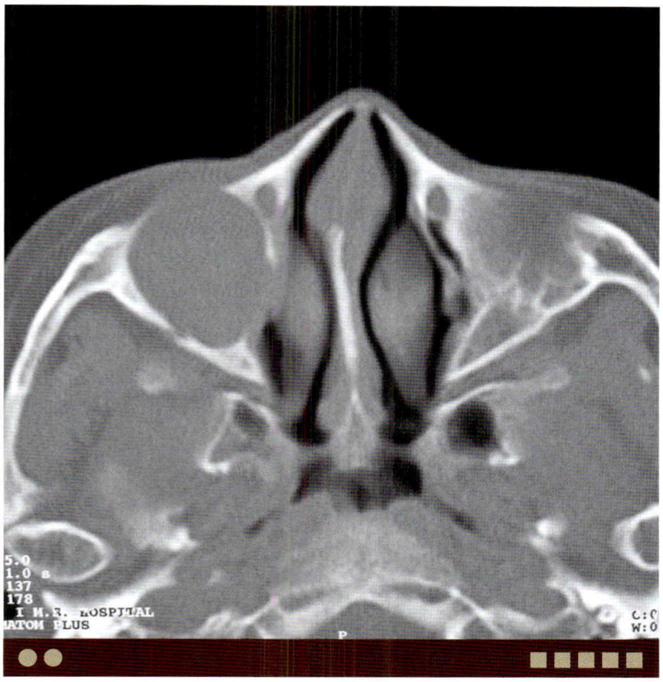

B. Postoperative mucocele, same patient as A. Axial bone window CT demonstrates bone remodeling/erosion in the obliterated right maxillary sinus.

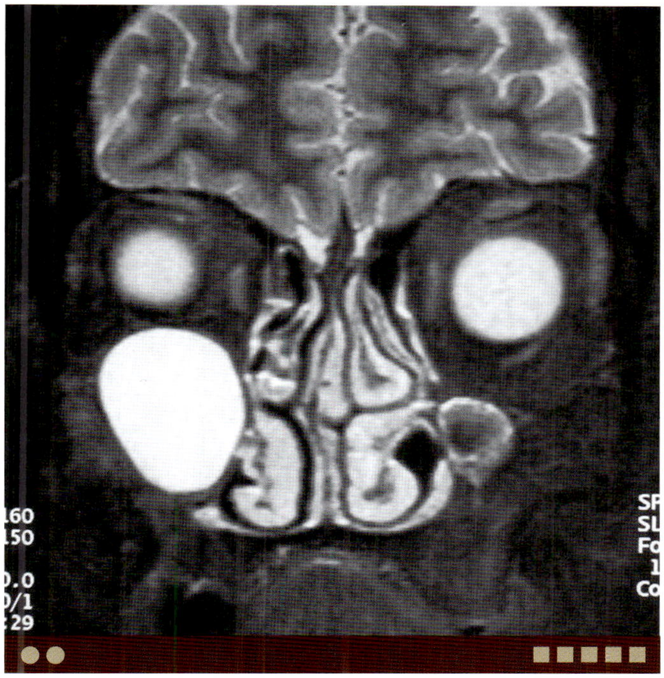

C. Postoperative mucocele, same patient as A. Coronal STIR MR image demonstrates homogeneous high signal from the cystic lesion in the right maxillary sinus. Note the left maxillary sinus lesion demonstrating low signal due to proteinaceous collection.

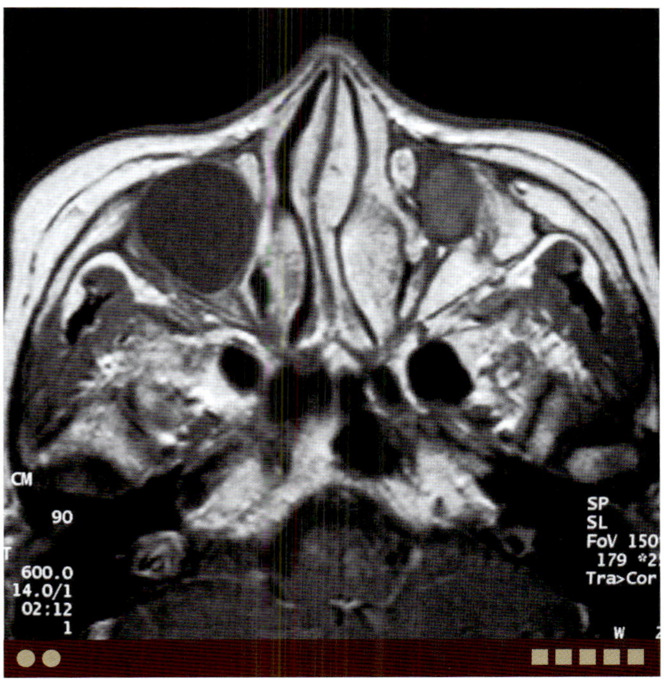

D. Postoperative mucocele, same patient as A. Axial postcontrast T1W MR image demonstrates cystic lesions in the maxillary sinuses, right larger than left. Note increased signal in the left maxillary cyst due to proteinaceous content.

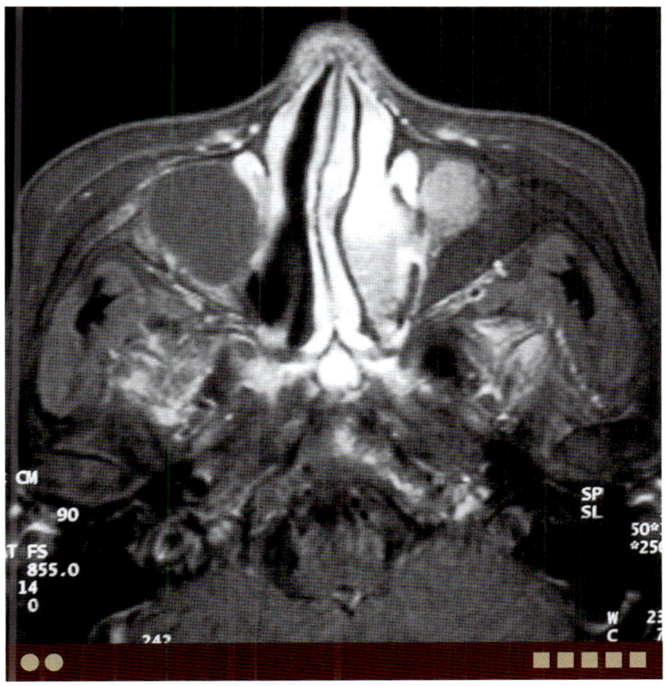

E. Postoperative mucocele, same patient as A. Axial postcontrast fat-suppressed T1W MR image demonstrates no enhancement in the cystic lesions in the maxillary sinuses. Increased signal is again seen in the left maxillary cyst due to proteinaceous content.

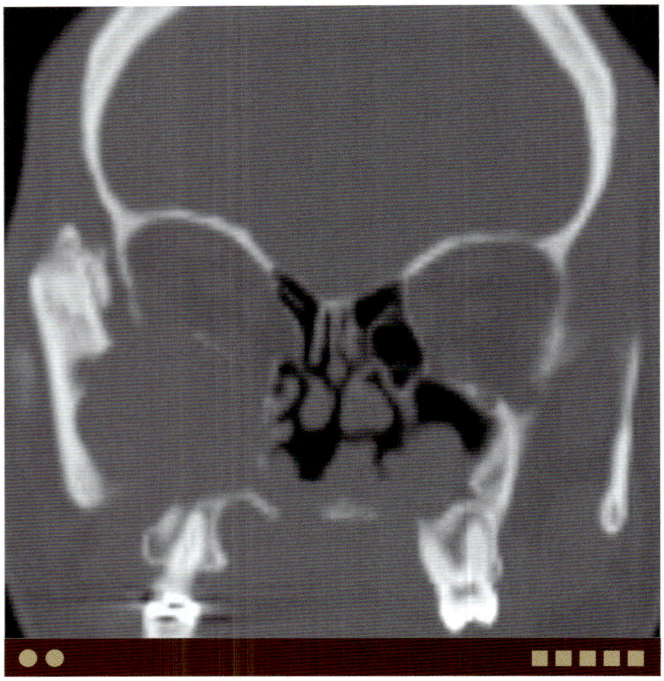

F. **Posttraumatic mucocele**. Coronal noncontrast CT demonstrates an expansile cystic lesion eroding walls of the right maxillary sinus.

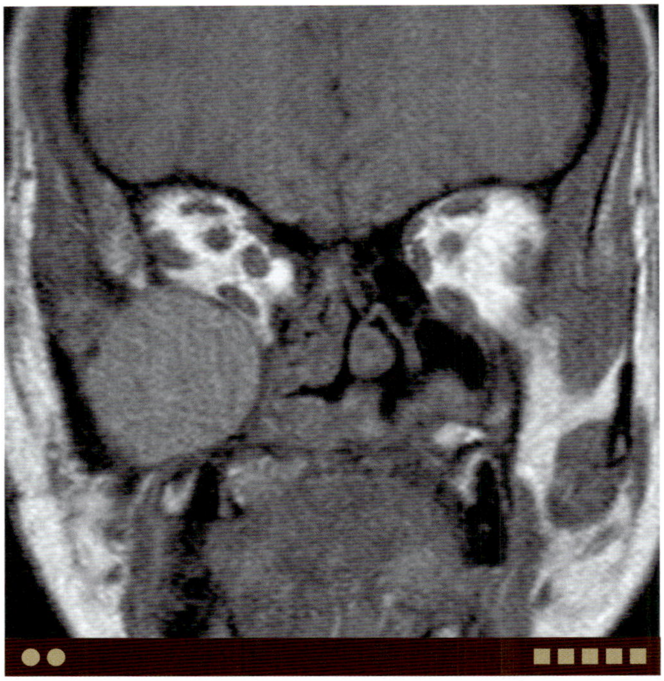

G. Posttraumatic mucocele, same patient as F. Coronal T1W MR demonstrates the expansile cystic lesion with homogeneous mildly increased signal in the right maxillary sinus.

DIFFERENTIAL DIAGNOSIS IMAGES (H-I)

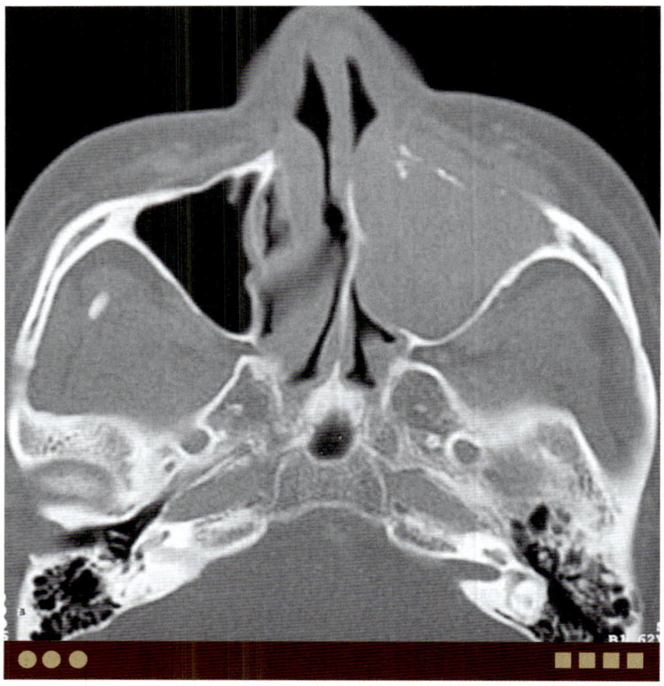

H. **Squamous cell carcinoma**. Axial bone window CT demonstrates total opacification of the left maxillary sinus with bowing of the medial wall. Note erosion/destruction of the anterior wall.

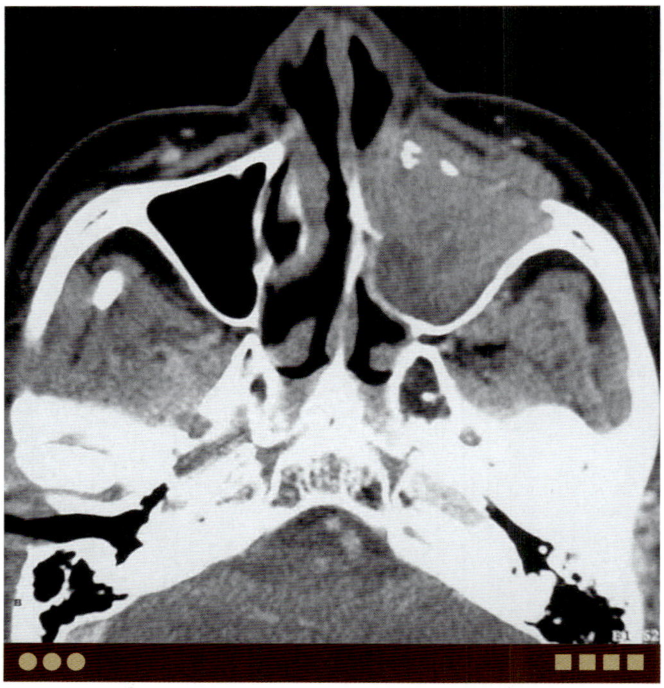

I. Squamous cell carcinoma, same patient as H. Axial soft tissue window contrast-enhanced CT demonstrates a heterogeneously enhancing tumor destroying the anterior wall of the maxillary sinus and extending to the overlying soft tissues.

Case 3–4 Sinonasal Melanoma

Osamu Sakai, Susmitha Reddy

PRESENTATION

Nasal mass.

FINDINGS

CT and MRI demonstrate an avidly enhancing, relatively low T2 signal lesion in the nasal cavity.

DIFFERENTIAL DIAGNOSIS

- Polyp: This usually demonstrates high signal on T2W images, although fibrotic lesions demonstrate decreased T2 signal.
- Squamous cell carcinoma (SCCA): SCCA is the most common malignant tumor in the sinonasal cavity and often demonstrates nonspecific heterogeneous density/signal with bone destruction.
- Lymphoma: Demonstrates relatively homogeneous intermediate T2 signal.
- Plasmacytoma: Demonstrates similar findings to lymphoma. Expansion of the marrow space is commonly seen.

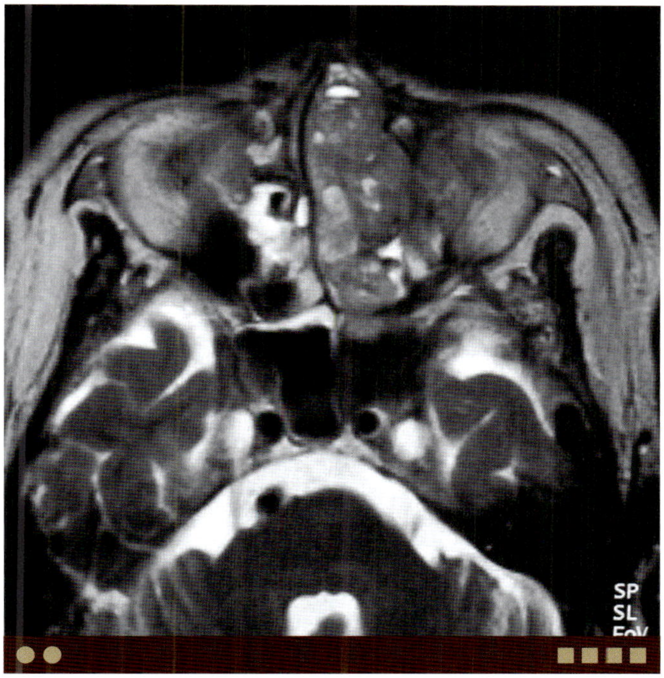

A. Melanoma. Axial T2W image demonstrates an intermediate-to-low signal lesion in the left nasal cavity and ethmoid.

COMMENTS

This is a 76-year-old woman with a dark nasal mass.

Sinonasal melanoma is a relatively rare tumor, comprising 3.6% of all sinonasal tumors and 2.5% of melanoma lesions throughout the body. It typically occurs in patients in their sixth to eighth decades, presenting with nasal obstruction and epistaxis. When it occurs in the nasal cavity, the nasal septum is commonly involved. Ten to thirty percent of sinonasal melanomas are amelanotic melanomas, and about 40% of patients have nodal metastases at the time of diagnosis. Over 60% patients have local recurrent disease or distant metastases within a year of diagnosis.

CT findings are often nonspecific; however bony remodeling is commonly seen. Tumors with high cellularity and melanin concentration show increased density. Avid enhancement is common on postcontrast images. Melanin has paramagnetic properties that can cause T1 and T2 shortening, therefore a characteristic intensity pattern of high signal on T1W and low signal on T2W images can be seen. However, amelanotic melanoma does not follow this signal pattern. Most melanomas demonstrate homogeneous intermediate signal on both T1W and T2W images and avid enhancement after intravenous contrast administration.

PEARLS

- **Melanoma classically demonstrates high signal on T1W and low signal on T2W images due to paramagnetic effect of melanin; however this is not always seen.**
- **Most melanomas demonstrate homogeneous intermediate signal on both T1W and T2W images and avid enhancement.**
- **CT findings are often nonspecific; however, bony remodeling is commonly seen. Tumors with high cellularity and melanin concentration show increased density.**

ADDITIONAL IMAGES (B-G)

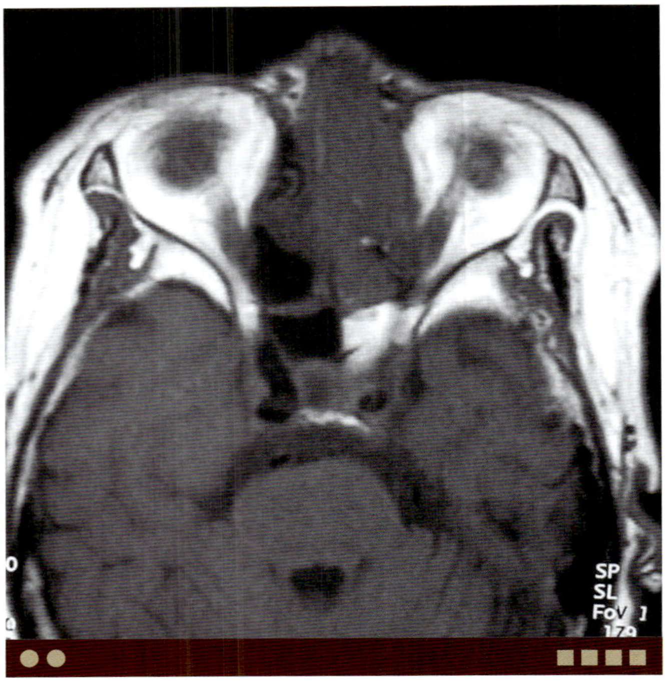

B. Melanoma, same patient as A. Axial T1W image demonstrates a low-signal lesion in the left nasal cavity and ethmoid.

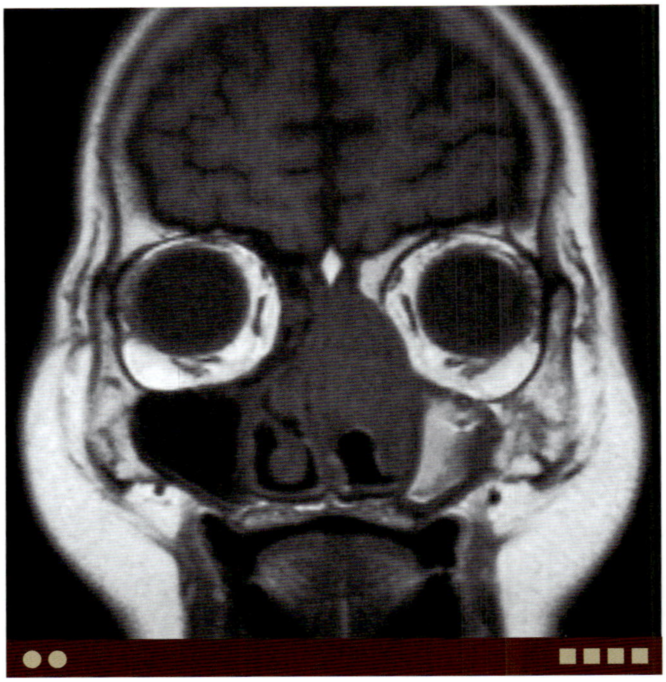

C. Melanoma, same patient as A. Coronal T1W image demonstrates an expansile lesion bowing the medial wall of the left orbit. Note proteinaceous mucus demonstrating high signal in the left maxillary sinus.

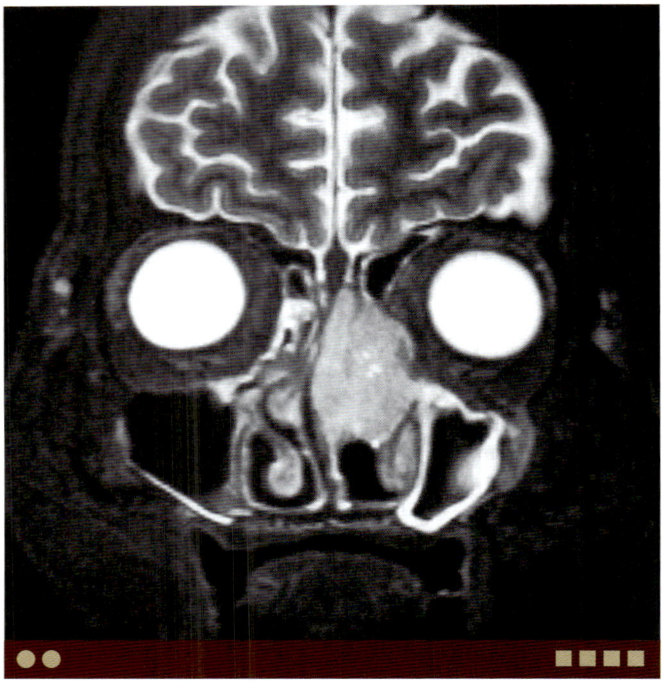

D. Melanoma, same patient as A. Coronal STIR image demonstrates slightly heterogeneous high signal in the lesion. Note the proteinaceous mucus in the left maxillary sinus is demonstrates low signal.

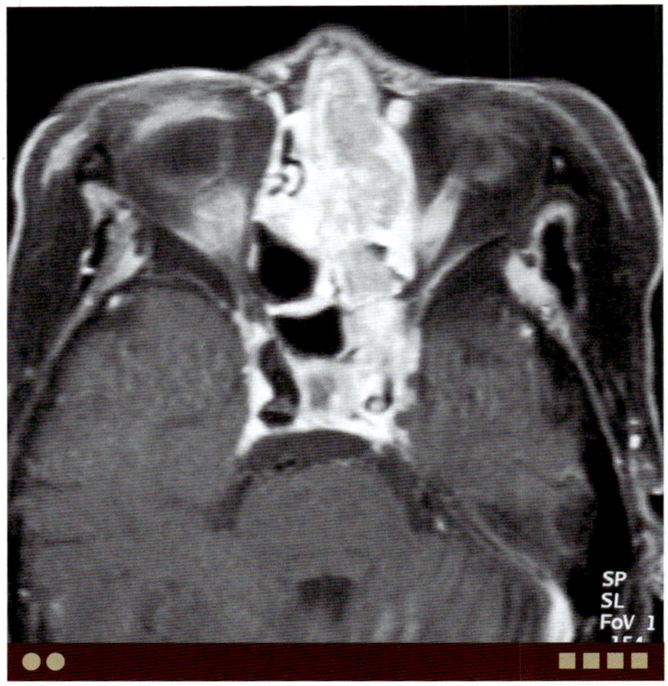

E. Melanoma, same patient as A. Axial postcontrast fat-suppressed T1W image demonstrates slightly heterogeneous enhancement of the tumor.

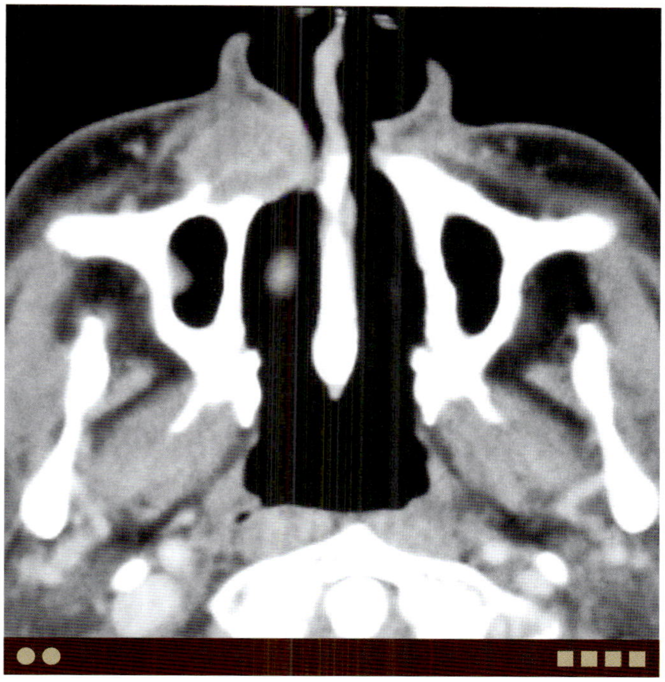

F. Melanoma, in a different patient. Axial postcontrast CT demonstrates an enhancing tumor involving the right nasal ala and the anterior wall of the right maxillary sinus.

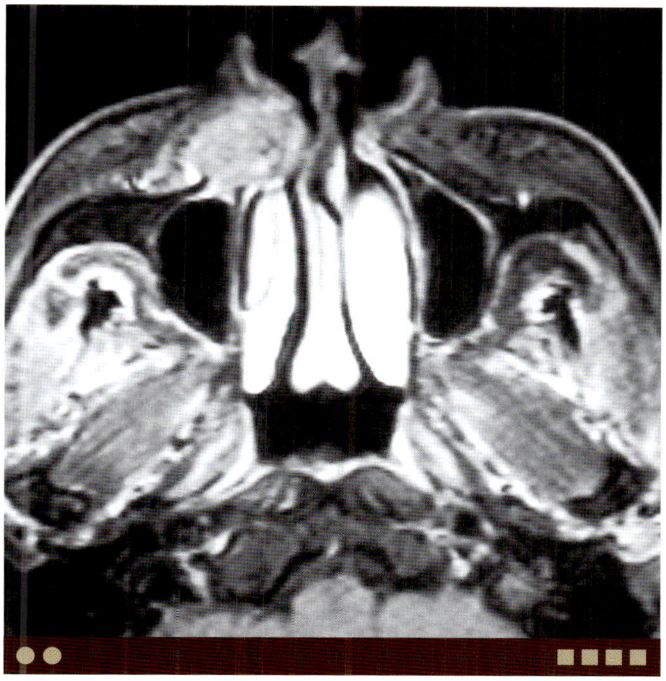

G. Melanoma, same patient as F. Axial postcontrast fat-suppressed T1W image demonstrates slightly heterogeneous enhancement of the tumor.

DIFFERENTIAL DIAGNOSIS IMAGES (H-I)

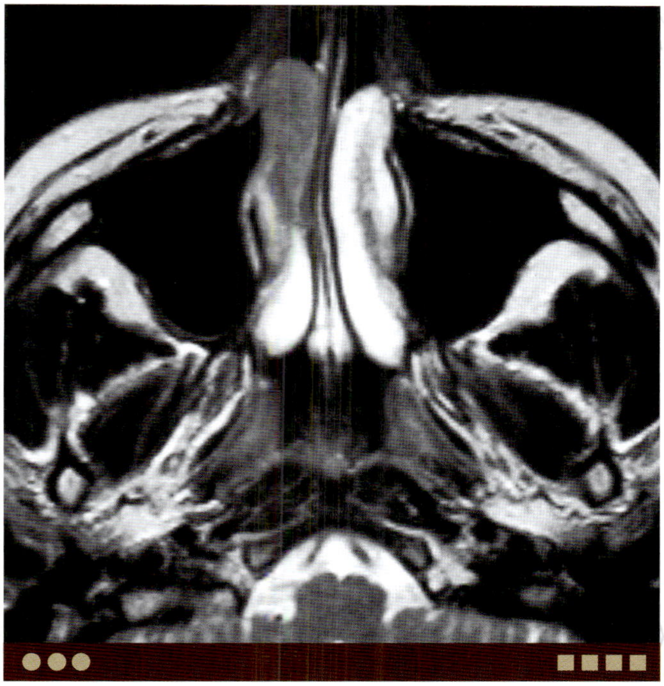

H. Lymphoma. Axial T2W image demonstrates an intermediate-to-low signal lesion in the anterior portion of the right middle turbinate.

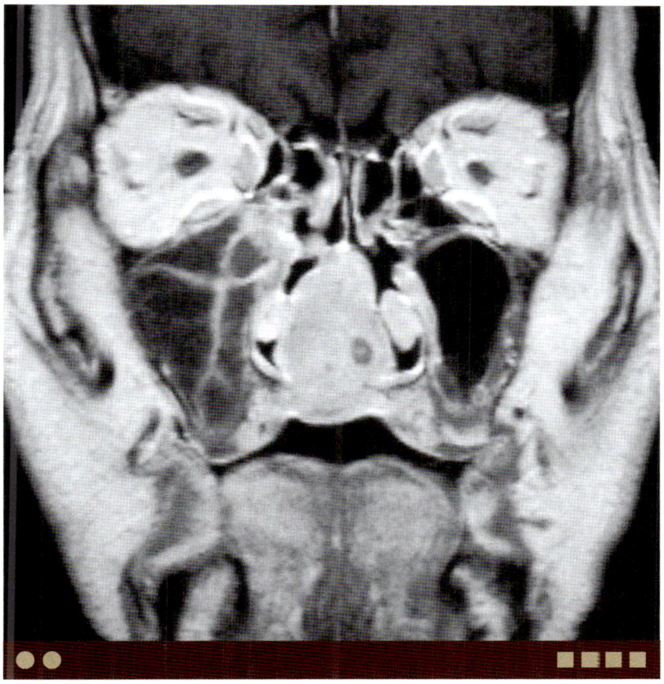

I. Plasmacytoma. Coronal postcontract T1W image demonstrates a relatively homogeneous enhancing tumor arising from the nasal septum. Note the lesion is centered in the marrow space of the septum and extends to the hard palate.

Case 3–5 Antrochoanal Polyp

Osamu Sakai, Elisa Flower

PRESENTATION

Nasal obstruction with a mass in the nasopharynx.

FINDINGS

CT demonstrates a polyp arising from the maxillary sinus extending posteriorly into the nasopharynx.

DIFFERENTIAL DIAGNOSIS

- Nasal polyp: This usually arises from the nasal cavity, along the turbinate and demonstrates variable density/signal.
- Inverted papilloma: This often arises from the lateral wall of the nasal cavity and extends into the maxillary sinus. The density is usually heterogeneously increased, often with calcification.
- Squamous cell carcinoma (SCCA): SCCA often demonstrates heterogeneous density/signal and enhancement, and aggressive bone destruction rather than benign remodeling or erosion.
- Lymphoma: This demonstrates homogeneous solid signal without necrosis or cystic change.

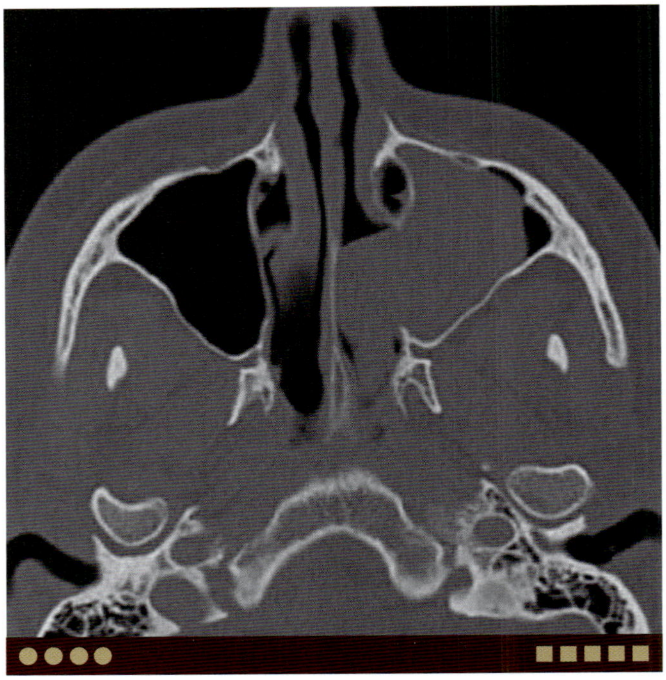

A. Antrochoanal polyp. Axial CT in bone window demonstrates soft tissue density nearly completely opacifying the left maxillary sinus with extension into the nasal cavity.

COMMENTS

This is a 31-year-old man with a polypoid lesion arising from the maxillary sinus extending posteriorly to the nasopharynx.

Antrochoanal polyp is a polypoid lesion arising from the maxillary sinus protruding into the nasal cavity through the ostium, then extending posteriorly to the nasopharynx. Clinically, it is recognized as a mass in the nasopharynx in addition to the polyp obstructing the nasal cavity. Usually, it is a unilateral lesion but occasionally bilateral, and often seen in young adults. The exact cause is still unknown, however it appears associated with allergy, chronic inflammation, and infection, and other possible causes are diabetes mellitus, cystic fibrosis, and aspirin allergy.

A polyp is initially very watery and demonstrates similar density or signal to water. Then, with increase of fibrotic components and protein concentration, it increases in density on CT and signal on T1W images and decreases in signal on T2W images. It generally demonstrates only peripheral enhancement with no central enhancement. If, however, there is significant neovascularity, enhancement and signal characteristic may become similar to that of juvenile angiofibroma, however it should be differentiated by the location.

Inverted papilloma often arises from the lateral wall of the nasal cavity and extends into the maxillary sinus, and may show similar appearance to antorochoanal polyp. However, they tend to show more heterogeneous higher density on CT, often with calcification. Further, presence of bone destruction suggests co-existing SCCA. MRI better demonstrates heterogeneity of the lesion.

PEARLS

- **Antrochoanal polyp arises in the maxillary sinus and extends posteriorly to the nasopharynx.**
- **On CT, it demonstrates relatively homogeneous low-to-intermediate density.**
- **On T2W MR images, it shows intermediate-to-high signal, higher than inverted papilloma.**
- **Bone remodeling is seen at the ostium.**

ADDITIONAL IMAGES (B-F)

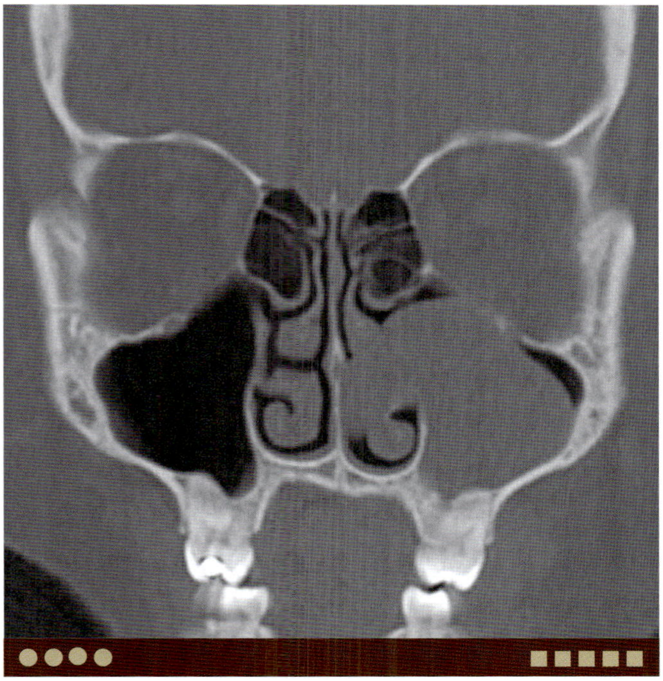

B. Antrochoanal polyp, same patient as A. Coronal CT demonstrates a polypoid lesion from the maxillary sinus with widening of the ostium and extension into the nasal cavity.

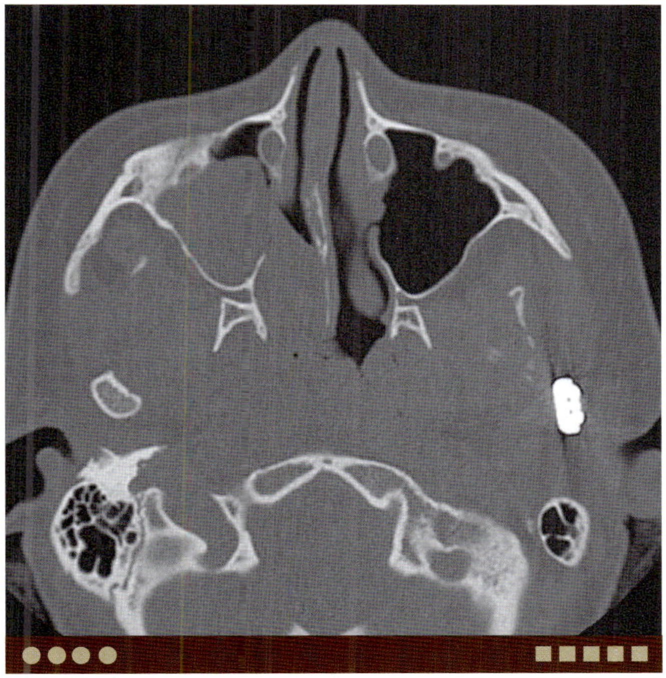

C. **Antrochoanal polyp** in a different patient. Axial CT demonstrates a polypoid lesion in the right maxillary sinus extending into the nasal cavity.

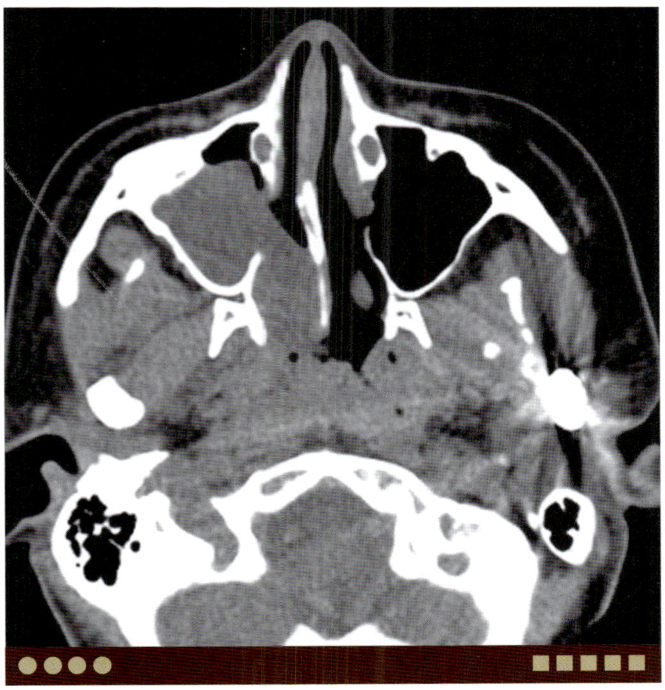

D. Antrochoanal polyp, same patient as in C. Axial soft tissue window CT demonstrates homogeneous watery density of the lesion.

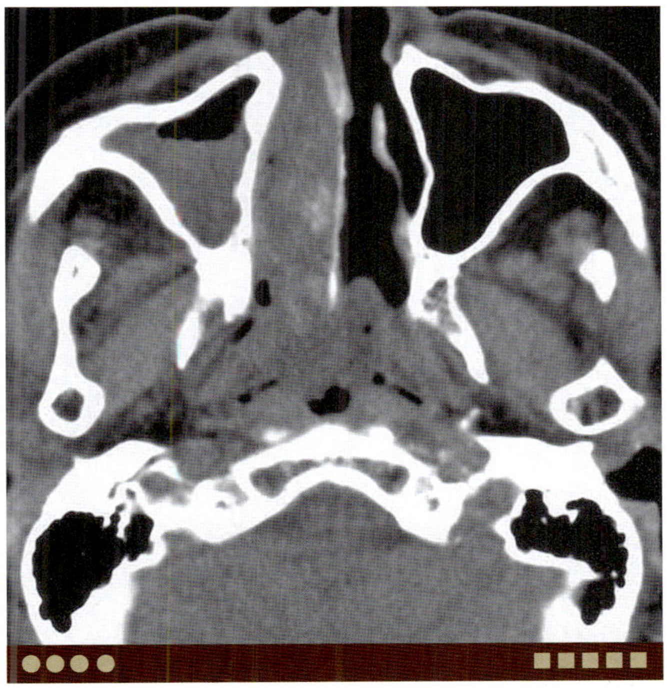

E. **Nasal polyp**. Axial soft tissue window CT demonstrates a slightly heterogeneous polypoid lesion in the right nasal cavity. Air-fluid level is seen in the right maxillary sinus.

DIFFERENTIAL DIAGNOSIS IMAGES (G-I)

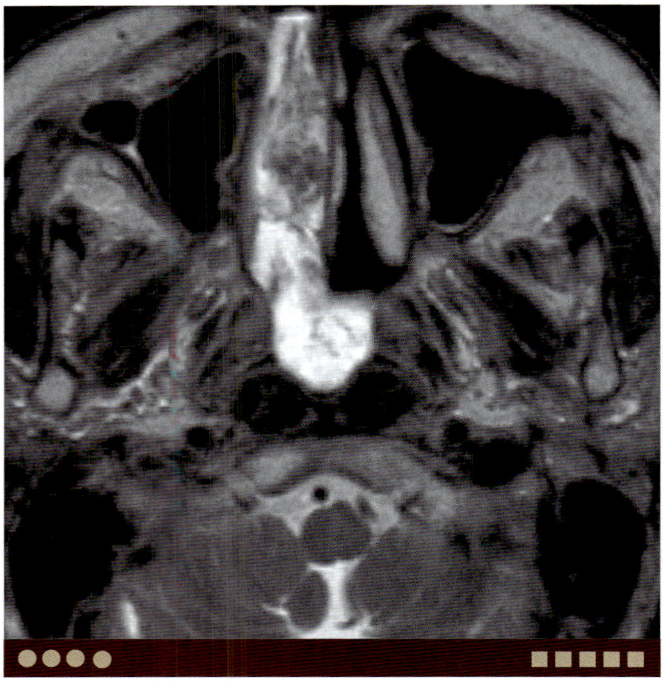

F. Nasal polyp, same patient as in E. Axial T2W MR image demonstrates slightly heterogeneous high signal within the lesion. The finding is similar to antorochoanal polyp, however no mass is seen in the maxillary sinus.

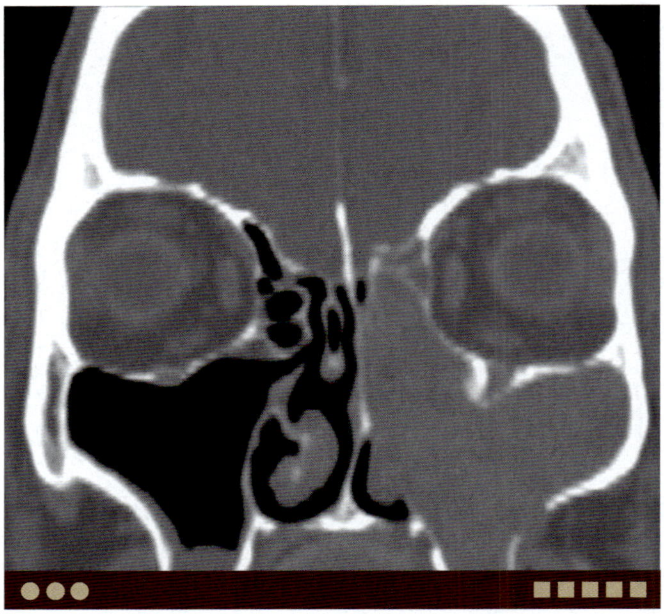

G. Inverted papilloma. Coronal bone window CT demonstrates complete opacification of the left ethmoid and maxillary sinuses with erosion of the medial and lateral walls of the left maxillary sinus.

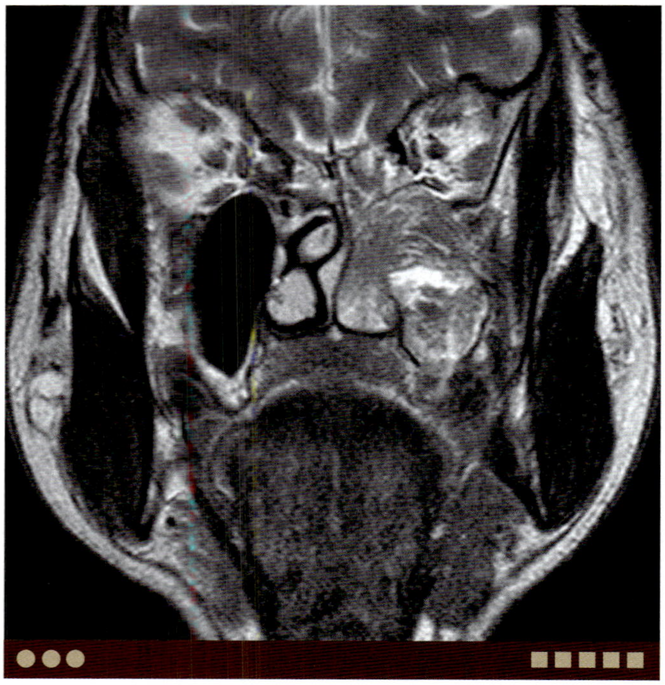

H. Inverted papilloma, same patient as G. Coronal T2W image demonstrates heterogeneous, intermediate signal within the lesion.

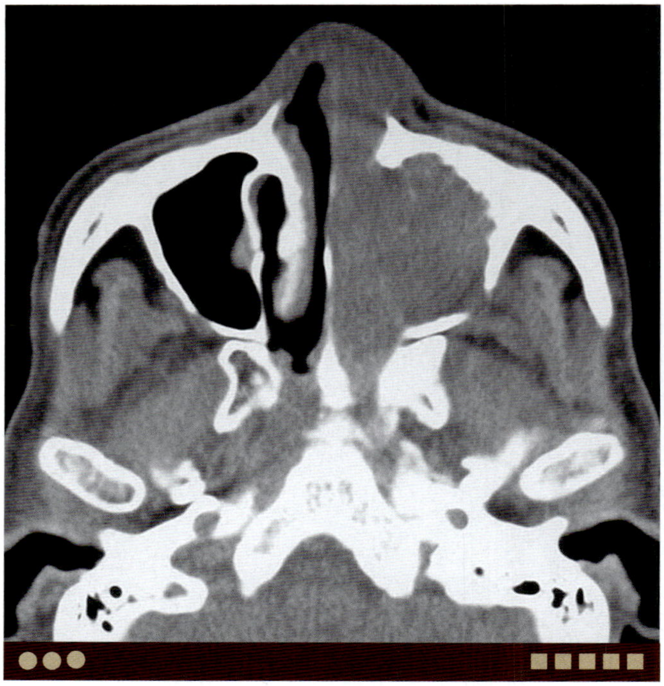

I. Inverted papilloma with SCCA in a different patient. Axial CT demonstrates a large tumor with bone destruction in the medial and posterior walls of the left maxillary sinus. Note involvement of the pterygopalatine fossa.

Case 3–6 Nasal Septal Deviation

Osamu Sakai, Rania Hito

PRESENTATION

Nasal obstruction.

FINDINGS

CT demonstrates deviation of the nasal septum.

DIFFERENTIAL DIAGNOSIS

- Nasal septal fracture: Fractures are usually accompanied by other signs to suggest trauma.
- Nasal septal hematoma: This is rare, however early diagnosis and treatment is required to avoid abscess formation, septal perforation, and saddle-nose deformity, potentially permanent complications from cartilage necrosis.
- Nasal septal tumors: Nasal septum has cartilage and bone. Chondroid or osseous tumors may arise from the nasal septum.
- Nasal septal perforation: Defect in the nasal septum may be seen secondary to trauma, vasculitis, cocaine use, and lymphoma.

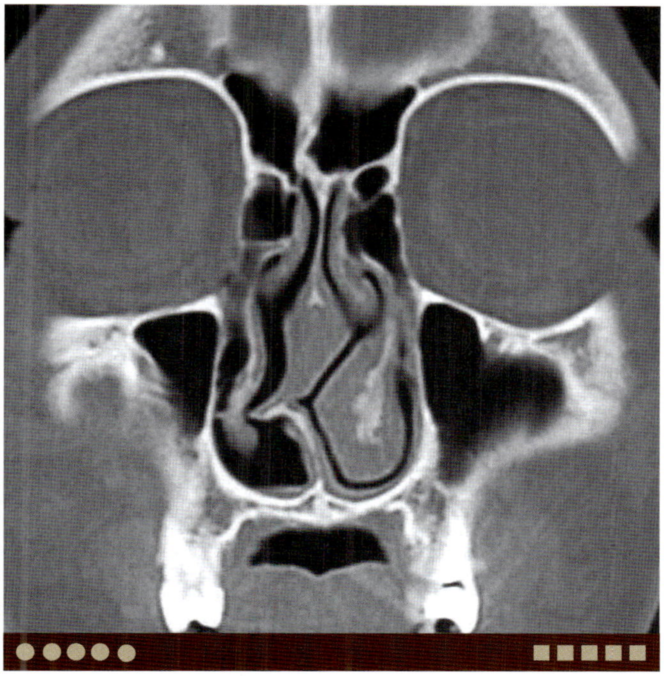

A. Nasal septal deviation. Coronal CT demonstrates nasal septal deviation to the right with a bony spur.

COMMENTS

This is a 35-year-old man who complains of nasal obstruction.

Nasal septal deviation is divergence of the septum from the midline and is a very common condition. The three components of the nasal septum are the vomer, perpendicular plate of the ethmoid, and septal cartilage. Disturbance in any of these structures can lead to nasal septal deviation. In most cases, exact etiology of septal deviation is unclear, but at times it is secondary to prior trauma. The deviation is most commonly broad based but can have an S-shaped configuration. Very few adults have a completely straight septum.

Nasal septal deviation may not have clinical significance. It has been postulated that mechanical obstruction of the ostiomeatal complex can occur if the deviation is severe. Some authors have proposed that sinus disease occurs due to an alteration of the ciliary activity secondary to a modified airflow. It has not been conclusively shown that there is a higher incidence of sinus disease in patients with septal deviation. If the septal deviation contacts the inferior turbinate, the patient may complain of significant pain and nasal obstruction. In such a case nasal septoplasty may be indicated.

Narrowing of the nasal passage can make intranasal intervention difficult. Therefore, the surgeon needs to know the anatomy before surgery, and nasal septoplasty is often performed at the time of sinus surgery for chronic sinusitis or sinonasal polyposis.

On CT, nasal septal deviation is easily seen on both coronal and axial images. A bony spur is often present pointing toward the side of the septal deviation. When there is pneumatization of middle turbinate or concha bullosa, the nasal septum deviates away from the pneumatized turbinate.

PEARLS

- **Nasal septal deviation is a very common condition.**
- **It can cause narrowing of the nasal passage and lead to inflammation.**
- **After identifying septal deviation one should assess for the presence or absence of bony spur, degree of the deviation, and relationship to the turbinates.**

ADDITIONAL IMAGES (B-C)

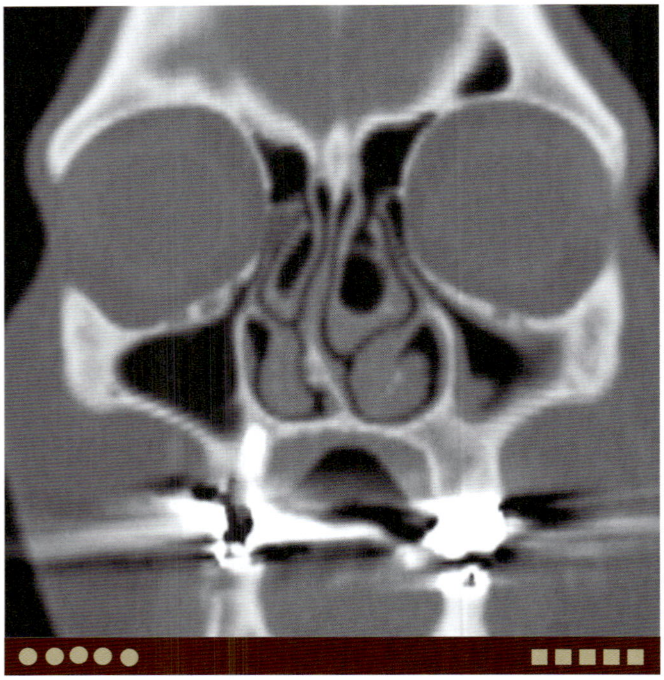

B. Nasal septal deviation in a different patient. Coronal CT demonstrates bilateral pneumatized middle turbinates, left larger than right, and nasal septal deviation to the right.

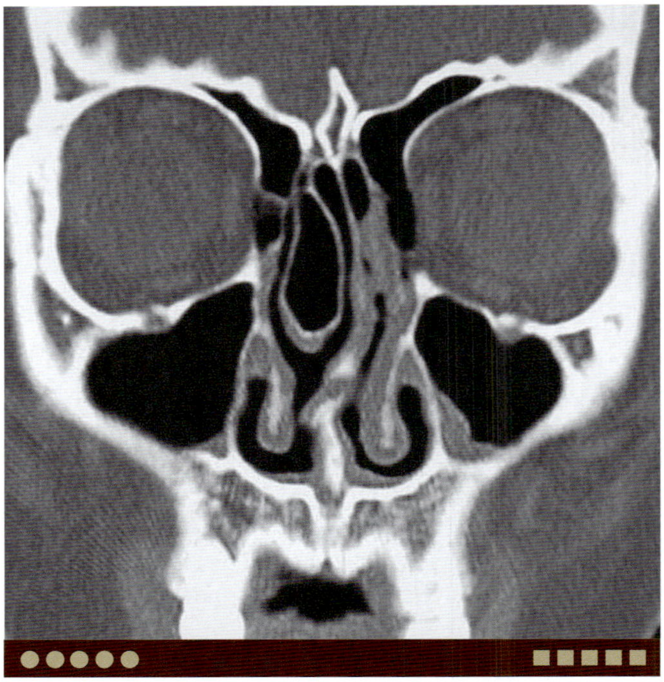

C. Nasal septal deviation in a different patient. Coronal CT demonstrates pneumatized right middle turbinate with an S-shaped nasal septal deviation.

DIFFERENTIAL DIAGNOSIS IMAGES (D-G)

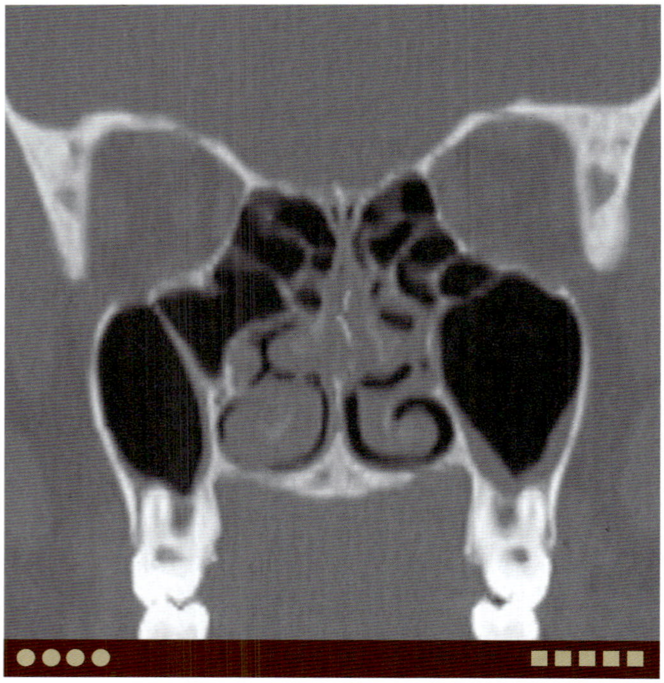

D. Nasal septal fracture. Coronal CT demonstrates fracture of the nasal septum and associated small hematoma along the septum.

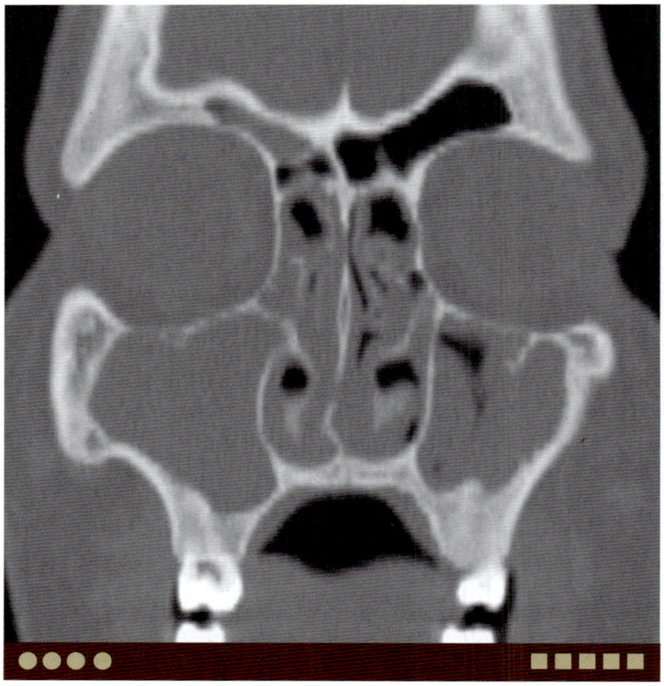

E. Nasal septal fracture in a different patient. Coronal CT demonstrates fracture of the inferior nasal septum.

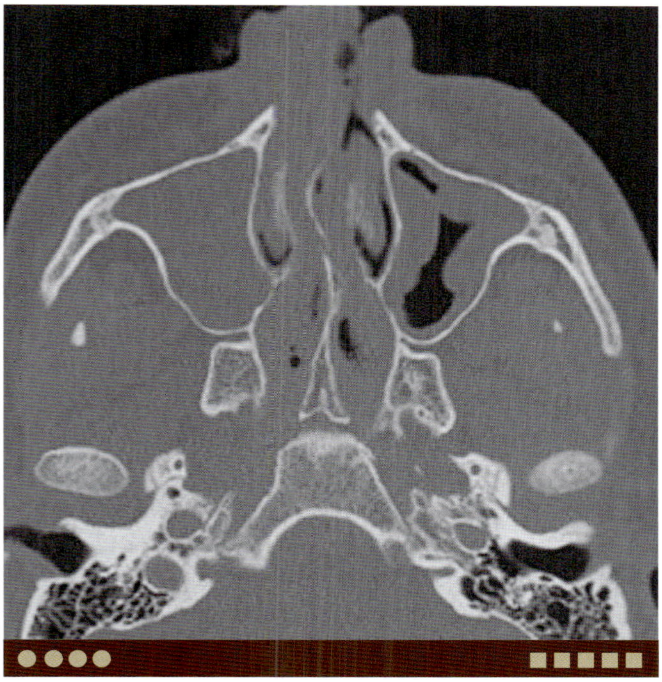

F. Nasal septal fracture, same patient as E. Axial CT demonstrates fracture of the nasal septum.

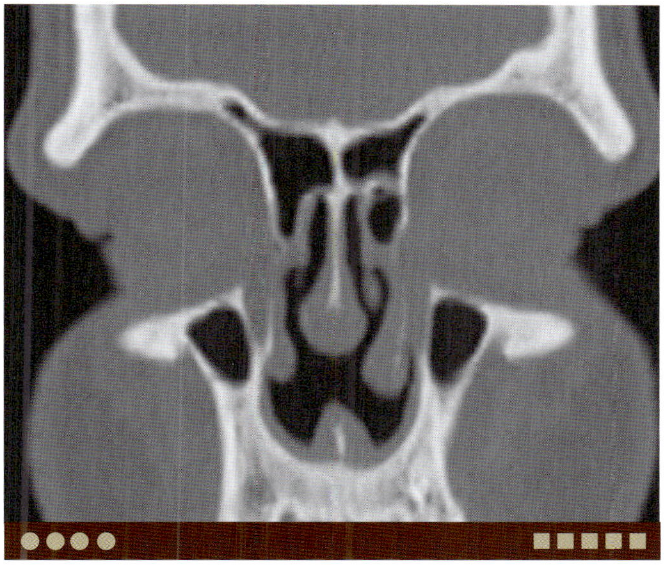

G. **Nasal septal perforation**. Coronal CT demonstrates a large defect in the nasal septum.

Case 3–7 Paradoxical Turbinate

Osamu Sakai, Rania Hito

PRESENTATION

Normal variant.

FINDINGS

CT demonstrates inward curling of the middle turbinate.

DIFFERENTIAL DIAGNOSIS

- Trauma/fracture: Trauma may result in alternate curvature of the turbinate, however usually accompanies other signs to suggest trauma.
- Nasal polyp: Polypoid lesions can narrow the middle meatus. However, there should be no osseous paradoxic curvature of the turbinate.

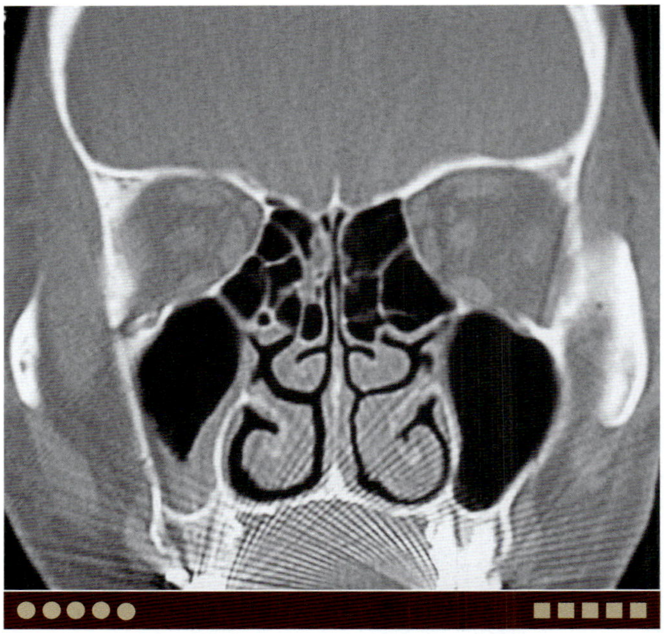

A. Paradoxical middle turbinate. Coronal CT demonstrates the middle turbinate is convex laterally and curls inward, slightly narrowing the middle meatus bilaterally.

COMMENTS

This is a 35-year-old man who complains of nasal obstruction.

Paradoxical turbinate, paradoxic curvature of the turbinate is a common normal variant, which is often significant in the middle turbinate. Usually, the middle turbinate is convex medially, however in a case with paradoxical middle turbinate, the middle turbinate is convex laterally and curls inward, narrowing the middle meatus. The prevalence of this variant has been reported at 26%.

The etiology is unclear, but the paradoxical turbinate is often seen where the mucosa is hyperplastic, and it is thought that overgrowth causes the mucosa to buckle and fold the turbinate inward with the resultant curve pointing toward the septum.

Clinical significance is not clear but it may worsen inflammatory process due to narrowing the middle meatus, although some authors have reported no statistical correlation between paradoxical turbinate and symptomatic sinusitis. The surgeon must know this variant anatomy before intervention.

On CT, the paradoxical middle turbinate demonstrates middle turbinate curling inward, convex laterally, best seen on coronal images. Most paradoxical middle turbinates are partial, which means it goes back to normal curvature posteriorly.

PEARLS

- **Paradoxical middle turbinate is a common normal variant.**
- **In paradoxical middle turbinate the middle turbinate curls inward and is convex laterally.**
- **Paradoxical middle turbinate narrows the middle meatus.**

ADDITIONAL IMAGES (B-D)

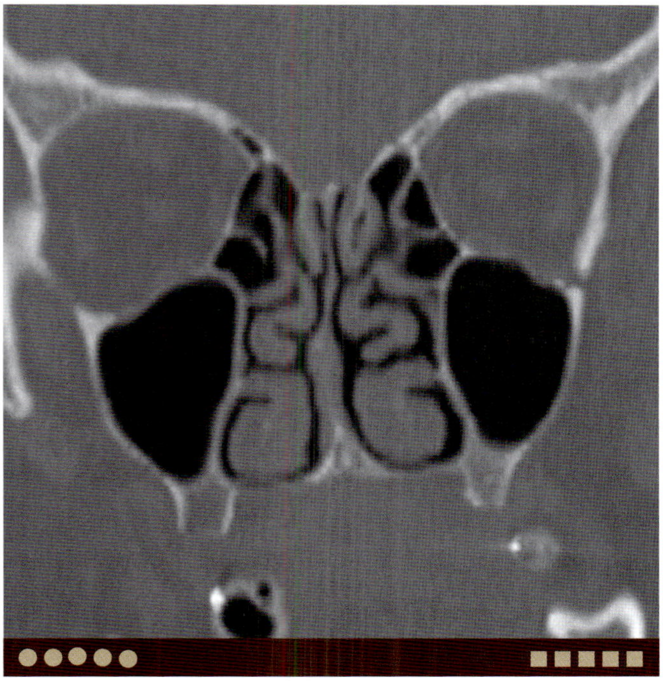

B. Paradoxical middle turbinate in a different patient. Coronal CT demonstrates the middle turbinate is convex laterally and curls inward, slightly narrowing the middle meatus bilaterally.

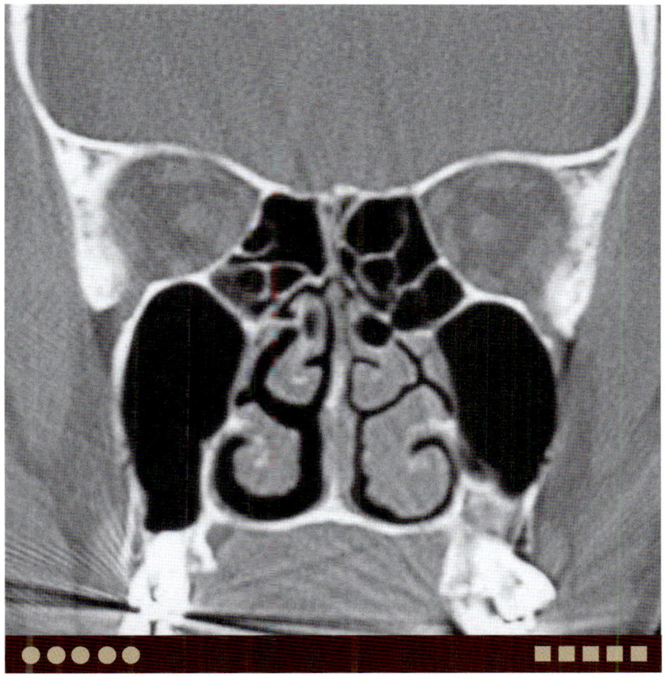

C. Paradoxical middle turbinate in a different patient. Coronal CT demonstrates the middle turbinate is convex laterally and curls inward, slightly narrowing the middle meatus bilaterally.

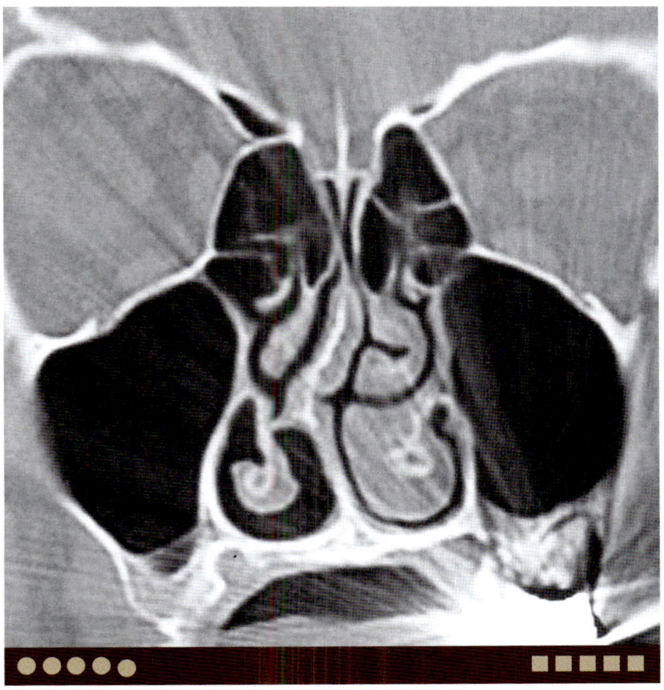

D. Paradoxical middle turbinate with nasal septal deviation in a different patient. Coronal CT demonstrates the left middle turbinate is convex laterally and curls inward. There is nasal septal deviation to the right with bony spur.

DIFFERENTIAL DIAGNOSIS IMAGES (E-F)

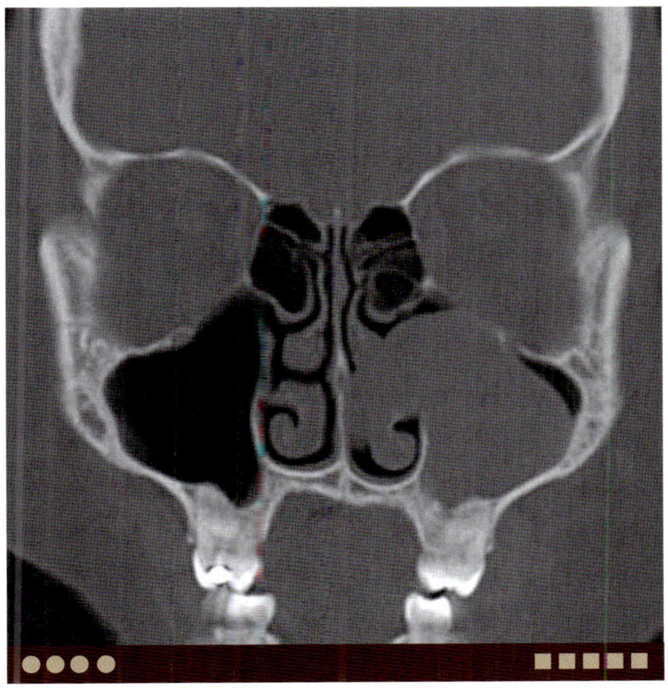

E. Antrochoanal polyp. Coronal CT demonstrates a polypoid lesion from the maxillary sinus with widening of the ostium and extension into the nasal cavity.

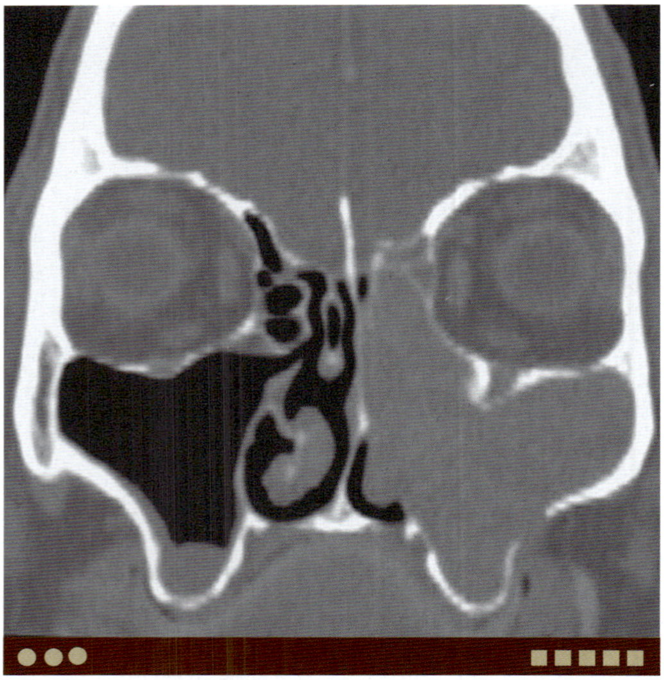

F. Inverted papilloma. Coronal CT demonstrates complete opacification of the left ethmoid and maxillary sinuses with erosion of the medial and lateral walls of the left maxillary sinus and narrowing the middle meatus.

Case 3–8 Haller Air Cell

Osamu Sakai, Rania Hito

PRESENTATION

Normal variant.

FINDINGS

CT demonstrates inferiorly and laterally extended ethmoid air cells.

DIFFERENTIAL DIAGNOSIS

- Ethmoid bulla: This is the largest air cell in the anterior ethmoid complex. It is almost always present, however may vary in size. It may prolapse into the middle nasal meatus or ethmoid infundibulum and narrow these structures, when it is enlarged.
- Agger nasi cell: This is pneumatization of the *agger nasi*, which means nasal eminence. It arises from the superior aspect of the infundibulum or the frontal recess.
- Onodi (sphenoethmoid) cell: This is highly pneumatized most posterior cell, extending posteriorly along the lamina papyracea into the anterior wall of the sphenoid sinus. The optic nerve may be adjacent to the posterior ethmoid air cell.

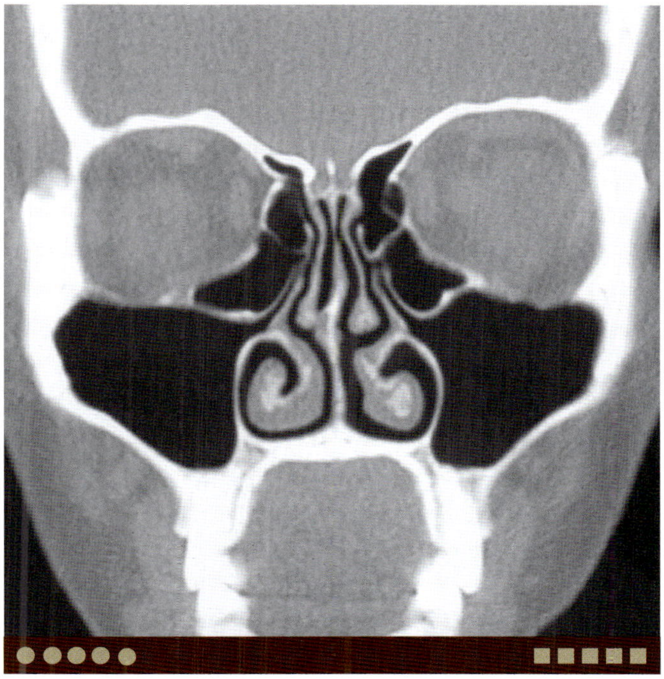

A. Haller air cells. Coronal CT shows large ethmoid air cells extending inferiorly and laterally along the inferior orbit bilaterally.

COMMENTS

This is a 34-year-old man who had a CT of the sinuses for nasal obstruction.

Haller air cell, also known as an infraorbital air cell, is a variant of the ethmoid air cells that extends inferiorly and laterally along the inferior aspect of the orbital floor. It is adjacent to the natural ostium of the maxillary sinus and forms the roof of the sinus. While it can originate from the anterior or posterior ethmoid air cells, extension from the anterior ethmoid air cells is far more common. This variant is found more frequently in women than in men.

An enlarged Haller air cell originating from the anterior ethmoid air cells may contribute to narrowing of the ostium or infundibulum. Pathology such as infection in the Haller air cell can cause obstruction of the ostiomeatal complex resulting in opacification of the maxillary sinus. Haller air cells have been implicated in recurrent maxillary sinusitis. As with any paranasal sinus variant, the surgeon must be aware of this before sinus surgery.

On CT, Haller air cell is best seen on coronal images along the inferior aspect of the floor of the orbit, forming the roof of the infundibulum. These air cells are often bilateral, thin walled, and seen in continuity with the ethmoid capsule.

PEARLS

- **Haller air cell is extension of the ethmoid air cells inferiorly and laterally forming the roof of the ostium.**
- **Enlargement of Haller air cells originating from the anterior ethmoid air cells has been implicated in recurrent maxillary sinus disease.**
- **Variant found in up to 10% of patients, important to identify preoperatively for sinus surgery.**

ADDITIONAL IMAGES (B-D)

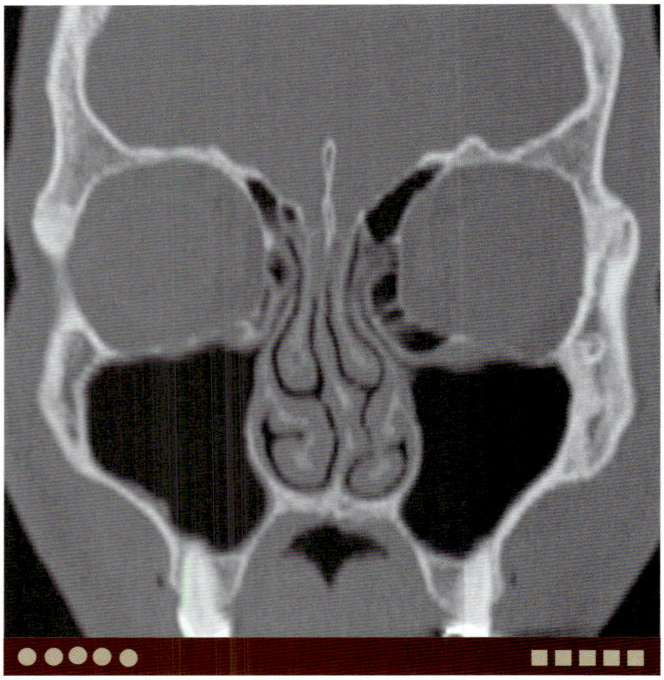

B. Haller air cells in a different patient. Coronal CT shows bilateral Haller air cells, left larger than right.

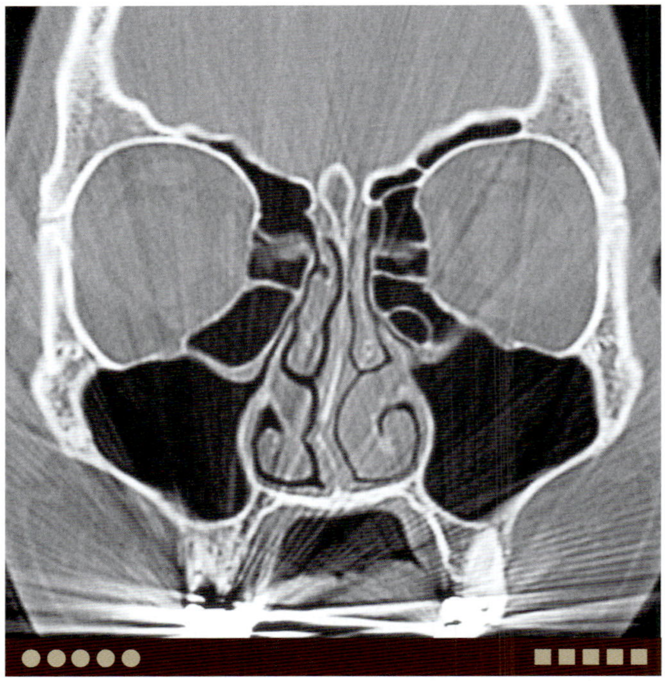

C. Haller air cells in a different patient. Coronal CT shows bilateral Haller air cells, right larger than left. Note is made of nasal septal deviation to the right.

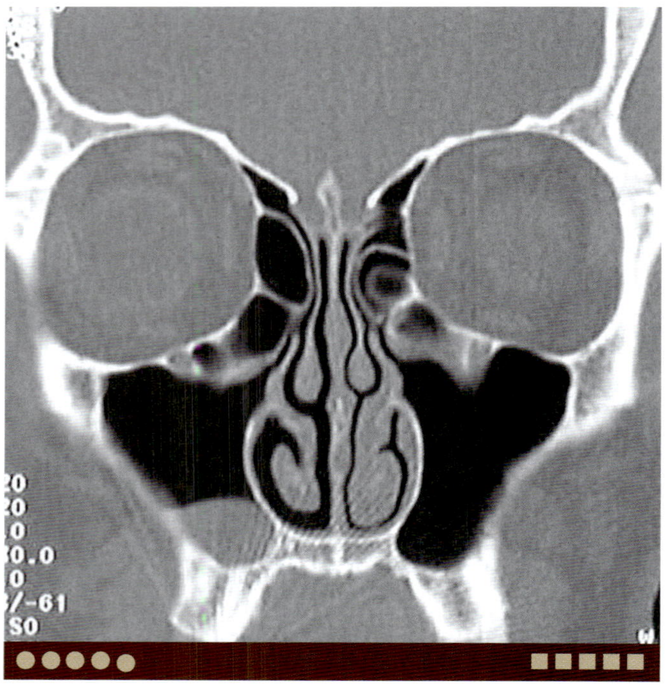

D. Haller air cells in a different patient. Coronal CT shows bilateral Haller air cells.

DIFFERENTIAL DIAGNOSIS IMAGES (E-F)

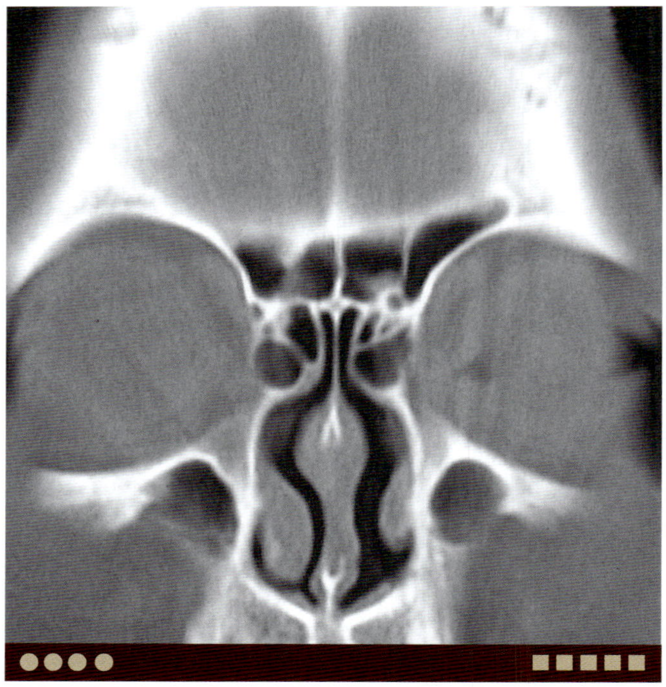

E. Agger nasi cells. Coronal CT shows air cells anterior to the frontal processes of the maxilla bilaterally.

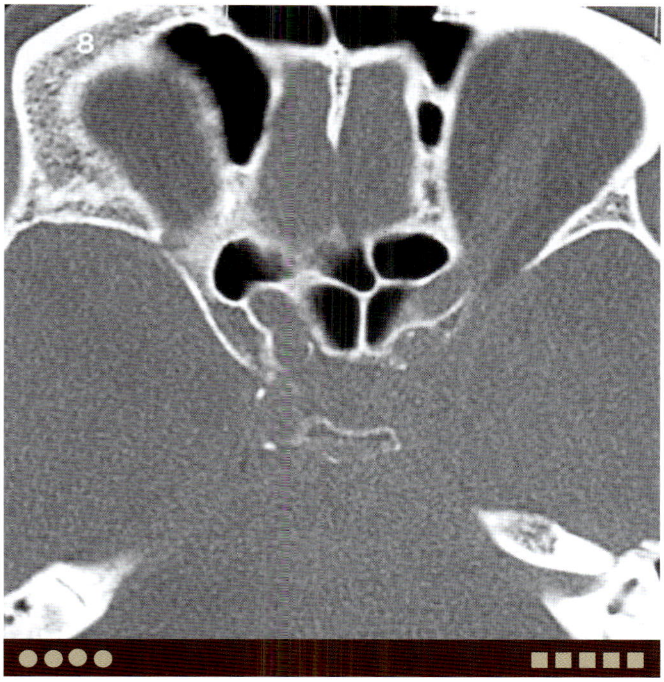

F. Onodi cells. Axial CT demonstrates pneumatized posterior ethmoid air cells, extending posterolaterally. The optic nerves are adjacent to the air cells.

Case 3–9 Wegener's Granulomatosis

Osamu Sakai, Gabriel Monagas

PRESENTATION

Sinus pain.

FINDINGS

CT and MRI demonstrate nasal septal perforation and nonspecific inflammatory changes along the sinuses.

DIFFERENTIAL DIAGNOSIS

- Chronic sinusitis: This condition shows nonspecific chronic inflammatory changes, such as opacification of the sinonasal cavities and thickening of sinus walls, without osseous destruction.
- Lymphoma: Lymphoma may demonstrate similar findings to Wegener's granulomatosis. So-called "midline lethal granuloma" is lymphoma, often natural killer/T-cell lymphoma. An infiltrative skull base lesion in an immunocompromised patient should raise suspicion for lymphoma.
- Cocaine abuse: Cocaine is a commonly used recreational drug worldwide and is a well documented cause of nasal septum perforation in abusers through intranasal administration. Case reports have also shown incidental C-ANCA antibody positivity in users with no histologic evidence of Wegener's granulomatosis which may cause confusion in diagnosis.

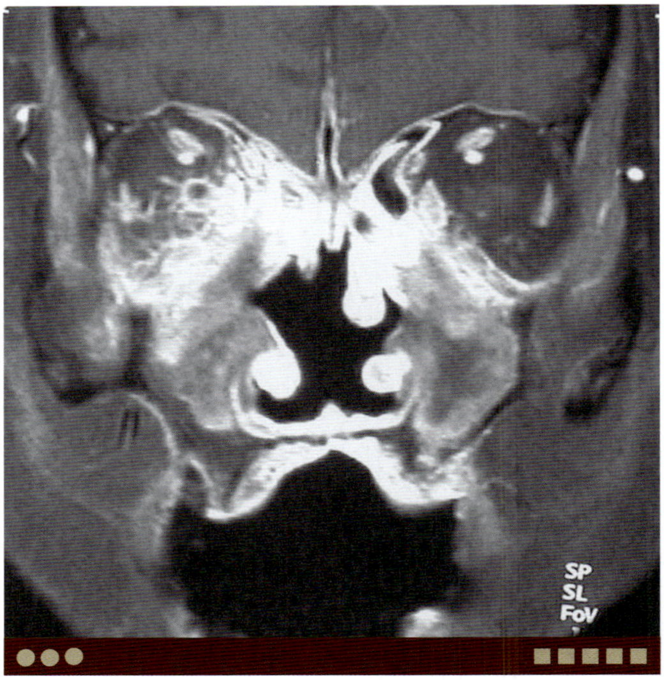

A. Wegener's granulomatosis. Coronal postcontrast fat-suppressed T1W image demonstrates diffuse enhancement in the maxillary sinuses and the inferomedial portion of the orbits bilaterally. Note large nasal septal perforation. Further, abnormal dural enhancement along the anterior skull base and falx is present.

COMMENTS

This is a 50-year-old man who complains of sinusitis symptoms and eye pain.

Wegener's granulomatosis is a form of vasculitis of unknown etiology but likely associated with autoimmune abnormality. C-ANCA is almost always positive and its positivity is highly suggestive of Wegener's granulomatosis. Wegener's granulomatosis can occur at any age, but more common between the ages of 30 and 50, with a male-to-female ratio of 2:1.

Wegener's granulomatosis shows various neurological and otolaryngological presentations. Neurological abnormalities are seen in 25%–54% of patients. Classic triads are: (1) respiratory tract granulomatous inflammation, (2) systemic small vessel vasculitis, and (3) necrotizing granuloma. In the head and neck, it is well-known as a cause of nasal septal perforation. However, it not only involves the sinonasal cavities but also the orbits and skull base. Its infiltrative or invasive extension pattern may resemble malignant neoplasms including lymphoma. Intracranial involvement is not rare and can be seen in up to 10% of patients. Commonly, meningeal thickening with abnormal enhancement is noted. Furthermore, white matter and pituitary gland/stalk abnormalities, as well as cerebellar atrophy may also be seen. Therefore, evaluation of the skull base and intracranial structures is important when the patient is scanned for sinus or orbital abnormalities.

PEARLS

- **Wegener's granulomatosis causes nasal septal perforation.**
- **Findings of Wegener's granulomatosis in the paranasal sinuses are nonspecific.**
- **Orbital and intracranial involvements are commonly seen.**

ADDITIONAL IMAGES (B-G)

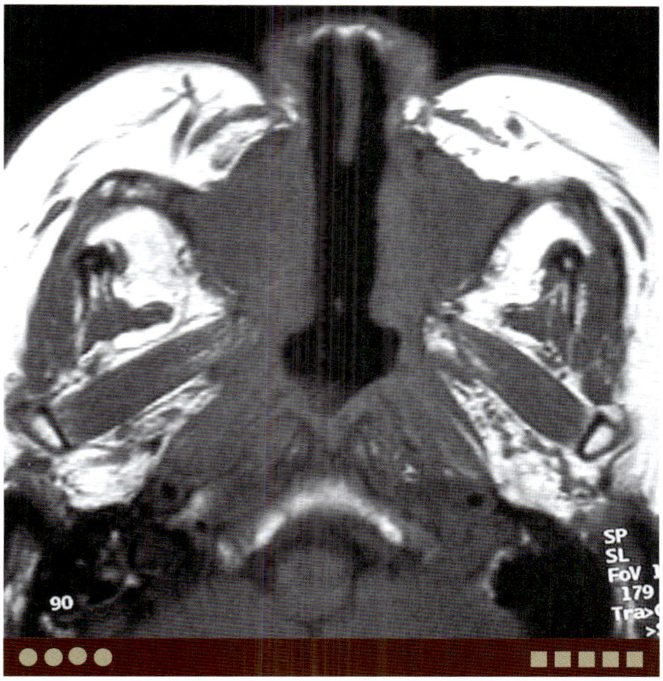

B. Wegener's granulomatosis, same patient as A. Axial T1W demonstrates opacified and contracted maxillary sinuses bilaterally. A large septal perforation is again seen.

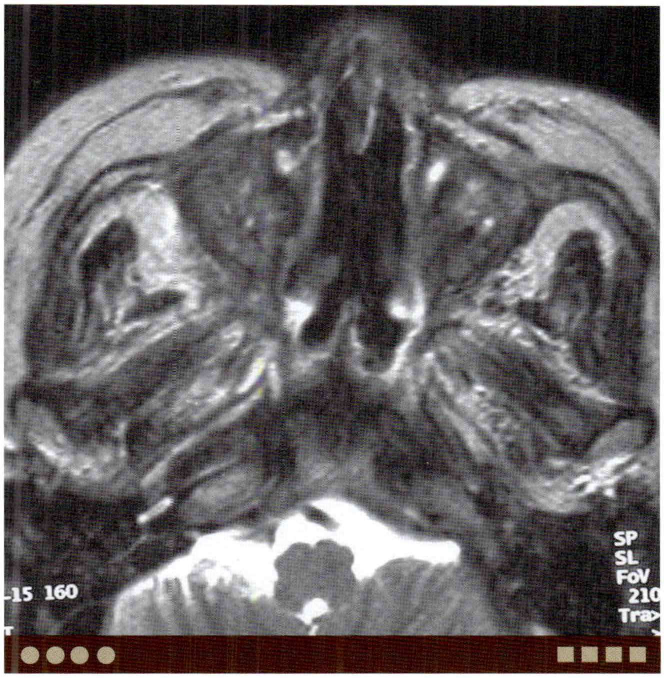

C. Wegener's granulomatosis, same patient as A. Axial T2W shows the opacified maxillary sinuses demonstrating decreased signal to suggest sclerosis from chronic inflammation.

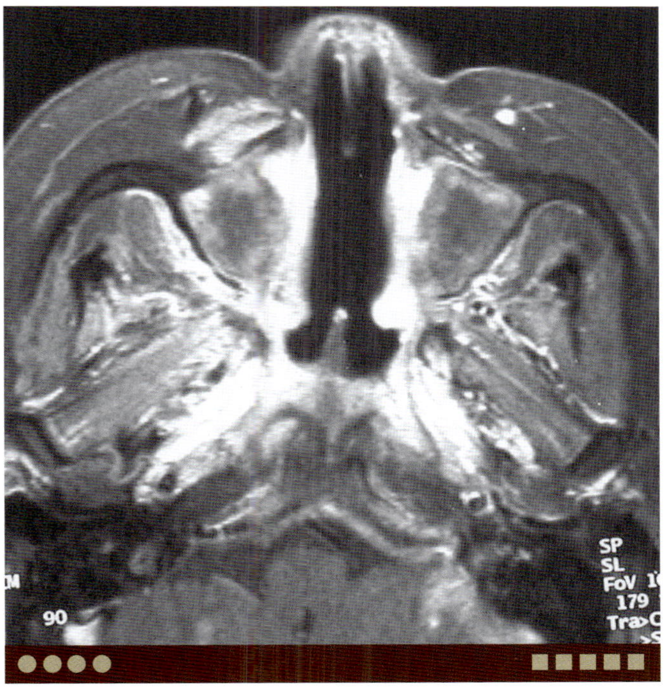

D. Wegener's granulomatosis, same patient as A. Axial postcontrast fat-suppressed T1W image demonstrates diffuse enhancement in the right buccal space, nasopharynx, longus colli muscles in addition to the sinonasal cavities consistent with infiltrative process.

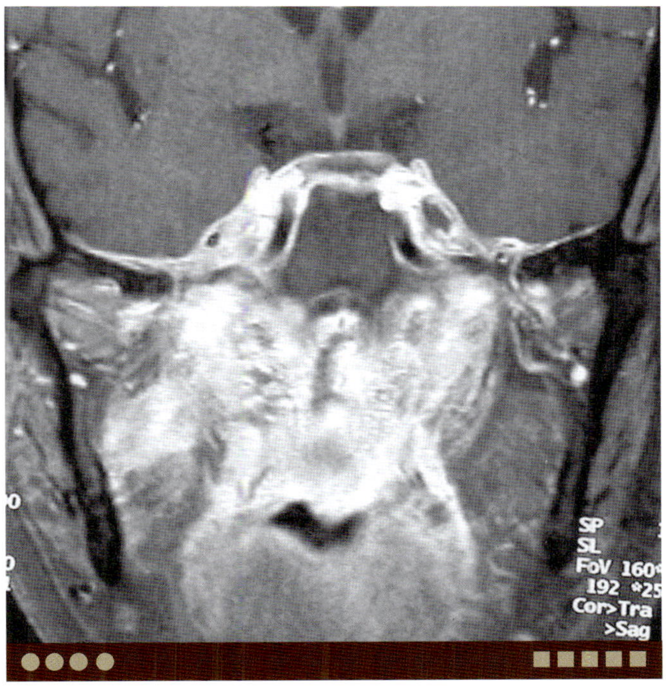

E. Wegener's granulomatosis, same patient as A. Coronal postcontrast fat-suppressed T1W image demonstrates enhancement of thickened dura in the middle cranial fossa and diffuse enhancement of the nasopharynx and part of the masticator space bilaterally.

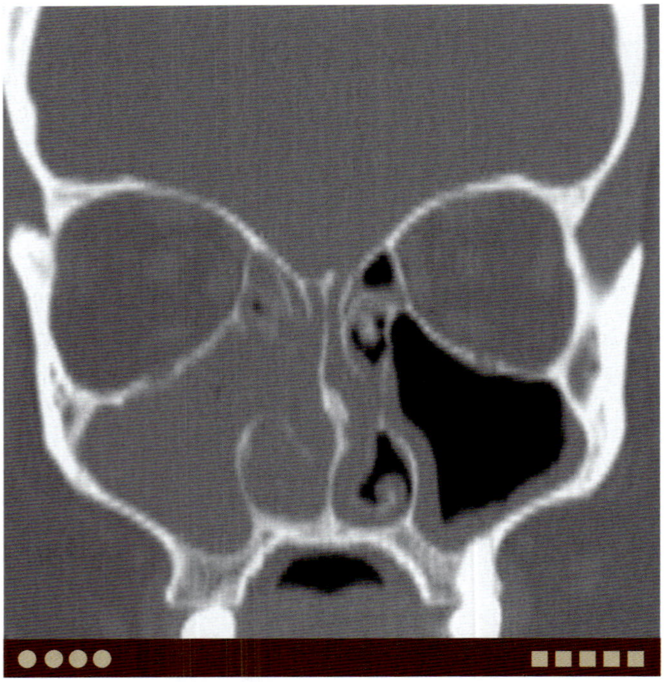

F. Wegener's granulomatosis in a different patient. Coronal bone window CT demonstrates opacified sinonasal cavities on the right, a nonspecific finding.

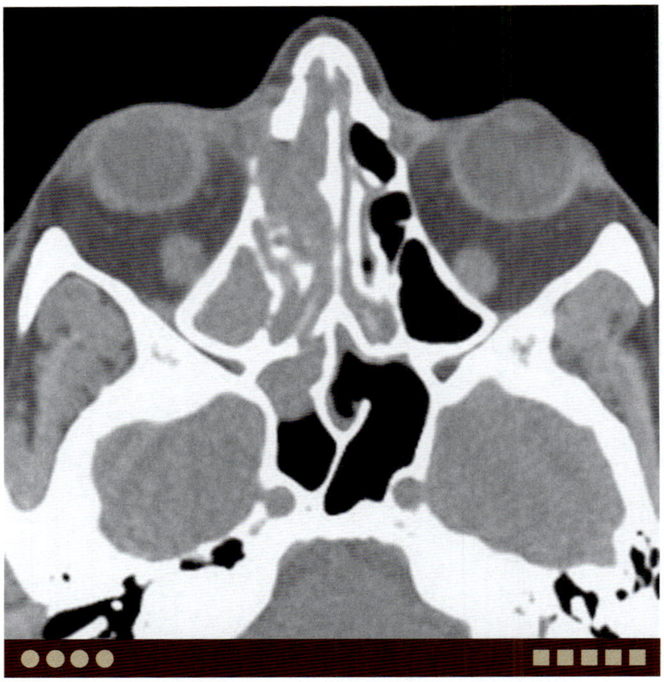

G. Wegener's granulomatosis, same patient as F. Axial soft tissue windowed noncontrast-enhanced CT demonstrates opacified right ethmoid air cells and sphenoid sinus. Note erosion of the anterior portion of the right medial orbital wall and infiltrative process extending to the lacrimal fossa.

DIFFERENTIAL DIAGNOSIS IMAGE

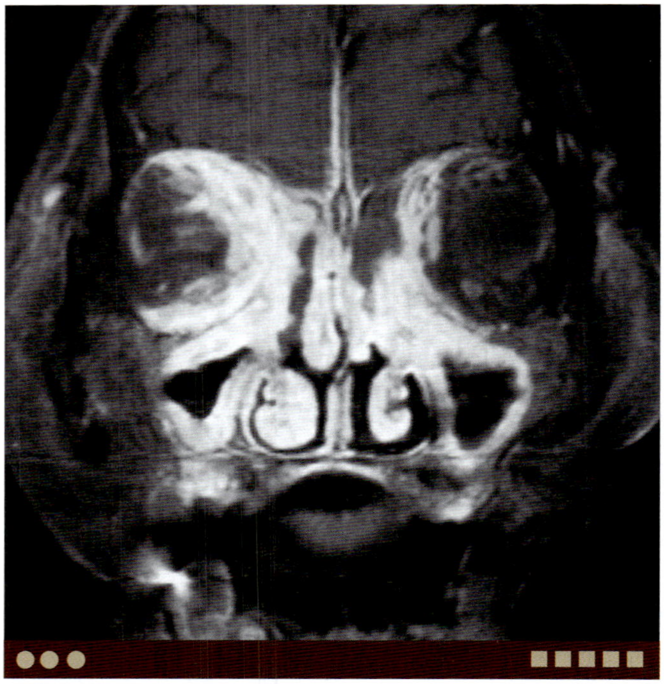

H. Lymphoma. Coronal postcontrast fat-suppressed T1W image demonstrates diffuse enhancement in the maxillary sinuses and the medial portion of the orbit bilaterally. Note abnormal dural enhancement along the anterior skull base and falx.

Case 3–10 Acute Sinusitis

Osamu Sakai, Susmitha Reddy, Rohini Nadgir

PRESENTATION

Sinus pain and fever.

FINDINGS

CT demonstrates mucosal thickening with air-fluid level in the sinuses.

DIFFERENTIAL DIAGNOSIS

- Chronic sinusitis: This usually shows osseous changes such as sclerosis, thickening as well as volume loss of the sinuses, and is often associated with polypoid lesions/polyposis. The retained secretions show variable density on CT and signal on MRI depending on the proteinaceous content or inspissated mucus.
- Squamous cell carcinoma (SCCA): This often shows bone destruction and a heterogeneously enhancing soft tissue mass if intravenous contrast is given. SCCA should be considered when sinus opacification is seen on one side.
- Lymphoma: A large, non-necrotic mass is a common finding. Among extranodal lymphoma in the head and neck, 40%–50% occurs in the sinonasal cavity, most commonly in the nasal cavity and maxillary sinus.

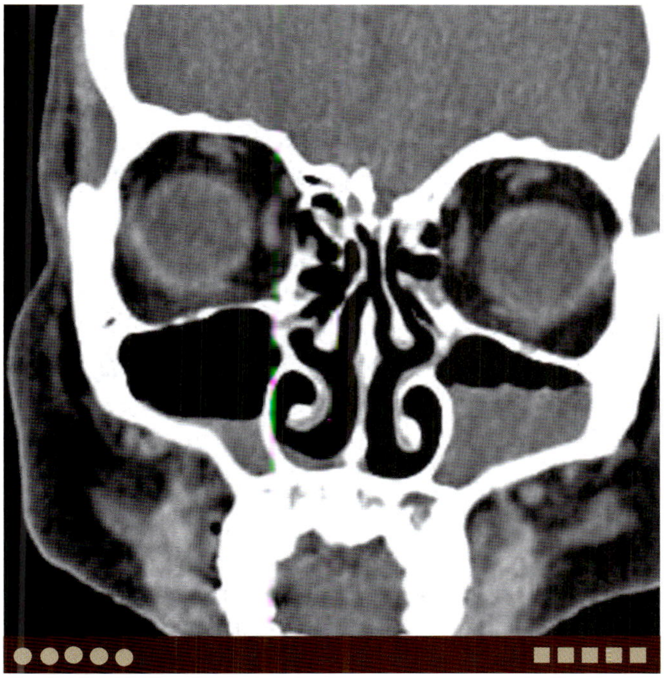

A. Acute sinusitis. Directly acquired coronal CT demonstrates air-fluid level in bilateral maxillary sinuses.

COMMENTS

This is a 35-year-old woman with acute sinus pain and fever.

Acute sinusitis is a clinical diagnosis and not a radiological diagnosis. Precise history and physical examination is the key to making this diagnosis.

In patients with sinusitis, mucosal thickening is seen on CT and MRI to variable degrees. Imaging findings are nonspecific and often it is difficult to determine acute or chronic inflammation/infection. In general, air-fluid level formation is the only finding to raise concern for an acute infection; however, air-fluid level can be seen without active inflammation or infection. Again, clinical findings are very important.

Direct coronal CT scan is rarely performed with the advent of spiral and multidetector CT capability. The advantages include lesser artifact from dental hardware and patient comfort during scanning. On reconstructed coronal images, the fluid level is not apparent. Axial (original) images should always be evaluated in conjunction with reconstructed images.

Plain films are still performed to evaluate for opacification of sinuses when acute sinus infection is suspected clinically. However, the role of plain film is minimal in evaluation for chronic sinusitis. CT should be performed for diagnosis as well as surgical planning when chronic sinusitis is suspected.

PEARLS

- **Sinusitis is a clinical diagnosis. Imaging findings are often nonspecific.**
- **Air-fluid level is a strong indicator of acute infection, although it can be seen without active inflammation or infection.**
- **Air-fluid level formation is not apparent on reconstructed coronal images, and "air-fluid level" on coronal reformatted images is not a real fluid level.**

ADDITIONAL IMAGES (B-F)

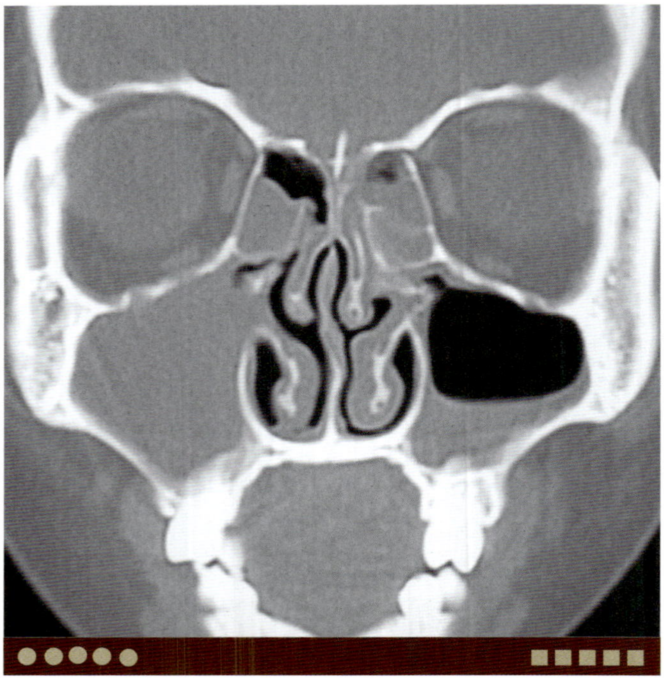

B. Acute sinusitis in a different patient. Directly acquired coronal CT demonstrates air-fluid level in the left and complete opacification of the right maxillary sinuses.

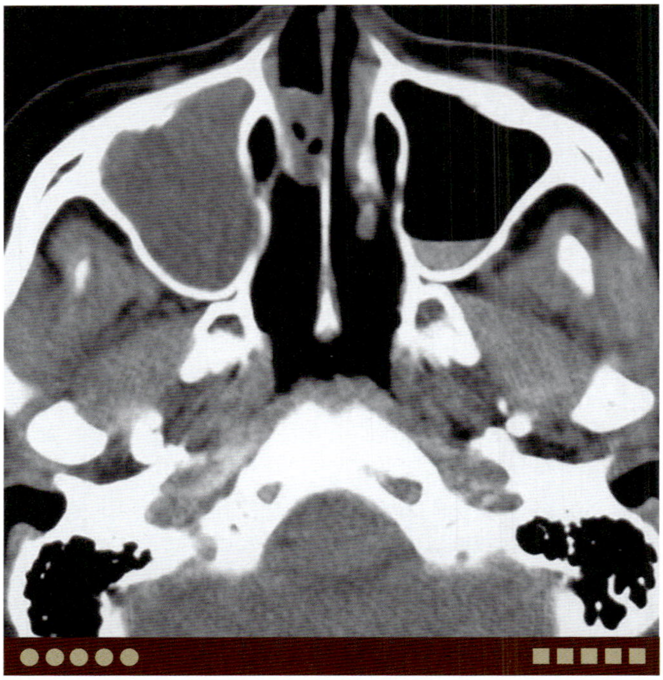

C. Acute sinusitis, same patient as B. Axial CT demonstrates total opacification of the right maxillary sinus and air-fluid level in the left maxillary sinus.

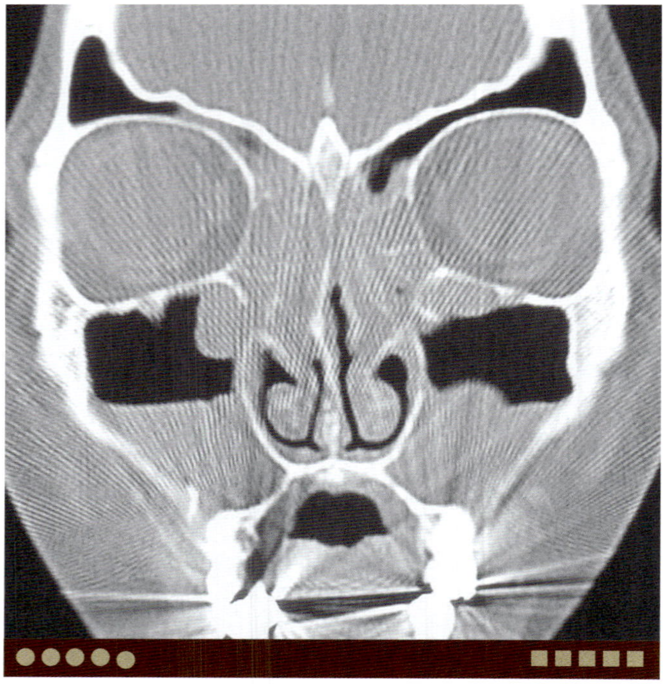

D. Acute sinusitis in a patient with sinonasal polyposis. Directly acquired coronal CT demonstrates apparent "air-fluid levels" in the maxillary sinuses bilaterally. The upper nasal cavities and ethmoid air cells are completely opacified.

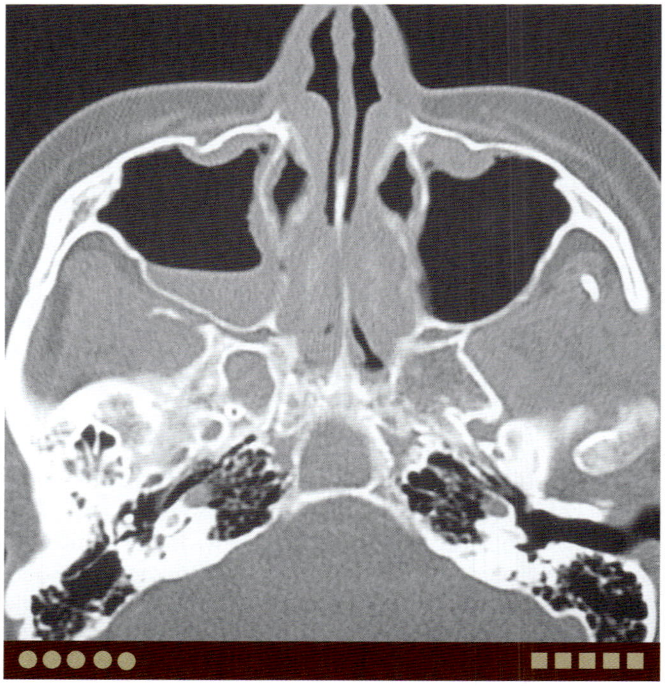

E. Acute sinusitis, same patient as D. Axial CT demonstrates air-fluid level in the maxillary sinus on the right side only. The left maxillary sinus opacity on coronal image was due to a retention cyst and mucosal thickening.

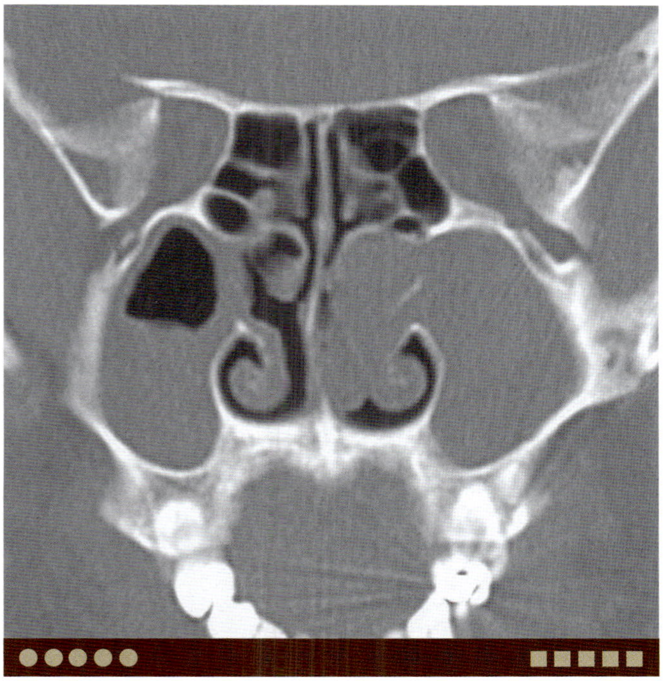

F. Acute sinusitis in a patient with a polypoid lesion. Directly acquired coronal CT demonstrates "air-fluid levels" in the right maxillary sinus with mucosal thickening. The left ostiomeatal complex is obstructed by a polypoid lesion and the left maxillary sinus is completely opacified.

DIFFERENTIAL DIAGNOSIS IMAGES (G-H)

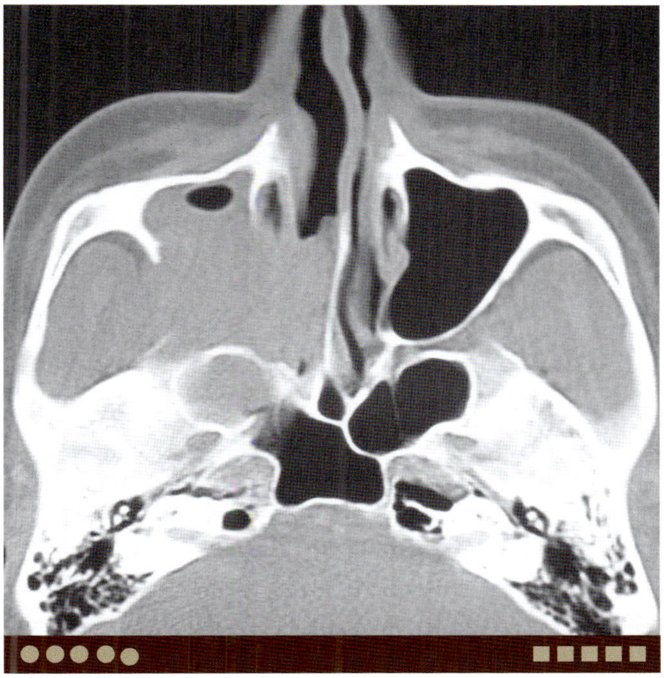

G. Squamous cell carcinoma. Axial CT demonstrates near complete opacification of the right maxillary sinus. Note destruction of the posterior and medial walls to suggest an aggressive lesion.

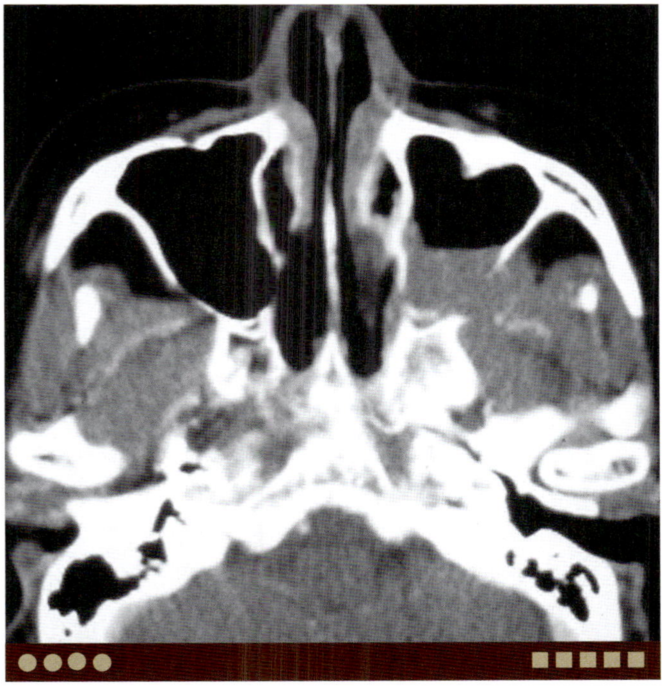

H. Lymphoma. Axial postcontrast CT demonstrates flat surface of the lesion in the left maxillary sinus. Note soft tissue density lesion extending to the left pterygomaxillary fissure and pterygopalatine fossa.

Case 3–11 Concha Bullosa

Osamu Sakai, Rania Hito

PRESENTATION

Normal variant

FINDINGS

CT demonstrates pneumatized and enlarged middle turbinate.

DIFFERENTIAL DIAGNOSIS

- Nasal polyp: A polyp is a polypoid mass arising from the nasal mucosa without osseous component.
- Submucosal tumors: Submucosal tumors show similar clinical findings to concha bullosa, however, they should be easily differentiated radiologically.

COMMENTS

This is a 63-year-old man with nasal obstruction.

Pneumatization of the turbinates is often seen as a normal variant. If the pneumatized turbinate shows an expansile change, it is called a Concha bullosa. It has been reported that this is seen in 4% to 17% of healthy adults, but is present in up to 80% of patients with sinus disease. Pneumatization most commonly occurs at the middle turbinate. Three types of pneumatization are described; pneumatization of the vertical lamella, bulbous segment, or whole turbinate.

This condition itself does not have clinical significance. Mucocele formation is uncommon but can result from obstruction of drainage of the concha bullosa. Concha bullosa can contain polyps, cysts, pyoceles, or mucoceles. It has been described that in cases where the middle turbinate is abnormally large, obstruction of the ostiomeatal complex can result in infection of the ethmoid, frontal and maxillary sinuses. The relationship between concha bullosa and chronic sinus disease is controversial as some authors report size of the concha bullosa is implicated in sinus disease whereas others report that contact of the mucosal surfaces is the pathologic factor. Other authors have found no correlation between location of concha bullosa and sinus disease. There is also a strong association between the presence of a concha bullosa and contralateral deviation of the nasal septum.

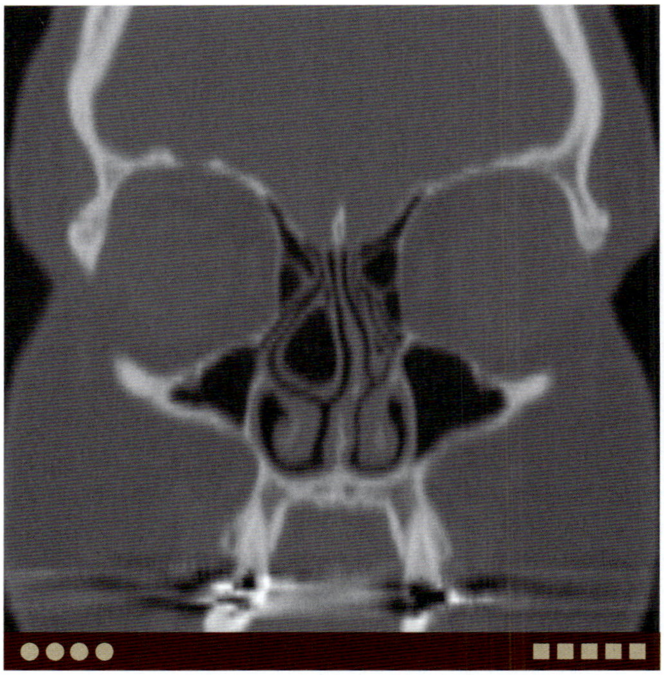

A. Concha bullosa. Coronal CT demonstrates a pneumatized and expanded right middle turbinate with mild nasal septal deviation to the left.

The surgeon must know this anatomical variant before surgery since this may mimic a polypoid or submucosal lesion endoscopically.

PEARLS

- **Pneumatization of the middle turbinate is a normal anatomic variant.**
- **It is commonly associated with nasal septal deviation.**
- **Role of concha bullosa in pathogenesis of sinus disease is controversial.**
- **Endoscopically may mimic a polypoid or submucosal lesion, thus knowledge of this variant prior to surgery is imperative.**

ADDITIONAL IMAGES (B-F)

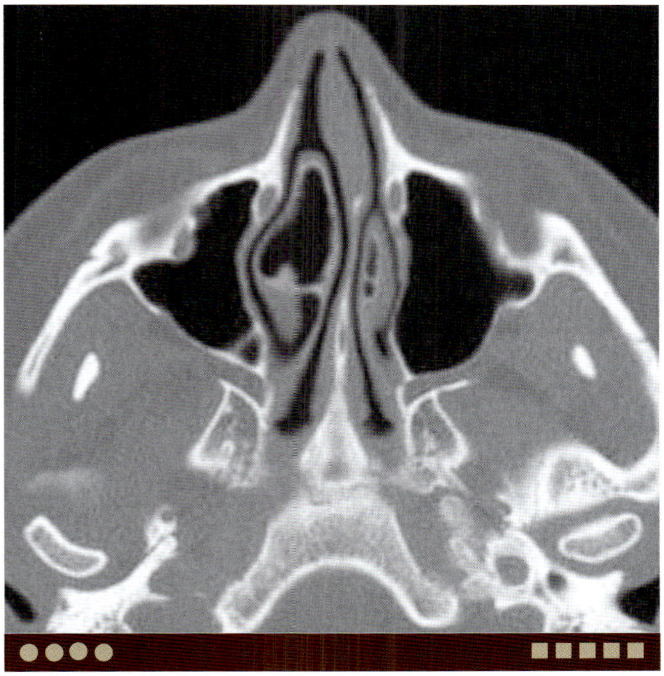

B. Concha bullosa, same patient as A. Axial CT demonstrates a pneumatized and expanded right middle turbinate.

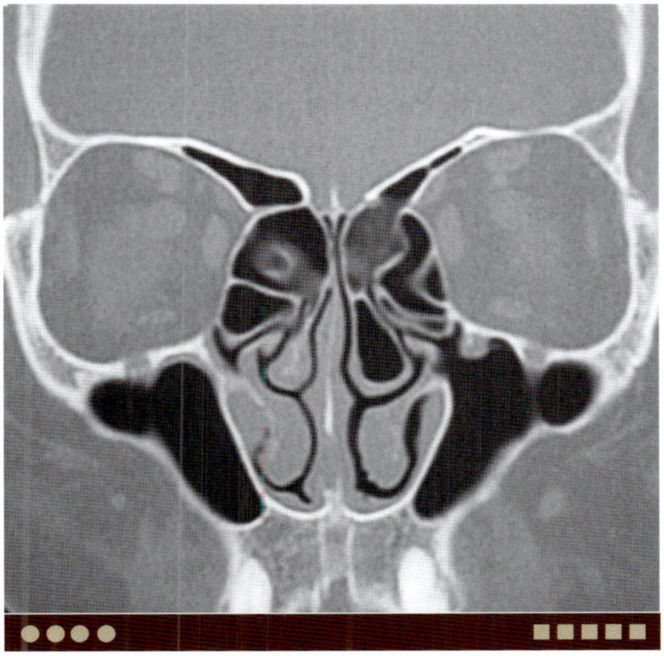

C. **Concha bullosa** in a different patient. Coronal CT demonstrates a pneumatized and mildly expanded left middle turbinate without nasal septal deviation.

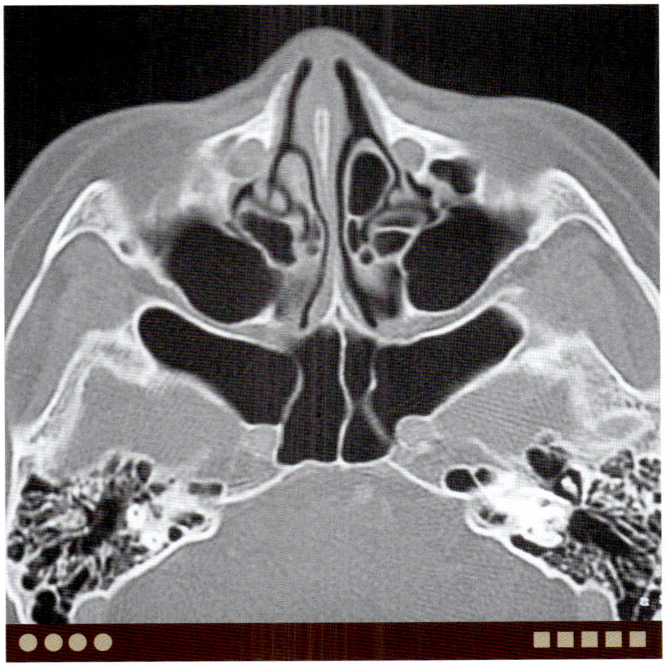

D. Concha bullosa, same patient as C. Axial CT demonstrates a pneumatized left middle turbinate. Note prominent pneumatization of the lateral recess of the sphenoid sinus bilaterally.

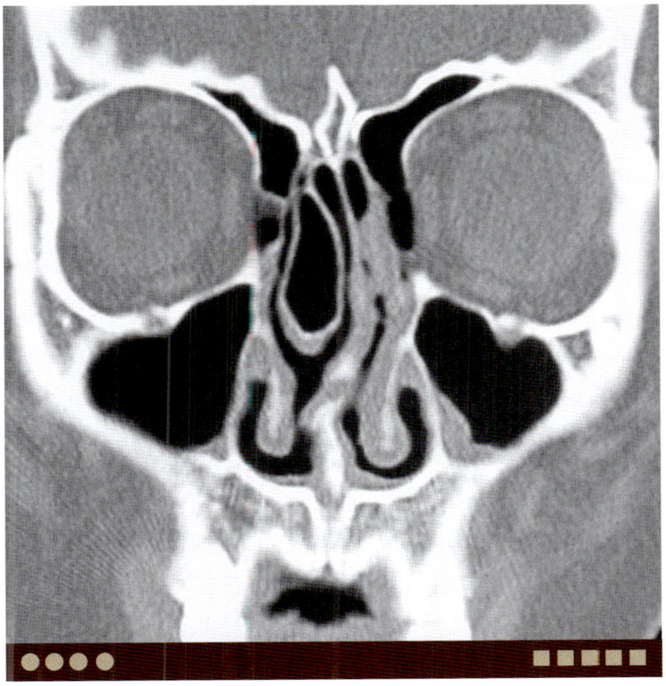

E. Concha bullosa in a different patient. Coronal CT demonstrates a pneumatized and expanded right middle turbinate with an S-shaped nasal septal deviation.

DIFFERENTIAL DIAGNOSIS IMAGES (G-H)

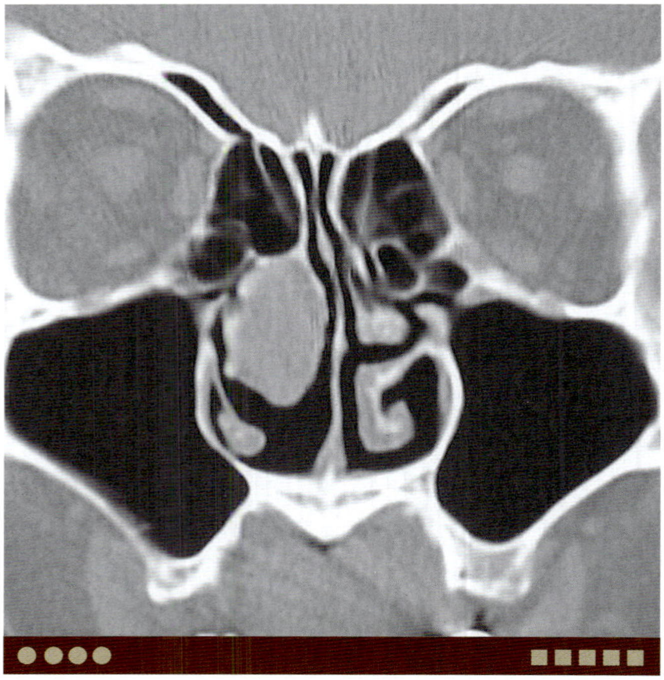

F. Concha bullosa with mucocele in a different patient. Coronal CT demonstrates a fluid-filled expanded right middle turbinate.

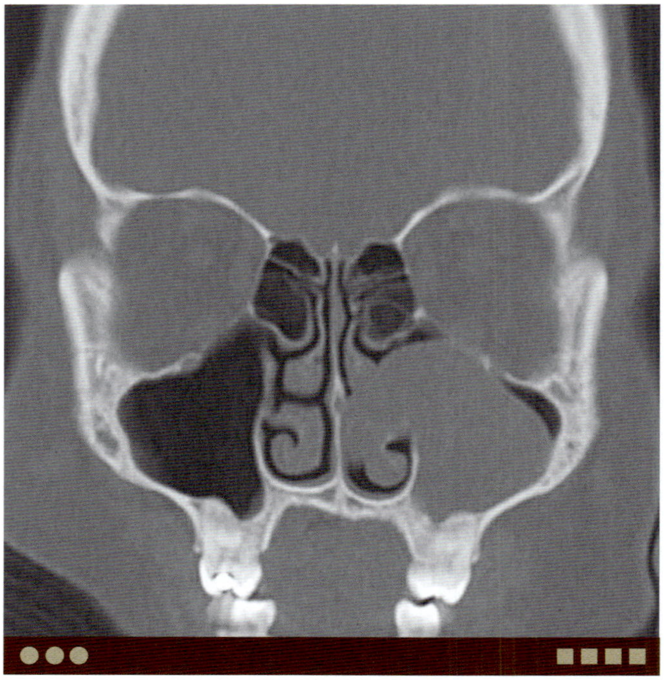

G Antrochoanal polyp. Coronal CT demonstrates a polyp extending into the nasal cavity from the maxillary sinus displacing the turbinates.

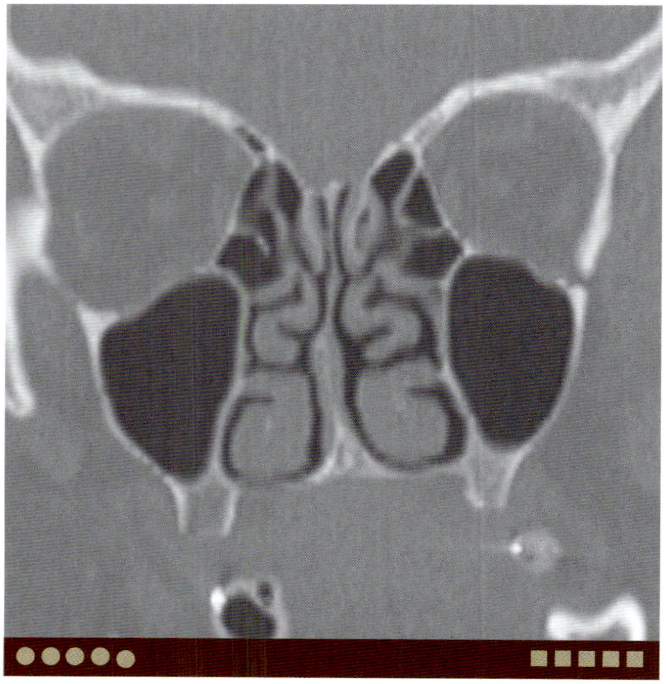

H. Paradoxical middle turbinate. Coronal CT demonstrates the middle turbinate is convex laterally and curls inward, slightly narrowing the middle meatus bilaterally.

Case 3–12 Squamous Cell Carcinoma—Maxillary Sinus

Osamu Sakai, Elisa Flower

PRESENTATION

Nasal obstruction and sinus pain.

FINDINGS

CT and MRI demonstrate opacified maxillary sinus with bone destruction.

DIFFERENTIAL DIAGNOSIS

- Sinusitis: Initial presentation of squamous cell carcinoma (SCCA) is often similar to sinusitis. Aggressive bone destruction should not be seen with sinusitis.
- Lymphoma: A large, non-necrotic mass is a common finding. Among extranodal lymphoma in the head and neck, 40% to 50% occurs in the sinonasal cavity, commonly in the nasal cavity and maxillary sinus.
- Adenoid cystic carcinoma: This is a malignant tumor which arises from the minor salivary gland. Perineural tumor spread is commonly seen.
- Adenocarcinoma and its variant: Adenocarcinoma is not common in the paranasal sinuses. Sinonasal undifferentiated carcinoma (SNUC) is very aggressive and has poor outcome.
- Inverted papilloma: Approximately 10% to 15% of inverted papillomas develop or are associated with SCCA. Careful evaluation for aggressive bone destruction is important.

COMMENTS

This is a 70-year-old man with nasal obstruction and sinus pain.

Squamous cell carcinoma (SCCA) is the most common malignant tumor in the sinonasal cavity as well as in the aerodigestive tract, and consists about 80% to 90% of all malignancy in this region. Thirty to sixty percent of these tumors occur in the maxillary sinus, and more than 80% tumors originated in other sinuses also involve the maxillary sinus. SCCA invades adjacent structures, therefore diagnosis of its extension is an important role of imaging. Ohngren line is a line crossing the medial cantus and mandibular angle, and divides the maxillary sinus into the posterosuperior and anteroinferior portions. Tumors involving the posterosuperior portion of the maxilla (above the Ohngren line) likely invade into the orbit and skullbase and extend intracranially, and have poor prognosis. About 20% of patients already have nodal metastasis at the time of diagnosis.

Perineural spread is well-known in adenoid cystic carcinoma and lymphoma, however, SCCA is the most common among the tumors presented with perineural spread because it is the most common malignancy in the head and neck. The fat planes in the pterygopalatine fossa, inferior orbital fissure, foramen rotundum, and Vidian (pterygoid) canal must be carefully evaluated in all cases for possible perineural tumor spread. To identify normal fat density or signal in these locations reassure that the tumor does not reach these structures.

It may be difficult to differentiate the tumor from secondary inflammatory change on noncontrast CT. Intravenous contrast is necessary to evaluate tumor extent. SCCA usually demonstrates lesser enhancement compared to normal or inflamed mucosa on CT and MRI, and can be easily differentiated. Additionally, SCCA demonstrates lower signal than normal or inflamed mucosa on T2W images.

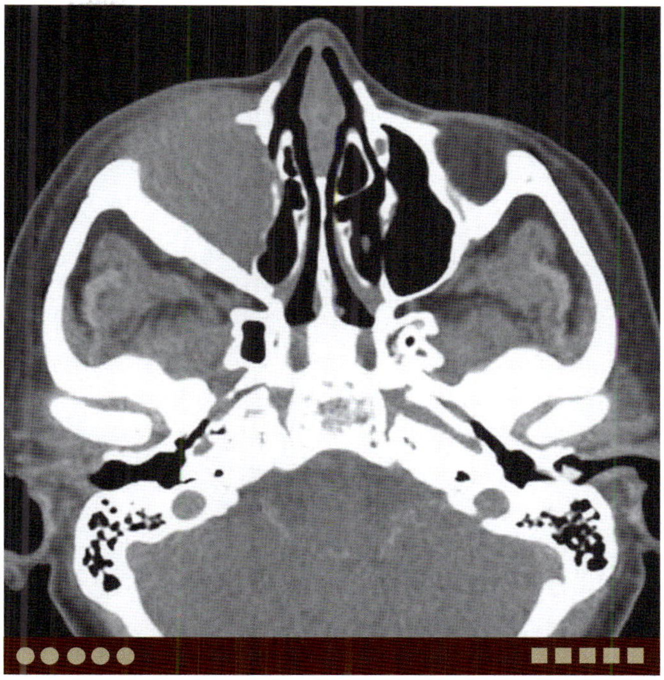

A. SCCA. Axial CT demonstrates a solid tumor occupying the right maxillary sinus, destructing the anterior wall and extending to the superficial soft tissue.

PEARLS

- **SCCA is the most common malignant tumor in the sinonasal cavities.**
- **SCCA is often seen in the maxillary sinus. Posterosuperior involvement suggests poor prognosis.**
- **Always evaluate fat planes in the pterygopalatine fossa, inferior orbital fissure, foramen rotundum, and Vidian (pterygoid) canal for possible perineural tumor spread.**

ADDITIONAL IMAGES (B-G)

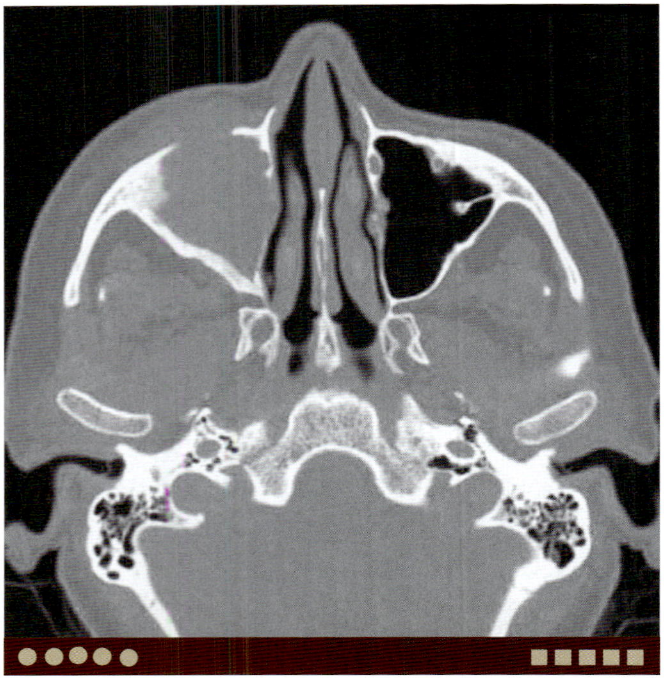

B. SCCA, same patient as A. Axial bone window CT demonstrates destruction of the anterior wall of the right maxillary sinus.

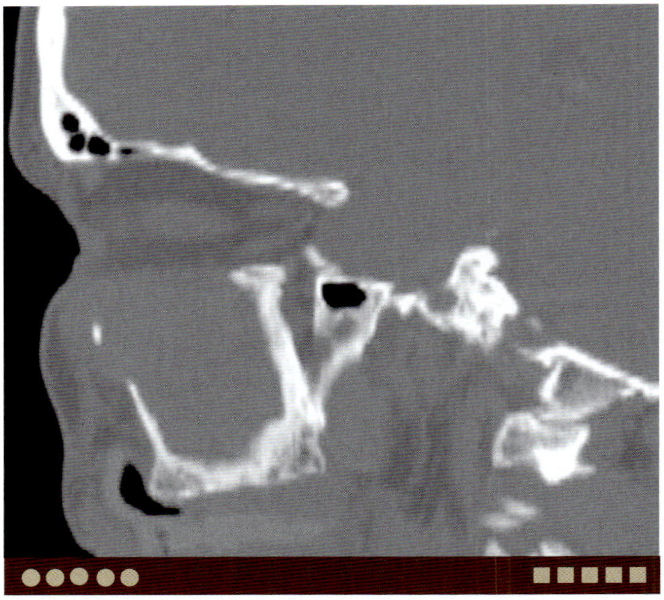

C. SCCA, same patient as A. Sagittal bone window CT demonstrates destruction of the anterior and superior walls of the maxillary sinus.

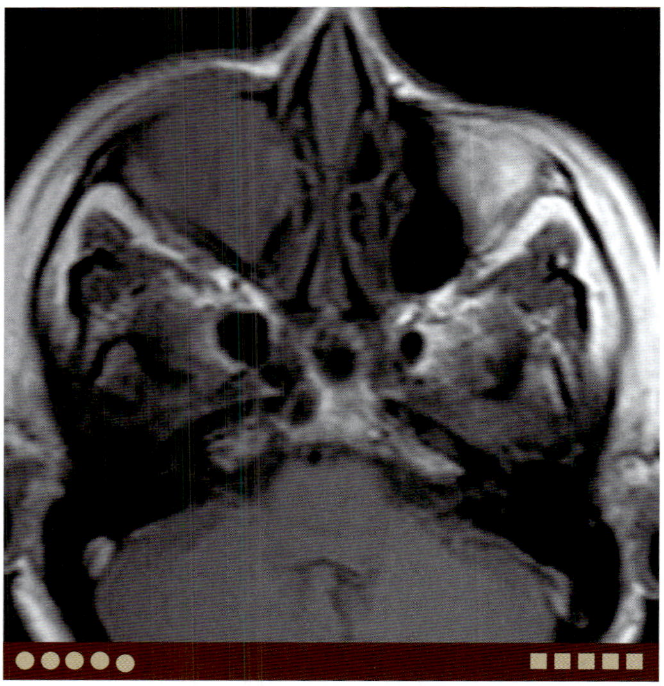

D. SCCA, same patient as A. Axial T1W MR image demonstrates a low-signal tumor extending beyond the anterior wall of the right maxillary sinus.

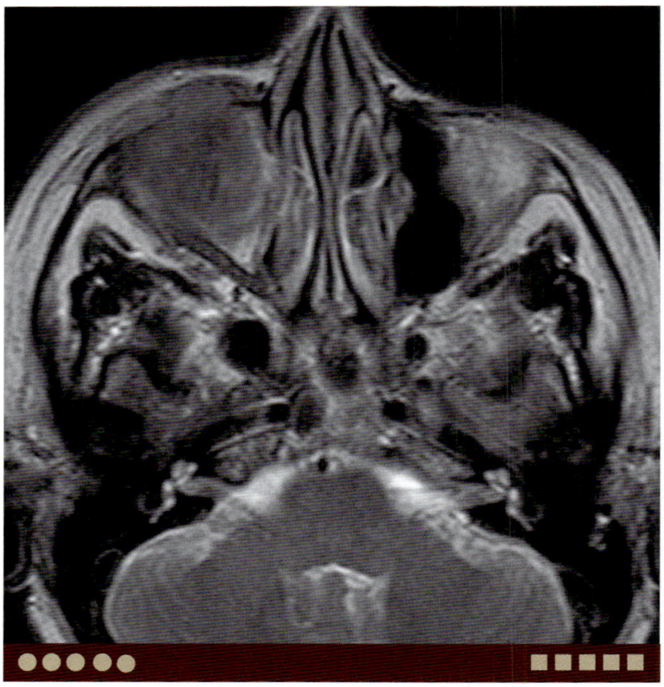

E. SCCA, same patient as A. Axial T2W MR image demonstrates intermediate-to-low signal in the tumor.

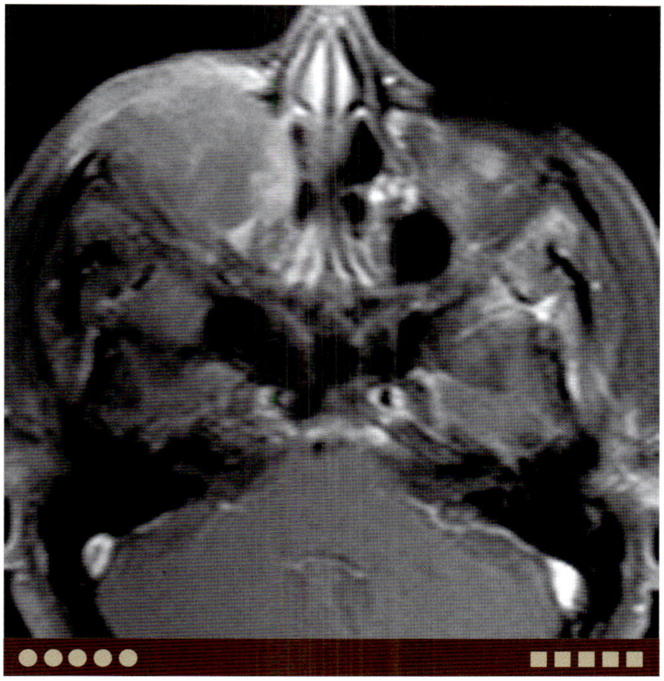

F. SCCA, same patient as A. Axial postcontrast fat-suppressed T1W MR image demonstrates mild enhancement of the tumor. Note more avid enhancement of the normal sinonasal mucosa.

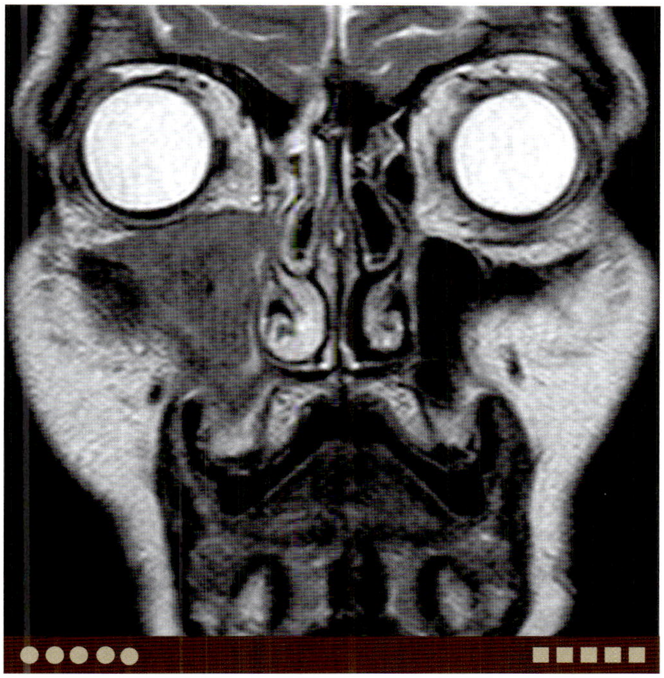

G. SCCA, same patient as A. Coronal T2W image demonstrates intermediate-to-low signal in the tumor. Note clear signal difference between the tumor and normal mucosa.

DIFFERENTIAL DIAGNOSIS IMAGES (H-J)

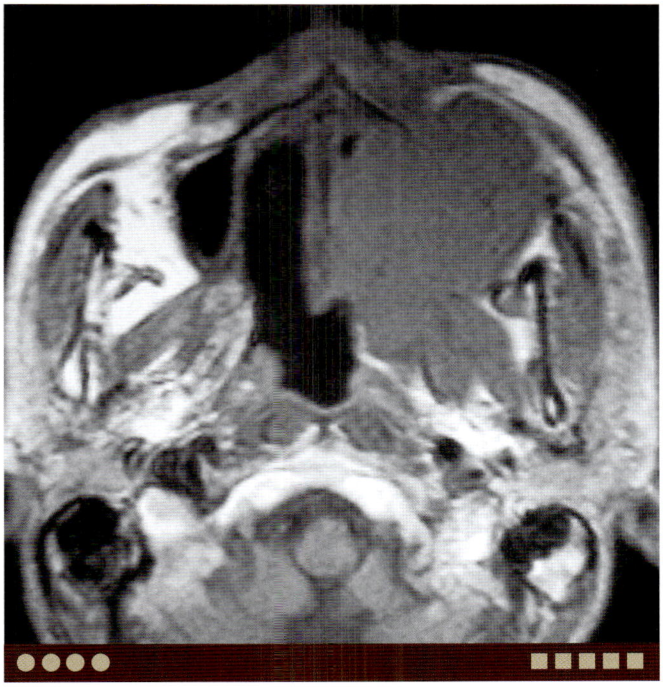

H. Lymphoma. Axial T1W MR image demonstrates a large, homogenous, and low-signal tumor in the left maxillary sinus.

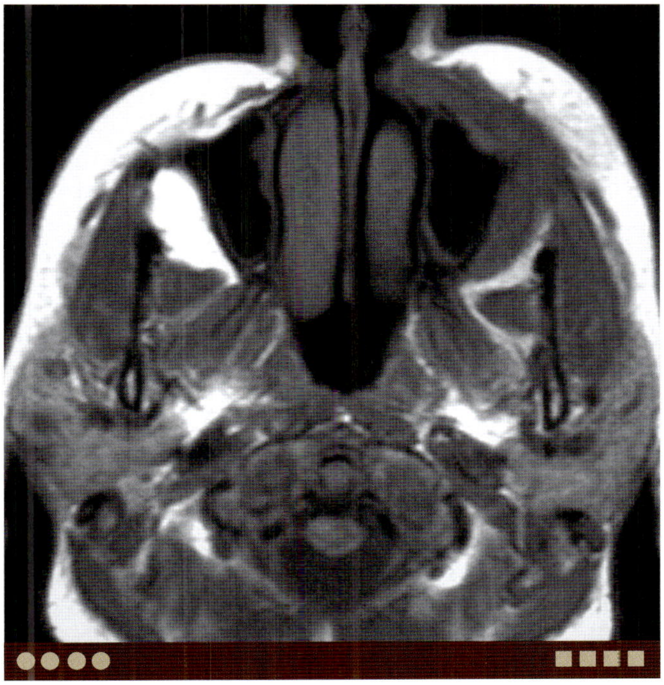

I. Lymphoma in a different patient. Axial T1W MR image demonstrates a homogenous, low-signal tumor extending along the left maxillary sinus wall.

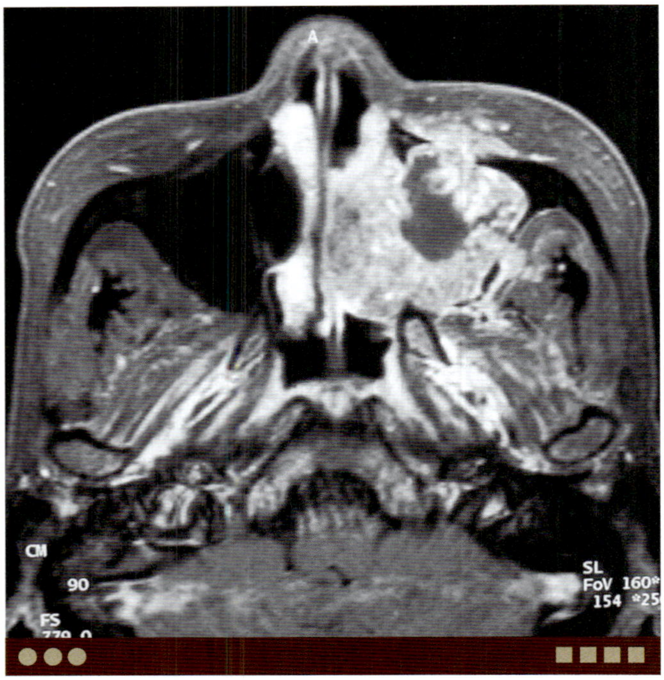

J. Adenosquamous cell carcinoma. Axial postcontrast fat-suppressed T1W MR image demonstrates a heterogeneously enhancing tumor destructing the walls of the left maxillary sinus and invading adjacent structures.

Case 3–13 Fungal Sinusitis—Allergic Fungal Sinusitis

Osamu Sakai, Brooke Devenney-Cakir

PRESENTATION

Nasal obstruction.

FINDINGS

CT demonstrates opacified ethmoid and maxillary sinuses with high-density material without osseous destruction.

DIFFERENTIAL DIAGNOSIS

- Acute sinusitis: This condition typically demonstrates water density opacification of the paranasal sinuses often with air-fluid levels.
- Chronic sinusitis: Heterogeneous density can be seen in the opacified sinuses with inspissated secretion and dystrophic calcification. Sclerotic changes of the osseous walls and contraction of the affected sinus is often seen.
- Wegener's granulomatosis: This condition demonstrates nonspecific inflammatory changes in the sinonasal cavities, however often aggressive findings such as nasal septal perforation and orbital involvement are seen. Intracranial extension of the disease occurs occasionally.

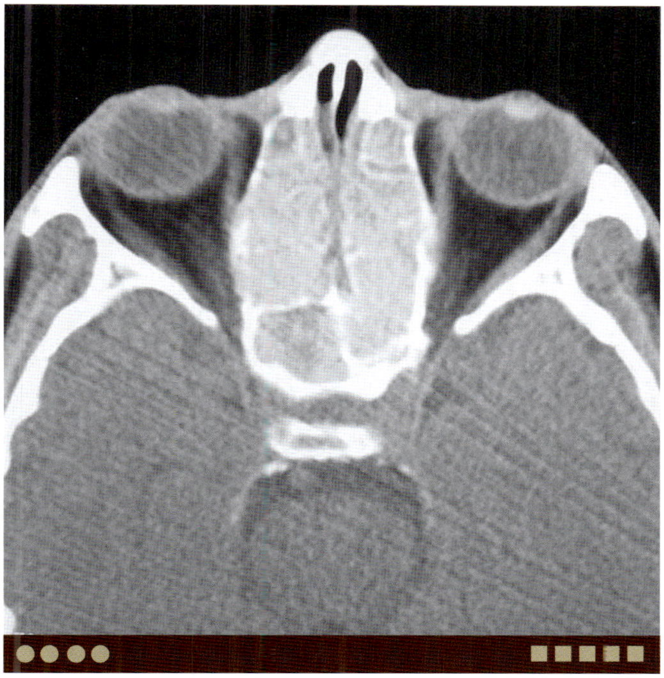

A. Allergic aspergillus sinusitis. Axial CT demonstrates high-density material within the ethmoid sinuses.

COMMENTS

This is a 50-year-old man with history of asthma, now presented nasal obstruction and sinus pain.

Fungal sinusitis can be divided into noninvasive and invasive forms. The noninvasive form of fungal sinusitis includes allergic fungal sinusitis and mycetoma/fungus ball. Allergic fungal sinusitis is the most common form of fungal infection in the paranasal sinuses and occurs as an allergic reaction to inhaled environmental fungi in the air, which causes thick mucinous debris in the sinuses. This condition is seen in patients with allergic rhinitis, asthma, and nasal polyps, who are not immunocompromised. Elevated total fungus-specific immunoglobulin E (IgE) concentration is seen. Allergic fungal sinusitis is commonly seen with *Aspergillus fumigatus*, *Curvularia lunata*, *Bipolaris*, and *Drechslera* infection.

CT commonly demonstrates diffusely opacified paranasal sinuses with high-density material. This high-density material has very dark signal on MRI, particularly on T2W images due to significant T2 shortening effect by inspissated secretions and manganese, which is characteristic for fungal infection. If MRI is performed prior to CT, opacified sinuses may demonstrate no signal mimicking air, and this condition could be completely missed. Therefore, CT should be performed first if sinusitis is suspected clinically, and the paranasal sinuses should be carefully evaluated on multiple sequences when MRI is performed prior to CT for other reasons. Bone destruction/erosion is rare in patients with allergic fungal sinusitis. However, preservation of bones and fat in the adjacent areas, such as the orbit, pterygopalatine fossa, and pterygomaxillary fissure should always be evaluated to identify aggressive, invasive processes associated with fungal infections which can manifest as bone destruction, orbital and intracranial extension, cavernous sinus invasion, hematogenous dissemination, and vasculitis, especially in the immunocompromised patient.

PEARLS

- **Allergic fungal sinusitis is seen in immunocompetent patients, often in conjunction with allergic rhinitis and asthma.**
- **Allergic fungal sinusitis causes high-density sinuses on CT and black sinuses on MRI.**
- **Proteinaceous or inspissated secretions are the most common cause of a high-density sinus. The high density is not pathognomonic for fungal infection.**
- **Invasive fungal sinusitis is typically seen in immunocompromised patients. Intraorbital or intracranial extension is common, and can cause cavernous sinus invasion, hematogenous dissemination, and vasculitis.**

ADDITIONAL IMAGES (B-D)

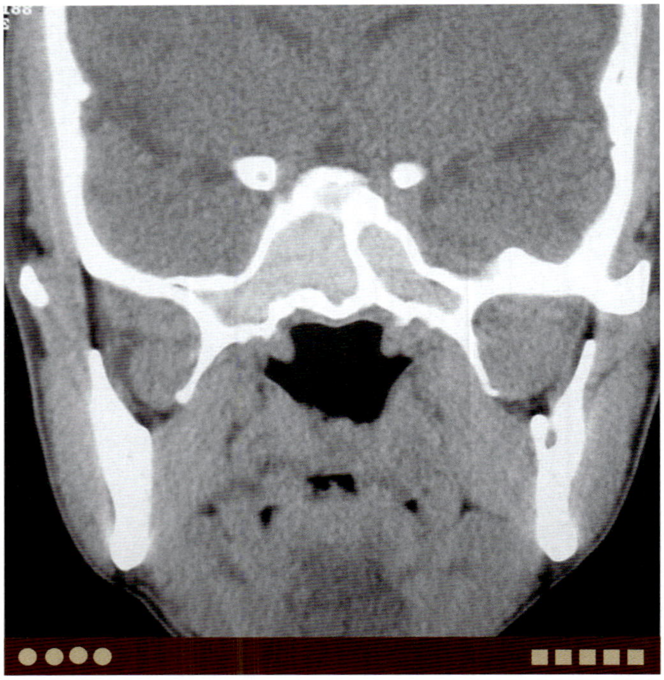

B. Allergic aspergillus sinusitis, same patient as A. Coronal CT shows high-density material within the sphenoid sinuses.

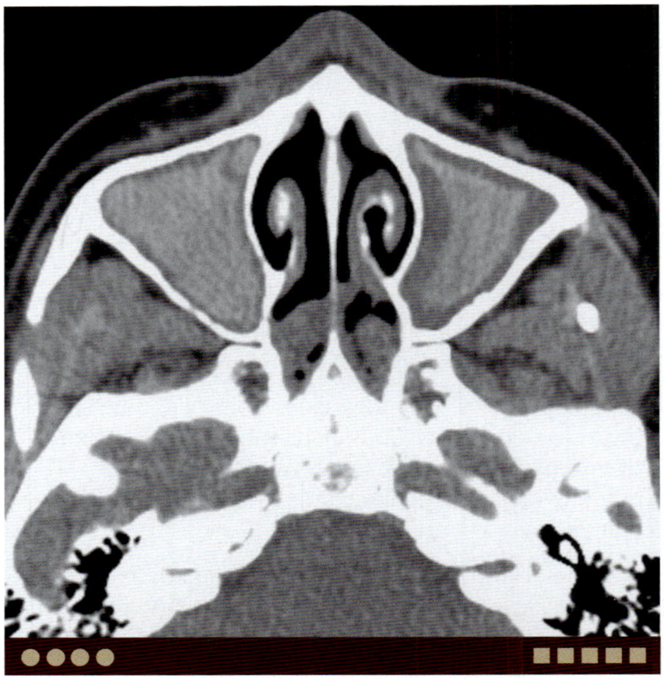

C. Allergic aspergillus sinusitis in a different patient. Axial CT soft tissue window shows low-density mucosal thickening/submucosal edema within the maxillary sinuses with central high-density opacification.

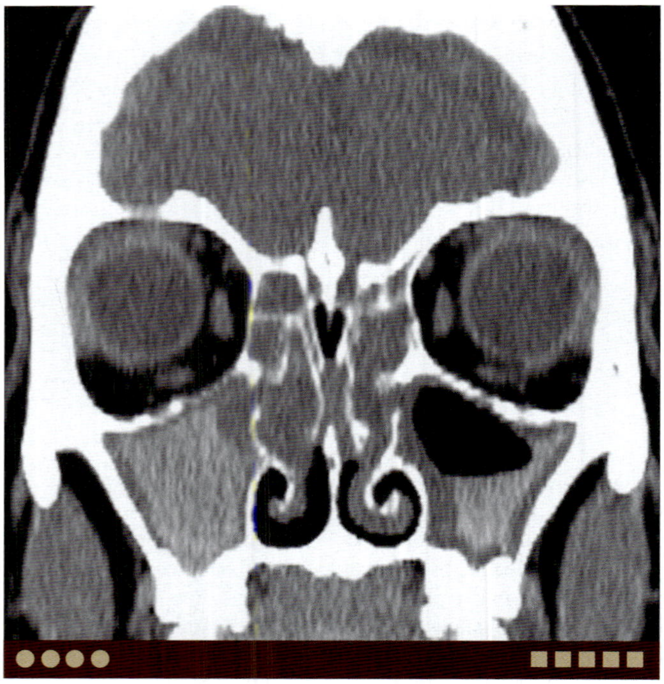

D. Allergic aspergillus sinusitis, same patient as C. Coronal CT shows low-density mucosal thickening/submucosal edema within the maxillary sinuses with central high-density opacification. Low-density opacification within the ethmoid air cells and nasal cavities consistent with sinonasal polyps.

DIFFERENTIAL DIAGNOSIS IMAGES (E-J)

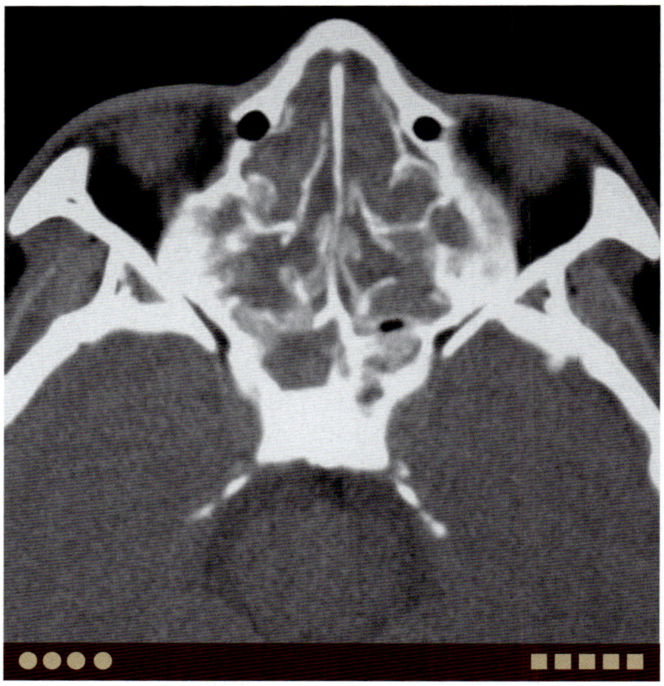

E. Polyposis with inspissated secretions. Axial CT shows opacification and mild expansion of the ethmoid sinuses with multiple foci of high density consistent with inspissated secretions.

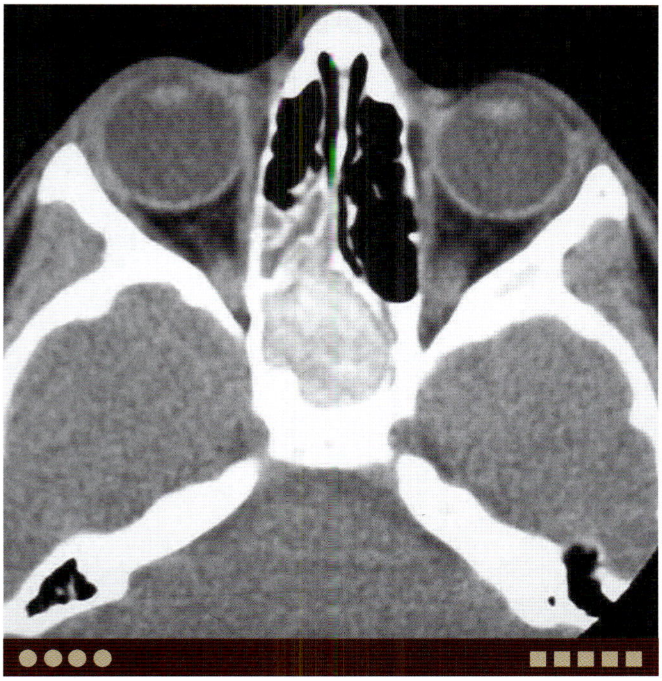

F. Mycetoma. Axial CT shows high-density opacification of the sphenoid sinus.

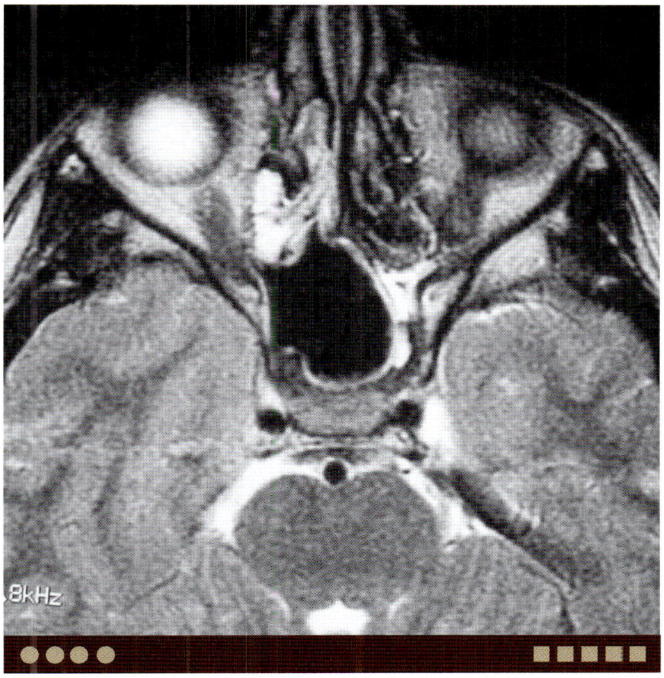

G. Mycetoma, same patient as F. Axial T2W MR image demonstrates signal-void in the sphenoid sinus due to significant T2 shortening effect by the opacified material.

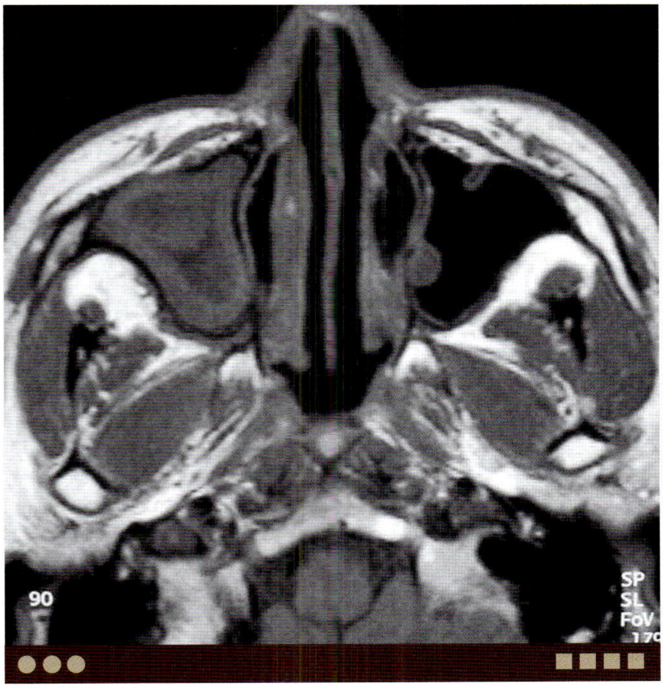

H. Acute invasive fungal sinusitis, aspergillus. Axial T1W MR image demonstrates opacified right maxillary sinus. Note abnormal signal posterior to the posterolateral wall of the maxillary sinus, in the pterygomaxillary fissure and pterygopalatine fossa.

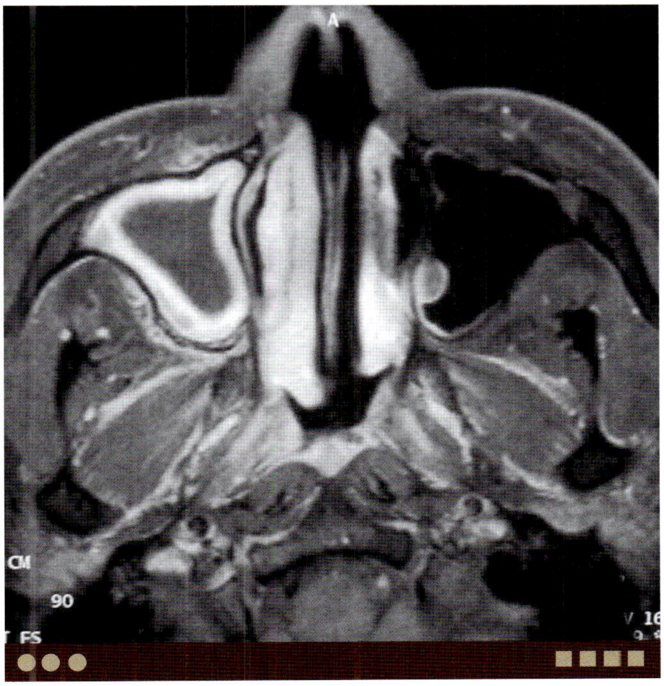

I. Acute invasive fungal sinusitis, same patient as H. Axial postcontrast fat-suppressed T1W MR image demonstrates abnormal enhancement in the pterygomaxillary fissure and pterygopalatine fossa, in addition to enhancement of the mucosa of the opacified right maxillary sinus.

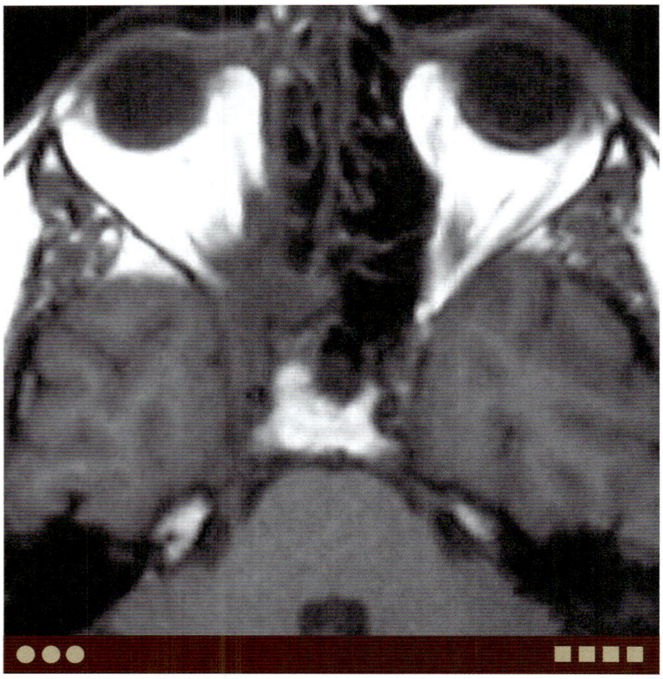

J. Invasive fungal sinusitis, *Mucor* infection. Axial T1W MR image demonstrates an abnormal low-signal lesion in the right posterior ethmoid air cell invading the orbital apex and paracavernous region, obliterating the normal fat.

Case 3–14 Osteoma

Osamu Sakai, Elisa Flower

PRESENTATION

Incidental finding.

FINDINGS

CT demonstrates osseous high density in the frontal sinus.

DIFFERENTIAL DIAGNOSIS

- Fibrous dysplasia: This is usually larger than osteoma and can involve multiple contiguous bones.
- Ossifying fibroma: This tumor shows a very similar appearance to fibrous dysplasia but generally presents with more aggressive features and requires radical surgical approach.
- Osteoblastoma: This is very rare in the paranasal sinuses and usually appears as a sclerotic lesion with a radiolucent rim.
- Osteochondroma: This contains a cartilaginous component and is very rare in the paranasal sinuses.
- Reactive osteoblastic changes: Malignant tumors, commonly squamous cell carcinoma can cause prominent osteosclerotic changes.

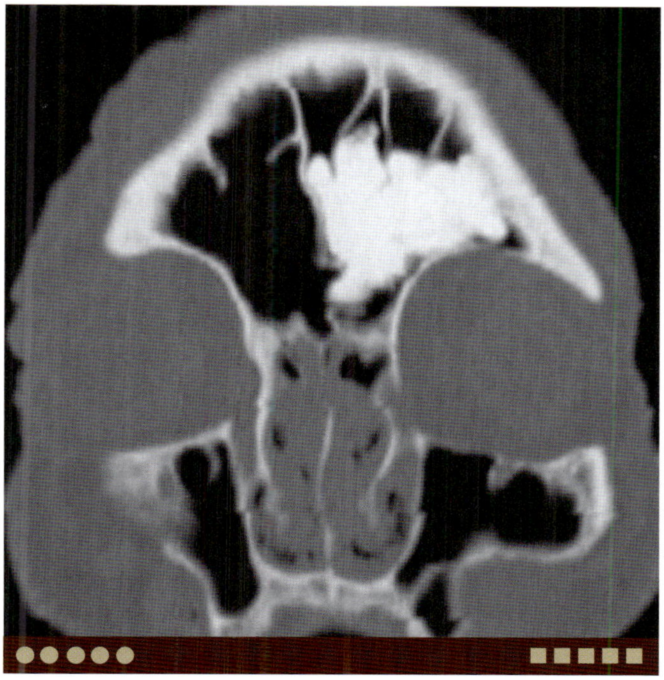

A. Osteoma. Coronal CT demonstrates a lobulated compact osseous lesion in the left frontal sinus without soft tissue density.

COMMENTS

This is a 50-year-old man with nasal obstruction scanned for chronic sinusitis.

Osteomas are commonly seen in the frontal sinus (70–80%), followed by the ethmoid, maxillary, and sphenoid sinuses in descending order of frequency. Incidence of osteoma has been reported at about 3%. The size varies from a few millimeters to a few centimeters. The density varies based on its histological components; compact bone like cortex, fatty marrow, and prominent fibrous component. It may be difficult to differentiate osteoma from ossifying fibroma or other benign fibro-osseous lesions. Multiple osteomas can be seen associated with Gardner's syndrome, one of the familial polyposis. In young patients, osteomas can be found before polyposis is diagnosed.

An osteoma is seen as a well-defined high-density lesion in the sinus on CT. On MRI it is generally seen as signal void, however, appearance on MRI varies depending on the matrix. If there is a portion of heterogeneity or soft tissue density/signal, other benign fibro-osseous lesion or osteochondroma should be suspected. Presence of bone destruction and large soft tissue component strongly suggests malignancy such as metastasis, osteosarcoma, or chondrosarcoma.

PEARLS

- **Osteomas are commonly seen in the frontal sinus, followed by the ethmoid, maxillary, and sphenoid sinuses in descending order of frequency.**
- **Multiple osteomas can be seen associated with Gardner's syndrome.**
- **Presence of bone destruction and large soft tissue component strongly suggests malignancy such as metastasis, osteosarcoma, or chondrosarcoma.**

ADDITIONAL IMAGES (B-F)

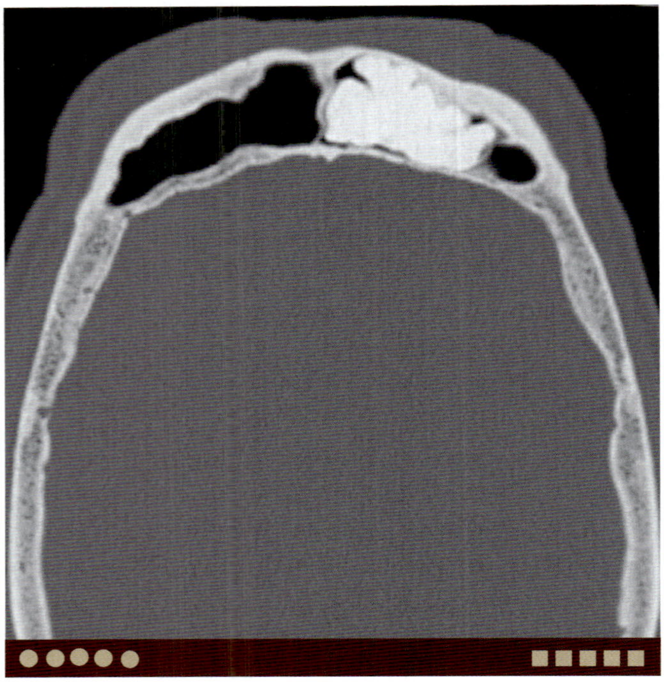

B. Osteoma, same patient as A. Axial CT demonstrates the lobulated compact osseous lesion in the left frontal sinus.

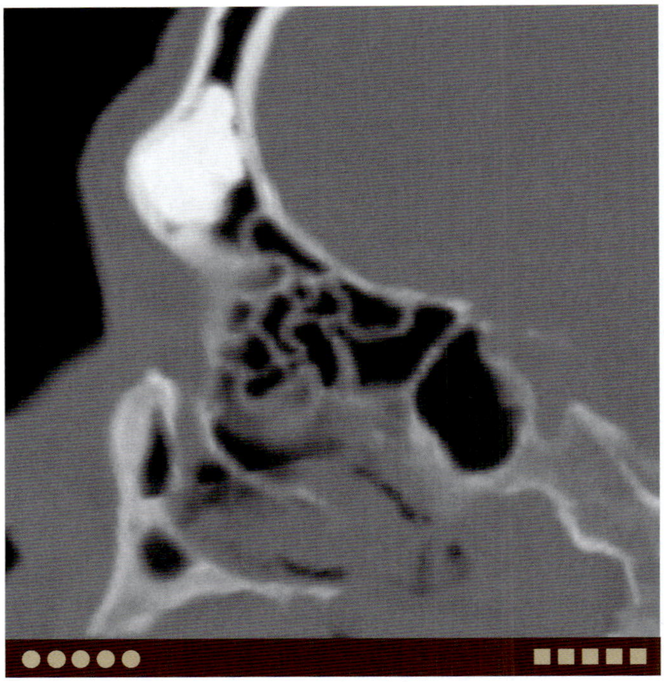

C. Osteoma, same patient as A. Sagittal CT demonstrates no obstruction of the frontoethmoid junction by the osteoma.

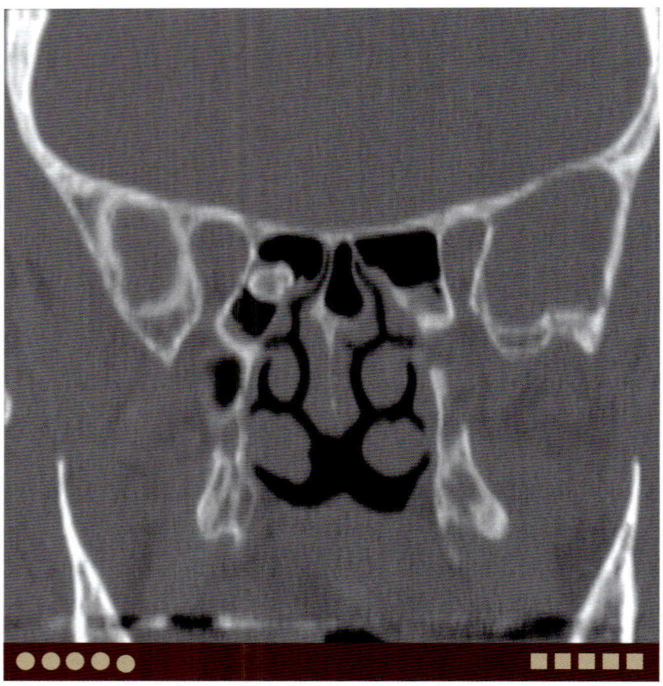

D. **Osteoma** in a different patient. Coronal CT demonstrates a small osteoma in the right posterior ethmoid. The lesion is well-corticated and contains bone marrow.

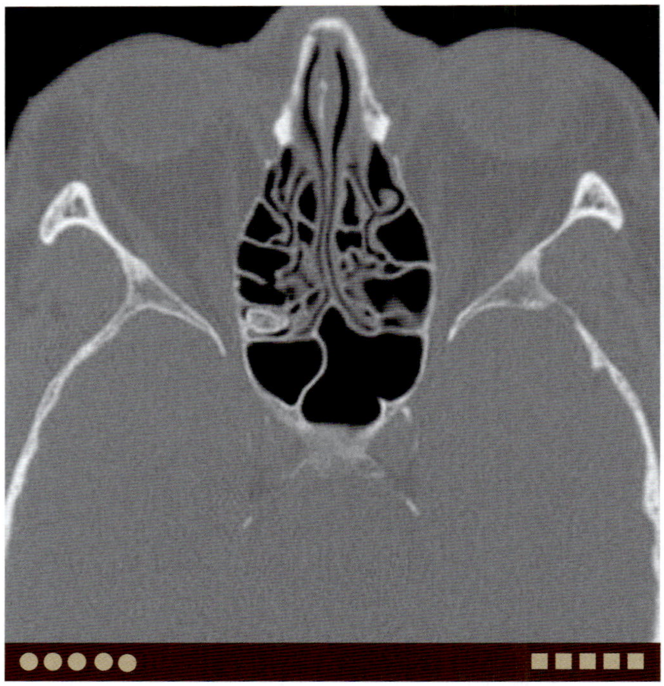

E. Osteoma, same patient as D. Axial CT demonstrates a small osteoma in the right posterior ethmoid. The lesion is well-corticated and contains bone marrow.

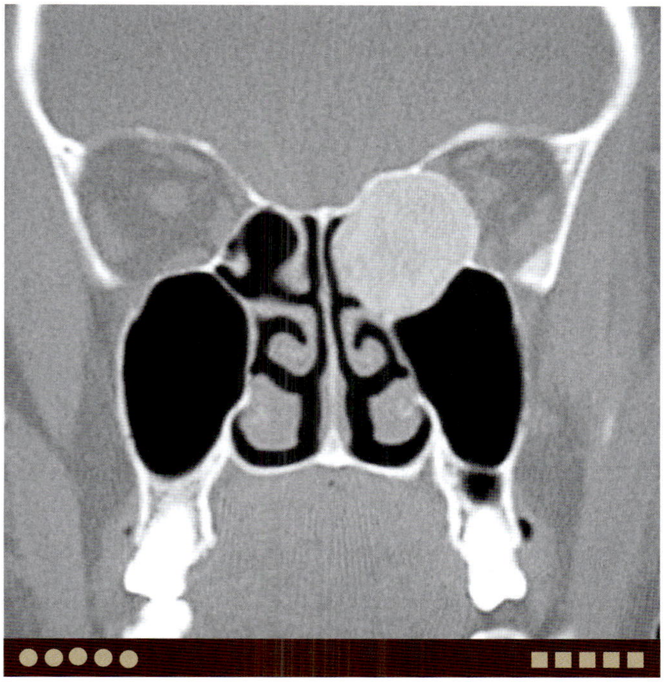

F. **Osteoma** in a different patient. Coronal CT demonstrates a large ground-glass density lesion in the left posterior ethmoid causing mass-effect onto the left orbit. Radiologically, this lesion cannot be differentiated from other benign fibroosseous lesions such as ossifying fibroma or fibrous dysplasia.

DIFFERENTIAL DIAGNOSIS IMAGES (G-I)

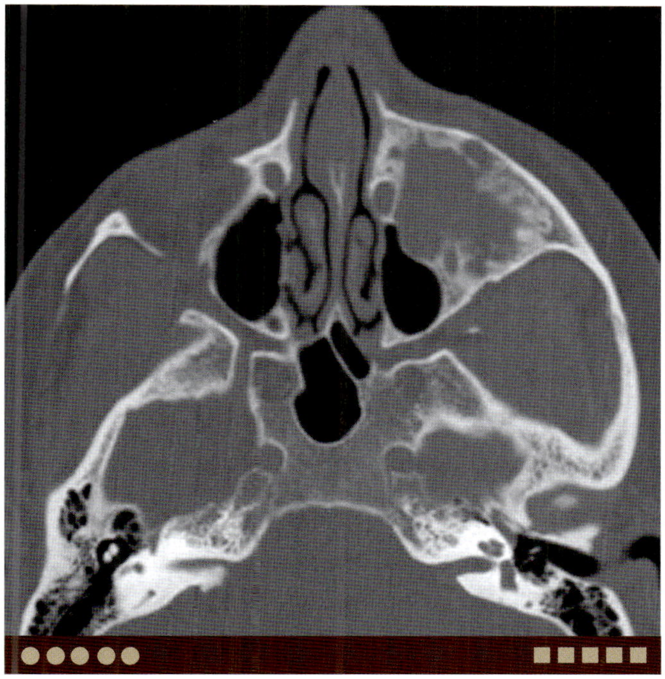

G. **Fibrous dysplasia**. Axial CT demonstrates a heterogeneous density osseous lesion in the left maxilla with internal soft tissue density.

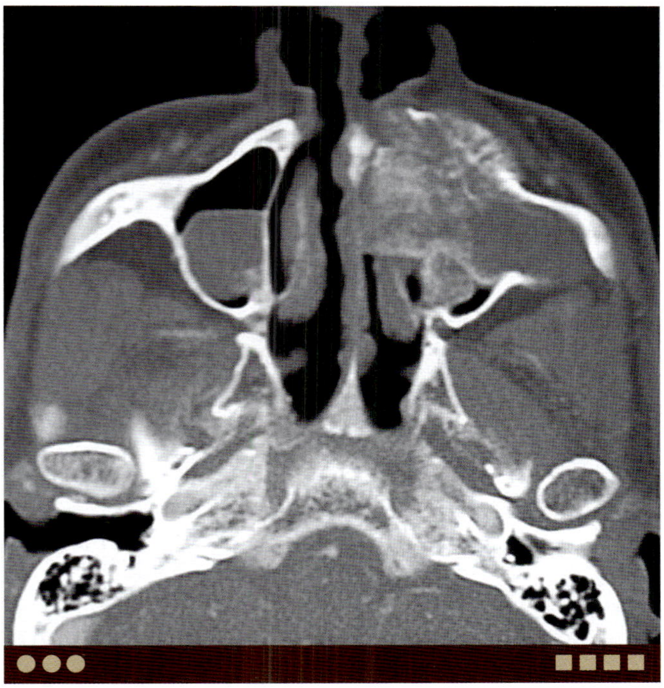

H. **Hemangioma**. Axial CT demonstrates an expansile osseous lesion with coarse trabeculation in the anteromedial portion of the left maxilla with secondary obstructive change.

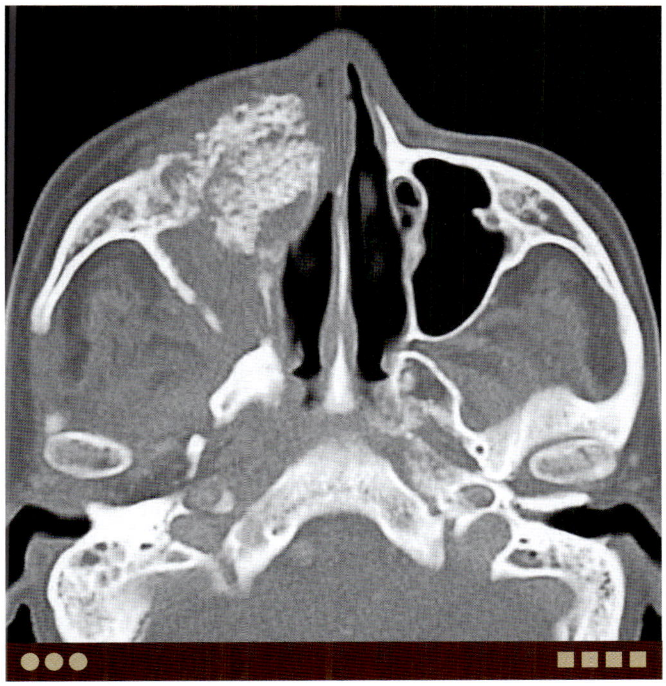

I. **Mucoepidermoid carcinoma**. Axial CT demonstrates a heterogeneous, sclerotic lesion centered in the anteromedial portion of the right maxillary sinus with soft tissue component. Note destructive and infiltrative change to suggest malignancy in the posterolateral wall of the right maxillary sinus.

Case 3–15 Adenoid Cystic Carcinoma

Osamu Sakai, Elisa Flower

PRESENTATION

Nasal obstruction and sinus pain.

FINDINGS

CT demonstrates a soft tissue mass destructing the sinus wall and obliterating the adjacent fat plane. MRI shows variable T2 signal depending on cellularity and avid enhancement of the tumor.

DIFFERENTIAL DIAGNOSIS

- Squamous cell carcinoma (SCCA): SCCA is the most common malignancy in the sinonasal cavity as well as in the rest of the head and neck. The density/signal and enhancement of the lesion is usually heterogeneous, and aggressive bone destruction is commonly seen.
- Lymphoma: Lymphoma is relatively rare in the sinonasal cavity, although it is the most common nonepithelial malignant tumor in this region. It tends to show homogeneous density/signal without necrosis.
- Mucoepidermoid carcinoma: This is a common minor salivary gland malignant tumor. Low-grade tumors tend to be cystic with a benign appearance, while high-grade tumors tend to be solid with infiltrative margins.

COMMENTS

This is a 71-year-old man with nasal obstruction and sinus pain.

Adenoid cystic carcinoma is a common minor salivary gland malignancy which often occurs in the palate and nasal cavity. However, it is relatively rare in the paranasal sinuses, and makes up to approximately 10% of malignant neoplasm in this region. Within the paranasal sinuses, the maxillary sinus is most frequently involved, followed in order by the ethmoid, sphenoid, and frontal sinuses. Adenoid cystic carcinoma is commonly seen in patients in their thirties through seventies and is rare in young patients under 20.

Imaging findings are often nonspecific; high signal on T2W, low signal on T1W images, and enhancement after intravenous contrast. Decreased T2 signal reflects higher cellularity of the tumor and suggests a worse prognosis.

Perineural tumor spread is often seen in adenoid cystic carcinoma. Its diagnosis is very important for staging and planning for treatment. Fat in the pterygopalatine fossa, pterygomaxillary fissure, and inferior orbital fissure should have pristine low density on CT and high signal on T1W images. Evaluation on precontrast T1W images is extremely important to diagnose perineural tumor spread in the skull base. Occasionally, skip lesions may be present, therefore it is important to assess the entire course of the nerve. Meckel's cave, foramen rotundum and Vidian canal should be extensively evaluated. Missing perineural tumor spread results in "early recurrence or metastasis" after surgery.

Nodal metastasis is not very common. Hematogeneous metastasis is seen in 20%–50% of patients with adenoid cystic carcinoma.

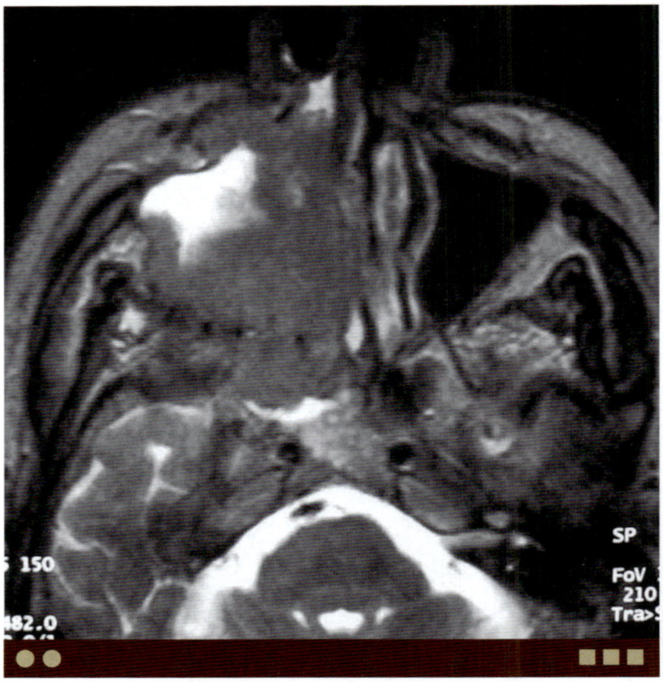

A. Adenoid cystic carcinoma. Axial T2W MR image demonstrates an intermediate-to-low signal lesion in the right maxillary sinus involving almost the entire wall of the maxillary sinus and invading the right pterygoid plate and pterygomaxillary fissure. Decreased T2 signal suggests higher cellularity and poor prognosis.

PEARLS

- **Adenoid cystic carcinoma is a common minor salivary gland malignancy and often occurs in the palate and nasal cavity. It is relatively rare in the paranasal sinuses, but when seen it most frequently involves the maxillary sinus.**
- **Imaging findings are often nonspecific; usually high on T2W and low on T1W images, however decreased T2 signal suggests higher cellularity and poor prognosis.**
- **Perineural tumor spread is common with adenoid cystic carcinoma.**

ADDITIONAL IMAGES (B-G)

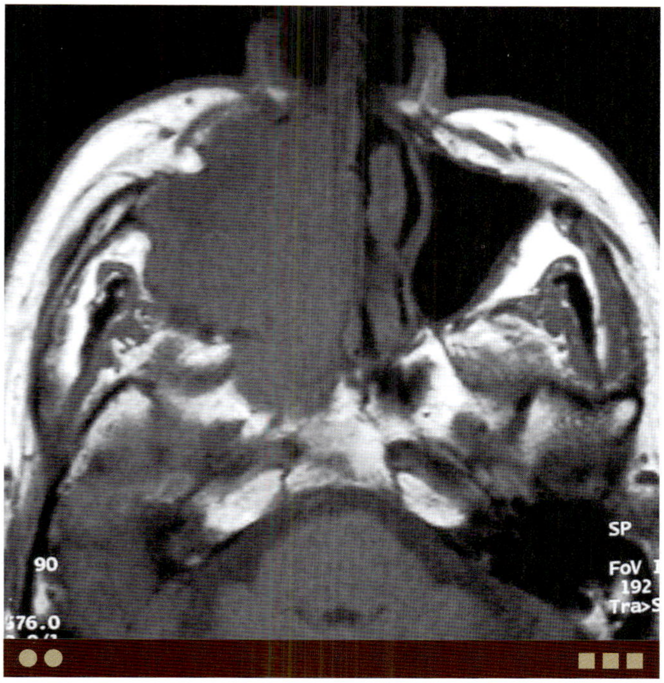

B. Adenoid cystic carcinoma, same patient as A. Axial T1W MR image demonstrates a homogeneously low-signal lesion in the right maxillary sinus extending to the right pterygoid plate and pterygomaxillary fissure obliterating the retroantral fat pad.

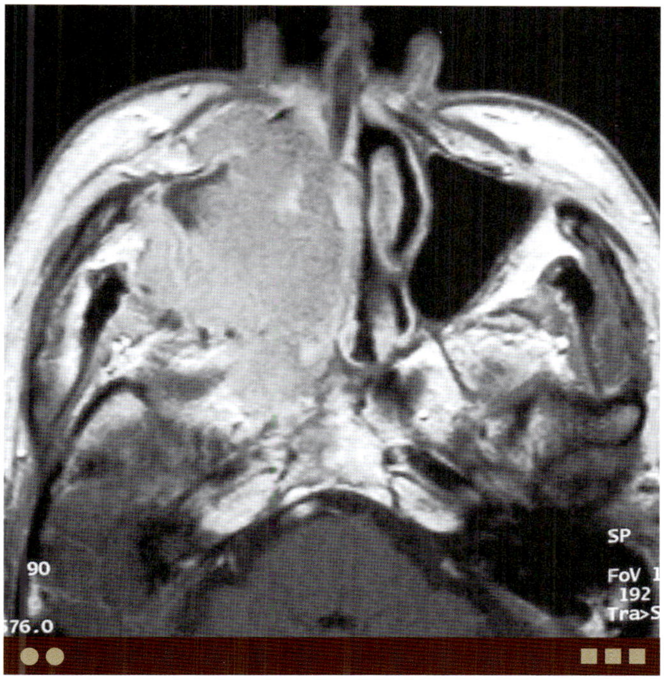

C. Adenoid cystic carcinoma, same patient as A. Axial postcontrast T1W MR image demonstrates homogeneous enhancement of the lesion.

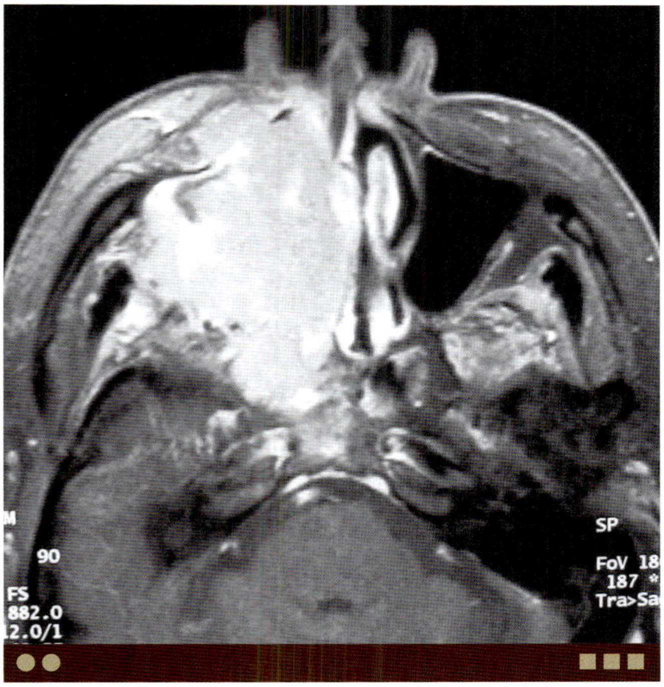

D. Adenoid cystic carcinoma, same patient as A. Axial postcontrast fat-suppressed T1W MR image demonstrates homogeneous enhancement of the lesion. In addition, there is abnormal enhancement in the subcutaneous soft tissue over the right maxilla due to denervation by tumor invasion of the infraorbital nerve/V2.

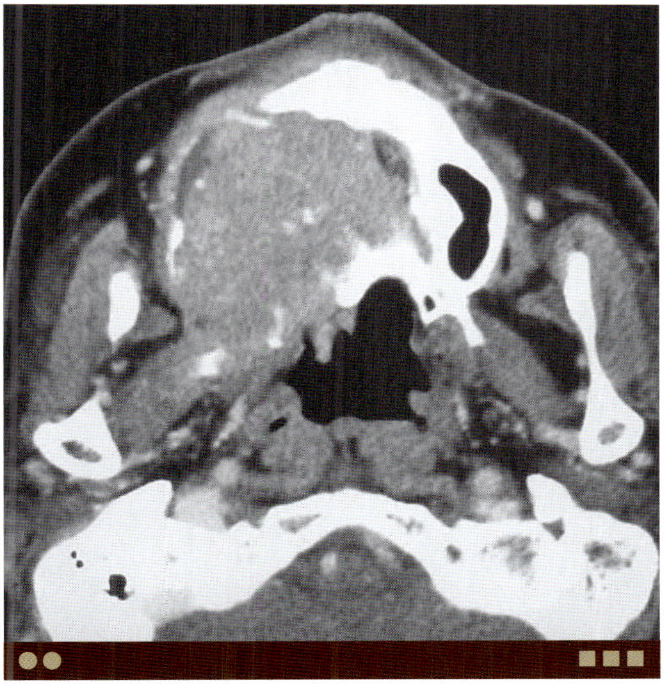

E. Adenoid cystic carcinoma, same patient as A. Axial postcontrast CT demonstrates a mildly enhancing large tumor in the right maxillary sinus. The tumor invades the hard palate and crosses the midline, and posteriorly invades the pterygoid plate and lateral pterygoid muscle.

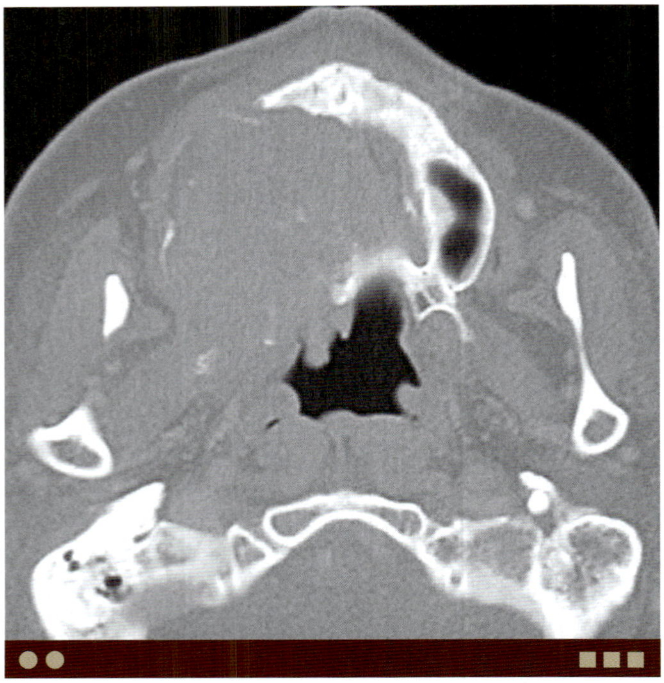

F. Adenoid cystic carcinoma, same patient as A. Axial bone window CT demonstrates significant bone destruction in the right maxilla, palate, and pterygoid plate.

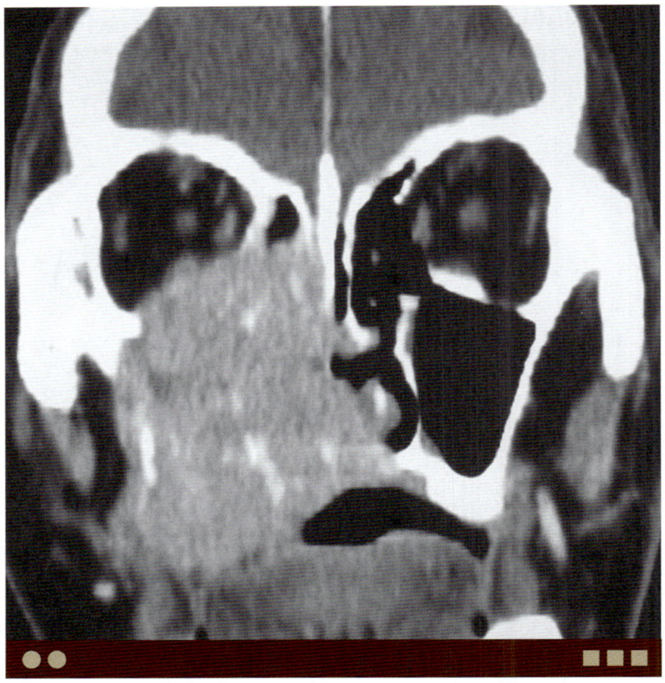

G. Adenoid cystic carcinoma, same patient as A. Coronal postcontrast CT demonstrates an enhancing large tumor in the right maxillary sinus invading the orbit, ethmoid, alveolar ridge, and hard palate crossing the midline.

DIFFERENTIAL DIAGNOSIS IMAGES (H-J)

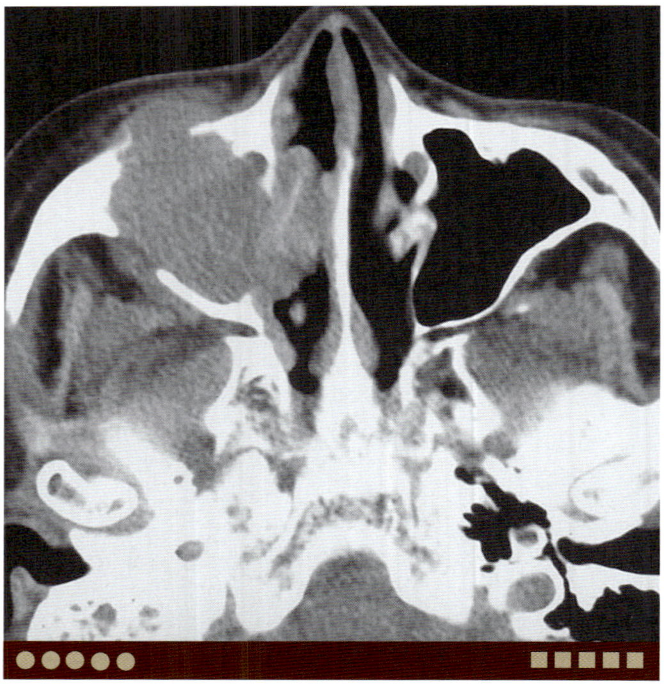

H. SCCA. Axial CT demonstrates a large tumor in the right maxillary sinus destructing the sinus walls and invading the superficial soft tissue as well as the retroantral fat.

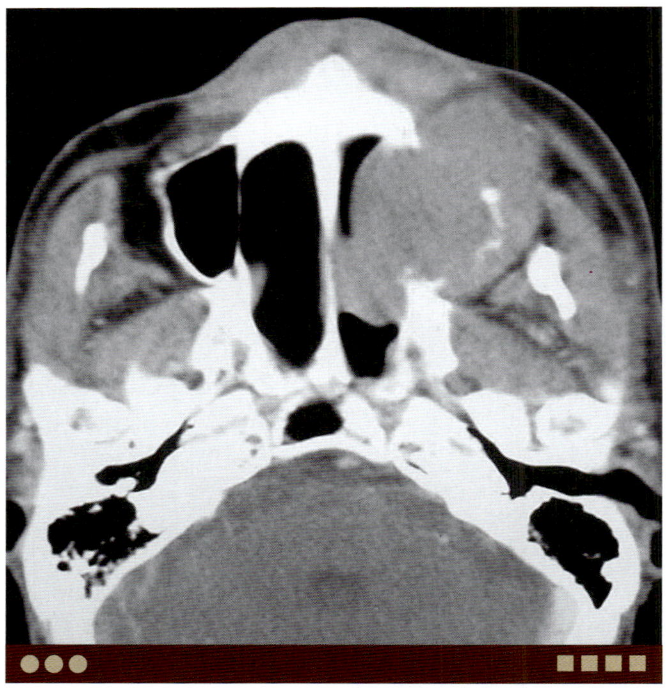

I. Lymphoma. Axial contrast-enhanced CT demonstrates a large homogeneous, mildly enhancing tumor in the left maxilla. Note spared "frame" of the sinus wall even with significant tumor extension outside of the sinus.

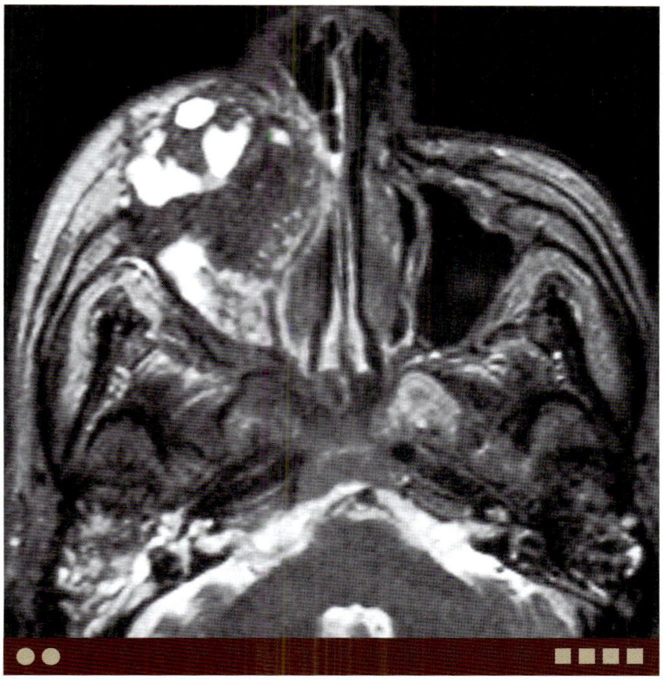

J. Mucoepidermoid carcinoma. Axial T2W MR image demonstrates a predominantly low-signal tumor with cystic components destructing the anterior wall of the right maxillary sinus.

Case 3-16 Lymphoma

Osamu Sakai, Elisa Flower

PRESENTATION

Nasal obstruction and cheek numbness.

FINDINGS

CT and MRI demonstrate a large tumor with homogeneous density/signal without necrosis.

DIFFERENTIAL DIAGNOSIS

- Squamous cell carcinoma (SCCA): This is the most common malignant tumor in the sinonasal cavities. SCCA often shows heterogeneous density/signal and enhancement, and aggressive bone destruction.
- Adenoid cystic carcinoma: This is a malignant tumor which arises from the minor salivary gland. Perineural tumor spread is commonly seen.
- Plasmacytoma: Plasmacytoma commonly involves the mandible, but it is rare in the paranasal sinuses. Moderate-to-marked enhancement is usually seen.

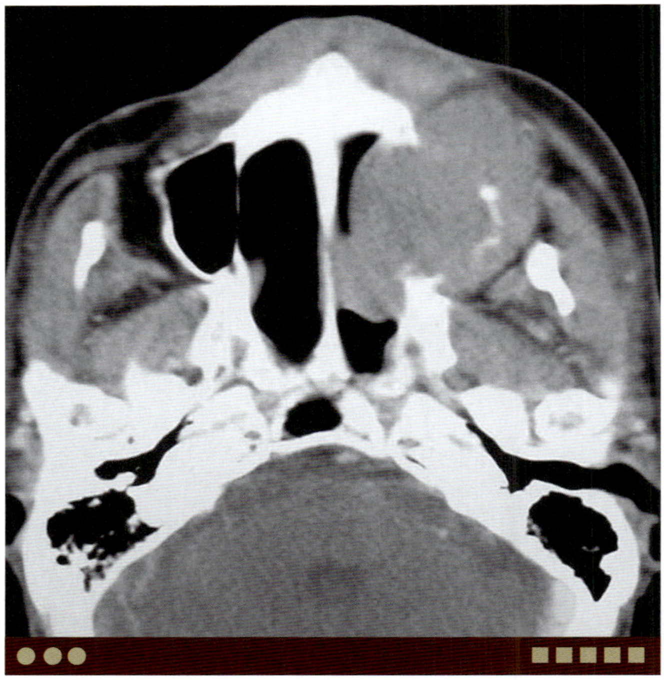

A. Lymphoma. Axial contrast-enhanced CT demonstrates a large homogenous density tumor extending beyond the anterior and posterolateral walls of the left maxillary sinus. No necrosis is noted despite the large tumor size.

COMMENTS

This is a 54-year-old woman with nasal obstruction and left cheek numbness.

Lymphoma in the neck usually occurs in lymph nodes, however, about 10% of lymphoma occur extranodally. Among extranodal lymphoma in the head and neck, 40%–50% occurs in the sinonasal cavity, commonly in the nasal cavity and maxillary sinus. If sinonasal lymphoma presents with nodal metastasis, 5-year survival will be halved.

Lymphoma usually demonstrates relatively large homogeneous mass demonstrating intermediate enhancement on CT. On MRI, lymphoma usually demonstrates intermediate signal on all sequences and be differentiated from normal or inflamed mucosa, which demonstrates higher signal on T2W images and postcontrast T1W images. Bone destruction can be seen, however, lymphoma shows a more infiltrative or permeative pattern sparing preexisting structures. Bone remodeling or erosion is not rare in lymphoma. We should remember that bone remodeling does not always suggest a benign process. As seen in adenoid cystic carcinoma, perineural tumor spread is common in lymphoma. Normal fat density or signal in the pterygopalatine fossa, pterygomaxillary fissure, inferior orbital fissure, foramen rotundum, and Vidian canal should be confirmed to rule out perineural tumor spread.

PEARLS

- **Lymphoma usually demonstrates homogeneous density on CT and homogenous signal which is intermediate on all MR sequences.**
- **Perineural tumor spread is common in lymphoma.**
- **Involvement of osseous structures may manifest as a permeative pattern sparing preexisting structures or remodeling/ erosion if lymphoma occurs adjacent to the bone.**

ADDITIONAL IMAGES (B-G)

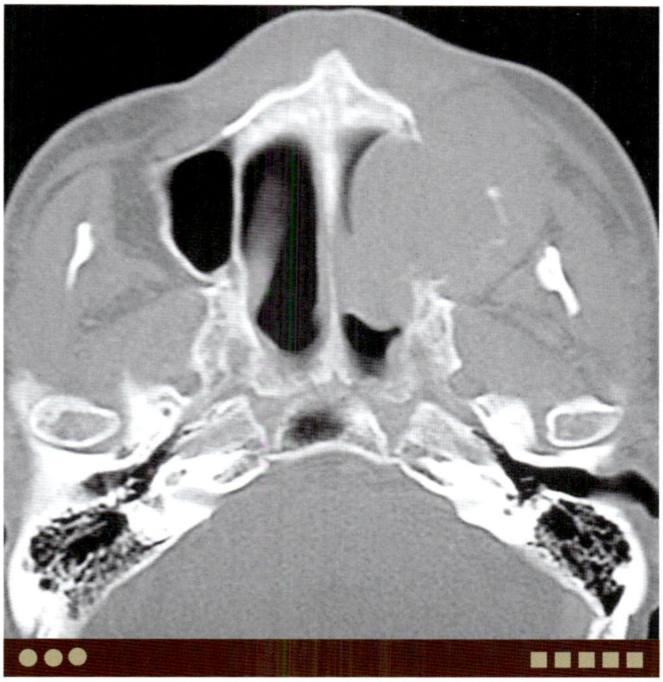

B. Lymphoma, same patient as A. Axial bone window CT demonstrates relatively preserved shape of the osseous walls of the left maxillary sinus.

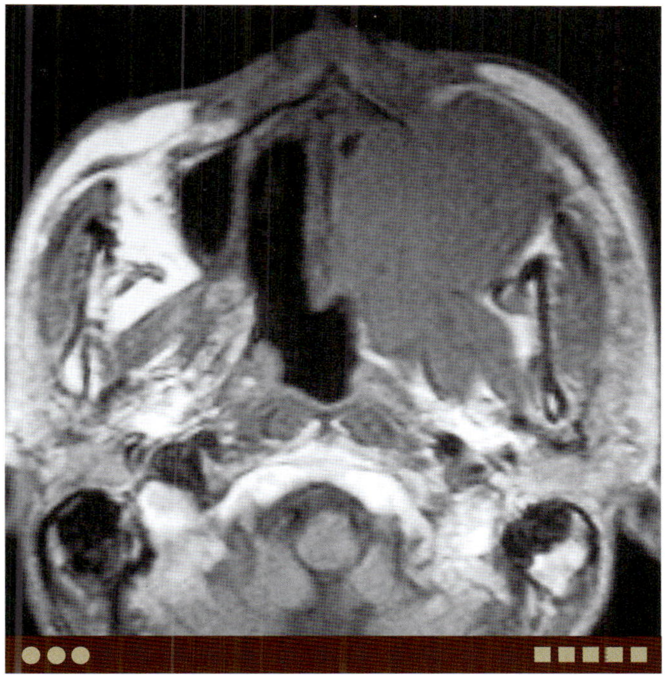

C. Lymphoma, same patient as A. Axial T1W image demonstrates homogeneous low signal in the tumor.

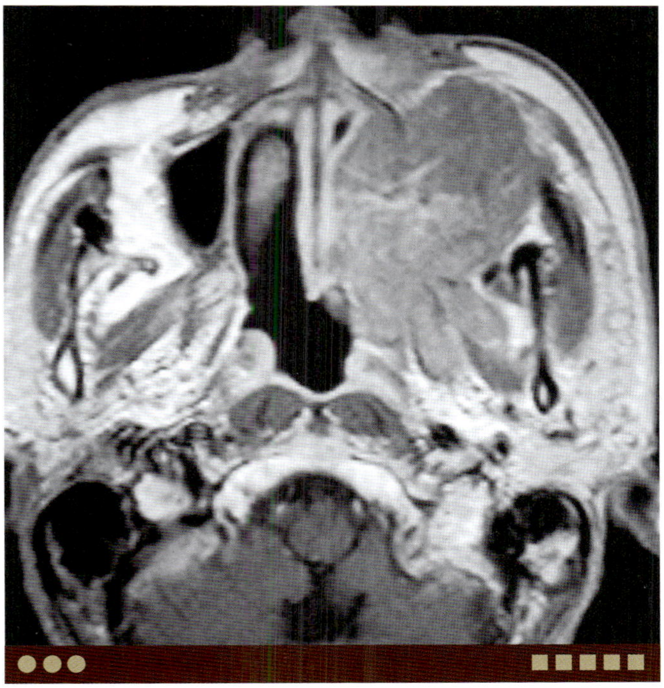

D. Lymphoma, same patient as A. Axial postcontrast T1W image demonstrates mild enhancement within the tumor. Note infiltrative tumor extension into the pterygoid muscles.

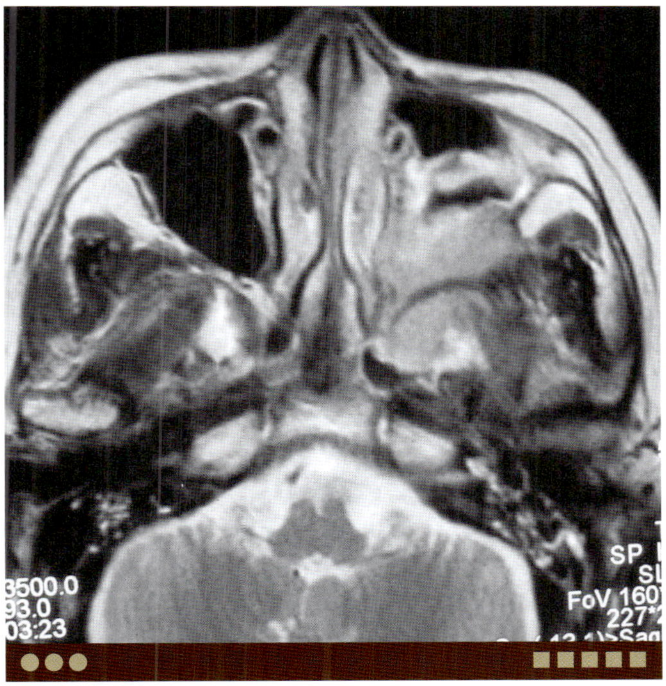

E. Lymphoma in a different patient. Axial T2W image demonstrates a homogenous intermediate-signal lesion centered in the pterygopalatine fossa and infiltrating into the pterygoid plate and remodeling the posterolateral wall of the maxillary sinus.

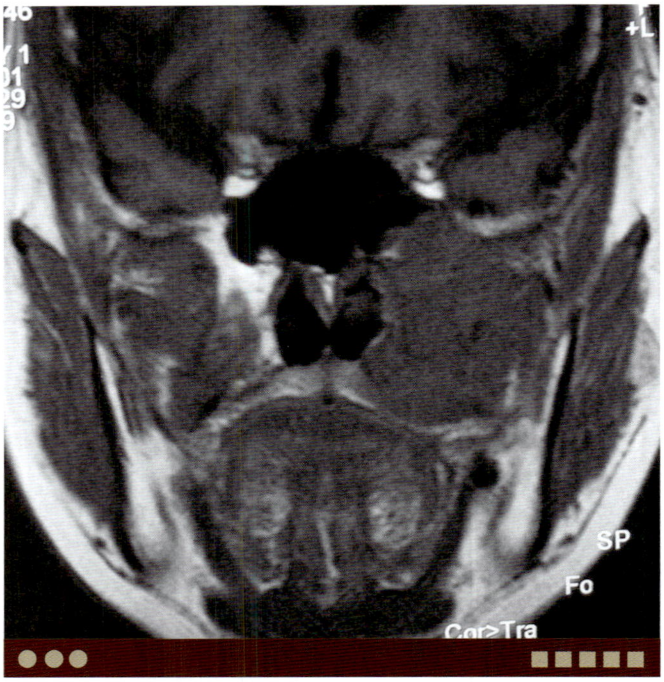

F. Lymphoma, same patient as E. Coronal T1W image demonstrates a large low-signal lesion infiltrating into the left pterygoid plate and muscles, and palate.

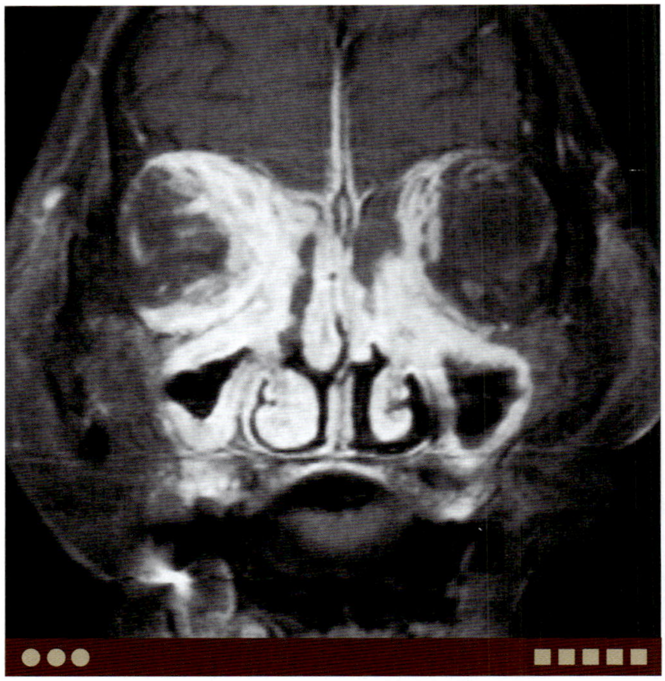

G. Lymphoma in a different patient. Coronal postcontrast fat-suppressed T1W image demonstrates diffuse enhancement in the maxillary sinuses and the medial portion of the orbit bilaterally. Note abnormal dural enhancement along the anterior skull base and falx.

DIFFERENTIAL DIAGNOSIS IMAGES (H-J)

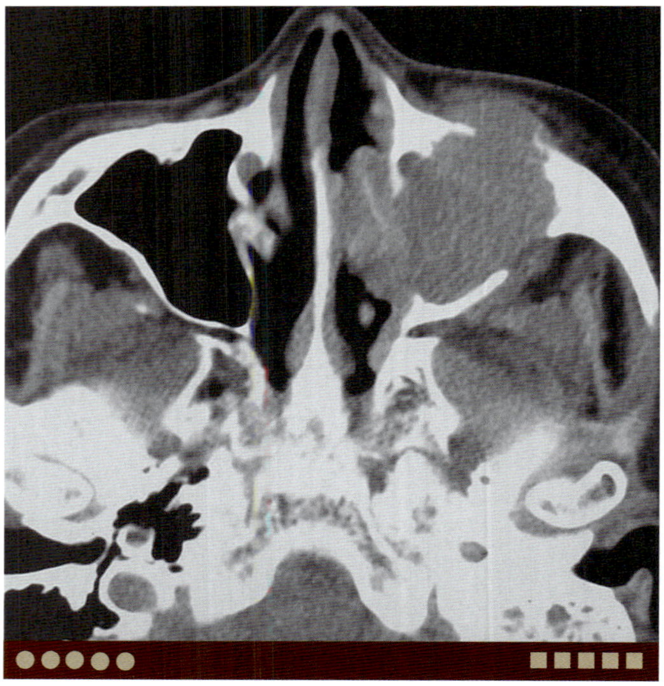

H. SCCA. Axial CT demonstrates a large tumor destructing the anterior, medial and posterolateral walls of the left maxillary sinus.

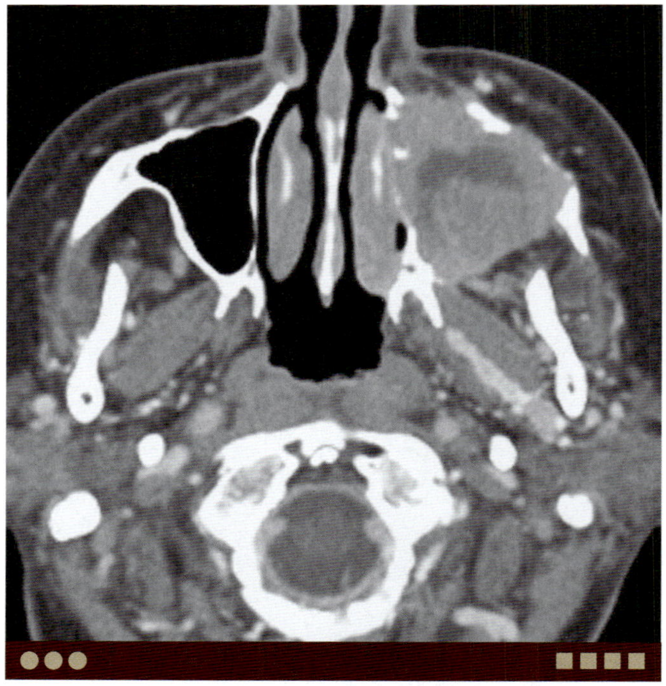

I. Sinonasal undifferentiated carcinoma. Axial contrast-enhanced CT demonstrates a mildly enhancing tumor with central low density destructing almost entire walls of the left maxillary sinus.

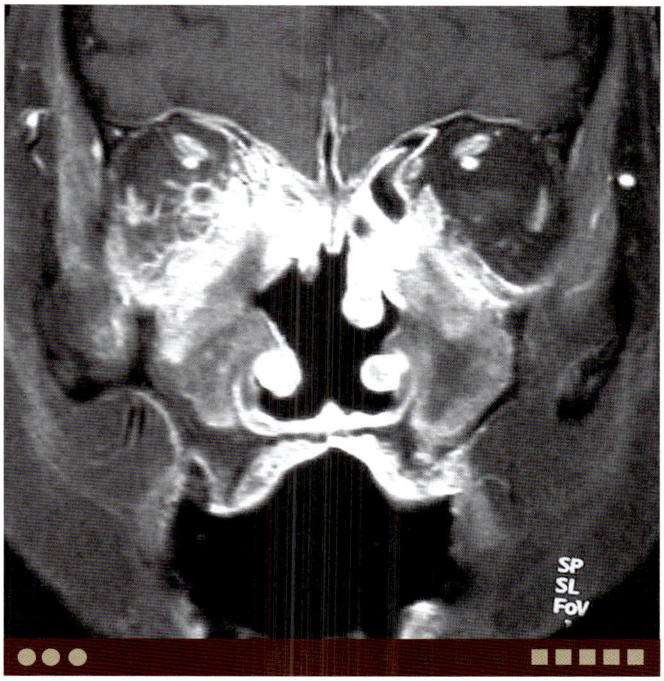

J. **Wegener's granulomatosis**. Coronal postcontrast fat-suppressed T1W image demonstrates diffuse enhancement in the maxillary sinuses and the inferomedial portion of the orbits bilaterally. Large nasal septal perforation is noted. Note abnormal dural enhancement along the anterior skull base and falx.

Case 3-17 Sinus Atelectasis

Osamu Sakai, Gabriel Monagas

PRESENTATION

Enophthalmos.

FINDINGS

CT demonstrates decreased volume of the unilateral maxillary sinus.

DIFFERENTIAL DIAGNOSIS

- Prior surgery: Postsurgical changes such as bone defect in the anterior and/or medial walls of the maxillary sinus are seen.
- Trauma: This demonstrates deformity of bones from prior fractures in the maxilla, zygoma, and orbit.
- Congenital hypoplasia: Nonpneumatized maxilla demonstrates normal trabeculation and fatty marrow. However, this may be difficult to be differentiated from chronic inflammation.
- Extramedullary hematopoiesis: Thalassemia and sickle cell anemia patients may have obliterated paranasal sinuses due to bone marrow space expansion and extramedullary hematopoiesis.

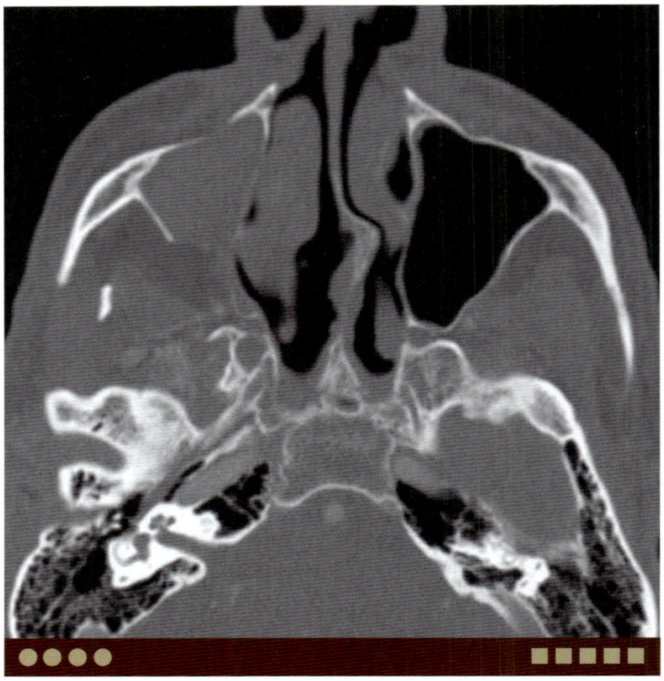

A. Sinus atelectasis. Axial CT demonstrates small opacified right maxillary sinus. The left maxillary sinus is normal.

COMMENTS

This is a 45-year-old man with sore throat, lymphadenopathy, and facial asymmetry.

Sinus atelectasis, also called "silent sinus syndrome," is collapse of the maxillary sinus, usually from chronic inflammation. It is thought that obstruction of the ostiomeatal complex causes negative pressure in the sinus, and then results in volume loss of the sinus. However, the actual cause is unknown and although chronic sinus inflammation may result in osseous thickening and sclerosis, it is thought that in these cases there is a low-grade inflammation which, along with the negative sinus pressure, results in thinning and osteolysis which permits the later remodeling. This condition can produce enophthalmos or "pseudoexophthalmos" of the contralateral side. This is also sometimes associated with diplopia and midfacial depression.

The medial wall of the maxillary sinus as well as the ostiomeatal complex is retracted laterally, the middle meatus is widened, and the orbital floor may be depressed. Atelectatic sinus often demonstrates increased density and signal on CT and T1W MR imaging, respectively, and decreased signal on T2W imaging reflecting inspissated mucus. Enophthalmos on axial images and craniocaudal elongation of the orbit on coronal images are often seen.

This condition usually develops in a chronic fashion. However, it can occur quickly in a few weeks to months. Surgical maxillary sinus ventilation, such as middle meatal antrostomy or nasal antral window can stop progression of retraction; however, it cannot reverse the phenomenon.

PEARLS

- **Sinus atelectasis, also called as "silent sinus syndrome," is a painless collapse of the maxillary sinus.**
- **It can cause enophthalmos of the affected side or "pseudoexophthalmos" of the contralateral side.**
- **The process is usually a result of chronic sinus obstruction and low-grade inflammation; however, it could also develop quickly.**

ADDITIONAL IMAGES (B-G)

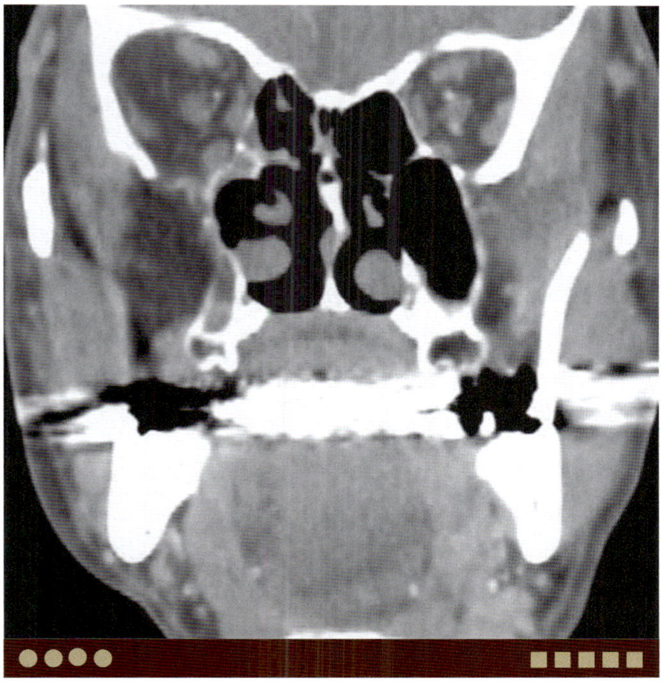

B. Sinus atelectasis, same patient as A. Coronal CT demonstrates almost completely collapsed right maxillary sinus with prominent buccal space fat.

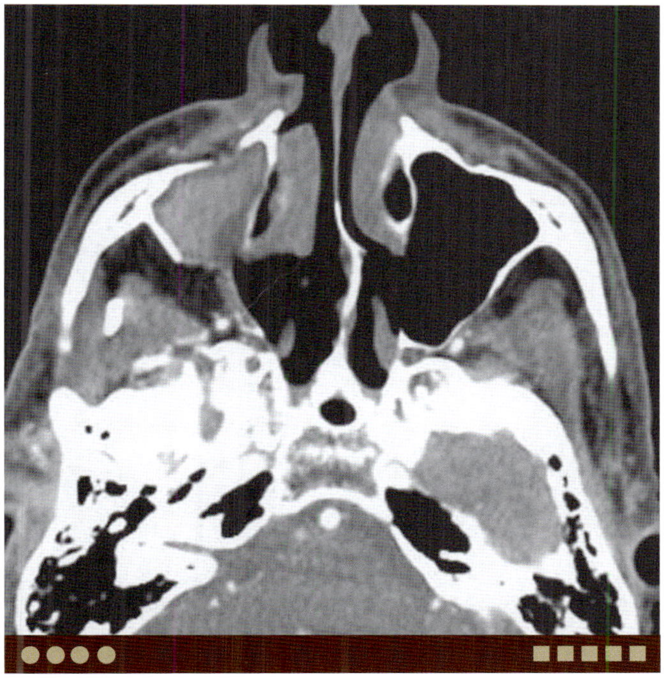

C. Sinus atelectasis, same patient as A. Axial CT demonstrates decreased volume of the right maxillary sinus. Inspissated mucus in the sinus demonstrates high density. Note widening of the retroantral fat pad.

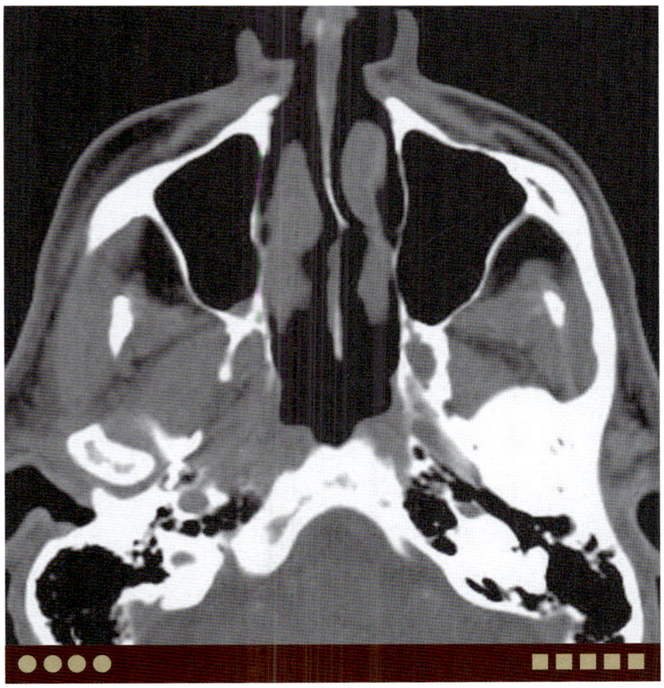

D. Same patient as A, 2 years ago. Axial CT demonstrates normal maxillary sinuses bilaterally.

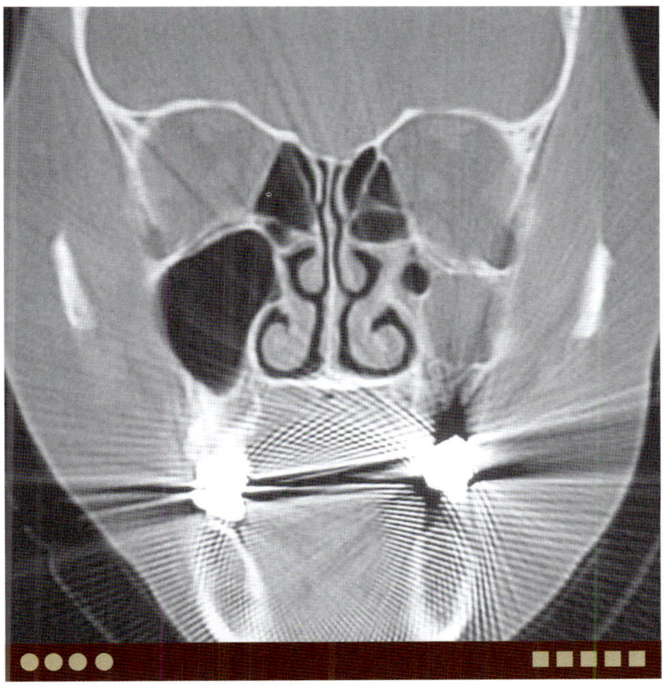

E. **Sinus atelectasis** in a different patient. Coronal CT demonstrates completely opacified, small left maxillary sinus. Note craniocaudal elongation of the left orbit.

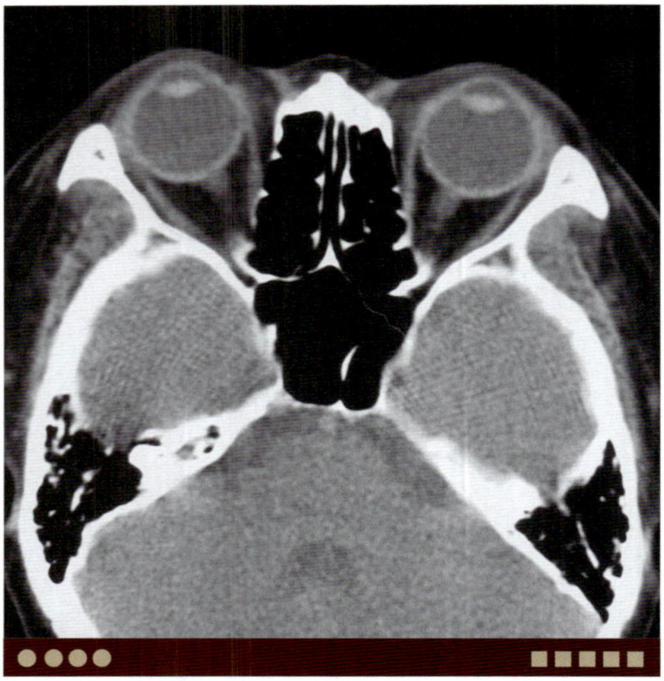

F. Sinus atelectasis, same patient as E. Axial CT through the orbits demonstrates enophthalmos on the left.

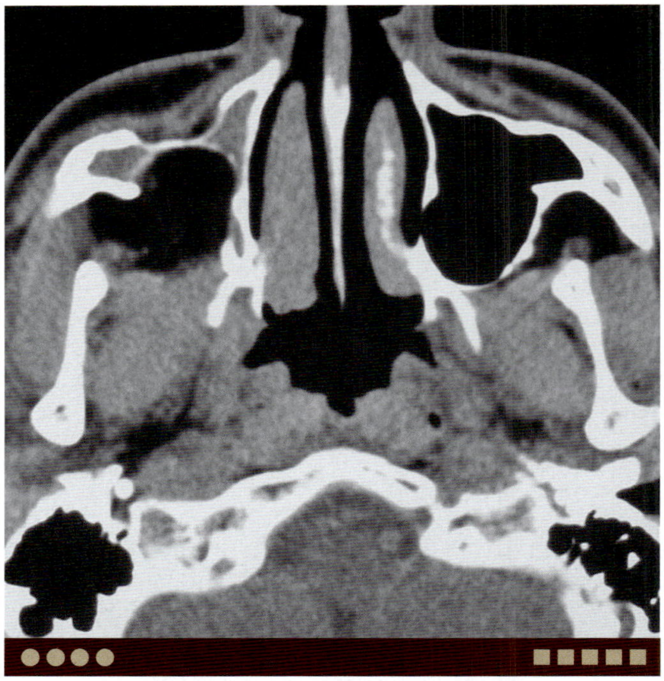

G. Sinus atelectasis in a different patient. Axial CT demonstrates nearly complete collapse of the right maxillary sinus.

DIFFERENTIAL DIAGNOSIS IMAGES (H-J)

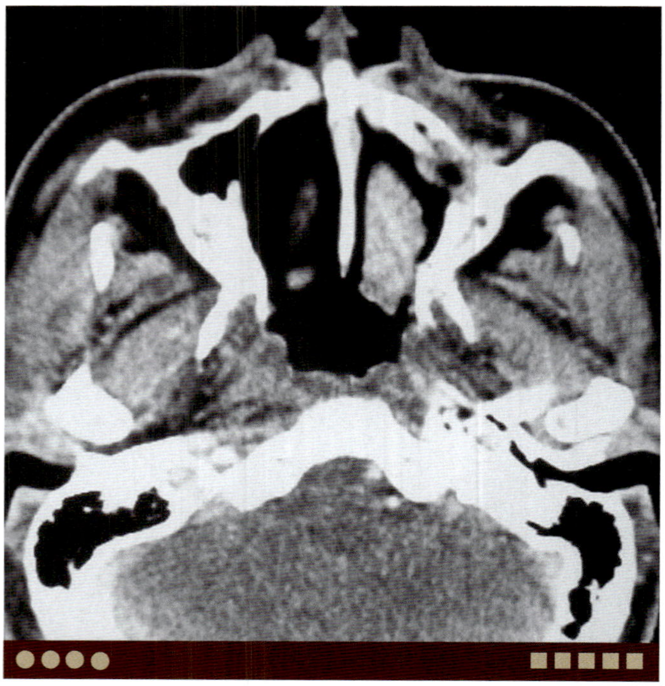

H. **Status post bilateral Caldwell-Luc surgery**. Axial CT demonstrates significantly decreased volume of the maxillary sinuses with bone defects.

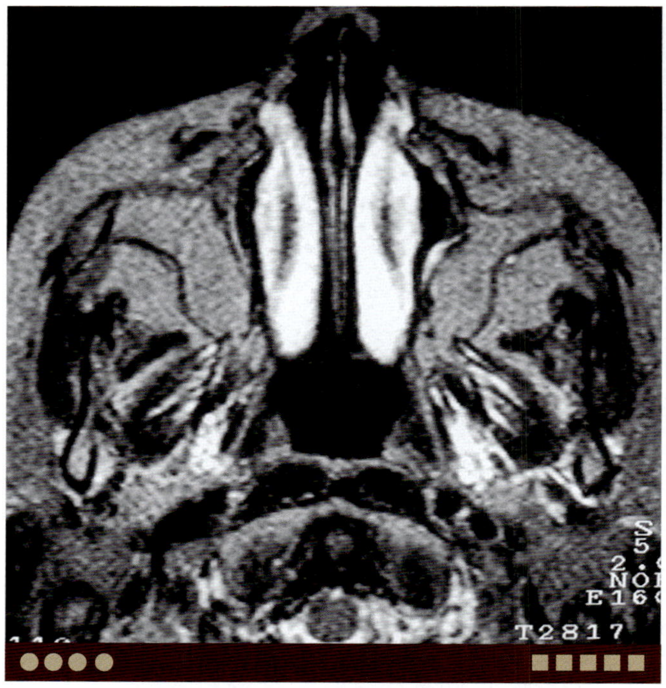

I. **Status post bilateral Caldwell-Luc surgery** in a different patient. Axial T2W MR image demonstrates complete loss of maxillary sinus lumen and thickened posterolateral walls.

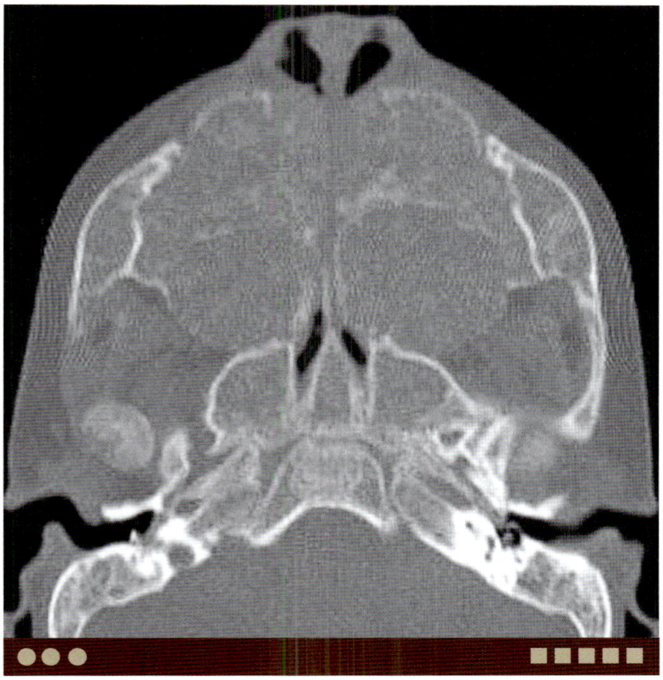

J. Thalassemia. Axial CT demonstrates significantly expanded bone marrow space and complete obliteration of the maxillary sinuses.

Case 3–18 Juvenile Angiofibroma

Osamu Sakai, Elisa Flower

PRESENTATION

Nasal obstruction, epistaxis.

FINDINGS

CT demonstrates an avidly enhancing nasal cavity/nasopharyngeal mass extending to the pterygopalatine fossa. MRI demonstrates flow-voids within the lesion.

DIFFERENTIAL DIAGNOSIS

- Vascular malformation: This condition has wider age range of presentation. High-flow type ones may demonstrate similar findings.
- Neurofibromatosis: This may be seen in a similar age group however it has less enhancement and no flow-voids.
- Antrochoanal polyp: This can be quite large and obstruct the nasopharynx, however does not involve pterygopalatine fossa. This may demonstrate milder peripheral enhancement without flow-voids.
- Squamous cell carcinoma: This is the most common malignant tumor in the sinonasal cavity, usually seen in the older patient group.
- Lymphoma: This is not common but the most common nonepithelial malignant tumor in this region. It demonstrates less avid enhancement without necrosis.

COMMENTS

This is a 15-year-old boy with epistaxis.

Juvenile angiofibroma is a hypervascular benign nonepithelial tumor. It usually occurs in adolescent boys, however occasionally occurs in girls and elderly people. Nasal obstruction and epistaxis are common first symptoms. Usually, it occurs in the superior, posterior, and lateral wall of the nasal cavity or nasopharynx. Histologically, it is benign, however locally aggressive and usually already invaded into the pterygopalatine fossa (PPF) at the time of diagnosis. Occasionally, it forms a large mass and completely occupies the nasopharynx. Intracranial extension can be seen in 20% to 35% of cases.

Biopsy in outpatient setting should be avoided due to risk of uncontrollable massive hemorrhage. Wide resection is the main stem of the treatment, although radiation and hormonal therapy have been attempted. Preoperative embolization can reduce intraoperative blood loss. Diagnosis of its extension is extremely important. Particularly, extent to the PPF, inferior orbital fissure, foramen rotundum, Vidian canal and superior orbital fissure should be carefully evaluated.

On CT, juvenile angiofibroma is seen as a mass arising from the nasal cavity and superolateral portion of the palate

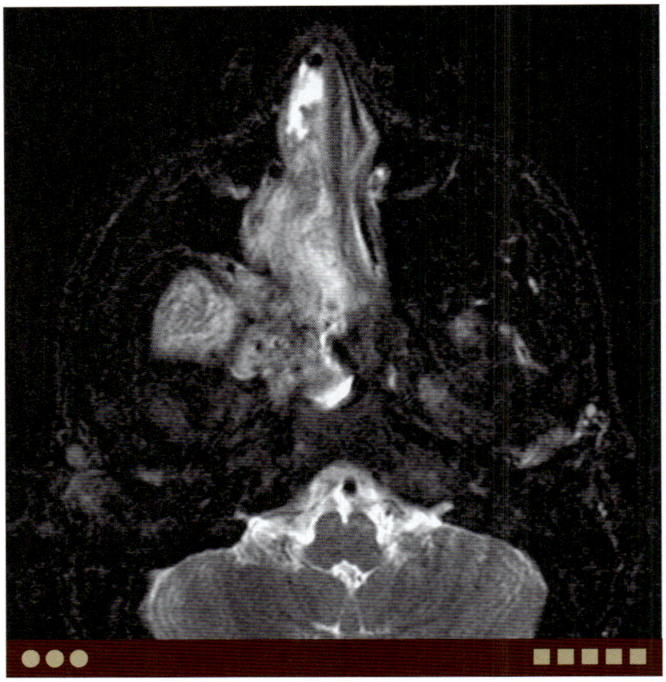

A. Juvenile angiofibroma. Axial T2W image demonstrates a T2 hyperintense tumor expanding the right pterygopalatine fossa with extension through the sphenopalatine foramen into the nasal cavity, and extension into the sphenoid sinus. There is also a lateral extension through the pterygomaxillary fissure. Note the flow-voids within the lesion.

extending to the nasopharynx and PPF. Destruction of the pterygoid plate and widening or remodeling of the PPF and pterygomaxillary fissure is commonly seen. The tumor shows avid enhancement.

On MRI, it usually demonstrates low-to-intermediate signal on T1W and intermediate-to-high signal on T2W images. Flow-voids are commonly seen in the lesion reflecting its hypervascularity, which is a very characteristic finding. Avid enhancement is seen in the solid portion with multiple flow-voids. Fat-suppression technique often causes blurring adjacent to the nasopharyngeal lumen and sinuses, obscuring the details. Therefore, it is important perform at least one sequence without fat suppression.

PEARLS

- **Juvenile angiofibroma is a hypervascular tumor commonly seen in adolescent boys.**
- **Avid enhancement on CT and multiple flow-voids on MRI are characteristic findings.**
- **The pterygopalatine fossa is often already involved at the time of diagnosis.**

ADDITIONAL IMAGES (B-F)

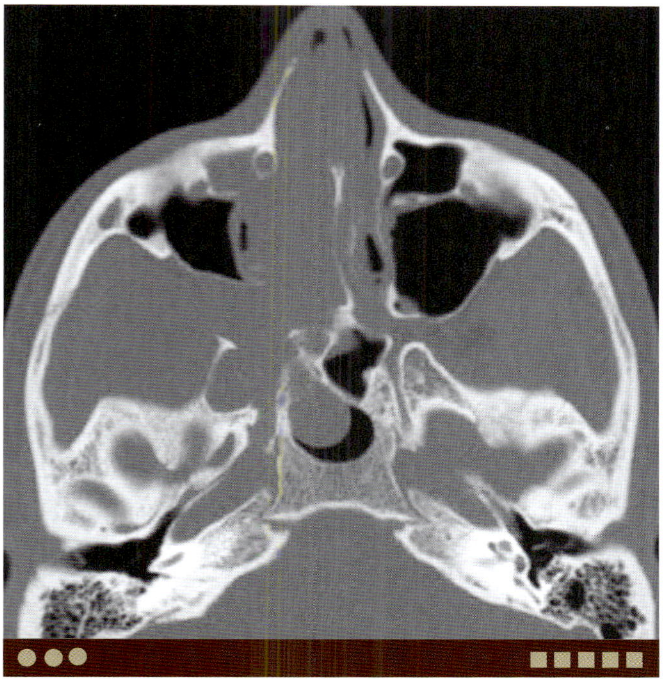

B. Juvenile angiofibroma, same patient as A. Axial CT scan in bony window demonstrates widening of the pterygopalatine fossa and the enlarged ipsilateral Vidian canal, suggesting growth through this canal. Note anterior displacement of the posterolateral wall of the right maxillary sinus.

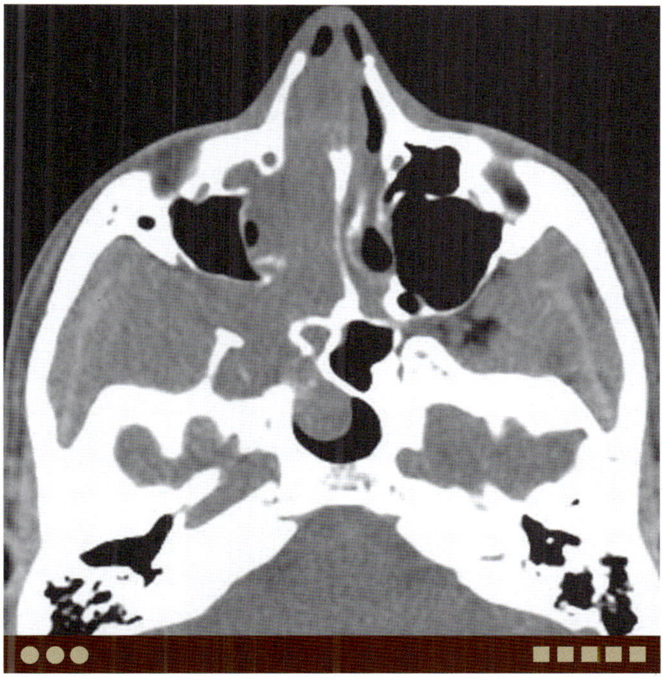

C. Juvenile angiofibroma, same patient as A. Axial CT scan in soft tissue window demonstrates a soft tissue density mass centered in the pterygopalatine fossa obliterating the normal fat and extending the nasal cavity and sphenoid sinus.

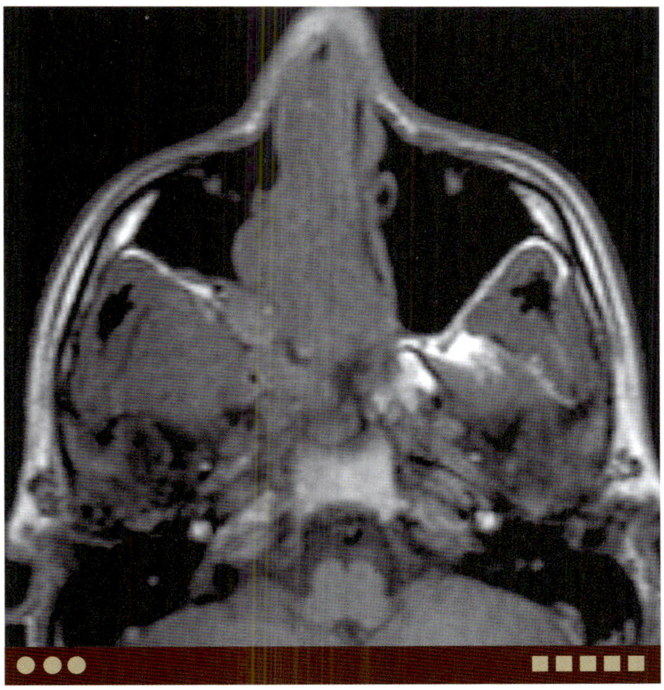

D. Juvenile angiofibroma, same patient A. Axial T1W image demonstrates an isointense lesion, obliterating the normal fat in the expanded pterygopalatine fossa.

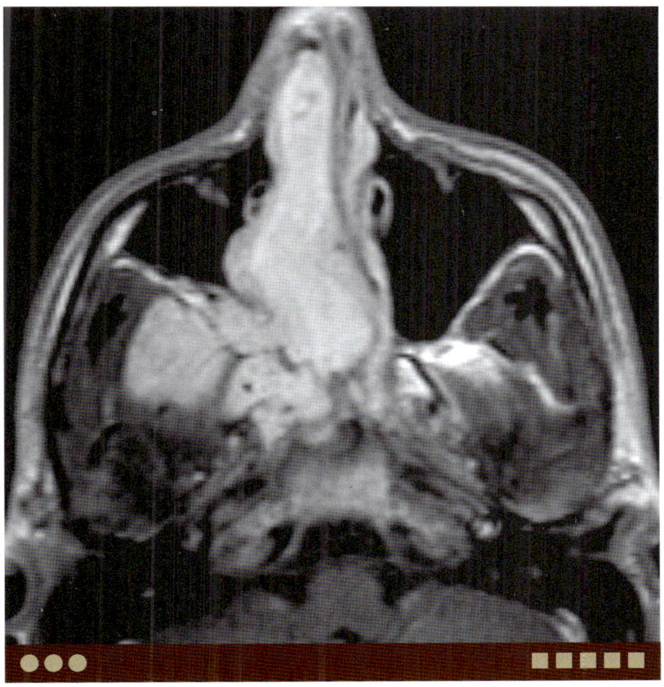

E. Juvenile angiofibroma, same patient A. Axial postcontrast T1W images demonstrate avid enhancement of the tumor which is seen to extend into the masticator space. Flow-voids are again noted.

DIFFERENTIAL DIAGNOSIS IMAGES (G-J)

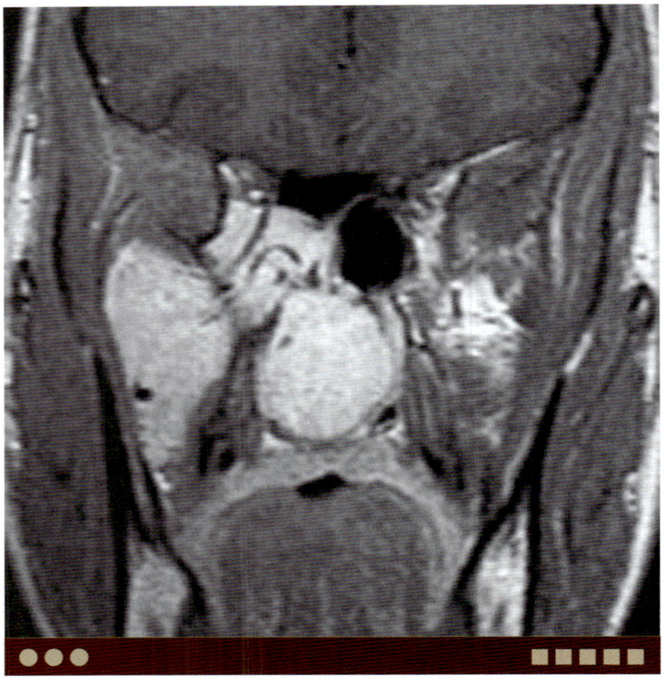

F. Juvenile angiofibroma, same patient A. Coronal postcontrast T1W images demonstrate avid enhancement of the tumor which is seen to extend into the masticator space. Note very prominent flow-voids in the tumor.

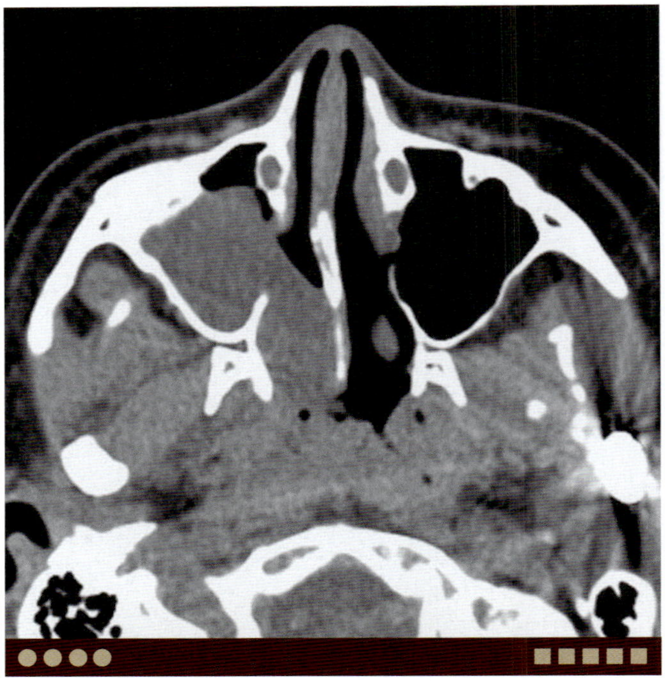

G. **Antrochoanal polyp**. Axial CT in bone window demonstrates soft tissue density near completely opacifying the right maxillary sinus with extension into the nasal cavity.

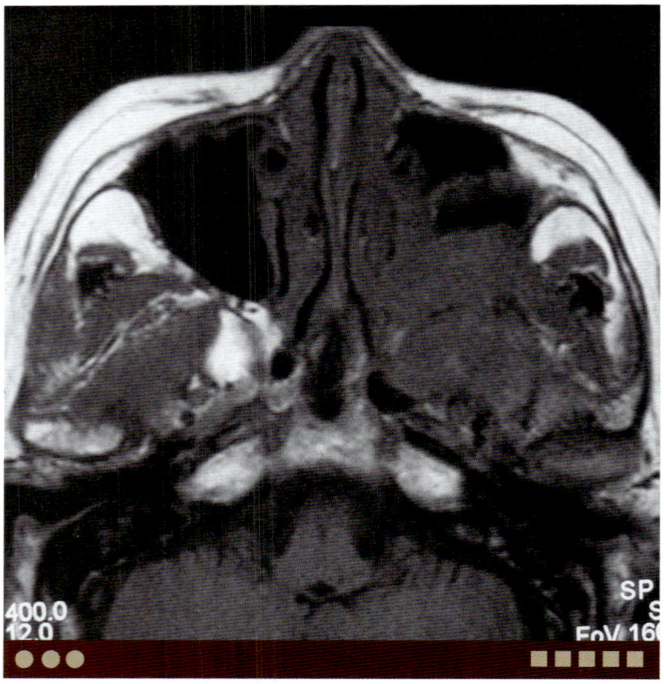

H. **Lymphoma**. Axial T1W image demonstrates a homogeneous low-signal lesion, obliterating the normal fat in the left pterygopalatine fossa.

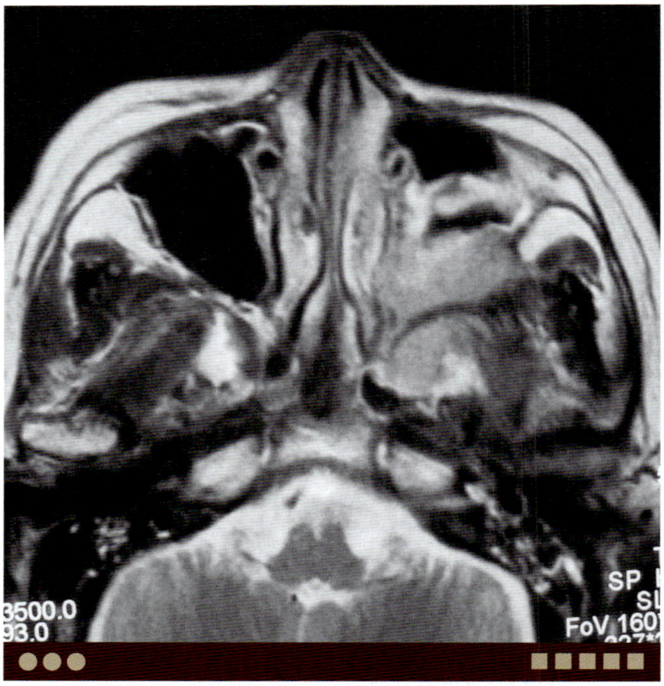

I. Lymphoma, same patient as H. Axial T2W image demonstrates homogeneous intermediate signal within the lesion without flow-voids.

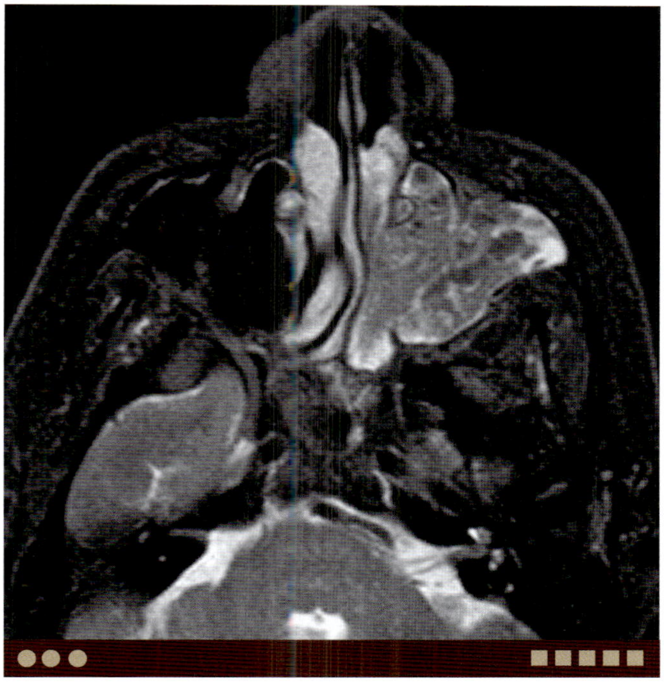

J. Inverted papilloma. Axial T2W image demonstrates a heterogeneous intermediate-signal lesion within the left nasal cavity extending into the maxillary sinus.

Case 3–19 Esthesioneuroblastoma

Osamu Sakai, Gabriel Monagas

PRESENTATION

Nasal obstruction, anosmia.

FINDINGS

CT demonstrates an enhancing upper nasal cavity mass extending intracranially.

DIFFERENTIAL DIAGNOSIS

- Neuroendocrine carcinoma: This is an epithelial tumor that often arises in the nasal cavity as well as in the larynx. Imaging findings are identical to esthesioneuroblastoma and difficult to differentiate. Histologically, it can be differentiated from esthesioneuroblastoma by epithelial markers.
- Squamous cell carcinoma (SCCA): SCCA is the most common malignant tumor in the sinonasal cavity. Most occur in the maxillary sinus. SCCA in the upper nasal cavity is not very common. However, an esthesioneuroblastoma could also arise from lower within the nasal cavity in a more common area for an SCCA.
- Metastatic tumor: Metastasis to the sinonasal cavity is not very common but occurs, often to the ethmoid from gastrointestinal and urogenital cancers.
- Meningioma: This is the most common benign intracranial tumor. The olfactory groove and planum sphenoidale are common sites. This tumor occurs intracranially and may extend extracranially.
- Fungal infection: Fungal infection may show aggressive skull base invasion.

COMMENTS

This is a 58-year-old man with epistaxis.

Esthesioneuroblastoma is also known as olfactory neuroblastoma, arising from the neurosensory body cell in the olfactory epithelium. The patient often complains of nasal obstruction and repeating epistaxis. With further progression of the tumor, local pain, nasal discharge, and headache is noted. There are two peaks in patients' age groups: second and sixth decades. Clinically, it is often misdiagnosed as an inflammatory or angiomatous polyp. The average delay between the appearance of the first symptom and the diagnosis is about 6 months.

Most of the olfactory neuroepithelium is located at the cribriform plate, therefore most esthesioneuroblastomas occur in the upper nasal cavity. However, islands of olfactory mucosa may be found in the upper turbinates and the upper one third of the nasal septum as well as on the entire middle turbinate. Therefore, occasionally, the tumor arises far from the cribriform plate. Pathologically, this tumor may be difficult to be differentiated from neuroendocrine carcinoma and sinonasal undifferentiated carcinoma (SNUC) without special stains.

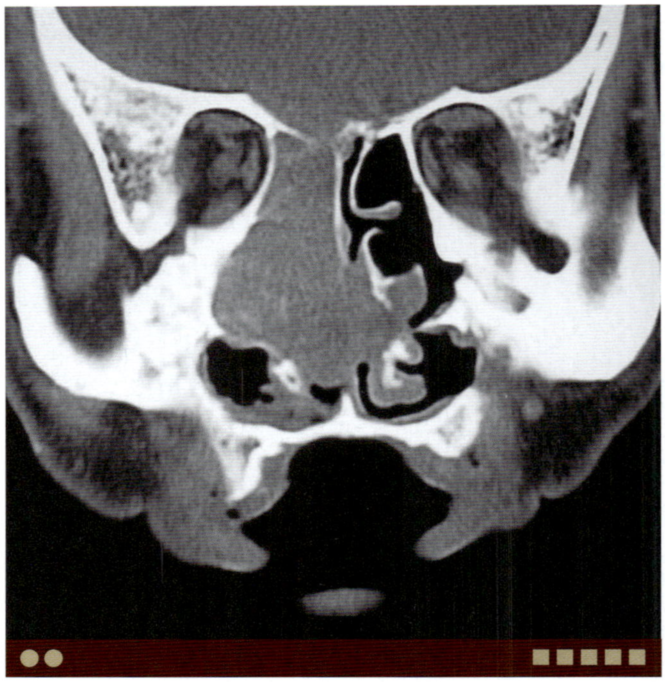

A. Esthesioneuroblastoma. Coronal noncontrast CT demonstrates a solid tumor in the right nasal cavity. Note erosion of the right cribriform plate and ethmoid roof and intracranial extension of the tumor.

On CT and MRI, esthesioneuroblastoma is seen as an avidly enhancing mass in the upper nasal cavity, just below the cribriform plate. Intracranial extension is commonly

PEARLS

- **Esthesioneuroblastoma is also known as olfactory neuroblastoma, arising from the neurosensory body cell in the olfactory epithelium.**
- **Esthesioneuroblastoma is seen as an avidly enhancing lesion in the upper nasal cavity invading the skull base.**
- **Differentiation of esthesioneuroblastoma from neuroendocrine carcinoma and other small round cell tumors by imaging is impossible.**
- **Peripheral cysts along the tumor–brain interface should raise suspicion of an esthesioneuroblastoma with intracranial extension.**

seen at the time of diagnosis, forming a mass at the anterior skull base with bone erosion and destruction. Bilateral involvement is common. Inferiorly, it extends into the ethmoid with bone destruction. On T2W images, it shows relatively low signal corresponding to high cellularity similar to other small round cell tumors. Differentiation of esthesioneuroblastoma from neuroendocrine carcinoma and other small round cell tumors by imaging alone is impossible except for melanoma, which can show increased signal on T1W by paramagnetic effect from melanin. Although not pathognomonic, peripheral cysts along the tumor–brain interface are more often seen with esthesioneuroblastomas compared with other tumors.

ADDITIONAL IMAGES (B-F)

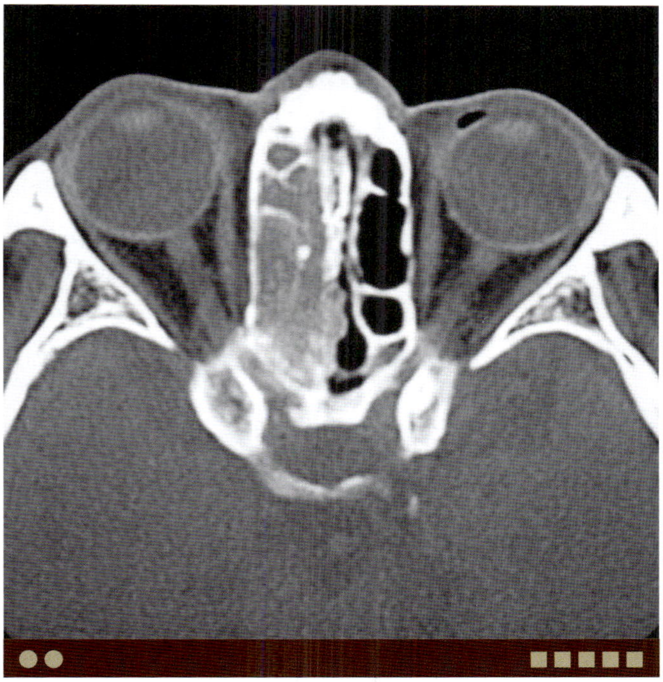

B. Esthesioneuroblastoma, same patient as A. Axial noncontrast CT demonstrates the tumor occupying the right upper nasal cavity as well as ethmoid air cells and destructing the bone.

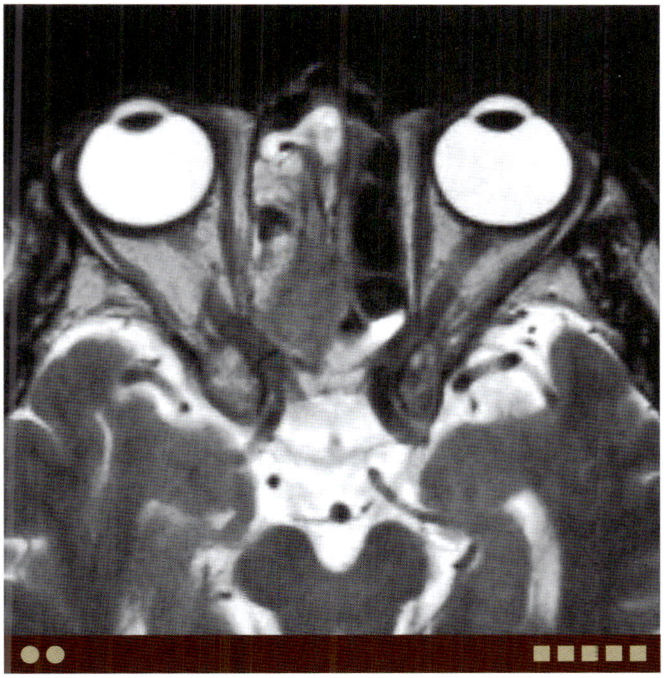

C. Esthesioneuroblastoma, same patient as A. Axial T2W MR image demonstrates intermediate-to-low signal of the tumor, consistent with a small round cell tumor.

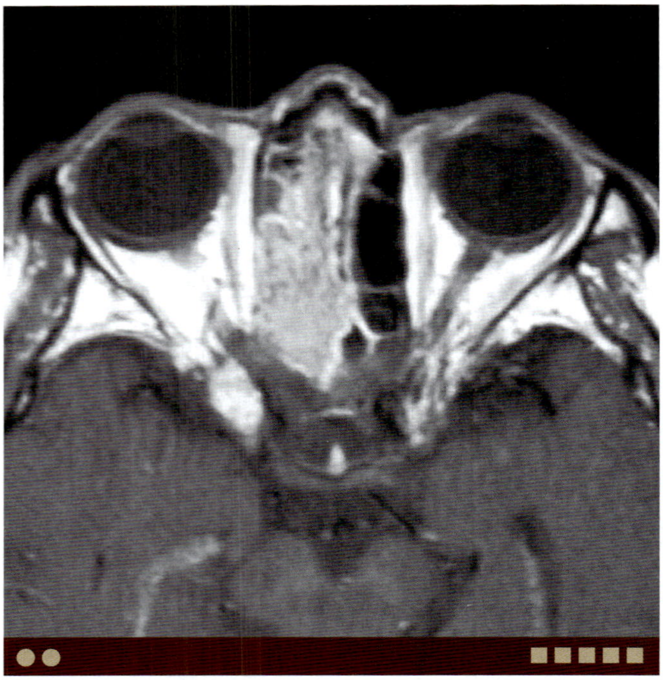

D. Esthesioneuroblastoma, same patient as A. Axial postcontrast T1W MR image demonstrates avid enhancement of the tumor.

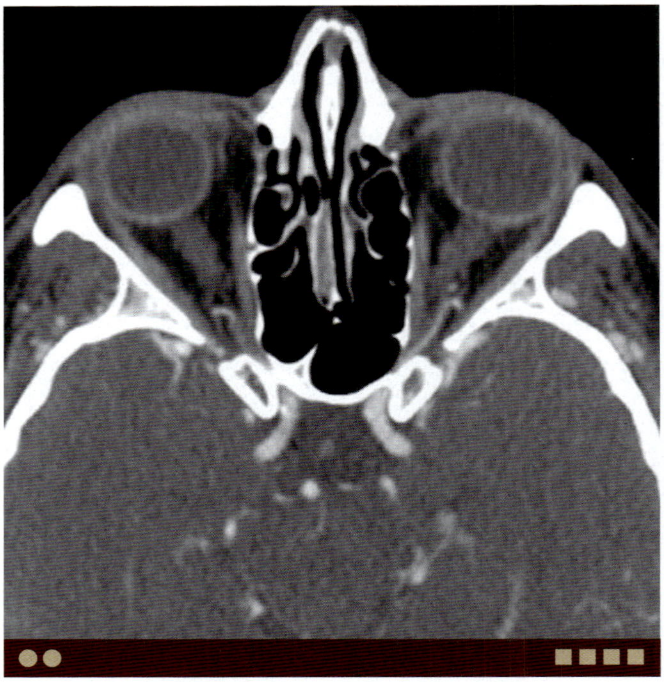

E. **Esthesioneuroblastoma** in a different patient. Axial postcontrast CT demonstrates an enhancing tumor in the right upper nasal cavity.

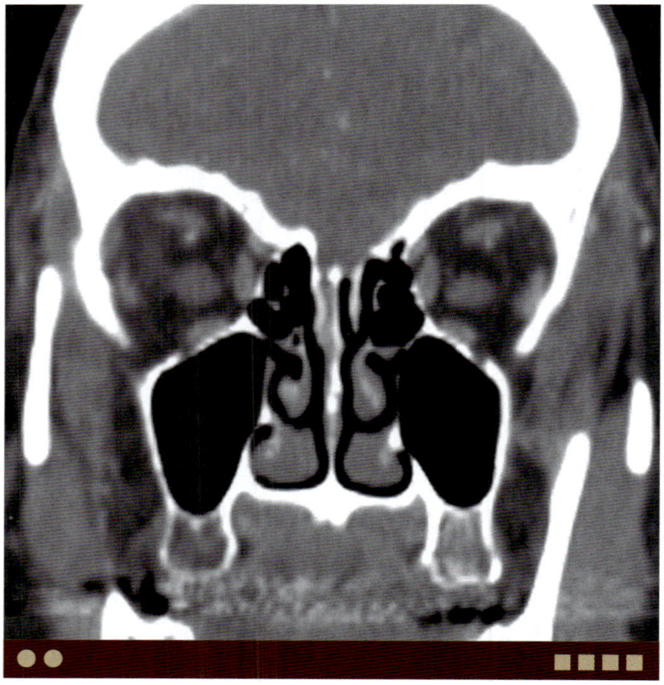

F. Esthesioneuroblastoma, same patient as E. Coronal postcontrast CT demonstrates an enhancing tumor in the right upper nasal cavity, just below the cribriform plate without bone destruction or intracranial extension.

DIFFERENTIAL DIAGNOSIS IMAGES (G-J)

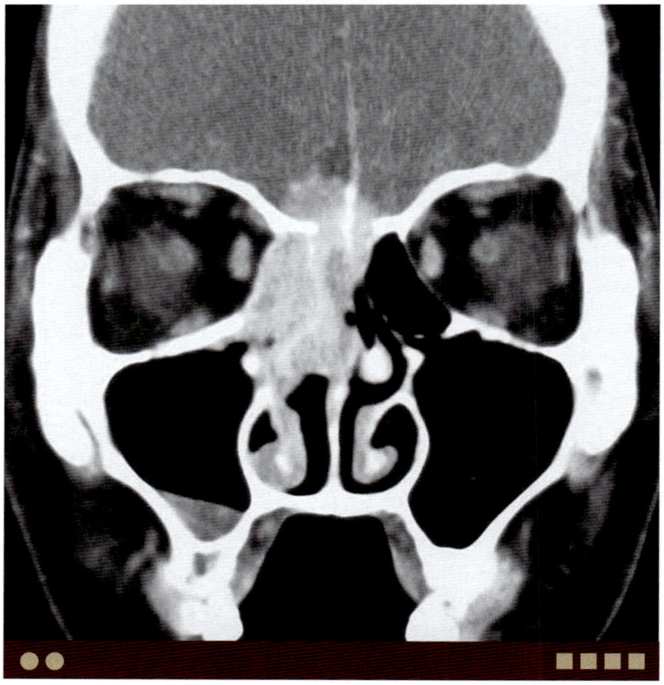

G. **Neuroendocrine carcinoma**. Coronal postcontrast CT demonstrates an avidly enhancing tumor centered in the right upper nasal cavity, crossing midline, destructing the bone and extending intracranially.

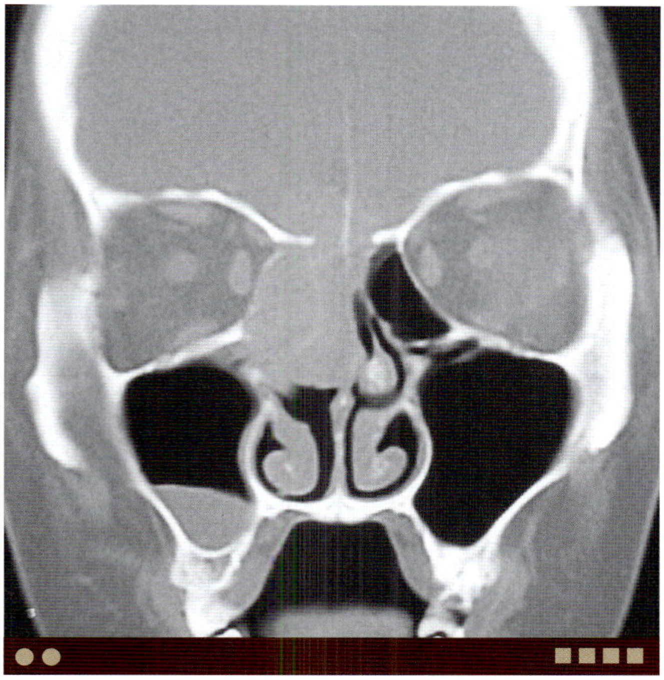

H. Neuroendocrine carcinoma, same patient as G. Coronal bone window CT demonstrates destruction of the cribriform plate.

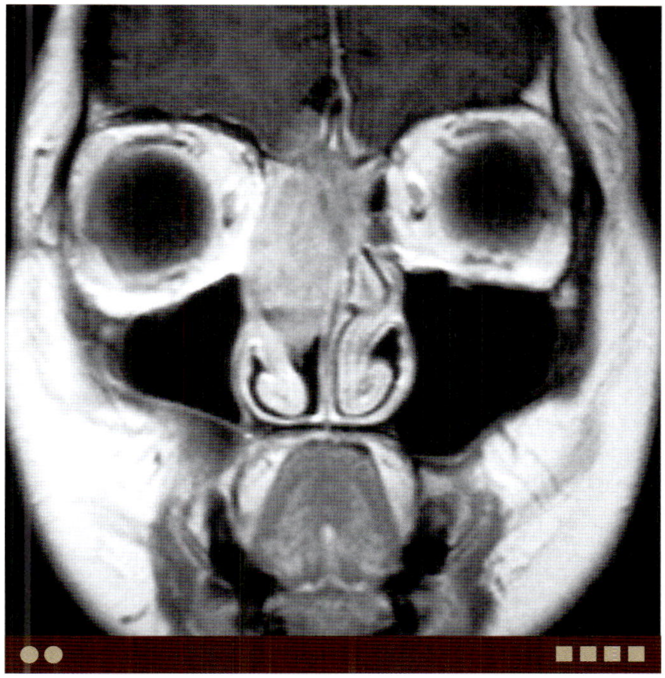

I. Neuroendocrine carcinoma, same patient as G. Coronal postcontrast T1W MR image demonstrates a heterogeneously enhancing tumor centered in the right upper nasal cavity crossing midline and invading the anterior skull base.

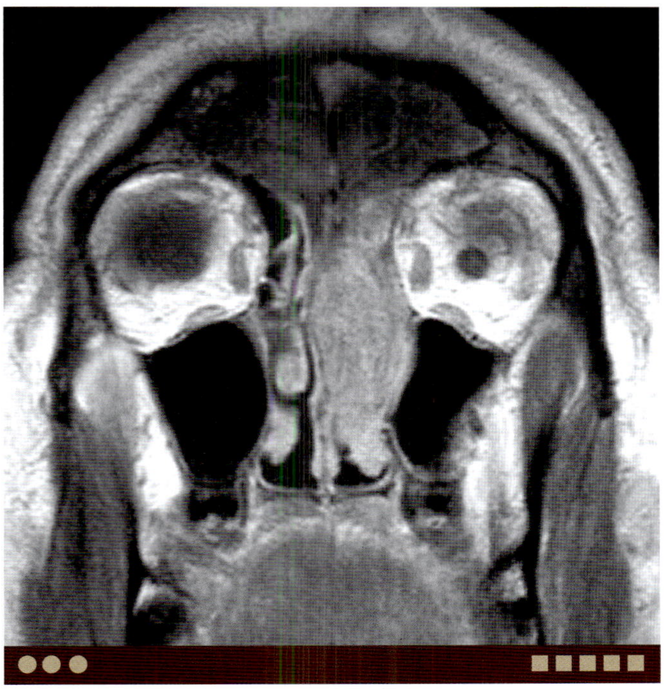

J. SNUC. Coronal postcontrast T1W MR image demonstrates a heterogeneously enhancing tumor centered in the left upper nasal cavity and invading the anterior skull base.

Case 3-20 Anosmia—Kallman Syndrome

Osamu Sakai, Gabriel Monagas

PRESENTATION

Anosmia.

FINDINGS

MRI demonstrates hypoplastic olfactory bulbs.

DIFFERENTIAL DIAGNOSIS

- Chronic rhinosinusitis: Blockage of the upper nasal cavity causes impaired perception of smell. CT should be performed to rule out sinonasal cavity pathology.
- Frontal contusion: This is a common cause of acquired central cause of anosmia. Encephalomalacia with post-traumatic change in the skull base is commonly seen.
- Meningioma: Meningiomas often occur in the anterior skull base and involve the olfactory groove. Other skull base lesions may also present with loss of smell.

COMMENTS

This is a 56-year-old woman with anosmia.

Anosmia is a lack of olfaction, which can be congenital or acquired, and either temporary or permanent. Temporary inability to perceive smells can be from nasal obstruction due to acute or chronic sinusitis, nasal polyposis and allergy, or sinonasal tumors. On the other hand, permanent anosmia is seen patients with brain injury, brain tumors, or neurodegenerative disorders. Rarely, anosmia can also be congenital, as seen with Kallman syndrome.

Kallman syndrome is commonly recognized by anosmia or severe hyposmia from hypoplasia of the olfactory bulb and tract as well as hypogonadism from low gonadotropin. It is thought to be due to gene abnormality involving chromosome Xp22.3 resulting in problems in migration of the gonadotropin releasing hormone cell from the olfactory stem to the hypothalamus. Patients may be unaware of lack of smell and should be tested appropriately if suspected. The prevalence is 1/10,000 in men and 1/50,000 in women. Other anomalies associated with this condition are cleft palate/lip, renal agenesis and hearing loss.

CT is usually performed first in a patient with anosmia to exclude abnormality in the sinonasal cavity because rhinosinusitis is a common cause of anosmia. It is important to evaluate the upper nasal cavity, just below the cribriform plate to rule out obstructive or destructive lesions. At the same time, intracranial structures should be evaluated. Olfactory meningioma or evidence of prior trauma such as contusion can be seen in patients with anosmia. However, although CT provides superior evaluation of osseous

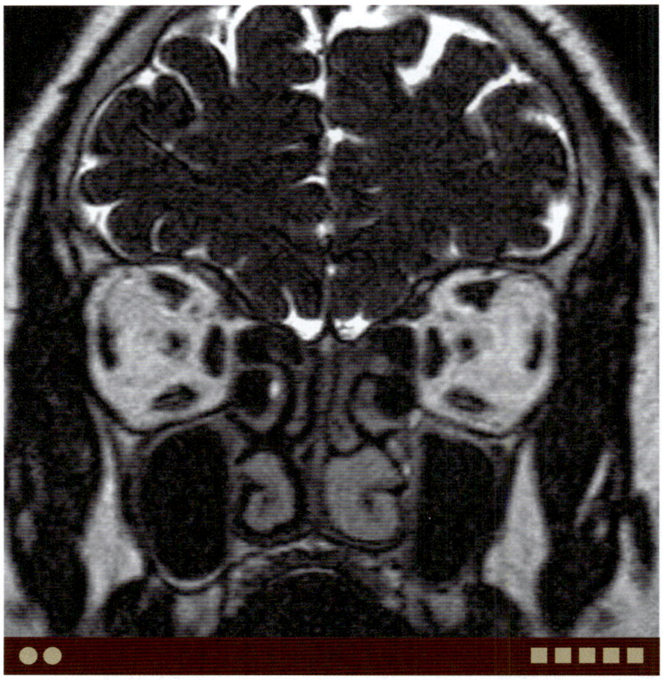

A. Hypoplastic olfactory bulbs. Coronal high-resolution T2W MR image demonstrates empty right olfactory groove. Very hypoplastic or remnant of the olfactory bulb is seen on the left.

structures, evaluation of the olfactory bulbs/tracts and other intracranial structures is rather limited on CT.

MRI, especially with high-resolution coronal sections, is a suitable modality to evaluate for hypoplasia or aplasia of the olfactory bulbs. Also, MRI easily demonstrates gliosis and encephalomalacia of the rectus gyri from prior trauma, as well as better characterization of other intracranial pathology.

PEARLS

- **Anosmia can be congenital or acquired, and temporary or permanent.**
- **First step is to rule out sinonasal pathology obstructing the upper nasal cavity. Relevant clinical history may aid in choosing an appropriate imaging modality.**
- **Any lesions obstructing or destructing the anterior skull base can cause anosmia. Common lesions include squamous cell carcinoma, esthesioneuroblastoma, meningioma, dermoid, cephalocele, and inverted papilloma.**
- **Kallman syndrome is a syndrome with anosmia or severe hyposmia due to hypoplasia or aplasia of the olfactory bulbs often associated with hypopituitarism and hypogonadism.**

ADDITIONAL IMAGES (B-D)

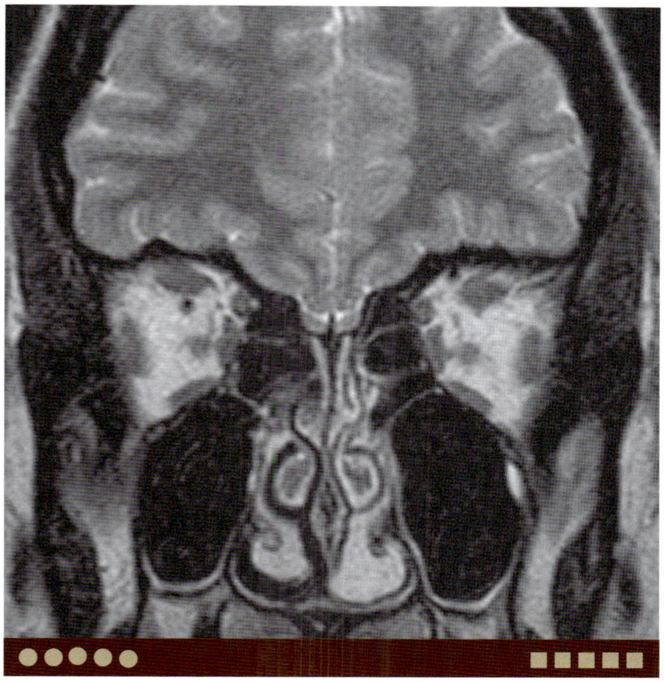

B. Normal olfactory bulbs. Coronal T2W MR image demonstrates normal size olfactory bulbs bilaterally.

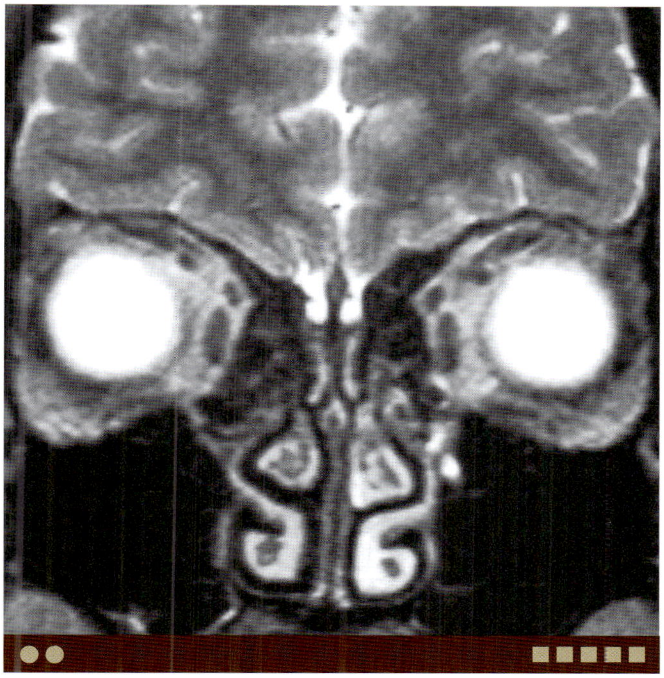

C. Kallman syndrome. Coronal T2W MR image demonstrates empty olfactory grooves bilaterally.

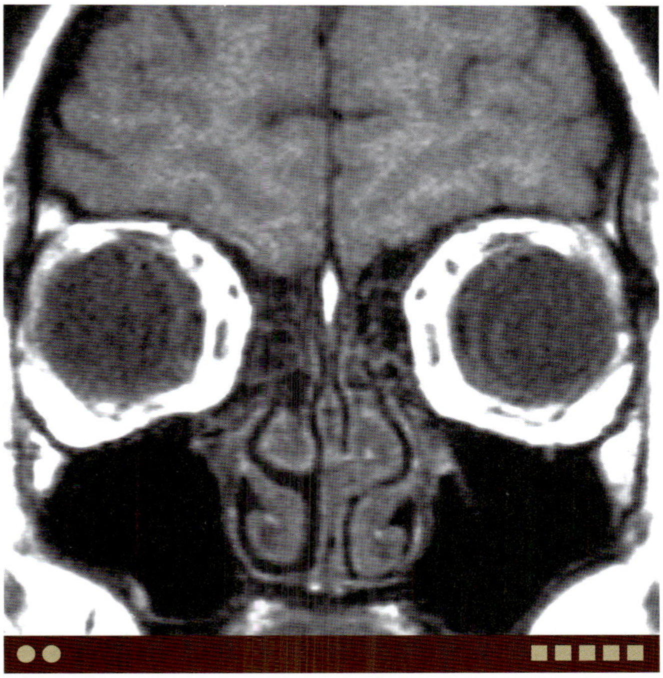

D. Kallman syndrome, same patient as C. Coronal T1W MR image is unremarkable.

DIFFERENTIAL DIAGNOSIS IMAGES (E-I)

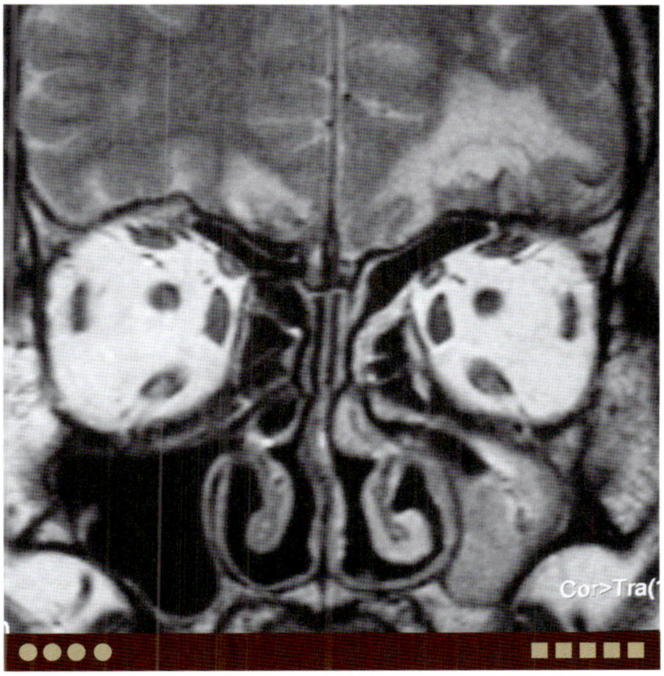

E. Frontal contusions. Coronal T2W MR image demonstrates encephalomalacia of the frontal lobes, left larger than right.

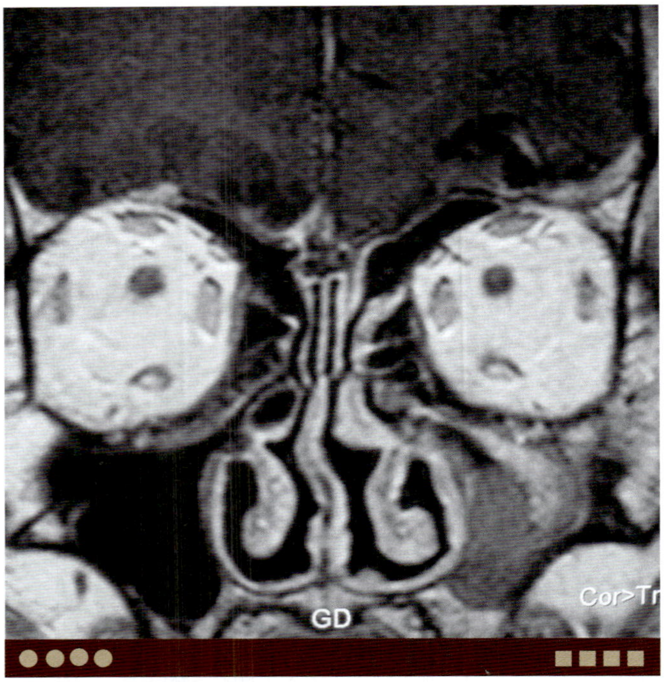

F. Frontal contusions, same patient as E. Coronal postcontrast T1W MR image demonstrates peripheral enhancement in areas of encephalomalacia in the frontal lobes.

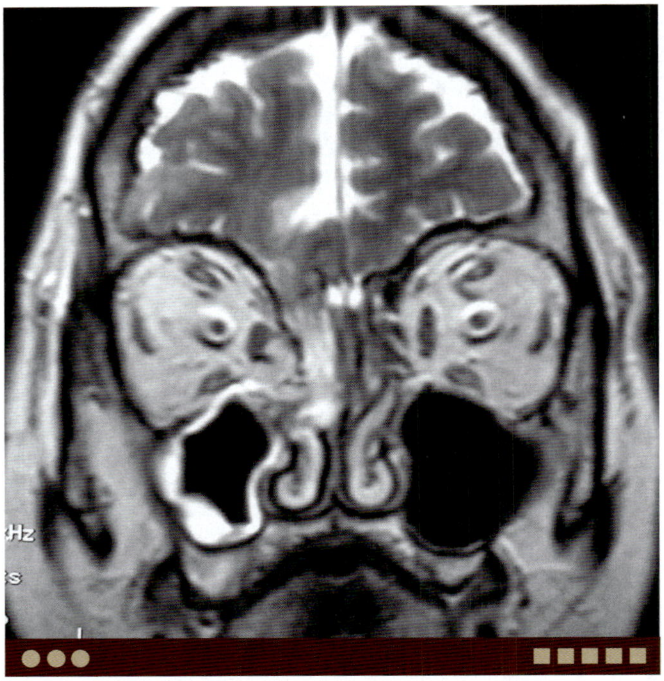

G. Cephalocele. Coronal T2W MR image demonstrates downward herniation of the brain parenchyma through the bone defect in the right ethmoid roof. Note the meninges containing the cerebrospinal fluid extend lower to the nasal cavity.

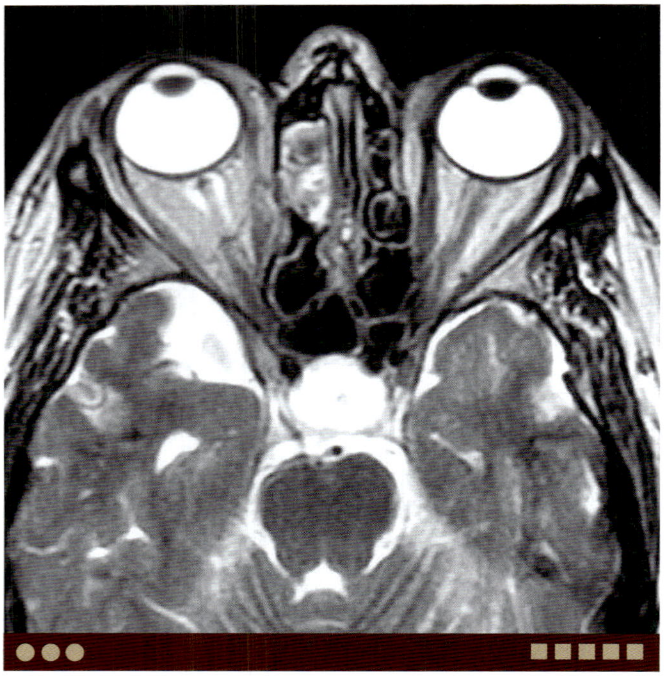

H. Cephalocele, same patient as G. Axial T2W MR image demonstrates brain parenchymal tissue in the right anterior ethmoid.

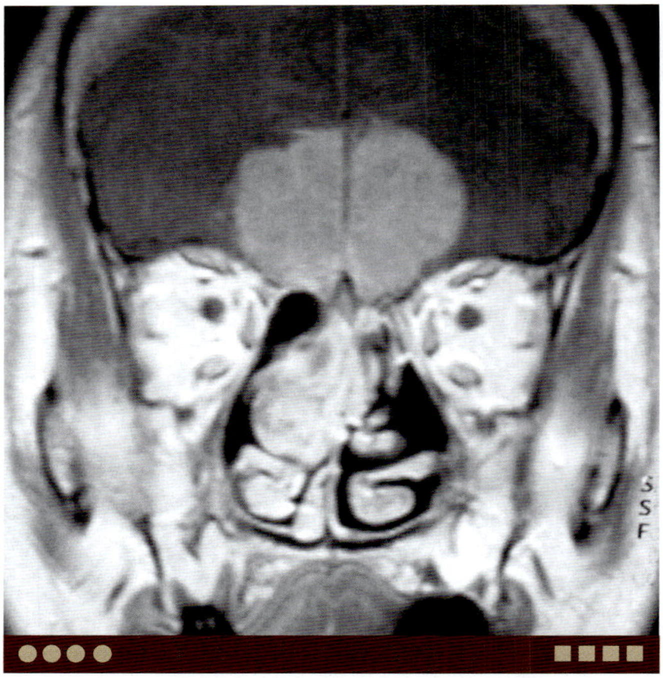

I. Meningioma. Coronal postcontrast T1W MR image demonstrates a large enhancing tumor in the anterior skull base involving the olfactory grooves.

Case 3–21 Intraosseous Hemangioma

Osamu Sakai, Gabriel Monagas

PRESENTATION

Subcutaneous cheek mass.

FINDINGS

CT demonstrates a mass with coarse trabeculation and avid contrast enhancement. T2W MR image demonstrates very high signal.

DIFFERENTIAL DIAGNOSIS

- Fibrous dysplasia: This shows bone expansion with a "ground-glass" matrix and is generally diagnosed in childhood or adolescence, before the age of 30.
- Ossifying fibroma: This is a benign fibro-osseous lesion composed of lamellar bone with prominent osteoblastic rimming in dense fibrous stroma demonstrating nearly identical radiological findings to fibrous dysplasia.
- Paget's disease: This is a common disease of unknown etiology, usually seen in elderly people and unusual before age 40. Involvement of the skull and skull base is common, although any bone can be affected. Spectrum of findings range from demineralization (early stage), "ground-glass" matrix (intermediate stage) to extreme thickening with diploic heterogeneity (late stage).
- Reactive sclerosis/calcification due to malignant tumors: Occasionally, prominent sclerotic change is seen with malignant tumors, often squamous cell carcinoma due to stimulation of osteoblasts by the tumor.

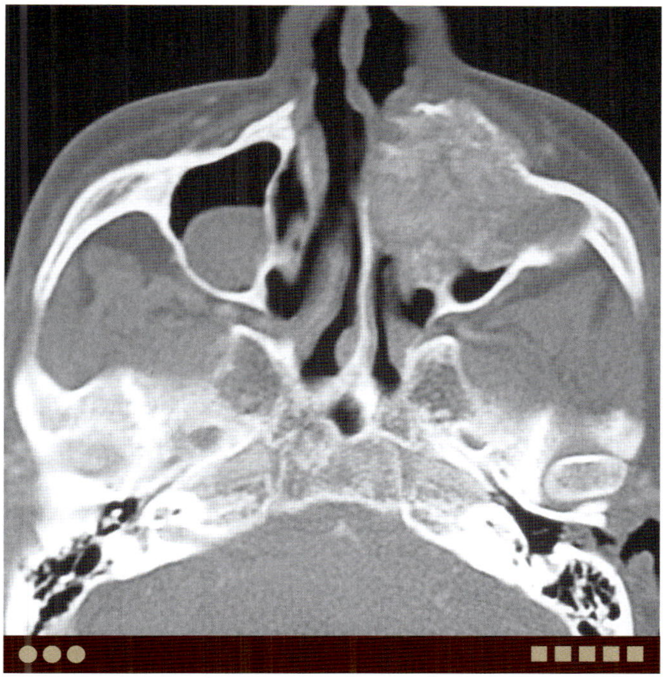

A. Hemangioma. Axial CT demonstrates an expansile osseous lesion in the left maxillary sinus with coarse heterogeneous internal density.

COMMENTS

This is a 48-year-old woman with nasal obstruction and left cheek mass.

Hemangioma of bone in the paranasal sinus is rare. It presents with a painless slow-growing swelling and may present with severe epistaxis.

Hemangiomas of bone often show substantial destructive changes and mimic malignant epithelial tumors. It is very important to suspect the vascular nature of these lesions prior to surgical intervention to avoid massive hemorrhage associated with the procedure.

Radiographic appearance of hemangiomas of the paranasal sinus is variable. They may show radiodense, expansile masses with destructive features. However, coarse trabeculation on CT is typically seen. On MRI, very high signal on T2W images is characteristic as seen in hemangiomas of other locations. Avid enhancement reflecting high vascularity is commonly seen.

PEARLS

- **Hemangioma of bone in the paranasal sinus is rare.**
- **Radiographic appearance of hemangiomas of the paranasal sinus is variable. They may show radiodense, expansile masses with destructive features similar to other osseous lesions.**
- **Coarse trabeculation on CT, high T2 signal on MRI, and avid enhancement are commonly seen.**

ADDITIONAL IMAGES (B-F)

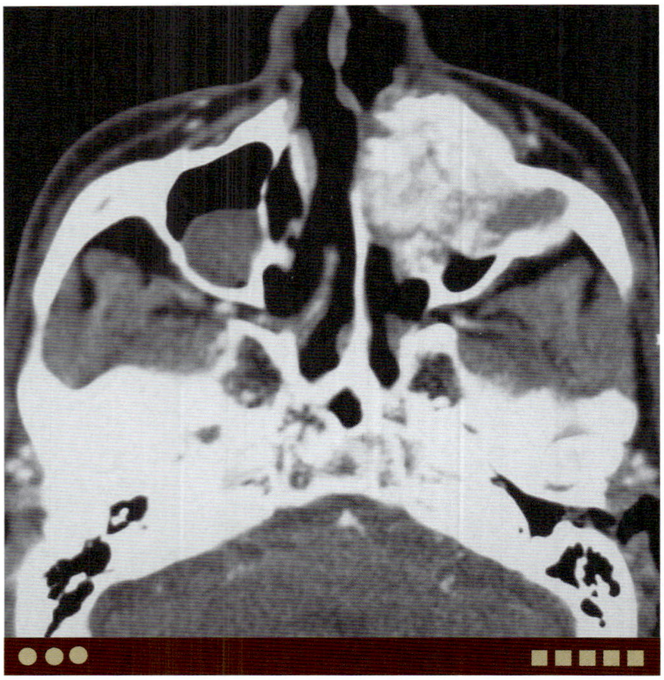

B. Hemangioma, same patient as A. Axial postcontrast CT demonstrates enhancement of the lesion in the left maxillary sinus.

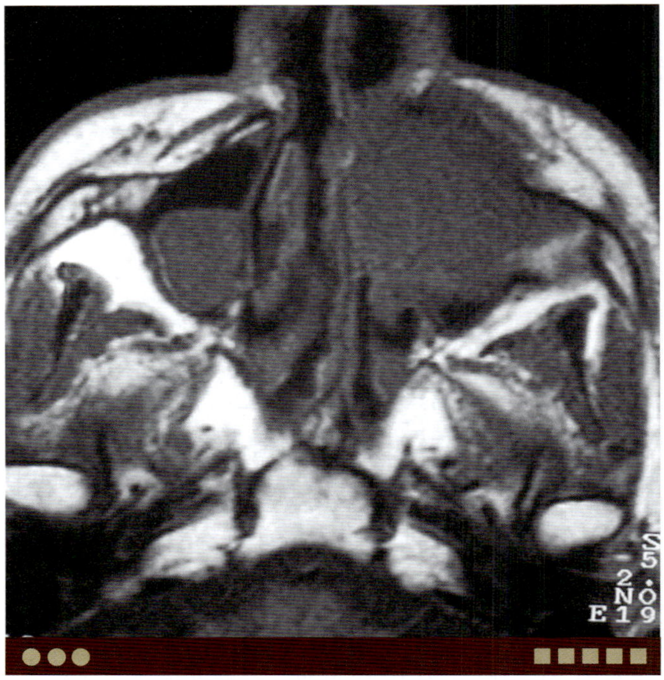

C. Hemangioma, same patient as A. Axial T1W image demonstrates homogeneous low signal in the lesion.

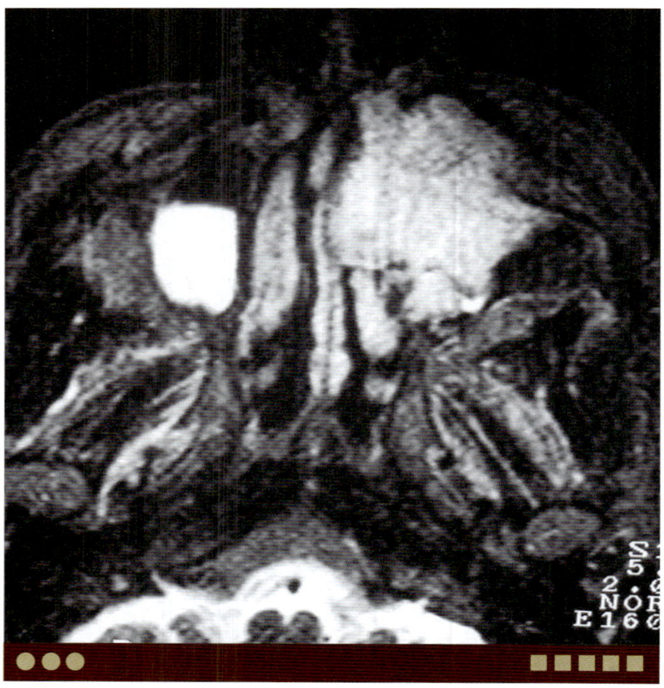

D. Hemangioma, same patient as A. Axial T2W image demonstrates very high signal in the lesion.

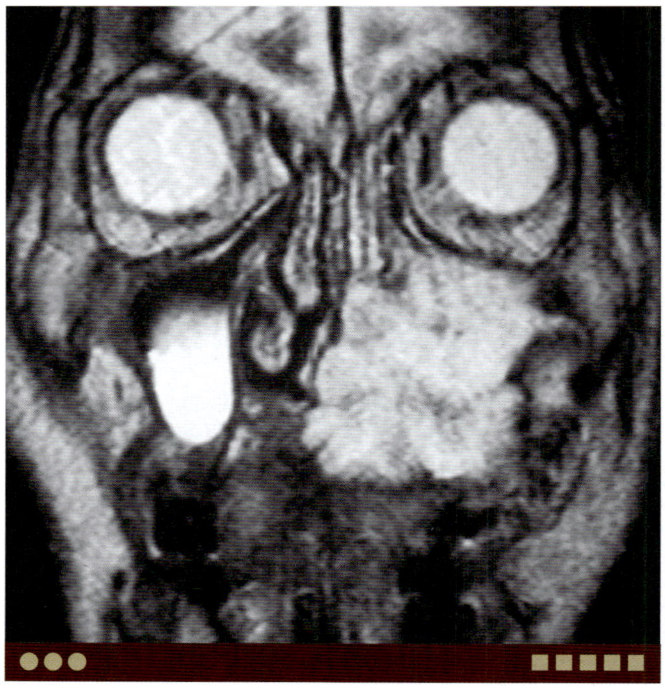

E. Hemangioma, same patient as A. Coronal T2W image demonstrates a lobulated left maxillary lesion with very high internal signal.

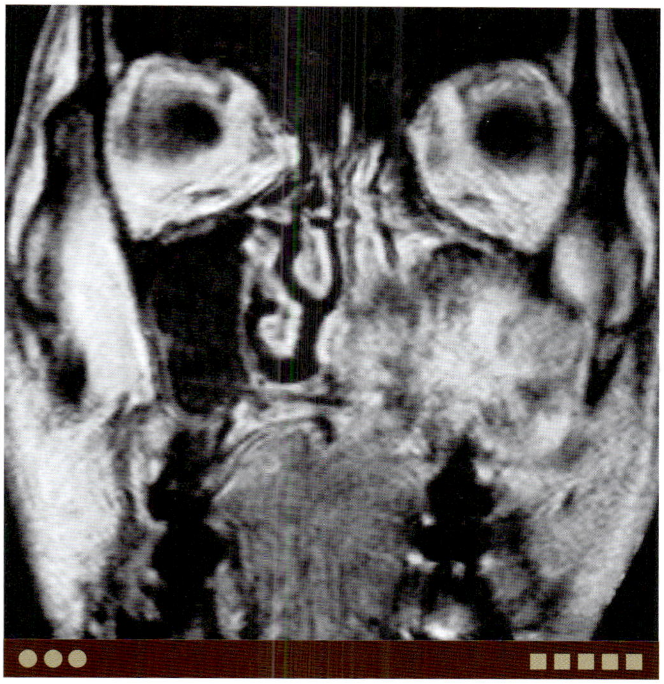

F. Hemangioma, same patient as A. Coronal postcontrast T1W image demonstrates heterogeneous enhancement of the lesion.

DIFFERENTIAL DIAGNOSIS IMAGES (G-J)

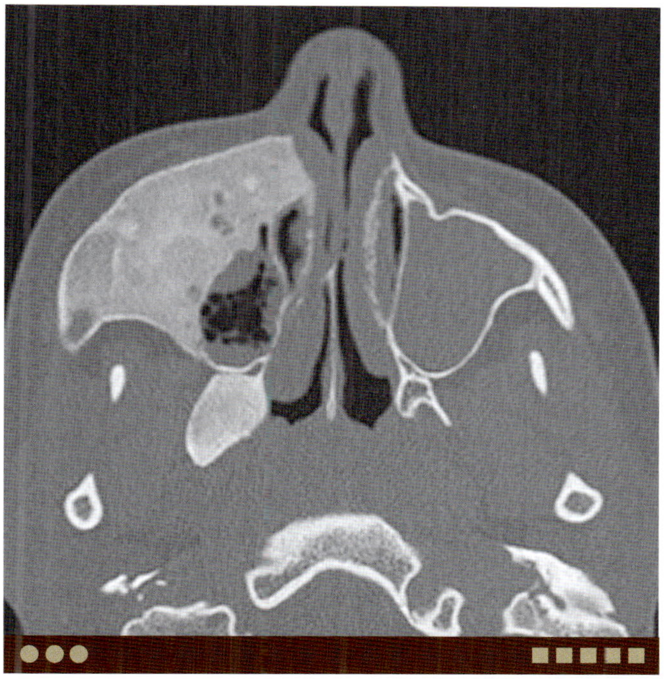

G. **Fibrous dysplasia**. Axial CT demonstrates expansion of the anterior and lateral walls of the right maxillary sinus with a "ground-glass" internal matrix. Also note involvement of the right pterygoid process.

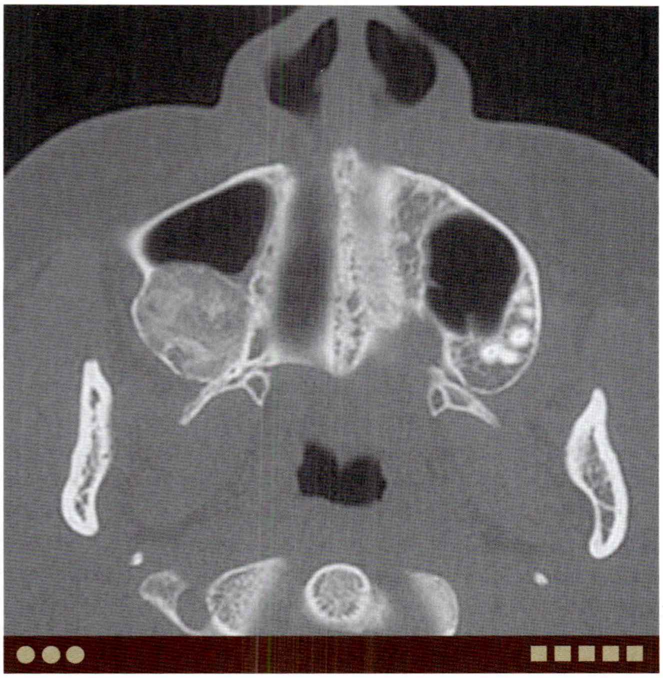

H. **Ossifying fibroma**. Axial CT demonstrates an expansile, radiodense mass in the posterolateral wall of the right maxillary sinus.

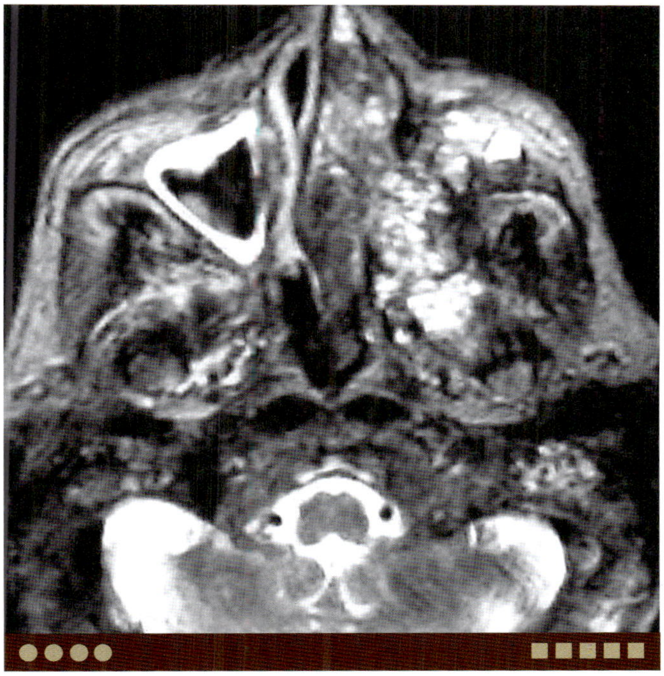

I. **Paget's disease**. Axial T2W image demonstrates a heterogeneous signal lesion in the left maxillary sinus obliterating the sinus lumen. Note expanded marrow space and heterogeneous signal through the skull base.

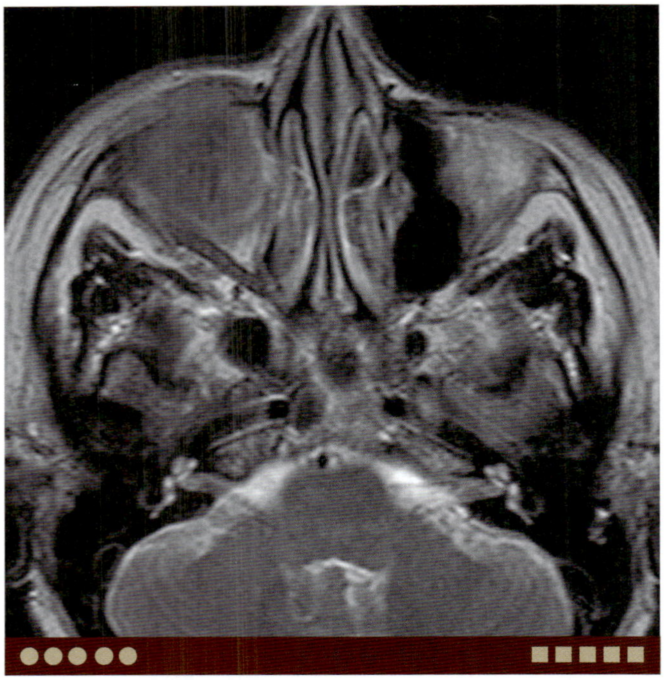

J. Squamous cell carcinoma. Axial T2W image demonstrates an intermediate-signal tumor in the right maxillary sinus. Note destruction of the anterior wall and invasion to the superficial soft tissue.

Case 3–22 Fibrous Dysplasia

Elisa Flower, Osamu Sakai

PRESENTATION

Facial asymmetry.

FINDINGS

CT demonstrates expansion of the bones of the skull base and paranasal sinus wall with a ground-glass internal matrix.

DIFFERENTIAL DIAGNOSIS

- Ossifying fibroma: This is a benign fibro-osseous lesion composed of lamellar bone with prominent osteoblastic rimming in dense fibrous stroma demonstrating nearly identical radiological findings to fibrous dysplasia.
- Paget's disease: This is a common disease of unknown etiology, usually seen in elderly people and unusual before age 40. Involvement of the skull and skull base is common, although any bones can be affected.
- Osteoma: This lesion is usually smaller, more focal and densely ossified. Multiple osteomas are associated with Gardner's syndrome.
- Reactive sclerosis/calcification due to malignant tumors: Occasionally, prominent sclerotic change is seen with malignant tumors, often squamous cell carcinomas due to stimulation of osteoblasts by the tumor.

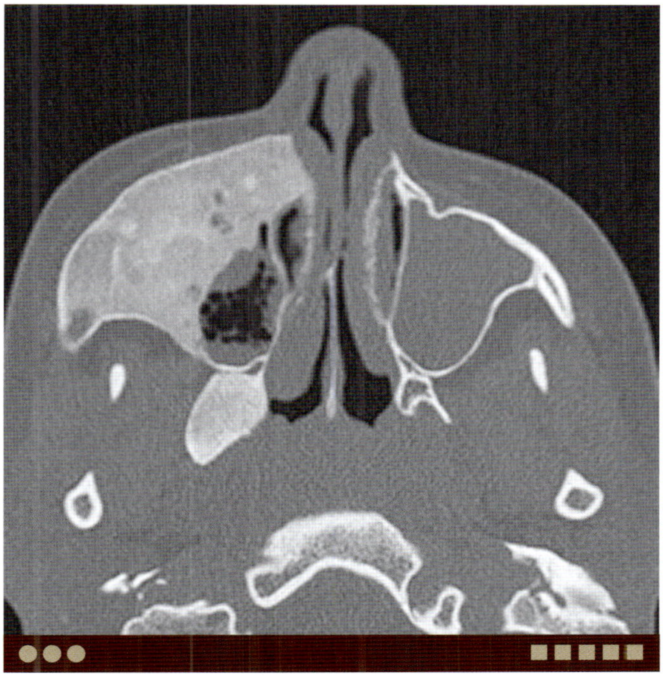

A. Fibrous dysplasia. Axial CT demonstrates expansion of the anterior and lateral walls of the right maxillary sinus with a "ground-glass" internal matrix. Also note involvement of the right pterygoid process.

COMMENTS

This is a 16-year-old girl with longstanding facial asymmetry.

Fibrous dysplasia is an idiopathic disorder where normal medullary bone is replaced by poorly organized weak fibroosseous tissue. As opposed to a neoplasm, it is a developmental anomaly. Fibrous dysplasia is generally diagnosed in childhood or adolescence, before the age of 30. In the sinonasal region it presents with painless swelling or sinus obstruction. Fibrous dysplasia can be monoostotic (~75% of cases with one quarter of which have head and neck involvement) or polyostotic (~25% with head and neck involvement seen over half of these cases). Mucoceles can be seen in association with sinonasal fibrous dysplasia. McCune-Albright syndrome is seen exclusively in females consists of polyostotic fibrous dysplasia, pigmented skin macules and precocious puberty.

The classic CT appearance is that of bony expansion with a "ground-glass" matrix. The diploic space is expanded generally with an intact rim of overlying cortex. Variable appearance is possible resulting from the inhomogeneity of bony and fibrous components. On MRI, the lesion tends to be both T1 and T2 hypointense and demonstrates intense enhancement.

Fibrous dysplasia is treated surgically if there is functional impairment. Radiation is not used as this causes increased risk of malignant transformation.

PEARLS

- **Fibrous dysplasia causes expansion of bone with a "ground-glass" matrix.**
- **Fibrous dysplasia can be difficult to distinguish from ossifying fibroma, and indeterminate lesions are often described as "benign fibroosseous lesion."**

ADDITIONAL IMAGES (B-F)

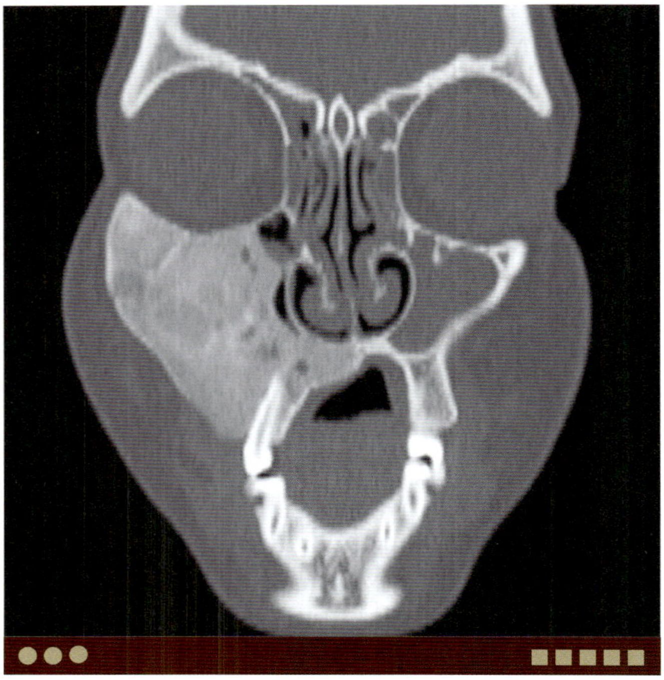

B. Fibrous dysplasia, same patient as A. Coronal CT demonstrates extension of the lesion to involve the palate and alveolar ridge.

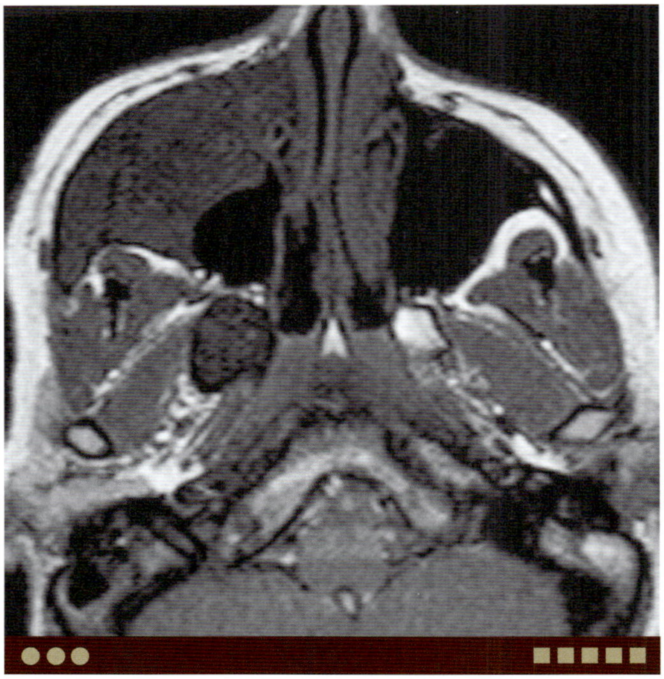

C. Fibrous dysplasia, same patient as A. Axial T1W MR image demonstrates low signal of the lesion when compared to normal marrow signal. Thin rim of low-density signal seen around the lesion from intact overlying cortex.

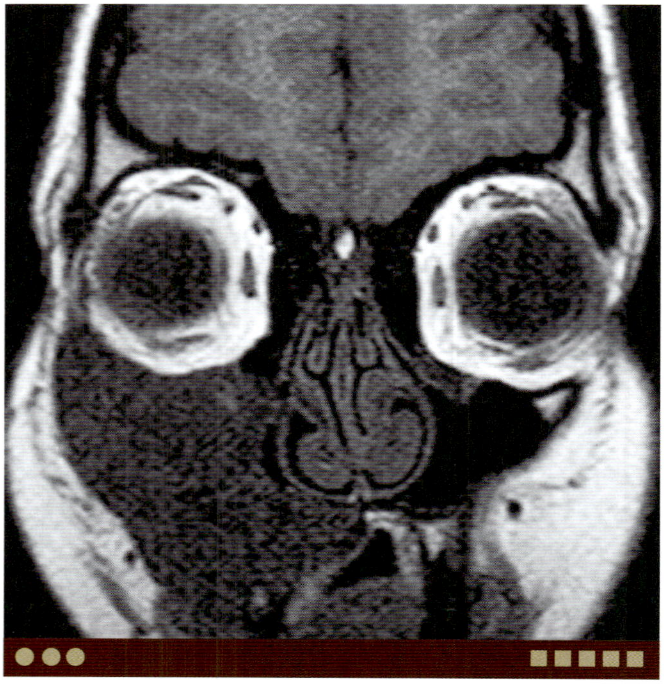

D. Fibrous dysplasia, same patient as A. Coronal T1W MR image demonstrates low signal of the lesion when compared to normal marrow signal.

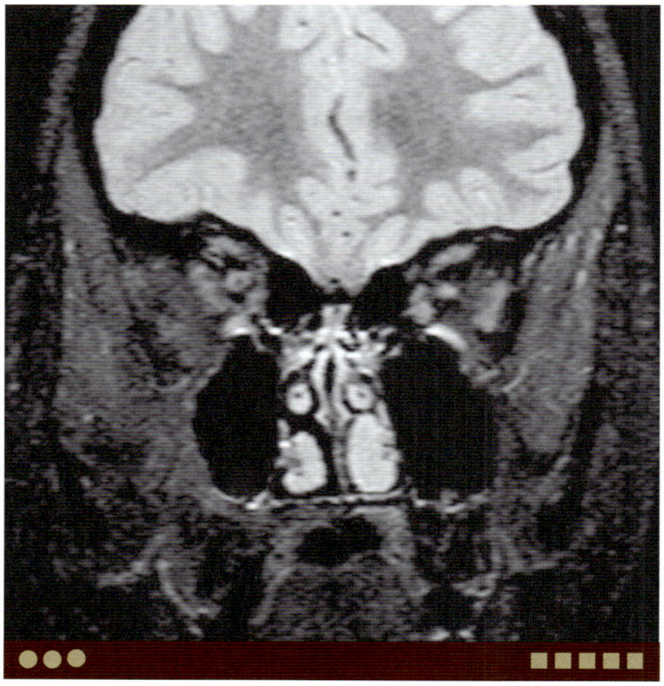

E. Fibrous dysplasia, same patient as A. Coronal STIR image demonstrates low signal of the lesion.

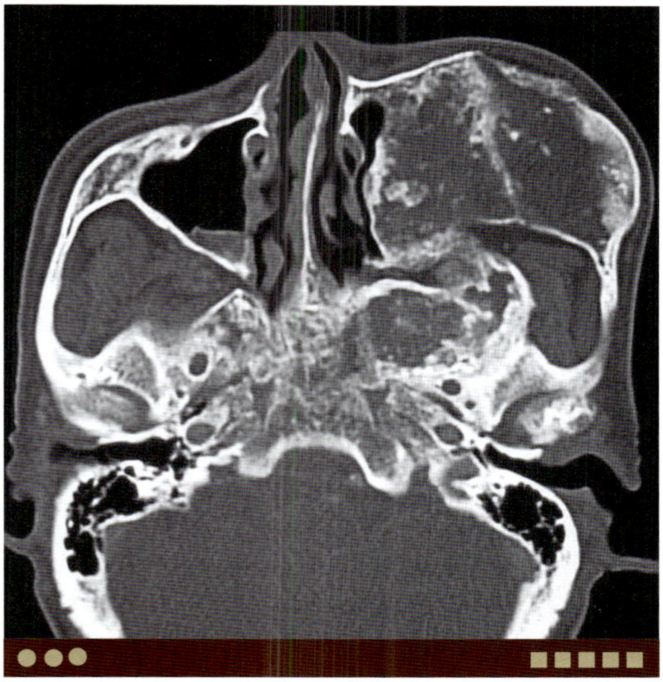

F. **Fibrous dysplasia** in a different patient. Axial CT demonstrates significant expansion of the anterior and lateral wall of the left maxillary sinus and pterygoid with foci of coarse calcification. The cortex is preserved.

DIFFERENTIAL DIAGNOSIS IMAGES (G-I)

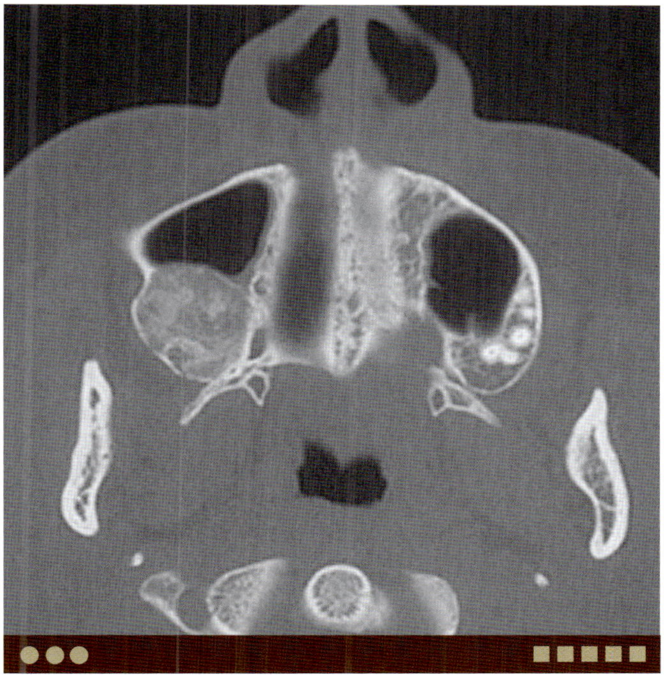

G. **Ossifying fibroma**. Axial CT demonstrates an expansile, radiodense mass in the posterolateral wall of the right maxillary sinus.

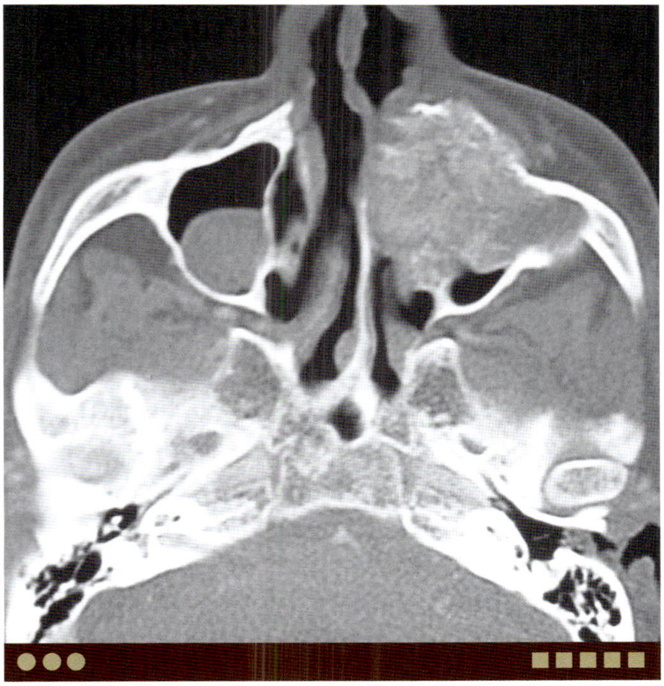

H. **Hemangioma**. Axial CT demonstrates an expansile osseous lesion in the left maxillary sinus with coarse heterogeneous internal density.

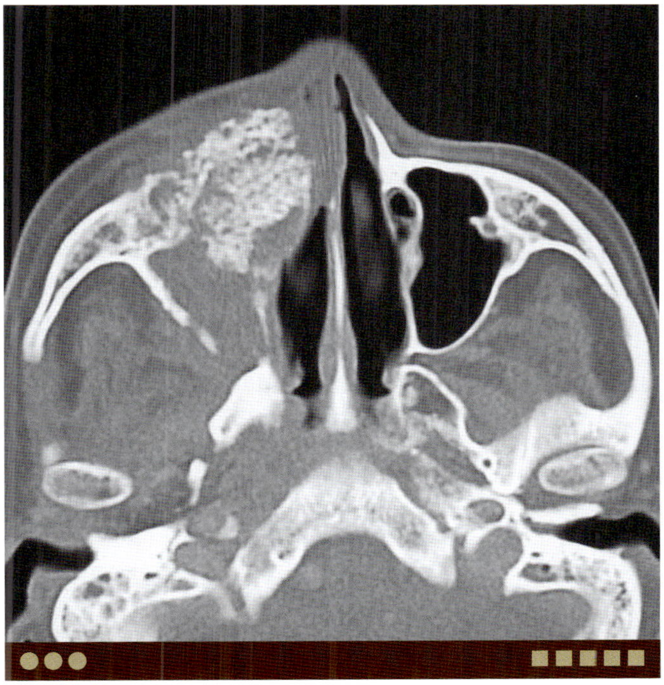

I. **Mucoepidermoid carcinoma**. Axial CT demonstrates a mass with irregular, coarse calcification in the anterior wall of the right maxillary sinus. Note a large soft tissue component.

Case 3–23 Inverted Papilloma

Osamu Sakai, Elisa Flower

PRESENTATION

Nasal obstruction, nasal mass.

FINDINGS

MR images show a convoluted cerebriform mass occupying the nasal cavity extending into the maxillary sinus.

DIFFERENTIAL DIAGNOSIS

- Antrochoanal polyp: Extent of the lesion may be similar to inverted papilloma, however this polyp starts from the maxillary sinus and extends to the nasal cavity and to the choana.
- Squamous cell carcinoma (SCCA): SCCA may coexist with inverted papilloma. SCCA shows more destructive or invasive changes to the adjacent structures, however it is often difficult to be differentiated by imaging alone.
- Lymphoma: Lymphoma shows homogeneous density/signal and enhancement without necrosis.

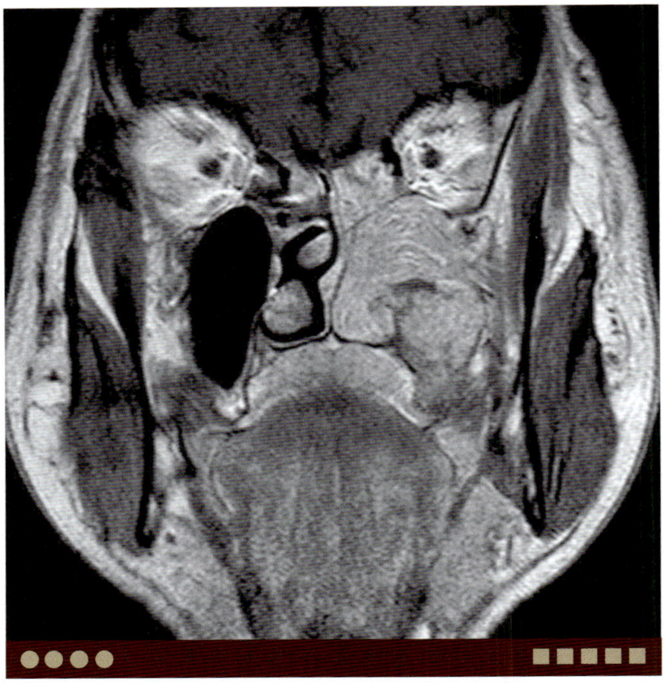

A. Inverted papilloma. Coronal postcontrast T1W image demonstrates a convoluted cerebriform enhancing mass in the left nasal cavity extending into the maxillary sinus.

COMMENTS

This is a 52-year-old man with nasal obstruction and mass in the left nasal cavity.

Sinonasal papillomas can be divided into three distinct forms: fungiform papilloma, inverted papilloma, and cylindric cell papilloma. Inverted papilloma accounts for 47% of all nasal papillomas, however nasal papillomas are uncommon, accounting for less than 5% of all sinonasal tumors. Inverted papilloma is a benign, however, locally aggressive epithelial neoplasm in the sinonasal cavity with significant malignant potential. Approximately 10% to 15% of inverted papillomas of the sinonasal cavity develop or are associated with SCCA. Inverted papillomas can occur anywhere in the sinonasal cavity, however, often arise from the lateral wall of the nasal cavity and extend into the maxillary sinus with bony remodeling. Bony destruction or invasion into the adjacent structures raises the possibility of transformation or coexisting SCCA.

CT is helpful to identify the lesion and to evaluate for bony remodeling or destruction. Calcification is often seen. MRI often demonstrates convoluted cerebriform appearance, which is very unique to inverted papilloma on T2W or postcontrast T1W images, although findings can be nonspecific. Imaging is very important for surgical planning and to evaluate for co-existing SCCA, skull base invasion or perineural tumor spread.

PEARLS

- **Inverted papilloma often arises from the lateral wall of the nasal cavity and extends into the maxillary sinus with bony remodeling.**
- **MRI often demonstrates convoluted cerebriform appearance, which is very unique to inverted papilloma on T2W and postcontrast T1W images.**
- **Ten to fifteen percent of inverted papillomas develop or are associated with squamous cell carcinoma. Bony destruction and invasion to the adjacent structures raise the possibility of malignancy.**

ADDITIONAL IMAGES (B-H)

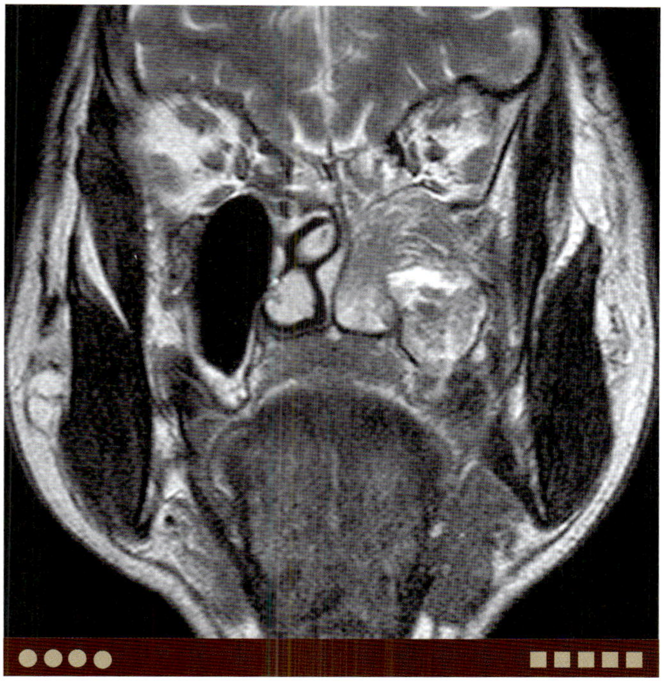

B. Inverted papilloma, same patient as A. Coronal T2W image demonstrates heterogeneous, intermediate signal within the lesion.

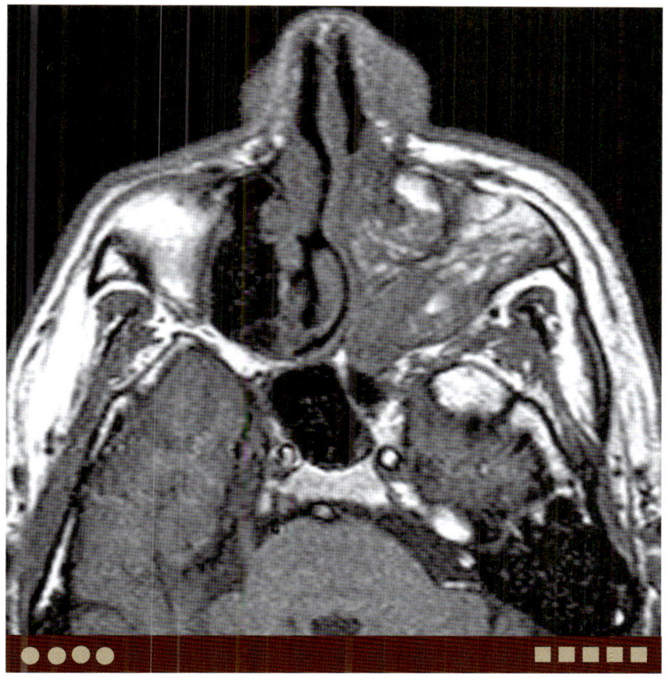

C. Inverted papilloma, same patient as A. Axial T1W image demonstrates a heterogeneous signal mass remodeling of the posterior wall of the left maxillary sinus. The heterogeneously increased signal is mostly from proteinaceous secretion and partially from microcalcification.

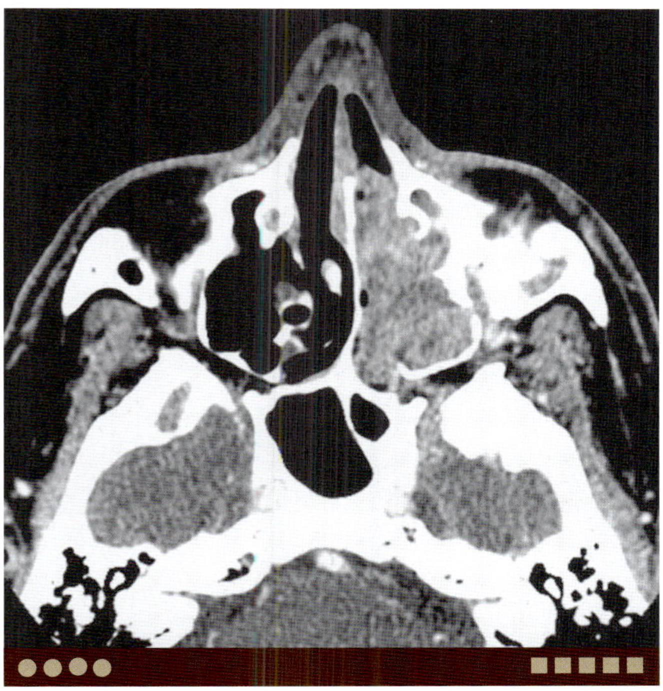

D. Inverted papilloma in a different patient. Axial CT demonstrates a heterogeneous mass in the left maxillary sinus.

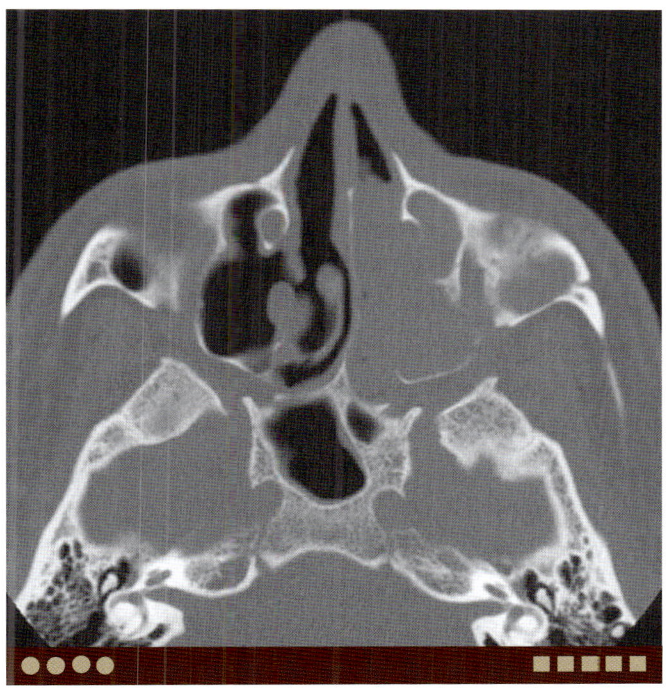

E. Inverted papilloma, same patient as D. Axial bone window CT demonstrates erosion of the medial wall of the left maxillary sinus.

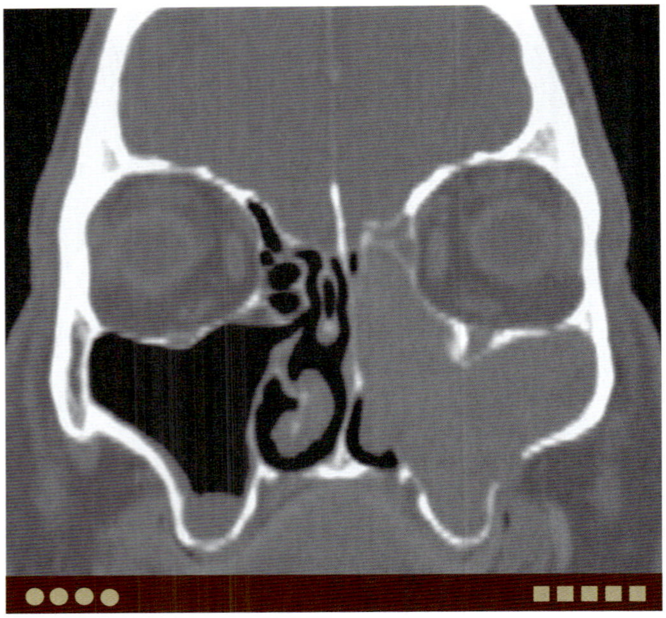

F. Inverted papilloma, same patient as E. Coronal bone window CT demonstrates erosion of the medial and lateral walls of the left maxillary sinus.

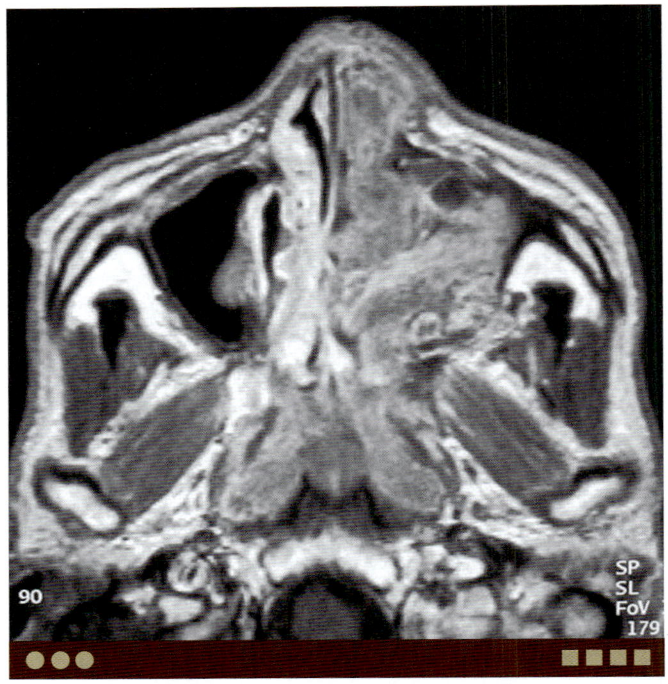

G. **Inverted papilloma with SCCA** in a different patient. Axial post-contrast T1W image demonstrates a heterogeneously enhancing tumor occupying the left maxillary sinus and nasal cavity. Note destruction of the posterolateral wall of the maxillary sinus and tumor invasion to the retroantral fat and pterygoid plate.

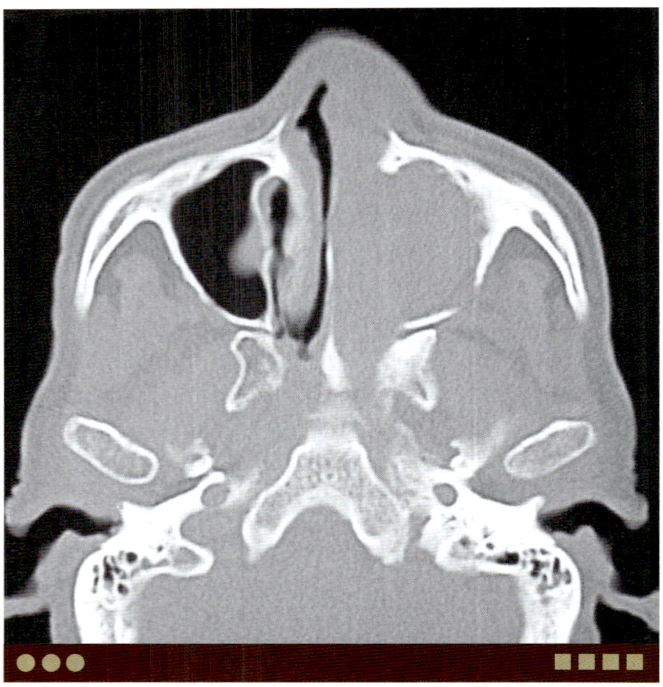

H. Inverted papilloma with SCCA, same patient as G. Axial bone window CT demonstrates disruption of the posterolateral wall of the left maxillary sinus and erosion and sclerotic change in the left pterygoid plate.

DIFFERENTIAL DIAGNOSIS IMAGES (I-J)

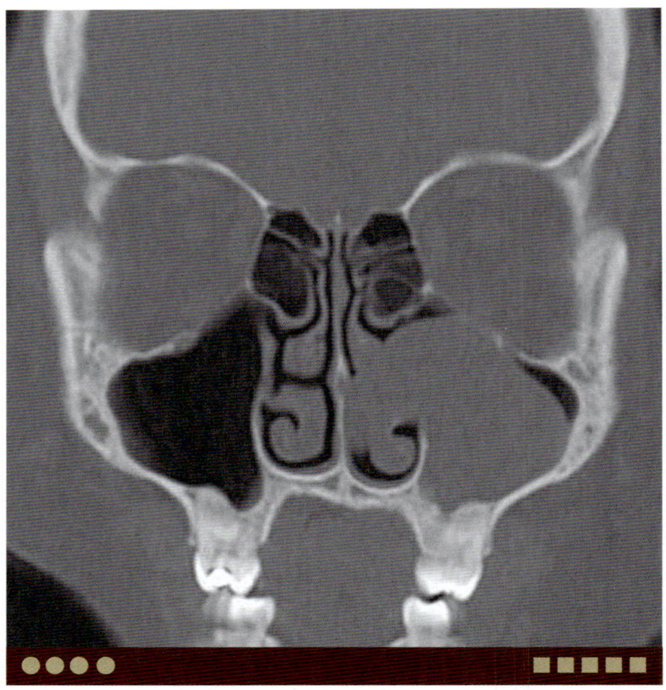

I. **Antrochoanal polyp**. Coronal CT demonstrates a polyp extending into the nasal cavity from the maxillary sinus with benign bone remodeling.

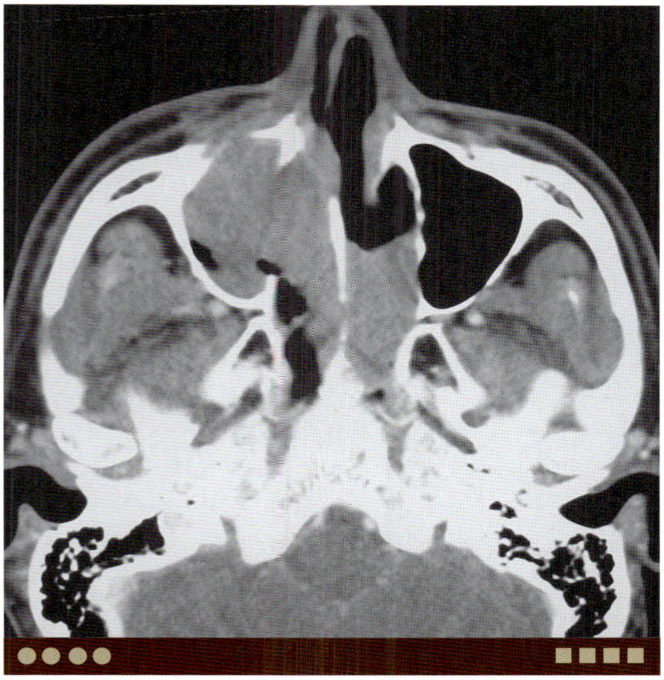

J. Lymphoma. Axial postcontrast CT demonstrates tumor extension beyond the anterior wall of the right maxillary sinus. The tumor also involves bilateral nasal cavities.

Case 3–24 Plasmacytoma

Osamu Sakai, Gabriel Monagas

PRESENTATION

A nasal mass.

FINDINGS

CT and MRI demonstrate an expansile nasal septal mass with homogeneous enhancement.

DIFFERENTIAL DIAGNOSIS

- Lymphoma: This is rare in the nasal cavity but may demonstrate relatively well-circumscribe margins and homogeneous density/signal. Bone expansion or infiltration is more common than erosion.
- Nasal polyp: This is a polypoid mass arising from the nasal mucosa.
- Squamous cell carcinoma (SCCA): SCCA is the most common malignant tumor in the sinonasal cavity. However, osseous involvement would show a more destructive pattern, rather than an expansile lesion.
- Adenoid cystic carcinoma: This is a malignant tumor arising from the minor salivary gland. High-grade tumors show higher cellularity and low signal on T2W images. Perineural tumor spread is common. Other malignancies arising from the minor salivary gland, which are spread throughout the nasal mucosa and sinuses, could potentially present in a similar manner. However, these are also unlikely to present as expansile osseous lesions.

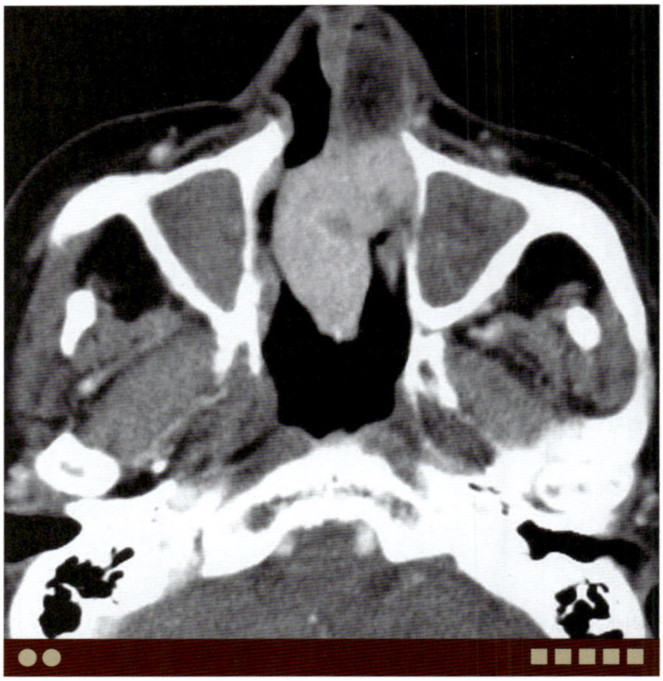

A. Plasmacytoma. Axial postcontrast CT demonstrates a homogeneously enhancing tumor centered in the nasal septum.

COMMENTS

This is an 82-year-old man with a nasal septal mass.

The nasal septum has cartilage and bone, therefore it is susceptible to chondroid and osseous tumors including hematological neoplastic lesions. Tumors arising from the marrow space within the septum show unique expansion of the septum rather than eccentric mass formation or destruction. Therefore, the differential diagnosis may be able to be narrowed by the imaging findings.

Plasmacytoma of the nasal septum is a rare neoplasm of B-lymphocyte populations, accounting less than 1% of all head and neck malignancy. This tumor usually occurs in the elderly population, usually 60 to 80 years, predominantly in men. Epistaxis, nasal obstruction and pain are common initial presentations. Diagnosis by the biochemical profile is often difficult because only 25% of the patients have increased M-protein levels in their blood or urine. Therefore, biopsy is required for the diagnosis.

CT shows expansion and remodeling of the bone. Expansile change of the osseous portion of the nasal septum strongly suggests a lesion arising from the marrow not mucosa. Plasmacytoma demonstrates intermediate signal on T1W and moderate-to-high signal on T2W images, and moderate-to-marked enhancement.

The differential diagnosis includes more common lesions in the sinonasal cavity, such as SCCA, lymphoma, adenoid cystic carcinoma, rhabdomyosarcoma, and Wegener's granulomatosis.

PEARLS

- **Plasmacytoma is rare in the sinonasal cavity.**
- **Expansile change of the osseous portion of the nasal septum strongly suggests a lesion arising from the marrow not mucosa.**
- **Imaging findings are similar to other small round cell tumors.**

ADDITIONAL IMAGES (B-F)

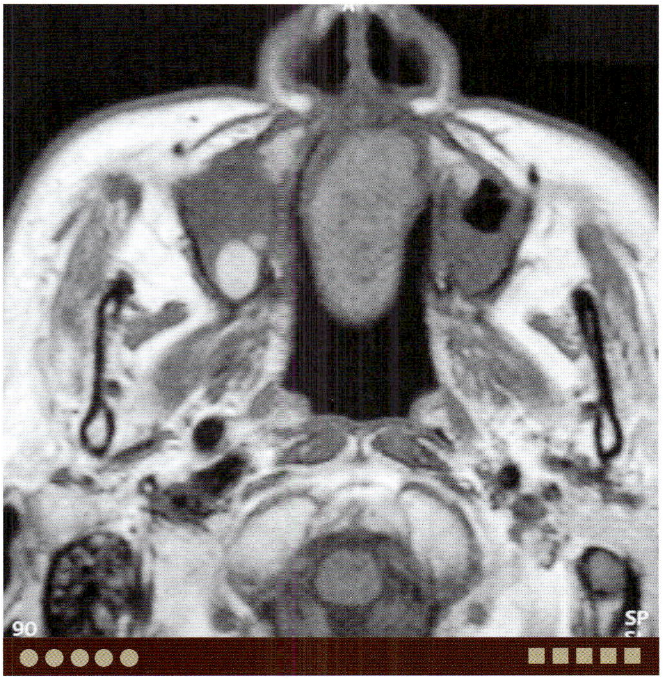

B. Plasmacytoma, same patient as A. Axial T1W image demonstrates an intermediate-signal lesion centered in the nasal septum.

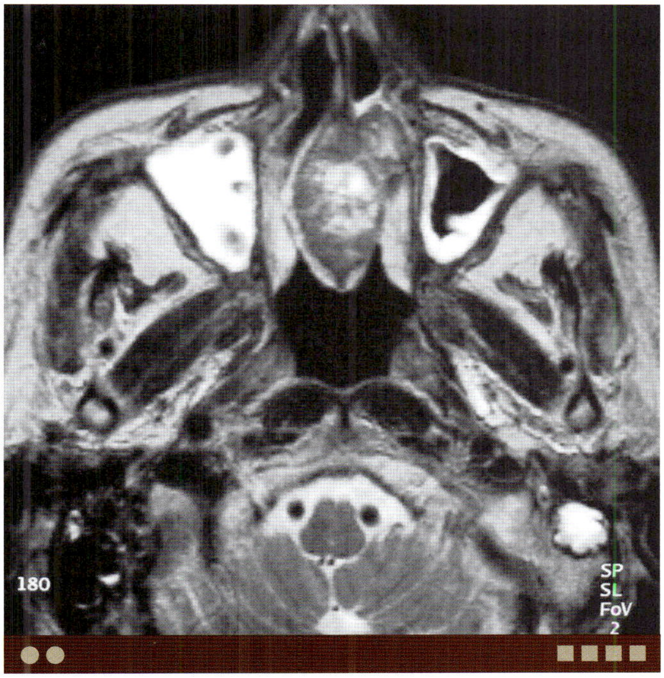

C. Plasmacytoma, same patient as A. Axial T2W image demonstrates a heterogeneous moderate-to-high signal lesion centered in the nasal septum.

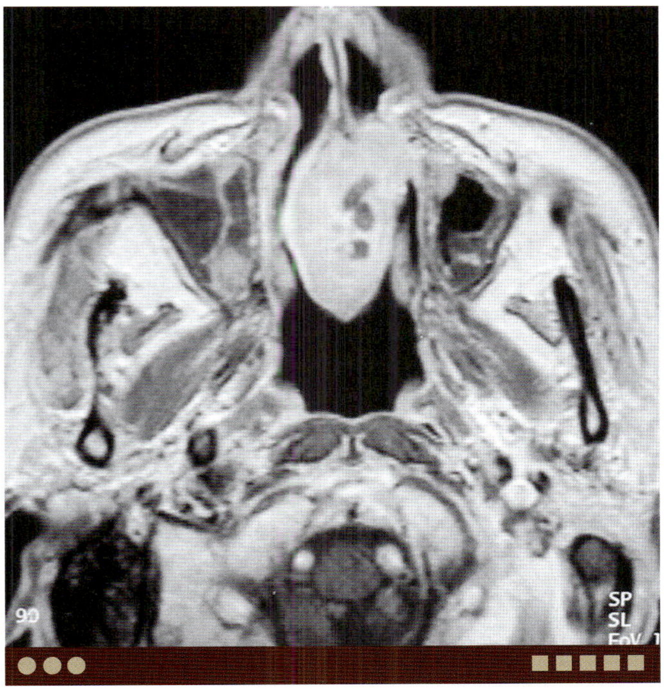

D. Plasmacytoma, same patient as A. Axial postcontrast T1W image demonstrates homogeneous enhancement of the lesion except the central cystic or necrotic portion.

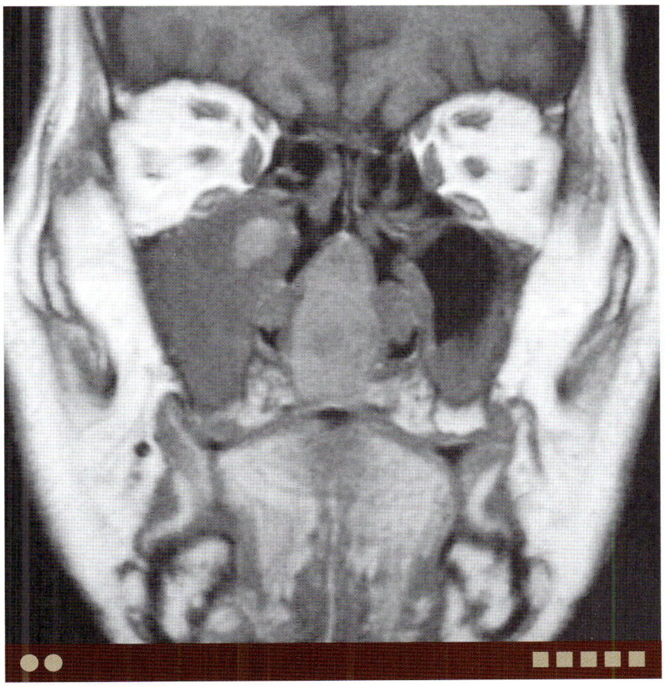

E. Plasmacytoma, same patient as A. Coronal T1W image demonstrates an intermediate-signal lesion centered in the nasal septum.

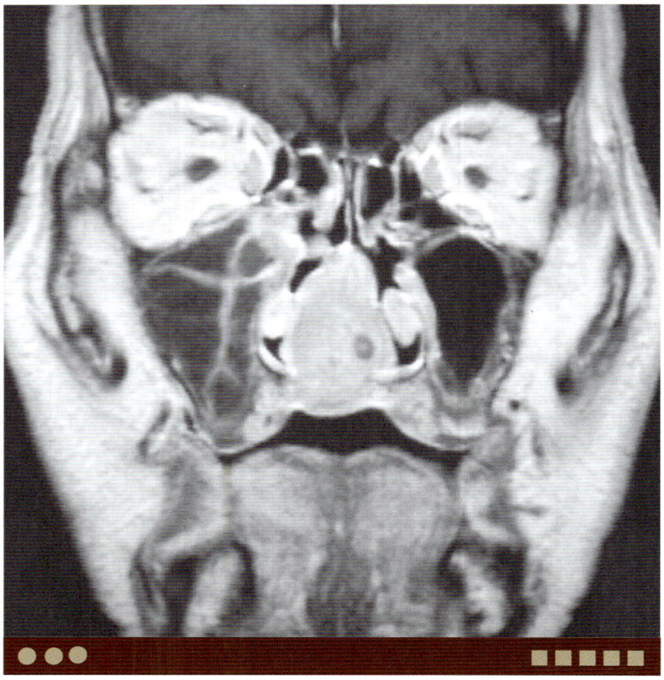

F. Plasmacytoma, same patient as A. Coronal postcontrast T1W image demonstrates homogeneous enhancement of the lesion.

DIFFERENTIAL DIAGNOSIS IMAGES (G-I)

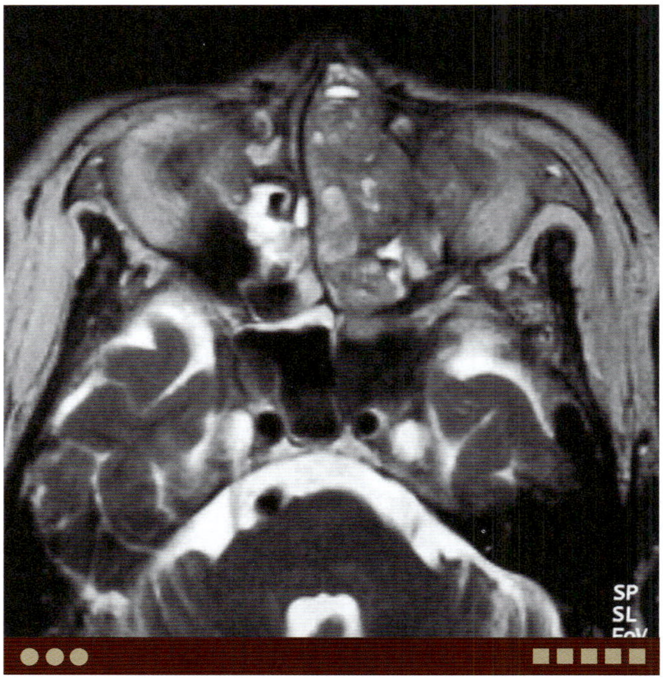

G. Melanoma. Axial T2W image demonstrates a heterogeneous intermediate-to-low signal lesion in the left nasal cavity and ethmoid.

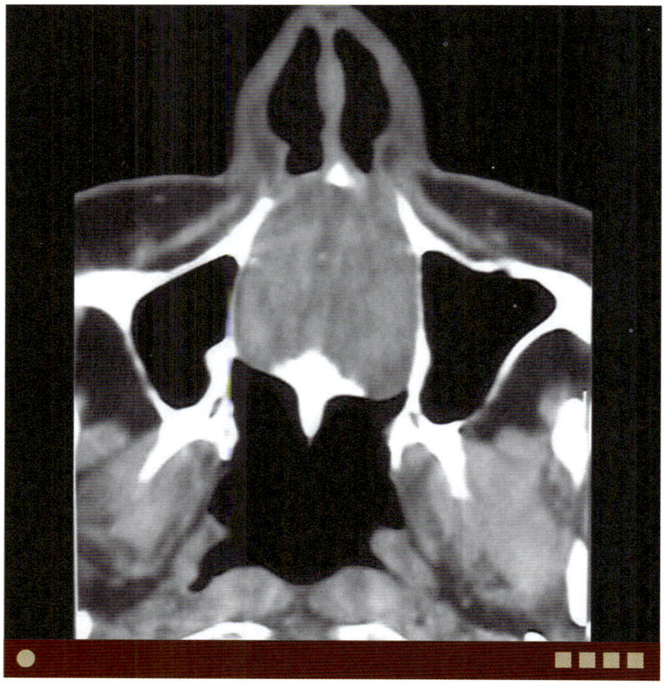

H. Chondromyxoid fibroma. Axial noncontrast CT demonstrates an expansile soft tissue density mass centered in the nasal septum.

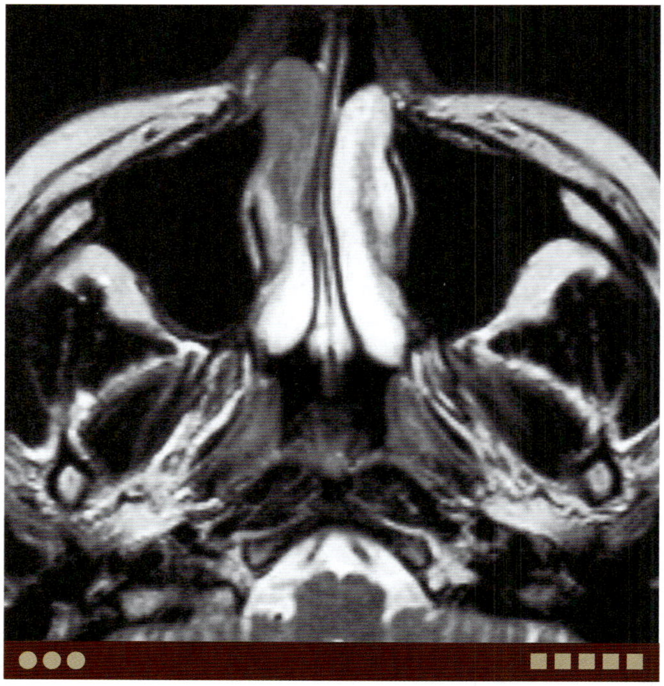

I. Lymphoma. Axial T2W image demonstrates a homogeneous intermediate-signal lesion in the right turbinate.

Case 3–25 Sinonasal Undifferentiated Carcinoma

Osamu Sakai, Daniel Weller

PRESENTATION

Nasal obstruction and sinus pain.

FINDINGS

CT and MRI demonstrate opacified sinus with aggressive bone destruction.

DIFFERENTIAL DIAGNOSIS

- Squamous cell carcinoma (SCCA): Most common sinonasal malignant tumor, most commonly occurs in the maxillary sinus.
- Lymphoma: A large, non-necrotic mass is a common finding. Among extranodal lymphoma in the head and neck, 40% to 50% occurs in the sinonasal cavity, commonly in the nasal cavity and maxillary sinus.
- Adenoid cystic carcinoma: Malignant tumor which arises from the minor salivary gland. Perineural tumor spread is commonly seen.
- Sinusitis: Initial presentation of SCCA is often similar to sinusitis. However, aggressive bone destruction should not be seen with sinusitis.
- Inverted papilloma: 10% to 15% of inverted papillomas develop from or are associated with SCCA. Careful evaluation to look for aggressive bone destruction is important.

COMMENTS

This is a 68-year-old man with nasal obstruction and sinus pain.

Sinonasal undifferentiated carcinoma (SNUC) is a rare and extremely aggressive neoplasm of the paranasal sinuses, first described in 1986 by Frierson et al. SNUC is characterized by rapid growth, a propensity for locoregional recurrence, distant metastases particularly to the lung and bone, and has very poor prognosis. SNUC consists of small to medium-sized undifferentiated cells, showing high mitotic rates and significant cellular pleomorphism with high nuclear to cytoplasmic ratios. Intratumoral necrosis and vascular invasion are commonly seen. Aggressive multimodality approach including surgery, radiation, and chemotherapy is needed for the best chance for locoregional control and cure.

Imaging findings of SNUC are nonspecific, however heterogeneous, avid enhancement, intratumoral necrosis, and aggressive invasion of the adjacent structures are commonly seen. These findings may be similar to that of esthesioneuroblastomas and neuroendocrine carcinomas, particularly when it occurs in the upper nasal cavity. Differentiation between SNUC and these tumors is often difficult, even histologically. Precise characterization of tumor extension is essential for appropriate treatment.

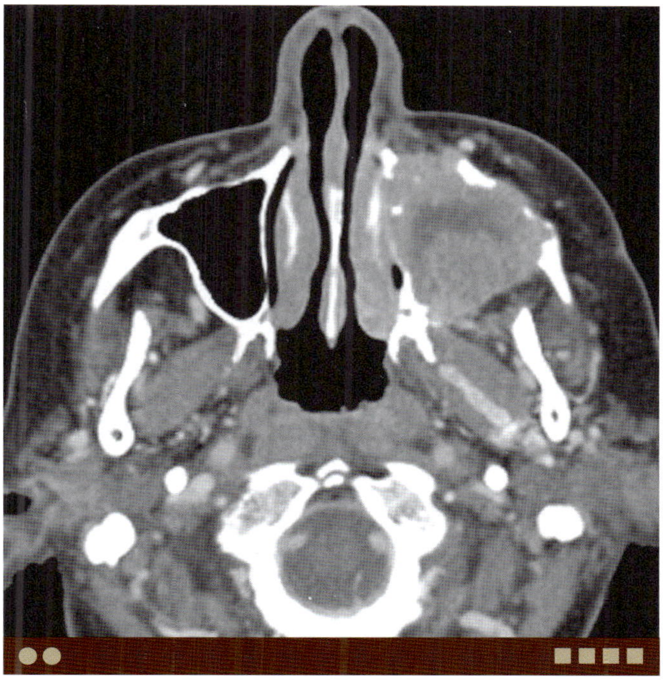

A. SNUC. Axial CT postcontrast demonstrates a solid enhancing tumor with necrosis, occupying the left maxillary sinus with evidence of destruction.

PEARLS

- **SNUC is a rare and extremely aggressive neoplasm of the paranasal sinuses**
- **Imaging findings are nonspecific, but aggressive, invasive, and destructive findings are seen.**
- **Differentiation between SNUC, esthesioneuroblastoma and neuroendocrine carcinomas is often difficult radiologically and histologically.**

ADDITIONAL IMAGES (B-G)

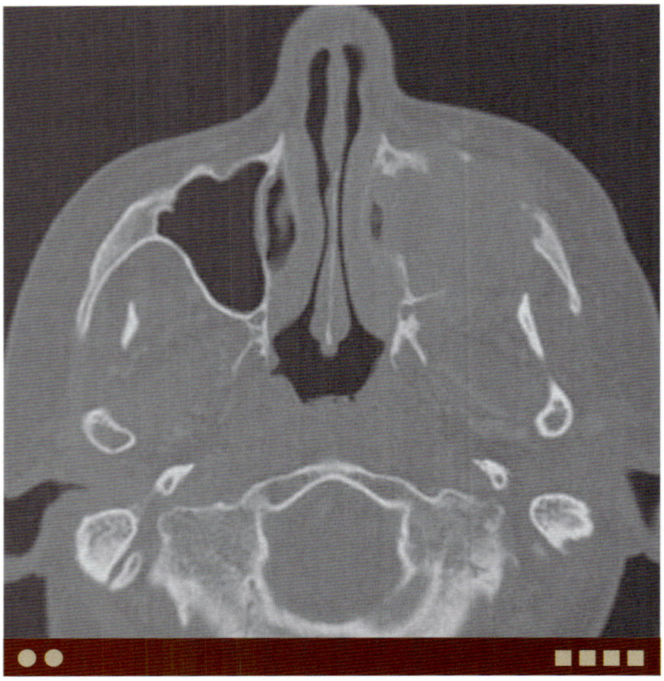

B. SNUC, same patient as A. Axial CT in bone window better demonstrates bone destruction by the tumor.

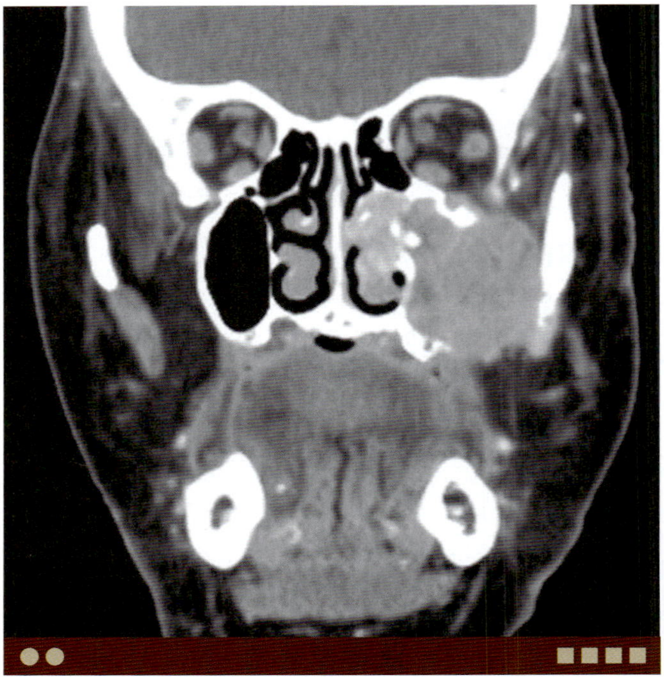

C. SNUC, same patient as A. Coronal postcontrast CT demonstrates tumor invading the buccal space and inferior orbital fissure with destruction of the lateral wall of the left maxillary sinus. Thickening of the infraorbital nerve suggests perineural tumor spread.

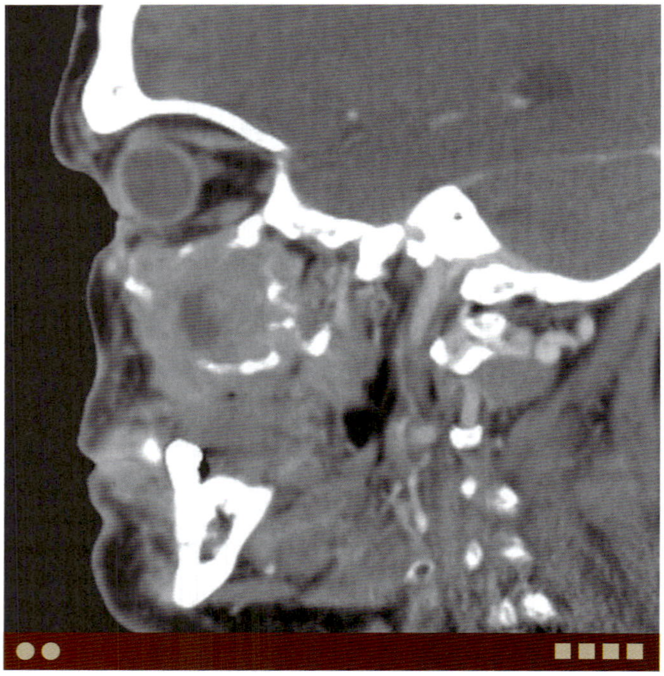

D. SNUC, same patient as A. Sagittal postcontrast CT demonstrates destruction of the maxillary sinus and tumor invasion to the buccal space and orbit.

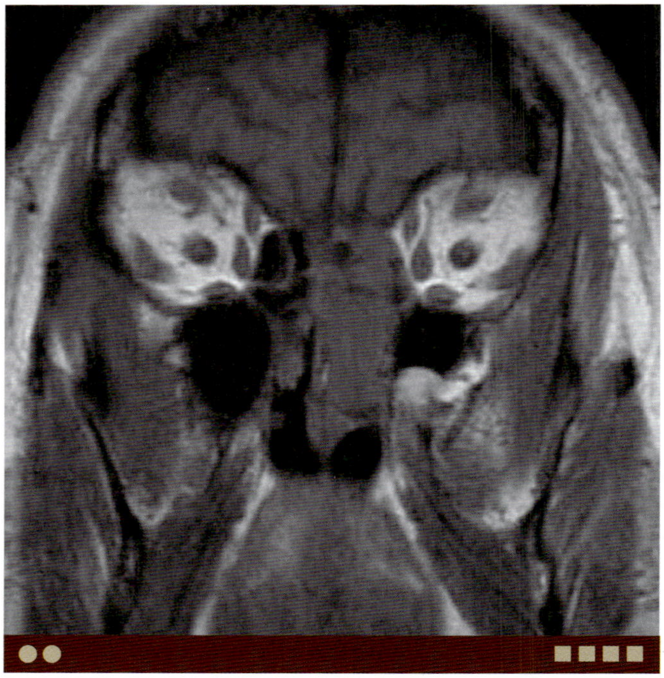

E. **SNUC** in a different patient. Coronal T1W MR image demonstrates a heterogeneously low-signal tumor occupying the left upper nasal cavity.

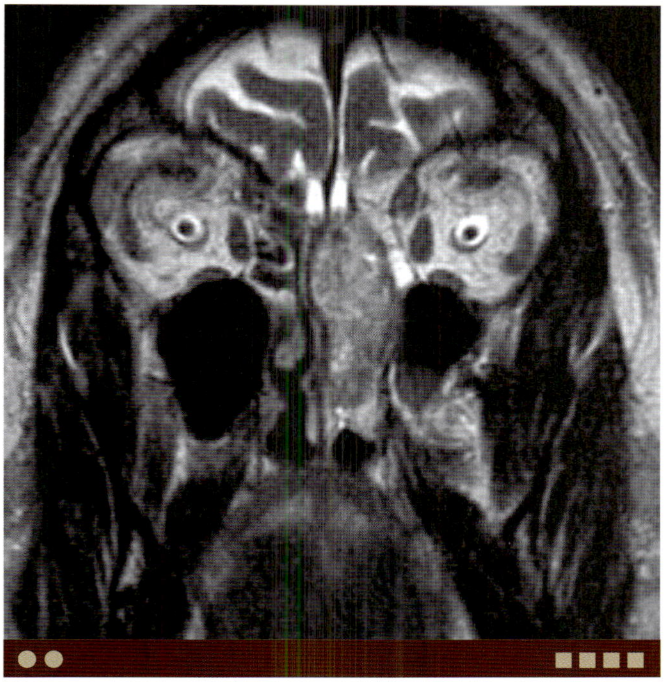

F. SNUC, same patient as E. Coronal T2W MR image demonstrates heterogeneous intermediate signal of the tumor.

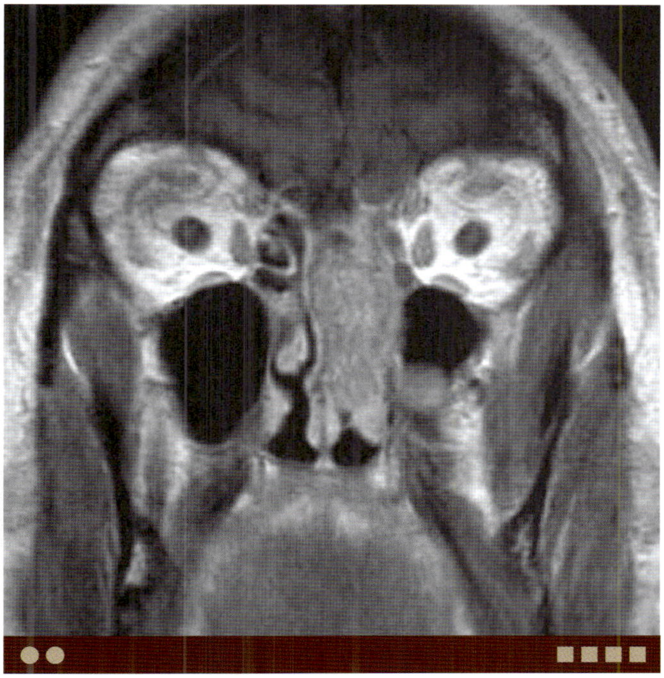

G. SNUC, same patient as E. Coronal postcontrast T1W MR image demonstrates heterogeneous enhancement of the tumor. Note enhancement along the left ethmoid roof suggesting skull base involvement.

DIFFERENTIAL DIAGNOSIS IMAGES (H-J)

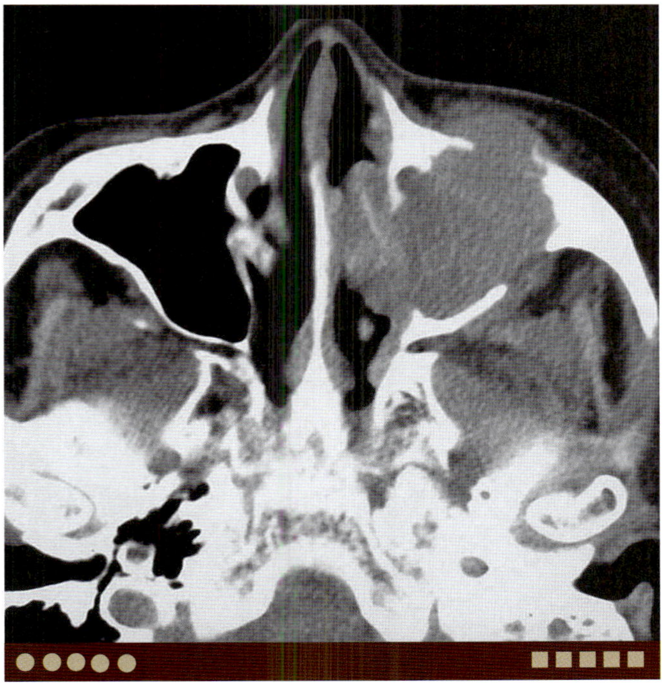

H. **SCCA**. Axial CT demonstrates a solid tumor occupying the left maxillary sinus, with destruction of the anterior wall and extension to the superficial soft tissue.

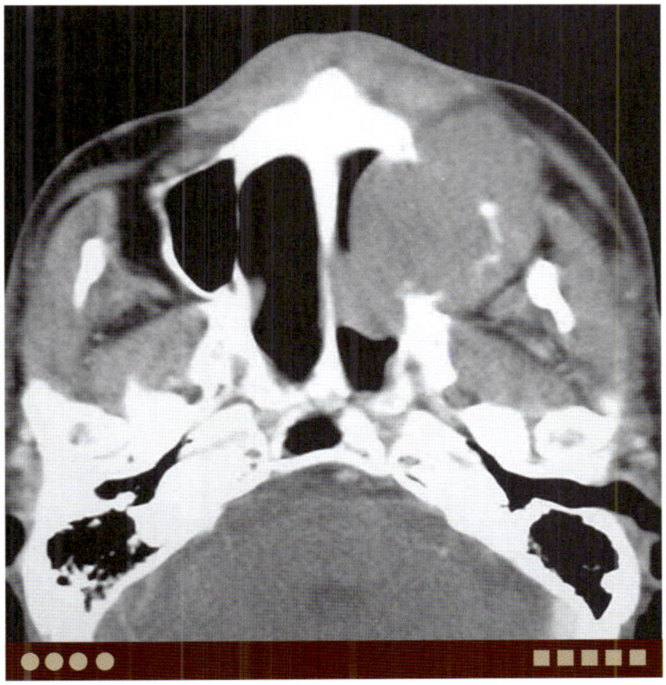

I. **Lymphoma**. Axial postcontrast CT demonstrates a large homogenous density tumor extending beyond the anterior and posterolateral walls of the left maxillary sinus. No necrosis is noted despite the large tumor size.

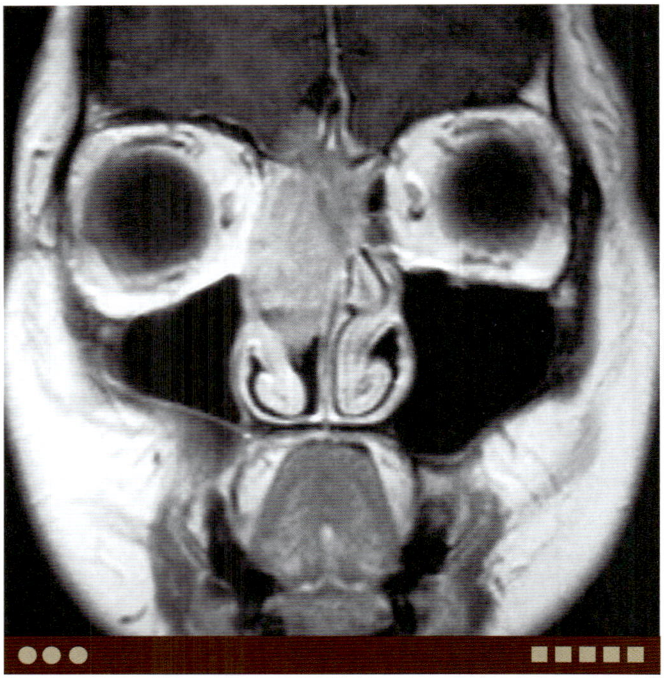

J. Neuroendocrine carcinoma. Coronal postcontrast T1W MR image demonstrates a heterogeneously enhancing tumor centered in the right upper nasal cavity crossing midline and invading the anterior skull base.

Case 3–26 Choanal Atresia

June Cheng, Osamu Sakai

PRESENTATION

Respiratory distress in a neonate and inability to pass a nasogastric tube.

FINDINGS

CT demonstrates narrowing or atresia of the posterior nasal passage.

DIFFERENTIAL DIAGNOSIS

- Nasal septum deviation: This is a very common condition causing narrowing of the nasal passage.
- Mucosal thickening/turbinate hypertrophy: This condition may cause soft tissue stenosis or obstruction of the choana.
- Dacryocystocele: This is the second most common cause of nasal obstruction in neonates after choanal atresia. There is an obstruction of the nasolacrimal duct, causing dilatation of the nasolacrimal sac.
- Pyriform aperture stenosis: This condition also may cause respiratory distress in a newborn. However, there is narrowing of the anterior nasal cavity, often associated with a central megaincisor.

COMMENTS

This is a 20-year-old woman with symptoms of sinusitis.

Choanal atresia is the most common congenital abnormality of the nasal cavity. The posterior nasal cavity (choana) is atretic or stenotic. Diagnosis in a neonate is often suspected with the inability to pass a nasogastric tube. However, imaging is necessary to confirm choanal atresia caused by a bony, membranous, or mixed obstruction. Neonates are obligate nasal breathers. Therefore, when choanal atresia is bilateral, patients present with severe respiratory distress. Unilateral choanal atresia is often not detected until adolescence and patients may present with a history of chronic purulent rhinorrhea and hyposmia.

CT demonstrates narrowing of the posterior choana and thickening of the vomer and posterior wall of the nasal cavity. Retained fluid is often detected in the involved nasal cavity. The posterior choanal width should be >0.5 cm in neonates and >2 cm in adolescents.

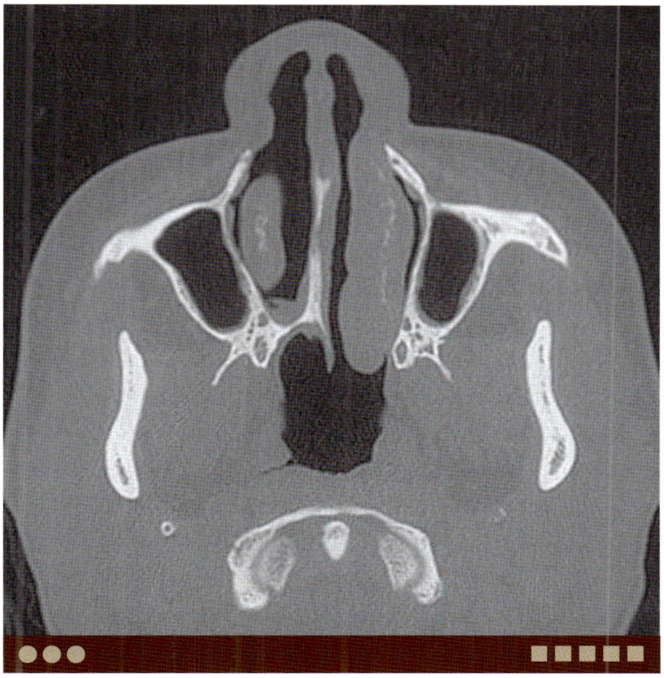

A. Choanal atresia. Axial CT demonstrates soft tissue and osseous closure of the right posterior nasal passage.

Patients with bilateral choanal atresia often have additional CNS and non-CNS congenital anomalies (75%), such as CHARGE syndrome. Therefore, MRI is useful in the evaluation of associated CNS anomalies.

PEARLS

- **CT demonstrates narrowing of the choana from a bony, membranous, or mixed obstruction and thickening of the vomer and posterior nasal cavity.**
- **Bilateral choanal atresia present in neonates with severe respiratory distress, while unilateral choanal atresia present in adolescents often with a history of purulent rhinorrhea and hyposmia, however the patient can be asymptomatic.**
- **Once bilateral choanal atresia is diagnosed, a search for additional anomalies should be performed.**

ADDITIONAL IMAGES (B-D)

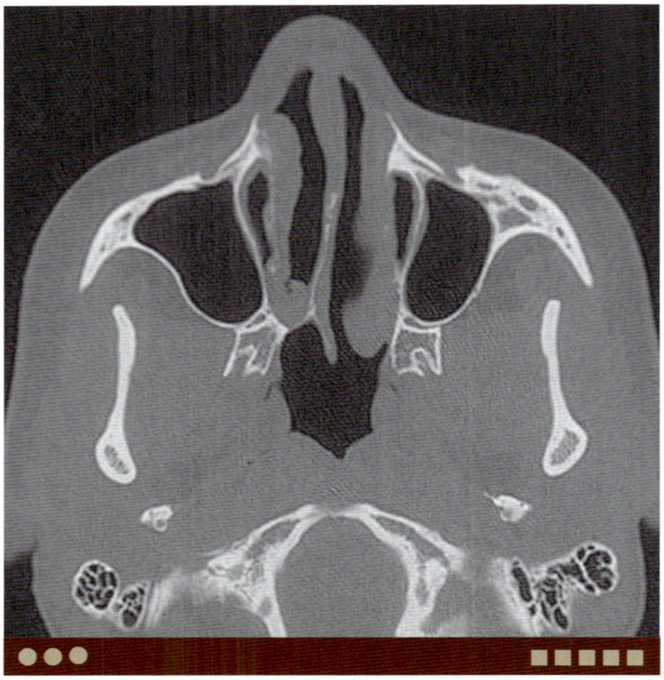

B. Choanal atresia, same patient as A. Axial CT through the slightly lower level again demonstrates soft tissue and osseous closure of the right posterior nasal passage.

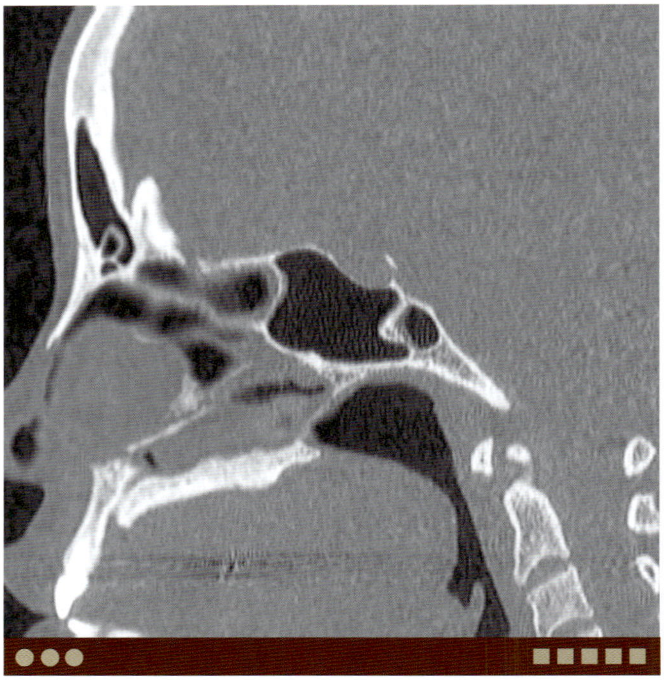

C. Choanal atresia, same patient as A. Sagittal CT demonstrates osseous closure of the choana.

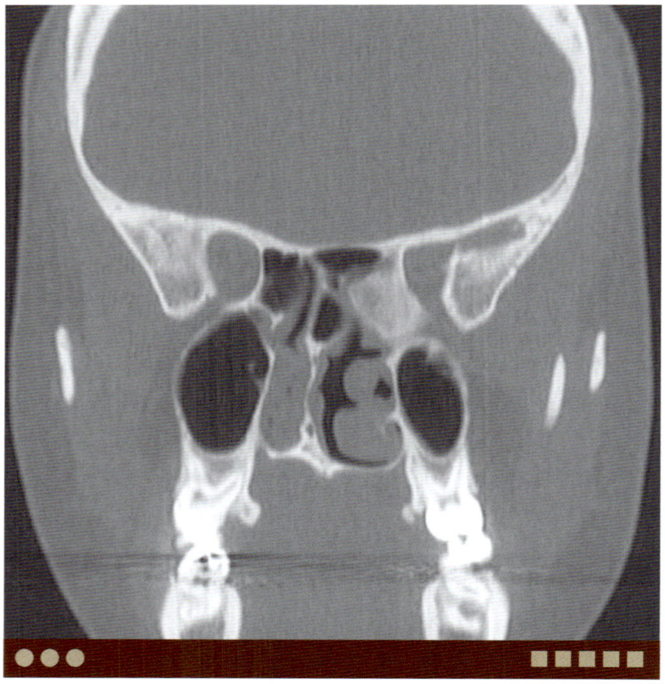

D. Choanal atresia, same patient as A. Coronal CT demonstrates debris in the right nasal cavity due to the atresia.

DIFFERENTIAL DIAGNOSIS IMAGES (E-F)

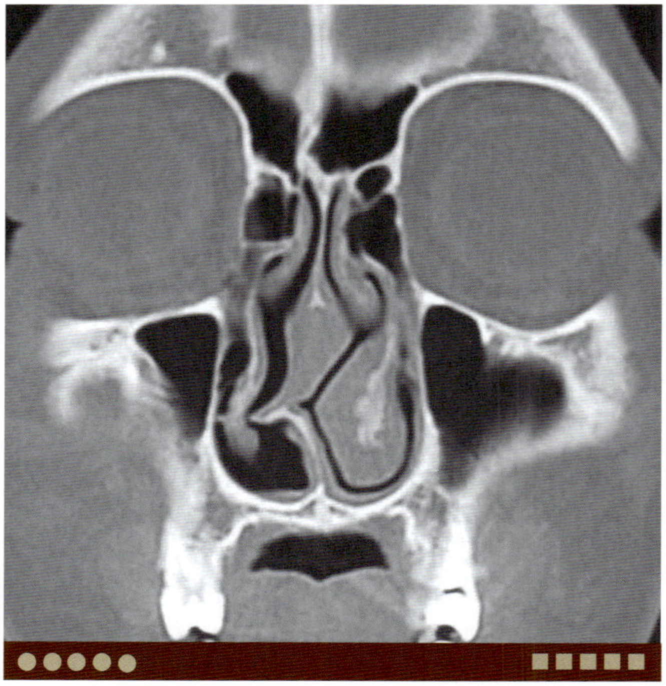

E. **Nasal septal deviation**. Coronal CT demonstrates nasal septal deviation to the right with a bony spur.

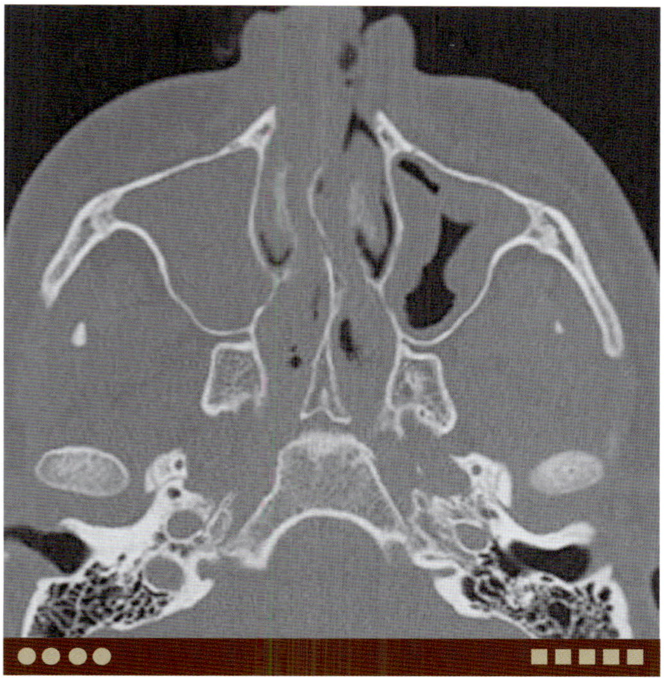

F. Nasal septal fracture. Axial CT demonstrates fracture of the nasal septum and swelling of the soft tissue obstructing the choana.

Case 3–27 Fungal Sinusitis—Mycetoma

Brooke Devenney-Cakir, Osamu Sakai

PRESENTATION

Sinusitis.

FINDINGS

CT demonstrates high-density opacification of the paranasal sinus with or without calcification. MRI demonstrates T2 low-signal opacification.

DIFFERENTIAL DIAGNOSIS

- Chronic sinusitis: Heterogeneous density can be seen in the opacified sinuses with inspissated secretion and dystrophic calcification. Sclerotic changes of the osseous walls and contraction of the affected sinus is often seen.
- Allergic fungal sinusitis: This is another form of noninvasive fungal sinusitis and typically involves multiple sinuses with high-density materials.
- Inverted papilloma: Inverted papilloma most often occurs in the lateral wall of the nasal cavity and grows into the maxillary sinus and causes unilateral high-density opacification.
- Acute sinusitis: This condition typically demonstrates water density opacification of the paranasal sinuses, often with air-fluid levels.
- Acute invasive fungal sinusitis: This condition is typically seen in immunocompromised patients. Intraorbital or intracranial extension is common, and can cause cavernous sinus invasion, hematogenous dissemination and vasculitis.

COMMENTS

This is a 55-year-old man with history of sinusitis.

Fungal sinusitis can be divided into noninvasive and invasive forms. The noninvasive form of fungal sinusitis includes allergic fungal sinusitis and mycetoma/fungus ball.

Sinus mycetoma usually involves unilateral maxillary sinus. Patients are usually immunocompetent, and clinical presentation of sinus mycetoma is similar to that of usual sinusitis. This condition is suspected by CT findings. Mucopurulent, cheesy, or claylike material is seen endoscopically or at the time of surgery. Allergic conditions and elevated fungus-specific IgE are less common compared with allergic fungal sinusitis.

CT commonly demonstrates high-density opacification with or without calcification. Sclerosis and thickening of the sinus wall is commonly seen due to chronic inflammation. Maxillary sinuses are most commonly involved, although mycetoma can be seen anywhere in the sinuses. This high-density material has very dark signal on MRI, particularly on T2W images due to the significant T2 shortening effect by inspissated secretions and manganese, which is characteristic for fungal infection. If MRI is performed prior to CT, opacified sinuses may show signal-void mimicking air, and this condition could be completely missed. Therefore, CT should be performed first if sinusitis is suspected clinically. Also, the paranasal sinuses should be carefully evaluated on multiple sequences when MRI is performed prior to CT for other reasons. Close attention should be paid to the adjacent structures for evidence of more aggressive and invasive processes associated with fungal infections, particularly in immunocompromised patients.

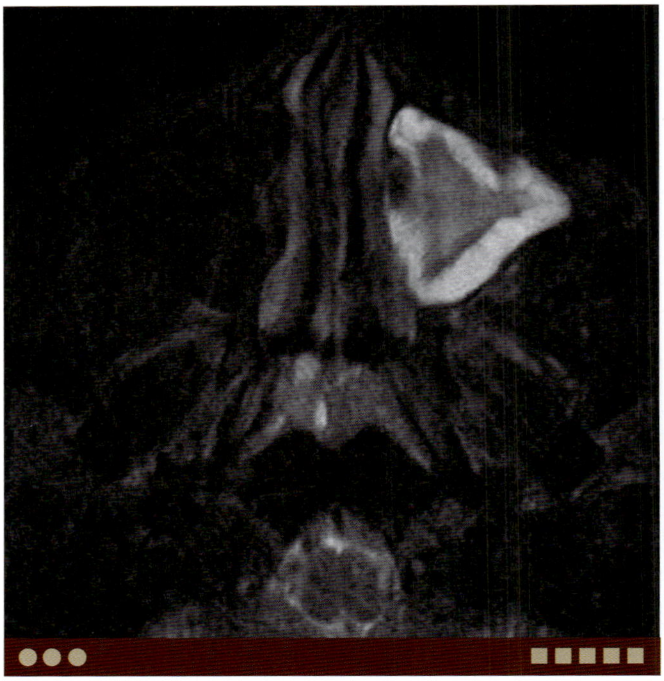

A. Sinus mycetoma. Axial fat-suppressed T2W MR image demonstrates opacified left maxillary sinus. Note decreased signal in the opacified lumen. Submucosal edema demonstrates homogeneous high signal.

PEARLS

- **Sinus mycetoma is seen in immunocompetent patients. The patient is often minimally symptomatic.**
- **Fungal sinus mycetoma causes a focal high-density mass within the sinus on CT and low signal on MRI.**
- **High density is characteristic, however not pathognomonic for fungal sinusitis. Proteinaceous or inspissated secretions are the most common cause of the high density.**

ADDITIONAL IMAGES (B-G)

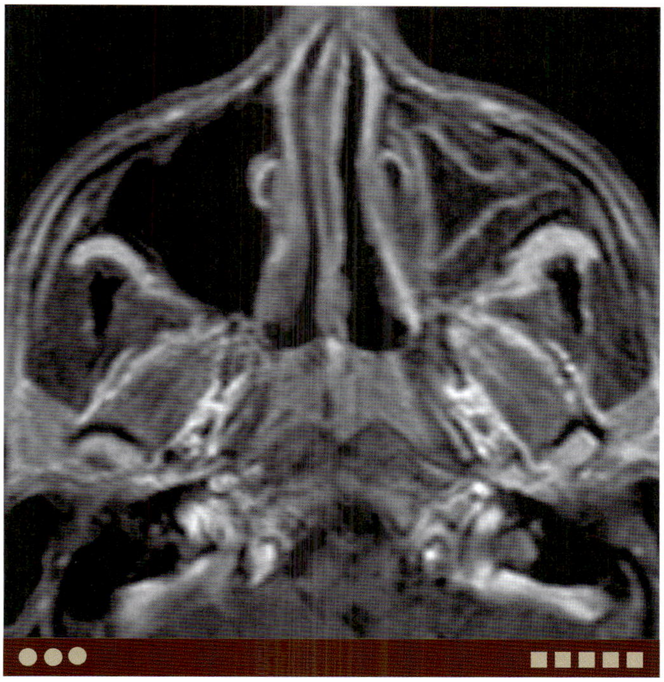

B. Sinus mycetoma, same patient as A. Axial postcontrast T1W MR image demonstrates linear enhancement of the mucosa in the left maxillary sinus. No enhancement is seen in the lumen or submucosal edema.

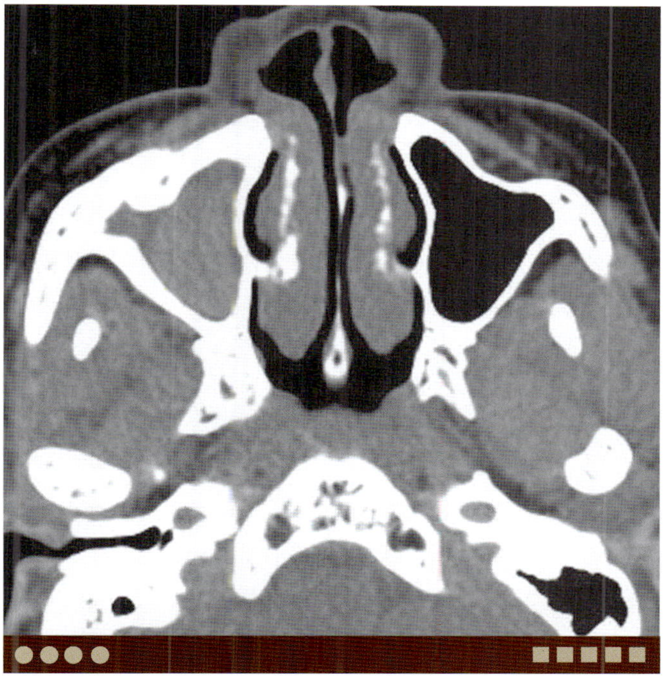

C. Sinus mycetoma in a different patient. Axial CT demonstrates high-density material within the opacified right maxillary sinus.

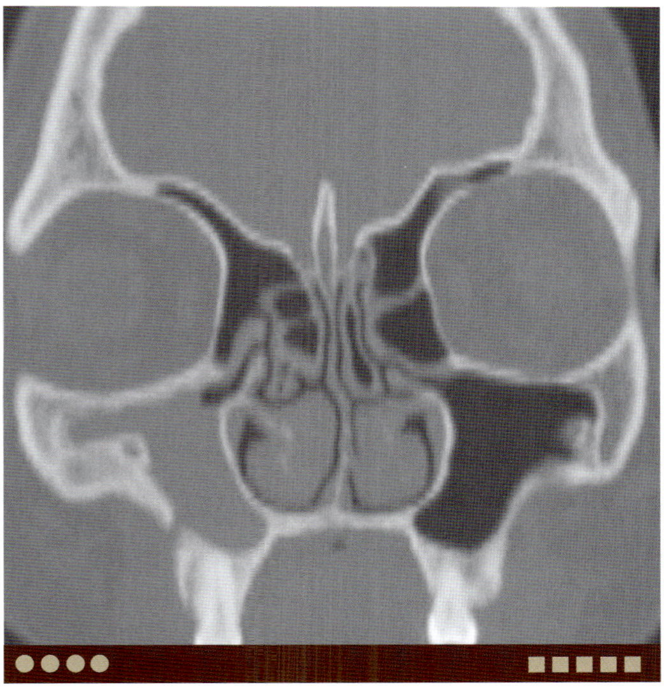

D. Sinus mycetoma, same patient as C. Coronal bone window CT demonstrates contraction of the right maxillary sinus with thickened walls consistent with chronic inflammation.

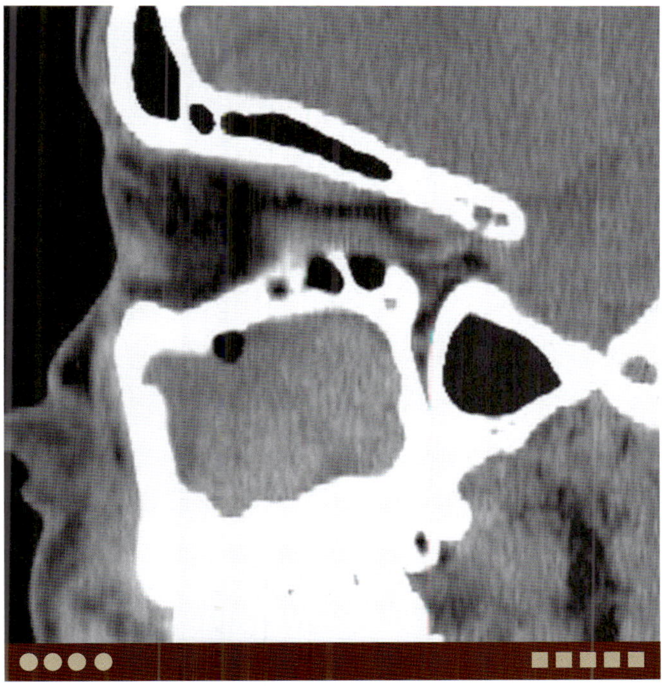

E. Sinus mycetoma, same patient as C. Sagittal soft tissue window CT demonstrates heterogeneously high-density materials in the maxillary sinus. Fat in the inferior orbital fissure and pterygopalatine fossa is preserved.

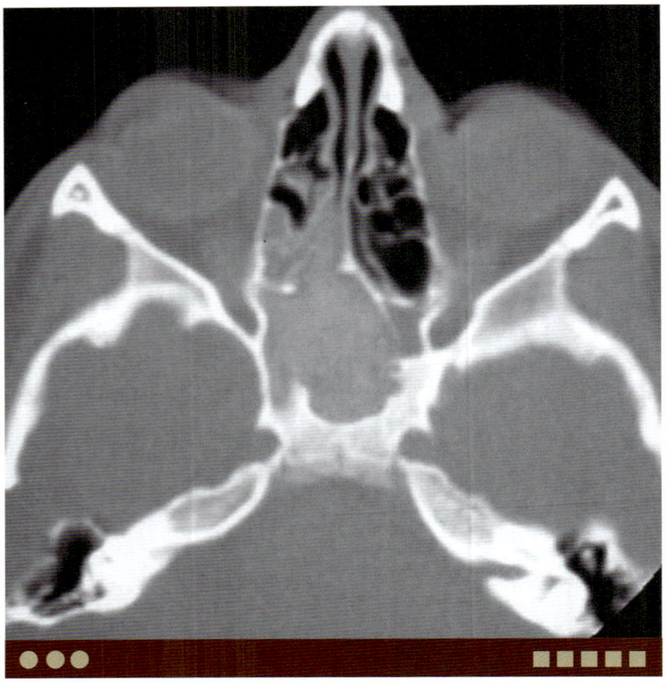

F. Sinus mycetoma in a different patient. Axial bone window CT demonstrates complete opacification of the sphenoid sinus with high-density materials. Note sclerosis and thickening of the sinus consistent with chronic inflammation.

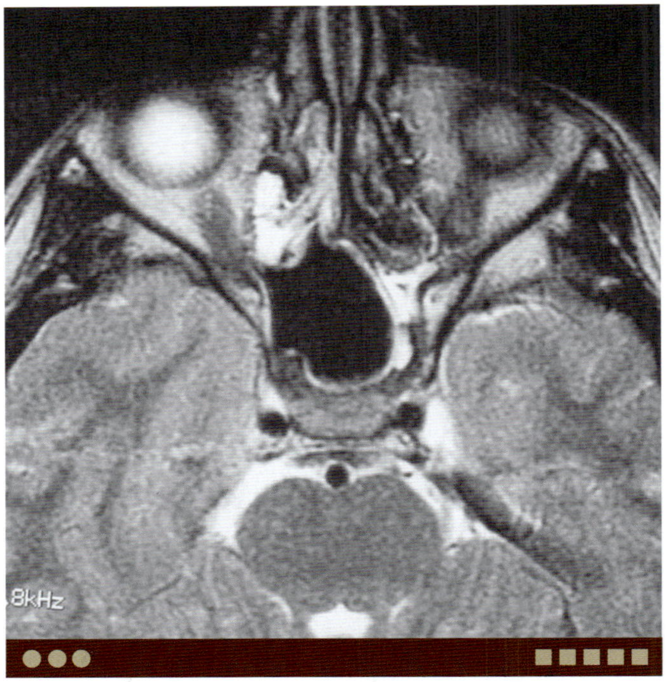

G. Sinus mycetoma, same patient as F. Axial T2W MR image demonstrates complete signal-void in the sphenoid sinus consistent with T2 shortening effect from inspissated secretions and manganese.

DIFFERENTIAL DIAGNOSIS IMAGES (H-J)

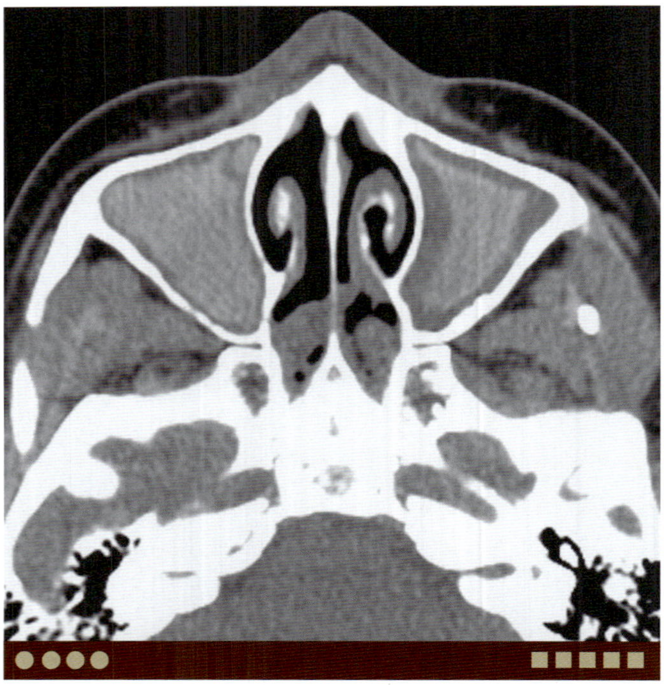

H. Allergic aspergillus sinusitis. Axial soft tissue window CT shows opacified maxillary sinuses with high-density material.

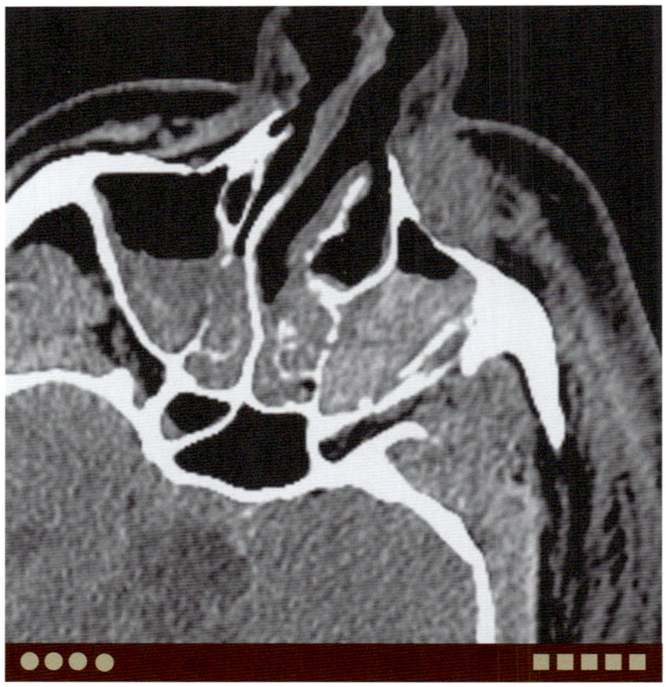

I. Maxillary sinus fracture with hemorrhage. Axial soft tissue window CT shows high-density materials forming air-fluid level in the left maxillary sinus. Note fracture of the posterolateral wall.

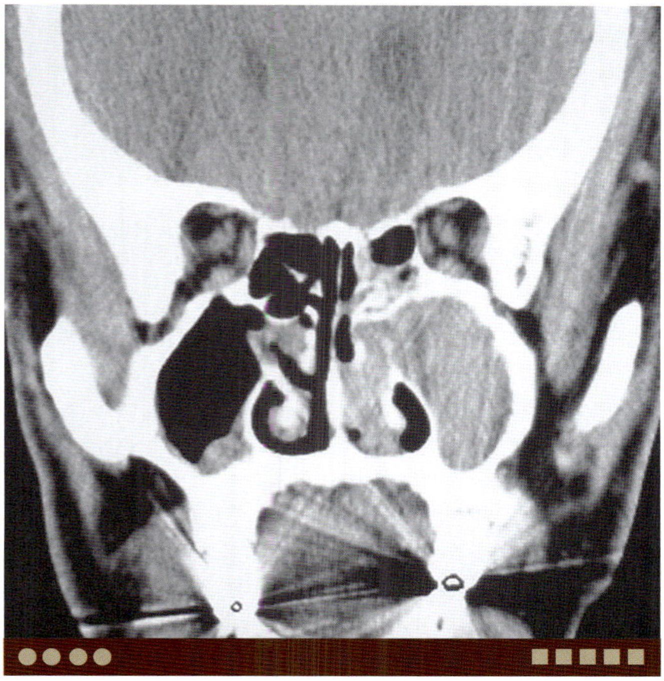

J. Inverted papilloma. Coronal soft tissue window CT demonstrates opacified left maxillary sinus with high density. Note a contiguous mass lesion in the left nasal cavity and bone remodeling of the ostium.

Case 3–28 Cephalocele (Meningocele and Meningoencephalocele)

Osamu Sakai, Daniel Weller

PRESENTATION

Nasal mass.

FINDINGS

CT demonstrates a cystic appearing mass in the nasal cavity extending from the anterior skull base through a bone defect.

DIFFERENTIAL DIAGNOSIS

- Nasal polyp: This is a solid lesion, but often demonstrates water density/signal. However, there should not be an associated bone defect at the skull base.
- Papilloma: This is a solid lesion and should not have an associated bone defect at the skull base.

COMMENTS

This is a 14-year-old girl scanned for a nasal mass.

Cephalocele is defined as a herniation of cranial contents through a bone defect in the skull. They are classified according to their contents [meningocele: meninges and cerebrospinal fluid (CSF), meningoencephalocele: brain parenchyma in addition to meninges and CSF]. These are congenital anomalies due to failure of neural tube closure. Despite many theories, the cause of cephalocele is not known. It is commonly seen in the occipital region (occipital cephalocele) and these are diagnosed earlier, often at birth. On the other hand, trans-ethmoid and trans-sphenoid cephaloceles are usually diagnosed later as a nasal obstruction, mass or CSF leak. Clinically, hypopituitarism and diabetes inspidus may be present. Unintentional injury to cephaloceles due to biopsy or resection can cause serious complications such as CSF leak, meningitis and hemorrhage. Therefore, biopsy or resection of polypoid or cystic lesions in the nasal cavity or nasopharynx, particularly in young patients, should not be performed without preoperative imaging evaluation. Cephalocele should always be in the differential diagnosis of nasal masses.

CT is useful to evaluate for a bone defect. Thin slices with multiplanar reformation are needed. In addition to a bone defect, smooth bone remodeling due to CSF pulsation can be seen in the skull base and paranasal sinuses. Cleft lip/palate and choanal atresia may be seen with cephaloceles. MRI is essential to evaluate contents of the protruded structures and other possible intracranial anomalies, such as agenesis of the corpus callosum, optic nerve/chiasmal anomalies, Chiari malformation, and hydrocephalus.

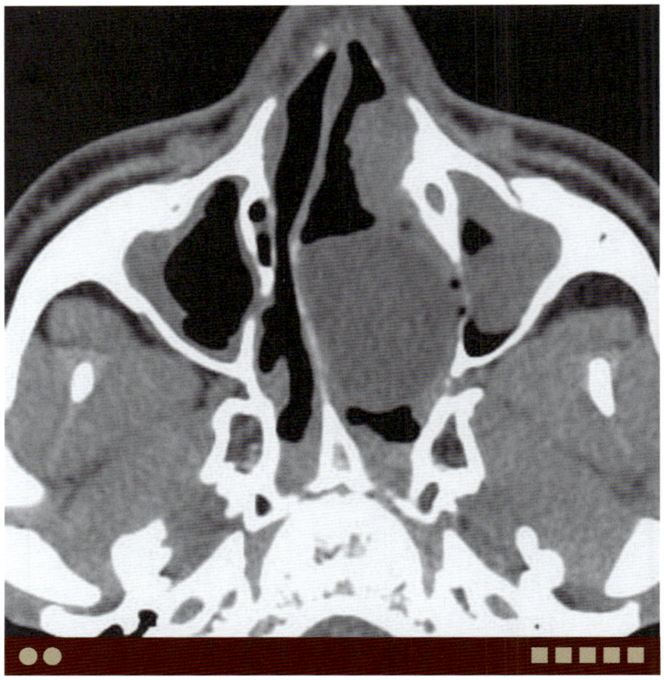

A. Cephalocele. Axial CT shows a large, water density lesion in the left nasal cavity mildly remodeling the nasal septum.

PEARLS

- **Cephalocele represents a failure of neural tube closure and herniation of the meninges and its contents (meningocele: meninges + CSF, meningo encephalocele: meninges + CSF + brain tissue).**
- **Trans-ethmoid and trans-sphenoid cephaloceles can present as a nasal mass later in life, while occipital cephalocele is usually diagnosed at birth.**
- **Cephalocele should always be included in the differential diagnosis of nasal masses, particularly in young patients.**

ADDITIONAL IMAGES (B-F)

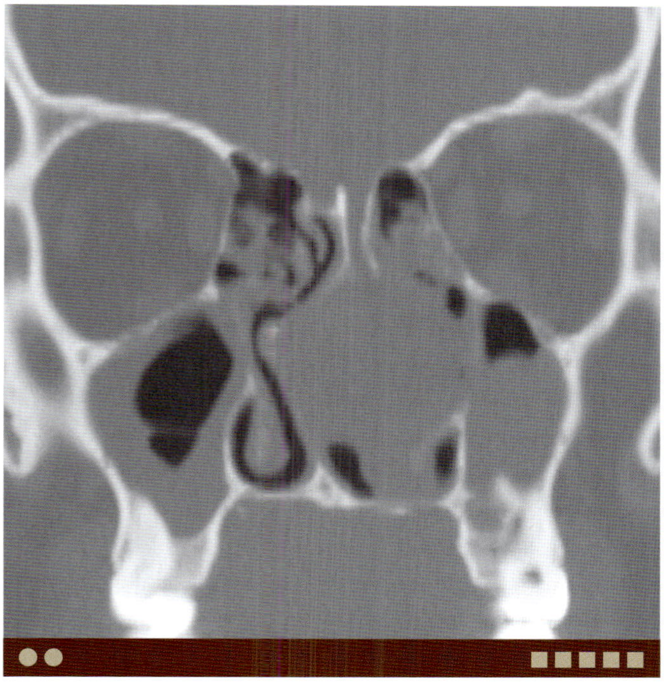

B. Cephalocele, same patient as A. Coronal CT shows a bone defect in the left cribriform plate and a large cystic lesion in the left nasal cavity. Note a relatively small bone defect with a large cephalocele.

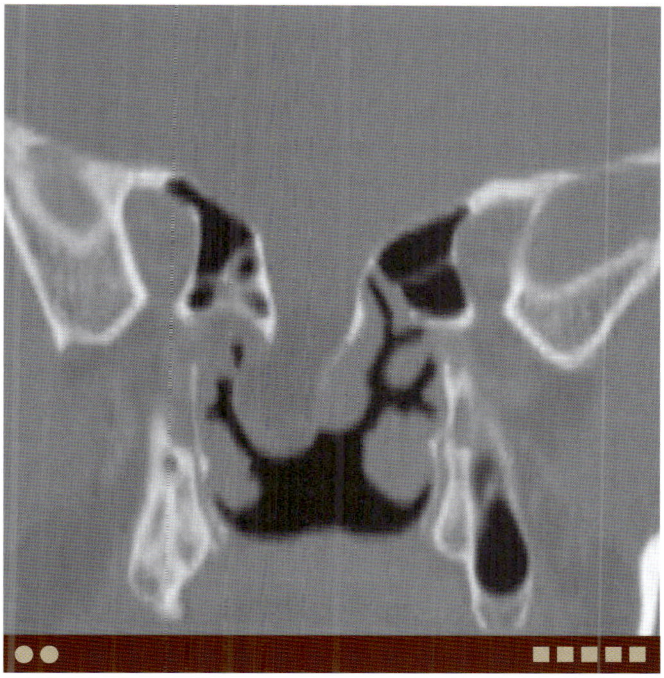

C. **Cephalocele, trans-ethmoid** in a different patient. Coronal CT shows a large bone defect in the right ethmoid roof.

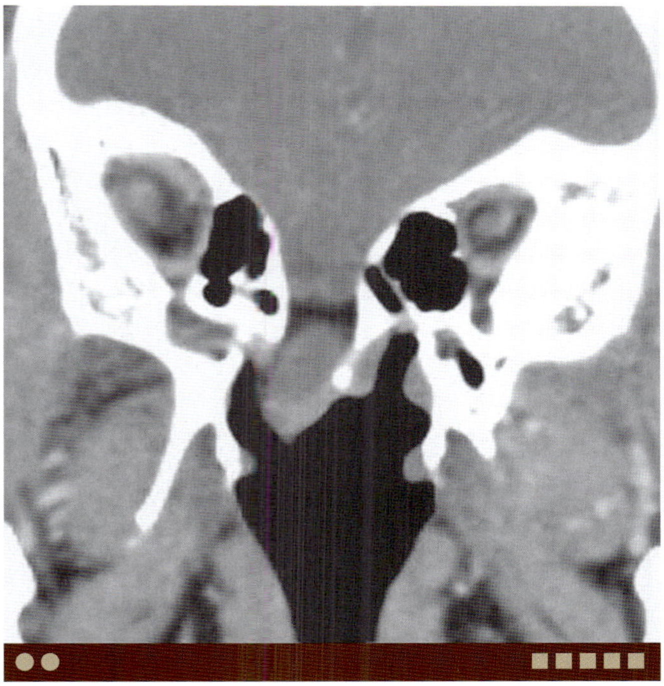

D. Cephalocele, trans-ethmoid, same patient as C. Coronal CT with soft tissue window shows herniation of brain parenchyma as well as hamartomatous fatty tissue through the bone defect.

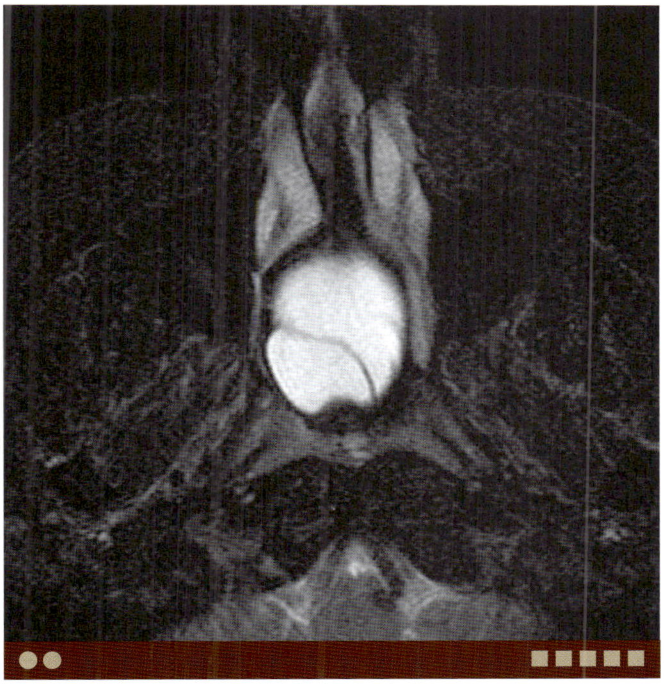

E. **Cephalocele, trans-ethmoid/sphenoid** in a different patient. Axial fat-suppressed T2W MR demonstrates a large, septated, cystic mass in the posterior nasal cavity and nasopharynx.

DIFFERENTIAL DIAGNOSIS IMAGES (G-I)

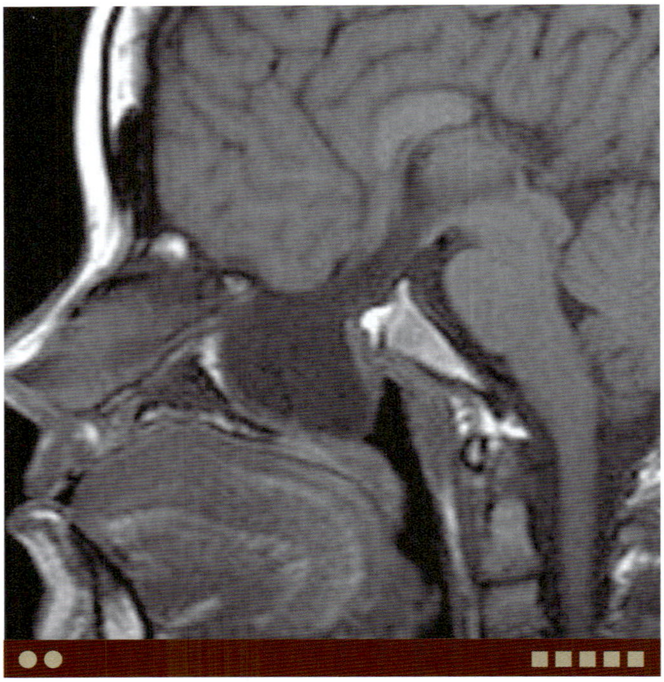

F. Cephalocele, trans-ethmoid/sphenoid, same patient as E. Sagittal T1W MR demonstrates a meningocele extending inferiorly to the posterior ethmoids and nasopharynx through a large defect in the posterior ethmoid.

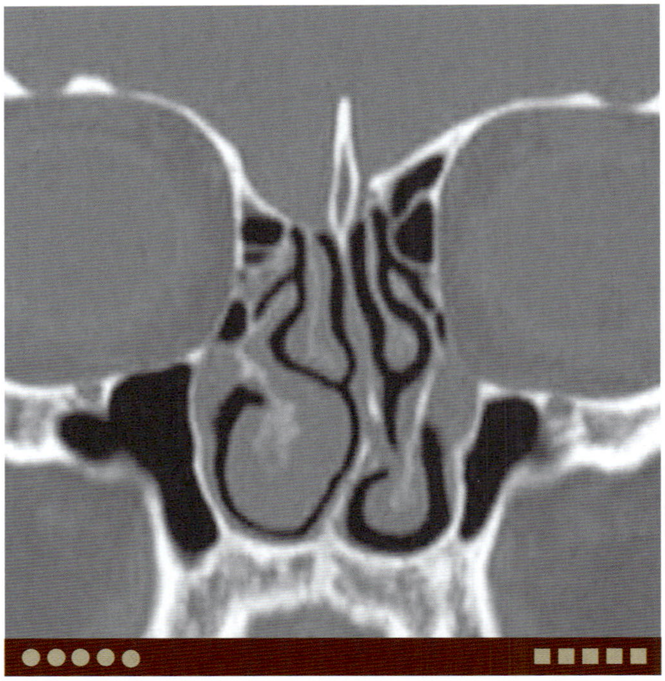

G. **Asymmetry of the cribriform plates**. Coronal CT demonstrates asymmetric shape and height of the ethmoid roofs and cribriform plates, right lower than left.

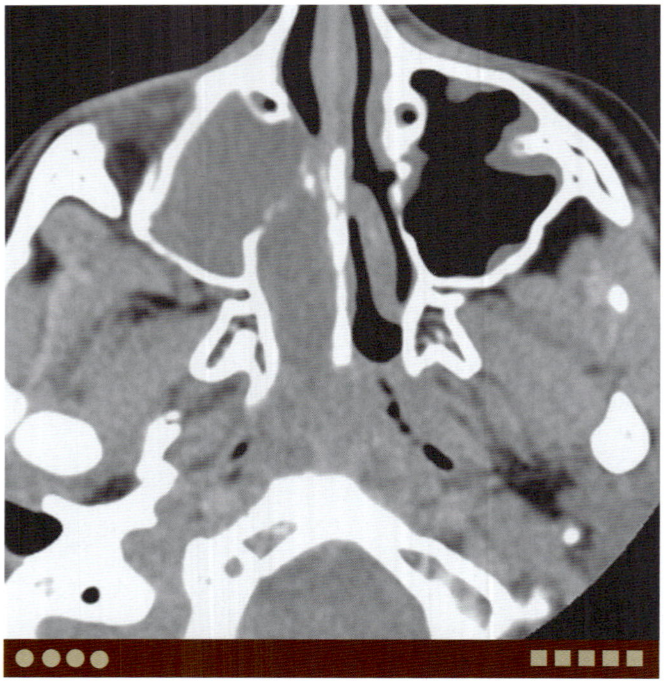

H. **Antrochoanal polyp**. Axial CT shows a large, water density lesion occupying the posterior right nasal cavity and right maxillary sinus.

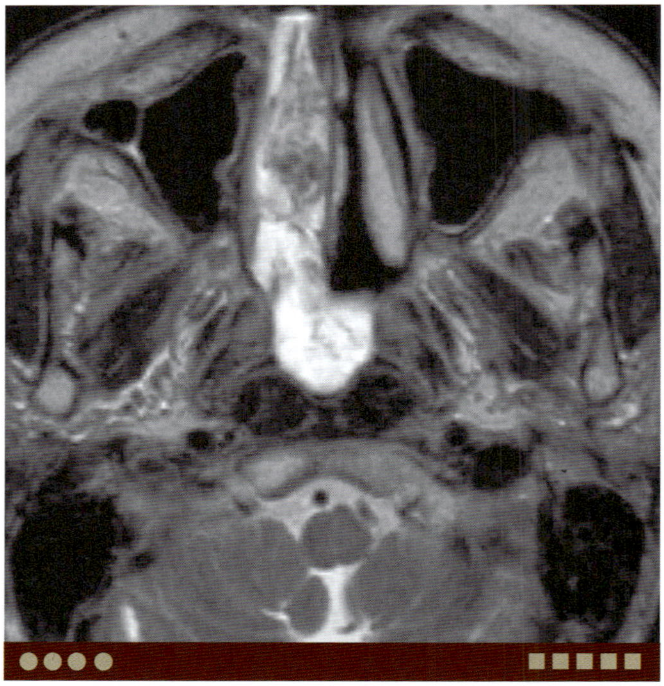

I. **Nasal polyp**. Axial T2W MR demonstrates a heterogeneously high-signal lesion in the right nasal cavity extending to and occupying the nasopharynx.

Case 3–29 Asymmetry of the Cribriform Plate

Osamu Sakai, Daniel Weller

PRESENTATION

Incidental finding.

FINDINGS

CT demonstrates asymmetry in height of the cribriform plates, often with asymmetry in height and shape of the roof of the ethmoid.

DIFFERENTIAL DIAGNOSIS

- Cephalocele: Herniation of cranial contents through a bone defect in the skull. Trans-ethmoid and trans-sphenoid cephaloceles are seen in the sinonasal cavity.
- Pseudocephalocele: This condition is a herniation of cranial contents through a bone defect secondary to prior trauma or surgery. Evidence of prior injury is often seen.
- Nasal polyp: This is a solid lesion, but often demonstrates water density/signal. However, this should not have a bone defect at the skull base.

COMMENTS

This is a 42-year-old man who underwent CT for chronic sinusitis.

Preoperative understanding of the anatomy of the paranasal sinuses in each patient is essential for endoscopic sinus surgery, even with image-guided surgery. Asymmetry of the cribriform plates and roofs of the ethmoid/fovea ethmoidalis is a common normal variant. The surgeon should be aware of this anomaly before surgery. If they are asymmetrically low-lying or thin, there is increased risk of injury during the surgery, which may result in serious complications, such as CSF leak, hemorrhage, and intracranial infection. Therefore, this anomaly should be described in the sinus CT report.

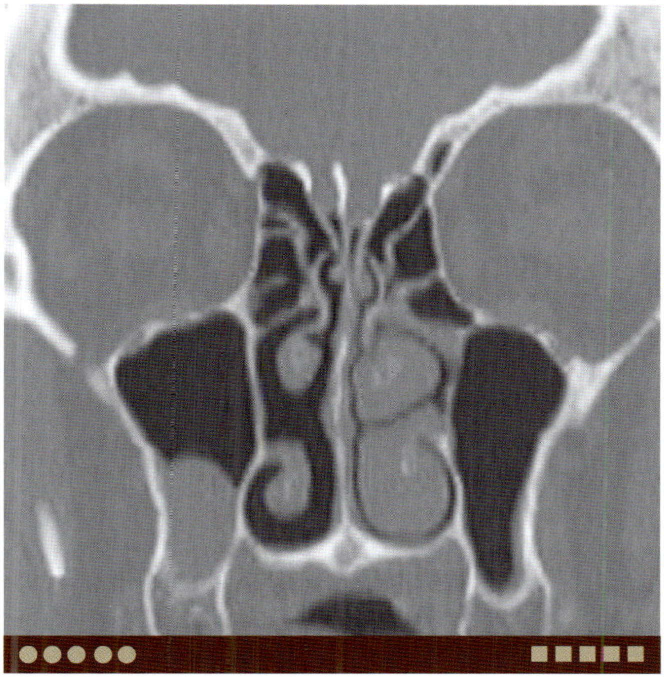

A. Asymmetry of the cribriform plates. Coronal CT demonstrates low-lying left cribriform plate compared with the right with asymmetry in ethmoid roofs.

PEARLS

- **Asymmetry of the cribriform plates and ethmoid roofs is a common anomaly.**
- **Asymmetrically low-lying or thin cribriform plates and ethmoid roofs increase the risk of injury during surgery.**

ADDITIONAL IMAGES (B-C)

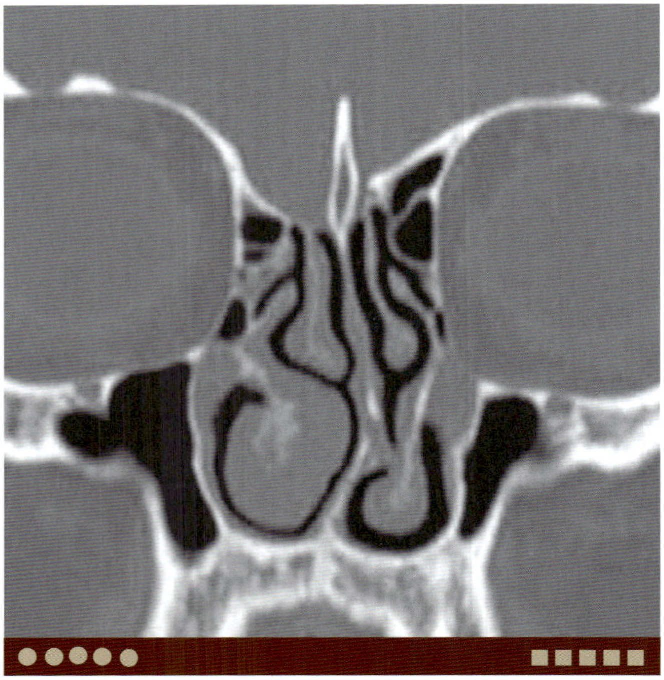

B. **Asymmetry of the cribriform plates** in a different patient. Coronal CT demonstrates asymmetry in shape and height of the ethmoid roofs. The right side is lower and wider than the left. The cribriform plate is also slightly lower on the right.

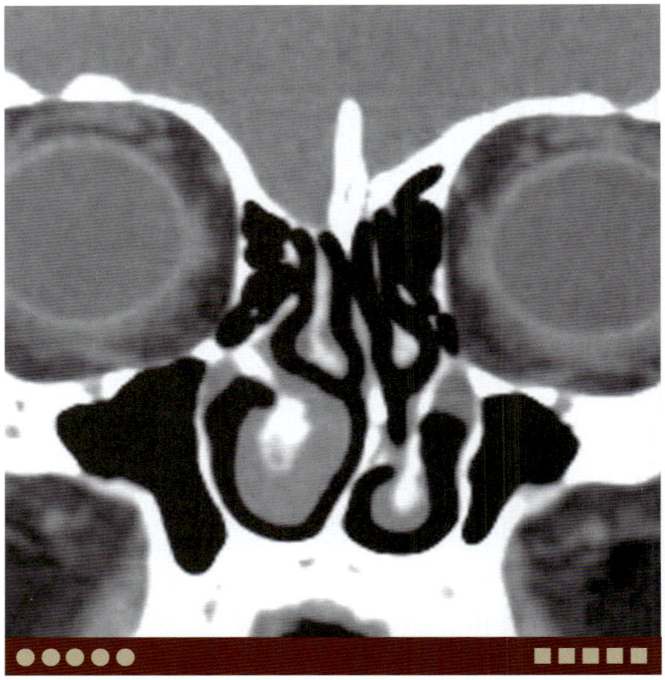

C. Asymmetry of the ethmoid roofs, same patient as B. Coronal soft tissue window CT demonstrates asymmetry in shape and height of the ethmoid roofs, right lower than left, with filling of the inferior frontal lobe.

DIFFERENTIAL DIAGNOSIS IMAGES (D-H)

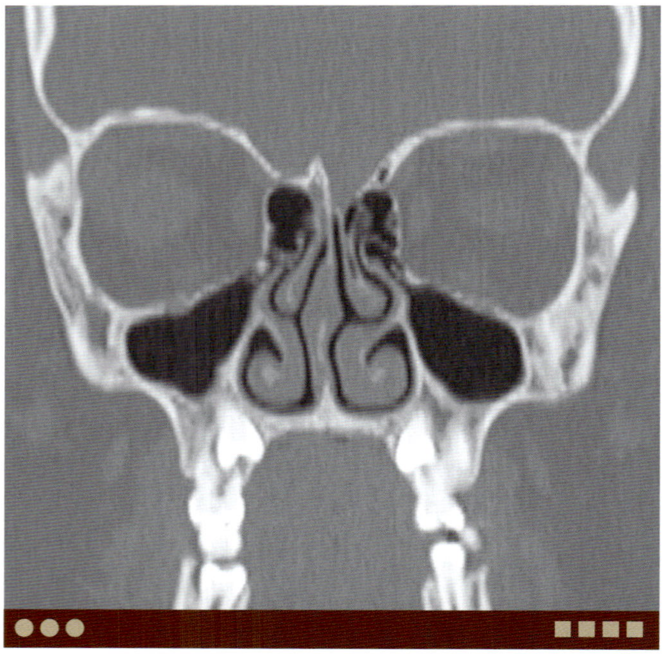

D. **Cephalocele, trans-ethmoid.** Coronal CT demonstrates bone dehiscence in the left ethmoid roof with a focal extension of the intracranial contents.

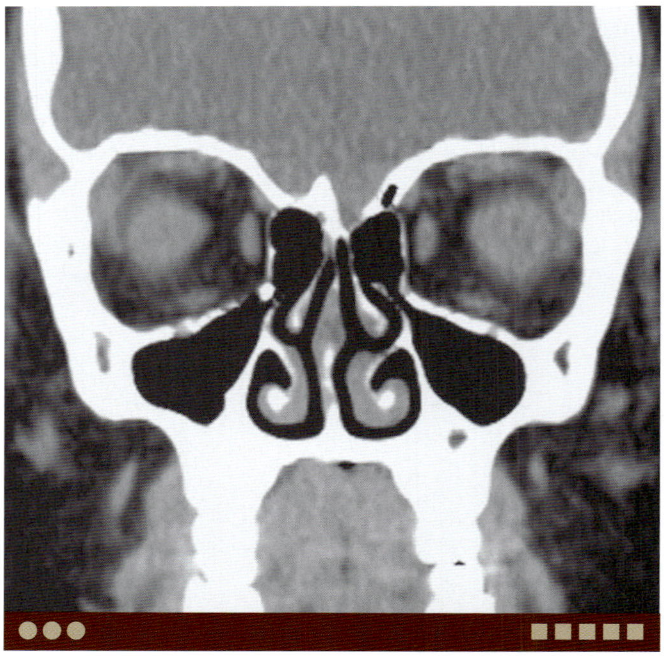

E. Cephalocele, trans-ethmoid, same patient as D. Coronal soft tissue window CT demonstrates focal region of inferior extension of the intracranial contents.

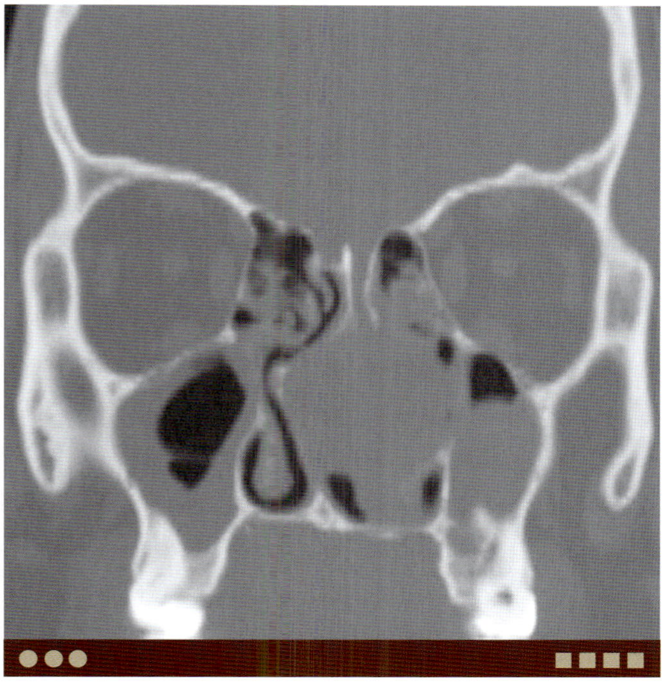

F. **Cephalocele** in a different patient. Coronal CT demonstrates a large cephalocele in the left nasal cavity through a small bone defect at the left cribriform plate.

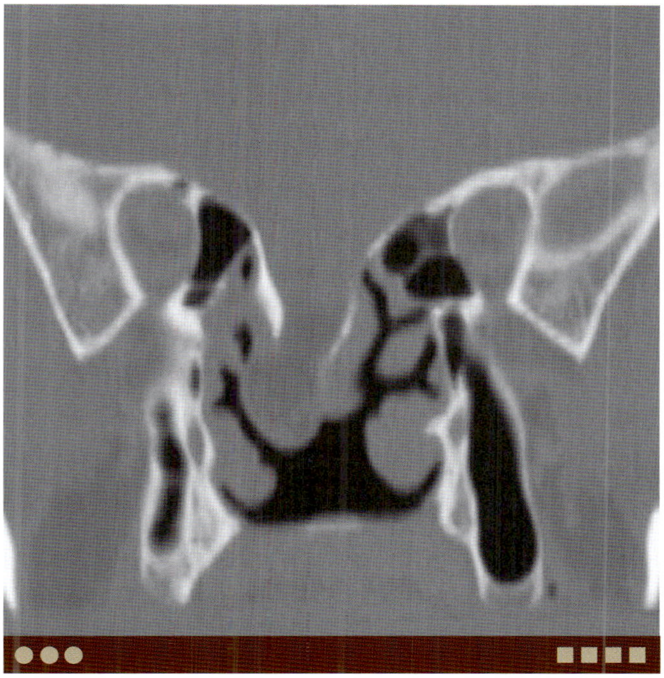

G. **Cephalocele** in a different patient. Coronal CT demonstrates a large bone defect in the right ethmoid roof.

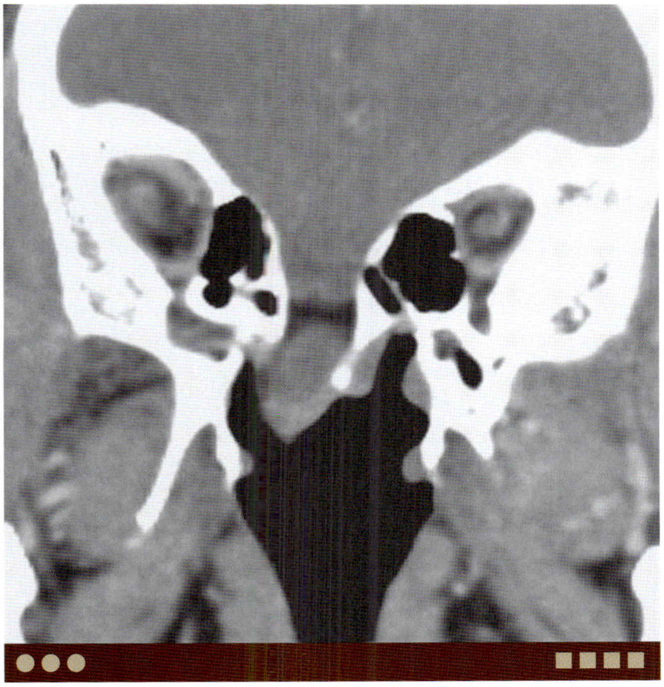

H. Cephalocele, same patient as G. Coronal CT with soft tissue window demonstrates inferior protrusion of the brain parenchyma as well as hamartomatous fatty tissue.

Case 3-30 Pleomorphic Adenoma—Sinonasal

Osamu Sakai, Daniel Weller

PRESENTATION

Nasal mass.

FINDINGS

CT and MRI demonstrate a well-circumscribed mass in the nasal cavity exerting some mass effect on the adjacent structures and bone erosion.

DIFFERENTIAL DIAGNOSIS

- Nasal polyp: Polypoid mass arising from the nasal mucosa.
- Squamous cell carcinoma (SCCA): SCCA is the most common malignant tumor in the sinonasal cavity, and usually shows ill-defined, infiltrative margins and heterogeneous density/signal and enhancement.
- Adenoid cystic carcinoma: Malignant tumor arising from the minor salivary gland. High-grade tumors show higher cellularity and low signal on T2W images. Perineural tumor spread is common.
- Mucoepidermoid carcinoma: Also a malignant tumor arising from the minor salivary gland. Low-grade tumors tend to be cystic and high-grade tumors tend to be more solid.
- Lymphoma: Rare tumor in the sinonasal cavity that may demonstrate relatively well-circumscribed margins and homogeneous density/signal. Bone expansion or infiltration is more common than erosion.

COMMENTS

This is a 19-year-old woman with a mass in the palate.

Pleomorphic adenoma, also known as a benign mixed tumor, occurs commonly in the major salivary glands, however rarely in the nasal cavity, pharynx, larynx, trachea, or lacrimal glands. Intranasal pleomorphic adenomas commonly occur between the third and sixth decades of life, and are seen more often in women. Nasal obstruction, painless mass, and epistaxis are common presentations. Clinically, a polypoid, smooth, gray mass is seen.

Similar to pleomorphic adenomas occurring elsewhere, they contain both mesenchymal and epithelial components. However, nasal cavity tumors often have higher cellularity, and epithelial elements rather than the stromal elements predominate. Infrequently, the chondroid, myxoid, or collagenous stroma predominate locally and present in a similar appearance to classic mixed tumors of the major salivary glands.

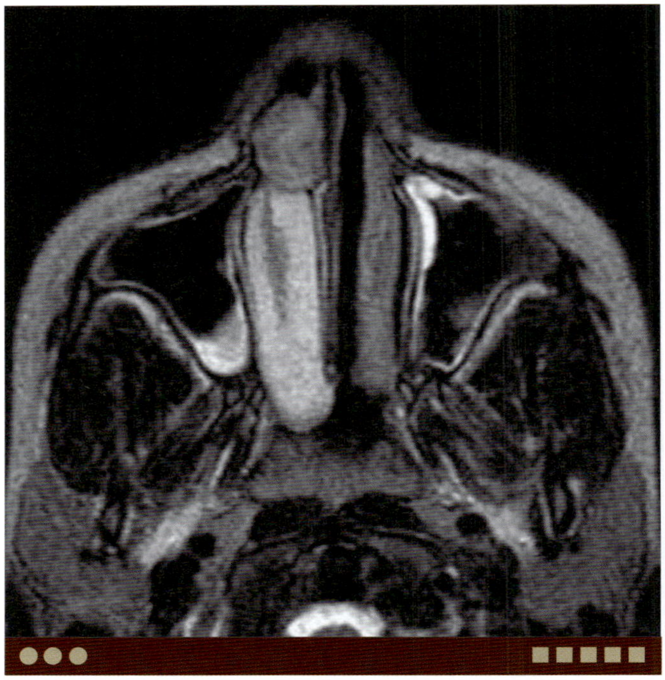

A. Pleomorphic adenoma. Axial T2W MR image demonstrates a well-circumscribed intermediate-signal mass in the anterior right nasal cavity.

CT demonstrates a solid lesion with variable enhancement. When present, pressure erosion/remodeling of bone suggests a benign, long-standing lesion, while aggressive bone destruction and calcification suggest a malignant neoplasm, including chondrosarcoma.

MRI shows a relatively homogeneous mass with low signal on T1W images, intermediate-to-high signal on T2W and STIR images, and enhancement, which is characteristically delayed and less pronounced than surrounding mucosa.

The differential diagnosis includes benign and malignant tumors, such as SCCA, adenocarcinoma, inverted papilloma, schwannoma, melanoma, benign or malignant minor salivary gland tumor, and cartilaginous tumor from the nasal septum.

PEARLS

- **Pleomorphic adenoma occurs commonly in the major salivary glands, however rarely in the nasal cavity.**
- **CT and MRI demonstrate a well-circumscribed mass. Benign-appearing bone remodeling may be present in the adjacent bone.**
- **Delayed enhancement is characteristic for pleomorphic adenoma.**

ADDITIONAL IMAGES (B-E)

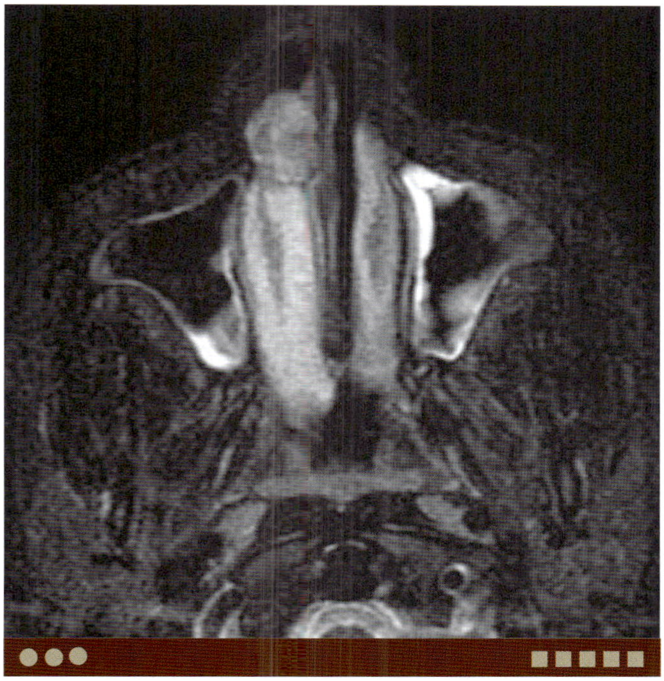

B. Pleomorphic adenoma, same patient as A. Axial fat-suppressed T2W image demonstrates a well-circumscribed intermediate-signal mass in the anterior right nasal cavity.

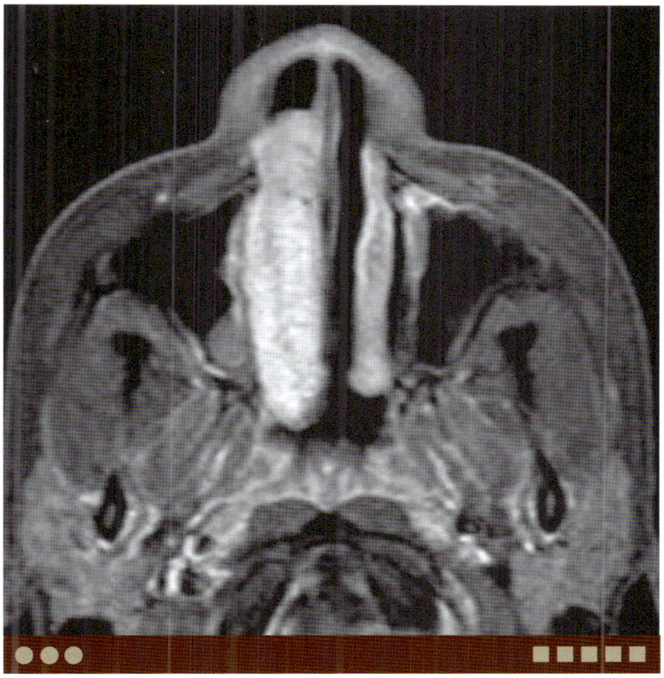

C. Pleomorphic adenoma, same patient as A. Axial postcontrast fat-suppressed T1W image demonstrates mild enhancement of the lesion.

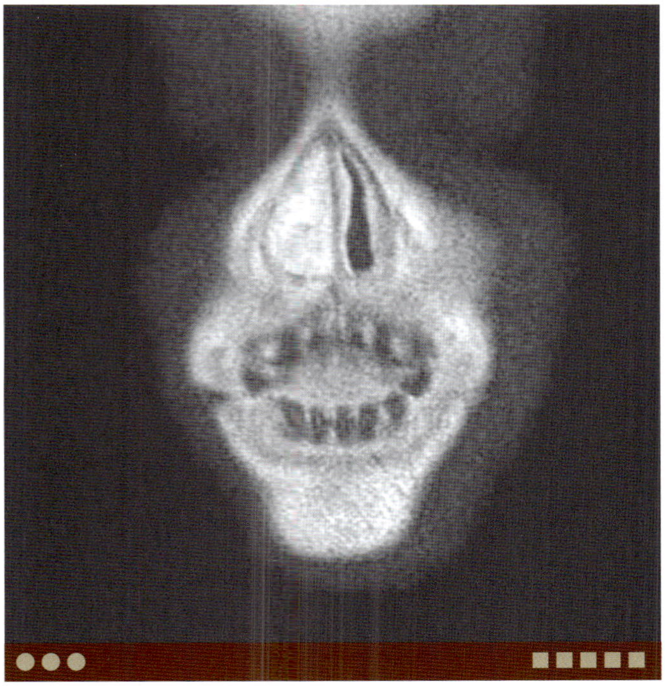

D. Pleomorphic adenoma, same patient as A. Coronal postcontrast T1W image demonstrates persistent enhancement of the lesion.

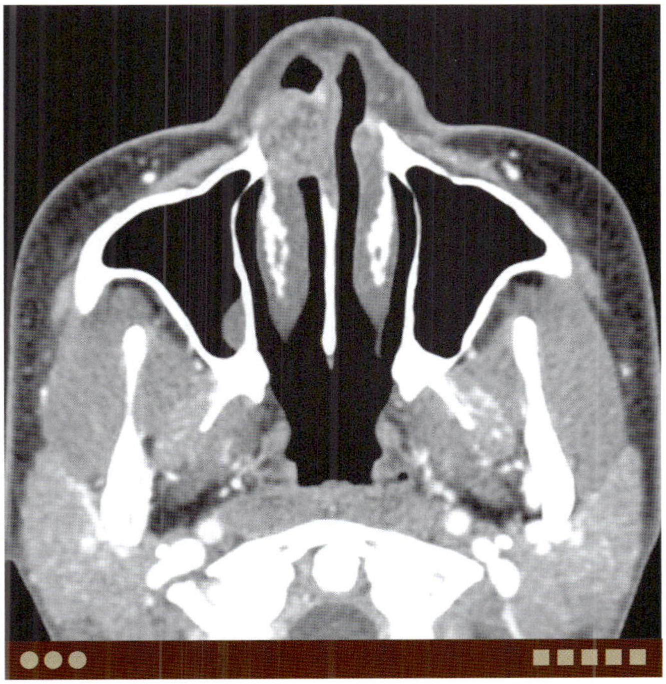

E. Pleomorphic adenoma, same patient as A. Axial postcontrast CT demonstrates a heterogeneously enhancing mass in the right nasal cavity.

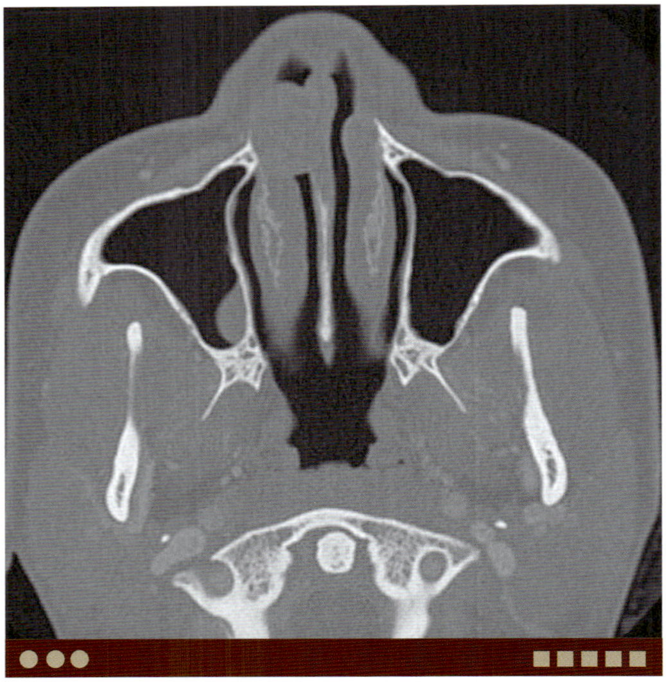

F. Pleomorphic adenoma, same patient as A. Axial bone window CT demonstrates benign appearing bone remodeling of the frontal process of the right maxilla. No calcification is seen in the tumor.

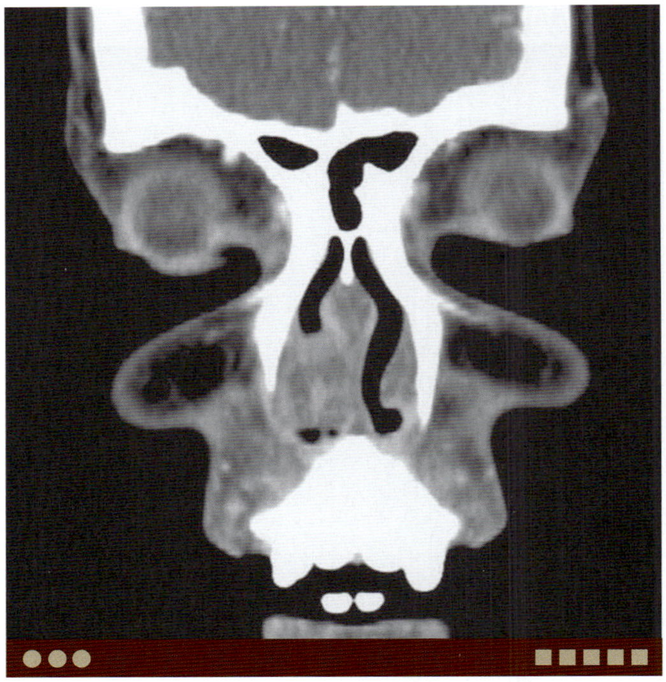

G. Pleomorphic adenoma, same patient as A. Coronal postcontrast CT demonstrates a heterogeneously enhancing mass in the right nasal cavity.

DIFFERENTIAL DIAGNOSIS IMAGES (H-J)

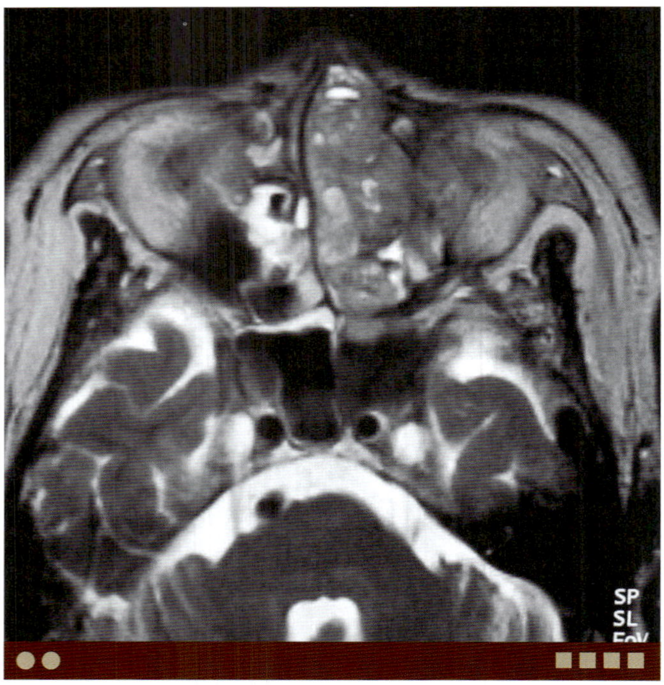

H. Melanoma. Axial T2W MR image demonstrates a heterogeneous, intermediate-to-low signal lesion in the left nasal cavity and ethmoid.

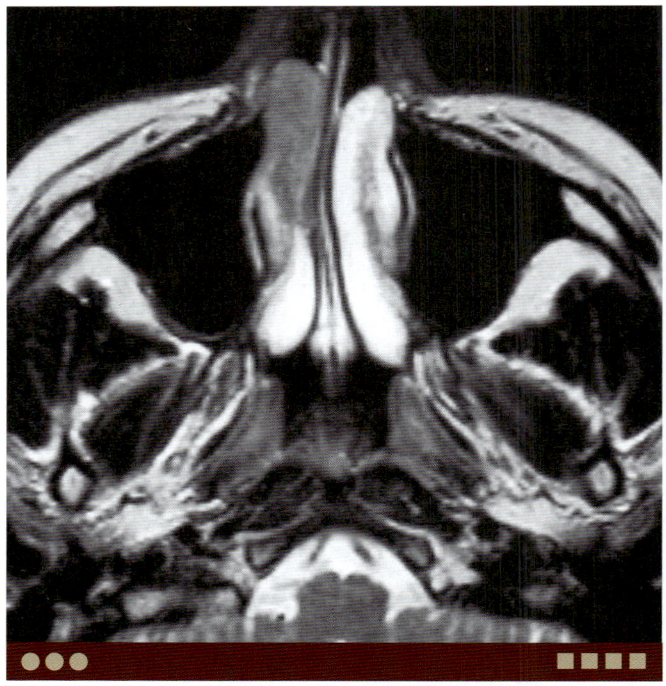

I. Lymphoma. Axial T2W MR image demonstrates a homogeneous, intermediate-to-low signal lesion in the anterior right nasal cavity.

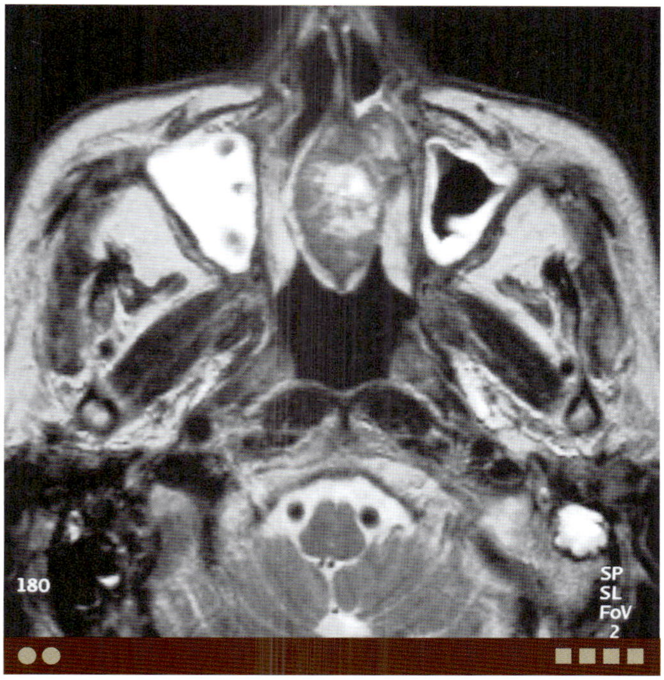

J. Plasmacytoma. Axial T2W MR image demonstrates a heterogeneous, intermediate-to-low signal lesion arising from the nasal septum.

Case 3–31 Sinonasal Organized Hematoma

Yosuke Sato, Akifumi Fujita, Osamu Sakai

PRESENTATION

Nasal obstruction and epistaxis.

FINDINGS

CT and MR show an expansile soft tissue mass in the maxillary sinus with smooth sinus wall erosion and heterogeneous enhancement.

DIFFERENTIAL DIAGNOSIS

- Squamous cell carcinoma: Bone destruction associated with adjacent soft tissue invasion is a hallmark of carcinoma.
- Inverted papilloma: It often arises from the lateral wall of the nasal cavity and extends into the maxillary sinus, and shows the characteristic convoluted cerebriform pattern on T2W and postcontrast T1W images.
- Mucocele, fungal infection, and cholesterol granuloma: These conditions usually do not show central enhancement.
- Hemangioma: Cavernous hemangioma is the most difficult tumor to differentiate from organized hematoma both clinically and radiologically.

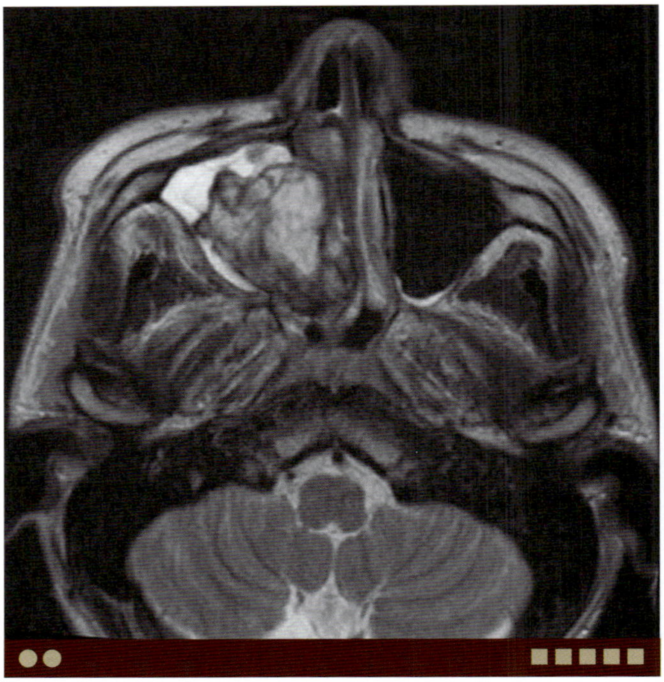

A. Organized hematoma. Axial T2W image demonstrates a heterogeneous signal mass in the right maxillary sinus. A dark peripheral rim surrounding the lesion is seen. High signal from inflamed mucosa in the involved sinus clearly defines the extent of the lesion.

COMMENTS

This is a 24-year-old man with right nasal obstruction and epistaxis.

Sinonasal organized hematoma is an uncommon, nonneoplastic benign condition that can be locally aggressive. It most commonly affects the maxillary sinus. Epistaxis and nasal obstruction are common symptoms. Without careful evaluation of all of the imaging features, this may be mistaken for a malignant lesion both clinically and radiologically. Accurate preoperative diagnosis is important for appropriate treatment planning because sinonasal organized hematoma is usually curative with complete surgical resection simply by endoscopic sinus surgery.

CT can demonstrate an expansile soft tissue mass with smooth erosion of the osseous sinus wall and patchy heterogeneous enhancement. MRI can demonstrate characteristic findings including heterogeneous signal with a peripheral rim of hypointensity on T2W images, and nodular or papillary enhancement on postcontrast T1W images.

Organized hematoma is a relatively rare condition; however, it should be included in the differential diagnosis of a unilateral sinonasal lesion with more common conditions such as mucocele, fungus ball (mycetoma), inflammatory polyp, inverted papilloma, hemangioma, and carcinomas.

PEARLS

- **Sinonasal organized hematoma may be mistaken for a malignant tumor because of an expansile soft tissue mass with erosion of the adjacent sinus walls.**
- **Characteristic CT and MR imaging findings include an expansile soft tissue mass with smooth sinus wall erosion, heterogeneous signal with a hypointense peripheral rim on T2W images, and irregular nodular or papillary enhancement.**

ADDITIONAL IMAGES (B-E)

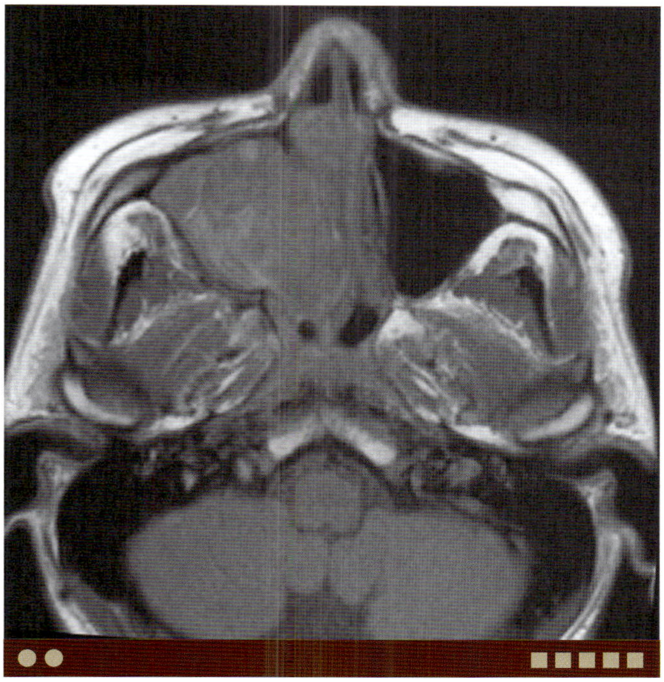

B. Organized hematoma, same patient as A. Axial T1W image demonstrates that the lesion is mostly isointense to the inferior turbinate interspersed with hyperintensity foci.

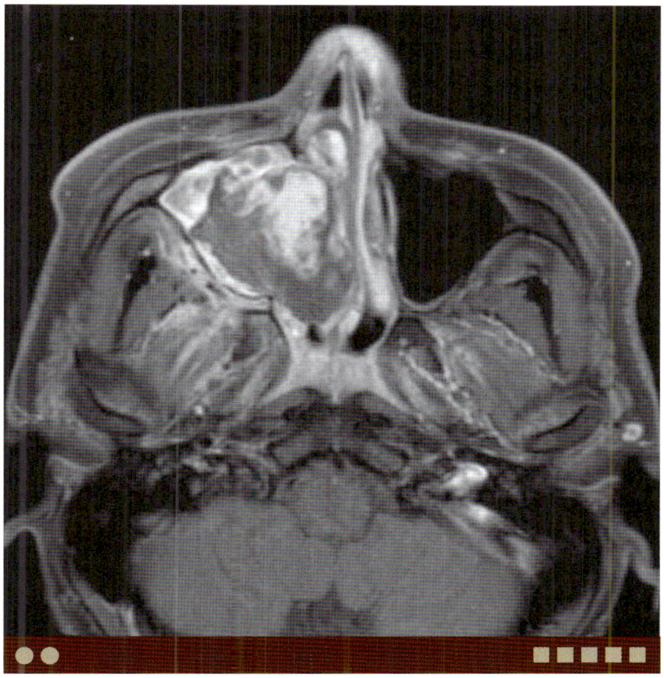

C. Organized hematoma, same patient as A. Axial postcontrast fat-suppressed T1W image demonstrates an irregular nodular, papillary enhancement within the lesion.

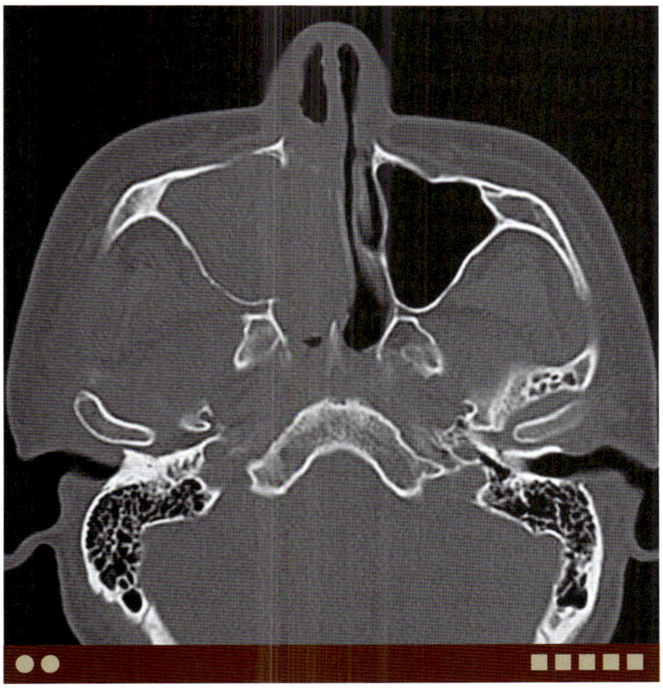

D. Organized hematoma, same patient as A. Axial bone algorithm CT demonstrates a large, expansile soft tissue lesion in the right maxillary sinus remodeling the osseous walls with significant bowing of the medial wall. The lesion completely occupies the ipsilateral nasal cavity and bows the nasal septum.

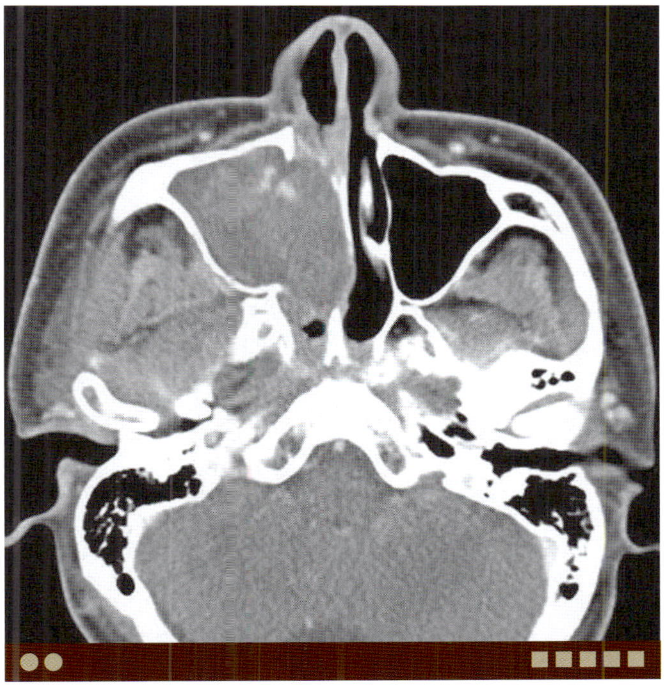

E. Organized hematoma, same patient as A. Axial postcontrast CT demonstrates irregular nodular enhancement within the lesion.

DIFFERENTIAL DIAGNOSIS IMAGES (F-I)

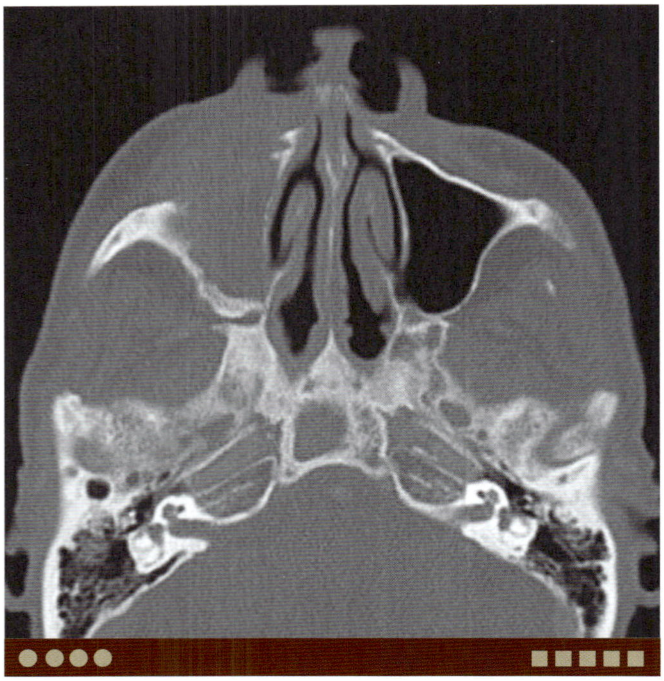

F. Squamous cell carcinoma. Axial bone algorithm CT demonstrates bone destruction, rather than smooth erosion, in the anterior wall of the right maxillary sinus.

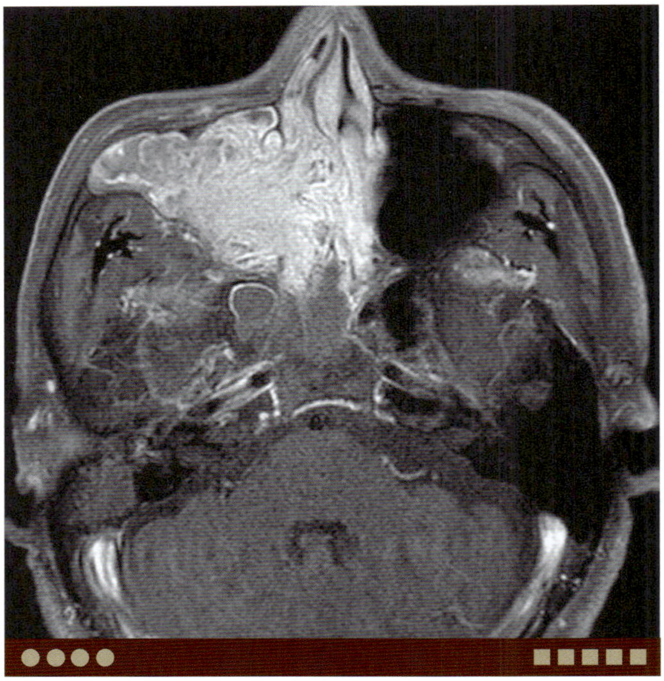

G. Inverted papilloma. Axial postcontrast fat-suppressed T1W image demonstrates a large expansile lesion with convoluted cerebriform enhancement in the right nasal cavity extending into the maxillary sinus.

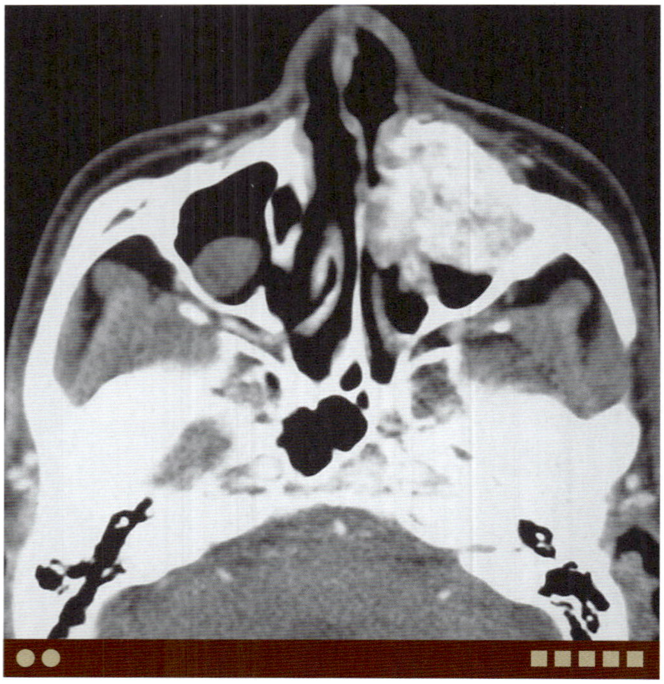

H. Hemangioma. Axial postcontrast CT demonstrates a heterogeneously enhancing lesion in the left maxillary sinus.

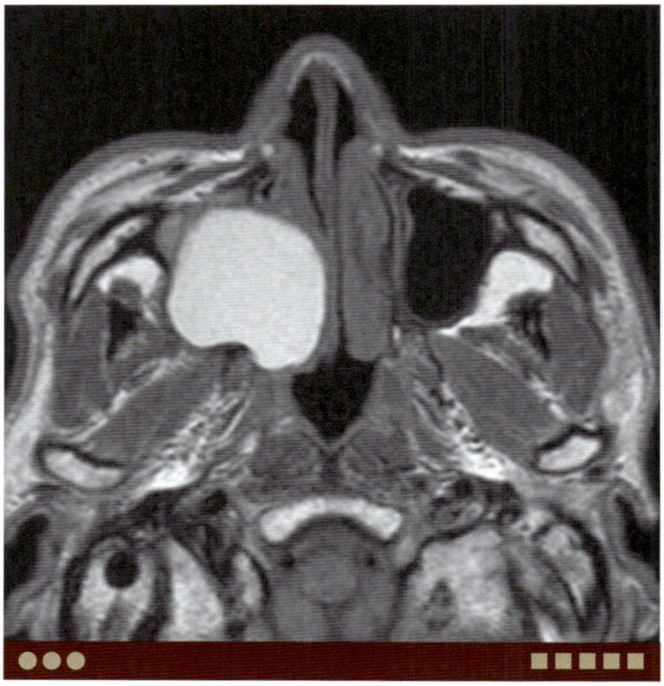

I. Mucocele. Axial T1W image demonstrates a high-signal cystic lesion with smooth margins in the right maxillary sinus. The increased T1 signal corresponds to the proteinaceous content. The mass does not enhance after contrast (not shown).

Case 3–32 Nasal Septal Perforation

Brooke Devenney-Cakir, Osamu Sakai

PRESENTATION

Intermittent episodes of epistaxis, whistling sound during nasal breathing.

FINDINGS

CT demonstrates perforation in the nasal septum.

DIFFERENTIAL DIAGNOSIS

- Trauma and prior surgery: Trauma and prior surgery, particularly septoplasty are common causes of nasal septal perforation.
- Cocaine use: Cocaine is a strong vasoconstrictor and causes necrosis.
- Wegener's granulomatosis: Systemic inflammatory diseases and collagen vascular diseases, such as Wegener's granulomatosis and sarcoidosis cause nasal septal perforation.
- Infection: Tuberculosis, syphilis, fungal disease. Typically see other systemic manifestations.
- Lymphoma: Midline lethal granulomatosis or natural killer/T-cell lymphoma often causes destructive lesions.

COMMENTS

This is a 45-year-old female with a history of heavy cocaine use.

Nasal septal perforation is commonly asymptomatic and the diagnosis is made incidentally. Symptoms however can include a history of nasal congestion or obstruction, nasal crusting and drainage, recurrent epistaxis, and a whistling sound from the nose.

The nasal septal mucoperichondrium provides the vascular supply to the septal quadrangular cartilage. Any physical, iatrogenic, or chemical insults can cause septal perforation. Congenital septal perforation occurs after the 9th gestational week resulting in cellular apoptosis which causes the disappearance of these membranes and the resultant configuration and patency of the posterior choanae.

Traumatic causes of septal perforation include external trauma such as nasal septal fracture, self-inflicted causes such as digital manipulation, foreign body or piercing, iatrogenic causes such as surgeries including septoplasty, nasal packing or cauterization for epistaxis, chronic nasal cannula use, and nasotracheal intubation. Chronic inhalational exposure to medications such as vasoconstrictive and steroid nasal sprays and illicit drugs such as cocaine are the common causes of septal perforation. Systemic inflammatory processes such as collagen diseases (systemic lupus erythematodes, rheumatoid arthritis, etc.), sarcoidosis, Wegener's granulomatosis and Crohn's disease can cause septal perforation. Systemic infections including tuberculosis, syphilis, HIV, and diphtheria are also rare causes. Neoplastic causes including sinonasal carcinoma, lymphomas including "lethal midline granuloma"/natural killer/T-cell lymphoma and cryoglobulinemia have been documented.

CT is useful to evaluate nasal septum, whereas MRI can be used to delineate lesion boundaries and to demonstrate possible intracranial and intraorbital extension particularly when neoplastic or systemic processes are suspected.

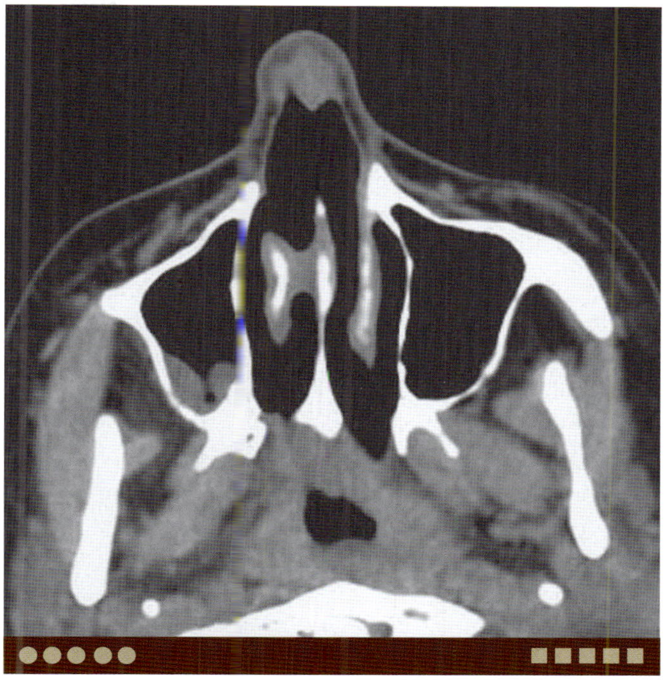

A. Nasal septal perforation, cocaine use. Axial CT image in soft tissue algorithm demonstrates loss of the mid nasal septum.

PEARLS

- **Nasal septal perforation can be congenital or acquired. Acquired lesions may be due to trauma, inflammation/infection, ischemia, or neoplasm.**
- **Due to the nonspecific nature of the imaging features, the diagnosis usually is supported by clinical history and histopathologic findings.**
- **It is important to exclude systemic disease processes as the cause. If systemic disease is present, MRI may provide additional information regarding intraorbital or intracranial involvement.**

ADDITIONAL IMAGES (B-G)

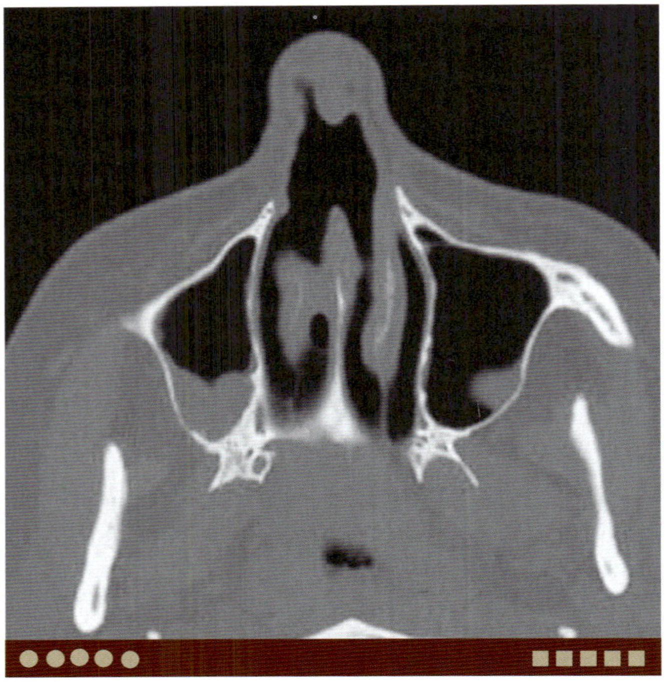

B. Nasal septal perforation, cocaine use, same patient as A. Axial CT image in bone tissue algorithm demonstrates loss of the mid nasal septum.

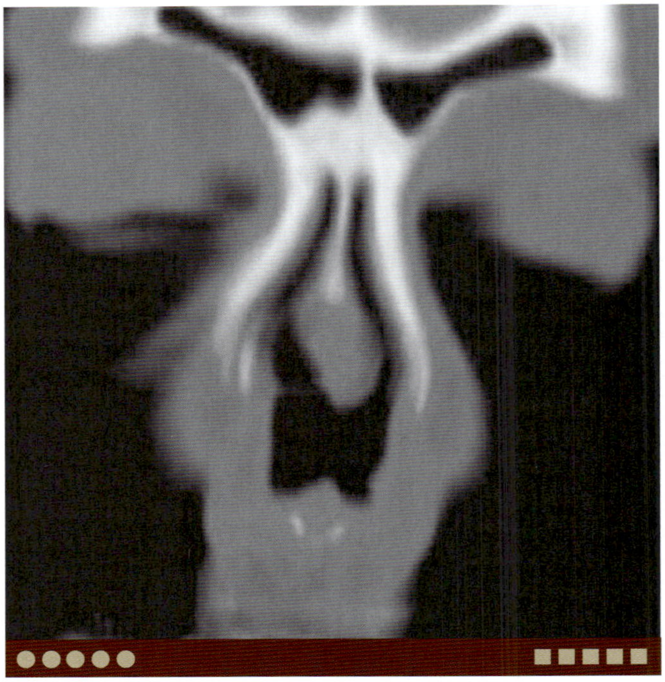

C. Nasal septal perforation, cocaine use, same patient as A. Coronal CT image in bone algorithm demonstrates loss of the mid nasal septum.

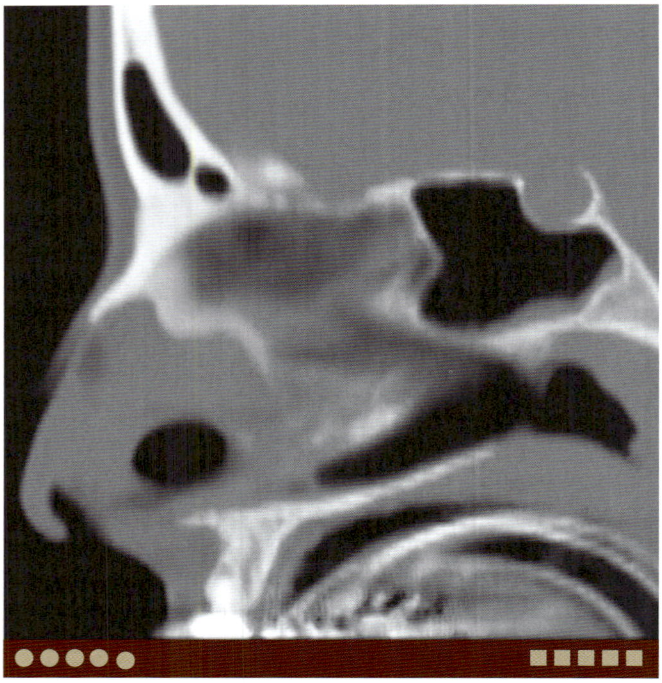

D. Nasal septal perforation, cocaine use, same patient as A. Sagittal CT image in bone algorithm demonstrates a well-circumscribed lucency in the mid nasal septum.

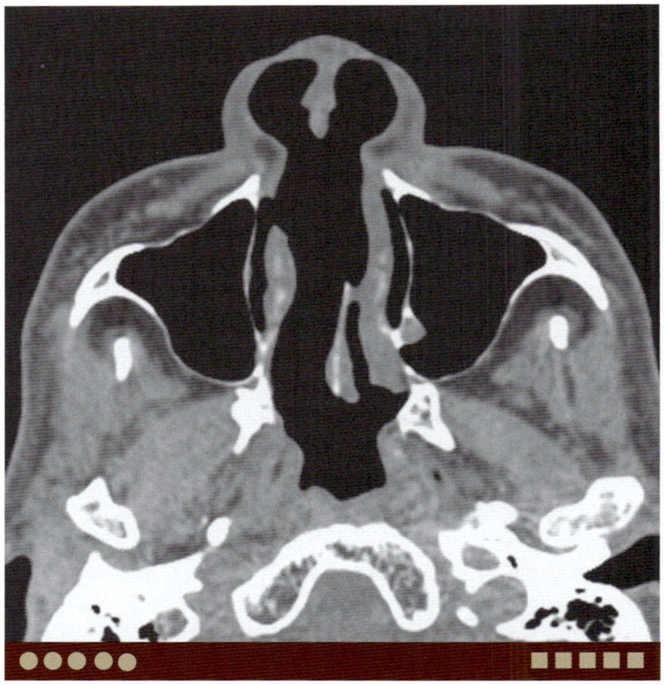

E. **Nasal septal perforation, cocaine use** in a different patient. Axial CT image in soft tissue algorithm demonstrates loss of the mid nasal septum.

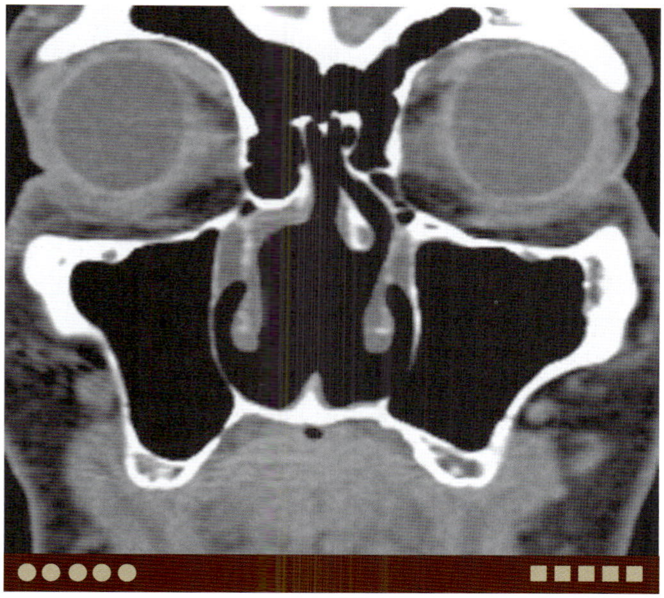

F. Nasal septal perforation, cocaine use, same patient as E. Coronal CT image in soft tissue algorithm demonstrates loss of the mid nasal septum.

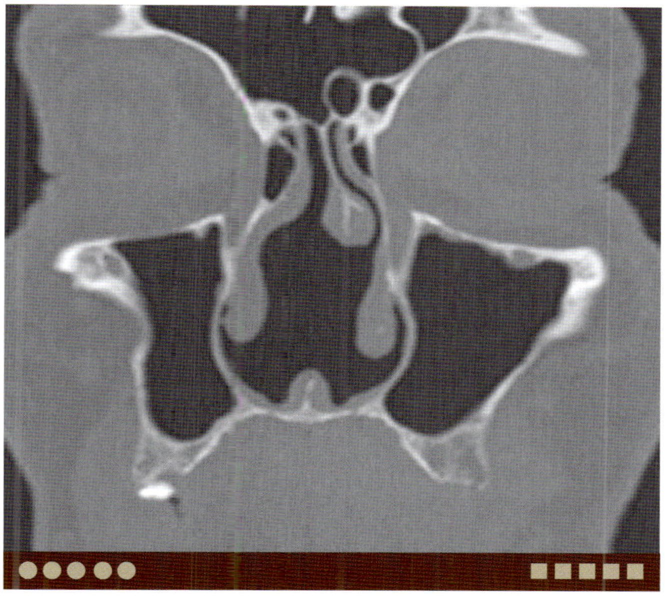

G. Nasal septal perforation, cocaine use, same patient as E. Coronal CT image in bone algorithm demonstrates loss of the mid nasal septum.

DIFFERENTIAL DIAGNOSIS IMAGE

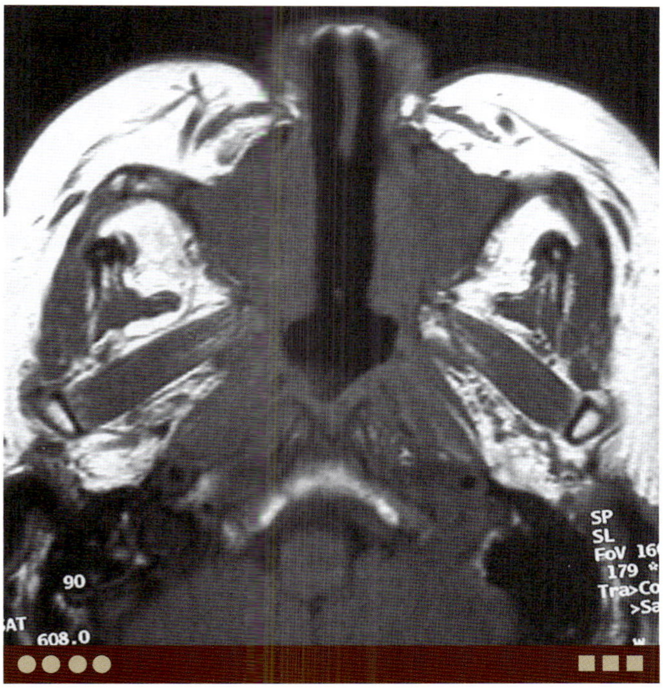

H. **Wegener's granulomatosis**. Axial T1W MR image demonstrates a large defect in the nasal septum.

Case 3–33 Extramedullary Hematopoiesis

Naoko Saito, Rohini Nadgir, Osamu Sakai

PRESENTATION

Incidental, asymptomatic. Laboratory analysis reveals anemia.

FINDINGS

CT and MRI demonstrate paranasal sinuses filled with soft tissue density/intensity masses.

DIFFERENTIAL DIAGNOSIS

- Chronic sinusitis: In addition to mucosal thickening, thickening of the osseous sinus wall is often observed with chronic inflammation.
- Lymphoma: Lymphoma demonstrates homogeneous density/signal and involves bone marrow. However, infiltration of tumor into adjacent structures such as retroantral fat pad and perineural extension are commonly seen.
- Squamous cell carcinoma (SCCA): SCCA is the most common malignancy in the sinonasal cavity. This usually demonstrates more focal and invasive findings and heterogeneous density/signal.
- Other benign and malignant tumors: Langerhans cell histiocytosis and rhabdomyosarcoma should be in the differential diagnosis of solid lesions in the maxillofacial and skull base regions in children.

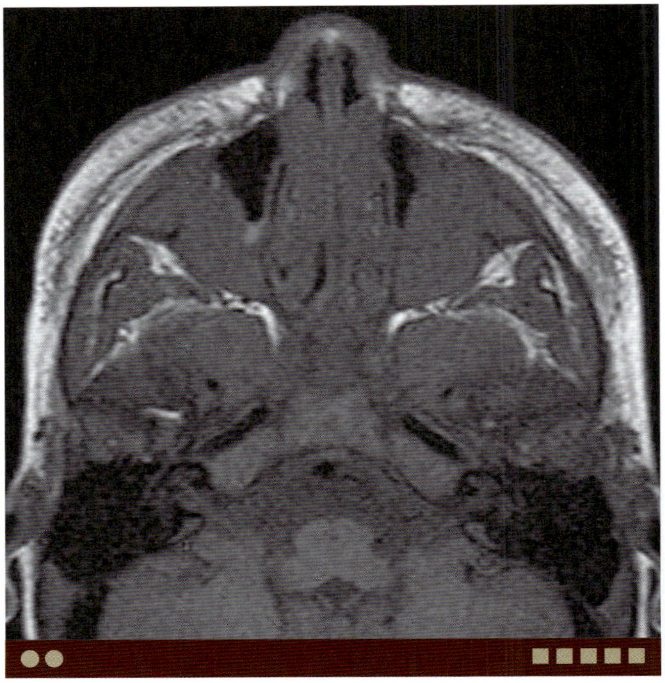

A. Extramedullary hematopoiesis (sickle cell disease). Axial T1W image demonstrates homogeneous hypointense masses filling the bilateral maxillary sinuses.

COMMENTS

This is a 2-year-old boy with sickle cell disease (Hb SS) who underwent MRI to evaluate for cerebral infarct.

Extramedullary hematopoiesis can be seen in the setting of chronic anemic conditions such as thalassemia, sickle cell disease, and myeloproliferative disorders. It is hypothesized that extramedullary hematopoiesis occurs as a compensatory response in the face of an increased need for blood production. Extramedullary hematopoiesis most commonly occurs in the liver and spleen, and other common sites include the paravertebral regions, kidneys, and adrenal glands. Extramedullary hematopoiesis in the head and neck is rare, however it has been reported in the paranasal sinuses, middle ear, thyroid gland, cervical lymph nodes, and lacrimal fossae in the literature.

On CT, soft tissue density mass or marrow is seen filling and expanding the maxilla. A markedly expanded diploic space protrudes into the sinus cavity and gives the radiologic appearance of the sinuses being filled with a soft tissue mass. Both CT and MRI demonstrate the same density and signal intensity mass as red bone marrow (intramedullary hematopoietic tissue) and homogeneous enhancement. In young children, sinus pneumatization is delayed because it only occurs in a bone once red marrow has converted to yellow marrow.

This condition is often asymptomatic and it may be identified as an incidental finding in the workup of other complaints. Progressive bilateral nasal obstruction has been reported when extramedullary hematopoiesis involves the paranasal sinuses.

PEARLS

- **Extramedullary hematopoiesis has been seen in chronic anemic conditions such as thalassemia, sickle cell disease, and myeloproliferative disorders.**
- **Extramedullary hematopoiesis is rare in the head and neck but may be seen in the paranasal sinuses, middle ear, thyroid gland, cervical lymph nodes, and lacrimal fossae.**
- **The lesion shows the same density/signal to red marrow.**

ADDITIONAL IMAGES (B-E)

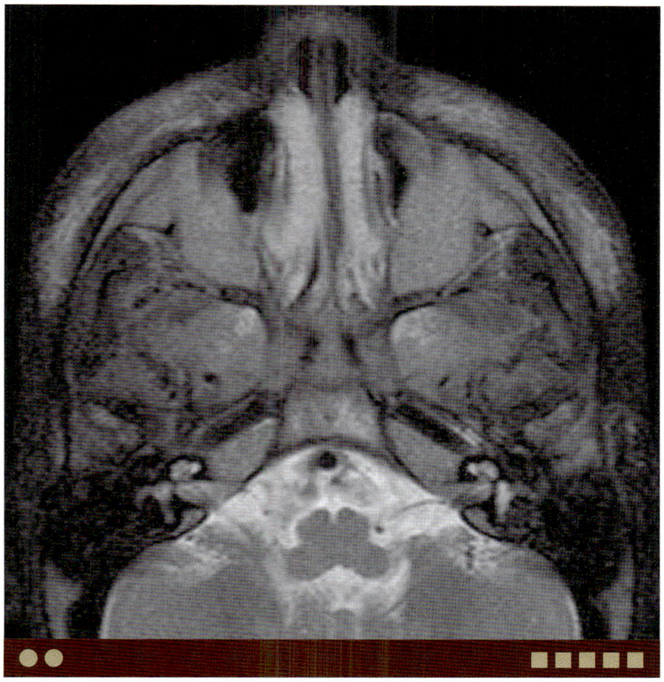

B. Extramedullary hematopoiesis (sickle cell disease), same patient as A. Axial fat-suppressed T2W image demonstrates homogeneous slight hyperintense masses filling the bilateral maxillary sinuses.

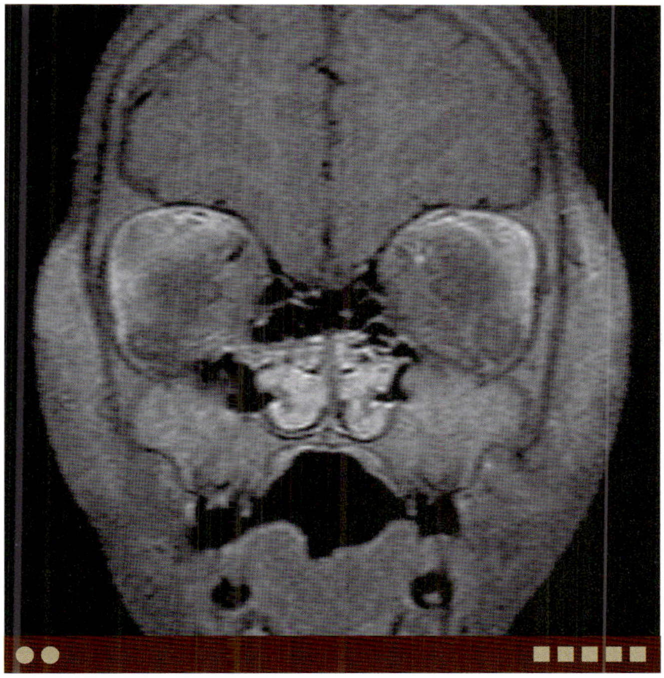

C. Extramedullary hematopoiesis (sickle cell disease), same patient as A. Coronal postcontrast fat-suppressed T1W image shows homogeneous enhancement of the masses.

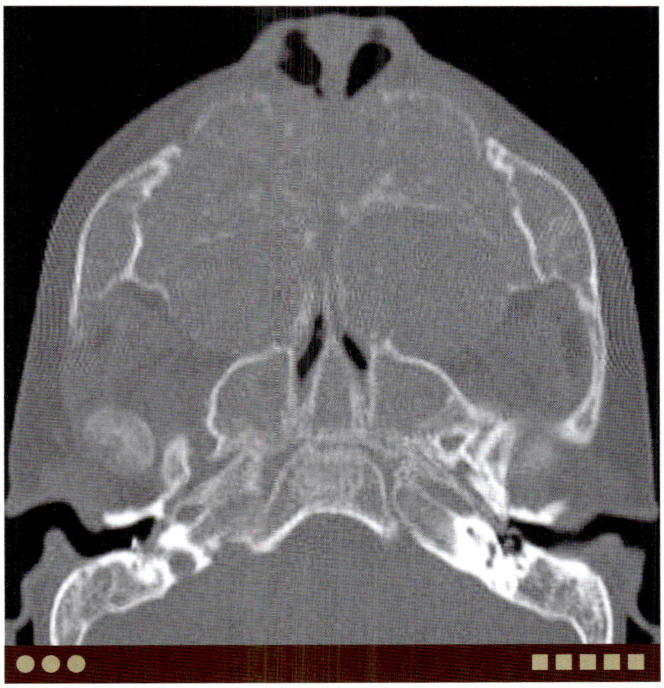

D. Extramedullary hematopoiesis (thalassemia). Axial CT demonstrates markedly expanded diploic space of the maxilla completely obliterating the sinus cavities.

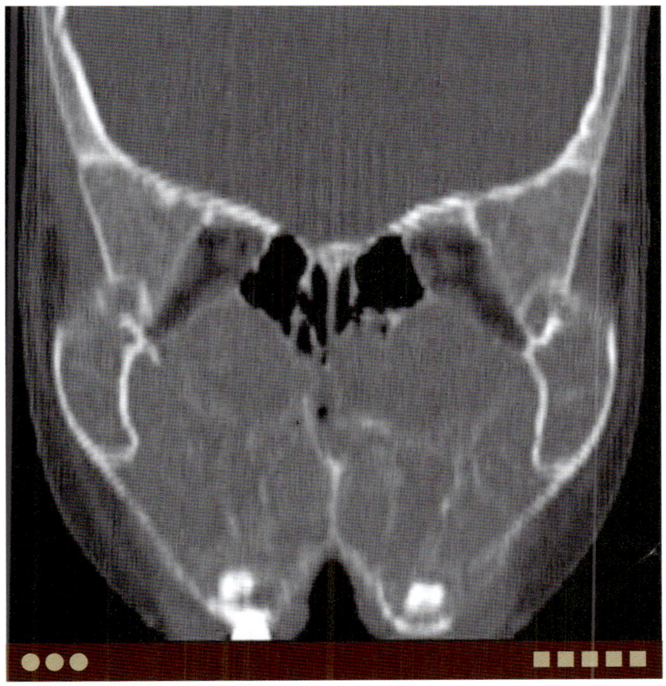

E. Extramedullary hematopoiesis (thalassemia), same patient as D. Coronal CT demonstrates marked expansion of the maxilla completely obliterating the sinus cavities. Expansion of diploic space is also seen in other bones.

DIFFERENTIAL DIAGNOSIS IMAGES (F-G)

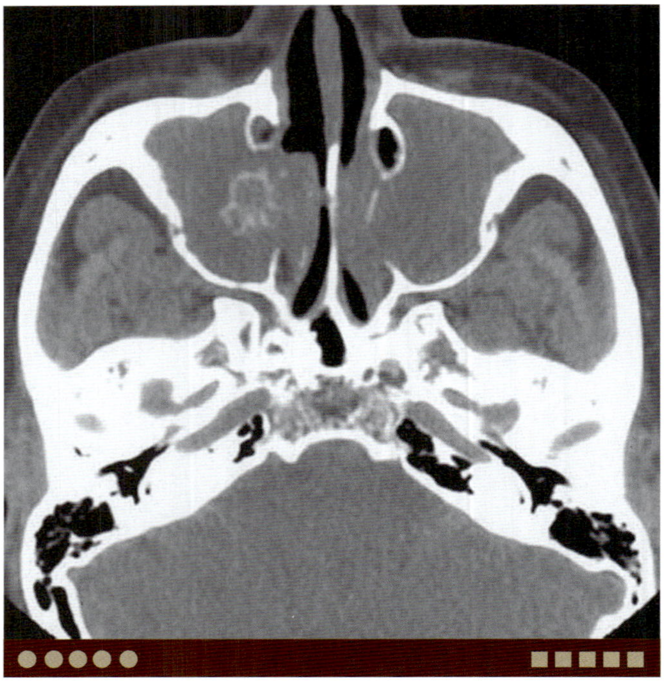

F. Chronic sinusitis. Axial CT demonstrates complete opacification of the bilateral maxillary sinuses. There is calcification within the right maxillary sinus, secondary to chronic inflammation.

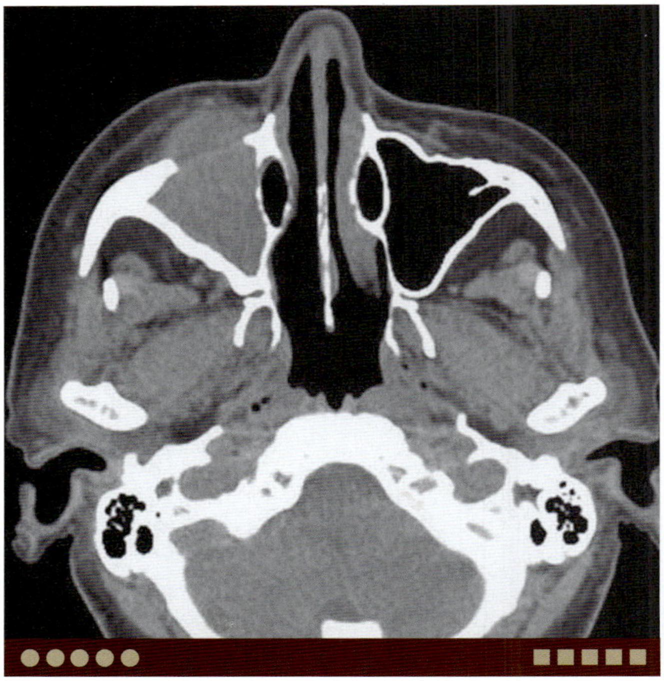

G. Squamous cell carcinoma. Axial CT demonstrates soft tissue density completely filling the right maxillary sinus. Note destruction of the anterior wall and soft tissue density extension into the overlying soft tissue.

Case 3–34 Sarcoidosis

Osamu Sakai, Daniel Weller

PRESENTATION

Nasal mass.

FINDINGS

CT and MRI demonstrate heterogeneously enhancing nodular lesions in the nasal cavity.

DIFFERENTIAL DIAGNOSIS

- Nasal polyposis: Polyp is the most common benign mass in the nasal cavity. Polyposis may be associated with allergy and fungal infection.
- Wegener's granulomatosis: A form of vasculitis of unknown etiology but likely associated with autoimmune abnormality. C-ANCA is almost always positive.
- Granulomatous infection: Tuberculosis and cryptococcosis demonstrate similar findings. These patients usually demonstrate symptoms of infection.

COMMENTS

This is a 65-year-old woman with nasal masses.

Sarcoidosis is a disease causing noncaseous epithelioid granulomas in multiple organs, such as lungs, lymphoid tissues, skin, and orbits. Pulmonary disease is the most common manifestation and affects nearly all patients. The incidence of sinonasal involvement with sarcoidosis is approximately 1%. Patients with sinonasal sarcoidosis can experience epistaxis, nasal congestion, polyps, rhinorrhea, and nasal crusts. Septal perforation may be seen. Serologically, increased angiotensin-converting enzyme (ACE) is common.

Imaging findings of sinonasal sarcoidosis are nonspecific and it is almost impossible to diagnose by imaging alone. Findings may be similar to those seen in Wegener's granulomatosis and other granulomatous diseases. Other systemic findings help the diagnosis, and histological evaluation is necessary to confirm the diagnosis.

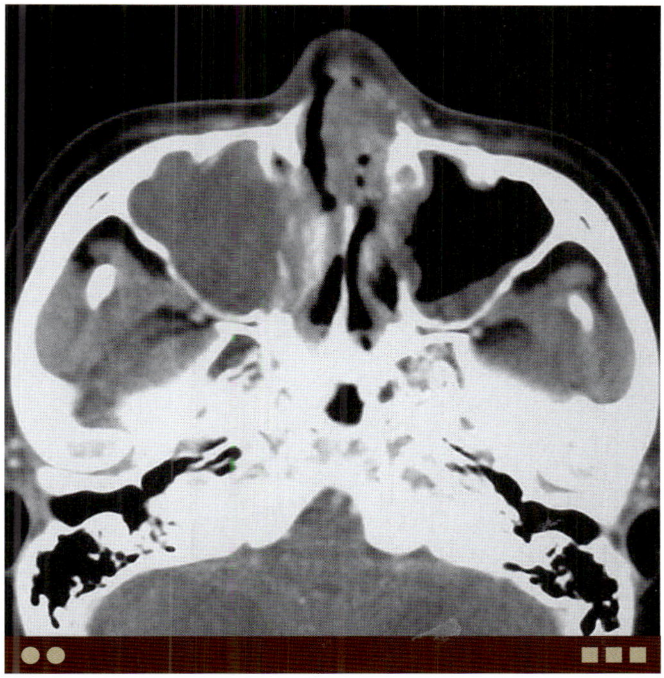

A. Sarcoidosis. Axial postcontrast CT demonstrates mildly enhancing polypoid lesions in the anterior nasal cavity. The right maxillary sinus is completely opacified.

About 5% of patients with sarcoidosis show CNS involvement, and rarely is the disease limited to the CNS. Therefore, it is important to evaluate the intracranial structures when interpreting the case.

PEARLS

- **Sinonasal sarcoidosis is rare, only involving about 1% of patients with sarcoidosis.**
- **Imaging findings are nonspecific and similar to Wegener's granulomatosis and other granulomatous disease.**
- **About 5% of patients with sarcoidosis show CNS involvement.**

ADDITIONAL IMAGES (B-E)

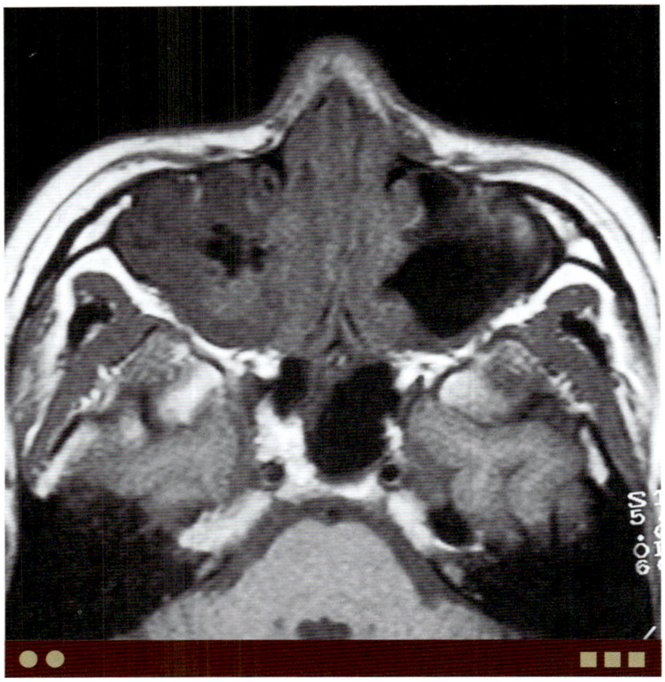

B. Sarcoidosis, same patient as A. Axial T1W MR shows polypoid lesions filling the nasal cavities bilaterally.

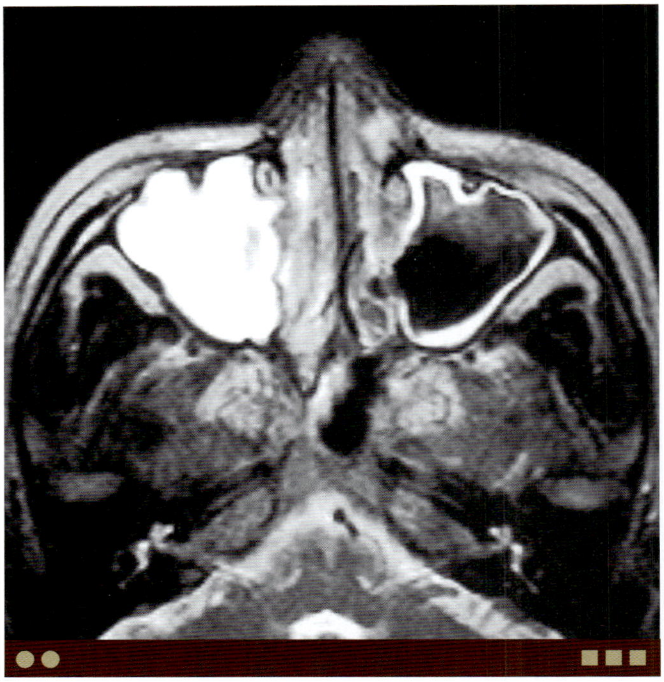

C. Sarcoidosis, same patient as A. Axial T2W MR shows polypoid lesions filling the nasal cavities bilaterally, demonstrating heterogeneous, intermediate signal, lower than the signal of submucosal edema seen in the maxillary sinuses.

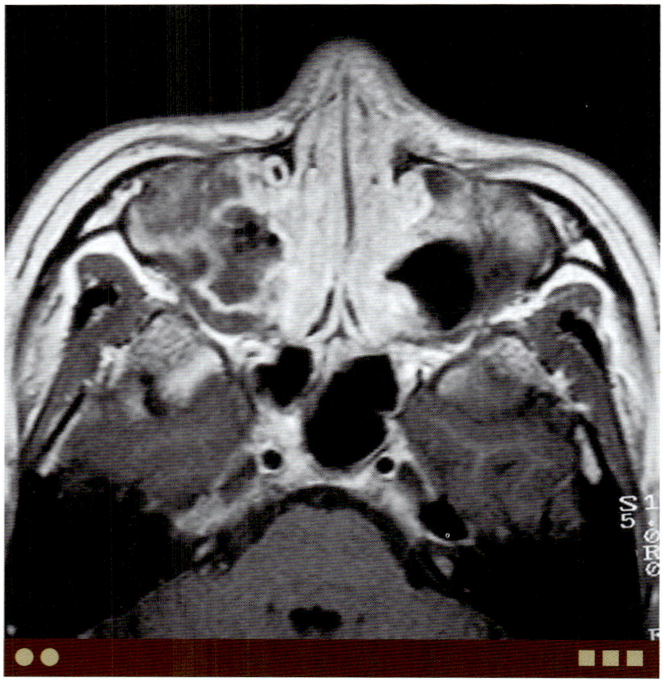

D. Sarcoidosis, same patient as A. Axial postcontrast T1W MR shows diffuse enhancement of the lesion.

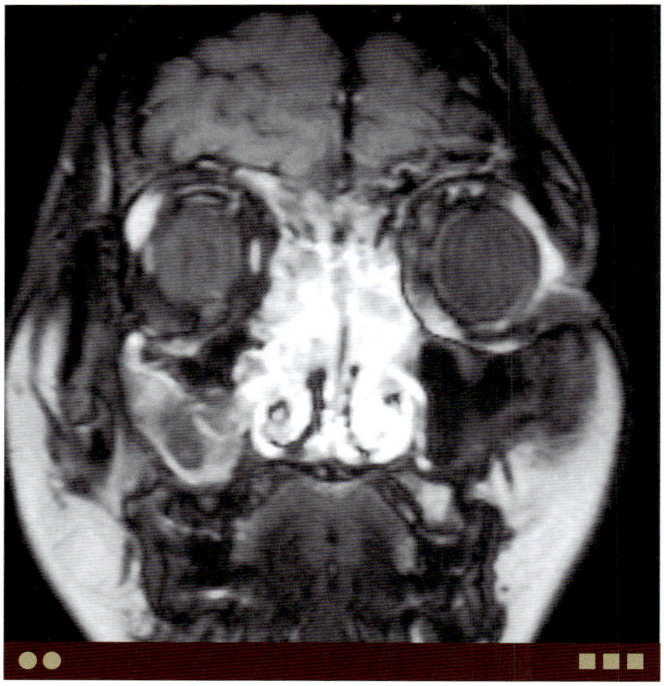

E. Sarcoidosis, same patient as A. Coronal postcontrast fat-suppressed T1W MR shows diffuse enhancement of the lesion.

DIFFERENTIAL DIAGNOSIS IMAGES (F-G)

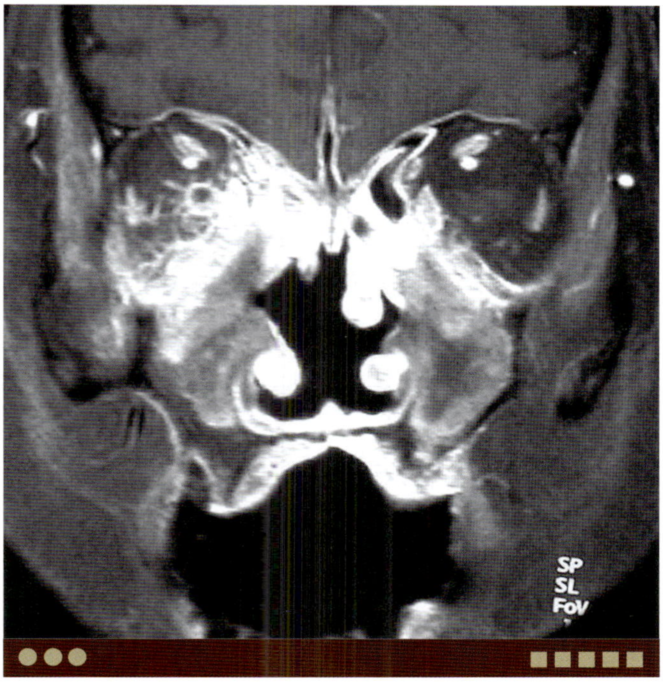

F. Wegener's granulomatosis. Coronal postcontrast fat-suppressed T1W MR demonstrates diffuse enhancement in the ethmoid and maxillary sinuses bilaterally and medial orbits. Large nasal septal perforation is present. Note abnormal dural enhancement.

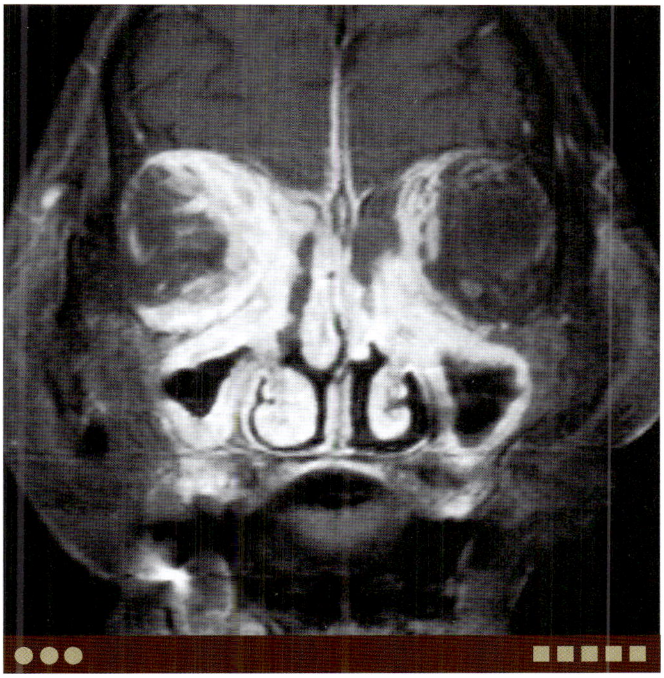

G. Lymphoma. Coronal postcontrast fat-suppressed T1W image demonstrates diffuse enhancement in the ethmoid and maxillary sinuses bilaterally and medial orbits. Note abnormal dural enhancement.

Case 3-35 Giant Cell Tumor

Elisa Flower, Osamu Sakai

PRESENTATION

Facial swelling.

FINDINGS

CT demonstrates a soft tissue mass arising from the wall of the maxillary sinus.

DIFFERENTIAL DIAGNOSIS

- Giant cell reparative granuloma: This condition is difficult to be distinguished from giant cell tumor (GCT) by imaging and histology but history of trauma or tooth extraction and younger age at presentation can help.
- "Brown tumor" of hyperparathyroidism: This condition demonstrates similar appearance to GCT; however, the history and clinical data support hyperparathyroidism.
- Fibrous dysplasia: This lesion often shows ground-glass matrix, although cystic type may demonstrate similar findings to GCT.
- Aneurysmal bone cyst (ABC): Soap bubble appearance with fluid–fluid level is a characteristic finding for ABC. ABC can be seen in association with GCT.
- Osteosarcoma: Osteosarcomas of the jaw occur in older patients compared with those arise from the long bones. They usually show aggressive findings such as periosteal reaction and extraosseous extension, and rapid growth.
- Metastasis: Metastasis to the maxillofacial bone is not rare, commonly seen in the posterior body of the mandible.

COMMENTS

This is an 82-year-old female who presented with facial swelling.

Giant cell tumors (GCTs) are histologically characterized by a large number of osteoclastic giant cells on a background of mononuclear spindled cells with similar nuclei. They generally demonstrate benign features but can be locally aggressive or metastasize. Their peak incidence is between the third and fourth decades, with a female predominance. GCT is most often seen at the epiphyses of long bones, with craniofacial lesions much less common. Cranial involvement is most common in the sphenoid bone. The most common clinical presentation is pain and swelling. Other associated symptoms such as cranial nerve palsies can be related to the location of the lesion, as opposed to the lesion itself.

Imaging appearances of GCT on CT include a well circumscribed, expansile mildly hyperdense mass with thin overlying cortical margin. Internal calcification can be seen but are not common. Lesions of the cranium can be purely lytic, commonly with cortical breakthrough and associated soft tissue extension. GCT demonstrates moderate enhancement. On MRI, GCT can show mixed signal, generally low on all sequences with hypointense rim and marked enhancement.

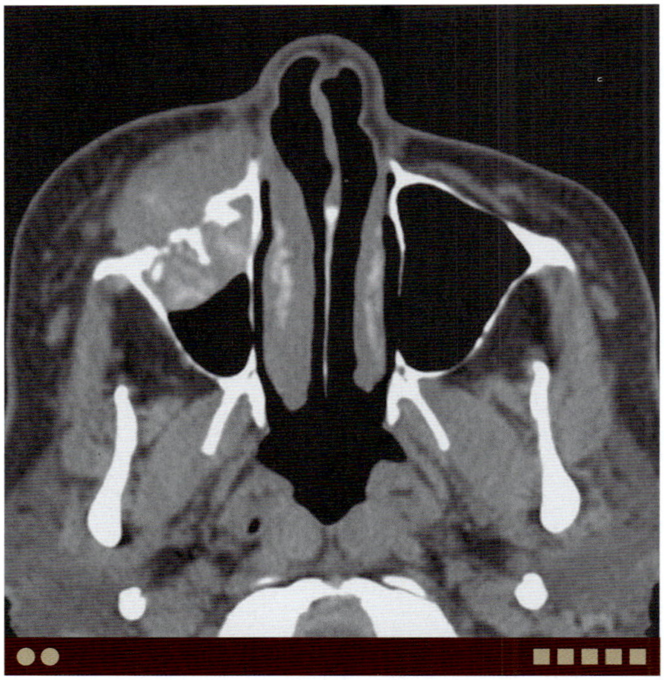

A. GCT. Axial CT demonstrates a relatively dense expansile soft tissue lesion with destruction of the anterior wall of the right maxillary sinus.

None of the radiologic characteristics are diagnostic and histology is required for definitive diagnosis. Unfortunately, giant cells can also be identified in histological analysis of giant cell reparative granuloma, "brown tumors," fibrous dysplasia, and ABCs. Both radiographic and histologic findings in the setting of the patient's clinical background are required for accurate diagnosis.

Treatment for GCT is possible preoperative embolization followed by complete surgical resection or curettage. Recurrence risk is 30-50% and mostly occurs within 2 years of treatment. Radiation therapy is reserved for inoperable lesions as GCT are generally not radiosensitive and this treatment results in increased risk of sarcomatous transformation.

PEARLS

- **GCT of the craniofacial bones is quite rare and for that reason not often a differential diagnostic consideration.**
- **Clinical, radiographic, and histology analysis must be evaluated together to make an accurate diagnosis.**

ADDITIONAL IMAGES (B-F)

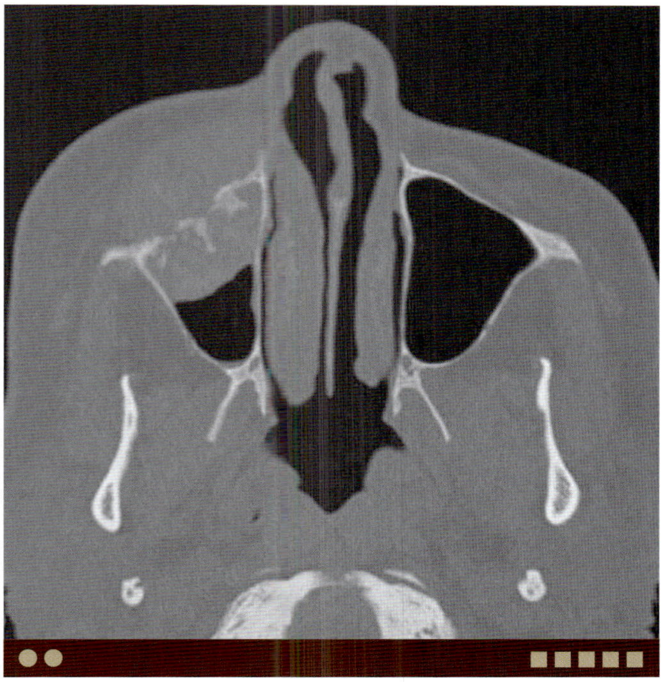

B. GCT, same patient as A. Axial CT in bony window demonstrates internal calcifications within the lesion.

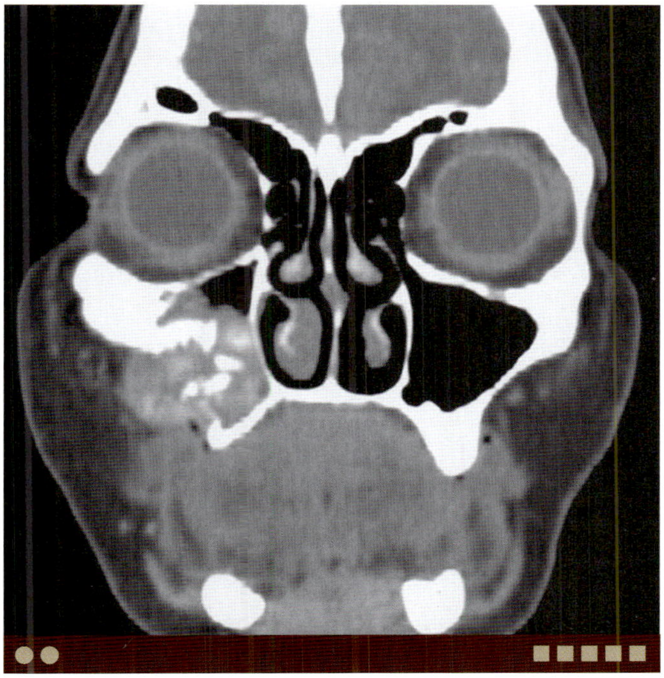

C. GCT, same patient as A. Coronal CT in soft tissue window demonstrates a destructive, expansile soft tissue lesion of the anterior right maxillary sinus wall. This lesion demonstrates heterogeneous increased density.

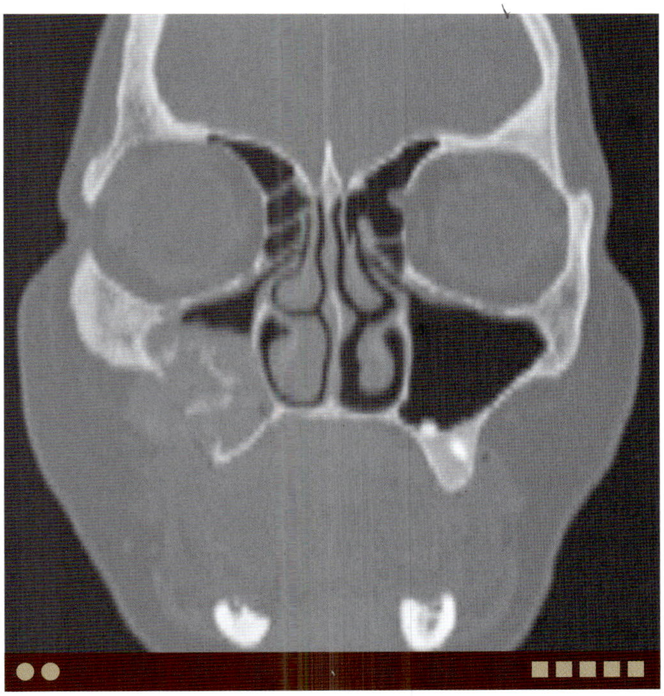

D. GCT, same patient as A. Coronal CT in bony window demonstrates osseous destruction of the anterior sinus wall with extension inferiorly into the alveolar ridge.

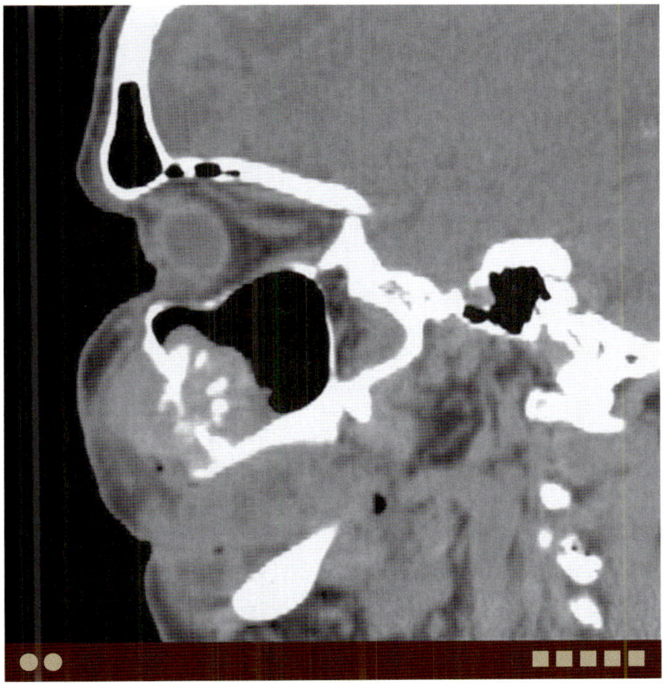

E. GCT, same patient as A. Sagittal CT in soft tissue window demonstrates a destructive, expansile soft tissue lesion of the anterior maxillary sinus wall. This lesion demonstrates heterogeneous increased density.

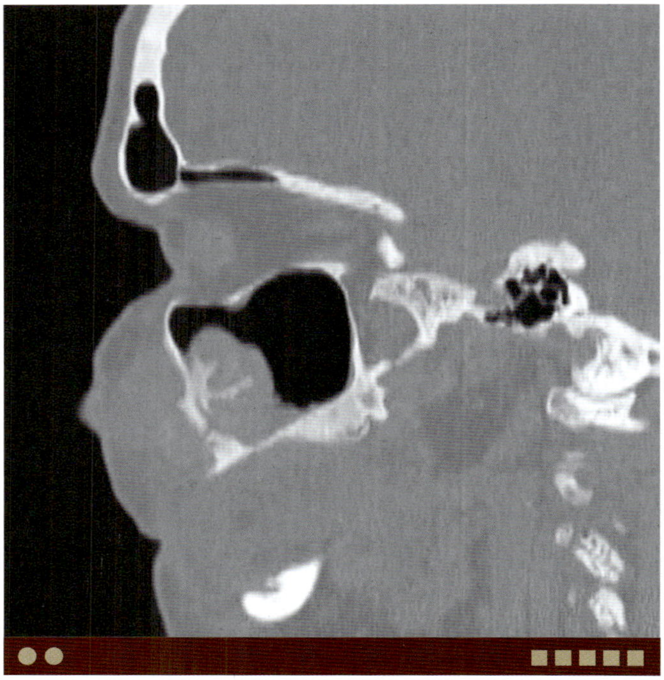

F. GCT, same patient as A. Sagittal CT in bony window demonstrates osseous destruction of the anterior sinus wall.

DIFFERENTIAL DIAGNOSIS IMAGES (G-I)

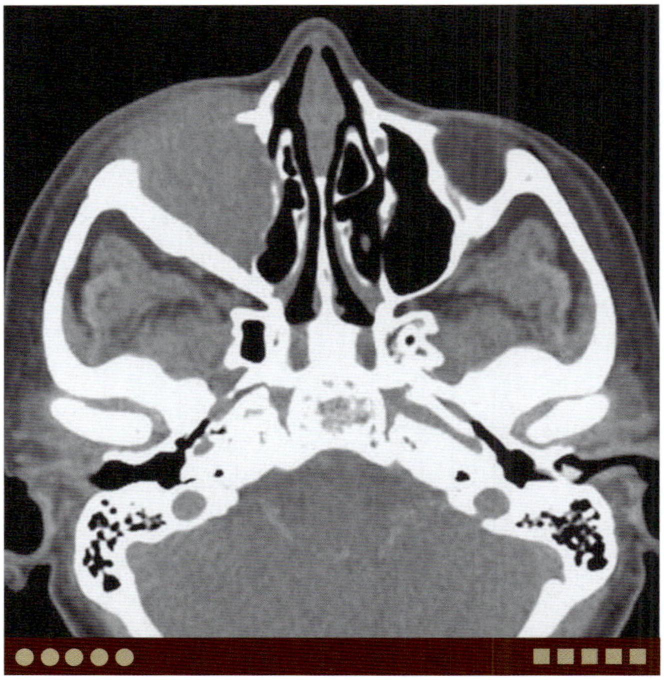

G. Squamous cell carcinoma. Axial CT demonstrates a solid tumor occupying the right maxillary sinus, destructing the anterior wall and extending to the superficial soft tissue.

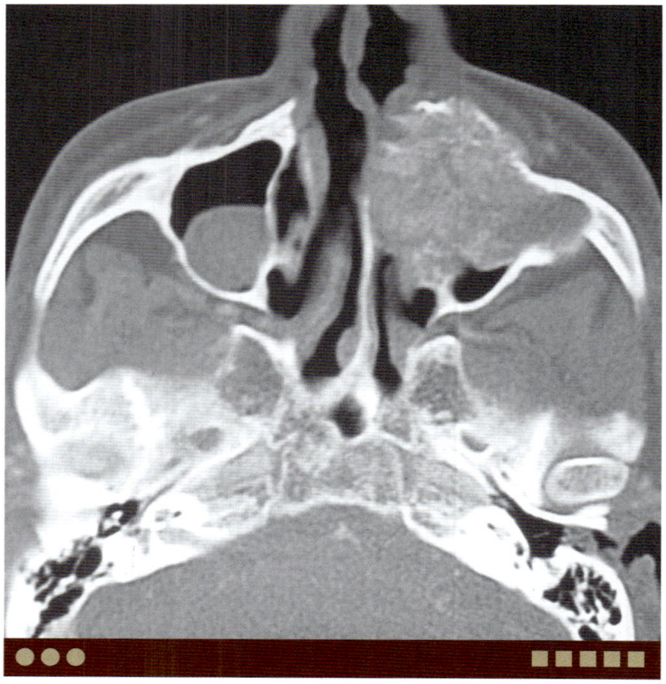

H. Hemangioma. Axial CT demonstrates an expansile osseous lesion in the left maxillary sinus with coarse heterogeneous internal density and destructive features.

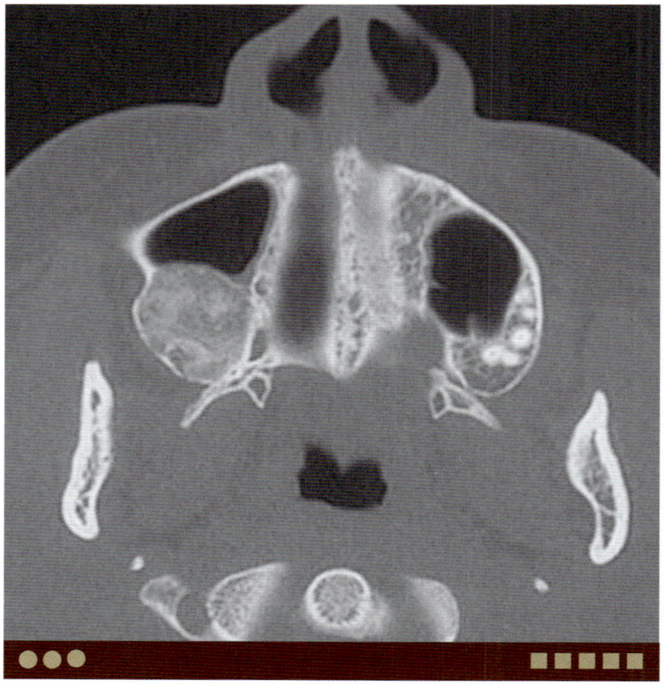

I. Ossifying fibroma. Axial CT demonstrates an expansile, radiodense mass in the posterolateral wall of the right maxillary sinus.

Case 3–36 Invasive Fungal Sinusitis

Hiroki Kato, Osamu Sakai

PRESENTATION

Nasal congestion or obstruction, nasal discharge, facial pain, facial swelling, headache, dental pain, and visual complaints.

FINDINGS

CT and MRI demonstrate an invasive and destructive sinonasal mass.

DIFFERENTIAL DIAGNOSIS

- Squamous cell carcinoma (SCCA): SCCA is the most common malignancy in the sinonasal cavity and often invades the orbit and skull base. Intratumoral necrosis is common in a large SCCA, which demonstrates heterogeneous enhancement and high signal on T2W images.
- Minor salivary gland tumors: Minor salivary gland tumors, such as mucoepidermoid carcinoma and adenoid cystic carcinoma occur in the sinonasal cavity. High-grade malignant salivary gland tumors tend to demonstrate low signal on T2W images reflecting the high cellularity.
- Lymphoma: In immunohistochemistry, sinonasal lymphomas have been separated into B-cell, T-cell, and most recently into natural killer (NK) cell phenotypes. Lymphomas tend to show homogeneous density/intensity, and enhancement. On diffusion-weighted MR images, low ADC value is a characteristic.

COMMENTS

This is a 56-year-old man with poorly controlled diabetes mellitus.

Fungal sinusitis can be divided into noninvasive and invasive forms. Acute fulminant invasive fungal sinusitis is a rapidly progressing, destructive process almost exclusively affecting immunocompromised patients as a result of systemic chemotherapy, bone marrow transplantation, immunosuppressive agents used after organ transplantation, acquired immunodeficiency syndrome, or long-term systemic steroid use. Poorly controlled diabetes mellitus, usually with diabetic ketoacidosis, is another common underlying cause in development of invasive fungal sinusitis. Intracranial or intraorbital extension is a true otolaryngologic emergency. In the absence of timely diagnosis and treatment, these diseases can be fatal. Treatment usually consists of aggressive surgical debridement and intravenous antifungal therapy.

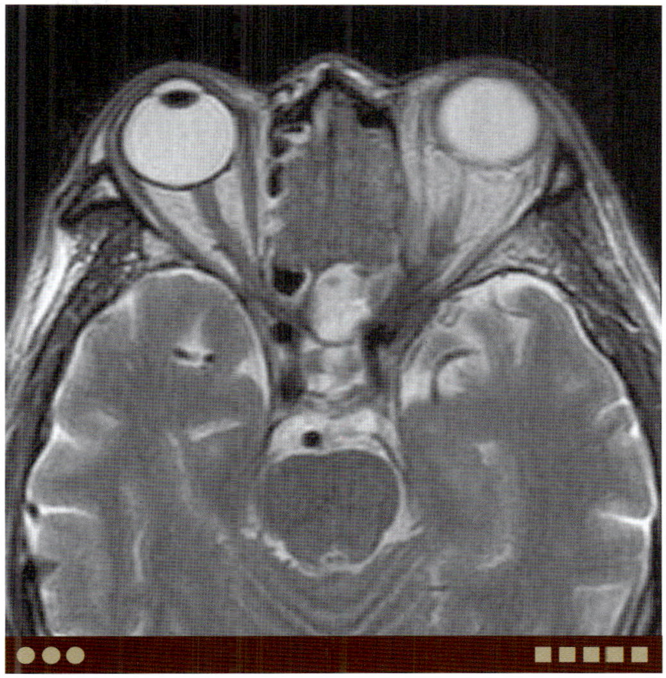

A. Invasive fungal sinusitis (Aspergillus). Axial T2W MR image demonstrates a hypointense lesion of the bilateral ethmoid air cells and the left orbital apex.

Unilateral involvement of the ethmoid and sphenoid sinuses is often seen in invasive fungal sinusitis. CT is better to assess bone changes, and MRI is superior in evaluating for intracranial and intraorbital extension. Aggressive bone destruction of the sinus walls rapidly results in intracranial and intraorbital extension of the infection. Dural or leptomeningeal enhancement may be seen with intracranial extension. Intracranial extension of fungal infection shows three major forms: (1) meningitis, (2) brain abscess, and (3) cerebral infarct due to involvement of large- and intermediate-sized vessels. Further, vascular involvement may result in a mycotic aneurysm and hemorrhage. On T2W images, fungal infections demonstrate remarkably low signal secondary to increased concentrations of iron and manganese. Strong contrast enhancement on CT and MRI may suggest development of fungal infection.

PEARLS

- **Invasive fungal sinusitis often demonstrates intracranial and intraorbital extension.**
- **CT is better to assess bone changes, and MR imaging is useful in evaluating for intracranial and intraorbital extension.**
- **Fungal infections demonstrate remarkably low signal on T2W images.**

ADDITIONAL IMAGES (B-E)

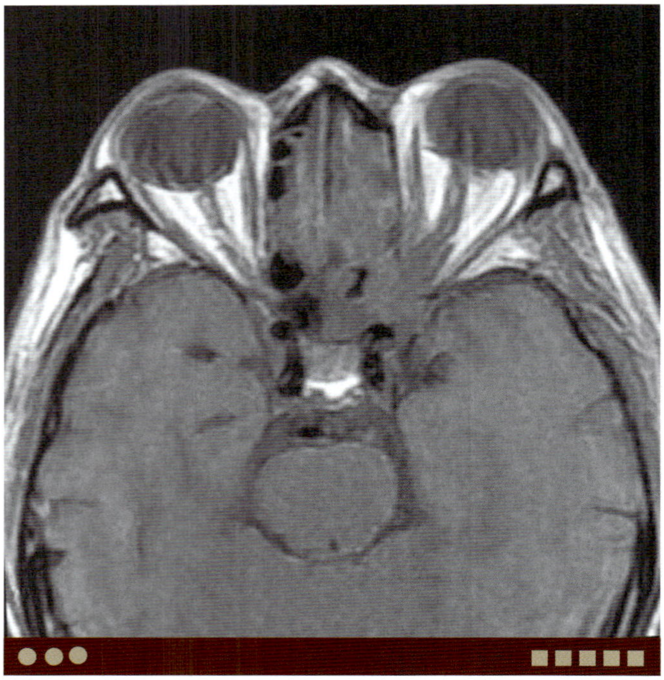

B. Invasive fungal sinusitis (Aspergillus), same patient as A. Axial T1W image demonstrates hypointensity with in the lesion.

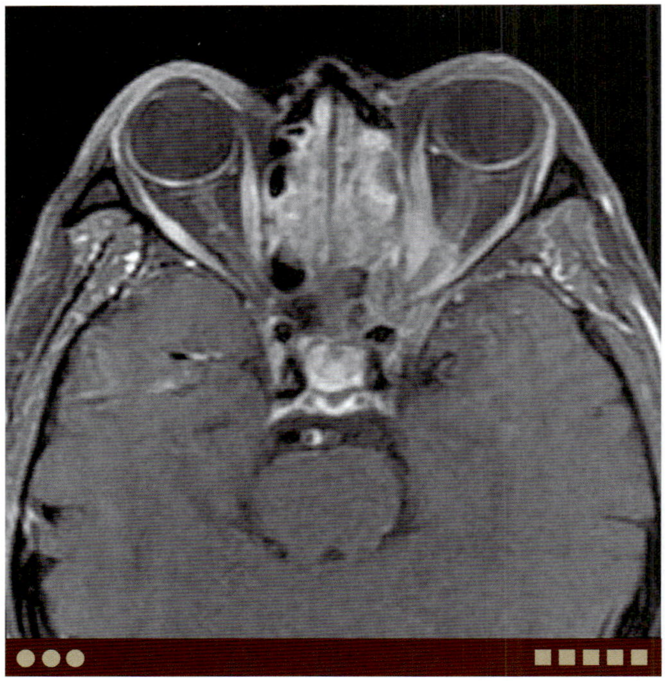

C. Invasive fungal sinusitis (Aspergillus), same patient as A. Axial postcontrast fat-suppressed T1W image demonstrates diffuse enhancement of the lesion.

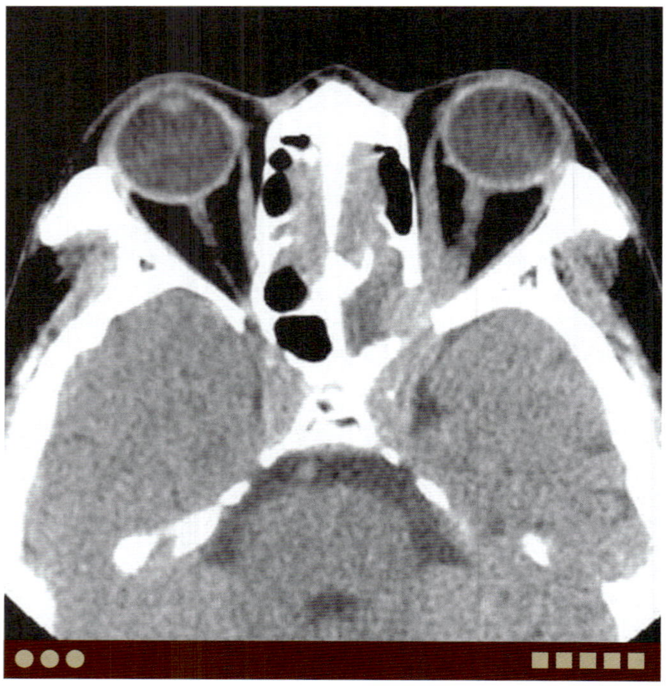

D. Invasive fungal sinusitis (Aspergillus), same patient as A. Axial postcontrast CT demonstrates an enhancing lesion in the bilateral ethmoid and left sphenoid sinuses. Note bone destruction and intra-orbital extension as well as cavernous sinus invasion on the left.

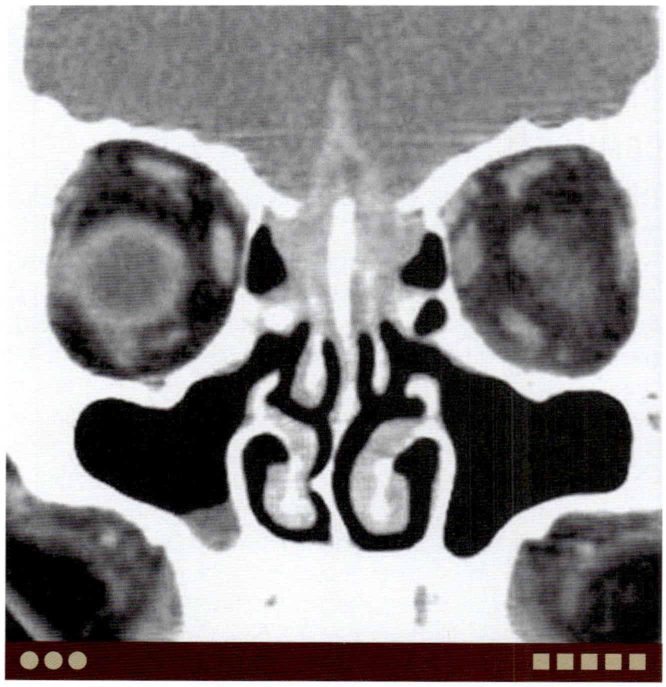

E. Invasive fungal sinusitis (Aspergillus), same patient as A. Coronal postcontrast CT demonstrates an enhancing lesion in the bilateral nasal cavity and ethmoid air cells with skull base destruction and dural enhancement.

DIFFERENTIAL DIAGNOSIS IMAGES (F-G)

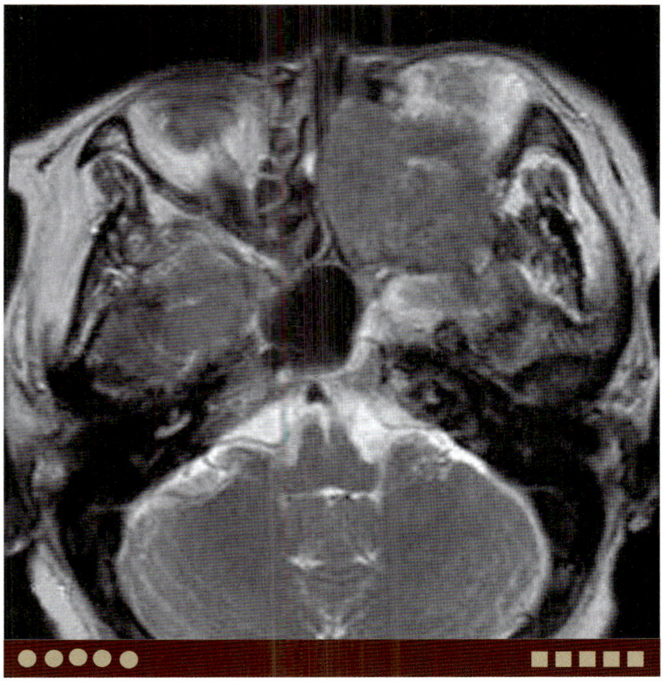

F. SCCA. Axial T2W MR image demonstrates a heterogeneous intermediate-signal tumor in the left maxillary sinus invading the left orbit.

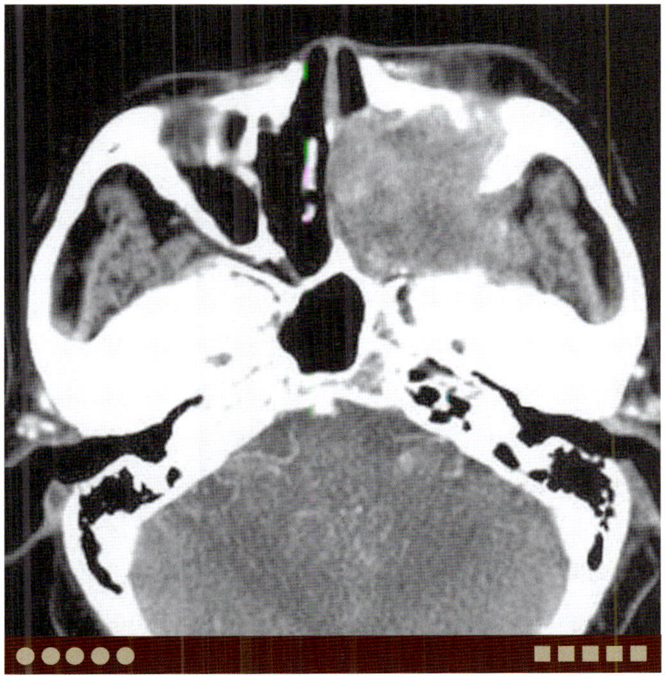

G. SCCA, same patient as F. Axial postcontrast CT demonstrates heterogeneous enhancement of the tumor destructing the posterolateral wall and invading the pterygopalatine fossa.

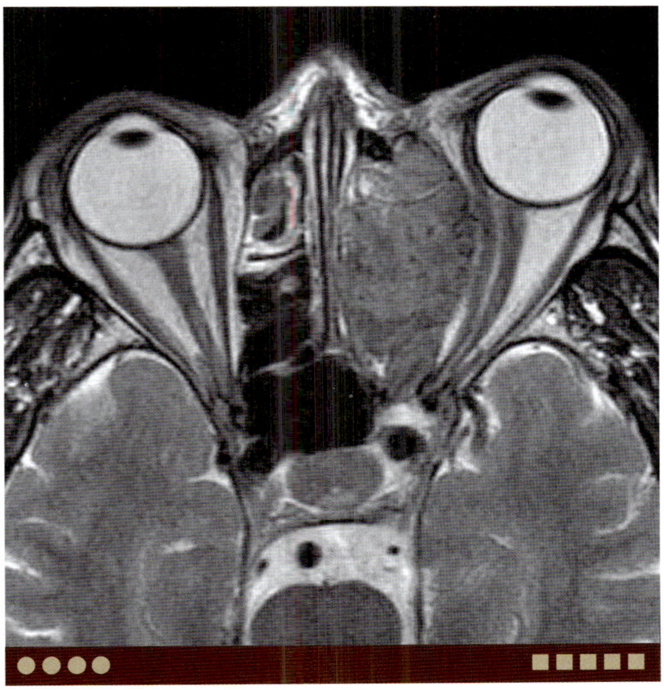

H. Lymphoma, B cell diffuse large. Axial T2W MR image demonstrates a heterogeneous intermediate-signal lesion in the left ethmoid with orbital extension.

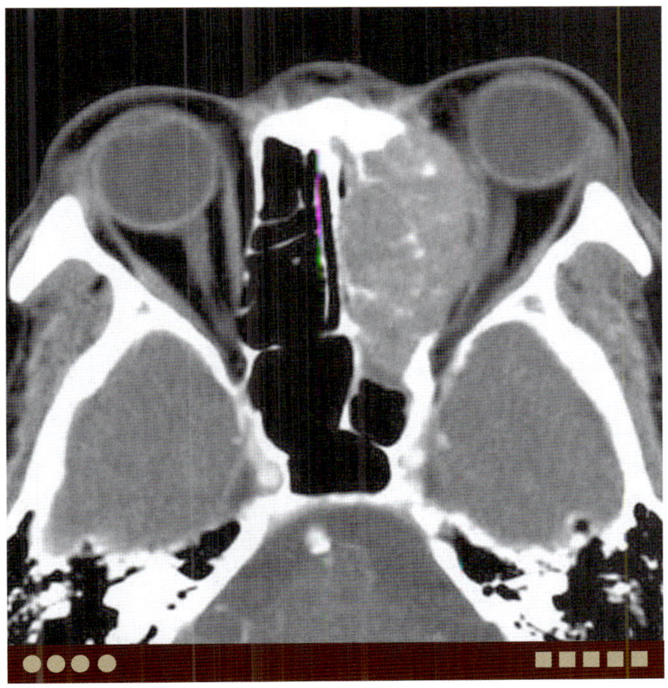

I. Lymphoma, B cell diffuse large, same patient as H. Axial postcontrast CT demonstrates mild enhancement of the lesion.

Case 3-37 Nasal Dermoid

Asim Mian, Osamu Sakai

PRESENTATION

Congenital midline nasal mass.

FINDINGS

CT and MRI demonstrate a well-defined, nonenhancing midline nasal mass that extends below the nasal bridge with possible intracranial extension.

DIFFERENTIAL DIAGNOSIS

- Frontoethmoidal cephalocele: This anomaly typically has large bony dehiscence along the cribriform plate or frontal bone with extension of dura and parenchyma through the defect.
- Nasal glioma: This is a solid mass of dysplastic neural tissue along the nasal dorsum with no intracranial connection. It may have a fibrous band that extends to the skull base but not intracranially.
- Non-ossified foramen cecum: Foramen cecum is located between the frontal bone and the crista galli and measures up to 10 mm in width (average, 4 mm). It contains fibrous tissue and shows soft tissue density on CT and low-to-intermediate signal on MRI.
- Prominent fatty marrow of crista galli: High signal from prominent crista galli may be confused with dermoid.

COMMENTS

This is a 4-year-old boy who underwent MRI for seizure.

Nasal dermoids are rare congenital midline nasal masses that typically occur because of failure of involution of the dural tract during embryologic development. It can occur as a cyst, sinus or fistula. Its incidence is 1:20000 to 1:40000 births. It affects boys and girls equally. Clinically it presents at birth or early infancy as a midline nasal mass along the dorsum. Occasionally, it can have a sinus tract that is typically found at the distal one-third with a tuft of hair. There is an association with discharge of sebaceous material and recurrent infections. Intracranial extension occurs in 20% and involves a tract that goes through the foramen cecum and cribriform plate and attaches itself to the dura. Involvement of the brain parenchyma has also been described.

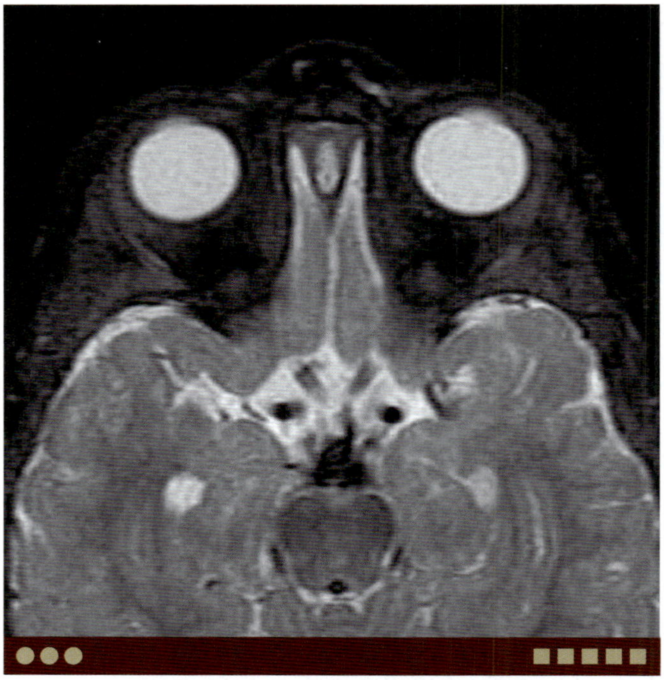

A. Nasal dermoid. Axial fat-suppressed T2W image demonstrates a high-signal midline mass at the anterior skull base below the crista galli.

CT demonstrates a midline nasal mass with a large foramen cecum, a bifid crista galli and occasionally deformity of the cribriform plate with soft tissue. MRI typically requires thin section imaging and demonstrates a mass with iso- to hyperintense signal on T1W and hyperintense signal on T2W images anywhere from the tip of the nose to the crista galli. There may be a sinus tract to the distal one-third of the nose and attachment to the dura intracranially.

PEARLS

- **Nasal dermoids are rare congenital lesions that occur along the midline of the nose with intracranial communication through a sinus tract.**
- **Nasal dermoid may have a sinus tract passing through enlarged foramen cecum with attachment intracranially to the dura and can have defects of the cribriform plate or bifid crista galli.**

ADDITIONAL IMAGES (B-F)

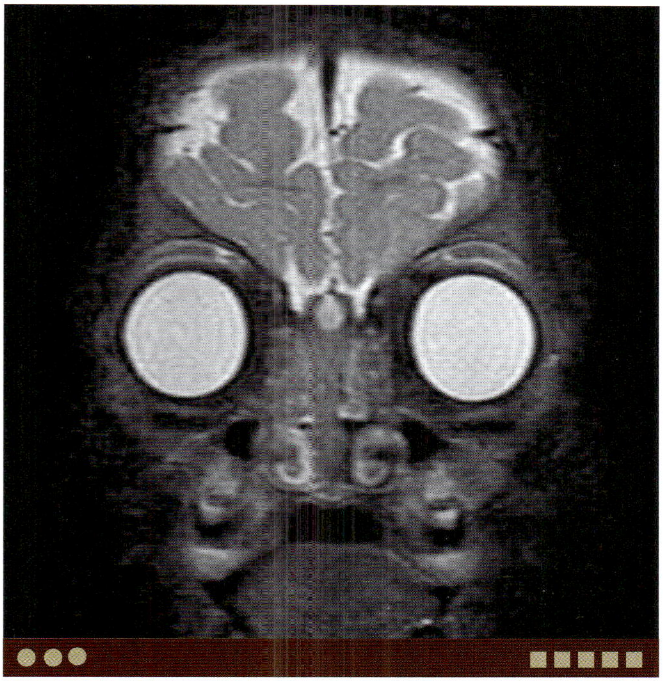

B. Nasal dermoid, same patient as A. Coronal fat-suppressed T2W image demonstrates a high-signal midline mass at the level of the cribriform plates.

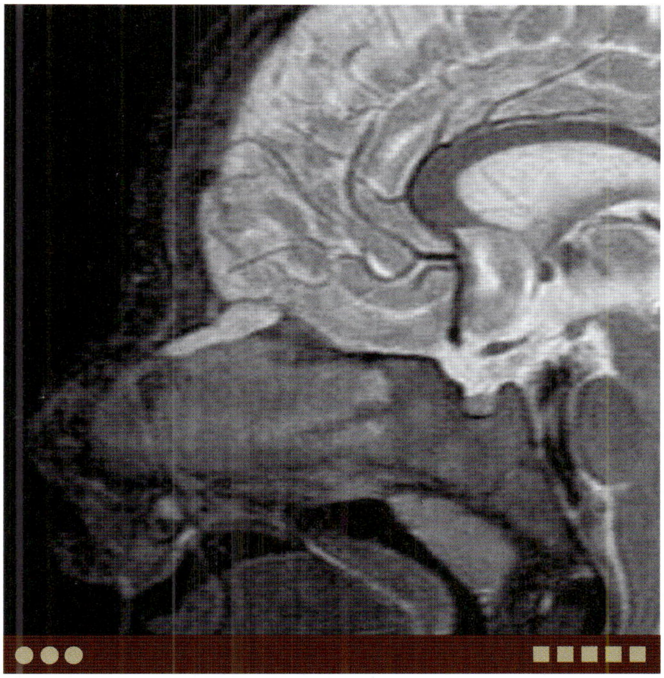

C. Nasal dermoid, same patient as A. Sagittal fat-suppressed T2W image demonstrates a high-signal tubular midline mass along the dorsum of the nasal bridge through an enlarged foramen cecum with intracranial extension and attachment to the dura.

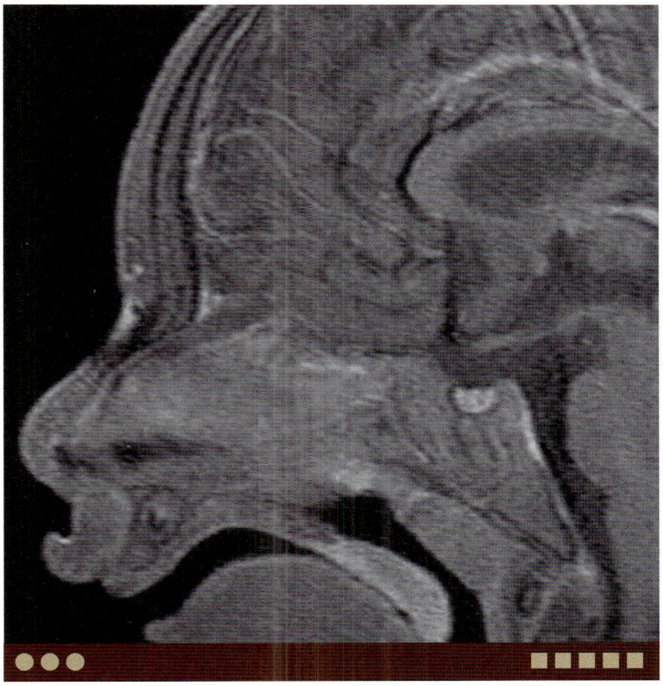

D. Nasal dermoid, same patient as A. Sagittal postcontrast T1W image demonstrates nonenhancement of the lesion.

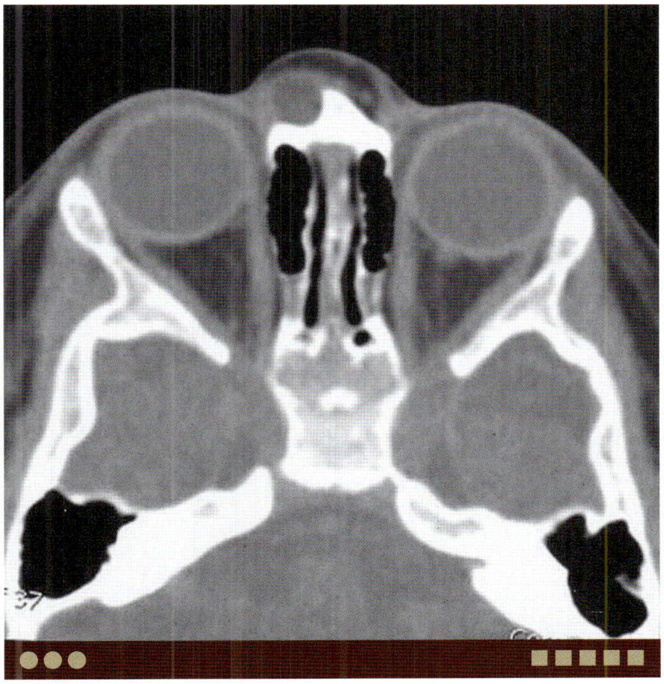

E. **Nasal dermoid** in a different patient. Axial CT demonstrates an off-midline cystic lesion at the right nasal bone.

DIFFERENTIAL DIAGNOSIS IMAGES (G-I)

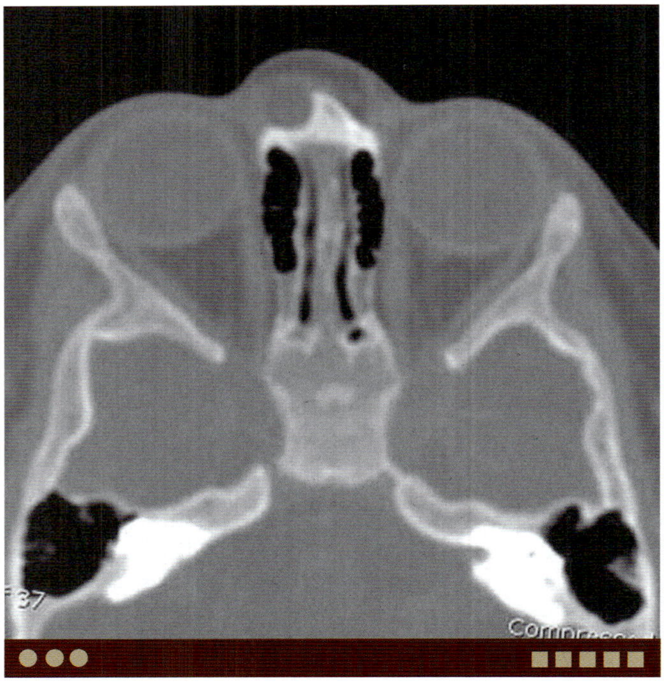

F. Nasal dermoid, same patient as E. Axial bone window CT demonstrates a cystic lesion eroding the nasal bone.

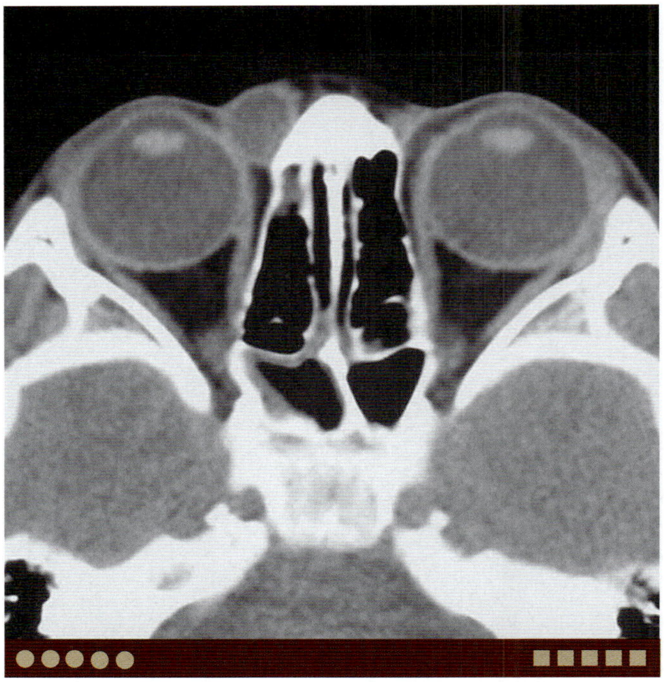

G. Orbital dermoid cyst. Axial CT demonstrates a water density cystic lesion in the medial portion of the right orbit.

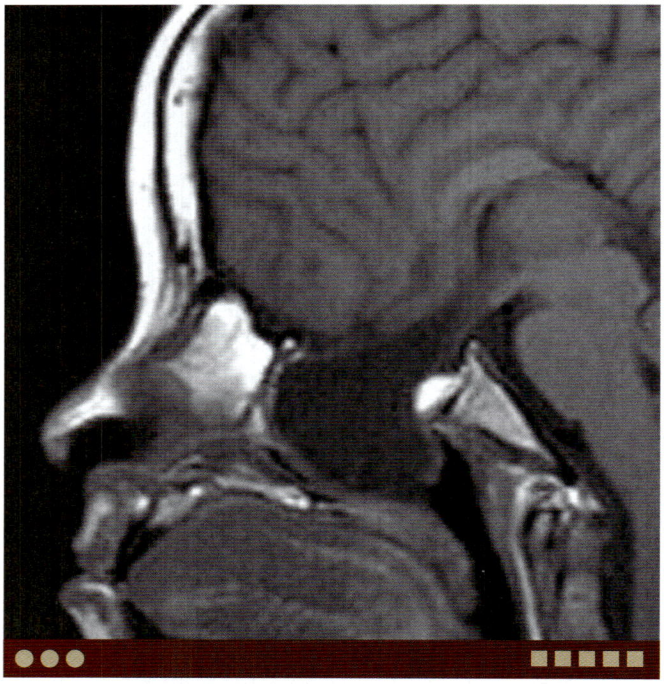

H. Cephalocele. Sagittal T1W image demonstrates a large trans-ethmoid meningocele.

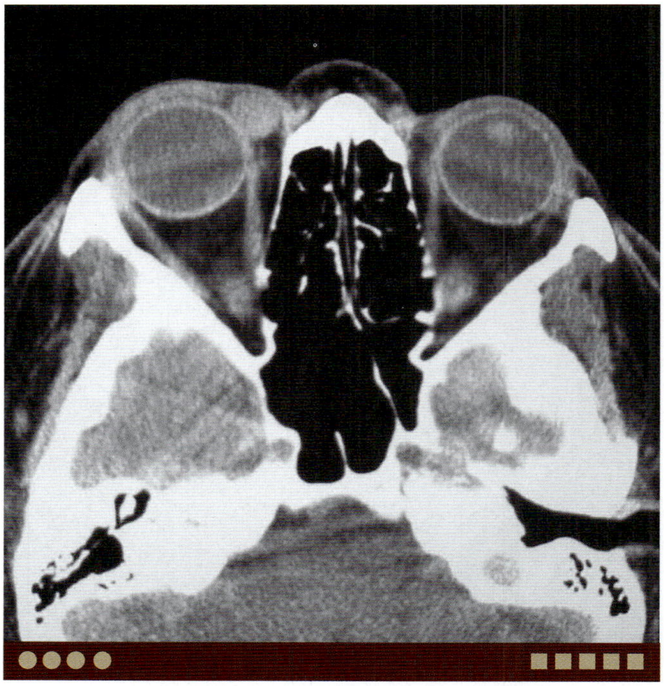

I. Moll's gland cyst. Axial CT demonstrates a slightly high-density cystic lesion in the medial portion of the right upper eyelid.

Case 3–38 Zygomaticomaxillary Complex Fracture

Carlos Gonzalez, Osamu Sakai

PRESENTATION

Facial pain and swelling

FINDINGS

CT demonstrates fractures through three main structures: (1) the frontozygomatic suture, (2) the maxillary process of the zygoma including the orbital floor, inferior orbital rim, and lateral wall of the maxillary sinus, and (3) the zygomatic arch.

DIFFERENTIAL DIAGNOSIS

- Fractures of the midface (Le Fort Fractures): These are of three types and differ in location of the fracture plane across the face. The fracture planes of Le Fort I, II, and III fractures are through the maxillary sinuses, the medial orbital and lateral maxillary walls, and through the orbits, respectively. These are all bilateral processes.
- Orbital floor blow-out fracture: Result from a direct blow to the eye. The sudden increase in intraorbital pressure leads to a comminuted fracture of the orbital floor, with herniation of orbital contents into the maxillary sinus. The orbital rim remains intact in this type of fracture.
- Nasoethmoidal complex fractures: Result from direct blow to the midface between the eyes. This term groups a wide variety of different fractures which may include the inferior, medial and supraorbital rims, orbital roof, ethmoid or frontal sinuses, sphenoid bone, nasal bone, and/or frontal process of maxilla. The zygomatic arch remains intact in this type of fractures.

COMMENTS

This is a 26-year-old man status post assault with facial pain and swelling, especially in the cheek and eyelid.

Zygomaticomaxillary complex (ZMC) fractures, also known as "tripod or quadripod" fractures, result from a direct blow to the malar eminence, body of zygoma. Knowledge of the anatomy is crucial for understanding the possible clinical findings which may be associated with this fracture. The zygoma articulates with the frontal, sphenoid, maxillary and temporal bones. Hence, it plays a key role in the structure, function, and aesthetic appearance of the facial skeleton. It also has a role in vision and mastication.

On CT, fractures are somewhat variable, but typically involve the frontozygomatic suture, the zygomatic arch, inferior orbital rim, orbital floor, lateral wall of the maxillary sinus, and lateral wall of the orbit. Many of these fractures can be also seen on plain films. Associated findings on plain films include opacification of the ipsilateral maxillary sinus and posterior displacement of the body of the zygoma, best visualized on the submental vertex view.

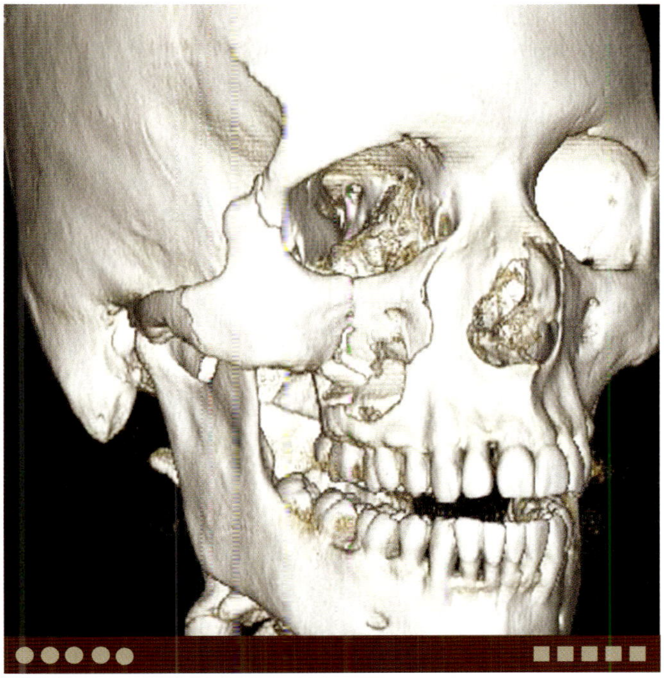

A. ZMC fractures. Volume rendered 3D CT image demonstrates fractures involving the right frontozygomatic suture, zygomatic arch, and inferior orbital rim.

Paresthesia of the cheek results from injury to the infraorbital nerve secondary to fracture of the inferiorbital rim at the infraorbital foramen. Limitation of jaw movement and flattening of the cheek are secondary to depressed fractures of the zygomatic process of the temporal bone or zygomatic arch. Unilateral epistaxis is a result of fractures of the zygomatic process of the maxilla or the floor of the orbit. Unequal pupil height and decreased extraocular muscle function with diplopia are caused secondary to fractures of the orbital or of the zygoma, frontal process of the zygoma or orbital floor.

The differential diagnoses include fractures of the midface, orbital floor blow-out fractures and nasoethmoidal complex fractures.

PEARLS

- **Zygomaticomaxillary complex plays an important role in the structure, function and aesthetic appearance of the facial skeleton, as well as in vision and mastication.**
- **The zygoma is one of the most common sites of injury involved when facial trauma occurs.**
- **A zygomaticomaxillary complex fracture should be suspected whenever there is trauma to the malar eminence. It typically involves the frontozygomatic suture, zygomatic arch, inferior orbital rim, orbital floor, lateral wall of maxillary sinus, and lateral wall of the orbit.**

ADDITIONAL IMAGES (B-E)

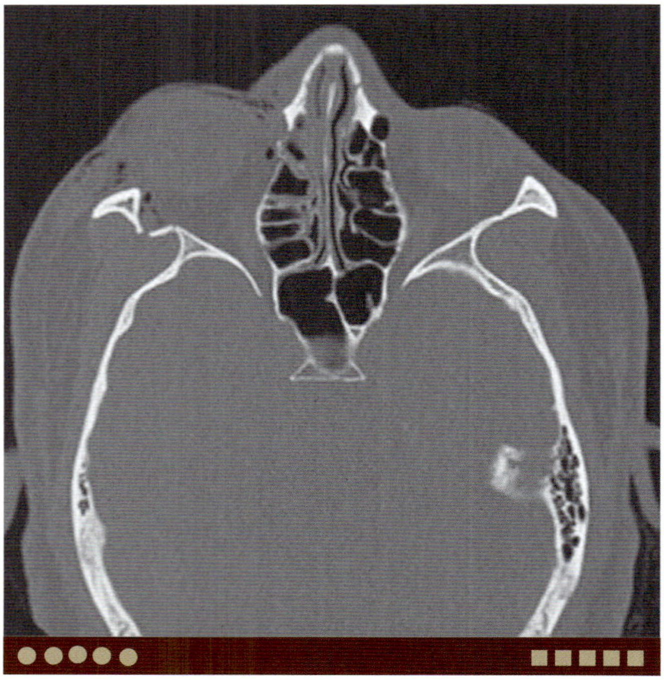

B. ZMC fractures, same patient as A. Axial CT image demonstrates a fracture through the right lateral orbital wall.

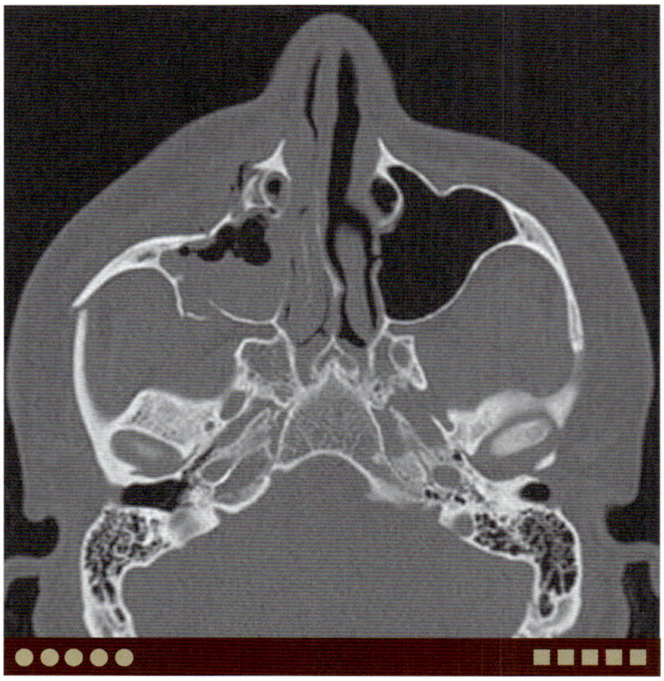

C. ZMC fractures, same patient as A. Axial CT image demonstrates fractures through the right zygomatic arch, as well as the anterior and posterolateral walls of the right maxillary sinus. Note involvement of right nasolacrimal duct (not part of the ZMC fracture).

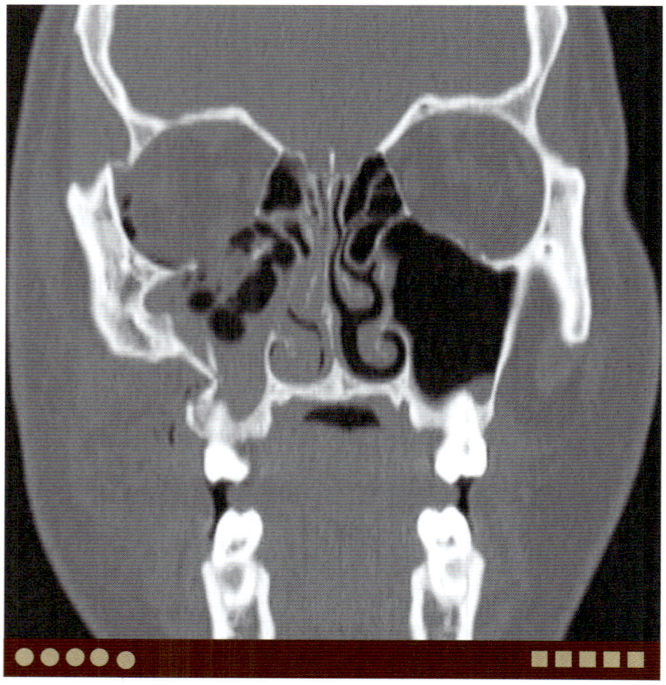

D. ZMC fractures, same patient as A. Coronal CT image demonstrates fractures through the right lateral and inferior orbital walls, as well as the lateral wall of the right maxillary sinus.

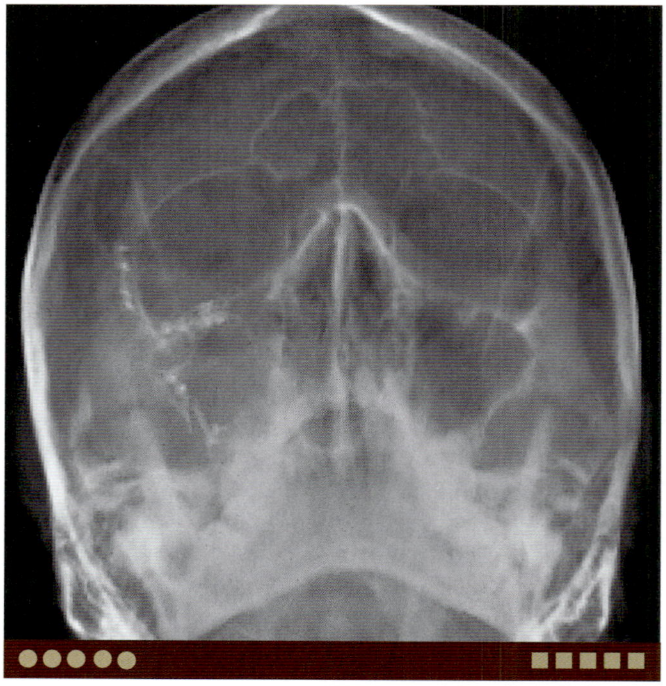

E. ZMC fractures, same patient as A. Waters view after surgery demonstrates three metallic plates fixing the fracture fragments.

DIFFERENTIAL DIAGNOSIS IMAGES (F-H)

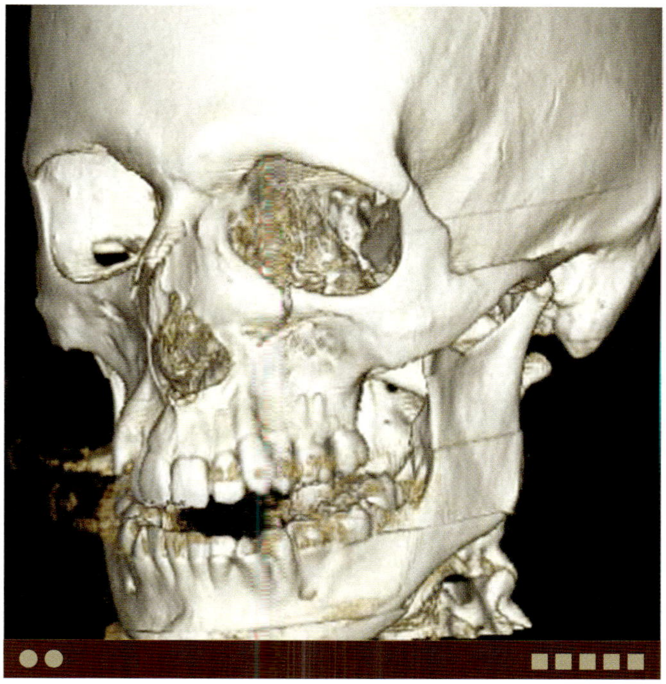

F. **Medial maxillary fracture**. Volume rendered 3D CT image demonstrates fractures involving the medial portion of the left maxillary sinus, preserving the frontozygomatic suture and zygomatic arch.

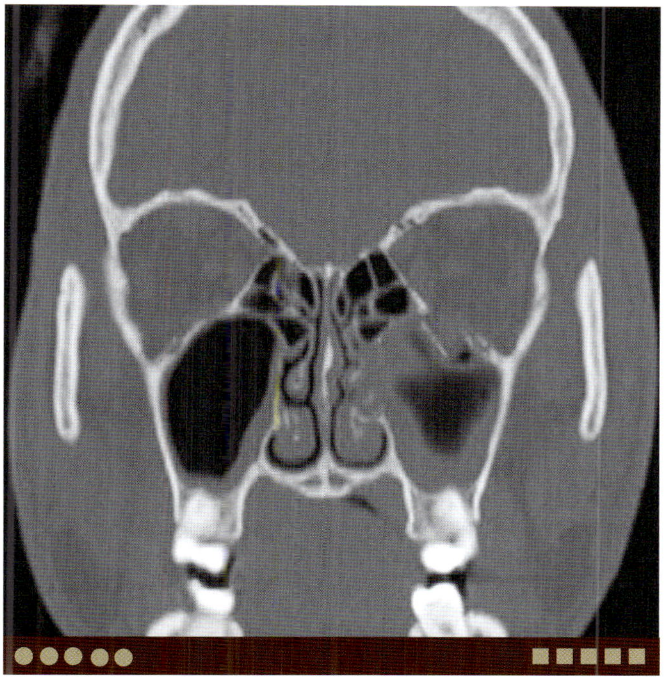

G. **Blow-out fracture**. Coronal CT demonstrates a fracture of the left orbital floor and inferior displacement of the fracture fragment.

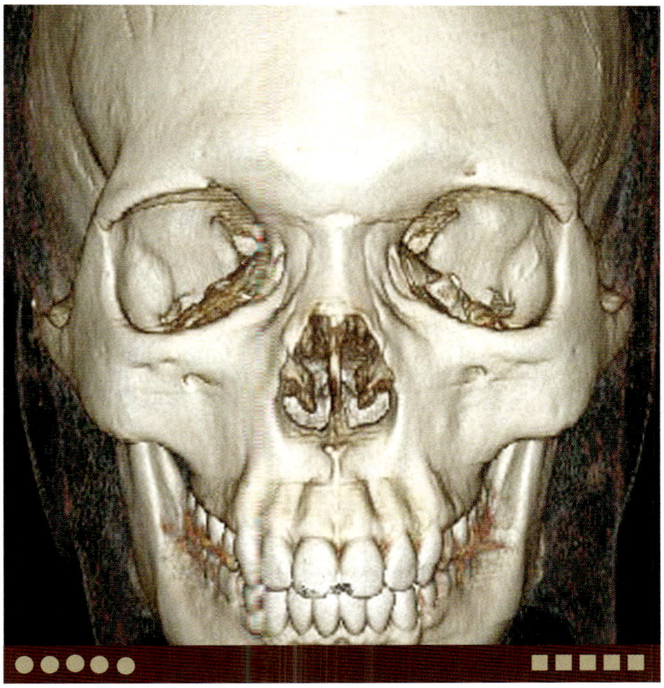

H. Blow-out fracture, same patient as G. Volume rendered 3D CT image demonstrates preservation of the left orbital rim.

Case 3–39 Pott's Puffy Tumor

Benjamin Ludwig, Osamu Sakai

PRESENTATION

Enlarging forehead mass.

FINDINGS

Sinus opacification with associated osseous destruction and subperiosteal collection.

DIFFERENTIAL DIAGNOSIS

- Mucocele: Mucocele is an obstructed sinus or air cell with bone remodeling/expansion, often seen in the frontal and ethmoid sinuses.
- Langerhans cell histiocytosis: This may present as an enhancing soft tissue mass with osseous erosion in its localized form, which commonly involves the skull.
- Dermoid/epidermoid: Subcutaneous lesions which commonly occur in midline and frontotemporal locations, often with skin ostia or sinus tracts.
- Cephalocele: Protrusion of intracranial tissue through a calvarial defect, which occurs in a similar location, especially the nasofrontal and frontoethmoidal subtypes. Usually swelling is present from birth, and nonprogressive.
- Cephalohematoma: This is most often results from birth trauma, with subperiosteal hematoma. Underlying osseous erosion and periosteal reaction are also characteristic.

COMMENTS

This is a 65-year-old woman with an enlarging forehead mass.

Pott's puffy tumor refers to a subperiosteal abscess associated with frontal bone osteomyelitis, and is most commonly secondary to frontal or ethmoid sinusitis. Sinus infection spreads via valveless veins, with subsequent osteomyelitis and subperiosteal abscess formation. The incidence has decreased with antibiotic treatment of sinusitis, however may result from untreated or incompletely treated sinus disease.

Spread of infection via emissary veins, which communicate between the frontal and dural sinuses, results in intracranial complications, including subdural or epidural empyema, cavernous sinus thrombosis, meningitis, or cerebral abscess.

Patients present with symptoms of sinusitis as well as an enlarging, fluctuant bump overlying the brow, which is "doughy" in consistency.

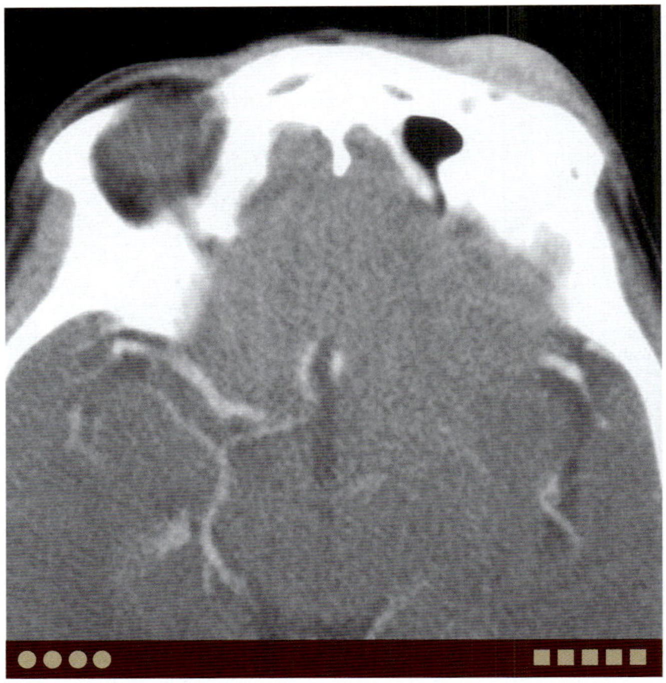

A. Pott's puffy tumor. Axial CT images demonstrate soft tissue swelling with heterogeneous enhancement in the left forehead.

Imaging findings on CT and MRI include sinus opacification, osteomyelitis with osseous destruction/fistula formation of the frontal bone, a frontal subgaleal fluid collection, and soft tissue swelling. MRI is more sensitive for intracranial complications including meningeal enhancement, epidural or subdural abscess, cerebritis, and cavernous sinus thrombosis.

Treatment includes surgical drainage, debridement of necrotic bone, and long-term intravenous antibiotics.

PEARLS

- **Pott's puffy tumor presents as a progressively enlarging, fluctuant, "doughy" mass overlying the brow.**
- **Pott's puffy tumor most commonly results from frontal sinusitis with frontal bone osteomyelitis and subperiosteal abscess.**
- **Intracranial complications include extra-axial empyema, meningitis, cavernous sinus thrombisis, and parenchymal abscess.**

ADDITIONAL IMAGES (3-H)

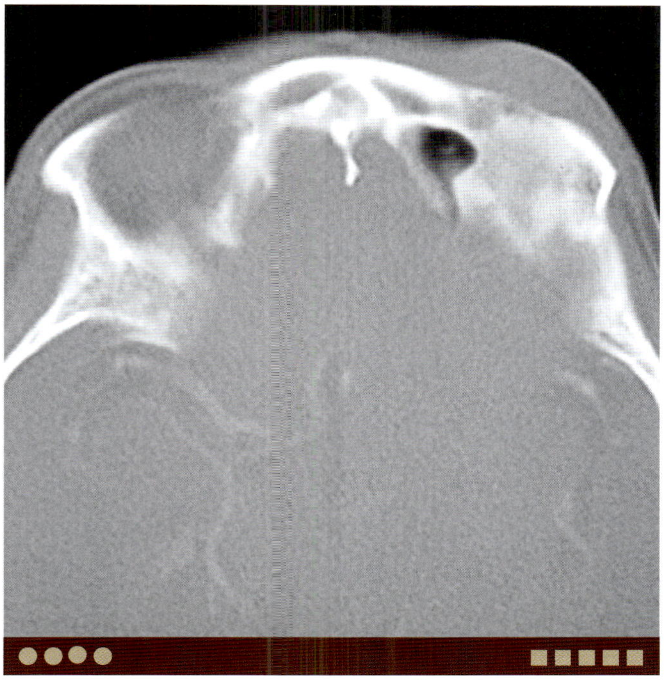

B. Pott's puffy tumor, same patient as A. Axial bone window CT demonstrates opacified frontal sinuses and focal osteolytic change.

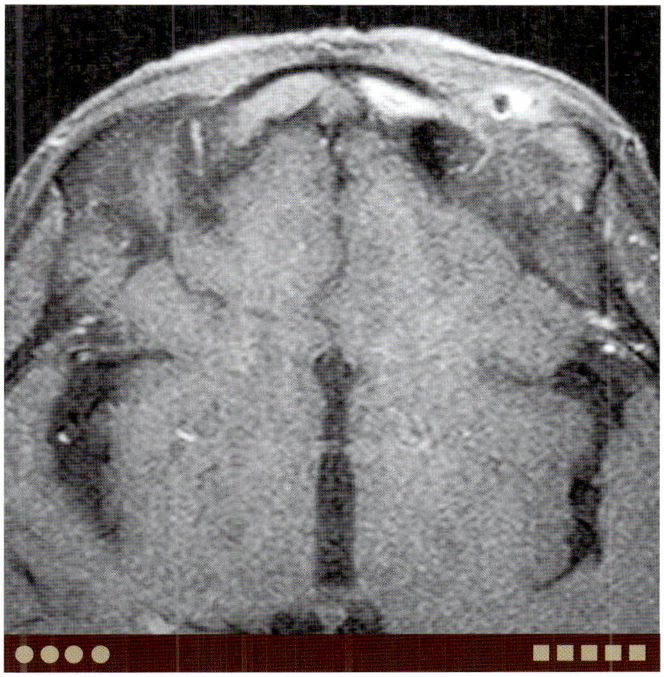

C. Pott's puffy tumor, same patient as A. Axial postcontrast fat-suppressed T1W image demonstrates opacified and enhancing left frontal sinus and a small rim-enhancing extraosseous collection with phlegmon. Note loss of normal signal-void of the bone cortex.

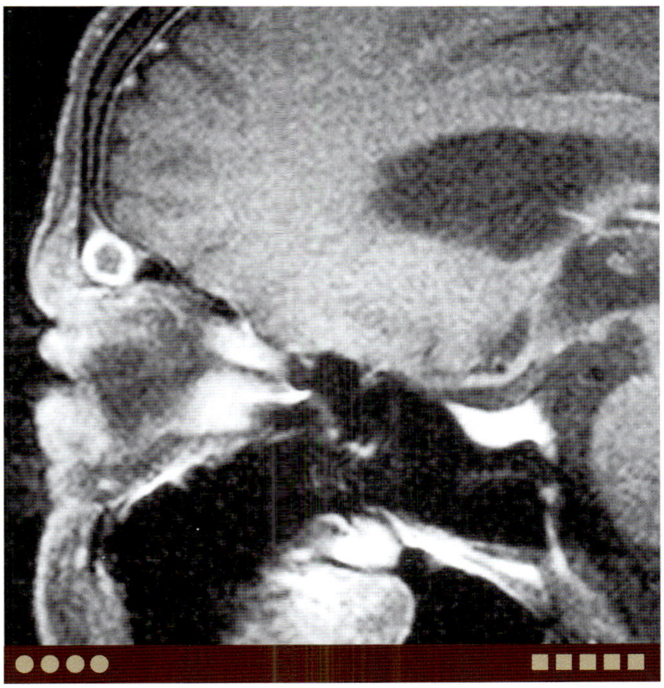

D. Pott's puffy tumor, same patient as A. Coronal postcontrast fat-suppressed T1W image demonstrates opacified and enhancing frontal sinus and phlegmon in the superficial soft tissue.

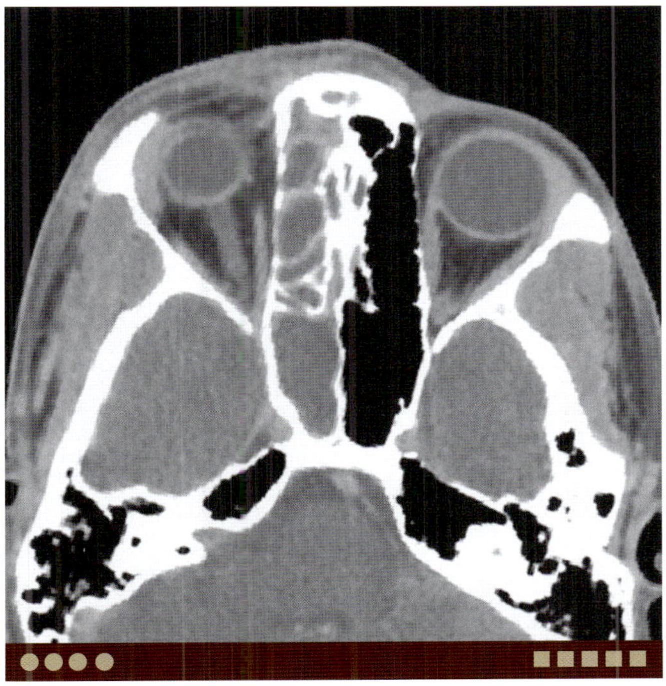

E. Pott's puffy tumor in a different patient. Axial postcontrast CT demonstrates ethmoid air cell opacification and right periorbital soft tissue swelling.

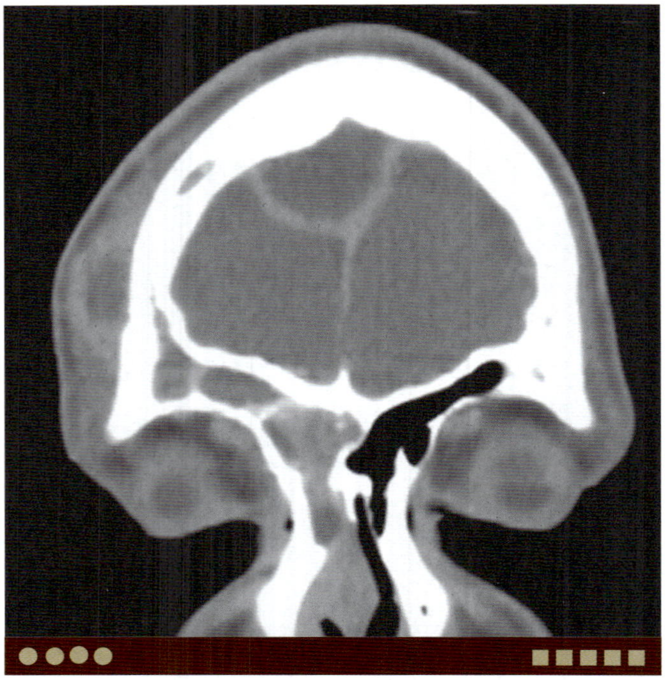

F. Pott's puffy tumor, same patient as E. Coronal postcontrast CT demonstrates opacification of the right frontal sinus with subgaleal abscess. Note epidural empyema.

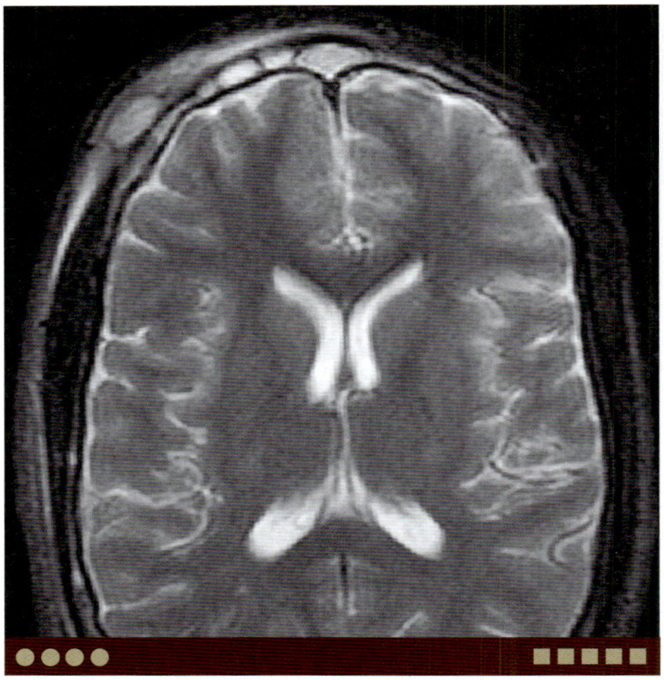

G. Pott's puffy tumor, same patient as E. Axial fat-suppressed T2W image demonstrates frontal sinus opacification and increased signal in the frontal bone marrow (osteomyelitis) as well as extracranial collection with phlegmon.

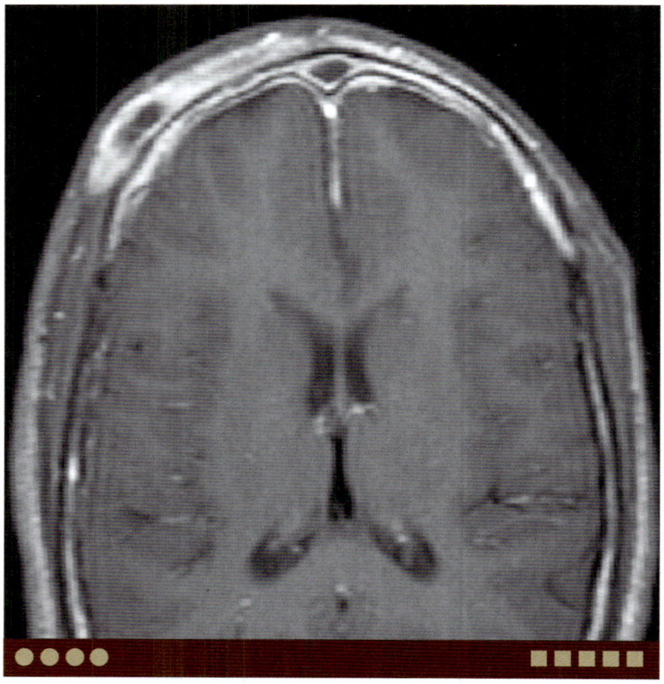

H. Pott's puffy tumor, same patient as E. Axial postcontrast T1W image demonstrates abnormal enhancement of the frontal bone marrow and dura, as well as soft tissue around the extracranial collection.

DIFFERENTIAL DIAGNOSIS IMAGE

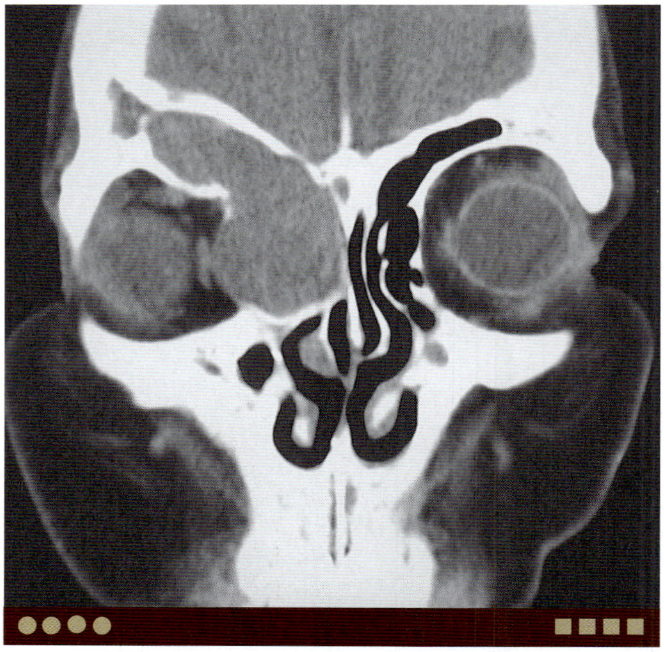

I. Mucocele. Coronal soft tissue windowed CT demonstrates obstructed right frontal sinus with bone remodeling. The increased density within the lesion compared with the left globe is suggestive of increased protein concentration.

Case 3–40 Chronic Sinusitis

Osamu Sakai, Rohini Nadgir

PRESENTATION

Episodes of recurrent sinusitis.

FINDINGS

CT demonstrates various degrees of mucosal thickening with sclerosis and thickening of the sinus wall.

DIFFERENTIAL DIAGNOSIS

- Acute sinusitis: The diagnosis should be made clinically, not radiologically. There is no specific sign for acute sinusitis, although presence of air-fluid levels is suggestive of acute infection/inflammation.
- Sinus mycetoma: Usually involves unilateral maxillary sinus. Patients are usually immunocompetent, and clinical presentation of sinus mycetoma is similar to that of usual sinusitis.
- Wegener's granulomatosis: This condition demonstrates nonspecific inflammatory changes in the sinonasal cavities, however often aggressive findings such as nasal septal perforation and orbital involvement are seen. Intracranial extension of the disease occurs occasionally.
- Squamous cell carcinoma (SCCA): This often shows bone destruction and heterogeneously enhancing soft tissue mass if intravenous contrast is given. SCCA should be considered when total sinus opacification is seen on one side.
- Lymphoma: Large, non-necrotic mass is a common finding. Among extranodal lymphoma in the head and neck, 40% to 50% occurs in the sinonasal cavity, commonly in the nasal cavity and maxillary sinus.

COMMENTS

This is a 45-year-old man with nasal congestion.

Sinusitis is a clinical diagnosis, not a radiological diagnosis. Precise history and physical examination is the key to making this diagnosis. In patients with sinusitis, variable degrees of mucosal thickening are seen on CT and MRI, however, imaging findings are nonspecific, and it is often difficult to determine whether or not acute or chronic inflammation is present. Air-fluid level can strongly suggest acute inflammation/infection, although this finding is not specific. With chronic sinusitis, osseous changes such as sclerosis, thickening as well as volume loss of the sinus are seen, often associated with mucosal thickening and polypoid lesions in the nasal cavity. The retained secretions within sinuses show variable density on CT and signal on MRI depending on its proteinaceous content.

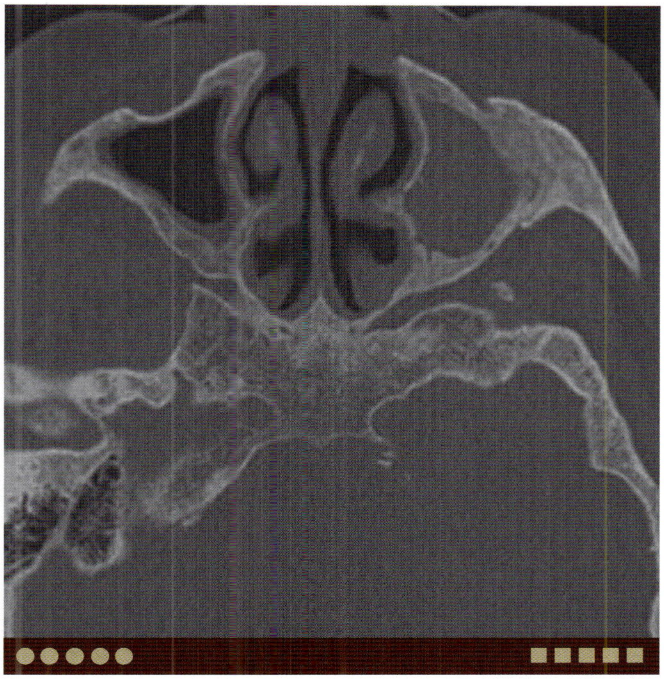

A. Chronic sinusitis. Axial CT demonstrates sclerosis and thickening of the maxillary sinus walls bilaterally with complete opacification of the left maxillary sinus.

The purpose of imaging is usually not to make the diagnosis but to provide detailed anatomy for surgical planning. Further, it is very important not to miss underlying tumors or other causes of sinus symptoms. A complete evaluation includes an assessment of teeth/teeth roots, retroantral fat pad, pterygopalatine fossa and osseous canals and foramina to look for possible perineural spread.

PEARLS

- **Sinusitis is a clinical diagnosis. Imaging findings are often nonspecific.**
- **Chronic sinusitis often shows variable degrees of mucosal and osseous changes such as sclerosis, thickening as well as volume loss of the sinuses.**
- **Careful observation of the fat pad, canal, and foramina is important not to miss other causes of sinus symptoms.**

ADDITIONAL IMAGES (B-G)

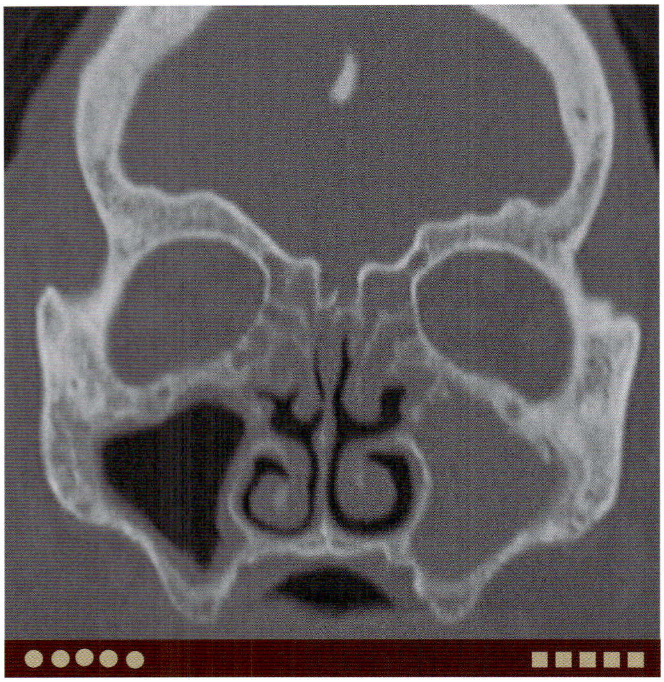

B. Chronic sinusitis, same patient as A. Coronal CT demonstrates sclerosis and thickening of the bilateral maxillary sinus walls with complete opacification of the left maxillary sinus. Ethmoid air cells are opacified and show sclerotic changes.

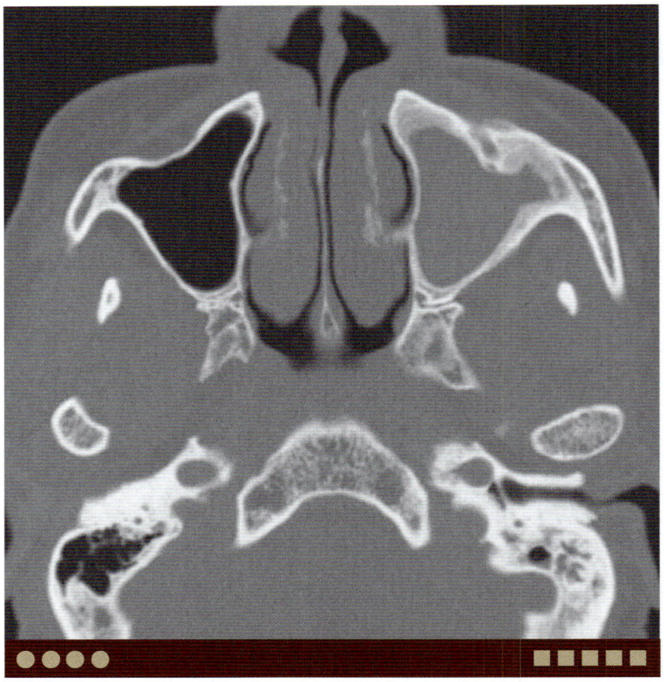

C. Chronic sinusitis, mycetoma. Axial CT demonstrates complete opacification of the left maxillary sinus, with sclerosis of the sinus wall.

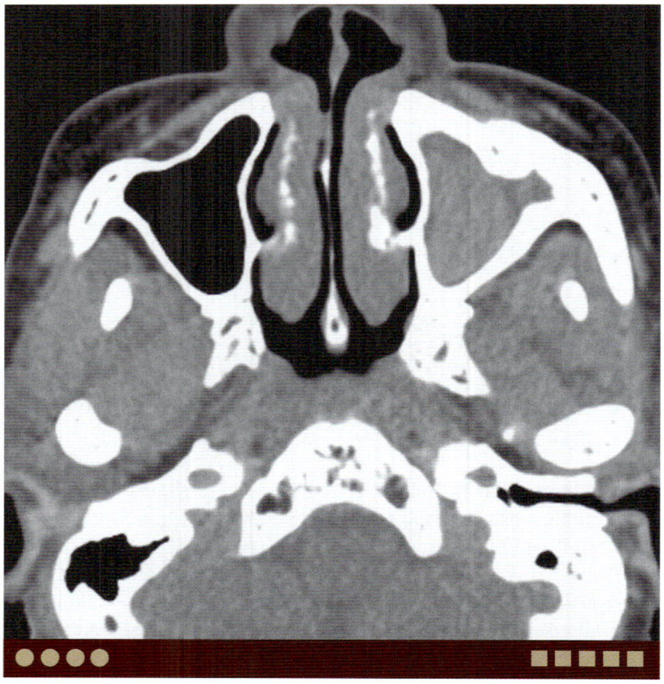

D. Chronic sinusitis, mycetoma, same patient as C. Axial CT with soft tissue window demonstrates increased density of the opacified left maxillary sinus.

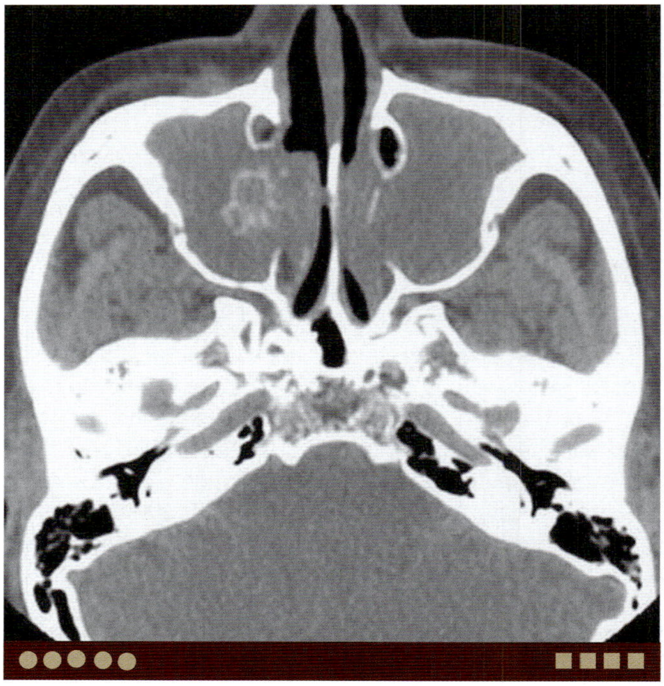

E. Chronic sinusitis in a different patient. Axial CT with soft tissue window demonstrates opacification of the bilateral maxillary sinuses. Calcification is seen in the right maxillary sinus.

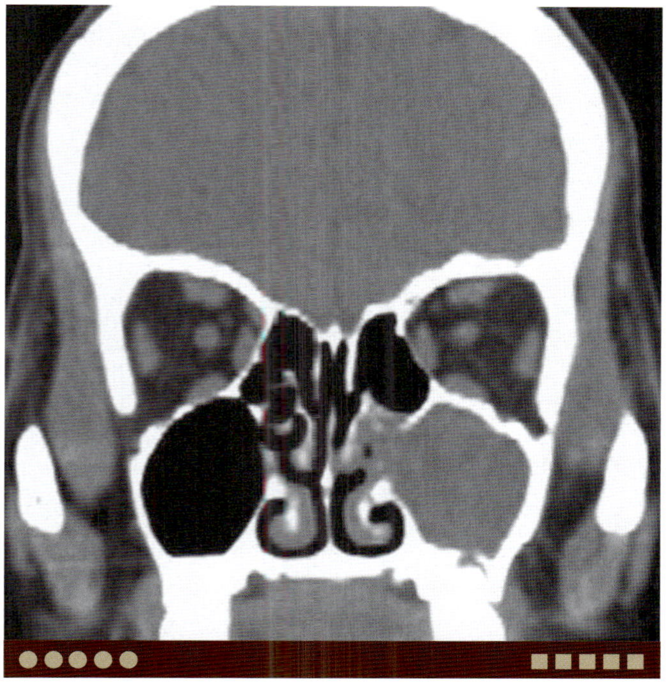

F. Chronic sinusitis, secondary to odontogenic infection. Coronal CT with soft tissue window demonstrates opacified left maxillary sinus.

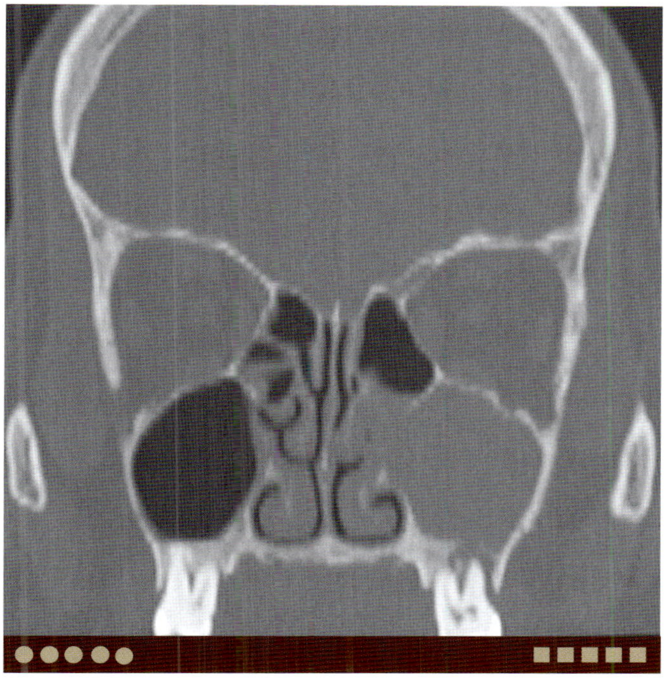

G. Chronic sinusitis, secondary to odontogenic infection, same patient as F. Coronal CT with bone window demonstrates periapical lucency with a focal defect of the floor of the maxillary sinus.

DIFFERENTIAL DIAGNOSIS IMAGES (H-J)

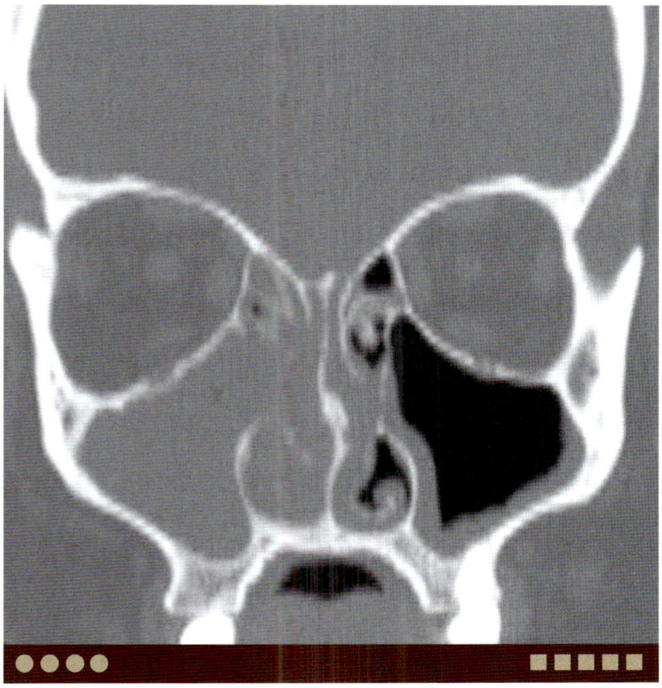

H. Wegener's granulomatosis. Coronal CT demonstrates opacified right maxillary sinus and ethmoid air cells and nasal cavity. Mild mucosal thickening is also seen in the left maxillary sinus, a nonspecific finding.

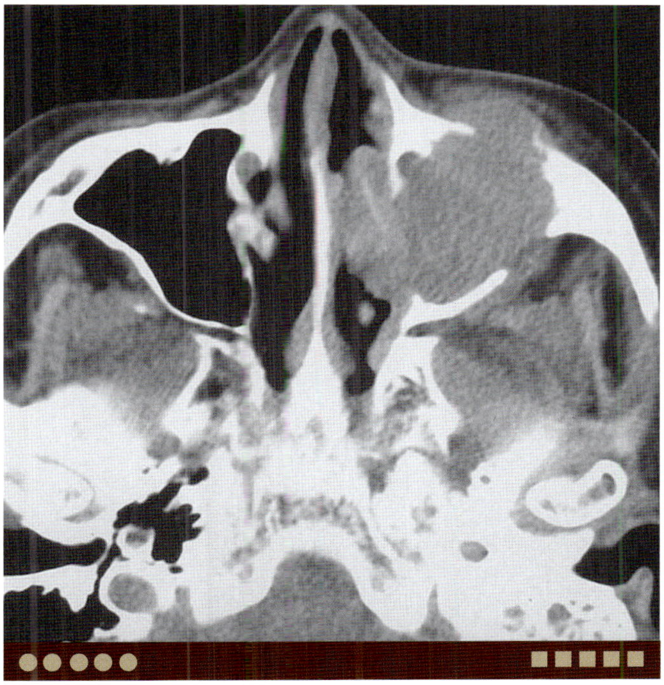

I. SCCA. Axial CT demonstrates a large tumor destroying the anterior, medial, and posterolateral walls of the left maxillary sinus.

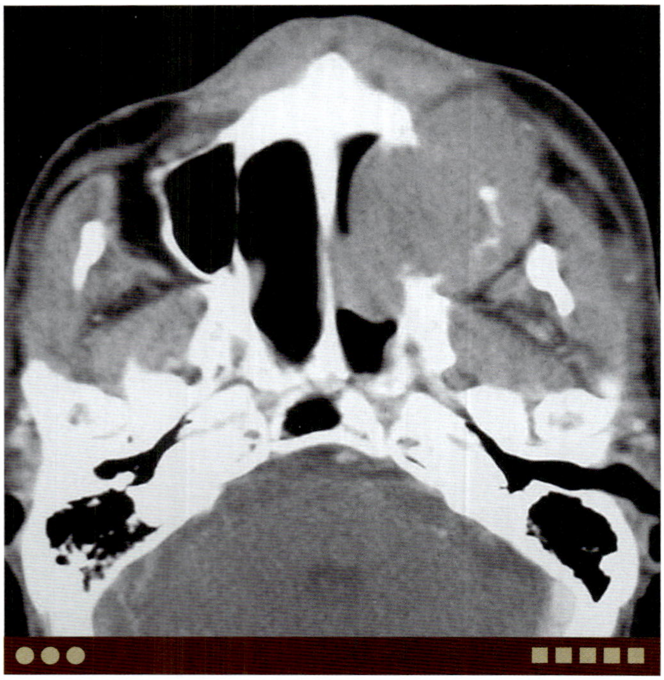

J. Lymphoma. Axial postcontrast CT demonstrates a large homogenous density tumor extending beyond the anterior and posterolateral walls of the left maxillary sinus. No necrosis is noted despite the large tumor size.

Case 3–41 Sinonasal Polyposis

Osamu Sakai, Rohini Nadgir

PRESENTATION

Nasal obstruction. Anosmia.

FINDINGS

CT demonstrates opacified sinuses with multiple polypoid lesions in the nasal cavity.

DIFFERENTIAL DIAGNOSIS

- Antrochoanal polyp: Polyp originating within the maxillary sinus and extending into the nasal cavity and choana, usually unilaterally.
- Inverted papilloma: Soft tissue mass arising from the lateral wall of the nasal cavity and extending into the maxillary sinus. The density is usually heterogeneously increased, often with calcification.
- Cephalocele: This anomaly has extension of dura and brain parenchyma through a bone defect in the cribriform plate or frontal bone. Sometimes the bone defect is not apparent.
- Chronic sinusitis: Heterogeneous density can be seen in the opacified sinuses with inspissated secretion and dystrophic calcifications. Sclerotic changes of the osseous walls and contraction of the affected sinus is often seen.

COMMENTS

This is a 47-year-old man with history of chronic sinusitis and anosmia.

Nasal polyps are the most common benign intranasal tumor. Patients often present with sinonasal obstruction, chronic sinusitis and anosmia. Patients with nasal polyps may also have asthma, aspirin intolerance and allergic aspergillosis. Nasal polyps are seen in patients of all ages, in about 2% of the population. Nasal polyps are relatively rare in children. When nasal polyps are seen in children, possibility of cystic fibrosis should be considered.

The diagnosis of polyposis is easily made clinically but CT is very helpful to evaluate extent of disease and for surgical planning and image guided procedures. Any significant normal variants, such as asymmetry in the cribriform plate, bone dehiscence of lamina papyracea, and onodi cells, should be documented in the radiological report to avoid surgical complication.

CT commonly demonstrates diffusely opacified paranasal sinuses with multiple polypoid lesions in the sinonasal cavities, which usually demonstrate relatively low density on CT, while obstructed, inspissated mucus demonstrates high density, particularly with fungal infection. With complete obstruction of the nasal cavities by polyps, expansion of the obstructed ethmoid air cells is often seen, which is called polypoid mucocele.

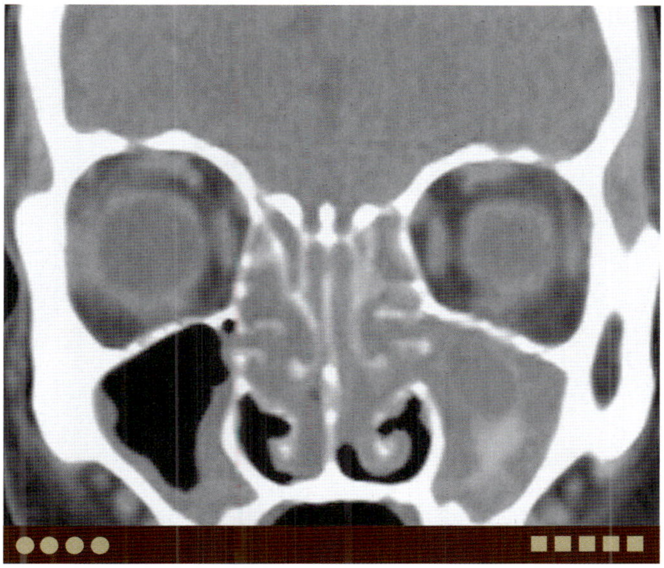

A. Sinonasal polyposis. Coronal CT demonstrates multiple polypoid lesions in the bilateral nasal cavities, ethmoid air cells and left maxillary sinus. Note high density inspissated secretion in the left maxillary sinus.

On MRI, polyps usually show intermediate to high signal on T2W images. Inspissated mucus demonstrates high density on CT, while on MRI, it shows very dark signal on T2W images due to the significant T2 shortening effect, particularly when there is fungal infection present. It is important to remember opacified sinuses may demonstrate no signal mimicking air, and this condition could be completely missed.

The differential diagnosis includes various sinonasal masses such as papillomas and squamous cell carcinoma. Neoplasms are usually unilateral and friable, and show spontaneous hemorrhage. Congenital and developmental abnormalities such as cephaloceles and dermoid cysts may present with features similar to nasal polyposis clinically.

PEARLS

- **Patients with nasal polyps may also have asthma, aspirin intolerance and allergic aspergillosis.**
- **In children, nasal polyps raise the possibility of cystic fibrosis.**
- **With complete obstruction of the nasal cavities, expansion of the obstructed ethmoid air cells is often seen.**

ADDITIONAL IMAGES (B-G)

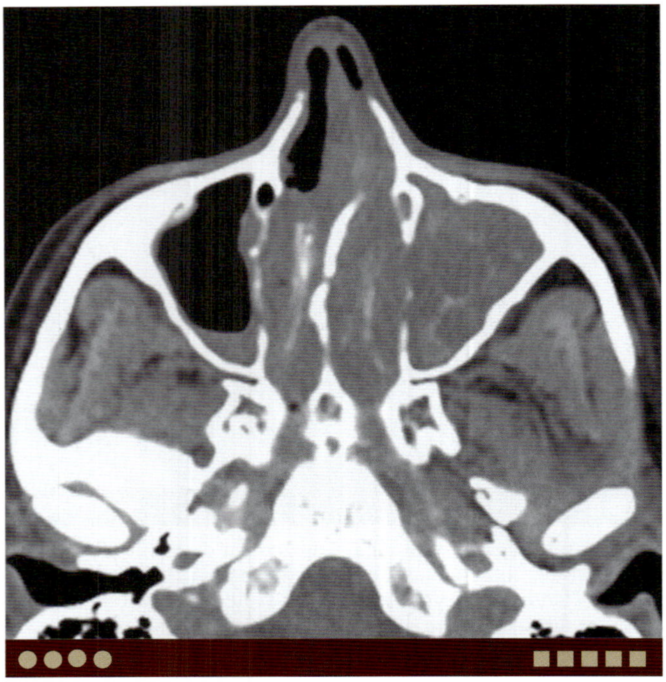

B. Sinonasal polyposis, same patient as A. Axial CT shows multiple polypoid lesions in the bilateral nasal cavities and left maxillary sinus.

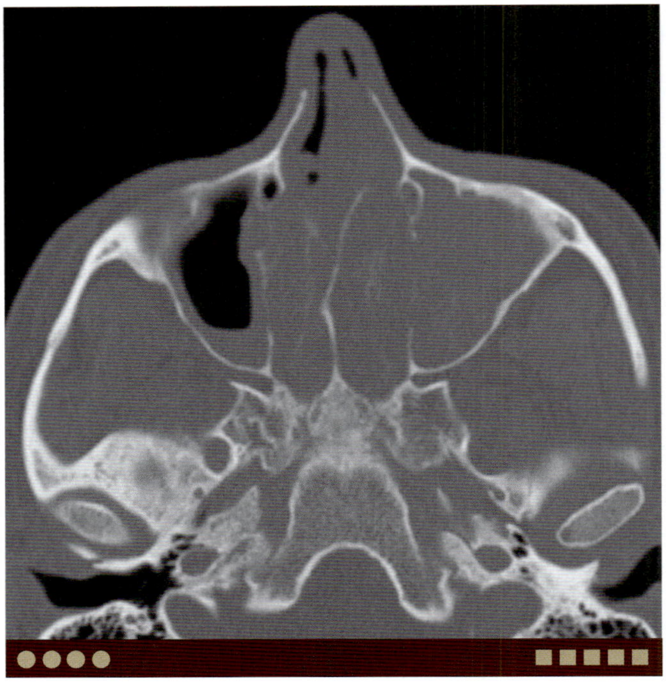

C. Sinonasal polyposis, same patient as A. Axial CT with bone window shows opacified nasal cavities and left maxillary sinus without bone destruction.

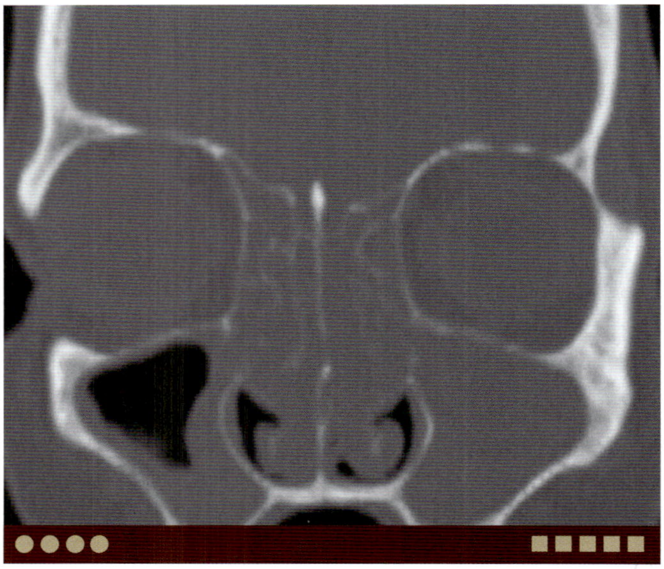

D. Sinonasal polyposis, same patient as A. Coronal CT with bone window shows opacified bilateral nasal cavities, ethmoid air cells and left maxillary sinus without bone destruction.

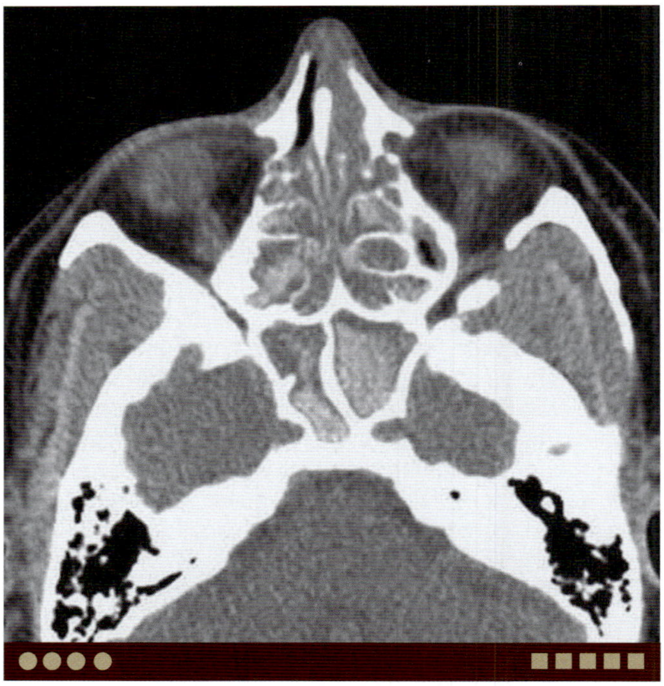

E. Sinonasal polyposis in a patient with asthma and allergic aspergillosis. Axial CT demonstrates high-density material within the ethmoid and sphenoid sinuses.

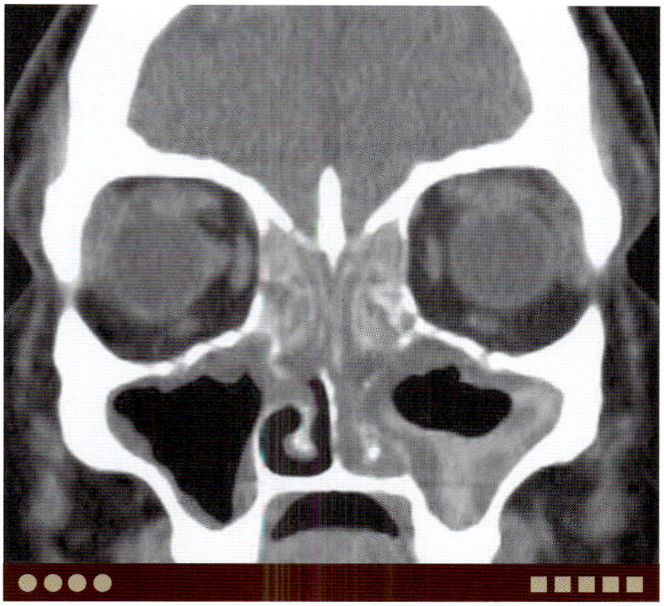

F. Sinonasal polyposis in a patient with asthma and allergic aspergillosis, same patient as E. Coronal CT shows polypoid lesions in the nasal cavities and high-density material within the ethmoid air cells and left maxillary sinus.

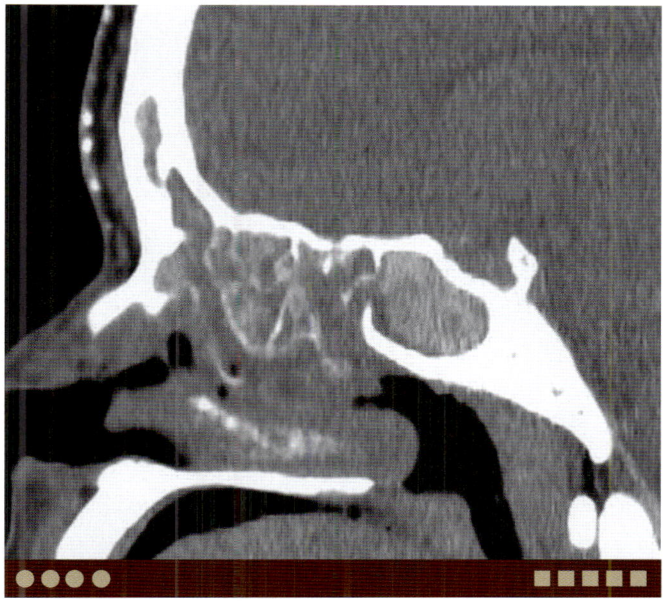

G. Sinonasal polyposis in a patient with asthma and allergic aspergillosis, same patient as E. Sagittal CT shows polypoid lesions in the ethmoid air cells and nasal cavity with high-density material. The sphenoid sinus is completely opacified with high-density material.

DIFFERENTIAL DIAGNOSIS IMAGES (H-J)

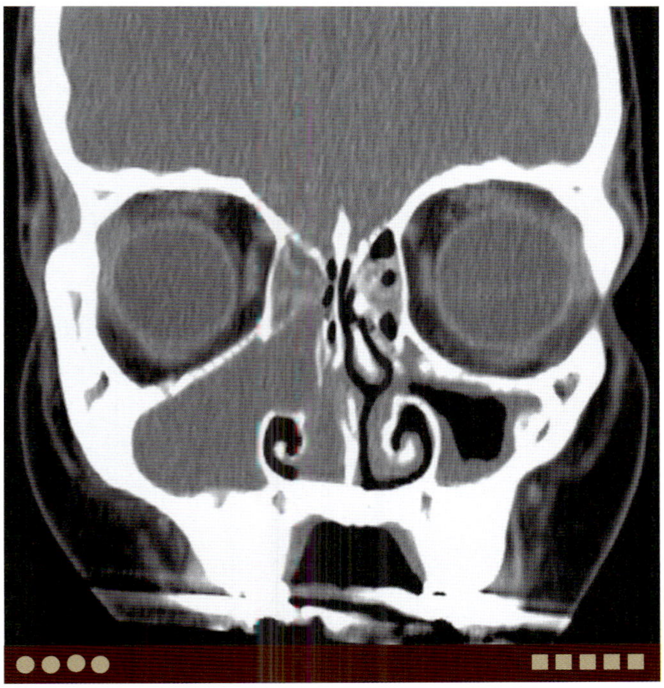

H. Antrochoanal polyp. Coronal CT demonstrates a polypoid lesion from the maxillary sinus with widening of the ostium and extension into the nasal cavity.

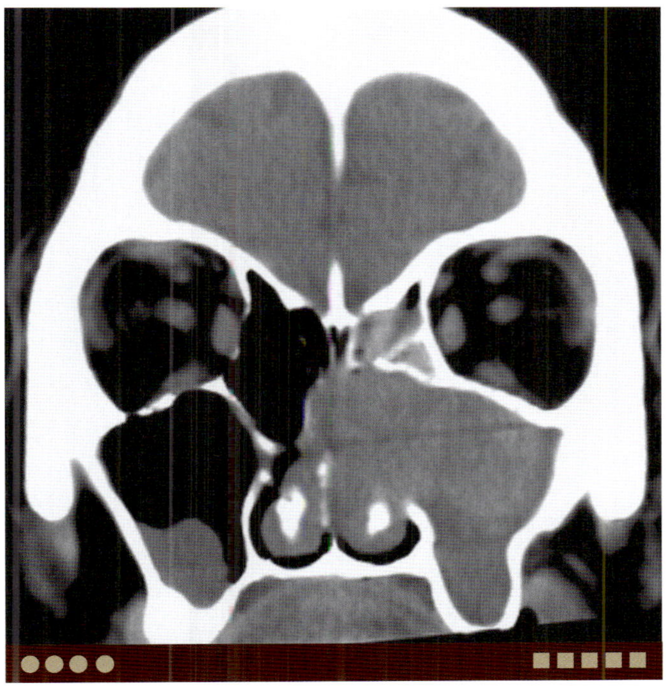

I. Inverted papilloma. Coronal CT demonstrates completely opacified left maxillary sinus with mild expansion. Note heterogeneous density in the sinus cavity.

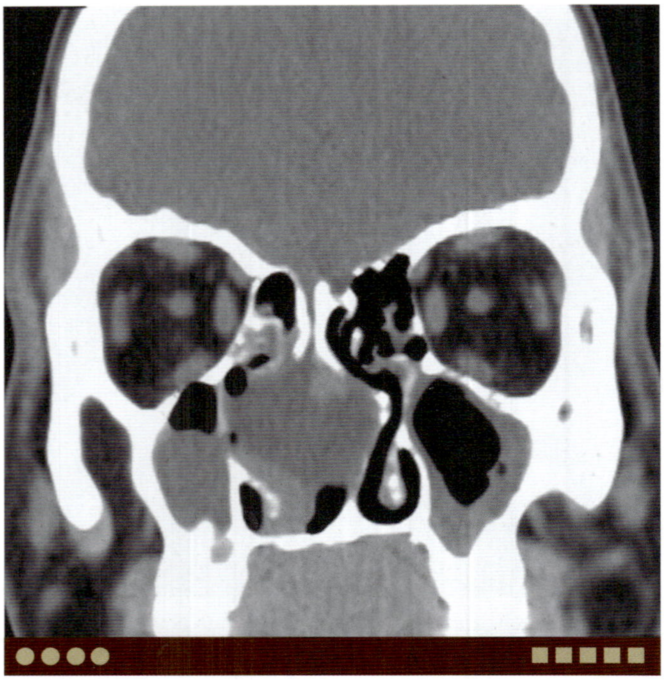

J. Cephalocele. Coronal CT demonstrates a heterogeneous, but mostly water density mass in the right nasal cavity, with bony remodeling.

Chapter 4

ORBIT

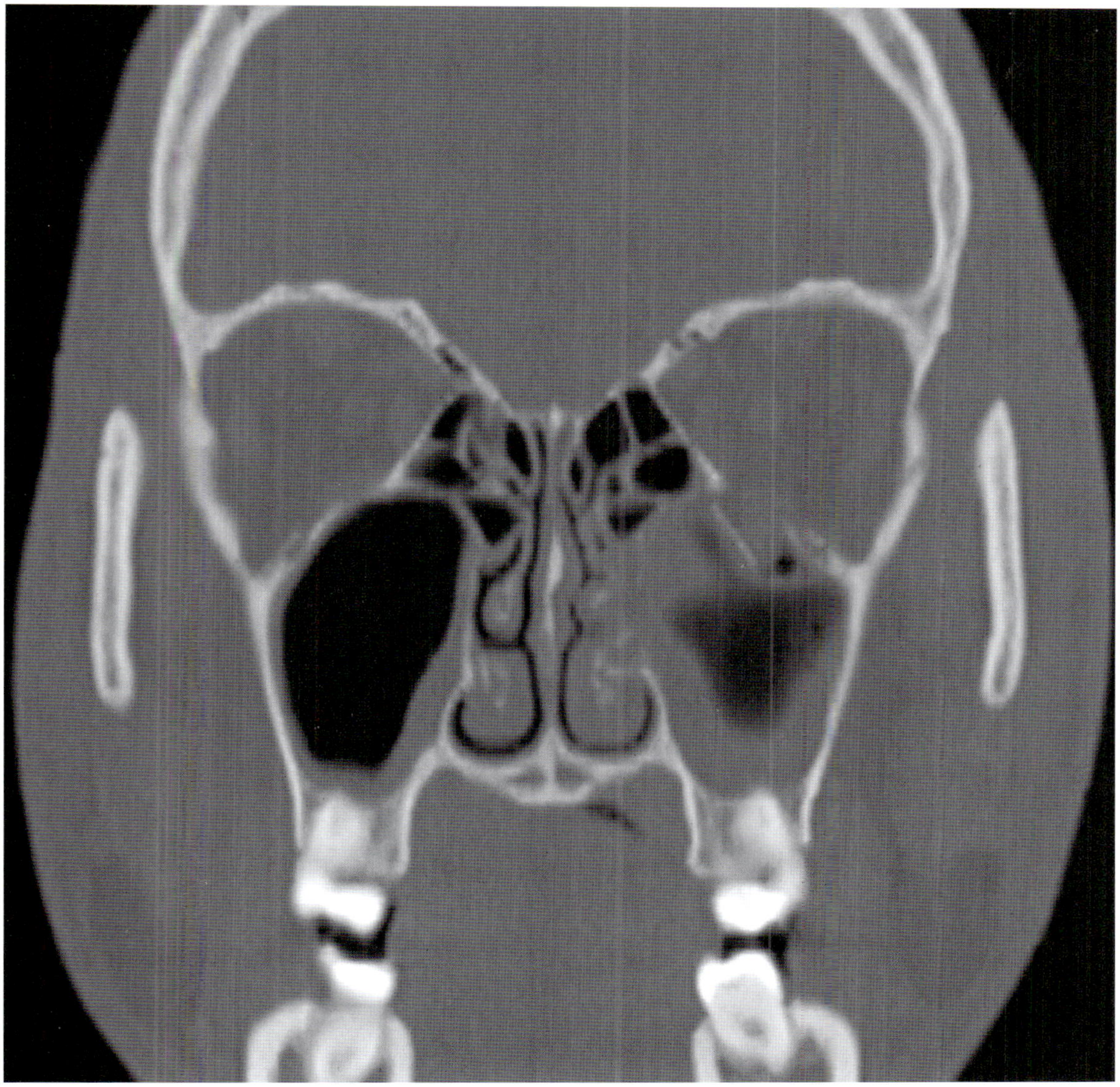

Case 4–1 Blow-Out Fracture

Osamu Sakai, Francisco Contreras

PRESENTATION

Punched in the eye.

FINDINGS

Coronal computed tomography (CT) demonstrates fracture of the floor of the orbit.

DIFFERENTIAL DIAGNOSIS

- Bony dehiscence of lamina papyracea: This can be seen without a history of trauma. Some investigators believe that this is a congenital anomaly; however, others think it is due to old trauma with unclear remembrance by the patient.

COMMENTS

This is a 20-year-old man after an assault.

Blow-out fractures are a disruption of the orbital wall secondary to increased intraorbital pressure, postulated to prevent globe rupture. By definition, the orbital rim must be preserved. Fractures are most commonly through the orbital floor, followed by those involving the medial wall/lamina papyracea. Intraorbital fat and extraocular muscles can be displaced or herniated into the maxillary sinus and/or the ethmoid air cells. Impingement of extraocular muscles causes restriction of eye movement and diplopia, which is an indication for surgery. The development of an optic nerve sheath hematoma is a true emergency requiring immediate decompression. Intraorbital air (orbital emphysema) is often seen with medial wall fractures. Extraocular muscle swelling from edema/hematoma is also a common finding. Blow-out fractures of the orbital roof are very rare.

CT is useful in evaluating fractures and soft tissue injuries. Coronal images are particularly useful to identify subtle floor fractures, which are often seen medial to the infraorbital groove. Medial wall/lamina papyracea fractures are seen in about 50% of patients with floor fractures. Impingement is usually diagnosed clinically, although occasionally, impinged muscle is identified on CT. Not all blow-out fractures require immediate surgery, however, emergent repair is indicated in patients with large bony defect, usually >2 cm^2 and extraocular muscle impingement.

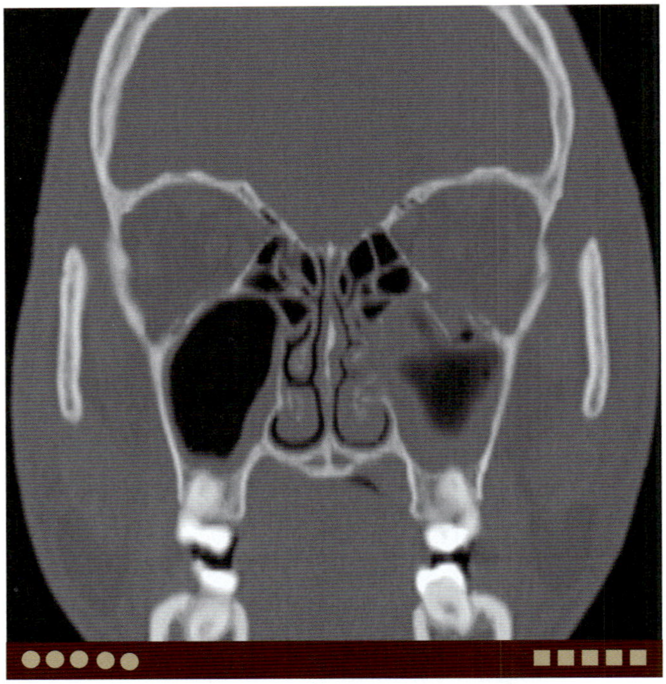

A. Blow-out fracture. Coronal CT demonstrates a fracture of the left orbital floor and inferior displacement of the fracture fragment. Mucosal thickening is present in the maxillary sinus.

Evaluation for other maxillofacial bone fractures and intracranial injury is critical for patient management. MRI is useful to evaluate for soft tissue injury and intracranial complications, although fractures are difficult to identify.

PEARLS

- **Blow-out fractures are most commonly seen in the medial aspect of the orbital floor, followed by those involving the medial wall/lamina papyracea. Medial wall fractures are seen in about 50% of patients with floor fractures.**
- **By definition, the orbital rim must be entirely preserved.**
- **Evaluation with bone and soft tissue windows is essential to look for intra- and extraorbital complications.**
- **Optic nerve sheath hematomas require emergent decompression.**

ADDITIONAL IMAGES (B-G)

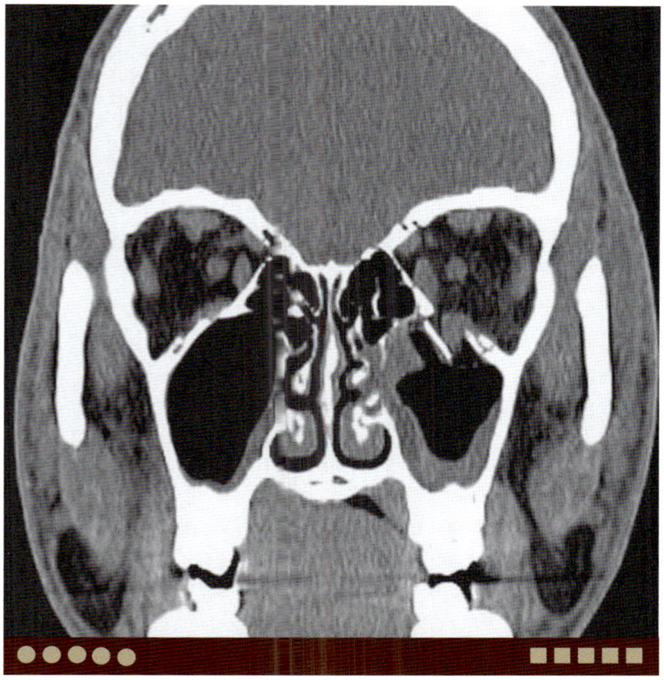

B. Blow-out fracture, same patient as A. Coronal CT in soft tissue window demonstrates distortion and partial herniation of the inferior rectus muscle into the maxillary sinus through the fracture defect.

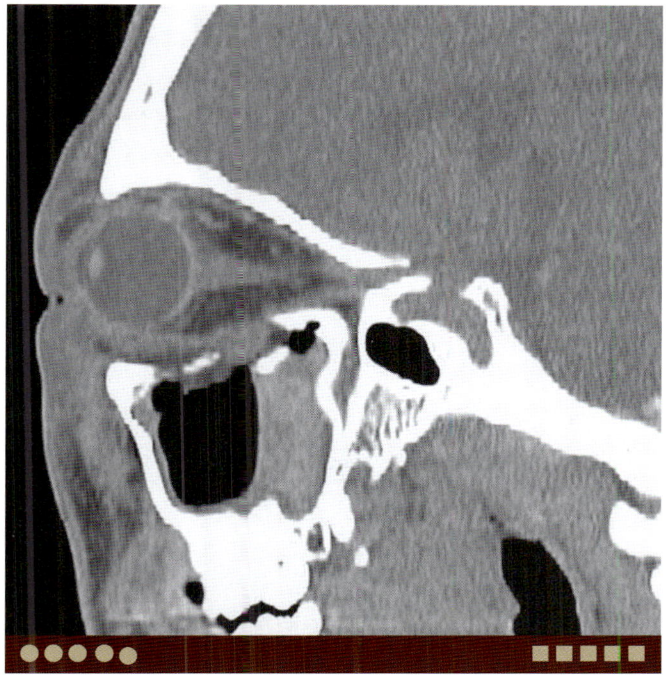

C. Blow-out fracture, same patient as A. Sagittal CT in soft tissue window demonstrates the inferior rectus muscle partially herniating into the maxillary sinus with inferiorly displaced fracture fragment. Note high-density air-fluid level formation consistent with acute hemorrhage associated with injury.

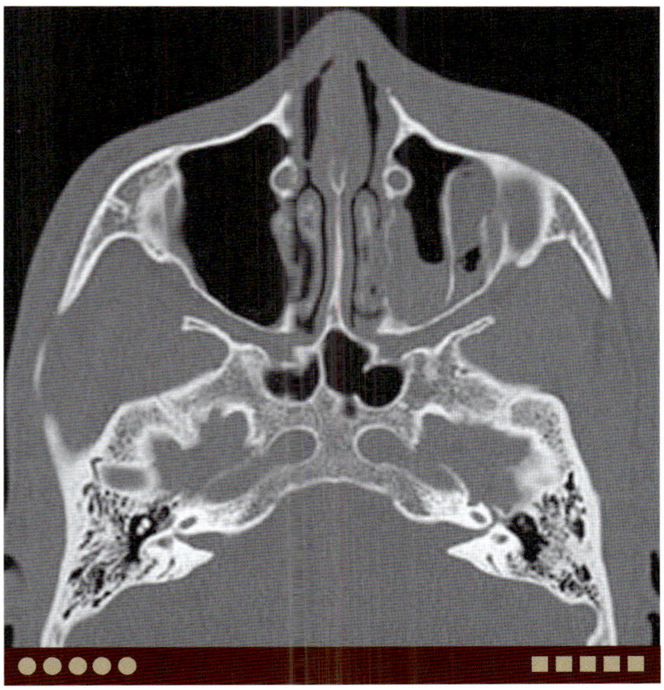

D. Blow-out fracture, same patient as A. Axial CT in bone window demonstrates asymmetry in the orbital floor, left lower than right, with displaced fracture fragment and hemorrhage in the left maxillary sinus.

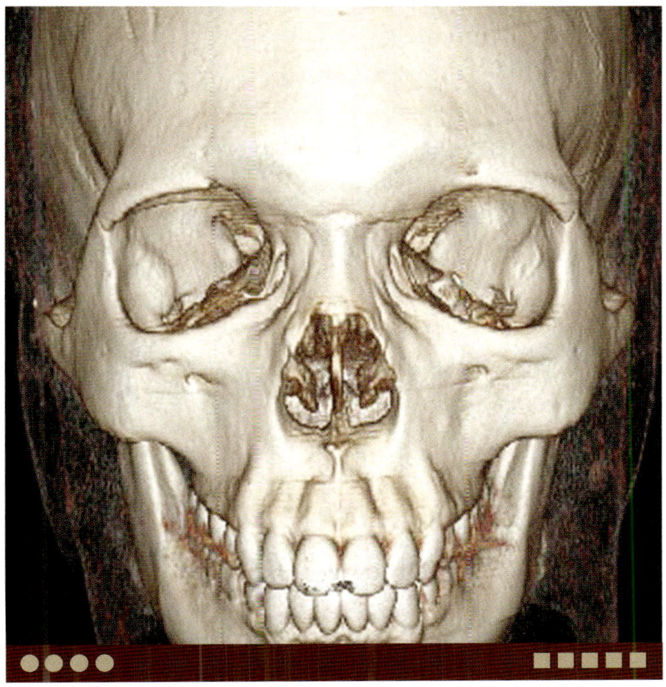

E. Blow-out fracture, same patient as A. Volume rendered 3D CT image demonstrates preservation of the left orbital rim.

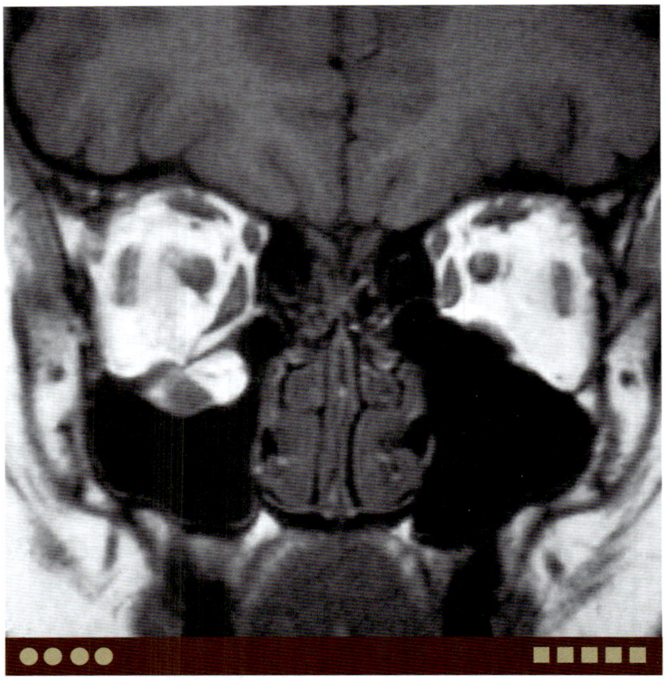

F. **Blow-out fracture** in a different patient. Coronal T1W MR image demonstrates herniation of the intraorbital fat and inferior rectus muscle into the right maxillary sinus.

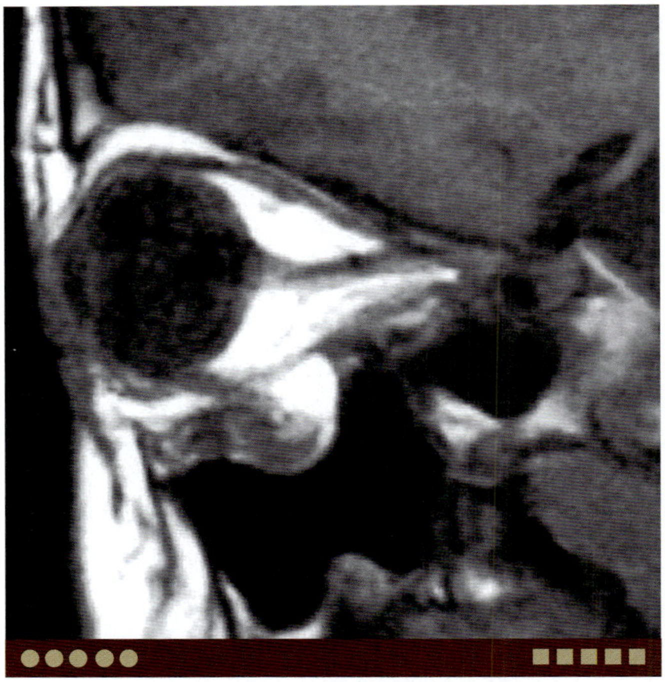

G. Blow-out fracture, same patient as F. Sagittal T1W MR image demonstrates intraorbital fat and inferior rectus muscle herniation into the maxillary sinus.

DIFFERENTIAL DIAGNOSIS IMAGES (H-I)

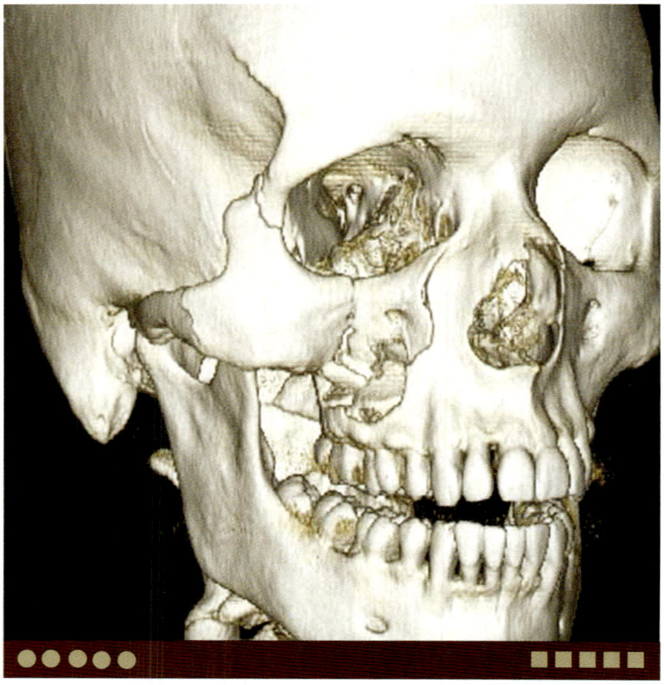

H. **Zygomaticomaxillary complex fractures**. Volume rendered 3D CT image demonstrates fractures involving the right frontozygomatic suture, zygomatic arch, and inferior orbital rim.

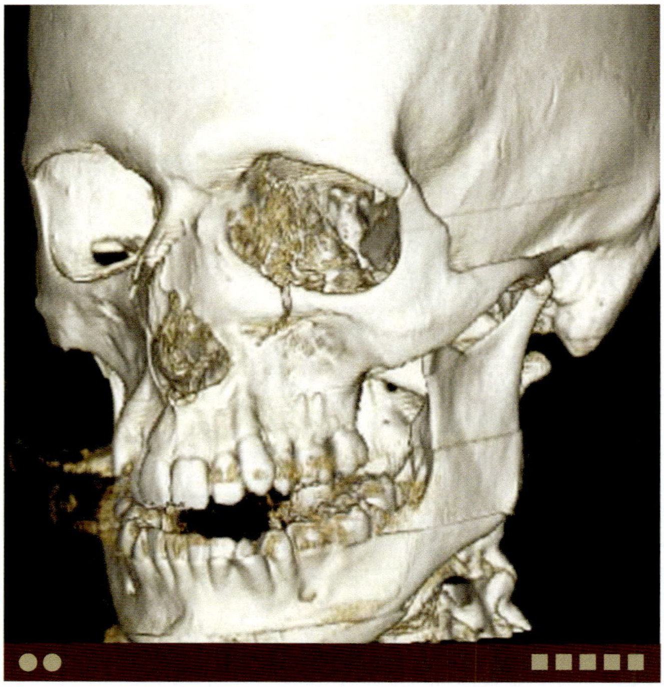

I. **Medial maxillary fracture**. Volume rendered 3D CT image demonstrates fractures involving the medial portion of the left maxillary sinus, preserving the frontozygomatic suture and zygomatic arch.

Case 4-2 Schwannoma

Osamu Sakai, Bhavya Shah

PRESENTATION

Painless unilateral proptosis.

FINDINGS

CT and MRI demonstrate an oval-shaped retrobulbar soft tissue mass in the orbit.

DIFFERENTIAL DIAGNOSIS

- Hemangioma: This is the most common intraorbital tumor found in adults. It is characterized as a low-flow lesion that demonstrates heterogeneous patchy central enhancement with homogenous enhancement on delayed images.
- Venous malformation: This is a low-flow vascular malformation and often presents with variable ophthalmoplegia. Phleboliths are the typical findings on CT.
- Idiopathic orbital inflammation (IOI) ("pseudotumor"): This may present as a poorly marginated mass-like enhancing soft tissue lesion involving any area of the orbit.
- Optic nerve sheath meningioma: This involves the optic nerve sheath and shows an enhancing mass that surrounds the optic nerve often with calcification.

COMMENTS

This is a 70-year-old man who presented with painless proptosis.

Neurogenic tumors account for approximately 4% of all orbital tumors. These tumors are usually schwannomas and neurofibromas with malignant neurogenic tumors being rare in the orbit. Schwannoma grows gradually and cause insidious proptosis. They typically arise from sensory nerves and may cause pain; however, eye movement and visual acuity are usually preserved. Schwannomas are most often seen in the superior portion of the orbit because of an increased distribution of sensory nerves within the superior portion of the orbit. Schwannoma typically has thin capsule and appears as a well-demarcated oval- or spindle-shaped intraconal mass within the orbit.

The optic nerve is an extension of the central nervous system and lacks Schwann cells, therefore, schwannoma does not arise from the optic nerve. Alternatively, lesions arising from the optic nerve most likely represent gliomas.

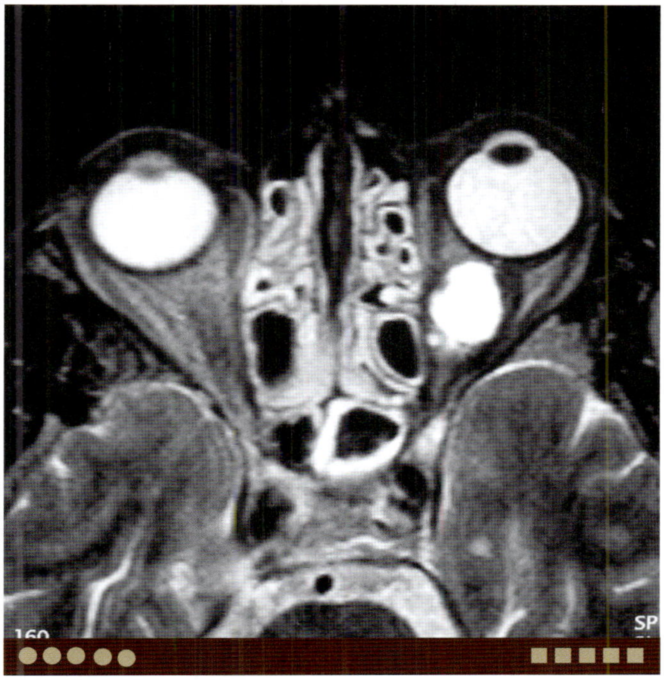

A Schwannoma. Axial T2W magnetic resonance (MR) image demonstrates a well-circumscribed, ovoid, high-signal mass with minimal septations in the retrobulbar space.

On CT, schwannoma is a well-demarcated soft tissue density mass that demonstrates subtle-to-intermediate enhancement. On magnetic resonance imaging (MRI), it demonstrates low signal on T1W images similar to the muscle and intermediate-to-high signal on T2W images. Apparent enhancement is usually seen after intravenous contrast administration. Cystic degeneration is proportional to the increasing size of the lesion.

PEARLS

- **Schwannoma is seen as a well-demarcated soft tissue density mass with subtle-to-intermediate enhancement on CT.**
- **Schwannoma demonstrates low signal on T1W and intermediate-to-high signal on T2W images and apparent enhancement.**
- **Cystic degeneration is common with increase in size.**

ADDITIONAL IMAGES (B-G)

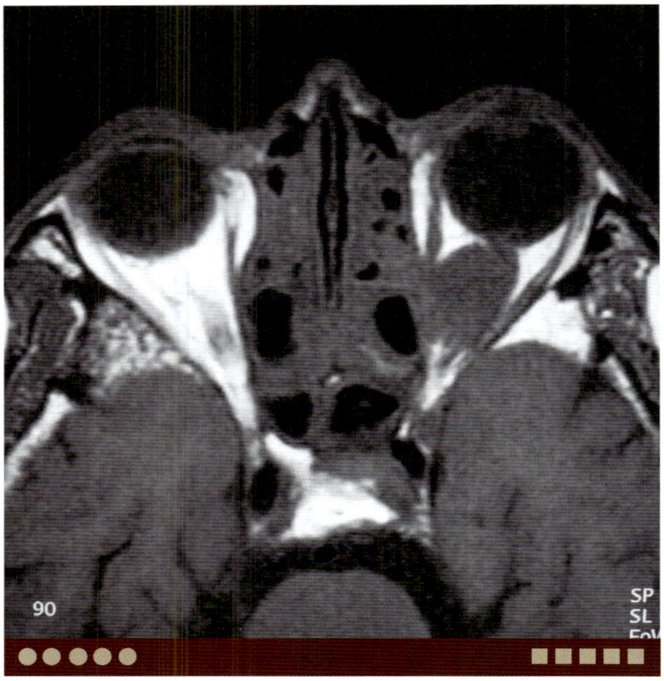

B. Schwannoma, same patient as A. Axial T1W MR image demonstrates an ovoid low-signal mass.

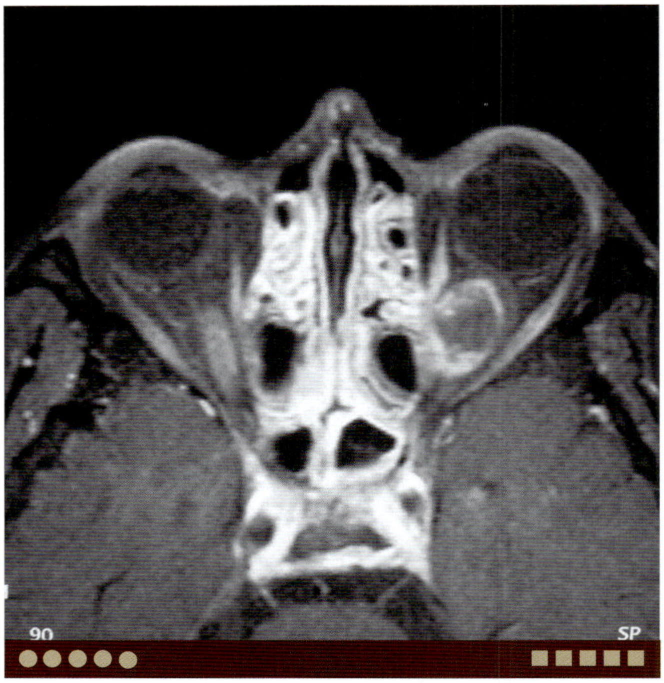

C. Schwannoma, same patient as A. Axial postcontrast fat-suppressed T1W MR image demonstrates peripheral enhancement of the lesion.

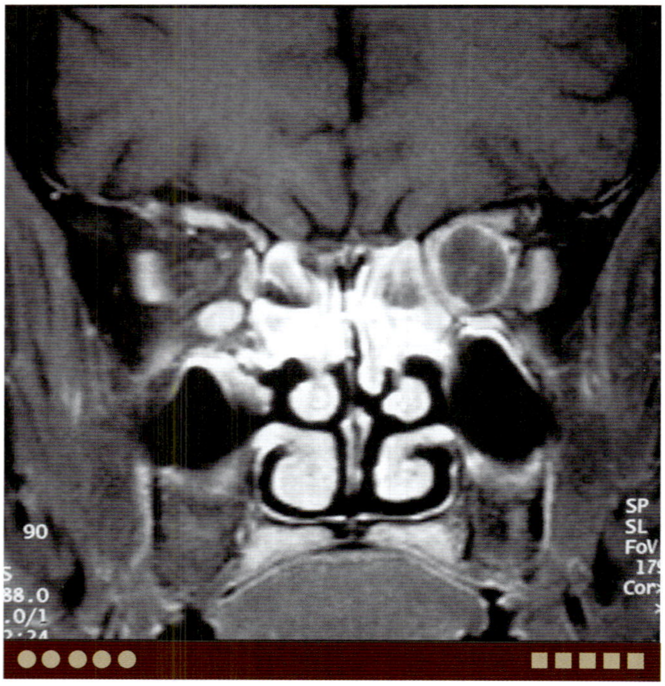

D. Schwannoma, same patient as A. Coronal postcontrast fat-suppressed T1W MR image demonstrates peripheral enhancement of the lesion.

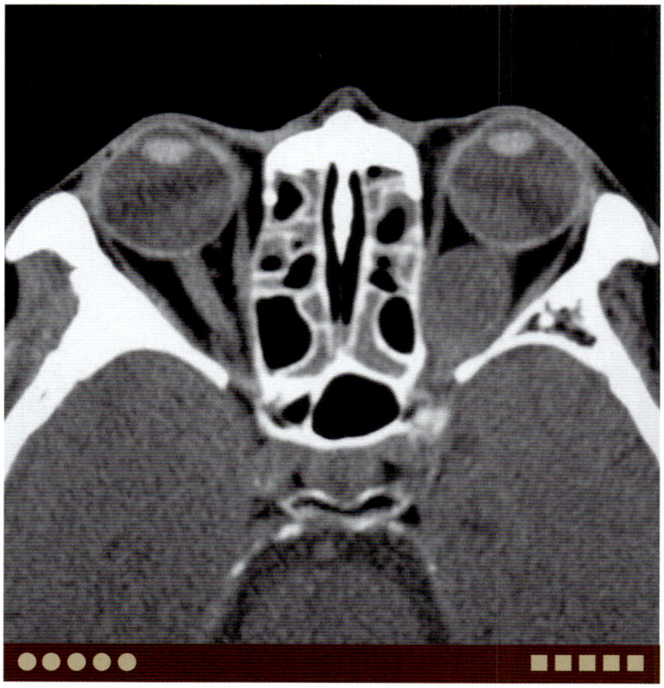

E. Schwannoma, same patient as A. Axial noncontrast-enhanced CT demonstrates a well-demarcated, low-density mass in the retrobulbar space.

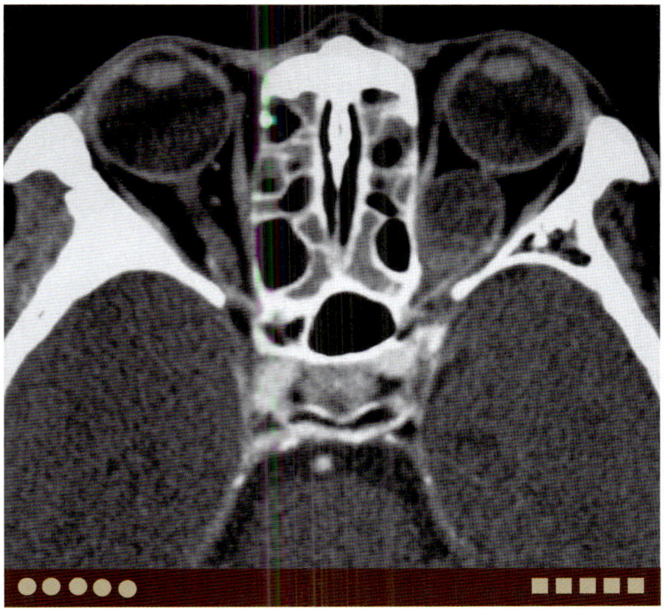

F. Schwannoma, same patient as A. Axial postcontrast CT demonstrates mild, predominantly peripheral enhancement of the lesion.

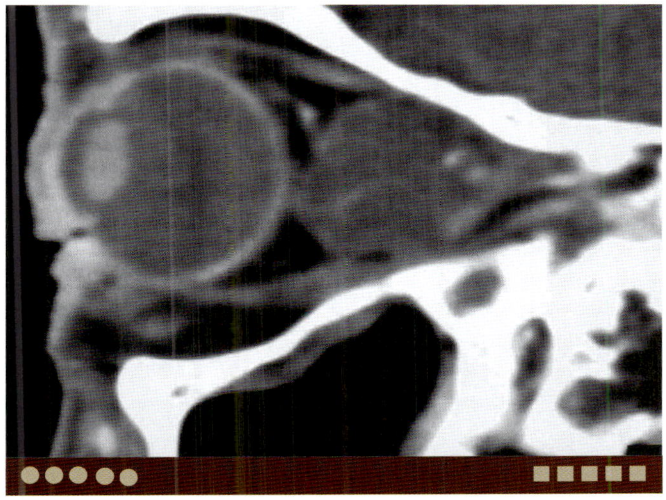

G. Schwannoma, same patient as A. Sagittal postcontrast CT demonstrates mild, predominantly peripheral enhancement of the lesion.

DIFFERENTIAL DIAGNOSIS IMAGES (H-J)

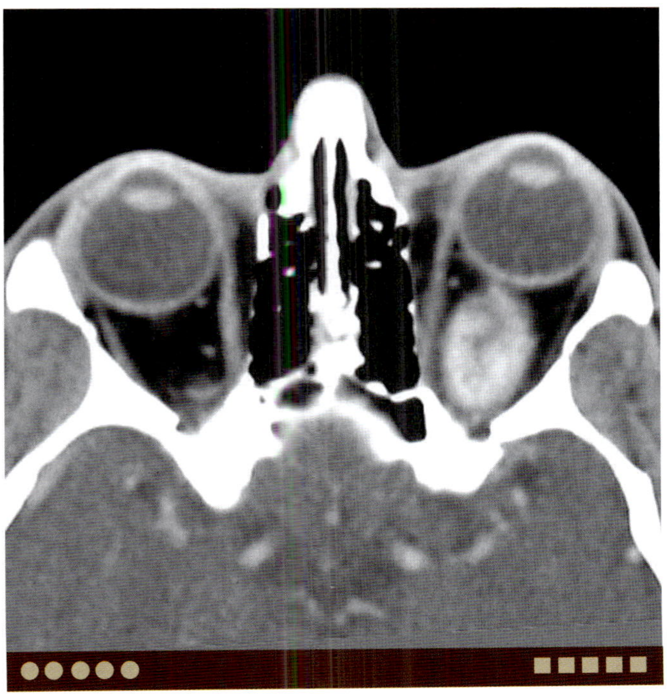

H. Hemangioma. Axial postcontrast CT demonstrates a well-marginated, ovoid enhancing lesion in the retrobulbar space of the left orbit.

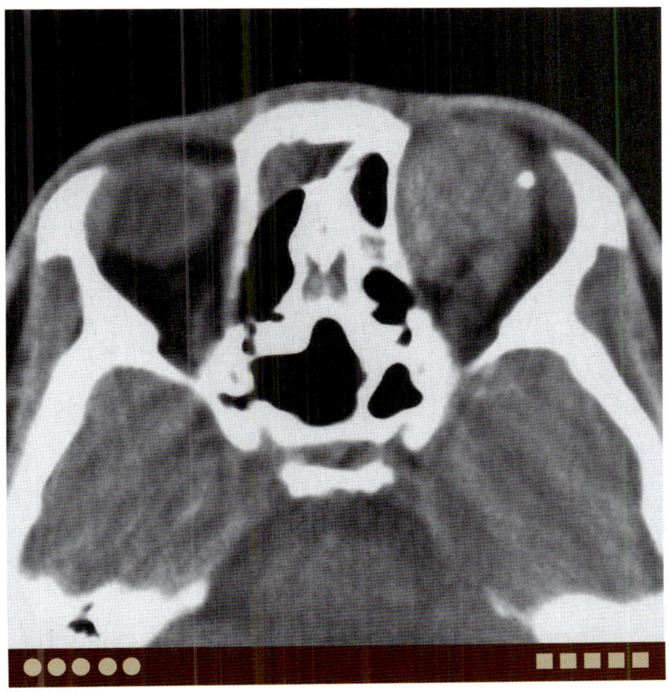

I. Venous malformation. Axial postcontrast CT demonstrates an enhancing lesion with phlebolith in the superior left orbit.

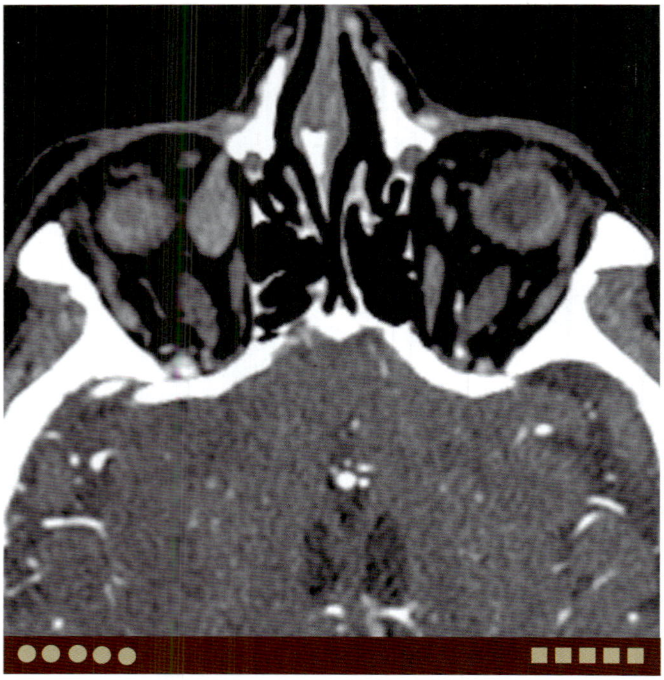

J. Varix. Axial postcontrast CT demonstrates an enhancing spindle-shaped lesion contiguous to the angular vein in the right orbit.

Case 4–3 Graves Disease, Thyroid Orbitopathy

Osamu Sakai, Bhavya Shah

PRESENTATION

Proptosis.

FINDINGS

CT and MRI demonstrate bilateral proptosis and symmetric enlargement of the extraocular muscles.

DIFFERENTIAL DIAGNOSIS

- Idiopathic orbital inflammation (IOI) ("pseudotumor"): This condition often involves the extraocular muscles (EOMs) and lacrimal glands, usually asymmetrically although bilateral involvement can be seen. IOI usually involves the tendinous insertions of the EOMs.
- Lymphoproliferative disorders and lymphoma: These show very similar findings to IOI. Differentiation is often difficult by imaging alone. Histological diagnosis is required.
- Infectious cellulitis-myositis: This is usually secondary to sinonasal infection involving the ethmoid sinuses and tends to affect the medial rectus muscle.
- Sarcoidosis: Sarcoidosis often involves the lacrimal gland; however, isolated EOM involvement is occasionally seen.
- Metastasis: Metastasis to the EOM is rare but does occur.

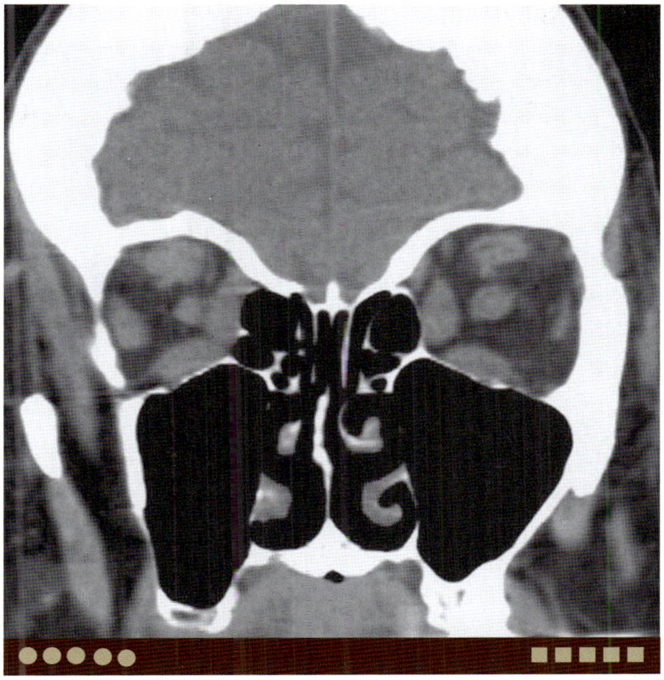

A. Thyroid orbitopathy. Coronal CT demonstrates symmetric swelling of the extraocular muscles bilaterally.

COMMENTS

This is a 55-year-old woman who presented with bilateral proptosis.

Endocrine or thyroid orbitopathy is the most common cause of exophtalmos, followed by idiopathic orbital inflammation (IOI), "pseudotumor." Although primarily associated with hyperthyroidism, the orbital abnormalities can also be seen in patients whose lab values suggest hypo- or euthyroidism.

In 90% of patients the condition is bilateral and in 70% of the patients the findings are symmetric. In the acute phase, the disease is characterized by increase in the amount of intraorbital fat, enlargement of the EOMs, which is mostly seen in the belly of the muscle sparing the tendinous portion, enlargement of the lacrimal gland, and infiltration of the fat adjacent to the posterior sclera, also known as "shaggy sclera." This is thought to be due to the infiltration by lymphocytes, glycoproteins, and mucopolysaccarides. In the chronic phase, the disease is characterized by fatty deposition and fibrotic changes within the EOMs, demonstrated by low attenuation regions on CT and high-signal intensity on T1W images.

The predilection of thyroid ophthalmopathy for specific muscles is remembered by the pneumonic, "I'M SLOW." The inferior rectus muscle is most commonly involved, followed by medial, superior, and lateral rectus muscles in descending orders. In 5% of all cases, the superior recti are the only muscles involved.

PEARLS

- **Thyroid orbitopathy is the most common cause of exophtalmos. This condition is usually bilateral, however unilateral involvement is not uncommon.**
- **The inferior rectus muscle is most commonly involved, followed by medial, superior, and lateral rectus muscles in descending order.**
- **Swelling is mostly seen in the belly of the muscle and the tendinous portion is usually spared.**

ADDITIONAL IMAGES (B-G)

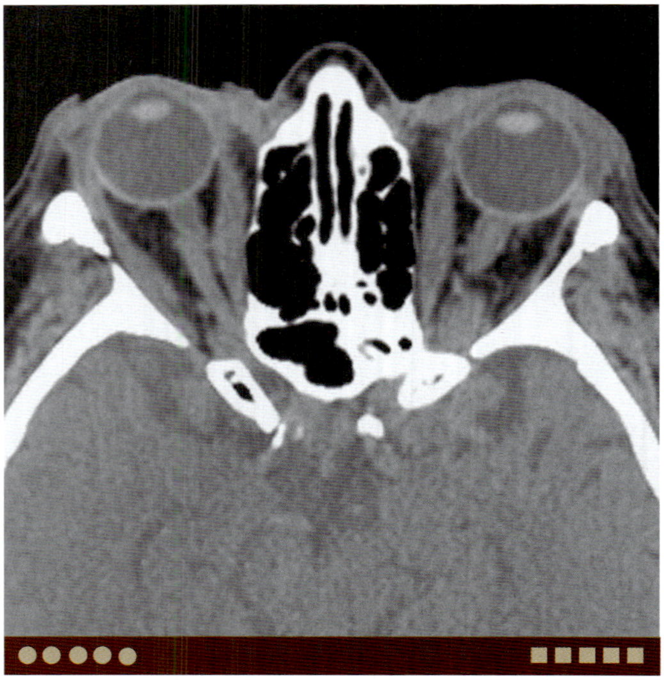

B. Thyroid orbitopathy, same patient as A. Axial CT demonstrates swelling of the bilateral EOMs sparing tendinous insertions.

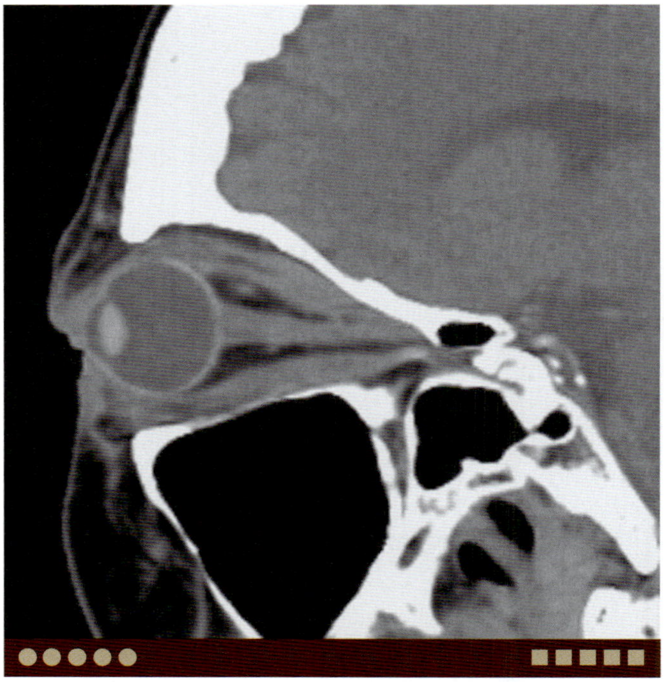

C. Thyroid orbitopathy, same patient as A. Sagittal CT demonstrates swelling of the levator palpebrae superioris and superior and inferior rectus muscles, sparing tendinous insertions.

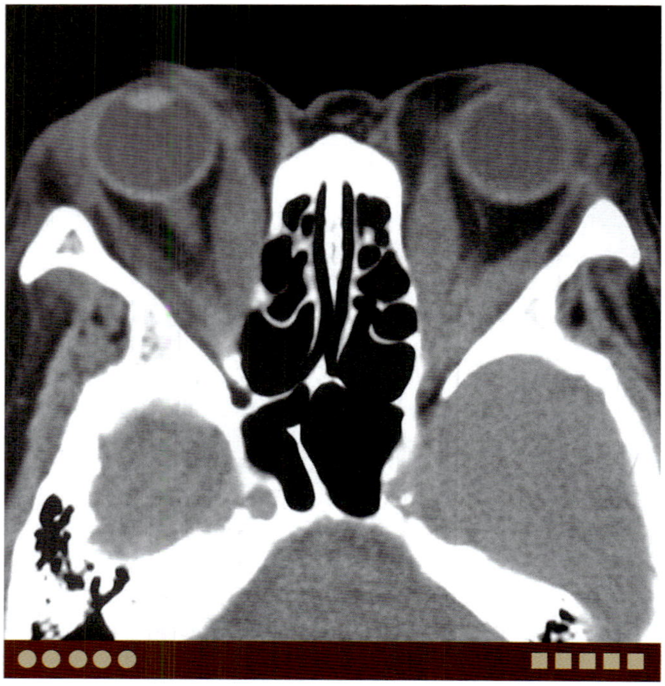

D. **Thyroid orbitopathy** in a different patient. Axial CT demonstrates swelling of the bilateral EOMs sparing tendinous insertions.

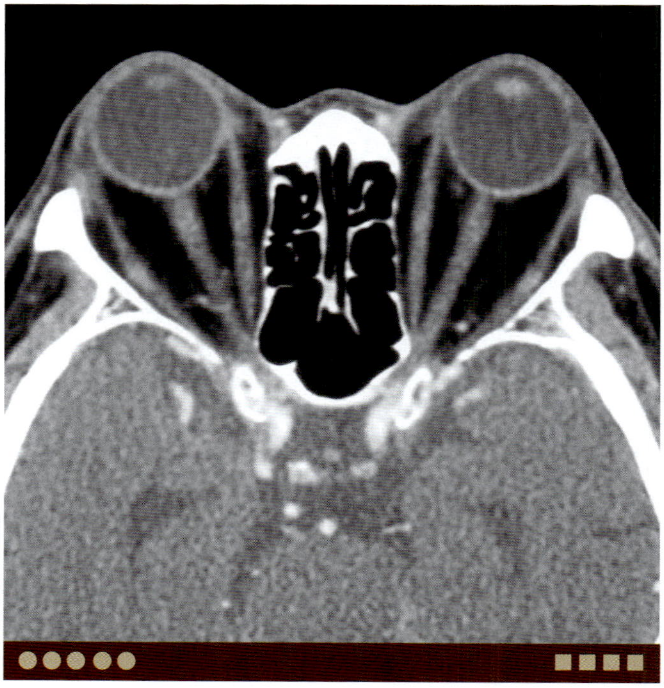

E. **Thyroid orbitopathy** in a different patient. Axial postcontrast CT demonstrates bilateral exophthalmos secondary to increase in volume of the retrobulbar fat without swelling of the EOMs.

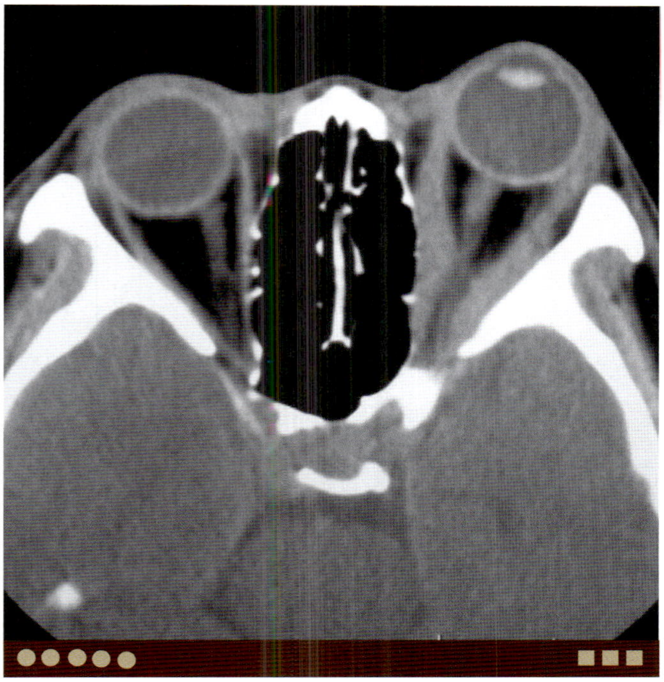

F. Unilateral thyroid orbitopathy. Axial CT demonstrates unilateral exophthalmos and swelling of the EOMs.

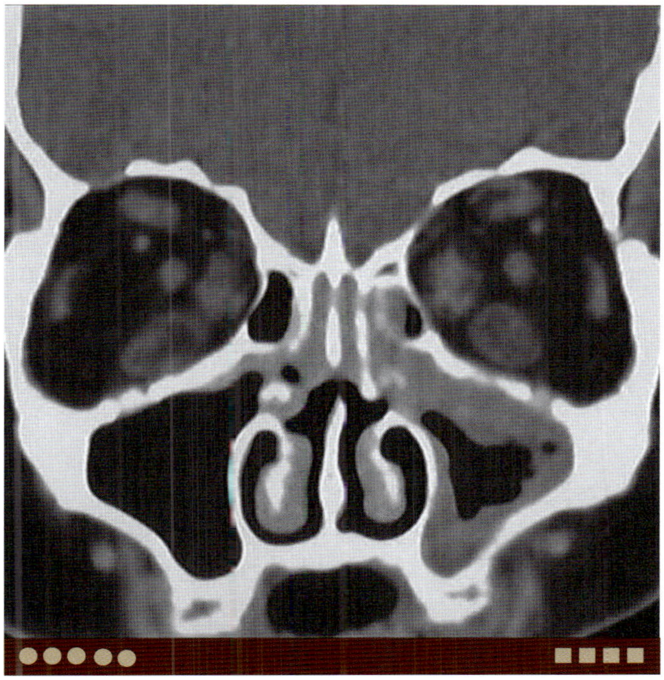

G. Chronic thyroid orbitopathy. Coronal CT demonstrates swelling and fat deposit of the inferior and medial rectus muscles bilaterally.

DIFFERENTIAL DIAGNOSIS IMAGES (H-J)

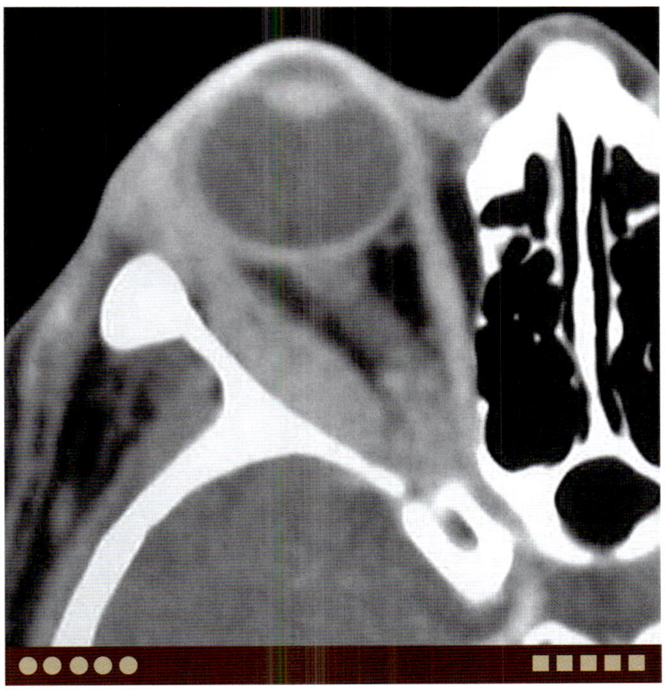

H. IOI. Axial postcontrast CT demonstrates swelling of the lateral rectus muscle involving the tendinous insertion.

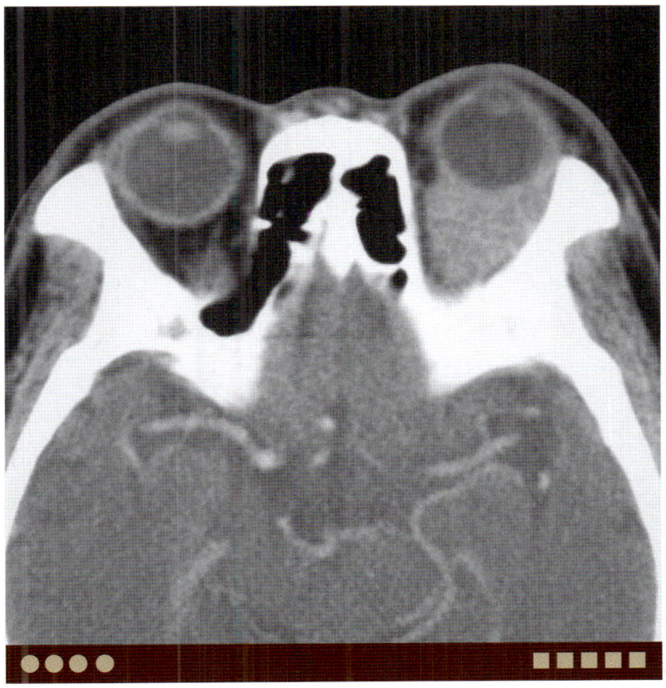

I. Lymphoma. Axial postcontrast CT demonstrates a mildly enhancing mass involving the superior rectus muscle.

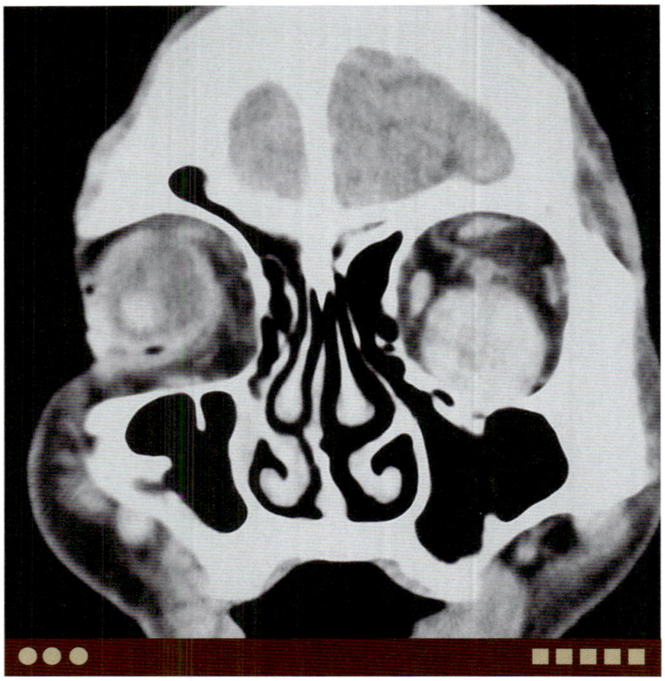

J. Metastasis, renal cell carcinoma. Coronal postcontrast CT demonstrates an avidly enhancing metastatic tumor replacing the inferior rectus muscle.

Case 4–4 Calcification of the Trochlea

Osamu Sakai, Bhavya Shah

PRESENTATION

Incidental finding.

FINDINGS

CT demonstrates punctuate calcification in the anterior, medial and superior corner of the orbit.

DIFFERENTIAL DIAGNOSIS

- Foreign body: High-density foreign bodies may mimic calcification of the trochlea. The location and density of the high-density structure as well as history is important.
- Phlebolith: Venous malformation may be seen with phlebolith. This can be seen anywhere in the orbit, however, a soft tissue mass is usually identified.

COMMENTS

This is a 50-year-old man who underwent CT for headache.

The trochlea is a cartilaginous structure with a synovium-lined sheath that permits unimpeded movement of the superior oblique muscle. The tendon of the superior oblique muscle passes through the trochlea before it inserts along the supero-lateral portion of the globe. Calcification of the trochlea is often seen in elderly patients (25-30% in persons over 50 years old) and considered as degenerative change without clinical significance. However, if the patient is younger than 40 years of age, there is a statistically significant correlation with diabetes and these findings should prompt an endocrine evaluation. Other less common causes of trochlear calcification are Brown's syndrome, traumatic and postsurgical changes.

On CT, punctuate calcification of the trochlea is seen in the anterior, medial, and superior corner of the orbit, usually bilateral. This location is important not to be mistaken as a high-density foreign body.

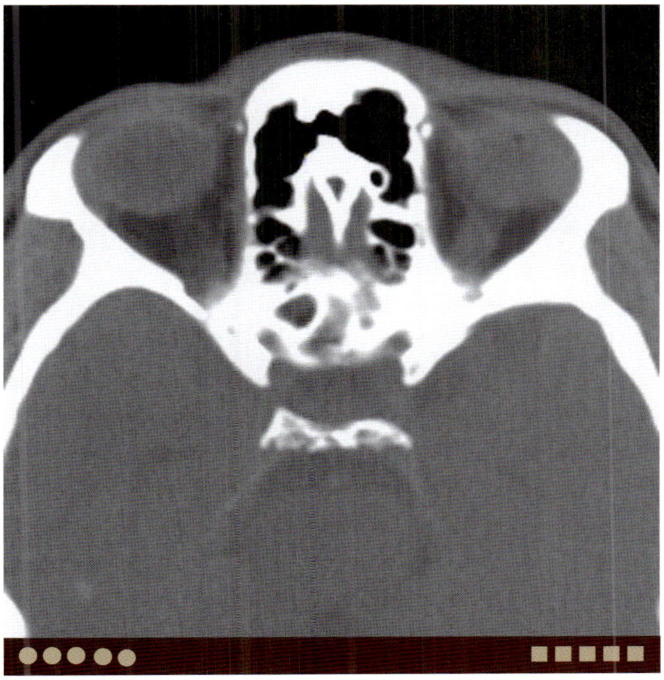

A. Calcification of the trochlea. Axial CT demonstrates punctate calcifications in the anteromedial portion of the orbit bilaterally.

PEARLS

- **Calcification of the trochlea is often seen in elderly persons and considered as degenerative change without clinical significance.**
- **Calcification of the trochlea in younger persons is strongly associated with diabetes.**

ADDITIONAL IMAGES (B-D)

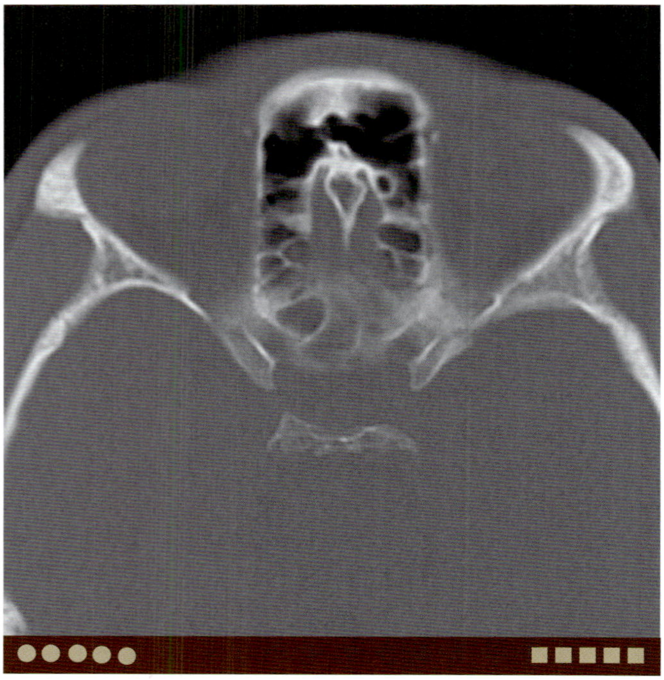

B. Calcification of the trochlea, same patient as A. Axial bone window CT confirms calcifications.

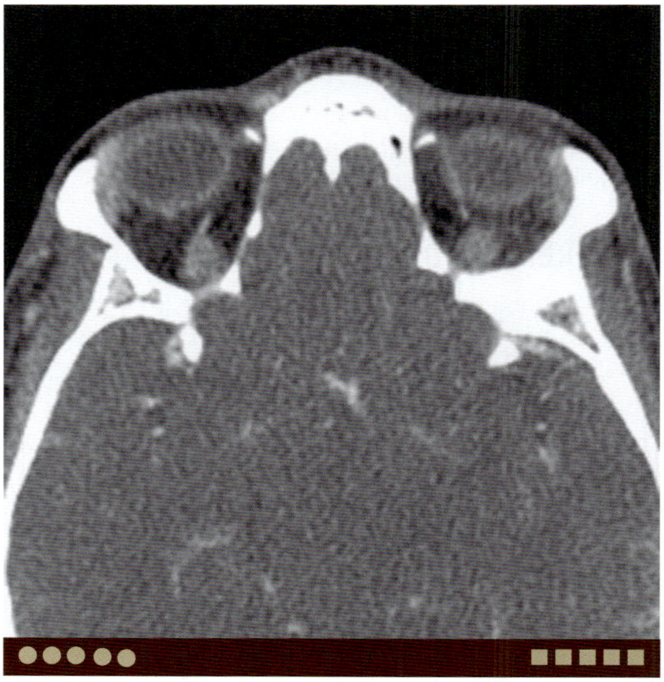

C. **Calcification of the trochlea** in a 31-year-old-man. Axial postcontrast CT demonstrates punctate calcifications in the anteromedial portion of the orbit bilaterally. This patient was found to be diabetic.

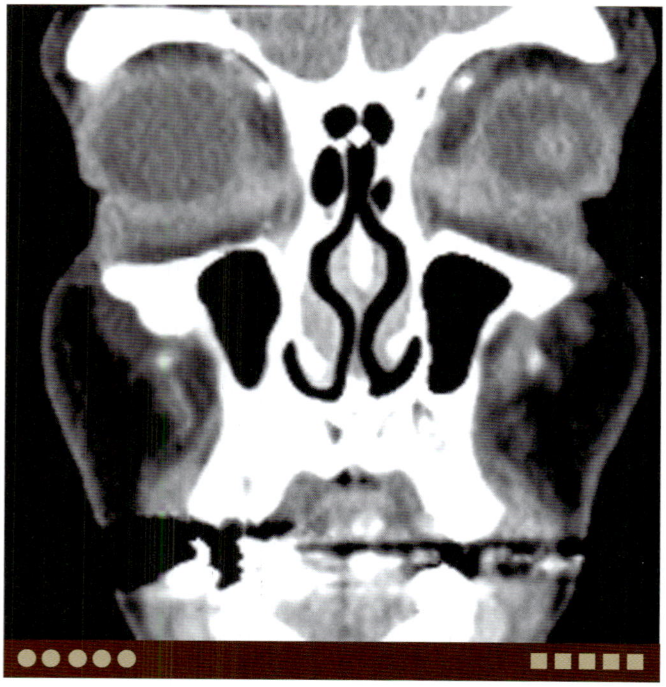

D. Calcification of the trochlea, same patient as C. Coronal postcontrast CT demonstrates punctate calcifications in the superomedial portion of the orbit bilaterally.

DIFFERENTIAL DIAGNOSIS IMAGES (E-F)

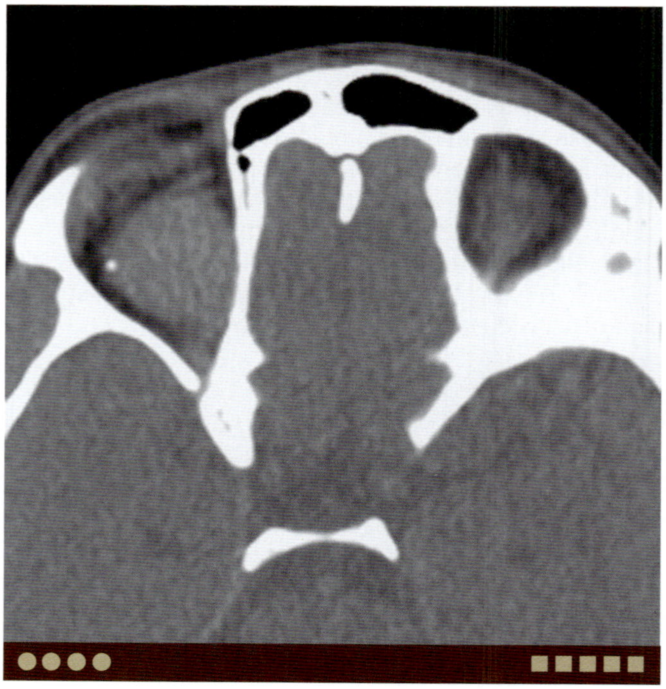

E. **Venous malformation**. Axial noncontrast CT demonstrates a punctate calcification with a soft tissue mass in the superolateral portion of the right orbit.

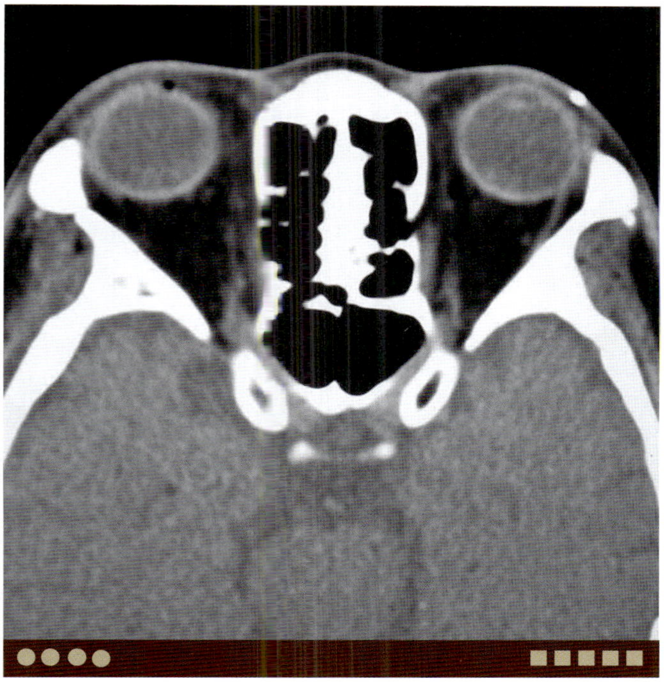

F. **Foreign body**. Axial noncontrast CT demonstrates a punctate high-density foreign body in the eyelid.

Case 4–5 Bone Dehiscence of the Lamina Papyracea

Osamu Sakai, Bhavya Shah

PRESENTATION

Incidental finding.

FINDINGS

CT and MRI demonstrate bone dehiscence of the lamina papyracea and protrusion of the intraorbital fat into the ethmoid air cells.

DIFFERENTIAL DIAGNOSIS

- Blow-out fracture: This is most commonly seen in the floor of the orbit. However, about 50% of floor fractures also have medial wall fractures. Further, isolated medial wall fractures are also common.

COMMENTS

This is a 48-year-old man who underwent MRI for headache.

The lamina papyracea is the thinnest portion of the orbital wall, and is located along the medial aspect of the orbit. Bone dehiscence of the lamina papyracea, medial wall of the orbit with intraorbital fat protrusion into the ethmoid air cells is often seen incidentally without mucosal thickening or edema. The patient has no history of prior trauma or eye symptoms.

Without the history of trauma, this condition can be congenital, although some investigators believe it is due to old forgotten trauma. The finding is identical to blow-out fracture of the lamina papyracea, and it is impossible to differentiate it from old fracture.

These findings become clinically relevant if the patient is to undergo endoscopic sinus surgery because resection of the protruded orbital fat from the ethmoid air cells may cause injury to the medial rectus muscle. The surgeon has to know this anatomical variant before surgery. Therefore, this finding must be described in the CT report.

On CT or MRI, protrusion of the fat and medial rectus muscle in the ethmoid air cells is clearly seen without edema or hemorrhage. Occasionally, mild mucosal thickening or partial opacification of the ethmoid air cells is seen due to the altered anatomy. The medial rectus muscle often appears thickened likely from focal decompression.

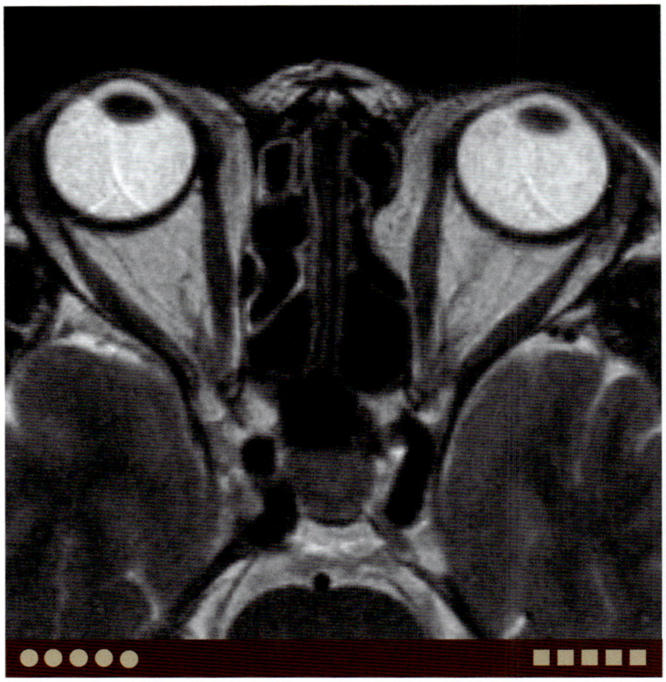

A. Lamina papyracea bone dehiscence. Axial T2W MR image demonstrates medial protrusion of the intraorbital fat into the ethmoid air cell through the bone dehiscence of the lamina papyracea.

PEARLS

- **Bone dehiscence of the lamina papyracea may be congenital variant or from old trauma.**
- **The surgeon must know this altered anatomy before endoscopic surgery to avoid complication.**

ADDITIONAL IMAGES (B-D)

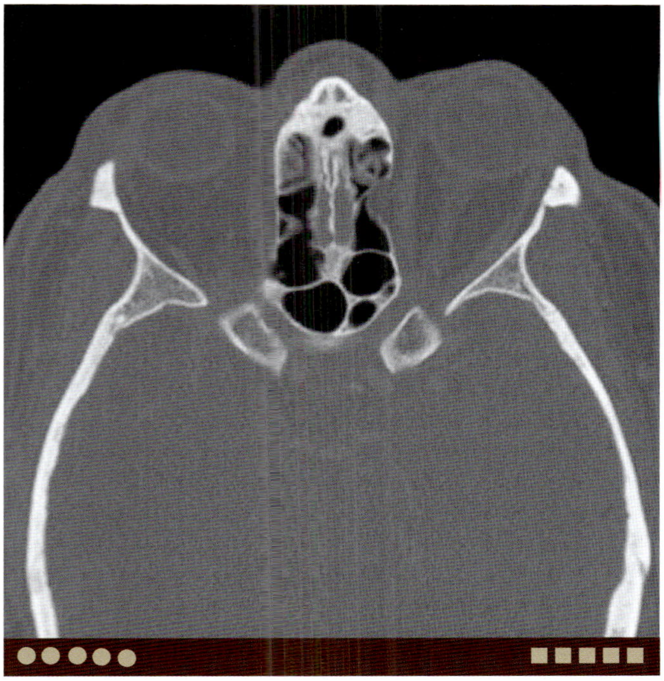

B. Lamina papyracea bone dehiscence in a different patient. Axial CT demonstrates a focal medial deviation of the left lamina papyracea.

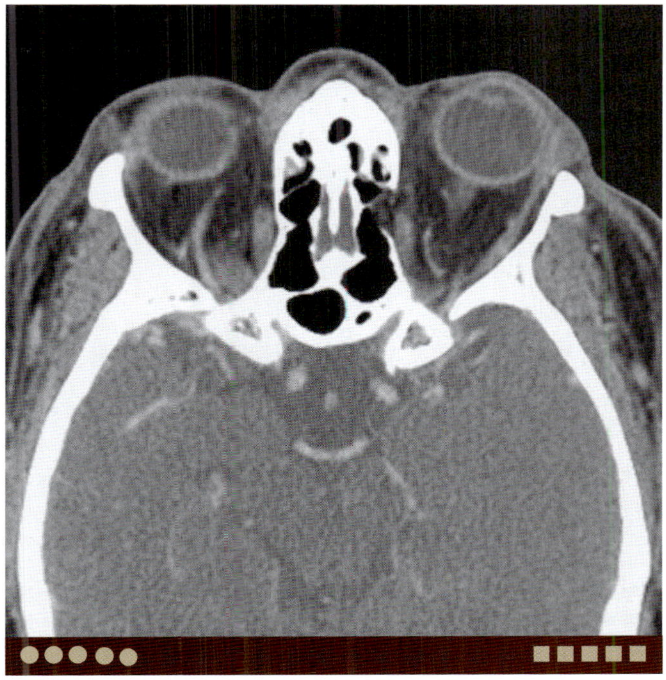

C. Lamina papyracea bone dehiscence, same patient as B. Axial postcontrast soft tissue window CT demonstrates medial protrusion of the intraorbital fat through the bone dehiscence.

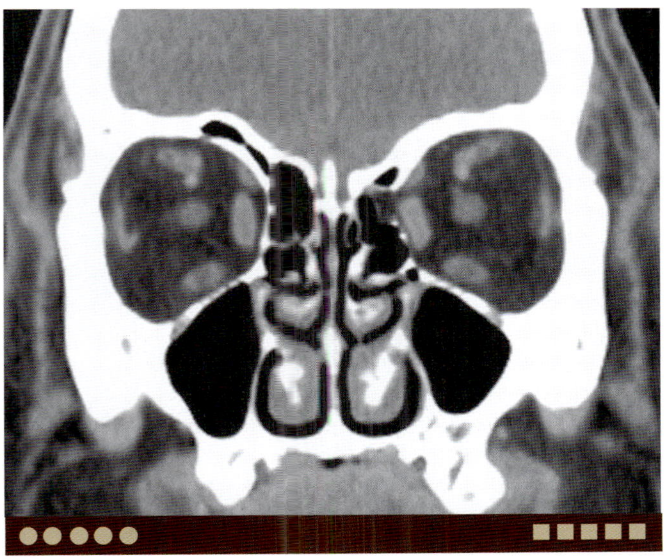

D. Lamina papyracea bone dehiscence, same patient as B. Coronal soft tissue windowed CT demonstrates medial protrusion of the intraorbital fat through the bone dehiscence. Note minimal distortion of the medial rectus muscle.

DIFFERENTIAL DIAGNOSIS IMAGES (E-G)

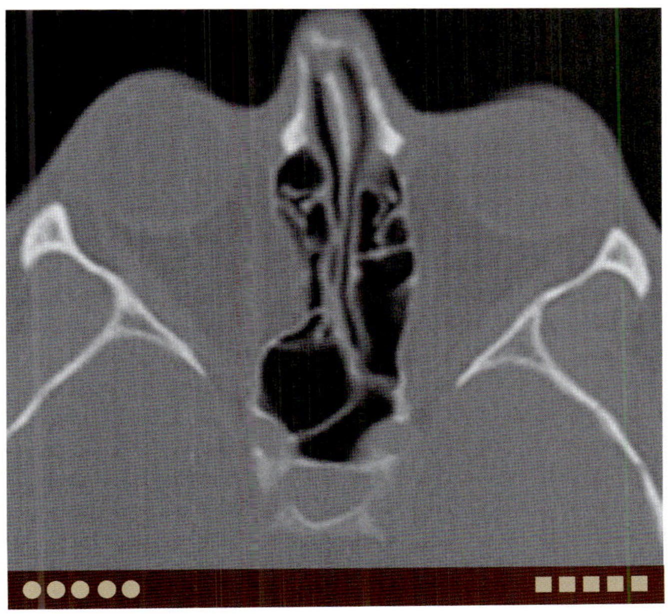

E. Blow-out fracture. Axial CT demonstrates fracture of the medial wall of the right orbit and medial protrusion of the intraorbital fat.

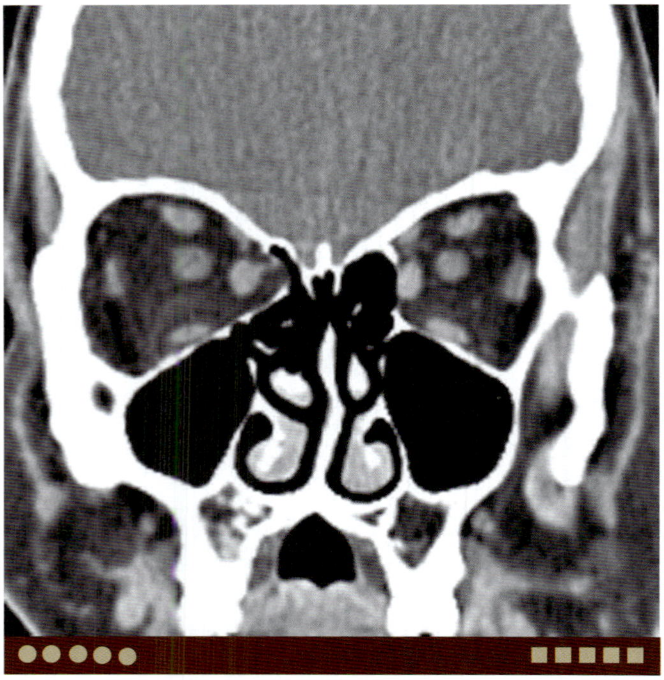

F. Blow-out fracture, same patient as E. Coronal soft tissue windowed CT demonstrates medial protrusion of the intraorbital fat and medial displacement of the medial rectus muscle.

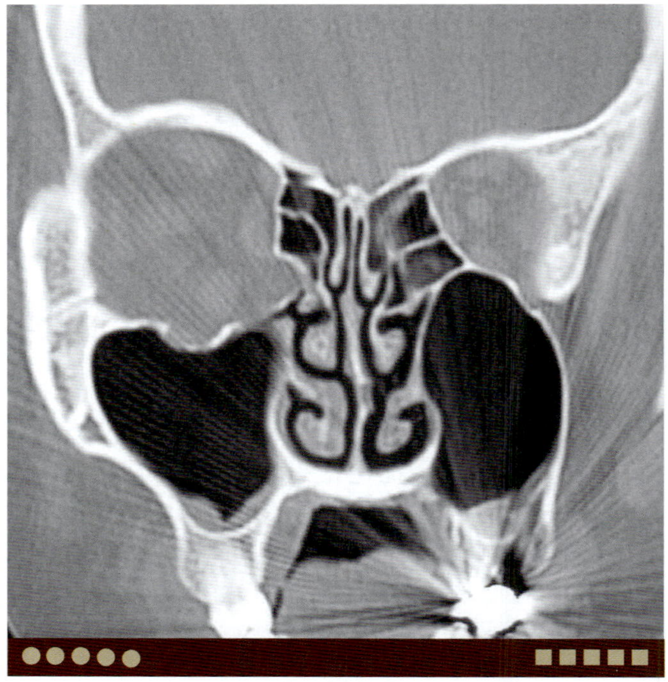

G. **Blow-out fracture** in a different patient. Coronal CT demonstrates fracture of the medial and inferior walls of the right orbit, typical locations for blow-out fractures.

Case 4–5 Artifact from Eye Makeup

Osamu Sakai, Bhavya Shah

PRESENTATION

Incidental finding.

FINDINGS

MRI demonstrates deformity and signal loss of the anterior globe.

DIFFERENTIAL DIAGNOSIS

- Metallic foreign body: Patients with intraorbital metallic foreign bodies are contraindicated to MRI. Careful screening should be performed for all patients who undergo MRI studies.
- Congenital anomaly: Globe deformity may be seen in colobomas and other conditions. However, image distortion from metallic substance should be also seen outside the globe.

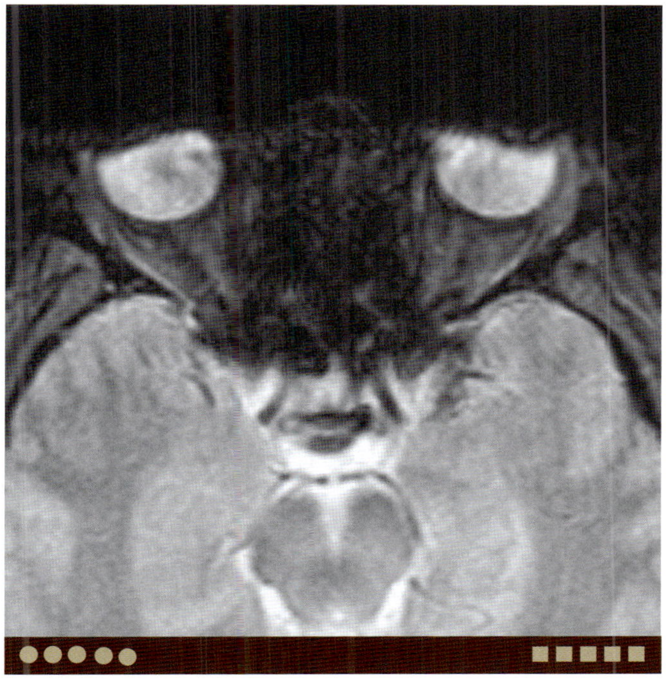

A. Eye makeup artifact. Axial fast field echo T2W MR image demonstrates signal loss and image distortion of the anterior portions of the eyes.

COMMENTS

This is a 45-year-old woman who underwent MRI for headache.

Eye makeup, both mascara and permanent makeup (tattoo eyeliner) can cause image distortion and signal loss associated with the use of iron oxide or other metal-based pigments. Therefore, the patient should be advised to remove eye makeups before MR exam, if possible, particularly when indicated to evaluate for abnormalities in the brain and face.

Slight "tingling" and sensation of "burning" have been reported in subjects who wear permanent cosmetics, however, the frequency and severity of soft tissue reactions or other problems related to MRI and permanent cosmetics is unknown. Therefore, permanent cosmetics should not prevent patients from undergoing MRI. Decorative tattoo has higher chance to cause worse complication compared to cosmetic tattoo. Radiologist or technician should be informed that the patient wears permanent makeup or tattoos before the exam and possible complication and artifact should be discussed with patients.

Image distortion is more significant with gradient echo (field echo) T2W imaging compared with other sequences.

PEARLS

- **Eye makeup, both mascara and permanent makeup (tattoo eyeliner) can cause image distortion and signal loss.**
- **"Tingling" and sensation of "burning" have been reported in subjects who wear permanent cosmetics.**

ADDITIONAL IMAGES (B-G)

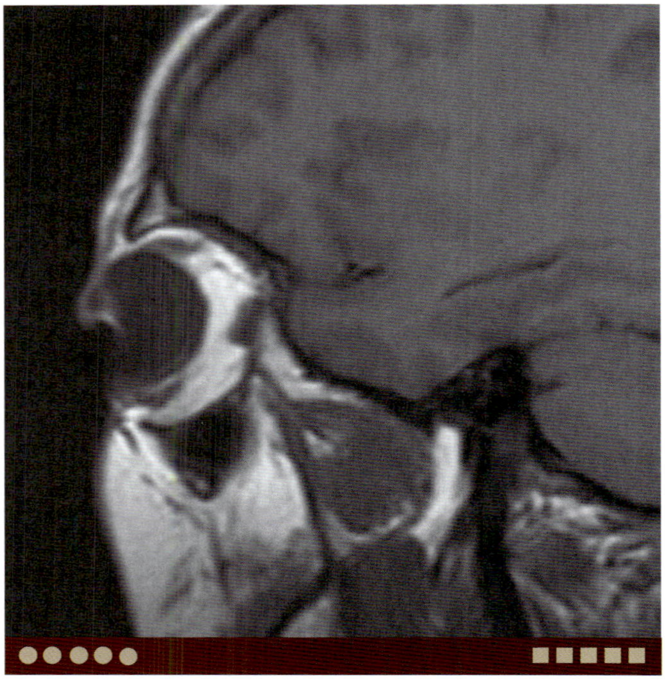

B. Eye makeup artifact, same patient as A. Sagittal T1W MR image demonstrates signal loss and image distortion of the anterior and lower portion of the eye and lower eyelid.

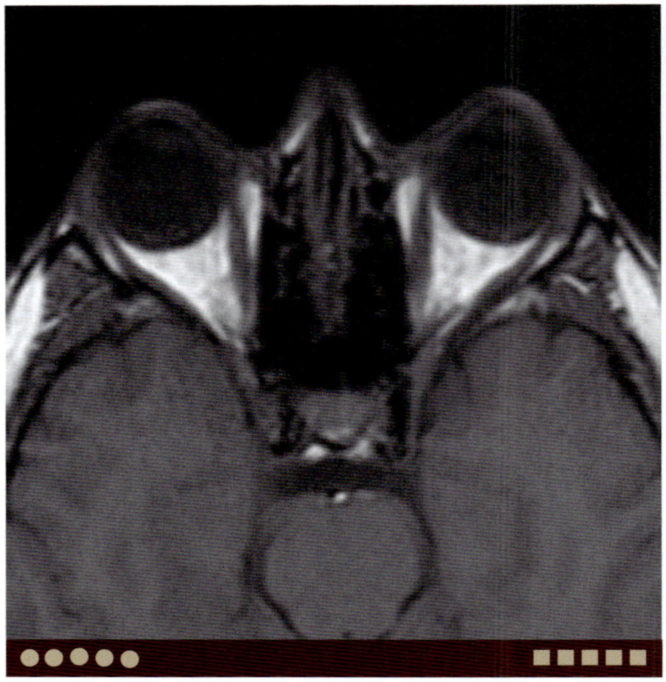

C. Eye makeup artifact, same patient as A. Axial T1W MR image demonstrates mild image distortion of the anterior portions of the eyes, however. significantly less compared with fast field echo T2W imaging (A).

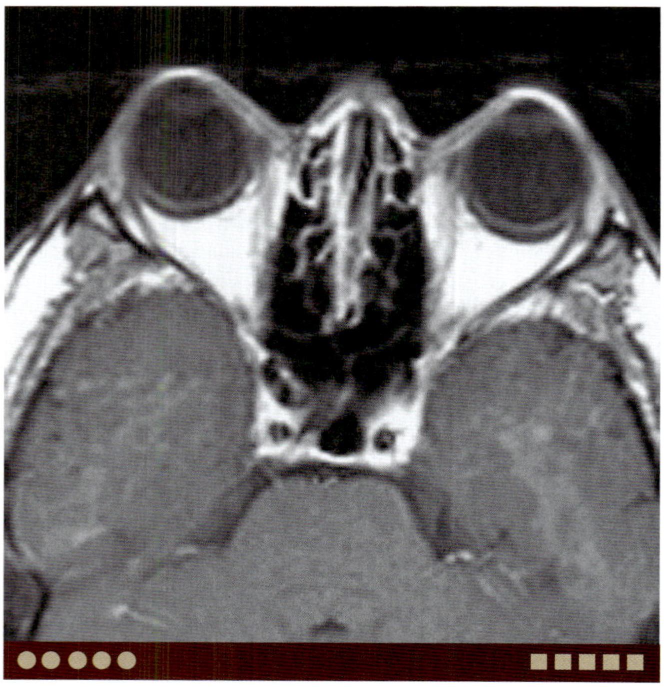

D. Eye makeup artifact, same patient as A. Axia postcontrast T1W MR image demonstrates mild image distortion of the anterior portions of the eyes similar to C.

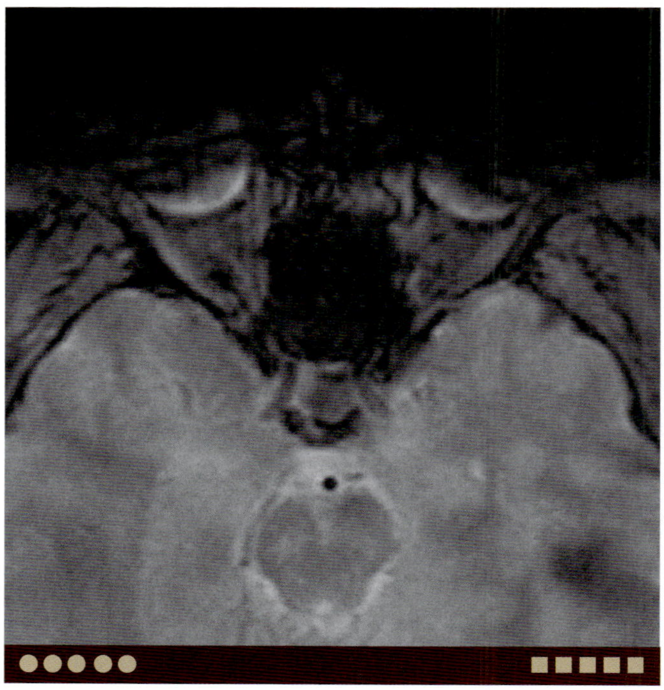

E. **Eye makeup artifact** in a different patient. Axial fast field echo T2W MR image demonstrates significant signal loss and image distortion of the eyes.

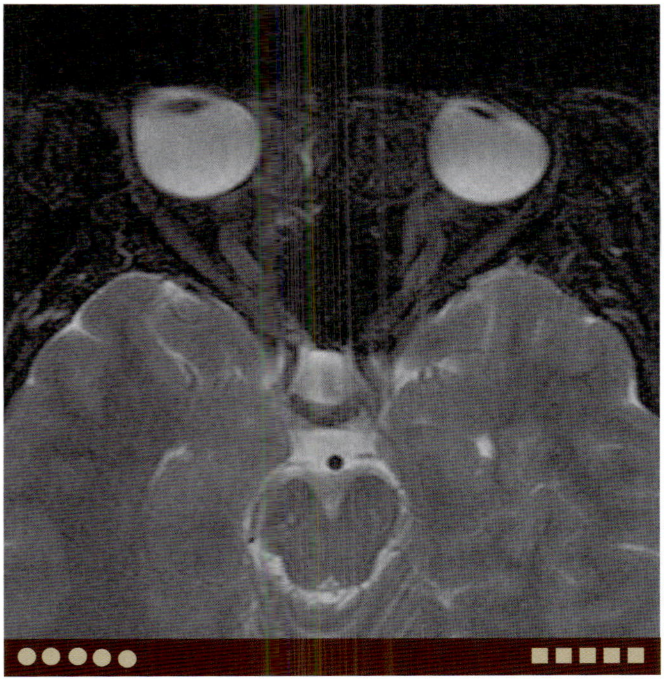

F. Eye makeup artifact, same patient as E. Axial TSE-based fat-suppressed T2W MR image demonstrates less severe image distortion.

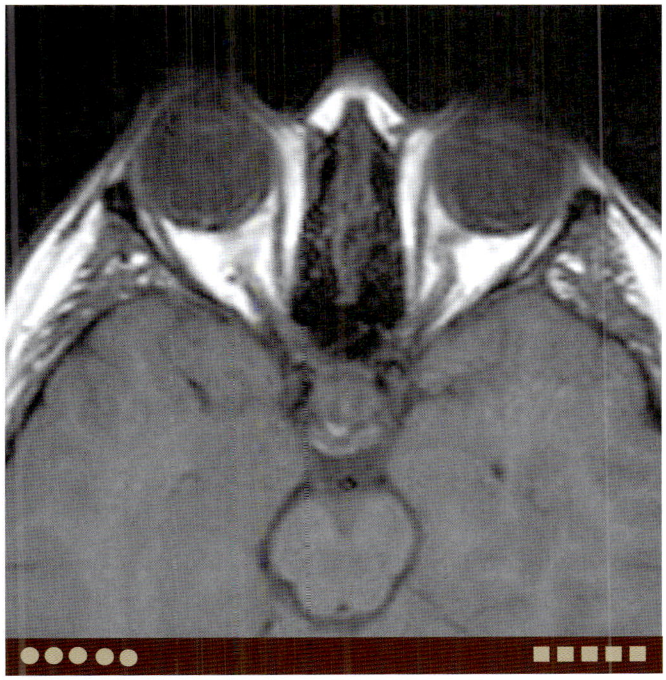

G. Eye makeup artifact, same patient as E. Axial SE T1W MR image demonstrates mild image distortion of the anterior portions of the eyes.

Case 4–7 Cavernous Hemangioma

Osamu Sakai, Susmitha Reddy

PRESENTATION

Proptosis.

FINDINGS

CT and MRI demonstrate an oval, well-demarcated mass showing high signal on T2W images.

DIFFERENTIAL DIAGNOSIS

- Schwannoma: This typically arises from sensory nerves and may cause pain. Eye movements and visual acuity are preserved. This tumor is most often seen in the superior portion of the orbit because of an increased distribution of sensory nerves in this area.
- Venous malformation: This is a low-flow vascular malformation and often presents with variable ophthalmoplegia. Phleboliths are typical findings on CT.
- Optic nerve sheath meningioma: This involves the optic nerve sheath and shows an enhancing mass surrounding the optic nerve often with calcification.
- Idiopathic orbital inflammation (IOI) ("pseudotumor"): This often presents as a poorly marginated mass-like enhancing soft tissue lesion involving any area of the orbit.

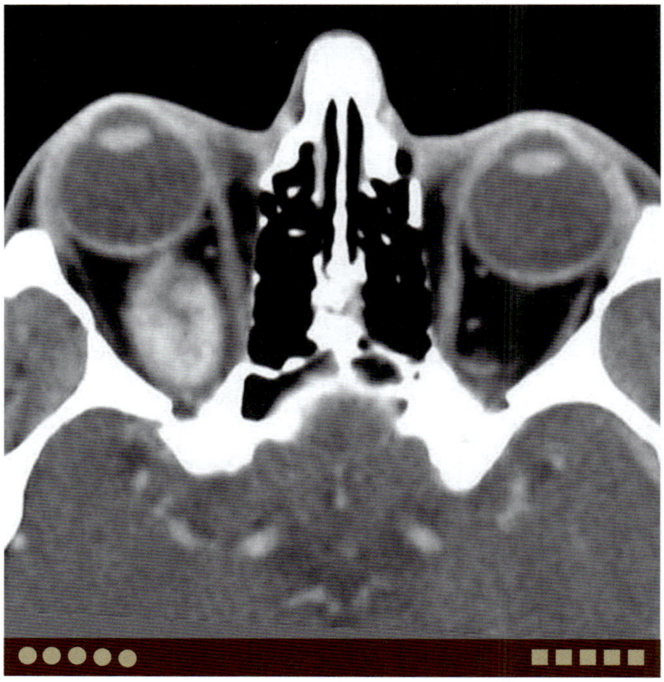

A. Cavernous hemangioma. Axial postcontrast CT demonstrates a well-marginated, ovoid enhancing lesion in the retrobulbar space of the right orbit.

COMMENTS

This is a 49-year-old woman with proptosis.

Cavernous hemangioma is the most common benign orbital tumor, often seen in middle-aged women. It is most commonly seen in the intraconal space, although can occur anywhere in the orbit. It has a thin capsule and is seen as a well demarcated, ovoid mass.

On CT, cavernous hemangioma demonstrates similar density to the vasculature. On MRI, it shows low signal similar to the muscle on T1W and very high signal on T2W images. After contrast, it may show peripheral or heterogeneous enhancement in the early phase, but homogeneous enhancement is usually seen in the late phase. The differential diagnosis includes schwannoma, hemangiopericytoma, and meningioma. Presence of very high T2 signal, ovoid shape, and homogeneous enhancement suggests cavernous hemangioma.

Capillary hemangioma occurs in infants. It usually grows in the first year of life, and then decreases in size. Most of them are seen in the superior and medial portion of the orbit, and can be intra- or extraconal. It demonstrates low signal on T1W and high signal on T2W images, and shows avid enhancement. The margins are often not clear. Postcontrast fat-suppressed sequence is useful to evaluate for extension. Venous malformation is a slow-flow vascular malformation and often seen with nodular calcifications, phleboliths.

PEARLS

- **Cavernous hemangioma is the most common benign orbital tumor in adults.**
- **Well-demarcated margin, ovoid shape, high T2 signal, and homogeneous delayed/prolonged enhancement are characteristic findings for cavernous hemangioma.**
- **Capillary hemangioma occurs in infants.**

ADDITIONAL IMAGES (B-D)

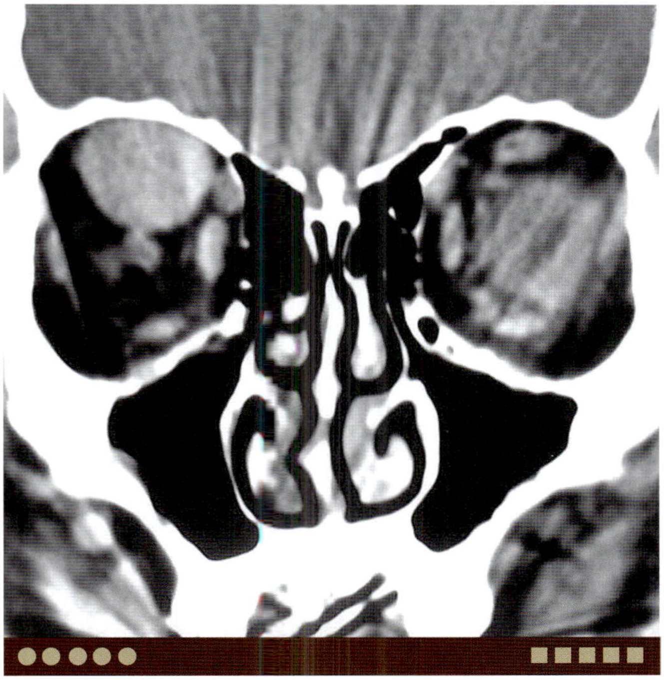

B. Cavernous hemangioma, same patient as A. Coronal postcontrast CT demonstrates a well-marginated, ovoid-enhancing lesion in the retrobulbar space of the right orbit.

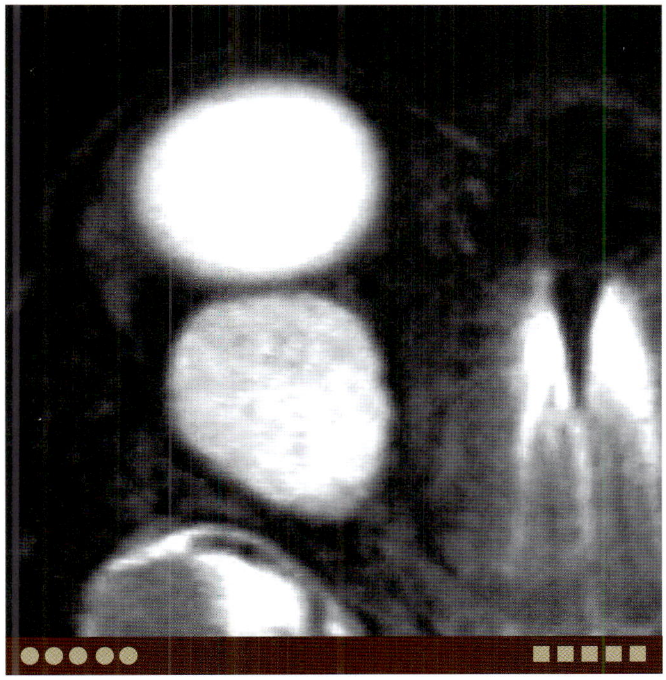

C. **Cavernous hemangioma** in a different patient. Axial T2W MR image demonstrates a well-marginated, high-signal lesion in the right orbit.

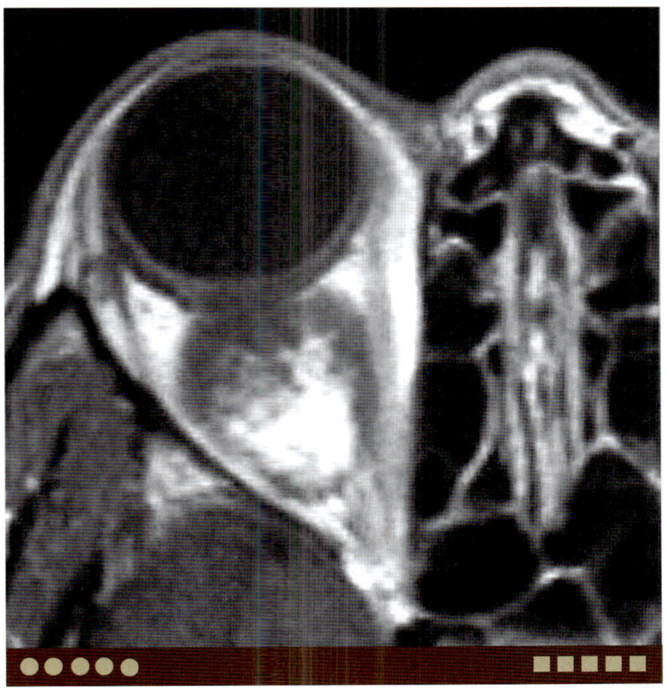

D. Cavernous hemangioma, same patient as C. Axial postcontrast T1W MR image demonstrates slightly heterogeneous enhancement of the lesion.

DIFFERENTIAL DIAGNOSIS IMAGES (E-J)

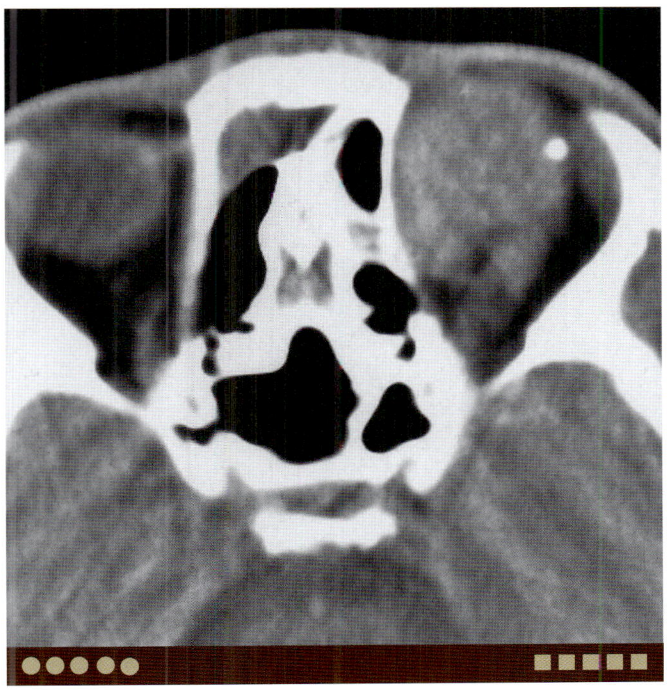

E. **Venous malformation**. Axial postcontrast CT demonstrates an enhancing lesion with phlebolith in the superior left orbit.

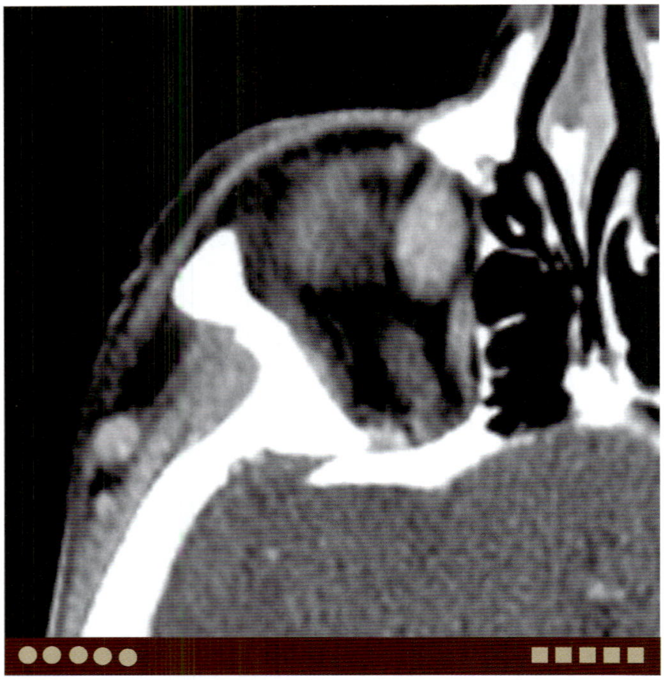

F. Varix. Axial postcontrast CT demonstrates an enhancing spindle-shaped lesion contiguous to the angular vein.

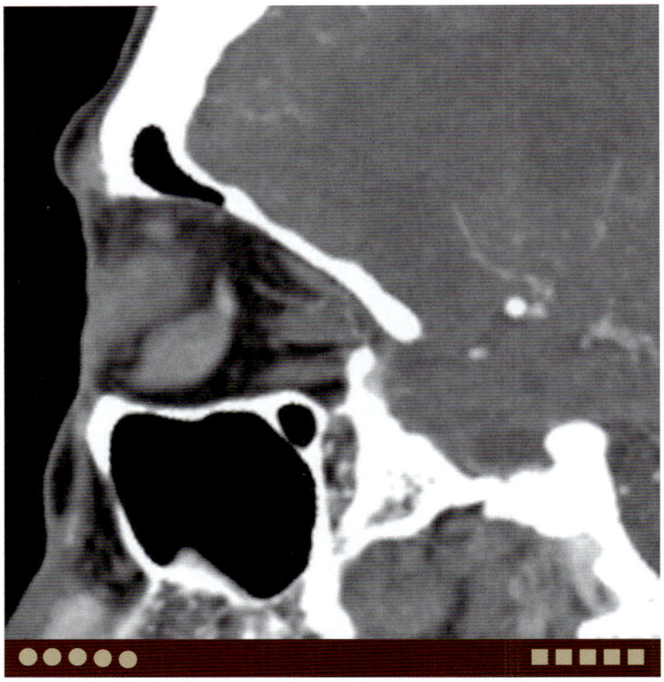

G. Varix, same patient as F. Sagittal postcontrast CT demonstrates an enhancing spindle-shaped lesion contiguous to the angular vein.

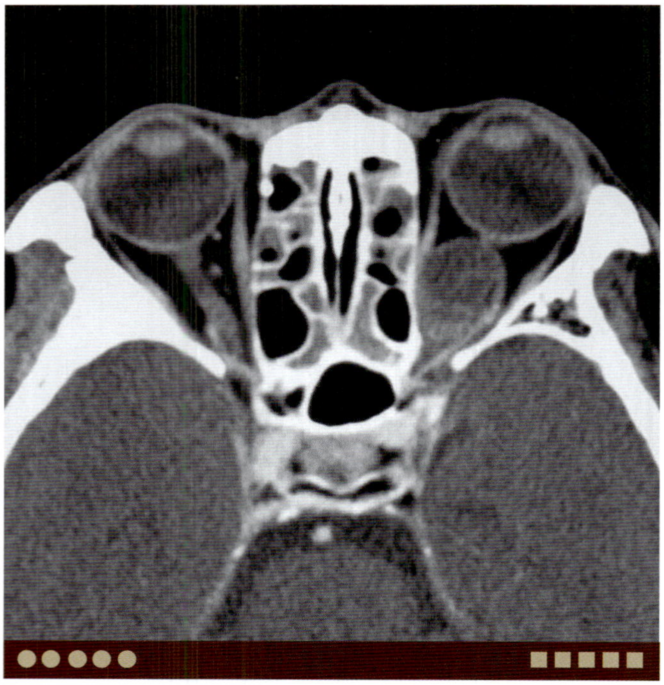

H. Schwannoma. Axial postcontrast CT demonstrates a well-marginated, ovoid-shaped lesion with predominantly peripheral mild enhancement in the left orbit.

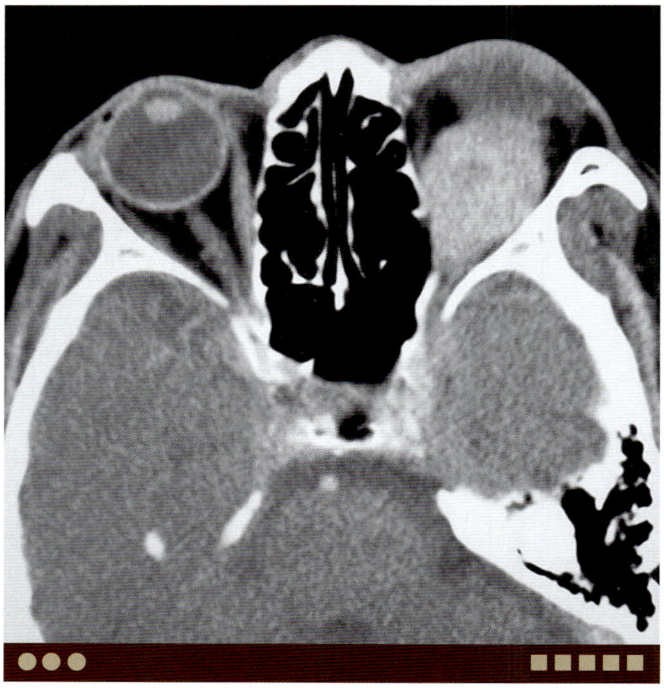

I. Metastasis from renal cell carcinoma. Axial postcontrast CT demonstrates an avidly enhancing tumor in the left orbit.

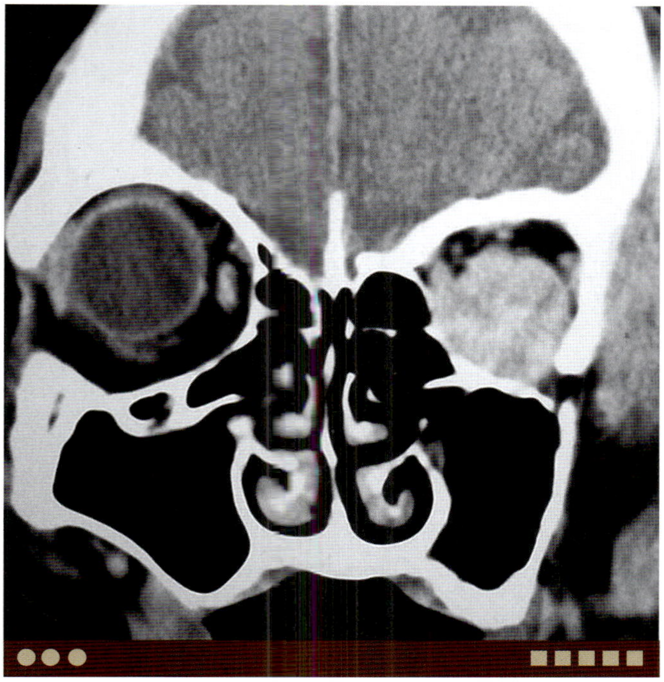

J. Metastasis from renal cell carcinoma, same patient as I. Coronal postcontrast CT demonstrates a round avidly enhancing tumor in the left orbit.

Case 4–8 Optic Glioma

Osamu Sakai, Francisco Contreras

PRESENTATION

Decreased vision.

FINDINGS

MRI demonstrates enlargement of the optic nerve.

DIFFERENTIAL DIAGNOSIS

- Optic neuritis: This entity is defined as inflammation of the optic nerve and typically presents as a classic triad consisting of loss of vision, eye pain, and dyschromatopsia. Optic neuritis can be the initial episode for multiple sclerosis. This condition typically manifests as T2W hyperintense foci within a minimally or nonexpanded nerve. These lesions will also typically enhance following gadolinium administration in the active phase.
- Meningioma: This is a benign tumor arising from arachnoid cells within the optic nerve sheath. This is typically a solid, tubular, enhancing, well-defined enlargement of the optic nerve sheath complex which classically demonstrates "tram-track" appearance caused by tumor enhancement or calcification on either side of the optic nerve.
- Metastatic tumor: CSF tumor dissemination can demonstrate abnormal enlargement and enhancement of the optic nerve sheath complex, and also typically manifest with extraorbital lesions as well as possible multifocal intraorbital lesions.
- Schwannoma: Schwannomas commonly arise in the superior portion of the orbit because more sensory nerves are present in that location. The optic never is an extension of the brain and does not have Schwann cells. Therefore, schwannoma should not arise from the optic nerve.

COMMENTS

This is an 11-year-old boy presenting with decreased vision. Optic gliomas account for 4% of orbital tumors and often occur between the ages of 2 and 8 years old. It can be seen in 15% to 40% of patients with neurofibromatosis type I. Bilateral optic gliomas are characteristic for neurofibromatosis type I. In general, optic gliomas extend both anteriorly and posteriorly along the optic nerve and often involve the optic chiasm. Optic gliomas in adults are rare but highly malignant and carry a much worse prognosis.

The three subtypes include: (1) childhood benign tumors associated with neurofibromatosis type I, which typically demonstrate a smooth, tubular, and tortuous enlargement of the optic nerve with moderate to patchy enhancement, (2) childhood benign tumors not associated with neurofibromatosis type I, which demonstrate a smooth, nodular enlargement of the optic nerve with cystic components and show moderate-to-intense enhancement, and (3) adult tumors that are typically malignant, which demonstrate diffuse enlargement of the optic nerve with invasive features as well as moderate irregular enhancement.

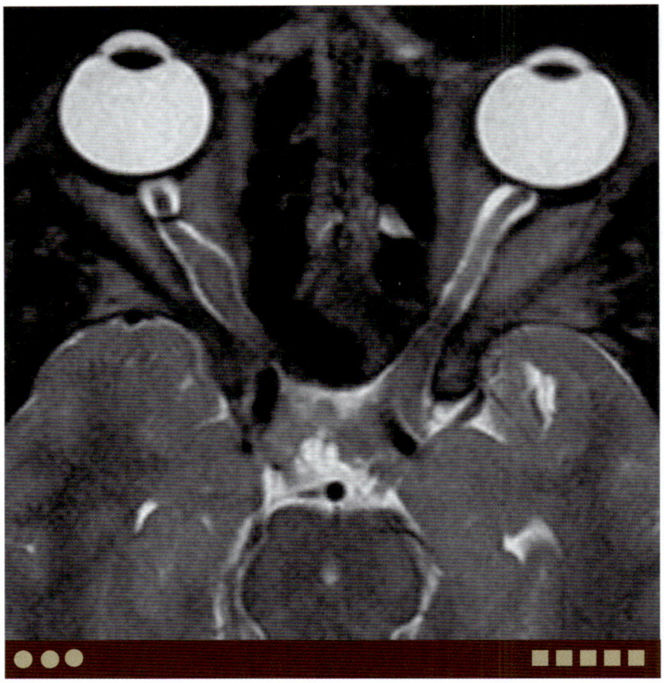

A. Optic glioma. Axial T2W MR image demonstrates enlargement of the right optic nerve at the orbital apex. Swelling is also seen in the intracanalicular portion of the left optic nerve.

CT demonstrates enlargement, tortuosity and kinking of the optic nerve. Unlike optic nerve sheath meningiomas, calcifications are rare. Cystic degeneration is often seen. If there is an intracranial extension, there will typically be some element of enlargement of the bony optic canal. MRI shows similar signal to the optic nerve on T1W, and intermediate signal, slightly higher than the gray matter on T2W images. In the setting of cystic degeneration, MRI shows heterogeneous signal intensity. Variable degrees of enhancement are seen after contrast administration, which is dependent on the lesion subtype.

PEARLS

- **Optic gliomas often occur between the ages of 2 and 8 years old. Bilateral optic gliomas are characteristic of neurofibromatosis type I.**
- **Optic gliomas extend anteriorly and posteriorly along the optic nerve and often involve the optic chiasm.**
- **Optic glioma in adults is rare but highly malignant and has a worse prognosis.**

ADDITIONAL IMAGES (B-G)

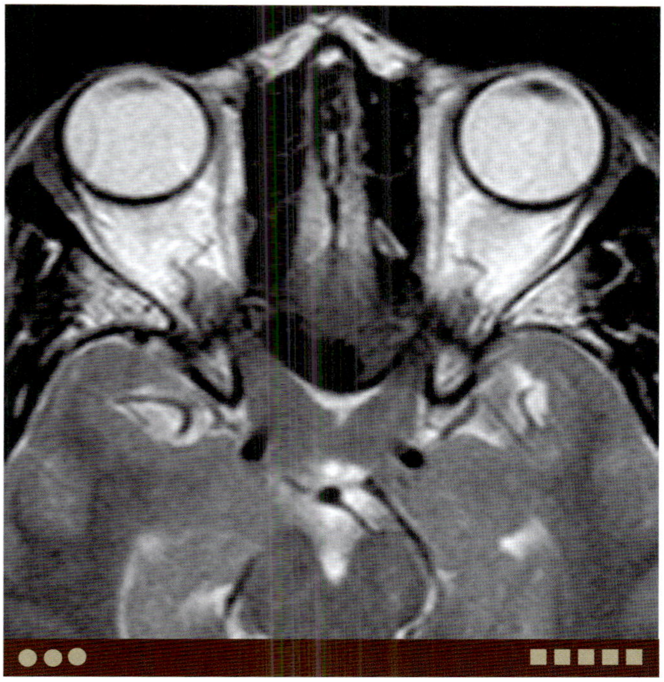

B. Optic glioma, same patient as A. Axial T2W MR image demonstrates enlargement of the cisternal portions of the bilateral optic nerves and chiasm.

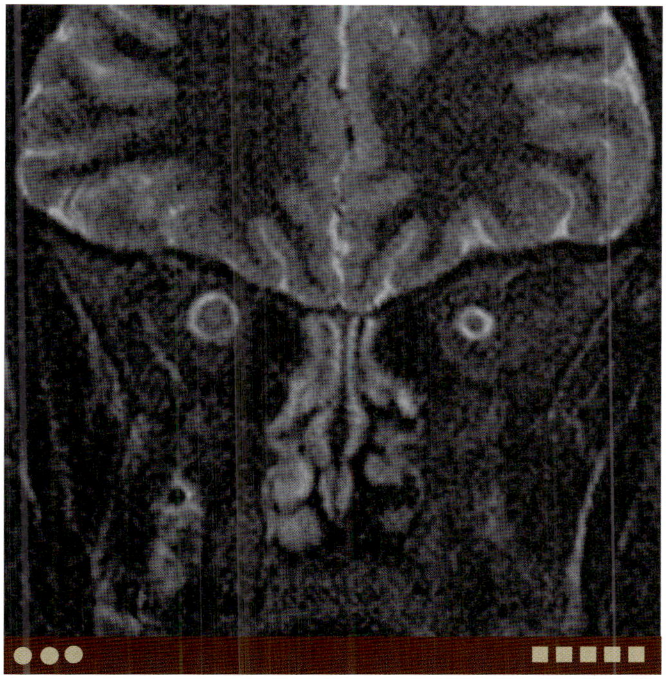

C. Optic glioma, same patient as A. Coronal fat-suppressed T2W MR image shows an asymmetric enlargement and increased signal of the right optic nerve.

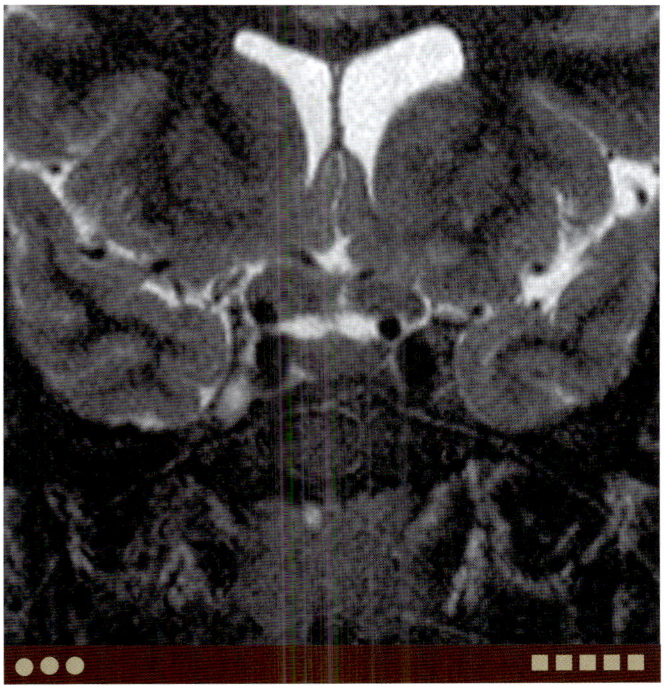

D. Optic glioma, same patient as A. Coronal fat-suppressed T2W MR image shows enlargement of the optic chiasm, right more than left.

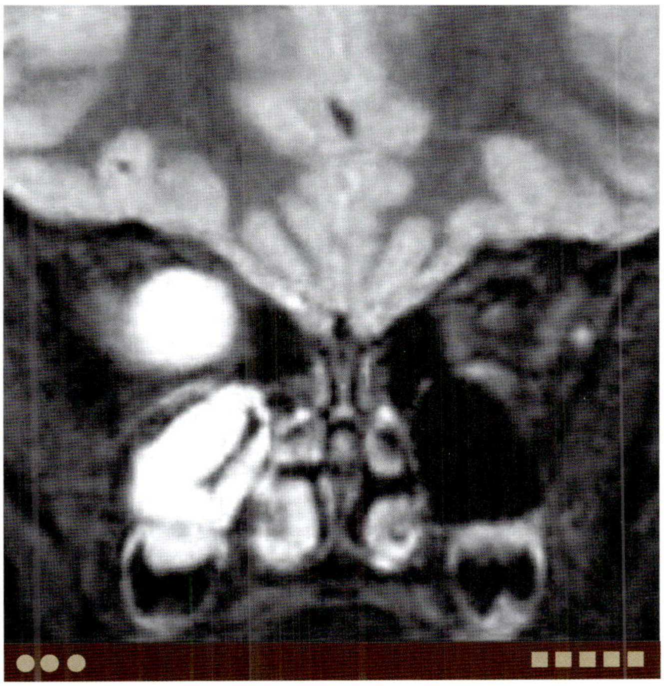

E. **Optic glioma** in a different patient. Coronal fat-suppressed T2W MR image shows significantly enlarged right optic nerve showing very high signal.

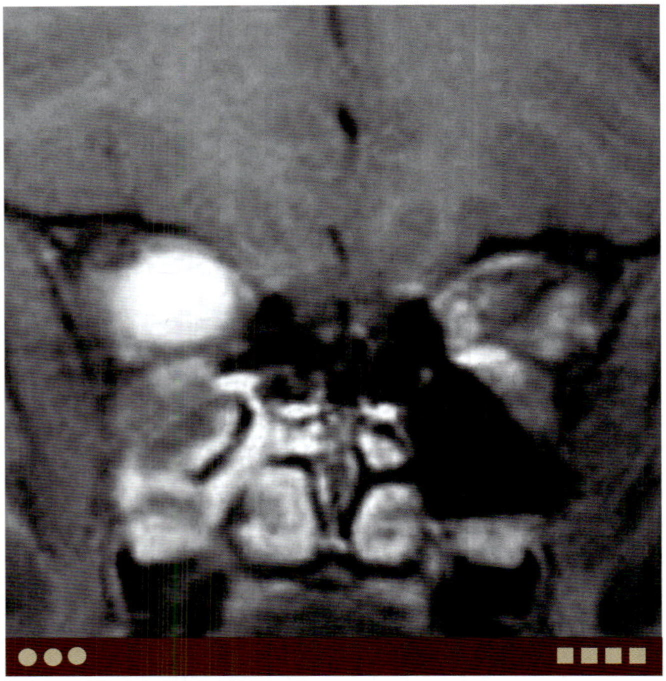

F. Optic glioma, same patient as E. Coronal postcontrast fat-suppressed T1W MR image shows avid enhancement of the lesion.

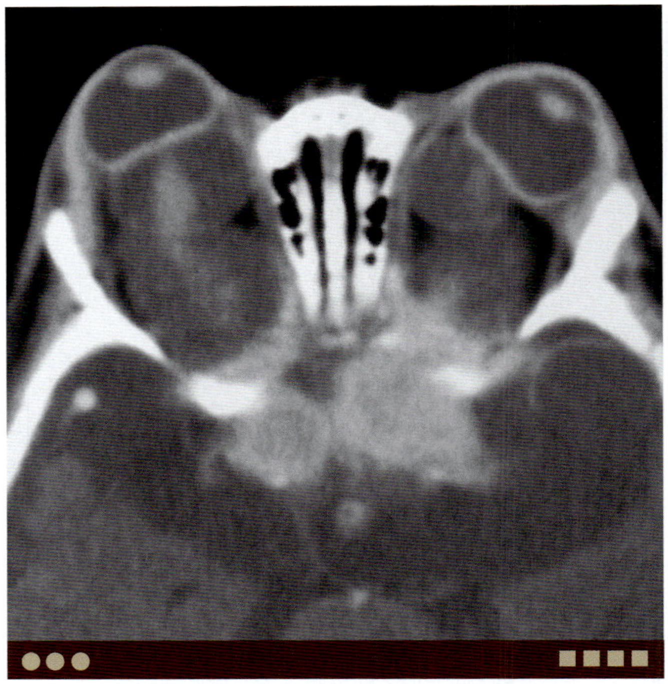

G. **Optic glioma** in a different patient. Axial contrast-enhanced CT shows tortuous, markedly enlarged bilateral optic nerves and chiasm demonstrating avid enhancement. Note the significant compression exerted on the posterior globes by the pseudo-CSF lesions.

DIFFERENTIAL DIAGNOSIS IMAGES (H-J)

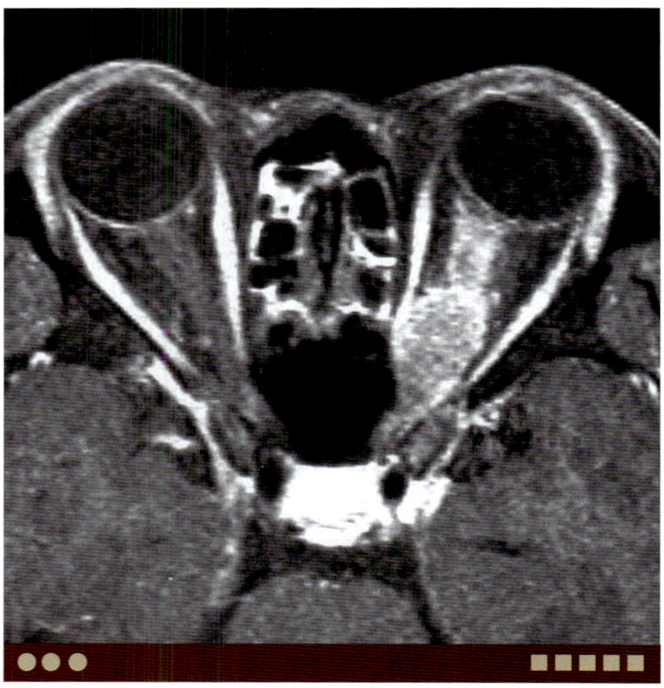

H. **Optic nerve sheath meningioma**. Axial contrast-enhanced fat-suppressed T1W MR image shows a well-defined tumor mass of the posterior left optic nerve sheath demonstrating "tram-track" enhancement.

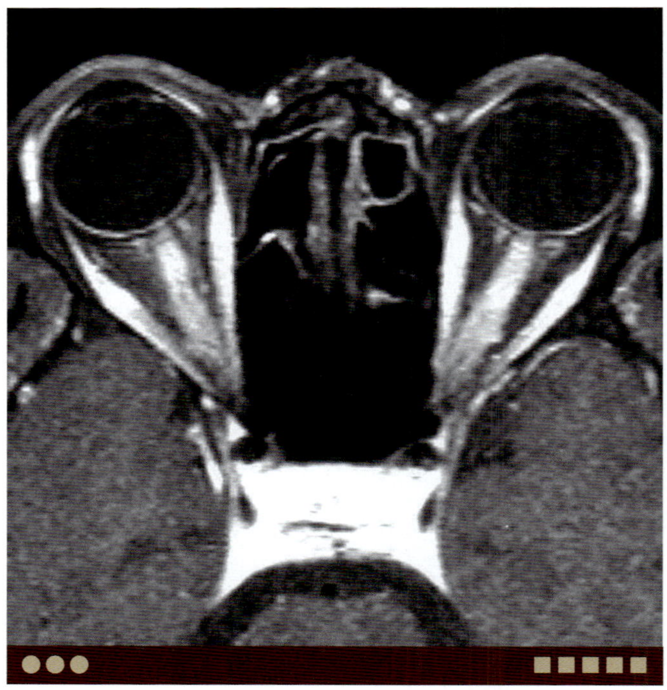

I. **Optic neuritis**. Axial contrast-enhanced fat-suppressed T1W MR image shows enhancement of the slightly enlarged optic nerves.

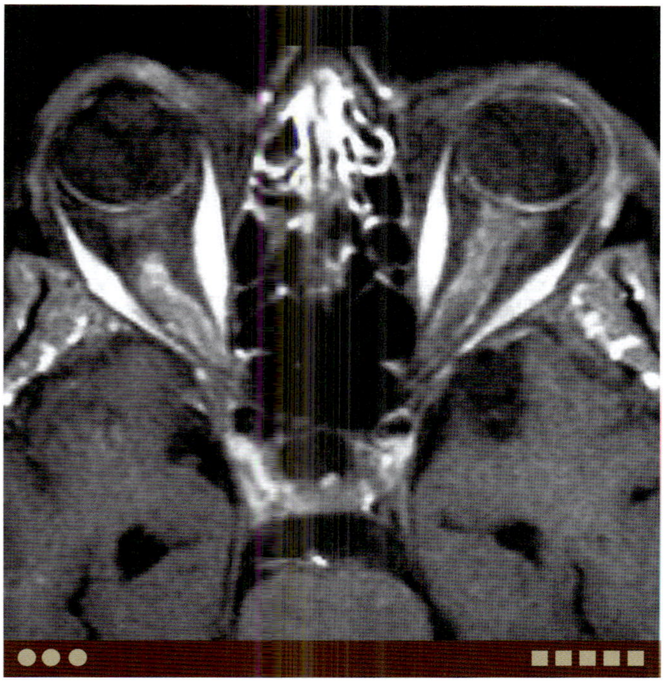

J. CSF dissemination of breast cancer. Axial contrast-enhanced fat-suppressed T1W MR images shows thickening of the optic nerve and sheath complex with peripheral enhancement.

Case 4-9 Optic Nerve Sheath Meningioma

Osamu Sakai, Brooke Devenney-Cakir

PRESENTATION

Decreased vision.

FINDINGS

CT and MRI demonstrate enlargement of the optic nerve sheath complex, often with calcification.

DIFFERENTIAL DIAGNOSIS

- Optic perineuritis: Enlarged enhancing optic nerve-sheath complex with inflammation involving other orbital structures. Additional findings include proptosis, diplopia, and restricted motility.
- Metastatic tumor, CSF dissemination: The optic nerve sheath is an extension of the dura which contains the CSF and susceptible to tumor implantation, most commonly due to malignancies from the breast and lung. Imaging findings may be similar to that of perineuritis, granulomatous diseases or meningioma.
- Sarcoidosis or other granulomatous disease: Granulomatous disease can involve the optic nerve and sheath complex and show similar findings to CSF tumor dissemination.
- Optic glioma: This causes enlargement and abnormal signal of the optic nerve itself rather than the optic nerve sheath. Calcifications are rare. Thirty to forty percent of patients have neurofibromatosis type I.
- Optic neuritis: This shows abnormal signal of the optic nerve. In actively demyelinating phase, the optic nerve demonstrates swelling and enhancement. Fifty to sixty percent of patients with optic neuritis ultimately develop multiple sclerosis. Also, this condition can be a part of manifestations of Devic's disease. In addition, ischemia can cause optic neuritis.

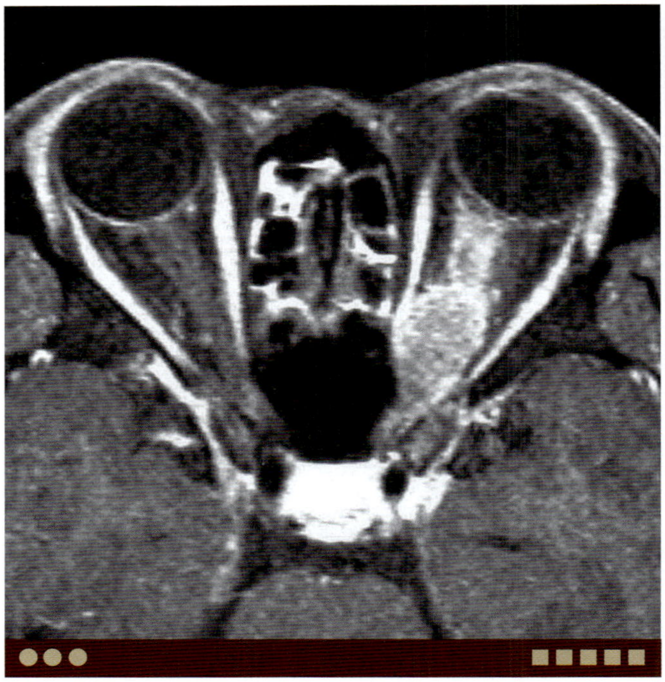

A. Optic nerve sheath meningioma. Axial postcontrast fat-suppressed T1W MR image demonstrates a fusiform-shaped lesion with peripheral enhancement. Note tram-track like enhancement extends to the optic nerve sheath anterior to the lesion.

COMMENTS

This is a 17-year-old girl presented with decreased vision.

Intraorbital meningioma can arise anywhere in the optic nerve sheath, but most commonly seen as orbital extension of the intracranial meningiomas. This is particularly true in adults, and typically seen in middle age women. On the other hand, primary optic nerve sheath meningioma is commonly seen in children and young adults.

Primary optic nerve sheath meningioma may be subdivided into two types: (1) long segment lesion resulting in tubular enlargement of the optic nerve sheath complex and (2) focal mass forming lesion, often at the orbital apex. Calcification is commonly seen and helpful to make the diagnosis, often demonstrating "tram-track appearance." After contrast, relatively homogeneous strong enhancement is seen in the lesion, sparing the optic nerve ("tram-track appearance") and is helpful to differentiate meningioma from optic glioma, in which the enlarged optic nerve enhances. However, peripheral enhancement is not pathognomonic for meningioma, and similar findings can

PEARLS

- **Intraorbital meningioma can arise anywhere in the optic nerve sheath, but most commonly seen as orbital extension of the intracranial meningiomas.**
- **Primary optic nerve sheath meningioma is often seen in children.**
- **Optic nerve sheath meningioma can be bilateral. Evaluation for contralateral as well as intracranial lesions is important.**

be seen in perineuritis, which can be a part of idiopathic orbital inflammation ("pseudotumor"), granulomatous disease, and CSF tumor dissemination.

Optic nerve sheath meningioma demonstrates isosignal intensity to the brain parenchyma both on T1W and T2W images and strong enhancement as intracranial meningioma. Precise evaluation for its extension is possible with postcontrast fat-suppressed T1W images, although careful evaluation is needed at the orbital apex because fat-suppressed images are often degraded by susceptibility artifacts due to air and bone interfaces. Bilateral involvement of the optic nerve sheath is not uncommon.

ADDITIONAL IMAGES (B-G)

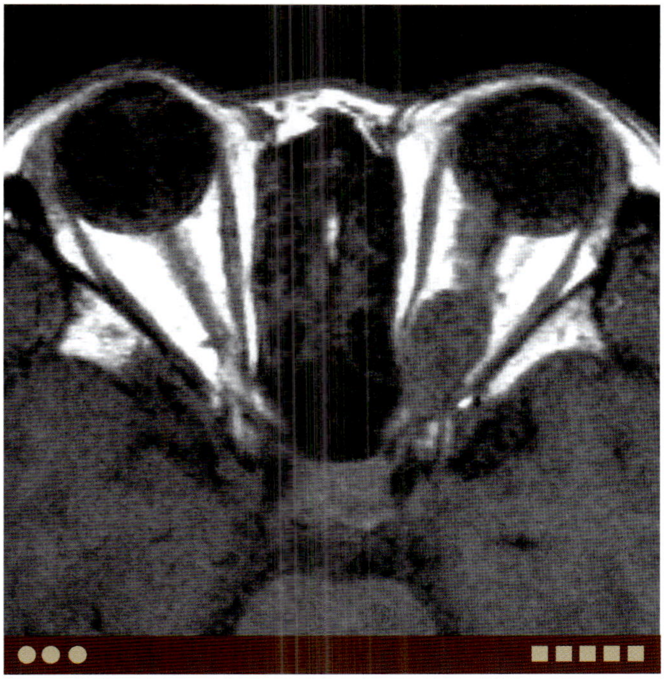

B. Optic nerve sheath meningioma, same patient as A. Axial T1W MR image demonstrates a fusiform-shaped low-signal lesion near the orbital apex with thickened optic nerve sheath complex anteriorly.

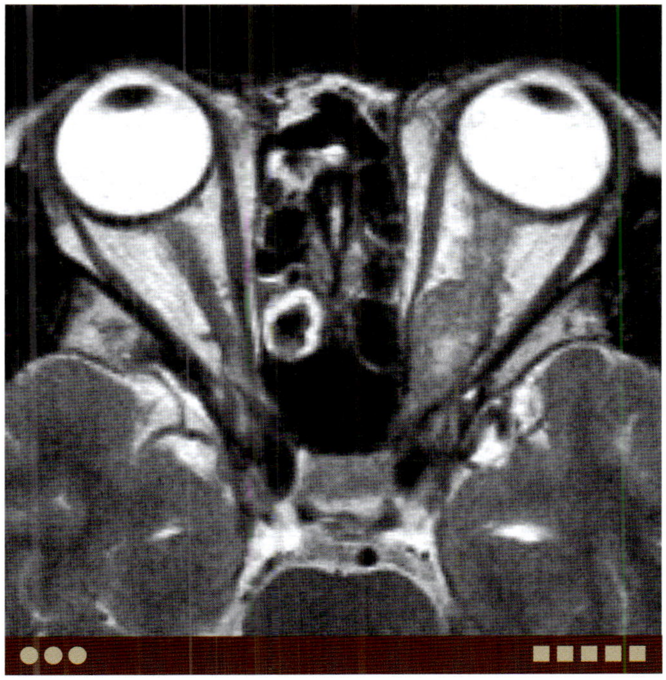

C. Optic nerve sheath meningioma, same patient as A. Axial T2W MR image demonstrates the lesion showing similar signal to the gray matter.

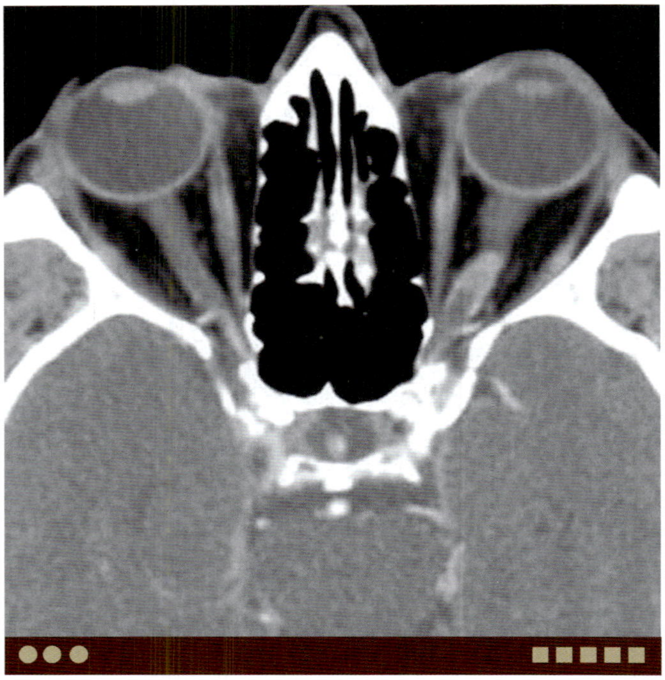

D. Optic nerve sheath meningioma in a different patient. Axial postcontrast CT demonstrates tram-track high density in the posterior portion of the intraorbital segment of the left optic nerve sheath. Note normal density of the optic nerve itself.

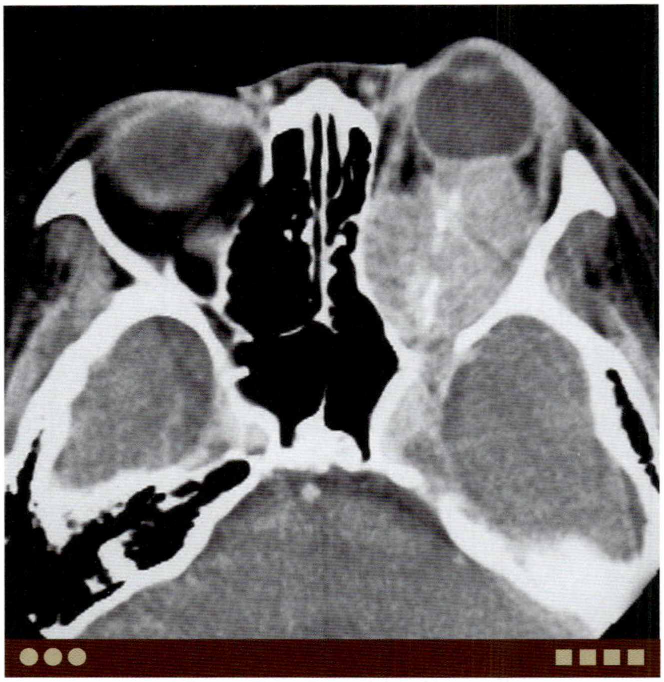

E. Optic nerve sheath meningioma in a different patient. Axial postcontrast CT demonstrates a large enhancing lesion in the retrobulbar space with central tram-track calcification. Left-sided proptosis is noted due to the mass-effect.

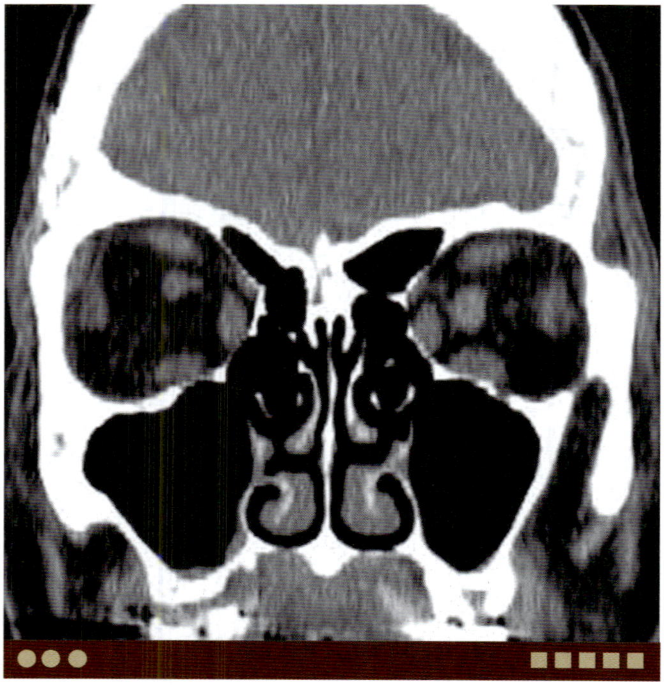

F. Optic nerve sheath meningioma in a different patient. Coronal noncontrast-enhanced CT demonstrates increased density and thickening of the left optic nerve and sheath complex.

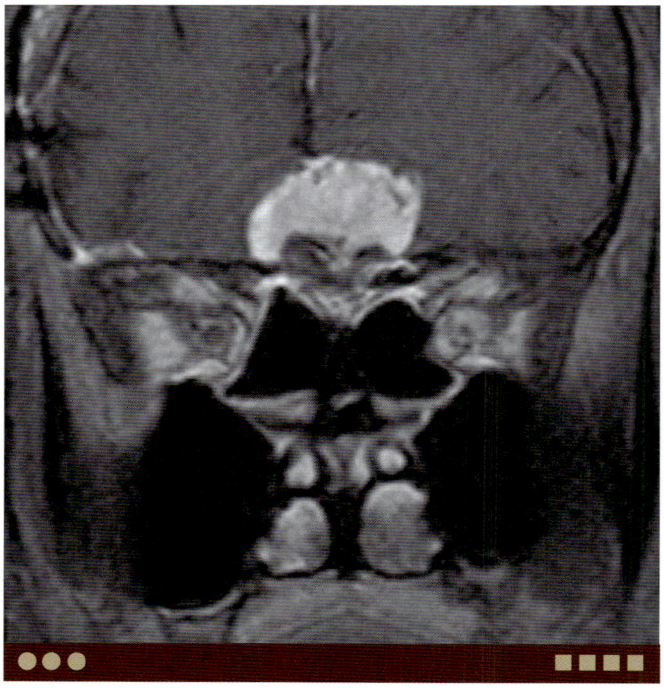

G. Bilateral optic nerve sheath and planum sphenoidale meningiomas, same patient as F. Coronal postcontrast fat-suppressed T1W image demonstrates enhancing thickened left optic nerve sheath squeezing the nerve as well as thin enhancement of the right optic nerve sheath. In addition, there is an enhancing dural based lesion in the anterior skull base with thickened bone ("blistering"), a typical finding for meningioma.

DIFFERENTIAL DIAGNOSIS IMAGES (H-J)

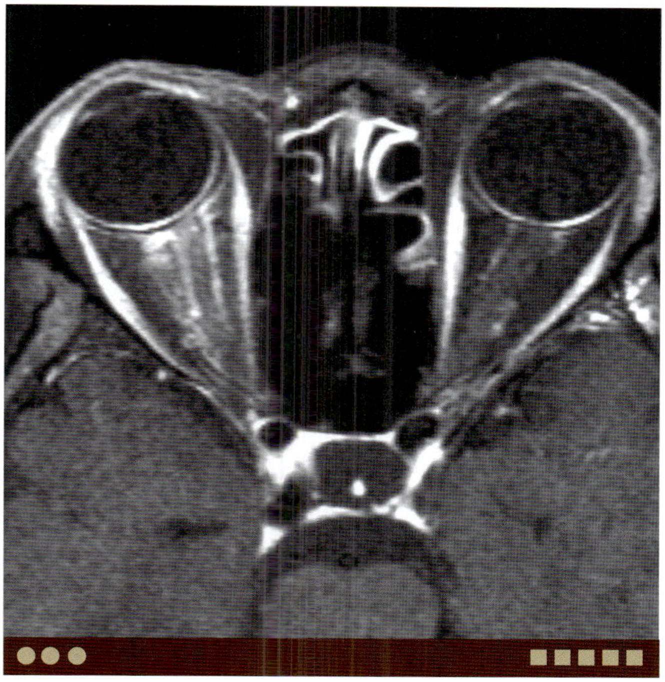

H. Perineuritis. Axial postcontrast fat-suppressed T1W MR image demonstrates peripheral enhancement of the right optic nerve sheath complex.

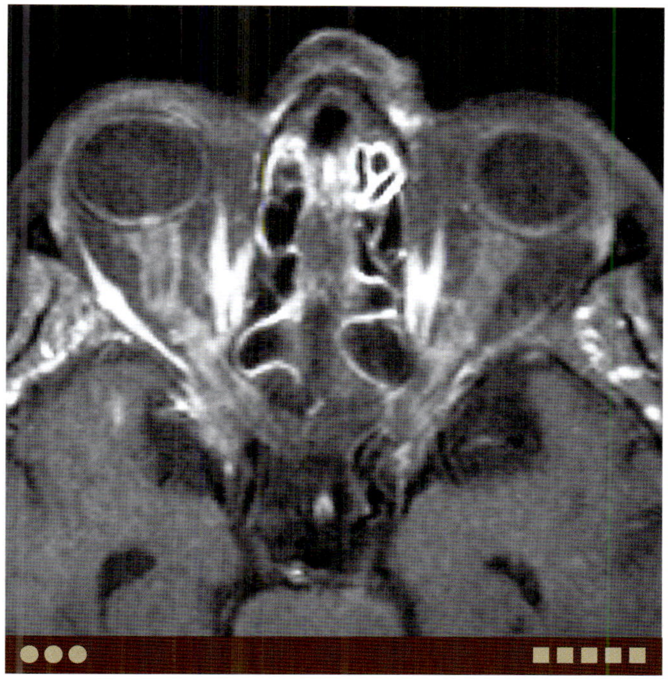

I. CSF tumor dissemination (breast cancer). Axial postcontrast fat-suppressed T1W MR image demonstrates peripheral enhancement of the right optic nerve sheath complex. Note faint enhancement along the left optic nerve sheath complex as well.

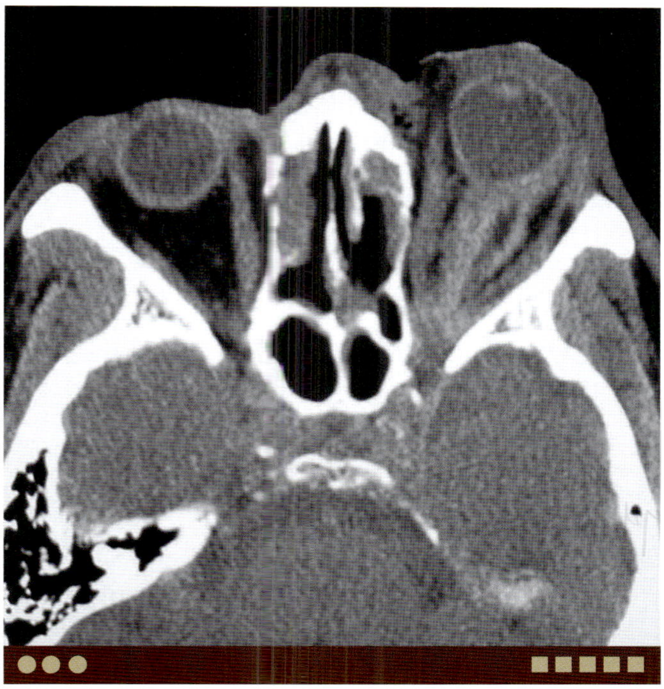

J. Optic nerve sheath hematoma. Axial noncontrast-enhanced CT demonstrates thickened left optic nerve sheath complex with increased density consistent with hemorrhage within the sheath.

Case 4–10 Optic Neuritis

Osamu Sakai, Bhavya Shah

PRESENTATION

Decreased vision.

FINDINGS

MRI demonstrates increased T2/STIR signal and enhancement of the optic nerve.

DIFFERENTIAL DIAGNOSIS

- Anterior ischemic optic neuropathy (AION): The patient population is elderly, usually male, with risk factors for ischemic disease elsewhere. MRI is normal in greater than 75% of patients with AION.
- Optic glioma: This is often associated with neurofibromatosis type 1, particularly when bilateral. This shows tubular enlarged enhancing optic nerves.
- Radiation-induced optic neuropathy: This shows similar appearance to usual optic neuritis. History of radiation is needed to be diagnosed.
- Optic perineuritis: Enlarged enhancing optic nerve-sheath complex with inflammation involving other orbital structures. Additional findings include proptosis, diplopia, and restricted motility.
- Meningioma: This is a histologically benign tumor; however, it is a serious disease when it involves the optic nerve sheath. Thickened enhancing optic nerve sheath with "tram-track appearance" often with calcifications is a typical finding.
- Metastatic tumor (CSF tumor dissemination): Because the optic nerve sheath is an extension of the dura, CSF tumor dissemination involves the optic nerve sheath complex and shows similar findings to optic perineuritis.

COMMENTS

This is a 45-year-old man presented with decreased vision.

The usual presentation of optic neuritis (ON) is a young-middle aged woman who presents with acute decrease in vision and pain with eye movement.

Acute optic neuritis can be subdivided into two types, multiple sclerosis (MS) associated ON, and idiopathic isolated monosymptomatic ON. Studies have identified that 50% to 70% of ON patients eventually develop MS, and in patients who have MS, 15% to 30% initially present with ON; hence imaging of the brain is important to evaluate for MS. Devic's disease is another type of demyelinating disease which preferably involves the optic nerve and spinal cord.

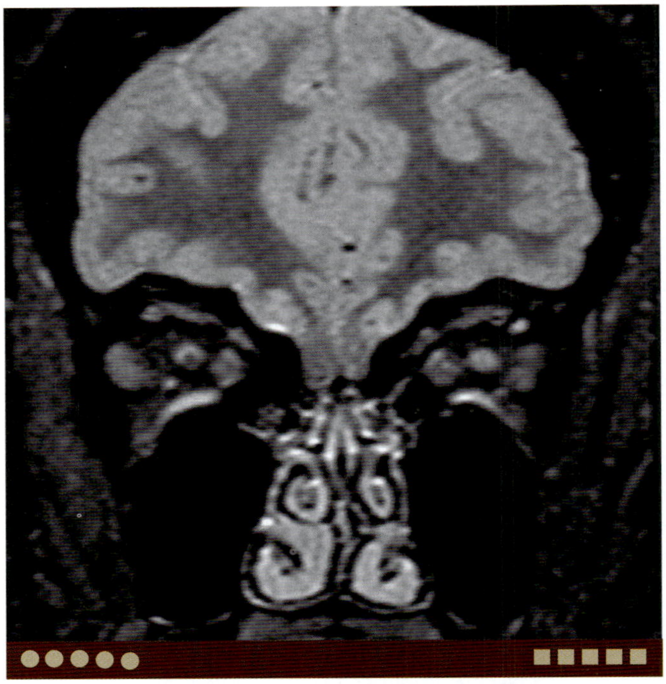

A. Optic neuritis. Coronal STIR image demonstrates increased signal of the left optic nerve.

MRI examination usually demonstrates a minimally enlarged enhancing optic nerve in the active phase. The majority of cases involve the mid-intraorbital segment of the optic nerve followed by the anterior intraoribital segment. Greater than 70% are unilateral and greater than 90% show optic nerve enhancement.

STIR sequence is a standard sequence to evaluate for optic nerve pathologies because inflammatory or demyelinating lesions demonstrate increased signal when compared to the brain white matter or extraocular muscle. Abnormal STIR signal is seen in both the acute phase and chronic phase, therefore, contrast-enhanced study with fat-suppression is needed to determine activity. Chronic ON shows high T2/STIR signal without enhancement, often with decreased caliber.

PEARLS

- **Optic neuritis is often seen as primary or secondary manifestation of multiple sclerosis.**
- **STIR sequence is very helpful and standard sequence to evaluate for optic nerve pathologies.**
- **Contrast enhancement using fat-suppressed technique is necessary to determine activity of the lesion.**

ADDITIONAL IMAGES (B-G)

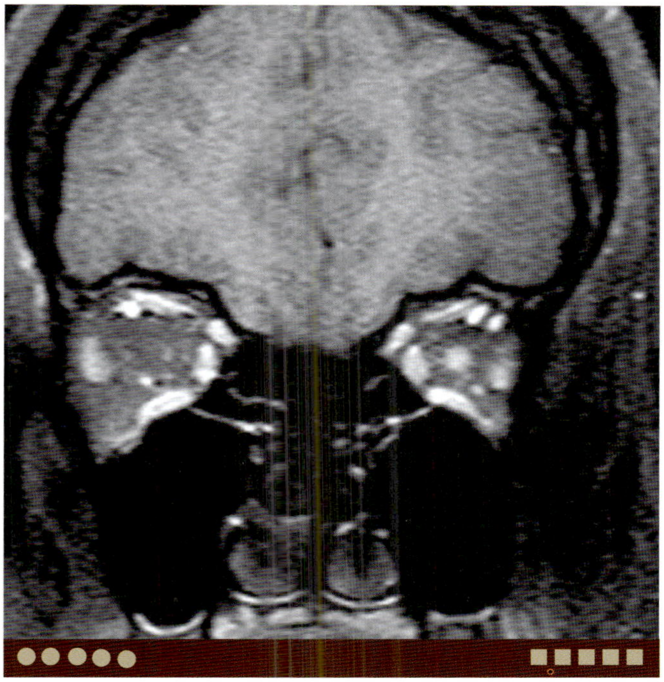

B. Optic neuritis, same patient as A. Coronal postcontrast fat-suppressed T1W image demonstrates abnormal enhancement of the left optic nerve, consistent with active demyelinating process.

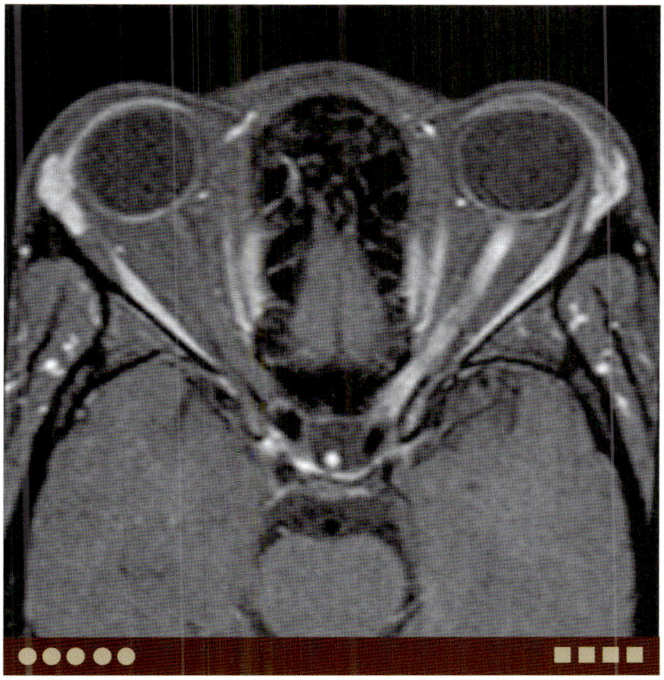

C. Optic neuritis, same patient as A. Axial postcontrast fat-suppressed T1W MR image demonstrates long segment enhancement of the left optic nerve.

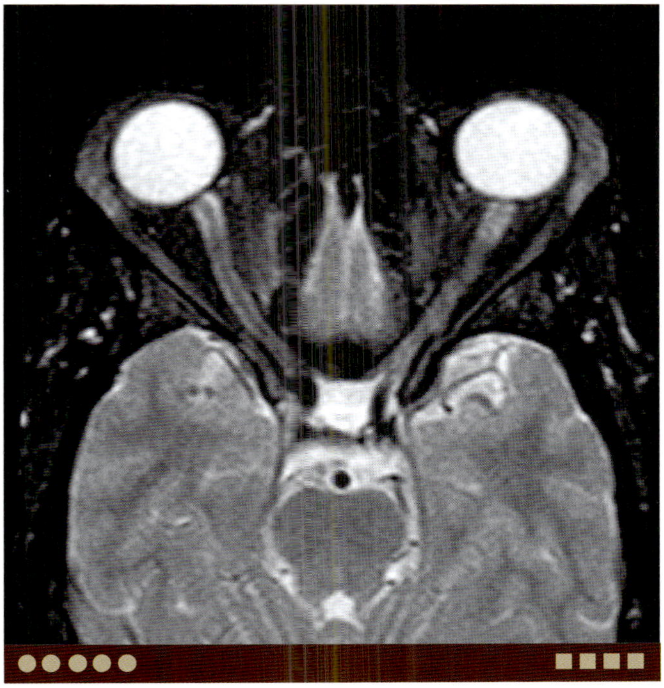

D. Optic neuritis, same patient as A. Axial T2W image demonstrates swelling of the left optic nerve.

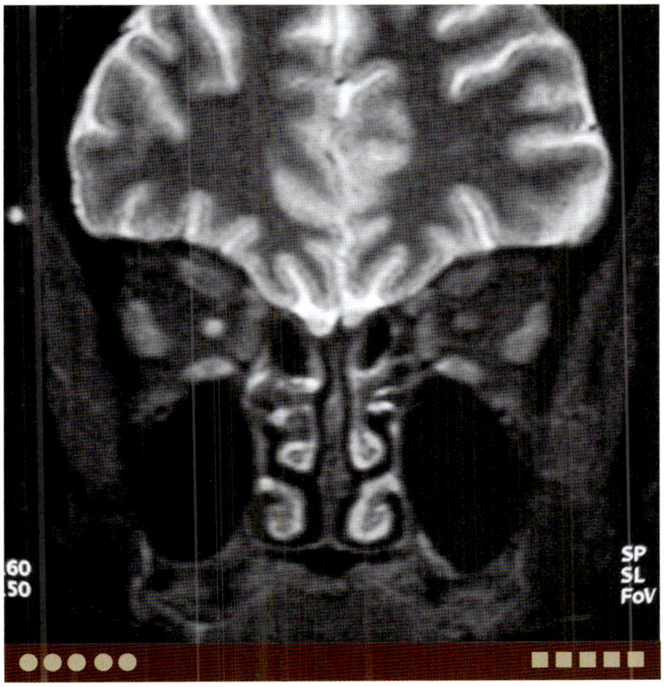

E. Optic neuritis, chronic. Coronal STIR image demonstrates increased signal of the right optic nerve.

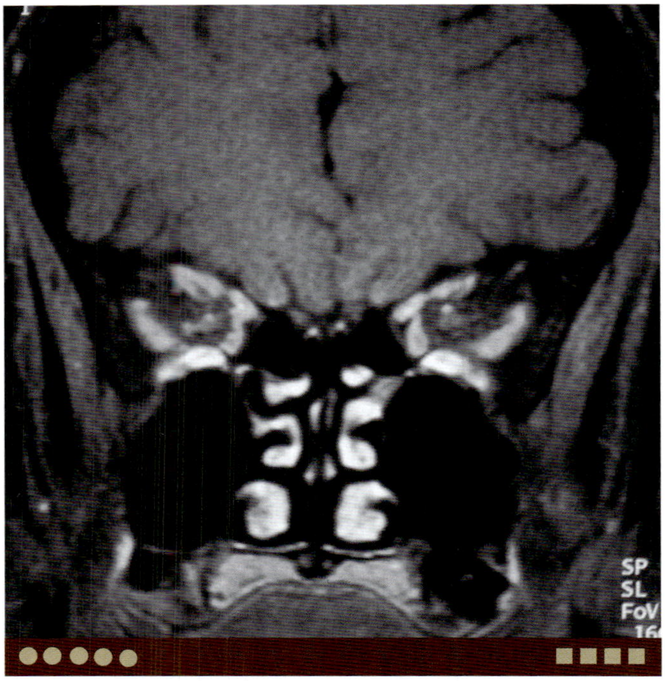

F. Optic neuritis, chronic, same patient as E. Coronal postcontrast fat-suppressed T1W image demonstrates no enhancement in the optic nerve.

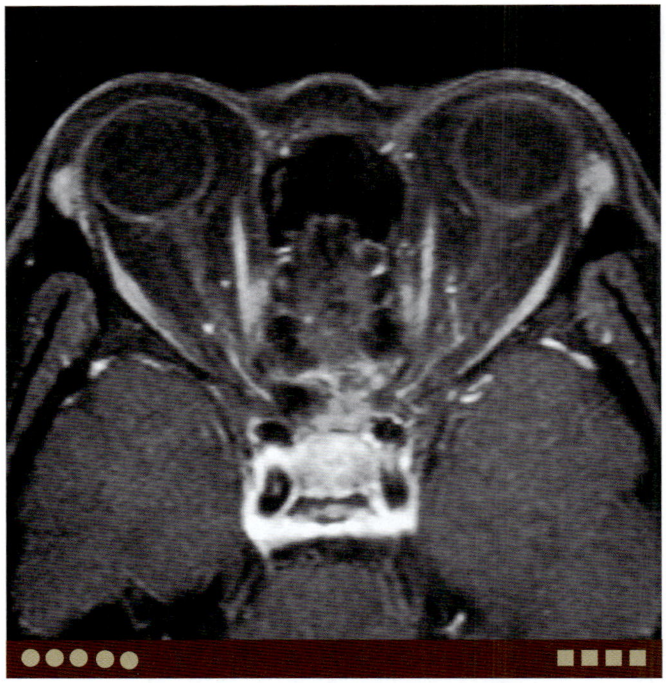

G. Optic neuritis, chronic, same patient as E. Axial postcontrast fat-suppressed T1W image demonstrates no enhancement in the optic nerve.

DIFFERENTIAL DIAGNOSIS IMAGES (H-J)

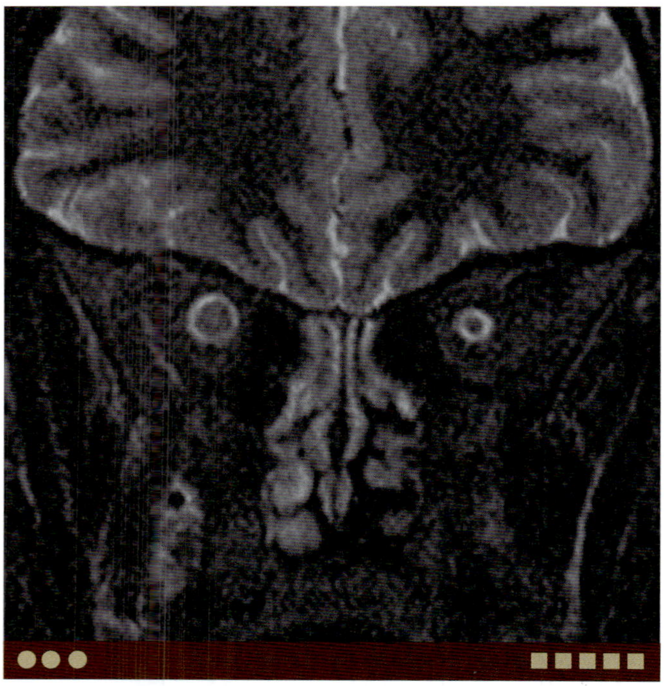

H. **Optic glioma**. Coronal STIR image demonstrates enlarged right optic nerve showing increased signal.

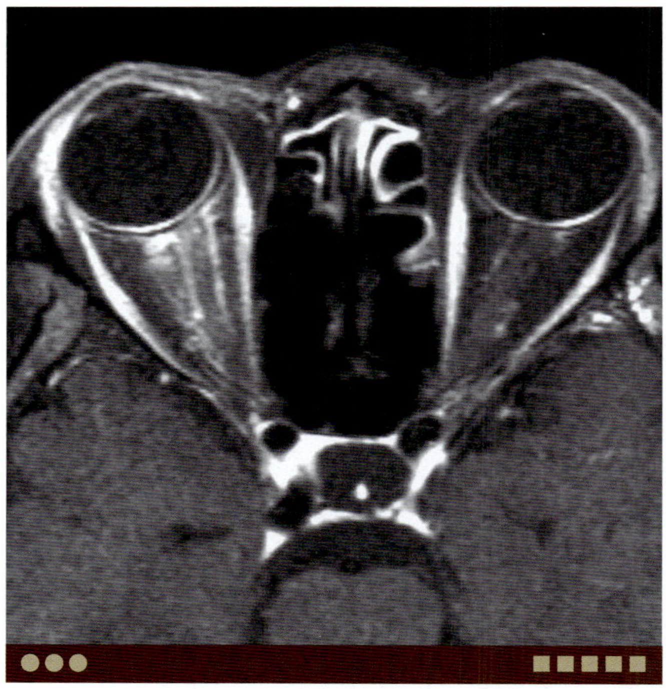

I. **Optic perineuritis.** Axial postcontrast fat-suppressed T1W image demonstrates tram-track-like peripheral enhancement of the right optic nerve sheath complex.

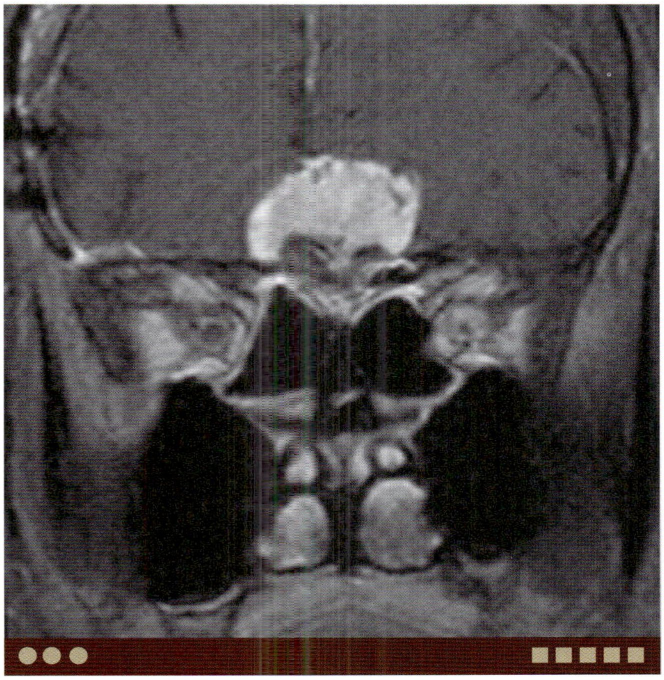

J. Optic nerve sheath meningioma. Coronal postcontrast fat-suppressed T1W image demonstrates peripheral enhancement of the optic nerve sheath complex, left greater than right. Note a large planum sphenoidale meningioma.

Case 4–11 Optic Perineuritis

Osamu Sakai, Bhavya Shah

PRESENTATION

Eye pain with decreased visual acuity.

FINDINGS

MRI demonstrates enlargement of the optic nerve sheath complex with peripheral enhancement.

DIFFERENTIAL DIAGNOSIS

- Sarcoidosis or other granulomatous disease: Granulomatous disease can involve the optic nerve sheath complex and show similar findings to perineuritis.
- Optic neuritis: This may be a part of manifestations of multiple sclerosis or Devic's disease. Minimally enlarged optic nerve with enhancement is seen in the active phase. Abnormal signal and enhancement is seen in the optic nerve center of the nerve sheath complex, not peripheral.
- Metastatic tumor (CSF tumor dissemination): Because the optic nerve sheath is an extension of the dura, CSF tumor dissemination involves the optic nerve sheath complex and shows similar findings to optic perineuritis.
- Meningioma: This is a histologically benign tumor; however, it is a serious disease when it involves the optic nerve sheath. Thickened enhancing optic nerve sheath with "tram-track appearance" often with calcification is a typical finding.

COMMENTS

This is a 50-year-old man presented with eye pain and decreased vision.

The usual presentation of optic perineuritis is a middle aged man who presents with painful proptosis, restricted motility, diplopia, and decrease in visual acuity. Optic perineuritis is an uncommon presentation of idiopathic orbital inflammatory syndrome and the inflammation typically involves other orbital structures, such as the lacrimal gland and extraocular muscles. Lymphoma may involve the optic nerve sheath complex and show similar findings. Granulomatous disease, such as sarcoidosis and Wegener's granulomatosis may demonstrate similar findings to optic perineuritis.

CT and MRI demonstrate enlargement of the optic nerve sheath complex with peripheral enhancement, enhancement of the sheath, not optic nerve itself.

Fat-suppressed T2W or STIR images and postcontrast fat-suppressed T1W images demonstrate peripheral high signal with enhancement while the signal of the optic nerve is preserved.

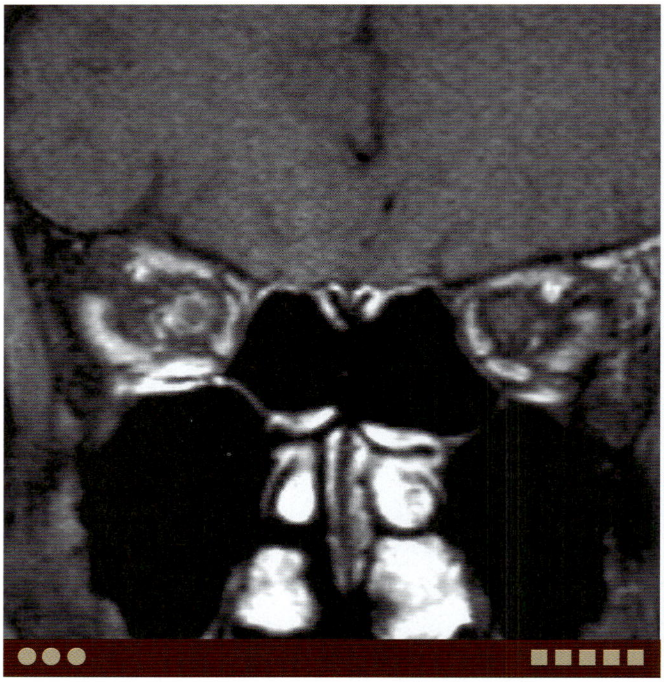

A. Optic perineuritis. Coronal postcontrast fat-suppressed T1W MR image demonstrates peripheral enhancement of the right optic nerve sheath complex.

PEARLS

- **Optic perineuritis is an unusual presentation of idiopathic orbital inflammatory syndrome.**
- **Abnormal signal and enhancement is seen in the optic nerve sheath. The signal of the optic nerve is preserved.**

ADDITIONAL IMAGES (B-D)

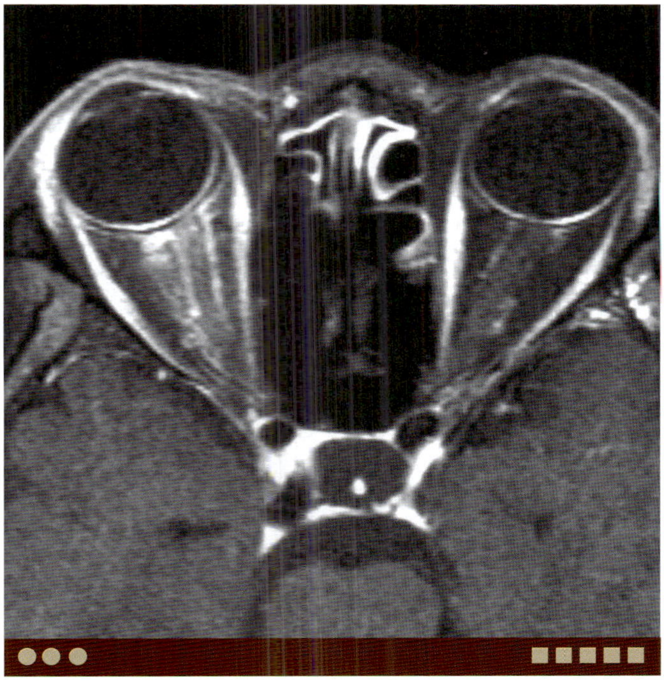

B. Optic perineuritis, same patient as A. Axial postcontrast fat-suppressed T1W MR image demonstrates tram-track-like peripheral enhancement of the right optic nerve sheath complex.

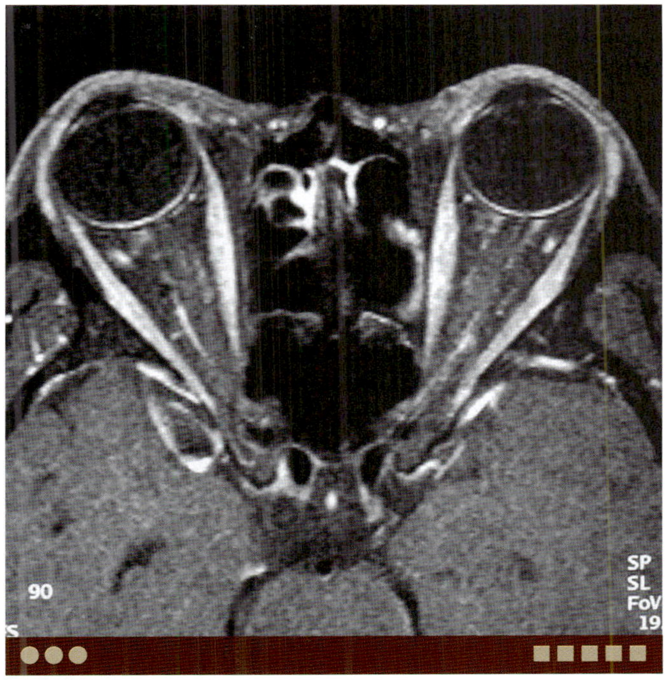

C. **Optic perineuritis** in a different patient. Axial postcontrast fat-suppressed T1W MR image demonstrates tram-track-like peripheral enhancement of the optic nerve sheath complex bilaterally.

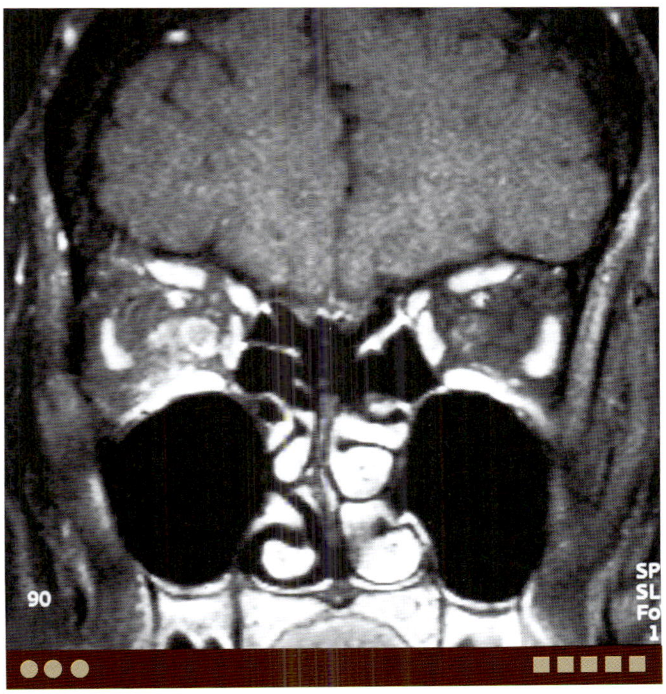

D. **Optic perineuritis** in a different patient. Coronal postcontrast fat-suppressed T1W MR image demonstrates thick peripheral enhancement of the right optic nerve sheath complex.

DIFFERENTIAL DIAGNOSIS IMAGES (E-G)

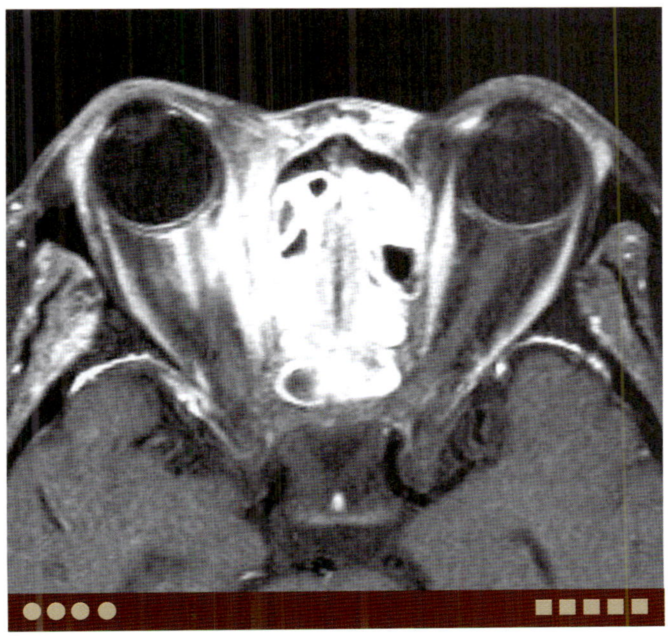

E. **Wegener's granulomatosis.** Coronal postcontrast fat-suppressed T1W MR image demonstrates tram-track-like peripheral enhancement of the right optic nerve sheath complex as well as abnormal enhancement involving the right medial rectus muscle and bilateral ethmoid air cells.

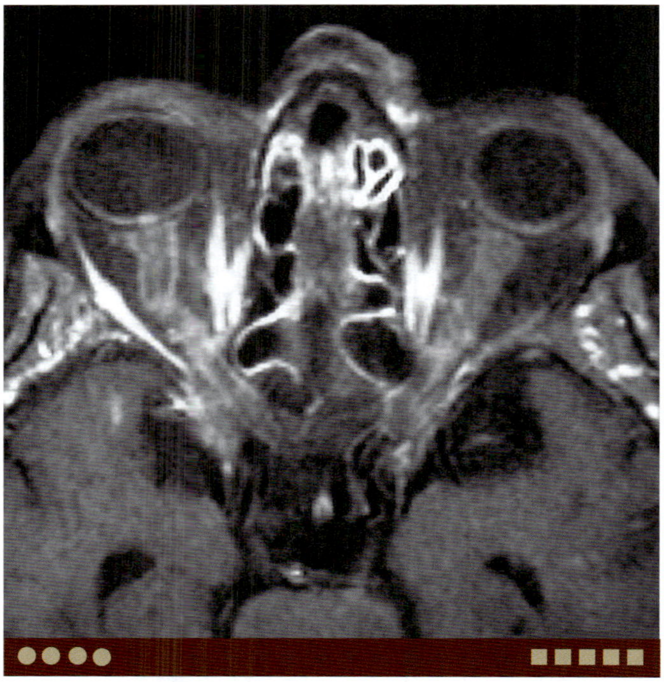

F. CSF tumor dissemination (breast cancer). Axial postcontrast fat-suppressed T1W MR image demonstrates peripheral enhancement of the right optic nerve sheath complex. Note faint enhancement along the left optic nerve sheath complex as well.

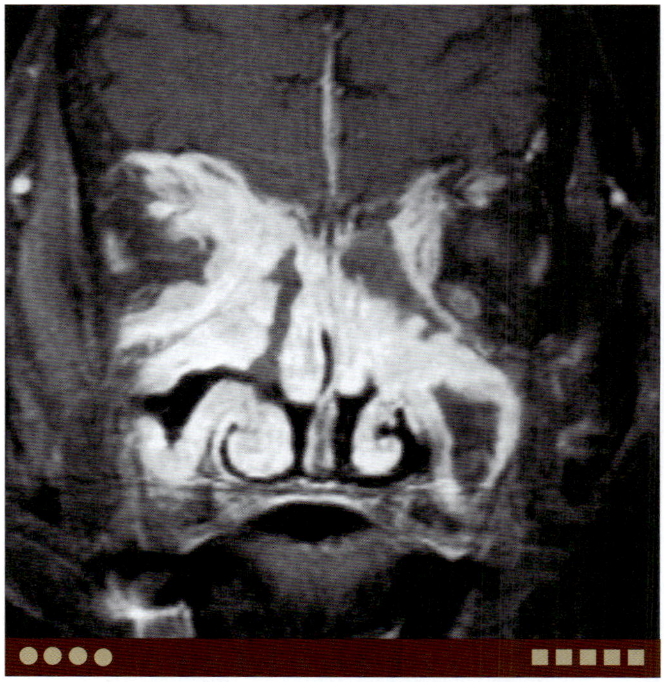

G. Lymphoma. Coronal postcontrast fat-suppressed T1W MR image demonstrates abnormal enhancement of the right optic nerve sheath in addition to diffuse enhancement in the bilateral orbits and paranasal sinuses. Note abnormal dural enhancement along the falx.

Case 4–12 Idiopathic Orbital Inflammation (Orbital Inflammatory Pseudotumor)

Osamu Sakai, Memi Watanabe

PRESENTATION

Eye pain and proptosis.

FINDINGS

CT and MRI demonstrate enlargement of the lateral rectus muscle and proptosis.

DIFFERENTIAL DIAGNOSIS

- Graves disease: This is the most common cause of exophthalmos. Radiological findings of this condition include enlargement of the extraocular muscles and lacrimal glands, and increase in volume and edema of the intraorbital fat. The inferior and medial rectus muscles are more commonly affected, however, their tendinous insertions tend to be spared.
- Sarcoidosis: Imaging findings of sarcoidosis are often similar to other inflammatory, granulomatous diseases, and neoplastic conditions, including idiopathic orbital inflammation (IOI), Wegener's granulomatosis, and lymphoma. The lacrimal gland is most commonly affected.
- Wegener's granulomatosis: This condition commonly affects men in their fifth decade with airway and renal involvement. This also presents with infiltration of the orbital soft tissues, mostly secondary to sinonasal involvement. Imaging findings are similar to IOI. Intracranial involvement is seen occasionally.
- Lymphoma: Imaging findings of lymphoma and other lymphoid tumors are similar to IOI and sarcoidosis. Histological diagnosis is required for differentiation.
- Leukemia: This rarely affects the orbit, however, it can present as orbital infiltration, involving the orbital fat, lacrimal glands and extraocular muscles.

COMMENTS

This is a 40-year-old woman with eye pain and proptosis.

Idiopathic orbital inflammation (IOI), also known as orbital inflammatory pseudotumor, is a non-granulomatous orbital inflammatory disorder of unknown etiology. This is the second most common cause of exophthalmos after Graves disease. In the acute phase, eye pain, swelling of the eyelids, proptosis, diplopia, and decrease in visual acuity can be seen. The lacrimal gland is often involved, however, IOI occurs anywhere in the orbit, and often also involves the extraocular muscles, intraorbital fat, optic nerve sheath complex, eyelid, and sclera. There is no specific imaging finding.

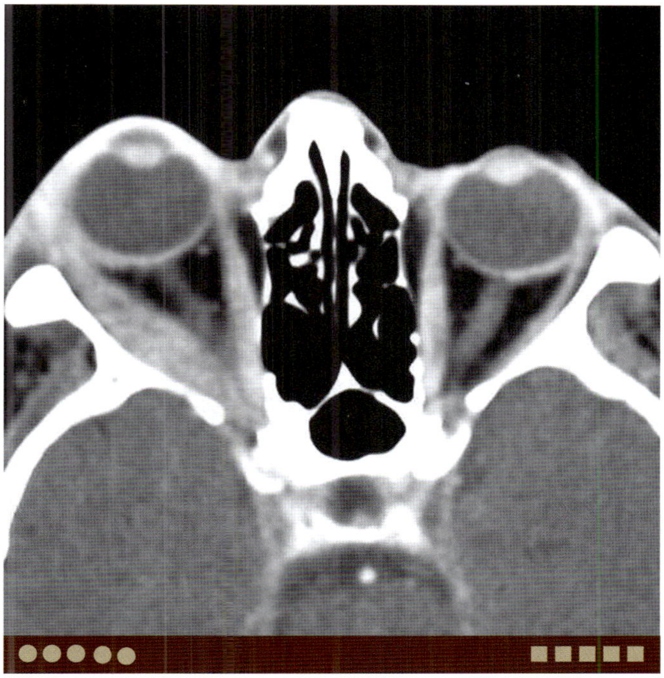

A. IOI. Axial contrast-enhanced CT demonstrates proptosis with enlargement and enhancement of the right lateral rectus muscle. Note tendinous insertion is also involved.

Extraocular muscle involvement can include single or multiple muscles, and can be unilateral or bilateral. IOI usually does not spare the tendinous insertions. The superior and lateral rectus muscles are often involved, which is different from Graves disease which typically involves the inferior and medial rectus muscles with sparing of the

PEARLS

- **Imaging findings of IOI are variable and nonspecific. IOI often involves the lacrimal gland, extraocular muscles, intraorbital fat, optic nerve sheath complex, eyelid, and sclera.**
- **Extraocular muscle involvement by IOI is often seen in the superior and lateral rectus muscles.**
- **Optic perineuritis has similar clinical symptoms to posterior scleritis, and may be a part of IOI.**
- **Abnormal signal and enhancement may be seen in the optic nerve sheath. The signal of the optic nerve is preserved.**

tendinous insertions. Mass formation and diffuse infiltration are also common. True neoplastic processes, such as lymphoma, should be always included in the differential diagnosis. Sarcoidosis and Wegener's granulomatosis demonstrate similar imaging findings as well.

Signal intensity of IOI on MRI is very variable and nonspecific. It usually shows low-signal intensity on T1W images, low- to high-signal intensity on T2W images, and moderate-to-strong enhancement following contrast administration. High T2 signal and strong enhancement suggest a better response to therapy. If the optic nerve sheath complex is involved, MR images usually demonstrate similar findings to perineuritis, with abnormal enhancement of the optic nerve sheath and preservation of the optic nerve signal.

ADDITIONAL IMAGES (B-G)

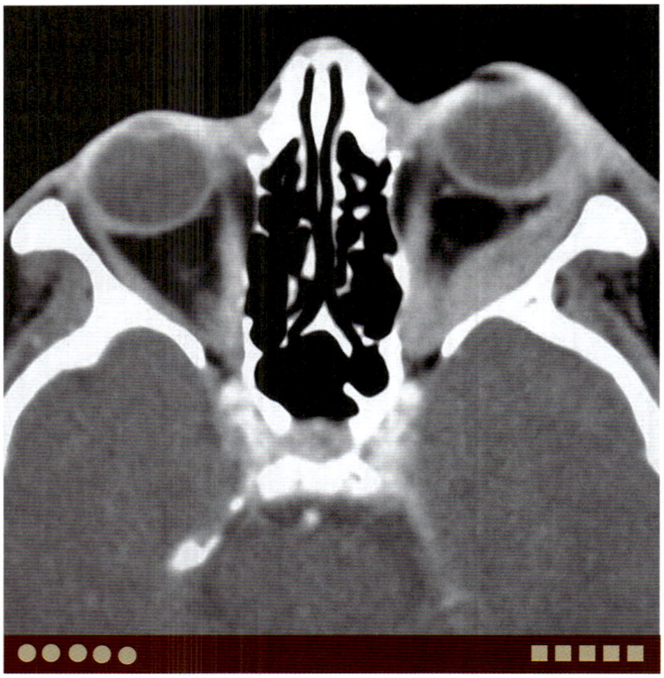

B. **IOI** in a different patient. Axial contrast-enhanced CT demonstrates proptosis with enlargement and enhancement of the left lateral rectus muscle with tendinous insertion involvement. Note periorbital soft tissue swelling.

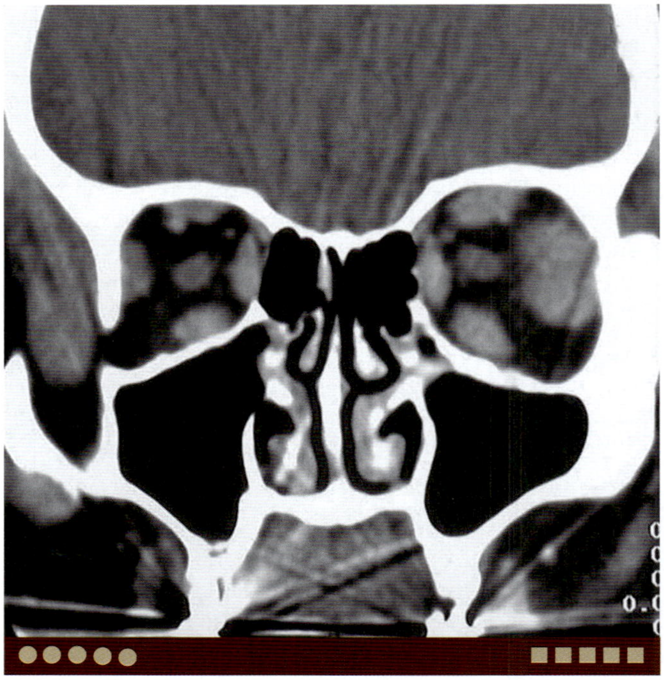

C. IOI, same patient as B. Coronal contrast-enhanced CT demonstrates enlargement of the left lateral rectus muscle.

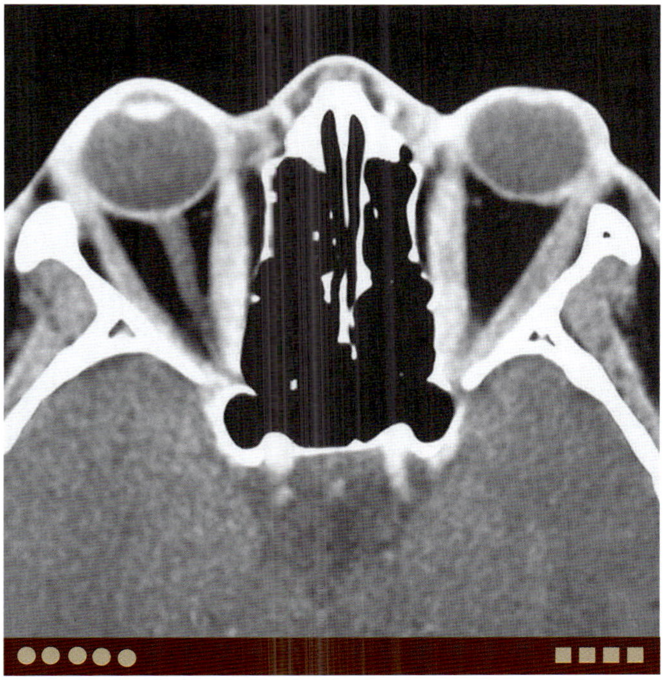

D. **IOI** in a different patient. Axial contrast-enhanced CT demonstrates diffuse enlargement and enhancement of the medial and lateral rectus muscles with tendinous insertion involvement.

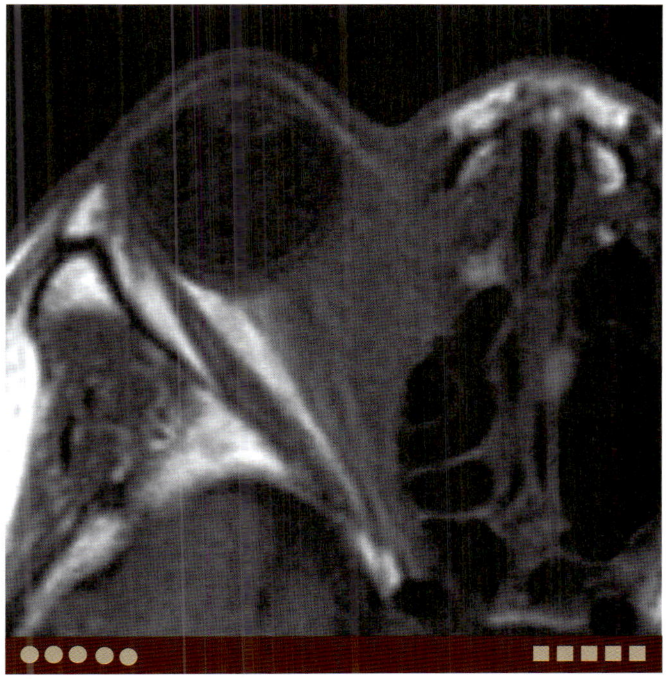

E. **IOI** in a different patient. Axial T1W image demonstrates proptosis with diffuse medial infiltration involving the right medial rectus muscle and optic nerve sheath complex.

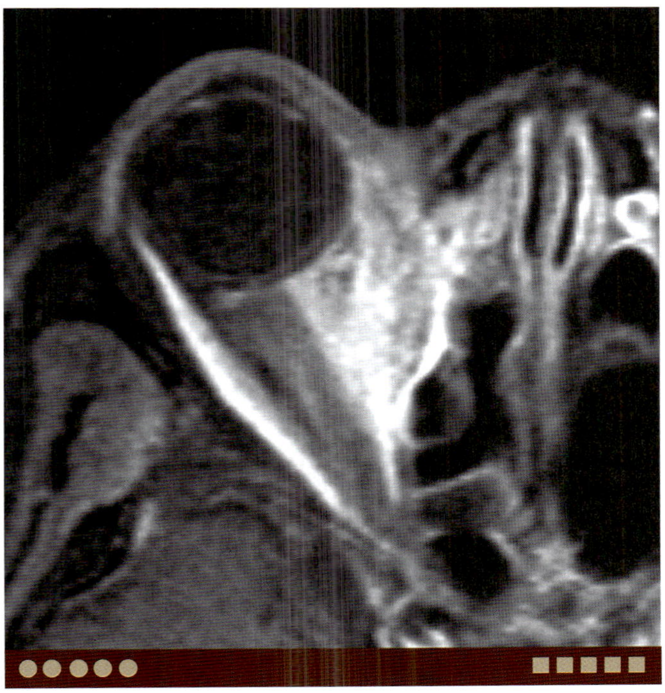

F. IOI, same patient as E. Axial postcontrast fat-suppressed T1W image demonstrates diffuse enhancement of the medial orbit, however, signal of the optic nerve is preserved.

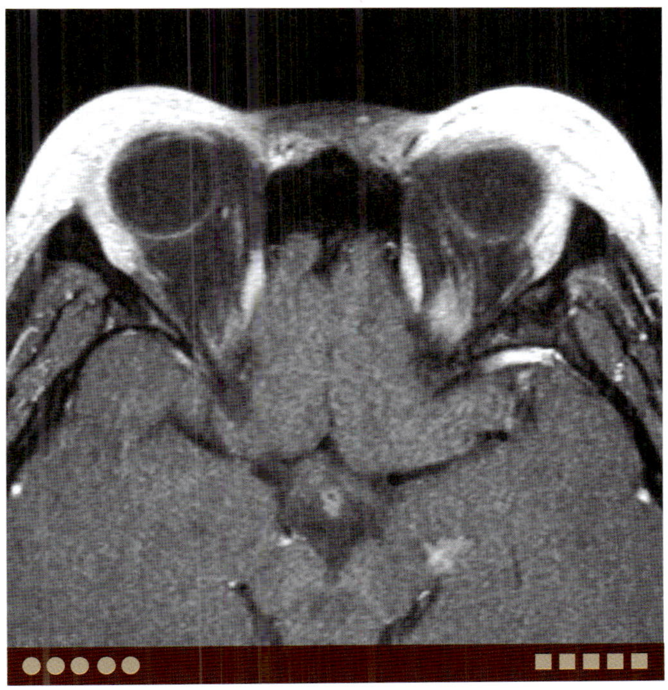

G. **IOI** in a different patient. Axial postcontrast fat-suppressed T1W image demonstrates marked swelling and enhancement of the periorbital soft tissues and lacrimal glands bilaterally.

DIFFERENTIAL DIAGNOSIS IMAGES (H-J)

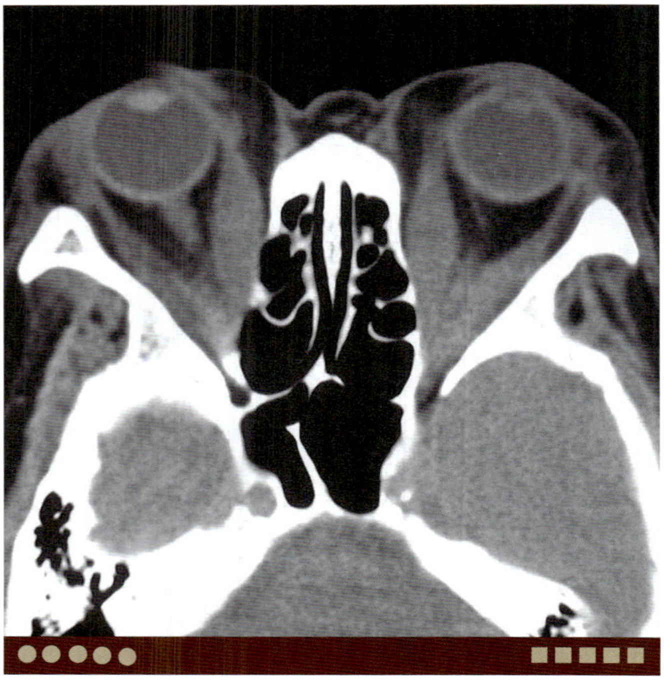

H. Thyroid orbitopathy. Axial CT demonstrates swelling of the bilateral extraocular muscles with sparing of the tendinous insertions.

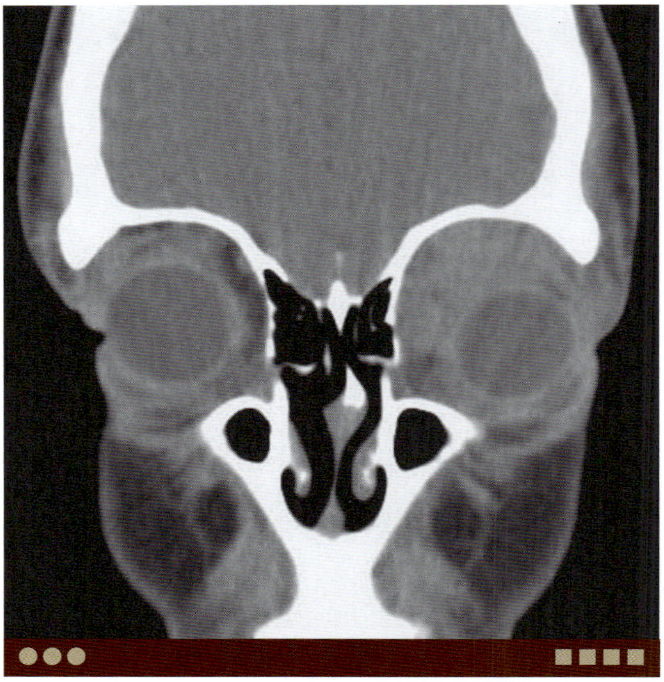

I. Sarcoidosis. Coronal CT demonstrates an ill-defined soft-tissue lesion in the superior left orbit displacing the globe inferiorly.

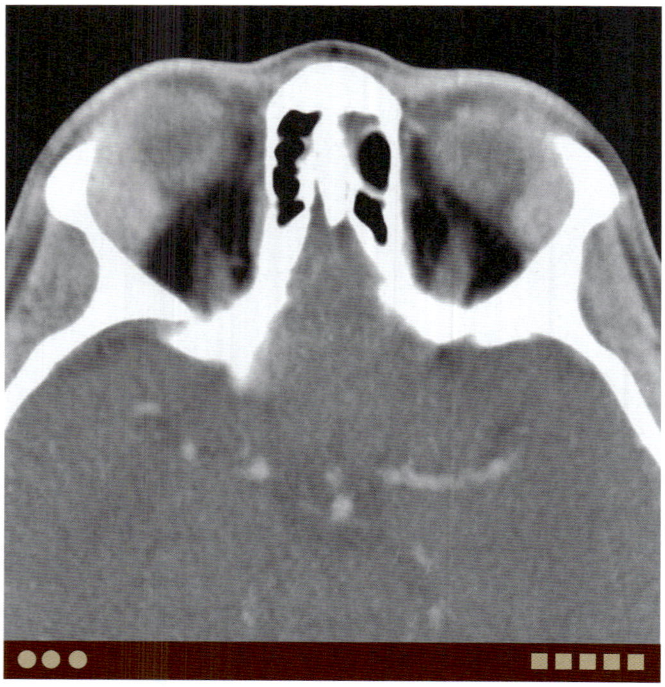

J. Wegener's granulomatosis. Axial contrast-enhanced CT demonstrates enlargement and abnormal enhancement of the lacrimal glands bilaterally.

Case 4–13 Carotid Cavernous Fistula

Memi Watanabe, Margaret Chapman, Osamu Sakai

PRESENTATION

Proptosis.

FINDINGS

CT and MRI demonstrate enlargement of the superior ophthalmic vein.

DIFFERENTIAL DIAGNOSIS

- Graves disease: This is the most common cause of proptosis. Imaging findings include enlargement of the extraocular muscles and edema within the retrobulbar fat. Dilatation of the superior ophthalmic vein may occur secondary to the enlarged extraocular muscles (EOMs).
- Idiopathic orbital inflammation (IOI) ("pseudotumor"): This is the second most common cause of proptosis. Imaging findings of IOI are variable and nonspecific, including enlargement of the EOMs and lacrimal glands, and ill-defined soft tissue density within the retrobulbar fat.
- Obstruction of cavernous sinus: Cavernous sinus thrombosis, cavernous sinus tumors such as meningioma or lymphoma, or cavernous sinus inflammation including Tolosa-Hunt syndrome can cause obstruction of the cavernous sinus resulting in dilatation of the superior ophthalmic vein and congestive enlargement of the EOMs.

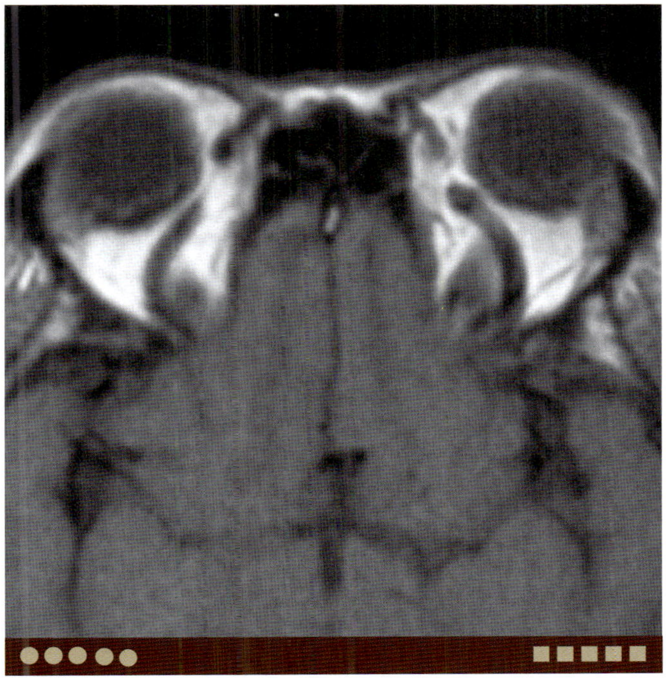

A. CCF. Axial T1W image demonstrates enlargement of the superior ophthalmic veins bilaterally.

COMMENTS

This is a 46-year-old woman presenting with proptosis.

Carotid cavernous fistula (CCF) is a condition characterized by shunt formation between the internal carotid artery and the cavernous sinus, and can be divided into direct and indirect types. The direct type demonstrates direct communication between these structures, and is often secondary to trauma or aneurysm rupture. The indirect type is shunting via dural arteriovenous fistula and is often idiopathic. The symptoms are less severe when compared with the direct type. The indirect type is further divided into three types; fistula formations via: (1) dural branches of the internal carotid artery, (2) dural branches of the external carotid artery, and (3) dural branches of both internal and external carotid arteries. The third type is the most common.

CT and MRI demonstrate dilatation of the cavernous sinus and superior ophthalmic vein. Since the right and left cavernous sinuses are contiguous, findings can be seen bilaterally, however, there is often some laterality. MRI can also show abnormal flow-voids within the cavernous sinus due to high-velocity inflow. The secondary findings seen on CT and MRI include enlargement of the EOMs, edema and congestion of the intraorbital fat. Dilatation of the superior ophthalmic vein may be a nonspecific finding and may not be apparent in some cases, therefore, when given an appropriate clinical history, careful evaluation for the secondary signs is important in making the diagnosis. In a case with a large fistula, abnormal flow-related signal can be seen in the cavernous sinus and superior ophthalmic vein on MRA. Catheter angiogram is often required to confirm the diagnosis.

PEARLS

- **Dilatation of the superior ophthalmic vein and cavernous sinus are typical findings for CCF.**
- **Dilatation of the superior ophthalmic vein may be a nonspecific finding and may not be apparent. Careful evaluation for secondary signs, such as enlargement of the EOMs, edema, and congestion of the intraorbital fat is important in making the diagnosis.**
- **Catheter angiogram is often required to confirm the diagnosis.**

ADDITIONAL IMAGES (B-G)

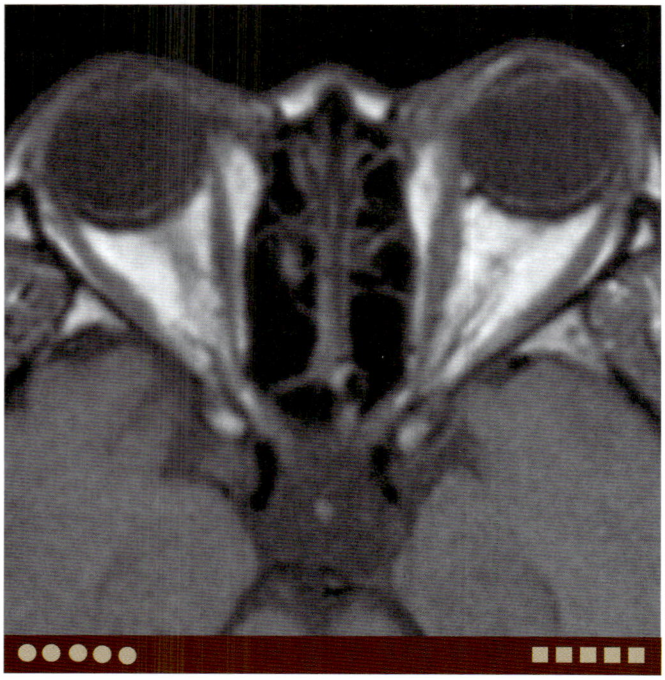

B. CCF, same patient as A. Axial T1W image demonstrates mild proptosis and enlargement of the EOMs, left greater than right.

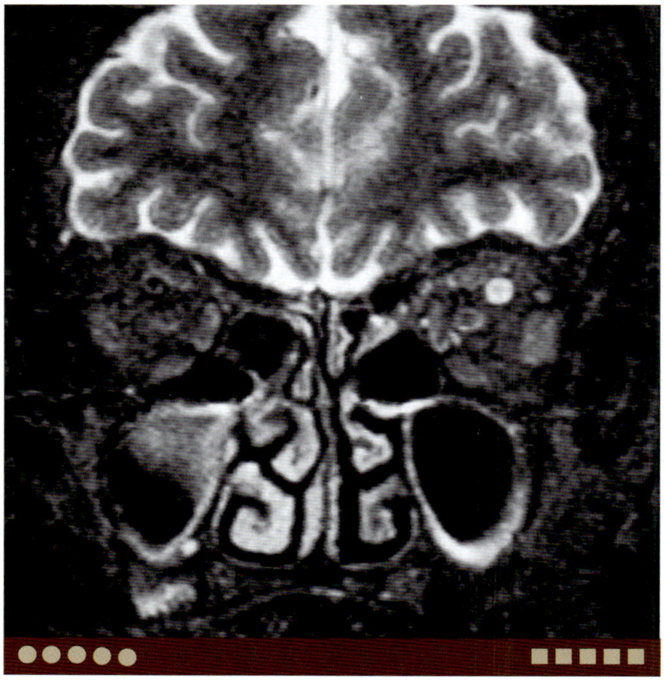

C. **CCF** in a different patient. Coronal fat-suppressed T2W image demonstrates enlargement of the left EOMs and superior ophthalmic vein, which demonstrates high-signal intensity.

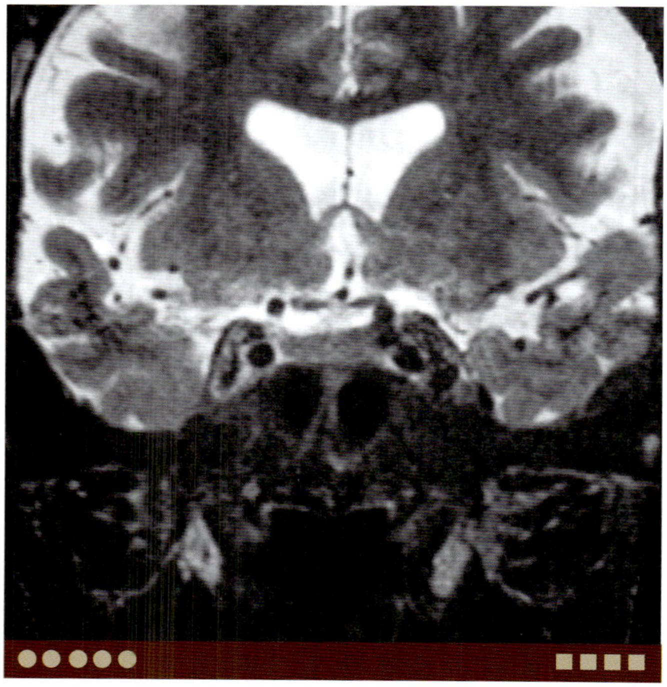

D. CCF, same patient as C. Coronal fat-suppressed T2W image demonstrates abnormal flow-voids within the cavernous sinuses, left greater than right, indicative of high-velocity inflow.

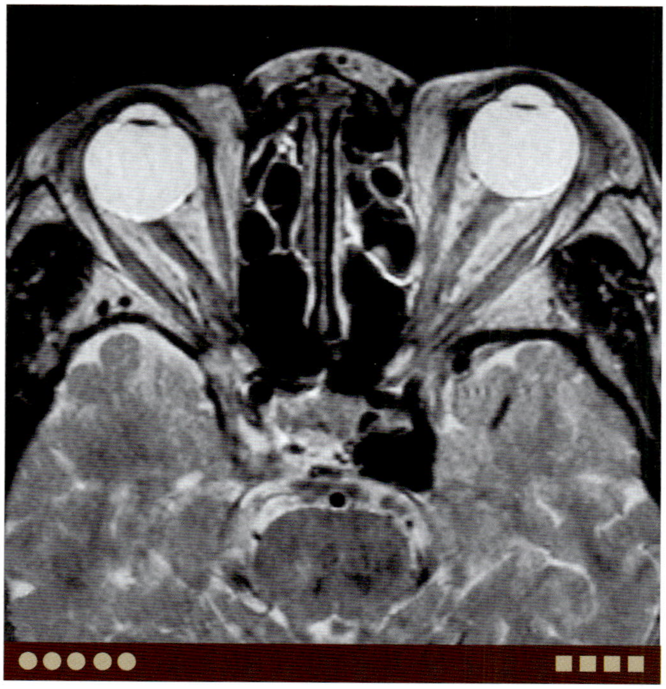

E. CCF, same patient as C. Axial T2W image demonstrates dilatation of the left cavernous sinus and large flow-voids. Note mild proptosis and mild swelling of the EOMs on the left.

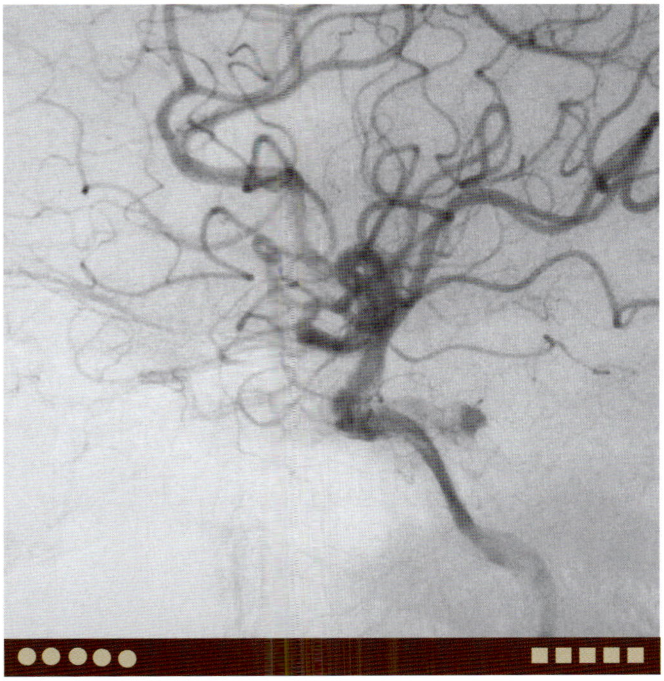

F. CCF, same patient as C. Internal carotid arteriogram demonstrates early visualization of the cavernous sinus in the arterial phase.

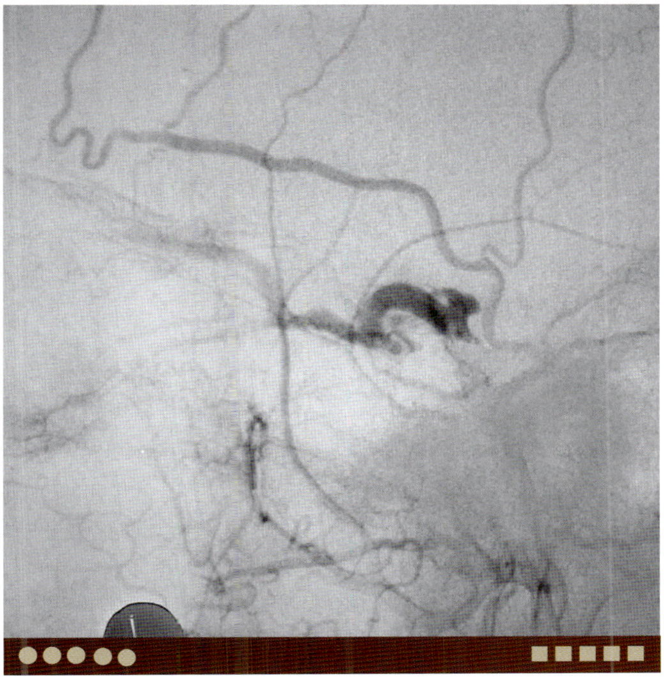

G. CCF, same patient as C. Late phase of carotid arteriogram demonstrates retrograde filling of the superior ophthalmic vein from the cavernous sinus.

DIFFERENTIAL DIAGNOSIS IMAGES (H-J)

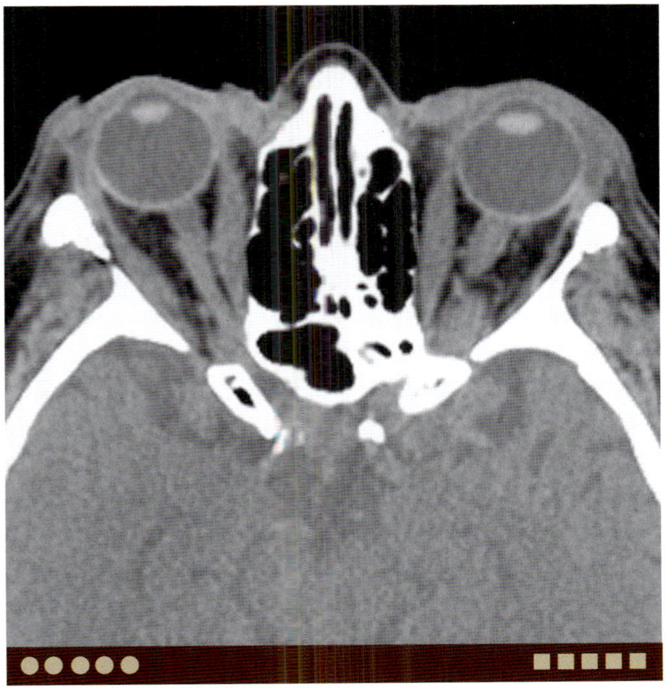

H. **Thyroid orbitopathy**. Axial CT demonstrates swelling of the bilateral EOMs with sparing of the tendinous insertions.

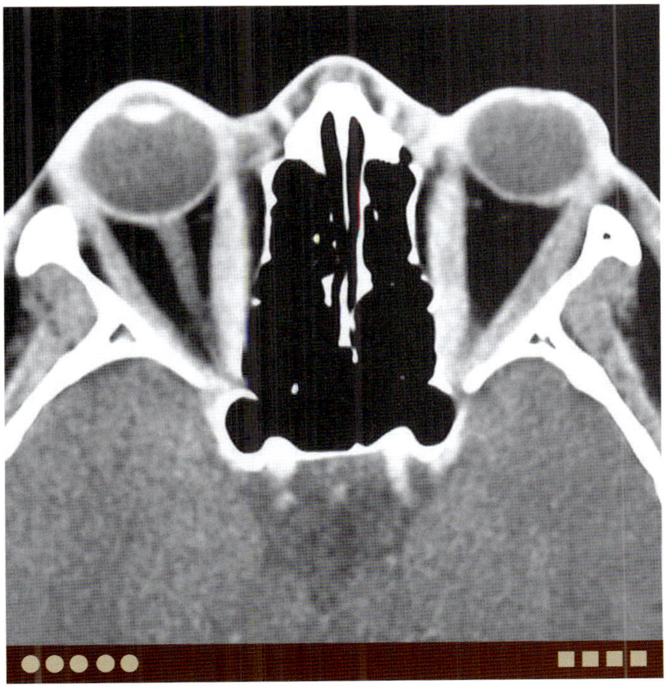

I. **IOI**. Axial contrast-enhanced CT demonstrates diffuse enlargement and enhancement of the medial and lateral rectus muscles with tendinous insertion involvement.

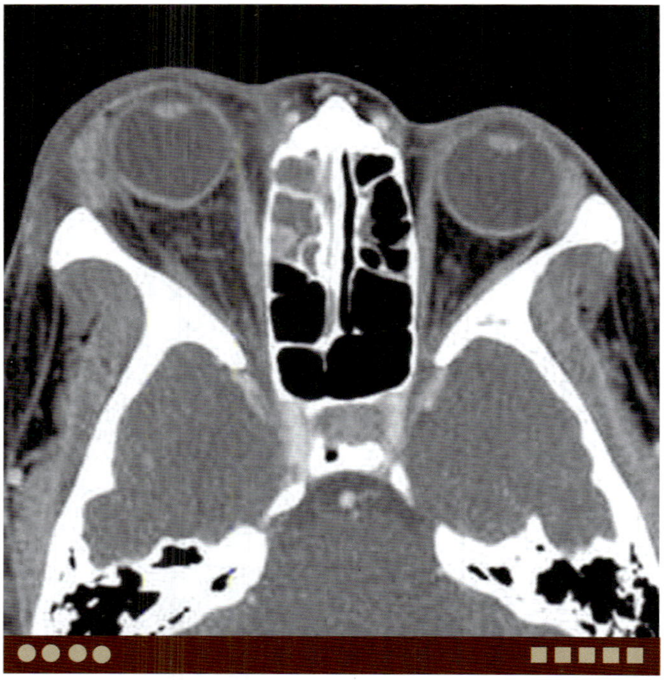

J. Orbital cellulitis. Axial contrast-enhanced CT demonstrates soft tissue swelling over the right orbit and increased density within the right retrobulbar fat without evidence of abscess formation.

Case 4–14 Dermoid, Epidermoid

Osamu Sakai, Elisa Flower

PRESENTATION

Fullness of the upper eyelid.

FINDINGS

CT and MRI demonstrate a round cystic appearing lesion.

DIFFERENTIAL DIAGNOSIS

- Retention cyst: A retention cyst from the meibomian gland or Moll's gland can be seen in the eyelid.
- Lacrimal gland tumor: Lymphoid or epithelial lesions occur from the lacrimal gland. Epithelial lesions may be predominantly cystic. Invasive, infiltrative change may be seen with malignant tumors.
- Conjunctival cyst: Cyst formation, fluid filled structure is seen in the conjunctiva, often with a history of prior trauma, surgery, or inflammation.
- Dacryocystocele (nasolacrimal duct cyst): This is a cyst formation caused by blockage of the nasolacrimal duct. The diagnosis can be made prenatally.

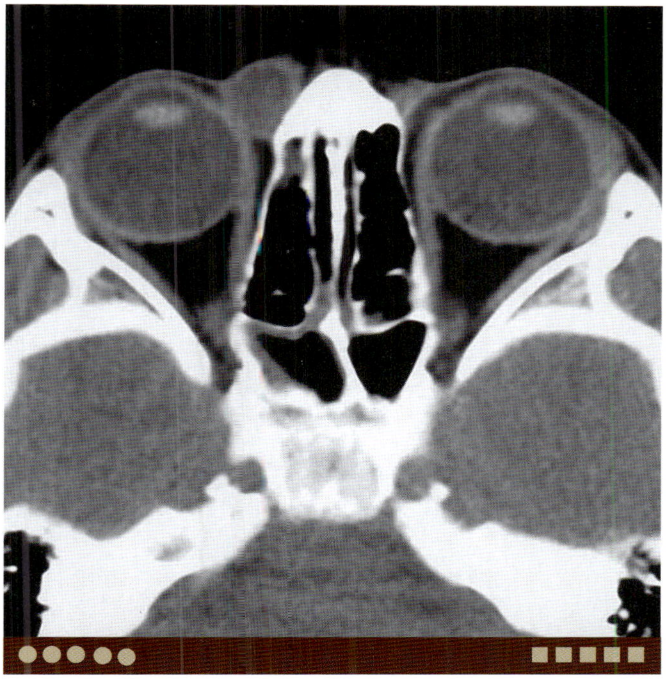

A. Dermoid cyst. Axial CT demonstrates a water density cystic lesion in the medial portion of the right orbit.

COMMENTS

This is a 4-year-old girl presented with an orbital mass.

Dermoid and epidermoid are also called as choristomas, and are aberrant ectodermal tissues migrated often between 3 and 5 weeks of gestation. Most are diagnosed in childhood; however, adult presentation is not rare. They often occur near the frontozygomatic and frontoethmoid sutures, and commonly seen in the upper outer quadrant of the orbit, and seen as a round cystic mass, occasionally with erosion of the adjacent osseous structure.

Epidermoid has a thin squamous lining and contains debris from epithelial desquamation, such as keratin, cholesterol, and some proteinaceous and lipid material. It usually demonstrates water density, and occasionally slightly negative attenuation values on CT, however, it usually does not demonstrate very low density like true fat, as seen in dermoids. On MRI, it shows slightly higher signal than water on T1W and variable signal on T2W images depending on its contents. Epidermoids will not be suppressed on FLAIR sequences and classically demonstrate restricted diffusion. Minimal thin peripheral enhancement can be seen. Calcification is rare.

Dermoid has more variable imaging characteristics due to more complex contents, such as apocrine glands, sweat glands, sebaceous glands, and hair follicles. The lining is usually thicker and often calcifies. Sebaceous, lipid materials in dermoids demonstrate similar density and signal intensity to fat on both CT and MRI, and a "lipid-water level," lighter lipid material layering on proteinaceous debris can be seen. Thin peripheral enhancement may also be noted.

Without apparent fat density or signal, it is difficult to differentiate dermoid from epidermoid radiologically. However, pathology can also misdiagnose dermoid as epidermoid due to failure to identify the dermal appendage structures from inadequate sampling or review.

PEARLS

- **Dermoid and epidermoid occur as a result of migration of aberrant ectodermal tissue.**
- **Dermoid often demonstrates calcification and fat density or signal. Without apparent fat, it is difficult to differentiate dermoid from epidermoid radiologically.**

ADDITIONAL IMAGES (B-G)

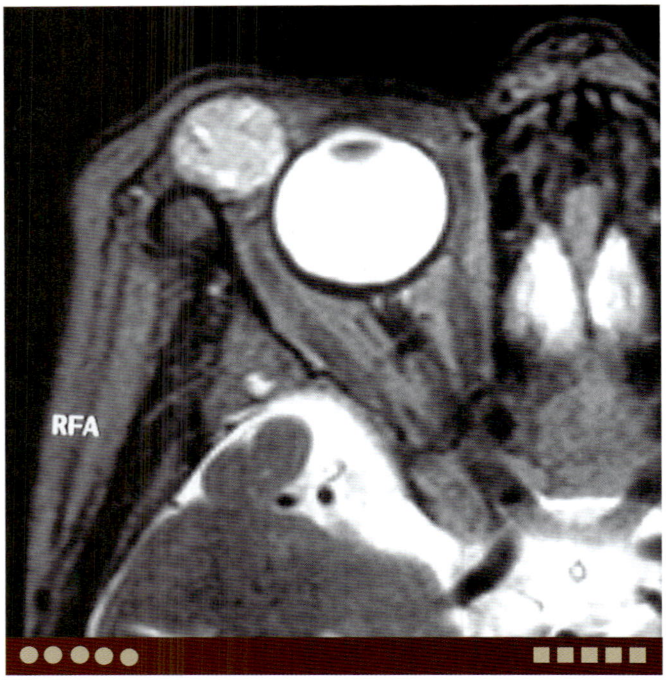

B. **Dermoid cyst** in a different patient. Axial T2W MR image demonstrates a round, slightly heterogeneous, high-signal lesion in the lateral portion of the right orbit.

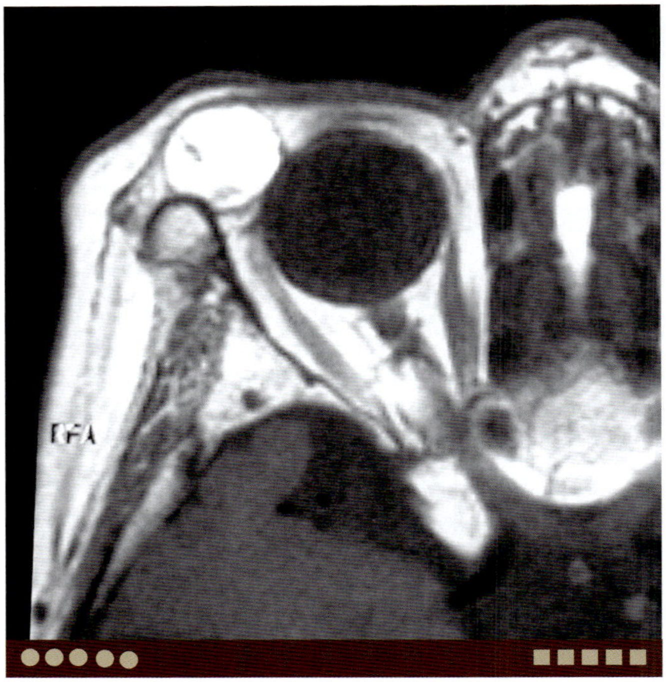

C. Dermoid cyst, same patient as B. Axial T1W MR image demonstrates high signal in the lesion.

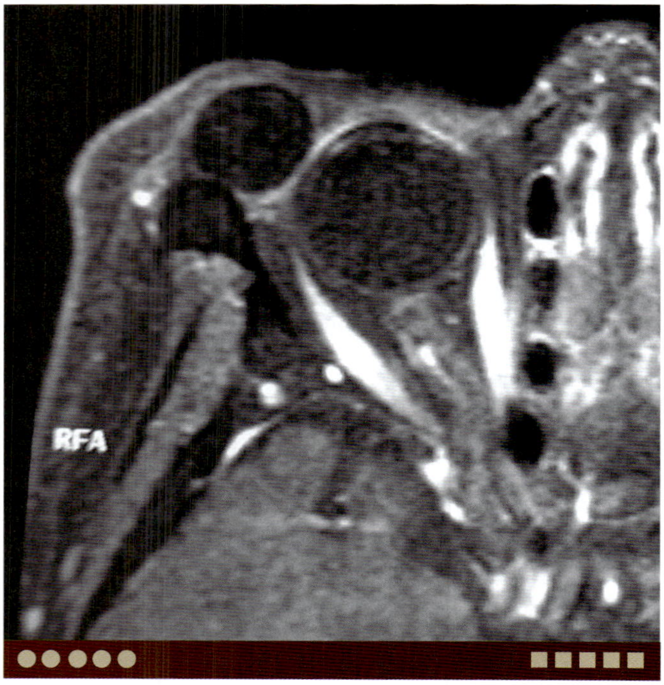

D. Dermoid cyst, same patient as B. Axial postcontrast fat-suppressed T1W MR image demonstrates complete signal suppression in the lesion.

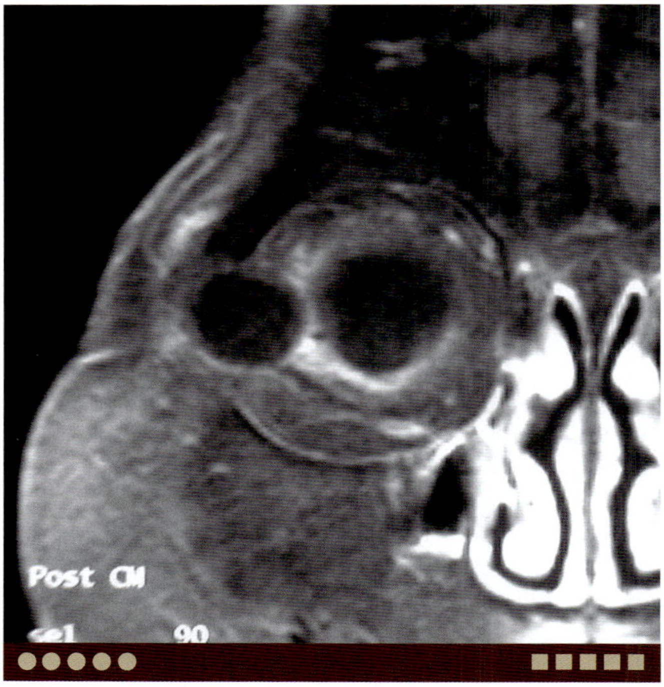

E. Dermoid cyst, same patient as B. Coronal postcontrast fat-suppressed T1W MR image demonstrates complete signal suppression in the lesion.

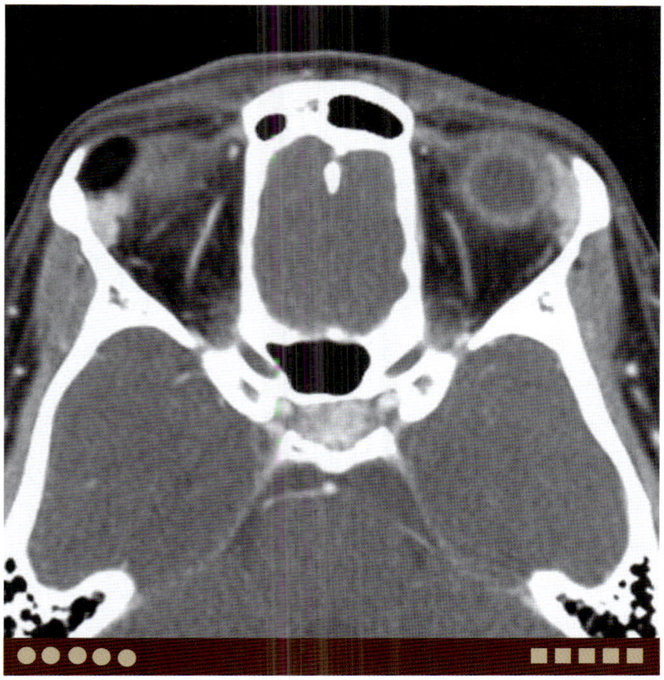

F. **Dermoid cyst** in a different patient. Axial CT demonstrates a fat density cystic lesion in the superolateral portion of the right orbit.

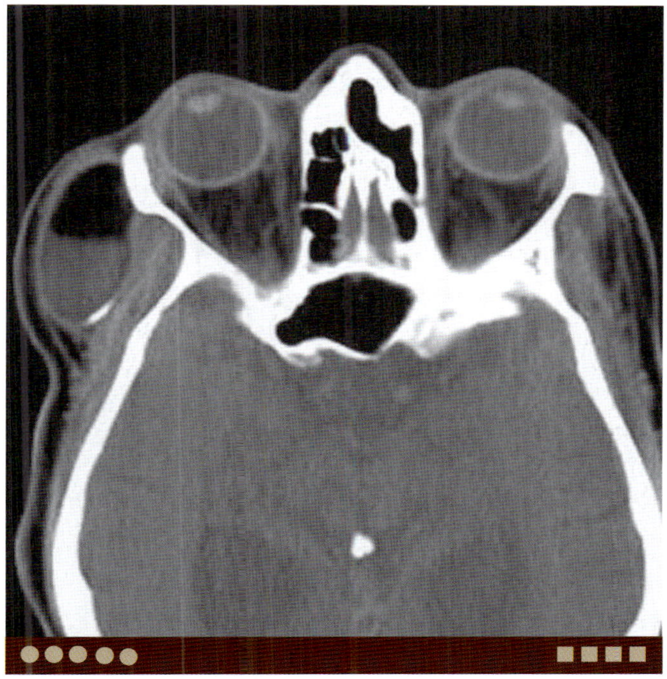

G. **Dermoid cyst** in a different patient. Axial CT demonstrates a large cystic lesion with lipid-fluid level formation lateral to the right orbit. A small calcification is noted in the wall.

DIFFERENTIAL DIAGNOSIS IMAGES (H-J)

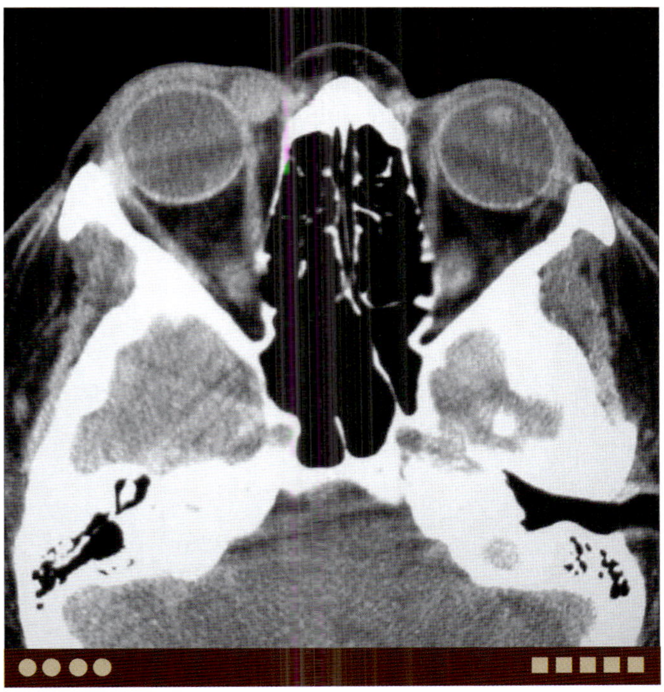

H. **Moll's gland cyst**. Axial CT demonstrates a slightly high-density cystic lesion in the medial portion of the right upper eyelid.

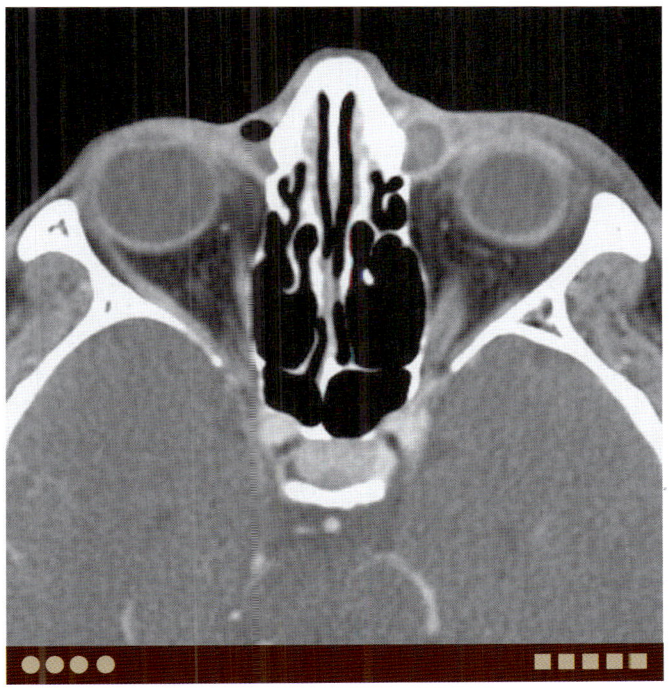

I. **Dacryocystitis**. Axial postcontrast CT demonstrates a rim-enhancing cystic lesion in the anteromedial portion of the orbit bilaterally, obstructed and inflamed lacrimal sacs.

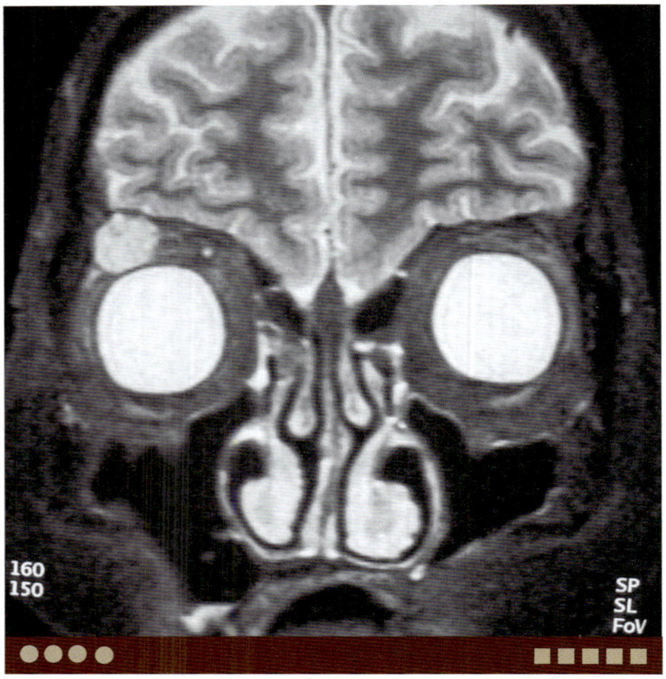

J. Pleomorphic adenoma of the lacrimal gland. Coronal fat-suppressed T2W image demonstrates a high-signal mass in the superolateral portion of the right orbit.

Case 4–15 Orbital Lymphoma

Osamu Sakai, Susmitha Reddy

PRESENTATION

Proptosis.

FINDINGS

CT and MRI demonstrate a mass with homogeneous density/signal and enhancement in the orbit.

DIFFERENTIAL DIAGNOSIS

- Idiopathic orbital inflammation (IOI) ("pseudotumor"): Imaging alone cannot differentiate IOI from lymphoma and histological diagnosis is required. IOI often demonstrates higher T2/STIR signal compared to lymphoma, although chronic inflammation shows decrease in T2 signal secondary to fibrosis.
- Wegener's granulomatosis: Imaging findings of orbital involvement are similar to IOI and lymphoma. This disease usually involves other structures such as paranasal sinuses, and the disease limited only to the orbit is rare.
- Sarcoidosis: Bilateral infiltration of lacrimal glands is common. The optic nerve may also be involved. Further, extraorbital involvement such as that of salivary gland is often seen.
- Leukemia: Chronic lymphocytic leukemia in adults and acute myelogenous leukemia in children commonly involve the orbit. Lacrimal gland enlargement and diffuse infiltration are seen, and imaging findings can be similar to lymphoma.
- Metastasis: Metastasis to the orbital soft tissue is not uncommon, and is often seen in patients with breast cancer and melanoma.

COMMENTS

This is a 66-year-old man presented with proptosis.

Lymphoma accounts for 10% of orbital tumors. Most are B-cell non-Hodgkin lymphomas. Lymphoma can occur in any structures in the orbit, including eyelids, conjunctiva, lacrimal glands, and extraocular muscles. They may vary in appearance; mass like, infiltrative, diffuse, or multifocal. It may present as scleritis or perineuritis. Although lymphoma is a systemic disease, orbital lymphoma can be an isolated presentation. It is important to search for extraorbital disease sites, particularly in the cranium.

On CT, lymphoma demonstrates homogeneous density similar to the muscle and shows variable degree of enhancement. On MRI, it shows intermediate-to-low signal on T1W images similar to the muscle, intermediate-to-high signal on T2W images and variable degree of enhancement after intravenous contrast administration. Significant overlaps in MR signal characteristics exist between lymphoma and IOI. Multiplicity, bilaterality and presence of extraorbital lesions suggest lymphoma; however, these can also be seen in IOI and non-neoplastic infiltrative conditions. Therefore, biopsy is necessary to make a diagnosis. However, even histologically it may be difficult to differentiate lymphoma from IOI or lymphoproliferative disorders.

The response to chemotherapy and radiotherapy is often dramatic with significant reduction in the size of the tumor mass. After treatment, heterogeneous density/signal and calcification may be seen in the residual mass.

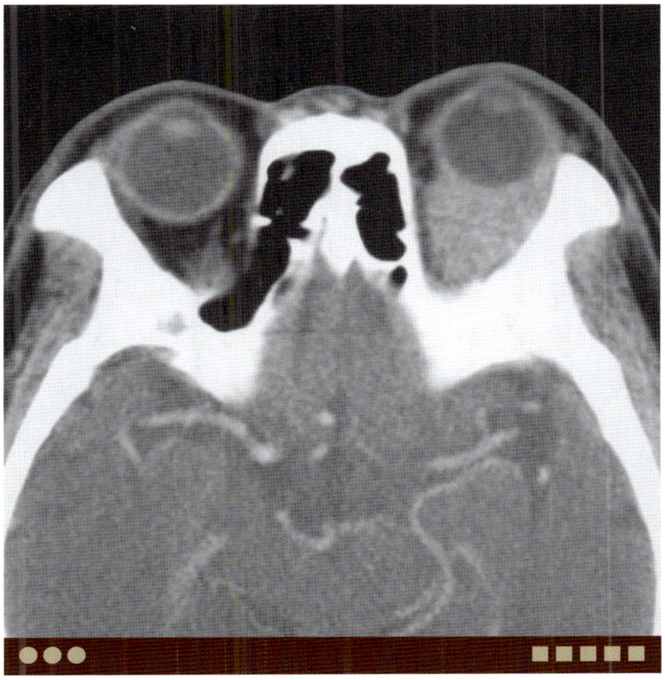

A. Lymphoma. Axial postcontrast CT demonstrates a homogeneously enhancing tumor in the left orbit.

PEARLS

- **Orbital lymphoma has similar imaging characteristics to IOI ("pseudotumor") or lymphoproliferative disorders.**
- **Multiplicity, bilaterality, and presence of extraorbital lesions suggest lymphoma; however, those can be also seen in IOI or non-neoplastic lymphoid lesions.**
- **The signal intensity can vary from low-to-intermediate signal on T1W and intermediate-to-high on T2W images. Homogeneous enhancement is commonly seen.**

ADDITIONAL IMAGES (B-G)

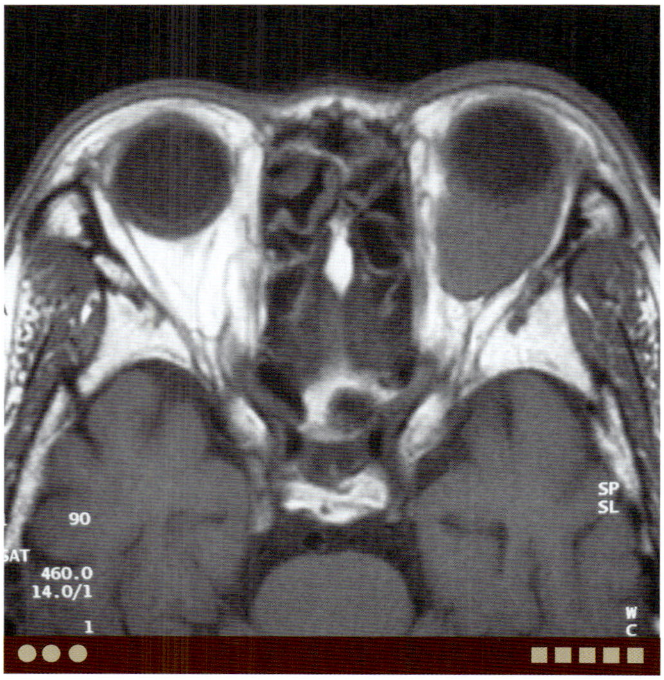

B. Lymphoma, same patient as A. Axial T1W MR image demonstrates a homogeneous low-signal lesion in the left orbit.

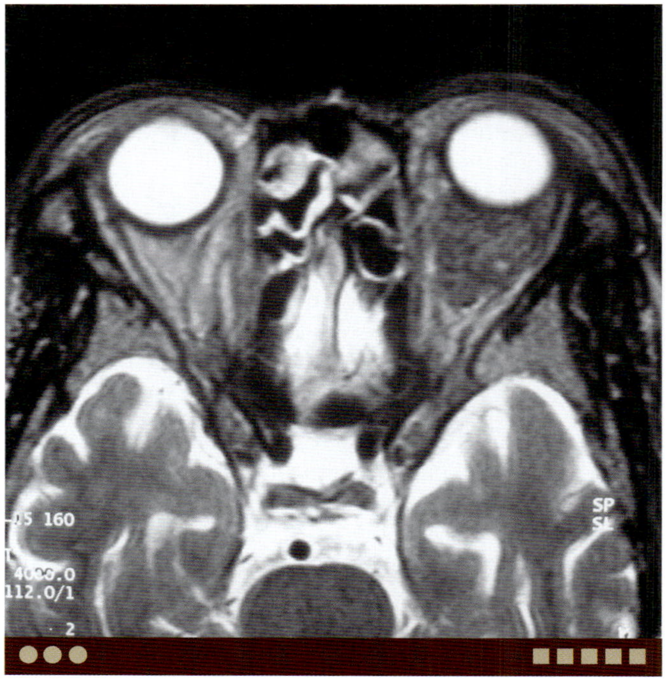

C. Lymphoma, same patient as A. Axial T2W MR image demonstrates an intermediate-to-low signal lesion in the left orbit.

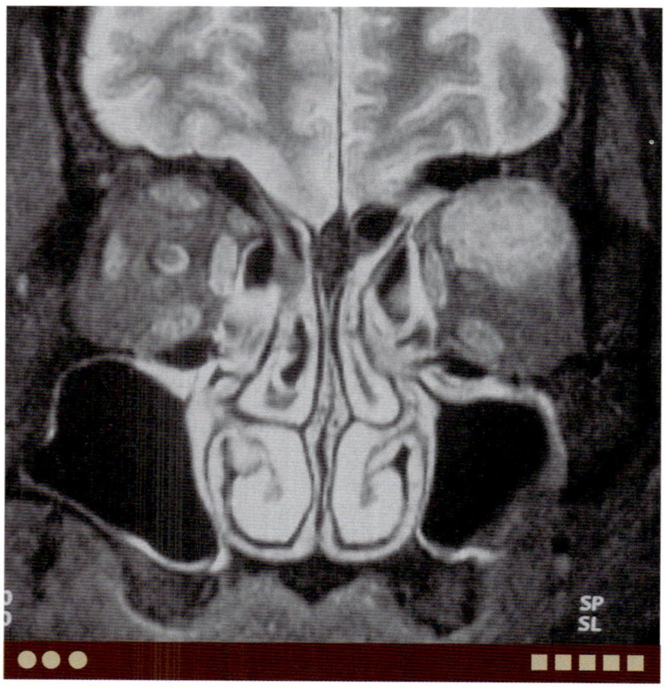

D. Lymphoma, same patient as A. Coronal STIR MR image demonstrates an intermediate-to-high signal lesion in the superior portion of the left orbit. The superior rectus muscle complex is involved and cannot be appreciated separately.

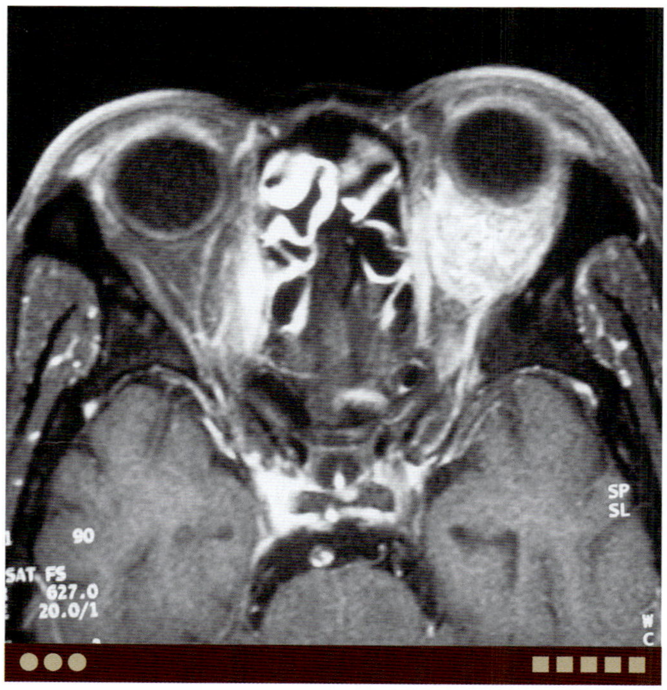

E. Lymphoma, same patient as A. Axial postcontrast fat-suppressed T1W MR image demonstrates enhancement in the tumor.

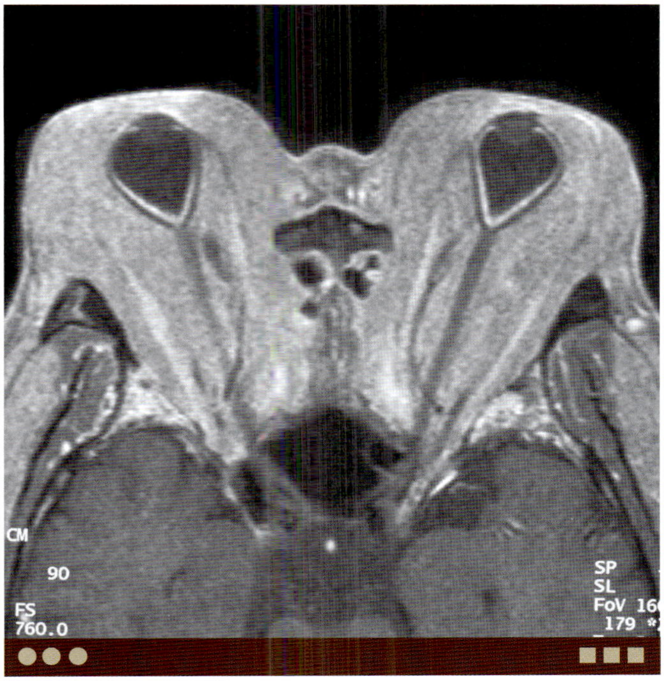

F. Lymphoma in a different patient. Axial postcontrast T1W MR image demonstrates diffuse involvement of the bilateral orbits resulting in significant exophthalmos. Note stretching of the optic nerve sheath complex and deformity of the globe bilaterally.

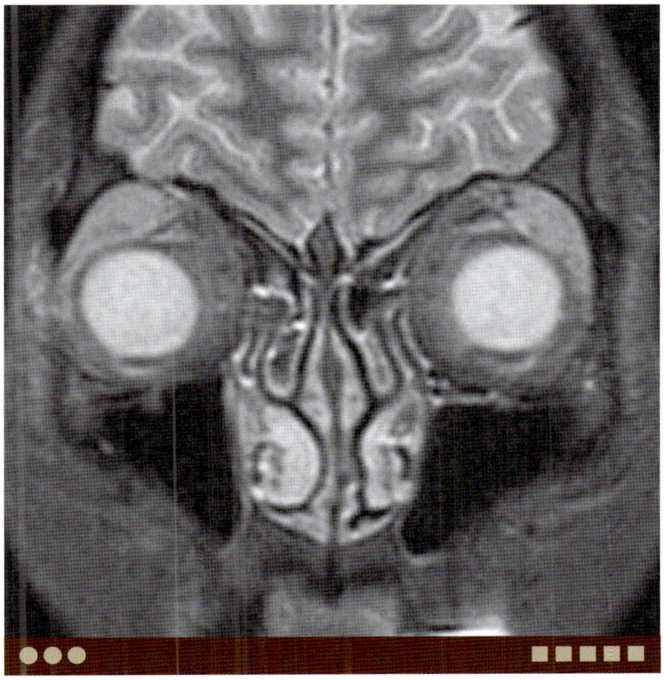

G. Lymphoma in a different patient. Coronal STIR MR image demonstrates enlargement of the bilateral lacrimal glands

DIFFERENTIAL DIAGNOSIS IMAGES (H-J)

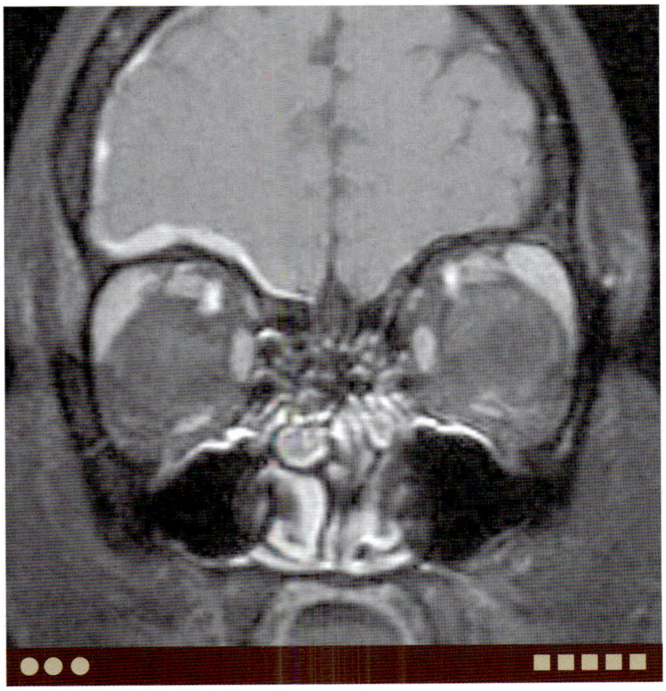

H. Sarcoidosis. Coronal postcontrast fat-suppressed T1W MR image demonstrates enlargement of the bilateral lacrimal glands. Note abnormal dural enhancement in the right frontal region.

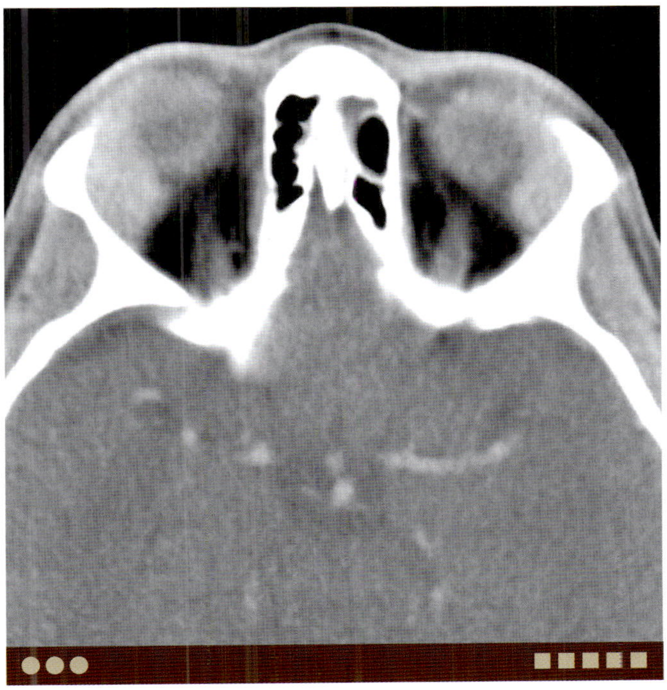

I. Wegener's granulomatosis. Axial postcontrast CT demonstrates homogeneously enhancing enlarged lacrimal glands bilaterally.

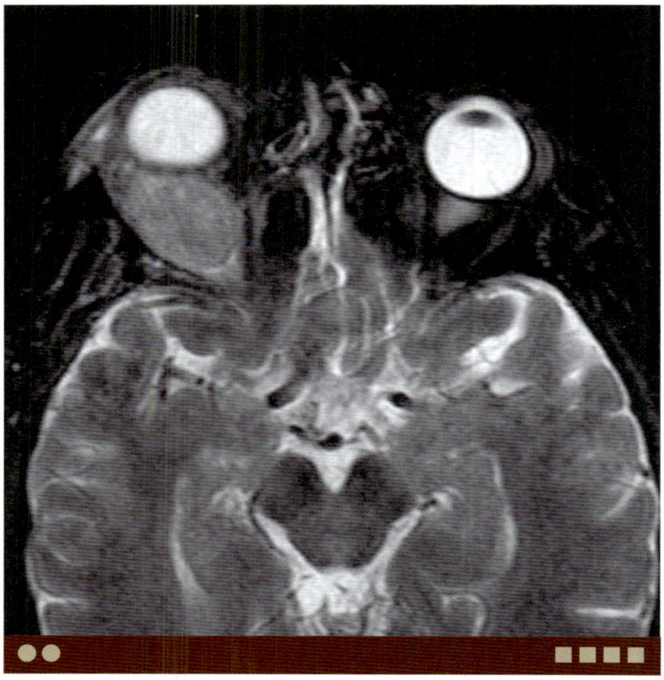

J. Metastatic melanoma. Axial T2W MR image demonstrates a large relatively homogeneous T2 intermediate-signal lesion displacing the right globe.

Case 4–15 Pleomorphic Adenoma in Lacrimal Gland

Memi Watanabe, Margaret Chapman, Osamu Sakai

PRESENTATION

Slowly progressing, painless swelling of the upper eyelid.

FINDINGS

CT and MRI demonstrate a well-circumscribed lesion in the lacrimal gland.

DIFFERENTIAL DIAGNOSIS

- Adenoid cystic carcinoma: This is the most common malignant epithelial tumor of the lacrimal gland. Imaging findings may be similar to pleomorphic adenoma, but more invasive features, such as bony destruction and a propensity for perineural spread that often result in severe pain may be seen. Calcification and hemorrhage may be present.
- Other malignant epithelial tumors: Other malignant epithelial tumors of the lacrimal gland include mucoepidermoid carcinoma, anaplastic carcinoma, and primary adenocarcinoma. These conditions present with similar imaging features and differentiation may only be possible histologically.
- Lymphoma and other lymphoid tumors: Secondary involvement from extraorbital origin is more common. MALT lymphoma is the most common primary lymphoma of the lacrimal gland. These conditions tend to affect the orbit diffusively.
- Sarcoidosis: Sarcoidosis frequently involves the lacrimal gland and other soft tissues in the orbit. Sarcoidosis tends toward a more infiltrative appearance.

COMMENTS

This is a 45-year-old woman with slowly progressing proptosis.

Pleomorphic adenoma accounts for half of the epithelial neoplasms of the lacrimal gland. This presents as painless proptosis, slowly progressive swelling of the upper eyelid, and downward displacement of the globe, most commonly in patients between the second and fifth decades of life. "Fifty percent rules" can be applied to lacrimal gland lesions. In the lacrimal gland, about half of the masses are epithelial neoplasms, and the other half are caused by lymphoproliferative or inflammatory disorders. Among the epithelial neoplasms, about half are benign, and the other half are malignant.

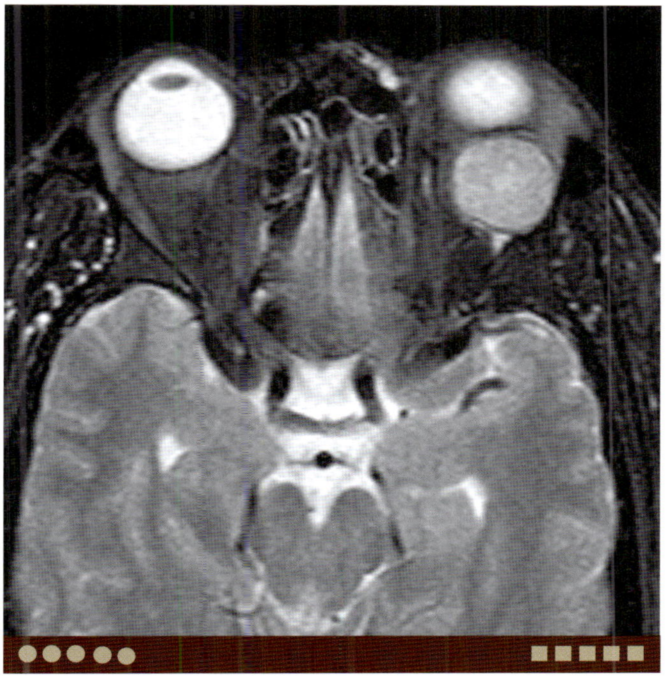

A. Pleomorphic adenoma. Axial T2W MR image demonstrates a well-circumscribed ovoid mass in the left lacrimal gland, which is isointense to the brain parenchyma.

Imaging findings of pleomorphic adenoma are often nonspecific and variable, reflecting its variable histological features; ductal epithelial cells and metaplastic epithelium forming a variable matrix (myxoid, fibrous, and cartilaginous). MRI demonstrates a well-circumscribed ovoid lesion with a moderately heterogenous appearance; low signal on T1W images, intermediate to high, often isointense

PEARLS

- **Pleomorphic adenoma most commonly presents between the second and fifth decades of life with slow-growing features.**
- **MRI demonstrates a well-circumscribed, moderately heterogenous lesion. Calcification or hemorrhage may be seen.**
- **Malignant transformation of pleomorphic adenoma and adenoid cystic carcinoma should be considered if rapid growth or invasive features are noted.**

to the brain parenchyma on T2W images, and moderate enhancement following contrast administration. CT may demonstrate expansion of the lacrimal fossa without aggressive bone destruction. Calcification and hemorrhage are rare, but have been reported.

In a follow-up series lasting over 20 years, 10% to 20% of pleomorphic adenomas undergo malignant transformation. Malignant transformation is suspected by an aggressive clinical course during follow-up. MRI demonstrates heterogeneous invasive tumors. Again, imaging findings of pleomorphic adenoma are often nonspecific and similar to other tumors, including malignant tumors such as malignant transformation of pleomorphic adenoma, adenoid cystic carcinoma, lymphoma, and metastases, and benign tumors such as neurogenic tumors. Histological diagnosis is therefore, essential for differentiation.

ADDITIONAL IMAGES (B-F)

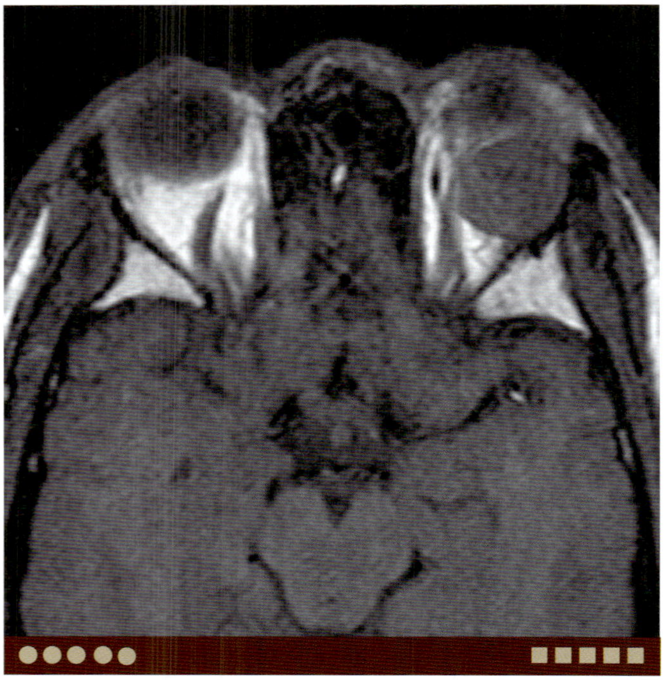

B. Pleomorphic adenoma, same patient as A. Axial T1W MR image demonstrates a low-signal lacrimal gland tumor.

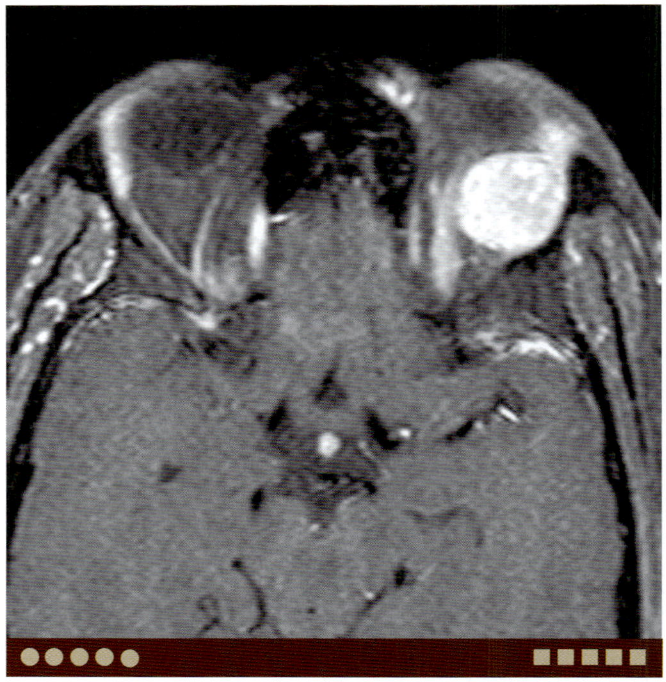

C. Pleomorphic adenoma, same patient as A. Axial postcontrast fat-suppressed T1W MR image demonstrates moderate enhancement of the lacrimal gland tumor.

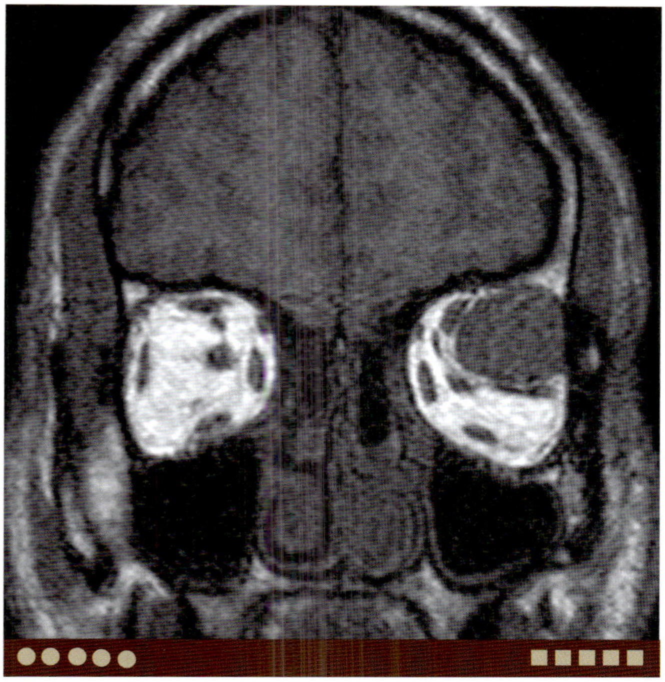

D. Pleomorphic adenoma, same patient as A. Coronal T1W MR image demonstrates a hypointense mass in the superolateral left orbit, which displaces adjacent structures.

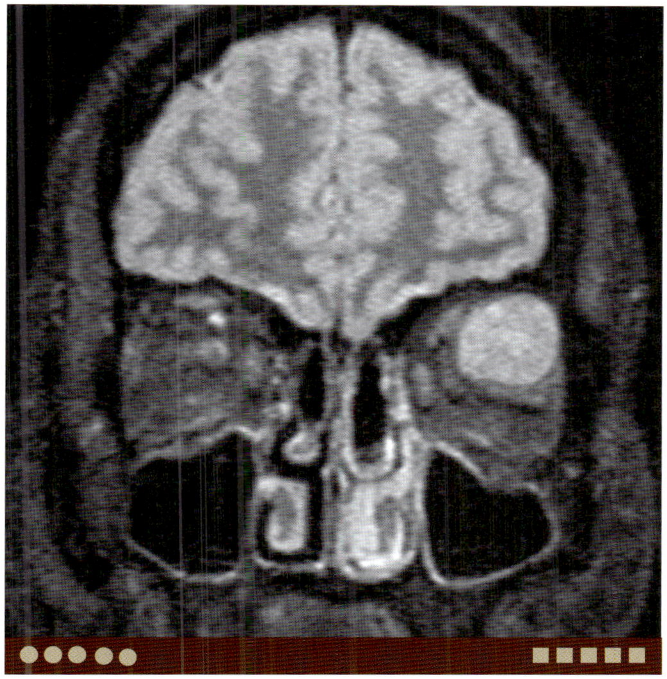

E. Pleomorphic adenoma, same patient as A. Coronal fat-suppressed T2W MR image demonstrates a well-demarcated ovoid mass in the lacrimal gland.

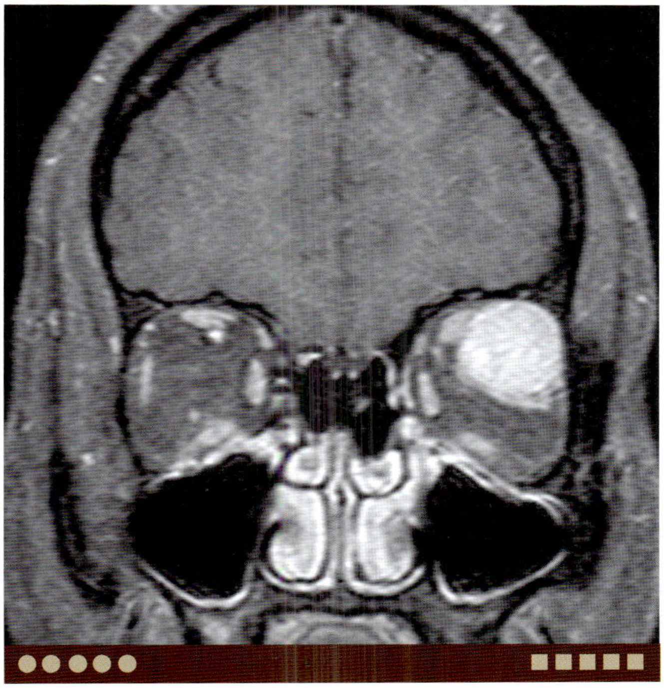

F. Pleomorphic adenoma, same patient as A. Coronal postcontrast fat-suppressed T1W MR image demonstrates a moderate enhancement of the tumor.

DIFFERENTIAL DIAGNOSIS IMAGES (G-J)

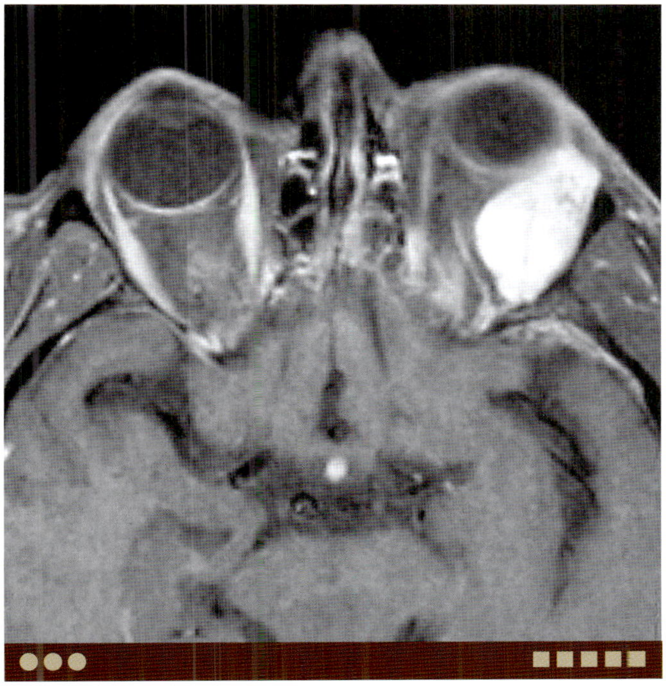

G. **Adenoid cystic carcinoma**. Axial postcontrast fat-suppressed T1W MR image demonstrates a homogeneously enhancing lacrimal gland tumor, which is well-defined but irregularly shaped.

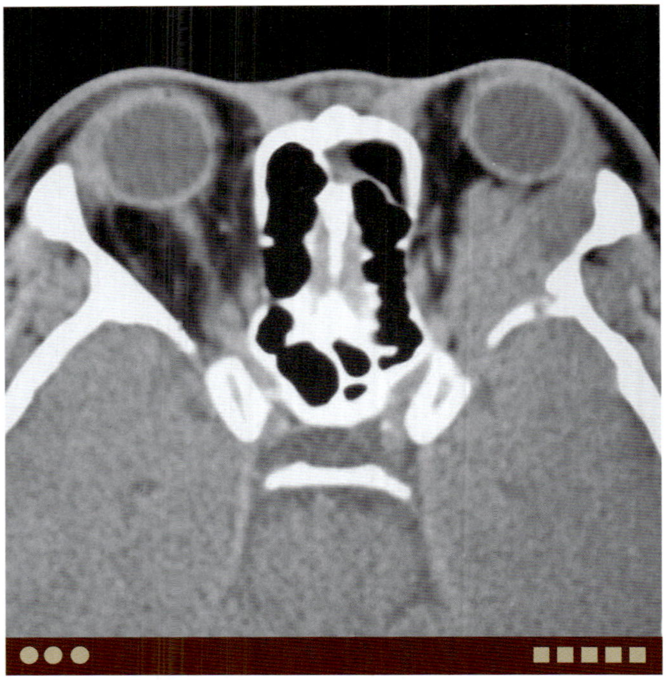

H. Adenoid cystic carcinoma in a different patient. Axial postcontrast CT demonstrates an infiltrating tumor in the superolateral portion of the left orbit with adjacent bony destruction.

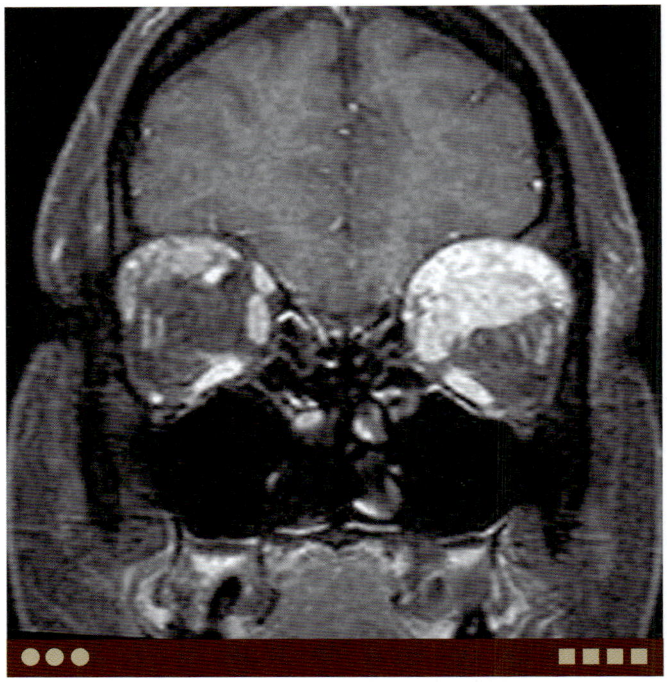

I. Sarcoidosis. Coronal postcontrast fat-suppressed T1W MR image demonstrates a poorly defined heterogeneously enhancing lesion involving the left lacrimal gland and extraocular muscles.

Case 4–17 Dacryocystitis

Bhavya Shah, Osamu Sakai

PRESENTATION

Epiphora.

FINDINGS

CT and MRI demonstrate a soft tissue or cystic mass in the inferomedial portion of the orbit, in the region of the medial epicanthus centered in the lacrimal sac.

DIFFERENTIAL DIAGNOSIS

- Dacryocystocele: This is dilatation of the lacrimal sac that is not infected.
- Squamous cell carcinoma (SCCA): SCCA accounts for 14% of all lacrimal sac tumors. They usually demonstrate low signal on T2W images and invasive appearance.
- Papilloma: Benign papilloma accounts for about 40% of all neoplasms of the lacrimal drainage system, and often present insidiously with symptoms of dacryostenosis or dacryocystitis.
- Dermoid: They often occur near the frontozygomatic and frontoethmoid sutures, not commonly seen near the lacrimal fossa.
- Lymphoproliferative disorders (lymphoid tumors): Lymphoid lesions occur in the lacrimal drainage system. They usually show intermediate signal on T2W images and relatively homogeneous enhancement. Infiltrative extension to both the orbit and sinonasal cavity is often seen.
- Granulomatous inflammation (sarcoidiosis or Wegener's granulomatosis): These lesions can occur anywhere in the orbit and show heterogeneously enhancing solid lesions.
- Moll's gland cyst: This is a retention cyst which occurs in the eyelid.

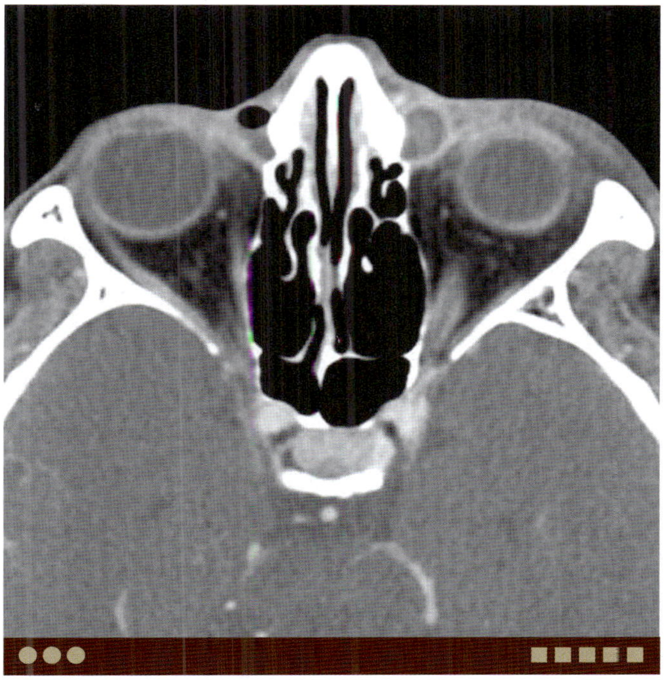

A. Dacryocystitis. Axial postcontrast CT demonstrates rim-enhancing cystic lesions in the anteromedial portion of the orbit, the region of the nasolacrimal sac, bilaterally. Note inflammation in the periorbital soft tissue.

COMMENTS

This is a 41-year-old woman with epiphora.

Dacryocystitis is inflammation of the lacrimal sac, demonstrated by soft tissue inflammation in the region of the medial epicanthus and lacrimal puncta as the result of infection of the nasolacrimal duct and lacrimal sac.

Clinically patients present with epiphora, pain, erythema, edema, and mucopurulent discharge from the puncta lacrimalia with associated conjunctivitis.

Dacryocystitis occurs in a bimodal distribution, it most commonly affect neonates and adults over the age of 40. In both cases inflammation of the lacrimal sac is secondary to obstruction of the outflow of tears. In neonates most cases are secondary to incomplete recanalization of the distal nasolacrimal duct in the region where it enters the nasal cavity. In adults greater than 40 years of age, the infections are related to acquired abnormalities that cause obstruction at the opening of the nasolacrimal duct into the inferior meatus.

The most common organisms identified in dacryocystitis are *Staphylococcus aureus* and *Pseudomonas aeruginosa*.

Treatment of acute dacryocystitis includes antibiotic therapy in the outpatient setting which may follow external dacryocystorhinostomy (DCR) or interventional procedures such as balloon dacryoplasty with stent placement at the site of obstruction.

PEARLS

- **Dacryocystitis is inflammation of the lacrimal sac secondary to obstruction of the nasolacrimal duct.**
- **Dacryocystitis most commonly affect neonates and adults over the age of 40.**

ADDITIONAL IMAGES (B-D)

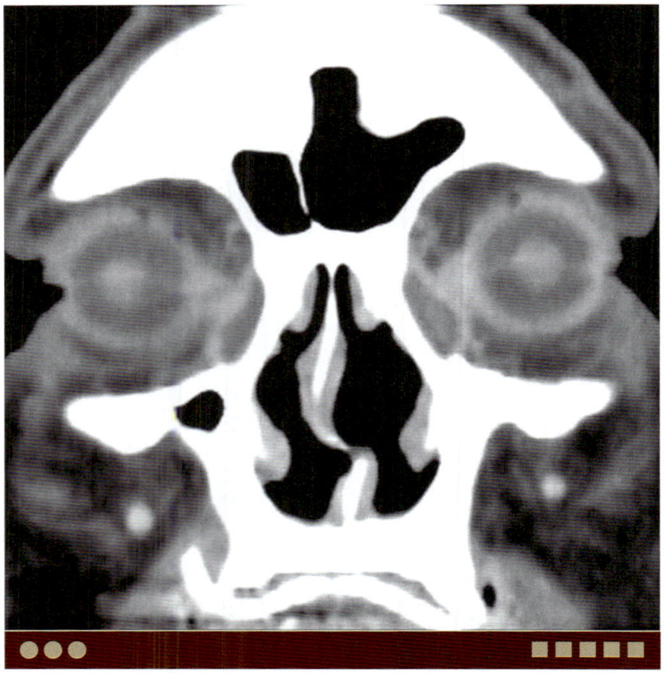

B. Dacryocystitis, same patient as A. Coronal postcontrast CT demonstrates rim-enhancing cystic lesions in the inferomedial portion of the orbit, the region of the lacrimal sac, bilaterally.

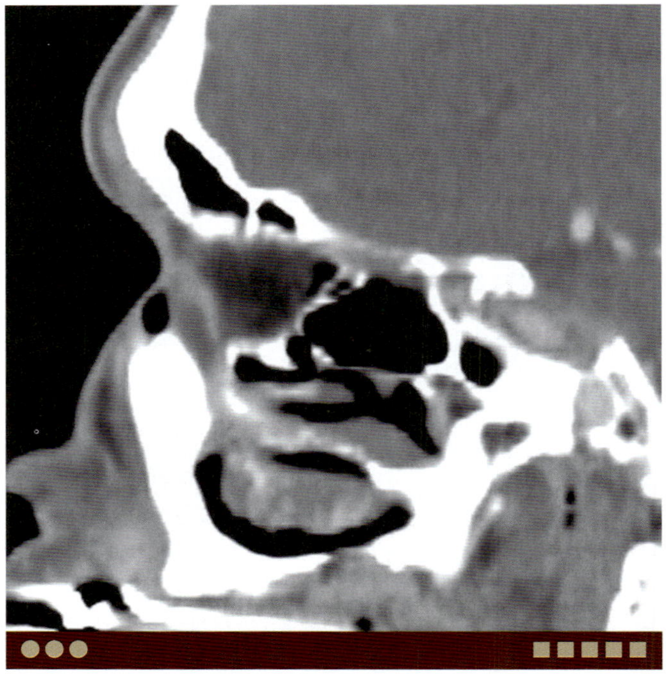

C. Dacryocystitis, same patient as A. Sagittal postcontrast CT of the right orbit demonstrates a rim-enhancing cystic lesion containing air in the anteroinferior portion of the orbit, the region of the lacrimal sac.

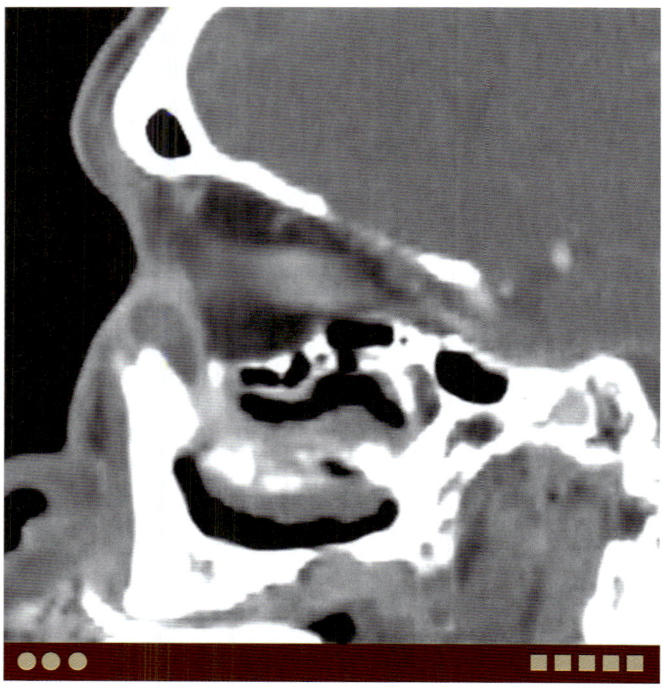

D. Dacryocystitis, same patient as A. Sagittal postcontrast CT of the left orbit demonstrates a rim-enhancing cystic lesion in the anteroinferior portion of the orbit, the region of the lacrimal sac. Note inflammation in the periorbital soft tissue.

DIFFERENTIAL DIAGNOSIS IMAGES (E-G)

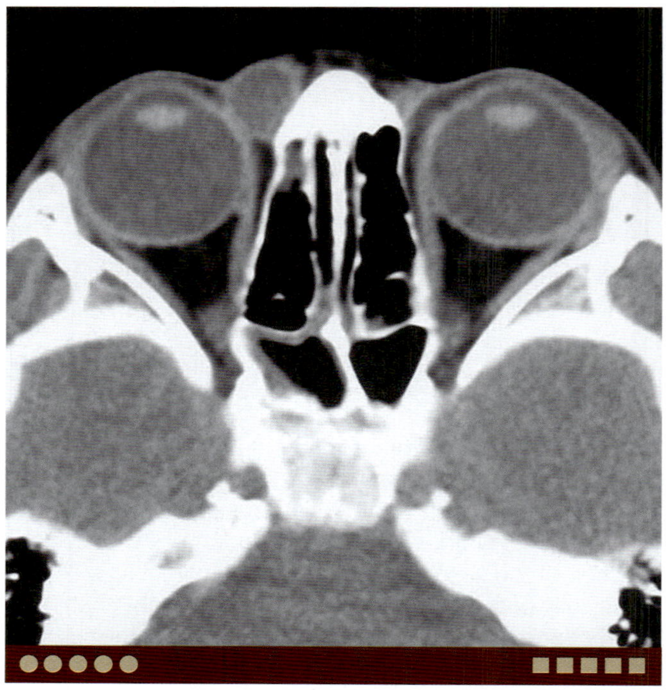

E. **Dermoid cyst**. Axial CT demonstrates a water density cystic lesion in the medial portion of the right orbit.

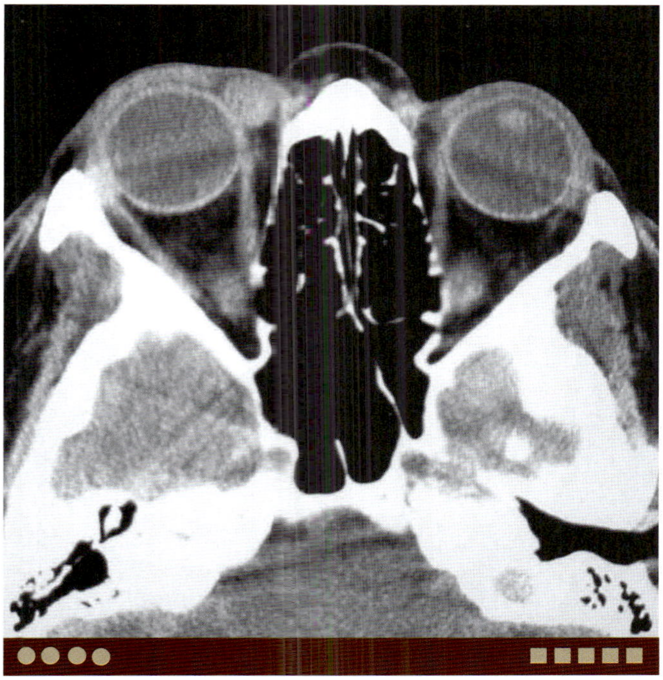

F. Moll's gland cyst. Axial CT demonstrates a slightly high-density cystic lesion in the medial portion of the right upper eyelid.

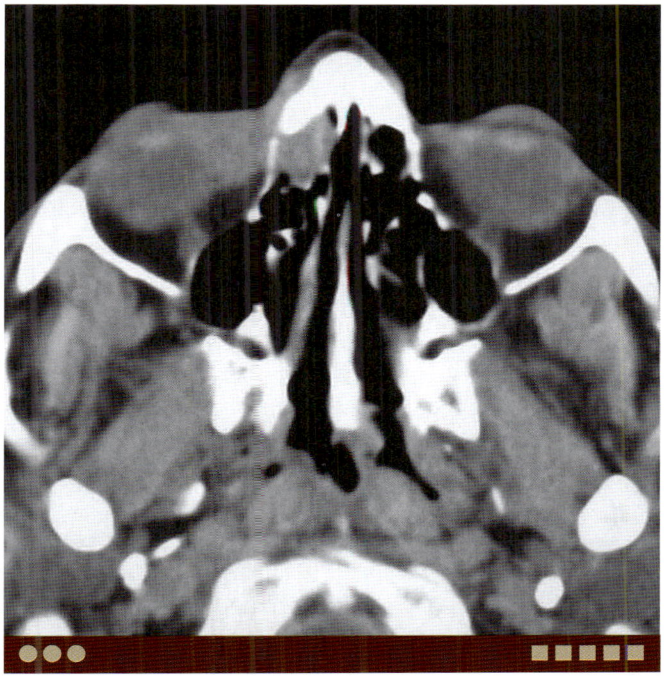

G. Lymphoma. Axial CT demonstrates a poorly marginated, soft tissue density lesion involving both the medial orbit and ethmoid without apparent destruction of the osseous structure.

Case 4–18 Sarcoidosis

Memi Watanabe, Margaret Chapman, Osamu Sakai

PRESENTATION

A slow-growing, periocular mass.

FINDINGS

CT and MRI demonstrate enlargement of the lacrimal gland or an intraorbital soft tissue mass with heterogeneous enhancement.

DIFFERENTIAL DIAGNOSIS

- Idiopathic orbital inflammation (IOI) ("pseudotumor"): This condition mimics sarcoidosis and lymphoid tumors such as lymphoma. Both the clinical and radiological presentations are nonspecific, and include diffuse infiltration, mass formation, and swelling of the lacrimal gland and extraocular muscles.
- Lymphoma: Imaging findings of lymphoma and other lymphoid tumors are similar to IOI and sarcoidosis. Histological diagnosis is required for differentiation.
- Wegener's granulomatosis: This condition commonly affects men in their fifth decade with airway and renal involvement. It can also present with diffuse infiltration of the orbital soft tissue, mostly secondary to sinonasal involvement. Imaging findings are similar to IOI.
- Thyroid orbitopathy: Radiological presentation of this condition includes enlargement of the extraocular muscles, lacrimal gland, and an increase in volume and edema of the intraorbital fat. When extraocular muscles are involved, the tendinous insertion tends to be spared.

COMMENTS

This is a 37-year-old woman presenting with left proptosis.

Sarcoidosis is a multisystem granulomatous disease of unknown etiology, typically diagnosed between the second and fourth decades of life. It may affect any organ system, but pulmonary, dermatologic, and ocular involvements are common manifestations. Ocular involvement is seen in 25% to 60% of cases, and can be the initial presentation. Findings include uveitis, chorioretinitis, and conjunctival and eyelid granulomas. Extraocular orbital tissue is affected less frequently, and may include the lacrimal gland, soft tissues of the orbit, and the optic nerve and sheath, with the lacrimal gland most commonly affected. The most common clinical presentation is an enlarging palpable mass. Other presentations include proptosis, globe displacement, and impairment of visual acuity secondary to optic nerve sheath involvement.

Imaging findings of sarcoidosis are often nonspecific and vary depending on the location and disease process. The lacrimal gland is most commonly affected and often demonstrates diffuse enlargement and homogenous enhancement, which may be associated with infiltrative changes to the adjacent structures. Diffuse enlargement of the affected extraocular muscles is often seen. Optic nerve involvement includes multiple nodular enhancing lesions similar to typical optic neuritis. Optic nerve sheath involvement demonstrates diffuse thickening of the optic nerve sheath, which may mimic dural metastasis and meningioma. Recurrent disease may be seen in the same location, in the contralateral orbit, or in other organ systems.

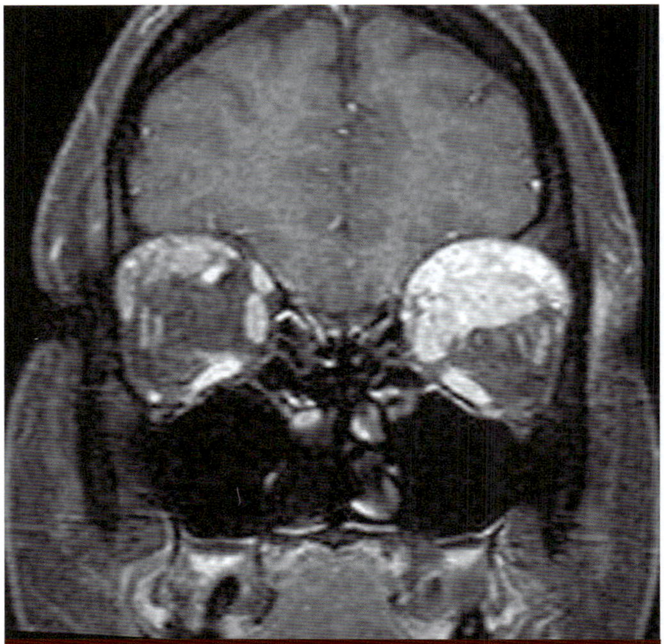

A. Sarcoidosis. Coronal postcontrast fat-suppressed T1W MR image demonstrates a poorly defined heterogeneously enhancing lesion involving the extraocular muscles and lacrimal gland in the superior left orbit.

PEARLS

- **Orbital involvement can be the initial presentation of sarcoidosis. Uveitis is the most common orbital presentation.**
- **Extraocular orbital sarcoidosis is less frequent compared with ocular involvement. The lacrimal gland is most commonly involved.**
- **Imaging findings of orbital sarcoidosis are nonspecific and similar to other inflammatory, granulomatous, and neoplastic conditions, including IOI, Wegener's granulomatosis, and lymphoma.**

ADDITIONAL IMAGES (B-G)

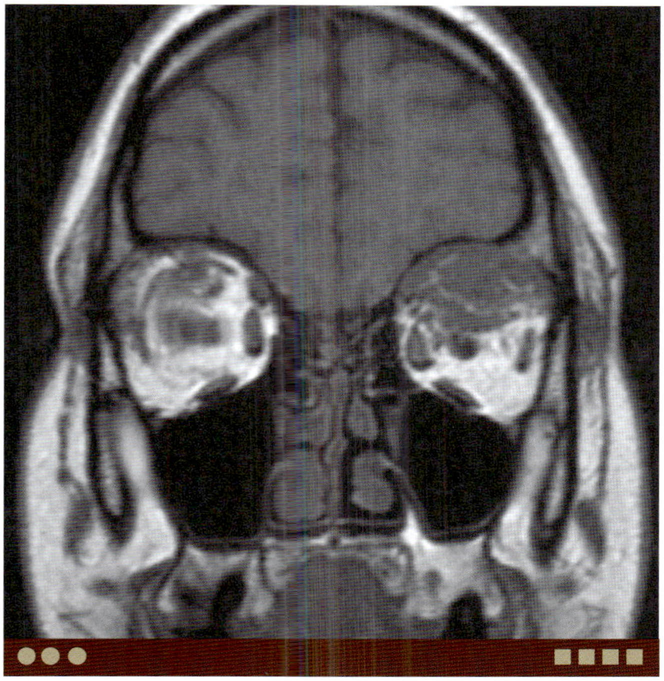

B. Sarcoidosis, same patient as A. Coronal T1W MR image demonstrates an infiltrative low-signal lesion.

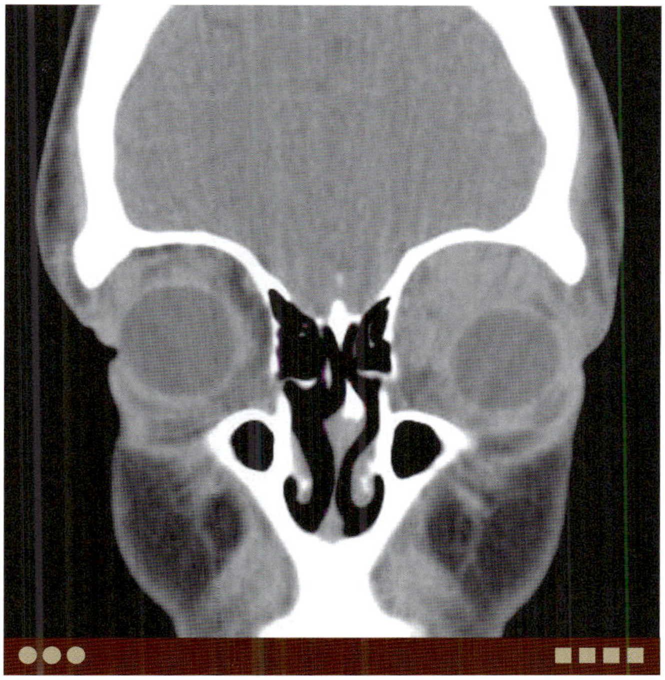

C. Sarcoidosis, same patient as A. Coronal CT demonstrates an ill-defined soft-tissue lesion in the superior left orbit displacing the globe inferiorly.

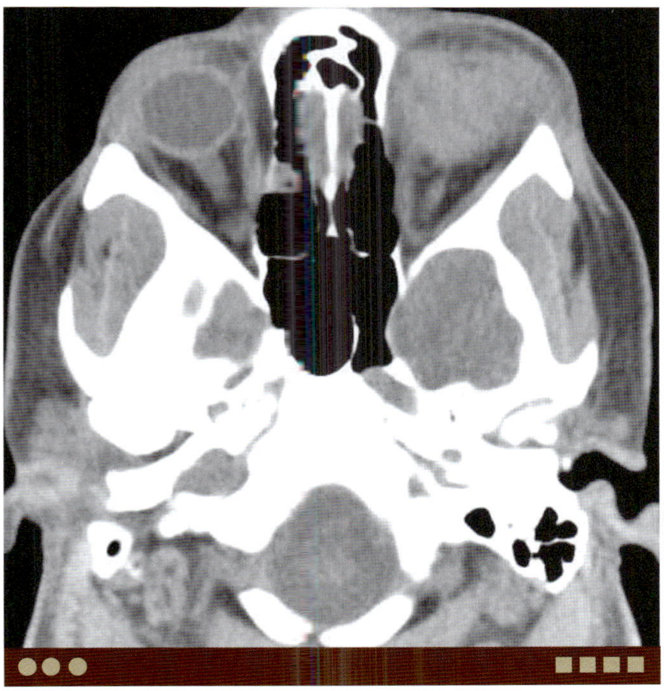

D. Sarcoidosis, same patient as A. Axial CT demonstrates diffuse soft-tissue infiltration in the superior left orbit extending to the periorbital soft tissues.

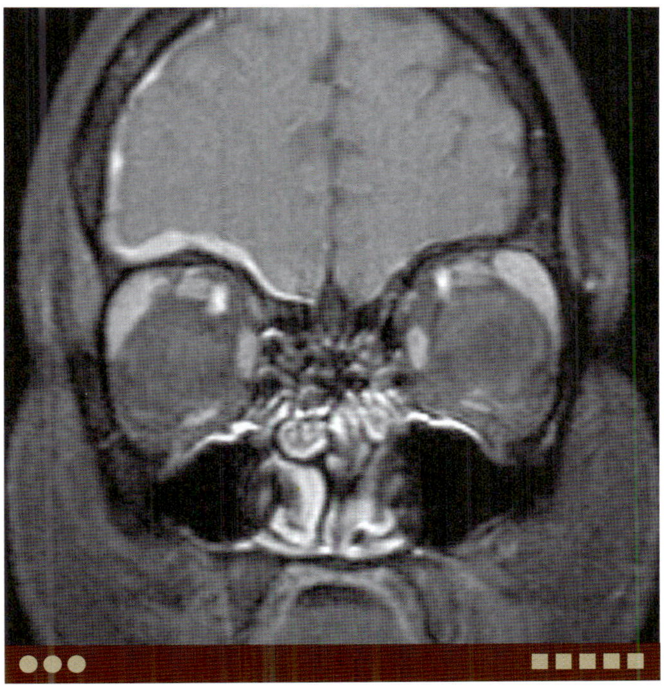

E. **Sarcoidosis** in a different patient. Coronal postcontrast fat-suppressed T1W MR image demonstrates enlargement and diffuse enhancement of the bilateral lacrimal glands. Note abnormal dural enhancement in the right frontal region.

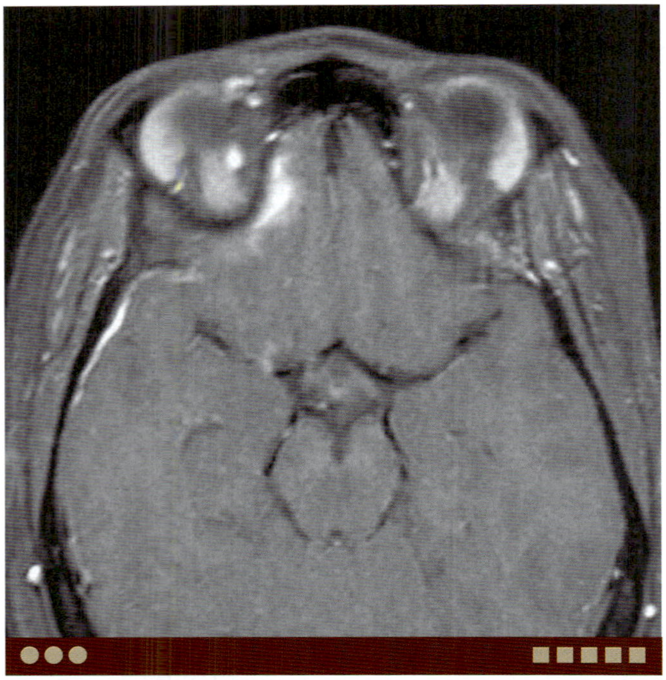

F. Sarcoidosis, same patient as E. Axial postcontrast fat-suppressed T1W MR image demonstrates homogenous enhancement of the lacrimal glands. Again, abnormal dural enhancement is seen in the right frontal region.

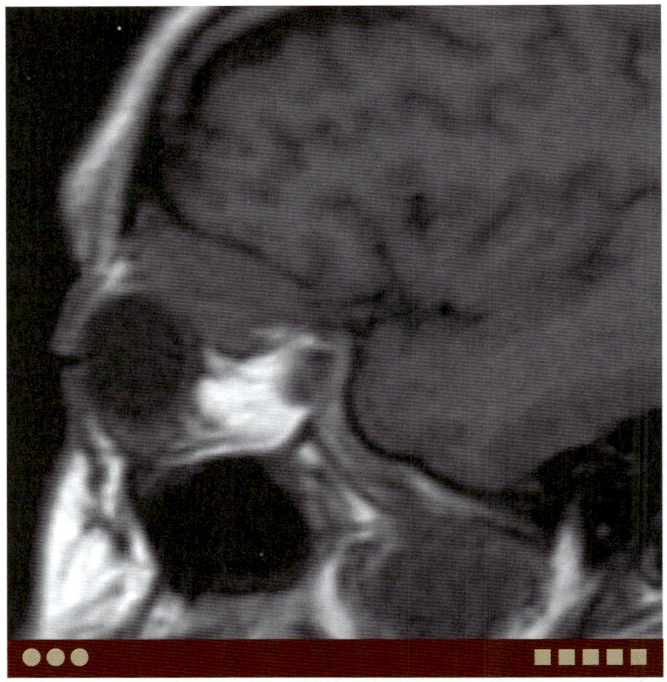

G. **Sarcoidosis** in a different patient. Sagittal T1W MR image demonstrates diffuse swelling of the superior rectus muscle complex.

DIFFERENTIAL DIAGNOSIS IMAGES (H-J)

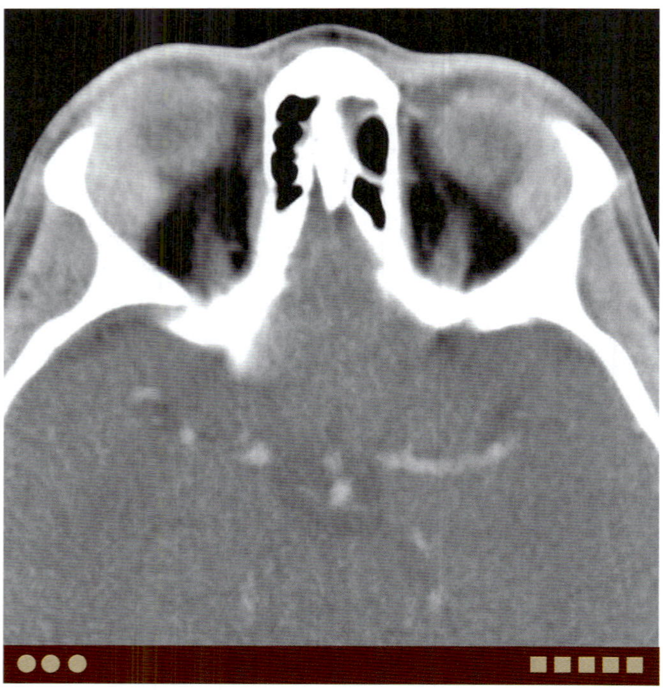

H. **Wegener's granulomatosis**. Axial postcontrast CT demonstrates enlargement and abnormal enhancement of the lacrimal glands bilaterally.

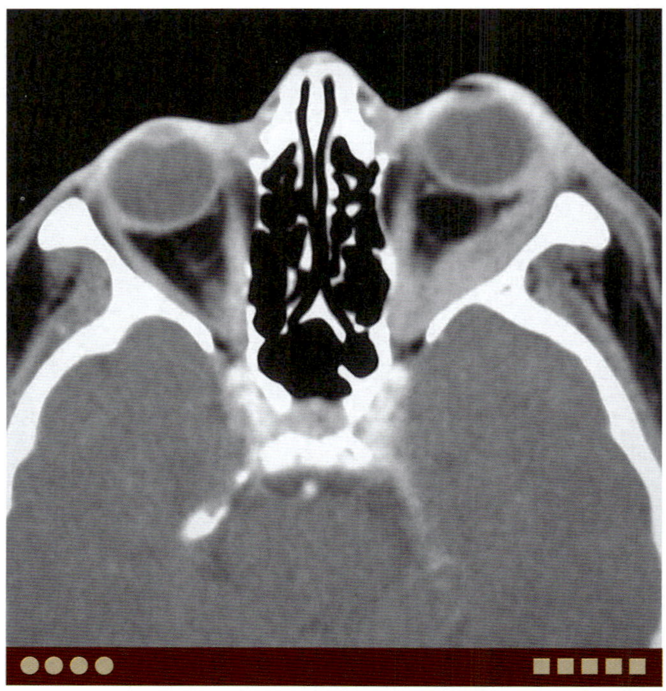

I. **Idiopathic orbital inflammation (IOI)**. Axial postcontrast CT demonstrates left-sided proptosis and enlargement of the lateral rectus muscle including the tendinous insertion. Isolated involvement of the lateral rectus muscle suggests IOI rather than thyroid orbitopathy.

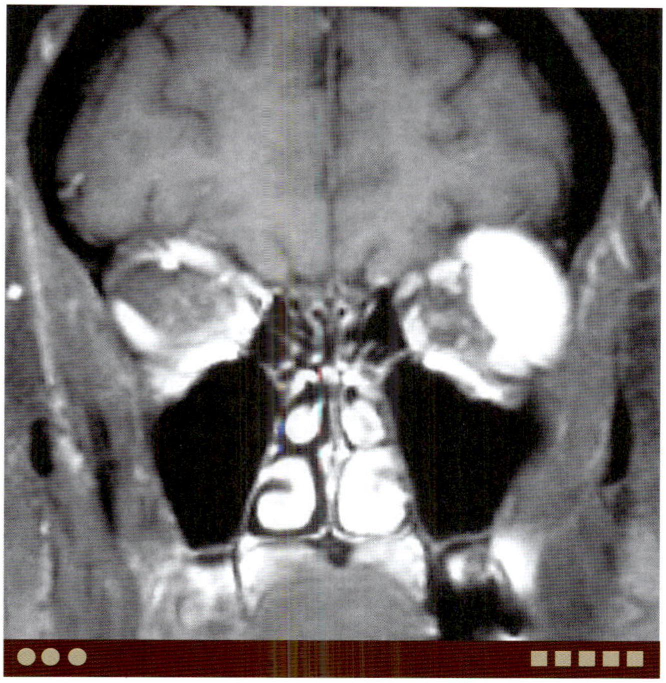

J. Adenoid cystic carcinoma. Coronal postcontrast fat-suppressed T1W MR image demonstrates an avidly enhancing lesion in the left lacrimal gland. Note the invasive appearance into the adjacent tissues.

Case 4–19 Orbital Capillary Hemangioma

Asim Mian, Osamu Sakai

PRESENTATION

Proptosis.

FINDINGS

CT demonstrates an avidly enhancing mass in the superior portion of the orbit.

DIFFERENTIAL DIAGNOSIS

- Venolymphatic malformation: Venolymphatic malformations usually consist of multiple cystic lesions that are prone to bleeding after minor trauma. On MRI, they are multicystic and may demonstrate fluid-fluid levels due to hemorrhage. The venous/capillary components show heterogeneous enhancement.
- Cellulitis: Cellulitis typically demonstrates inflammatory changes in the periorbital and orbital fat with or without a peripherally enhancing abscess. It is commonly associated with ethmoid sinusitis. Complications include superior ophthalmic vein and cavernous sinus thrombosis, meningitis and intracranial abscesses.
- Neuroblastoma: This is the most common metastatic tumor in children.
- Hematopoietic neoplasms: Leukemia and Langerhans cell histiocytosis are seen in children. Lymphoma in young children is relatively rare.

COMMENTS

This is a 7-year-old boy with proptosis.

Orbital capillary hemangioma is the most common orbital tumor of infancy and is thought to be a hamartomatous proliferation of vascular endothelial cells. They usually occur in the superior aspect of the orbit, eyelids, and supranasal region. It is uncommonly seen in a retrobulbar location (<10%). Orbital capillary hemangioma can range from 2 cm to 8 cm in size. It typically presents within the first 6 months of life. Orbital capillary hemangioma affects girls greater than boys by a ratio of 3:1. About 50% of lesions will involute by age 5 years, and 75% by age 7 years.

Treatments for lesions that do not resolve spontaneously include corticosteroids, surgery, and radiation depending on the aggressive nature of the lesion.

Ultrasound can provide rapid diagnosis by demonstrating a mass with prominent blood flow. CT demonstrates a homogeneous, avidly enhancing lobulated mass without

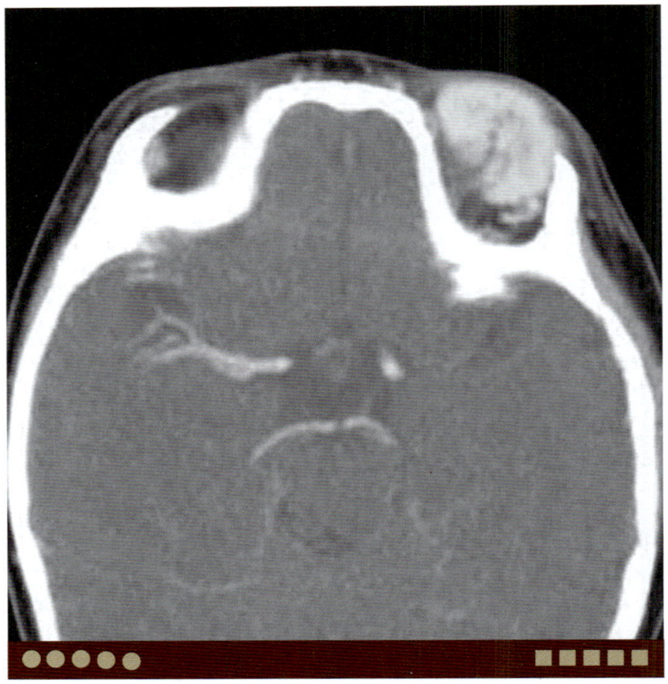

A. Orbital capillary hemangioma. Axial postcontrast CT demonstrates an avidly enhancing mass in the superior portion of the left orbit with partial extension into the preseptal space.

calcifications. MRI demonstrates a lobulated, hyperintense mass with flow voids on T2 W sequences. As on CT, there is avid enhancement of the lesion.

PEARLS

- **Capillary hemangioma is the most common orbital tumor of infancy.**
- **Capillary hemangioma typically presents within first 6 months of life and most involute after the first year.**
- **Ultrasound is useful for rapid diagnosis by demonstrating prominent blood flow.**
- **CT shows a lobulated, avidly enhancing mass without calcifications.**
- **On MRI, it shows a lobulated mass with high signal and flow-voids on T2W sequences and avid enhancement.**

ADDITIONAL IMAGE

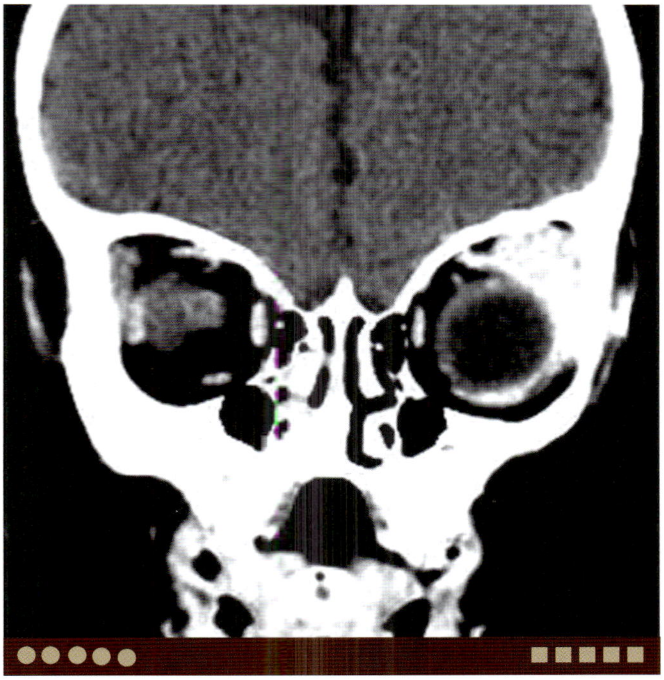

B. Orbital capillary hemangioma, same patient as A. Coronal postcontrast CT demonstrates an avidly enhancing mass in the superolateral portion of the left orbit displacing the globe.

DIFFERENTIAL DIAGNOSIS IMAGES (C-F)

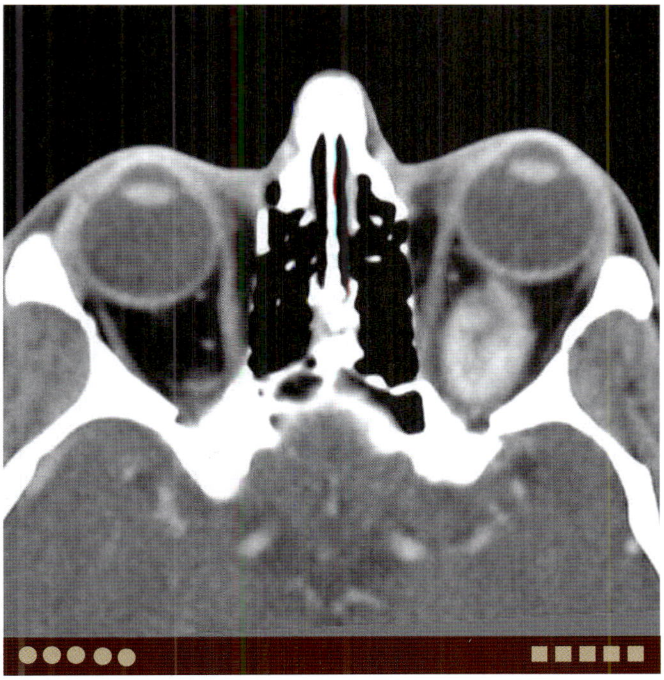

C. **Cavernous hemangioma**. Axial postcontrast CT demonstrates a well-marginated, ovoid enhancing lesion in the retrobulbar space of the left orbit.

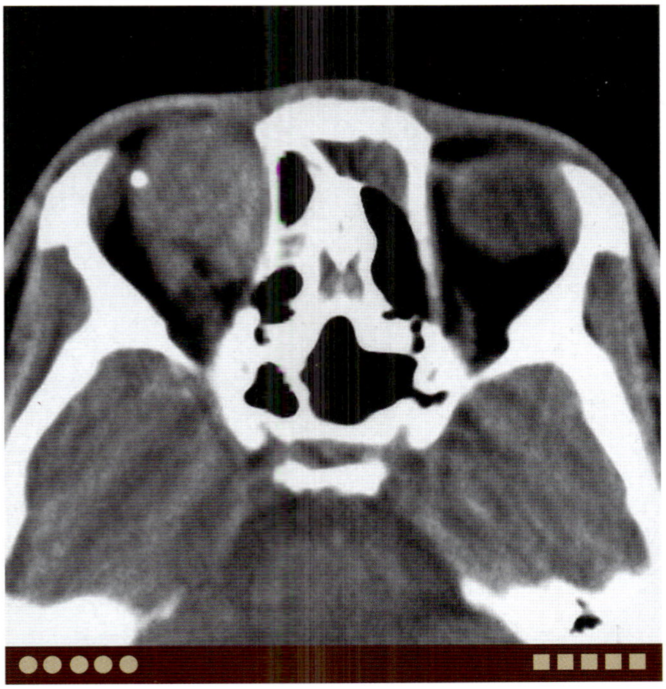

D. **Venous malformation**. Axial postcontrast CT demonstrates an enhancing lesion with phlebolith in the superior right orbit.

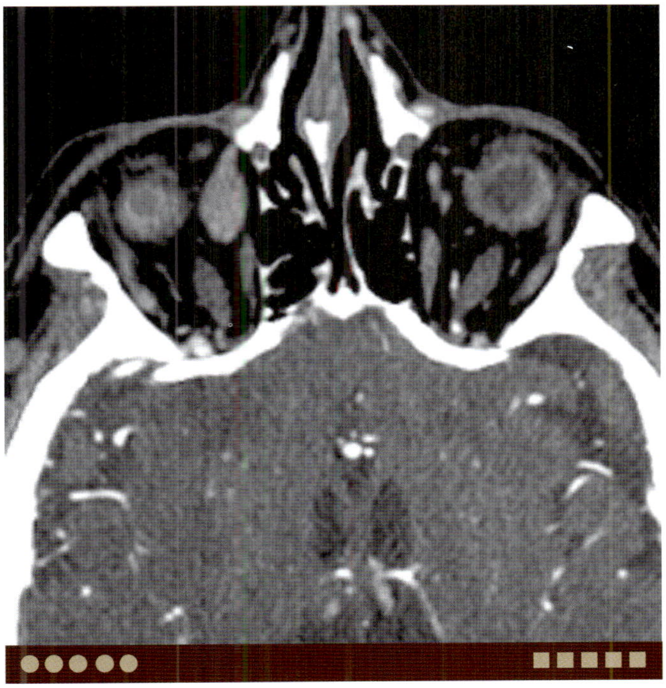

E. **Varix**. Axial postcontrast CT demonstrates an enhancing spindle-shaped lesion contiguous to the angular vein in the right orbit.

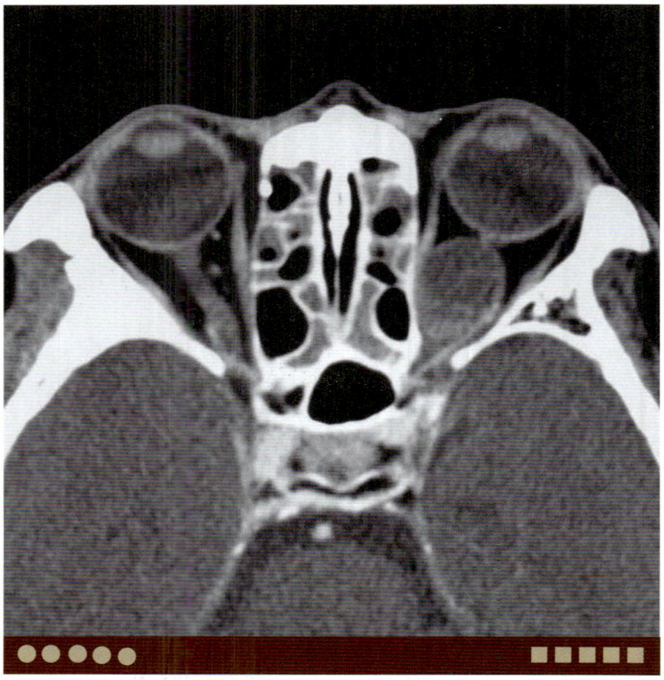

F. Schwannoma. Axial postcontrast CT demonstrates a mild, predominantly peripheral enhancement of the lesion in the left orbit.

Case 4–20 Subperiosteal Hematoma—Orbit

Hiroki Kato, Margaret Chapman, Osamu Sakai

PRESENTATION

Proptosis and downward displacement of the globe after trauma.

FINDINGS

CT demonstrates a well-defined, homogeneous, high attenuating mass located along the roof of the orbit.

DIFFERENTIAL DIAGNOSIS

- Lymphoma: Lymphoma can involve various structures of the orbit. A lesion along the orbital roof may mimic subperiosteal hematoma.
- Idiopathic orbital inflammation (IOI) ("pseudotumor"): IOIs are relatively common accounting for 12% to 15% of all orbital diseases. They commonly involve the lacrimal gland, extraocular muscles, and orbital fat. The mass forming type may demonstrate findings similar to subperiosteal hematoma.

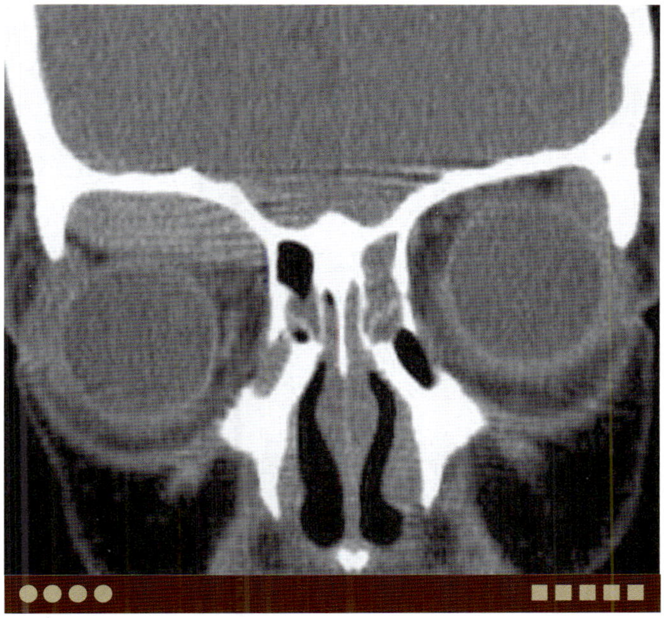

A. Traumatic subperiosteal hematoma. Coronal unenhanced CT demonstrates a well-defined, homogeneously high attenuating mass along the right orbital roof.

COMMENTS

This is an 8-year-old boy with slowly progressive proptosis after facial trauma.

Orbital hematomas are classified as either intraorbital or subperiosteal. Intraorbital (often retrobulbar) hematomas are common following maxillofacial trauma and orbital surgery, whereas subperiosteal hematomas are encountered less frequently. The etiology of subperiosteal hematoma is either traumatic or spontaneous. Traumatic subperiosteal hematomas occur more commonly in young males as a result of direct facial or orbital trauma. These usually occur either immediately following or within days of orbital trauma, as the hematoma develops secondary to rupture of the subperiosteal blood vessels. On the other hand, spontaneous subperiosteal hematoma can occur at any age after the sudden elevation of intracranial venous pressure.

Subperiosteal hematomas often involve the orbital roof, as the frontal bone comprises the largest surface area of the orbit. The orbit can compensate for small increases in orbital volume by proptosis. In fact, proptosis and downward displacement of the globe are commonly seen, even without apparent ecchymosis, chemosis, or subconjuctival hemorrhage. Increasing hematoma size and rapid increases in orbital tissue pressure can result in impairment of motility of the globe and a decrease in visual acuity due to acute compressive optic neuropathy.

CT is essential for the accurate diagnosis of orbital subperiosteal hematomas. Their extent can be delineated with coronal and sagittal reformatted images. Typical CT findings of acute and subacute subperiosteal hematomas include a well-defined, homogeneous, high attenuation mass along the roof of the orbit with inferior displacement of the orbital contents. Chronic subperiosteal hematomas show a heterogeneous, relatively low attenuation mass. MR images demonstrate characteristic signals of an evolving hematoma.

PEARLS

- **Subperiosteal hematomas are relatively rare when compared to intraorbital (retrobulbar) hematomas, and may develop either spontaneously or following trauma.**
- **CT is essential for the accurate diagnosis of orbital subperiosteal hematomas, particularly with coronal and sagittal reformatted images.**
- **Acute and subacute subperiosteal hematomas typically demonstrate a well-defined, homogeneous, high attenuation mass along the orbital roof with displacement of the orbital contents inferiorly.**

ADDITIONAL IMAGES (B-D)

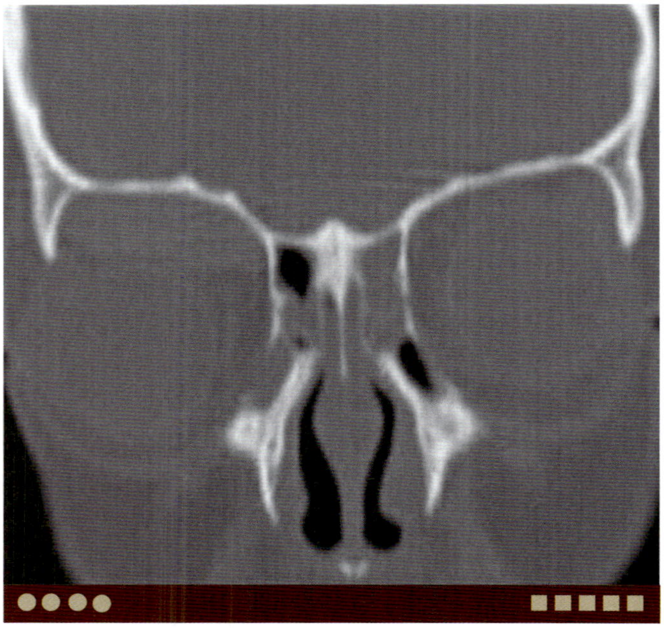

B. Subperiosteal hematoma, same patient as A. Coronal unenhanced CT (bone algorithm) demonstrates a hematoma without a fracture of the right orbital roof.

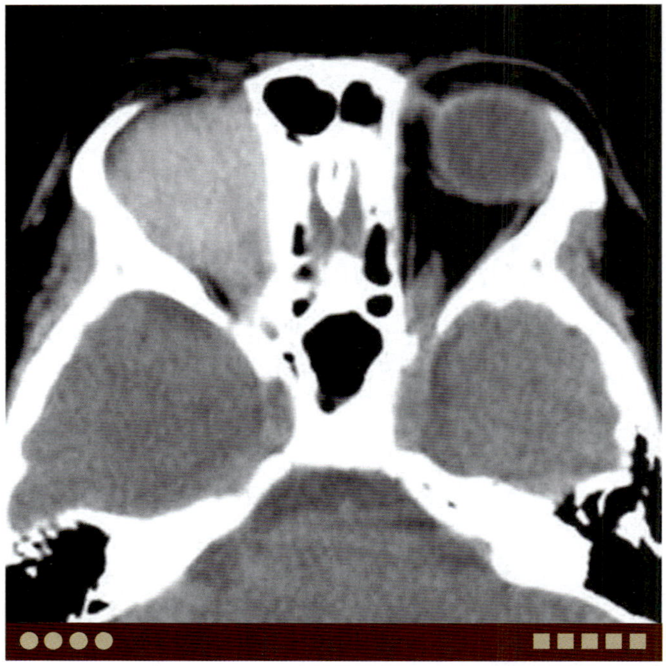

C. Subperiosteal hematoma, same patient as A. Axial unenhanced CT demonstrates a homogeneously hyperdense lesion in the superior right orbit.

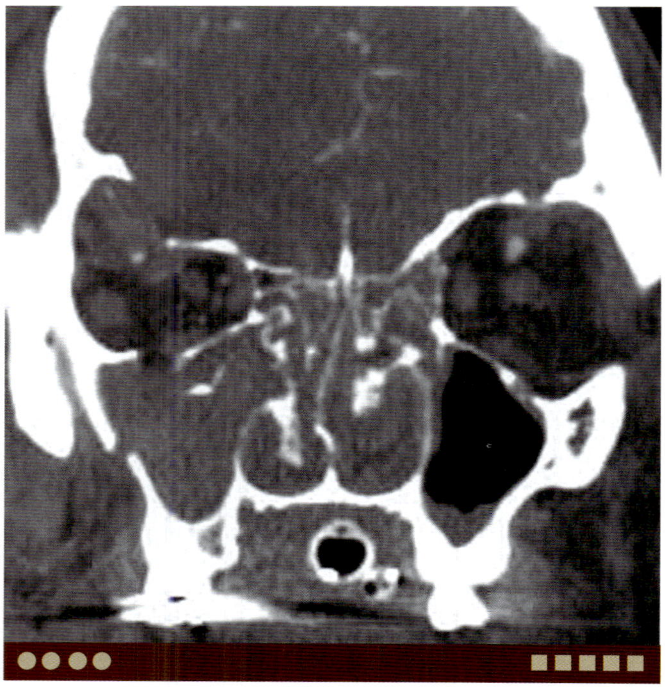

D. **Orbital fracture and hematoma**. Coronal postcontrast CT demonstrates a hematoma along a right orbital roof fracture. Fractures are also seen in the orbital floor and maxillary sinus wall.

DIFFERENTIAL DIAGNOSIS IMAGES (F-J)

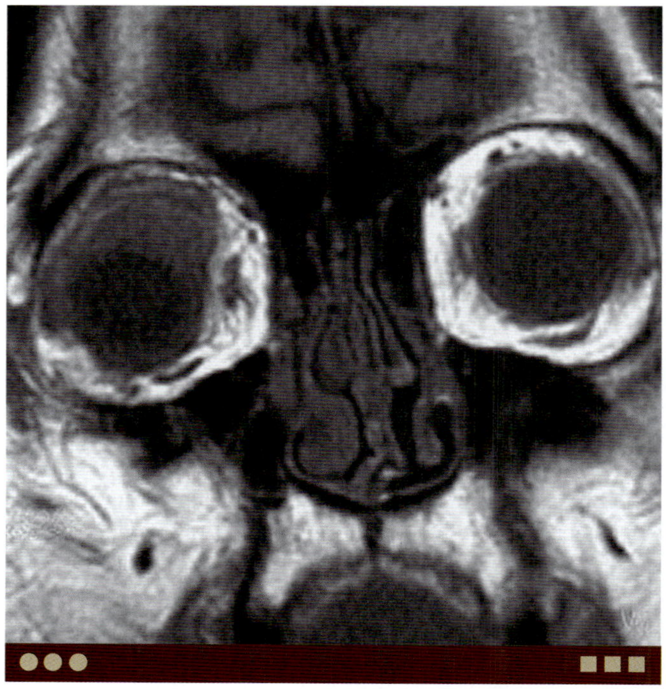

E. **IOI**. Coronal T1W image demonstrates a hypointense lesion in the superior portion of the right orbit.

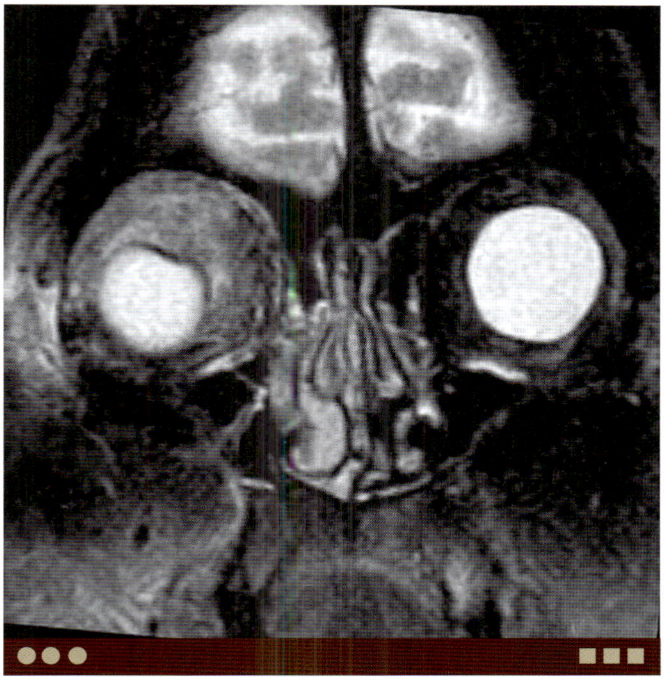

F. IOI, same patient as E. Coronal fat-suppressed T2W image demonstrates a relatively high-signal intensity lesion with ill-defined margins.

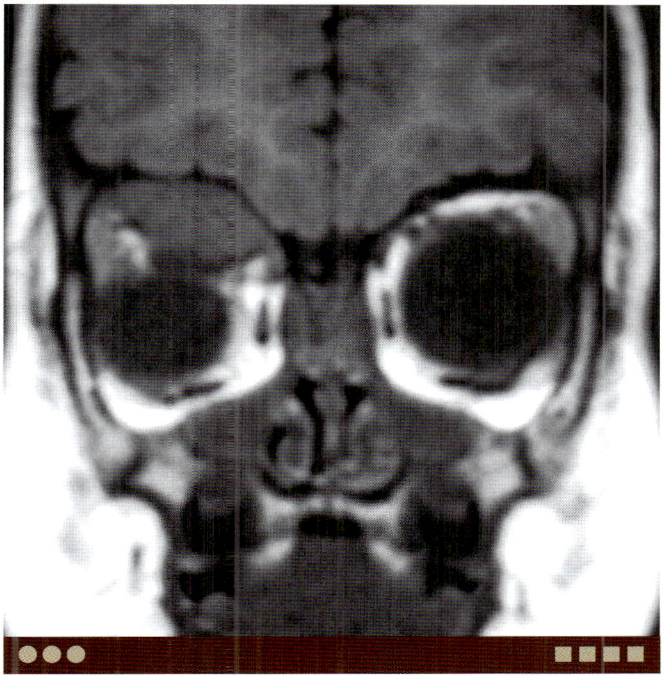

G. Langerhans cell histiocytosis. Coronal T1W image demonstrates a hypointense lesion along the roof of the right orbit.

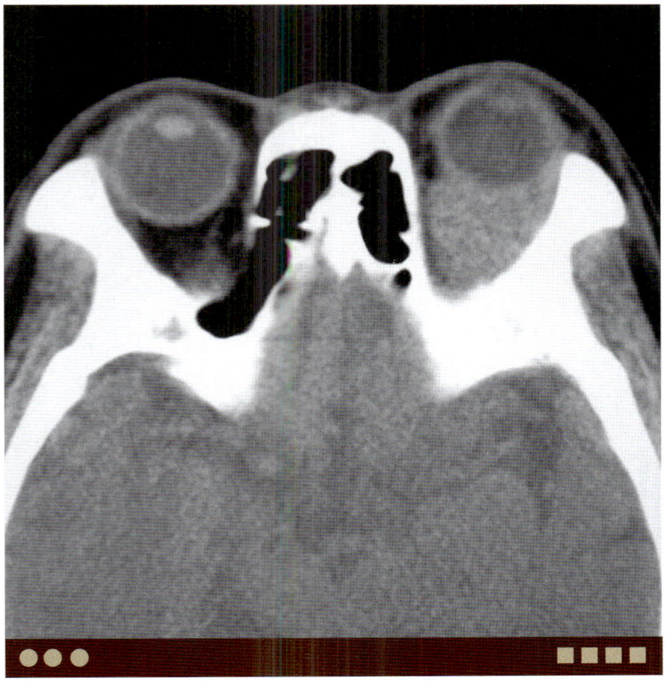

H. Lymphoma, B-cell large. Axial noncontrast CT demonstrates a homogeneous density soft tissue mass in the superior left orbit.

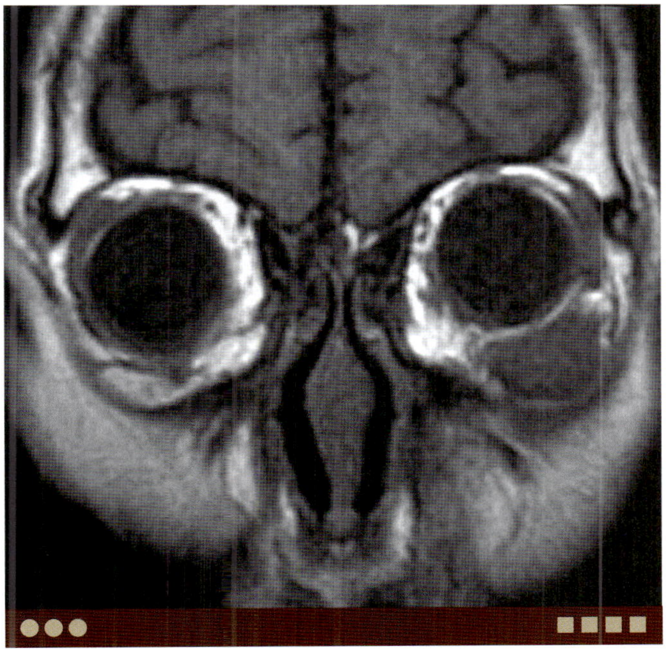

I. Lymphoma, mucosa associated lymphoid tissue (MALT). Coronal T1W image demonstrates a hypointense tumor in the inferior aspect of the right eyelid.

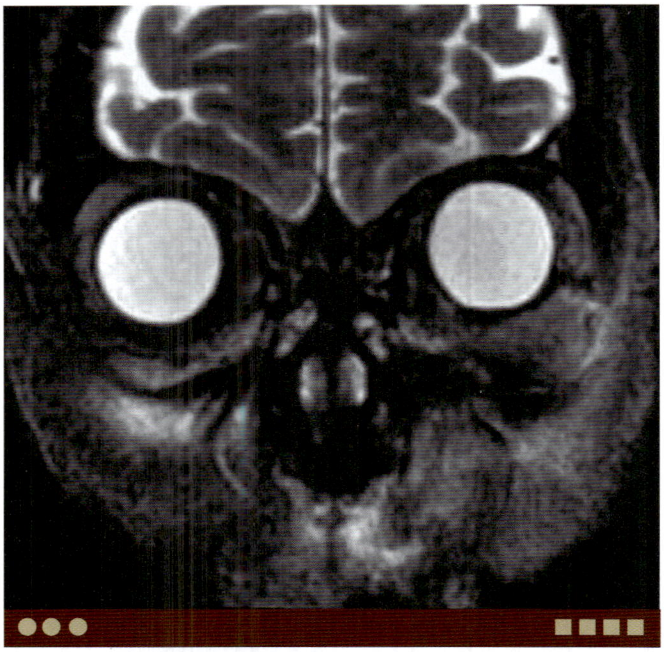

J. Lymphoma, MALT, same patient as I. Coronal fat-suppressed T2W image demonstrates low-to-intermediate signal intensity of the lesion.

Case 4–21 Retrobulbar Hemorrhage

Memi Watanabe, Margaret Chapman, Osamu Sakai

PRESENTATION

Sudden onset of painful proptosis and decreased visual acuity.

FINDINGS

CT demonstrates an ill-defined, irregularly shaped soft-tissue density in the retrobulbar space.

DIFFERENTIAL DIAGNOSIS

- Orbital cellulitis: This is infection/inflammation of the orbit proper, and requires intravenous antibiotics administration. Surgical drainage can be performed for abscess formation.
- Idiopathic orbital inflammation (IOI) ("pseudotumor"): This may present as an irregular soft-tissue density in the retrobulbar space, usually with enhancement after contrast administration.
- Lymphoma: Imaging findings of lymphoma may be similar to retrobulbar hemorrhage; however, clinically this condition does not progress within minutes or hours.
- Optic nerve sheath meningioma: A high density "tram-track sign" is seen with optic nerve sheath meningioma. However, the clinical scenario is quite different; there is no history of trauma and the decrease in visual acuity is gradual.

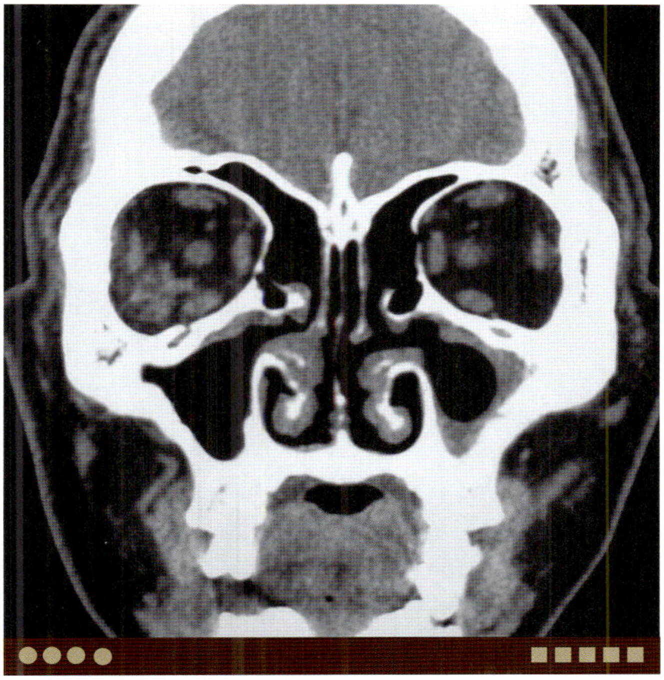

A. Retrobulbar hemorrhage. Coronal CT demonstrates poorly defined intermediate-density areas in the retrobulbar fat on the right.

COMMENTS

Retrobulbar hemorrhage is rare but may occur after maxillofacial trauma, such as zygomaticomaxillary complex and blow-out fractures, orbital and periorbital surgery, and retrobulbar injections. Trauma may be relatively subtle, and further hemorrhage can occur spontaneously. The early clinical features of retrobulbar hemorrhage are decreasing visual acuity, pain, and proptosis, while late signs include ophthalmoplegia, lid ecchymosis, chemosis, mydriasis, and loss of the direct light reflex. Fundoscopy may reveal a pale optic disc. Delayed onset of retrobulbar hemorrhage occurring days after facial injury has been reported.

Retrobulbar hemorrhage causes ischemia of the anterior optic nerve by direct compression of the nerve or vasculature, or by increasing the intraorbital pressure resulting in compression or occlusion of the central retinal artery (compartment syndrome). Because this condition can lead to serious complications including irreversible blindness, prompt recognition and decompression is critical.

CT is usually performed for the initial assessment of maxillofacial trauma and is very helpful in diagnosing retrobulbar hemorrhage, although it can be strongly suspected by clinical evaluation. CT usually demonstrates poorly marginated intermediate-to-high density areas in the retrobulbar fat with various degree of proptosis. Less frequently, hemorrhage confined to the optic nerve sheath is seen.

PEARLS

- **Acute retrobulbar hemorrhage is a sight-threatening condition which requires prompt decompression.**
- **Common clinical presentations include impairment of visual acuity, proptosis, ophthalmoplegia, and pain. Retrobulbar hemorrhage may present days after the injury.**
- **Retrobulbar hemorrhage is often seen as poorly defined densities in the retrobulbar fat. Less frequently, hemorrhage confined to the optic nerve sheath is seen.**

ADDITIONAL IMAGES (B-G)

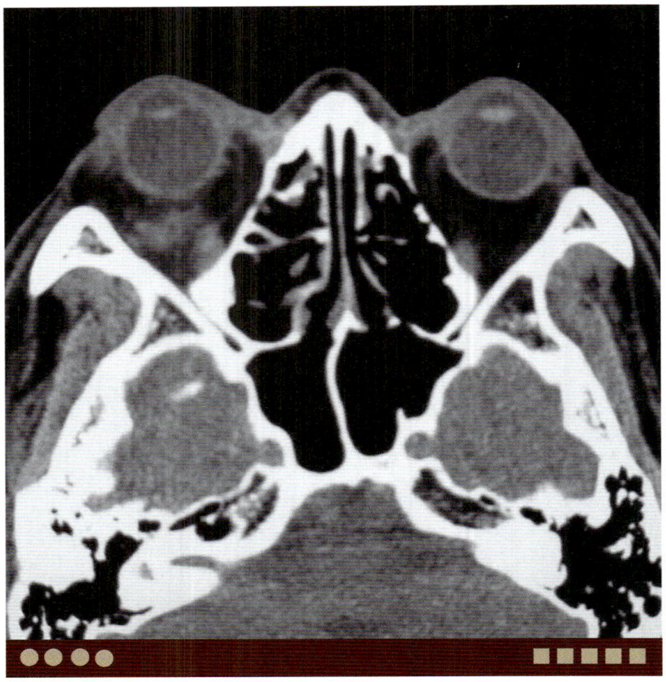

B. Retrobulbar hemorrhage, same patient as A. Axial CT demonstrates poorly defined densities in the retrobulbar space with slight proptosis on the right.

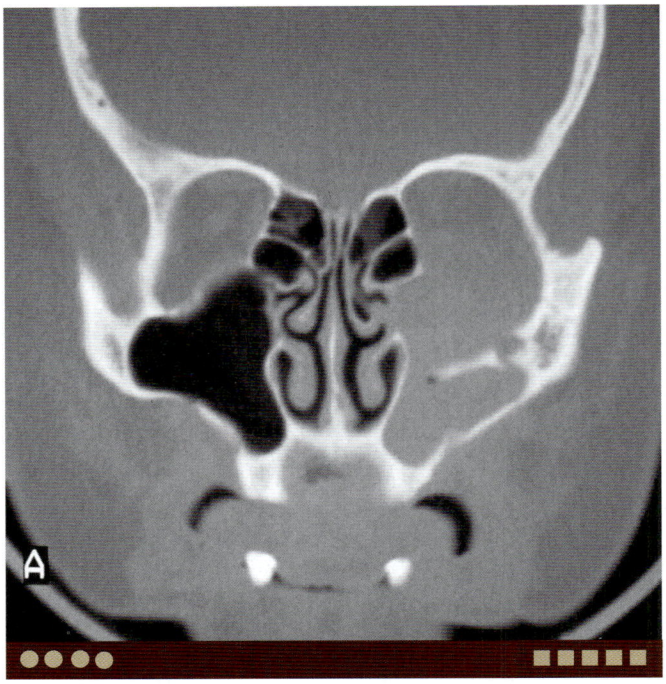

C. **Blow-out fracture and retrobulbar hemorrhage**. Coronal CT demonstrates fractures of the inferior and medial walls of the left orbit.

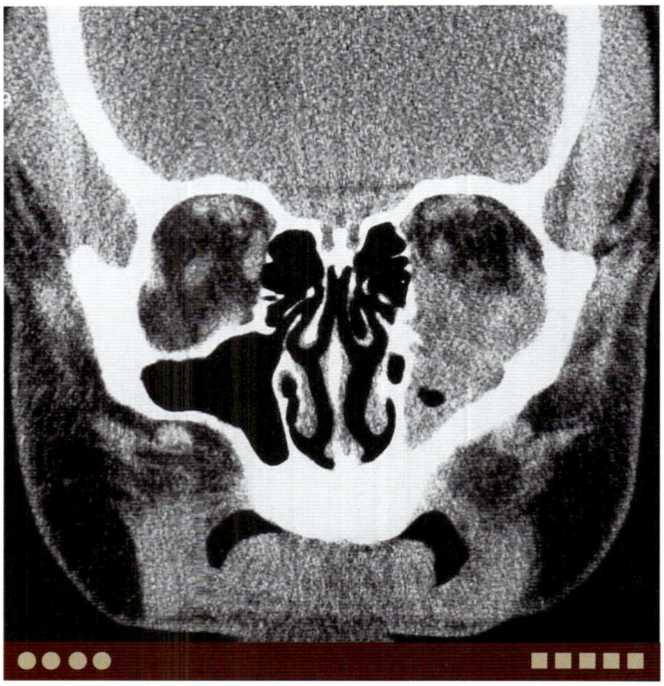

D. Blow-out fracture and retrobulbar hemorrhage, same patient as C. Coronal CT in soft tissue window demonstrates heterogeneous densities in the inferior retrobulbar space on the left.

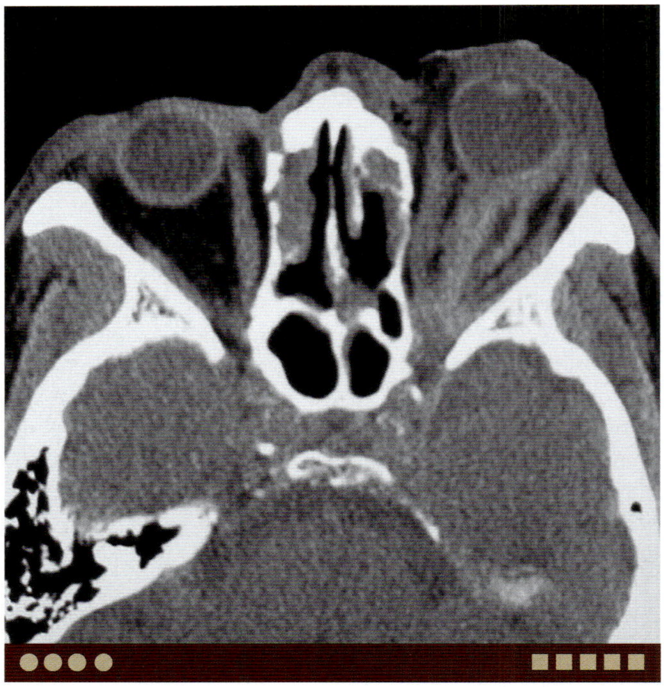

E. **Retrobulbar hemorrhage** in a different patient. Axial CT demonstrates proptosis, thickening and increased density of the left optic nerve sheath complex suggestive of hematoma. Note flattening of the posterior wall of the globe secondary to increased intraorbital pressure.

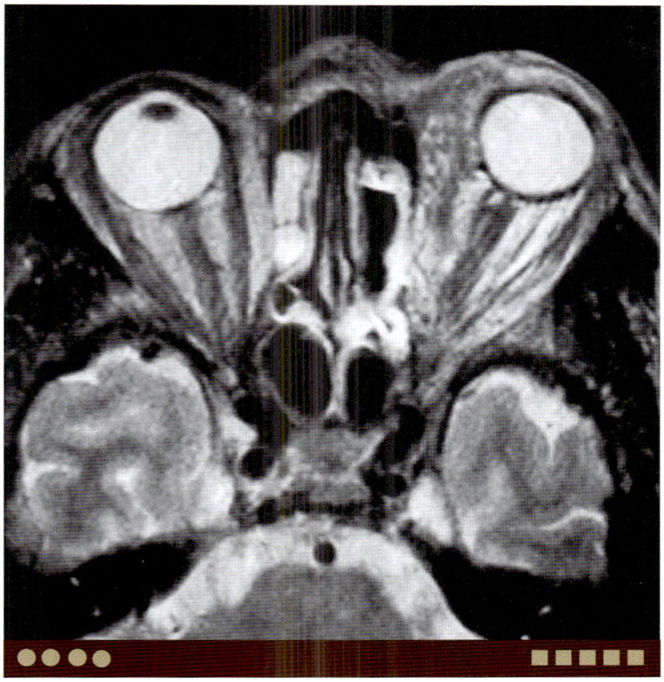

F. Retrobulbar hemorrhage, same patient as E. Axial T2W image demonstrates diffuse heterogeneous signal in the left retrobulbar fat. Thickened optic nerve sheath complex shows heterogeneous low signal likely from deoxyhemoglobin.

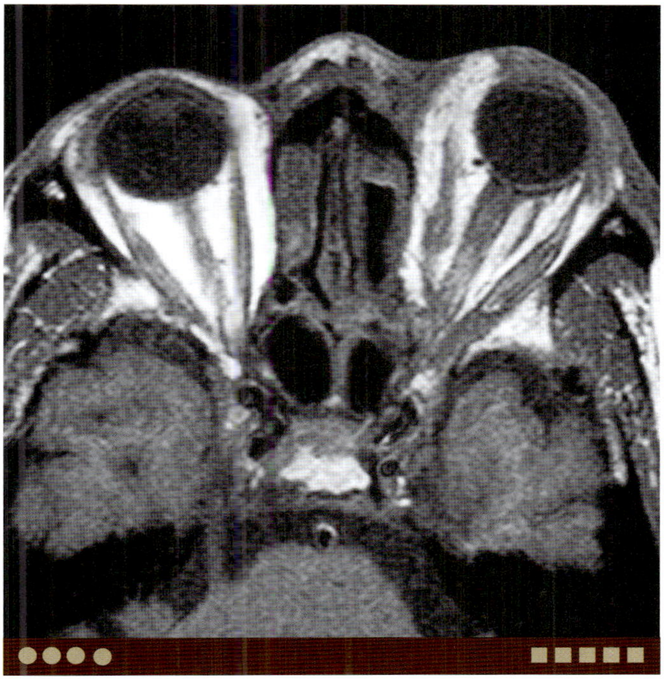

G. Retrobulbar hemorrhage, same patient as E. Axial T1W image demonstrates thickening of the left optic nerve sheath complex and the extraocular muscles.

DIFFERENTIAL DIAGNOSIS IMAGES (H-J)

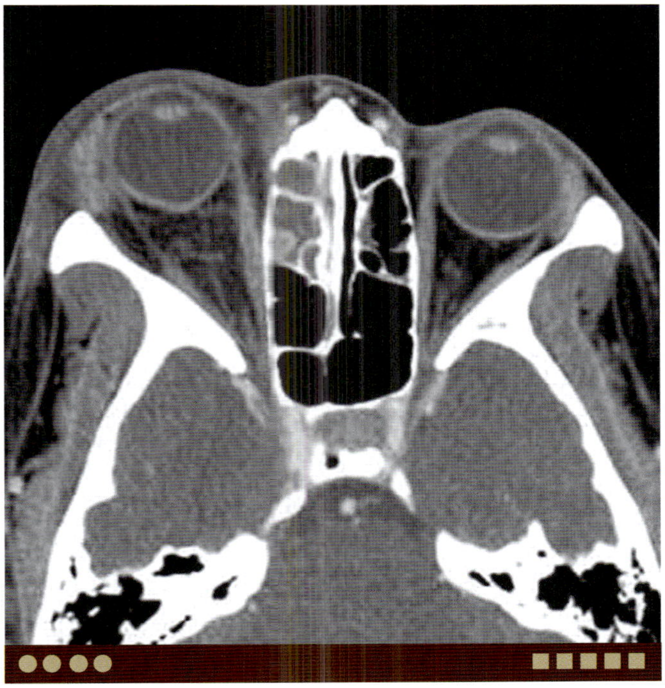

H. **Orbital cellulitis**. Axial contrast-enhanced CT demonstrates increased density in the right retrobulbar fat as well as soft tissue swelling over the right orbit.

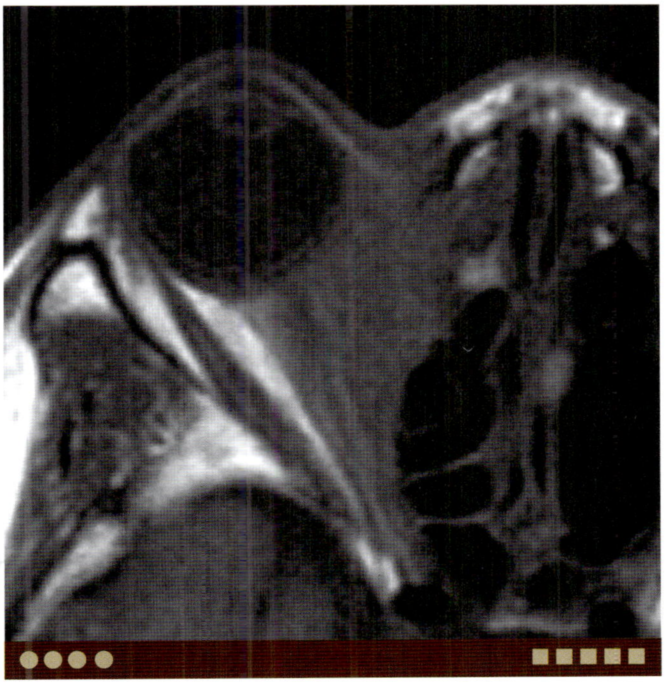

I. **IOI**. Axial T1W image demonstrates proptosis with diffuse medial infiltration that involves the optic nerve sheath complex.

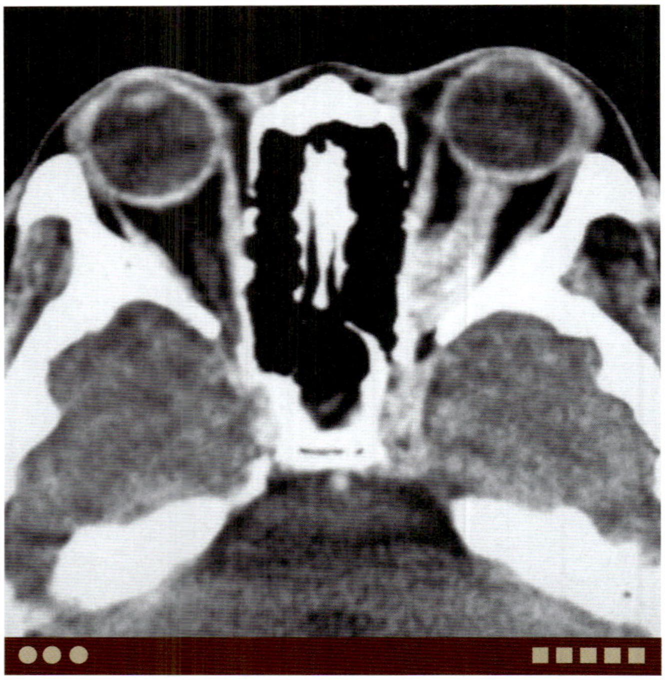

J. Optic nerve sheath meningioma. Axial postcontrast CT demonstrates "tram-track" high density in the posterior portion of the intraorbital segment of the left optic nerve sheath complex.

Case 4–22 Leukemia—Lacrimal Gland

Hiroki Kato, Asim Mian, Osamu Sakai

PRESENTATION

Rapid onset of proptosis and inflammation.

FINDINGS

CT and MRI demonstrate enlargement of the lacrimal gland.

DIFFERENTIAL DIAGNOSIS

- Lymphoma: Orbital lymphomas account for 5% to 14% of all extranodal lymphomas. In the largest reported series, approximately 20% of orbital lymphomas were located in the lacrimal gland followed by the conjunctiva and then the eyelid.
- Idiopathic orbital inflammation (IOI) ("pseudotumor"): IOI is often difficult to distinguish from lymphoma. This can be a solid or diffuse infiltrative lesion.
- Pleomorphic adenoma: Pleomorphic adenoma is the most common epithelial tumor of the lacrimal gland accounting for half of all epithelial lesions in the lacrimal fossa. Malignant mixed tumor (carcinoma ex pleomorphic adenoma) also occurs in the lacrimal gland.
- Adenoid cystic carcinoma: Adenoid cystic carcinoma is the most common malignant epithelial neoplasm in the lacrimal gland accounting for about 50% of malignant lacrimal gland tumors and 25% of all lacrimal gland tumors. Other malignant epithelial tumors of the lacrimal gland include mucoepidermoid carcinoma, adenocarcinoma, squamous cell carcinoma and undifferentiated carcinoma

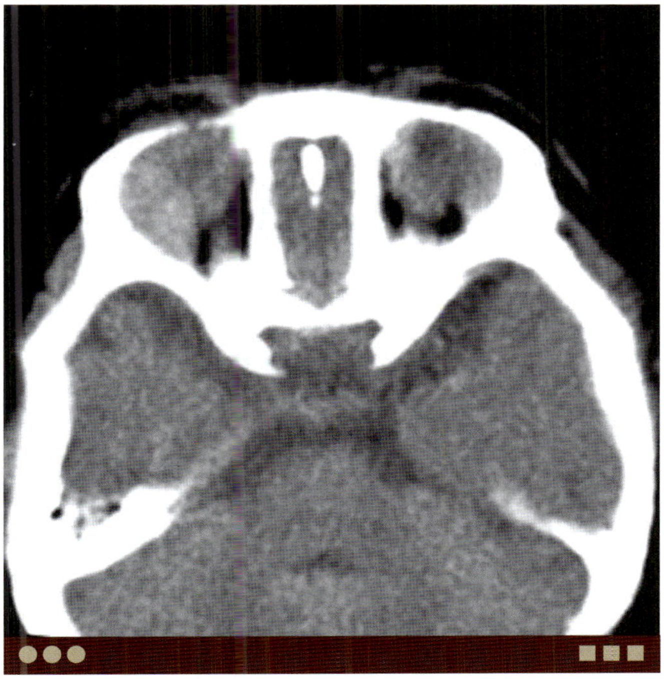

A. Acute myelogenous leukemia. Axial unenhanced CT demonstrates an enlargement of the right lacrimal gland.

COMMENTS

This is a 7-month-old girl who presented with right proptosis and painless enlargement of the right lacrimal gland.

Orbital involvement of leukemia is not uncommon. In children it is often by acute myelogenous leukemia (AML) and in adults chronic lymphocytic leukemia (CLL). The orbit is typically affected by malignant leukemic cells during the course of the disease. Orbital involvement is seen in about 10% of patients with systemic leukemia at autopsy. Orbital involvement is more common in children and is often bilateral. Signs of orbital disease include a rapid onset of proptosis and inflammation that may resemble orbital cellulitis. Spontaneous orbital hemorrhage has also been reported with leukemia. Granulocytic sarcoma, also known as "chloroma," is an orbital complication of AML. The orbital granulocytic sarcoma may cause progressive proptosis before or after the onset of systemic leukemia. This tumor primarily involves the orbital fat and it can extend to the lacrimal gland. If it extends into the temporal or anterior cranial fossa, dural or leptomeningeal enhancement is observed on enhanced CT and MRI.

Mikulicz's disease is benign and chronic dacryoadenitis which demonstrates swelling of the lacrimal gland and salivary gland. It usually involves the bilateral lacrimal glands and impairs lacrimation without pain. The term, Mikulicz's syndrome may be used if this condition occurs secondary to leukemia, lymphoma, IOI, sarcoidosis, tuberculosis and other granulomatous diseases.

PEARLS

- **Orbital involvement of leukemia is not uncommon. AML in children and CLL in adults commonly involve the orbit.**
- **Orbital involvement of leukemia is more common in children and is often bilateral.**
- **Granulocytic sarcoma is an orbital complication of AML.**

DIFFERENTIAL DIAGNOSIS IMAGES (B-G)

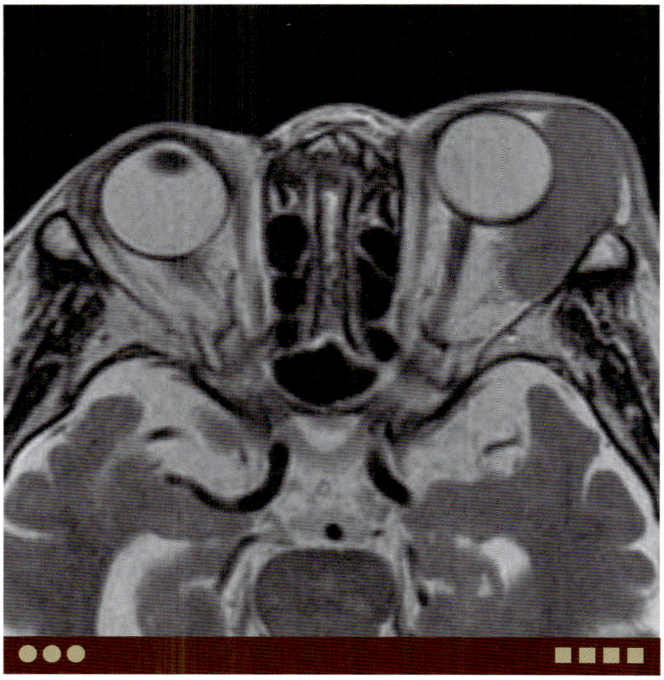

B. Mucosa-associated lymphoid tissue (MALT) lymphoma. Axial T2W image demonstrates a bulky, homogeneous intermediate signal mass in the left lacrimal gland.

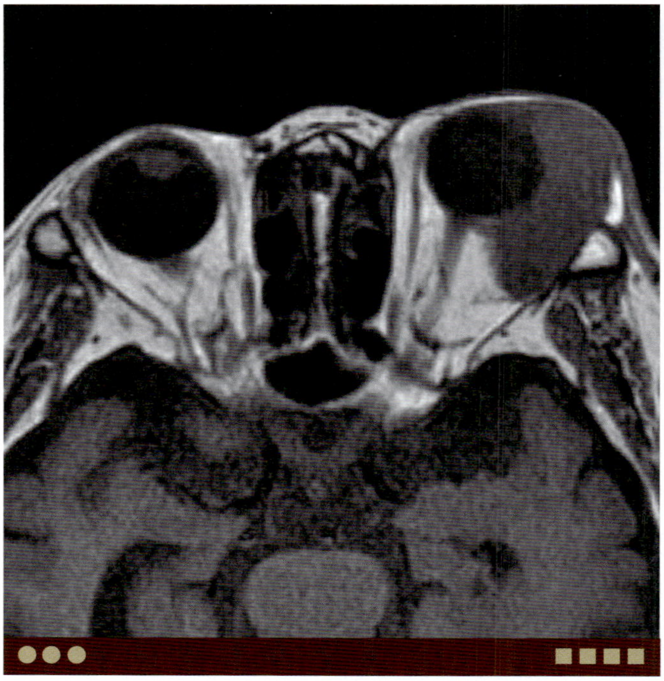

C. MALT lymphoma, same patient as B. Axial T1W image demonstrates a homogeneously low-signal lesion in the left lacrimal gland.

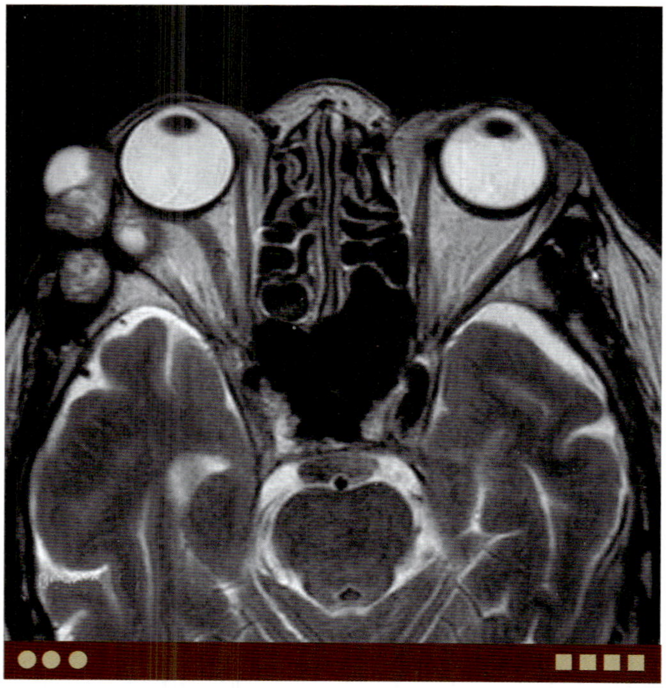

D. Recurrent pleomorphic adenoma. Axial T2W image demonstrates multicystic lesions centered in the region of the right lacrimal gland.

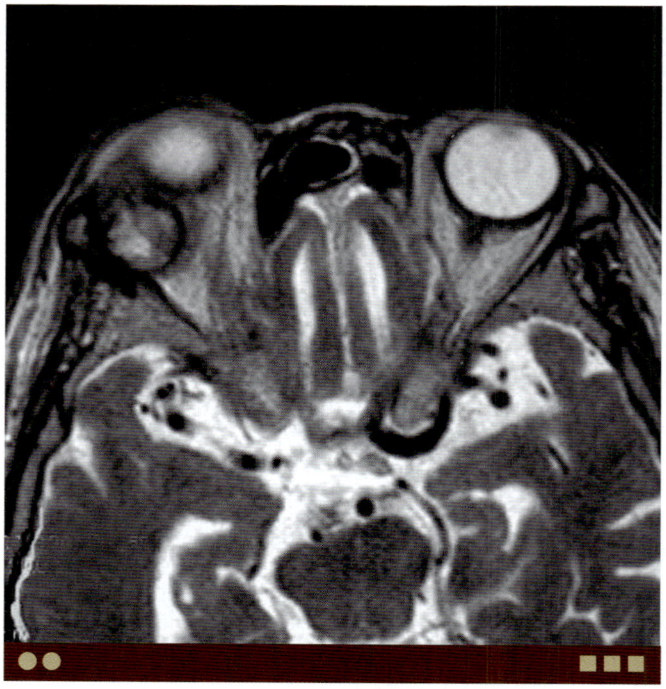

E. Adenocarcinoma. Axial T2W image demonstrates a poorly defined heterogeneously hyperintense tumor arising from the right lacrimal gland.

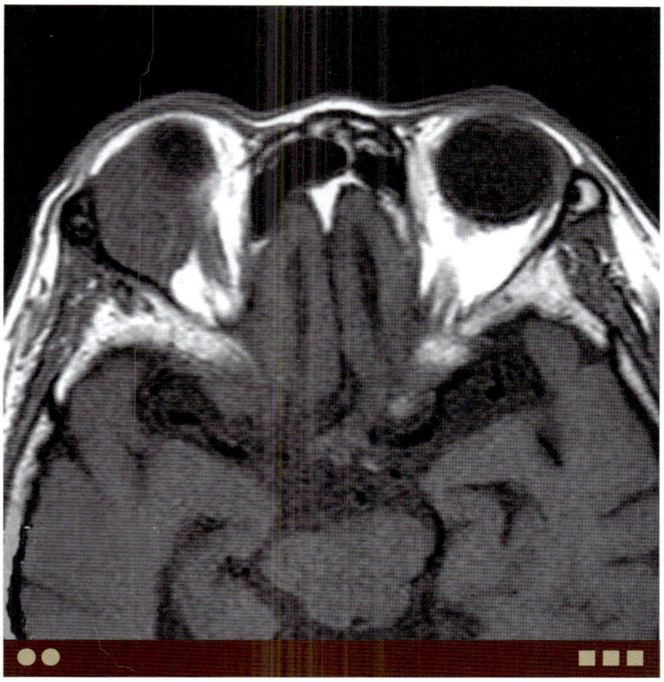

F. Adenocarcinoma, same patient as E. Axial T1W image demonstrates a low-signal lesion in the right lacrimal gland.

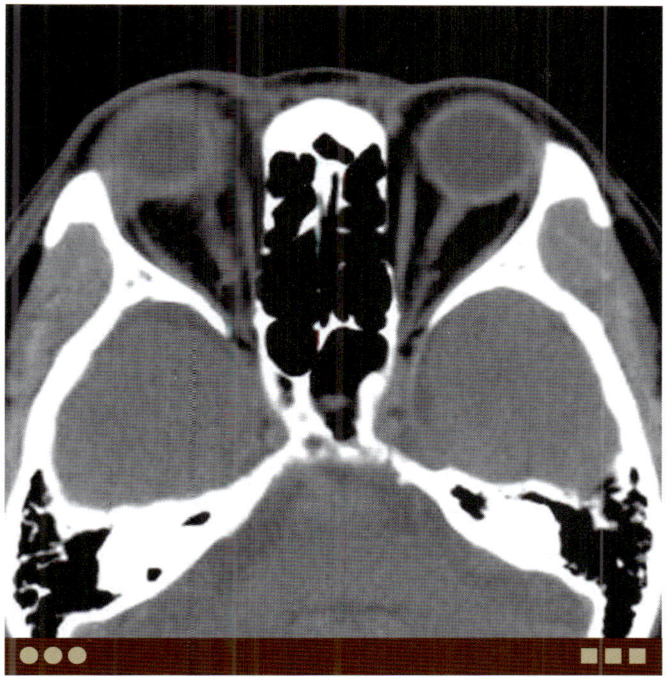

G. **IOI**. Axial unenhanced CT demonstrates a poorly defined soft tissue density lesion in the right orbit.

Case 4–23 Sjögren's Syndrome—Lacrimal Gland

Hiroki Kato, Margaret Chapman, Osamu Sakai

PRESENTATION

Enlargement of the lacrimal glands.

FINDINGS

CT and MRI demonstrate either symmetric or asymmetric enlargement of the bilateral lacrimal glands.

DIFFERENTIAL DIAGNOSIS

- Sarcoidosis: Ophthalmologic involvement in sarcoidosis is frequent, and is seen in 20% to 25% of affected patients. Uveitis is the most common ocular manifestation; however, sarcoidosis may involve any part of the orbit, including the lacrimal gland. Enlargement of the bilateral lacrimal glands is commonly seen.
- Lymphoma: Lymphoma of the lacrimal gland demonstrates diffuse enlargement with oblong contouring of the gland. These tumors are usually bulky, frequently exhibiting anterior and posterior extension.
- Idiopathic orbital inflammation (IOI) ("pseudotumor"): IOI often involves the lacrimal gland, although it can be seen in any part of the orbit.

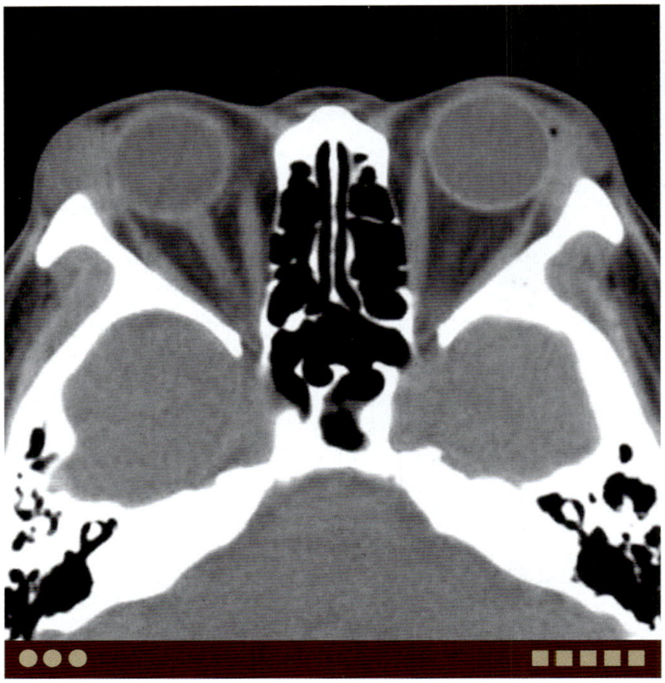

A. Sjögren's syndrome. Axial unenhanced CT demonstrates symmetric enlargement of the bilateral lacrimal glands.

COMMENTS

This is a 38-year-old woman presenting with bilateral symmetric enlargement of the lacrimal gland.

Sjögren's syndrome is a chronic autoimmune disease characterized by keratoconjunctivitis sicca and xerostomia. It has long been recognized that there is a spectrum of lymphoproliferative activity ranging from benign typical Sjögren's syndrome with local disease of glandular tissue (lymphoepithelial disease), to pseudolymphoma with extraglandular spread of the benign lymphoproliferation, and lymphoreticular malignancy. Lymphoma is reported to develop in up to 6% of patients per year in those with Sjögren's syndrome. The risk of patients developing lymphoma has been calculated to be approximately 44 times greater than that in a comparable unaffected population.

The lacrimal gland is one of the major targets of autoimmune diseases, including Sjögren's syndrome. Affected patients usually demonstrate bilateral symmetric or asymmetric enlargement of the lacrimal glands, reflecting a granulomatous inflammatory process composed of epithelial cells surrounded by macrophages and lymphocytes. The lacrimal gland in patients with Sjögren's syndrome exhibits varying signal on T1W and T2W images irrespective of lacrimal flow rates. Lacrimal glands in patients with Sjögren's syndrome can be categorized as hypertrophic, normal-sized, or atrophic. Hypertrophic glands are often moderately impaired in lacrimal function. Normal-sized glands show more heterogeneous lacrimal gland function, ranging from slightly to severely impaired lacrimal flow rates, and atrophic glands are the most severely impaired.

Although it is important to diagnose lymphoma in a patient with Sjögren's syndrome, it is often very difficult to differentiate between benign lymphoproliferative disorders and lymphoma because of their nonspecific imaging features.

PEARLS

- **Sjögren's syndrome usually demonstrates bilateral symmetric or asymmetric enlargement of the lacrimal glands, reflecting a granulomatous inflammatory infiltration.**
- **The lacrimal glands in patients with Sjögren's syndrome are categorized as hypertrophic, normal-sized, or atrophic.**
- **It is difficult to differentiate between benign lymphoproliferative disorders and lymphoma because of their nonspecific imaging features.**

ADDITIONAL IMAGES (B-D)

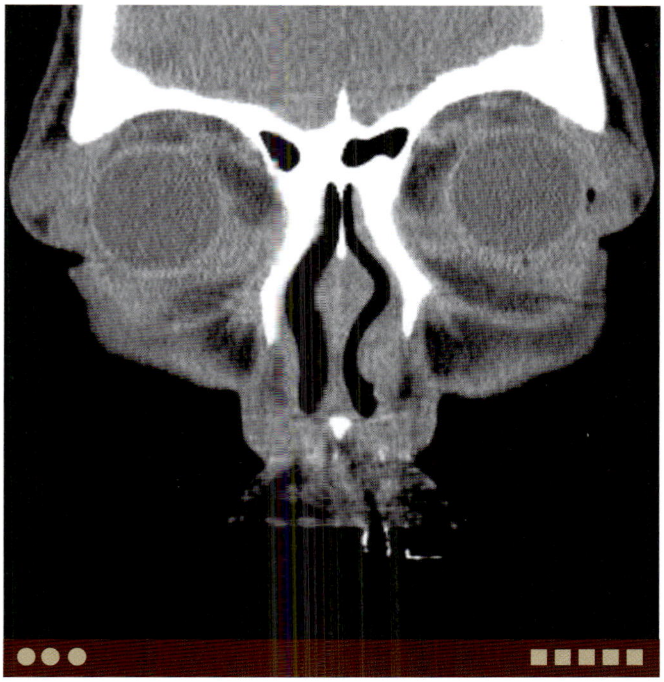

B. Sjögren's syndrome, same patient as A. Coronal unenhanced CT demonstrates symmetrical enlargement of the bilateral lacrimal glands.

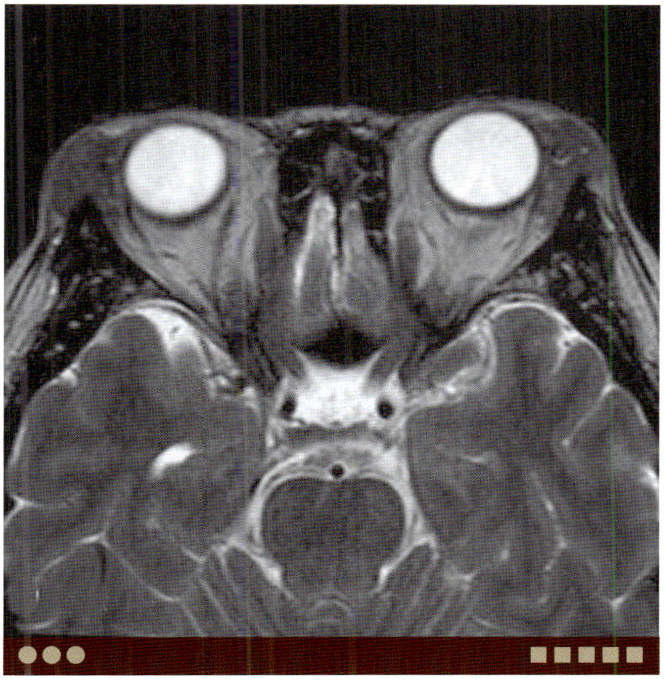

C. Sjögren's syndrome, same patient as A. Axial T2W image demonstrates intermediate signal in the enlarged lacrimal glands.

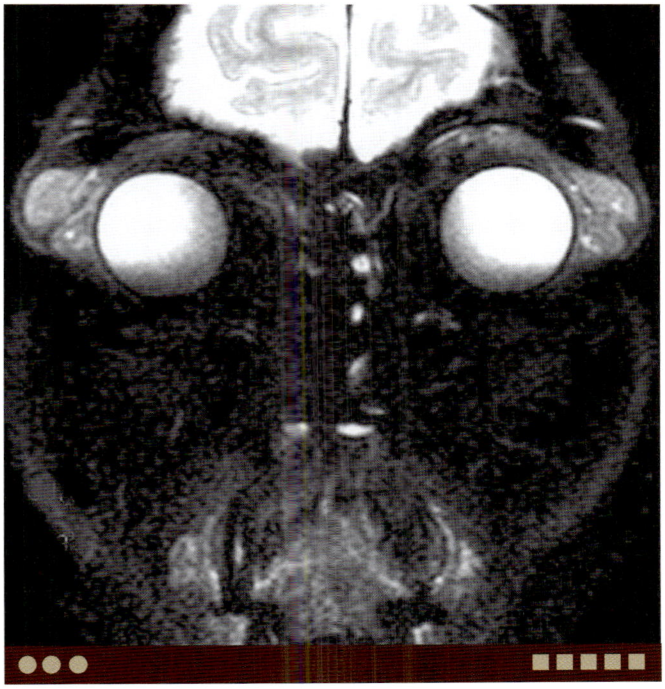

D. Sjögren's syndrome, same patient as A. Coronal fat-suppressed T2W image demonstrates relatively high signal in the enlarged lacrimal glands.

DIFFERENTIAL DIAGNOSIS IMAGES (E-G)

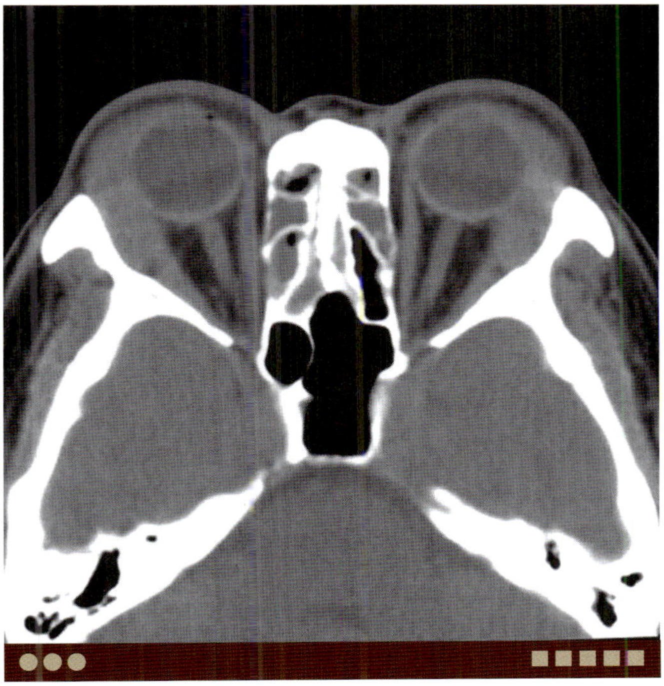

E. **Sarcoidosis**. Axial unenhanced CT demonstrates symmetrical enlargement of the bilateral lacrimal glands.

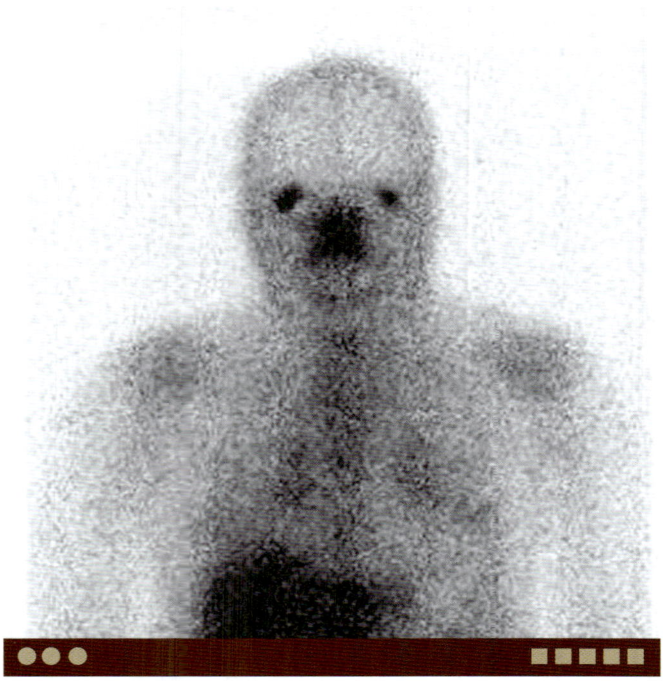

F. Sarcoidosis, same patient as E. 67-Gallium scintigraphy demonstrates diffusely increased uptake of the bilateral lacrimal glands.

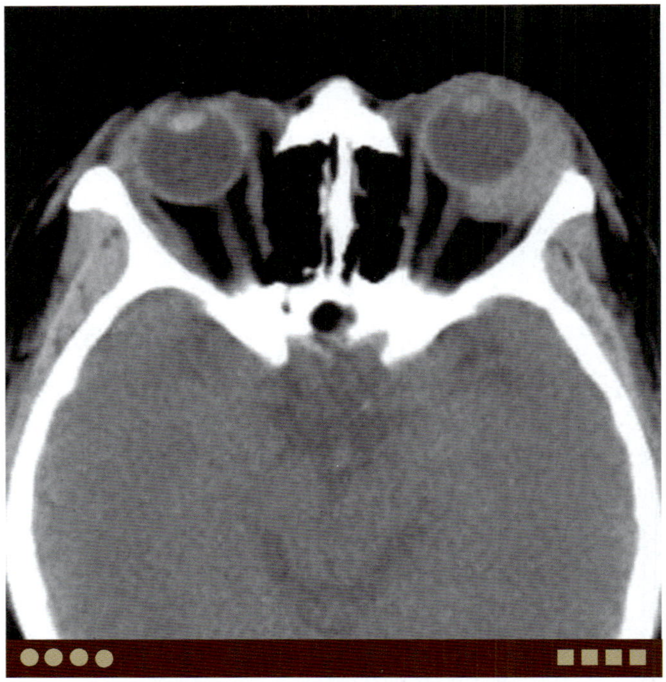

G. **Lymphoma**. Axial unenhanced CT demonstrates unilateral asymmetric enlargement of the left lacrimal gland.

Case 4–24 Orbital Subperiosteal Abscess

Asim Mian, Akifumi Fujita, Osamu Sakai

PRESENTATION

Painful erythematous eye swelling and fevers.

FINDINGS

CT demonstrates peripherally enhancing collection along the medial wall of the orbit with opacified ethmoid air cells.

DIFFERENTIAL DIAGNOSIS

- Subperiosteal hematoma: This occurs after trauma or spontaneously in patients with coagulopathy.
- Mucocele: This is usually caused by prolonged obstruction of the air cell or sinus which leads to accumulation of inspissated secretions and expansion. Ethmoid mucocele leads to bowing of the lamina papyracea. This is a slowly progressive process that does not demonstrate signs of infection.
- Dacryocystocele: This is dilatation of the lacrimal sac and seen as a cystic mass in the medial canthus, often due to congenital anomaly of the nasolacrimal apparatus. If infected and the cyst ruptures, the findings may be similar to orbital abscess.

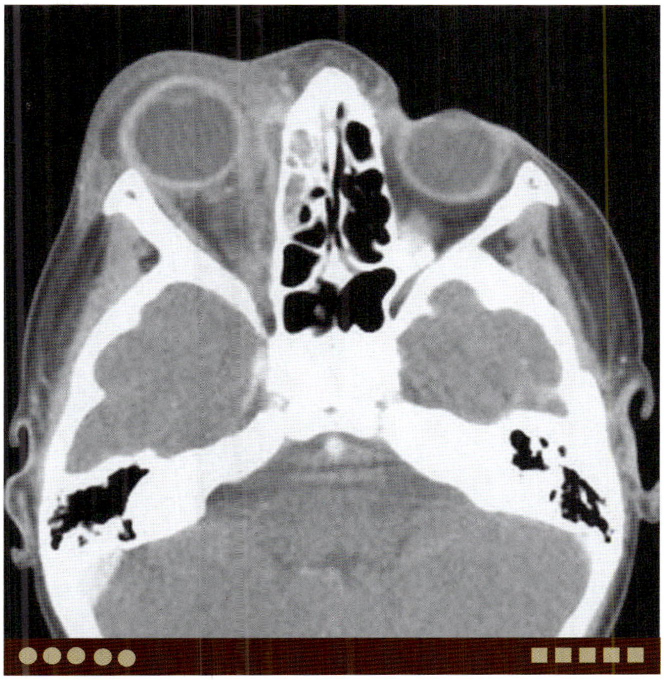

A. Subperiosteal abscess. Axial contrast-enhanced CT demonstrates a rim-enhancing collection in the medial right orbit along the lamina papyracea with preseptal and postseptal inflammatory changes. Significant proptosis is present. Note opacified right anterior ethmoid air cells.

COMMENTS

This is an 8-year-old boy with eye pain and proptosis.

Infection of the paranasal sinus spreads to the orbit often via a perivascular pathway. Thus, bone destruction is not usually seen. This pattern of spread from the sinus is commonly seen in children and young adults. Orbital subperiosteal abscess is a collection of pus that is typically located in the subperiosteal space adjacent to the lamina papyracea as a complication of ethmoid sinusitis.

Contrast-enhanced CT is the imaging study of choice. On CT, it is seen as a peripherally enhancing lentiform collection typically located in the medial extraconal orbit with inflammatory changes of the orbital fat, with opacified ethmoid air cells. The medial rectus muscle is displaced laterally and often shows edema.

Drainage of the abscess may be necessary to avoid a rapid elevation of intraorbital pressure and resultant visual impairment. Complications also include intracranial extension of the collection leading to subdural empyema and meningitis. Cavernous sinus thrombosis is an uncommon but potentially fatal complication. MRI should be performed if there is a concern for intracranial complications.

PEARLS

- **Subperiosteal abscess is typically seen associated with ethmoid sinusitis.**
- **Subperiosteal abscess shows a lentiform, rim-enhancing collection in the medial orbit, along the lamina papyracea, with displacement of the medial rectus muscle and inflammatory changes in the orbital fat.**
- **CT is the modality of choice if there is suspicion. MRI should be performed if there is concern for intracranial extension of the infectious process.**

ADDITIONAL IMAGES (B-D)

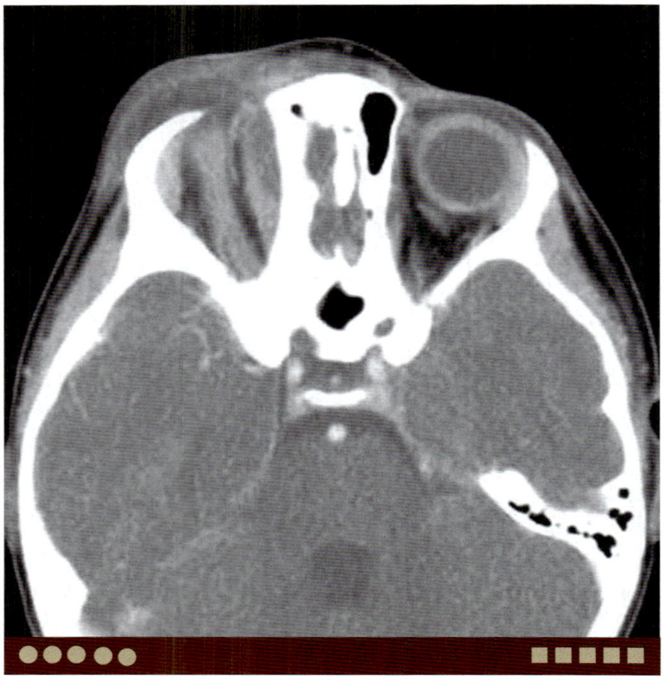

B. Subperiosteal abscess, same patient as A. Axial contrast-enhanced CT demonstrates superior extension of the subperiosteal abscess, lifting the superior oblique muscle, which is swollen due to edema.

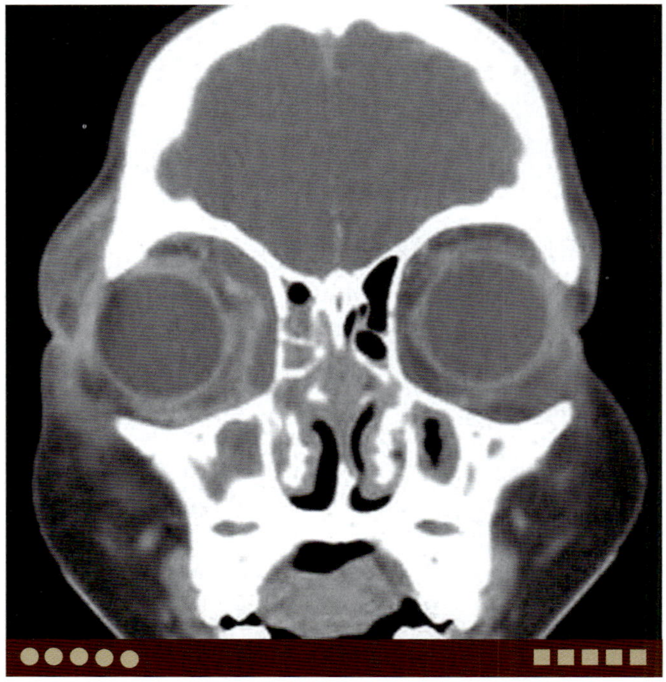

C. Subperiosteal abscess, same patient as A. Coronal contrast-enhanced CT demonstrates craniocaudal extension of the subperiosteal abscess, displacing the medial rectus muscle.

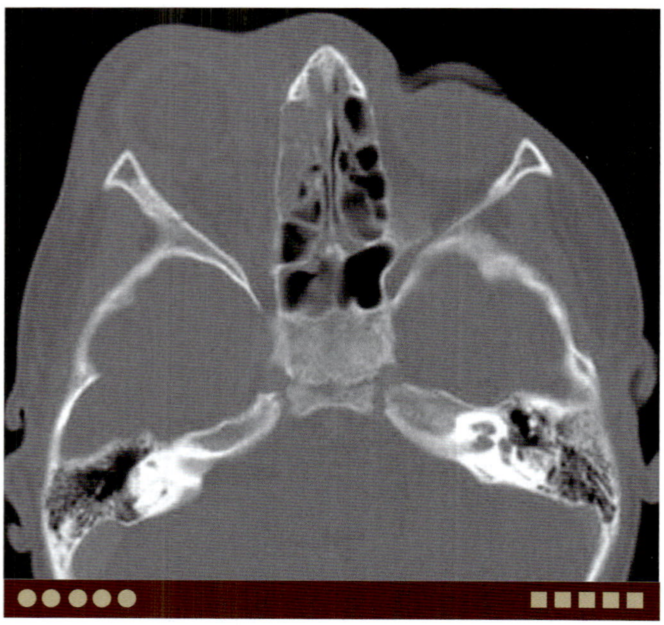

D. Subperiosteal abscess, same patient as A. Axial bone window CT demonstrates opacified right anterior ethmoid air cells. Note no apparent bone destruction in the lamina papyracea.

DIFFERENTIAL DIAGNOSIS IMAGES (E-G)

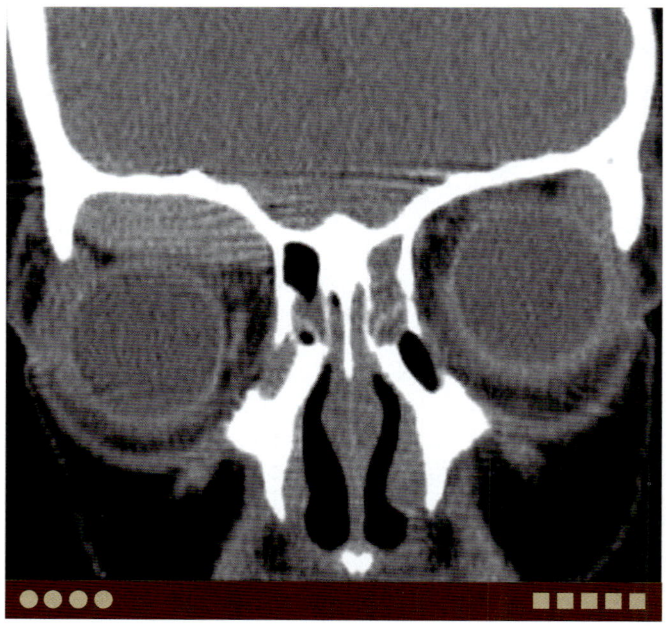

E. Traumatic subperiosteal hematoma of the orbit. Coronal unenhanced CT demonstrates a well defined, homogeneous high attenuating mass along the right orbital roof.

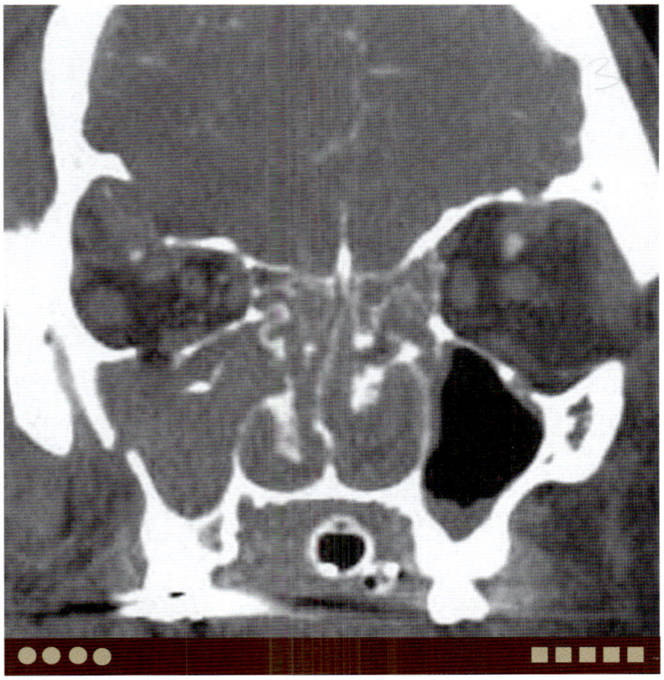

F. Orbital fracture and hematoma. Coronal postcontrast CT demonstrates hematoma along the orbital roof fracture. Fractures are also seen in the orbital floor and maxillary sinus wall.

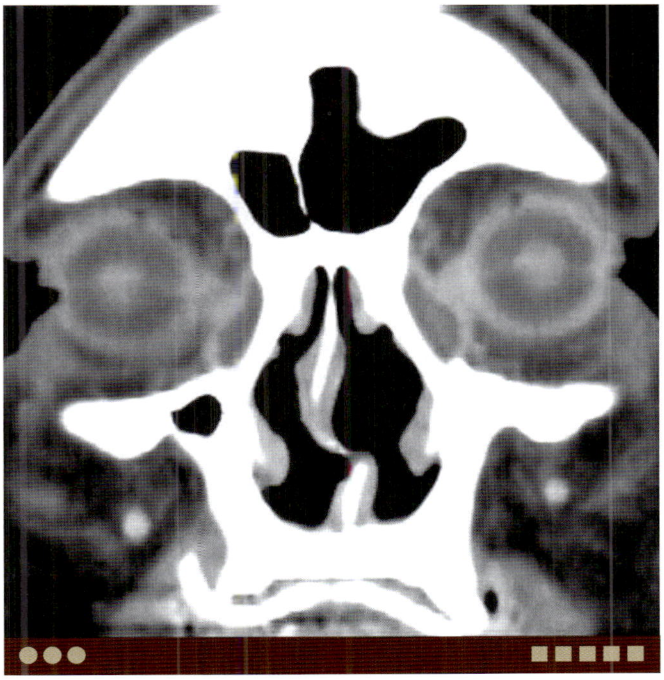

G. Dacryocystitis. Coronal postcontrast CT demonstrates rim-enhancing cystic lesions in the inferomedial portion of the orbit and the region of the lacrimal sac bilaterally.

Case 4–25 Orbital Venolymphatic Malformation

Asim Mian, Osamu Sakai

PRESENTATION

Proptosis.

FINDINGS

MRI demonstrates a predominately T2 hyperintense mass with cysts of variable size that demonstrate heterogeneous enhancement located in the intraconal and extraconal spaces.

DIFFERENTIAL DIAGNOSIS

- Cavernous hemangioma: This is the most common benign tumor of the orbit in adults. Usually, it is seen as a well-demarcated mass in the retrobulbar space showing high signal on T2W images and enhancement.
- Varix: This is a low-flow vascular lesion, and typically seen in the retrobulbar and extraconal region, although it can be present anywhere in the orbit. The size can change dramatically with venous pressure. It has well-defined margins and can be tubular or tortuous.
- Hemangiopericytoma: This is a rare vascular tumor of the orbit (0.2–1.2% of orbital tumors) that usually occurs between 20 and 70 years of age. The tumor typically occurs in the superior aspect of the orbit. CT and MRI demonstrate heterogeneous enhancement.

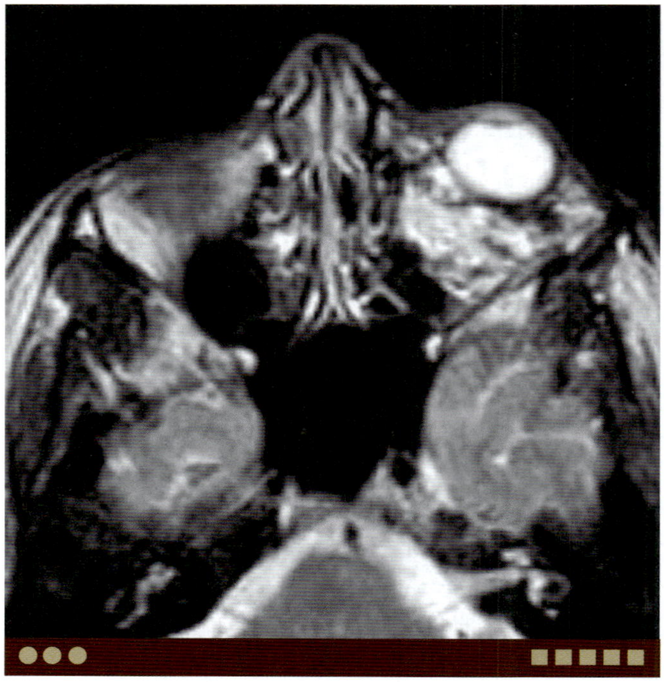

A. Venolymphatic malformation. Axial T2W image shows a heterogeneously high-signal lesion with poorly defined margins in the interior left orbit.

COMMENTS

This is a15-year-old boy with proptosis.

Venolymphatic malformation is one of the low-flow type vascular malformations and contains both lymphatic and venous vascular malformations, that is, so-called lymphangioma and hemangioma components. Reflecting these components, often there is a mixture of enhancing and nonenhancing portions after intravenous contrast administration.

Venolymphatic malformations of the orbit are rare lesions that typically occur in children before the age of 16. They usually consist of multiple cystic lesions that are prone to bleeding after minor trauma. They can be extraconal or multicompartmental. They usually occur sporadically, however there has been reported to be an association with Turner's syndrome and fetal alcohol syndrome.

On MRI, venolymphatic malformations demonstrate multicystic, predominantly high signal on T2W images. Some of the cysts can demonstrate fluid-fluid levels due to hemorrhage, or difference in lipid or protein concentration. Heterogeneous enhancement is seen in the venous/capillary components.

PEARLS

- **Venolymphatic malformation is a low-flow type vascular malformation and contains components of both lymphatic and venous malformations**
- **Enhancement is seen in the venous malformation component.**
- **Fluid-fluid levels may be present due to hemorrhage or difference in lipid or protein concentration.**

ADDITIONAL IMAGES (B-E)

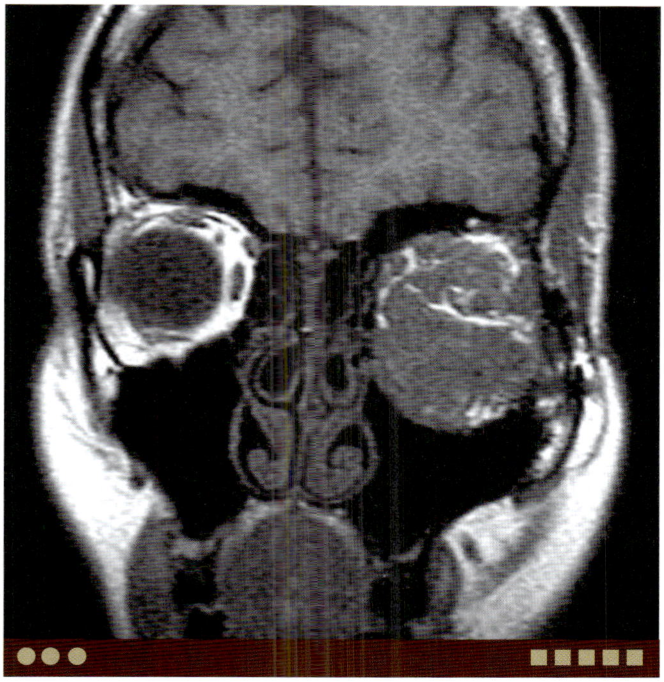

B. Venolymphatic malformation, same patient as A. Coronal T1W image shows a poorly defined low-signal lesion predominantly in the inferior portion of the left orbit with extension involving the entire orbit.

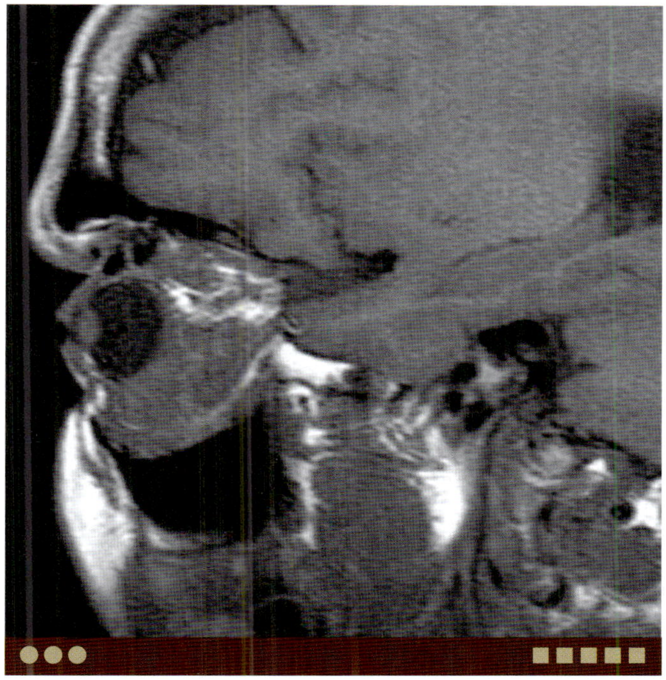

C. Venolymphatic malformation, same patient as A. Sagittal T1W image shows a poorly defined low-signal lesion.

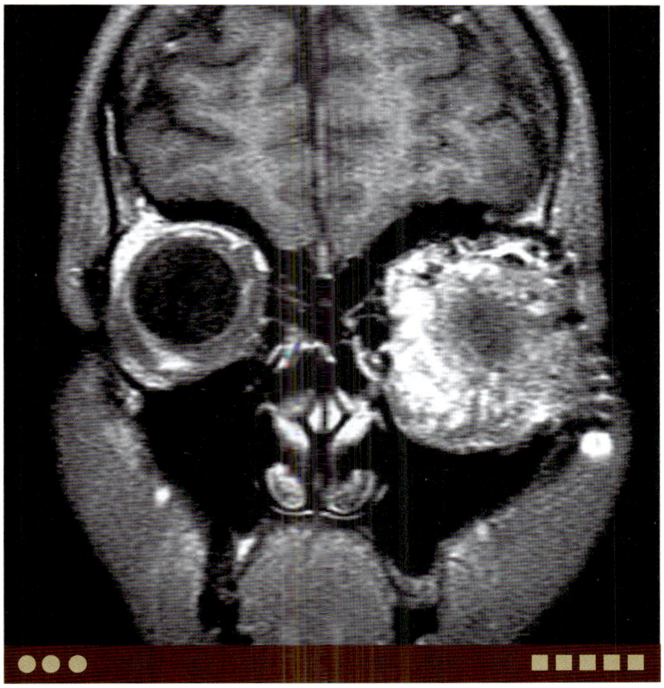

D. Venolymphatic malformation, same patient as A. Coronal post-contrast fat-suppressed T1W image shows heterogeneous enhancement of the lesion.

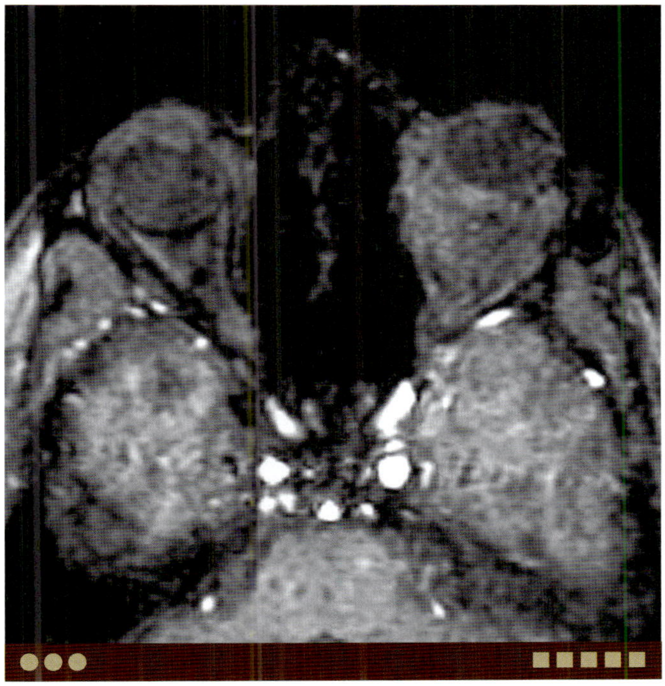

E. Venolymphatic malformation, same patient as A. Axial time-of-flight MR angiogram shows no flow-related signal within the lesion.

DIFFERENTIAL DIAGNOSIS IMAGES (F-H)

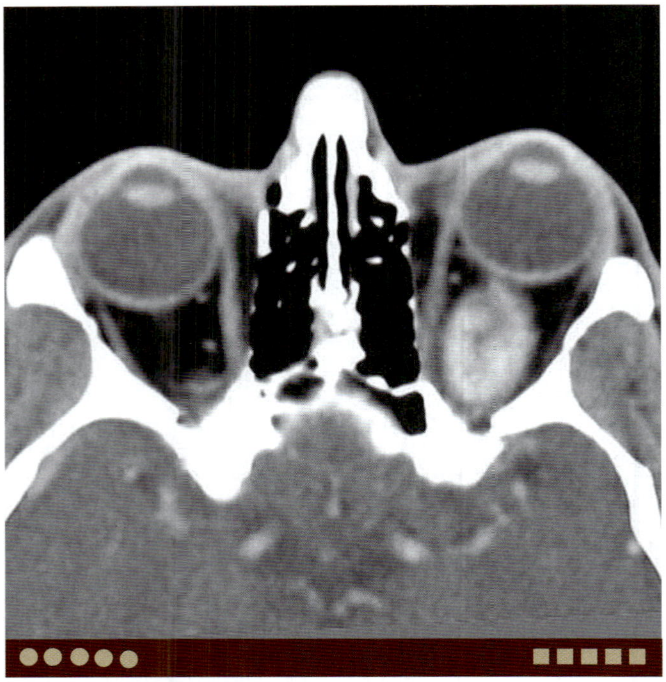

F. Hemangioma. Axial postcontrast CT demonstrates a well-marginated, ovoid enhancing lesion in the retrobulbar space of the left orbit.

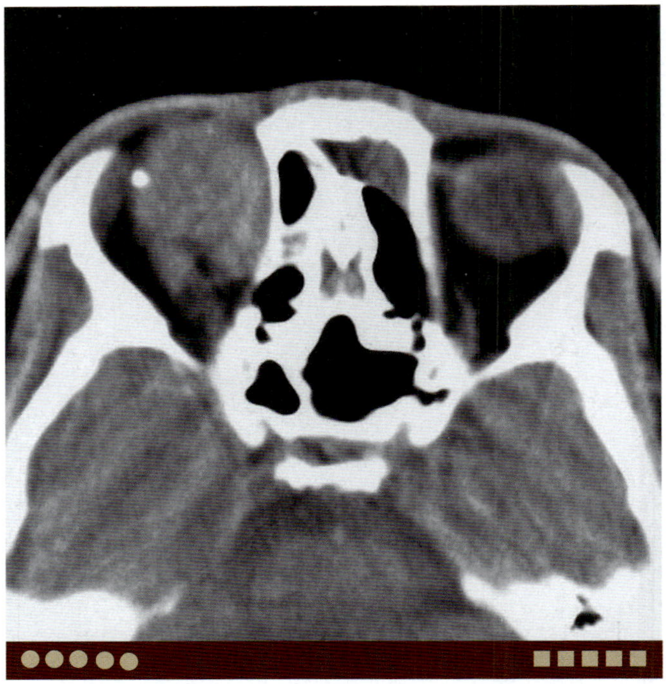

G. Venous malformation. Axial postcontrast CT demonstrates an enhancing lesion with phlebolith in the superior right orbit.

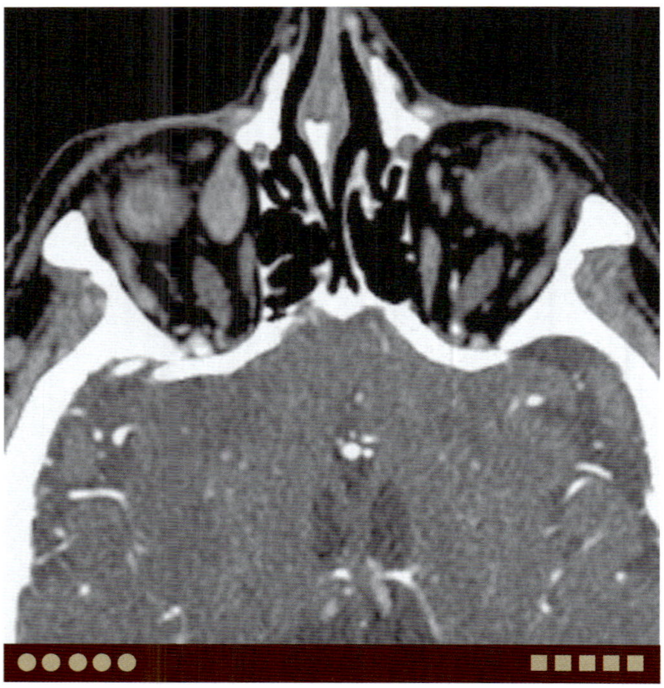

H. Varix. Axial postcontrast CT demonstrates an enhancing spindle-shaped lesion contiguous to the angular vein in the right orbit.

Case 4–26 Orbital Cellulitis

Hiroki Kato, Margaret Chapman, Osamu Sakai

PRESENTATION

Periorbital swelling and pain.

FINDINGS

CT and MRI demonstrate abnormal soft tissue swelling overlying the orbit and abnormal density/signal in the orbit proper.

DIFFERENTIAL DIAGNOSIS

- Idiopathic orbital inflammation (IOI) ("pseudotumor"): There is a significant overlap of clinical and CT/MRI findings of IOI, cellulitis, and lymphoid tumors. It is often difficult to make a definitive diagnosis without histology.
- Graves disease (thyroid orbitopathy): Imaging usually demonstrates extraocular muscle (EOM) swelling, most commonly involving the inferior and medial rectus muscles, although diffuse orbital inflammation without apparent EOM swelling is occasionally encountered. The enlarged EOMs typically demonstrate sharply defined and regular muscle edges that taper at their insertion into the globe.
- Lymphoma: Both clinical and imaging findings of orbital lymphoma are often very similar to that of IOI and cellulitis. Histological evaluation is necessary to make a definitive diagnosis.

COMMENTS

This is a 57-year-old woman presenting with right proptosis and ocular pain.

Periorbital cellulitis is a preseptal process limited to the soft tissues anterior to the orbital septum. It commonly arises from the contiguous spread of infection from adjacent structures, including the face, teeth, and ocular adnexa, or secondary to local trauma. The symptoms include swelling and erythema of the eyelids, chemosis, and in severe cases, eye movement limitation without proptosis. CT and MRI demonstrate diffuse soft-tissue thickening anterior to the orbital septum without abscess formation. In adults, periorbital cellulitis is typically treated with antibiotics on an outpatient basis.

Orbital cellulitis is a postseptal process commonly caused by sinusitis, which spreads to the orbit via a perivascular pathway. Symptoms at presentation are often similar to those of periorbital cellulitis; however, patients with orbital cellulitis may present with proptosis. Treatment typically requires the intravenous administration of antibiotics. Development of an orbital abscess often needs surgical drainage. Imaging therefore, plays an important role in guiding appropriate therapy as contrast-enhanced studies are necessary to identify abscesses. Additional complications of orbital cellulitis include thrombosis of the superior ophthalmic vein and cavernous sinuses, and intracranial complications, including bacterial meningitis, epidural and subdural abscess formation, and parenchymal brain abscess formation.

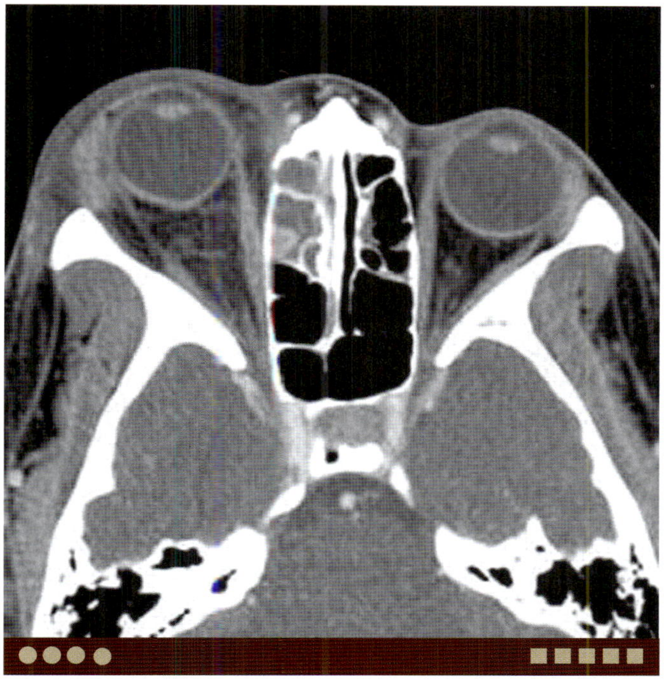

A. Orbital cellulitis. Axial contrast-enhanced CT demonstrates soft tissue swelling over the right orbit as well as increased density in the right retrobulbar fat without abscess. Opacified right anterior ethmoid air cells are noted.

Occasionally, IOI and lymphoid tumors may present with similar symptoms to cellulitis. If the condition does not respond to antibiotic therapy, histological diagnosis may be required for further evaluation. A recent report suggests that diffusion-weighted MR imaging may help differentiate IOI from lymphoid lesions and cellulitis.

PEARLS

- **Orbital cellulitis is often caused by infection of the orbital soft tissues by extension of infection from periorbital structures (especially the ethmoid air cells).**
- **CT and MRI are important diagnostic tools for the assessment of both the extent of infection and in the evaluation of sinusitis.**
- **Contrast-enhanced CT and MRI is necessary to differentiate edema, cellulitis, phlegmon, and abscess.**

ADDITIONAL IMAGES (B-E)

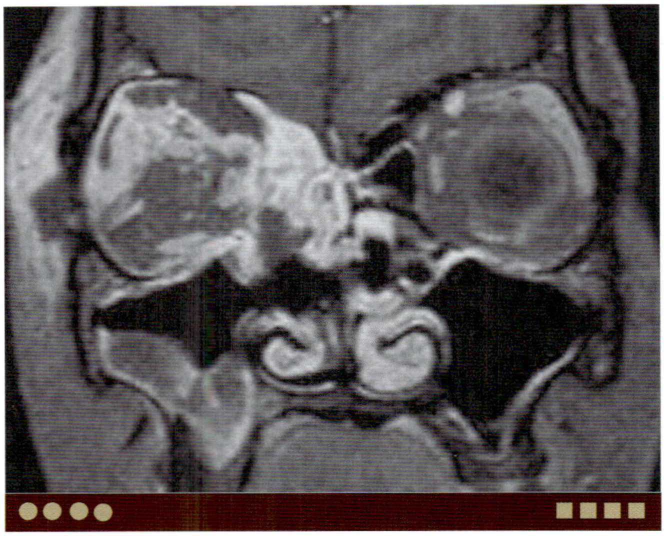

B. **Orbital cellulitis** in a different patient. Coronal postcontrast fat-suppressed T1W MR image demonstrates heterogeneous enhancement in the right retrobulbar fat as well as abnormal enhancement in the right ethmoid.

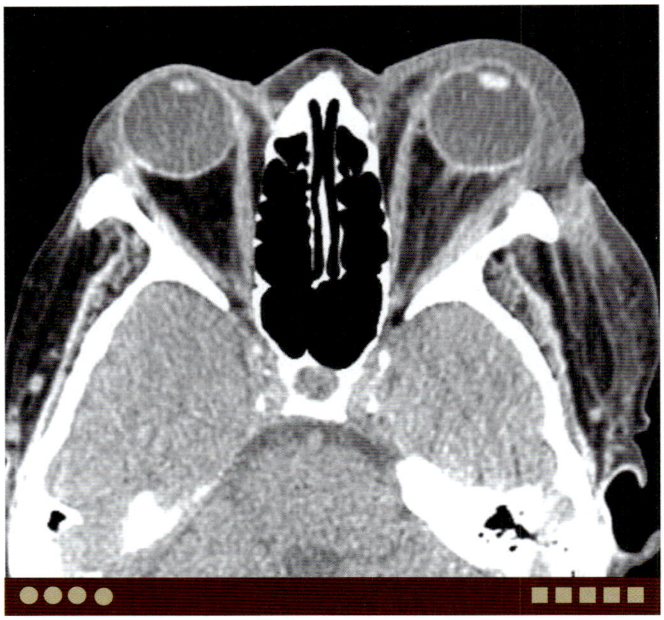

C. **Orbital cellulitis** in a different patient. Axial unenhanced CT demonstrates abnormally increased density in the left retrobulbar fat as well as periorbital soft tissue swelling.

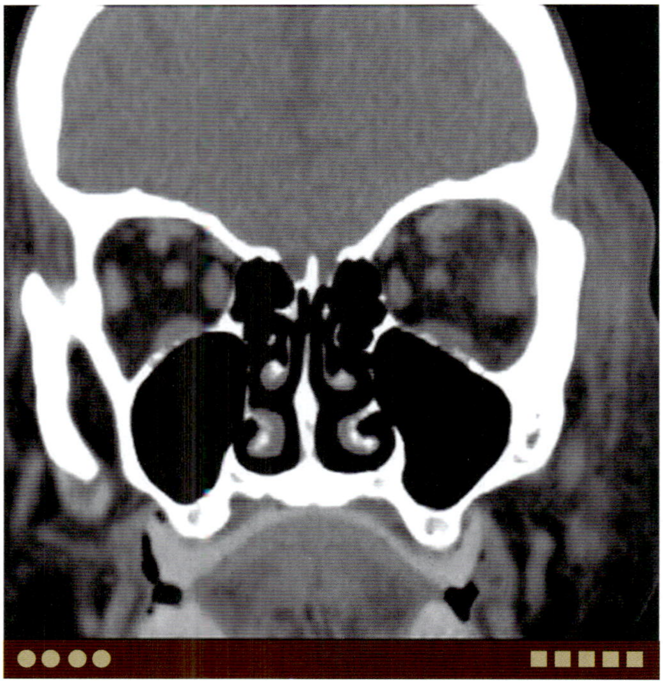

D. Orbital cellulitis, same patient as C. Coronal unenhanced CT demonstrates increased density in the left retrobulbar fat and swelling of the lateral rectus muscle. Left periorbital soft tissue swelling is also present.

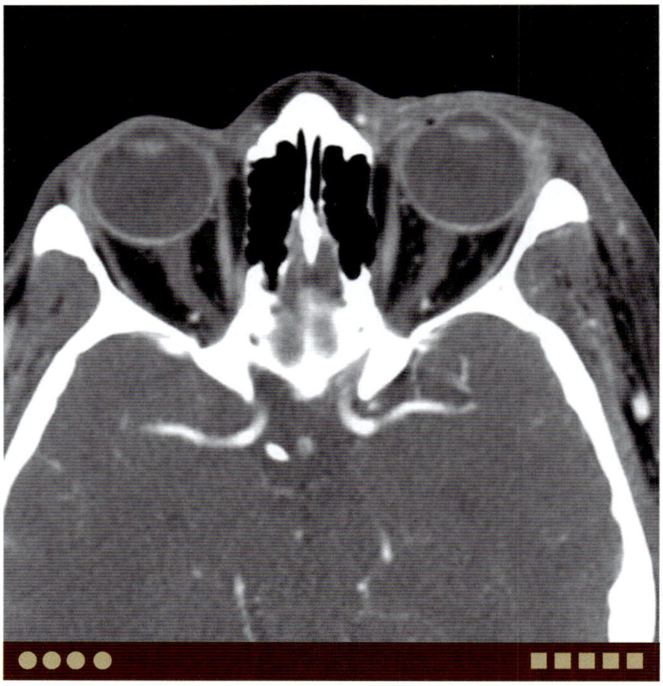

E. **Periorbital cellulitis**. Axial contrast-enhanced CT demonstrates soft tissue swelling over the left orbit without abnormality in the retrobulbar fat.

DIFFERENTIAL DIAGNOSIS IMAGES (F-J)

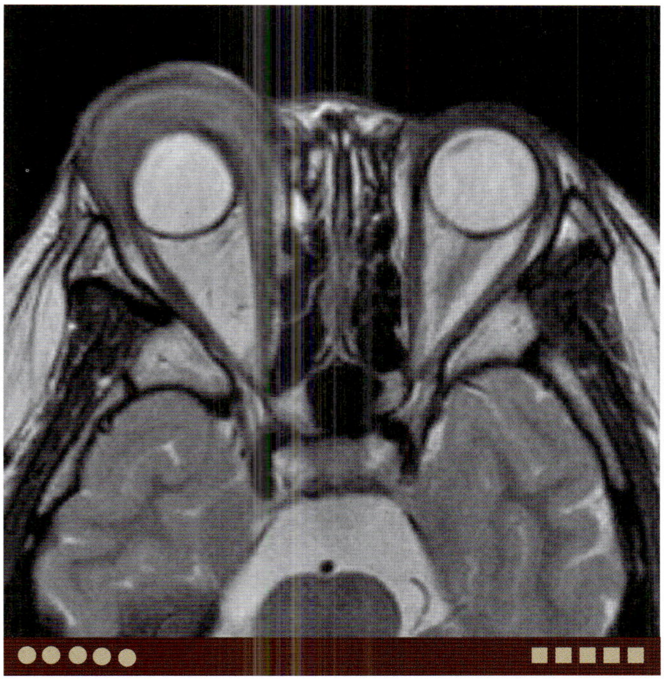

F. Lymphoma, diffuse B cell. Axial T2W image demonstrates a homogeneous intermediate-signal lesion in the right orbit.

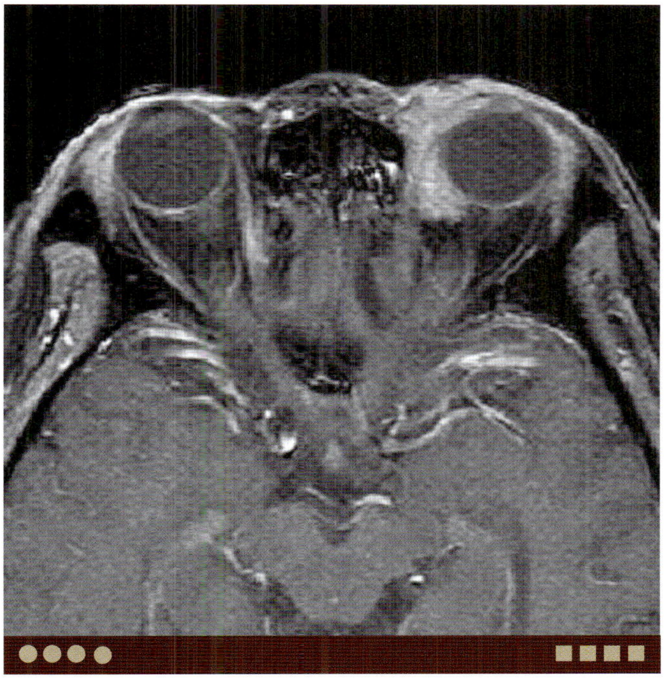

G. IOI. Axial postcontrast fat-suppressed T1W image demonstrates an enhancing lesion with poorly defined margins posterior and medial to the left globe.

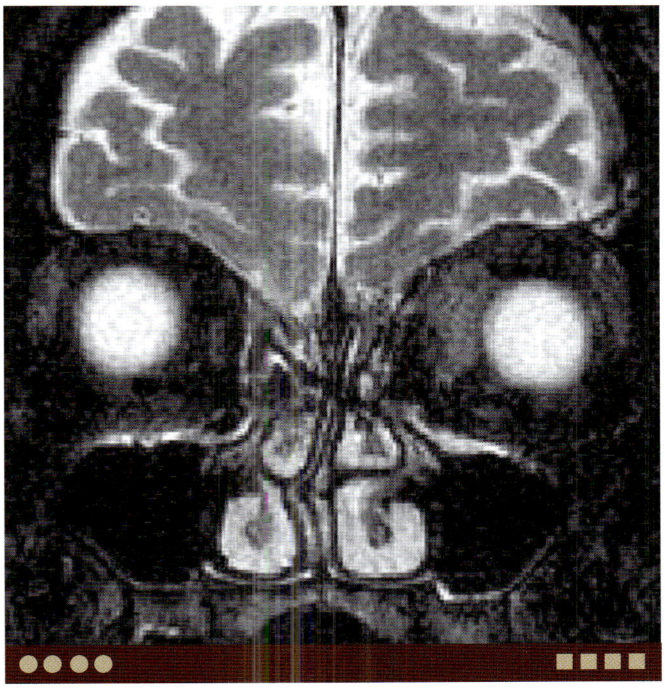

H. IOI, same patient as H. Coronal fat-suppressed T2W image demonstrates intermediate-signal within the lesion.

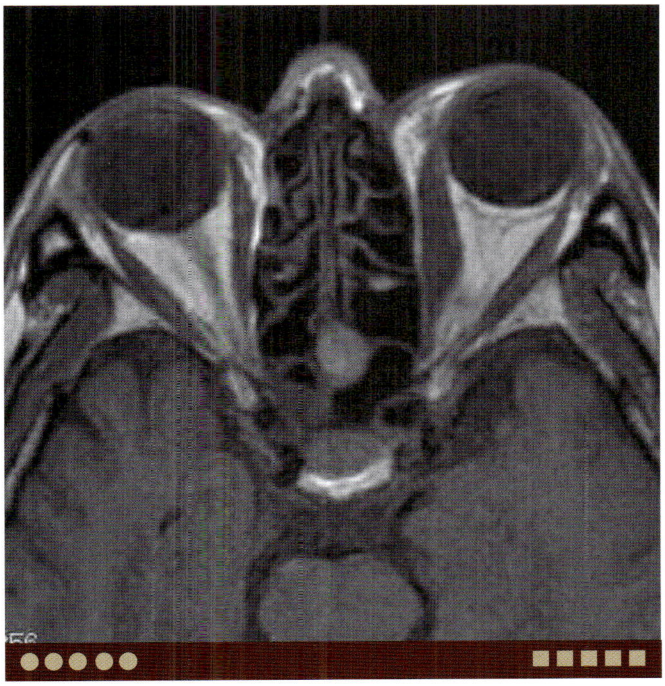

I. Graves disease. Axial T1W image demonstrates spindle-shaped swelling of the left medial rectus muscle with sparing of the tendinous insertion.

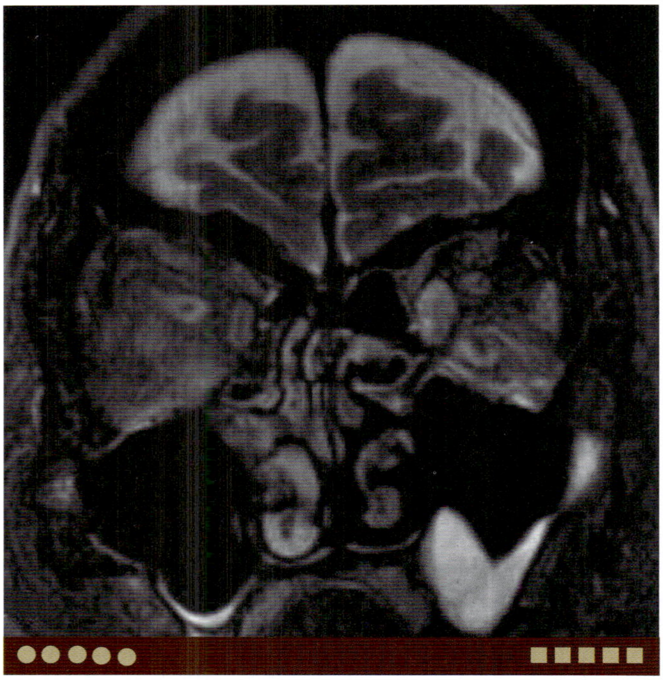

J. Graves disease, same patient as I. Coronal fat-suppressed T2W image demonstrates swelling of the left inferior and medial rectus muscles and diffusely increased signal of the bilateral retrobulbar fat.

Case 4–27 Fibrous Dysplasia

Memi Watanabe, Margaret Chapman, Osamu Sakai

PRESENTATION

Facial asymmetry.

FINDINGS

CT demonstrates bone expansion with "ground-glass" appearance.

DIFFERENTIAL DIAGNOSIS

- Ossifying fibroma and other fibro-osseous lesions: These demonstrate very similar findings to fibrous dysplasia and are often difficult to differentiate. Fibrous dysplasia tends to involve multiple bones.
- Paget's disease: This condition affects elderly patients usually with diffuse involvement of the skull. This tends to show heterogeneous density, with a mixture of sclerosis and lysis. MRI shows expanded marrow space with heterogeneous fatty changes.
- Osteoma: This is the most common benign tumor of the paranasal sinuses and may extend to the orbit. Osteoma is more focal and dense when compared with fibrous dysplasia. Primary orbital osteoma is very rare.
- Meningioma: So-called intraosseous meningioma often involves the sphenoid triangle. It tends to show irregular margins and dural enhancement.
- Metastasis: The sphenoid triangle has abundant bone marrow and is a common location for metastasis.

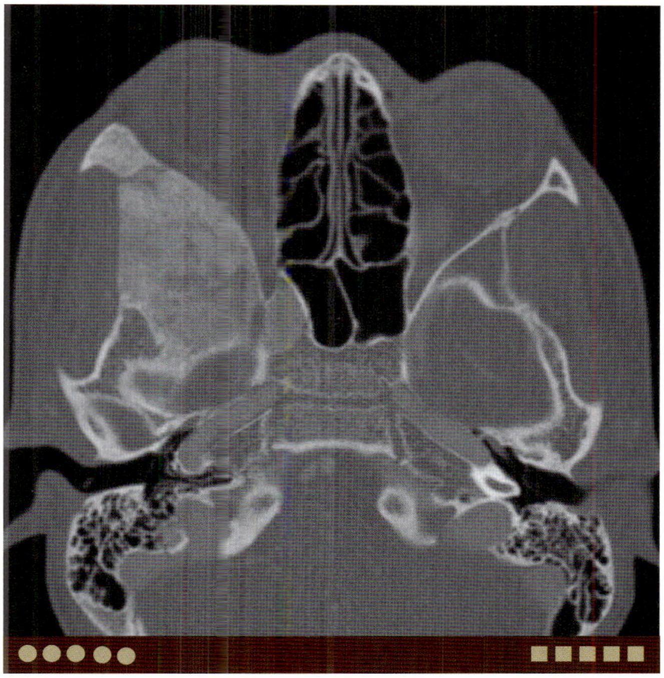

A. Fibrous dysplasia. Axial CT demonstrates an expansile lesion with "ground-glass" appearance in the right sphenoid bone.

COMMENTS

This is a 25-year-old woman with facial asymmetry.

Fibrous dysplasia is a developmental anomaly of the bone marrow. Typically seen in adolescents and young adults, normal bone marrow becomes replaced with fibroosseous tissue. Fibrous dysplasia may affect a single bone (monostotic) or multiple bones (polyostotic).

Clinically, small monostotic lesions may be asymptomatic and identified incidentally. Clinical presentations are nonspecific and include pain, swelling, tenderness, and pathologic fracture. Periorbital fibrous dysplasia may present as proptosis or diplopia, and can cause narrowing of the optic canal leading to visual impairment. Early decompression of the optic nerve is essential to preserve visual function.

Café-au-lait spots may be seen in one-third to one-half of patients with polyostotic fibrous dysplasia. Fibrous dysplasia has been reported in association with endocrine disorders, such as precocious puberty, hyperthyroidism, hyperparathyroidism, acromegaly, diabetes mellitus, and Cushing syndrome. Albright syndrome is known as the triad of fibrous dysplasia, café-au-lait spots, and endocrine dysfunction.

Radiological presentation of fibrous dysplasia demonstrates characteristic "ground-glass" appearance of bone on radiograph and CT. MRI demonstrates decreased signal intensity on both T1W and T2W images, occasionally with cystic components. Hemorrhage and dense fibrosis may be seen. Enhancement is common.

PEARLS

- **Fibrous dysplasia is typically identified in the first or second decades of life. Periorbital fibrous dysplasia may cause narrowing of the optic canal and may lead to visual impairment.**
- **CT demonstrates characteristic "ground-glass" appearance of bone, and MRI demonstrates hypointensity on both T1W and T2W images.**
- **Malignant transformation may be seen in 0.5% cases. Radiological findings such as osteolytic change or soft tissue mass suggest this condition.**

Fibrous dysplasia may rarely (0.5%) undergo malignant transformation in both monostotic and polyostotic types. The most common malignant transformation is osteosarcoma, followed by fibrosarcoma and chondrosarcoma. Clinically this may present with increasing pain, and enlargement of a soft tissue mass. Malignant transformation may be suspected by radiological changes such as osteolysis, marked periosteal reaction, or cortical disruption with an associated soft-tissue mass.

ADDITIONAL IMAGES (B-G)

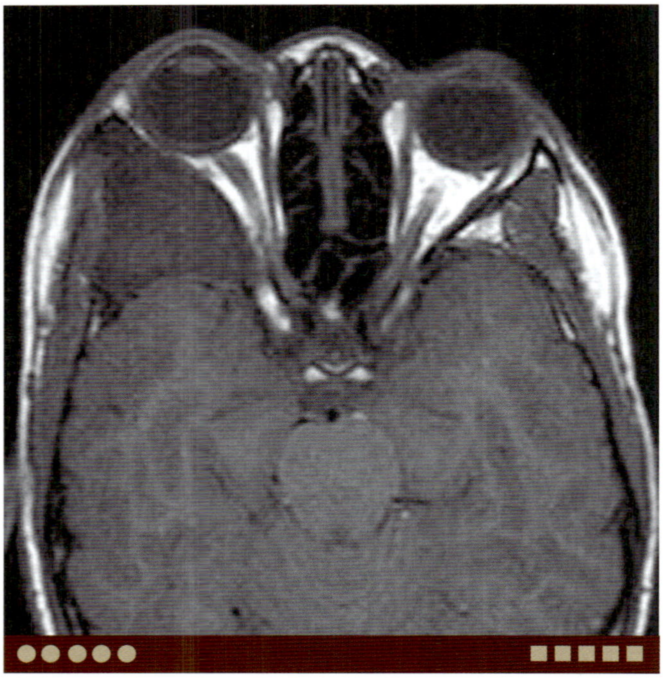

B. Fibrous dysplasia, same patient as A. Axial T1W MR image demonstrates an expansile lesion with low-signal centered in the right sphenoid triangle.

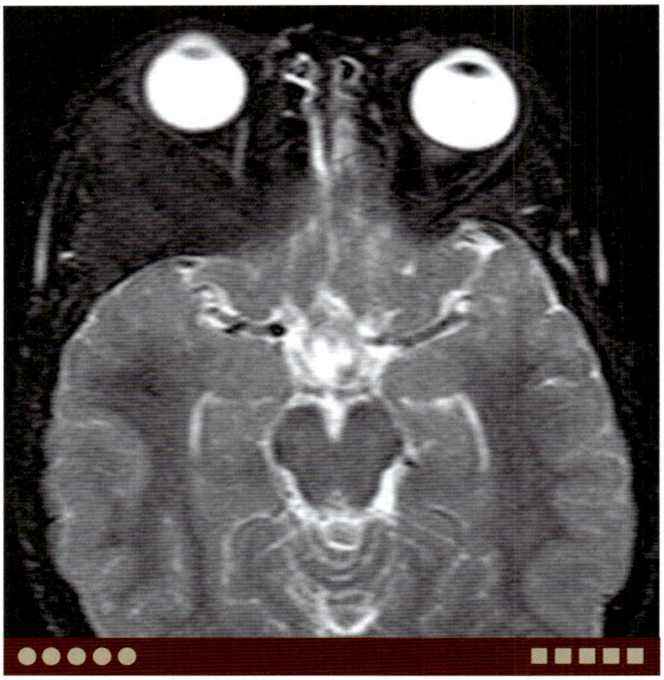

C. Fibrous dysplasia, same patient as A. Axial T2W image demonstrates homogeneous low signal of the lesion.

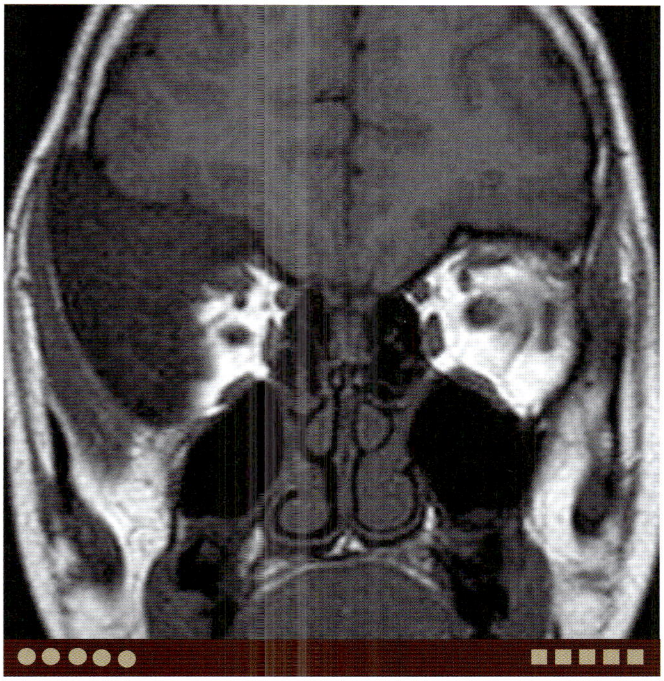

D. Fibrous dysplasia, same patient as A. Coronal T1W image demonstrates an expansile low-signal intensity lesion involving the lateral and superior walls of the right orbit.

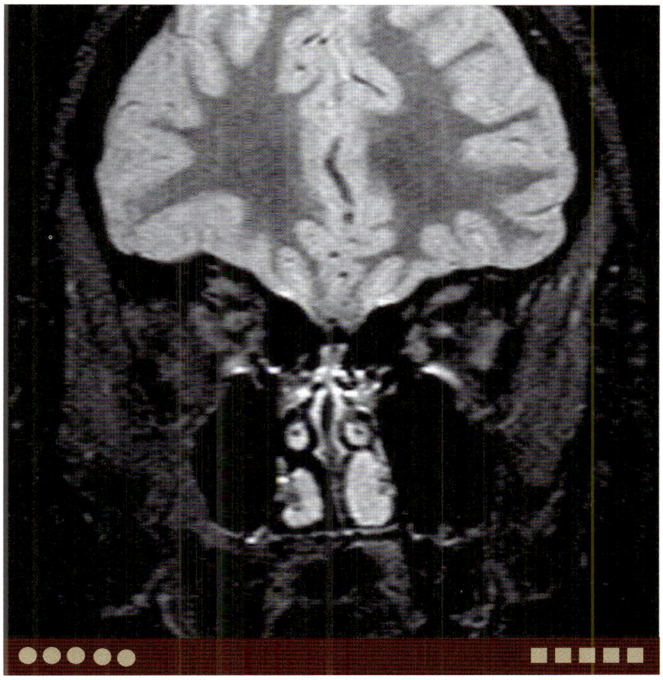

E. Fibrous dysplasia, same patient as A. Coronal fat-suppressed T2W image demonstrates slightly heterogeneous low-signal intensity of the lesion.

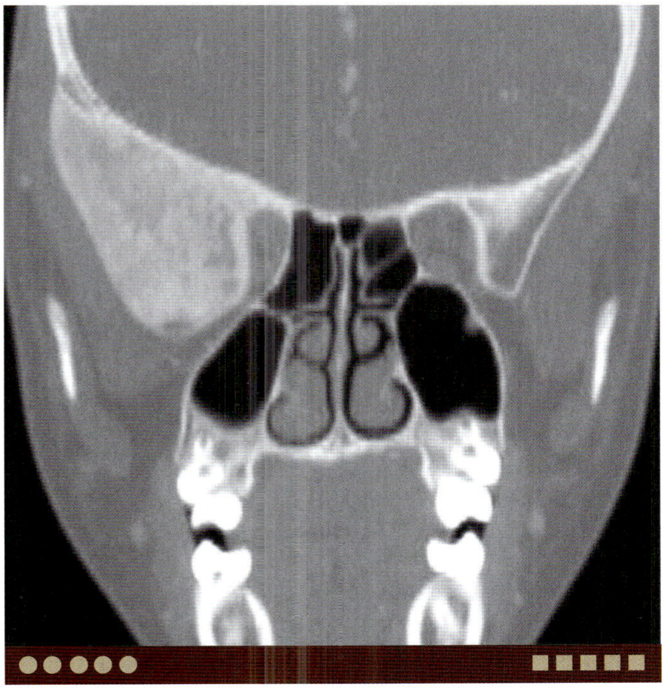

F. Fibrous dysplasia, same patient as A. Coronal CT demonstrates marked thickening of the lateral orbital wall narrowing the orbital apex.

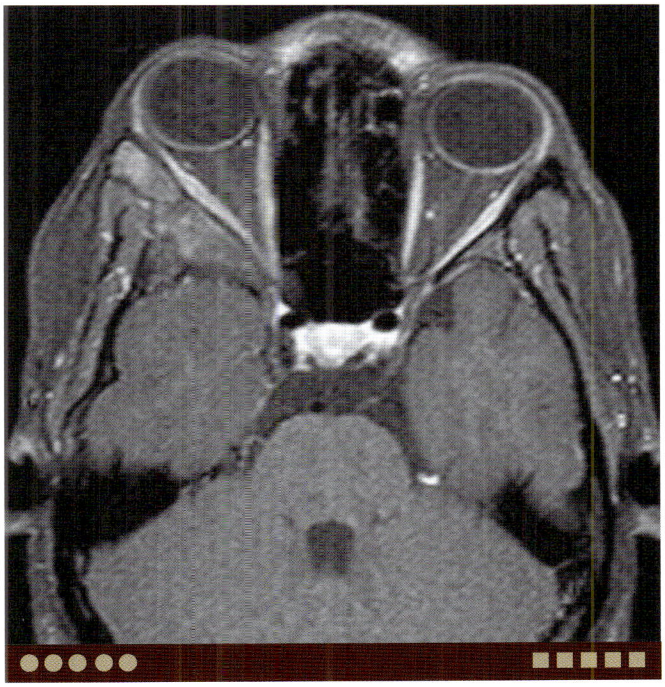

G. **Fibrous dysplasia** in a different patient. Axial fat-suppressed T1W image demonstrates a mildly enhancing, slightly expansile lesion in the right sphenoid triangle.

DIFFERENTIAL DIAGNOSIS IMAGES (H-J)

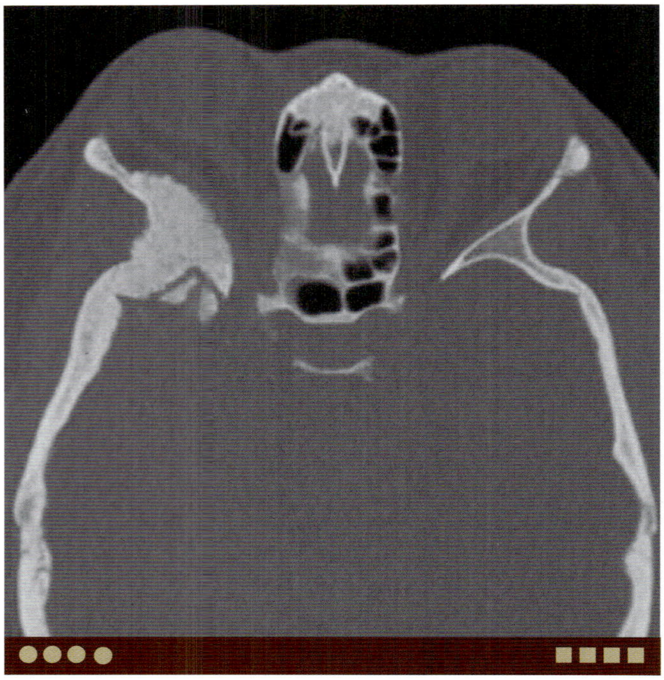

H. Meningioma. Axial CT demonstrates irregular hyperostosis of the right sphenoid triangle.

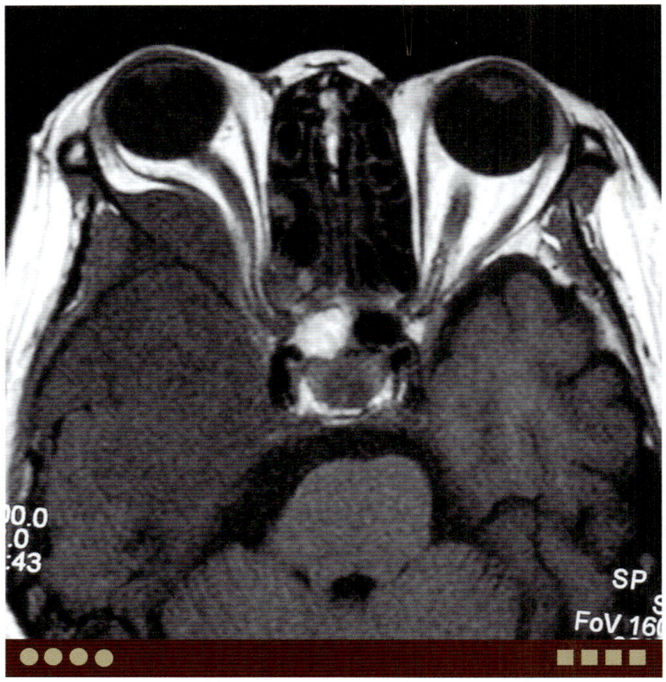

I. Metastasis from urethral cancer. Axial T1W image demonstrates a low-signal intensity expansile lesion centered in the right sphenoid triangle.

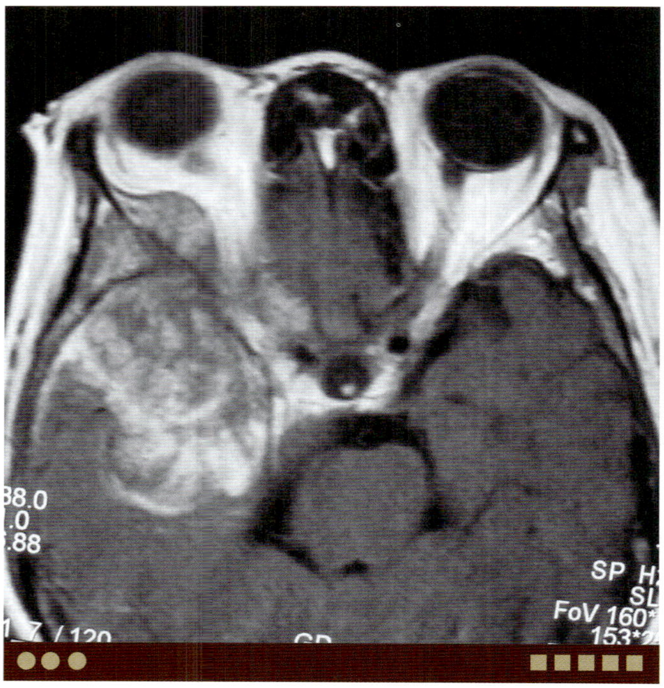

J. Metastasis from urethral cancer, same patient as I. Axial post-contrast T1W image demonstrates heterogeneous enhancement of the lesion. Note a large intracranial component of the lesion.

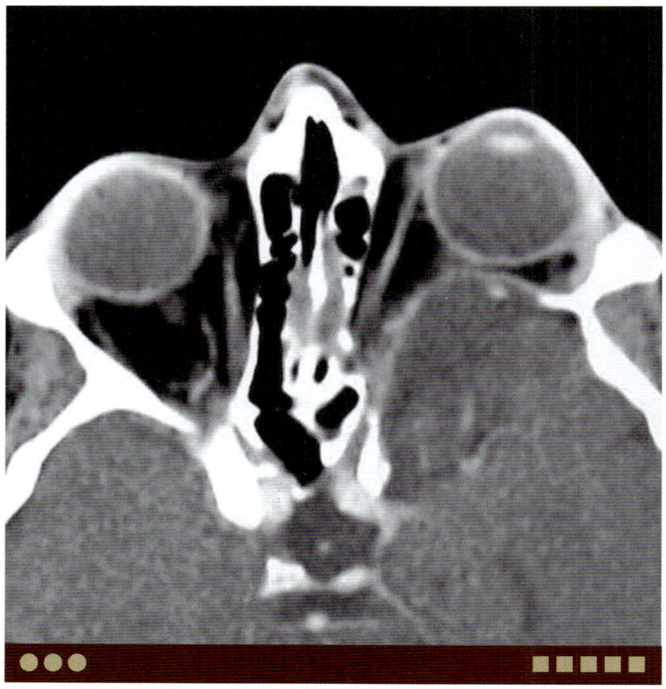

K. Neurofibromatosis. Axial CT demonstrates hypoplastic left sphenoid bone and dural dilatation extending into the left orbit resulting in proptosis.

Case 4–28 Adenoid Cystic Carcinoma—Lacrimal Gland

Memi Watanabe, Margaret Chapman, Osamu Sakai

PRESENTATION

Palpable mass of the upper eyelid with severe pain.

FINDINGS

CT and MRI demonstrate a heterogeneous lesion in the lacrimal gland with invasive features.

DIFFERENTIAL DIAGNOSIS

- Pleomorphic adenoma: This is the most common benign epithelial tumor of the lacrimal gland. Imaging findings may be similar to adenoid cystic carcinoma (ACC). CT may demonstrate erosion or scalloping of the orbital wall without aggressive bone destruction.
- Other malignant epithelial tumors: Other malignant epithelial tumors of the lacrimal gland include mucoepidermoid carcinomas, anaplastic carcinomas, and primary adenocarcinomas. Imaging findings are nonspecific and similar to ACC. Histological differentiation is essential.
- Lymphoma and other lymphoid tumors: Mucosa-associated lymphoid tissue (MALT) lymphoma is the most common type of primary lymphoma of the lacrimal gland, although secondary involvement from extraorbital origin is more common. Lymphomas affect the lacrimal gland diffusively while epithelial tumors commonly arise from the orbital lobe of the gland and spread posteriorly.

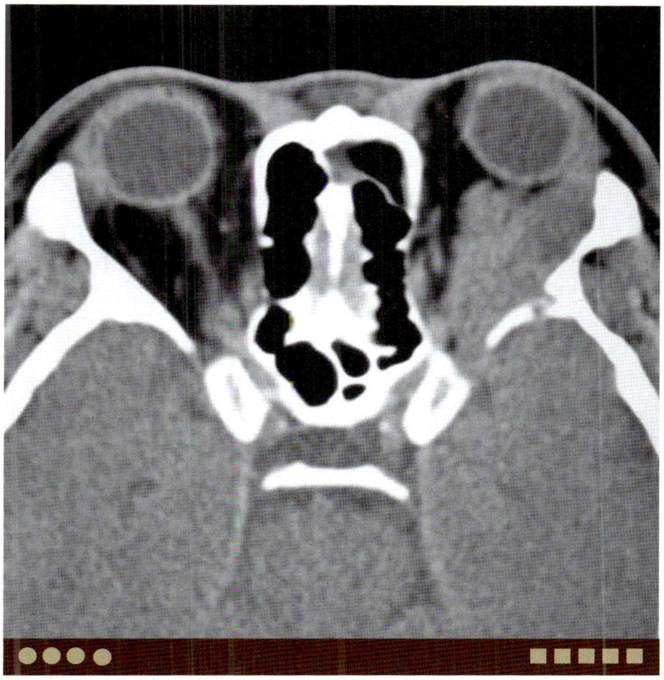

A. **ACC**. Axial CT demonstrates a poorly marginated mass in the lateral portion of the left orbit with bone destruction.

COMMENTS

This is a 40-year-old man with proptosis and pain of the left orbit.

Although adenoid cystic carcinoma (ACC) is rare, it is the most common malignant tumor of the lacrimal gland. It most frequently presents in the forth decade. Clinical presentation may mimic pleomorphic adenoma, but ACC typically demonstrates rapid growth and bony involvement. Its propensity for perineural or intraneural spread often results in severe pain and sometimes paresthesia.

Radiologically, ACC presents as a mass or infiltrative lesion with invasion into adjacent structures. Destruction of the adjacent bone is a highly typical feature. Perineural tumor extension through the superior orbital fissure into the paracavernous region results in more extensive neurological involvement. Calcification is rarely seen. MRI demonstrates a mass with low signal on T1W and intermediate-to-high signal on T2W images with diffuse enhancement after contrast administration. Low-signal intensity on T2W images suggests high cellularity of the lesion and worse prognosis. Intratumoral hemorrhage and necrosis may be seen.

ACC has a poor prognosis. Extensive disease with perineural spread is associated with difficulty in surgical management. Local recurrence is common, and distant metastases, usually to the lungs, may occur.

PEARLS

- **ACC is rare, but is the most common malignant tumor of the lacrimal gland most frequently presenting in the fourth decade.**
- **ACC is seen as a poorly marginated mass with bone destruction. Perineural tumor spread is common.**

ADDITIONAL IMAGES (B-E)

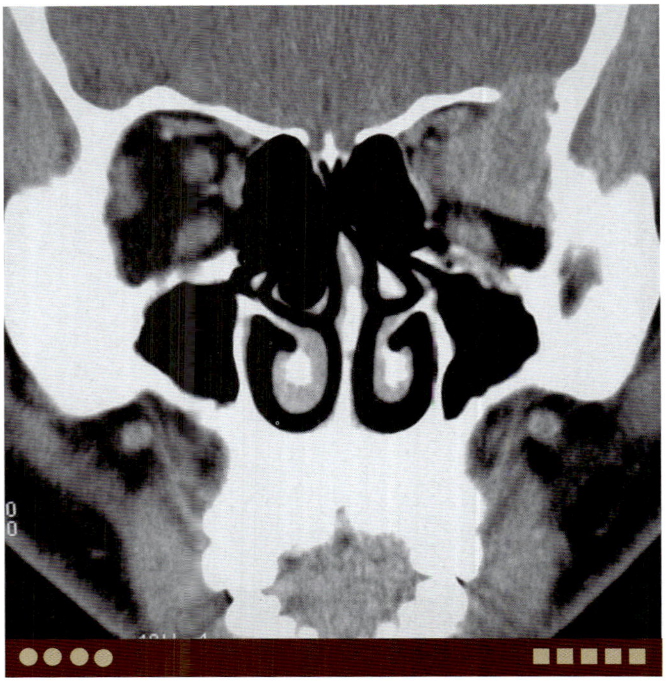

B. ACC, same patient as A. Coronal CT demonstrates a large lacrimal gland mass destructing the roof and lateral wall of the left orbit.

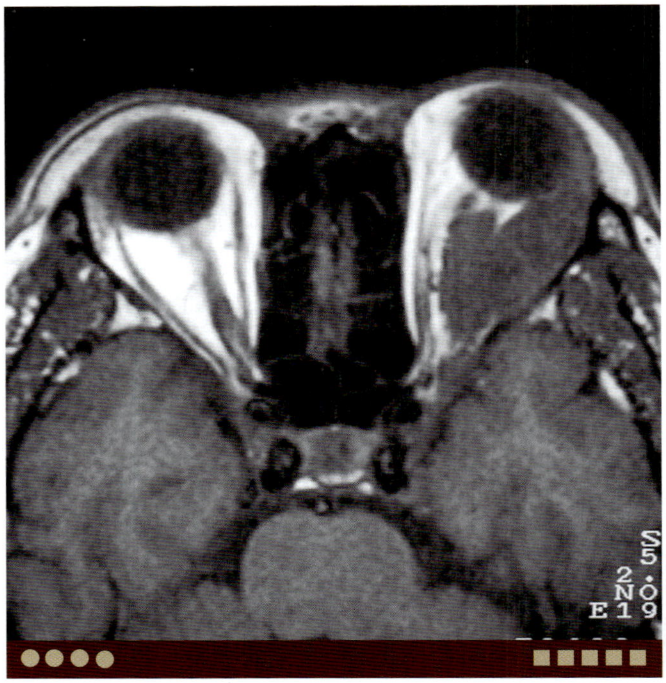

C. ACC, same patient as A. Axial T1W MR image demonstrates a low-signal lesion in the lateral portion of the left orbit extending to the orbital apex.

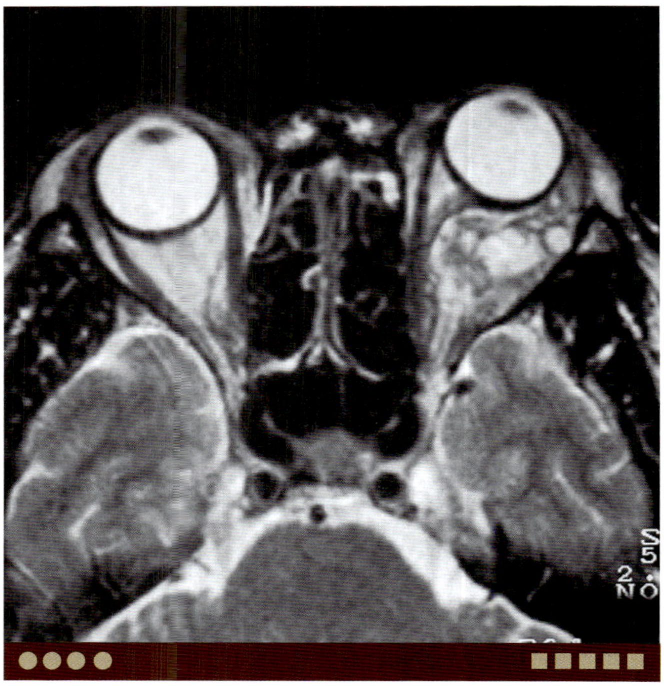

D. ACC, same patient as A. Axial T2W image demonstrates heterogeneous signal of the lesion. High-signal regions may represent cystic component or necrosis.

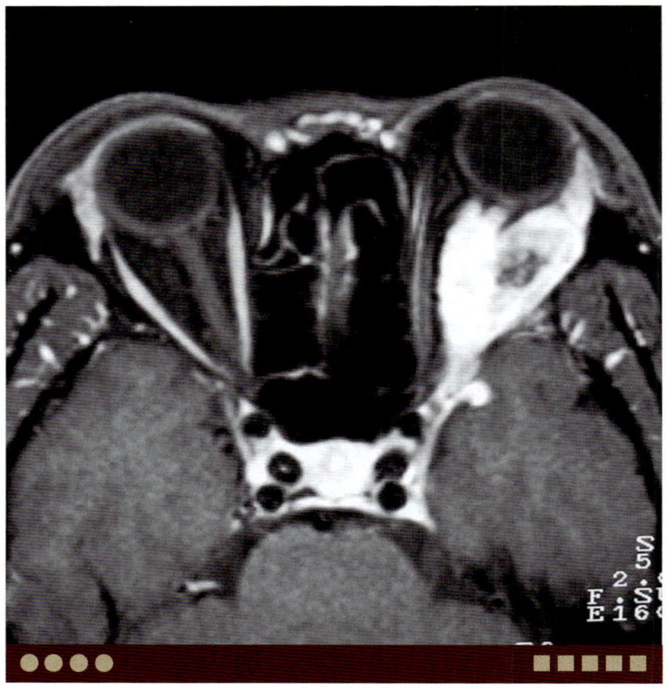

E. ACC, same patient as A. Axial postcontrast T1W image demonstrates diffuse enhancement of the lesion with a central area of nonenhancement suggestive of cystic component or necrosis. Note tumor extension into the paracavernous region.

DIFFERENTIAL DIAGNOSIS IMAGES (F-H)

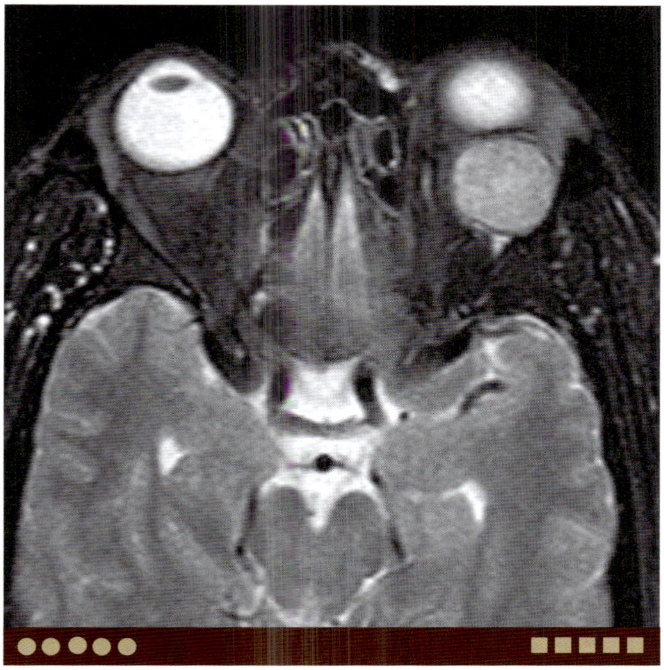

F. **Pleomorphic adenoma**. Axial T2W image demonstrates a well-circumscribed ovoid mass in the left lacrimal gland, which is isointense to the brain parenchyma.

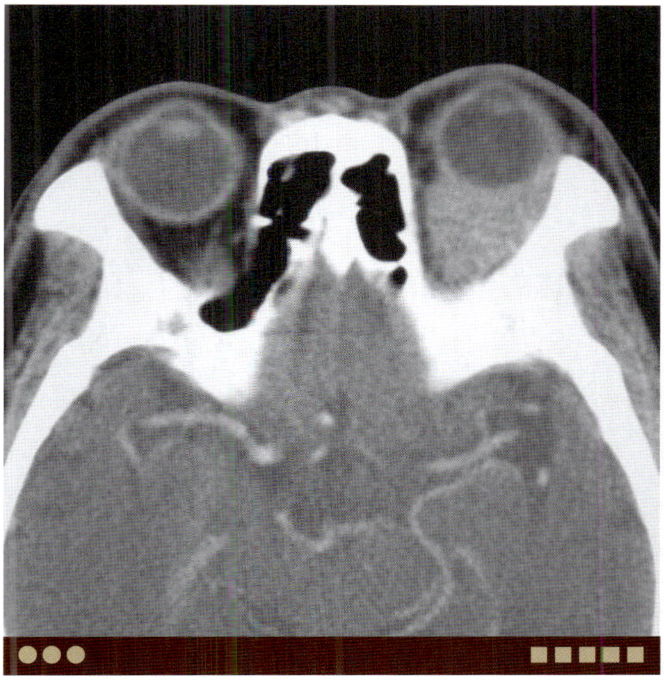

G. **Lymphoma**. Axial postcontrast CT demonstrates a poorly marginated, homogeneously enhancing tumor in the left orbit.

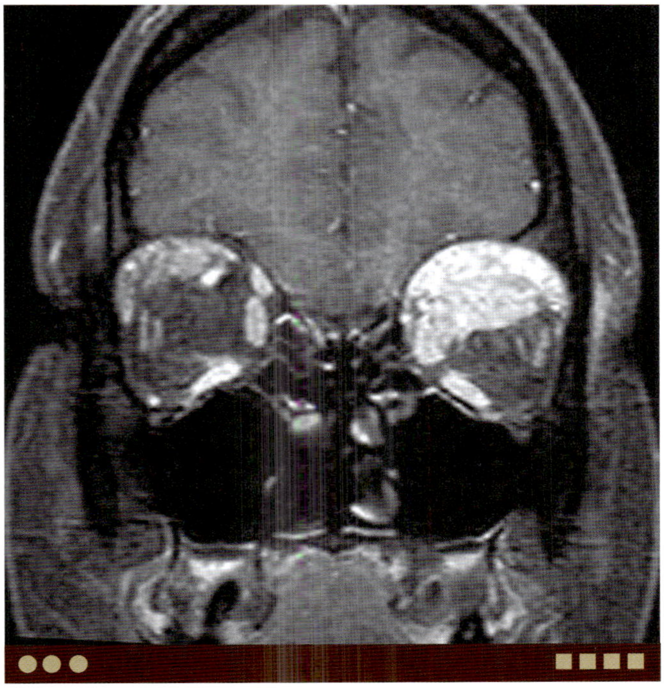

H. **Sarcoidosis**. Coronal postcontrast fat-suppressed T1W image demonstrates a poorly defined heterogeneously enhancing lesion involving the left lacrimal gland and extraocular muscles.

Case 4–29 CSF Dissemination

Osamu Sakai, Susmitha Reddy

PRESENTATION

Decreased visual acuity in a patient with history of malignancy.

FINDINGS

MRI scan demonstrates enlargement of the optic nerve sheath complex with peripheral enhancement.

DIFFERENTIAL DIAGNOSIS

- Optic perineuritis: This can be seen as a manifestation of idiopathic orbital inflammation (IOI). Enlarged optic nerve sheath complex with peripheral enhancement and inflammation of other orbital structures is seen. Additional findings include proptosis, diplopia, and restricted motility.
- Granulomatous diseases: Granulomatous diseases, such as sarcoidosis and Wegener's granulomatosis can involve the optic nerve sheath complex and show thickening and peripheral enhancement.
- Optic nerve sheath meningioma: This is a histologically benign tumor; however, it is a serious disease when it involves the optic nerve sheath. Thickened enhancing optic nerve sheath with "tram-track" appearance often with calcifications is a typical finding.
- Optic glioma: This is often associated with neurofibromatosis type I, particularly when bilateral. This shows tubular enlarged enhancing optic nerves.
- Optic neuritis: This condition may be a part of manifestation of multiple sclerosis or Devic's disease. Minimally enlarged optic nerve with enhancement is seen in the active phase. In later phases, it shows high T2/STIR signal without enhancement, often with decreased caliber.

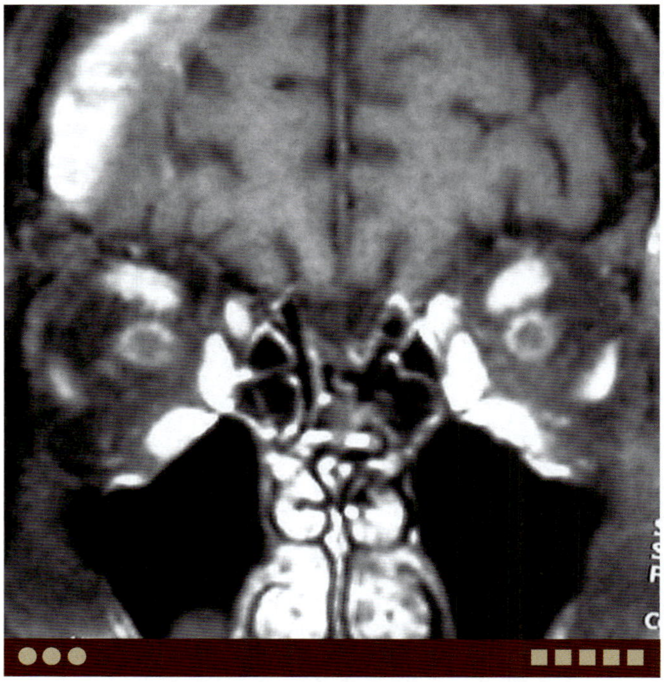

A. CSF dissemination in a patient with breast cancer. Coronal postcontrast fat-suppressed T1W MR image demonstrates peripheral enhancement of the bilateral optic nerve sheath complex.

COMMENTS

This is a 49-year-old woman with history of breast cancer, now presented with decreased visual acuity.

The optic nerve sheath is an extension of the dura which contains the cerebrospinal fluid (CSF) and therefore, susceptible to tumor implantation if the tumor is disseminated through the CSF. This condition is most commonly seen in patients with breast and lung cancers but can occur with other malignancies.

Imaging findings may be similar to that of perineuritis including idiopathic orbital inflammation (IOI), granulomatous diseases, such as sarcoidosis and Wegener's granulomatosis, optic nerve sheath meningioma, and lymphoma.

CT and MRI demonstrate enlargement of the optic nerve sheath complex and enhancement of the sheath, not the optic nerve itself. T2W or STIR images and postcontrast fat-suppressed T1W images demonstrate peripheral high signal with enhancement while the signal of the optic nerve is preserved. Careful evaluation of the intracranial structures as well as CSF analysis is crucial for the patient care.

PEARLS

- **The optic nerve sheath is an extension of the dura and susceptible to tumor implantation.**
- **Thickening of the optic nerve sheath complex and peripheral enhancement is seen.**
- **Careful evaluation of the intracranial structures as well as CSF analysis is crucial for the patient care.**

ADDITIONAL IMAGES (B-C)

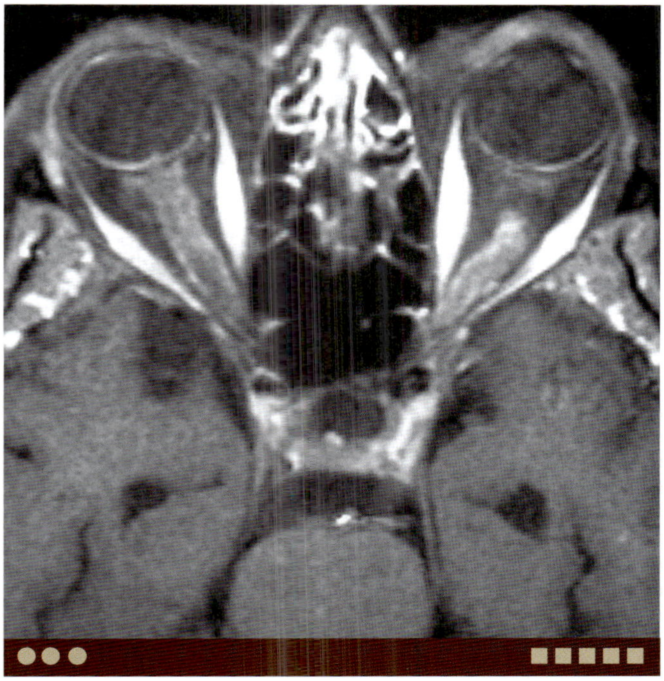

B. CSF dissemination, same patient as A. Axial postcontrast fat-suppressed T1W MR image demonstrates "tram-track like" peripheral enhancement of the optic nerve sheath complex bilaterally.

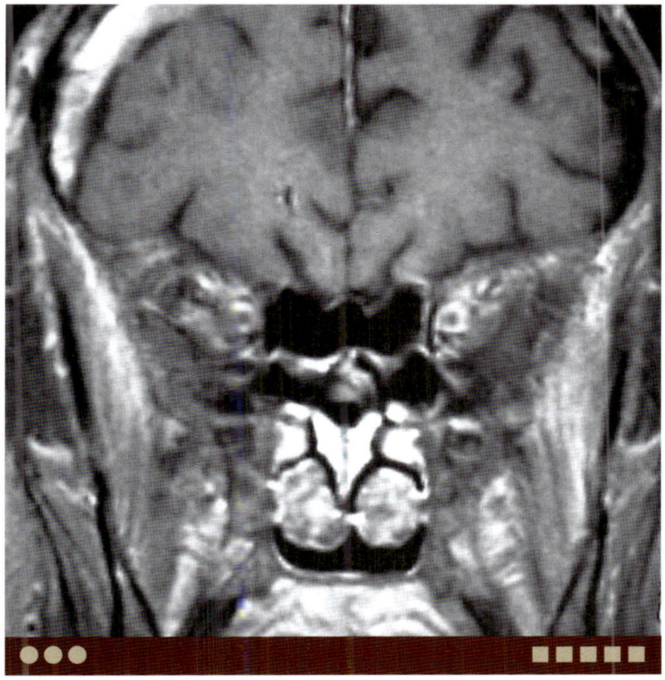

C. CSF dissemination, same patient as A. Coronal postcontrast fat-suppressed T1W MR image through the orbital apex demonstrates peripheral enhancement of the optic nerve sheath complex bilaterally.

DIFFERENTIAL DIAGNOSIS IMAGES (D-G)

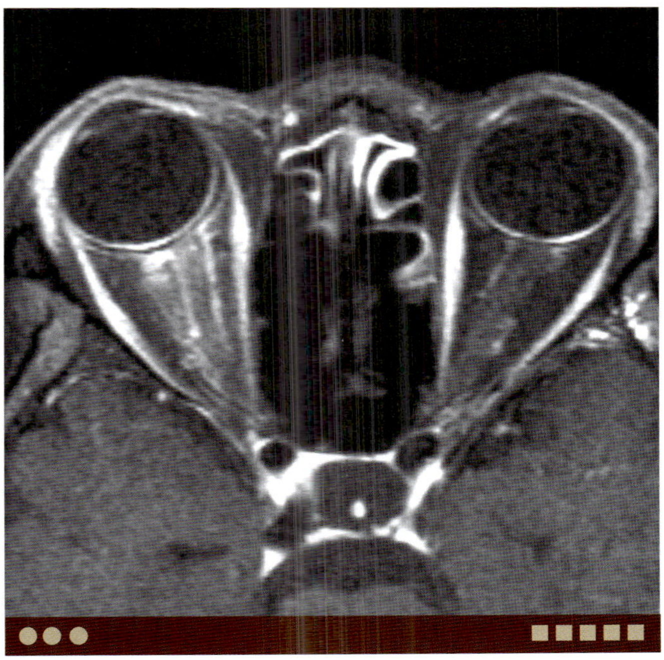

D. **Optic perineuritis**. Axial postcontrast fat-suppressed T1W MR image demonstrates "tram-track like" peripheral enhancement of the right optic nerve sheath complex.

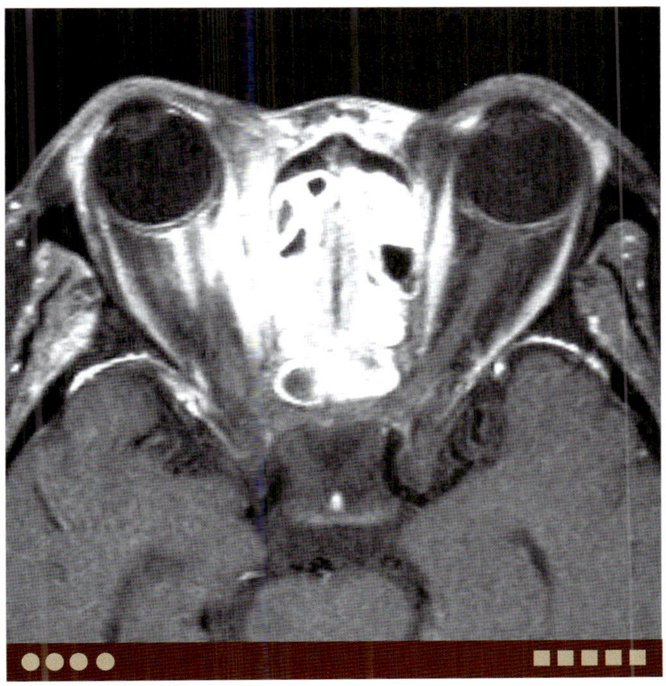

E. **Wegener's granulomatosis**. Axial postcontrast fat-suppressed T1W MR image demonstrates "tram-track like" peripheral enhancement of the right optic nerve sheath complex as well as abnormal enhancement involving the right medial rectus muscle and bilateral ethmoid air cells.

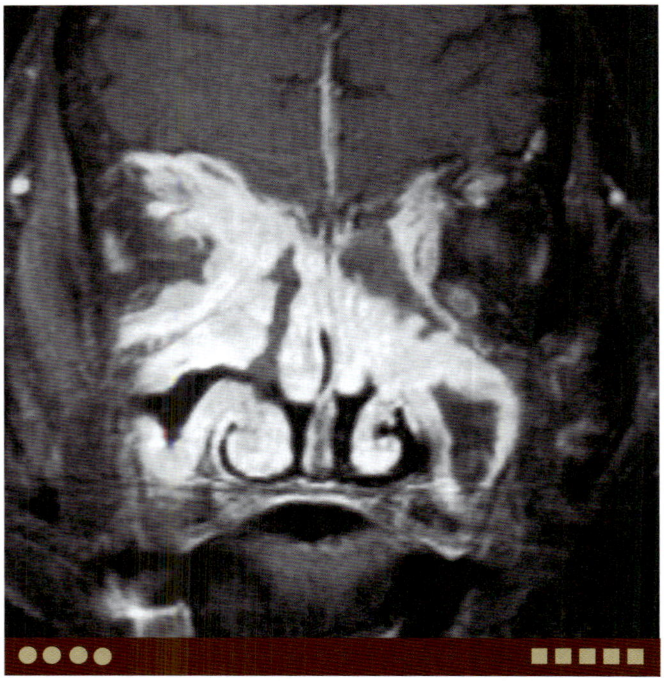

F. Lymphoma. Coronal postcontrast fat-suppressed T1W MR image demonstrates abnormal enhancement of the right optic nerve sheath in addition to diffuse enhancement in the bilateral orbits and paranasal sinuses. Note abnormal dural enhancement along the falx.

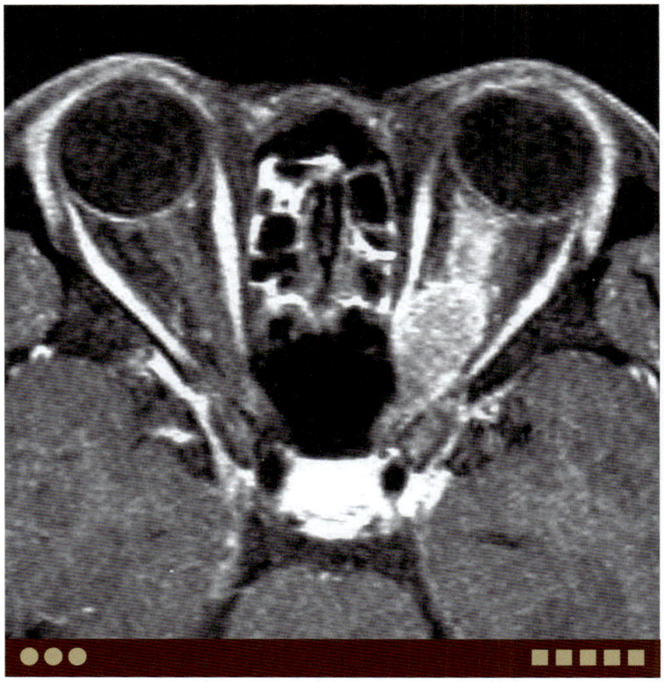

G. Optic nerve sheath meningioma. Axial postcontrast fat-suppressed T1W MR image demonstrates a fusiform-shaped lesion with peripheral enhancement. Note "tram-track like" enhancement extends to the optic nerve sheath anterior to the lesion.

Case 4–30 Orbital Varix

Osamu Sakai, Susmitha Reddy

PRESENTATION

Proptosis.

FINDINGS

CT and MRI demonstrate a fusiform or globular-shaped mass with high T2 signal and intense enhancement, which distends with Valsalva maneuver.

DIFFERENTIAL DIAGNOSIS

- Venous malformation: This is a low-flow vascular malformation and often presents with variable ophthalmoplegia. Phleboliths are the typical findings on CT.
- Venolymphatic malformation: Venolymphatic malformations usually consist of multiple cystic lesions that are prone to bleeding after minor trauma. On MRI, they are multicystic and may demonstrate fluid-fluid levels due to hemorrhage. The venous/capillary components show heterogeneous enhancement.
- Cavernous hemangioma: This is the most common benign tumor of the orbit in adults. Usually, it is seen as a well-demarcated mass in the retrobulbar space showing high signal on T2W images and enhancement.
- Hemangiopericytoma: This is a rare vascular tumor of the orbit that usually occurs between 20 and 70 years of age. The tumor typically occurs in the superior aspect of the orbit. CT and MRI demonstrate heterogeneous enhancement.

COMMENTS

This is a 55-year-old man with periodical bilateral proptosis.

Orbital varix is a low-flow congenital venous vascular lesion characterized by the proliferation of venous elements and by massive dilatation of one or more orbital veins. Most orbital varices have a large communication with the venous system, resulting in orbital varix distention and increased proptosis during the Valsalva maneuver or postural change. The size can change dramatically with change in venous pressure. Varices are typically seen in the retrobulbar and extraconal region, although they can be present anywhere in the orbit. Orbital varices that have small communications with the venous system are prone to thrombosis and hemorrhage. Orbital varices may be bilateral.

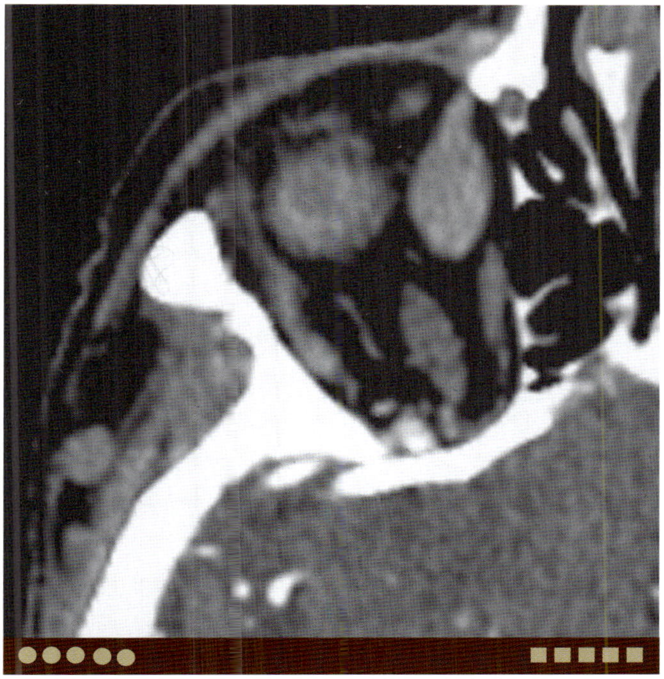

A. Varix. Axial postcontrast CT demonstrates an enhancing spindle-shaped lesion contiguous to the angular vein.

Imaging findings of orbital varices may be subtle, and imaging during the Valsalva maneuver may be necessary to elicit the characteristic appearance. Varices show tubular or tortuous appearance with well-defined margins. The lesions usually enhance intensely after intravenous contrast administration. Tubular or fusiform T2 hyperintense lesion is characteristic for varix.

PEARLS

- **Orbital varix is a low-flow congenital venous vascular lesion characterized by the proliferation of venous elements and by massive dilatation of one or more orbital veins.**
- **Dramatic increase in size of varices can be seen with increased venous pressure due to Valsalva maneuver or postural change.**
- **Varices show tubular or tortuous appearance with well-defined margins. Intense enhancement and high T2 signal is usually seen.**

ADDITIONAL IMAGES (B-D)

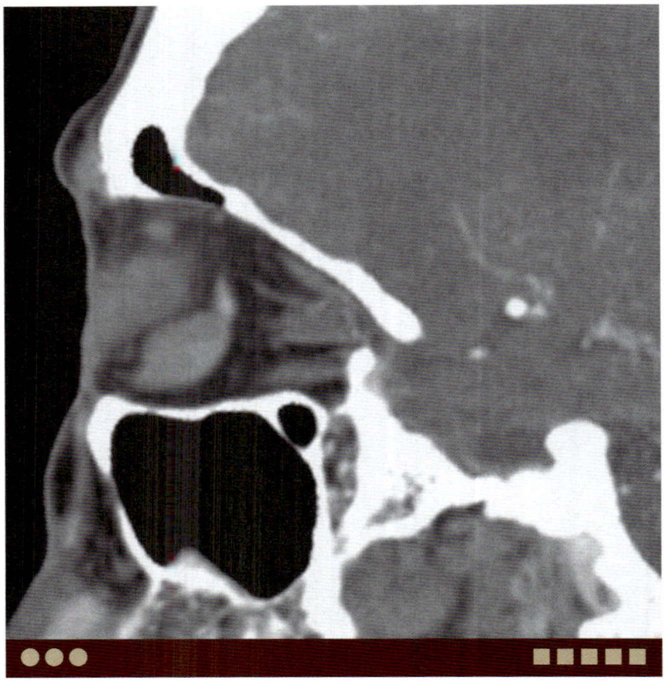

B. Varix, same patient as A. Axial postcontrast CT demonstrates an enhancing spindle-shaped lesion contiguous to the angular vein.

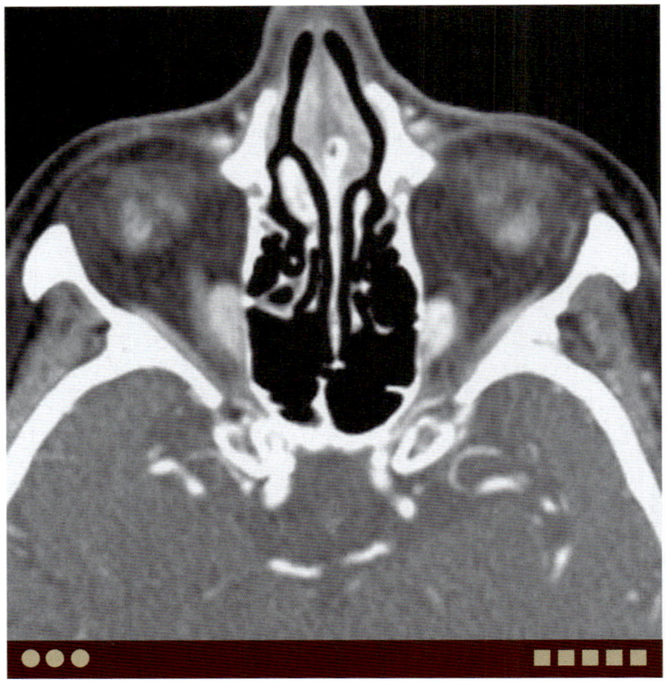

C. **Bilateral varices**. Axial postcontrast CT demonstrates avidly enhancing spindle-shaped lesions with well-defined margins in the medial orbit bilaterally.

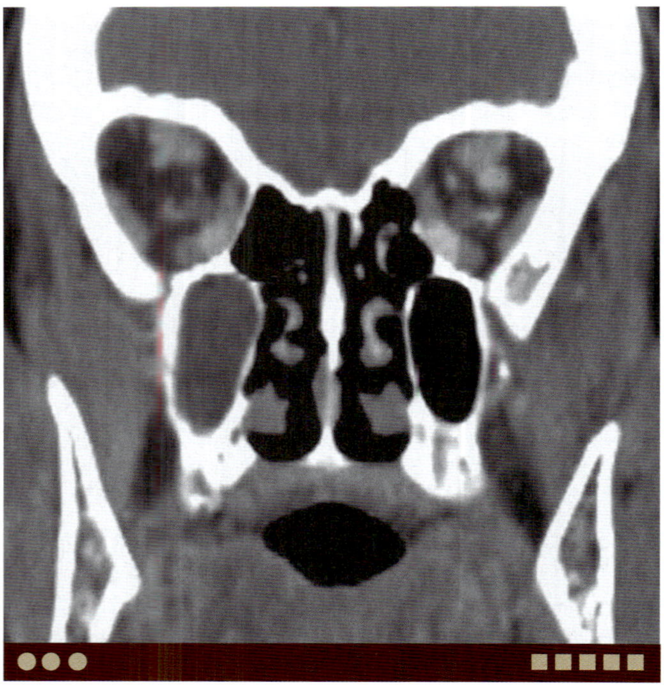

D. Bilateral varices, same patient as C. Coronal postcontrast CT demonstrates avidly enhancing lesions between the medial and inferior rectus muscles bilaterally.

DIFFERENTIAL DIAGNOSIS IMAGES (E-G)

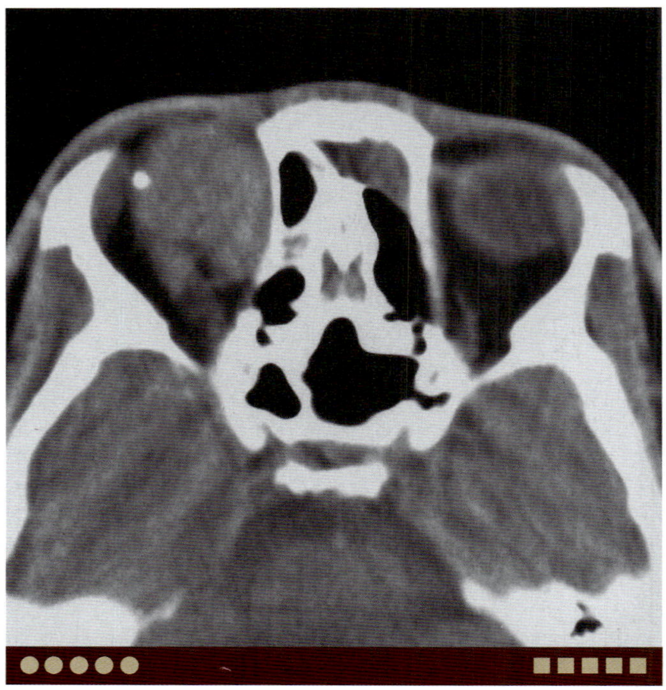

E. **Venous malformation**. Axial postcontrast CT demonstrates an enhancing lesion with phlebolith in the superior right orbit.

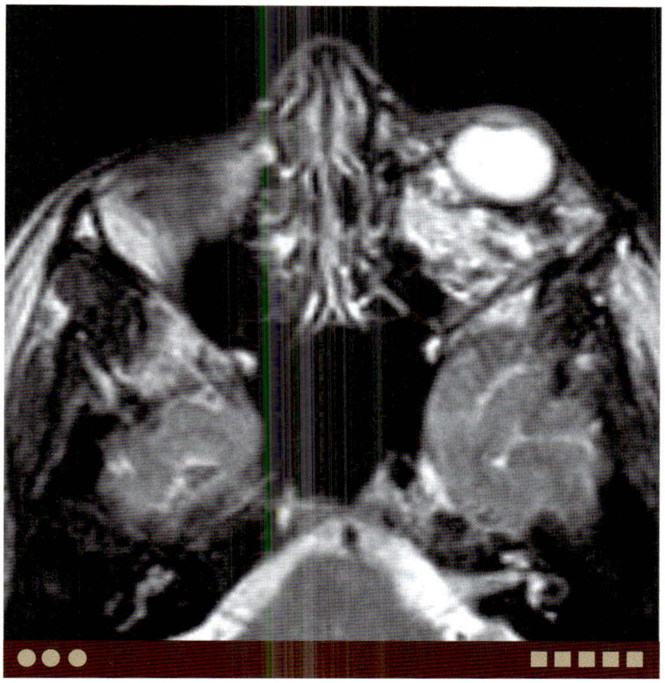

F. Venolymphatic malformation. Axial T2W image shows a heterogeneously high-signal lesion with poorly defined margins in the interior left orbit.

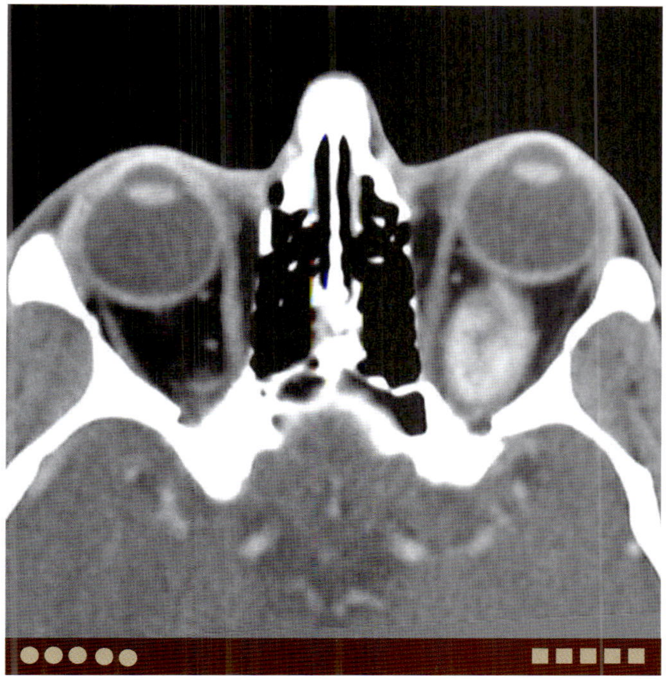

G. Hemangioma. Axial postcontrast CT demonstrates a well-marginated, ovoid enhancing lesion in the retrobulbar space of the left orbit.

Case 4–31 Orbital Meningioma

Brooke Devenney-Cakir, Osamu Sakai

PRESENTATION

Proptosis.

FINDINGS

CT demonstrates a well-circumscribed enhancing lesion at the orbital apex along the bone.

DIFFERENTIAL DIAGNOSIS

- Metastatic tumors: The sphenoid triangle is rich in bone marrow, making it susceptible to metastatic tumors or other marrow related lesions. Imaging findings can be similar to that of meningiomas.
- Lymphoma: It usually arises from the intraorbital soft tissue, however, bone involvement is not uncommon. It typically demonstrates homogeneous density or signal, and molds itself to adjacent structures without apparent destruction.
- Fibrous dysplasia (FD): FD commonly involves the sphenoid triangle and demonstrates "ground-glass" appearance. The cortex should be preserved in FD.

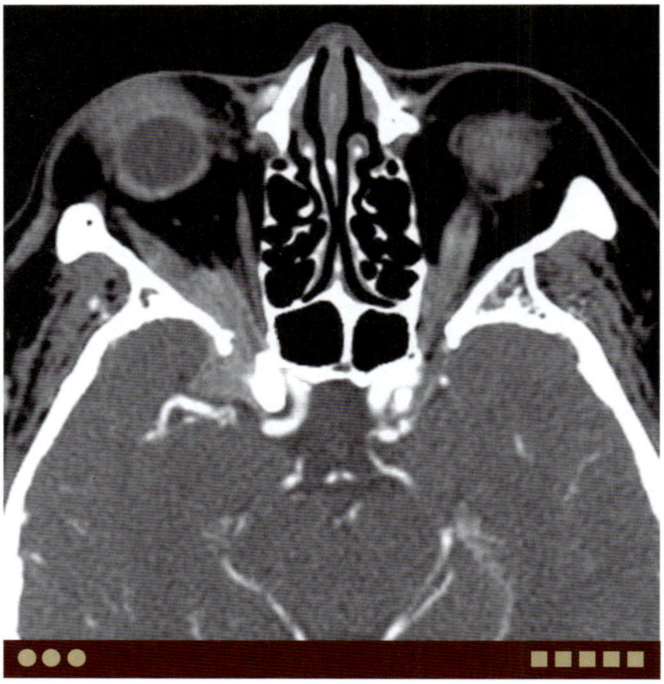

A. Orbital apex meningioma. Axial postcontrast CT soft tissue algorithm demonstrates a well-circumscribed homogenously enhancing mass at the right orbital apex.

COMMENTS

This is a 69-year-old woman with decreasing visual acuity.

Orbital meningiomas can arise from the optic nerve sheath, which is an extension of the dura. However, most orbital meningiomas actually represent intraorbital extension of intracranial meningiomas, and are often seen in mddle age women, whereas primary optic nerve sheath meningiomas are often seen in children and young adults. Meningiomas are commonly seen along the sphenoid bone, often involving the sphenoid triangle, which is also a common location for metastatic lesions. Therefore, bone or dural metastases should be always considered as differential diagnoses. Other differential considerations include lymphoproliferative disorders, lymphoma, and fibrous dysplasia.

On noncontrast CT, meningiomas appear as well-demarcated relatively homogeneous iso- to hyperdense lesions. Postcontrast CT demonstrates homogeneous strong enhancement of the lesion. Hyperostosis/sclerosis of the adjacent bone, "blistering" is commonly seen, which is characteristic of a meningioma. MRI can provide additional details regarding histological diagnosis and extension of the lesion. Just like typical intracranial meningiomas, orbital meningiomas demonstrate iscintense signal to the brain parenchyma on both T1W and T2W images with strong enhancement. Evaluation of lesion extension can be best obtained with postcontrast fat-suppressed T1W images, although careful evaluation is needed at the orbital apex because fat-suppressed images are often degraded by susceptibility artifacts due to air and bone interfaces.

PEARLS

- **Most orbital meningiomas represent orbital extension of intracranial meningiomas.**
- **Primary optic nerve sheath meningioma is often seen in children and young adults rather than middle age women.**
- **Metastatic tumors should be in the differential diagnosis of orbital meningioma when the lesion involves the sphenoid triangle.**

ADDITIONAL IMAGES (B-F)

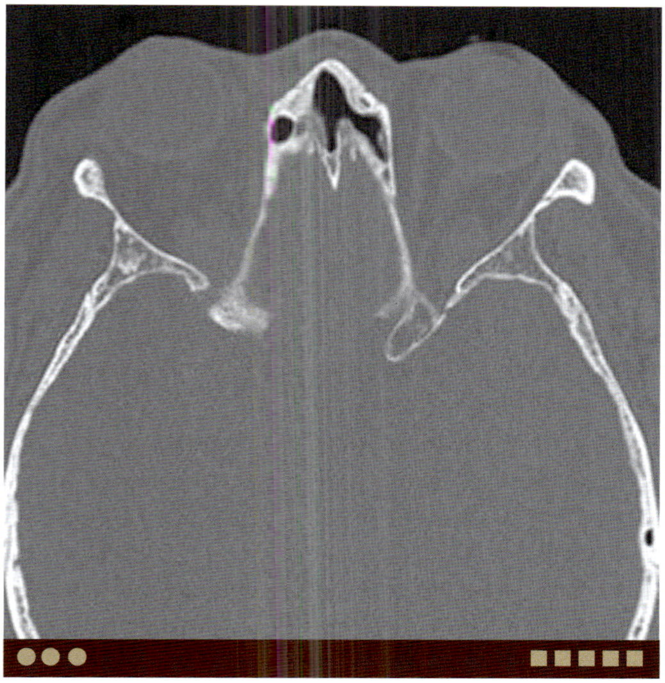

B. Orbital apex meningioma, same patient as A. Axial postcontrast CT bone algorithm demonstrates hyperostosis/sclerotic change of the anterior clinoid.

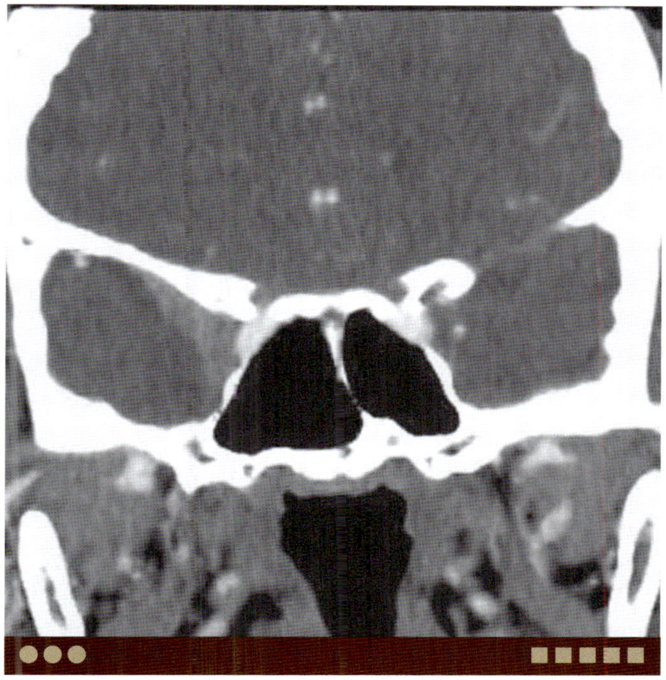

C. Orbital apex meningioma, same patient as A. Coronal postcontrast CT soft tissue algorithm demonstrates homogeneous enhancement of the dural based tumor.

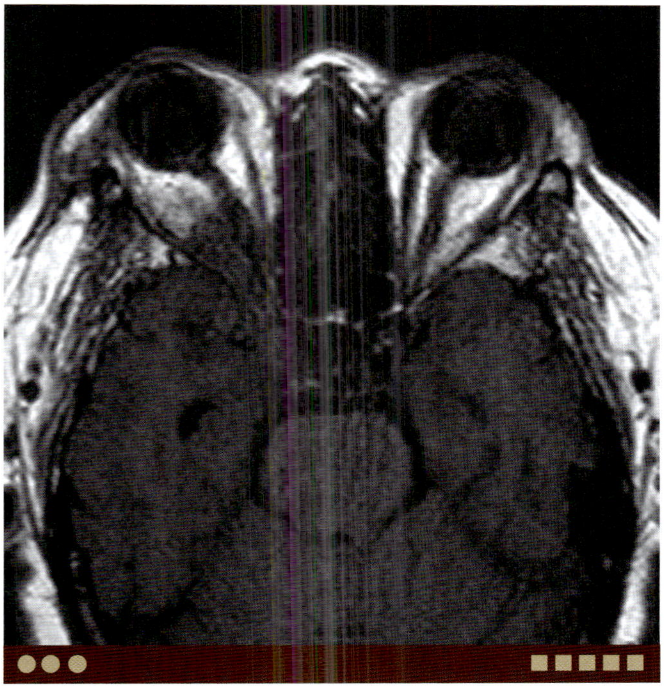

D. Orbital apex meningioma, same patient as A. Axial T1W MR image demonstrates a low-signal mass occupying the right orbital apex.

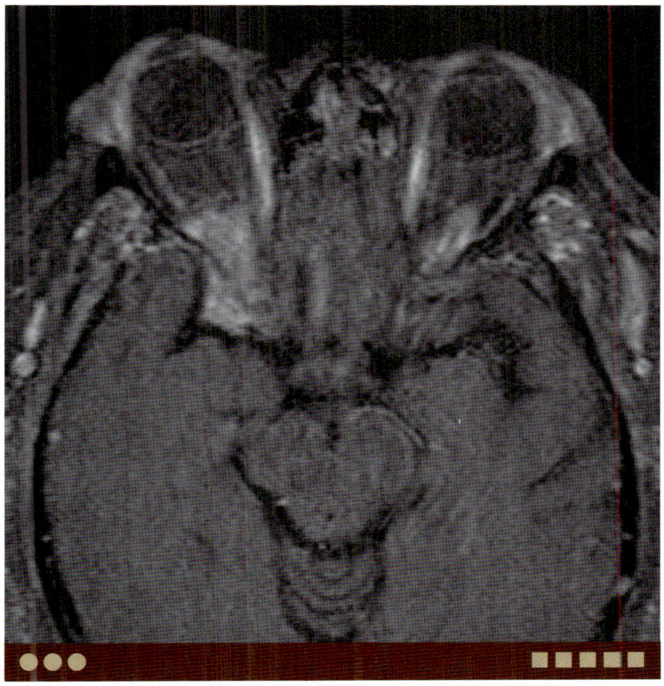

E. Orbital apex meningioma, same patient as A. Axial postcontrast fat-suppressed T1W MR image demonstrates relatively homogenous enhancement of the lesion.

DIFFERENTIAL DIAGNOSIS IMAGES (G-J)

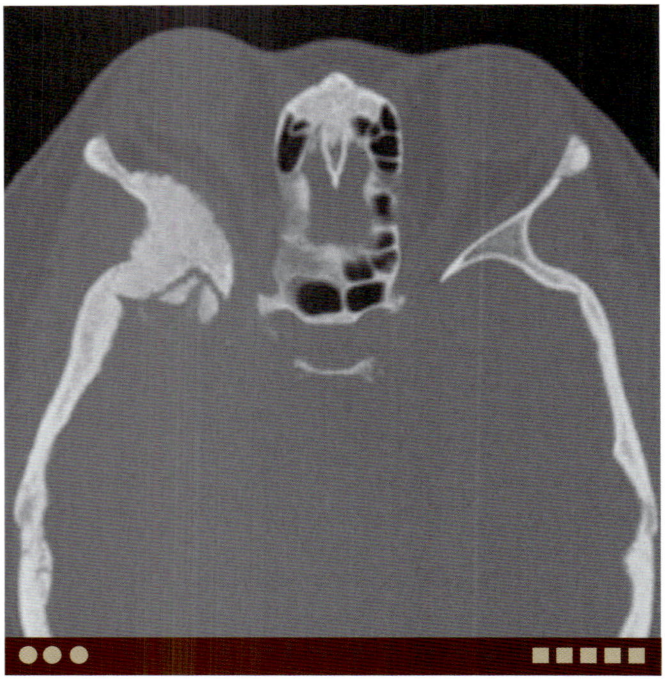

F. Sphenoid triangle meningioma in a different patient. Axial CT demonstrates irregular hyperostosis of the right sphenoid triangle.

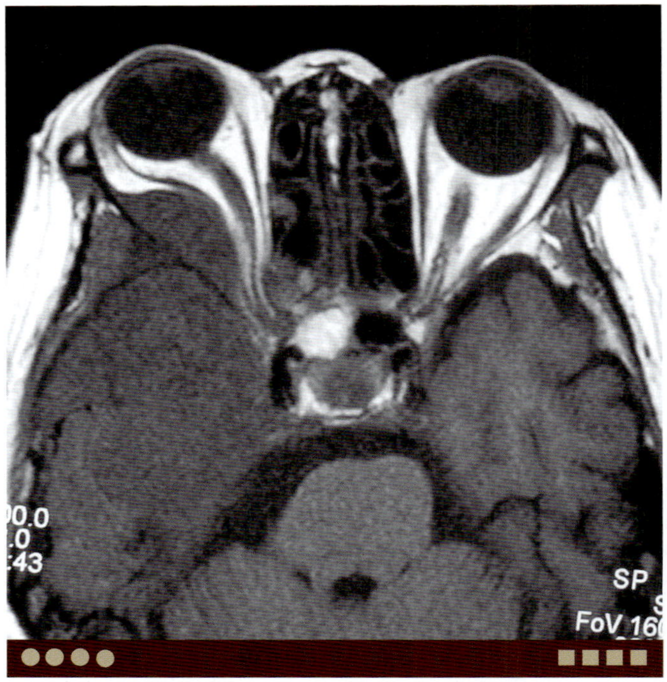

G. Metastasis from urethral cancer. Axial T1W image demonstrates a heterogeneous low-signal lesion along the lateral wall of the right orbit. Note a large intracranial component of the lesion.

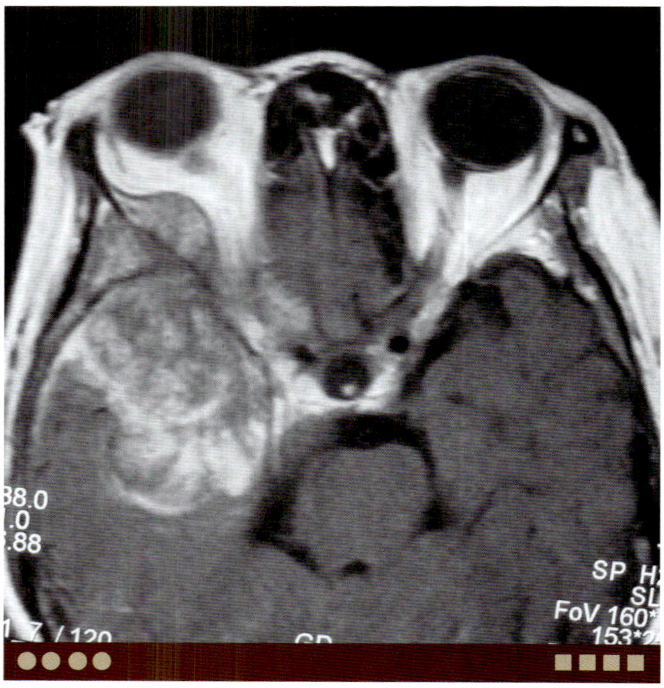

H. Metastasis from urethral cancer, same patient as G. Axial postcontrast T1W image demonstrates heterogeneous enhancement of the lesion.

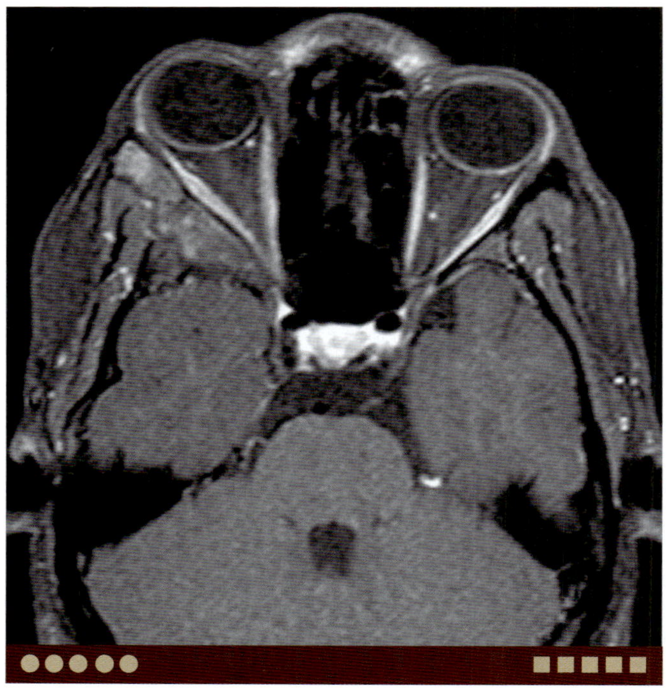

I. Fibrous dysplasia. Axial postcontrast fat-suppressed T1W image demonstrates a mildly enhancing, slightly expansile lesion in the right sphenoid triangle. No extraosseous mass is present.

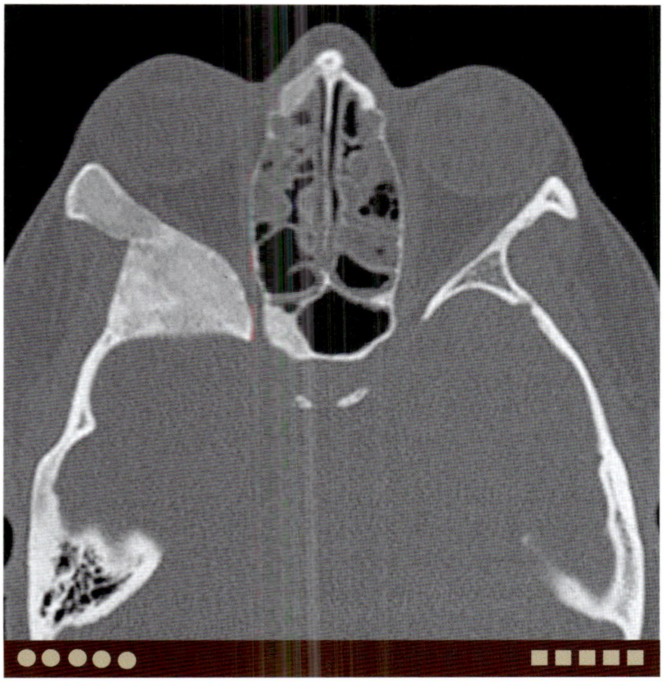

J. Fibrous dysplasia in a different patient. Axial CT demonstrates typical ground-glass appearance of the lesion. Note preserved cortex.

Chapter 5

GLOBE

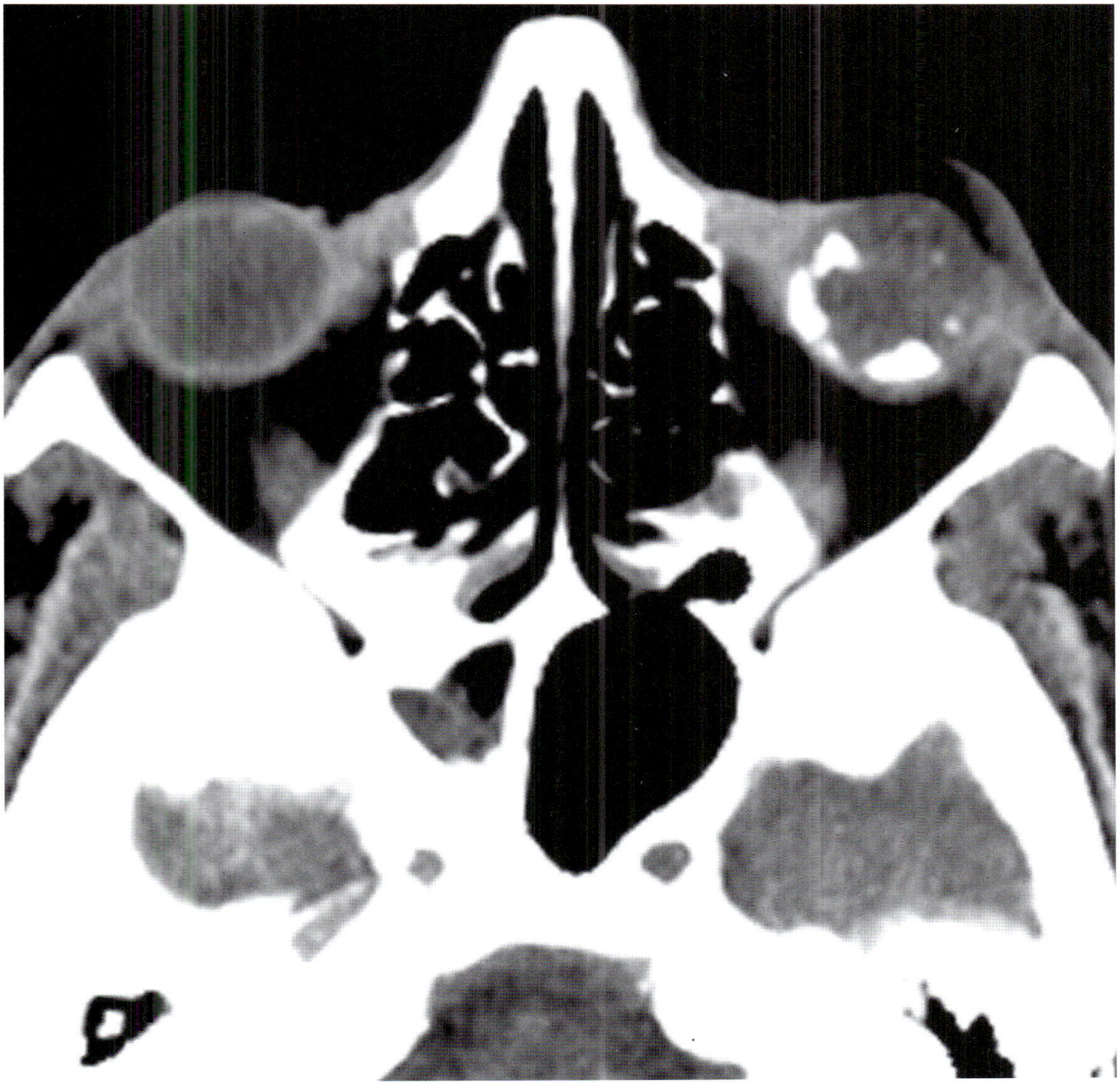

Case 5–1 Phthisis Bulbi

Osamu Sakai, Christina LeBedis

PRESENTATION

History of eye infection, inflammation, or trauma.

FINDINGS

CT and MR images demonstrate deformity and shrinkage of the globe with calcification.

DIFFERENTIAL DIAGNOSIS

- Ruptured globe with foreign body: Penetrating globe injury shows deformity/shrinkage of the globe. Obviously, this is an acute condition usually with a clinical history of trauma.
- Hyaline plaque: Focal calcification is seen at the insertion of medial and lateral rectus muscles without globe deformity. This is degenerative change and seen in elderly populations, usually over 80 years old.
- Optic drusen: Drusen is the accumulation of mucopolysaccharides and proteinaceous material in the surface of the optic disc, which become calcified with advancing age. The shape of the globe is normal.
- Choroidal osteoma: Choroidal osteoma is a benign, ossifying, choroidal tumor of unknown etiology. It occurs predominantly in young females with no history of systemic or ocular disease. The shape of the globe is also normal.

COMMENTS

This is a 75-year-old man with a history of eye trauma.

Phthisis means "wasting away" in Greek. Phthisis bulbi is the term used to describe a shrunken, nonfunctioning globe with ocular calcification or ossification that is the sequela of a wide variety of ocular pathology, including infection, inflammation, or trauma.

This condition usually includes deformity/shrinkage of the globe, a thickened sclera, exudates, and/or blood products in the potential spaces (ciliary body-sclera, choroid-sclera, etc.), chronic retinal detachment, atrophy of the optic nerve, and intraocular calcification or ossification, which is believed to be secondary to osseous metaplasia of the retinal pigment epithelium.

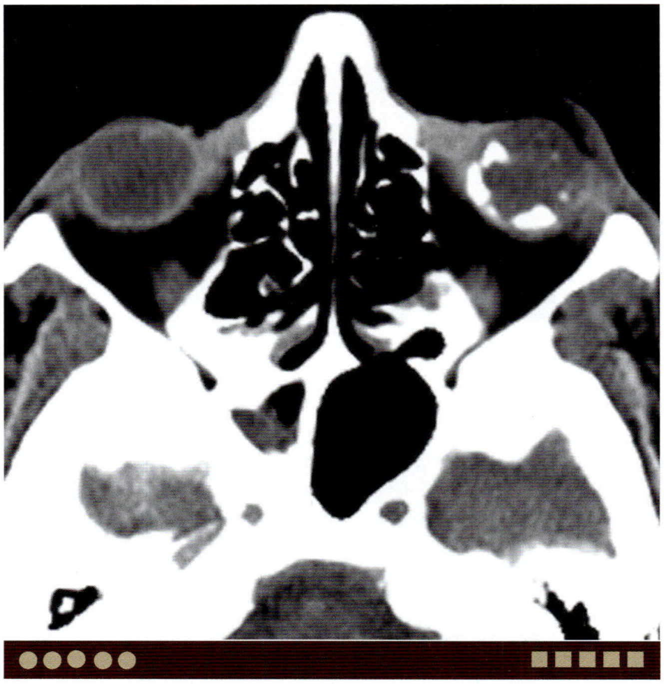

A. Phthisis bulbi. Axial noncontrast CT demonstrates calcifications and deformity of the left globe.

CT and MRI demonstrate severe deformity or shrinkage of the globe with thickened sclera and intraocular calcification. The density or signal within the globe is variable depending on the contents and chronicity of the findings.

PEARLS

- **Phthisis bulbi is the term used to describe a shrunken, nonfunctioning globe with ocular calcification or ossification.**
- **Phthisis bulbi is the sequela of a wide variety of ocular pathology, including infection, inflammation, or trauma.**

ADDITIONAL IMAGES (B-E)

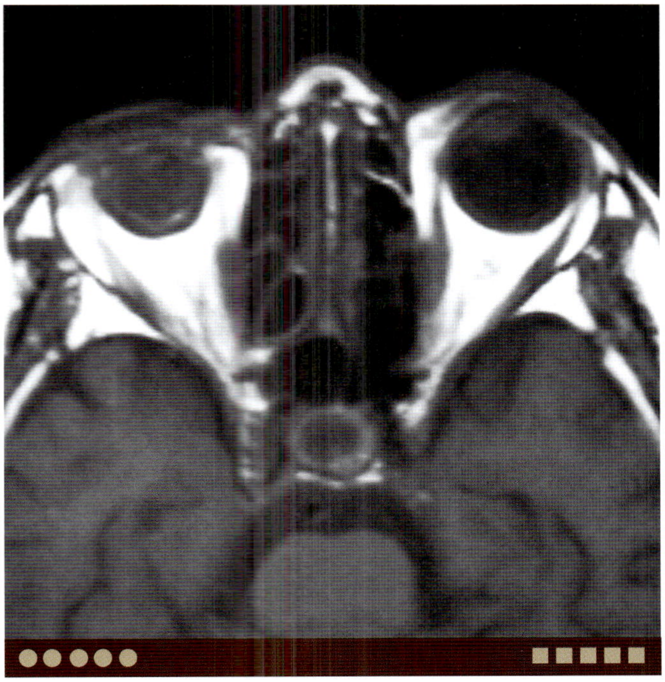

B. Phthisis bulbi in a different patient. Axial T1W MR image demonstrates a shrunken right globe with slightly increased internal signal likely representing increased protein contents.

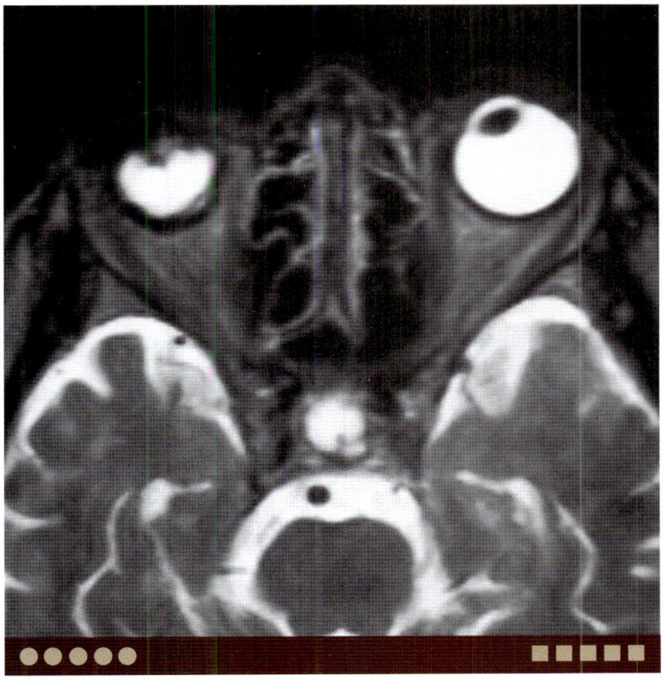

C. Phthisis bulbi, same patient as B. Axial T2W image demonstrates a shrunken right globe.

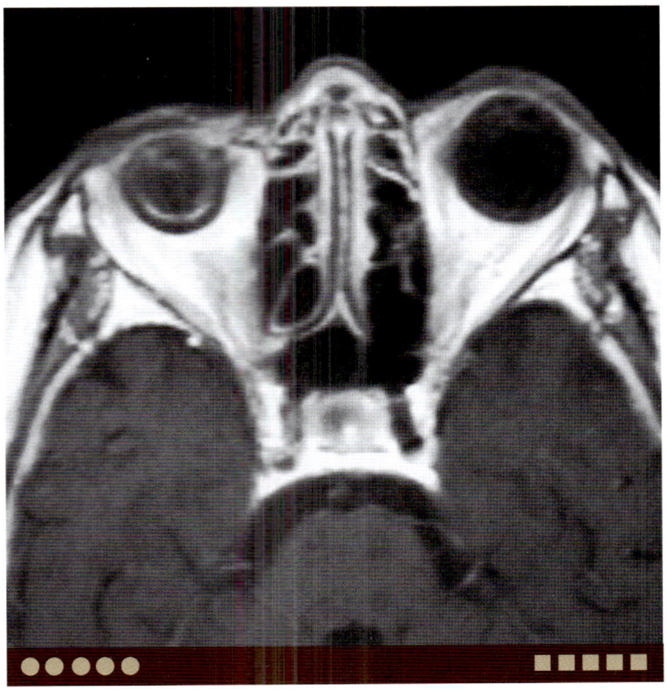

D. Phthisis bulbi, same patient as B. Axial postcontrast T1W image demonstrates no abnormal enhancement in the shrunken right globe.

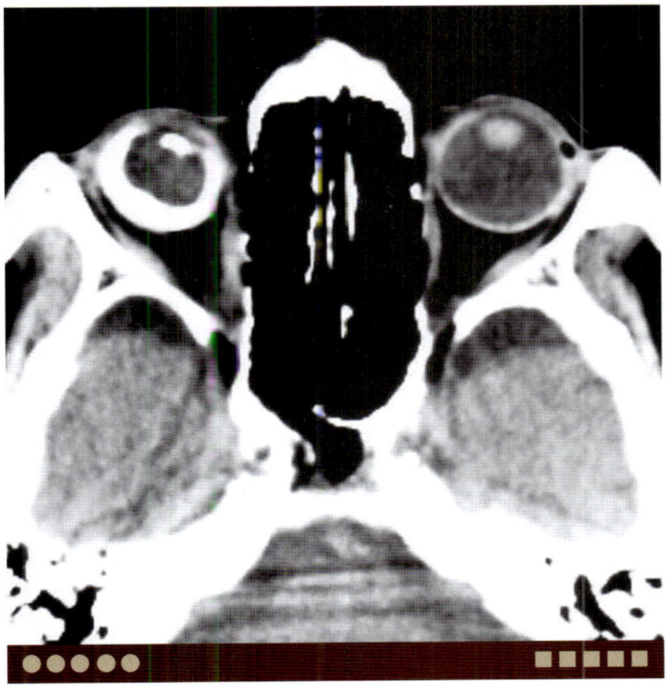

E. Phthisis bulbi in a different patient. Axial noncontrast CT demonstrates densely calcified sclera of the right globe.

DIFFERENTIAL DIAGNOSIS IMAGES (F–H)

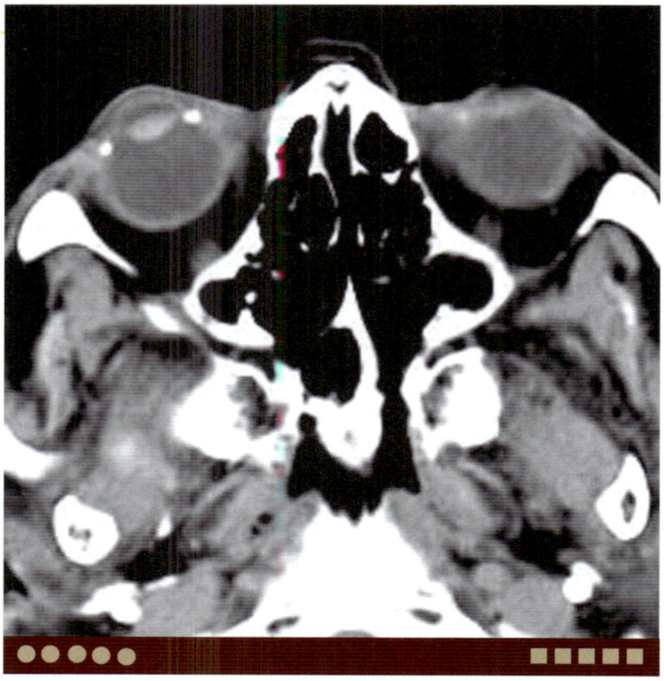

F. Hyaline plaque. Axial noncontrast CT in soft tissue window demonstrates punctate calcifications on the surface of the right globe at the insertion of the medial and lateral rectus muscles in the typical 3 and 9 o'clock positions.

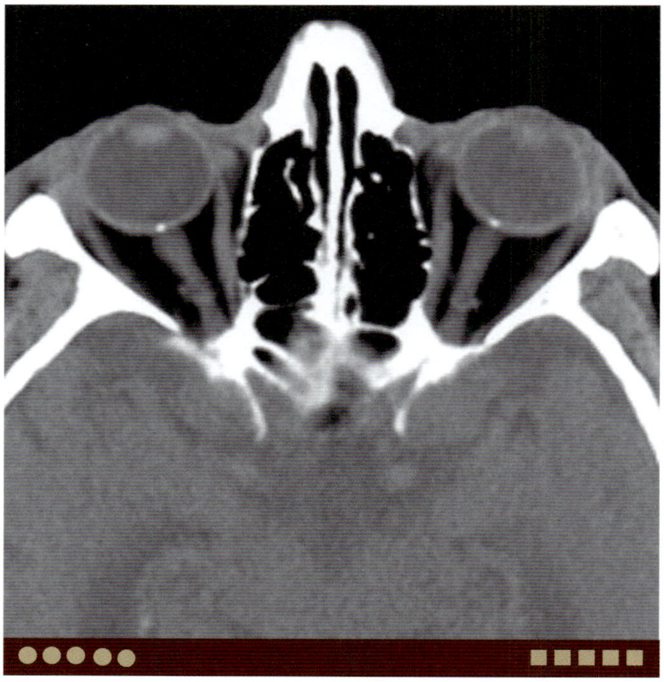

G. Optic drusen. Axial noncontrast CT demonstrates punctate calcifications at the optic discs bilaterally.

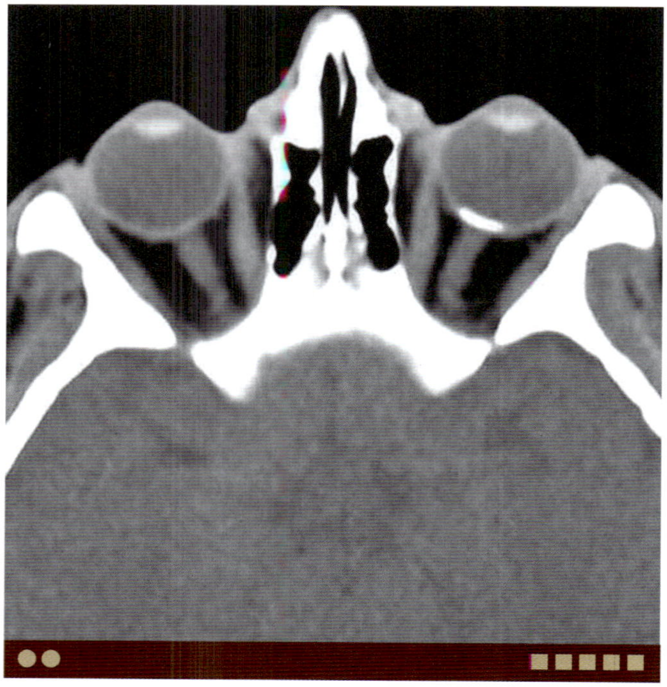

H. Choroidal osteoma. Axial noncontrast CT image demonstrates a plaque-like calcification along the posterior wall of the left globe.

Case 5-2 Lens Implant, Lens Removal

Osamu Sakai, Christina LeBedis

PRESENTATION

Incidental finding.

FINDINGS

CT and MR images demonstrate a slit-like structure in the anterior aspect of the globe

DIFFERENTIAL DIAGNOSIS

- Lens rupture/lens capsule disruption: This is due to a penetrating traumatic injury which manifests as a decrease in density and thinning of the lens.
- Lens dislocation: Dislocated lens can be seen sinking or floating in the vitreous body.
- Lens removal: No lens or lens implant is identified in the globe.

COMMENTS

This is a 68-year-old man with a past history of cataract and lens replacement.

Cataracts are very common in the elderly population, and lens removal and replacement are performed for treatment. Therefore, artificial lens implants are commonly encountered on imaging studies of the brain.

On CT, the artificial lens is seen as a thin, slit-like high-density structure in the anterior globe, at the location of the native lens. On MRI, it is seen as a slit-like signal-void on T2W images, and hardly appreciated on T1W images because of the decreased conspicuity of this hypointense structure against the hypointense background of the anterior chamber and vitreous body.

An absent lens can be a sequela of prior surgery or trauma. Occasionally, lens removal is performed without insertion of an artificial lens. The cause of lens dislocation is a direct blow or sudden motion. Sometimes, a dislocated lens is seen within the vitreous body. Dislocation of lens implants can also be seen both incidentally and in the setting of trauma. In capsule-supported lenses, the lens implant dislocates toward the anterior chamber, however, in iris-supported lenses, the dislocation occurs posteriorly.

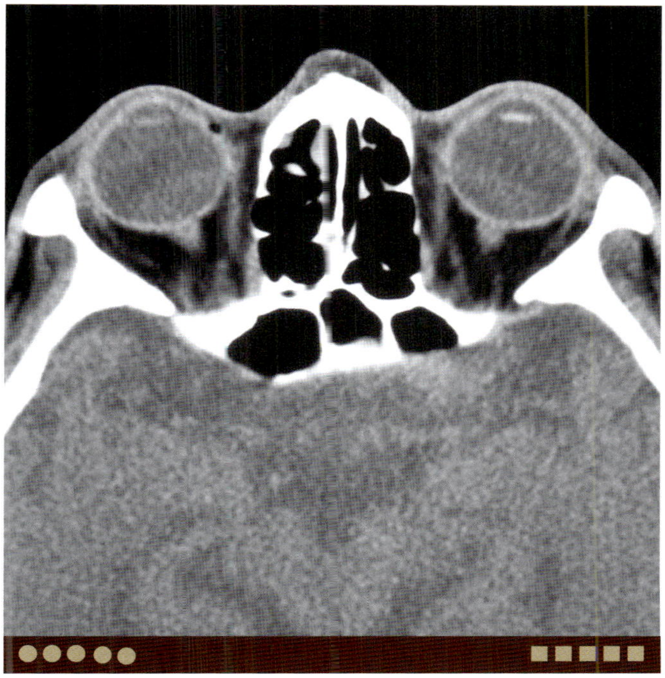

A. Bilateral lens replacement. Axial CT demonstrates slit-like high-density structures in the anterior globes bilaterally.

Imaging is usually not performed to evaluate for the lens, however, familiarity with theses findings is important so as not to misdiagnose the lens as a foreign body or congenital anomaly.

PEARLS

- **Cataracts are very common among the elderly population, and lens removal and replacement are performed for treatment.**
- **Lens implant is seen as a thin, slit-like high density on CT and a low-signal intensity structure on MR images in the anterior globe.**
- **An absent lens can be a sequela of prior surgery or trauma. A dislocated lens may be seen within the vitreous body.**

ADDITIONAL IMAGES (B-E)

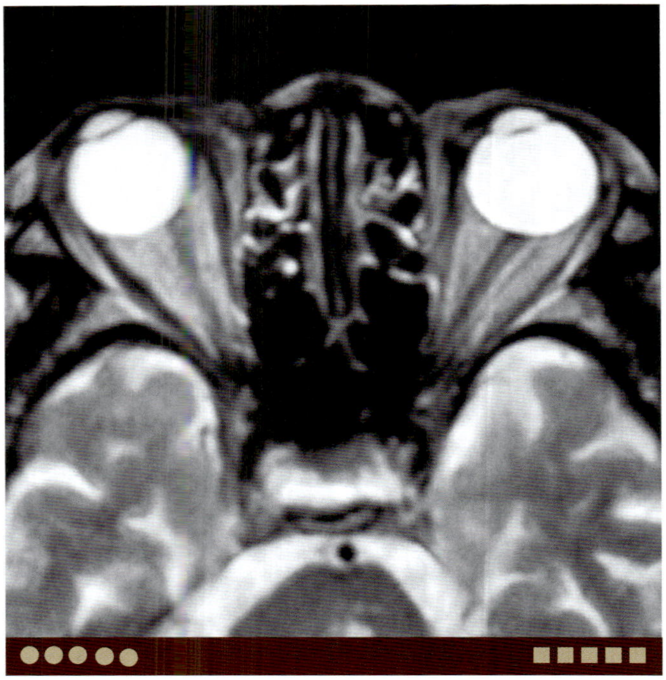

B. Bilateral lens replacement in a different patient. Axial T2W MR image demonstrates slit-like low-signal intensity structures in the anterior globes bilaterally.

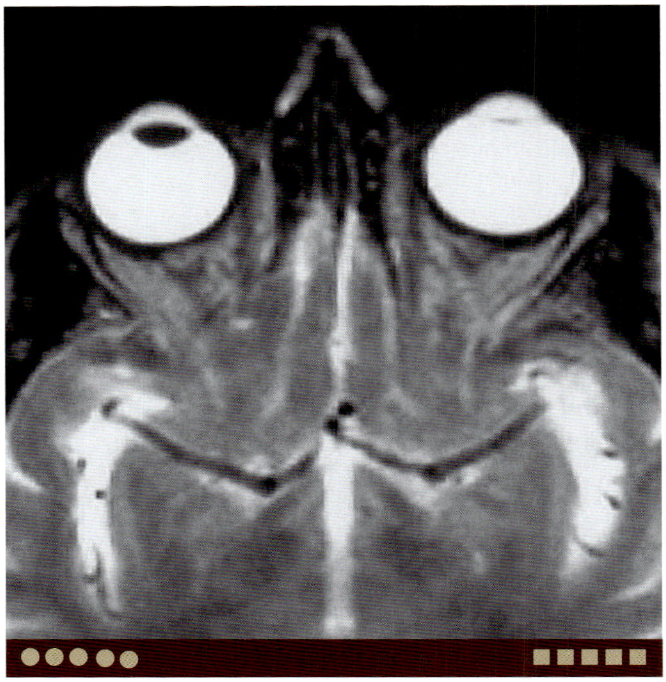

C. Unilateral lens replacement. Axial T2W MR image demonstrates a slit-like low-signal intensity structure in the anterior left globe. The right globe shows a native "lentiform" lens.

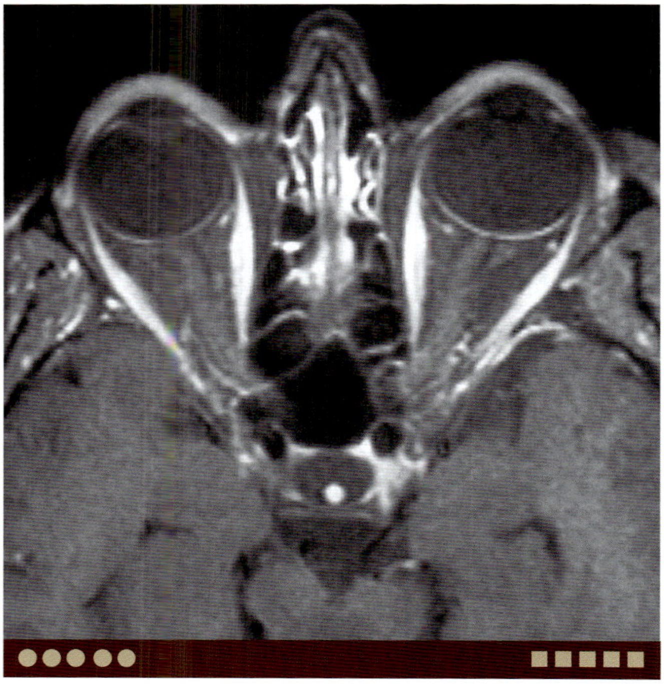

D. Unilateral lens replacement, same patient as C. Axial postcontrast fat-suppressed MR image demonstrates a slit-like signal-void in the anterior left globe. Note how subtle the lens replacement is when compared to the T2W image from the same patient in C. The native right lens is faintly visualized on the right.

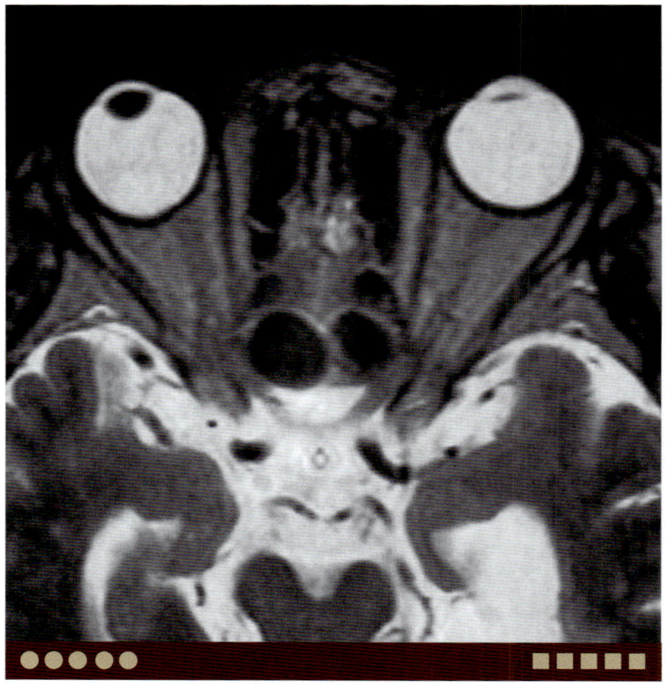

E. Unilateral lens replacement in a different patient. Axial T2W MR image demonstrates a slit-like low signal in the anterior left globe. The right globe shows a native "lentiform" lens.

DIFFERENTIAL DIAGNOSIS IMAGES (F-G)

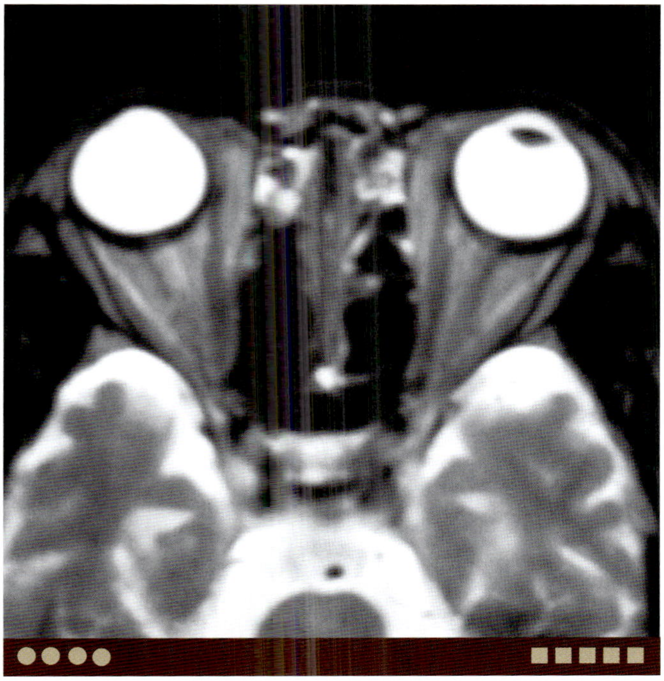

F. Unilateral lens removal Axial T2W MR image demonstrates an empty right anterior globe. The left globe shows a native lens.

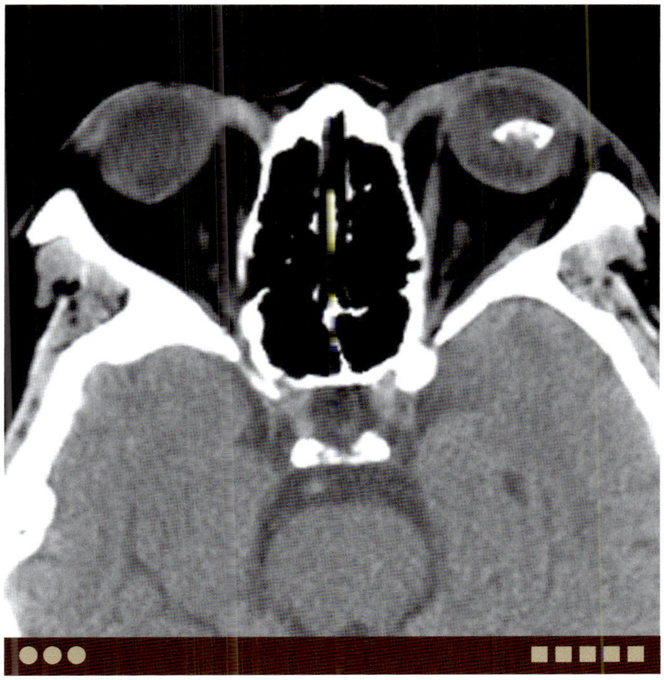

G. Dislocated calcified lens. Axial CT demonstrates a calcified lens dislocated into the vitreous body on the left.

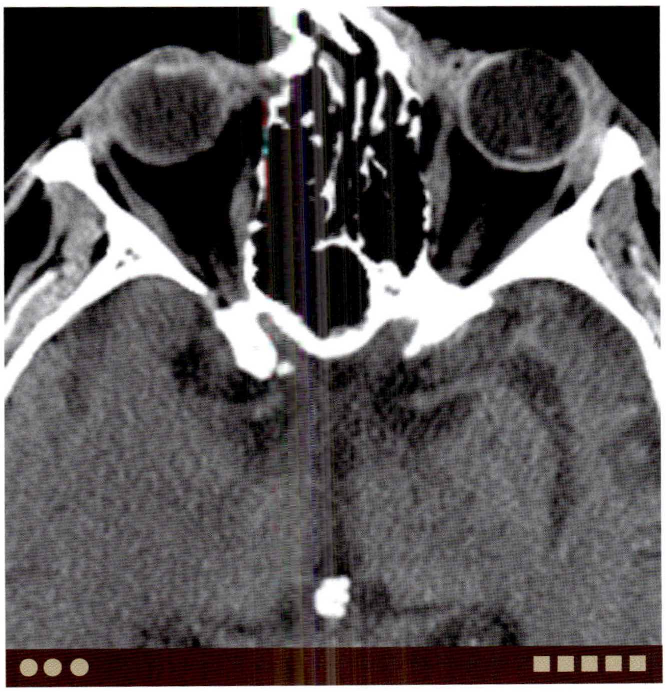

H. Dislocated lens implant. Axial CT demonstrates a dislocated lens implant sunk in the vitreous body on the left.

Case 5–3 Retinal Detachment

Osamu Sakai, Christina LeBedis

PRESENTATION

Decreased visual acuity.

FINDINGS

CT and MRI demonstrate a V-shaped intraocular collection.

DIFFERENTIAL DIAGNOSIS

- Choroidal detachment: This spares posterior aspect of the globe with the detached choroidal leaves having a parallel appearance on cross-sectional imaging.
- Posterior hyaloid detachment: This can cause a fluid-fluid level along the posterior aspect of the globe.

COMMENTS

This is a 74-year-old man who underwent a brain MRI for stroke.

Retinal detachment is seen as a small focal crescent-shaped thickening of the ocular wall when it is small. As the detachment becomes larger, it assumes a typical V-shaped appearance with its apex at the posterior pole (optic disc). Subretinal fluid is usually similar or slightly higher in signal intensity on T1W images and lower in signal intensity on T2W images compared to the vitreous body. However, the signal intensity of the subretinal fluid varies depending on the presence of proteinaceous fluid or hemorrhage. Hemorrhage demonstrates variable signal intensities depending on its acuity. CT is much less sensitive than MRI in the detection of small retinal detachment or simple subretinal fluid collections that do not contain significant amounts of protein or hemorrhage.

Retinal detachment is routinely diagnosed ophthalmologically. The role of imaging in this setting is not for the detection or characterization of the retinal detachment, but rather to evaluate for an underlying neoplastic process. Imaging is also helpful for intraocular inspection when fundoscopic examination is difficult due to opacity of the lens and/or vitreous body. Contrast-enhanced MRI can differentiate solid tumors from a subretinal fluid collection.

Choroidal detachment has a parallel configuration of the detached choroidal leaves with sparing of the posterior third of the globe due to the anchoring effects of the short posterior ciliary arteries, veins, and nerves. Hemorrhagic choroidal detachment is often seen in the setting of trauma and significantly affects the clinical outcome.

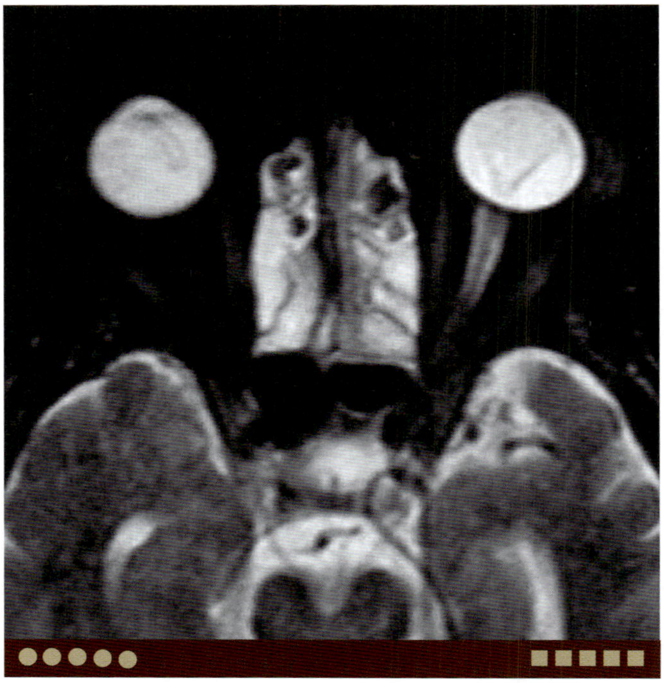

A. Retinal detachment. Axial T2W MR image demonstrates a left intraocular V-shaped appearance with the apex of the detachment at the optic disc. This serous subretinal fluid shows high signal similar to the vitreous body.

Subhyaloid effusion is freely mobile and is seen as a fluid-fluid level along the posterior aspect of the globe.

PEARLS

- **Retinal detachment has a V-shaped appearance with the apex of the detachment at the optic disc.**
- **Imaging can be performed to evaluate for underlying tumors.**
- **Choroidal detachment is seen as parallel detachments sparing the posterior third of the globe.**
- **Subhyaloid effusion is freely mobile and demonstrates a fluid-fluid level along the posterior aspect of the globe.**

ADDITIONAL IMAGES (B-E)

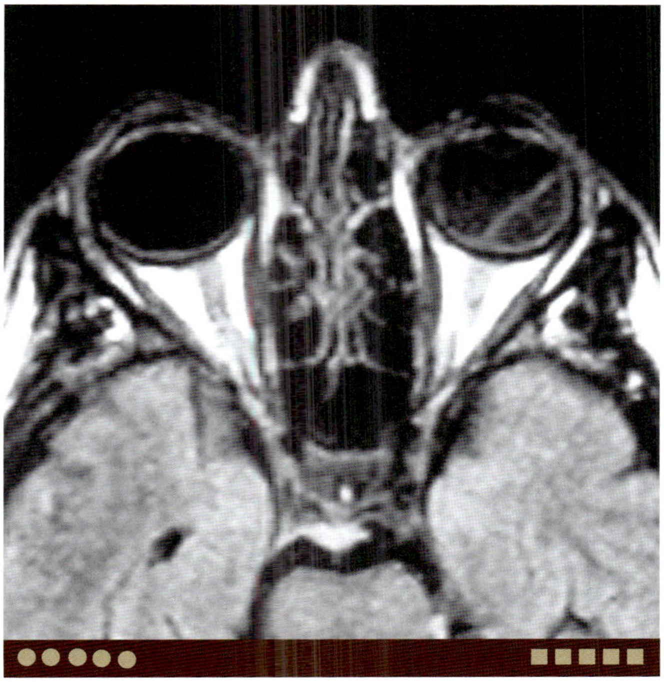

B. Retinal detachment in a different patient. Axial FLAIR MR image demonstrates a left retinal detachment. Note that the subretinal fluid shows minimally increased signal indicating slightly higher protein concentration compared with the vitreous body.

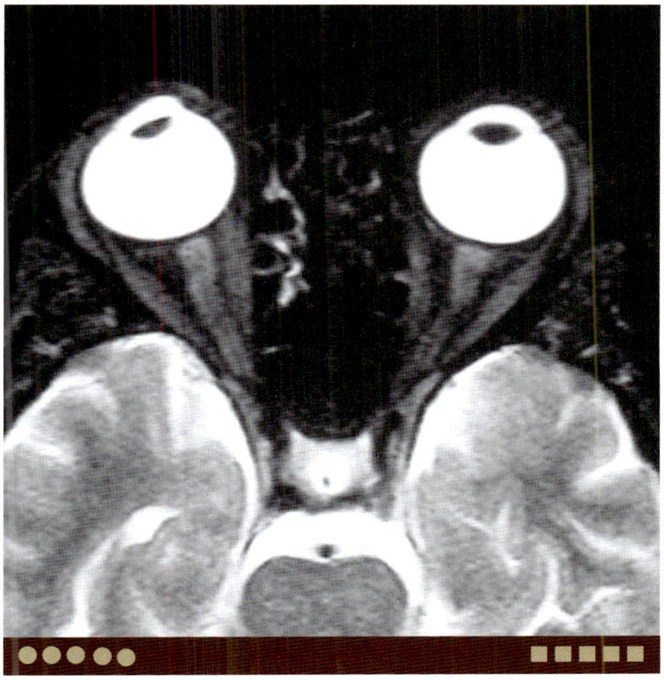

C. Retinal detachment, same patient as B. Axial T2W MR image fails to demonstrate detachment because of serous subretinal fluid showing similar signal to the vitreous body.

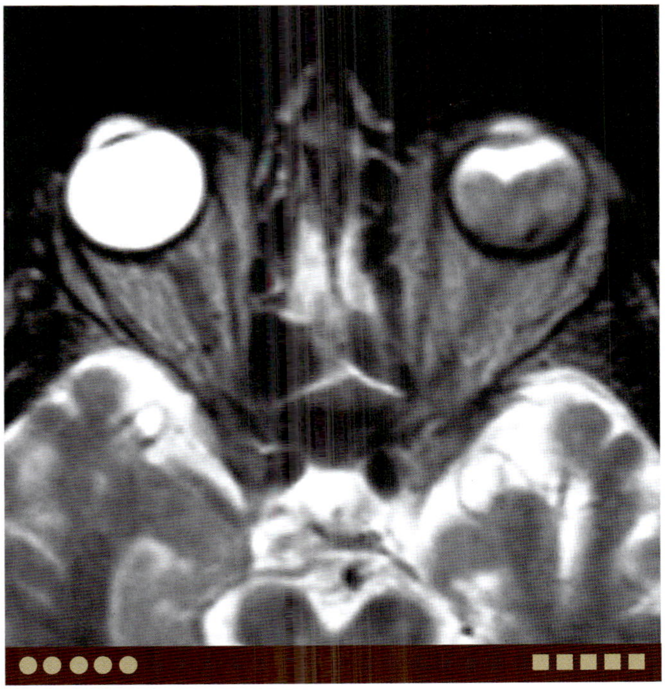

D. Retinal detachment in a different patient. Axial T2W MR image demonstrates a left retinal detachment with low-signal subretinal fluid secondary to hemorrhage.

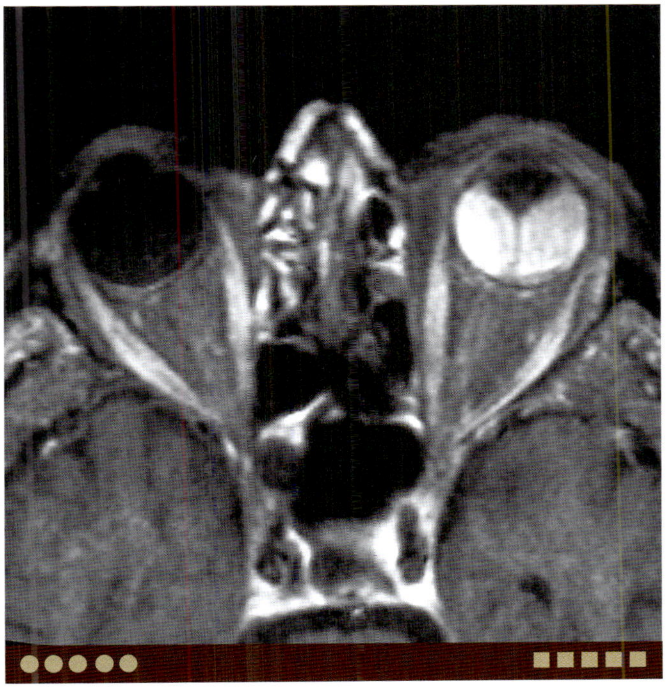

E. Retinal detachment, same patient as D. Axial postcontrast fat-suppressed T1W MR image demonstrates high-signal hemorrhagic subretinal fluid in the setting of a left retinal detachment.

DIFFERENTIAL DIAGNOSIS IMAGES (F-G)

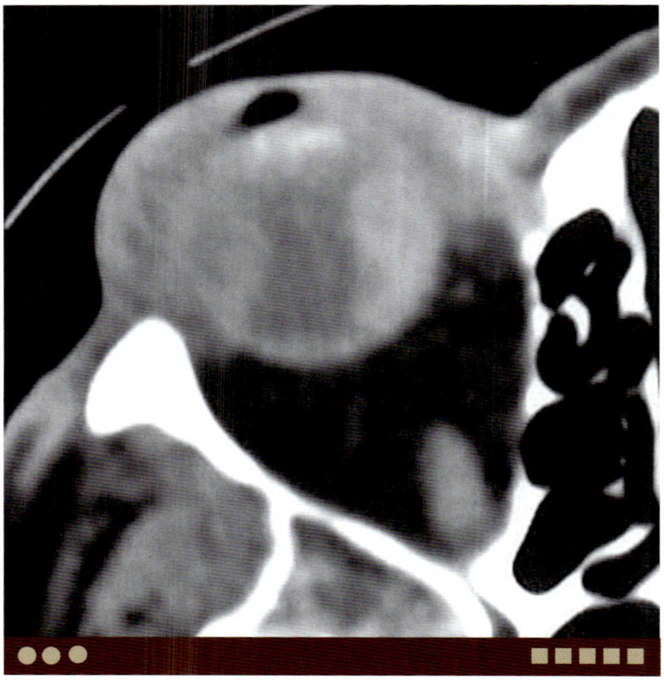

F. Choroidal hemorrhage. Axial CT demonstrates high-density parallel detachments sparing the posterior third of the globe.

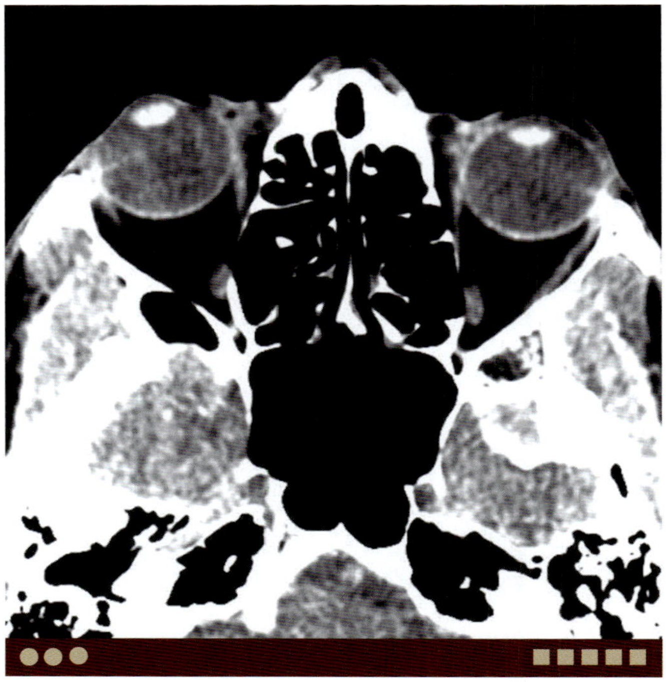

G. Choroidal detachment. Axial CT demonstrates parallel detachments sparing the posterior third of the right globe, a very subtle finding.

Case 5-4 Posttherapeutic Changes of Retinal Detachment

Osamu Sakai, Christina LeBedis

PRESENTATION

Incidental finding.

FINDINGS

Cross-sectional imaging demonstrates an abnormal structure around the globe and an unusual density (CT) and signal intensity (MRI) of the vitreous body.

DIFFERENTIAL DIAGNOSIS

- Intraocular hemorrhage: This condition is usually obvious from the clinical scenario and physical findings, such as can be seen in trauma.
- Intraocular abscess: This condition usually causes visible inflammatory change which is also obvious on imaging.
- Foreign body: Scleral buckle, band, and clip should be seen in expected locations. Otherwise, foreign bodies should be suspected

COMMENTS

This is a 56-year-old man with past medical history of retinal detachment.

Scleral buckle/banding is a common treatment for retinal detachment. A silicone band is usually used, which can be seen as either a radiopaque or a radiolucent structure. Sometimes a metallic clip, often located at the superior and lateral aspect of the globe is seen. If there is a history of retinal detachment and treatment, these findings are easily recognized. However, these posttreatment changes can be misinterpreted as a foreign body. The scleral band is most frequently seen as signal-void on MRI. Cystic degeneration of the scleral band is a relatively common complication. Occasionally, a subconjunctival cyst is formed in association with the scleral buckle.

Silicone oil injection is another common procedure used in the treatment of retinal detachment. The silicone oil is usually seen on CT as intraocular hyperattenuating material floating on top of the residual vitreous body. Recognition of this entity is crucial so as not to misdiagnose the imaging findings as hemorrhage. Another diagnostic clue of intraocular silicone oil is that on MRI it follows the signal intensity pattern of fat including signal suppression on fat-saturated sequences.

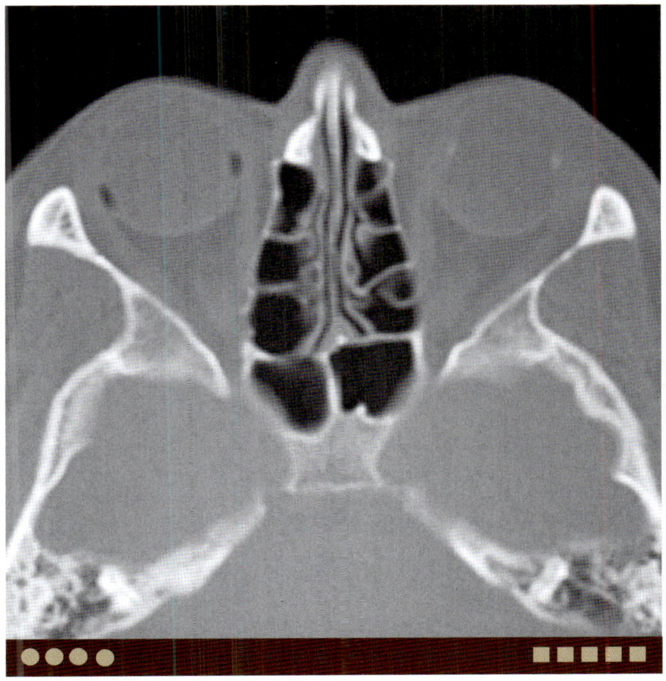

A. Scleral buckle. Axial CT demonstrates two different types of scleral buckles. The one on the right is low density while the one on the left is high density.

Pneumatic retinopexy, the injection of gas into the globe, is an alternative treatment for retinal detachment and is seen as intraocular air on CT.

PEARLS

- **Scleral buckle/banding is a common procedure for retinal detachment. Silicone bands can be seen as either a radiopaque or a radiolucent structure. A metallic clip may be present at the superolateral aspect of the globe.**
- **Cystic degeneration of the scleral band is a common complication.**
- **Silicone oil injection demonstrates high density in the globe on CT and follows fat-signal intensity on all MRI sequences, including signal suppression on fat-saturated sequences.**

ADDITIONAL IMAGES (B-E)

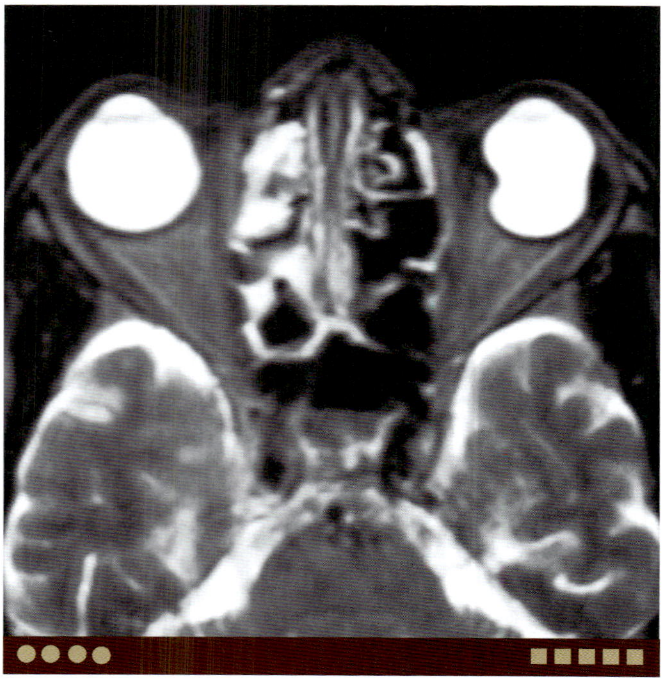

B. Scleral buckle in a different patient. Axial T2W MR image demonstrates a low-signal intensity scleral buckle on the left.

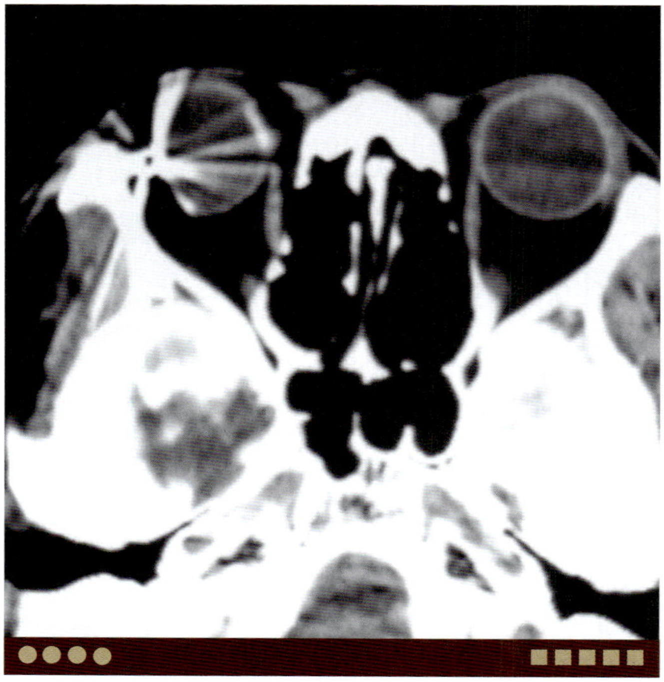

C. Scleral banding. Axial CT demonstrates streaking artifact from the titanium clip for scleral banding on the right.

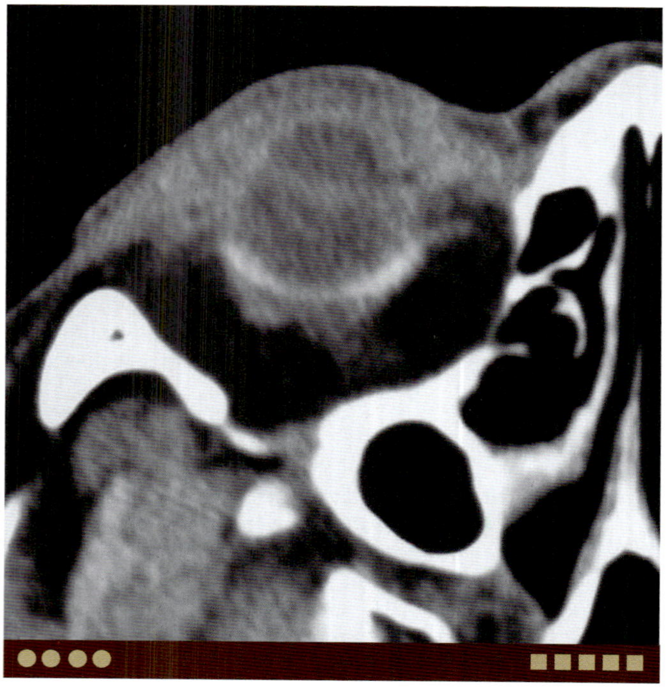

D. Scleral buckle, periorbital cellulitis. Axial CT demonstrates preseptal inflammatory change after a scleral buckle procedure. Note the hyperattenuating curvilinear scleral buckle.

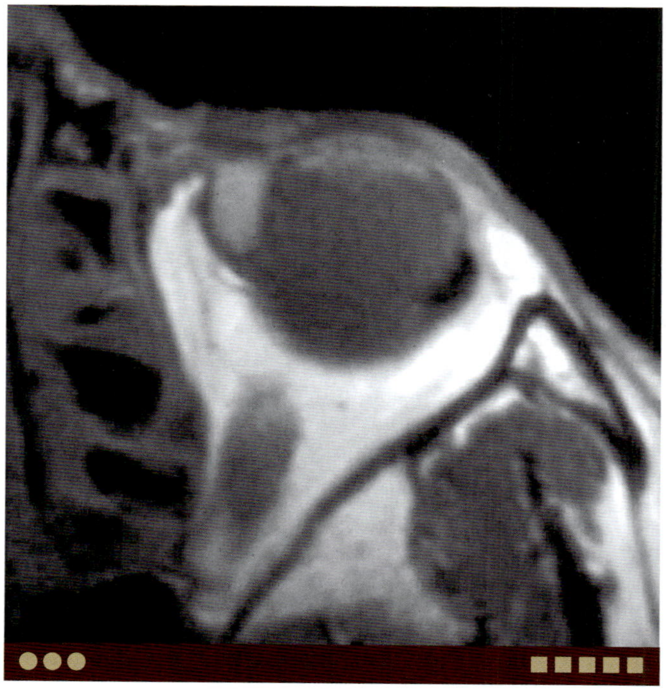

E. Scleral buckle, cystic degeneration. Axial T1W MR image demonstrates cystic degeneration of the medial portion of the scleral buckle.

DIFFERENTIAL DIAGNOSIS IMAGES (F-G)

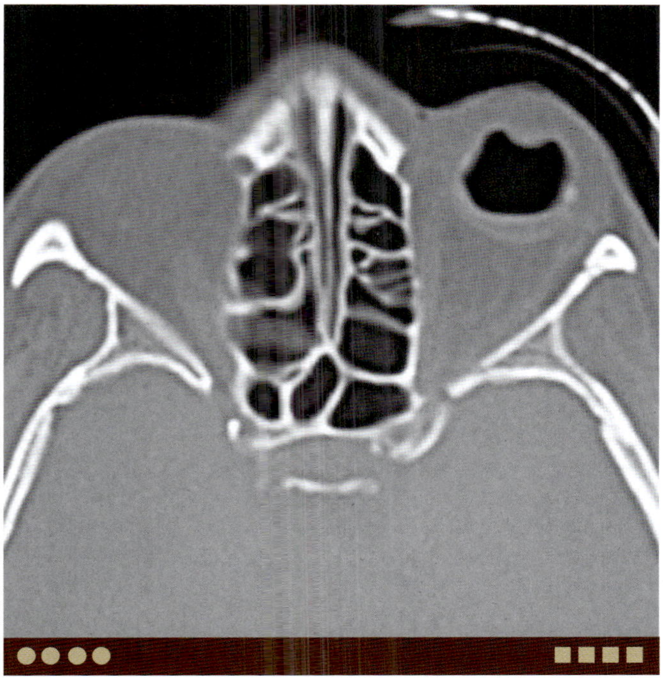

F. Pneumopexy. Axial CT demonstrates injected gas in the left globe for the treatment of retinal detachment.

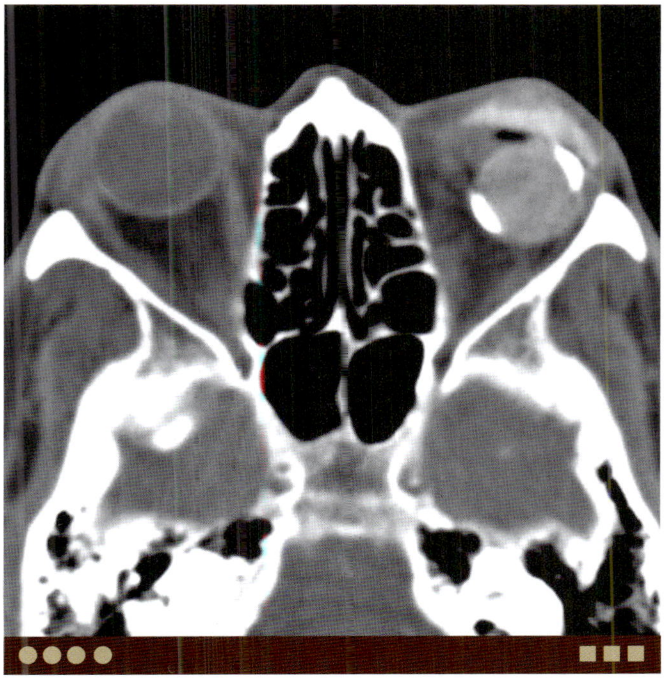

G. Ocular prosthesis. Two-piece prosthesis, the shell, and spacer is placed in the left orbit. The band-like high density of the spacer mimics scleral buckle.

Case 5-5 Posttherapeutic Changes of Retinal Detachment: Silicone Oil Injection

Christina LeBedis, Osamu Sakai

PRESENTATION

Incidental findings.

FINDINGS

CT demonstrates abnormal high-density material in the vitreous body. Silicon oil follows the signal pattern of fat on MRI.

DIFFERENTIAL DIAGNOSIS

- Intraocular hemorrhage: This can be seen primarily in trauma and is usually clinically evident.
- Ocular prosthesis: A two-piece prosthetic globe can have a confusing hyperattenuating appearance if not familiar with its appearance.

COMMENTS

This is a 59-year-old woman who underwent CT for dizziness.

Silicone oil injection is used for the treatment of retinal detachment. Silicone oil is usually seen on CT as intraocular hyperattenuating material floating on top of the residual vitreous body. Recognition of this entity is crucial so as not to misdiagnose the imaging findings as hemorrhage. An intraocular silicone injection can be distinguished from an intraocular hemorrhage by measuring the CT attenuation numbers (that of silicone is >100 Hounsfield unit [HU]; that of blood <90 HU) or by detecting a silicone-related chemical shift artifact on MR images. Another diagnostic clue of intraocular silicone oil on MRI is that it follows the signal intensity pattern of fat including signal suppression on fat-saturated sequences.

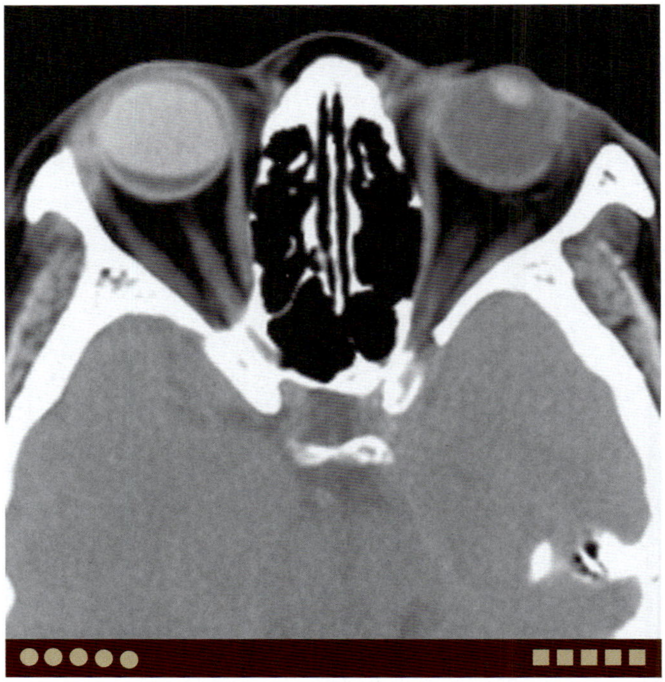

A. Intraocular silicone oil. Axial CT demonstrates hyperattenuating material in the right globe consistent with intraocular silicone oil injection for the treatment of retinal detachment.

PEARLS

- **Silicone oil injection is used for the treatment of retinal detachment.**
- **On CT, the attenuation values of silicone oil are >100 HU, whereas blood is <90 HU. On MRI, silicone oil can be detected by chemical shift artifact and signal suppression on fat-saturated sequences.**
- **Recognition of this entity is crucial not to mistake it for intraocular hemorrhage.**

ADDITIONAL IMAGES (B-E)

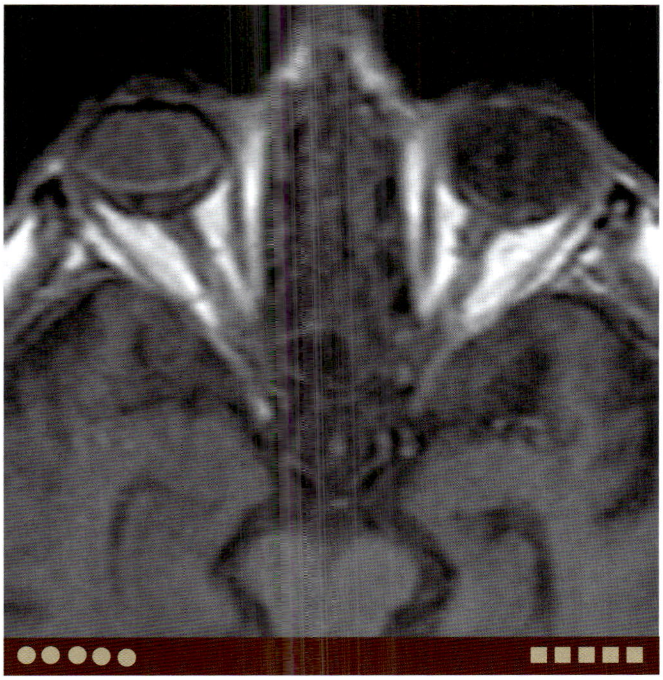

B. Intraocular silicone oil in a different patient. Axial T1W MR image demonstrates high-signal intensity right intraocular silicone oil used for the treatment of retinal detachment.

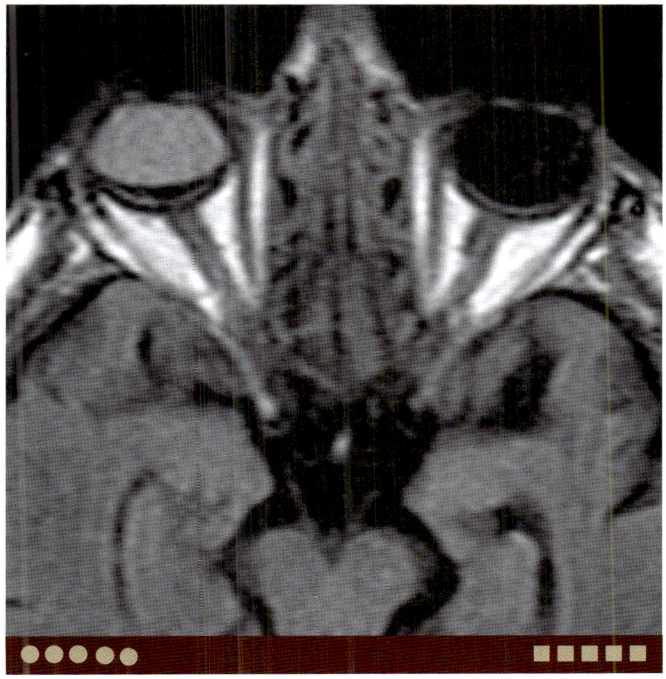

C. Intraocular silicone oil, same patient as B. Axial FLAIR MR image demonstrates hyperintense material in the right vitreous body.

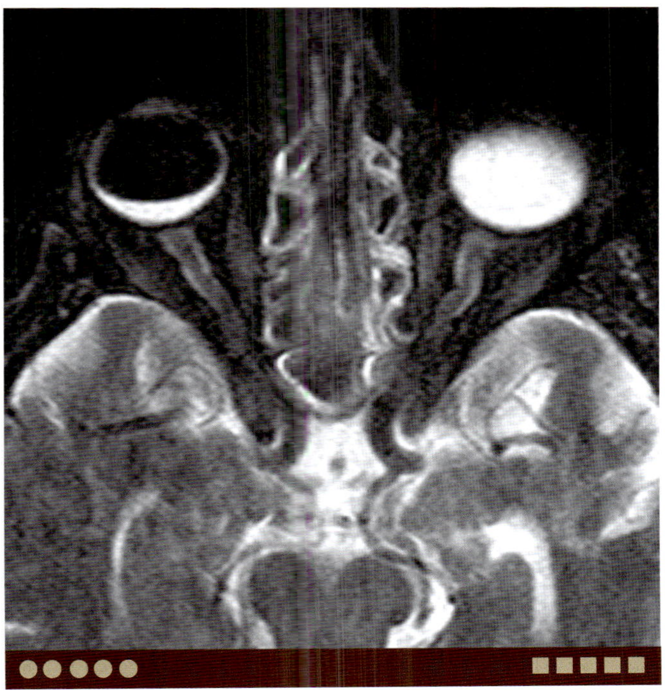

D. Intraocular silicone oil, same patient as B. Axial fat-suppressed T2W MR image demonstrates signal suppression of the right intraocular silicone oil used for the treatment of retinal detachment.

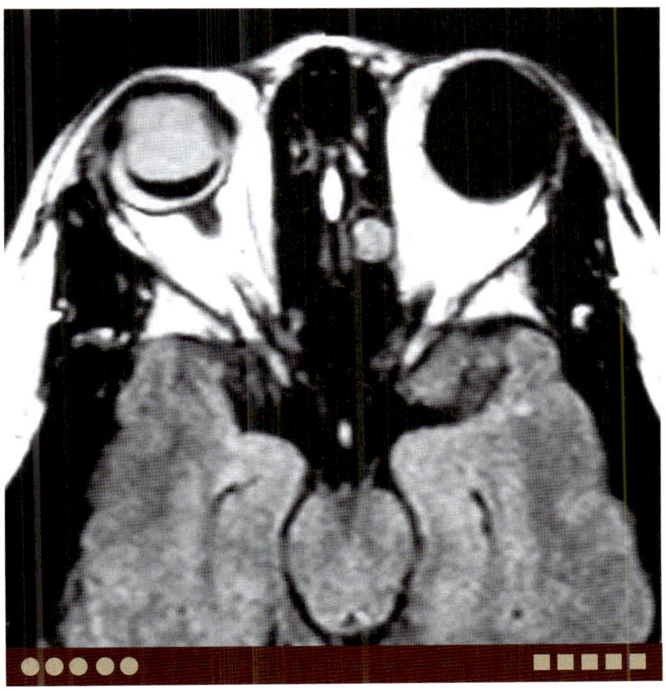

E. Intraocular silicone oil in a different patient. Axial FLAIR MR image demonstrates high-signal intensity silicone oil in the right globe.

DIFFERENTIAL DIAGNOSIS IMAGES (F-G)

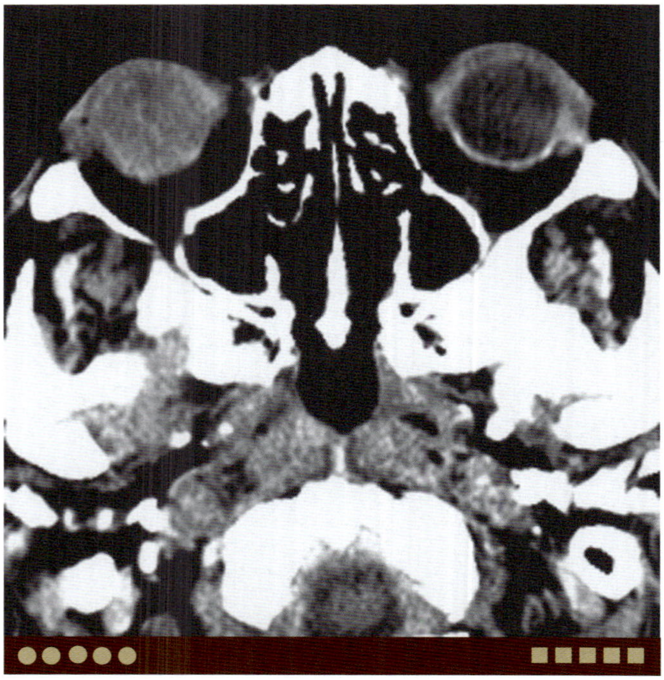

F. Vitreous hemorrhage. Axial CT demonstrates increased density within the right globe.

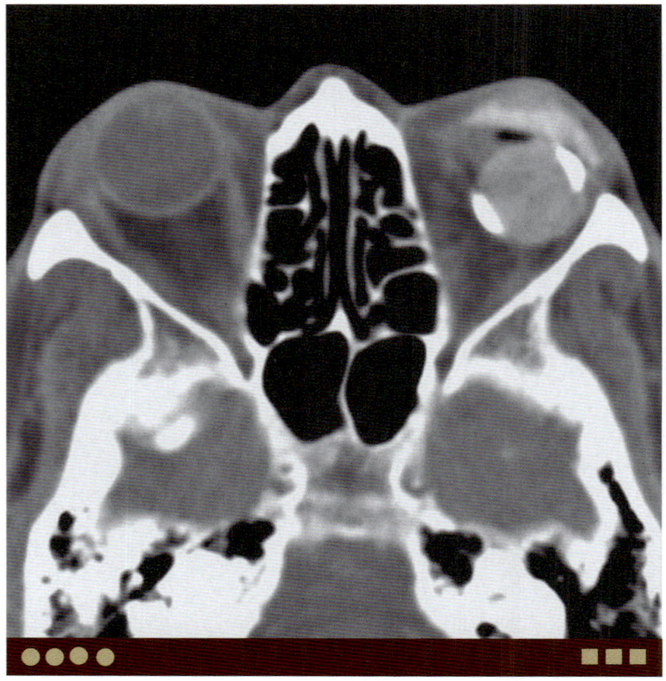

G. Ocular prosthesis. Axial CT demonstrates a two-piece prosthesis, the shell and spacer is placed in the left orbit. The spacer demonstrates high density and the band-like high density of the spacer mimics scleral buckle.

Case 5–6 Ocular Trauma: Penetrating Injury

Osamu Sakai, Christina LeBedis

PRESENTATION

Eye injury.

FINDINGS

CT demonstrates deformity of the globe with intraocular hemorrhage.

DIFFERENTIAL DIAGNOSIS

- Retinal detachment/hemorrhage: This demonstrates V-shaped appearance of the detachment with the apex at the optic disc.
- Choroidal detachment/hemorrhage: This entity spares the posterior globe with the detached choroid having a parallel appearance.
- Posterior hyaloid detachment/hemorrhage: This can cause fluid-fluid level along the posterior aspect of the globe.

COMMENTS

This is a 22-year-old man who sustained a left eye injury.

Although MRI is usually the first-line imaging modality for evaluation of the globe, CT should be performed in the setting of trauma due to its superior ability to delineate injury to the bony orbits, paranasal sinuses, and skull base. In addition, MRI is contraindicated when metallic foreign body is suspected. Severe penetrating globe injury and globe rupture result in globe deformity and collapse which are easily diagnosed. The "flat tire sign" describes flattening of the posterior wall due to decreased intraocular pressure. Intraocular foreign bodies and air are conclusive findings of penetrating globe injury. The measurement of decreased intraocular pressure is the gold standard for penetrating globe injury, however, subtle injuries may be difficult to diagnose clinically due to severe pain and inflammatory changes. Subtle change in the depth of the anterior chamber and a decrease in density of the lens can be an important radiologic clue for penetrating injuries.

Intraocular hemorrhage is commonly seen in trauma and can be vitreous, choroidal or subretinal in nature. MRI is not commonly used to evaluate for orbital trauma, however, it can demonstrate subtle intraocular hemorrhage and retinal or choroidal detachment which are not seen well on CT.

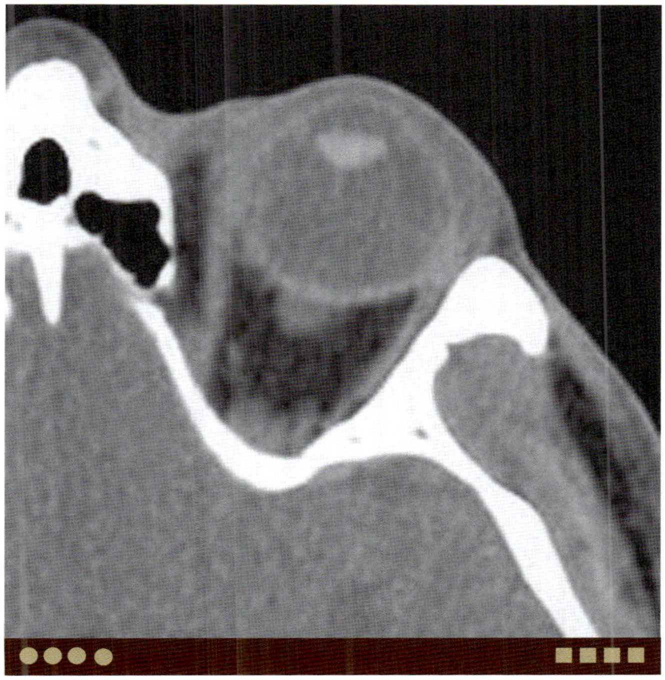

A. Penetrating injury. Axial CT demonstrates deep anterior chamber, "sinking lens" due to decreased intraocular pressure secondary to penetrating injury.

Attention must also be paid to evaluate for extraocular orbital and intracranial injuries when interpreting orbital imaging studies for trauma.

PEARLS

- **CT is the first-line modality to evaluate for orbital injury. MRI is contraindicated when metallic foreign body is suspected.**
- **Penetrating globe injury and globe rupture result in deformity and collapse of the globe. Flattening of the posterior wall of the globe is referred as the "flat tire sign."**
- **Subtle change in the depth of the anterior chamber and a decrease in density of the lens suggest penetrating globe injury.**

ADDITIONAL IMAGES (B-E)

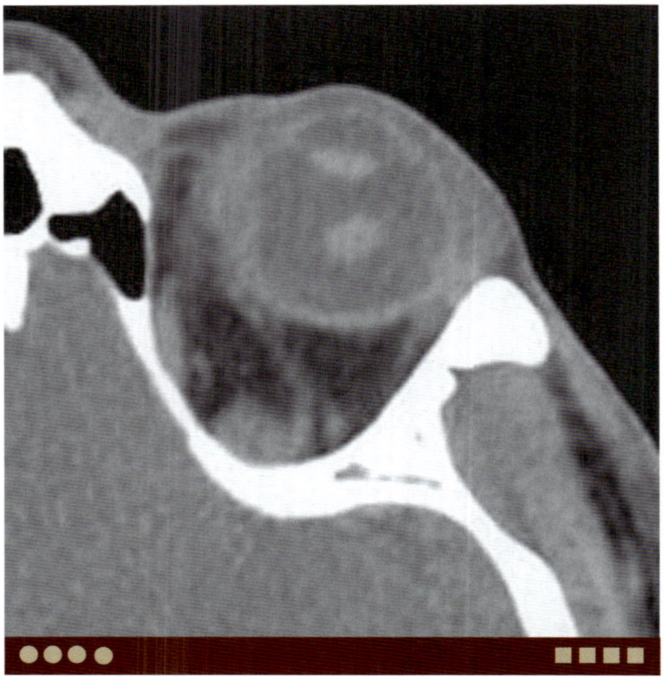

B. Penetrating injury, same patient as A. Axial CT demonstrates vitreous hemorrhage and choroidal hemorrhage along the medial aspect of the globe. The deep anterior chamber is again noted.

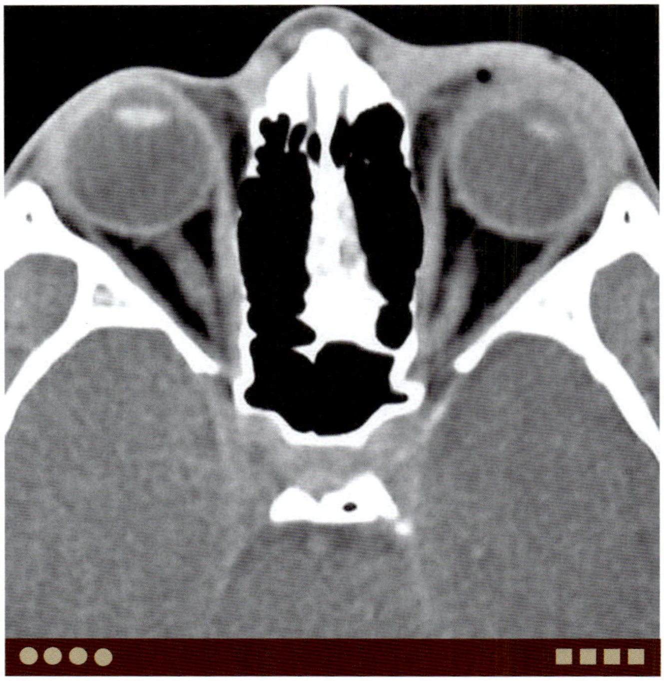

C. Penetrating injury in a different patient. Axial CT demonstrates decreased attenuation of the lens and deep anterior chamber secondary to lens rupture and decreased intraocular pressure.

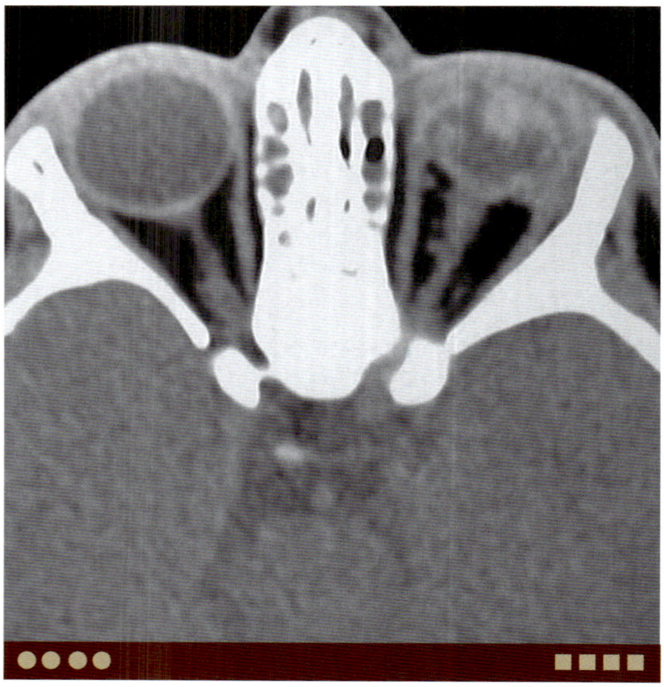

D. Globe rupture. Axial CT demonstrates shrinkage and irregular contour of the globe.

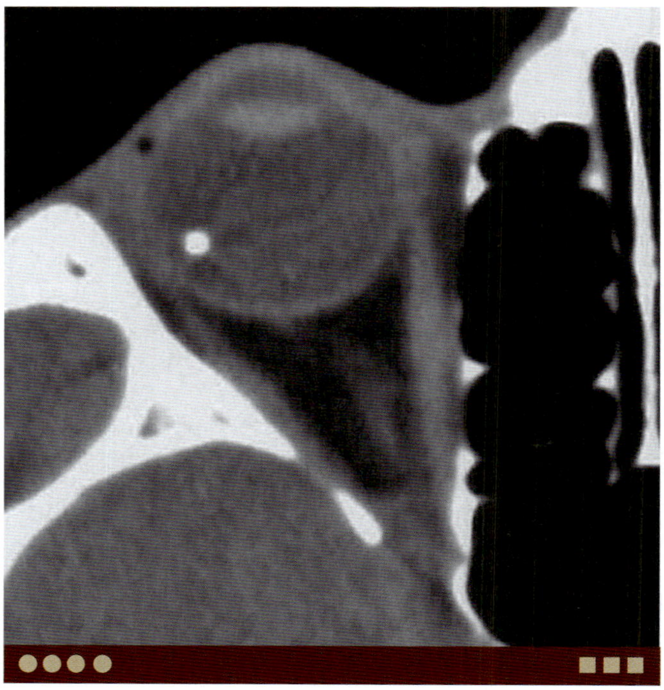

E. Intraocular foreign body. Axial CT demonstrates a high-density foreign body in the globe, conclusive findings of penetrating globe injury.

DIFFERENTIAL DIAGNOSIS IMAGE

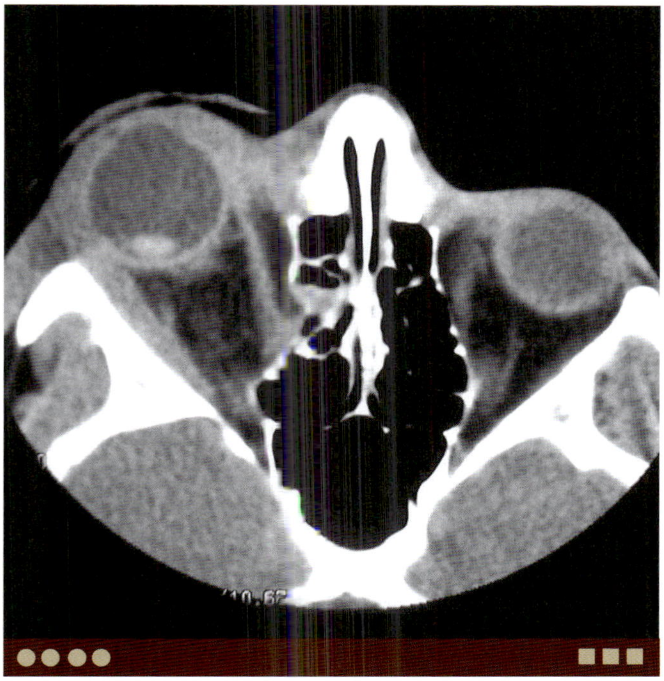

F. Lens dislocation. Axial CT demonstrates a dislocated lens in the posterior globe.

Case 5–7 Lens Dislocation

Osamu Sakai, Christina LeBedis

PRESENTATION

Incidental finding.

FINDINGS

Cross-sectional imaging demonstrates no lens in its normal location in the anterior globe and abnormal structure in the vitreous body.

DIFFERENTIAL DIAGNOSIS

- Intraocular hemorrhage: This condition is usually obvious from the clinical scenario and physical findings, such as can be seen in trauma.
- Intraocular foreign body: Presence of foreign body in the globe is a conclusive finding of penetrating globe injury, usually with apparent history of trauma.
- Intraocular abscess: This condition usually causes visible inflammatory change which is also obvious on imaging.

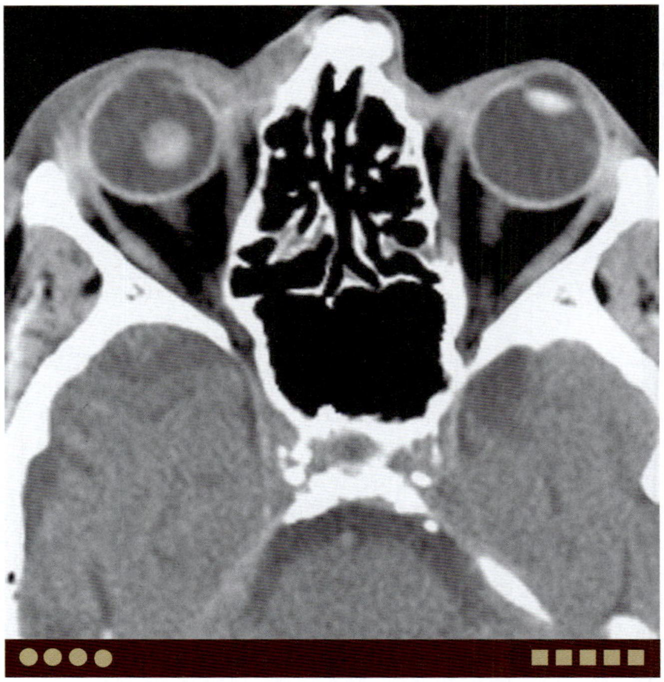

A. Lens dislocation. Axial CT demonstrates a dislocated lens floating in the right vitreous body.

COMMENTS

This is a 67-year-old man with right eye injury.

Lens dislocation may occur after trauma or can be a manifestation of congenital abnormalities, such as Marfan syndrome, homocystinuria, and Weill-Marchesani syndrome. Familial lens dislocation also known as ectopia lentis is congenital dislocation of the lens which is commonly associated with Marfan syndrome. There are, however different forms of familial ectopia lentis that do not manifest the other features of Marfan syndrome. Further, ectopia lentis can be associated with metabolic disease such as homocystinuria, or severe ocular complications such as glaucoma. Clinical symptoms of lens dislocation include myopia, astigmatism, and fluctuating or blurred vision.

Diagnosis of lens dislocation on physical examination can only be made by an ophthalmologic slit-lamp eye examination after fully dilating the pupil. On imaging, however, lens dislocation is conspicuous on both CT or MRI. A dislocated lens may manifest as a slight tilt of the lens in the anterior globe. When completely dislocated, the lens may either float or sink in the vitreous body. Lens dislocation may be complicated by cataract formation. If the patient is asymptomatic, the dislocated lens is best left untreated. If a dislocated lens becomes opaque, surgical removal may be indicated.

PEARLS

- **Lens dislocation may occur after trauma or can be a manifestation of congenital abnormalities.**
- **A dislocated lens may be visible as a slight tilt of the lens in the anterior globe. When completely dislocated, the lens may either float or sink in the vitreous body.**

ADDITIONAL IMAGES (E-F)

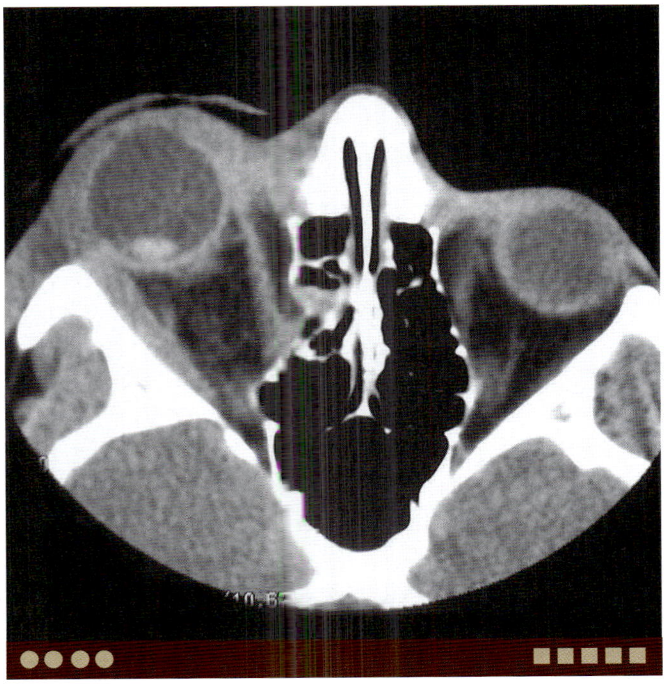

B. Lens dislocation in a different patient after trauma. Axial CT demonstrates a dislocated right lens that has sunk dependently in the vitreous body.

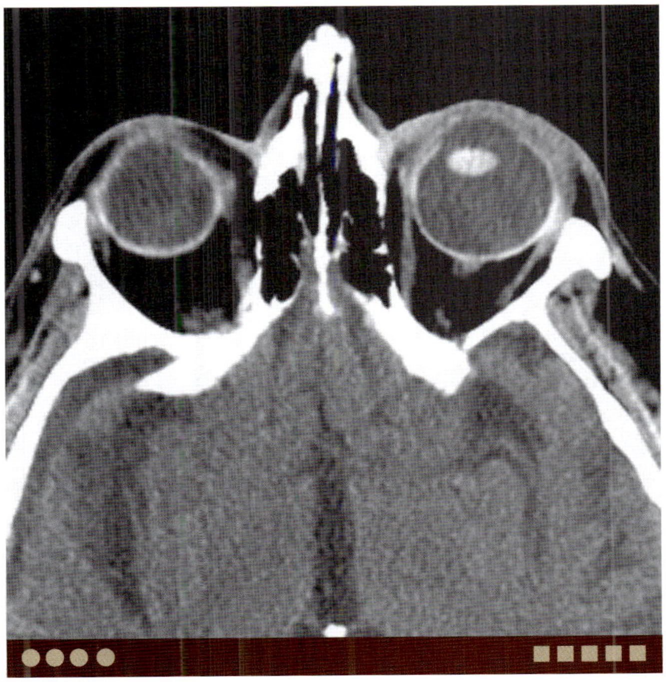

C. Lens dislocation in a different patient after trauma. Axial CT demonstrates a tilted left lens. The right lens has been surgically removed.

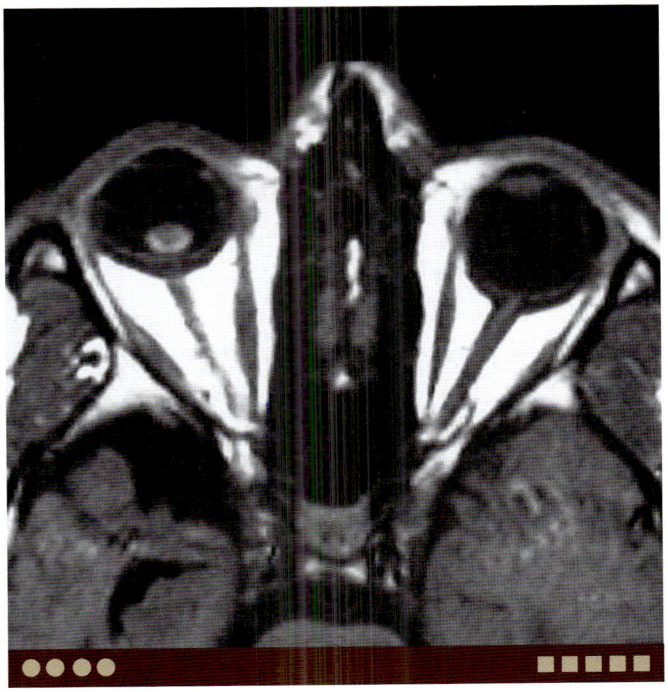

D. Lens dislocation in a different patient after trauma. Axial T1W MR image demonstrates a dislocated right lens that has sunk dependently in the vitreous body.

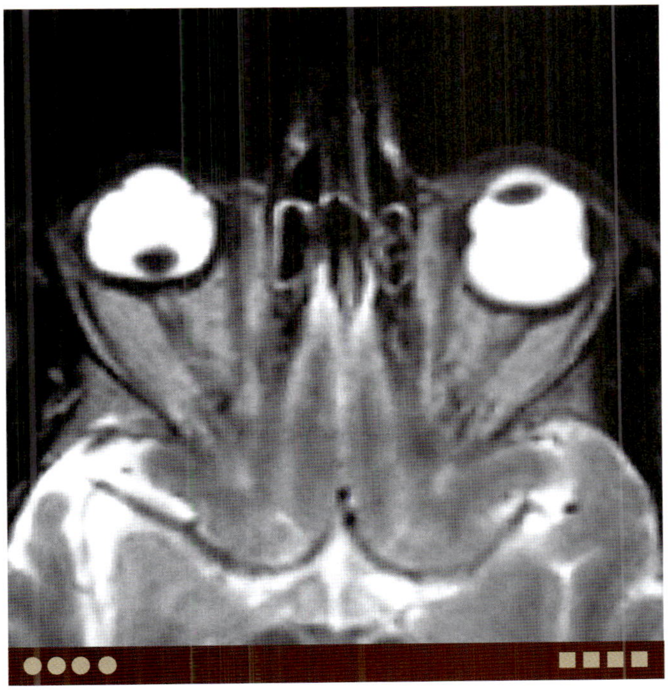

E. Lens dislocation, same patient as D. Axial T2W MR image again demonstrates a dislocated right lens that has sunk dependently in the vitreous body. Note scleral buckle on the left.

DIFFERENTIAL DIAGNOSIS IMAGE

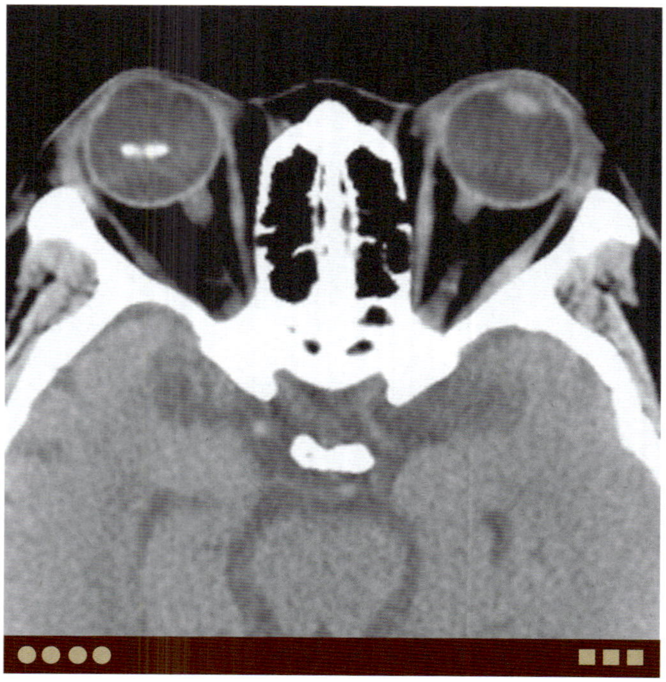

F. Lens dislocation. Axial CT demonstrates a dislocated calcified lens floating in the vitreous body.

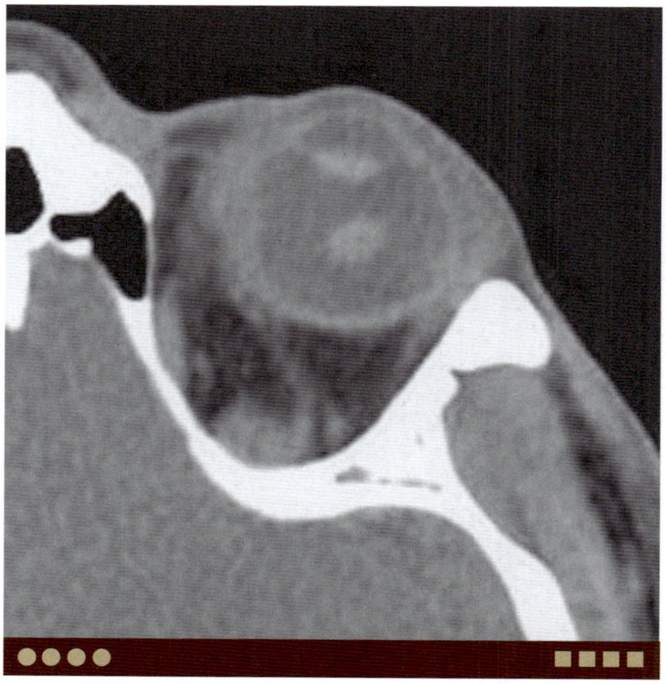

G. Vitreous hemorrhage after penetrating injury. Axial CT demonstrates an oval high density in the vitreous body corresponding to vitreous hemorrhage. Note the deep anterior chamber secondary to decreased intraocular pressure.

Case 5–8 Scleral Calcification: Hyaline Plaque

Osamu Sakai, Francisco Contreras

PRESENTATION

Incidental finding.

FINDINGS

CT demonstrates punctuate calcifications on the surface of the globe at the 3 and 9 o'clock locations.

DIFFERENTIAL DIAGNOSIS

- Glass or metallic foreign body: Foreign bodies can be seen in any age group and in random locations within or outside of the globe. A history of trauma and associated soft tissue injury are often present.
- Optic drusen: Drusen is accumulation of mucopolysaccharides and proteinaceous material in the surface of the optic disc, which become calcified with advancing age. However, drusen can be seen in relatively young patients.
- Choroidal osteoma: Choroidal osteoma is a benign, ossifying, choroidal tumor of unknown etiology. It occurs predominantly in young females with no history of systemic or ocular disease and usually unilateral.

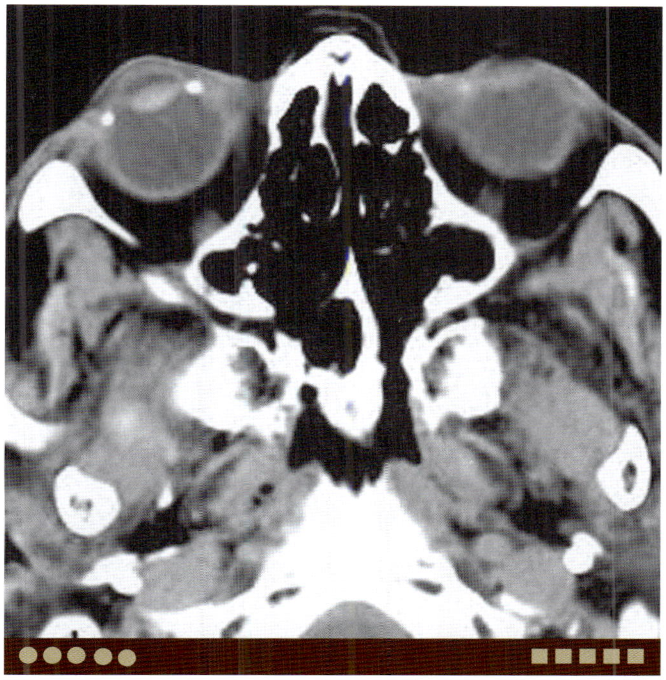

A. Hyaline plaque. Axial noncontrast CT image in soft tissue window demonstrates punctate calcifications on the surface of the right globe at the insertion of the medial and lateral rectus muscles in the typical 3 and 9 o'clock positions.

COMMENTS

This is an 82-year-old man who underwent CT for headache.

Punctate calcifications are often seen in elderly patients along the anterior surface of the globe at the 3 and 9 o'clock locations, and are usually bilateral. Common areas of degenerative hyaline plaque formation are at the insertions of the medial and lateral rectus muscles. It is thought that these calcific deposits are of no clinical significance. These patients are usually older than 80 years of age; however, this condition can be seen earlier in patients with a history of cataract surgery or other infectious or inflammatory conditions.

On CT, there is a clearly defined focal high-density lesion at the insertions of the medial and lateral rectus muscle, again typically at 3 and 9 o'clock locations. These lesions are difficult to visualize on MRI, although a signal-void can occasionally be identified.

Metallic or glass foreign bodies can show a similar appearance. Therefore, careful evaluation of the location of high-density lesions is critical. Hyaline plaques are seen in the typical surface locations in elderly patients, and should be easily distinguished from high-density foreign bodies.

PEARLS

- **Hyaline plaques are seen in very unique locations, at the 3 and 9 o'clock positions, at the insertions of the medial and lateral rectus muscles.**
- **Foreign body is an important differential consideration, which is typically associated with a history of trauma and/or associated soft tissue injury.**

ADDITIONAL IMAGE

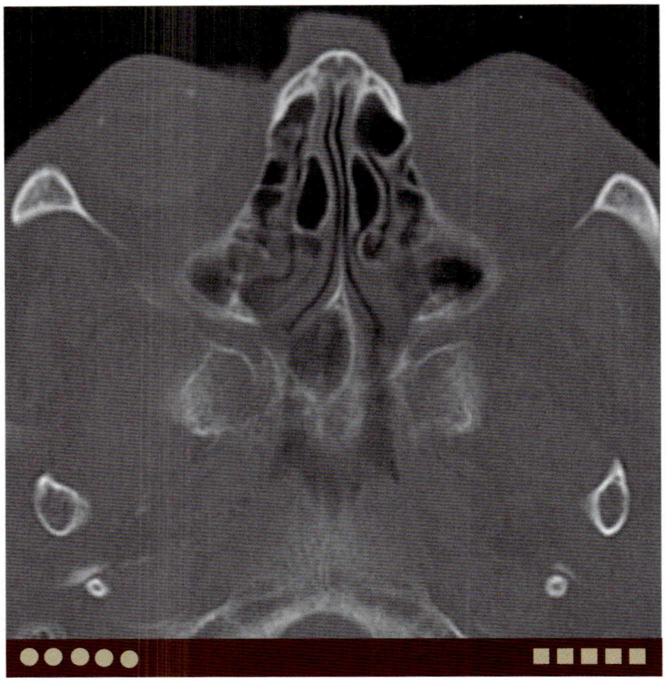

B. Hyaline plaque, same patient as A. Axial noncontrast CT in bone window demonstrates punctate calcifications on the surface of the right globe at the insertion of the medial and lateral rectus muscles in the typical 3 and 9 o'clock positions.

DIFFERENTIAL DIAGNOSIS IMAGES (C-F)

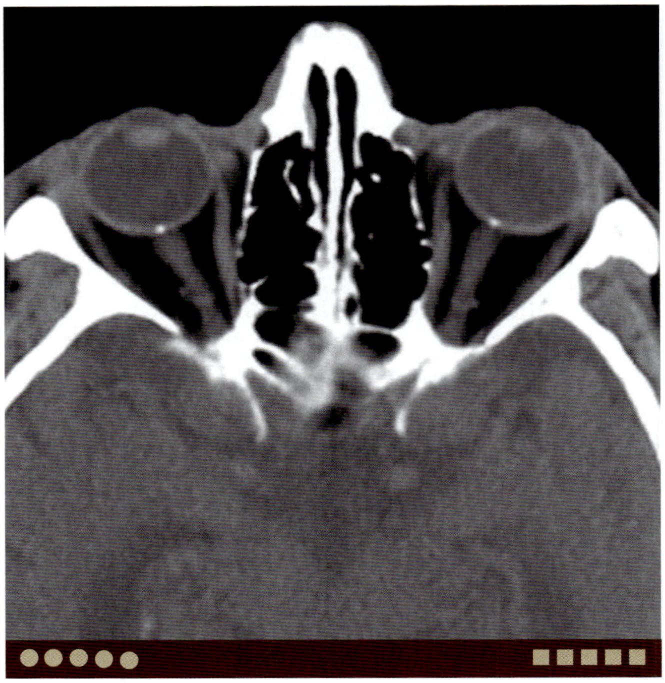

C. Optic drusen. Axial noncontrast CT demonstrates punctate calcifications at the optic discs bilaterally.

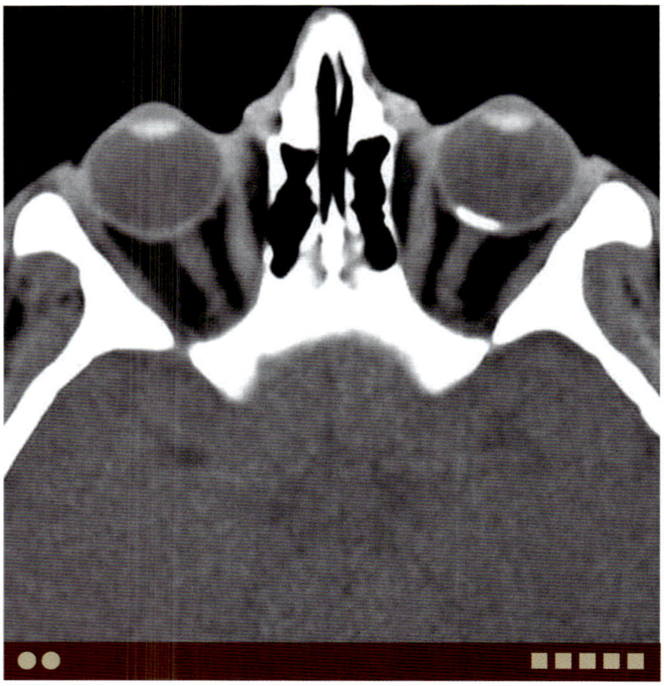

D. Choroidal osteoma. Axial noncontrast CT demonstrates a plague-like calcification along the posterior wall of the left globe.

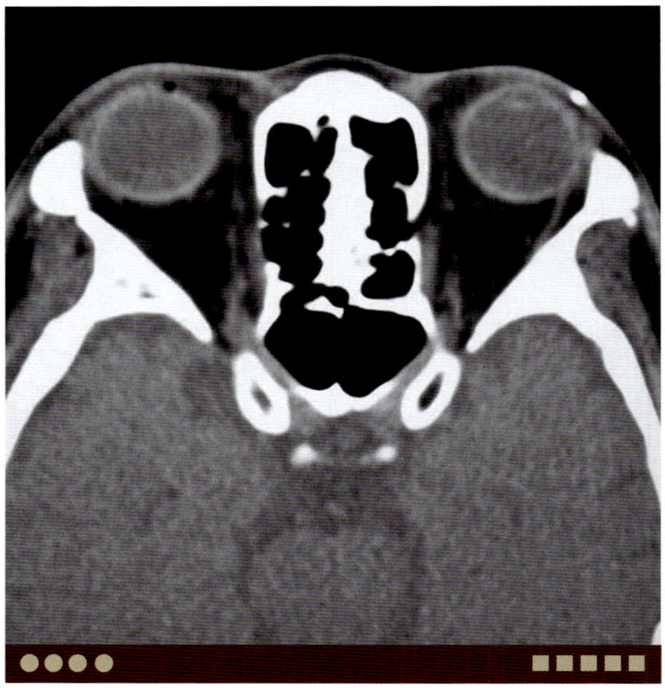

E. Foreign body. Axial noncontrast CT demonstrates a punctate high density in the left upper eyelid.

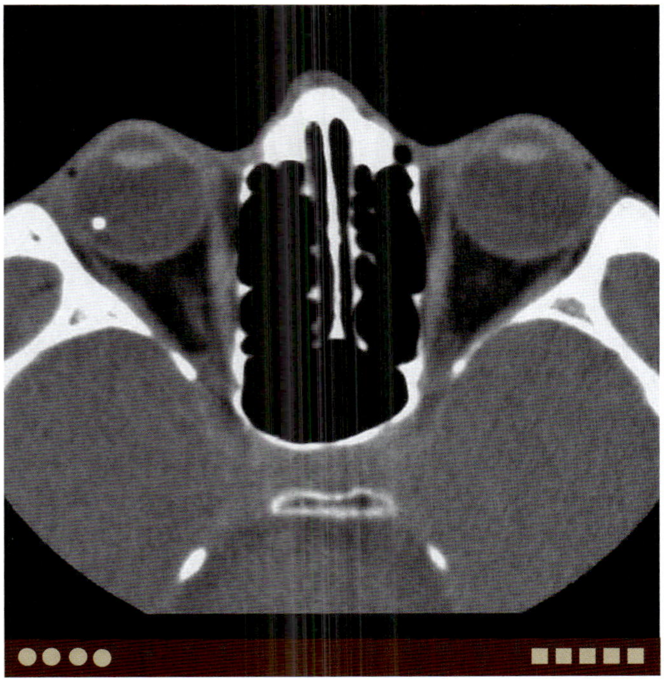

F. Foreign body. Axial noncontrast-enhanced CT demonstrates a radiopaque foreign body within the right globe.

Case 5–9 Choroidal Metastasis

Osamu Sakai, Francisco Contreras, Akifumi Fujita

PRESENTATION

Vision impairment.

FINDINGS

CT demonstrates irregular posterior wall thickening of the globe.

DIFFERENTIAL DIAGNOSIS

- Melanoma: This malignant tumor can occur anywhere in the uvea; it is not limited to the posterior one third of the affected globe. A characteristic high T1 and low T2 signal intensity is due to the paramagnetic effects from melanin.
- Choroidal or retinal detachment: Although irregularity of the posterior globe may also be noted, there is no enhancing mass detected after contrast administration.
- Hemangioma: This benign lesion is limited to the posterior half of the globe and usually does not grow rapidly. It is typically asymptomatic, but may present as a large retinal detachment.
- Hematoma: Ophthalmologically, this may show a similar appearance to metastasis, but typically demonstrates a crescent shape and does not enhance after contrast administration.

COMMENTS

This is a 43-year-old woman with a history of choriocarcinoma.

Metastases to the eye are not uncommon. The choroid is a richly vascular structure and therefore a common site for hematogeneous metastasis. Patients are often asymptomatic until the lesion involves the macula. Visual field defects or other ophthalmological symptoms can be the first clinical presentation of malignancy. This condition often accompanies retinal detachment, which is difficult to differentiate from intraocular tumors on CT, even with contrast enhancement. For this reason, MRI has become necessary to make the diagnosis. Contrast enhancement is usually necessary for MRI as well. Metastases from mucin-producing adenocarcinomas demonstrate increased T1 signal, similar to melanotic lesions. However, bilaterality, location near the posterior pole, morphologically flat and diffuse extension with irregular surfaces preferentially favor the diagnosis of metastatic tumors. The lung, breast, and gastrointestinal tract are the most common primary sites; however, it is often the case that the primary malignancy cannot be identified.

On CT, these lesions are usually seen as irregular thickening of the posterior wall of the globe. With increase in lesion size, retinal detachment becomes apparent and often leads to complete detachment. Proteinaceous or hemorrhagic subretinal effusion is detected as increased density.

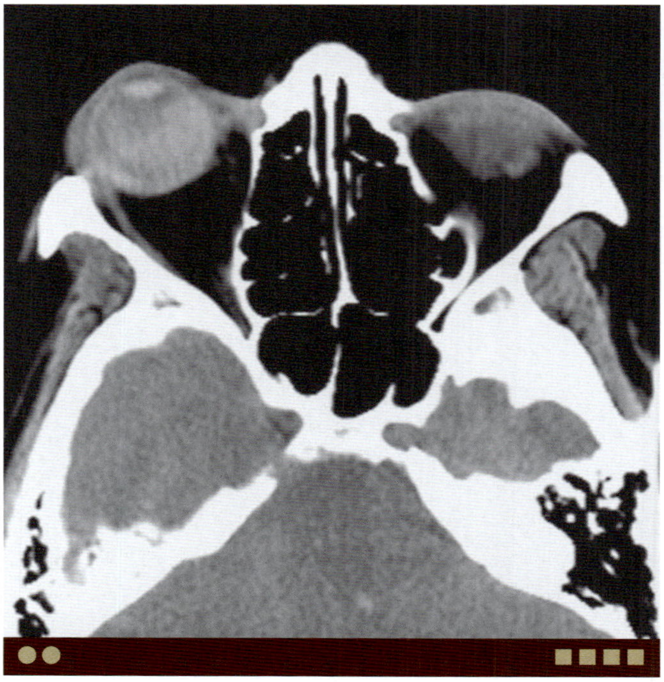

A. Choroidal metastasis, choriocarcinoma. Axial noncontrast CT shows an irregularly shaped high density in the right globe consistent with hemorrhagic metastasis.

On MRI, the tumor is better differentiated from the subretinal effusion. Proteinaceous or hemorrhagic subretinal effusion demonstrates increased T1 signal intensity, while unlike the effusion, the tumor enhances after contrast administration.

Metastasis to other sites, such as soft tissue and bony orbits, skull, dura/meninges, and brain is not common. Careful observation is necessary in order not to miss other metastatic lesions.

PEARLS

- **Metastases to the eyes are not uncommon. The richly vascular choroid is a common site for hematogeneous metastasis.**
- **Bilaterality, location within the posterior one third of the globe, flat irregular surfaces should lean the diagnosis toward metastatic tumors when compared with uvela melanoma.**
- **The lung, breast, and gastrointestinal tract are common primary sites for metastases.**

ADDITIONAL IMAGES (B-G)

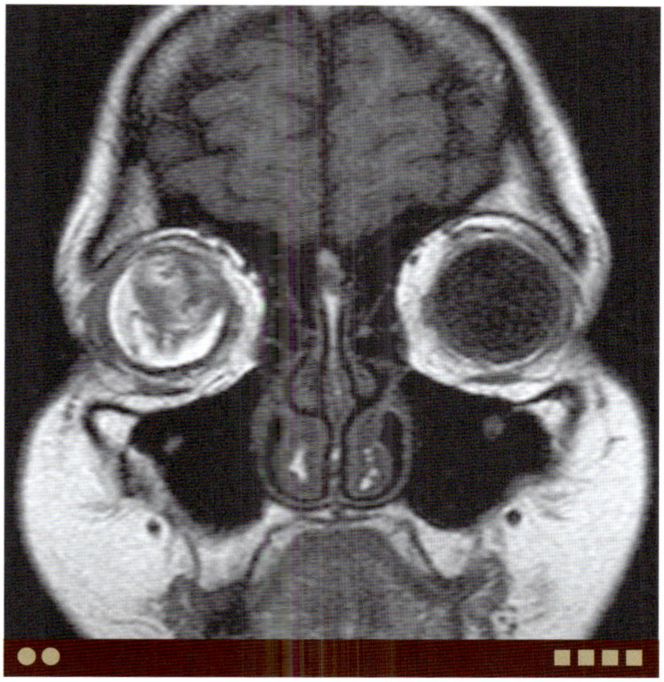

B. Choroidal metastasis, same patient as A. Coronal T1W MR image shows an irregularly shaped heterogeneous mass in the right globe.

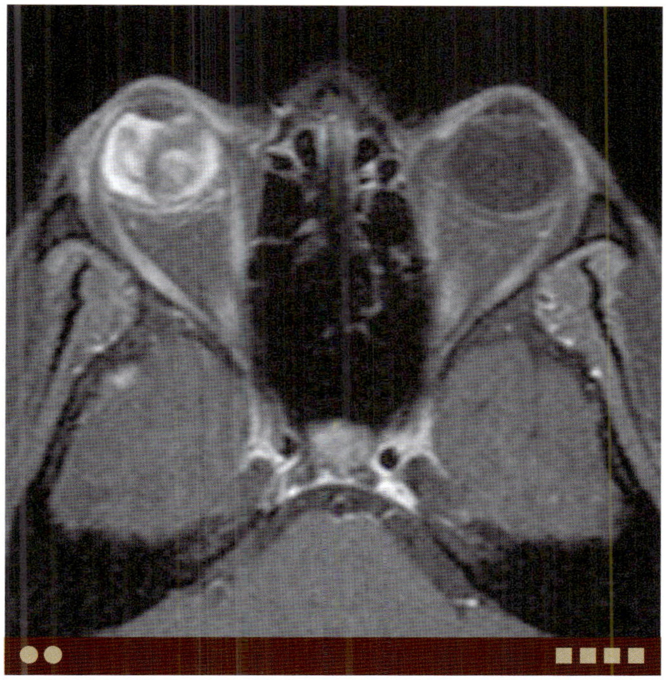

C. Choroidal metastasis, same patient as A. Axial postcontrast fat-suppressed T1W MR image shows a heterogeneous high-signal lesion in the right globe.

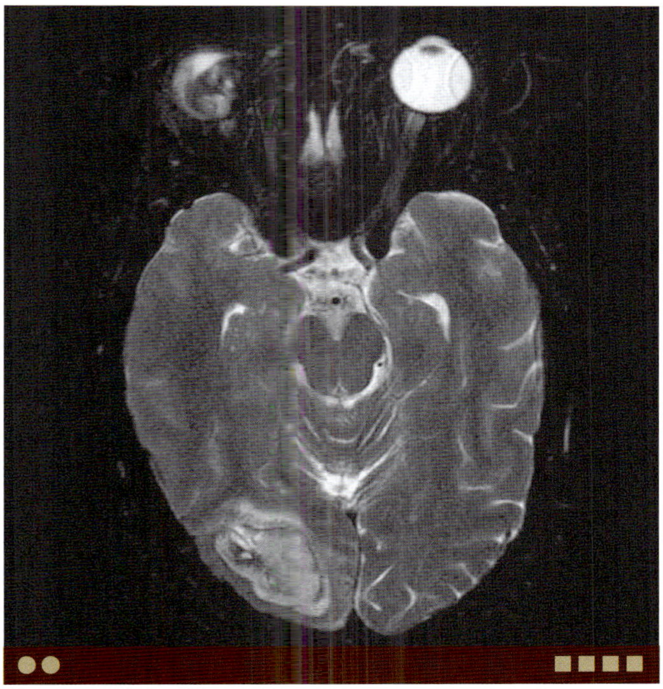

D. Choroidal metastasis, same patient as A. Axial fat-suppressed T2W MR image shows an irregularly shaped hemorrhagic mass with surrounding vasogenic edema in the right occipital lobe in addition to the hemorrhagic lesion within the right globe.

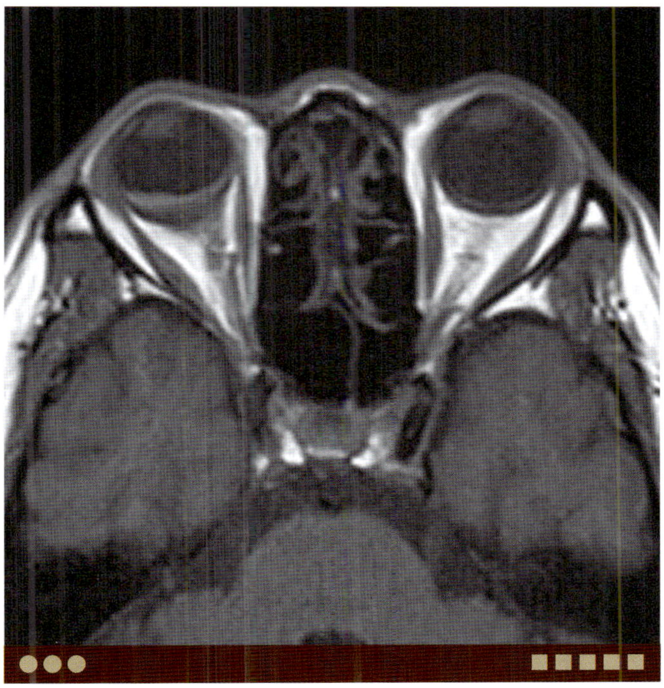

E. Choroidal metastasis in a different patient with lung cancer. Axial T1W MR image shows an irregularly shaped flat lesion along the posterior globe with retinal detachment.

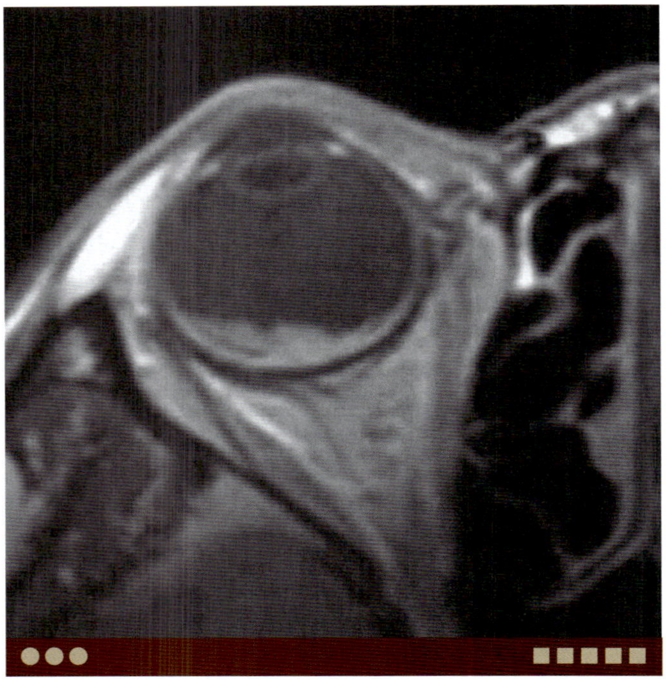

F. Choroidal metastasis in a different patient with breast cancer. Axial postcontrast T1W MR image shows an enhancing irregularly shaped flat lesion along the posterior globe.

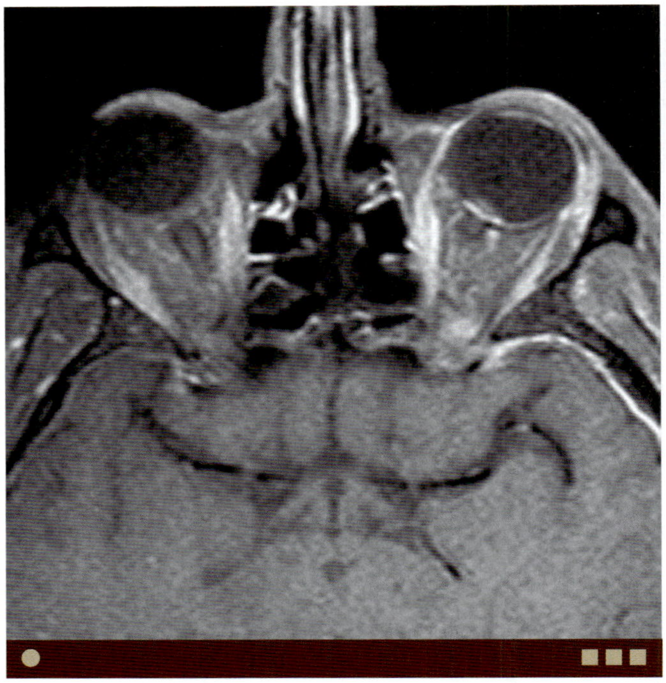

G. Intraocular lymphoma. Axial contrast-enhanced fat-suppressed T1W MR image demonstrates a small enhancing lesion in the left posterior globe. Note dural involvement by lymphoma in the left middle cranial fossa.

DIFFERENTIAL DIAGNOSIS IMAGES (H-J)

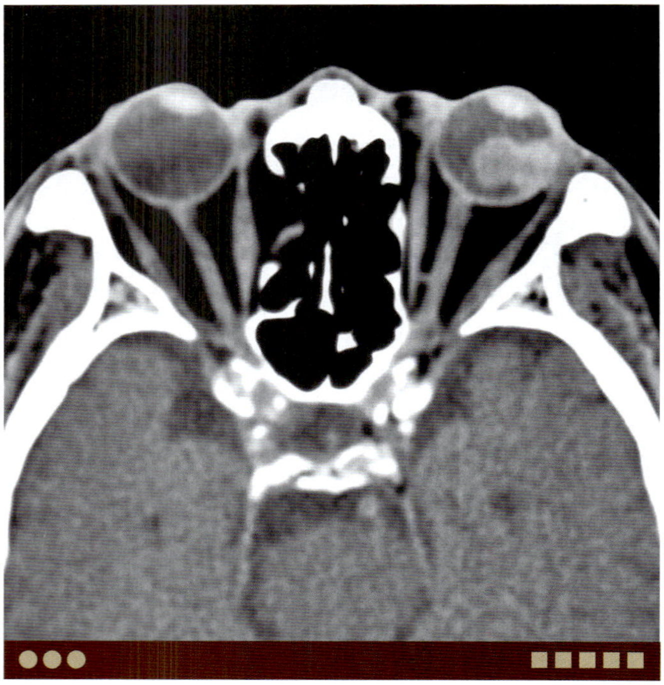

H. Choroidal melanoma. Axial contrast-enhanced CT demonstrates an enhancing mushroom-shaped lesion in the lateral wall of the left globe.

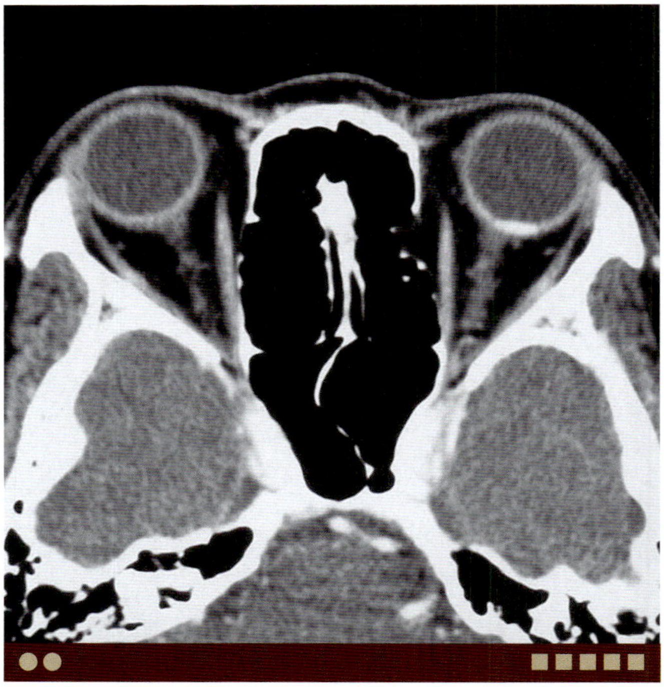

I. Choroidal hemangioma. Axial contrast-enhanced CT demonstrates an avidly enhancing lenticular lesion in the posterior wall of the left globe.

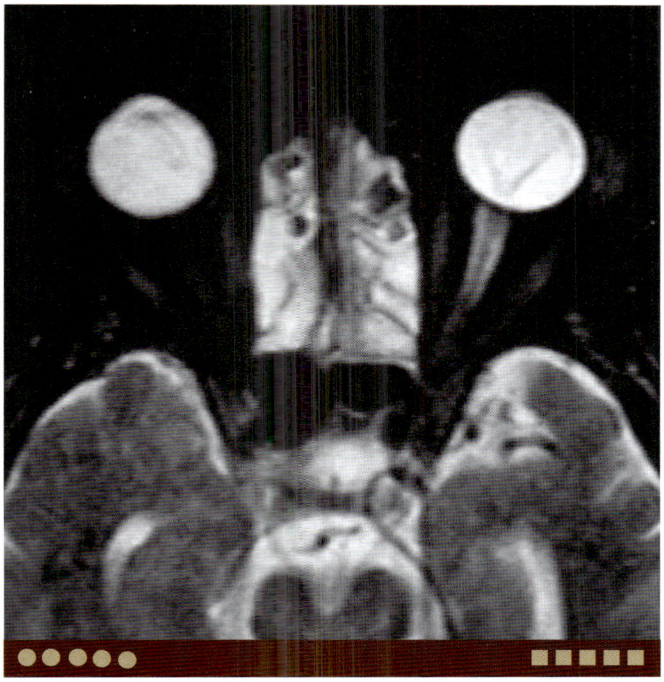

J. Retinal detachment. Axial T2W MR image demonstrates a left intraocular V-shaped appearance with the apex of the detachment at the optic disc. This serous subretinal fluid shows high signal similar to the vitreous body.

Case 5–10 Retinoblastoma

June Cheng, Ilse Castro-Aragon, Osamu Sakai

PRESENTATION

Leukocoria.

FINDINGS

CT demonstrates an intraocular mass with calcification.

DIFFERENTIAL DIAGNOSIS

- Persistent hyperplastic primary vitreous (PHPV): This condition demonstrates microphthalmos and subretinal or subhyaloid collection without calcification. PHPV is associated with an intracranial abnormality, particularly when bilateral.
- Coats disease: This is a congenital primary vascular anomaly of the retina, causing exudative retinal detachment secondary to dilatation of the retinal arterioles and disruption of the blood-retina barrier. The hyperdense subretinal collection is seen without a mass or calcification.
- Retinopathy of prematurity (retrolental fibroplasia): This condition demonstrates bilateral microphthalmos and hyperdense globes, rarely with calcification. The clinical history of prematurity with prolonged oxygen therapy is necessary in the diagnosis.
- Coloboma: This is a congenital focal defect in the wall of the globe, often near the optic nerve head insertion. However, different structures within the globe, including the choroid, iris, lens, optic nerve, and retina, may be involved. This condition may be bilateral and associated with various congenital malformation syndromes.

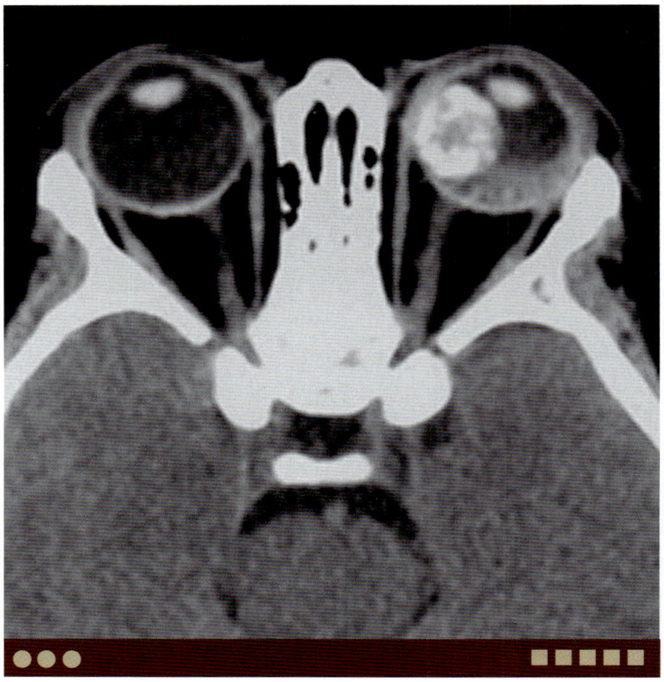

A. Retinoblastoma. Axial CT demonstrates a large predominantly calcified mass in the medial portion of the left globe. Note secondary retinal detachment with high-density subretinal fluid along the posterior wall of the globe.

COMMENTS

This is an 11-month-old infant with leukocoria.

Retinoblastoma is the most common intraocular malignancy in children, usually occurring before the age of 5 years, and is the most important cause of leukocoria. Other causes of leukocoria include PHPV, Coats disease, congenital cataract, coloboma, retinopathy of prematurity (retrolental fibroplasia), and *Toxocara canis*.

Retinoblastoma is highly malignant and its outcome depends on the degree of extension of tumor. When localized, overall long-term survival is better. Therefore, early diagnosis and therapy is essential for a favorable outcome. Biopsy should be avoided in the diagnosis of retinoblastoma due to the risk of seeding. Therefore, radiological diagnosis is crucial.

Retinoblastoma is usually unilateral (90%) and caused by mutations in the retinoblastoma gene (13q14). However, familial, autosomal dominant retinoblastoma (10%) is usually bilateral (90%). Upon diagnosis of retinoblastoma, evaluation of the central nervous system is important. Trilateral retinoblastoma is well known and occurs with lesions in both globes and in the pineal gland. Occasionally, quadrilateral retinoblastoma occurs with suprasellar lesions in addition to bilateral ocular and pineal lesions. Three main growth patterns of retinoblastoma have been described: endophytic, exophytic, and diffuse infiltrating.

Because intraocular calcification is very common (>95%), CT is the most useful imaging modality in differentiating retinoblastoma from other conditions presenting with leukocoria.

PEARLS

- **Retinoblastoma is the most common intraocular malignancy in children.**
- **Calcification is very common (>95%).**
- **Retinoblastoma can be bilateral (both eyes), trilateral (+ pineal), or quadrilateral (+ suprasellar).**

MRI is less sensitive in the detection of calcification. However, MRI has improved soft tissue contrast resolution and is particularly useful in the evaluation of extraocular tumor extension, intracranial involvement, pineal and suprasellar lesions, and cerebrospinal fluid dissemination. Lesions are often T1 hyperintense and T2 hypointense and demonstrate heterogeneous enhancement.

ADDITIONAL IMAGES (B-G)

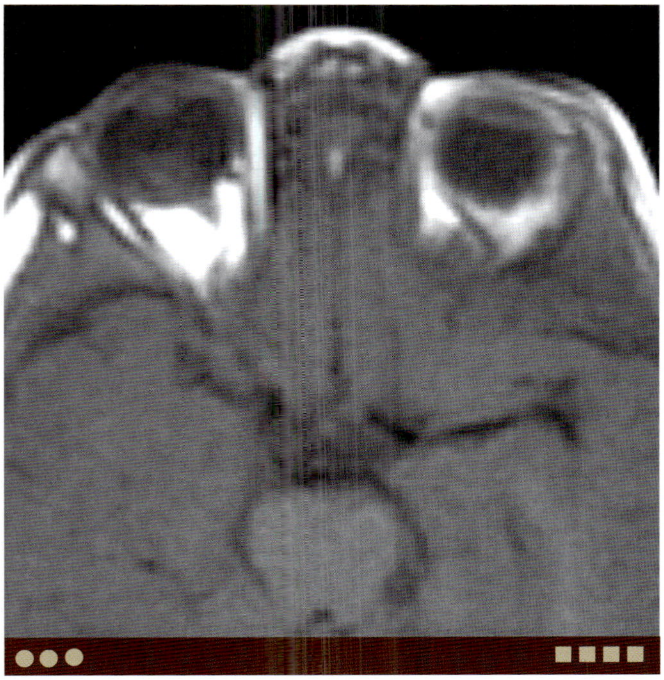

B. Retinoblastoma in a different patient. Axial T1W MR image demonstrates a slightly hyperintense mass relative to the vitreous body within the right globe.

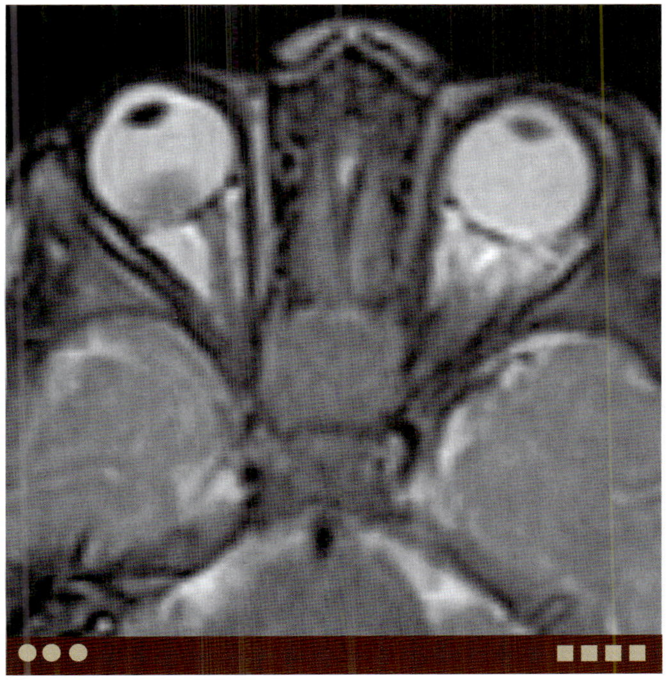

C. Retinoblastoma, same patient as B. Axial T2W MR image demonstrates a hypointense mass relative to the vitreous body within the right globe.

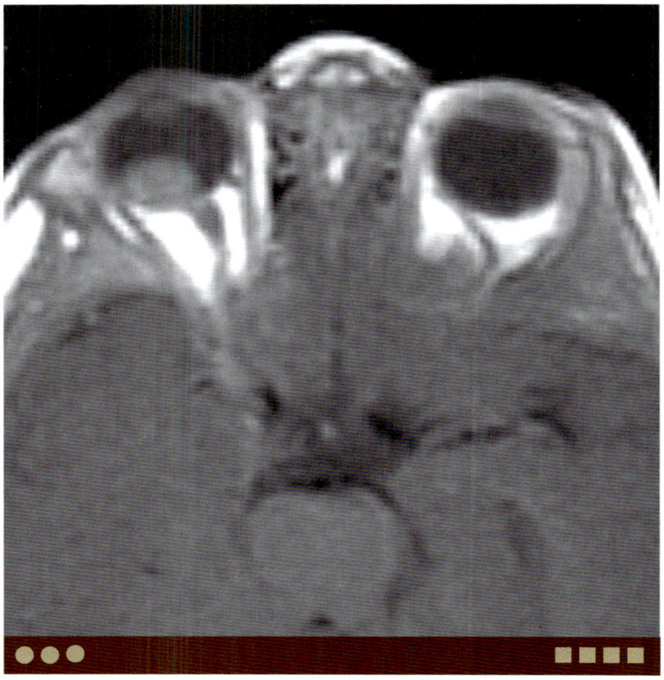

D. Retinoblastoma, same patient as B. Axial postcontrast T1W MR image demonstrates enhancement of the right intraocular mass.

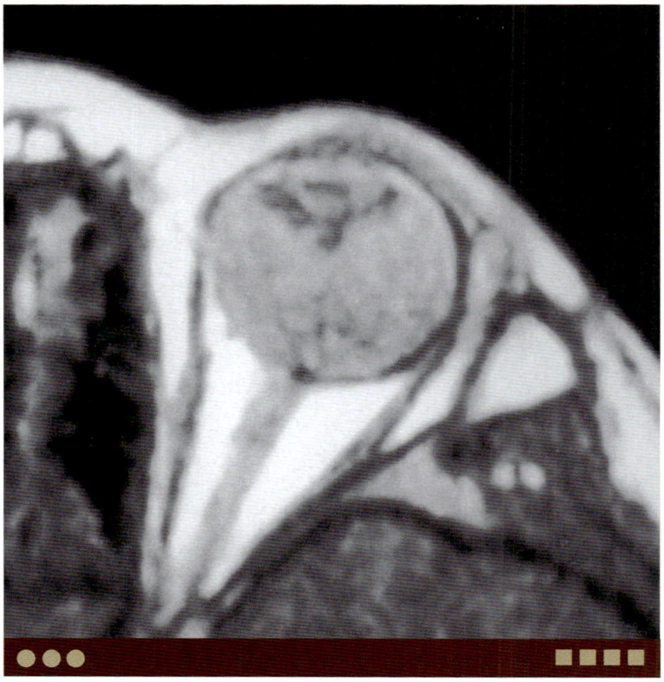

E. Retinoblastoma in a different patient. Axial T1W MR image demonstrates retinal detachment and increased signal throughout the globe.

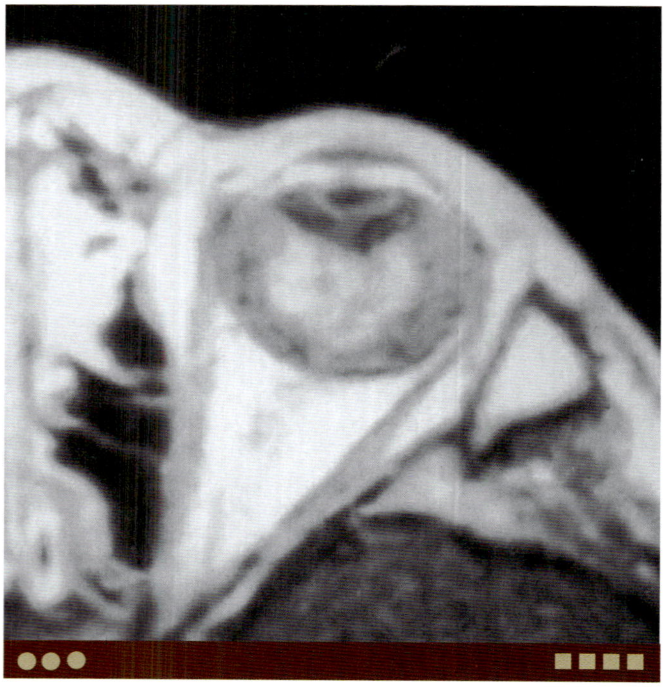

F. Retinoblastoma, same patient as E. Axial postcontrast T1W MR image demonstrates enhancement of the centrally located intraocular tumor.

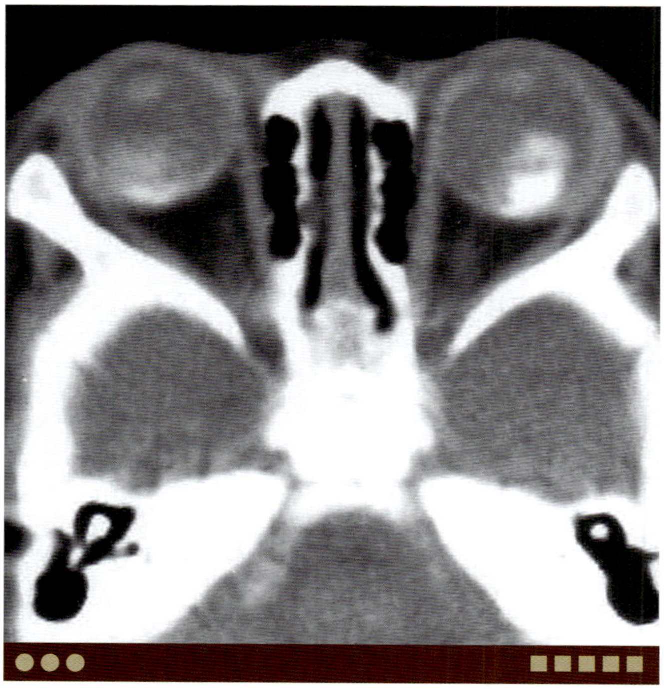

G. Bilateral retinoblastomas. Axial CT image demonstrates bilateral calcified intraocular tumors.

DIFFERENTIAL DIAGNOSIS IMAGES (H-J)

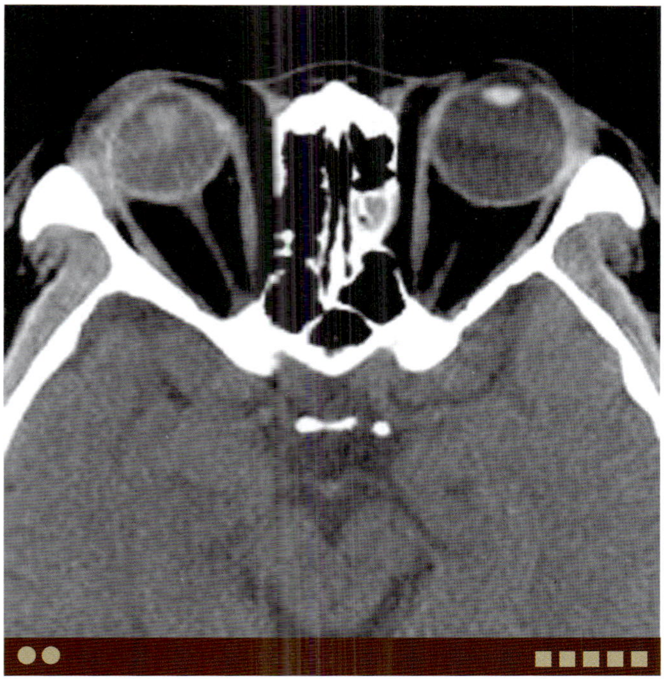

H. PHPV. Axial CT demonstrates right microphthalmos and a hyperdense vitreous body with retinal detachment. No intraocular calcification is present.

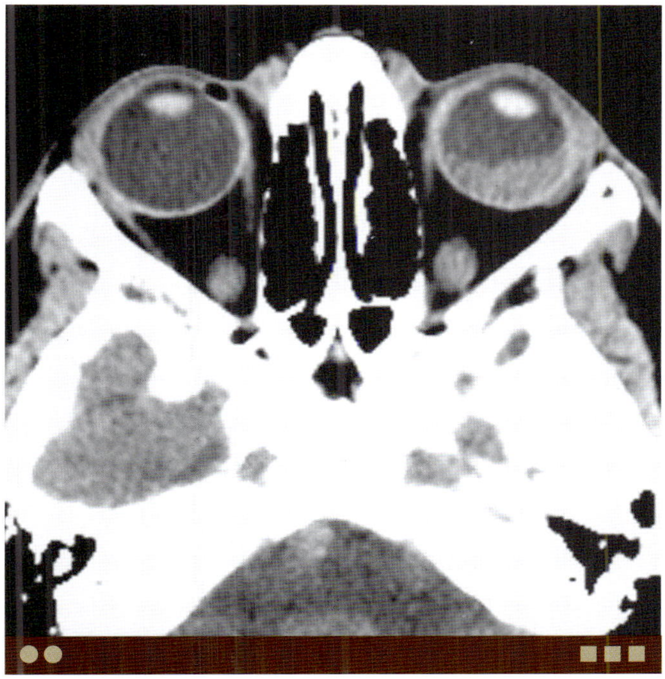

I. Coats disease. Axial CT demonstrates hyperdensity along the posterior wall of the left globe, representing proteinaceous or hemorrhagic subretinal exudate, and no calcification.

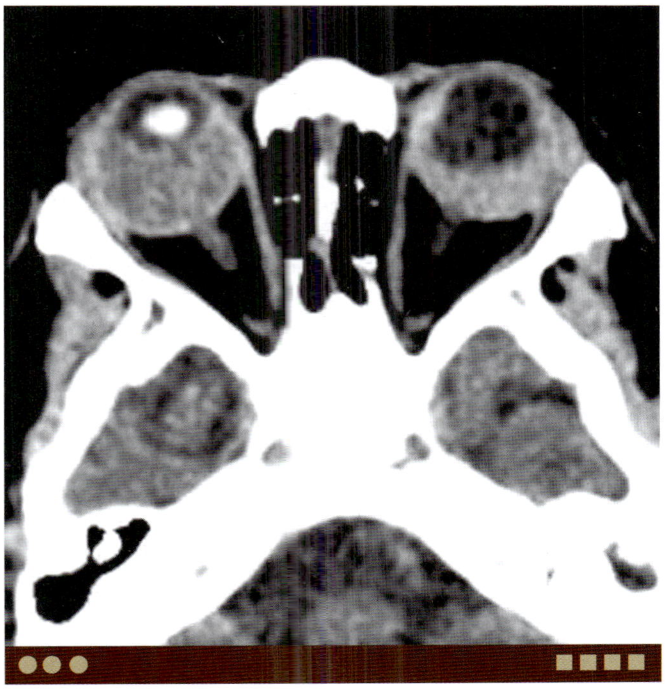

J. Retinopathy of prematurity. Axial CT demonstrates bilateral retinal detachment with high density subretinal collection and no calcification.

Case 5–11 Uveal Melanoma

Osamu Sakai, Benjamin Ludwig, Akifumi Fujita

PRESENTATION

Decrease in visual acuity.

FINDINGS

CT demonstrates a mushroom-shaped high-density mass in the globe. The tumor demonstrates high signal on T1W and low signal on T2W images.

DIFFERENTIAL DIAGNOSIS

- Metastatic disease: Choroidal metastases are fairly common, and typically seen as flat lesions in the posterior one third of the globe, where the choroidal arteries penetrate the wall and tumor cells are entrapped.
- Hemangioma: This entity mimics melanoma on fundoscopy, however, usually does not grow rapidly or has associated retinal detachment. Avid enhancement after contrast is characteristic.
- Hemorrhage (subretinal): May show a similar appearance to melanoma on fundoscopic examination, but on imaging, is crescentic in shape, and does not enhance after contrast administration.

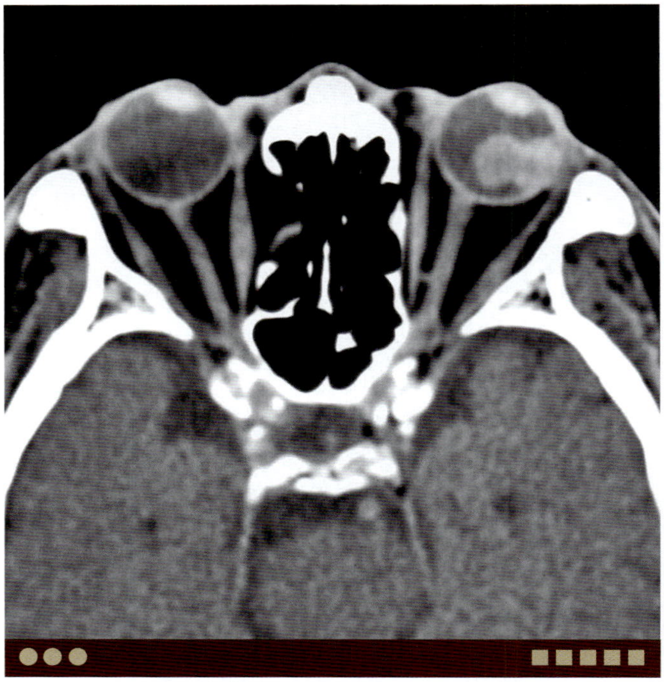

A. Choroidal melanoma. Axial CT demonstrates a high-density mushroom-shaped tumor in the left globe.

COMMENTS

This is a 69-year-old man with recent decrease in visual acuity of the left eye.

Uveal melanoma is the most common malignant primary ocular tumor, and occurs anywhere in the uvea; including the choroid, ciliary body, and iris. The most common location is within the posterior third of the choroid.

Patients most commonly present with decreased visual acuity in the absence of pain. Clinically, early melanomas can be difficult to differentiate from other tumors. When the lesion grows and penetrates the tight Bruch membrane, the typical mushroom-like appearance is seen. From its intraocular origin, the lesion can invade beyond the sclera or extend along the optic nerve. Large tumor size and invasive tumor extension suggest poor prognosis.

On CT, melanoma is hyperattenuating relative to vitreous humor due to its cellular composition and melanin content, and enhances after contrast administration. Similarly, on MRI, T1 hyperintensity and T2 hypointensity are characteristic, although the signal can be variable depending on melanin content. Avid enhancement is also seen after contrast administration. Retinal detachment with proteinaceous subretinal fluid is often present, demonstrating increased density on CT and hyperintensity on T1W MRI.

PEARLS

- **Melanoma is the most common malignant primary ocular tumor in adults.**
- **Melanoma typically demonstrates high density on CT, T1 hyperintense and T2 hypointense signal on MRI, and enhances after contrast administration. However, density and signal can be variable depending on melanin content.**
- **The "mushroom-shaped" growth pattern is characteristic of intraocular melanoma.**

ADDITIONAL IMAGES (B-G)

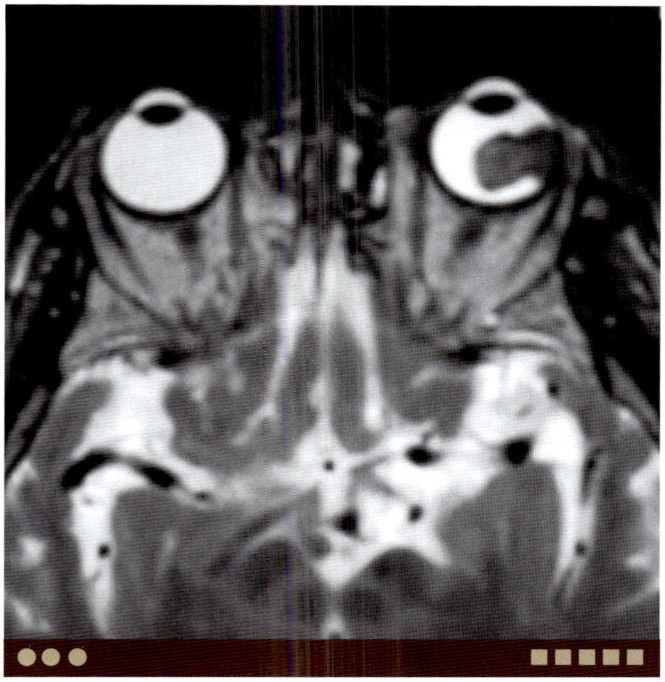

B. Choroidal melanoma, same patient as A. Axial T2W image demonstrates a low-signal intraocular tumor.

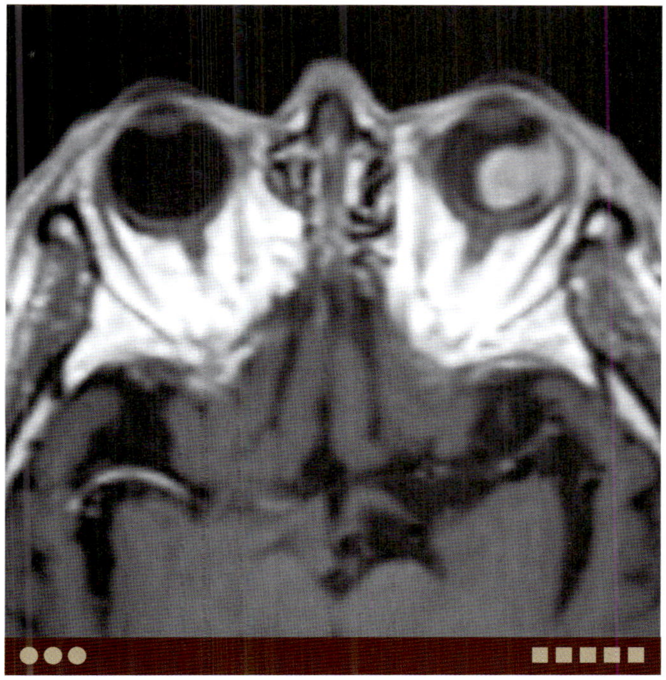

C. Choroidal melanoma, same patient as A. Axial postcontrast T1W image shows enhancement of the tumor.

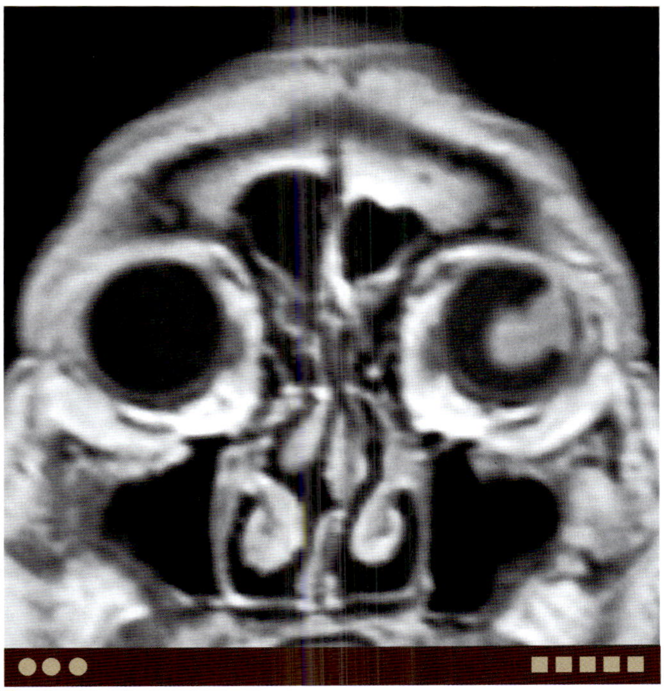

D. Choroidal melanoma, same patient as A. Coronal postcontrast T1W image shows enhancement of the tumor.

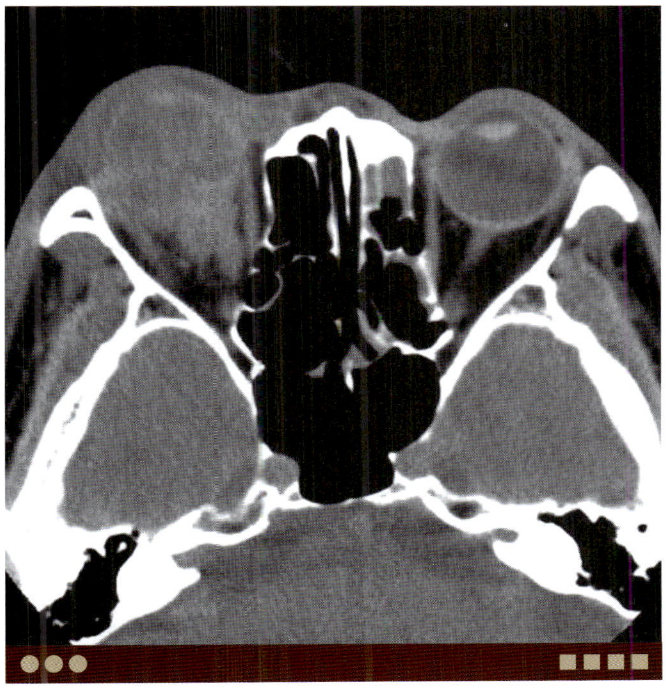

E. Choroidal melanoma in a different patient. Axial CT demonstrates exophthalmos and heterogeneously increased density of the right globe. Note the retrobulbar tumor extension.

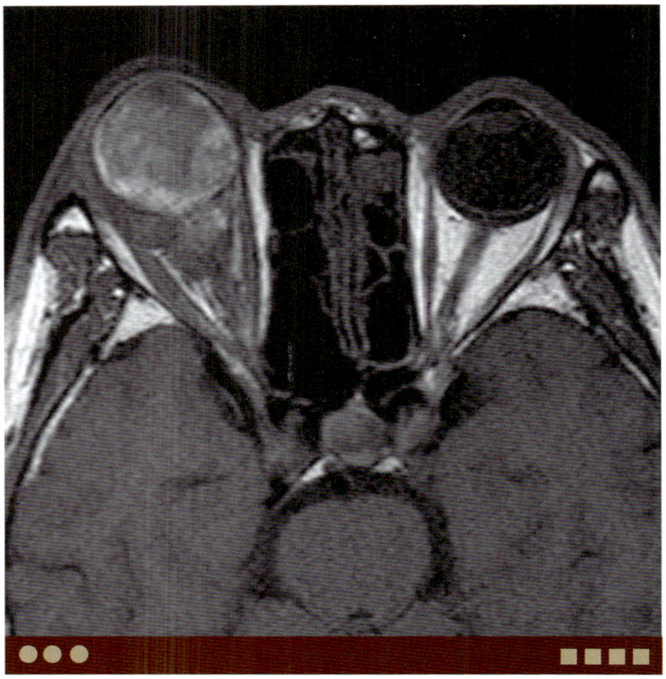

F. Choroidal melanoma, same patient as E. Axial T1W image shows a heterogeneously high-signal tumor within the right globe with retrobulbar extension. Increased T1 signal represents melanin and hemorrhage.

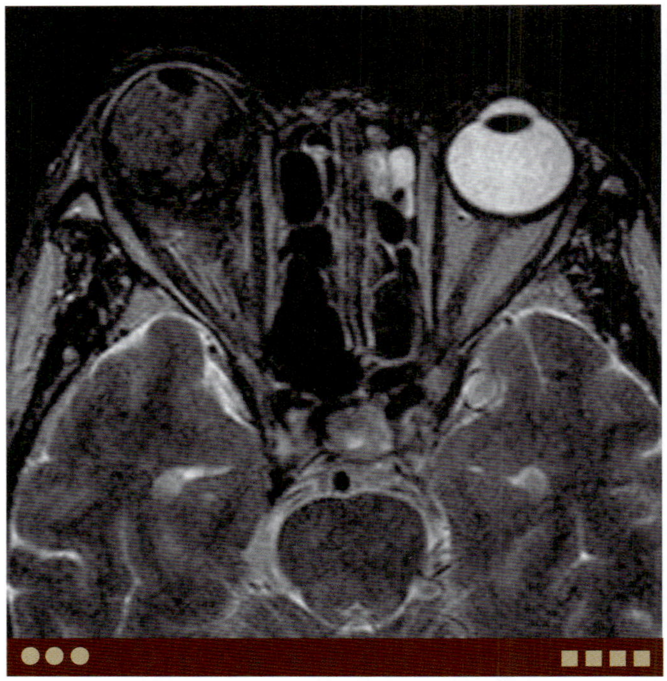

G. Choroidal melanoma, same patient as E. Axial T2W image shows a low-signal tumor within the right globe invading the retrobulbar fat and spreading along the optic nerve.

DIFFERENTIAL DIAGNOSIS IMAGES (H-I)

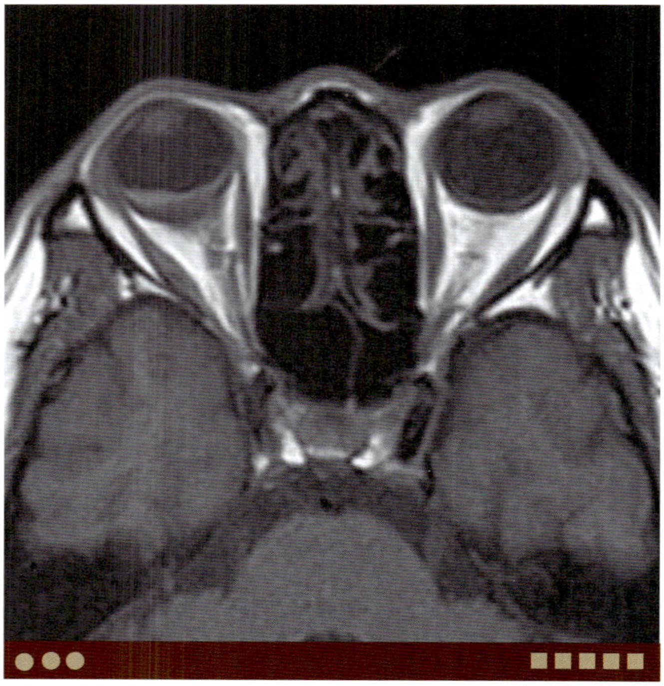

H. Choroidal metastasis. Axial T1W image demonstrates a broad-based high-intensity lesion in the posterior right globe. A primary lung neoplasm was subsequently identified.

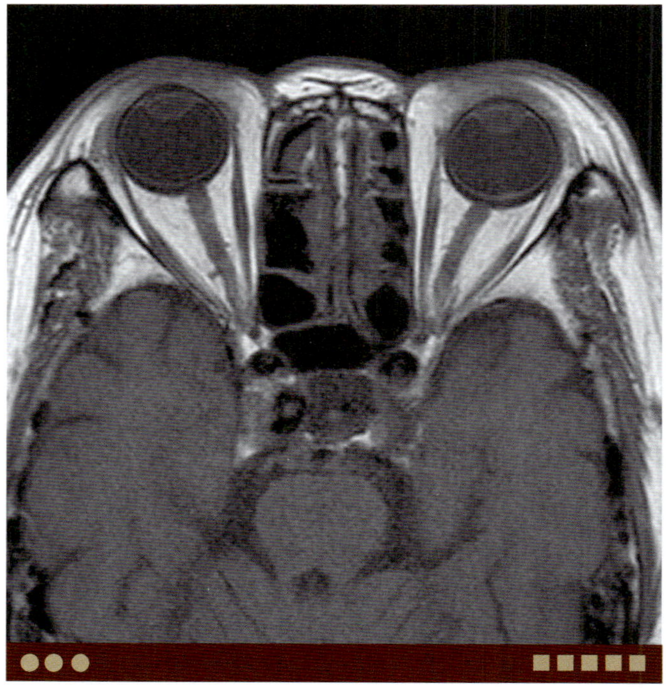

I. Subretinal hematoma. Axial T1W image demonstrates a small, flat, high-signal lesion in the posterior left globe, consistent with hemorrhage.

Case 5–12 Scleritis/Episcleritis

Osamu Sakai, Francisco Contreras, Akifumi Fujita

PRESENTATION

Eye pain.

FINDINGS

CT demonstrates thickened wall with inflammatory change in the adjacent fat.

DIFFERENTIAL DIAGNOSIS

- Idiopathic orbital inflammation (IOI) ("pseudotumor"): Scleritis may be a manifestation of IOI or lymphoproliferative disorders.
- Lymphoma and other lymphoid lesions: Intraocular lymphoma is rare, however, extraocular intraorbital lymphomatous involvement is common.
- Sarcoidosis: This condition typically shows bilateral ocular involvement of the uvea, but retinal detachment is rare. Extraocular orbital involvement is also common such as dacryoadenitis, orbital myositis, and optic neuritis.
- Metastatic tumors: Choroidal metastasis is often seen as a flat mass in the posterior one third of the globe, where the choroidal arteries penetrate the wall and tumor cells are entrapped.
- Vogt-Koyanagi-Harada (VKH) syndrome: VKH syndrome is a bilateral granulomatous panuveitis, which is an autoimmune disorder, with a melanocyte tyrosinase-related-protein being the most likely target antigen, and T-cells, the perpetrators.

COMMENTS

This is a 50-year-old woman with right eye pain.

Scleritis is a general term for scleral inflammation and includes both episcleritis and scleritis. Episcleritis is commonly a self-limiting process that responds well to topical therapy. On the other hand, scleritis more commonly manifests as a painful, destructive, and potentially blinding condition. Scleritis can be seen as an isolated finding, but is associated with a systemic process in up to 50% of patients. Common underlying systemic illnesses include multiple rheumatic diseases and infectious etiologies.

Anterior scleritis is common (occurring in approximately 90% of cases) and is usually easily diagnosed clinically. Patients complain of severe pain and inflammatory changes are evident clinically. There are three distinct subtypes of anterior scleritis, which include: diffuse, nodular, and necrotizing. These entities can be distinguished from one another by their variable presentations and distinctive physical manifestations.

Posterior scleritis is less common and more difficult to diagnose clinically. Pain is usually less compared to anterior scleritis.

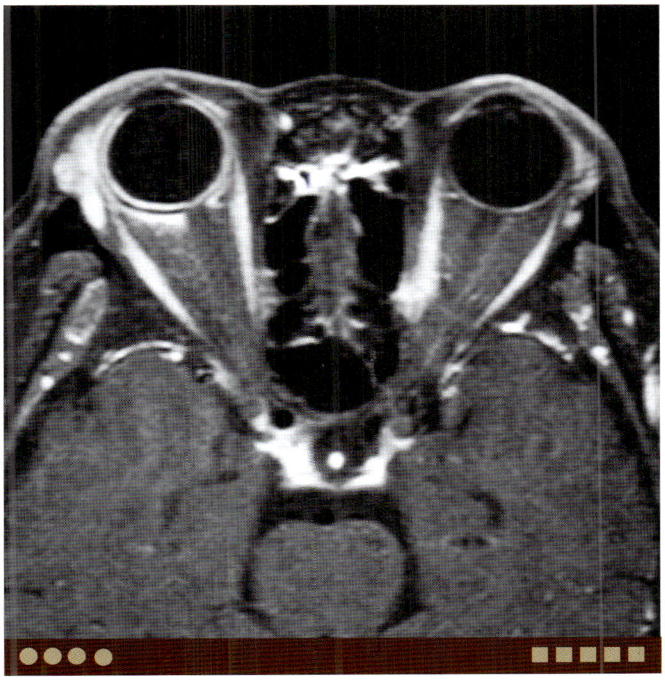

A. Scleritis. Axial postcontrast fat-suppressed T1W MR image demonstrates thickening and abnormal enhancement of the sclera of the right globe. Note abnormal enhancement of the right lacrimal gland as well as in the region of the Tenon's capsule, immediately posterior to the globe.

Fundoscopic examination may demonstrate papilledema, choroidal folds, and retinal hemorrhage or detachment. Imaging can be performed to rule out tumors. Posterior scleritis is also seen as a part of systemic diseases such as systemic lupus erythematosus (SLE) and other connective tissue disorders. It can also be one of the manifestations of idiopathic orbital inflammation ("pseudotumor") and lymphoproliferative disorders. Bilateral involvement is more common.

CT and MRI demonstrate thickening and abnormal enhancement of the sclera. Retinal or choroidal detachment and inflammatory changes adjacent to the sclera (episcleritis) are often seen. Edema and fluid is often noted in the Tenon's capsule.

PEARLS

- **Scleritis is a general term describing inflammatory conditions of the sclera and includes various subtypes, most commonly associated with an underlying systemic illness.**
- **Posterior scleritis, although less common, is seen as a part of systemic diseases such as SLE and other connective tissue disorders, idiopathic orbital inflammation ("pseudotumor"), and lymphoproliferative disorders.**
- **Bilateral involvement is common.**

ADDITIONAL IMAGES (B-G)

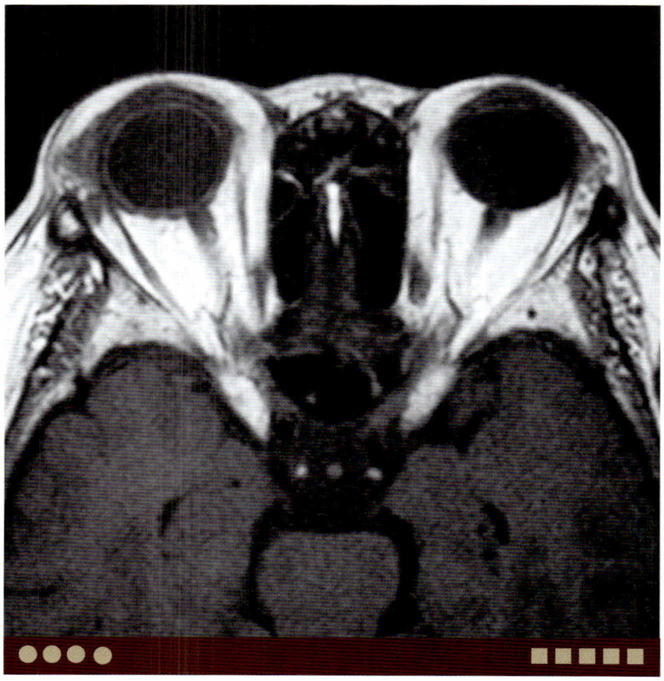

B. Scleritis, same patient as A. Axial T1W MR image demonstrates thickening of the sclera of the right globe with poorly defined posterior boundary. Mild enlargement of the right lacrimal gland is present.

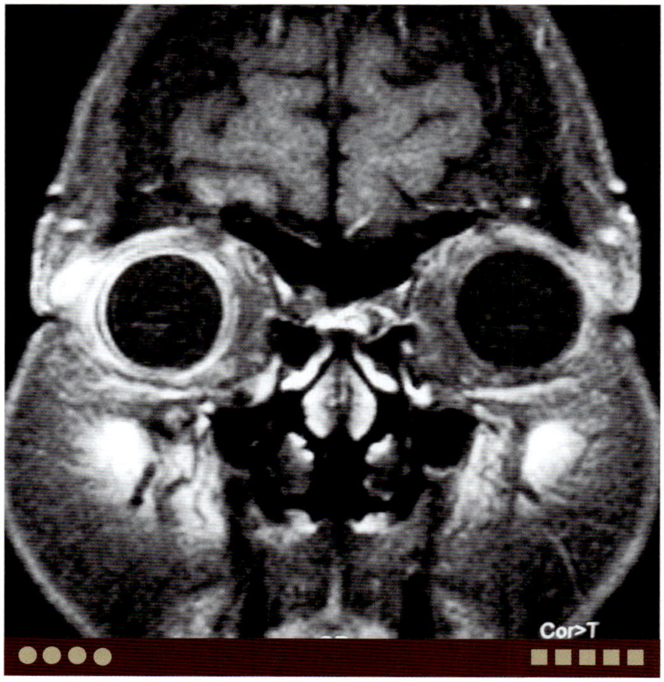

C. Scleritis in a different patient. Coronal postcontrast fat-suppressed T1W MR image demonstrates thickening and abnormal enhancement of the sclera of the right globe. Note abnormal enhancement of the right lacrimal gland as well as periorbital soft tissue.

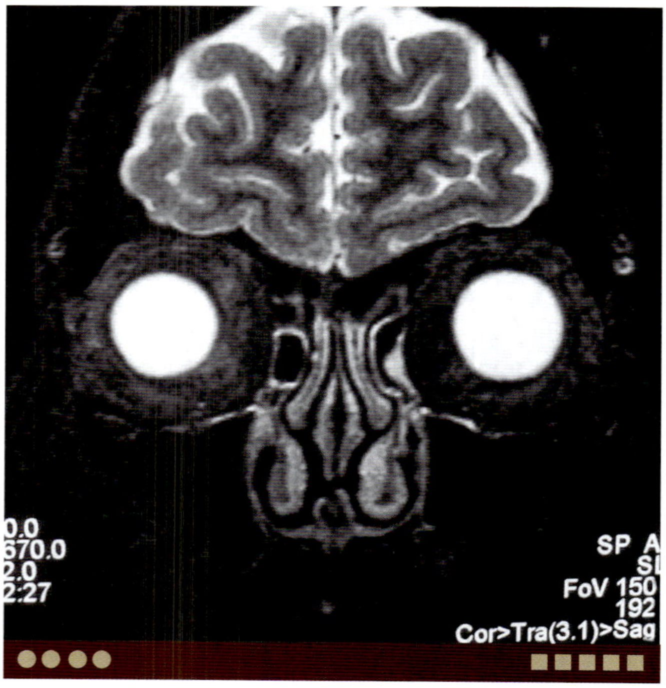

D. Scleritis, same patient as C. Coronal fat-suppressed T2W MR image demonstrates diffusely increased signal around the right globe compared with left.

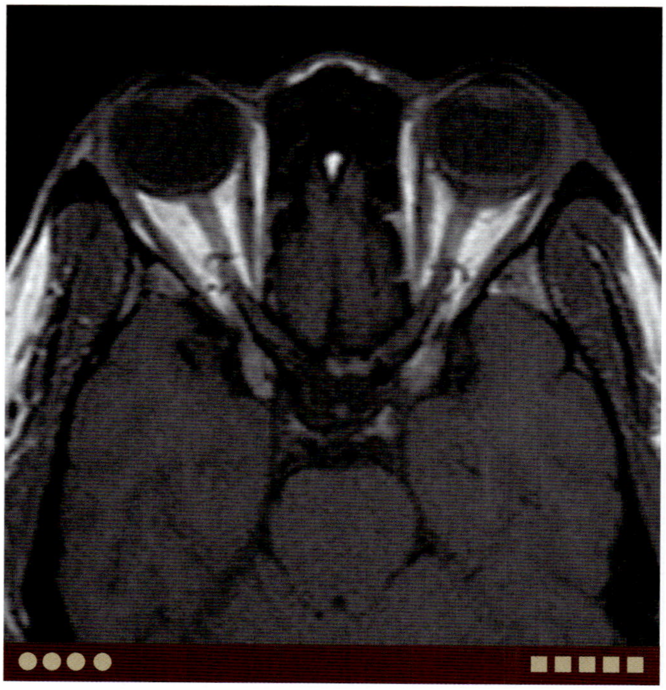

E. Posterior scleritis. Axial T1W MR image demonstrates thickening of the posterior sclera of the left globe with widening of the Tenon's capsule.

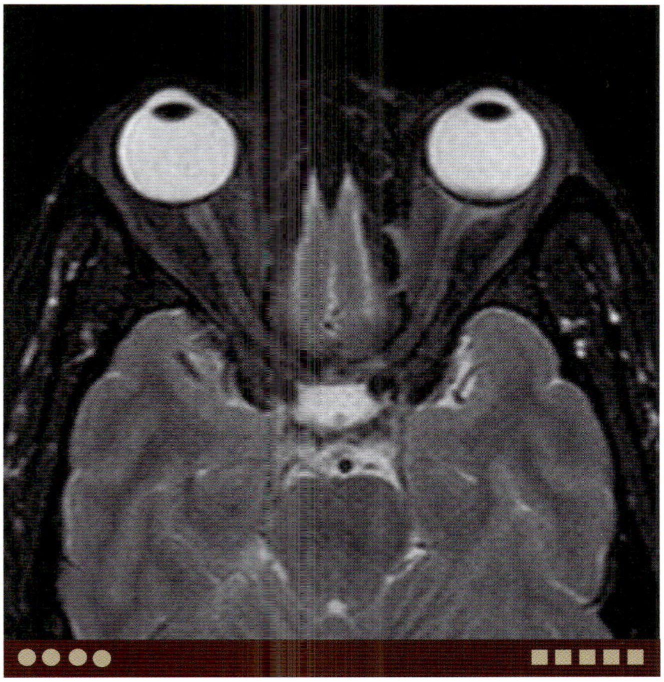

F. Posterior scleritis, same patient as E. Axial fat-suppressed T2W MR image demonstrates thickening of the posterior sclera with fluid signal in the widened Tenon's capsule on the left.

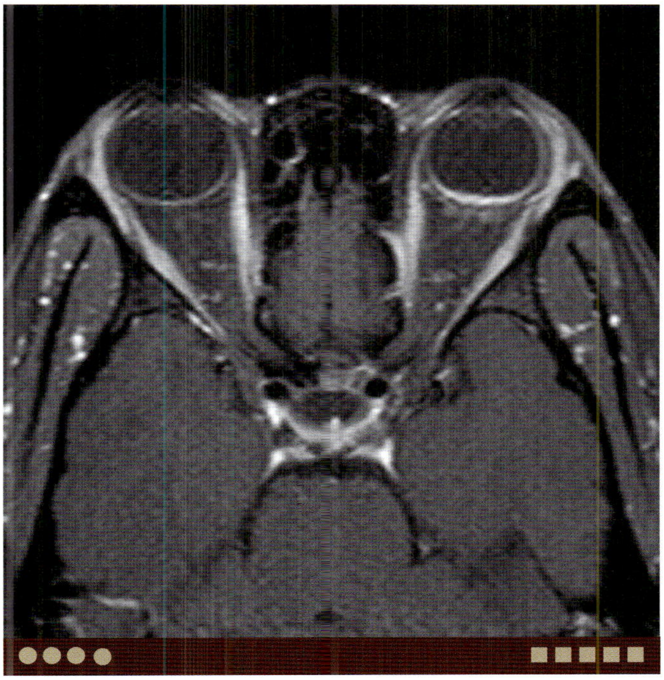

G. Posterior scleritis, same patient as E. Axial postcontrast fat-suppressed T1W MR image demonstrates abnormal enhancement of the thickened posterior sclera of the left globe.

DIFFERENTIAL DIAGNOSIS IMAGES (H-J)

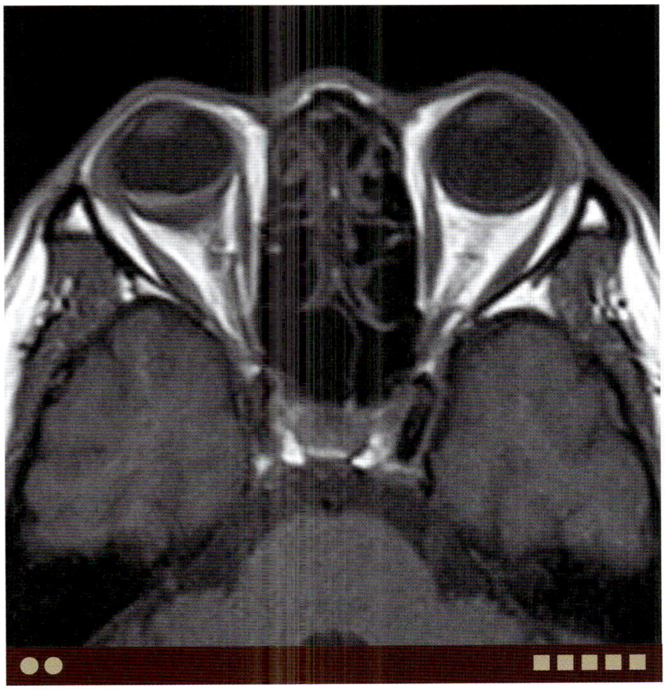

H. Choroidal metastasis. Axial T1W image demonstrates a broad-based high-signal mass in the posterior part of the right globe. Lung cancer was found after further evaluation.

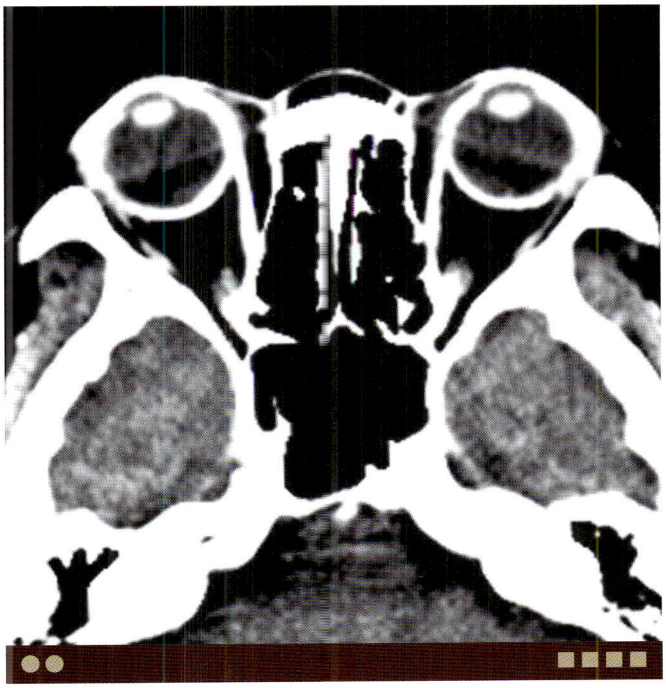

I. VKH syndrome. Axial postcontrast CT demonstrates diffuse bilateral choroidal thickening with marked enhancement.

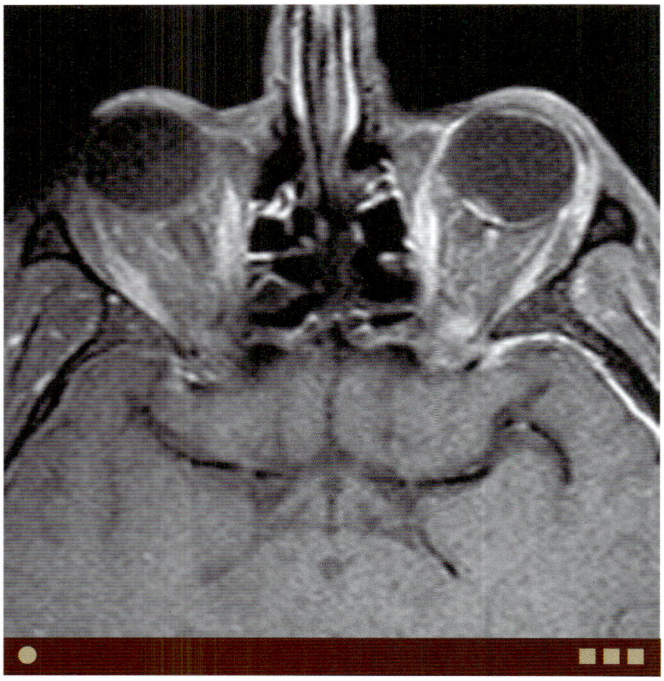

J. Intraocular lymphoma. Axial contrast-enhanced fat-suppressed T1W MR image demonstrates a small enhancing lesion in the left posterior globe. Note dural involvement by lymphoma in the left-middle cranial fossa.

Case 5–13 Persistent Hyperplastic Primary Vitreous

June Cheng, Ilse Castro-Aragon, Osamu Sakai

PRESENTATION

Leukocoria.

FINDINGS

CT demonstrates a small and hyperdense globe without calcification.

DIFFERENTIAL DIAGNOSIS

- Retinoblastoma: This is the most common intraocular malignancy in children. Intratumoral calcification is a key imaging finding. Usually, no microphthalmos is present.
- Coats disease: This is a congenital primary vascular anomaly of the retina, causing exudative retinal detachment secondary to dilatation of the retinal arterioles and disruption of the blood-retina barrier. The hyperdense subretinal collection is seen without a mass or calcification.
- Retinopathy of prematurity (retrolental fibroplasia): This condition demonstrates bilateral microphthalmos and hyperdense globes, rarely with calcification. The clinical history of prematurity with prolonged oxygen therapy is necessary in the diagnosis.
- Coloboma: This is a congenital focal defect in the wall of the globe, often near the optic nerve head insertion. However, different structures within the globe, including the choroid, iris, lens, optic nerve, and retina, may be involved. This condition may be bilateral and associated with various congenital malformation syndromes.

COMMENTS

This is a 5-month-old infant with leukocoria.

Persistent hyperplastic primary vitreous (PHPV) is the second most common cause of leukocoria and is important to differentiate from retinoblastoma. PHPV is a congenital, vascular lesion caused by persistence of the embryonic ocular blood supply (hyaloid artery) and hyperplasia of fibrovascular connective tissue.

On CT, the affected eye is small in size (microphthalmos) and the vitreous body appears dense due to proteinaceous and hemorrhagic debris. Retinal detachment is common. There is no definite calcification. These findings differentiate PHPV from retinoblastoma, which usually demonstrates a normal-sized globe with intraocular calcification.

On MRI, the vitreous body demonstrates increased signal on both T1W and T2W images due to proteinaceous and hemorrhagic debris. Fluid-fluid levels are often identified in

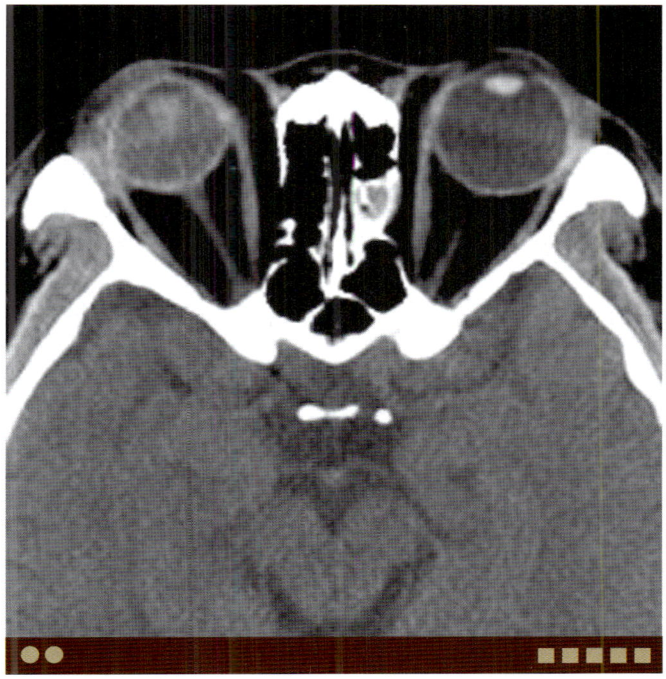

A. PHPV. Axial CT demonstrates right microphthalmos and a hyperdense vitreous body with retinal detachment.

the vitreous body due to repeated hemorrhages. A linear structure is often seen posterior to the lens, particularly on high-resolution MRI, which may represent the Cloquet canal or a detached retina. Postcontrast images may demonstrate enhancement of the retrolental tissue. A contrast-enhanced study is also useful to exclude neoplasm.

PHPV usually presents unilaterally. However, when PHPV occurs bilaterally, it is closely associated with CNS anomalies, such as Norrie disease and Warburg syndrome. Therefore, when PHPV is suspected, a thorough evaluation of the central nervous system (CNS) is crucial.

PEARLS

- **PHPV demonstrates microphthalmos and a hyperdense globe without calcification**
- **PHPV demonstrates increased signal within the globe on both T1W and T2W images due to proteinaceous and hemorrhagic debris.**
- **PHPV may be associated with CNS anomalies, such as Norrie disease and Warburg syndrome.**

ADDITIONAL IMAGES (B-G)

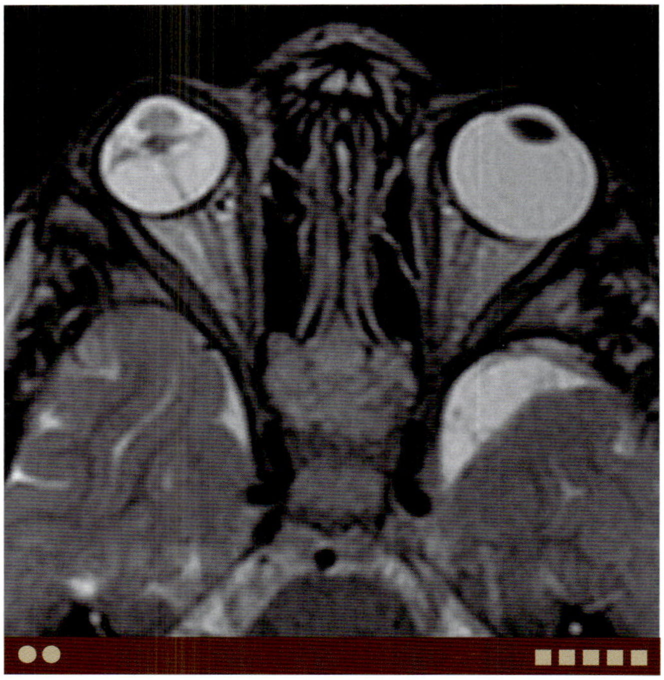

B. PHPV in a different patient. Axial T2W MR image demonstrates right microphthalmos, retinal detachment, and low-signal retrolental tissue, which likely represents a persistent hyaloid artery in the Cloquet canal.

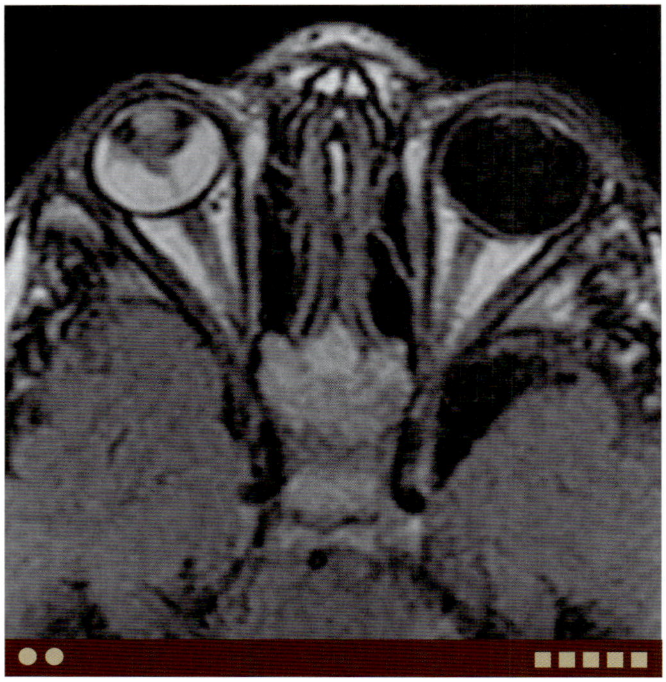

C. PHPV, same patient as B. Axial FLAIR MR image demonstrates right microphthalmos and retinal detachment with high-signal proteinaceous subretinal fluid.

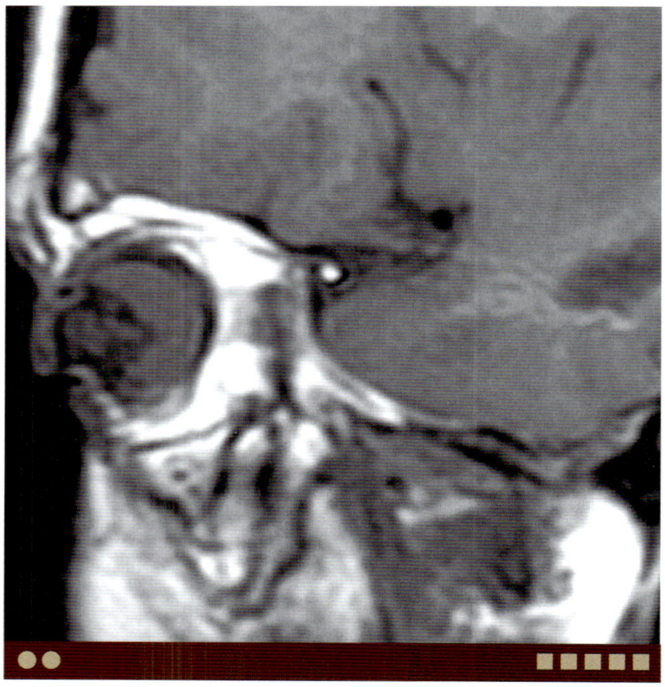

D. PHPV, same patient as B. Sagittal T1W MR image demonstrates retinal detachment and proteinaceous subretinal fluid.

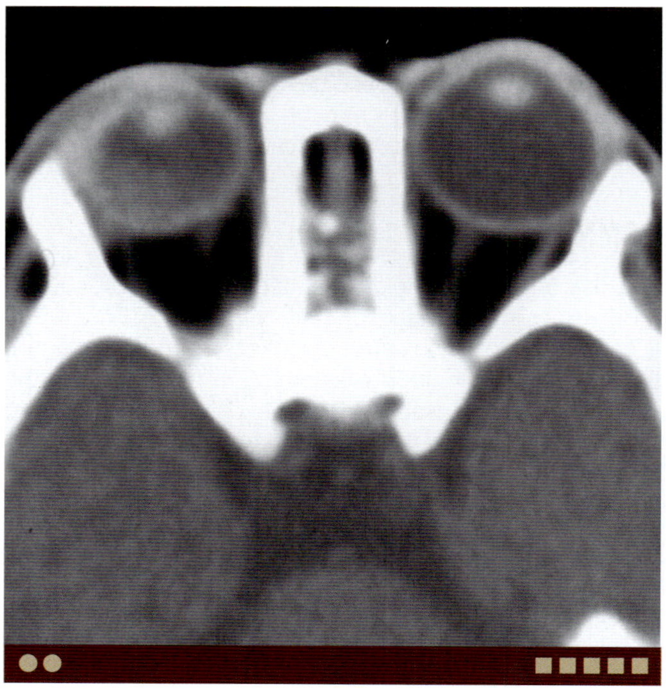

E. PHPV in a different patient. Axial CT image demonstrates right microphthalmos and increased density in the posterior globe.

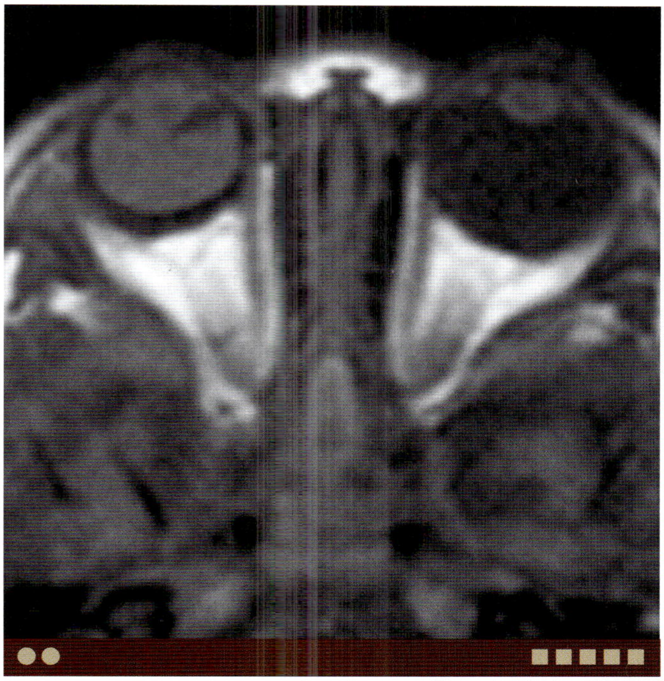

F. PHPV, same patient as E. Axial T1W MR image demonstrates right microphthalmos and increased T1 signal in the globe, consistent with subretinal proteinaceous or hemorrhagic material.

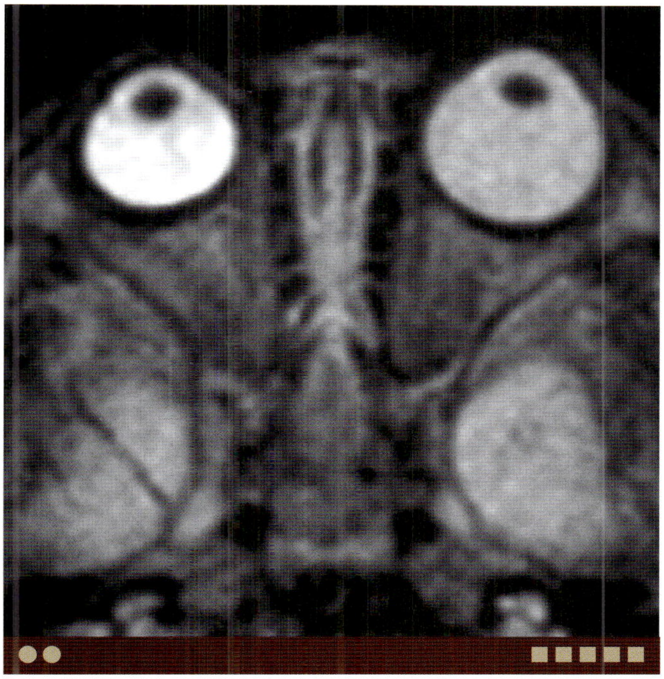

G. PHPV, same patient as E. Axial T2W MR image demonstrates right microphthalmos and increased T2 signal in the globe, consistent with subretinal proteinaceous or hemorrhagic material.

DIFFERENTIAL DIAGNOSIS IMAGES (H-J)

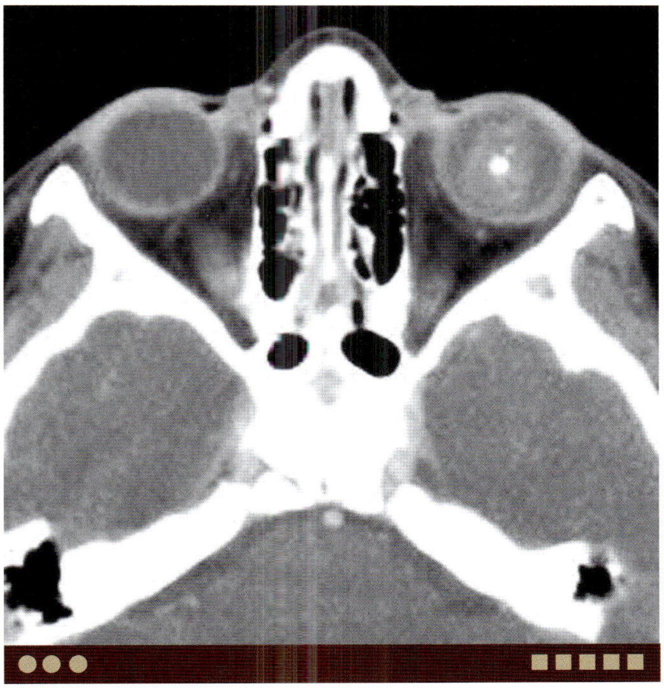

H. Retinoblastoma. Axial CT demonstrates a high-density mass with calcification in the normal-sized left globe.

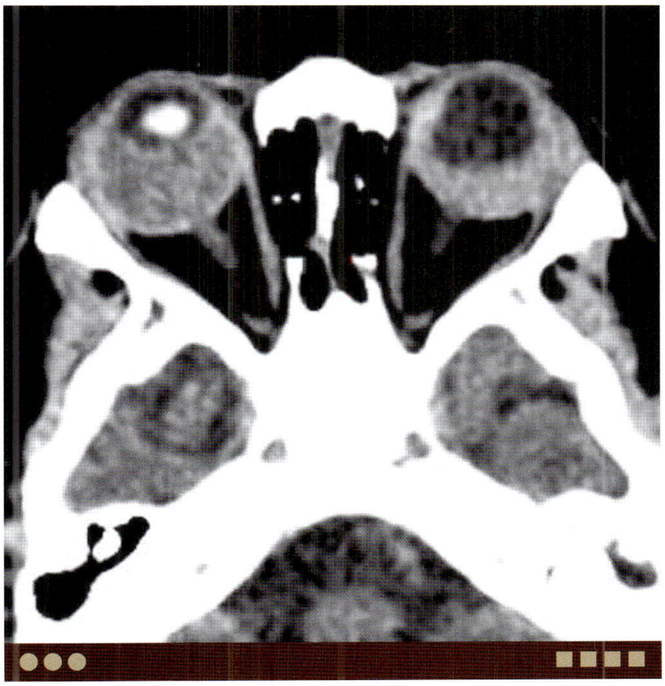

I. Retinopathy of prematurity. Axial CT demonstrates bilateral retinal detachment with high-density subretinal collection without calcification. No microphthalmos is idenitified.

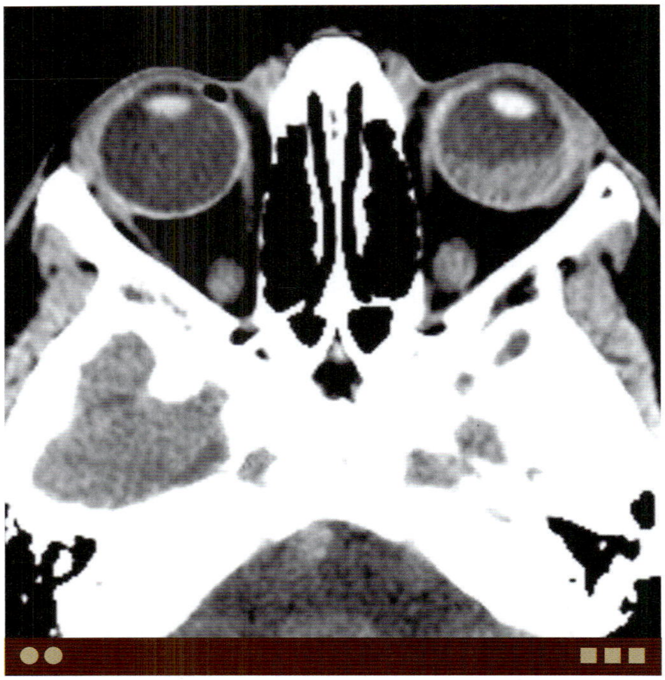

J. Coats disease. Axial CT demonstrates hyperdensity along the posterior wall of the left globe, representing proteinaceous or hemorrhagic subretinal exudate. There is no microphthalmos.

Case 5–14 Coats Disease

June Cheng, Ilse Castro-Aragon, Osamu Sakai

PRESENTATION

Leukocoria.

FINDINGS

CT and MRI demonstrate retinal detachment with lipoproteinaceous subretinal fluid collection.

DIFFERENTIAL DIAGNOSIS

- Retinoblastoma: This is the most common intraocular malignancy in children. Intratumoral calcification is a key imaging finding.
- Persistent hyperplastic primary vitreous (PHPV): This condition demonstrates microphthalmos and subretinal or subhyaloid collection without calcification. PHPV is associated with an intracranial abnormality, particularly when bilateral.
- Retinopathy of prematurity (retrolental fibroplasia): This demonstrates bilateral microphthalmos and hyperdense globes, rarely with calcification. The clinical history of prematurity with prolonged oxygen therapy is necessary in the diagnosis.
- Coloboma: This is a congenital focal defect in the wall of the globe, often near the optic nerve head insertion. However, different structures within the globe, including the choroid, iris, lens, optic nerve, and retina, may be involved. This condition may be bilateral and associated with various congenital malformation syndromes.

COMMENTS

This is a 5-year-old boy with leukocoria.

Coats disease is a congenital primary vascular anomaly of the retina, causing exudative retinal detachment secondary to dilatation of the retinal arterioles and disruption of the blood-retina barrier. The vessels leak lipoproteinaceous products into the retina and subretinal space, which may eventually obliterate the vitreous body. Presentation is usually gradual, and may not occur until complete retinal detachment and blindness. The age of diagnosis is most common between 6 and 8, slightly older than those presenting with retinoblastoma. Interestingly, boys are affected twice as often as girls.

CT demonstrates a hyperdense globe due to proteinaceous or hemorrhagic subretinal exudate. In addition, typically only one globe is affected, which is normal to small in size. Calcification is rare, distinguishing it from retinoblastoma.

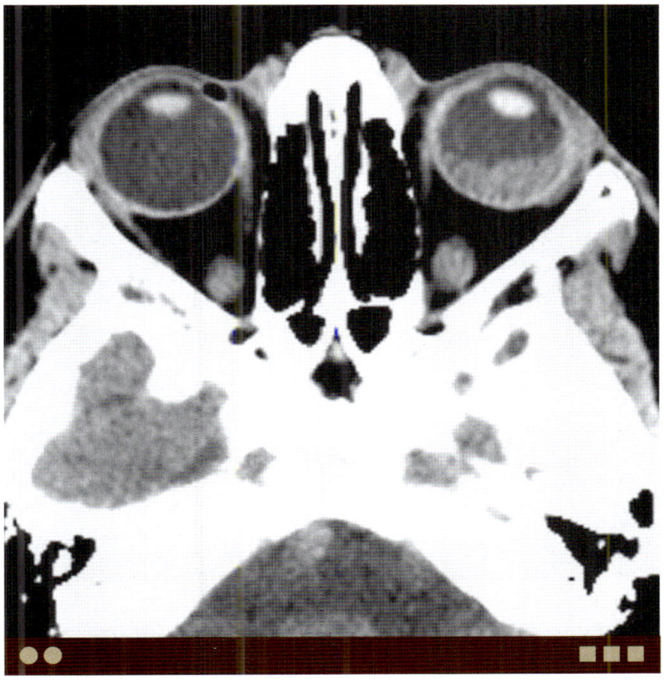

A. Coats disease. Axial CT demonstrates hyperdensity along the posterior left globe, representing proteinaceous or hemorrhagic subretinal exudate.

Coats disease demonstrates variable appearance on MRI depending on the stage of the disease. Total retinal detachment is often seen in patients with advanced disease. Subretinal fluid in patients with Coats disease demonstrates high signal on both T1W and T2W images secondary to high fat and protein content, while retinoblastoma usually demonstrates slightly decreased signal on T2W images. Heterogeneous signal on T2W images may also be secondary to hemorrhage from the abnormal retinal vessels. Upon administration of contrast, there is linear enhancement of the detached retina and no enhancing intraocular mass lesion is present.

PEARLS

- **Coats disease causes exudative retinal detachment due to dilatation of the retinal arterioles and disruption of the blood-retina barrier.**
- **Total retinal detachment is often seen in patients with advanced disease.**
- **Subretinal fluid in patients with Coats disease demonstrates high signal on both T1W and T2W images.**

ADDITIONAL IMAGES (B-D)

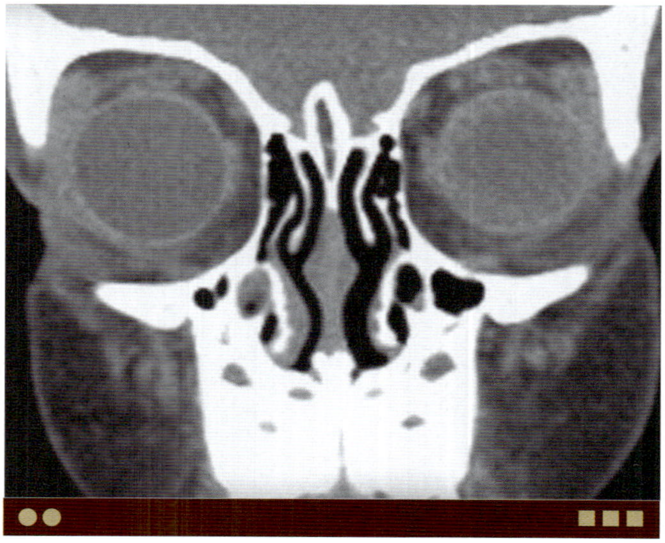

B. Coats disease same patient as A. Coronal CT image demonstrates increased density within the left globe. No calcification is identified.

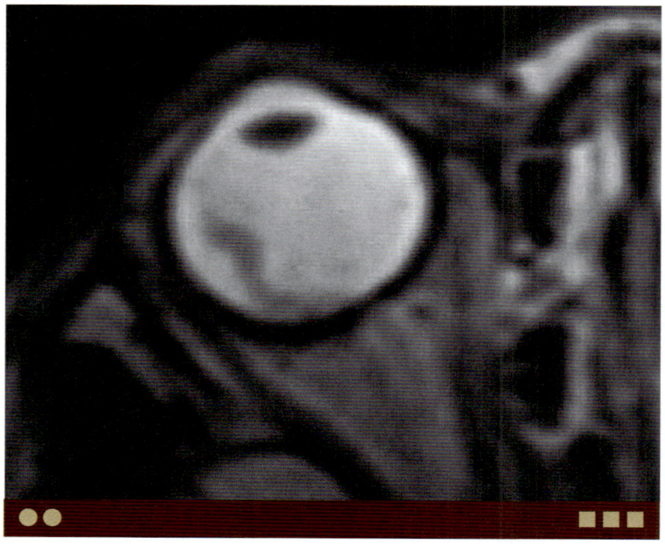

C. Coats disease in a different patient. Axial T2W MR image demonstrates a curvilinear focus of decreased signal at the lateral aspect of the globe, corresponding to retinal detachment. Subretinal fluid shows high signal.

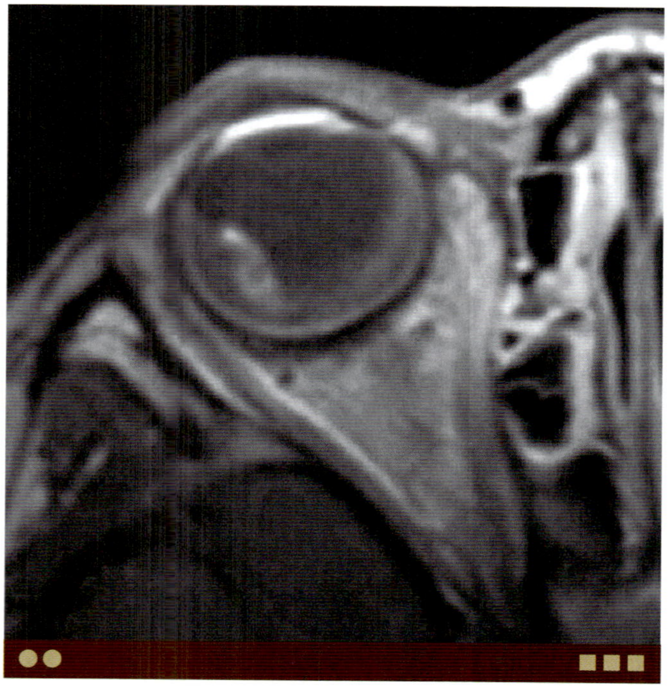

D. Coats disease same patient as C. Axial postcontrast T1W MR image demonstrates curvilinear enhancement involving the detached retina. Increased signal along the posterior aspect of the globe represents an exudative subretinal collection.

DIFFERENTIAL DIAGNOSIS IMAGES (E-G)

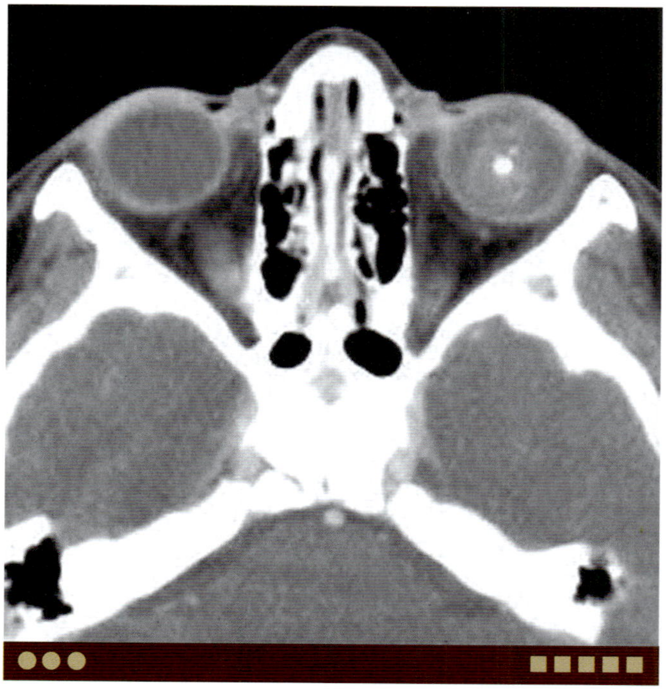

E. Retinoblastoma. Axial CT demonstrates a high-density mass with calcification within the left globe.

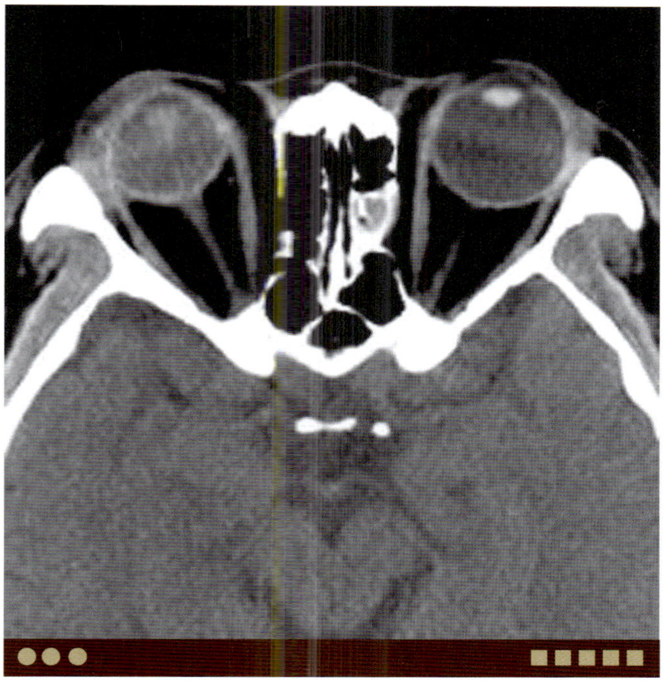

F. PHPV. Axial CT demonstrates right microphthalmos and a hyperdense vitreous body without calcification within the right globe.

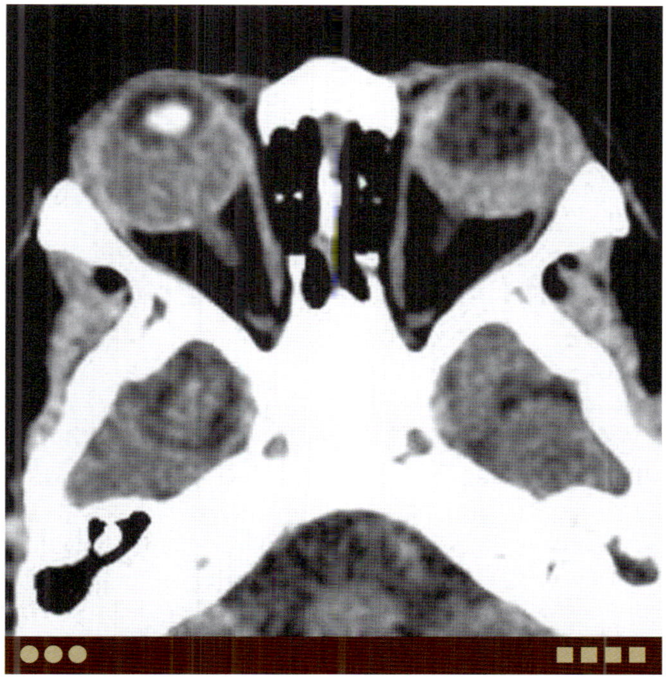

G. Retinopathy of prematurity. Axial CT demonstrates bilateral retinal detachment with high-density subretinal collection without calcification.

Case 5–15 Drusen

Osamu Sakai, Francisco Contreras

PRESENTATION

Incidental finding.

FINDINGS

CT demonstrates a punctuate calcification at the optic disc.

DIFFERENTIAL DIAGNOSIS

- Choroidal osteoma: Choroidal osteoma is a benign, ossifying, choroidal tumor of unknown etiology. It occurs predominantly in young females with no history of systemic or ocular disease, and usually unilateral.
- Choroidal hemangioma: Choroidal hemangioma is a benign vascular tumor. However, this may be difficult to differentiate from melanoma by ophthalmologic examination. Isointensity to the vitreous on T2W images combined with strong and early contrast enhancement are helpful to differentiate it from uveal melanoma.
- Choroidal metastases: Metastatic choroidal tumors are not rare, although they are not very often appreciated clinically. Most common primary sites are breasts and lungs.
- Hyaline plaque: This is degenerative change and seen in elderly populations, usually more than 80 years old. Focal calcification is seen at the insertion of medial and lateral rectus muscles.

COMMENTS

This is a 68-year-old man who underwent CT for headache.

Drusen is caused by the accumulation of mucopolysaccharides and proteinaceous material on the surface of the optic disc, which can become calcified with advancing age. There is an inherited form with an autosomal trait with irregular penetrance. Drusens are commonly asymptomatic and incidentally found on CT performed for other reasons. These lesions can cause visual field defects and rarely can also lead to deficits in central acuity. Approximately 75% of drusen are bilateral. They are usually seen in elderly patients, and are rare in children. They are also believed to cause headaches.

The diagnosis of drusen is simplified when these lesions lie on the surface of the optic disk, where they can be easily detected on fundoscopic examination. When drusen lie deep within the tissue of the optic nerve, however, the typical fundoscopic appearance may not be evident. When these small lesions develop within the nerve tissue, they can lead to elevation of the disc, which can be diagnosed as papilledema (pseudopapilledema). Under these circumstances, CT or MRI can be performed to look for conditions that may cause elevated intracranial pressure.

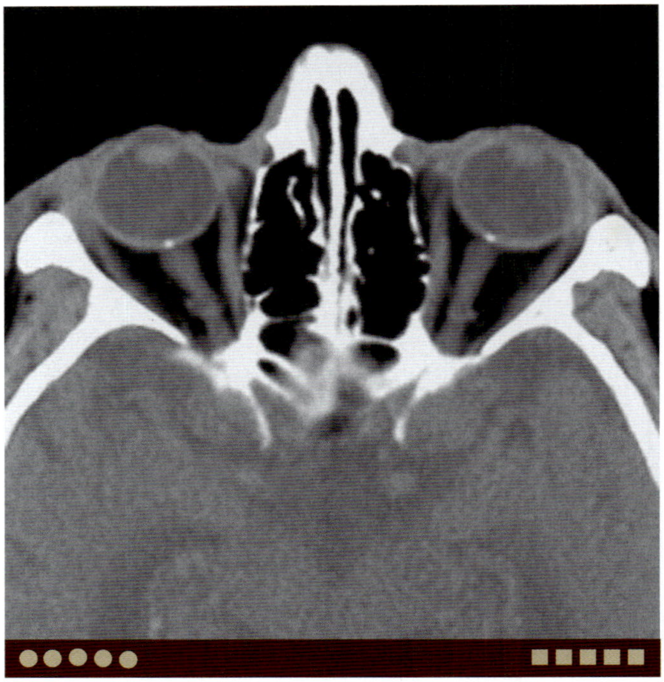

A. Optic drusen. Axial noncontrast CT demonstrates punctate calcifications at the optic discs bilaterally.

PEARLS

- **Drusen, which are typically bilateral, are benign calcifications at the optic disc.**
- **They are usually incidentally found and typically of no clinical significance. Rarely, they can cause defects in the visual fields or central acuity.**
- **When drusen are located deep within the optic nerve, they can cause elevation of the optic disc and lead to the diagnosis of papilledema (pseudopapilledema).**

ADDITIONAL IMAGES (B-C)

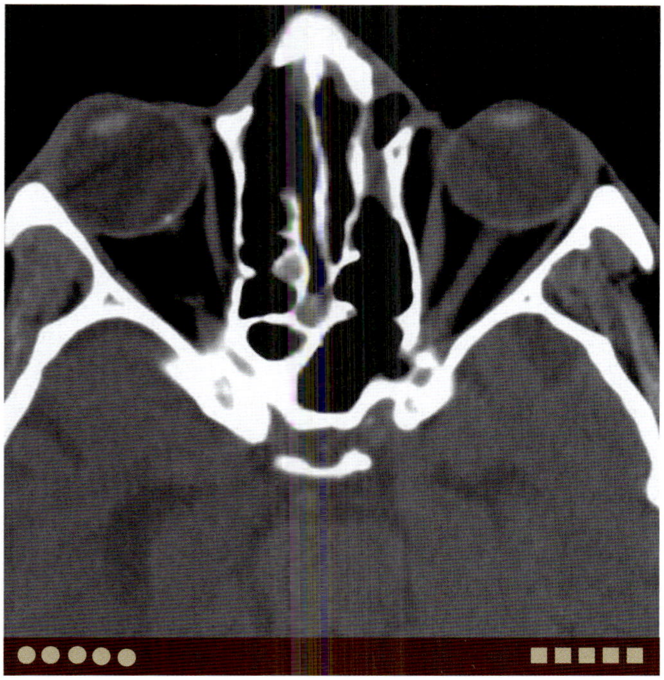

B. Optic drusen in a different patient. Axial noncontrast CT demonstrates a punctate calcification within the optic disc in the right globe.

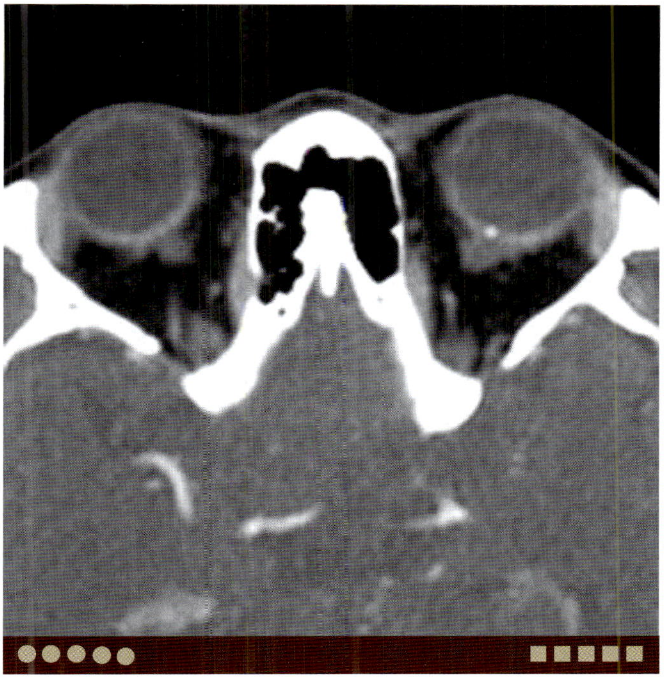

C. Optic drusen in a different patient. Axial contrast-enhanced CT demonstrates a punctate calcification at the optic disc within the left globe.

DIFFERENTIAL DIAGNOSIS IMAGES (D-G)

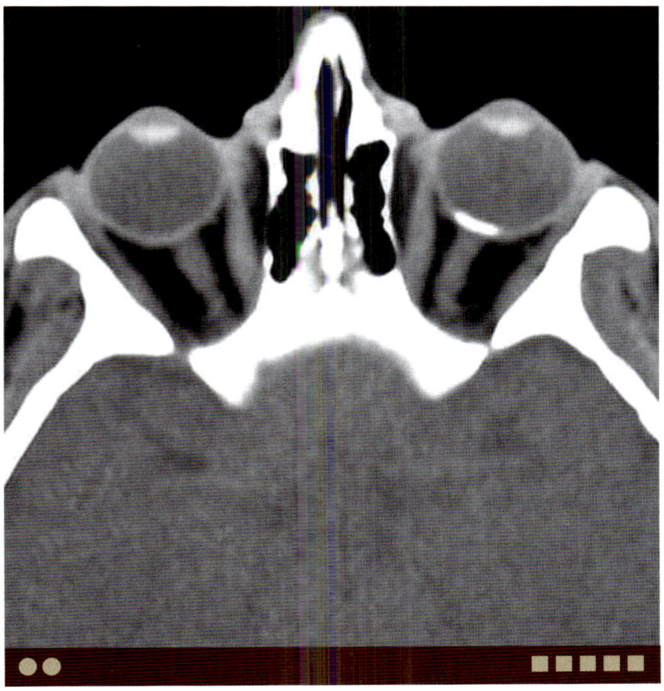

D. Choroidal osteotoma. Axial noncontrast CT image demonstrates a plaque-like calcification along the posterior left globe.

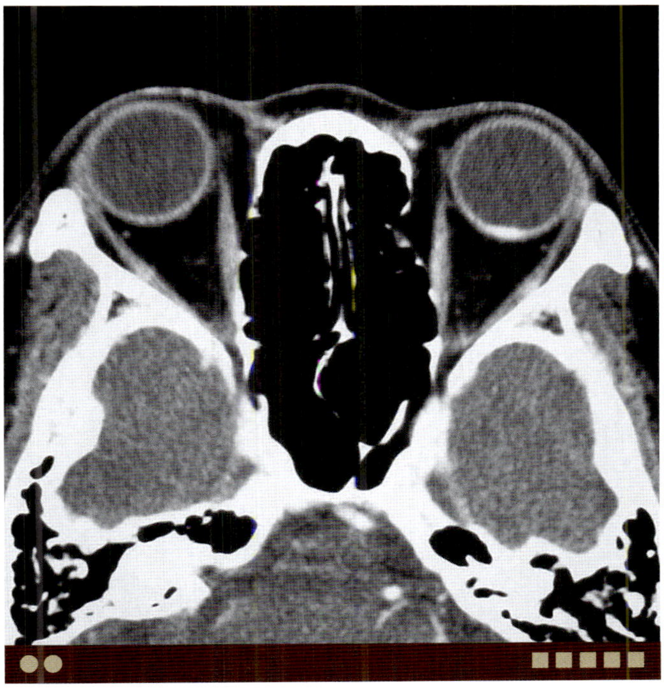

E. Choroidal hemangioma. Axial contrast-enhanced CT demonstrates an avidly enhancing lenticular lesion in the posterior wall of the left globe.

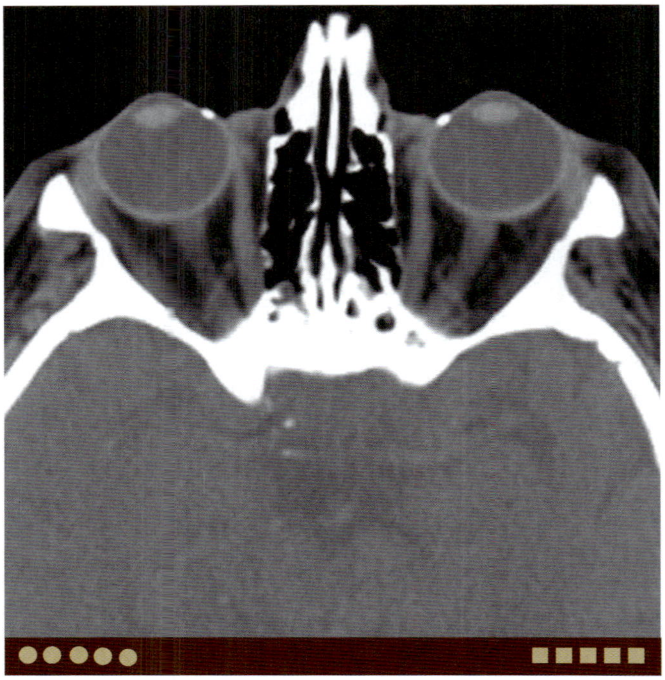

F. Hyaline plaque. Axial noncontrast-enhanced CT demonstrates punctate calcifications at the insertion of the medial rectus muscles bilaterally.

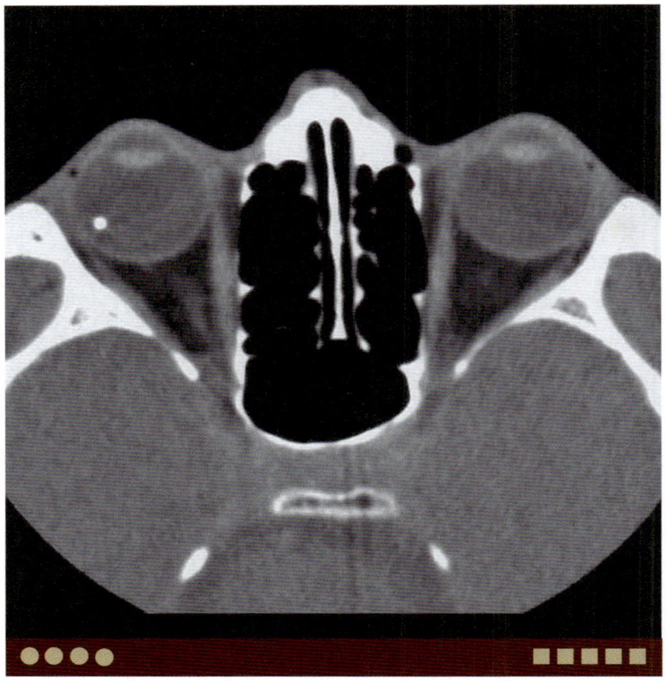

G. Foreign body. Axial noncontrast-enhanced CT demonstrates a radiopaque foreign body within the right globe.

Case 5–16 Choroidal Hemangioma

Francisco Contreras, Osamu Sakai, Akifumi Fujita

PRESENTATION

Blurred vision.

FINDINGS

Contrast-enhanced CT shows homogenous, lentiform, enhancement of the posterior globe.

DIFFERENTIAL DIAGNOSIS

- Choroidal osteoma: This plaque-like, benign ossifying lesion of the choroid layer does not demonstrate enhancement.
- Optic drusen: This is a punctuate calcification at the optic disc and does not demonstrate enhancement.
- Choroidal melanoma: This is the most common primary malignant ocular tumor in adults. Although avid enhancement is seen on CT, tumors typically also show increased attenuation on noncontrast CT.

COMMENTS

This is a 53-year-old man with blurred vision.

Choroidal hemangioma is an uncommon benign hamartomatous vascular tumor confined to the choroidal layer of the globe. They can be circumscribed or diffuse. Circumscribed choroidal hemangiomas are often diagnosed between the second and fourth decades of life when they cause visual disturbance secondary to an exudative retinal detachment. These tumors occur sporadically, without any associated local or systemic abnormalities. Diffuse choroidal hemangiomas occur as a part of neuro-oculo-cutaneous hemangiomatosis (Sturge-Weber syndrome), and are usually diagnosed at birth.

On fundoscopic examination, choroidal hemangioma appears as a dome-shaped, smoothly demarcated mass of a reddish-orange color that can sometimes blend into the surrounding choroid. The three histological classifications of choroidal hemangiomas include capillary, cavernous, or mixed. Asymptomatic lesions are usually not treated unless associated with a retinal detachment. In such cases, the treatment of choice is laser photocoagulation.

It is important to differentiate benign hemangiomas from potentially malignant melanomas in the choroid. Choroidal hemangiomas are identifiable on CT as ill-defined masses with avid enhancement and typically found on the posterior half of the globe. When a nonenhancing, calcified lesion is encountered in the choroid layer of the globe; both choroidal osteoma and optic disc drusen should be in the differential consideration.

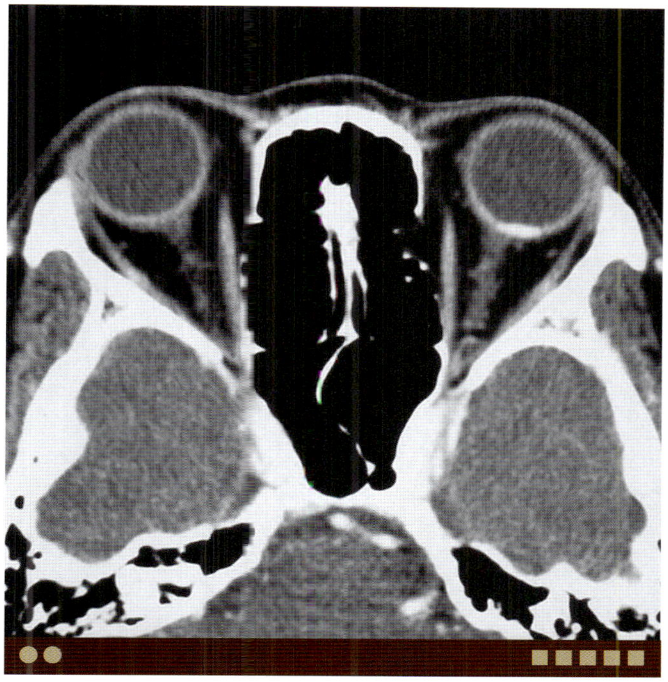

A. Choroidal hemangioma. Axial contrast-enhanced CT demonstrates an avidly enhancing lenticular lesion in the posterior wall of the left globe.

MRI is helpful in distinguishing choroidal hemangiomas from melanomas. The typical MR appearance of choroidal hemangioma includes T1W and T2W hyperintensity compared to the surrounding vitreous and avid enhancement. In contrast, melanomas typically demonstrate T1W hyperintensity and T2W hypointensity because of shortening T1 and T2 relaxation times by the paramagnetic effect of melanin.

PEARLS

- **Choroidal hemangiomas demonstrate avid lenticular-shaped enhancement confined to the choroidal layer of the globe.**
- **Circumscribed choroidal hemangiomas occur sporadically, while diffuse choroidal hemangiomas occur as a part of neuro-oculo-cutaneous hemangiomatosis (Sturge-Weber syndrome).**
- **MRI is helpful in distinguishing choroidal hemangiomas (high on T1W and T2W) from choroidal melanomas (high on T1W and low on T2W).**

ADDITIONAL IMAGES (B-E)

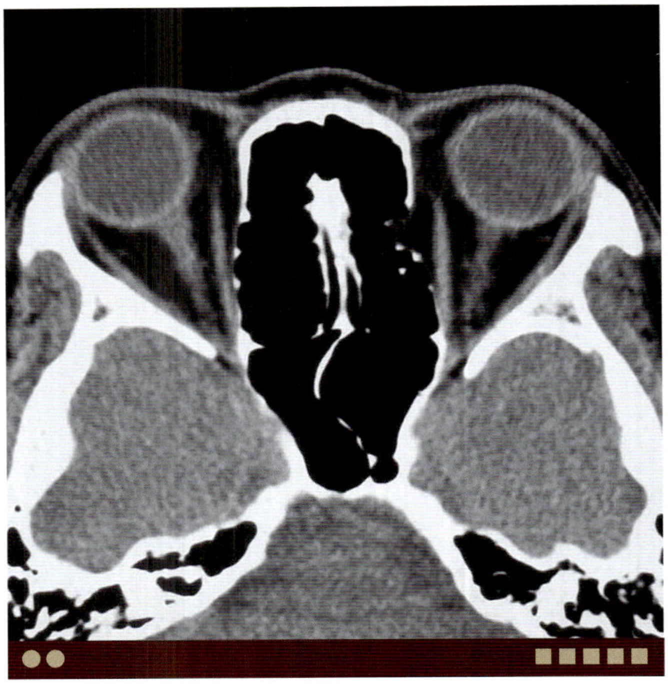

B. Choroidal hemangioma, same patient as A. Axial noncontrast-enhanced CT demonstrates a noncalcified lesion in the posterior wall of the left globe.

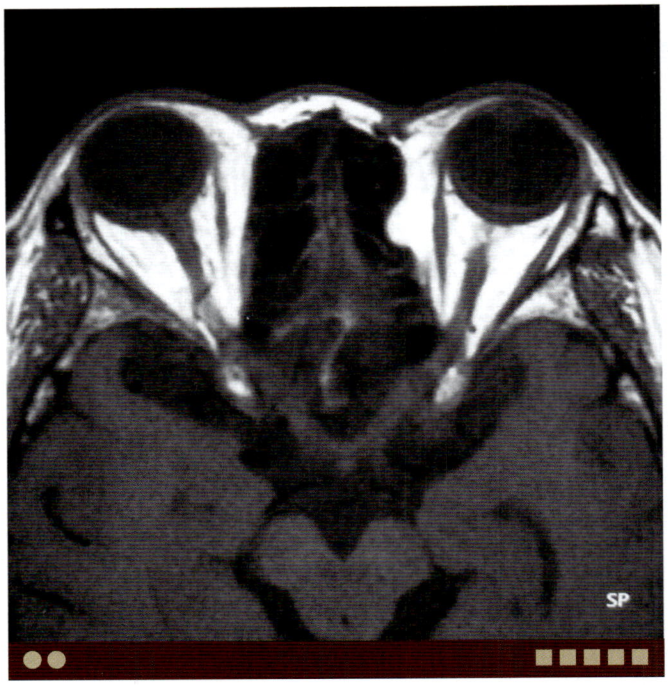

C. Choroidal hemangioma, same patient as A. Axial T1W MR image demonstrates subtle hyperintensity in the left posterior choroid.

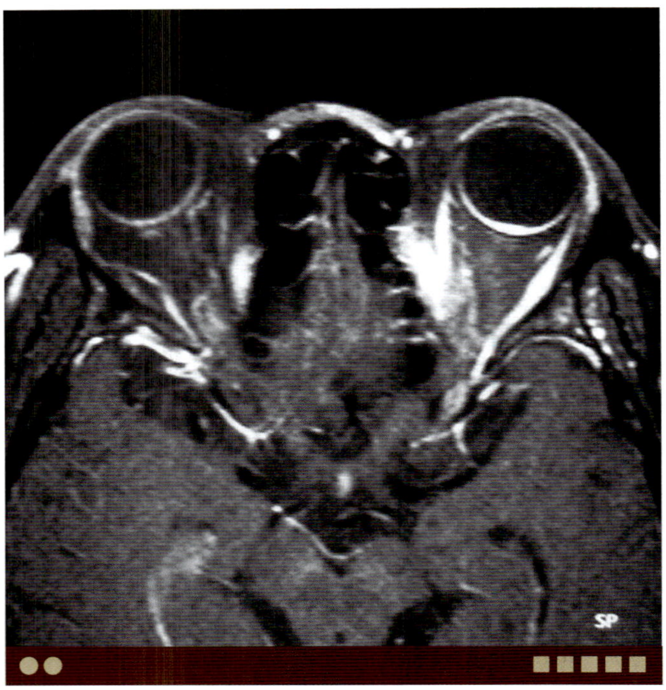

D. Choroidal hemangioma, same patient as A. Axial contrast-enhanced T1W MR image demonstrates avid lenticular enhancement in the left posterior choroid.

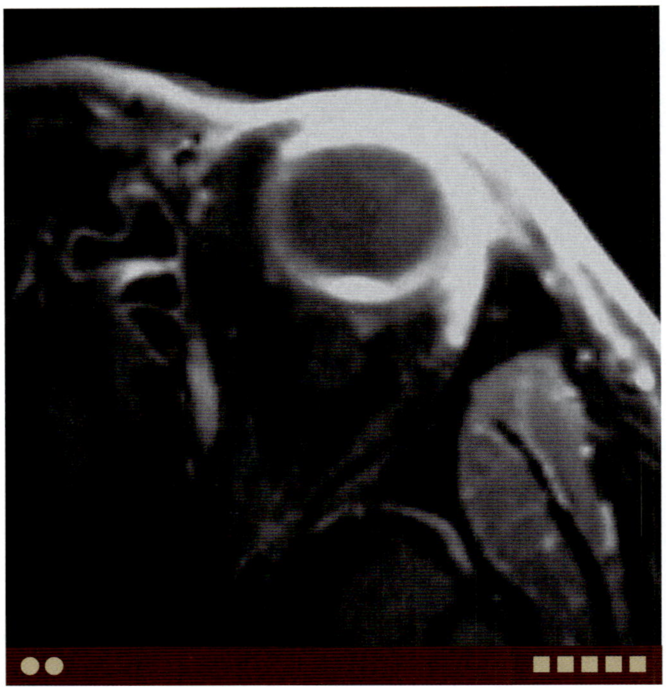

E. Choroidal hemangioma in a different patient. Axial contrast-enhanced fat-suppressed T1W MR image demonstrates avid lenticular enhancement in the posterior choroid.

DIFFERENTIAL DIAGNOSIS IMAGES (F-I)

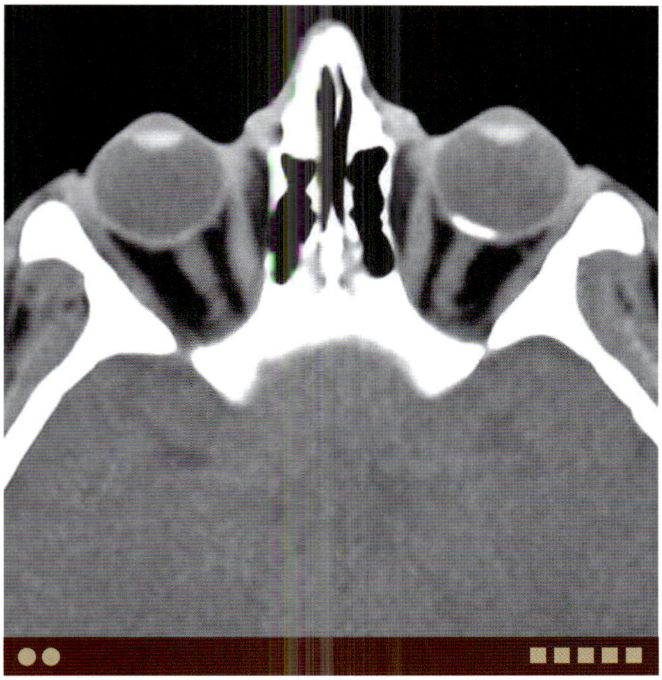

F. Choroidal osteoma. Axial noncontrast-enhanced CT demonstrates a plaque-like calcified lesion in the posterior wall of the left globe.

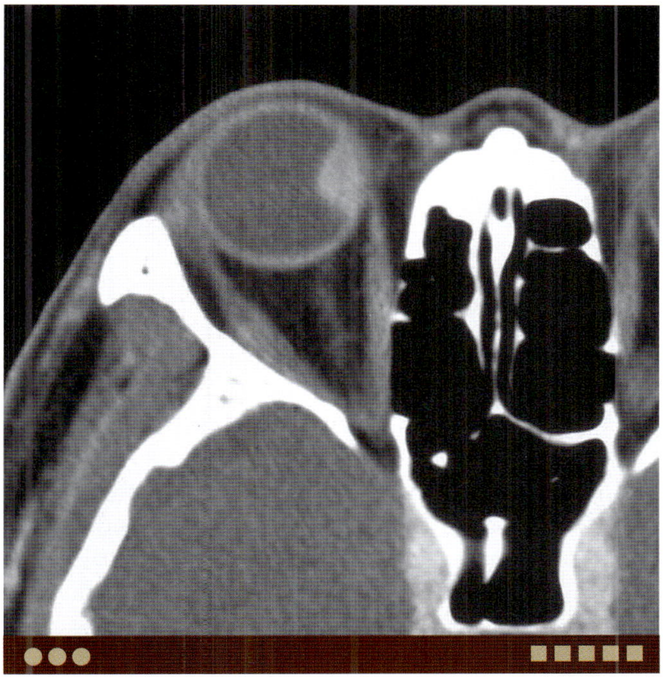

G. Choroidal melanoma. Axial contrast-enhanced CT demonstrates an enhancing elevated lesion in the medial wall of the right globe.

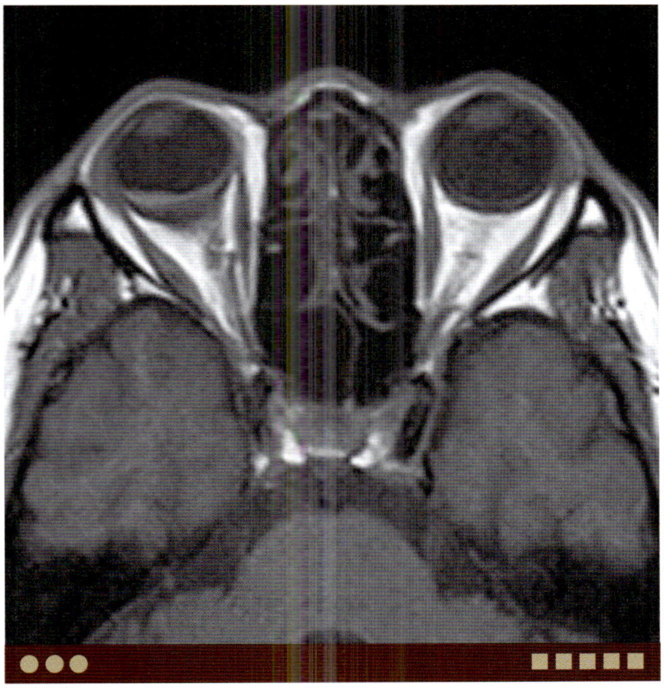

H. Choroidal metastasis from lung cancer. Axial T1W MR image demonstrates a broad-based high-intensity lesion in the posterior right globe.

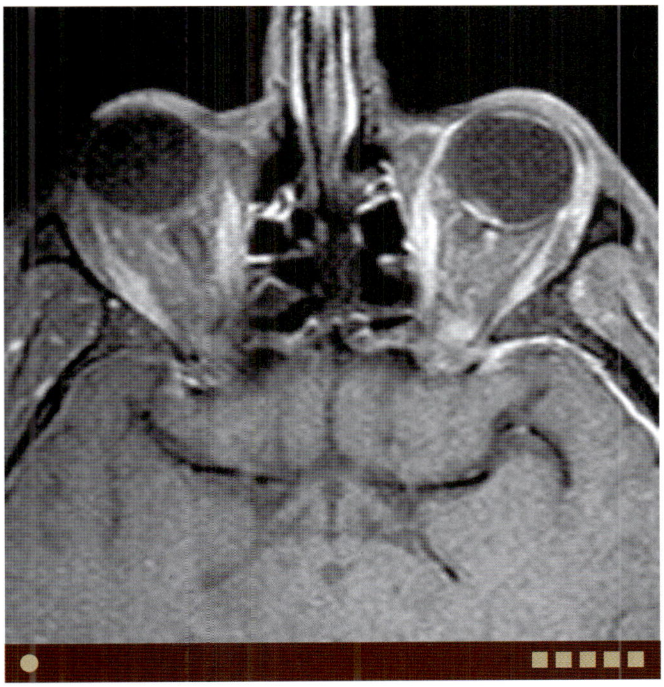

I. Lymphoma. Axial contrast-enhanced fat-suppressed T1W MR image demonstrates a curvilinear-enhancing lesion in the left posterior globe. Note dural involvement by lymphoma in the left middle cranial fossa.

Case 5–17 Retinopathy of Prematurity

June Cheng, Ilse Castro-Aragon, Osamu Sakai

PRESENTATION

Leukocoria.

FINDINGS

CT and MRI demonstrate bilateral microphthalmos and hyperdense globes, rarely with calcification. The clinical history of prematurity with prolonged oxygen therapy is necessary in the diagnosis.

DIFFERENTIAL DIAGNOSIS

- Retinoblastoma: This is the most common intraocular malignancy in children. Intratumoral calcification is a key imaging finding and typically microphthalmos is not present.
- Persistent hyperplastic primary vitreous (PHPV): This condition demonstrates microphthalmos and subretinal or subhyaloid collection without calcification. PHPV is associated with an intracranial abnormality, particularly when bilateral.
- Coats disease: This is a congenital primary vascular anomaly of the retina, causing exudative retinal detachment secondary to dilatation of the retinal arterioles and disruption of the blood-retina barrier. The hyperdense subretinal collection is seen without a mass or calcification.
- Coloboma: This is a congenital focal defect in the wall of the globe, often near the optic nerve head insertion. However, different structures within the globe, including the choroid, iris, lens, optic nerve, and retina, may be involved. This condition may be bilateral and associated with various congenital malformation syndromes.

COMMENTS

This is an infant, prematurely born at 25 weeks, with leukocoria.

Retinopathy of prematurity, previously known as retrolental fibroplasia, develops in premature infants with surfactant deficiency after excessive exposure to supplemental oxygen therapy. This condition was once the leading cause of blindness in children in the United States. However, advancements in surfactant and respiratory therapy have decreased the prevalence of retinopathy of prematurity. Diagnosis is usually made in early infancy and severity depends on the degree of prematurity, birth weight, and oxygen therapy. It is thought that hyperoxygenation causes narrowing and spasm of the retinal vessels. Then, after oxygen therapy is stopped, the retinal vessels dilate and new vessels develop in the periphery of the retina and grow into the vitreous body. This neovascularization spontaneously regresses in some patients. However, in other patients, an advanced, cicatricial stage may develop, in which fibrovascular scar tissue forms behind the lens causing retinal detachment. The neovascularization may also lead to vitreous hemorrhage.

On CT, the globe demonstrates increased density secondary to the proliferation of vessels in the retina and

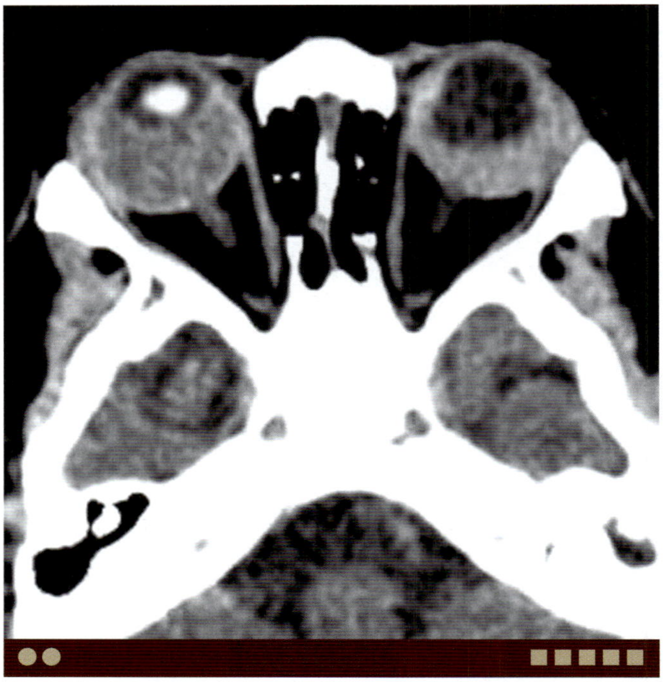

A. Retinopathy of prematurity. Axial CT image demonstrates bilateral microphthalmos. Layering hyperdensity along the posterior globes represent subretinal hemorrhages. Also, a dislocated left lens is identified.

PEARLS

- **Retinopathy of prematurity typically demonstrates bilateral microphthalmos and retinal detachment.**
- **Increased density within the globes occurs secondary to the neovascularization of the retina and vitreous body. Dystrophic calcification may be seen in advanced cases.**
- **The finding of periventricular leukomalacia may be helpful in the diagnosis.**

vitreous body. Typically, bilateral microphthalmos is identified. Calcification is uncommon, except in advanced stages when dystrophic calcification may develop. While this condition is almost always bilateral, the eyes may be affected asymmetrically.

On MRI, increased signal on T2W and T1W images occurs from chronic subretinal hemorrhages. A low-signal retrolental mass may be identified, representing retinal detachment. Evaluation of the brain often demonstrates associated findings of periventricular leukomalacia. There is no or minimal enhancement.

ADDITIONAL IMAGES (B-G)

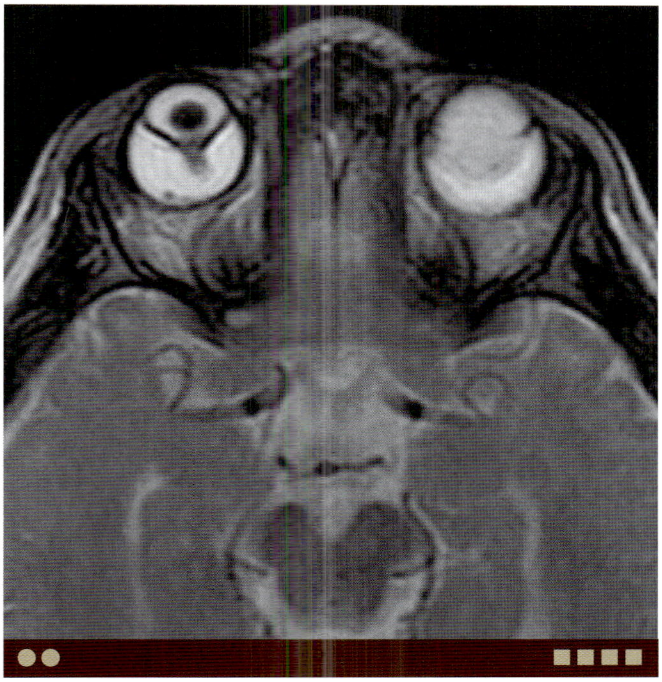

B. Retinopathy of prematurity, same patient as A. Axial T2W MR image demonstrates bilateral microphthalmos. The right globe demonstrates retinal detachment. Bilateral, asymmetric, subretinal hemorrhages are also identified, right larger in size than the left.

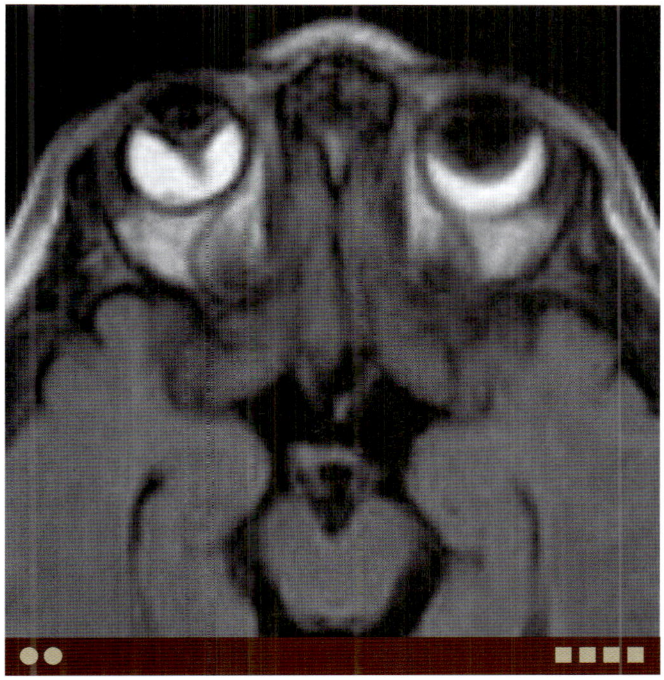

C. Retinopathy of prematurity, same patient as A. Axial FLAIR MR image demonstrates bilateral microphthalmos and increased signal in the posterior globes, representing subretinal hemorrhages.

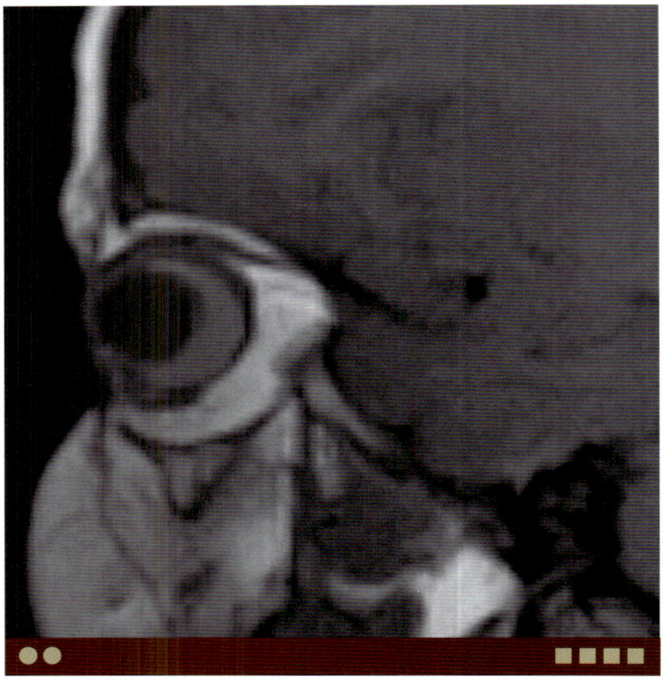

D. Retinopathy of prematurity, same patient as A. Sagittal T1W MR image demonstrates subretinal hemorrhage.

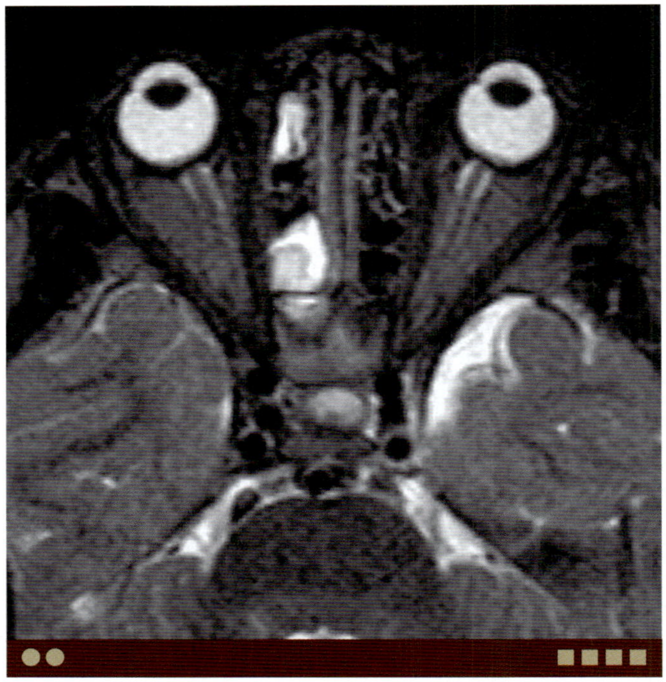

E. Retinopathy of prematurity in a different patient. Axial T2W MR image demonstrates bilateral microphthalmos.

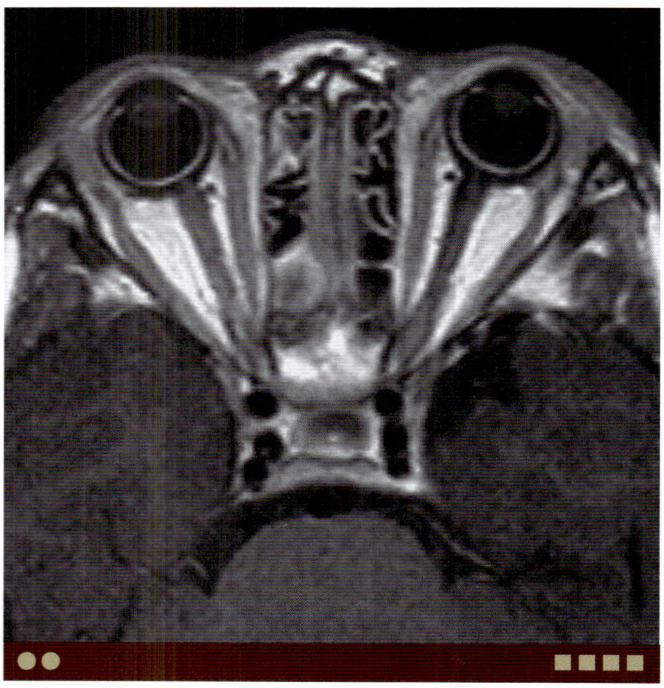

F. Retinopathy of prematurity, same patient as E. Axial postcontrast T1W MR image demonstrates mild enhancement along the retina. No enhancing intraocular mass identified.

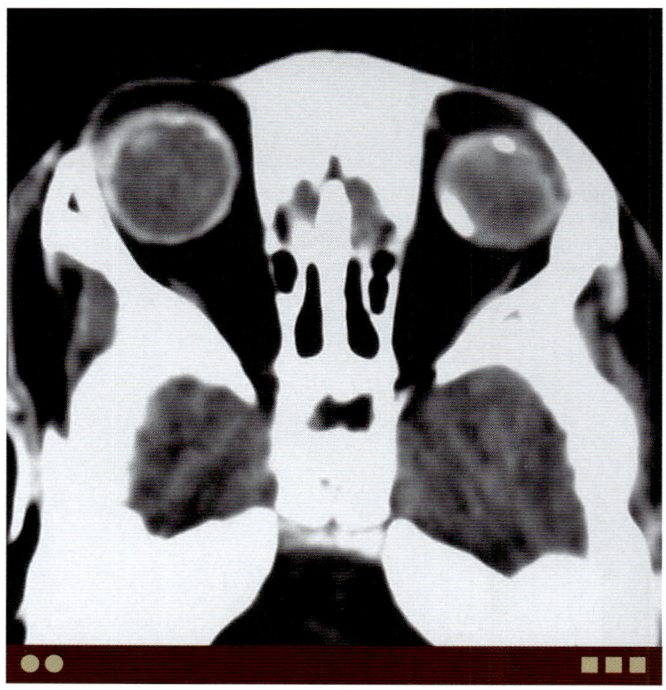

G. Retinopathy of prematurity in a different patient. Axial CT demonstrates dystrophic calcifications in the globes, left more than right.

DIFFERENTIAL DIAGNOSIS IMAGES (H-J)

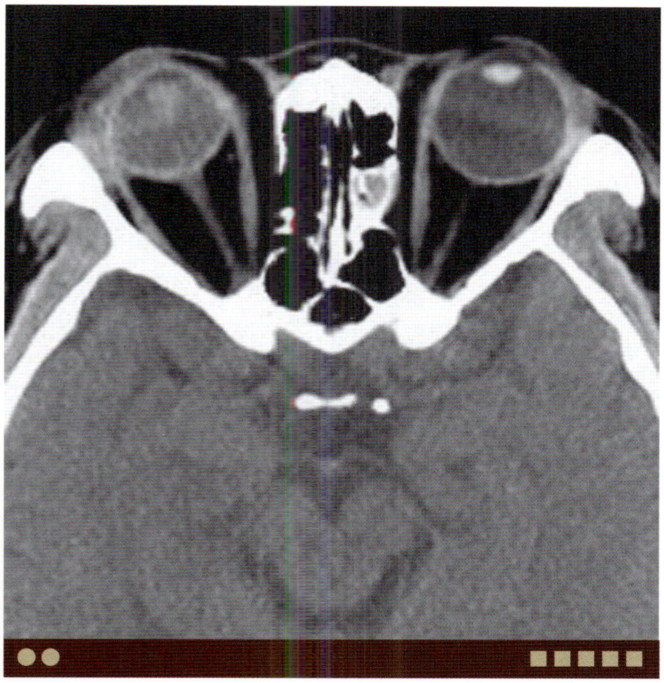

H. PHPV. Axial CT demonstrates right microphthalmos and a hyperdense vitreous body with retinal detachment. No intraocular calcification is present.

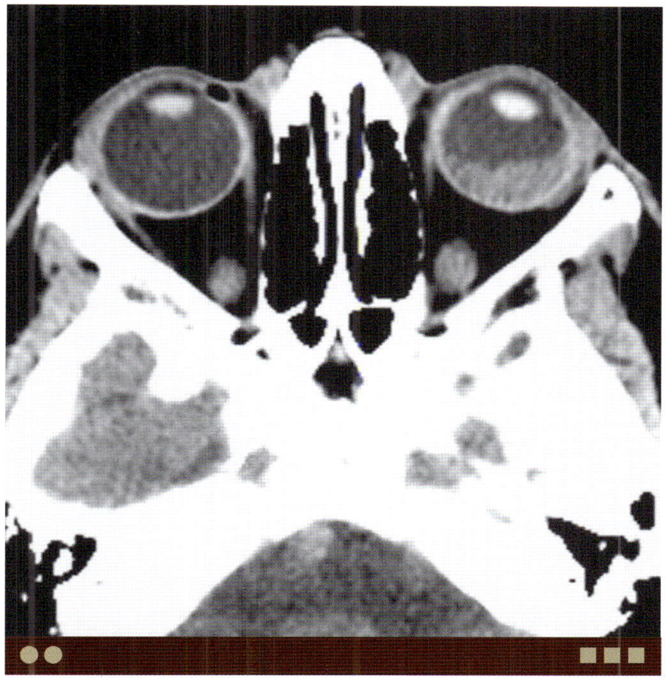

I. Coats disease. Axial CT demonstrates hyperdensity along the posterior wall of the left globe, representing proteinaceous or hemorrhagic subretinal exudate, and no calcification.

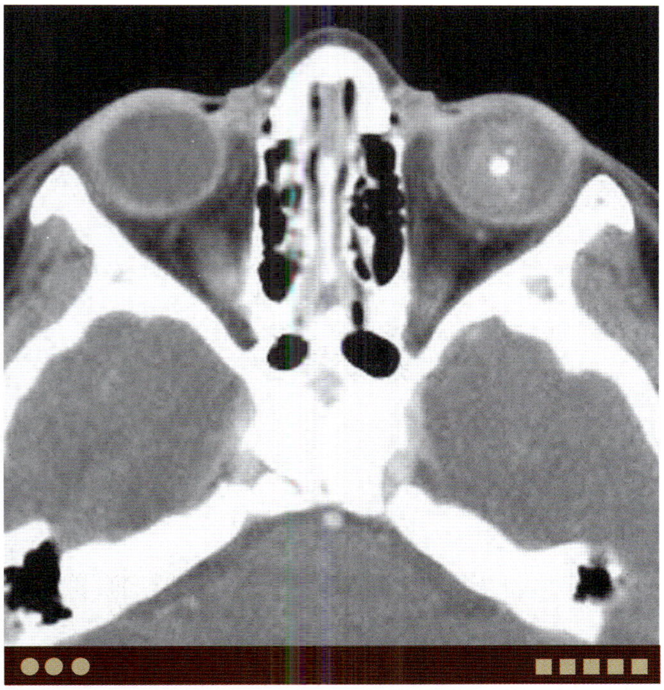

J. Retinoblastoma. Axial CT demonstrates a high-density mass with calcification in the normal-sized left globe.

Case 5–18 Choroidal Osteoma

Hiroki Kato, Benjamin Ludwig, Osamu Sakai

PRESENTATION

New onset of blurry, distorted vision.

FINDINGS

CT demonstrates a plaque-like calcification in the posterior pole of the affected eye.

DIFFERENTIAL DIAGNOSIS

- Optic drusen: Refers to accumulation of mucopolysaccharides and proteinaceous material within the optic disc, which calcifies with advancing age. Optic drusen, however, can also be seen in younger patients.
- Choroidal metastases: Choroidal metastases are fairly common, and typically seen as flat lesions in the posterior one third of the globe. The most common primary sites include breast and lung.
- Choroidal hemangioma: Benign vascular tumor, which is often difficult to distinguish from melanoma on ophthalmologic examination. Isointensity to the vitreous on T2W images combined with strong and early contrast enhancement are helpful in differentiation from uveal melanoma.
- Hyaline plaque: Refers to focal calcification at the insertion of the medial and lateral rectus muscles, which is dystrophic in etiology and seen in older patients.

COMMENTS

This is a 16-year-old adolescent who presented with slowly progressive vision loss in the left eye.

Choroidal osteomas are rare, benign, ossifying, choroidal tumors of unknown etiology. Histopathologic evaluation reveals mature bone with marrow space containing loose fibrovascular tissue. They occur predominantly in young females (90%) without a history of systemic or ocular disease, and are usually unilateral (75%). On ophthalmologic examination, they appear as yellow-white to orange-red plaques and are generally located in the macula or juxtapapillary region around the optic disc extending toward the macula. Variability in color occurs secondary to thinning, depigmentation, and hyperplasia of the overlaying retina pigment epithelium. They are typically oval in shape with well-defined scalloped margins. They may display progressive growth patterns, although regression in size has also been reported. Complications include choroidal neovascularization (CNV), which can result in vision loss and subretinal hemorrhage. Retinal detachment is also common.

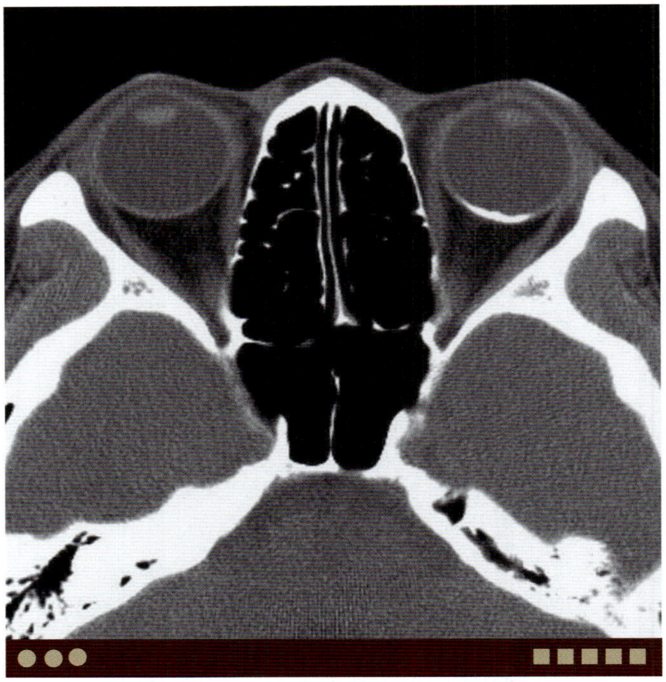

A. Choroidal osteoma. Axial unenhanced CT demonstrates a plaque-like calcification in the posterior pole of the left eye.

Ultrasound and CT are of particular value in diagnosing choroidal osteoma. With B-mode sonography, choroidal osteoma shows increased echogenicity posteriorly within the globe, with posterior acoustic shadowing, creating the "pseudo-optic nerve appearance." On CT, choroidal osteomas are flat calcified lesions, less than 2 mm in thickness, within the posterior pole of the globe. They are typically located in the juxtapapillary region, and typically do not involve the center of the optic disc, which aids in differentiation from optic drusen.

Given their benign nature, choroidal osteomas are typically followed clinically. Identification of complications, particularly choroidal neovascularization, warrants treatment given the risk of vision loss.

PEARLS

- **Choroidal osteoma occurs predominantly in young females and is typically unilateral.**
- **B-mode ultrasound demonstrates increased echogenicity within the posterior globe, with posterior acoustic shadowing.**
- **CT demonstrates a flat calcified lesion within the juxtapapillary region of the posterior globe.**

ADDITIONAL IMAGE

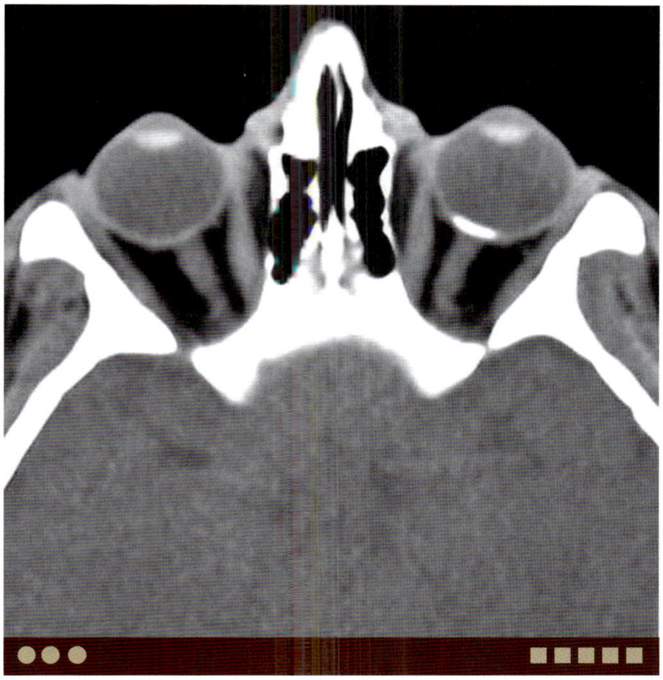

B. Choroidal osteoma in a different patient. Axial unenhanced CT demonstrates a plaque-like calcification in the posterior pole of the left eye.

DIFFERENTIAL DIAGNOSIS IMAGES (C-G)

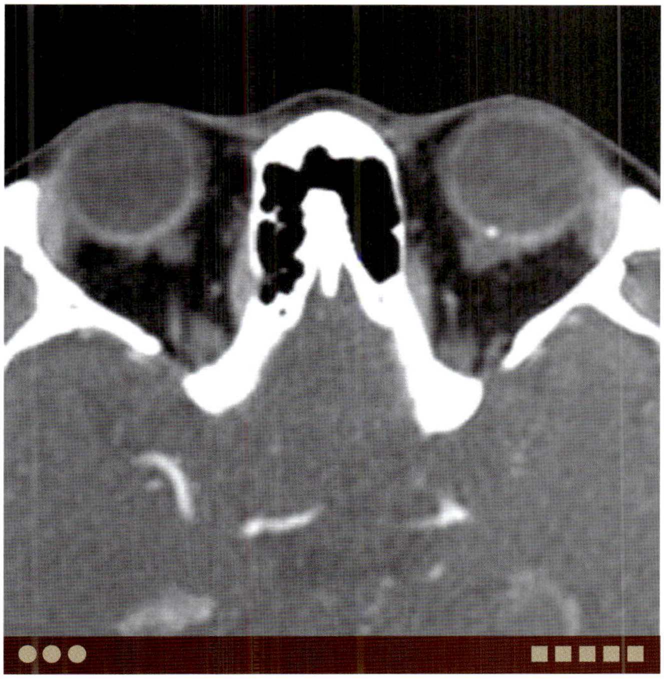

C. Optic drusen. Axial contrast-enhanced CT demonstrates a focal calcification within the optic disc in the posterior pole of the left eye.

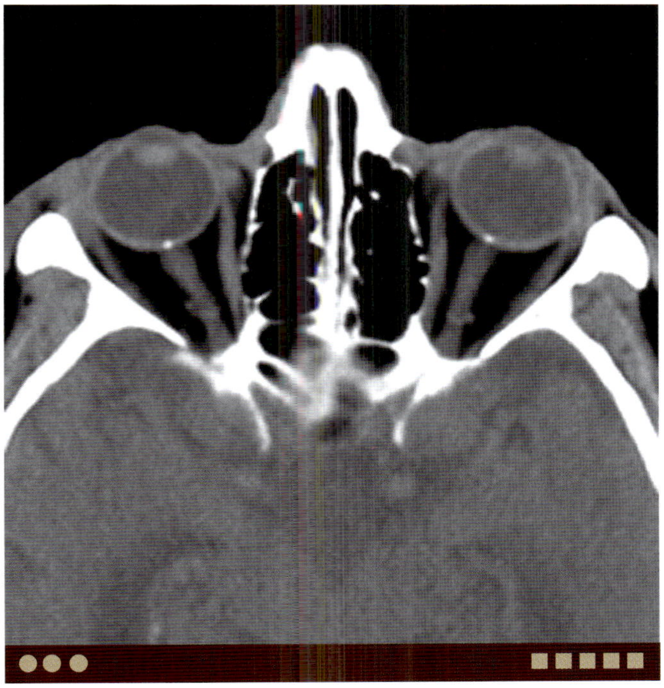

D. Optic drusen in a different patient. Axial unenhanced CT demonstrates a focal calcification within the optic discs in the posterior pole of the globes bilaterally.

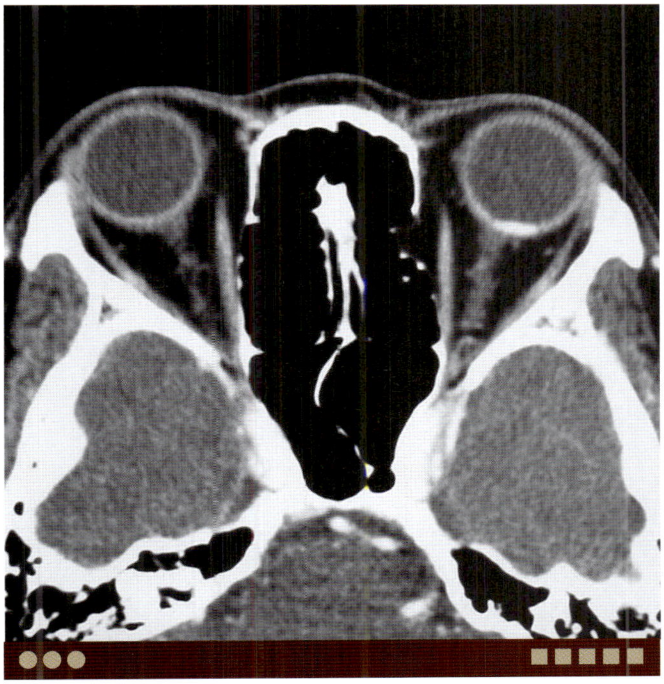

E. Choroidal hemangioma. Axial contrast-enhanced CT demonstrates a flat, avidly enhancing lesion in the posterior pole of the left eye.

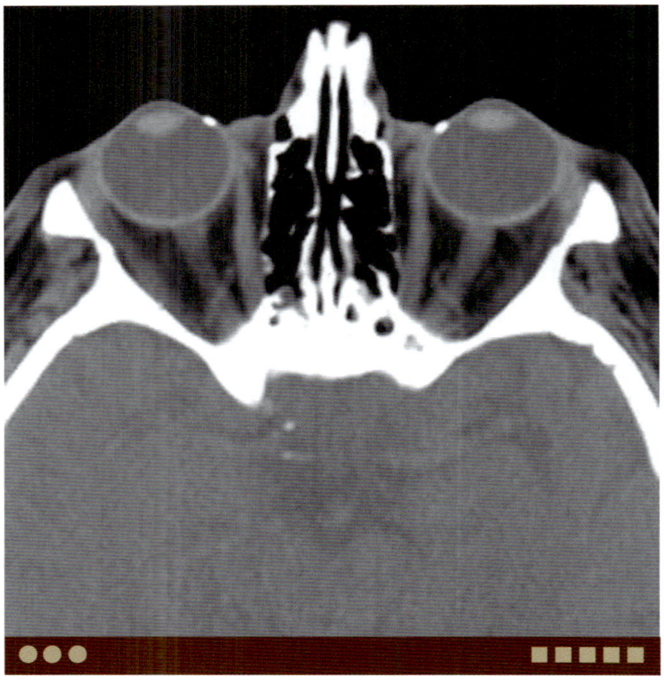

F. Hyaline plaque. Axial unenhanced CT demonstrates a focal calcification at the insertion of the medial rectus muscle bilaterally.

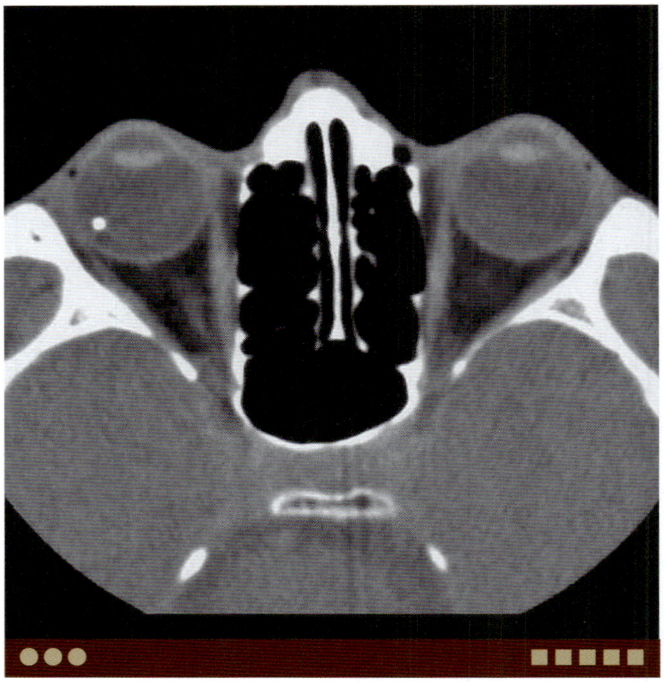

G. Foreign body. Axial unenhanced CT demonstrates a high-density foreign body in the right globe.

Case 5–19 Vogt-Koyanagi-Harada Syndrome

Akifumi Fujita, Benjamin Ludwig, Osamu Sakai

PRESENTATION

Visual disturbance due to retinal detachment.

FINDINGS

Postcontrast CT shows diffuse enhancement of the thickened choroid. MRI shows bilateral choroidal thickening and mild retinal detachment.

DIFFERENTIAL DIAGNOSIS

- Uveitis: Uveitis secondary to infection is typically unilateral. Other systemic etiologies of uveitis may involve both eyes, including autoimmune and inflammatory conditions.
- Sarcoidosis: This condition typically shows bilateral ocular involvement of the uvea, but retinal detachment is rare. Extraocular findings are also common, including dacryoadenitis, orbital myositis, and optic neuritis.
- Metastatic tumors: Choroidal metastases are often seen as a flat mass in the posterior one third of the globe, where the choroidal arteries penetrate the wall and tumor cells are entrapped.

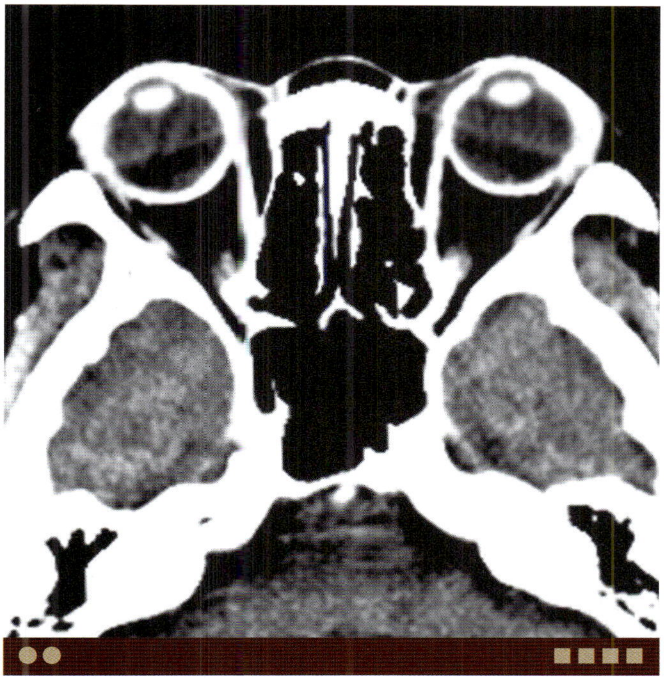

A. VKH syndrome. Axial postcontrast CT demonstrates diffuse bilateral choroidal thickening with marked enhancement.

COMMENTS

This is a 47-year-old woman with visual disturbance due to retinal detachment. Although neurological, auditory, and cutaneous findings of the condition were not clinically apparent, bilateral ocular involvement is compatible with diagnostic criteria of Vogt-Koyanagi-Harada (VKH) syndrome.

VKH syndrome affects melanocyte-containing structures, and is idiopathic, but thought to be potentially autoimmune in nature. Patients are most commonly of Asian descent, and present with neurologic symptoms (including fever, headache, vertigo, etc), followed by visual (vision loss, pain) and auditory complaints (hearing disturbance, tinnitus, vertigo), and, later, cutaneous manifestations (vitiligo, alopecia).

Imaging findings in VKH syndrome include bilateral symmetric choroidal thickening with enhancement on postcontrast images, secondary to chorioretinitis. VKH syndrome typically causes retinal detachment or pigment epithelial detachment, or both, and subretinal fibrosis and choroidal neovascularization. On MRI, retinal detachments are characterized as areas of hyperintensity on T1W images, with variable intensity on T2W images.

Uveitis may be infectious in etiology secondary to tuberculosis, toxoplasmosis, or cytomegalovirus. Sarcoidosis and other systemic diseases are also important differential considerations.

PEARLS

- **VKH syndrome results from bilateral granulomatous panuveitis, and is most likely autoimmune in etiology.**
- **Diffuse choroidal thickening, choroidal enhancement, and bilateral retinal detachments are common imaging findings.**

ADDITIONAL IMAGES (B-D)

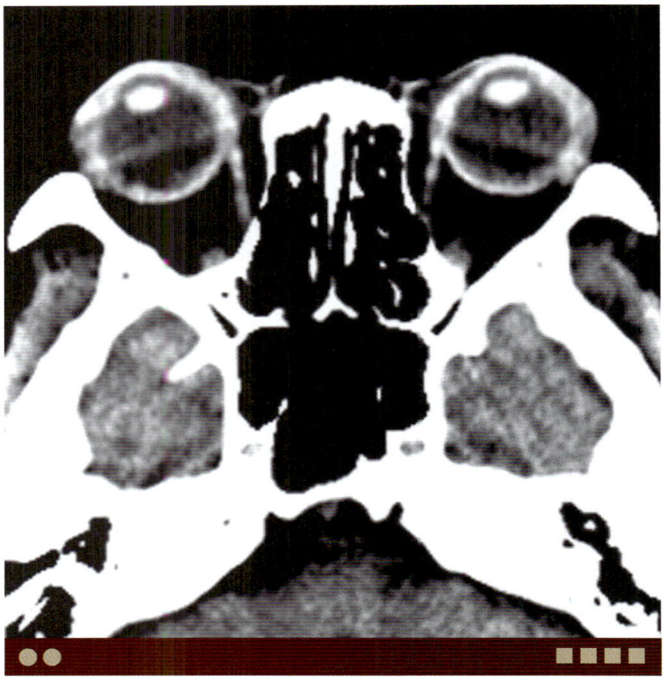

B. VKH syndrome, same patient as A. Axial noncontrast CT demonstrates diffuse bilateral choroidal thickening.

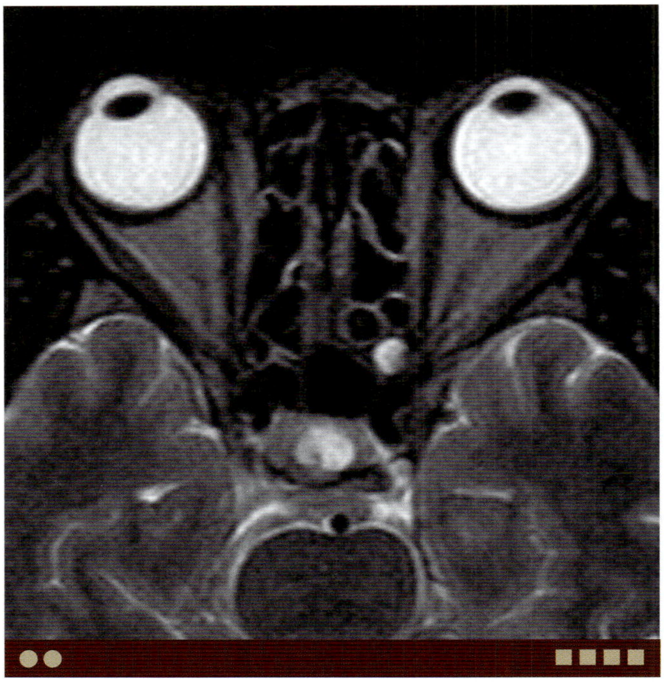

C. VKH syndrome, same patient as A. Axial T2W image demonstrates diffuse choroidal thickening bilaterally.

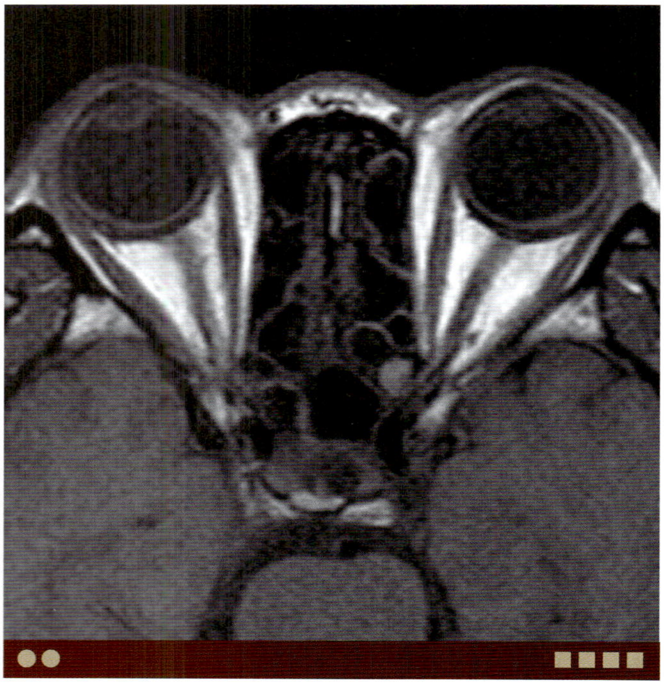

D. VKH syndrome, same patient as A. Axial T1W image demonstrates diffuse choroidal thickening bilaterally. Mild retinal detachment is also noted.

DIFFERENTIAL DIAGNOSIS IMAGES (E-G)

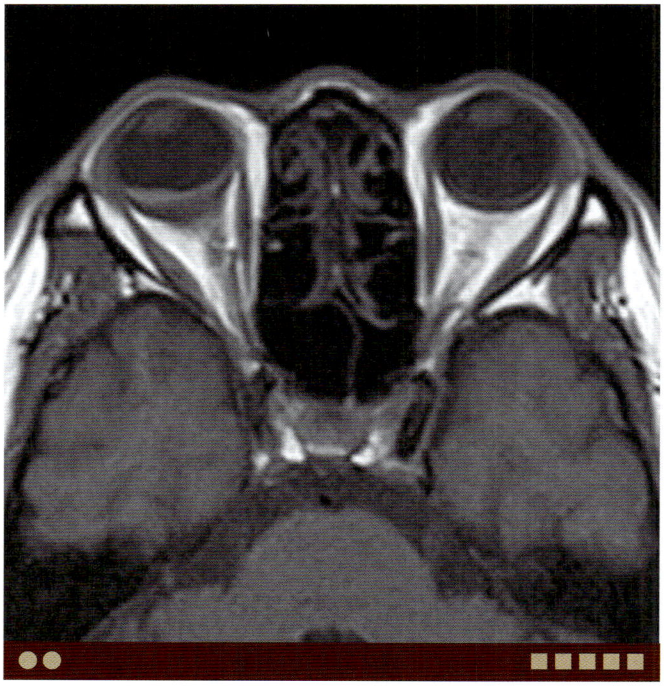

E. Choroidal metastasis. Axial T1W image demonstrates a broad-based high-signal mass in the posterior aspect of the right globe. A primary lung neoplasm was subsequently identified.

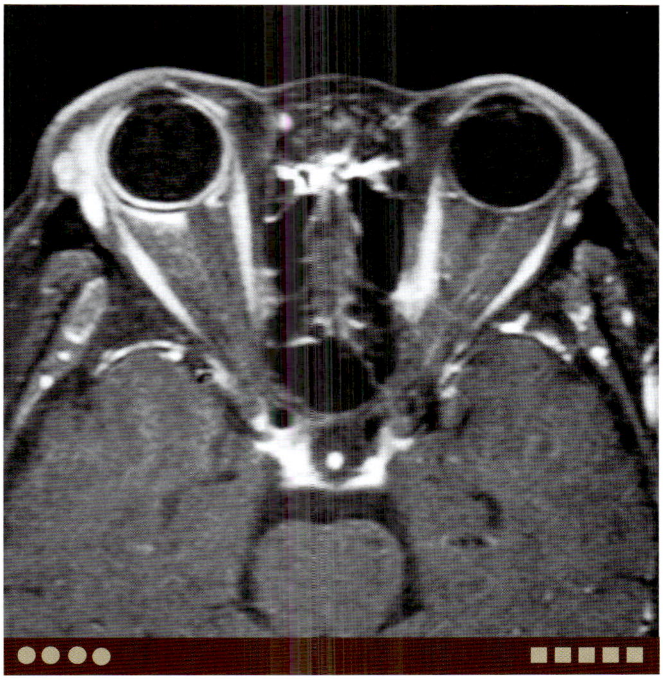

F. Scleritis. Axial postcontrast fat-suppressed T1W MR image demonstrates thickening and abnormal enhancement of the sclera of the right globe. Note abnormal enhancement of the right lacrimal gland as well as in the region of the Tenon's capsule, immediately posterior to the globe.

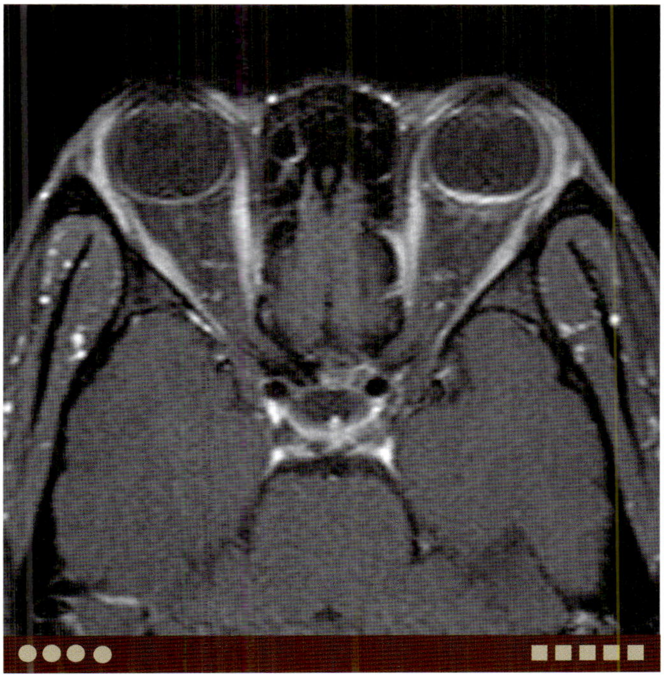

G. Posterior scleritis. Axial postcontrast fat-suppressed T1W MR image demonstrates abnormal enhancement of the thickened posterior sclera of the left globe.

Case 5–20 Coloboma

Osamu Sakai, Francisco Contreras

PRESENTATION

Leukocoria.

FINDINGS

CT and MRI demonstrate a focal defect of the globe, often in the posterior wall, and with an out-pouching vitreous.

DIFFERENTIAL DIAGNOSIS

- Morning glory anomaly: Morning glory disc anomaly is a congenital anomaly of the optic disc that is typically unilateral.
- Staphyloma: Staphyloma is an abnormal protrusion through a weak point in the globe due to weakening of outer layer of the globe (cornea or sclera) by an inflammatory or degenerative condition. Posterior staphyloma is commonly seen and associated with myopia.
- Trauma: Deformity of the globe and protrusion of the vitreous can be seen as a result of trauma, usually with apparent history of trauma.
- "Leukocoria" differential diagnoses: Retinoblastoma, persistent hyperplastic primary vitreous, retinopathy of prematurity, congenital cataract, and Coats disease are major diseases or conditions causing leukocoria. Imaging has an important role to exclude retinoblastoma.

COMMENTS

This is a 4-year-old boy with leukocoria.

Coloboma is a congenital defect of the optic disc manifesting as an out-pouching of the vitreous through a focal defect of the wall of the globe; often in the posterior wall near the optic nerve, head insertion. However, different structures within the globe, including the choroid, iris, lens, optic nerve, and retina, may be involved. This is typically caused by a lack of fusion of the superior embryonic fissures. This condition may be bilateral and other eye abnormalities may be present, such as microphthalmia, glaucoma, nystagmus or strabismus.

The most common presenting symptom is decreased visual acuity which can lead to microphthalmos, optic atrophy, and strabismus. In patients presenting with leukocoria, imaging is performed to exclude retinoblastoma and also to differentiate this from other conditions that can cause leukocoria.

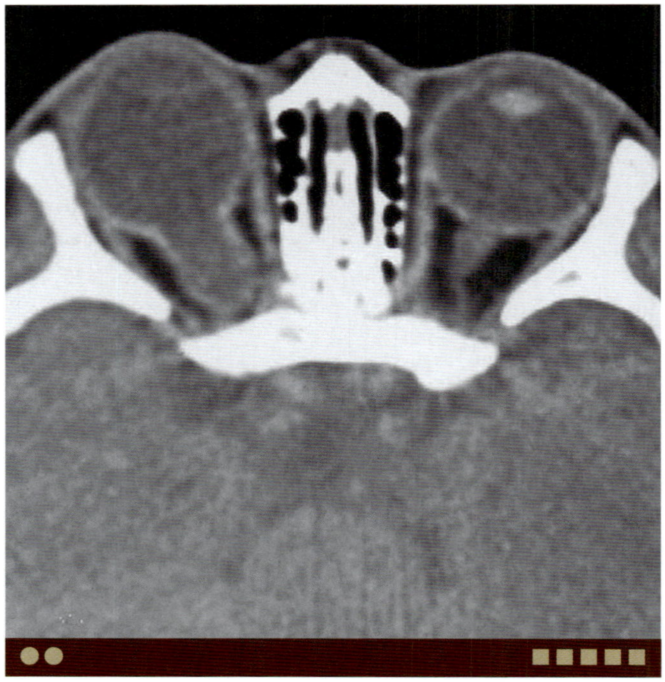

A. Coloboma. Axial noncontrast CT demonstrates a defect of the posterior wall of the right globe resulting in the characteristic vitreous-containing funnel-shaped deformity in the posterior right glove oriented along the axis of the optic nerve.

Colobomas are associated with various congenital malformation syndromes, and can be associated with a mutation in the PAX2 gene. Particularly, coloboma is closely associated with CNS anomalies, often mid-line anomalies. Imaging evaluation of the brain is, therefore, necessary to identify extraorbital pathology.

CT and MRI demonstrate a typical funnel-shaped defect oriented along the axis of the optic nerve. The appearance of a posterior wall defect or cystic-appearing

PEARLS

- **Coloboma is a congenital focal defect in the wall of the globe, often near the optic nerve head insertion.**
- **Colobomas are associated with various congenital malformation syndromes, and can be associated with a mutation in the PAX2 gene.**
- **Imaging of the brain is necessary to look for CNS anomalies, which are often associated with colobomas.**
- **In patients presenting with leukocoria, it is important to exclude retinoblastoma as the cause.**

lesion (retrobulbar colobomatous cyst) is helpful in excluding a neoplastic process. In addition to these findings, MRI can demonstrate irregularity/deformity of the surface of the retina, which commonly corresponds to the fundoscopic findings.

Morning glory disc anomaly is a congenital anomaly of the optic disc that is typically unilateral. The term "morning glory" was coined for its ophthalmoscopic resemblance to the morning glory flower. It is more common in women than men and is less common in African-Americans than Caucasians. This variant also demonstrates a funnel-shaped excavation, but is typically larger than colobomas and will usually demonstrate a central tuft, a glial tissue within the defect.

ADDITIONAL IMAGES (B-G)

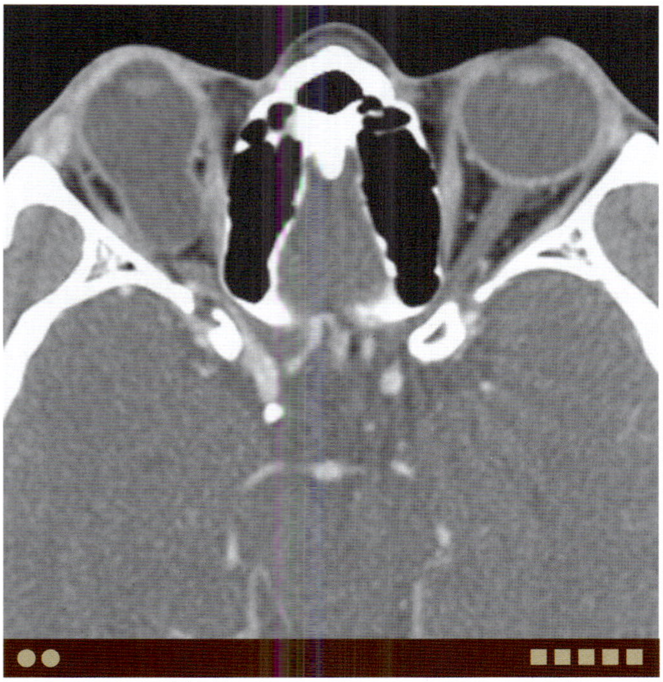

B. Coloboma in a different patient. Axial contrast-enhanced CT demonstrates a funnel-shaped defect in the posterior right globe oriented along the axis of the optic nerve.

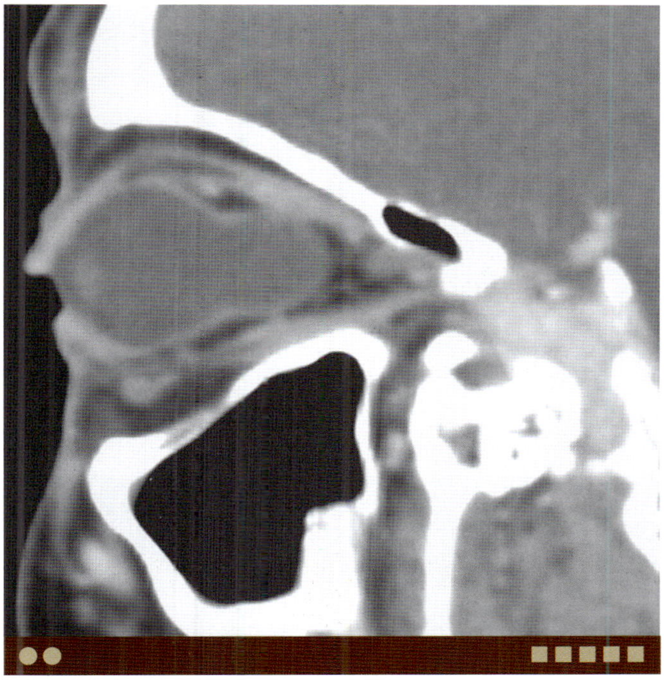

C. Coloboma, same patient as B. Sagittal contrast-enhanced CT demonstrates a funnel-shaped defect in the posterior globe oriented along the axis of the optic nerve.

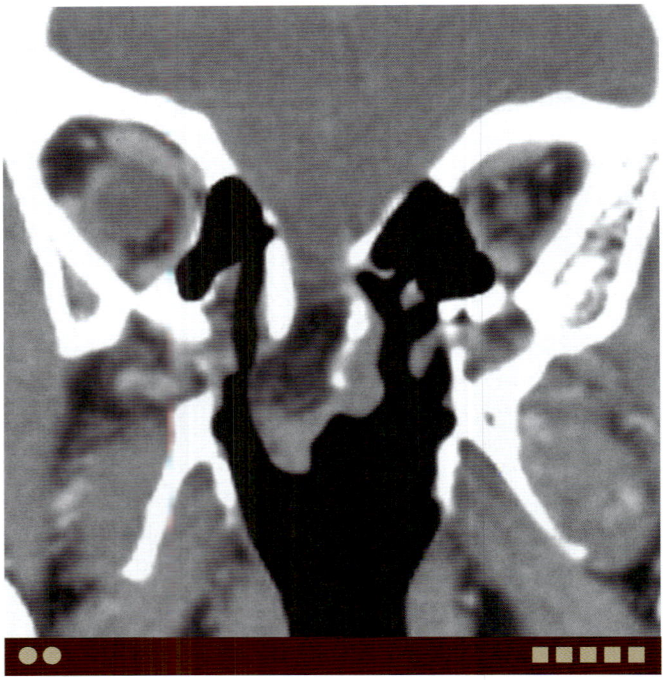

D. Coloboma, same patient as B. Coronal contrast-enhanced CT demonstrates a funnel-shaped defect in the anterior skull base and protrusion of the intracranial structures, cephalocele.

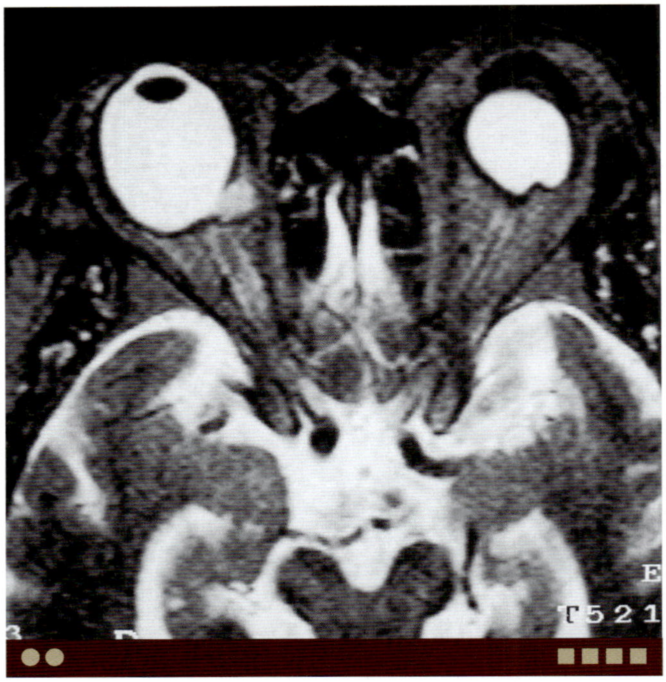

E. Coloboma in a different patient. Axial T2W MR image demonstrates AP elongation of the right globe with a retrobulbar colobomatous cyst, medial to the optic nerve. Note that the deformity is also present in the left globe.

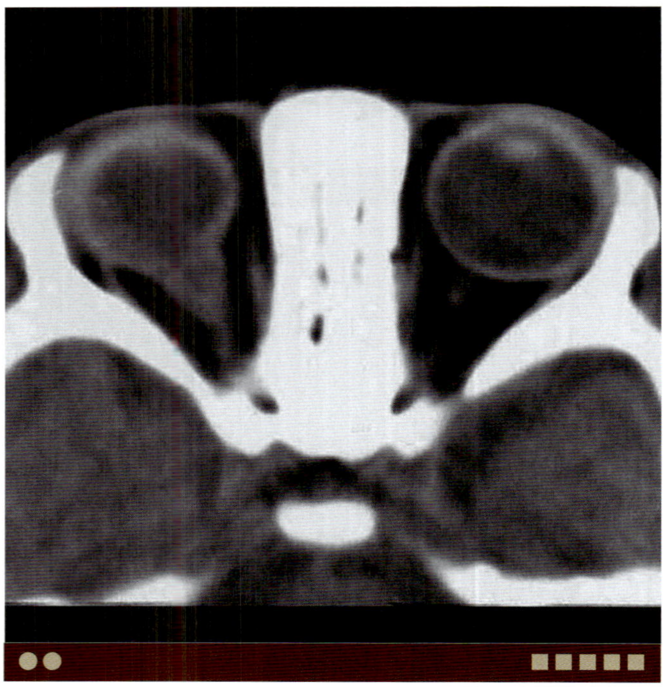

F. Morning glory anomaly. Axial noncontrast-enhanced CT demonstrates a funnel-shaped deformity of the right globe oriented along the axis of the optic nerve. Note the thickening of the retinal surface along the globe.

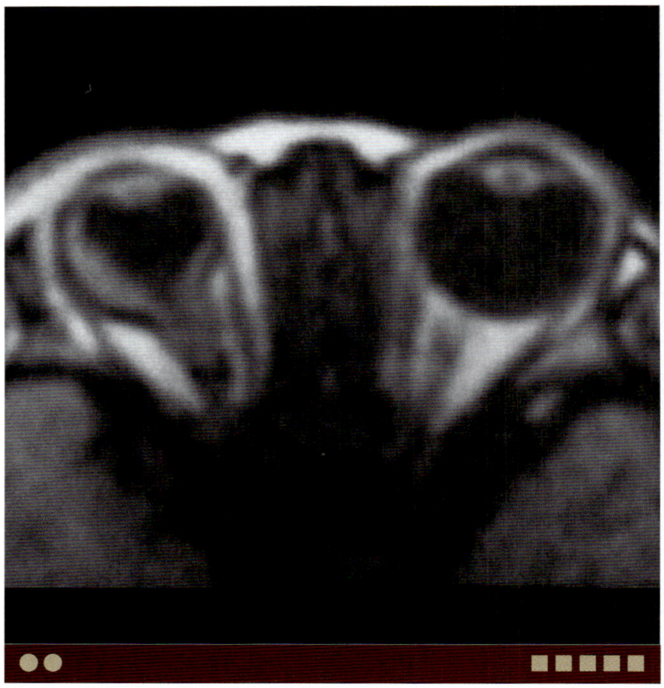

G. Morning glory anomaly, same patient as F. Axial T1W MR image demonstrates a funnel-shaped defect in the posterior right globe oriented along the axis of the optic nerve with thickening/irregularity of the retinal surface.

DIFFERENTIAL DIAGNOSIS IMAGE

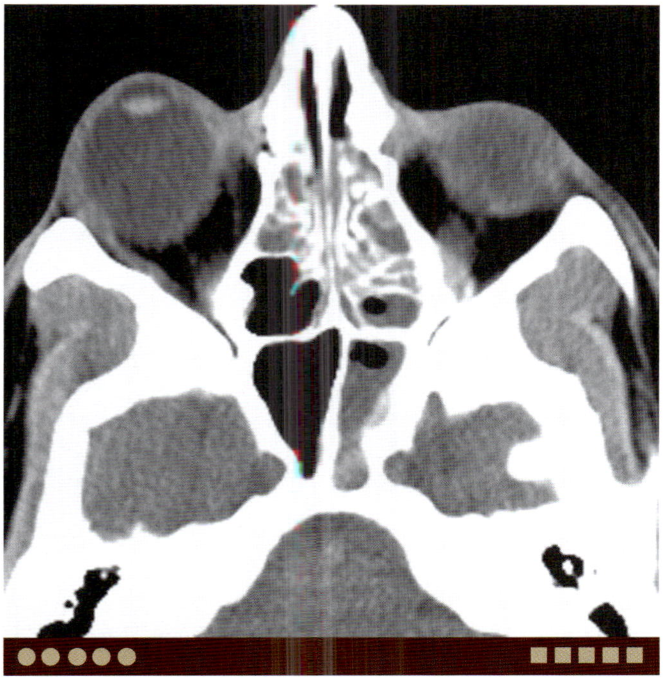

H. Staphyloma. Axial noncontrast-enhanced CT demonstrates AP elongation of the right globe.

Chapter 6

SUPRAHYOID NECK

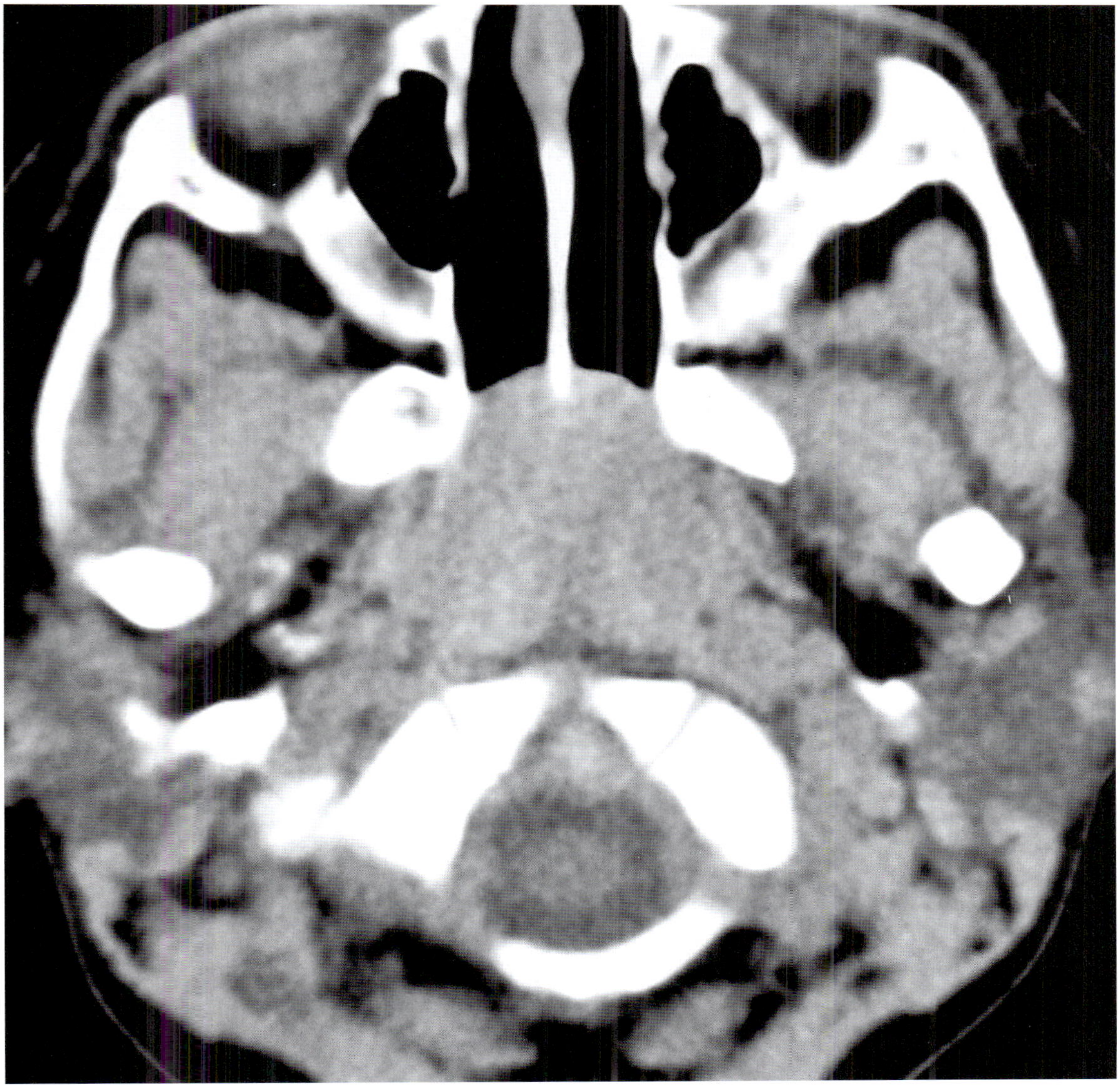

Case 6–1 Adenoid Hypertrophy

Osamu Sakai, Cory Siegel

PRESENTATION

Mouth breathing.

FINDINGS

Computed tomography (CT) demonstrates enlarged adenoids.

DIFFERENTIAL DIAGNOSIS

- Nasopharyngeal carcinoma: This is a common malignant tumor in people from south Asia and Africa. This tumor often causes significant submucosal extension. Ipsilateral mastoid opacification raises possibility of an underlying tumor.
- Lymphoma: Lymphoma in the nasopharynx is usually B-cell non-Hodgkin type. Imaging findings are often very similar to enlarged adenoids and nasopharyngeal carcinoma. Bone marrow signal abnormality is often seen in the clivus.

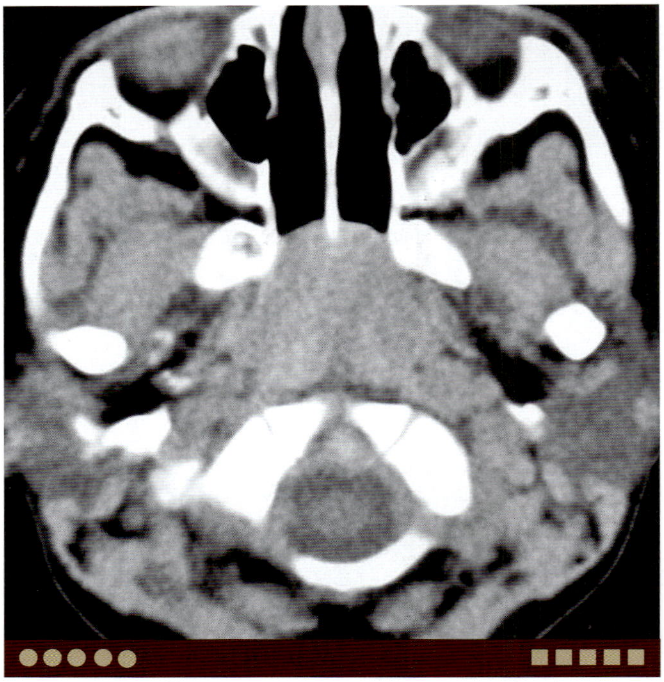

A. Adenoid hypertrophy. Axial noncontrast CT demonstrates enlarged adenoids.

COMMENTS

This is a 3-year-old girl with difficulty in breathing through the nose.

Adenoids, nasopharyngeal tonsils are located in the roof of the nasopharynx. Very little lymphoid tissue is present in the nasopharynx at birth, but these structures start increasing in size during the first year of life. Sometimes, they can fill the entire nasopharynx extending to the choana, and subsequently can cause difficulty in breathing through the nose. The adenoids usually reach their greatest size around 5 years of age, and then decrease in size. In fourth and fifth decades, they become very small, however, they still can be seen even in sixth or seventh decades. If adenoids are not seen in children, immunodeficiency has to be suspected. Enlarged adenoids can obstruct the nasal airway and eustachian tubes and therefore, may cause sinusitis and otitis media, respectively.

Adenoids demonstrate similar density to the muscles on CT, however, they enhance after contrast and thus are differentiated from the prevertebral muscle. On magnetic resonance imaging (MRI), they are isointense to muscle on T1W and hyperintense with respect to muscle on T2W, and show enhancement after contrast administration. In children, enlargement of the lateral retropharyngeal node (node of Rouvière) is commonly seen with adenoid hypertrophy. Lateral retropharyngeal nodes larger than 8 mm in diameter in adults are abnormal.

Lymphoma and other lymphoproliferative disorders show similar density and signal to adenoid hypertrophy. Preserved striated pattern within the enlarged adenoids suggest non-neoplastic hypertrophy. However, endoscopy and biopsy are needed to make a definitive diagnosis. Enlarged adenoids, bilateral multiple lymphoepithelial cysts in the parotid gland and cervical lymphadenopathy are the triad for imaging findings of HIV infection.

PEARLS

- **Prominent adenoids are often seen as a normal finding in children.**
- **Imaging findings of adenoid hypertrophy are similar to lymphoma and other lymphoproliferative disorders. Preserved striated pattern within the enlarged adenoids suggests non-neoplastic hypertrophy.**
- **Nasopharyngeal carcinoma and lymphoma may be almost completely submucosal lesions without apparent mucosal abnormality.**

ADDITIONAL IMAGES (B-F)

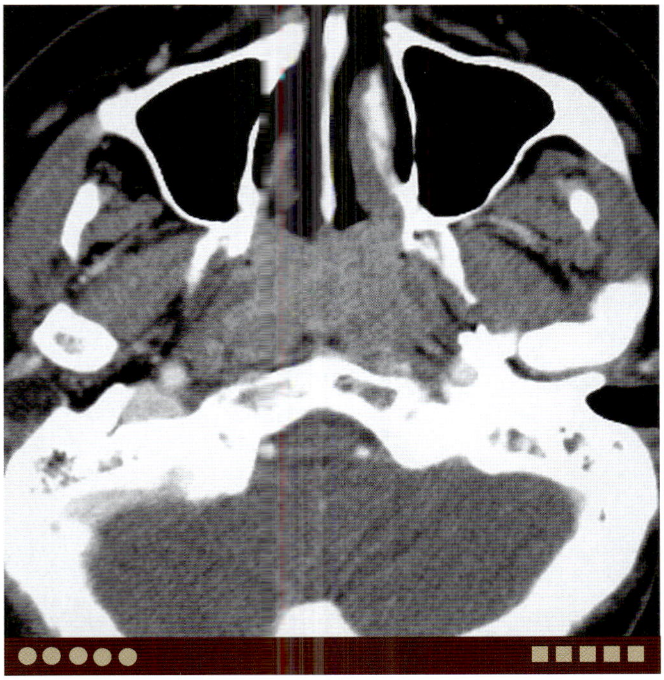

B. **Adenoid hypertrophy** in a different patient. Axial contrast-enhanced CT demonstrates mildly enhancing enlarged adenoids.

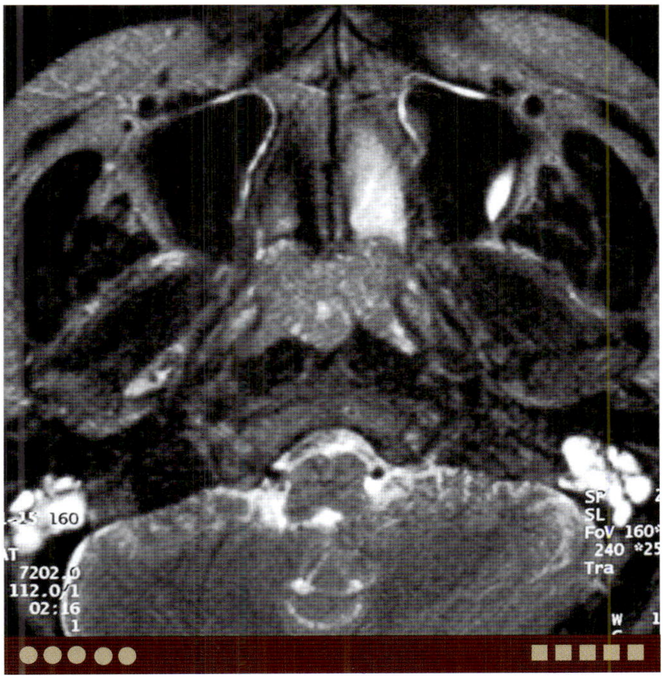

C. Adenoid hypertrophy, same patient as B. Axial T2W MR image demonstrates enlarged adenoids without invasive changes. Note opacified mastoid air cells bilaterally.

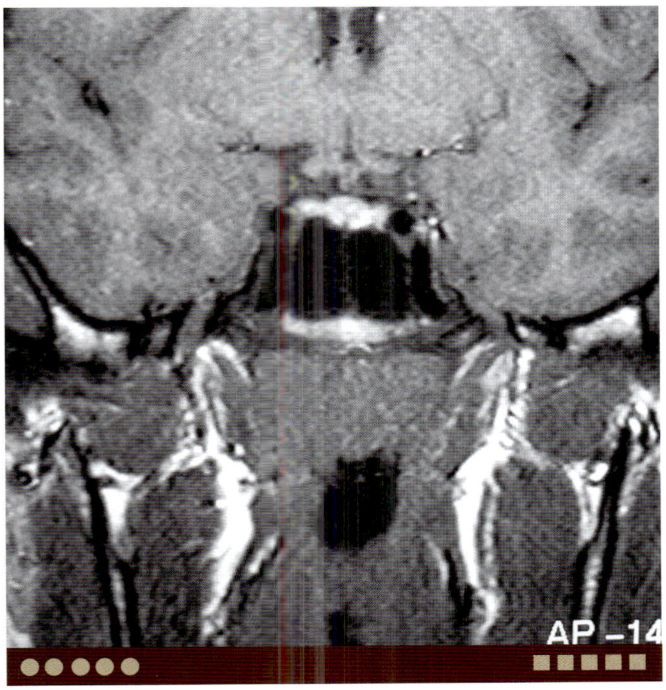

D. **Adenoid hypertrophy** in a different patient. Coronal T1W MR image demonstrates enlarged adenoids isointense to the muscle.

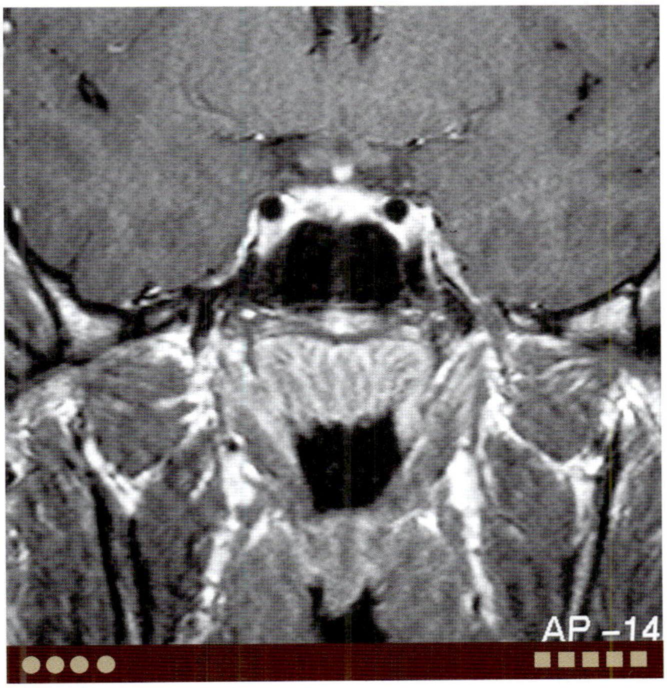

E. Adenoid hypertrophy, same patient as D. Coronal postcontrast T1W MR image demonstrates striated appearance of the enlarged adenoids.

DIFFERENTIAL DIAGNOSIS IMAGES (G-J)

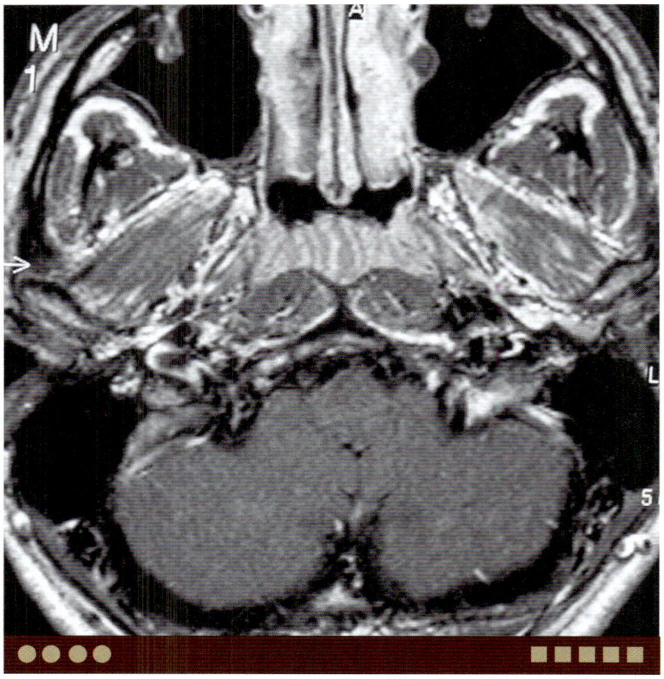

F. Adenoid hypertrophy, same patient as D. Axial postcontrast T1W MR image also demonstrates preserved striation within the enlarged adenoids.

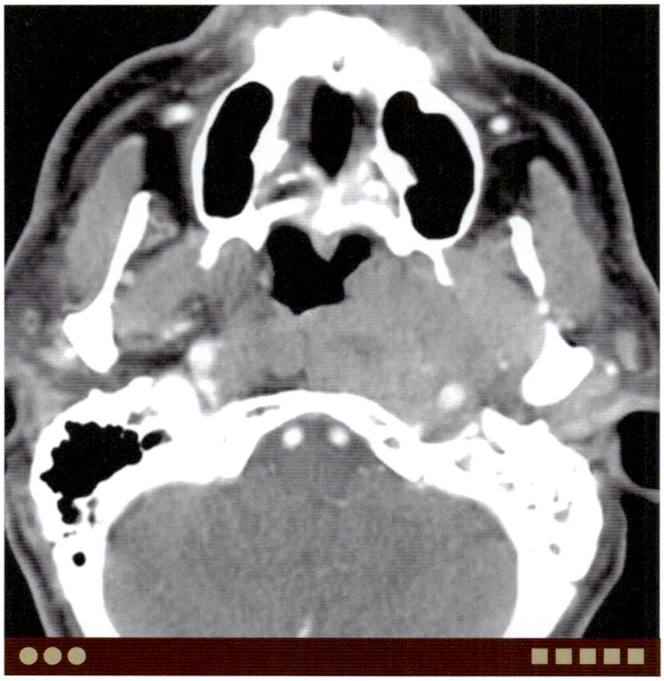

G. **Nasopharyngeal carcinoma**. Axial contrast-enhanced CT demonstrates fullness of the left nasopharynx and obliteration of the fossa of Rosenmüller. Note opacification of the left mastoid air cells. Loss of the left parapharyngeal fat indicates tumor invasion.

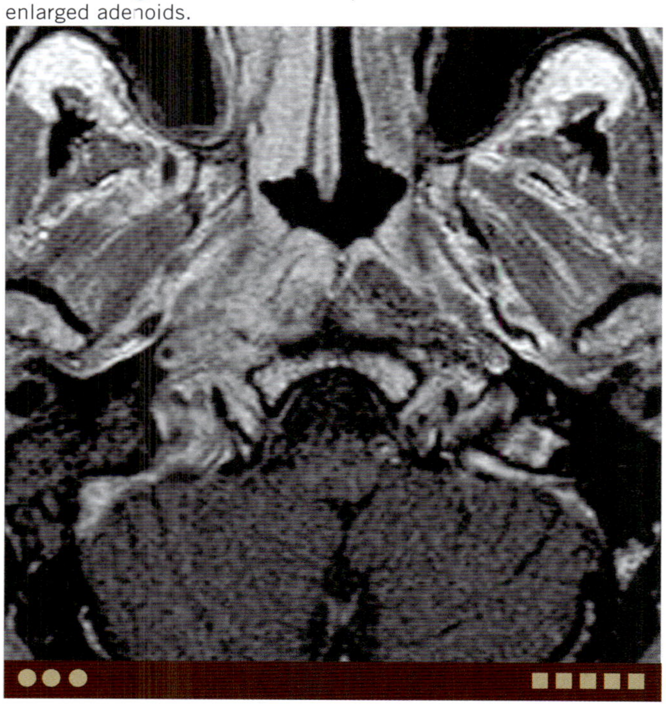

H. **Nasopharyngeal carcinoma** in a different patient. Axial postcontrast T1W MR image demonstrates an ill-defined enhancing lesion in the right nasopharynx centered in the fossa of Rosenmüller and involving the torus tubarius and eustachian tube. Note invasion to the right longus colli muscle and encasement of the right internal carotid artery.

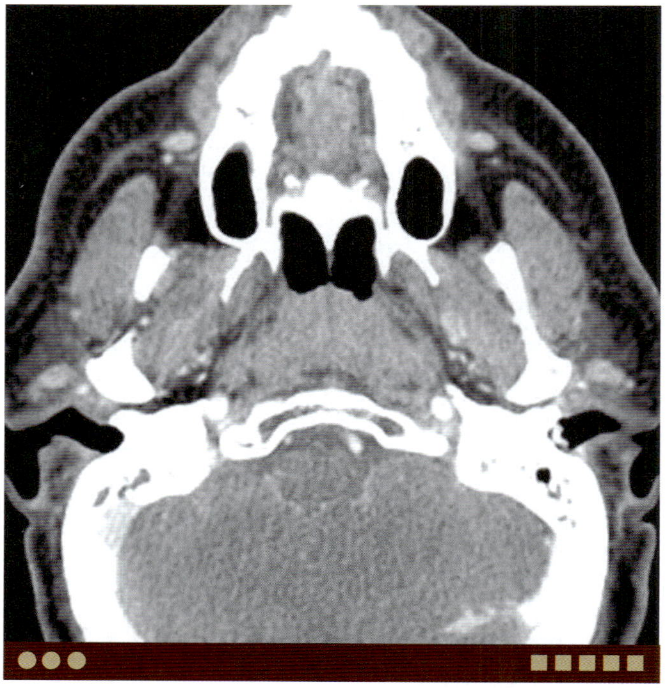

I. **Lymphoma**. Axial contrast-enhanced CT demonstrates symmetric fullness of the nasopharynx, almost identical finding to non-neoplastic lymphoid hypertrophy.

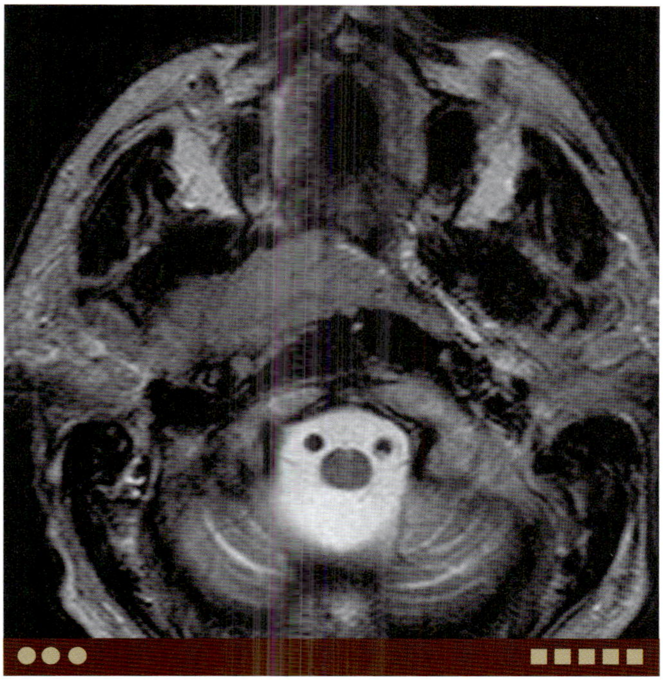

J. Lymphoma in a different patient. Axial T2W MR image demonstrates an intermediate homogeneous signal lesion centered in the right fossa of Rosenmüller. Note involvement of the right parapharyngeal and masticator spaces as well as prevertebral space.

Case 6–2 Tornwaldt Cyst

Osamu Sakai, Cory Siegel

PRESENTATION

An incidental finding.

FINDINGS

CT and MRI demonstrate a cystic lesion in the nasopharynx in midline.

DIFFERENTIAL DIAGNOSIS

- Mucous retention cyst: This usually locates off-midline.
- Pleomorphic adenoma: Its appearance on noncontrast-enhanced CT and MRI may be similar to Tornwaldt cyst. However, this shows enhancement after contrast administration.

COMMENTS

This is a 62-year-old woman originally referred for a headache.

Tornwaldt cyst is a cystic lesion seen in the nasopharynx in the midline. It is a notochord remnant and is seen in about 3% of adults. It is usually asymptomatic, however, sometimes it becomes infected and results in suppurative discharge, halitosis, pain, and odynophagia, at which point it is called Tornwaldt disease.

Tornwaldt cyst is located in the midline superficial to the superior constrictor muscles and between the longus colli muscles. It can be differentiated from a mucous retention cyst and epithelial tumors by location because the latter tend to occur off-midline.

On CT, Tornwaldt cyst usually demonstrates low density, however, it may be difficult to be identified if it is small. On MRI, it is easily seen as a cystic lesion between the longus colli muscles, demonstrating high signal on T2W images and low-to-intermediate signals on T1W images. They range in size from 2 to 10 mm in diameter. With increase in protein concentration, it shows higher signal on T1W and lower signal on T2W images, and higher density on CT. In this region, punctuate calcification in the pharyngeal bursa is often seen, which usually has no clinical significance.

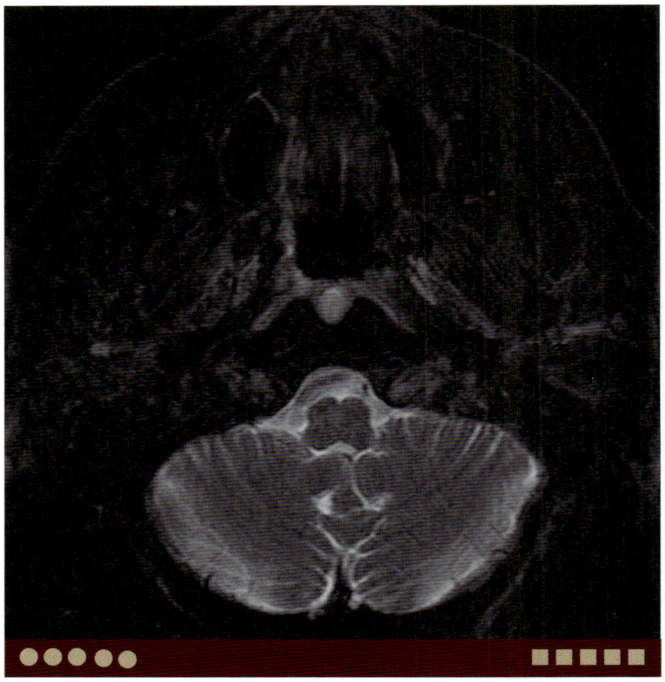

A. Tornwaldt cyst. Axial fat-suppressed T2W MR image demonstrates a round high-signal lesion in the nasopharynx in midline, between the longus colli muscles.

PEARLS

- **Tornwaldt cyst is a developmental cystic lesion seen in the midline of the nasopharynx.**
- **It shows variable signal on MRI and density on CT depending on protein concentration of its content.**
- **Usually there is no clinical significance, however, sometimes it is infected and causes suppurative discharge, halitosis, pain, and odynophagia.**

ADDITIONAL IMAGES (B-G)

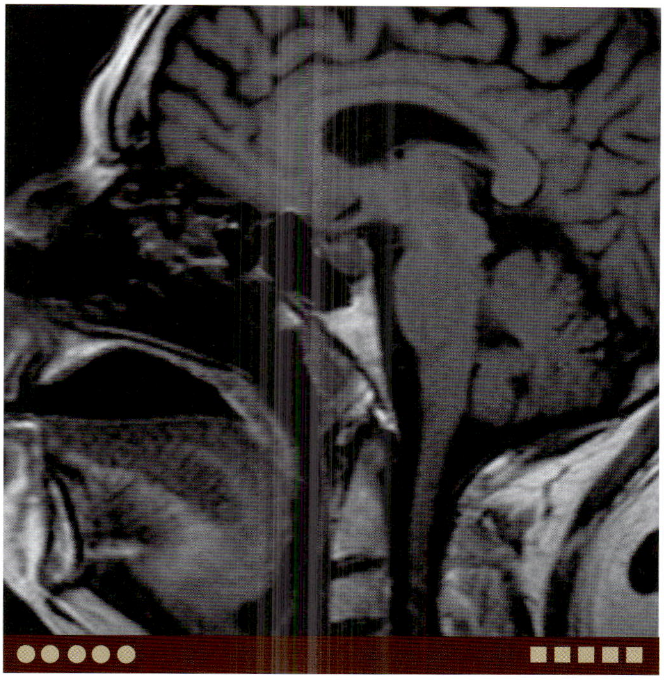

B. Tornwaldt cyst, same patient as A. Sagittal T1W image demonstrates the lesion showing low signal.

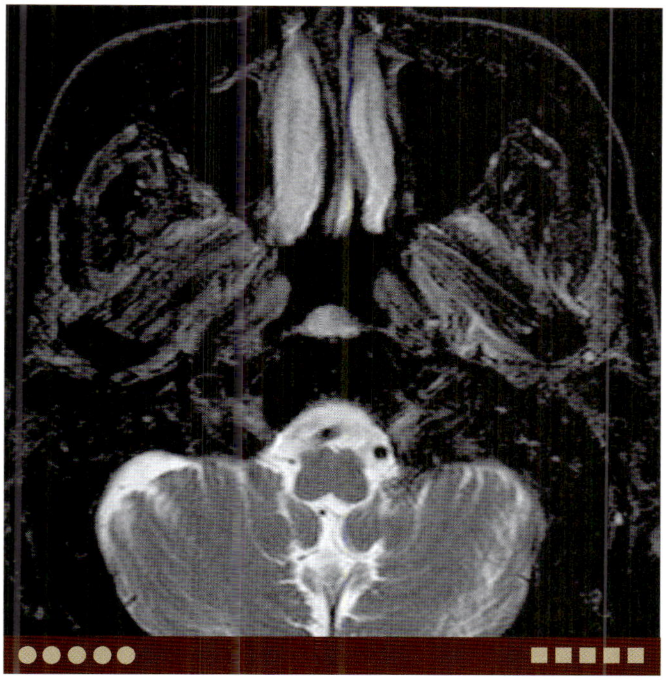

C. **Tornwaldt cyst** in a different patient. Axial fat-suppressed T2W MR image demonstrates a round high-signal lesion in the nasopharynx in midline.

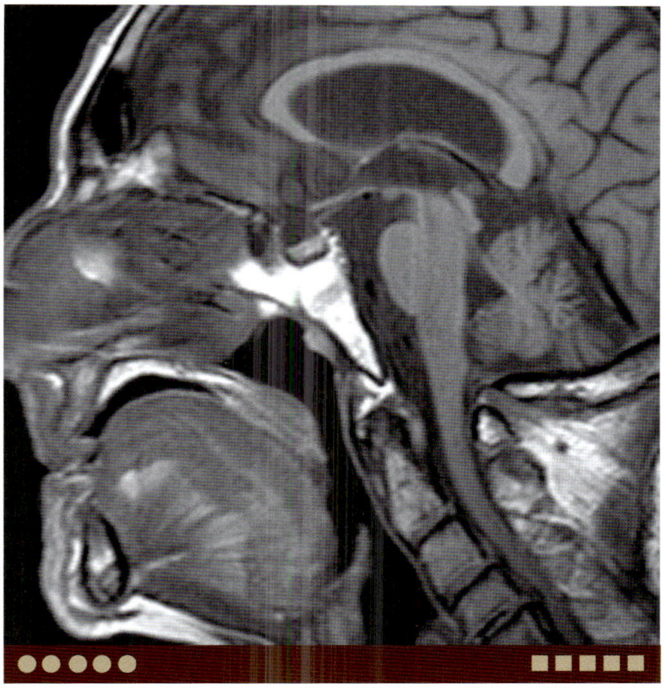

D. Tornwaldt cyst, same patient as C. Sagittal T1W image demonstrates the lesion showing intermediate signal.

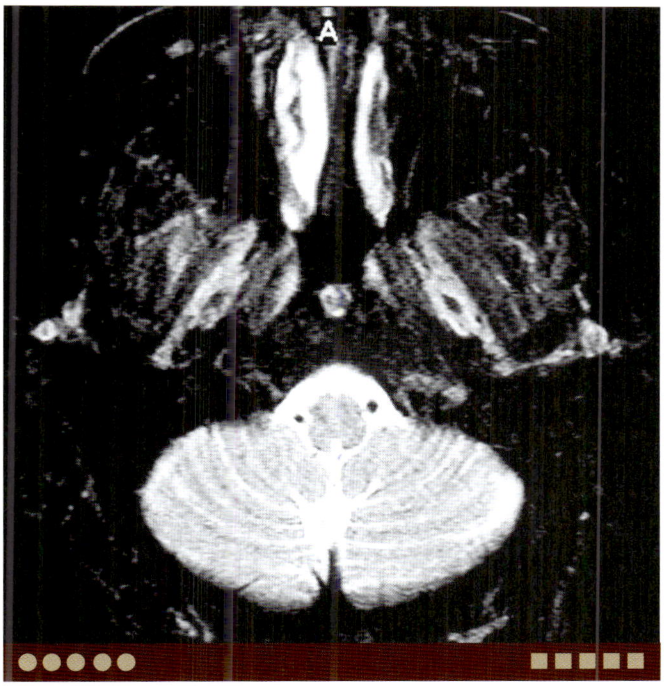

E. **Tornwaldt cyst** in a different patient. Axial fat-suppressed T2W MR image demonstrates a round heterogeneous signal lesion in the nasopharynx in midline.

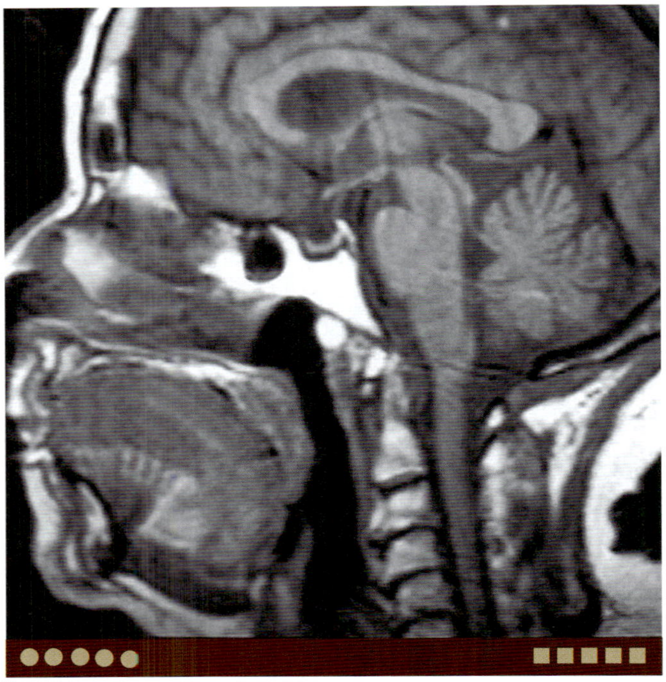

F. Tornwaldt cyst, same patient as E. Sagittal T1W image demonstrates the lesion showing high signal.

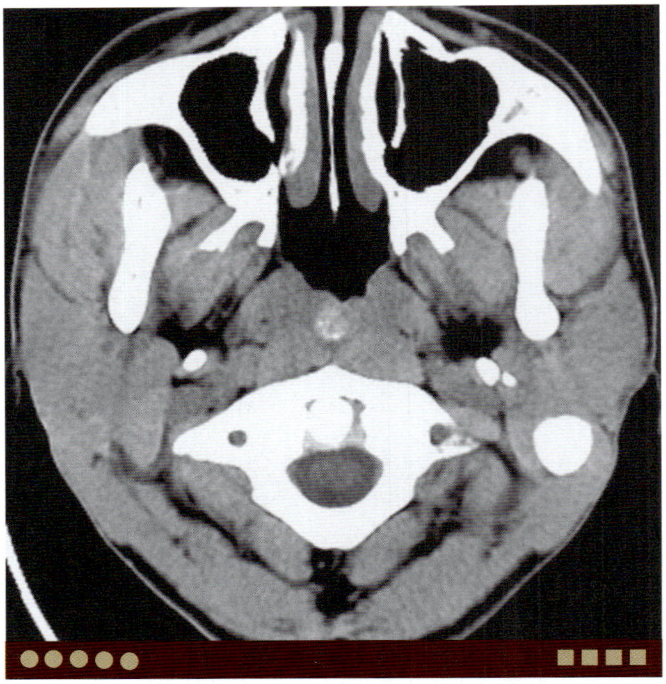

G. **Tornwaldt cyst** in a different patient. Axial noncontrast CT demonstrates a round high-density lesion in the nasopharynx in midline to suggest proteinaceous contents.

DIFFERENTIAL DIAGNOSIS IMAGES (H-J)

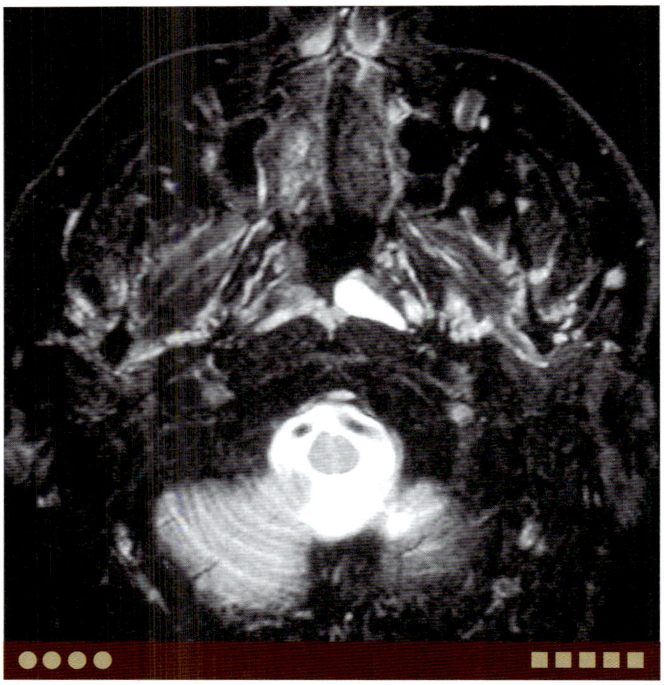

H. **Retention cyst**. Axial fat-suppressed T2W MR image demonstrates an ovoid-shaped high-signal lesion in the nasopharynx off-midline on the left.

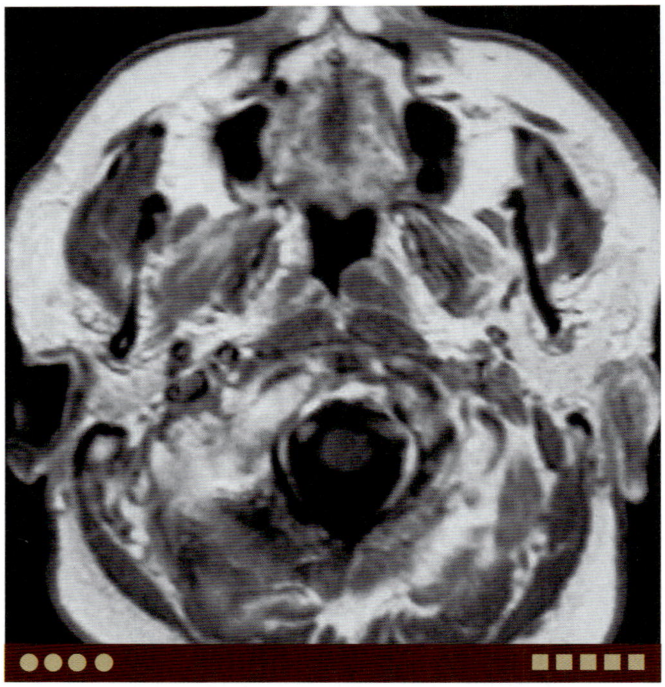

I. Retention cyst, same patient as H. Axial postcontrast T1W image demonstrates the lesion showing no enhancement.

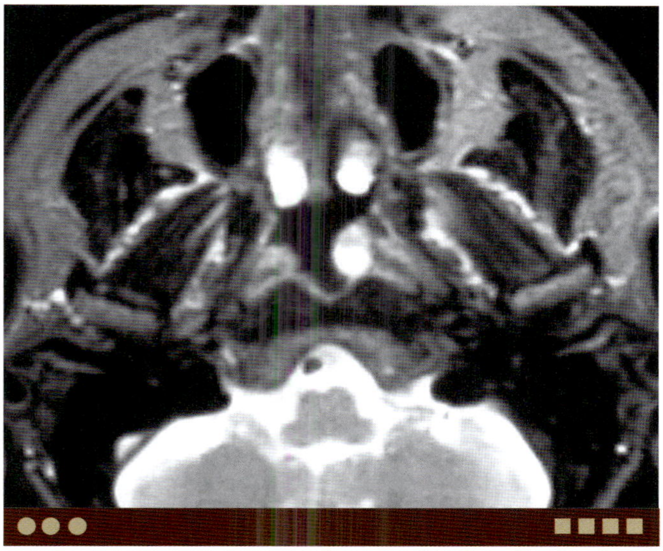

J. Pleomorphic adenoma. Axial T2W MR image demonstrates an ovoid-shaped high-signal lesion in the left nasopharynx.

Case 6–3 Nasopharyngeal Carcinoma

Osamu Sakai, Cory Siegel

PRESENTATION

Serous otitis media and conductive hearing loss.

FINDINGS

CT and MRI demonstrate a mass or abnormal signal involving the fossa of Rosenmüller with opacified mastoid air cells.

DIFFERENTIAL DIAGNOSIS

- Lymphoma: Lymphomas show very similar imaging findings to nasopharyngeal carcinoma (NPC), particularly WHO type III, and is very difficult to be differentiated from NPC. Lymphoma may show more homogeneous signal and infiltrative invasion rather than destruction.
- Enlarged adenoids: Proliferation of lymphoid tissue without involvement of the prevertebral muscles or clivus.
- Minor salivary gland tumors: More focal or localized, mass formation initially.

COMMENTS

This is a 65-year-old man with recent history of otitis media, conductive hearing loss and tinnitus.

According to WHO classification, nasopharyngeal carcinoma (NPC) can be divided into three types; type I: well-to-moderately differentiated squamous or transitional cell carcinoma with keratin production, type II: nonkeratinizing carcinoma, and type III: undifferentiated carcinoma, including lymphoepithelioma consists of malignant epithelial cells with lymphocytic infiltration. A strong genetic factor is suggested in NPC. The frequency of NPC is nearly 100-fold higher in southern Chinese than in most European populations. Males are more frequently affected. Epstein-Barr virus may be implicated. Typically, NPC arises from the posterolateral wall of the nasopharynx and involves the fossa of Rosenmüller. Obstruction of the eustachian tube results in opacification of the mastoid air cells and serous otitis media, which is a typical finding at presentation. Around the eustachian tube, there is a defect of the fascia, which is termed as the sinus of Morgani. Through this fascial defect, the tumor can invade into the deeper structures. Metastasis to the lateral retropharyngeal node (node of Rouvière) is common. Submucosal tumor extension is very common. Invasion to the clivus is often seen even with a very small, or almost no mucosal lesion. The nasopharynx is one of the primary sites for unknown primary cervical nodal metastasis. Therefore, imaging has an important role in diagnosis and management of the patient.

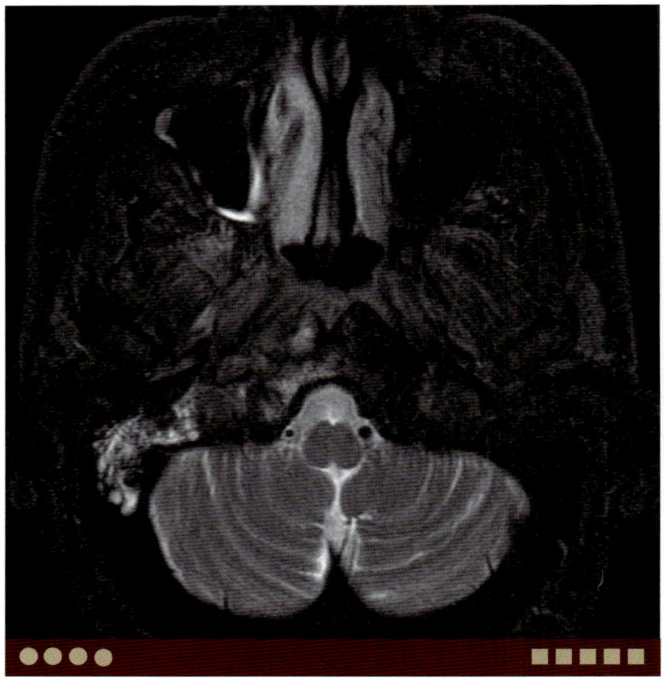

A. NPC. Axial fat-suppressed T2W MR image demonstrates abnormal signal involving the right fossa of Rosenmüller and longus colli muscle with opacified mastoid air cells. Note enlarged right lateral retropharyngeal node and abnormal signal in the clivus.

PEARLS

- **NPC often arises from the posterolateral wall of the nasopharynx, particularly around the fossa of Rosenmüller.**
- **Careful evaluation of the nasopharynx is essential in adults with serous otitis to diagnose NPC.**
- **The nasopharynx is one of the primary sites for unknown primary cervical nodal metastasis.**
- **Submucosal tumor extension is very common even with a small mucosal lesion.**

ADDITIONAL IMAGES (B-G)

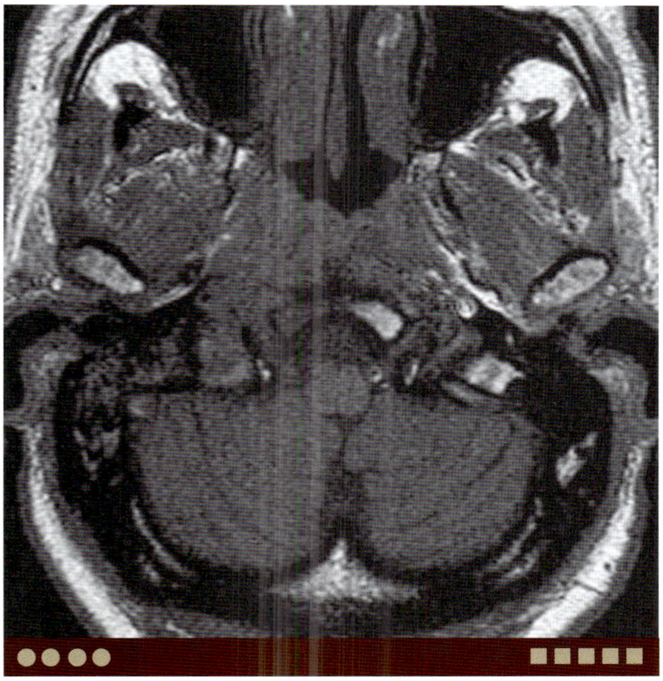

B. NPC, same patient as A. Axial T1W image demonstrates ill-defined low-signal lesion in the right nasopharynx which obscures margins of the longus colli muscle. Note abnormal low signal in the clivus consistent with tumor invasion.

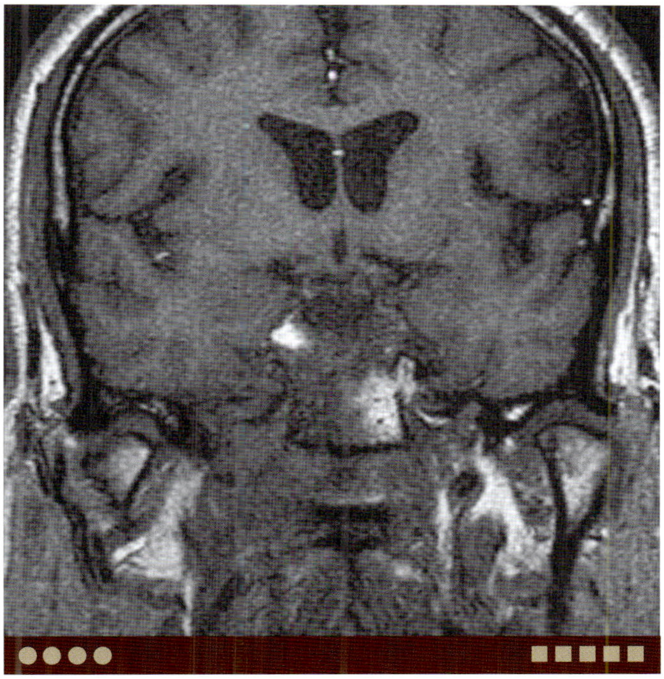

C. NPC, same patient as A. Coronal T1W image demonstrates tumor invasion to the petroclival synchondrosis with extension to the clivus and petrous apex of the temporal bone. Note loss of normal fatty marrow in these bones.

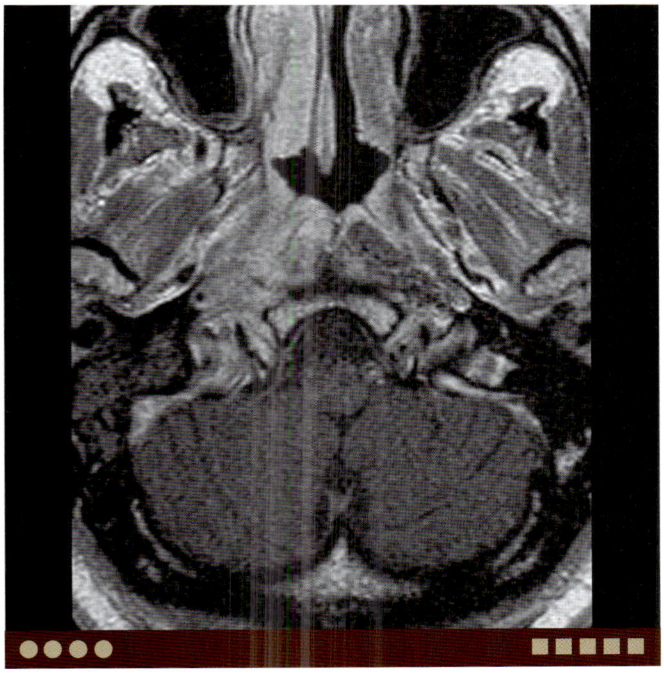

D. NPC, same patient as A. Axial postcontrast T1W image demonstrates abnormal enhancement in the lesion. Note invasion of the right longus colli muscle and encasement of the right internal carotid artery.

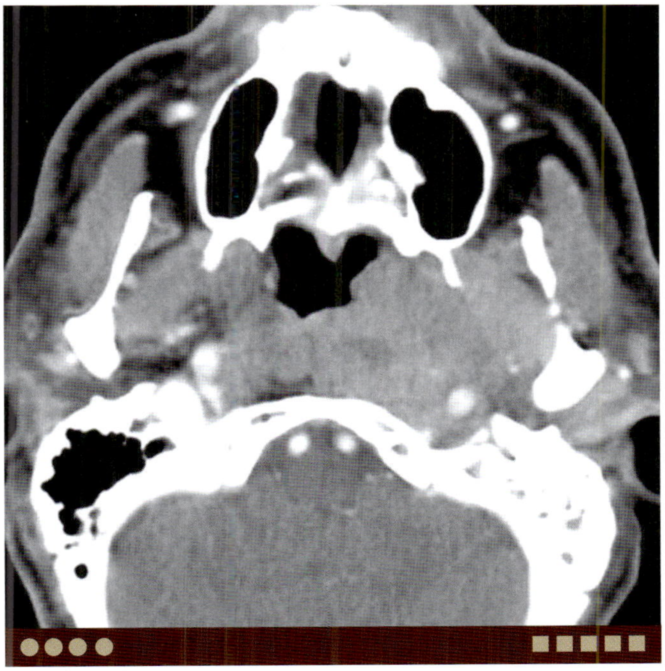

E. NPC in a different patient. Axial contrast-enhanced CT demonstrates fullness of the left nasopharynx and obliteration of the fossa of Rosenmüller. Note opacification of the left mastoid air cells. Loss of the left parapharyngeal fat indicates tumor invasion.

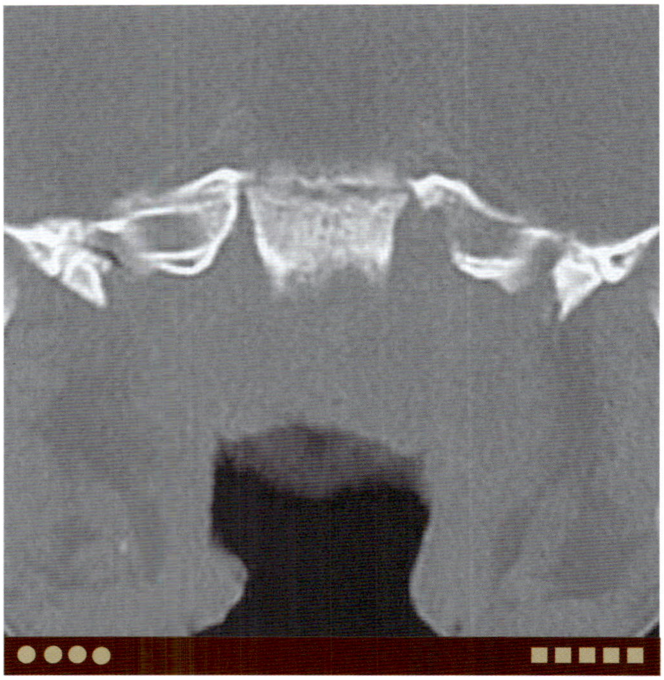

F. NPC in a different patient. Coronal bone window CT demonstrates widening of the left petroclival fissure. Note loss of the cortical bone to indicate tumor invasion.

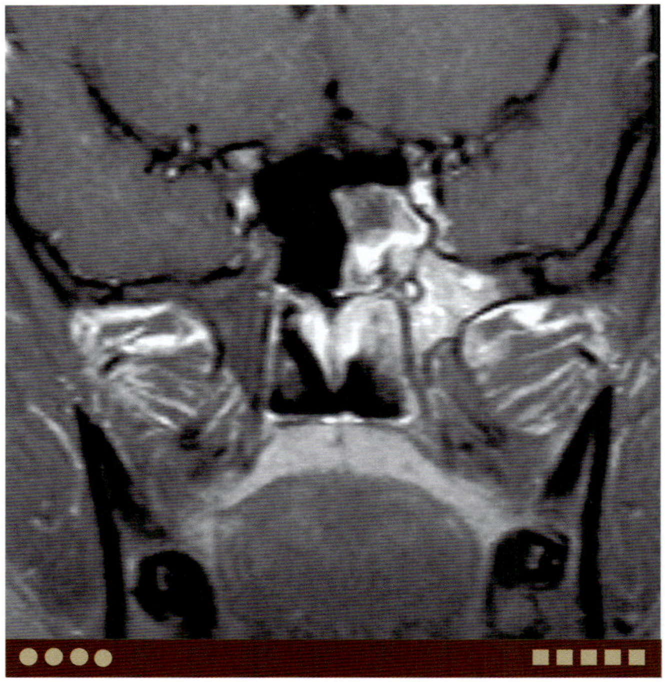

G. NPC in a different patient. Coronal postcontrast fat-suppressed T1W image demonstrates abnormal enhancement of the left pterygoid and mass formation in the left sphenoid sinus in addition to the relatively small tumor in the left nasopharyngeal mucosa. Note widened and enhancing Vidian canal to suggest perineural tumor spread.

DIFFERENTIAL DIAGNOSIS IMAGES (H-J)

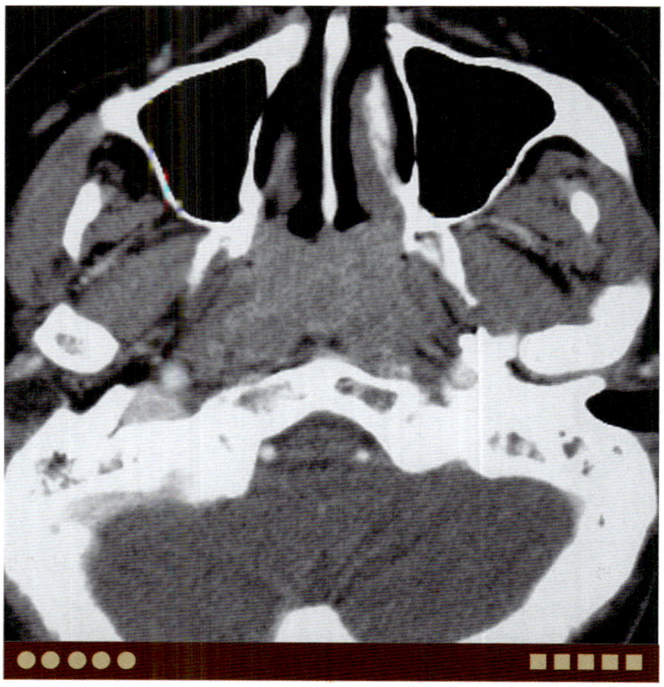

H. Adenoid hypertrophy. Axial contrast-enhanced CT demonstrates mildly enhancing enlarged adenoids.

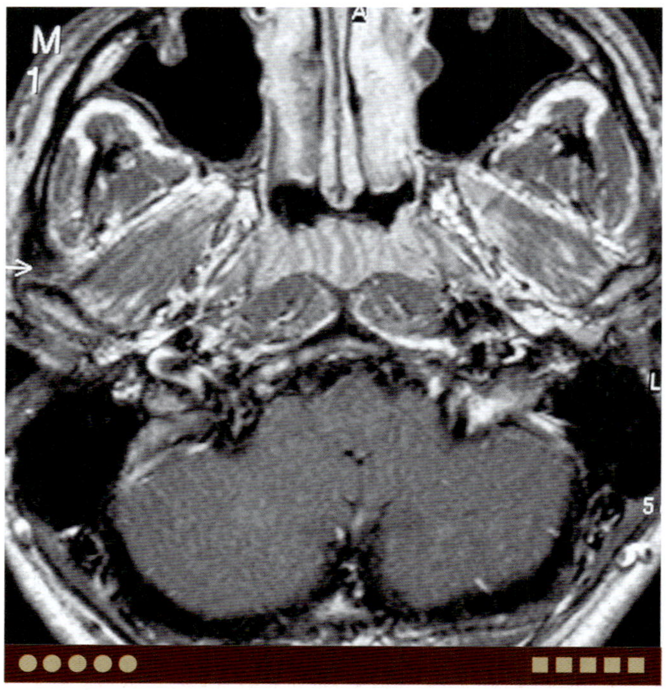

I. Adenoid hypertrophy in a different patient. Axial postcontrast T1W MR image demonstrates enlarged adenoids with preserved striation.

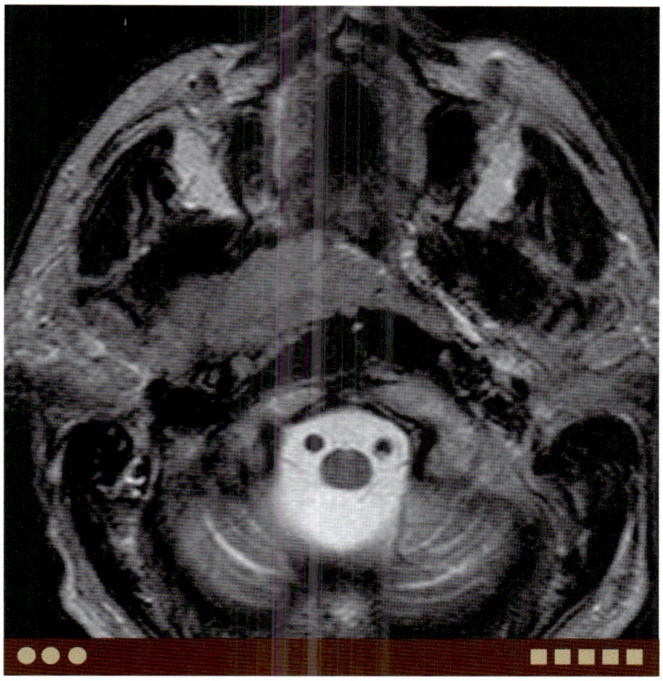

J. Lymphoma. Axial T2W MR image demonstrates an intermediate homogeneous signal lesion centered in the right fossa of Rosenmüller. Note involvement of the right parapharyngeal and masticator spaces as well as prevertebral space.

Case 6-4 Lymphoma

Osamu Sakai, Cory Sieger

PRESENTATION

Nasopharyngeal mass.

FINDINGS

CT and MRI demonstrate a nasopharyngeal mass with homogeneous density and signal.

DIFFERENTIAL DIAGNOSIS

- Nasopharyngeal carcinoma (NPC): NPC demonstrates very similar findings, however, may show a more heterogeneous and aggressive appearance with invasion and destruction of the adjacent structures.
- Adenoid hypertrophy: Proliferation of lymphoid tissues without involvement of the prevertebral muscles or clivus. This usually preserves linear structures within the enlarged adenoids.
- Minor salivary gland tumors: More focal or localized, mass formation initially.

COMMENTS

This is a 60-year-old woman with recent history of otitis media and conductive hearing loss.

Among lymphomas arising from the Waldeyer's ring, the nasopharynx is the second most common site following the palatine tonsils. Lymphoma is a relatively soft tumor and invades and infiltrates into the adjacent organs while preserving preexisting structures. Vessels are often involved, however, complete occlusion is rare. This finding is also seen in nasopharyngeal carcinoma (NPC) WHO type III.

Imaging findings of lymphoma is similar to that of NPC, particularly WHO type III, and often is impossible to differentiate each other. On noncontrast CT, lymphoma usually shows low-to-intermediate density similar to the muscle, and slight to intermediate enhancement after intravenous contrast administration. On MRI, lymphoma shows relatively low signal, slightly higher than the muscle on T1W images, and intermediate-to-high signal on T2W and STIR images. After contrast, it shows homogeneous intermediate enhancement. Similar to NPC, degree of enhancement is less compared to the adjacent normal or inflamed mucosa. With increase in size of the primary lesion as well as nodal metastasis, internal inhomogeneity is seen more often.

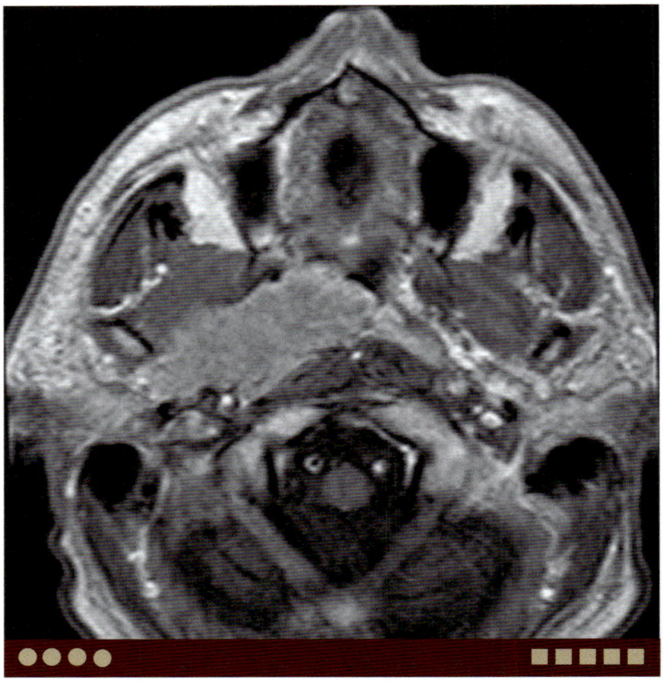

A. Lymphoma. Axial postcontrast T1W image demonstrates a homogeneously enhancing lesion in the right nasopharynx involving the right longus colli muscle, parapharyngeal space, and pterygoid muscles.

In young patients, it may be difficult to differentiate lymphoma from adenoid hypertrophy. In benign adenoid hypertrophy, striation within the adenoids is often preserved.

PEARLS

- **Lymphoma demonstrates homogeneous density on CT and signal on MRI without necrosis.**
- **Imaging findings of lymphoma are similar to that of NPC, particularly WHO type III.**
- **Lymphoma tends to show submucosal extension and infiltrates into the adjacent organs preserving preexisting structures.**

ADDITIONAL IMAGES (B–G)

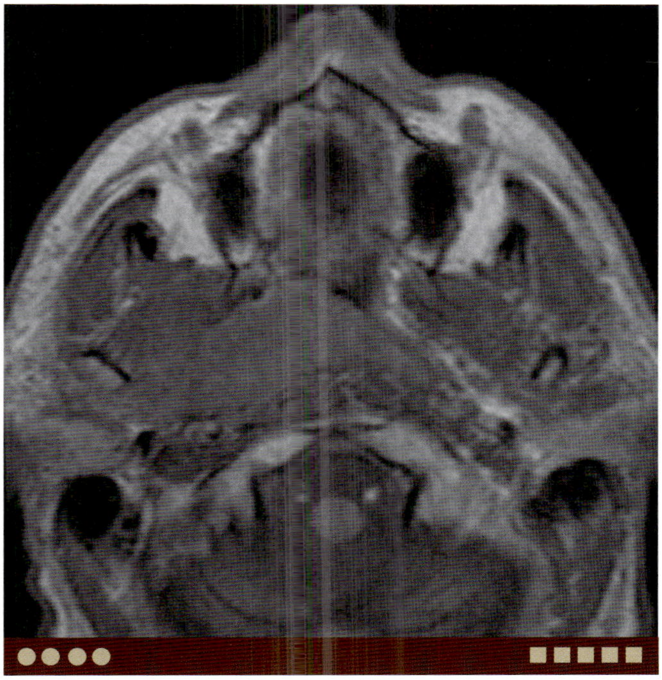

B. Lymphoma, same patient as A. Axial T1W image demonstrates a poorly defined low-signal lesion in the right nasopharynx obscuring the margins of the right longus colli muscle and pterygoid muscles. The right parapharyngeal space fat is completely obliterated.

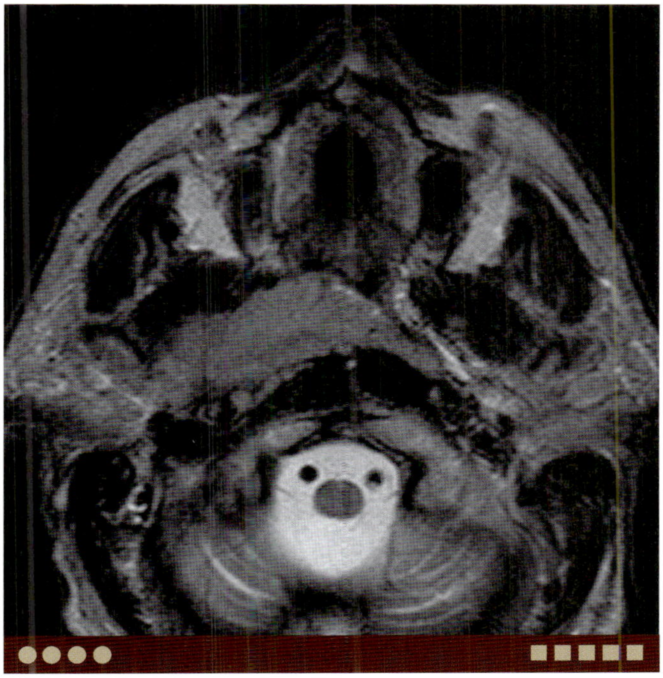

C. Lymphoma, same patient as A. Axial T2W image demonstrates the lesion showing intermediate signal.

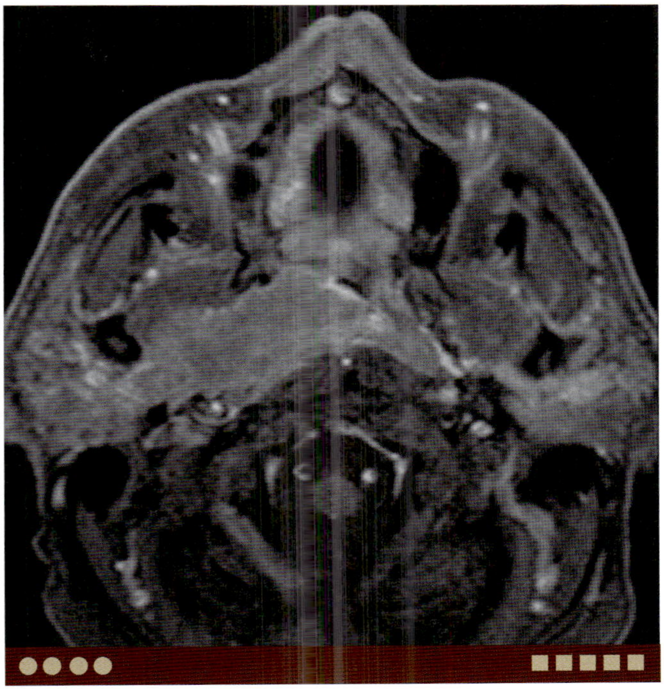

D. Lymphoma, same patient as A. Axial postcontrast fat-suppressed T1W image demonstrates homogeneous enhancement of the lesion.

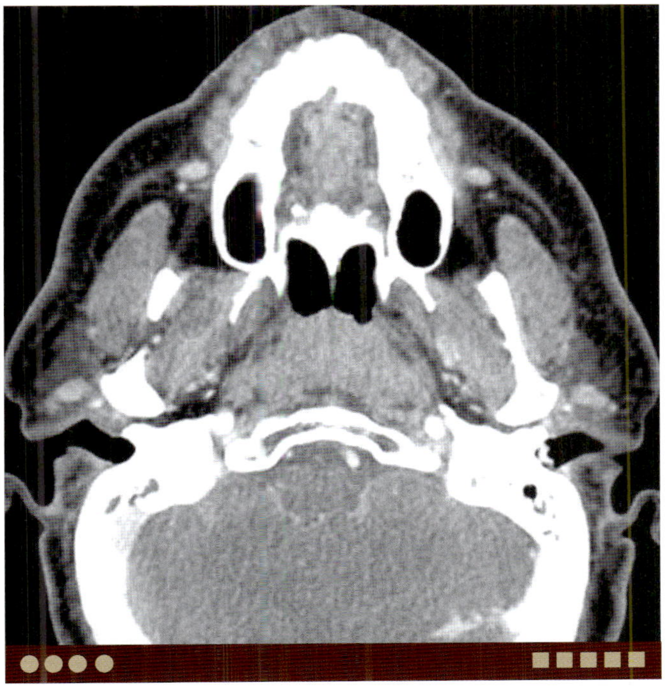

E. **Lymphoma** in a different patient. Axial postcontrast CT demonstrates homogeneously enhancing enlarged adenoids, similar to adenoid hypertrophy. Note opacified mastoid air cells.

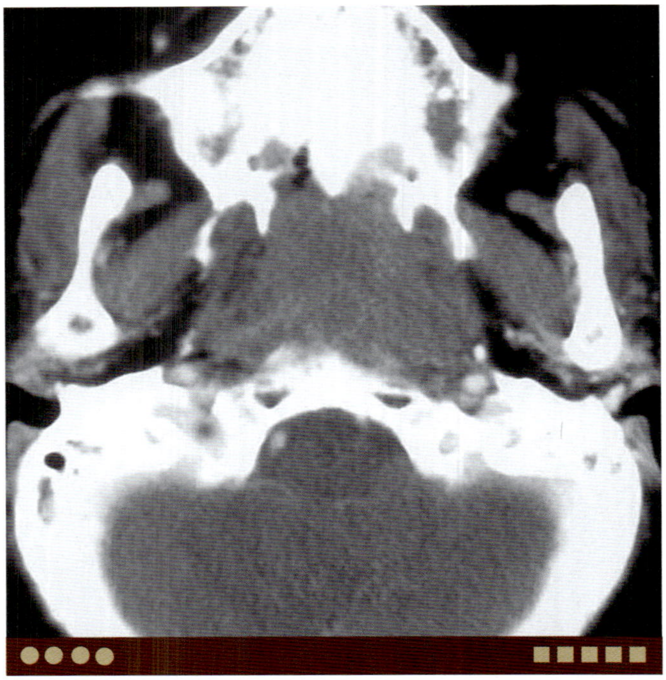

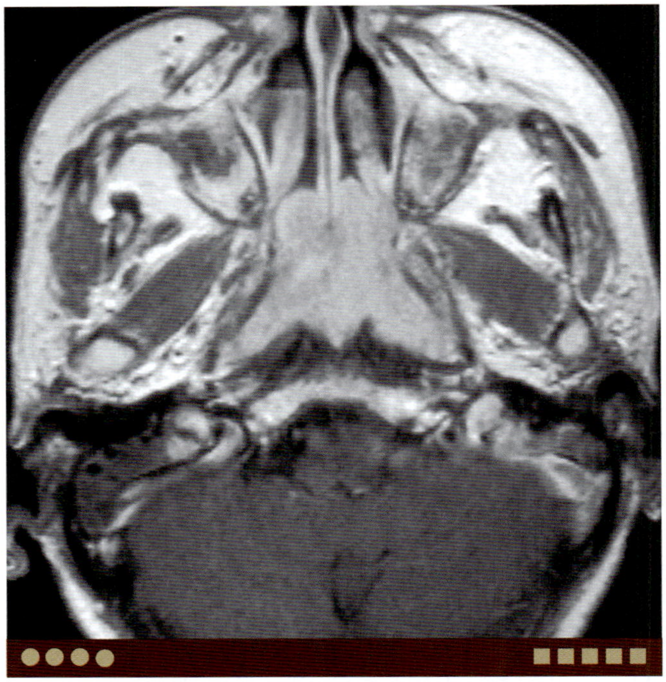

F. Lymphoma in a different patient. Axial postcontrast CT demonstrates significantly enlarged adenoids completely obstructing the nasopharynx. Mastoid air cells are opacified.

G. Lymphoma, same patient as F. Axial postcontrast T1W image demonstrates homogeneous enhancement of the lesion.

DIFFERENTIAL DIAGNOSIS IMAGES (H-J)

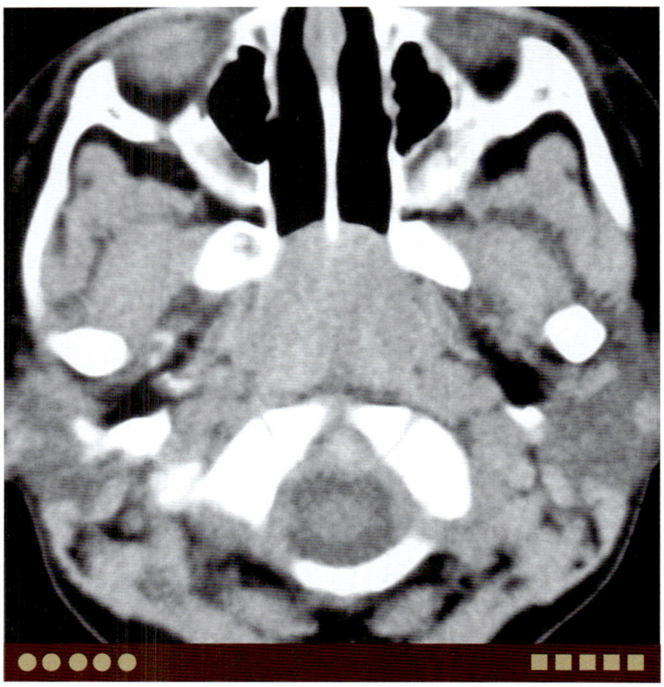

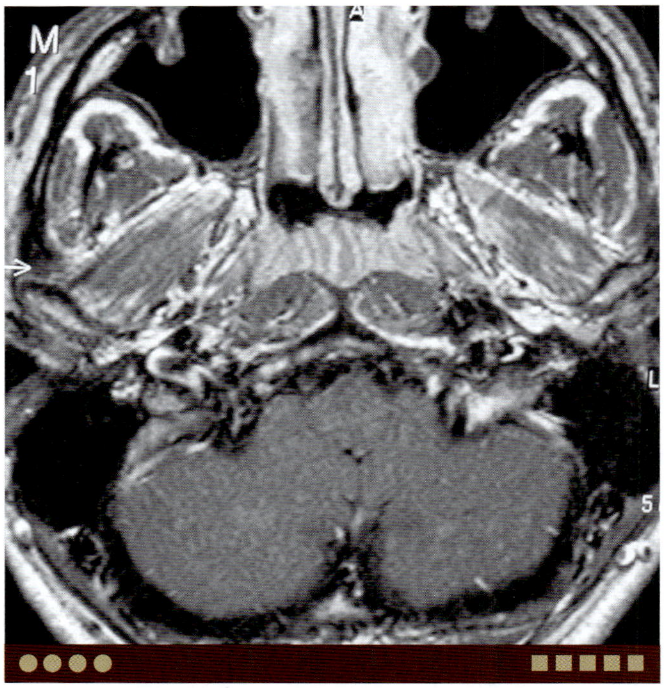

H. Adenoid hypertrophy in a 3-year-old girl. Axial noncontrast CT demonstrates enlarged adenoids.

I. Adenoid hypertrophy in a different patient. Axial postcontrast T1W image demonstrates preserved striation within the enlarged adenoids.

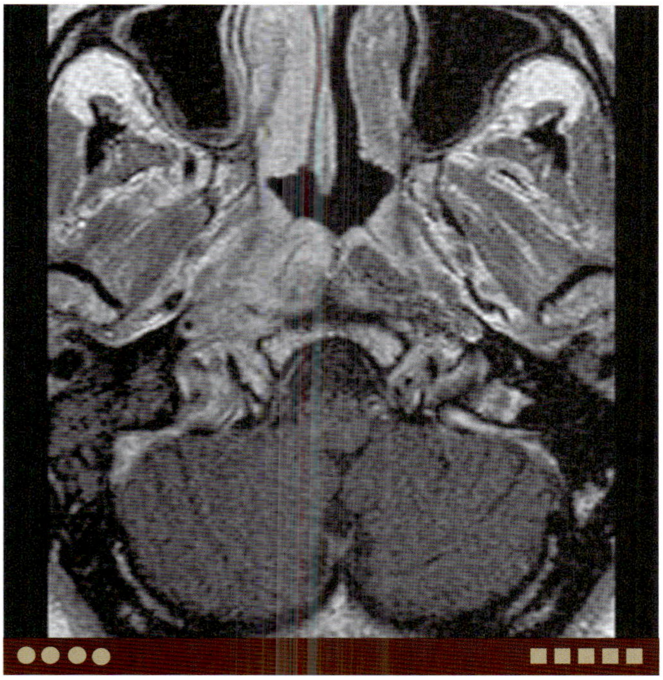

J. NPC. Axial postcontrast T1W image demonstrates a poorly defined, enhancing lesion in the right nasopharynx, centered in the fossa of Rosenmüller. Note invasion of the right longus colli muscle and encasement of the right internal carotid artery.

Case 6–5 Adenoid Hypertrophy in HIV-Positive Patients

Osamu Sakai, Cory Siegel

PRESENTATION

HIV infection.

FINDINGS

CT demonstrates enlarged adenoids in an HIV-positive patient.

DIFFERENTIAL DIAGNOSIS

- Adenoid hypertrophy: Proliferation of lymphoid tissue without involvement of the prevertebral muscles or clivus. This usually preserves linear structures within the enlarged tissue; is very common in children and young adults.
- Nasopharyngeal carcinoma (NPC): NPC demonstrates very similar findings but may show a more heterogeneous and aggressive appearance and can invade and destroy adjacent structures.
- Minor salivary gland tumors: More focal or localized, mass formation initially.

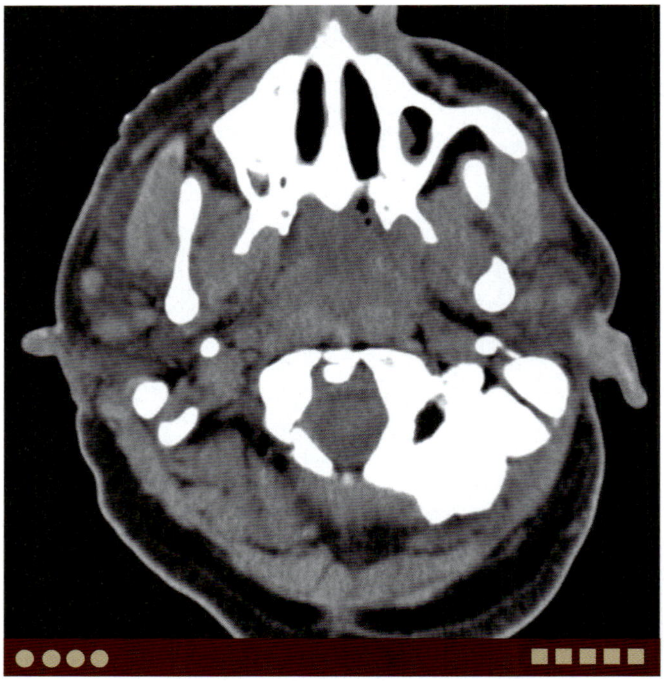

A. Adenoid hypertrophy in an HIV-positive patient. Axial noncontrast CT image demonstrates diffusely enlarged adenoids. Prominent intraparotid nodes are seen bilaterally.

COMMENTS

This is a 40-year-old man with HIV infection.

Adenoid hypertrophy in children and adolescents usually does not have clinical significance, however, neoplastic process should be always ruled out when enlarged adenoids are seen in adults. Enlarged adenoids are often seen in HIV-positive patients with bilateral multiple enlarged cervical lymph nodes and bilateral multiple lymphoepithelial cysts in the parotid glands. Enlarged lateral retropharyngeal nodes (nodes of Rouvière) are also common findings. These findings are often seen in asymptomatic patients and can be the first manifestation of HIV infection.

In HIV-infected patients, prevalence of malignancy such as lymphoma is significantly increased and opportunistic infection is commonly seen. When encountering enlarged adenoids, surrounding fat planes should be carefully evaluated because infiltrative changes are often seen in malignancy and aggressive fungal infection. Opacification of the mastoid air cells due to obstruction of the eustachian tube is often seen with neoplastic process in the nasopharynx, although benign adenoid hypertrophy can also block the eustachian tube.

Diffuse abnormal bone marrow signal is commonly seen in HIV-infected patients. White matter signal changes suggestive of HIV encephalopathy are also often encountered.

PEARLS

- **Enlarged adenoids are often seen in HIV-positive patients with bilateral multiple enlarged cervical lymph nodes and bilateral multiple lymphoepithelial cysts in the parotid glands.**
- **HIV-infected patients have higher risk for malignancy such as lymphoma and opportunistic infection.**

ADDITIONAL IMAGES (B-D)

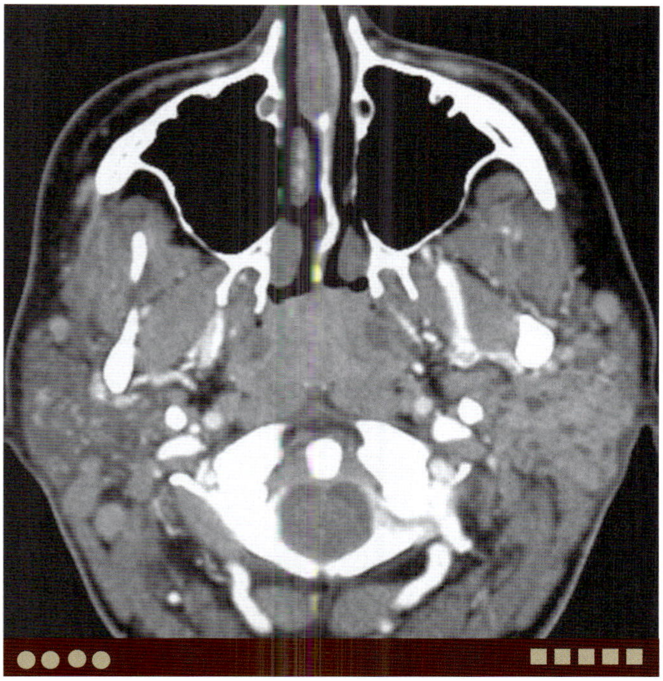

B. **Adenoid hypertrophy in an HIV-positive patient** in a different patient. Axial postcontrast CT demonstrates diffusely enlarged adenoids. Note heterogeneous nodular enhancement of the left parotid gland.

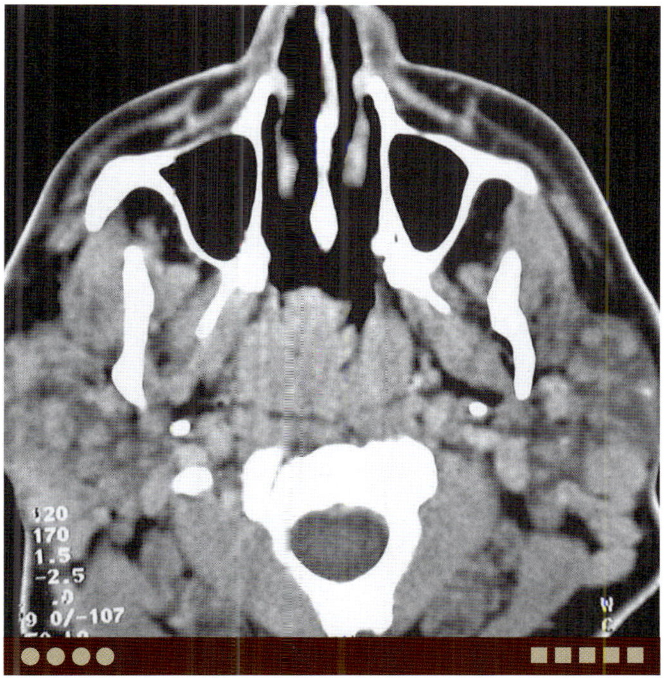

C. **Adenoid hypertrophy in an HIV-positive patient** in a different patient. Axial postcontrast CT demonstrates exophytic enlarged adenoids. Note prominent nodular lesions in the bilateral parotid glands.

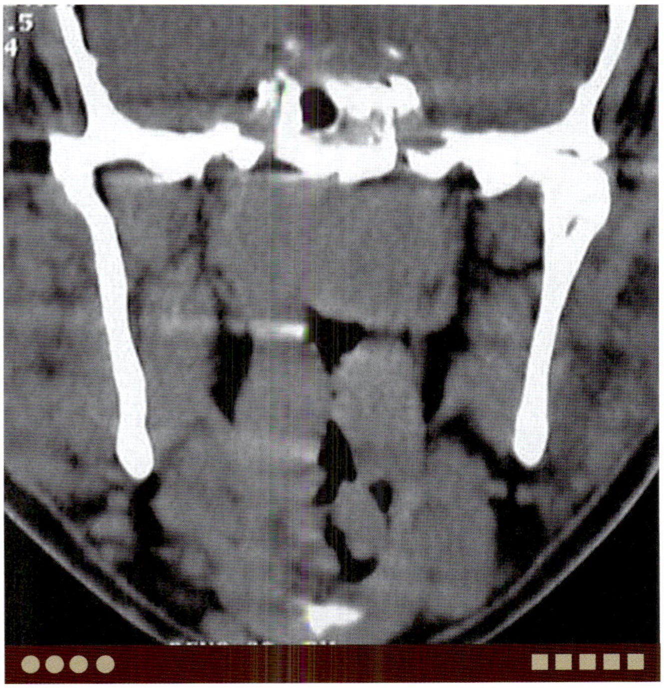

D. Adenoid hypertrophy in an HIV-positive patient, same patient as C. Coronal postcontrast CT demonstrates enlarged adenoids and palatine tonsils.

DIFFERENTIAL DIAGNOSIS IMAGES (E-I)

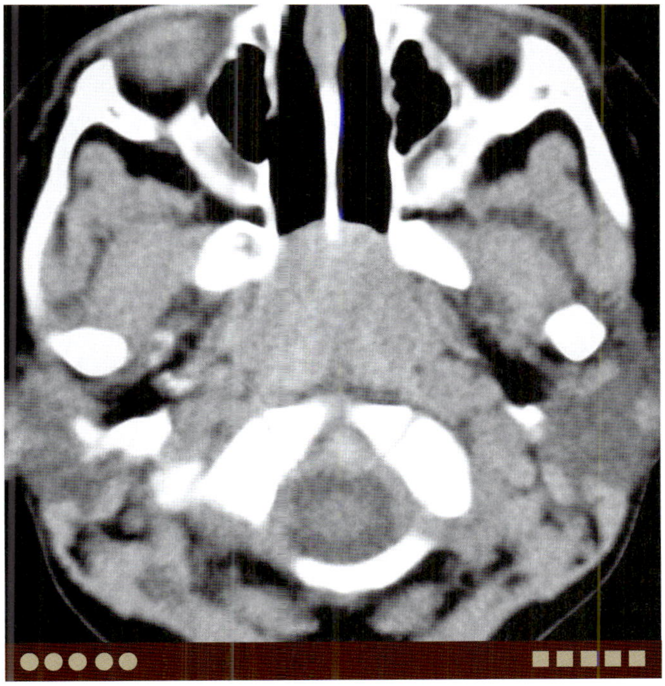

E. **Adenoid hypertrophy in an HIV-negative 3-year-old girl.** Axial noncontrast CT demonstrates enlarged adenoids.

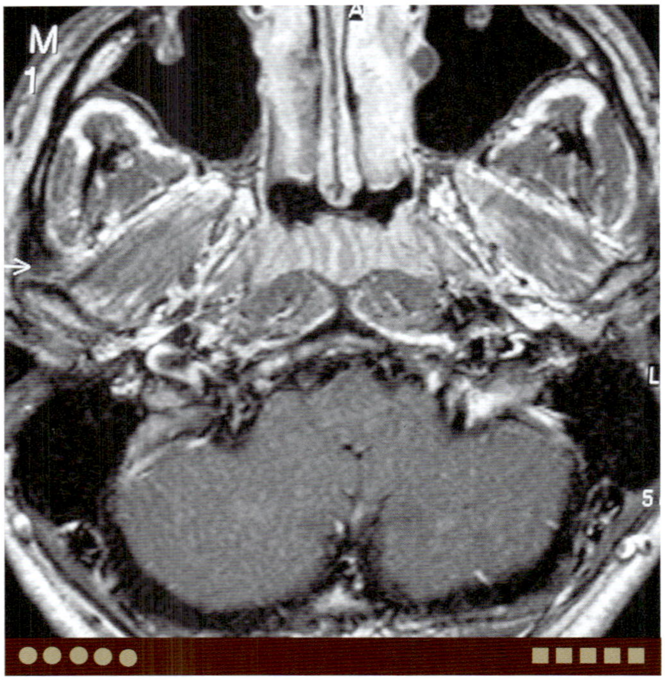

F. Adenoid hypertrophy, in an HIV-negative 27-year-old man. Axial postcontrast T1W image demonstrates preserved striation within the enlarged adenoids. Mastoid air cells are clear.

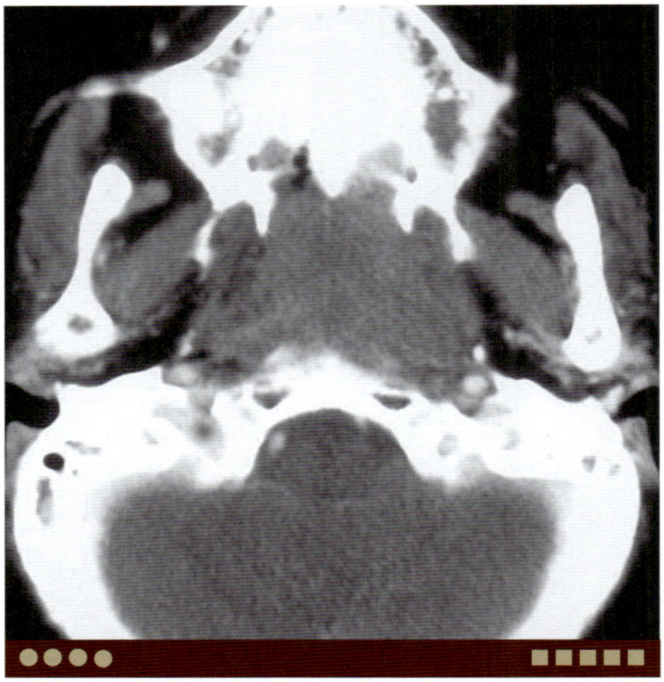

G. Lymphoma. Axial postcontrast CT demonstrates significantly enlarged adenoids completely obstructing the nasopharynx. Note opacified bilateral mastoid air cells.

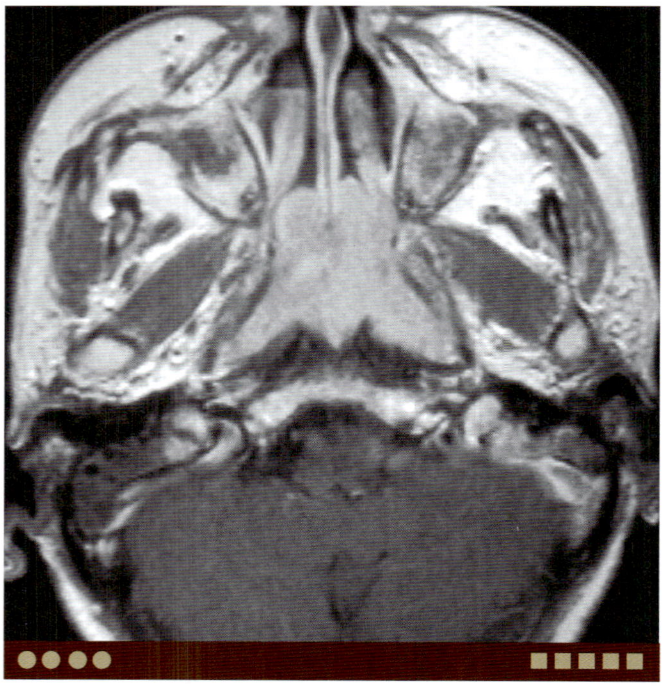

H. Lymphoma, same patient as G. Axial postcontrast T1W image demonstrates homogeneous enhancement of the lesion. Mastoid air cells are opacified.

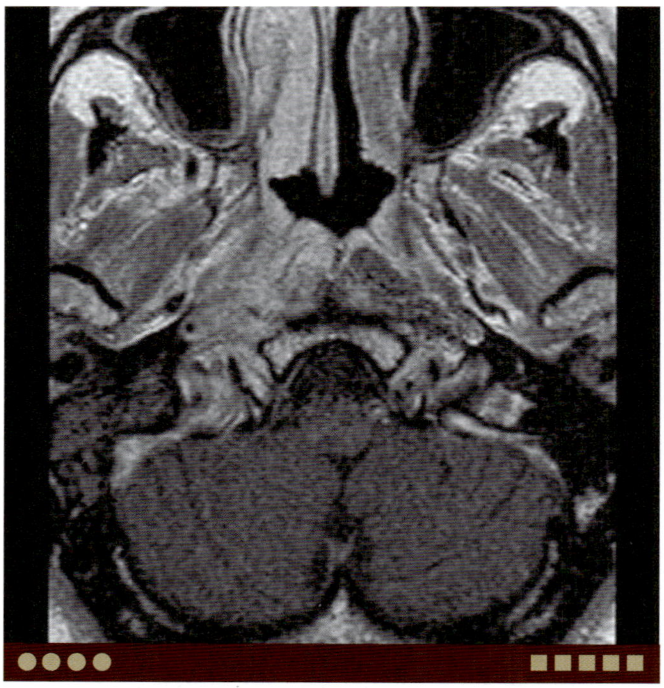

I. NPC. Axial postcontrast T1W image demonstrates abnormal enhancement in the lesion. Note invasion of the right longus colli muscle and encasement of the right internal carotid artery.

Case 6–6 Pharyngeal Amyloidosis

Akira Murakami, Osamu Sakai

PRESENTATION

Sensation of pharyngeal fullness.

FINDINGS

CT and MRI demonstrate irregular thickening of the pharyngeal mucosa.

DIFFERENTIAL DIAGNOSIS

- Nasopharyngeal carcinoma: This is the most common malignant epithelial tumor in the nasopharynx. This is more common among southern Chinese than most European populations. Epstein-Barr virus may be implicated.
- Lymphoma: This may show very similar findings to nasopharyngeal carcinoma. Usually lymphoma shows homogeneous signal and infiltrative extension rather than destruction. Calcification is rare without treatment.
- Extramedullary plasmacytoma: This has similar distribution to amyloidosis, and produces amyloid, and can coexist with amyloidoma.

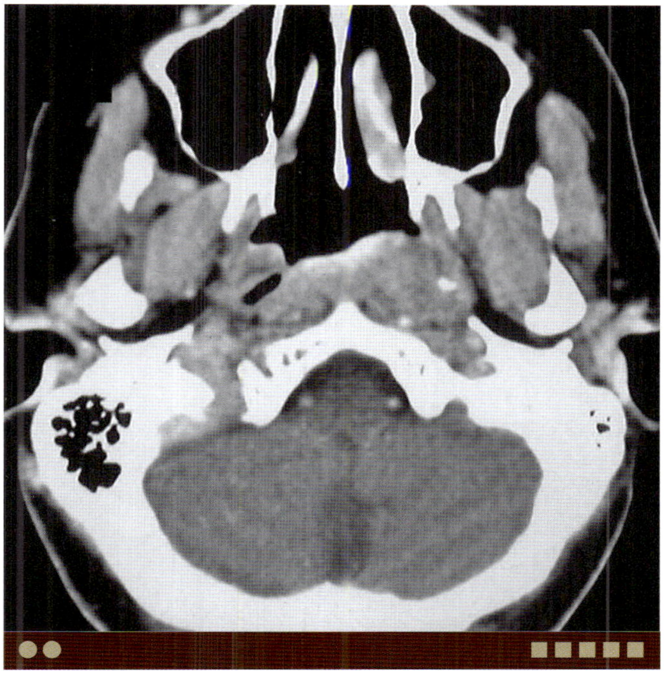

A. Amyloidosis. Axial postcontrast CT demonstrates fullness of the left nasopharynx obliterating the fossa of Rosenmüller with punctate calcifications.

COMMENTS

This is a 51-year-old woman with sensation of pharyngeal fullness.

Amyloidosis is a rare disorder of deposition of abnormal amount of proteins in various organs. Amyloidosis is collection of diseases which have in common the deposition of insoluble fibrillar proteins in the extracellular space. All fibrils are arranged in a beta pleated sheet conformation which produces the classic apple-green birefringence under polarized light microscopy.

Clinically, amyloidosis can be categorized into either systemic or localized disease. The majority of head and neck amyloidosis is secondary to local deposition of a precursor immunoglobulin light chain by a clone of plasma cells that are confined to that location. Oropharyngeal and nasopharyngeal amyloidomas represent up to 26% of cases, however these lesions can be found anywhere in the aerodigestive tract. Macroglossia is the most common head and neck manifestation of systemic amyloidosis, seen in 15% to 20% of patients.

The deposits are submucosal, homogenous, and soft tissue attenuating on CT and often have calcifications. There is generally little to no enhancement after contrast administration. On MRI, amyloidomas are often isointense with skeletal muscle. There is no evidence of bone destruction or intracranial extension. Lymphadenopathy is not typical in the localized form and should increase suspicion of systemic amyloid disease or more commonly head and neck malignancy.

Extramedullary plasmacytoma has similar distribution to amyloidosis, and produces amyloid, and can coexist with amyloidoma. Prominent enhancement may suggest plasmacytoma rather than amyloidosis alone.

PEARLS

- **The majority of head and neck amyloidosis is localized type.**
- **Amyloid deposits can be diffuse submucosal deposit or focal nodular deposit. Calcification is common.**
- **Bony destruction and lymphadenopathy are not typical for localized amyloidosis and should increase suspicion of more common squamous cell carcinomas.**
- **Amyloidoma shows low signal on T1W and T2W MR images, and no or minimal enhancement.**

ADDITIONAL IMAGES (B-F)

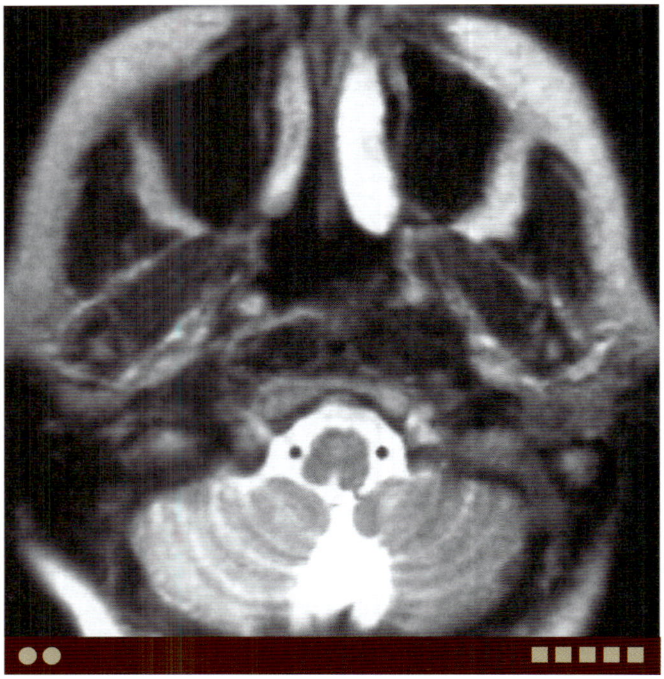

B. Amyloidosis, same patient as A. Axial T2W MR image shows low signal in the lesion.

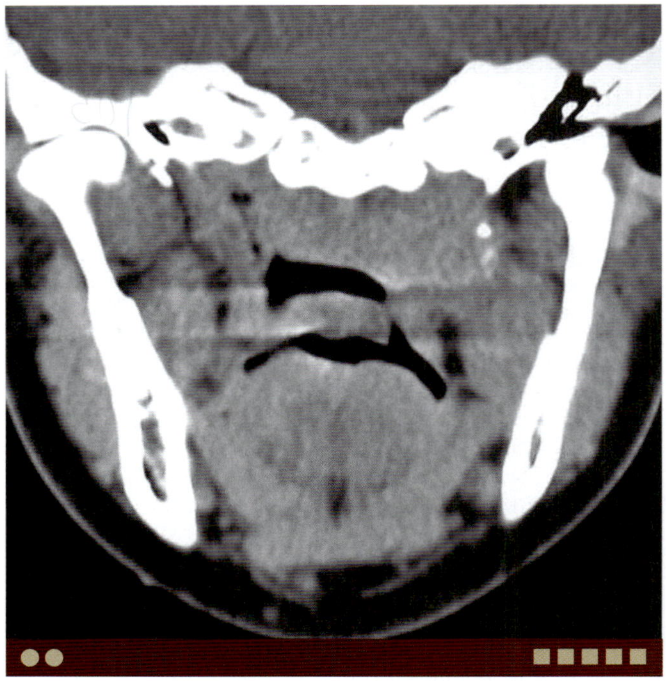

C. Amyloidosis, same patient as A. Coronal CT demonstrates fullness of the left nasopharynx with punctate calcifications.

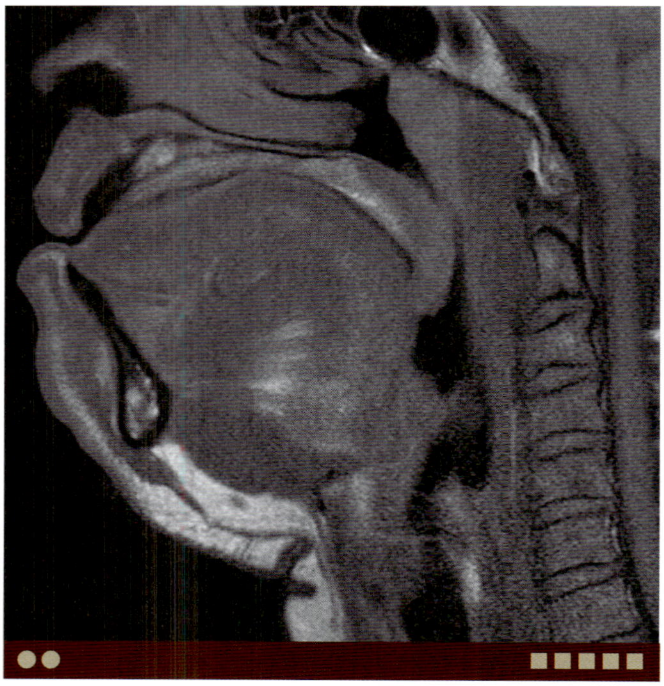

D. **Amyloidosis** in a different patient. Sagittal T1W mage shows macroglossia consistent with systemic amyloidosis.

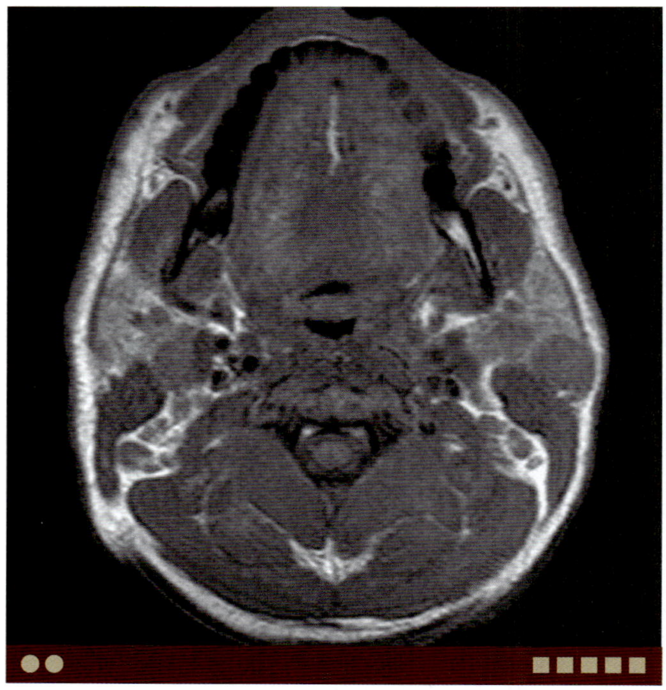

E. **Amyloidosis** in a different patient. Axial T1W image shows enlarged intraparotid nodes. Systemic amyloidosis.

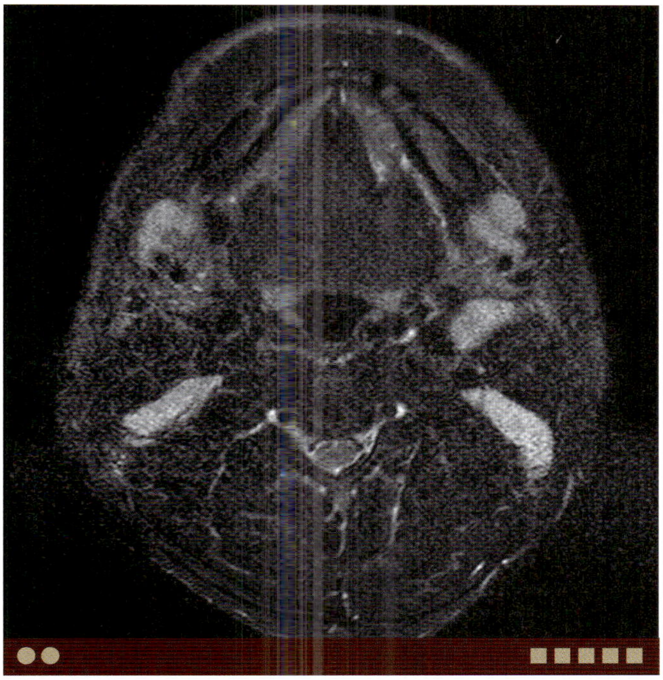

F. Amyloidosis, same patient as E. Axial fat-suppressed T2W image shows enlarged level I and II lymph nodes. Systemic amyloidosis.

DIFFERENTIAL DIAGNOSIS IMAGES (G-H)

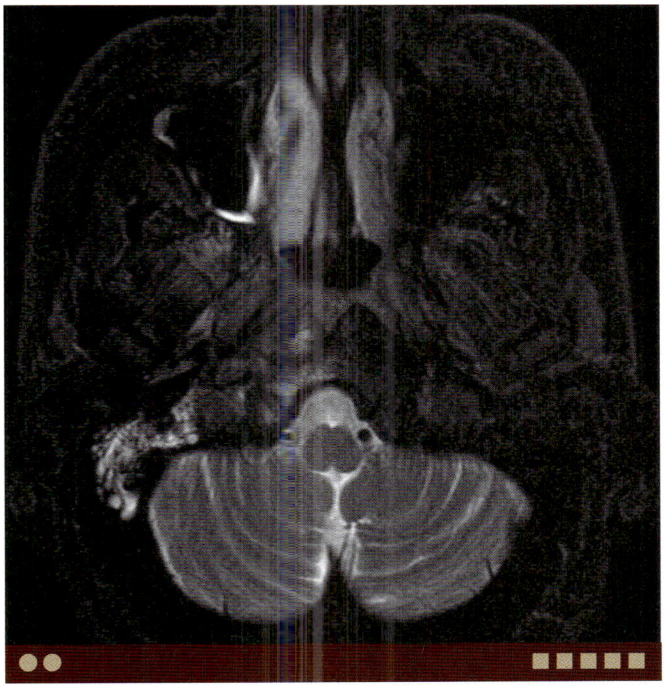

G. **Nasopharyngeal carcinoma**. Axial fat-suppressed T2W image demonstrates abnormal signal involving the right fossa of Rosenmüller and longus colli muscle with opacified mastoid air cells. Note enlarged right lateral retropharyngeal node and abnormal signal in the clivus.

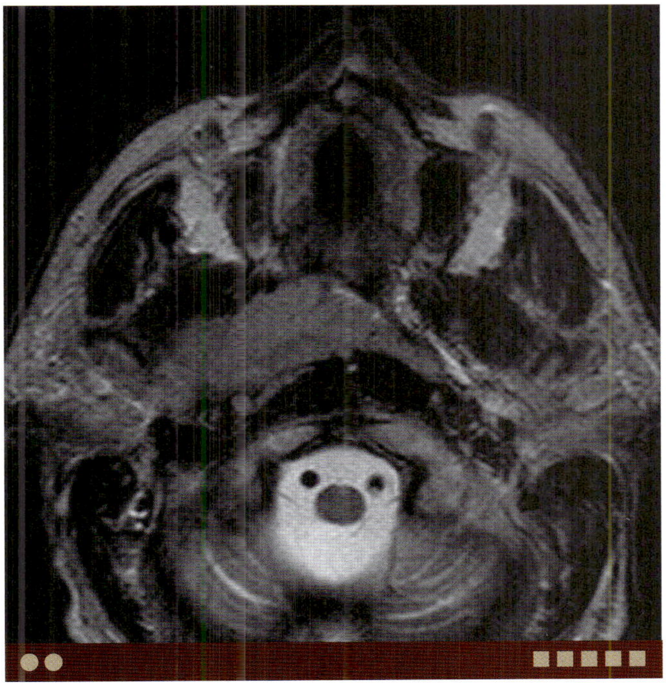

H. **Lymphoma**. Axial T2W image demonstrates homogeneous intermediate mass in the nasopharynx, right more than left, infiltrating into the right longus colli muscle and parapharyngeal space.

Case 6–7 Retropharyngeal Abscess

Osamu Sakai, Benjamin Ludwig

PRESENTATION

Fever, dysphagia, neck pain.

FINDINGS

CT demonstrates a rim-enhancing fluid collection in the retropharyngeal space.

DIFFERENTIAL DIAGNOSIS

- Retropharyngeal edema/effusion: This condition results in simple fluid density within the retropharyngeal space (RPS), without peripheral rim-enhancement, and is often difficult to differentiate from early abscess.
- Retropharyngeal lymphadenopathy: Enlargement of the medial or lateral retropharyngeal nodes causes thickening of the prevertebral and retropharyngeal soft tissue. Hypodense, peripherally enhancing nodes reflect nodal necrosis, which may be secondary to infection or metastatic disease.
- Retropharyngeal fibrosis: This is often seen after radiation therapy, usually with reticulation of the subcutaneous fat and thickening of the platysma, larynx, and pharynx.

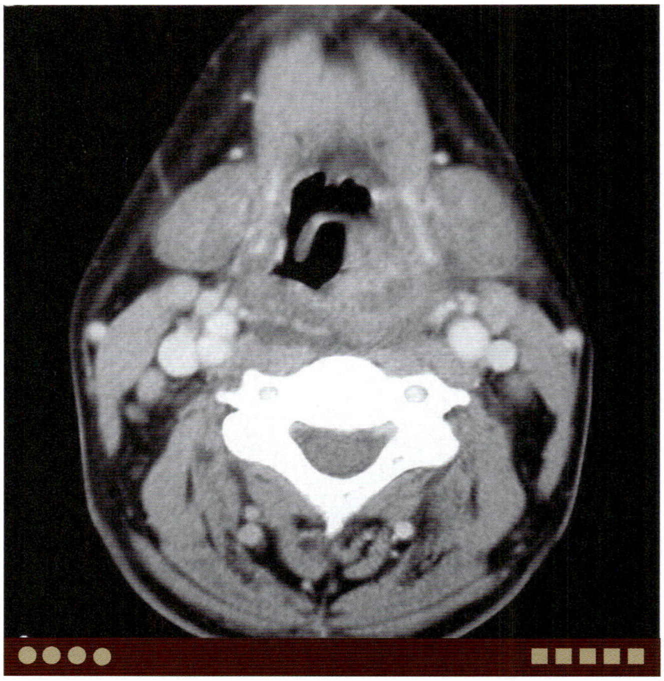

A. Retropharyngeal abscess. Axial postcontrast CT demonstrates a rim-enhancing fluid collection centered in the left hypopharynx as well as fluid collection with mild rim-enhancement in the RPS.

COMMENTS

This patient is a 27-year-old man with throat and neck pain and fever.

Retropharyngeal abscesses result from spread of infection from retropharyngeal lymph nodes, which drain the middle ear, sinuses, and upper respiratory tract. Abscesses are historically more common in children under 6 years old, as retropharyngeal nodes atrophy with age. Additional etiologies of abscess include foreign body ingestion/trauma or may be iatrogenic secondary to intervention.

The importance of recognizing this entity lies in the potentially life-threatening nature given potential for spread to adjacent deep spaces of the neck and possible airway compromise or mediastinitis.

The RPS is a potential space between the prevertebral and visceral spaces, between the middle and deep layers of the deep cervical fascia. With underlying pathology, the space is widened, resulting in the classic "bow-tie" appearance, with concave lateral borders laterally with the internal carotid arteries.

The clinical presentation is variable, but commonly involves fever, neck pain, and dysphagia.

On lateral neck radiographs, retropharyngeal abscesses demonstrate retropharyngeal/prevertebral soft tissue swelling, typically greater than one-third of vertebral body width from the C1 to C3 levels, and greater than the vertebral body width from the C4 level caudally. A common pitfall in pediatric patients is "pseudothickening" secondary to neck flexion or incomplete inspiration.

On contrast-enhanced CT, a peripherally enhancing fluid collection is present within the RPS. Similarly, on MRI, high-signal intensity on T2W images and rim-enhancement on postcontrast T1W images are typical. In the absence of rim-enhancement, it can be difficult to differentiate small abscesses from edema/cellulitis/effusion. Ultrasound may also be beneficial in demonstrating retropharyngeal fluid in pediatric patients.

PEARLS

- **The retropharyngeal space is a potential space, with a classic "bow-tie" morphology on CT or MRI in the presence of underlying pathology.**
- **On cross-sectional imaging, a rim-enhancing fluid collection within the retropharyngeal space is consistent with an abscess.**
- **It is imperative to recognize retropharyngeal abscess, as airway compromise and mediastinal spread of infection are life-threatening complications.**
- **In absence of rim-enhancement, it is difficult to differentiate abscesses from retropharyngeal edema/cellulitis/effusion.**

ADDITIONAL IMAGES (B-G)

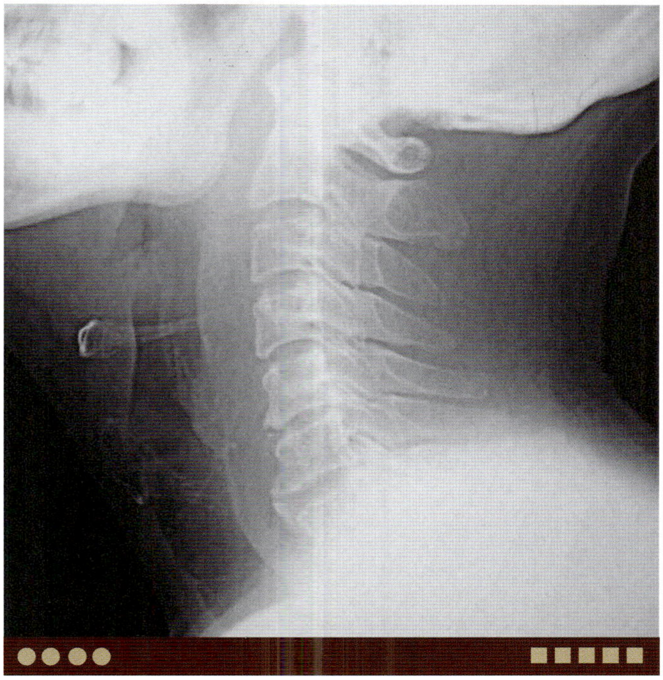

B. Retropharyngeal abscess, same patient as A. Lateral soft tissue neck radiograph demonstrates diffuse, marked thickening of the prevertebral soft tissues.

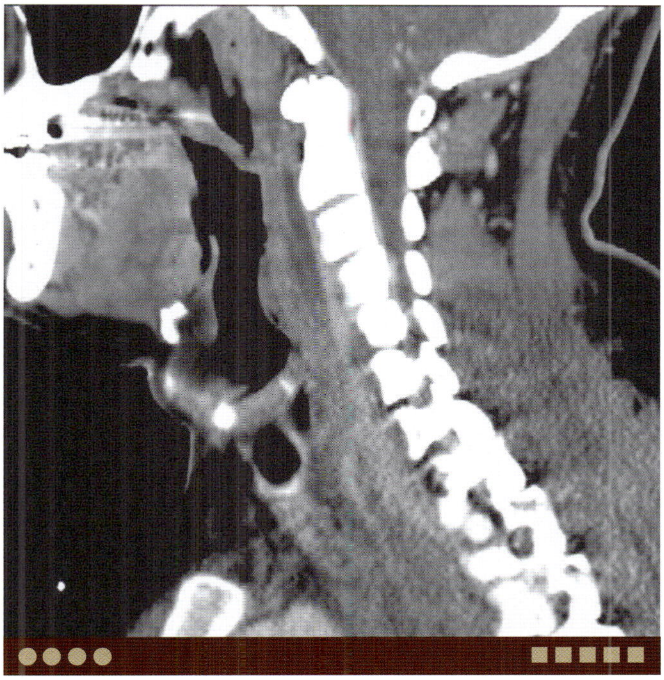

C. **Retropharyngeal abscess** in a different patient. Sagittal postcontrast CT demonstrates fluid collection in the RPS with extension in the craniocaudal dimension.

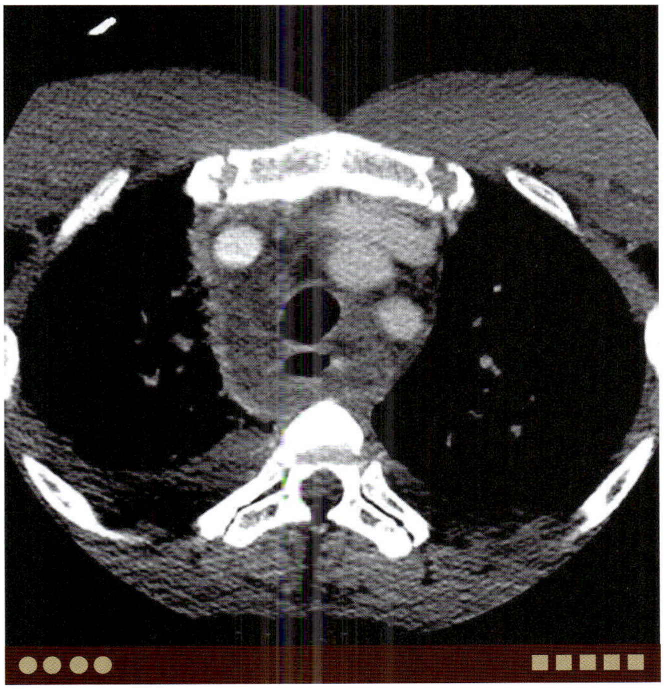

D. Retropharyngeal abscess, same patient C. Axial postcontrast CT demonstrates enhancing soft tissue within the middle and posterior mediastinum, consistent with mediastinitis. Note right pleural effusion.

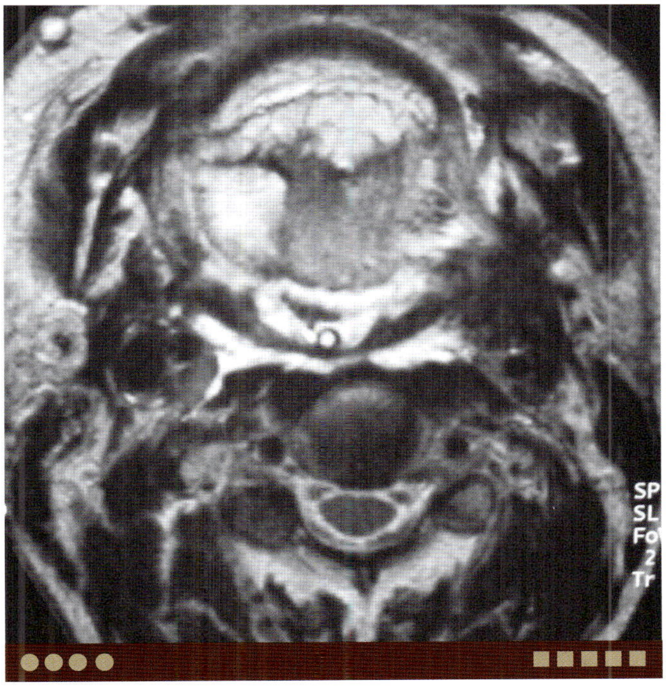

E. **Retropharyngeal abscess** in a different patient. Axial T2W MR image demonstrates fluid collection with "bow-tie" appearance in the RPS.

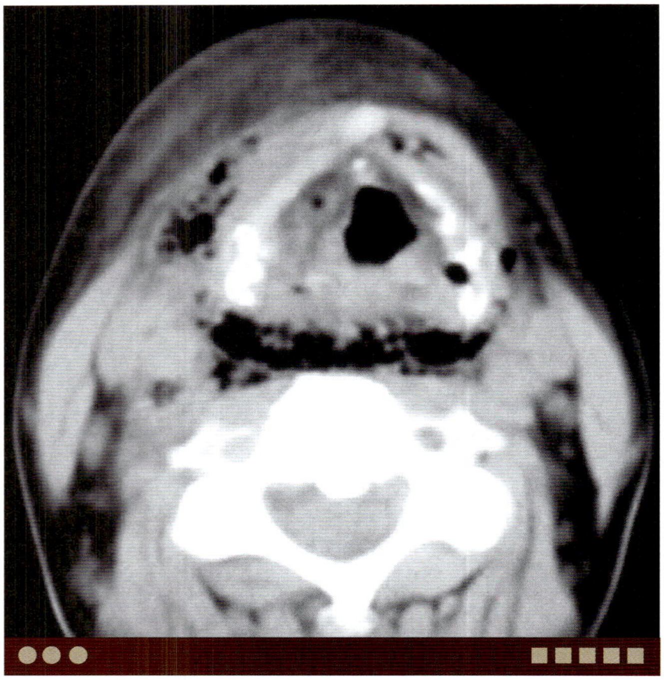

F. Retropharyngeal abscess in a different patient. Axial postcontrast CT demonstrates foci of gas within the RPS, consistent with gas-forming abscess.

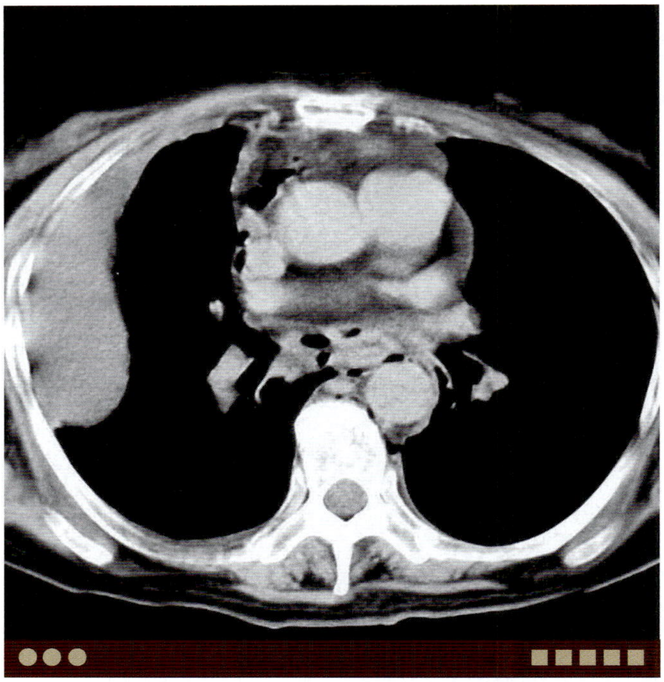

G. Retropharyngeal abscess, same patient F. Axial postcontrast CT demonstrates gas densities in the mediastinum and loculated right-sided pleural effusion.

DIFFERENTIAL DIAGNOSIS IMAGES (H-J)

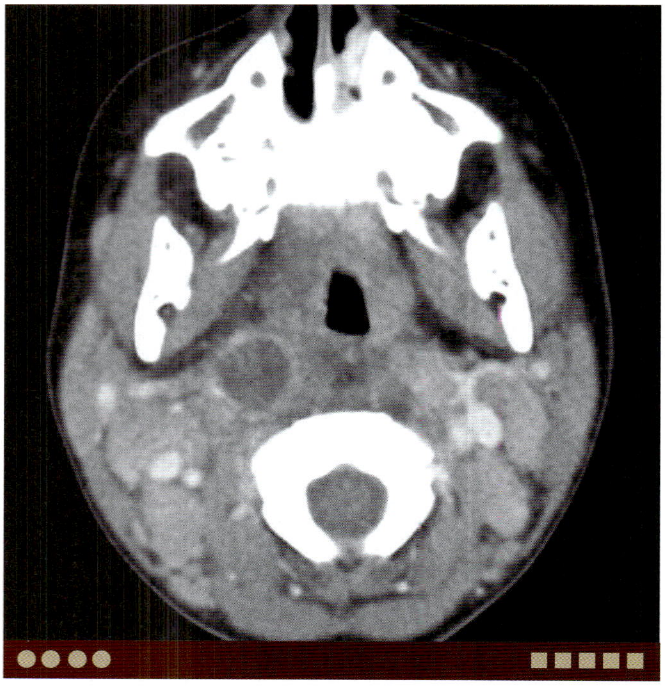

H. Lateral retropharyngeal intranodal abscess. Axial postcontrast CT demonstrates an enlarged, rim-enhancing right lateral retropharyngeal node (node of Rouvière) with adjacent phlegmon.

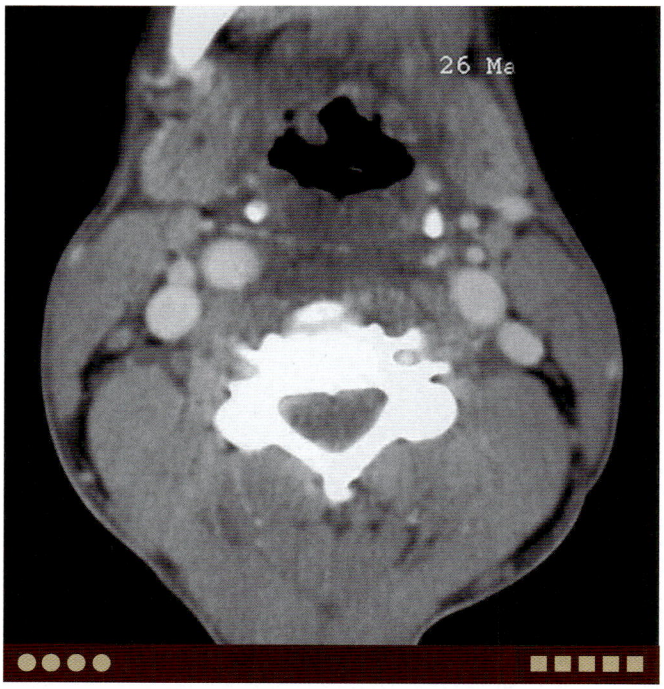

I. Prevertebral abscess. Axial postcontrast CT demonstrates fluid collection anterior to the longus colli muscles, which displaces the retropharyngeal fat anteriorly.

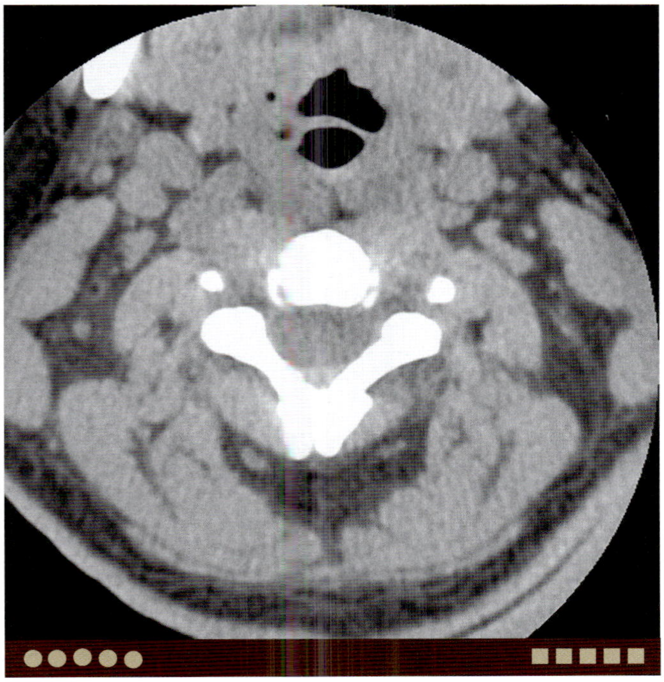

J. Retropharyngeal internal carotid arteries. Axial noncontrast CT demonstrates retropharyngeal course of the bilateral internal carotid arteries, which can result in apparent prevertebral/retropharyngeal thickening on radiographs.

Case 6–8 Arteriovenous Malformation

Osamu Sakai, Cory Siegel

PRESENTATION

Bleeding gums.

FINDINGS

CT demonstrates numerous tortuous vessels around and within the mandible.

DIFFERENTIAL DIAGNOSIS

- Venous malformation: Lobulated soft tissue "mass" often containing phleboliths, with variable enhancement after contrast. T2 high signal without flow-voids is characteristic.
- Lymphatic malformation: Imperceptible wall, uni-/multi-loculated, nonenhancing mass, which extends between vessels/normal structures.
- Plexiform neurofibroma: Usually demonstrates tortuous rope-like expansion within a major nerve distribution. Enhancement is seen more centrally than peripherally. Enlargement/remodeling of the neural foramina or canal is often seen.

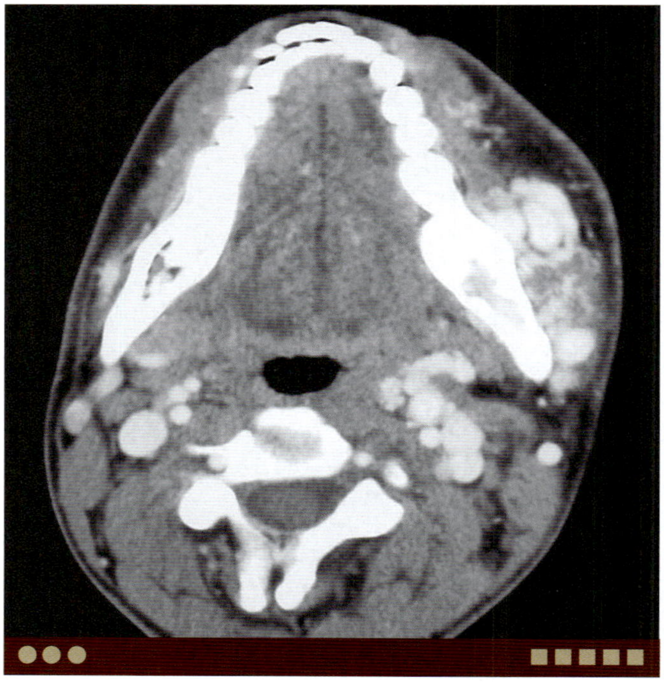

A. AVM. Axial postcontrast CT in soft tissue window demonstrates enhancing tortuous vessels adjacent to the left mandible with a heterogeneously enhancing soft tissue "mass."

COMMENTS

This is a 16-year-old adolescent with uncontrollable bleeding after tooth extraction.

Arteriovenous malformation (AVM) can occur anywhere in the body, however, is often seen in the face. It can be an arteriovenous fistula or mixture of arterial and venous anomalous vessels, that is, a mixture of high-flow and low-flow components.

Vascular malformations previously were often labeled as separate entities such as arteriovenous malformations, hemangiomas and lymphangiomas. However, more recently, they are categorized into a single entity and divided based on flow velocity; high-flow and low-flow types. The high-flow type includes arteriovenous malformation and fistula, and the low-flow type includes venous malformation (often called a hemangioma or venous angioma), venolymphatic malformation, and lymphatic malformation (often called a lymphangioma or cystic hygroma). Phleboliths are typically seen in venous malformations.

AVM is seen on enhanced CT as a vascular mass with enlarged feeding arteries and dilated tortuous draining veins. High-velocity blood flow from arterialized lesions result in flow-voids on MRI. Demineralization of the adjacent bone is common in high-flow lesions and abnormally dilated tortuous vessels are commonly seen in the bone marrow. Therefore, evaluation with both soft tissue and bone algorithm reconstructed images is important.

CT angiogram is useful to fully characterize the lesion because both arteries and veins are opacified, although it cannot separate the artery from the vein, which often makes it difficult to diagnose the exact location of the nidus or fistula.

Time-of-flight MR angiogram only demonstrates very high-flow components and often underestimates the extent of the lesion, while contrast-enhanced dynamic MRA can better demonstrate the lesion's features.

Catheter angiogram is performed to identify the exact location of shunting and for intervention.

Vascular malformation in the face also may be associated with intracranial vascular malformation, therefore, evaluation for an intracranial abnormality is important.

PEARLS

- **AVM can occur anywhere in the body, however, is often seen in the face.**
- **AVM can often cause demineralization of the adjacent bone with bone marrow involvement.**
- **Time-of-flight MR angiogram only demonstrates very high-flow components and often underestimates the lesion.**

ADDITIONAL IMAGES (B-H)

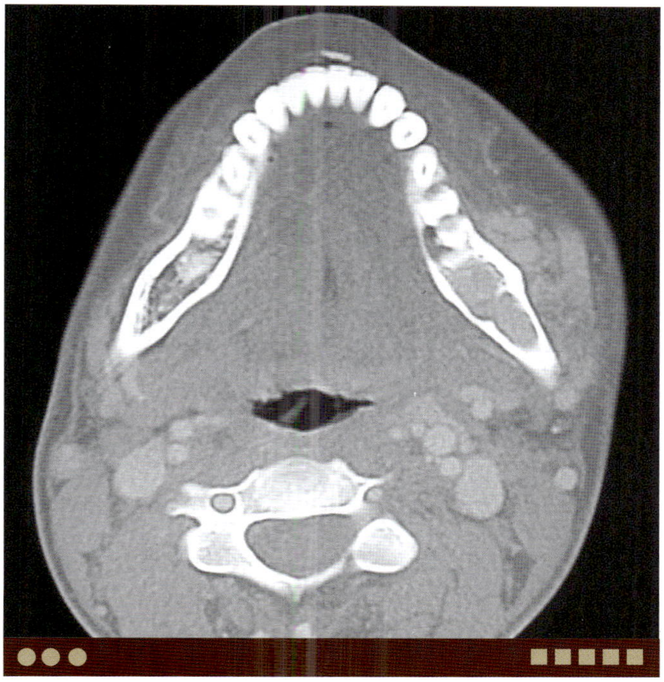

B. AVM, same patient as A. Axial postcontrast CT in bone window demonstrates loss of normal trabeculation, bony expansion with cortical thinning within the left mandible.

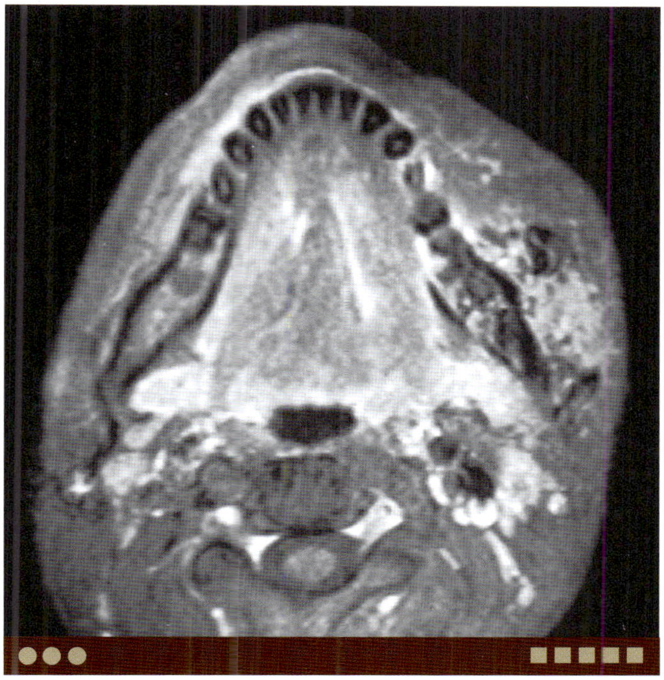

C. AVM, same patient as A. Axial postcontrast fat-suppressed T1W MR image demonstrates a heterogeneously enhancing "mass" lateral to the left mandible.

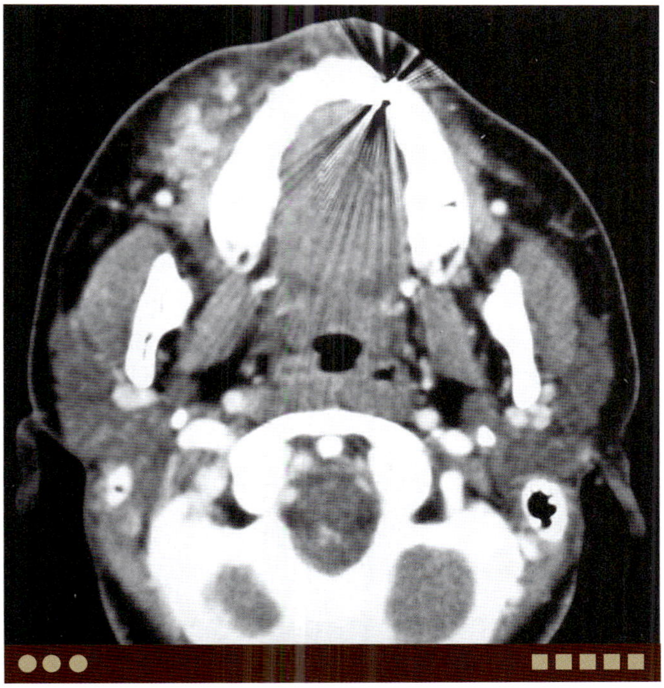

D. **AVM** in a different patient. Axial postcontrast CT in soft tissue window shows an ill-defined enhancing lesion over the right maxillary alveolus.

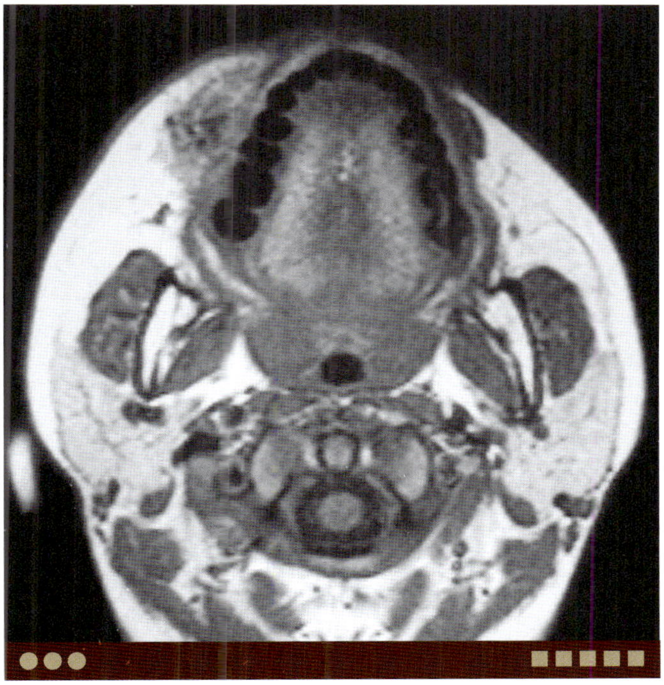

E. AVM, same patient as D. Axial T1W MR image demonstrates the lesion showing heterogeneous intermediate signal with multiple punctate hypointensities and flow-voids.

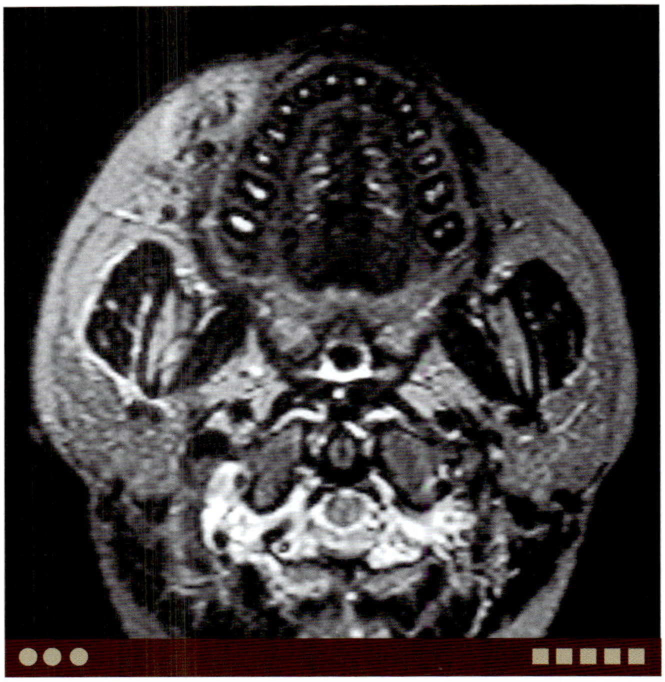

F. AVM, same patient as D. Axial T2W MR image demonstrates the lesion showing heterogeneous high signal with multiple punctate hypointensities and flow-voids.

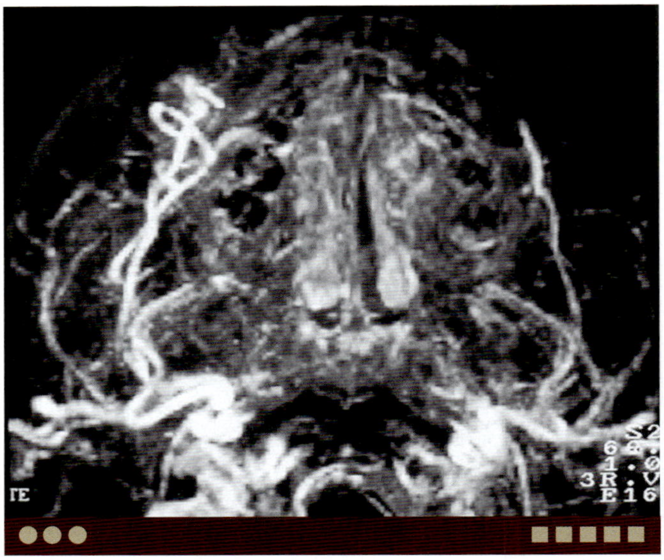

G. AVM, same patient as D. Axial MIP reconstruction of time-of-flight MRA demonstrates enlarged right internal maxillary and facial arteries.

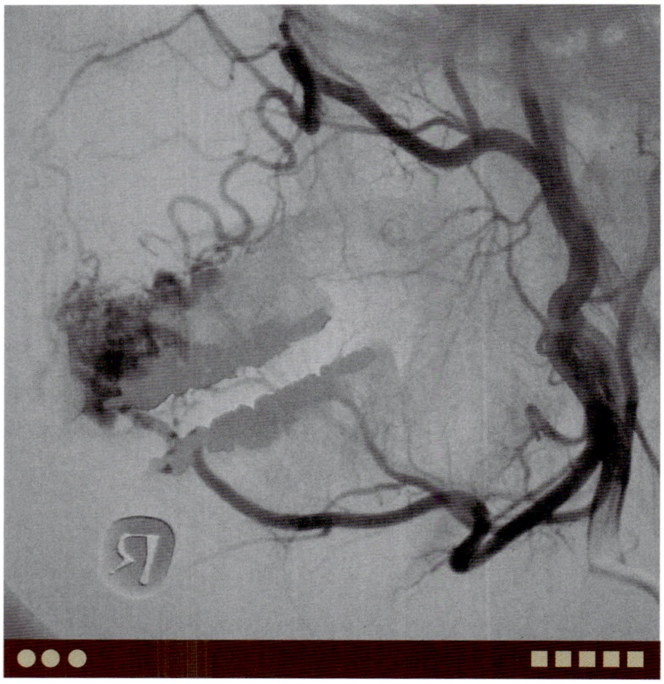

H. AVM, same patient as D. Lateral view of right external carotid arteriogram demonstrates tortuous vessels over the alveolus fed by the branches of the facial and internal maxillary arteries.

DIFFERENTIAL DIAGNOSIS IMAGES (I-J)

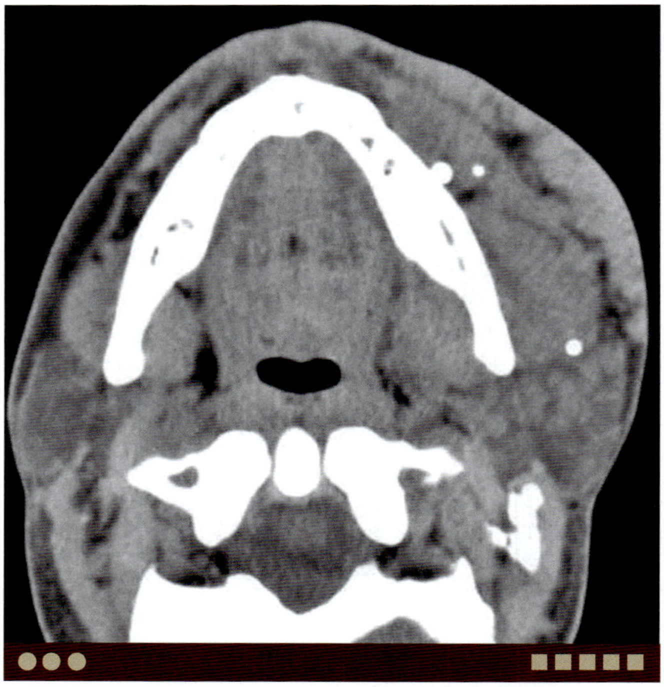

I. **Venous malformation**. Axial noncontrast CT demonstrates soft tissue density lesions with phlebolith involving the left masseter as well as subcutaneous tissues.

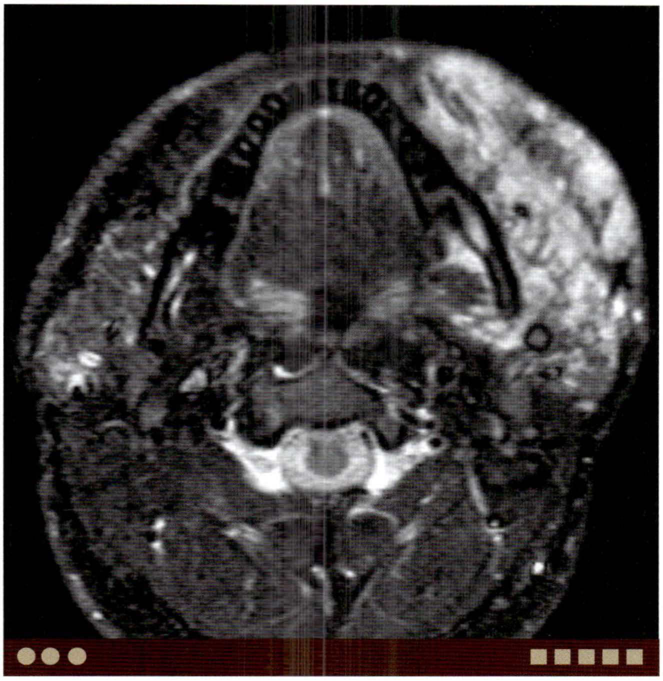

J. Venous malformation, same patient as I. Axial fat-suppressed T2W image demonstrates diffuse high-signal lesions involving the left masseter muscle, parotid gland and subcutaneous tissues.

Case 6–9 Lymphatic Malformation (Lymphangioma)

Osamu Sakai, Cory Siegel

PRESENTATION

Neck mass.

FINDINGS

CT demonstrates a cystic mass in the posterior triangle.

DIFFERENTIAL DIAGNOSIS

- Branchial cleft cyst: This usually arises from the second branchial cleft and locates anterolateral to the carotid vessels.
- Dermoid/epidermoid: Usually this is a unilocular cystic lesion. Presence of fat density suggests dermoid.
- Necrotic lymph node: This usually shows thick and irregular wall which enhances after contrast, with central hypoattenuating regions suggesting necrosis.

COMMENTS

This is a 5-year-old boy with a posterior neck mass.

Lymphatic malformation is one of the low-flow type vascular malformations also known as a lymphangioma or cystic hygroma. This malformation can be seen anywhere in the body, however, often occurs in the neck, particularly in the posterior cervical space. This can be unilocular or multilocular, and is very important as a differential diagnosis for congenital/developmental cystic masses in the neck.

In the past, due to limitations in resolution, small septi could not be demonstrated well and the lesion often appeared as a unilocular cyst. However, recent advances in imaging modalities have permitted the demonstration of these septi and compartmental differences in protein content on MRI or ultrasound.

After contrast administration, focal enhancement suggesting a venous component is often seen. The wall and septi also show subtle enhancement. If there is a significant amount of venous component then it is called as venolymphatic malformation.

On CT, it usually shows a unilocular appearance with water density because thin septi may not be demonstrated well. On MRI, it shows water signal which can be variable depending on protein concentration in each compartment; increased T1 and decreased T2 signal with an increase in protein concentration. MRI demonstrates subtle enhancement in the wall and septi compared to CT.

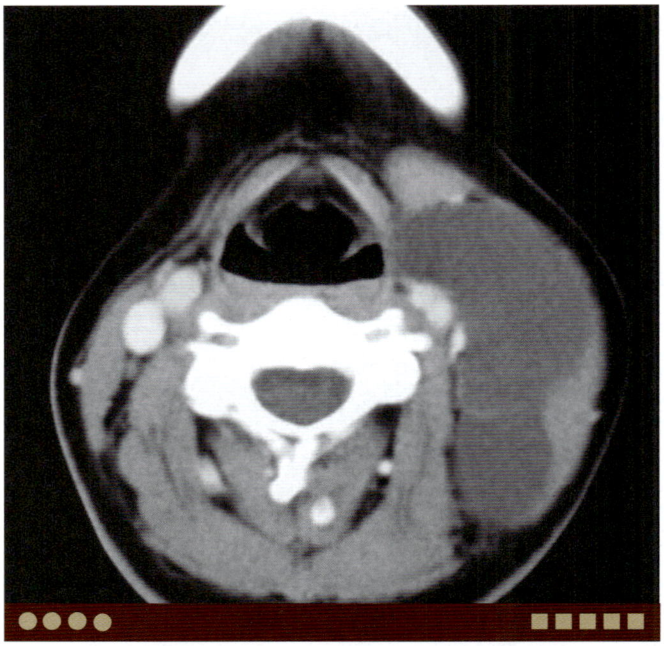

A. Lymphatic malformation. Axial postcontrast CT demonstrates a large thin-walled cystic lesion with some septation in the left neck, medial to the sternocleidomastoid muscle.

PEARLS

- **Lymphatic malformation is one of the low-flow type vascular malformations and is also called a lymphangioma or cystic hygroma.**
- **It can be unilocular or multilocular. Thin septi can be easily seen on modern MRI and ultrasound.**
- **It usually shows water density and signal, however, signal on MRI may be variable depending on protein concentration in each compartment.**

ADDITIONAL IMAGES (B-G)

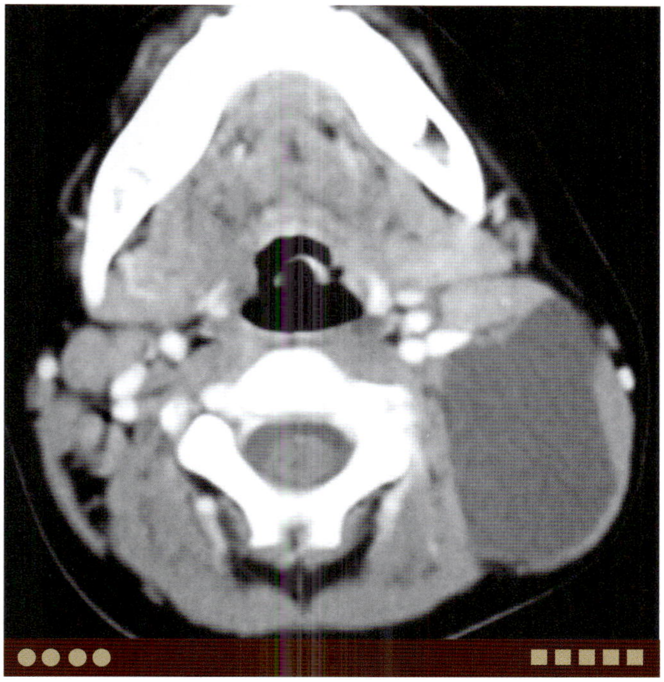

B. Lymphatic malformation in a different patient. Axial postcontrast CT demonstrates a hypoattenuating nonenhancing unilocular cystic lesion in the left posterior triangle.

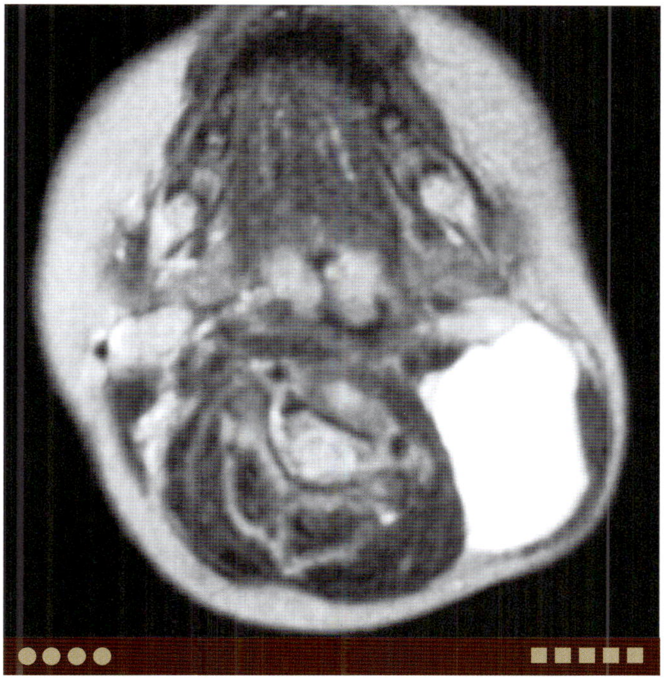

C. Lymphatic malformation, same patient as B. Axial T2W image shows this unilocular lesion to have homogeneous high signal.

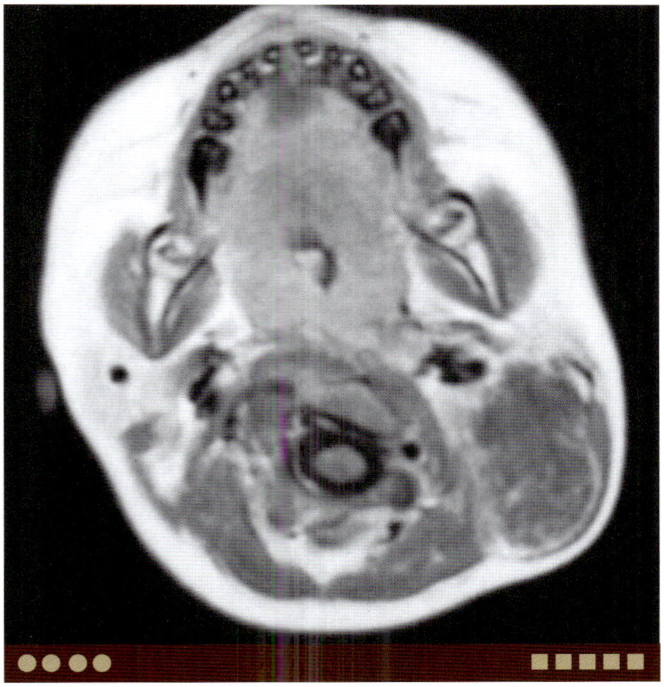

D. Lymphatic malformation, same patient as B. Axial postcontrast T1W image demonstrates mild enhancement of thin wall and septi.

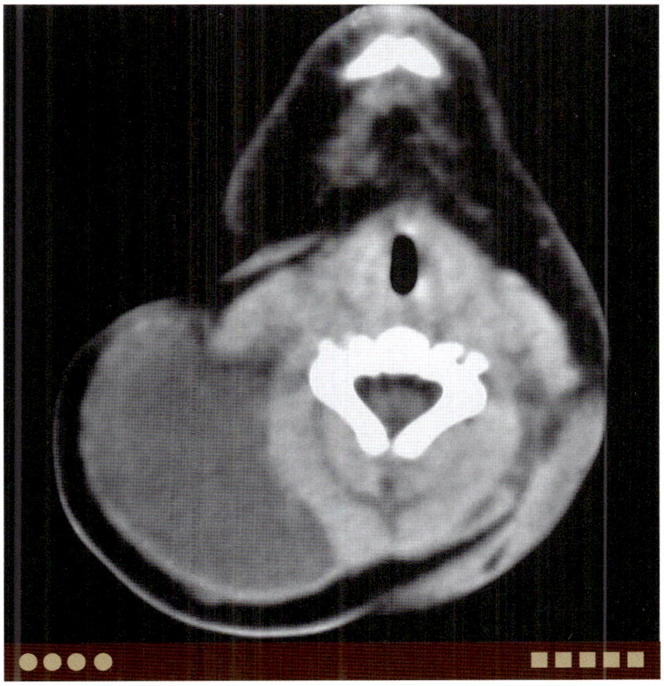

E. Lymphatic malformation in a different patient. Axial noncontrast CT demonstrates a large thin-walled cystic lesion in the right posterior triangle.

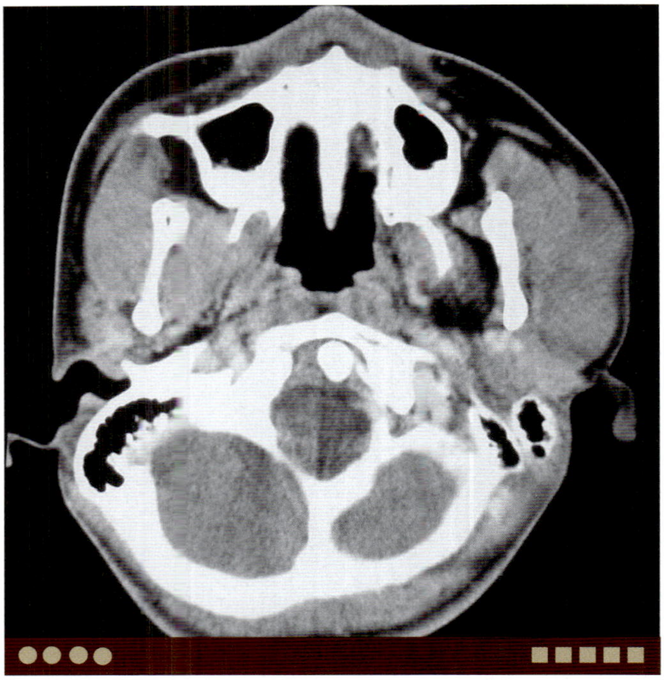

F. Lymphatic malformation in a different patient. Axial noncontrast CT demonstrates a lobulated soft tissue density lesion in the left cheek, over the masseter muscle.

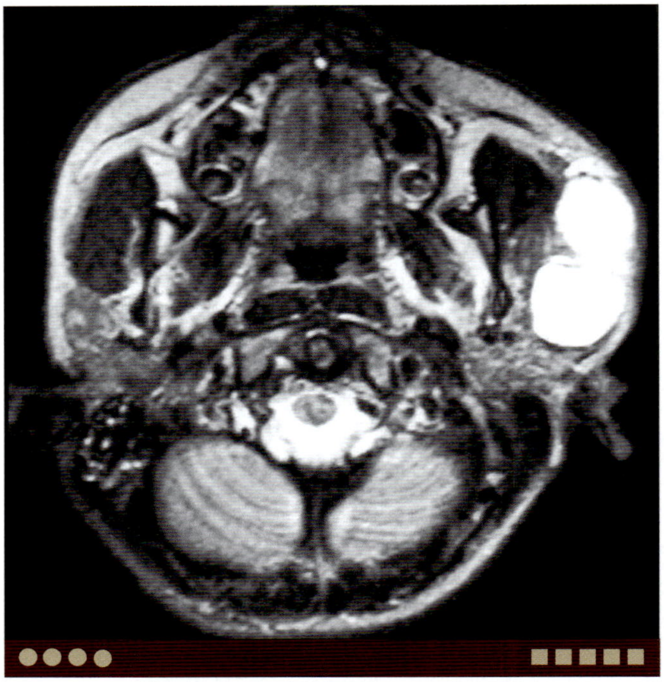

G. Lymphatic malformation, same patient as F. Axial T2W image shows the lobulated lesion to have high signal, suggesting fluid component, and well-demarcated margins.

DIFFERENTIAL DIAGNOSIS IMAGES (H-J)

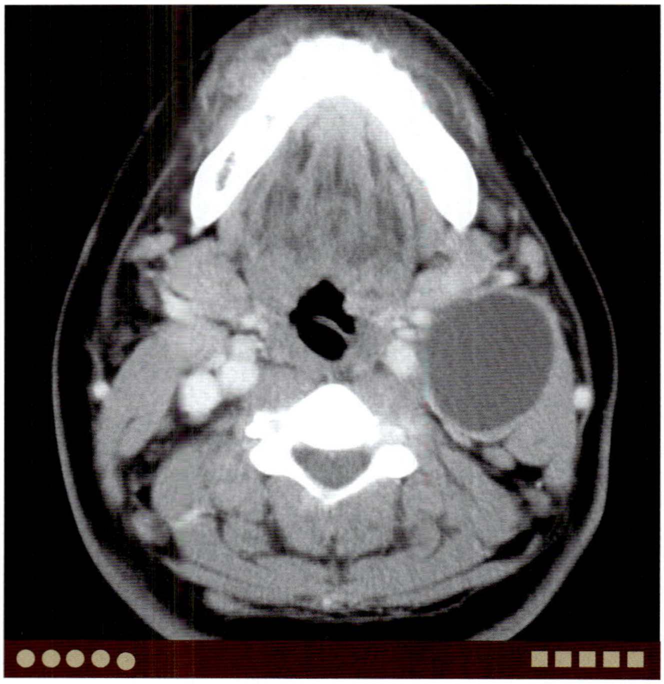

H. Second branchial cleft cyst. Axial postcontrast CT demonstrates a simple cystic lesion posterior to the left submandibular gland and anteromedial to the sternocleidomastoid muscle.

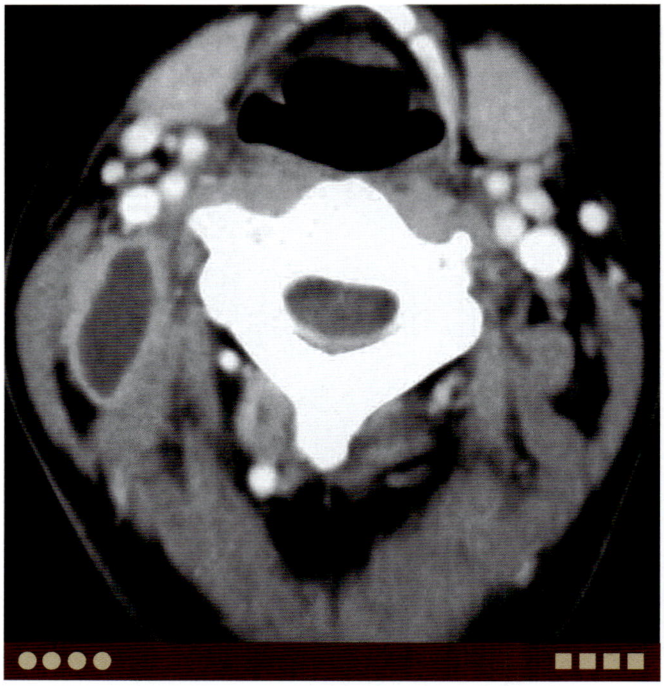

I. Tuberculosis. Axial postcontrast CT demonstrates a cystic nodal lesion with thick enhancing wall, posterior to the right internal jugular vein and medial to the sternocleidomastoid muscle.

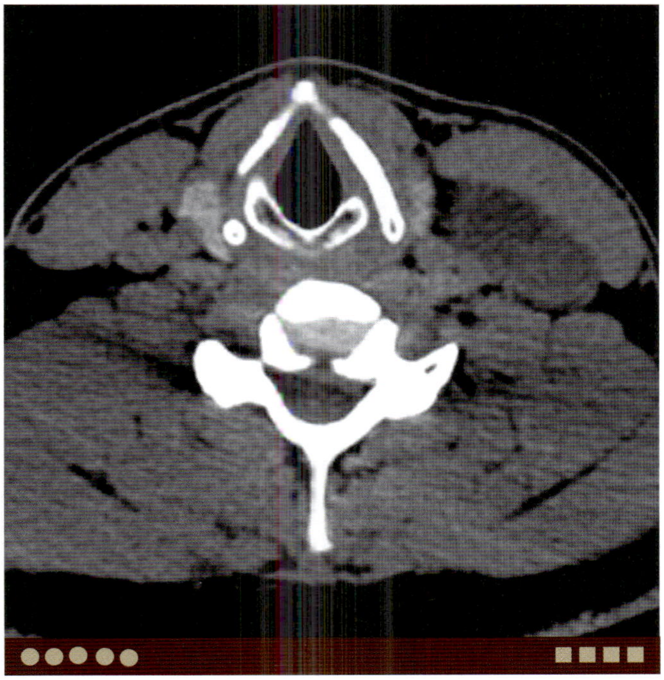

J. Papillary thyroid carcinoma. Axial noncontrast CT shows an ovoid cystic-appearing lesion deep to the left sternocleidomastoid muscle.

Case 6–10 First Branchial Cleft Anomaly

Akifumi Fujita, Benjamin Ludwig, Osamu Sakai

PRESENTATION

Parotid swelling and otorrhea.

FINDINGS

CT and MRI show a cystic mass with peripheral enhancement in the parotid region. Fistula draining into the external auditory canal may be also demonstrated.

DIFFERENTIAL DIAGNOSIS

- Lymphatic malformation (lymphangioma): This condition is difficult to differentiate by imaging alone, but lymphatic malformations are usually multilocular and involve multiple neck spaces. Rim-enhancement is typically absent.
- Benign lymphoepithelial cyst: This entity is usually seen in patients with HIV, characterized by multiple cysts of varying sizes within both parotid glands.
- Suppurative parotid lymph node: This condition usually results from bacterial infection, and presents with marked tenderness and fever. Cross-sectional imaging shows a thick-walled, rim-enhancing cystic mass in the parotid gland.
- Parotid gland tumor: Benign and malignant parotid neoplasms may contain cystic components/degeneration, and can be difficult to differentiate from other cystic lesions.

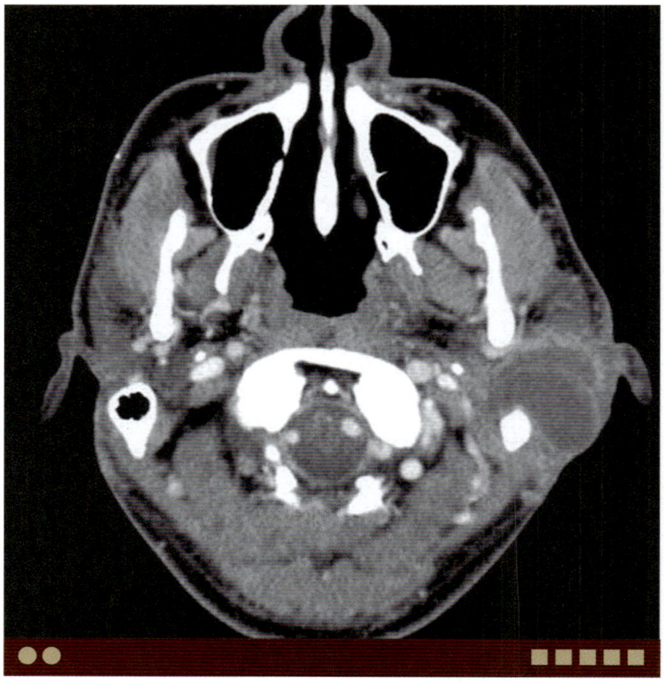

A. First branchial cleft cyst. Axial postcontrast CT image demonstrates a cystic mass with peripheral enhancement in the region of the left parotid gland.

COMMENTS

This is a 30-year-old man who presented with left parotid swelling and otorrhea, and a history of left parotid swelling requiring multiple surgical drainage as an adolescent.

Anomalies of the branchial complex are vestigial remnants, resulting from incomplete obliteration of the branchial apparatus or buried epithelial cell rests. First branchial complex anomalies are uncommon and account for 8% of all branchial anomalies. Periauricular and periparotid anatomic subtypes exist.

The most common presenting symptom is a painless soft mass in the periauricular or periparotid region. Recurrent swelling, tenderness, fever, and purulent ear drainage may be present if the lesion is infected or if an external auditory canal fistula or sinus tract is present. Most patients present in the first decade of life, but recurrent infections in young adults is also common.

Imaging aids in determining the anatomic location, size of the cyst, and relationship to adjacent structures. CT shows a thin-walled uni- or multilocular cystic lesion. When infected, the fluid may be complex in attenuation, or the cyst may demonstrate thick, rim-enhancement.

Multiplanar contrast-enhanced CT or MRI may assist in detecting clinically suspected fistulae and sinus tracts.

PEARLS

- **First branchial cleft anomalies are periauricular or periparotid thin-walled cystic lesions.**
- **Patients typically present when young, with parotid swelling and fever.**
- **Superinfection may result in complex fluid within the cyst, or thick, rim-enhancement on postcontrast CT or MRI.**

ADDITIONAL IMAGES (B–E)

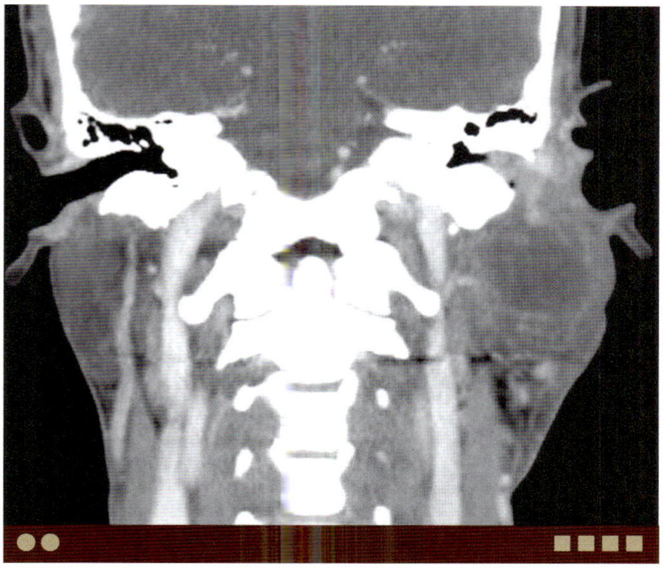

B. First branchial cleft cyst, same patient as A. Coronal postcontrast CT image demonstrates a cystic, periparotid mass with peripheral enhancement. Fistula to the external auditory canal is also noted.

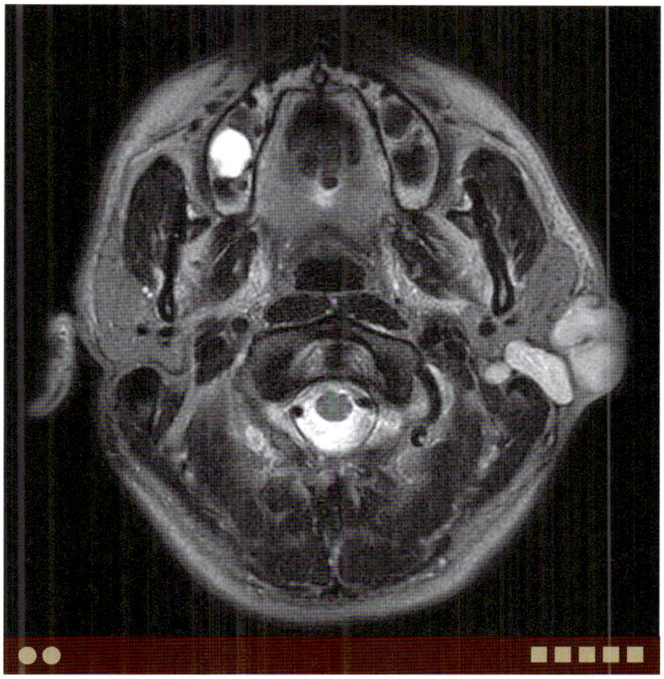

C. First branchial cleft cyst, same patient as A. Axial T2W image demonstrates a multilocular cystic mass in the region of the left parotid.

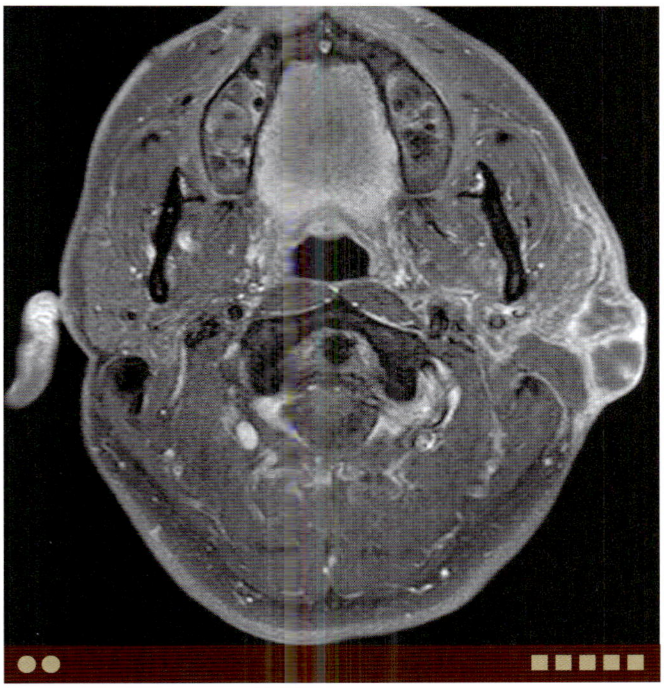

D. First branchial cleft cyst, same patient as A. Axial postcontrast fat-suppressed T1W image demonstrates a multilocular cystic mass with peripheral enhancement in the region of the left parotid.

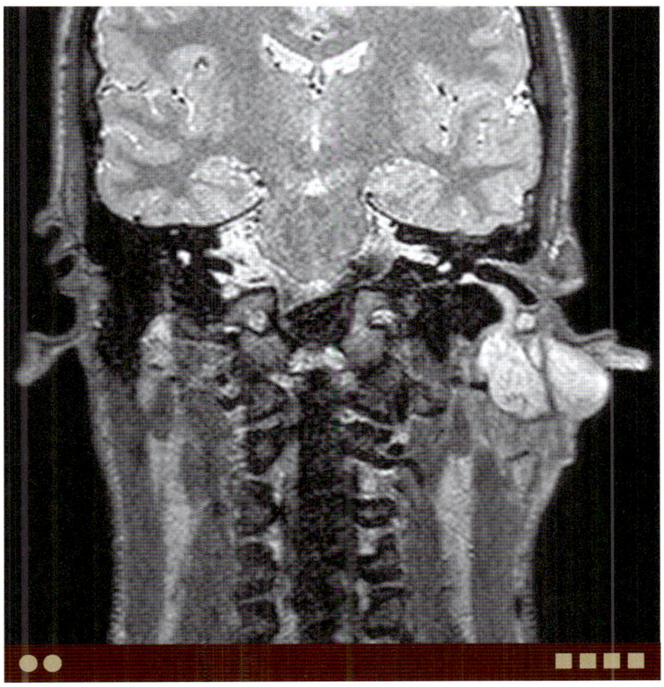

E. First branchial cleft cyst, same patient as A. Coronal reformatted 3D T2W image shows a multilocular, periparotid cystic mass. Fistula to the external auditory canal is clearly demonstrated.

DIFFERENTIAL DIAGNOSIS IMAGES (F-I)

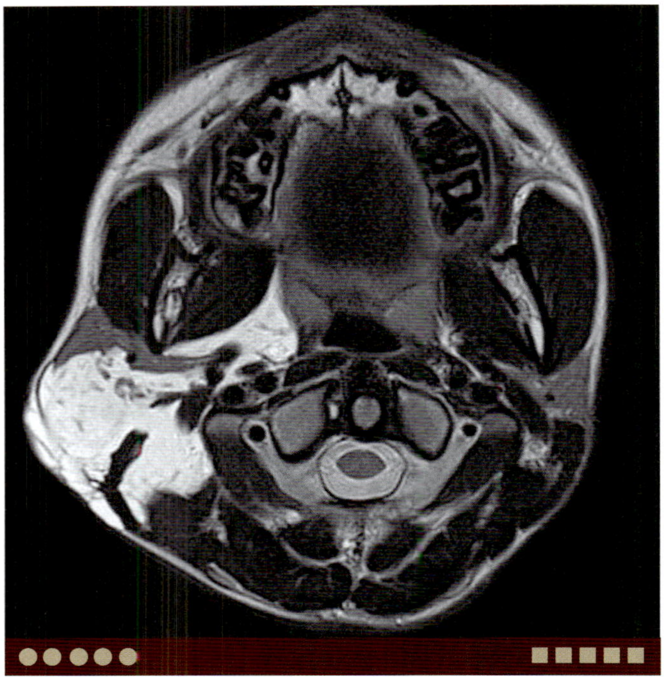

F. Lymphatic malformation. Axial T2W image demonstrates a multilocular cystic mass in the region of the right parotid, extending to posterior cervical and parapharyngeal spaces.

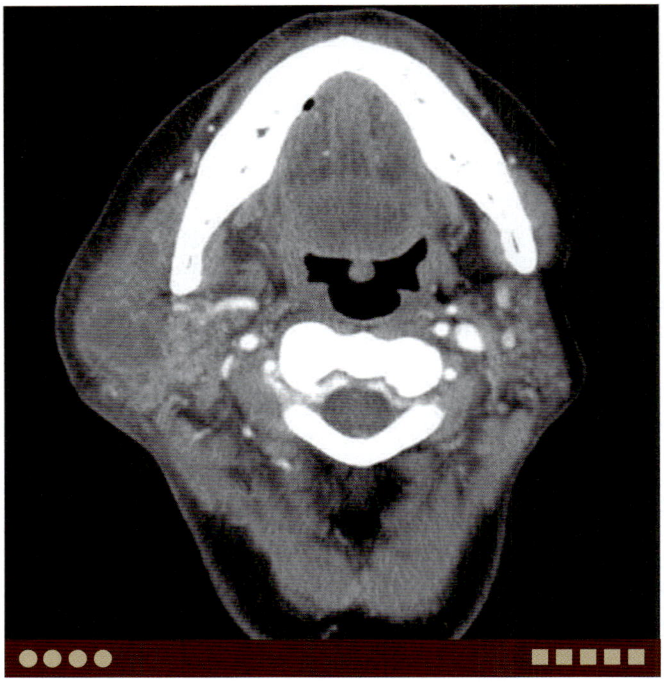

G. Suppurative parotid node. Axial postcontrast CT demonstrates a cystic mass with peripheral enhancement in the right parotid gland.

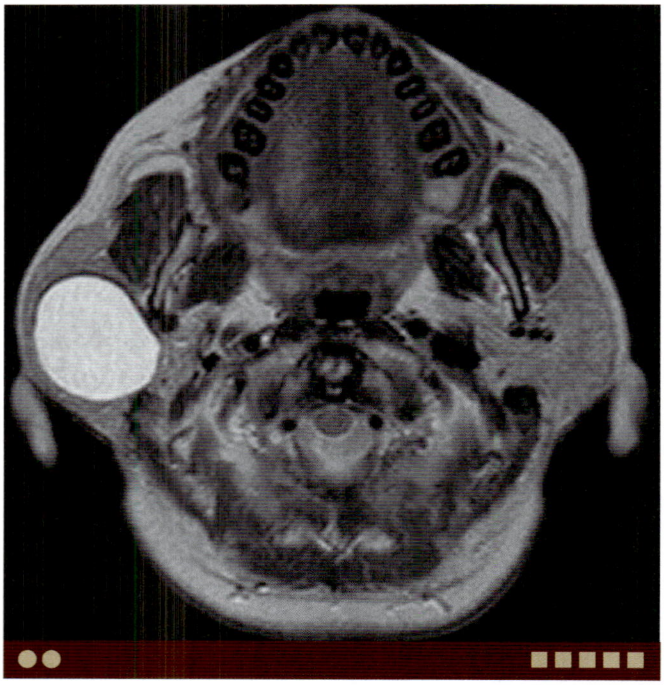

H. Lymphoepithelial cyst. Axial T2W image demonstrates a well-circumscribed unilocular cystic mass in the right parotid gland.

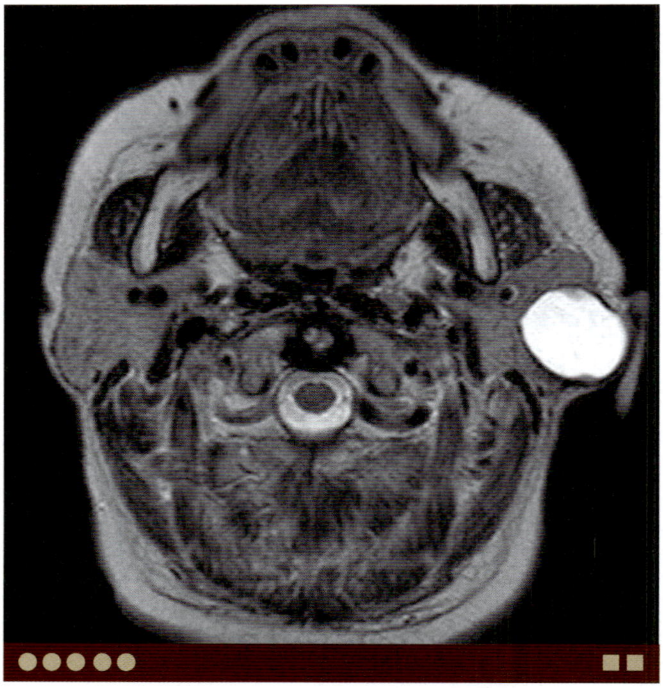

I. Pleomorphic adenoma. Axial T2W image demonstrates a well-circumscribed unilocular cystic mass with a mural nodule in the left parotid gland.

Case 6–11 Masticator Space Infection

Brooke Devenney-Cakir, Osamu Sakai

PRESENTATION

Painful cheek swelling.

FINDINGS

CT demonstrates enlarged heterogeneously enhancing masseter muscle.

DIFFERENTIAL DIAGNOSIS

- Venous malformation/hemangioma: This is the most common benign tumor in the masticator space. Presence of phlebolith suggests venous malformation.
- Squamous cell carcinoma (SCCA): SCCA of the oral cavity and oropharynx invades the masticator space. Then, it can extend intracranially along the V3 through the foramen ovale (perineural spread).
- Benign masseteric hypertrophy: This is a benign condition, usually bilateral, however, can be unilateral and mimic a mass lesion. This condition is commonly seen in young men.
- Mandibular osteonecrosis: Patients with histories of prior radiation therapy or bisphosphonate therapy can have osteonecrosis of the mandible. There may be associated soft tissue swelling and clinical findings may be similar to infection.

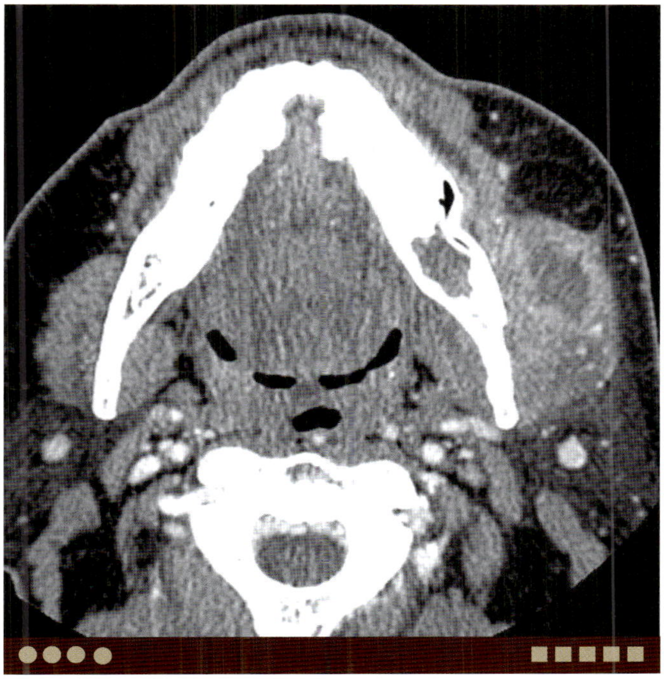

A. Masticator space abscess. Axial contrast-enhanced CT demonstrates a multiloculated low density peripherally enhancing collection in the left masseter muscle with inflammatory change in the surrounding soft tissues.

COMMENTS

This is a 69-year-old man with cheek swelling and pain.

Infection is the most common abnormality in the masticator space. It is usually odontogenic and seen in patients with dental caries and history of recent dental procedures. However, occasionally a patient is presented with a mass, suspected for neoplastic process because infectious process may not be apparent in a patient with chronic inflammation. Actinomycosis, a normal flora in the mouth can cause localized invasive change resulting in severe fibrotic change and fistula formation.

On CT, heterogeneous enhancement is seen in inflamed areas in the muscles of mastication with inflammatory changes in the adjacent fatty tissue. The diagnosis of an abscess, demonstrated by rim-enhancing fluid collection is important to determine the necessity of surgical intervention. Evaluation with bone algorithm reconstructed images is extremely important to identify the exact cause of the infectious process. Multiplanar reconstruction is helpful to demonstrate relationship between the dental cavity, periapical abscess, cortical fistula, and soft tissue abscess. MRI is not the first modality of choice, however, it is very useful to evaluate for abnormalities in the muscle and bone marrow. Imaging is important to make a diagnosis and to plan the access for the surgical intervention.

PEARLS

- **Odontogenic infection is the most common abnormality in the masticator space.**
- **CT is the modality of choice, and both soft tissue and bone algorithm reconstructed images should be carefully evaluated to identify the exact cause of infection.**
- **In a patient with chronic inflammation, clinical findings to suggest infection may be minimal.**

ADDITIONAL IMAGES (B-G)

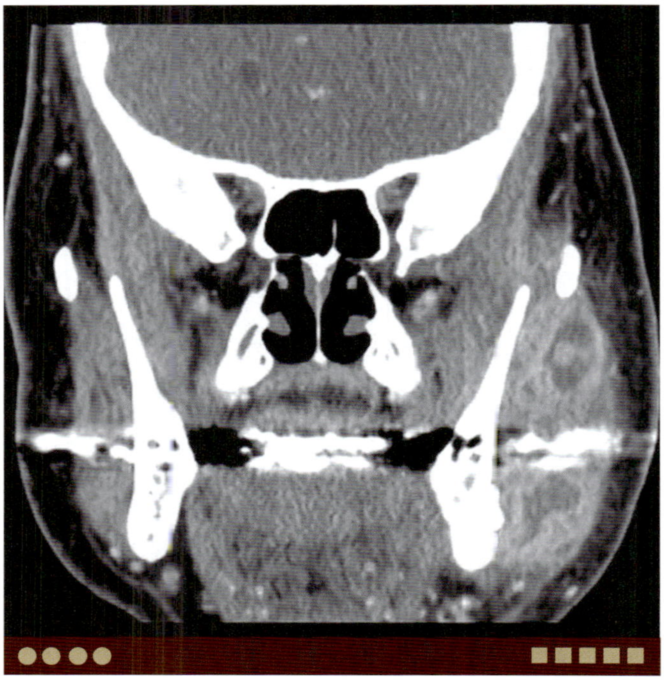

B. Masticator space abscess, same patient as A. Coronal contrast-enhanced CT demonstrates multiple peripherally enhancing collections in the left masseter muscle. Note significant inflammatory change in the surrounding soft tissues.

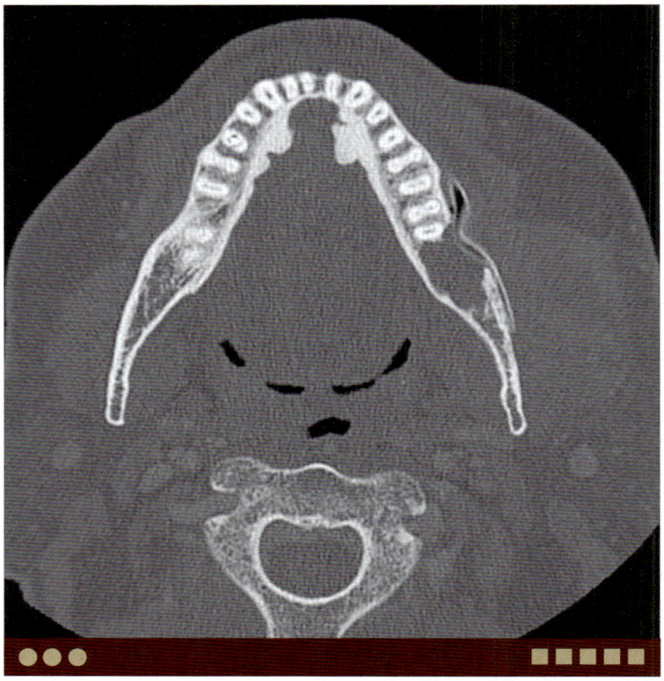

C. Masticator space abscess, same patient as A. Axial bone algorithm CT demonstrates a large bone defect, osteolytic change in the left posterior mandible consistent with status post molar extraction with infection.

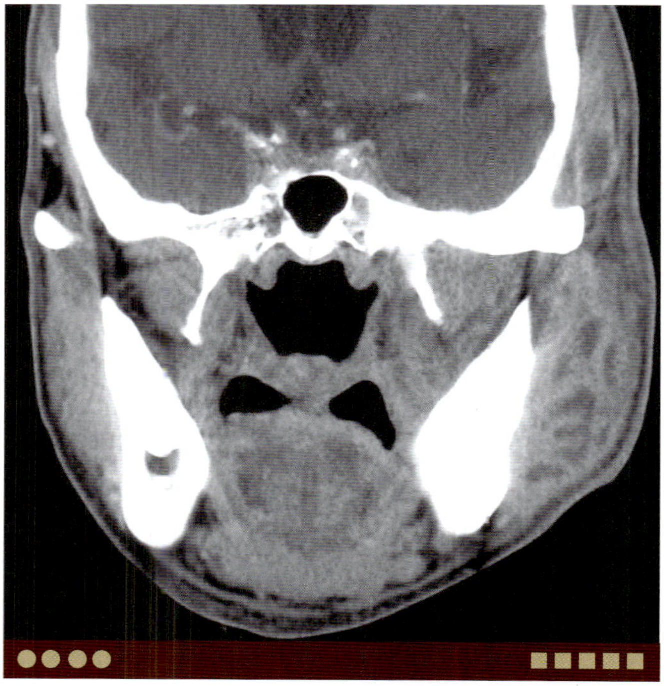

D. **Masticator space abscess** in a different patient. Coronal contrast-enhanced CT demonstrates multiple peripherally enhancing collections in the left masseter muscle. Note rim-enhancing collection is also seen in the left temporalis muscle.

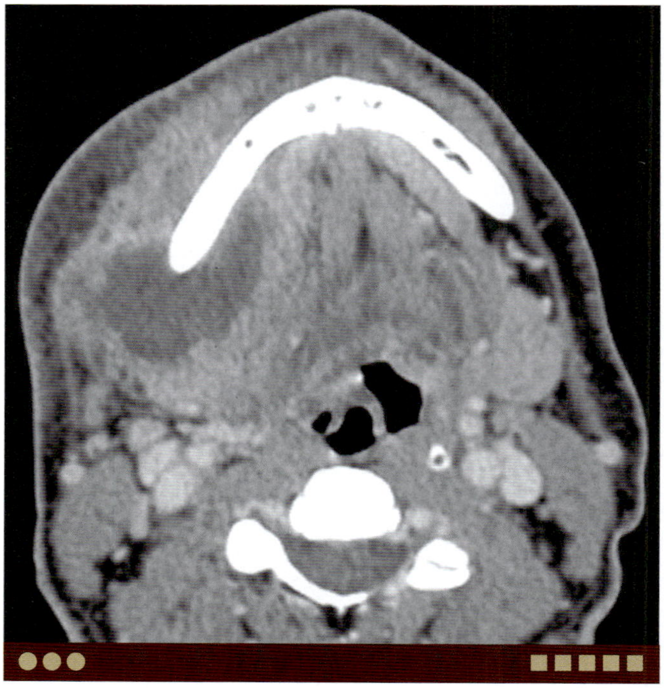

E. **Masticator space abscess** in a different patient. Axial contrast-enhanced CT demonstrates a large abscess at the right mandibular angle.

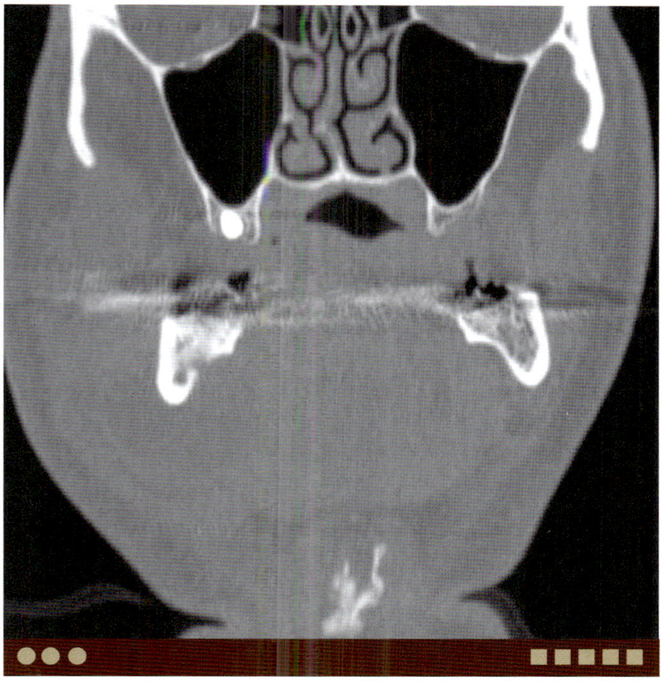

F. Masticator space abscess, same patient as E. Coronal bone algorithm CT demonstrates sclerotic change in the right mandible, and fistula formation in the lingual cortex.

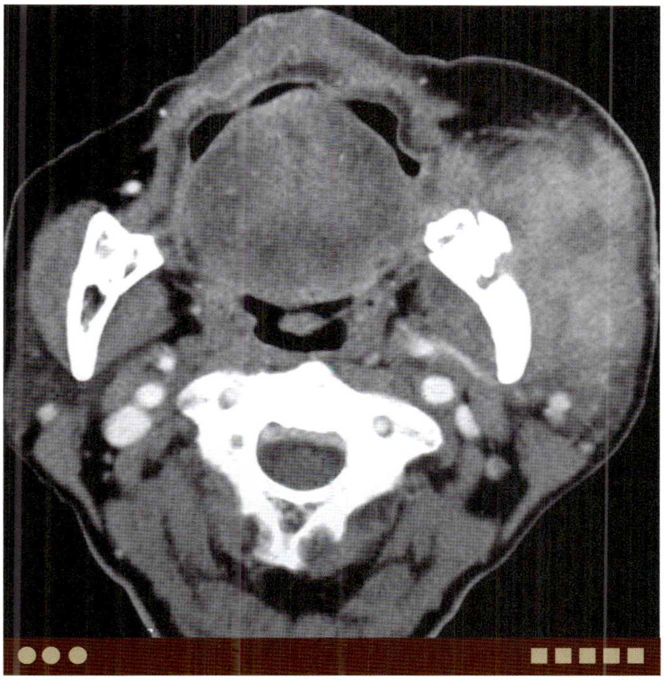

G. Masticator space abscess in a different patient, Actinomycosis. Axial contrast-enhanced CT demonstrates significant enlargement and heterogeneous enhancement of the left masseter muscle with small low-density foci consistent with abscesses. Note fistula formation in the mandible.

DIFFERENTIAL DIAGNOSIS IMAGES (H-J)

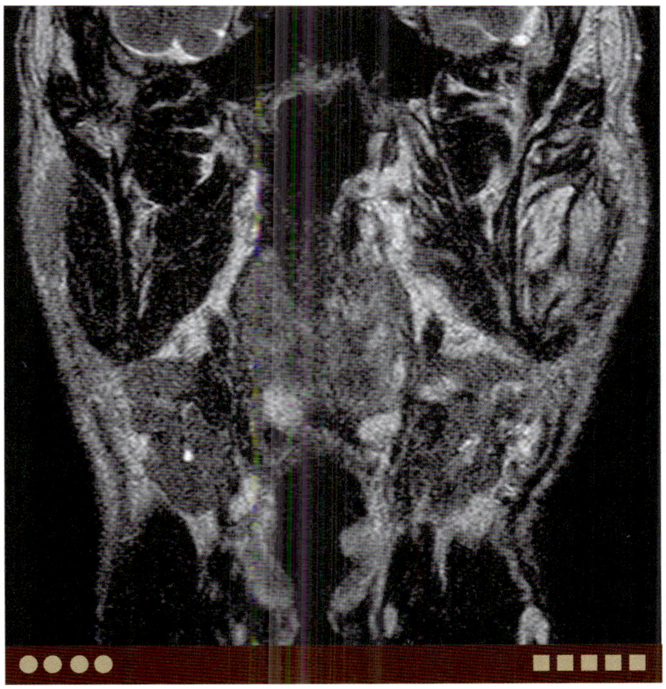

H. Venous malformation. Coronal T2W MR image demonstrates multiple areas of high signal in the left masseter muscle.

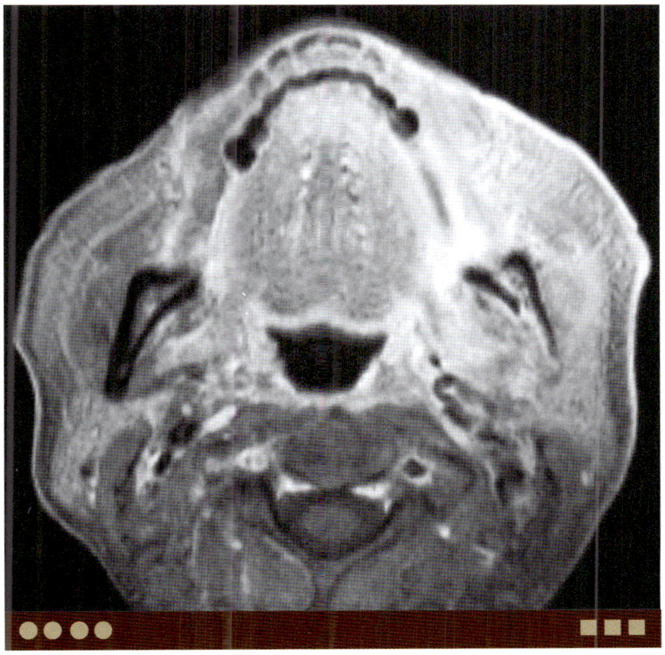

I. SCCA. Axial postcontrast fat-suppressed T1W MR image demonstrates abnormal enhancement centered in the left retromolar trigon. Note diffuse enhancement of the pterygoid and masseter muscles, as well as bone destruction and abnormal marrow enhancement in the left mandible, consistent with direct tumor invasion and denervation myositic change from V3 injury.

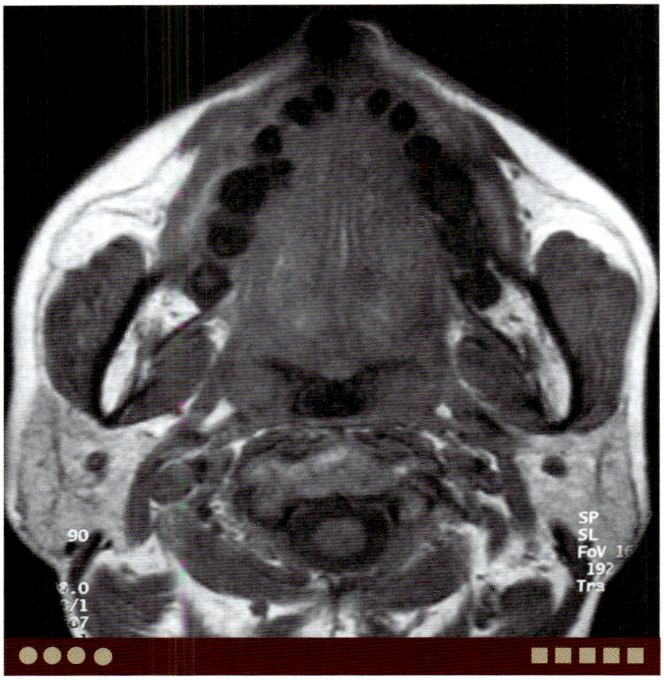

J. Benign masseteric hypertrophy. Axial T1W MR image demonstrates thickening of the left masseter muscle without signal abnormality.

Case 6–12 Venous Malformation

Osamu Sakai, Carlos Gonzalez, Susmitha Reddy

PRESENTATION

Painless cheek swelling.

FINDINGS

T2W MR image demonstrates very high-signal lesions infiltrating in the masticator space. CT demonstrates a lobulated or infiltrating soft tissue density mass with nodular calcification in the masticator space.

DIFFERENTIAL DIAGNOSIS

- Lymphatic malformation: These are cystic structures lined with endothelium and filled with protein-rich fluid, chyle, and most commonly occur in the neck and axilla. These cystic structures show high signal in T2W MR images but do not exhibit central enhancement with gadolinium. Fluid-fluid levels are often present.
- High-flow vascular malformations: Include arteriovenous malformations and arteriovenous fistulas. These are much less common than are low-flow vascular malformations. Appear as a tangle of multiple serpiginous "flow-voids" on T1W and T2W MR images with no focal discrete soft tissue mass.

COMMENTS

This is a 25-year-old woman with painless cheek swelling and discoloration.

Venous malformation is the most common vascular malformation of the head and neck. It is a slow-flow postcapillary lesion composed of endothelial-lined vascular sinusoids. This type of vascular malformations is often called hemangioma, which is recently avoided to be used because this is a developmental anomaly, not a neoplastic process. Their endothelial cell proliferation and turnover characteristics are normal, and they demonstrate a slow, steady growth pattern proportionate with the growth of the child, and further, they also never involute. This vascular anomaly often contains nodular calcification and phlebolith. Presence of phlebolith as well as the identification of discrete areas of homogeneous high-signal intensity, which represent venous lakes, strongly suggests venous malformation. This malformation is seen anywhere in the body, however, often occurs in the face, involving the masticator space. By definition, it is present at birth; however, it clinically manifests in children, adolescents or young adults.

On CT, it usually shows slightly lobulated appearance with density similar to the vasculature. Nodular calcification and phlebolith strongly suggests venous malformation. Enhancement is seen in venous malformation. However, enhancement may not be seen immediately after contrast administration due to slow flow. Catheter angiogram is not necessary for diagnosis. Just like other vascular malformations, venous malformation also extends beyond the fascia-defined space, involving multiple spaces. Bone erosion or remodeling can be seen.

On MRI, it shows low signal on T1W and very high signal on T2W images, and enhancement after contrast. Phlebolith can be seen as rounded or ovoid signal void. Like other vascular anomalies, this is often accompanied with increased fatty tissue, seen as high signals on T1W images and low density on CT.

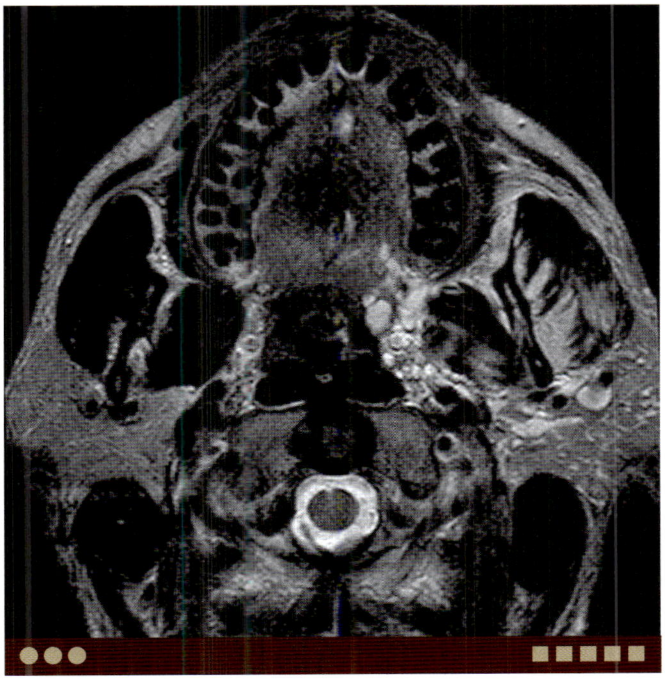

A. Venous malformation. Axial T2W image demonstrates high-signal lesions in the left masseter and pterygoid muscles.

PEARLS

- **Venous malformation is one of the low-flow type vascular malformations and used to be often called as hemangioma.**
- **It shows a lobulated appearance with similar density to the vasculature on CT, and low signal on T1W and very high signal on T2W MR images and enhancement.**
- **Presence of phlebolith strongly suggests venous malformation.**
- **Vascular malformations involve multiple fascia-defined spaces.**

ADDITIONAL IMAGES (B-G)

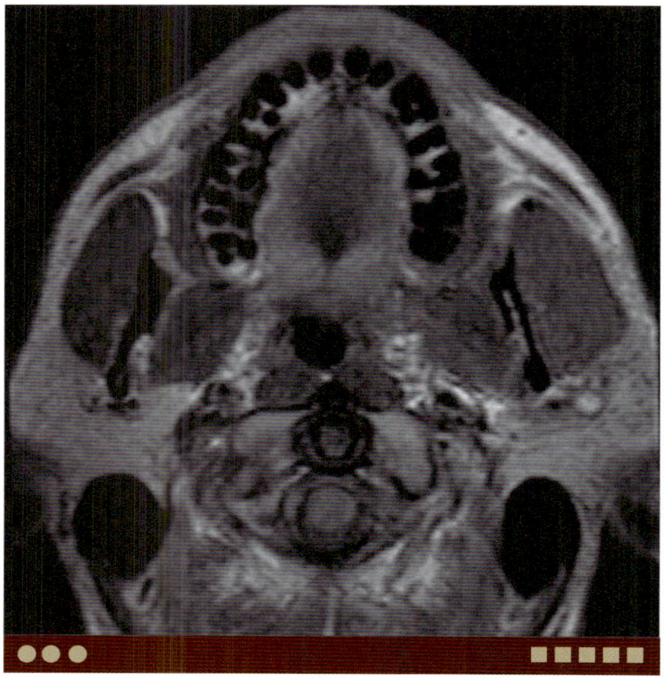

B. Venous malformation, same patient as A. Axial T1W images demonstrates slight thickening of the left masseter and pterygoid muscles.

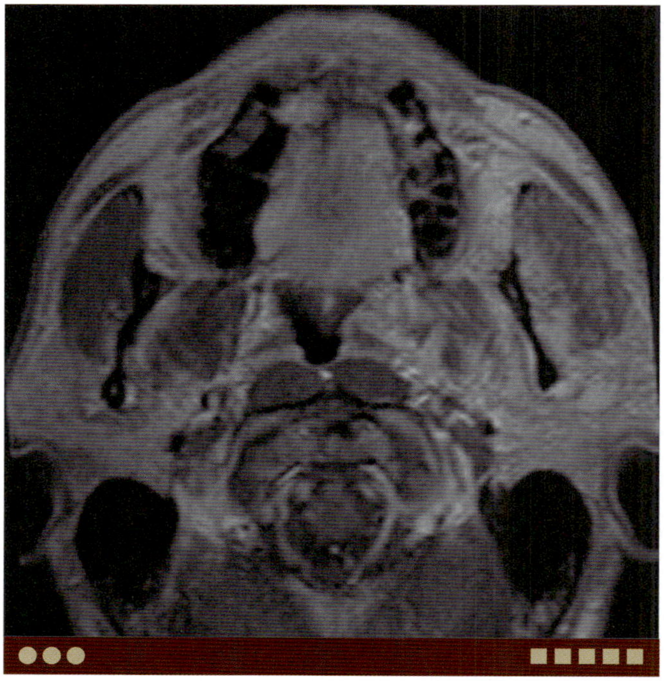

C. Venous malformation, same patient as A. Axial postcontrast T1W images demonstrates heterogeneous enhancement within the left masseter and pterygoid muscles.

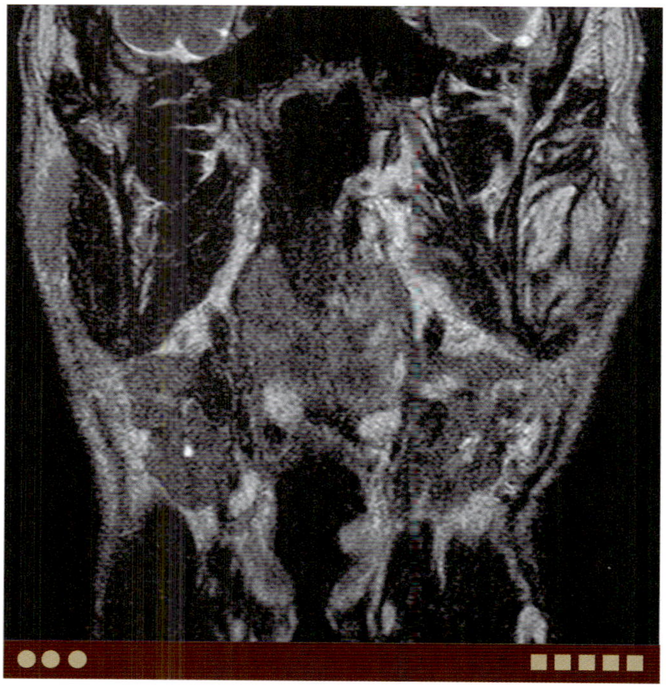

D. Venous malformation, same patient as A. Coronal T2W image demonstrates diffuse high-signal lesions involving the left masseter and medial pterygoid muscles.

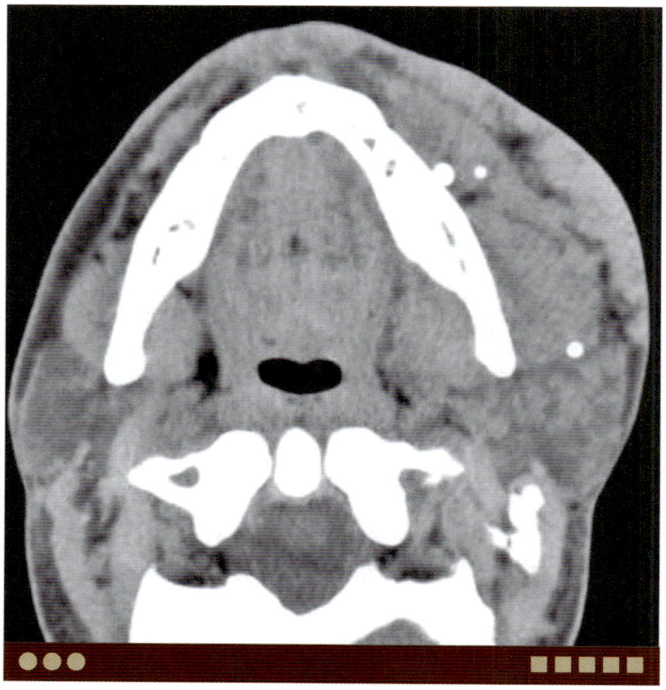

E. **Venous malformation** in a different patient. Axial noncontrast CT demonstrates soft tissue density lesions with phlebolith involving the left masseter as well as subcutaneous tissues.

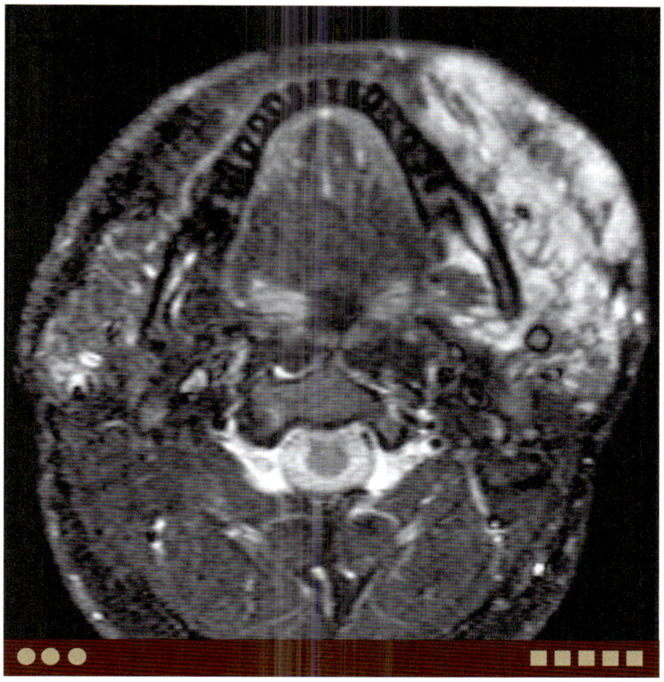

F. Venous malformation, same patient as E. Axial STIR image demonstrates diffuse high-signal lesions involving the left masseter muscle, parotid gland and subcutaneous tissues.

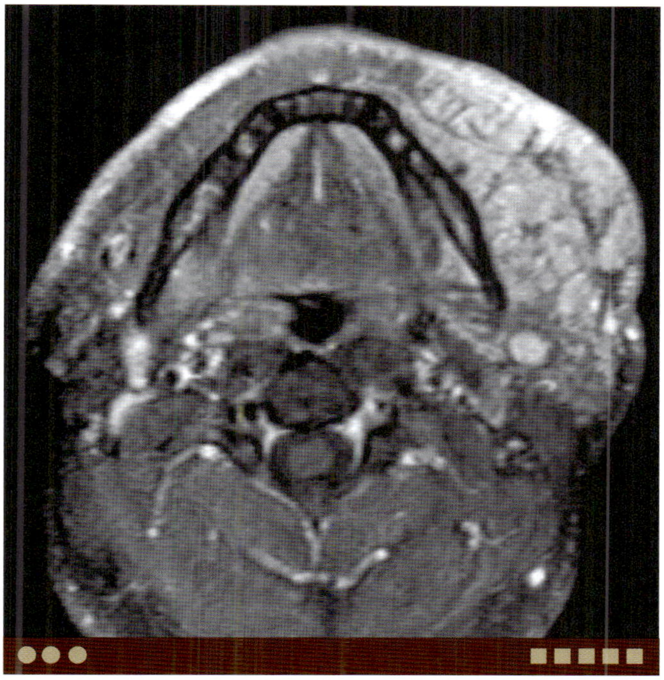

G. Venous malformation, same patient as E. Axial postcontrast fat-suppressed T1W image demonstrates enhancement of the lesion.

DIFFERENTIAL DIAGNOSIS IMAGES (H-J)

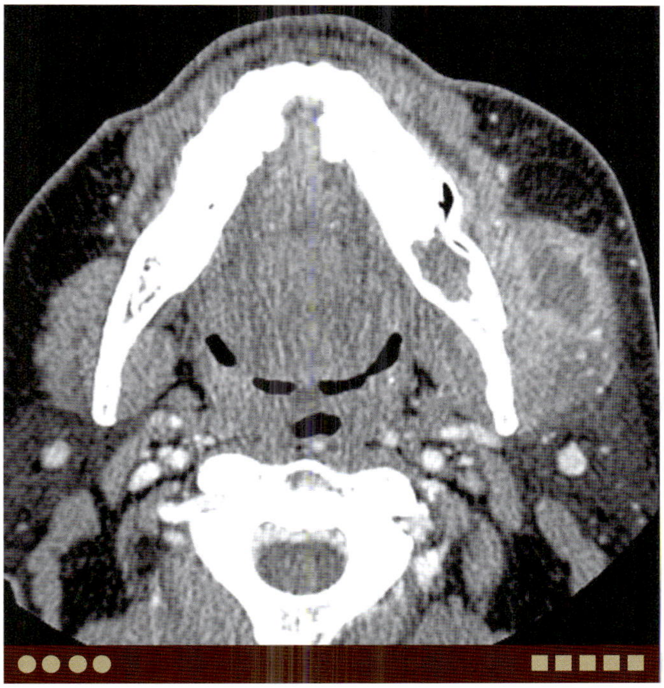

H. Masticator space abscess. Axial contrast-enhanced CT demonstrates a multiloculated low density, peripherally enhancing collection in the left masseter muscle with inflammatory change in the surrounding soft tissues.

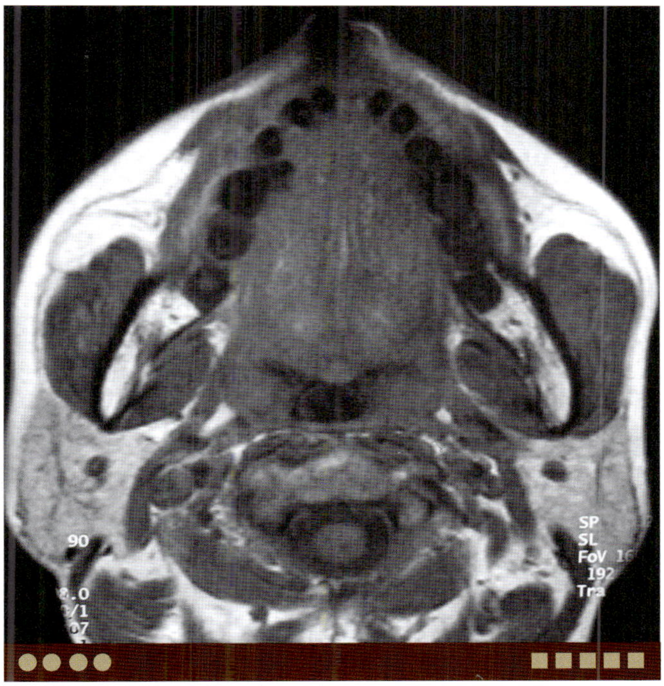

I. Benign masseteric hypertrophy. Axial T1W MR image demonstrates thickening of the left masseter muscle without signal abnormality.

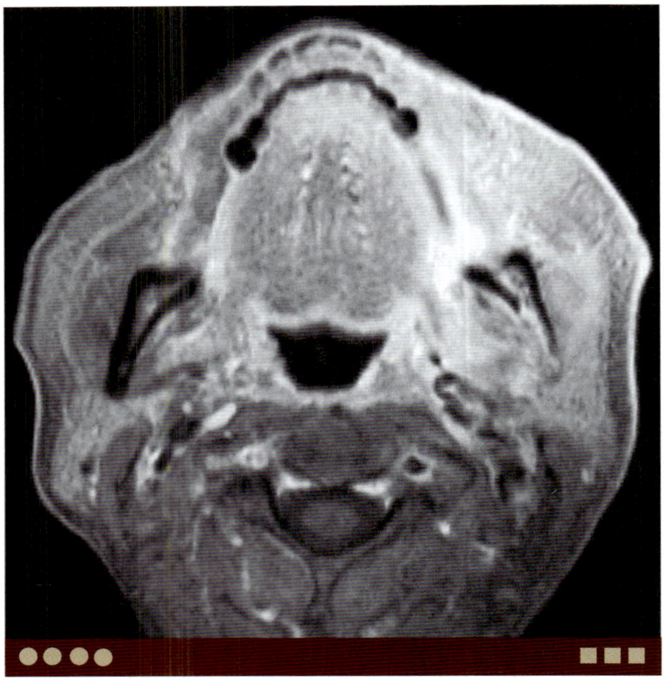

J. SCCA. Axial postcontrast fat-suppressed T1W MR image demonstrates abnormal enhancement centered in the left retromolar trigon. Bone destruction and denervation myositic change from V3 injury is seen in the masseter and pterygoid muscles.

Case 6–13 Hemangiopericytoma

Osamu Sakai, Susmitha Reddy

PRESENTATION

Painless cheek swelling.

FINDINGS

CT and MRI demonstrate an enhancing soft tissue mass in the masticator space.

DIFFERENTIAL DIAGNOSIS

- Infection: Odontogenic infection is the most common pathology in the masticator space. Partially treated infection may mimic neoplastic process, although diagnosis of infection is usually easily made by clinical information.
- Slow-flow vascular malformation: The imaging presentation varies with the type of vascular malformation that is, lymphatic, venolymphatic, and venous malformation. These are lobulated masses which show variable signal intensity areas on MRI depending on the constituents within the lesion. Phleboliths may be seen and are suggestive of venous malformation.
- Neurogenic tumors: These includes schwannoma and neurofibroma, and are usually well-demarcated tumors along the course of the mandibular branch of the trigeminal nerve, often with intermediate-to-low signal on T1W images compared to the adjacent muscles.
- Malignant fibrous histiocytoma and other sarcomas: Malignant tumors often show heterogeneous density/signal and invasive findings, and may show erosion/destruction of the mandible.
- Benign masseteric hypertrophy: This is a benign condition, usually bilateral, however, can be unilateral and mimic a mass lesion. This condition is commonly seen in young men.

COMMENTS

This is a 51-year-old man with painless mass in the right cheek.

Hemangiopericytoma is a rare vascular mesenchymal tumor arising from the pericyte of Zimmermann in the walls of the capillaries. They show generally low-grade malignant potential. These tumors are highly cellular and proliferation of the capillary vessels is seen often with arteriovenous shunting. Hemangiopericytoma is not common in the head and neck, therefore venous/venolymphatic/lymphatic vascular malformations (hemangioma/lymphangioma) or neurogenic tumors should be suspected first when very high-signal lesions are seen in the masticator space. However, thick, irregular capsule or wall, internal necrosis and rapid growth of the lesion are signs to suggest hemangiopericytoma or other malignancy.

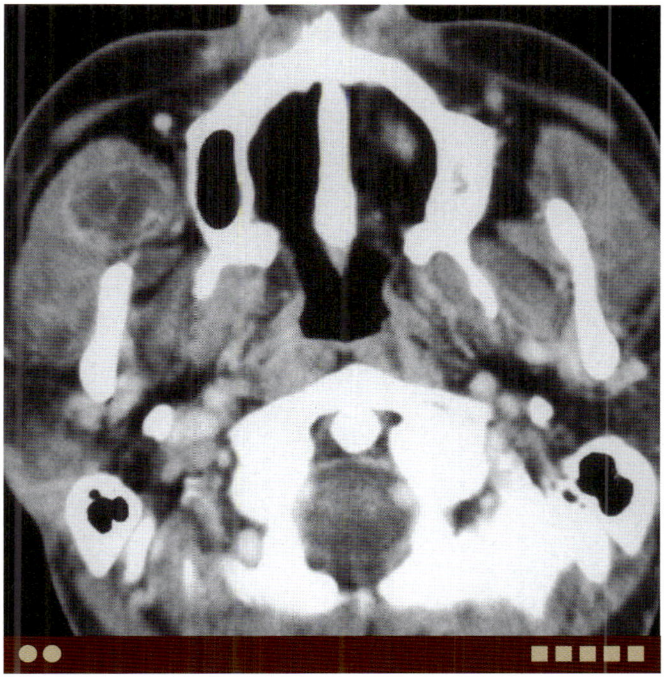

A. Hemangiopericytoma. Axial postcontrast CT shows a heterogeneously enhancing lesion in the anterior portion of the right masseter muscle; central necrosis and peripheral rim-enhancement. There is a further satellite lesion in the posterior aspect of the right masseter.

On CT, cystic appearing areas within the tumor are often seen reflecting necrosis. Avid enhancement is common reflecting rich vascular proliferation. On MRI, hemangiopericytoma often show very high signal on T2W and variable signal on T1W images, from low signal similar to the muscle to relatively high signal depending on its contents. Avid enhancement is seen after contrast.

Surgical resection is the treatment of choice; however, local recurrence is not uncommon. The prognosis depends on the tumor stage at presentation and complete primary resection. With recurrence, malignant appearance becomes more obvious on imaging and histology, however accurate grading of malignancy is difficult on either imaging or histology.

PEARLS

- **Hemangiopericytoma is a rare vascular mesenchymal tumor arising from the pericyte of Zimmermann.**
- **Avid enhancement is seen after contrast.**
- **Intratumoral necrosis is common.**

ADDITIONAL IMAGES (B-C)

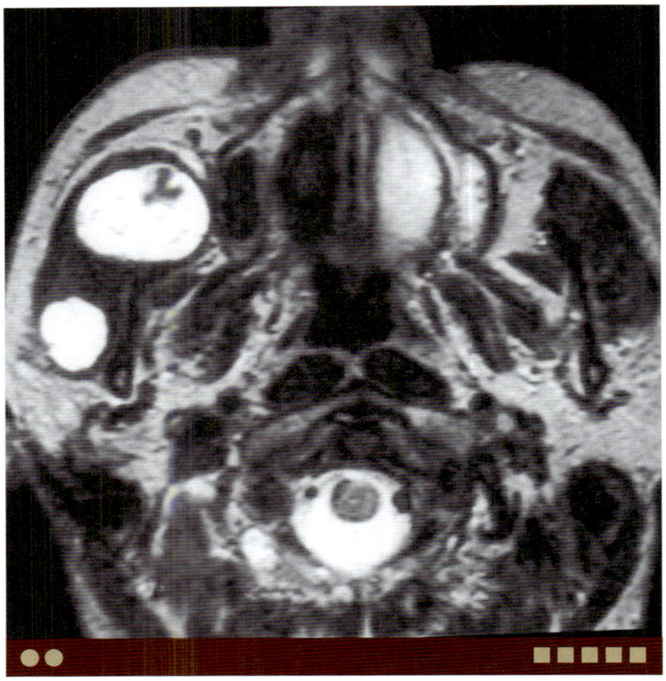

B. Hemangiopericytoma, same patient as A. Axial T2W MR image shows two very high-signal intensity lesions.

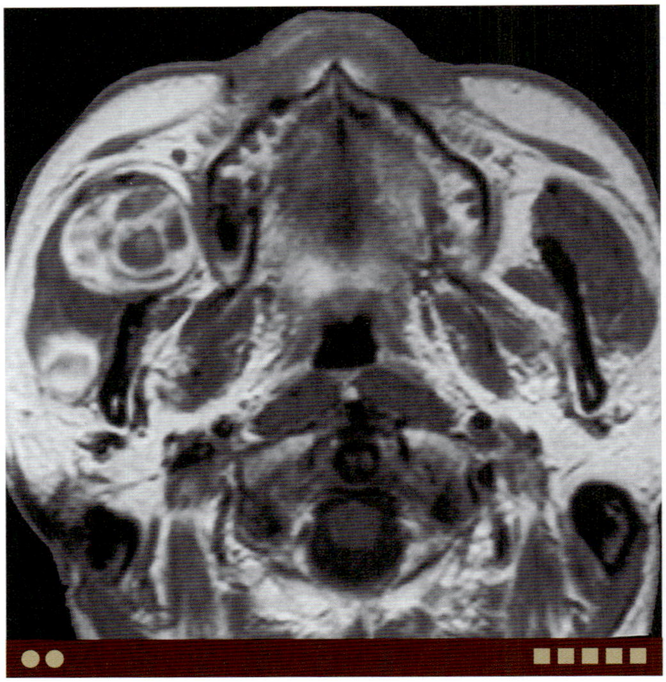

C. Hemangiopericytoma, same patient as A. Axial postcontrast T1W image shows avidly enhancing tumors with central necrosis.

DIFFERENTIAL DIAGNOSIS IMAGES (D-G)

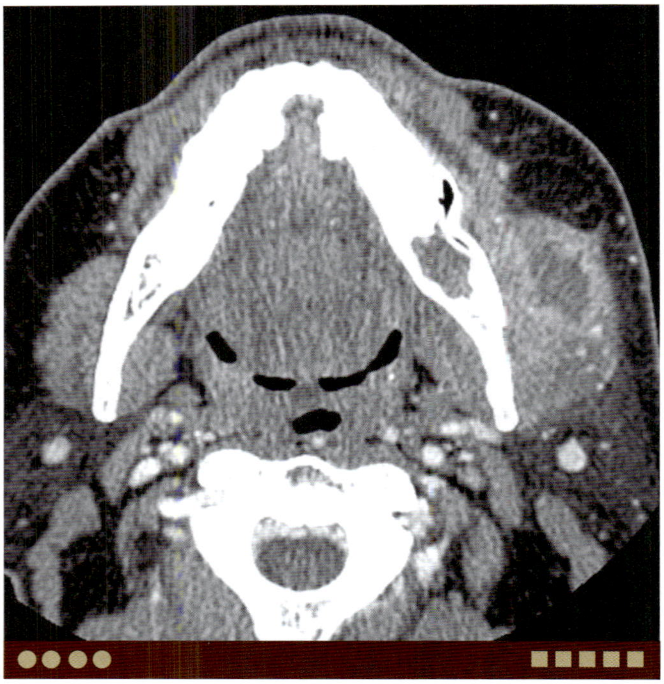

D. **Masticator space abscess**. Axial contrast-enhanced CT demonstrates a multiloculated low-density, peripherally enhancing collection in the left masseter muscle with inflammatory change in the surrounding soft tissues.

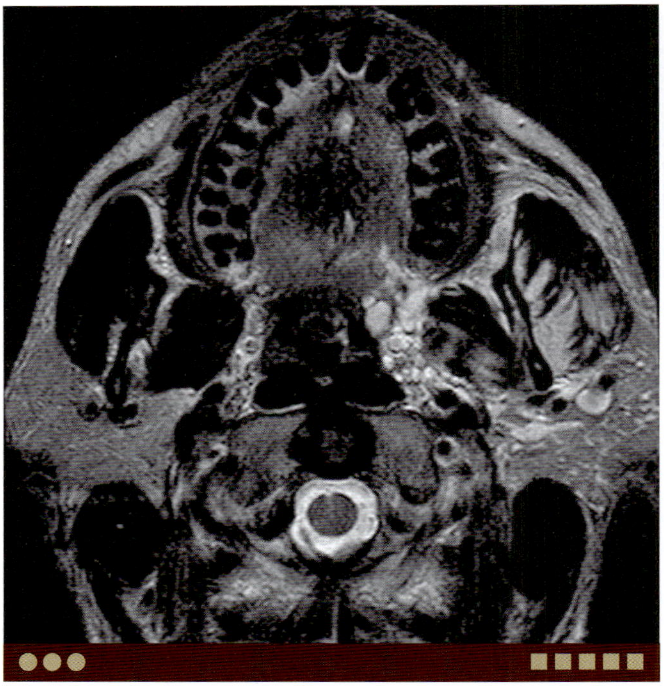

E. **Venous malformation**. Axial T2W image demonstrates high-signal lesions in the left masseter and pterygoid muscles.

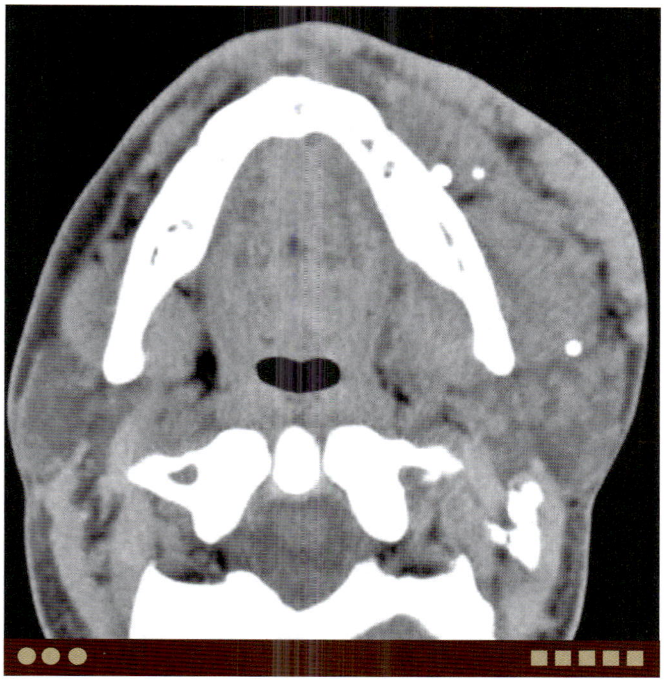

F. Venous malformation in a different patient. Axial noncontrast CT demonstrates soft tissue density lesions with phlebolith involving the left masseter as well as subcutaneous tissues.

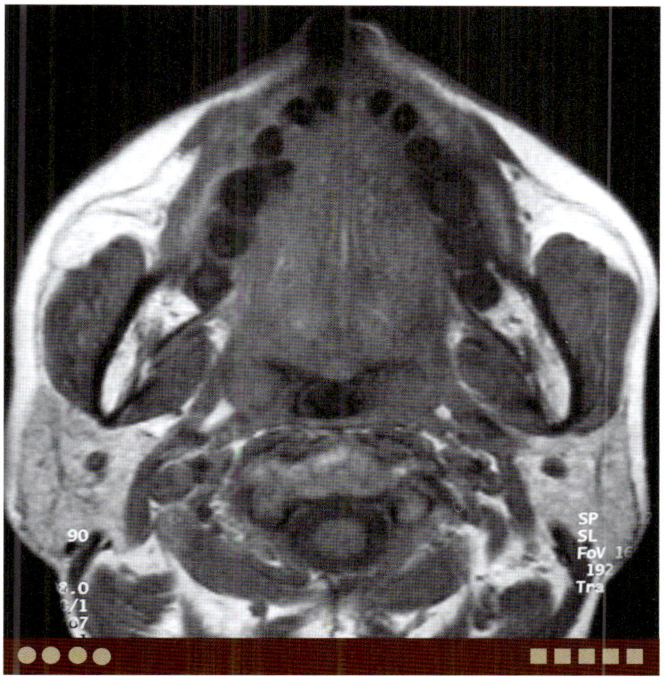

G. Benign masseteric hypertrophy. Axial T1W MR image demonstrates thickening of the left masseter muscle without signal abnormality.

Case 6–14 Benign Masseteric Hypertrophy

Osamu Sakai, Carlos Gonzalez

PRESENTATION

Painless bilateral or unilateral cheek swelling.

FINDINGS

CT and MRI demonstrate enlarged masseter muscles.

DIFFERENTIAL DIAGNOSIS

- Masticator space abscess: Usually as a result of molar tooth infection or following dental procedure. Contrast-enhanced CT demonstrates focal fluid density within the muscles of mastication with a thick enhancing rim. Evaluation of the mandible is necessary to identify the cause of infection and evaluate for osteomyelitis.
- Venous vascular malformation: Multilobulated mass with similar density to the vasculature on CT; low signal on T1W and very high signal on T2W MR images, and enhancement on postcontrast images. Presence of phlebolith strongly suggests venous malformation.
- Lymphoma: This is rare, however, more frequently seen in patients infected with HIV than in the general population. CT demonstrates an infiltrating homogenous mass isodense to normal musculature. MRI demonstrates a homogenous mass isointense to normal muscles on T1W and hyperintense on T2W images, and diffuse homogenous enhancement after contrast.
- Sarcoma: Imaging will demonstrate an aggressive, poorly marginated, heterogeneously enhancing mass within the muscles of mastication, with bone destruction and invasion of adjacent fascial planes/spaces.

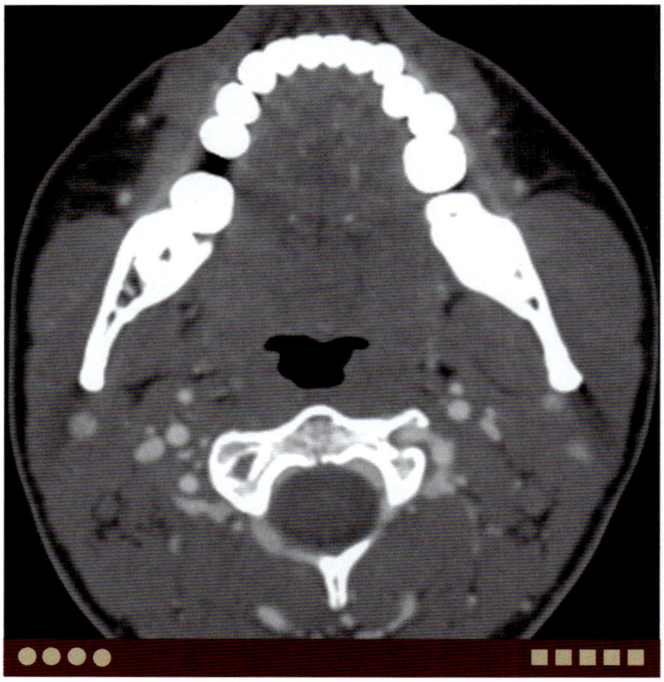

A. Benign masseteric hypertrophy. Axial postcontrast CT demonstrates asymmetric enlargement of the left masseter muscle without abnormal enhancement.

COMMENTS

This is a 30-year-old man with bilateral painless cheek swelling.

Benign masseteric hypertrophy is an asymptomatic enlargement of the masseter muscle. It is a relatively rare condition. It is thought to be related to "tooth gliding" and eating habits, however, exact cause is unknown. It is seen among all age or gender groups, however, most commonly seen in relatively young males, and usually bilateral, however, it can be unilateral.

On CT or MRI, enlargement of either one or both masseter muscles is seen without any density or signal abnormality, or enhancement. Lack of enhancement is helpful to exclude neoplasms and infection, particularly when it is unilateral. Bone spur development at the mandible angle may be seen in association with these findings.

The differential diagnosis includes infection/inflammation, vascular malformation, lymphoma, rhabdomyosarcoma, and expansile lesions of the mandible.

PEARLS

- **Benign masseteric hypertrophy is an enlargement of the masseter muscles, without any density or signal abnormality, or enhancement on CT and MRI.**
- **Lack of enhancement is helpful to exclude other diagnosis such as infection or neoplasms.**

ADDITIONAL IMAGES (B-F)

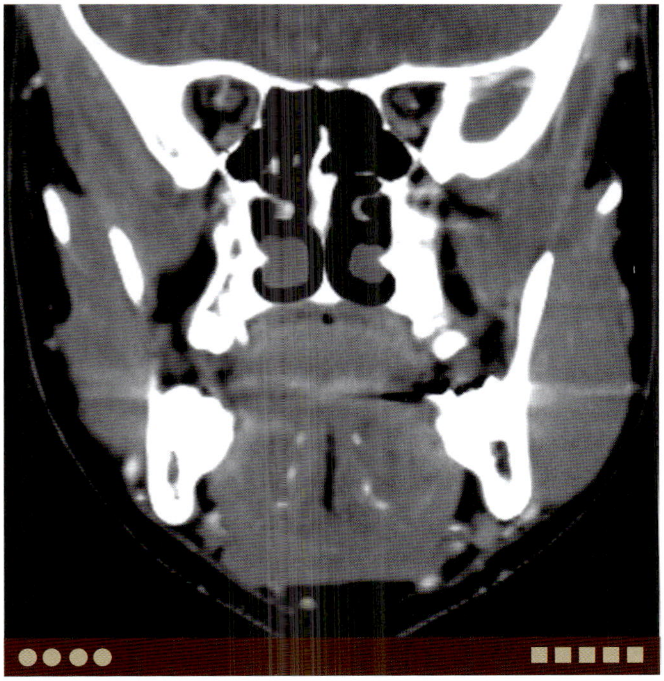

B. Benign masseteric hypertrophy, same patient as A. Coronal post-contrast CT demonstrates asymmetric enlargement of the left masseter muscle. There is also hypertrophy of the left pterygoid muscles.

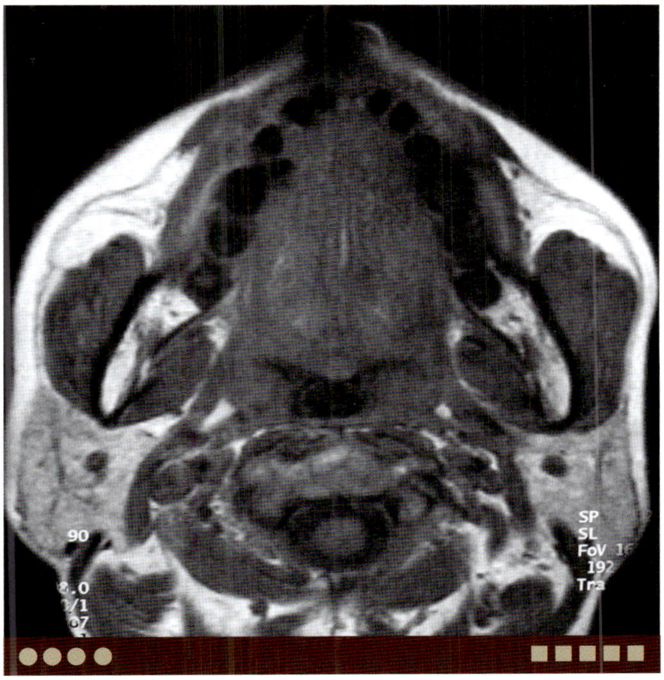

C. **Benign masseteric hypertrophy** in a different patient. Axial T1W MR image shows asymmetric enlargement of the left masseter muscle.

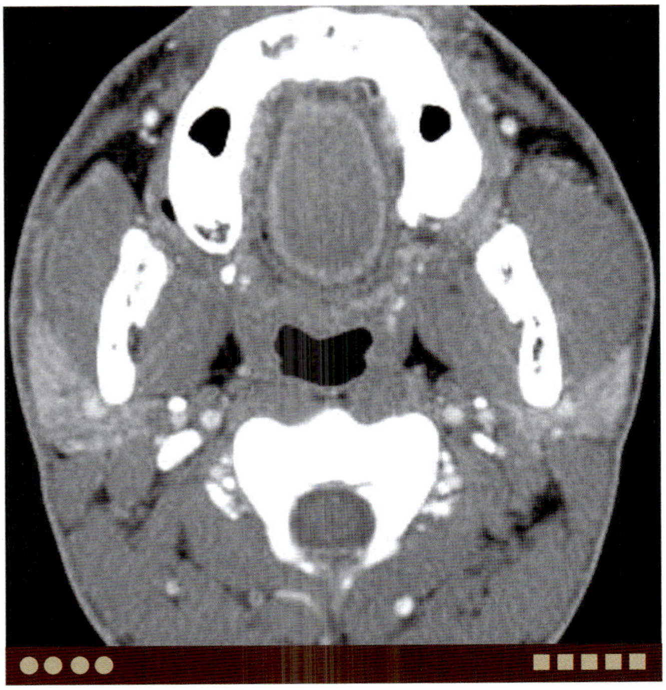

D. **Benign masseteric hypertrophy** in a different patient. Axial postcontrast CT demonstrates asymmetric enlargement of the left masseter muscle without abnormal enhancement. There is also hypertrophy of the left pterygoid muscles.

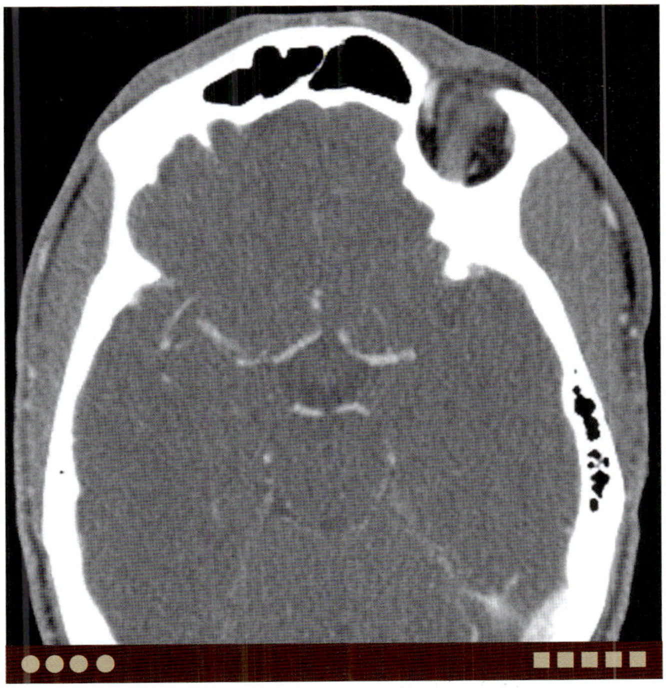

E. Benign masseteric hypertrophy, same patient as D. Axial post-contrast CT demonstrates asymmetric enlargement of the left temporalis muscle.

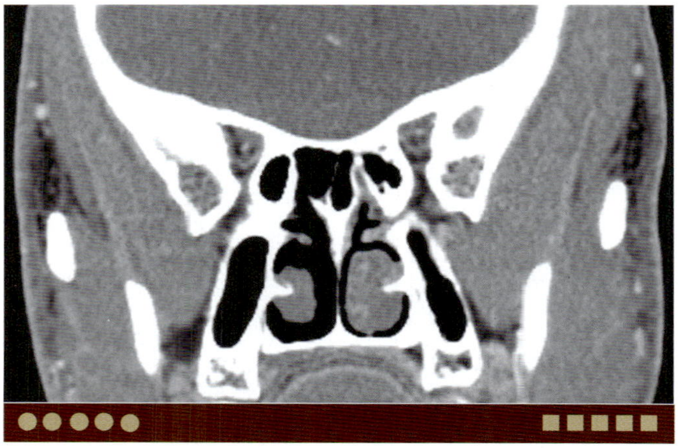

F. Benign masseteric hypertrophy, same patient as D. Coronal postcontrast CT demonstrates asymmetric enlargement of the left masseter and temporalis muscles.

DIFFERENTIAL DIAGNOSIS IMAGES (G-J)

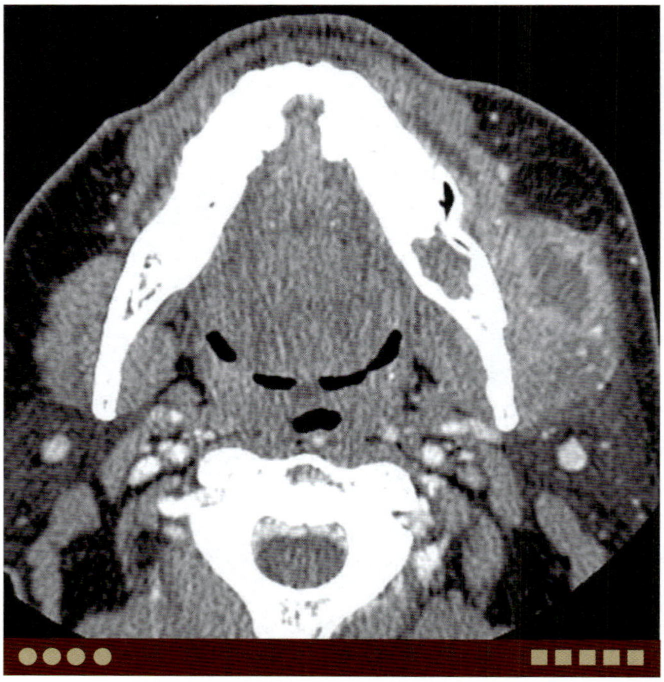

G. **Masticator space abscess**. Axial contrast-enhanced CT demonstrates a multiloculated low density, peripherally enhancing collection in the left masseter muscle with inflammatory changes in the surrounding soft tissues.

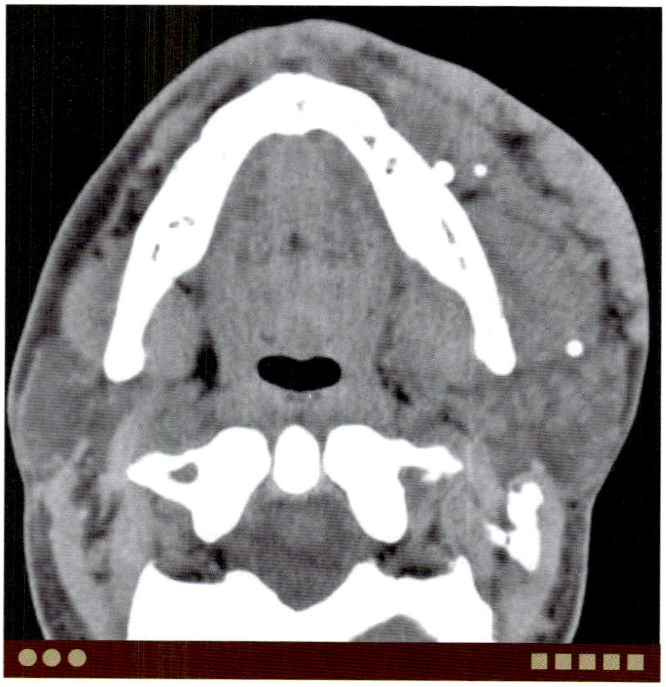

H. **Venous malformation.** Axial noncontrast CT demonstrates soft tissue density lesions with phlebolith involving the left masseter as well as subcutaneous tissues.

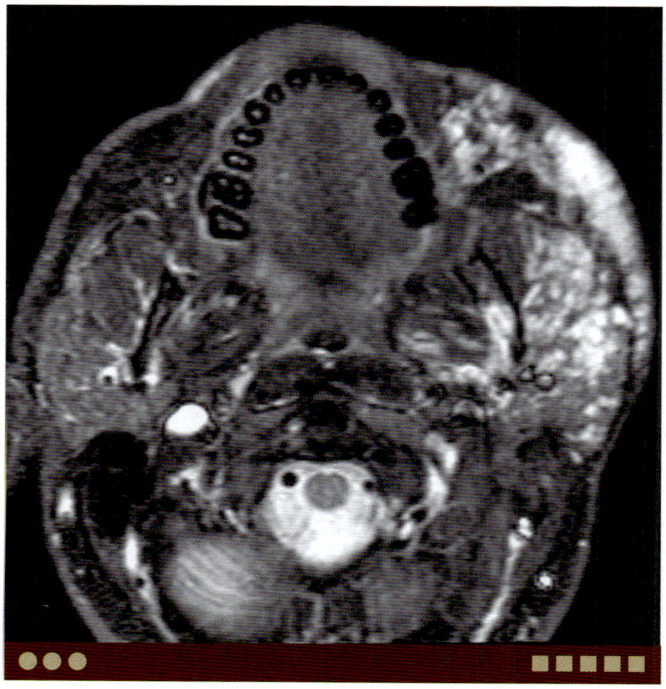

I. Venous malformation, same patient as H. Axial STIR image demonstrates diffuse high-signal lesions involving the left masseter muscle, parotid gland, and subcutaneous tissues.

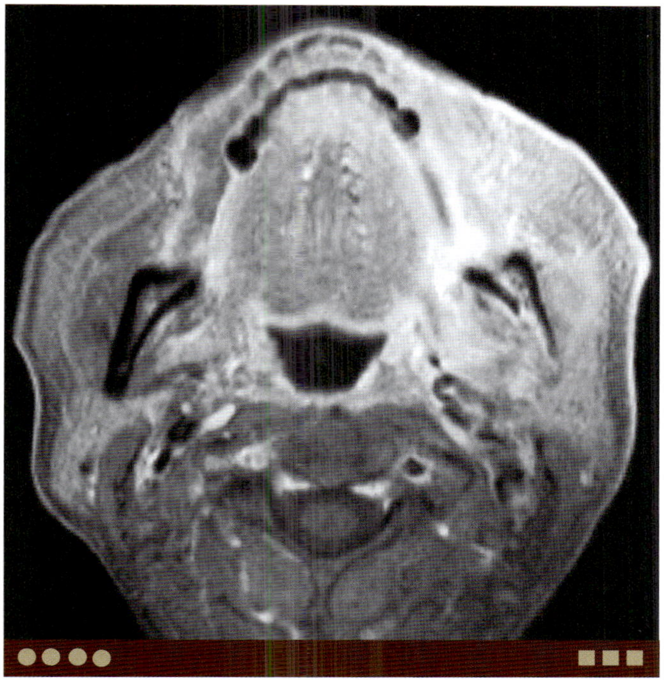

J. SCCA. Axial postcontrast fat-suppressed T1W MR image demonstrates abnormal enhancement centered in the left retromolar trigon. Note diffuse enhancement of the pterygoid and masseter muscles, as well as bone destruction and abnormal marrow enhancement in the left mandible, consistent with direct tumor invasion and denervation myositic change from V3 injury.

Case 6–15 Neurofibroma

Susmitha Reddy, Benjamin Ludwig, Osamu Sakai

PRESENTATION

Non-pulsatile neck mass.

FINDINGS

MRI demonstrates a circumscribed T2 high-signal lesion adjacent to the carotid vessels.

DIFFERENTIAL DIAGNOSIS

- Schwannoma: May appear similar to neurofibromas on imaging, however, schwannomas are encapsulated, located eccentric to the nerve, and may have cystic, fatty, or hemorrhagic components.
- Paraganglioma: This hypervascular tumor demonstrates avid enhancement, and classically has a "salt-and-pepper" appearance on MRI, with multiple punctate signal-voids and hyperintense foci on T2W and postcontrast T1W images.
- Castleman disease: This entity is a rare benign nodal lymphoproliferative disease. Enlarged nodes demonstrate marked, homogeneous enhancement.
- Nodal metastasis: Metastases are usually multiple and may be hypervascular. They are usually enlarged, with loss of normal nodal morphology, and heterogeneous density or signal.

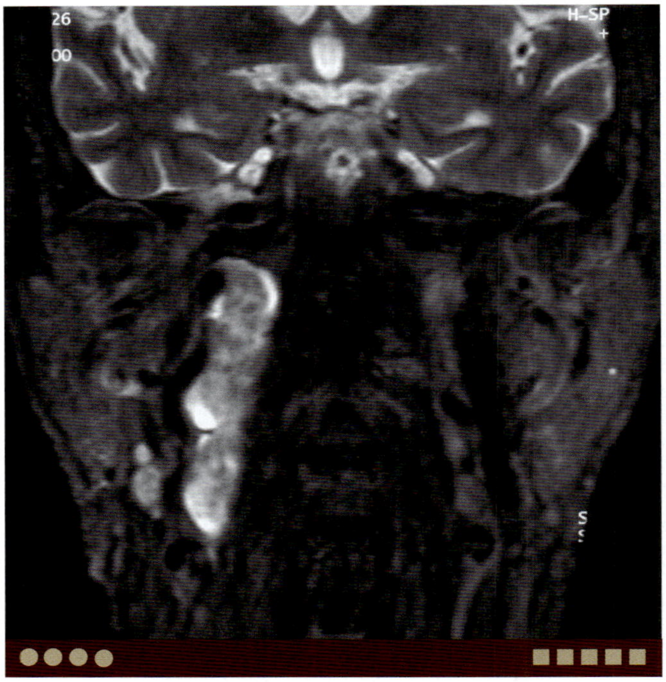

A. Neurofibroma. Coronal STIR MR image shows a slightly lobulated high-signal lesion extending craniocaudally along the right internal carotid artery (ICA). Note the decreased T2 signal centrally, referred to as the "central core sign" or "target sign."

COMMENTS

This is a 73-year-old man with a right neck mass.

Neurofibromas are seen in patients with neurofibromatosis type I (NFI), or von Recklinghausen disease, but this condition only accounts for 10% of all neurofibromas. The majority of neurofibromas is sporadic in origin, and may involve any nerve in the body. When associated with NFI, neurofibromas have a higher risk of malignant transformation.

Localized neurofibromas are often seen in fourth or fifth decades, while plexiform neurofibromas are usually diagnosed in childhood. Plexiform neurofibromas are highly suggestive of neurofibromatosis type I, but they may not be pathognomonic as previously claimed.

Neurofibromas are often seen as circumscribed masses near the carotid vessels or spine. Typically, they demonstrate fluid density on CT, low signal on T1W and intermediate-to-high signal on T2W images. Mild enhancement is usually seen. Often, the central portion of the lesion demonstrates slightly low signal on T2W images, referred to as "central core sign" or "target sign," although this finding can also be seen in other nerve sheath tumors. Plexiform neurofibromas are usually ill-defined lesions and extend across multiple spaces in the neck. The imaging finding may be similar to that of lymphatic malformations (lymphangiomas).

PEARLS

- **Neurofibromas are seen in patients with neurofibromatosis type I, however, these account for only about 10% of all neurofibromas.**
- **Plexiform neurofibromas are highly suggestive of neurofibromatosis type I, lack a capsule, and often involve multiple spaces.**
- **Neurofibromas may be difficult to differentiate from schwannomas on imaging, however, schwannomas are encapsulated and more commonly have cystic, fatty, or hemorrhagic components.**

ADDITIONAL IMAGES (B-G)

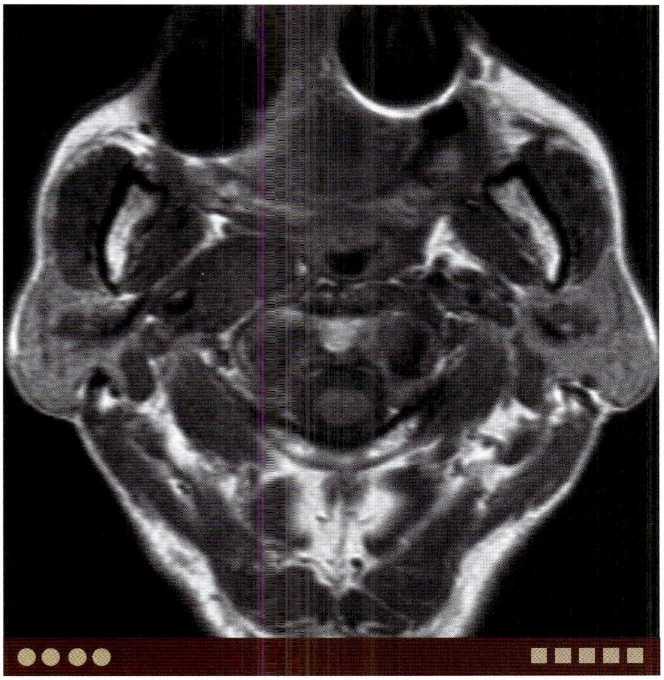

B. Neurofibroma, same patient as A. Axial T1W image demonstrates a well-demarcated, low-signal lesion, medial to the right ICA.

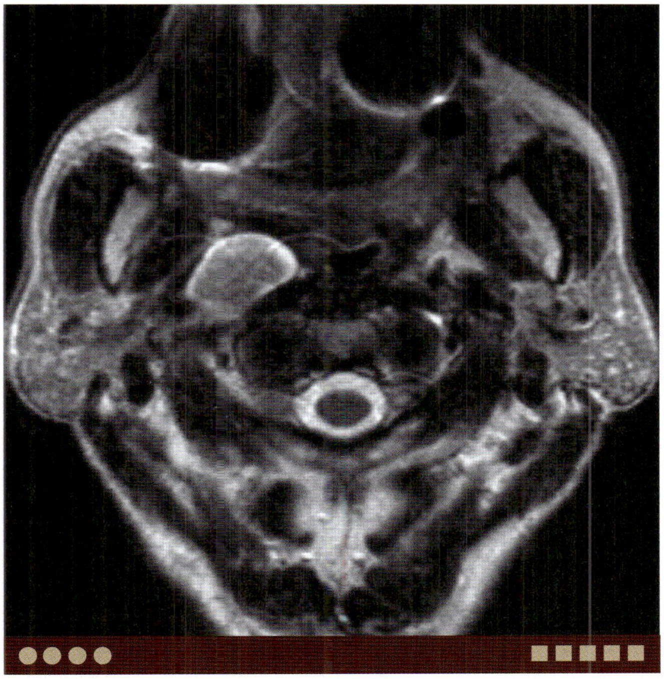

C. Neurofibroma, same patient as A. Axial T2W image demonstrates a high-signal lesion with low signal centrally.

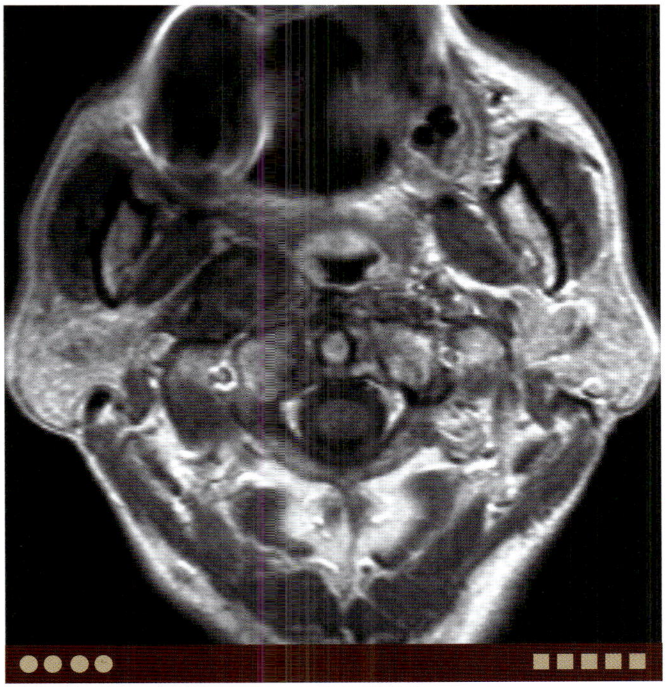

D. Neurofibroma, same patient as A. Axial postcontrast T1W image shows mild enhancement within the central portion of the lesion.

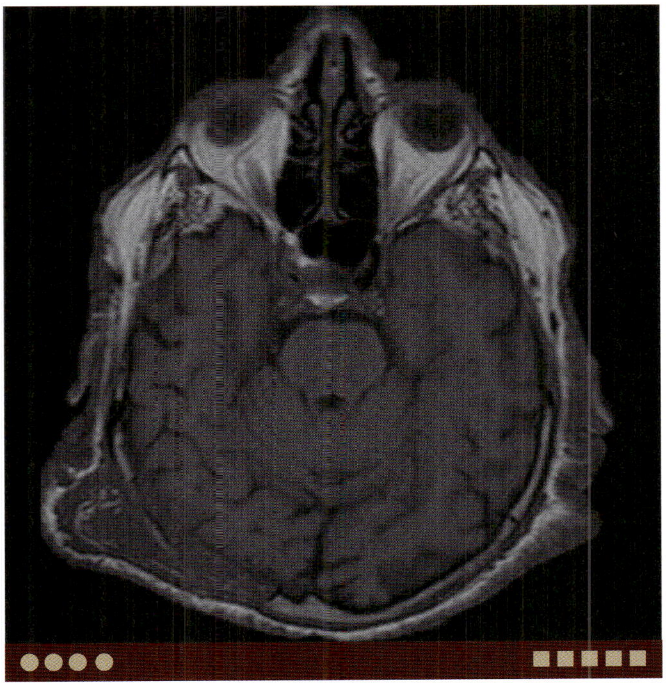

E. **Neurofibroma** in a different patient. Axial T1W image shows numerous cutaneous and subcutaneous lesions.

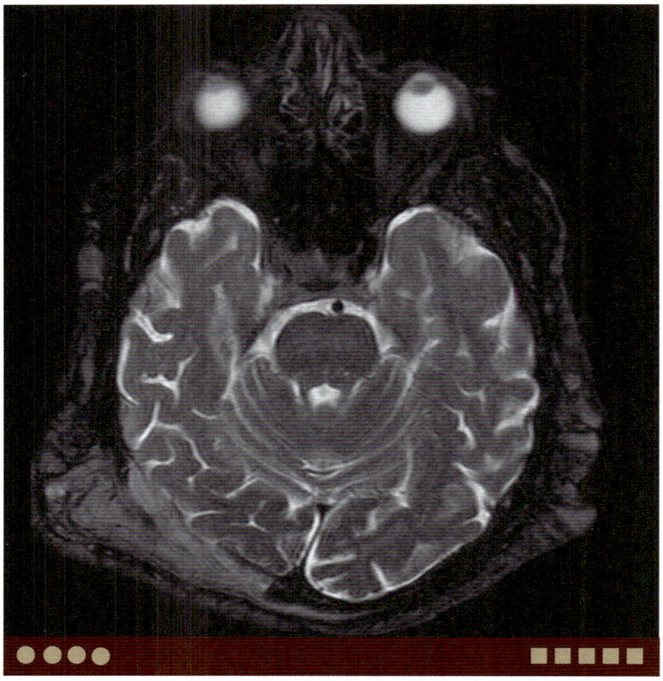

F. Neurofibroma, same patient as E. Axial fat-suppressed T2W image intermediate-to-high signal of the lesions.

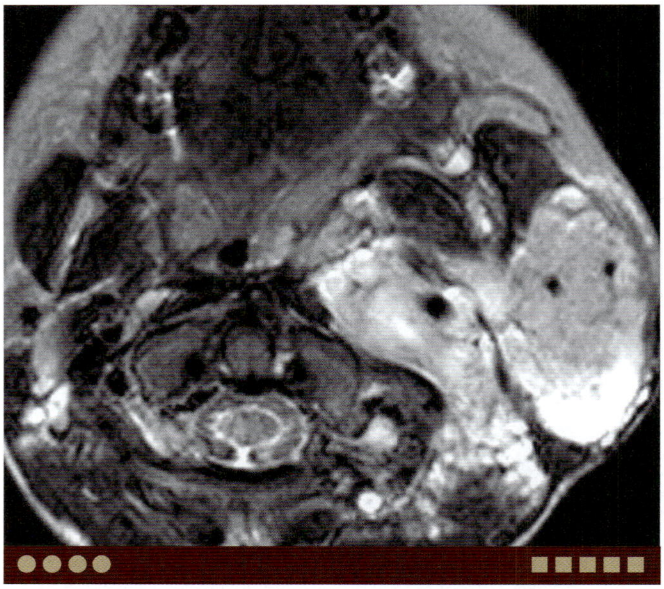

G. Plexiform neurofibroma. Axial T2W image demonstrates a large, lobulated high-signal lesion centered in the left retrostyloid parapharyngeal space. Note involvement of the parotid gland and paravertebral space.

DIFFERENTIAL DIAGNOSIS IMAGES (H-J)

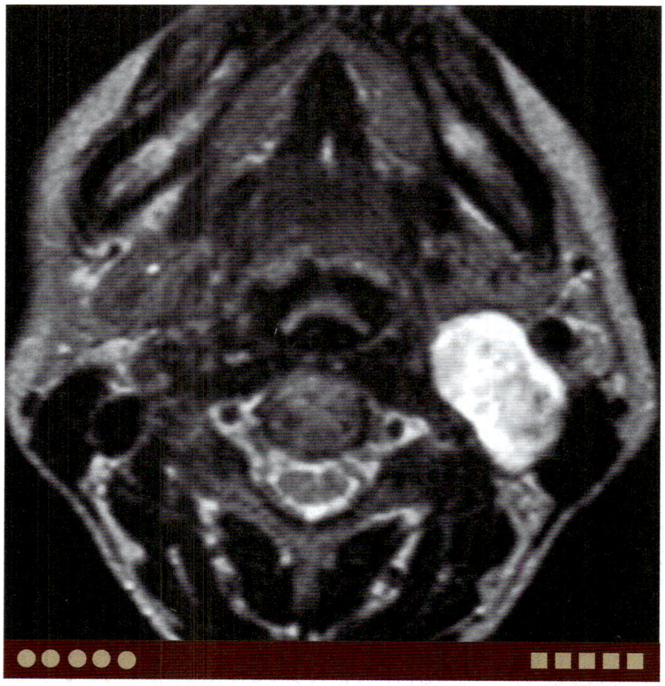

H. Schwannoma. Axial T2W image shows a slightly heterogeneous high-signal lesion displacing the left ICA laterally.

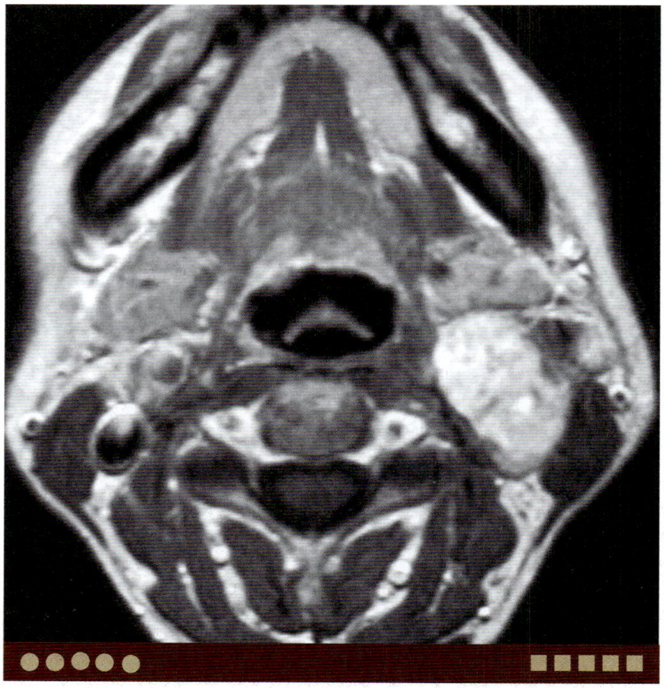

I. Schwannoma, same patient as H. Axial postcontrast T1W image shows enhancement of the lesion.

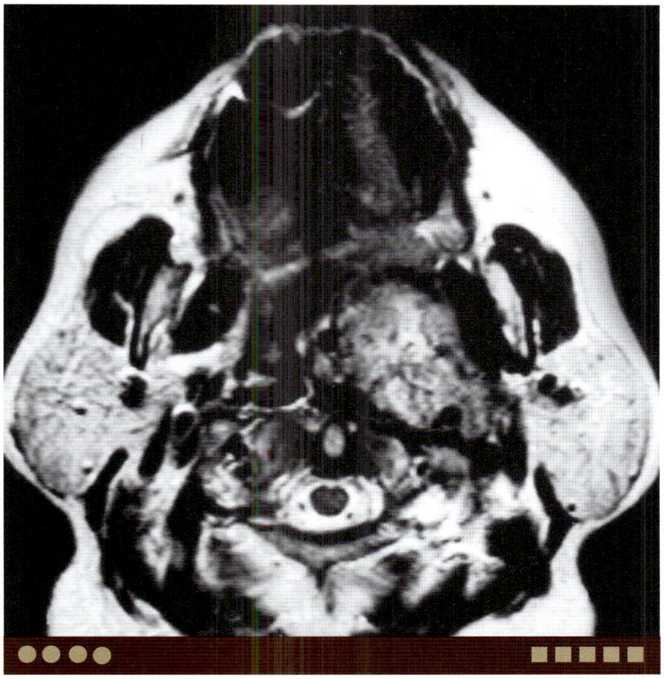

J. Paraganglioma (glomus vagale). Axial T2W MR image demonstrates a large heterogeneous signal lesion displacing the ICA anteromedially. Note "salt-and-pepper" appearance within the lesion.

Case 6–16 Second Branchial Cleft Cyst

Cory Siegel, Osamu Sakai

PRESENTATION

Neck mass.

FINDINGS

CT and MRI demonstrate a cystic lesion posterior to the left submandibular gland and anteromedial to the sternocleidomastoid muscle.

DIFFERENTIAL DIAGNOSIS

- Necrotic lymph node: This usually demonstrates rim-enhancement with a thick and irregular cyst wall.
- Dermoid/epidermoid: If the cystic lesion contains fat density, a diagnosis of dermoid is easily made. Often occurs in midline.
- Lymphatic malformation (lymphangioma/cystic hygroma): This is often seen in the posterior triangle or deep to the sternocleidomastoid muscle. Internal septation can be seen.
- Thyroglossal duct cyst: This usually occurs in midline, and is embedded in the strap muscle.
- Thymic cyst: Usually a cystic mass in lateral infrahyoid neck, adjacent to the carotid sheath, nonenhancing.

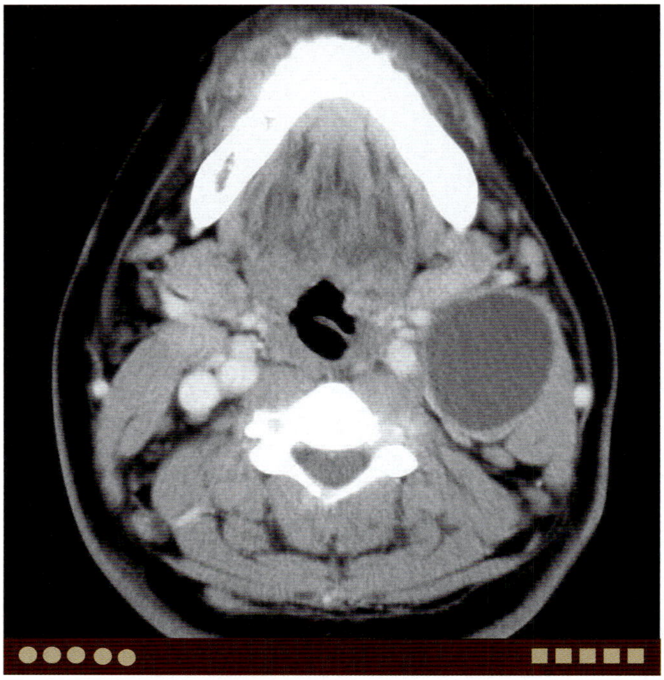

A. Second branchial cleft cyst. Axial postcontrast CT demonstrates a simple cystic lesion posterior to the left submandibular gland and anteromedial to the sternocleidomastoid muscle.

COMMENTS

This is a 25-year-old woman with recent increase in size of the left neck mass.

Branchial cleft cyst is a congenital/developmental cystic lesion associated with the branchial arch. Most of theses lesions originate from the second branchial cleft, and occasionally first branchial cleft cysts are also seen in the parotid region, which may have connection to the external auditory canal. Third and forth branchial cysts are rare.

These are developmental anomalies, and present as solitary, painless masses in the neck in children or young adults. A history of intermittent swelling and tenderness of the lesion during upper respiratory tract infection is common. However, presentation of these lesions in later of life is not uncommon. There is no gender predilection.

Second branchial cleft cyst is typically seen as a water density cystic mass with smooth, thin wall, posterior to the submandibular gland, anterolateral to the carotid vessels and anteromedial to the sternocleidomastoid muscle. With infection, the lesion often demonstrates increased internal density or signal, and a thick irregular enhancing wall.

Necrotic lymph node is the most important as a differential diagnosis, and should be always considered in adult patients, prompting a search for possible primary lesions. Nodes are likely located along the carotid vessels and deep to the sternocleidomastoid muscle.

PEARLS

- **Second branchial cleft cyst is the most common branchial cleft cyst and typically is seen posterior to the submandibular gland and anteromedial to the sternocleidomastoid muscle.**
- **The cyst is usually water density with smooth, thin wall, however, with infection, the lesion often demonstrates increased internal density or signal, and thick irregular enhancing wall.**
- **Necrotic lymph node is most important as a differential diagnosis, and should be always considered in adult patients, prompting a search for possible primary lesions.**

ADDITIONAL IMAGES (B-E)

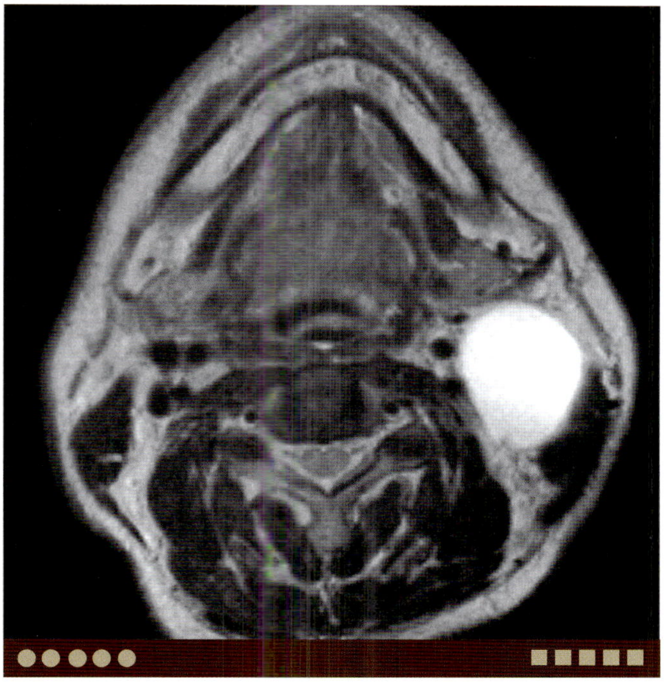

B. **Second branchial cleft cyst** in a different patient. Axial T2W MR image shows a cystic lesion in a similar location.

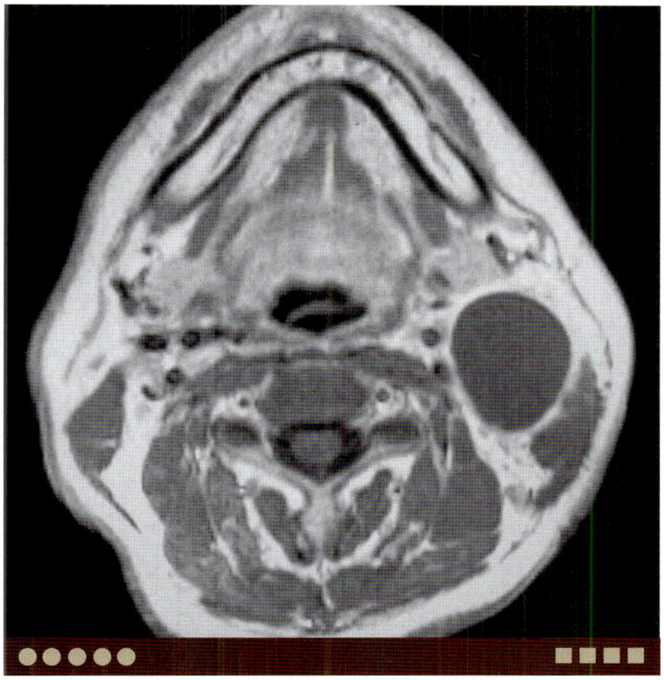

C. Second branchial cleft cyst, same patient as B. Axial postcontrast T1W MR image demonstrates mild enhancement of the cyst wall.

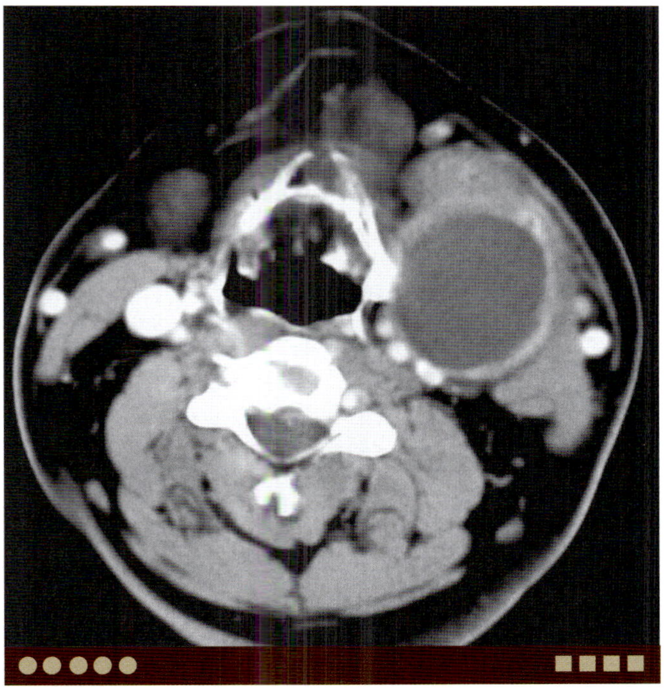

D. **Infected second branchial cleft cyst** in a different patient. Axial postcontrast CT demonstrates a cystic lesion posterior to the left submandibular gland and anteromedial to the left sternocleidomastoid muscle. Note thickened and enhancing wall to suggest infection.

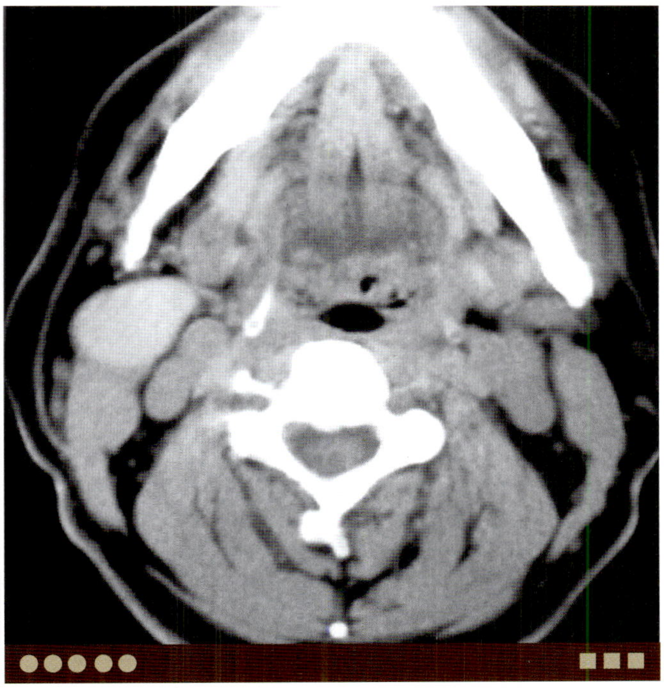

E. **Complicated second branchial cleft cyst** in a different patient. Axial noncontrast CT demonstrates a hyperdense cystic lesion anteromedial to the right sternocleidomastoid muscle, representing a hemorrhagic and proteinaceous cyst.

DIFFERENTIAL DIAGNOSIS IMAGES (F-J)

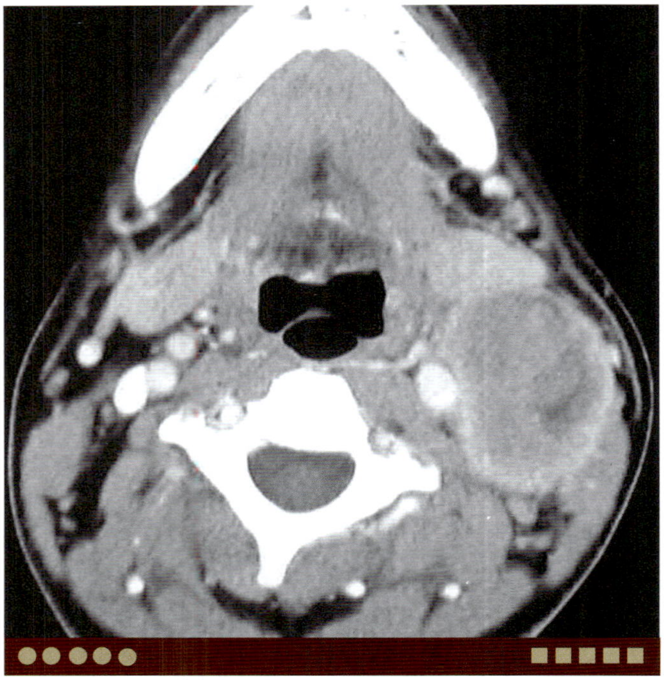

F. Necrotic metastatic node. Axial postcontrast CT demonstrates a heterogeneously enhancing, cystic-appearing lesion, posterior to the submandibular gland and anteromedial to the sternocleidomastoid muscle, similar in location to second branchial cleft cyst.

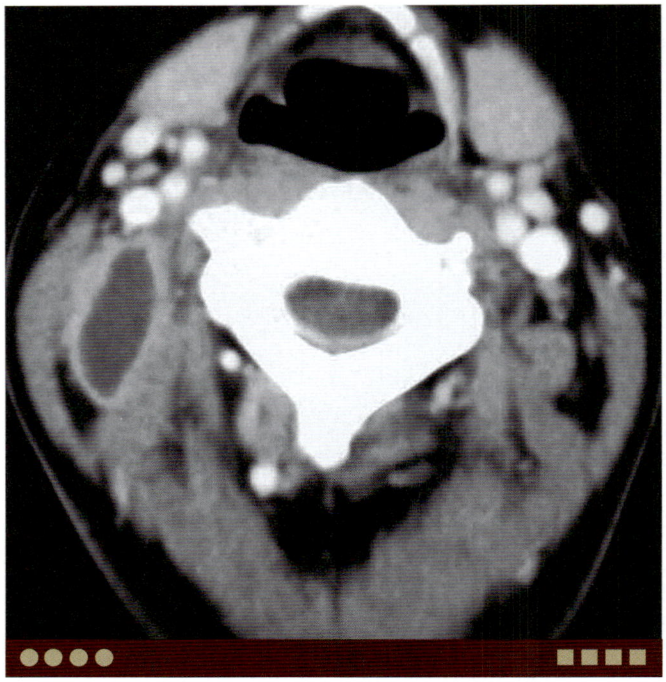

G. Tuberculosis. Axial postcontrast CT demonstrates a cystic nodal lesion with thick enhancing wall, posterior to the right internal jugular vein and medial to the sternocleidomastoid muscle.

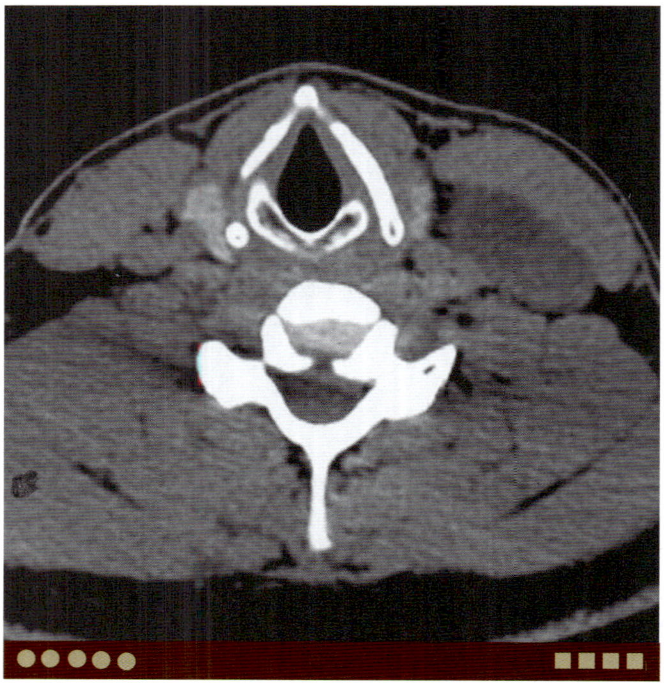

H. Papillary thyroid carcinoma. Axial noncontrast CT shows an ovoid cystic-appearing lesion deep to the left sternocleidomastoid muscle.

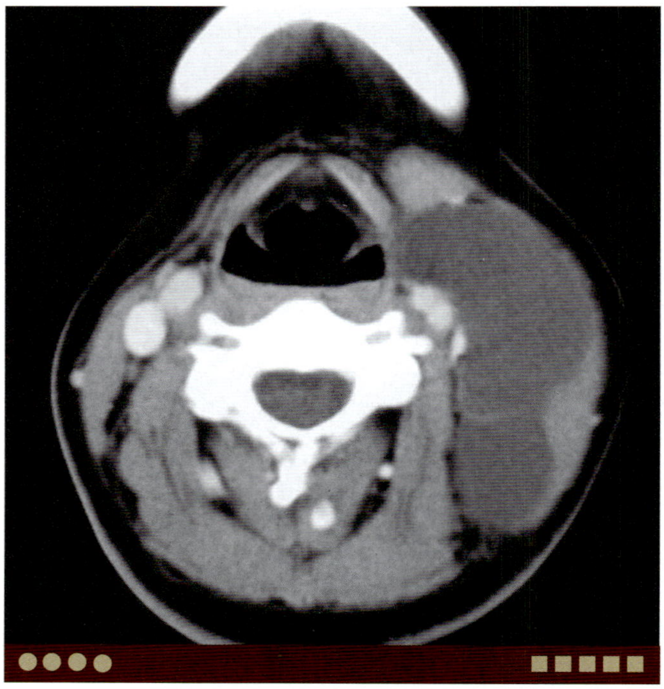

I. Lymphatic malformation. Axial postcontrast CT shows a lobulated rimless hypoattenuating lesion in the left neck. Note suggestion of an internal septation.

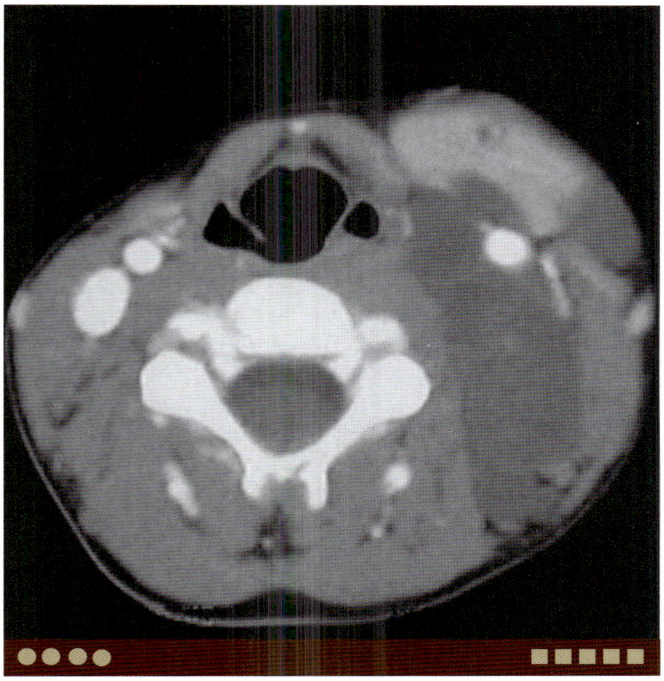

J. Neurofibroma. Axial postcontrast CT shows a hypoattenuating lesion medial to the left sternocleidomastoid muscle with anterior and posterior extension. The lesion surrounds the common carotid artery without narrowing.

Case 6–17 Paraganglioma—Carotid Body Tumor

Osamu Sakai, Brooke Devenney-Cakir

PRESENTATION

Pulsatile neck mass.

FINDINGS

CT demonstrates an avidly enhancing mass at the carotid bifurcation, splaying the internal and external carotid arteries.

DIFFERENTIAL DIAGNOSIS

- Schwannoma: This may occur in similar locations, however, enhancement on CT is less compared to paraganglioma. No flow-voids are seen within the lesion on MRI.
- Castleman disease: This is a nodal lymphoproliferative disease and usually very vascular. This usually displaces the vessels but does not encase them.
- Aneurysm: Normal carotid artery is usually missing with this condition, however, pseudoaneurysm is seen with normal appearing carotid artery.
- Nodal metastasis: Metastases from renal cell carcinoma, hepatocellular carcinoma and thyroid cancer can be very vascular. These metastatic lesions are usually multiple.

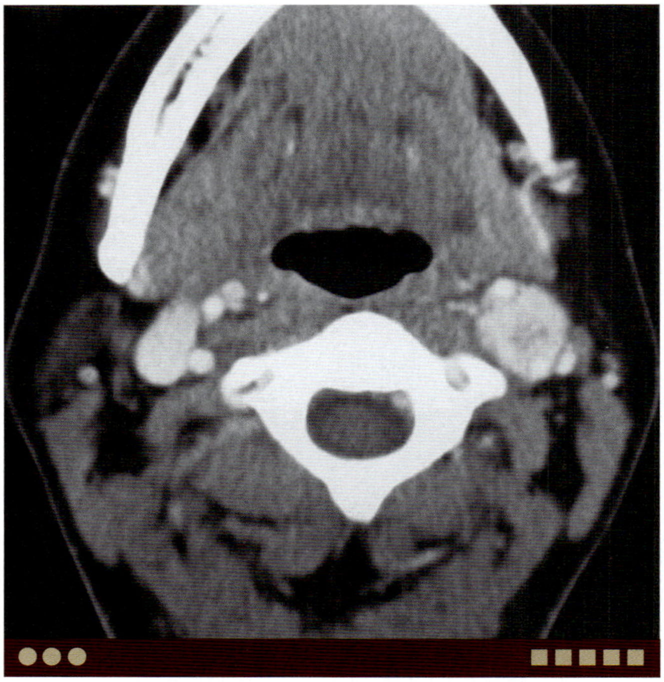

A. Carotid body tumor. Axial postcontrast CT demonstrates an avidly enhancing mass splaying the external and internal carotid arteries at the left carotid bifurcation.

COMMENTS

This is a 46-year-old woman with pulsatile right left neck mass.

Paraganglioma is a benign tumor originated in the neural crest, and occurs anywhere from the skull base to the aortic arch, along the carotid vessels. They are called differently based on locations; glomus jugulare at the skull base/jugular foramen, glomus vagale at the naso-oropharyngeal level, and carotid body tumor at the carotid bifurcation.

Paragangliomas are usually very hypervascular and demonstrate avid enhancement on CT. Vascularity is easily assessed by dynamic study. On MRI, characteristic "salt-and-pepper" appearance is seen corresponding to significantly increased vascularity on T2W images and postcontrast T1W images. Note due to prominent flow-voids, the tumor may not demonstrate very high signal on regular postcontrast T1W images. Prior to surgical resection, embolization is often performed, however, catheter angiogram is not needed for diagnosis.

Carotid body tumor splays the carotid bifurcation, which is very characteristic for this tumor, although displacement with slight splaying can be seen with schwannoma arising near the carotid bifurcation. However, schwannoma enhances less than paraganglioma on CT and should be easily differentiated. In addition, carotid body tumors often encase carotid arteries, more often external carotid arteries, while schwannomas just displace the vessels.

Similar to pheochromocytoma, paragangliomas can be bilateral, multiple, familial, and malignant. The entire neck should be evaluated for possible other lesions.

PEARLS

- **Paraganglioma occurs anywhere from the skull base to the aortic arch in the neck, along the carotid vessels.**
- **Paraganglioma demonstrates avid enhancement on CT. On MRI, characteristic "salt-and-pepper" appearance is often seen.**
- **Carotid body tumors splay the carotid bifurcation.**
- **Paragangliomas can be bilateral, multiple, familial, and malignant.**

ADDITIONAL IMAGES (B-G)

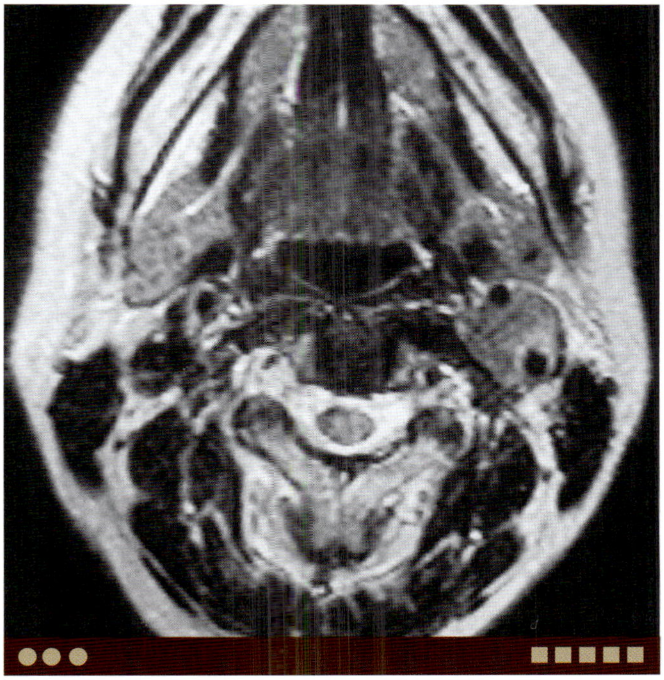

B. Carotid body tumor, same patient as A. Axial T2W MR image demonstrates a lesion with heterogeneous signal, "salt-and-pepper" appearance, splaying the external and internal carotid arteries. Note encasement of the arteries.

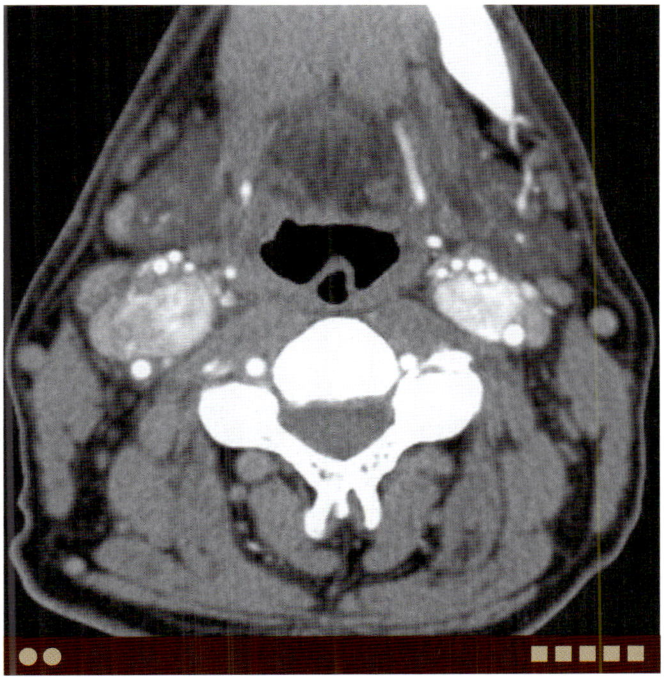

C. **Bilateral carotid body tumors**. Axial postcontrast CT demonstrates bilateral avidly enhancing masses splaying the external and internal carotid arteries.

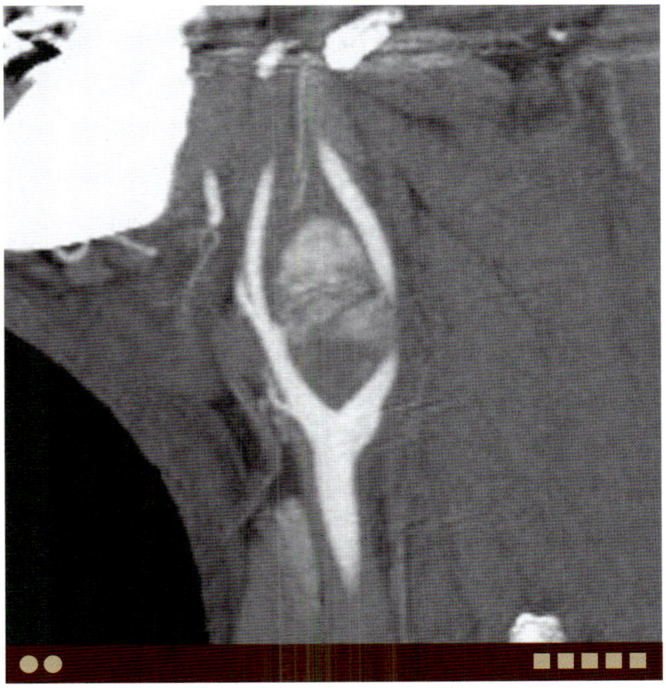

D. Bilateral carotid body tumors, same patient as C. Sagittal contrast-enhanced CT with MIP reconstruction demonstrates an enhancing lesion between the external and internal carotid arteries.

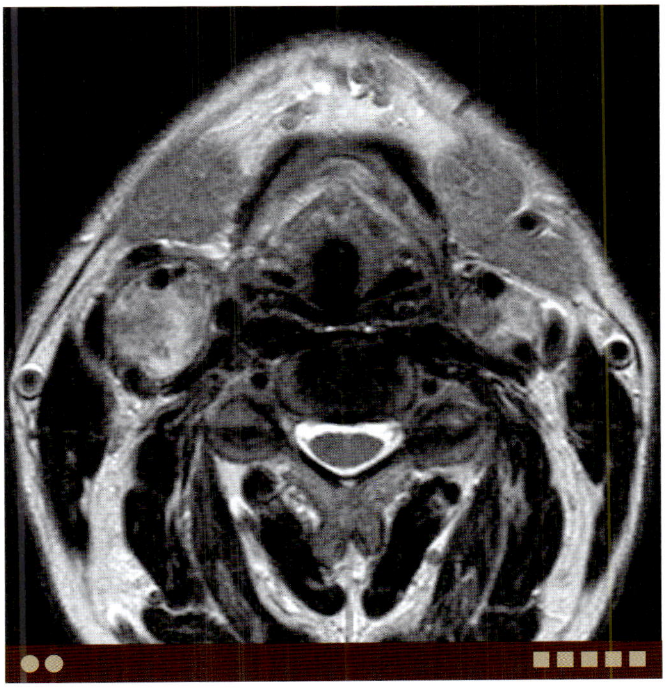

E. Bilateral carotid body tumors, same patient as C. Axial T2W demonstrates bilateral lesions with heterogeneous signal, "salt-and-pepper" appearance, splaying the external and internal carotid arteries.

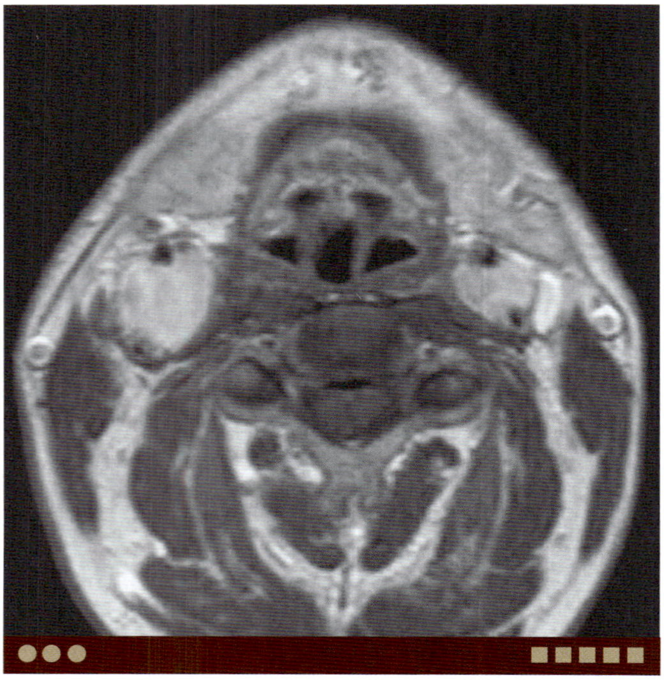

F. Bilateral carotid body tumors, same patient as C. Axial postcontrast T1W image demonstrates bilateral lesions with avid enhancement.

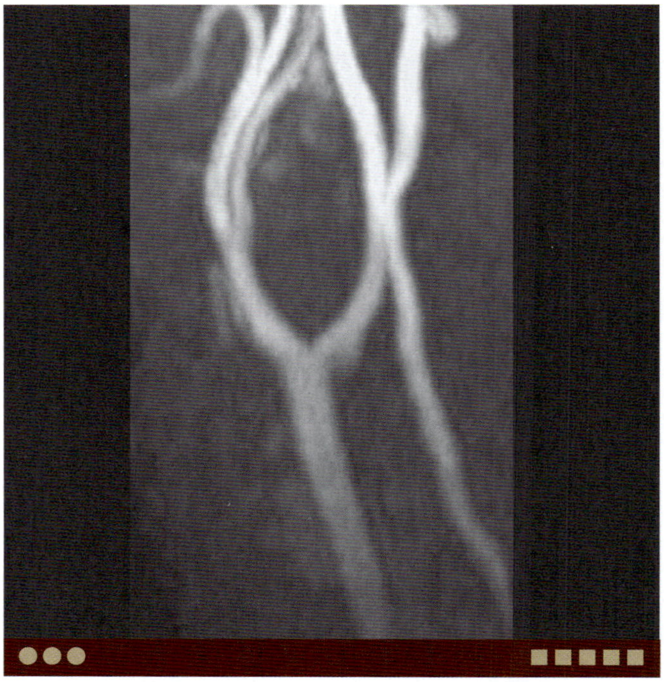

G. Bilateral carotid body tumors, same patient as C. Lateral projection image of time-of-flight MRA MIP reconstruction demonstrates splaying the external and internal carotid arteries at the bifurcation. Compared to CTA (D), time-of-flight MRA does not show high signal within the lesion.

DIFFERENTIAL DIAGNOSIS IMAGES (H-J)

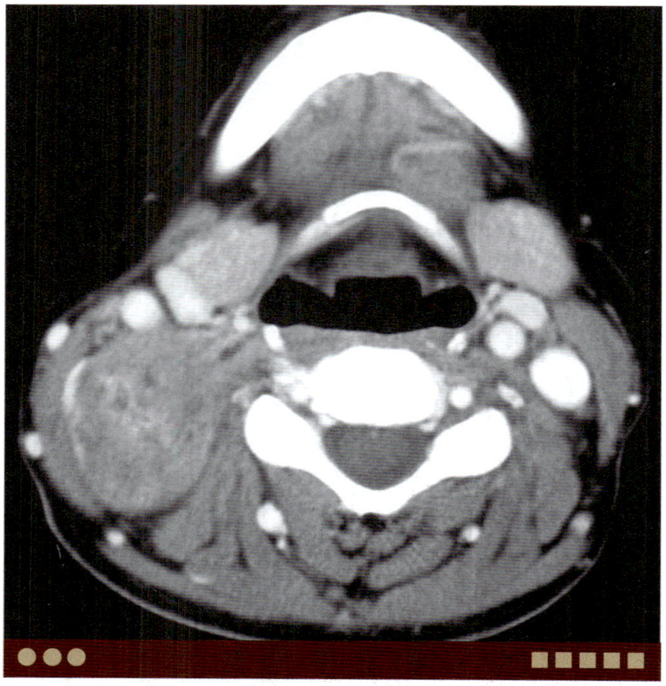

H. **Schwannoma**. Axial postcontrast CT demonstrates a mildly enhancing tumor displacing the internal and external carotid arteries anteriorly. Note less enhancement of this lesion compared with paraganglioma.

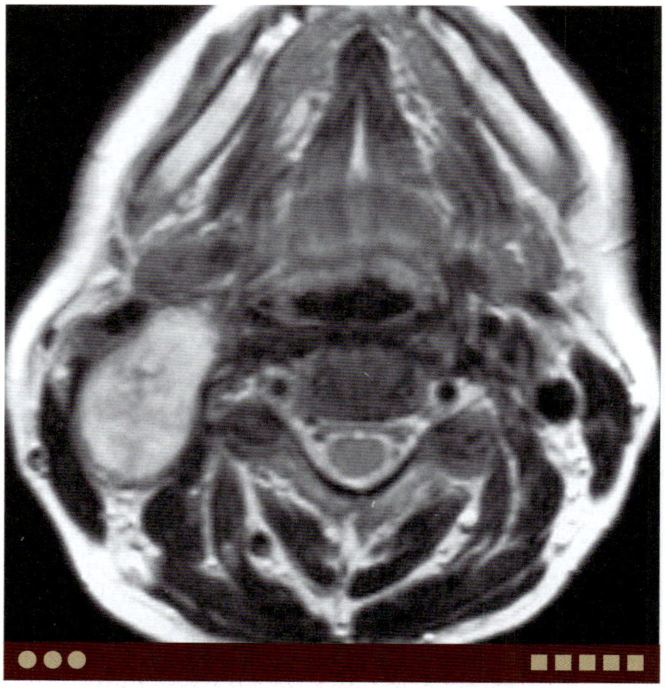

I. **Schwannoma** in a different patient. Axial T2W MR image demonstrates a high-signal smooth mass displacing the internal and external carotid arteries anterolaterally.

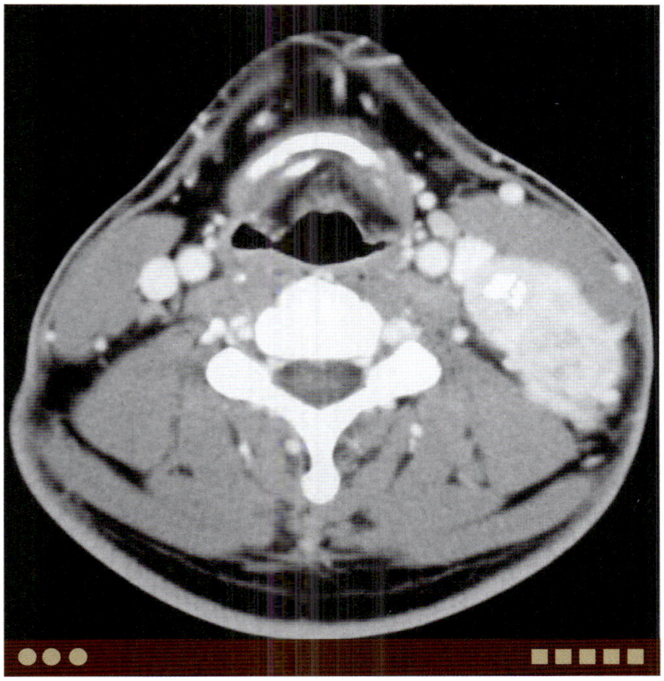

J. Castleman disease. Axial contrast-enhanced CT demonstrates an avidly enhancing lesion posterolateral to the carotid vessels.

Case 6–18 Extracranial Carotid Artery Aneurysm

Osamu Sakai, Cory Siegel

PRESENTATION

Pulsatile neck mass.

FINDINGS

CT demonstrates a well-demarcated avidly enhancing mass near the carotid bifurcation.

DIFFERENTIAL DIAGNOSIS

- Carotid body tumor: This is a very hypervascular lesion that demonstrates avid enhancement on CT, a "salt-and-pepper" appearance on MRI, and splays the carotid bifurcation.
- Castleman disease: This is a rare lymphoproliferative nodal disease that is usually very vascular.
- Nodal metastasis: Metastases are usually multiple and more heterogeneous in density or signal.
- Carotid pseudoaneurysm: Often secondary to trauma, surgery, or carotid dissection, and may be difficult to discern from true aneurysm on cross sectional imaging.

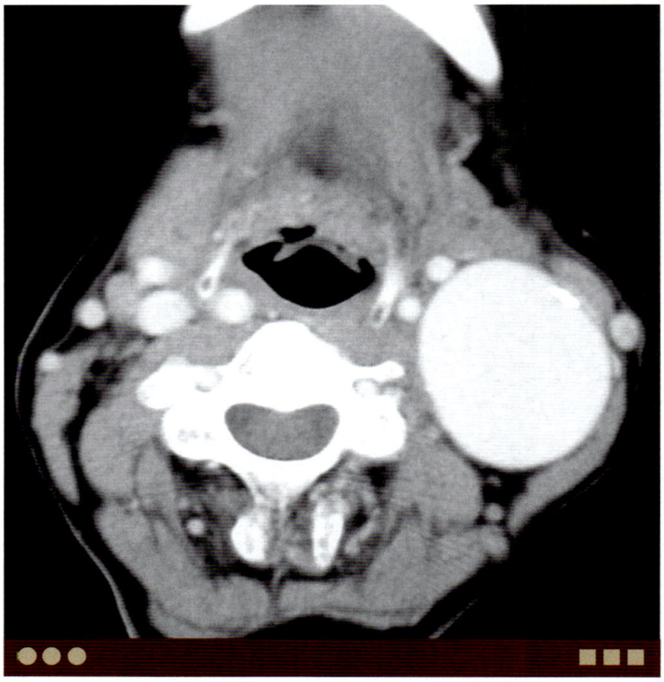

A. Internal carotid artery aneurysm. Axial postcontrast CT demonstrates a well-demarcated round avidly enhancing lesion posterolateral to the left internal and external carotid arteries.

COMMENTS

This is a 67-year-old woman with a pulsatile left neck mass.

An extracranial carotid artery aneurysm is a relatively rare entity when compared with the intracranial type. It is often seen near the carotid bifurcation as a pulsatile mass.

On CT, the aneurysm demonstrates strong enhancement like other vasculature, although a partially thrombosed aneurysm can be heterogeneous in density. Calcification is common. Diagnosis is usually easily made because of its enhancement and contiguity to the artery. However, partially thrombosed aneurysm may mimic a necrotic node or schwannoma with cystic degeneration. Also, on MRI, heterogeneous signal from turbulent flow or thrombosis may also mimic necrotic tumors or nodal lesions. It is important to identify normal carotid arteries when an avidly enhancing lesion is noted in the neck so as not to miss a carotid artery aneurysm. However, a pseudoaneurysm may be seen separated from the normal appearing carotid artery.

The differential diagnosis of a clinically suspected aneurysm with a pulsatile mass includes tortuous vessels, which is commonly seen with the subclavian artery in the supraclavicular fossa, retropharyngeal course of the internal/common carotid artery, schwannoma or lymph node adjacent to the artery transmitting the pulsation. CT and MRI are very useful to differentiate these conditions.

PEARLS

- **Extracranial carotid artery aneurysm is rare compared with an intracranial location, and is often seen at the carotid bifurcation.**
- **Partially thrombosed aneurysms can demonstrate heterogeneous density on CT or signal intensity on MRI. Turbulent flow causes heterogeneous signal on MRI.**
- **Calcification is commonly seen in the wall of the aneurysm.**

ADDITIONAL IMAGES (B-G)

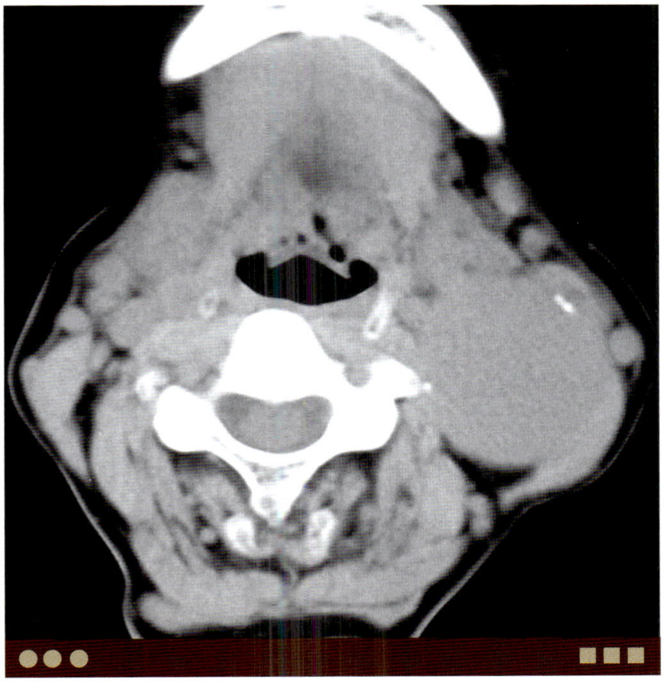

B. Internal carotid artery aneurysm, same patient as A. Axial non-contrast CT demonstrates a well-demarcated round lesion posterolateral to the internal and external carotid arteries. The lesion shows same density as the vasculature.

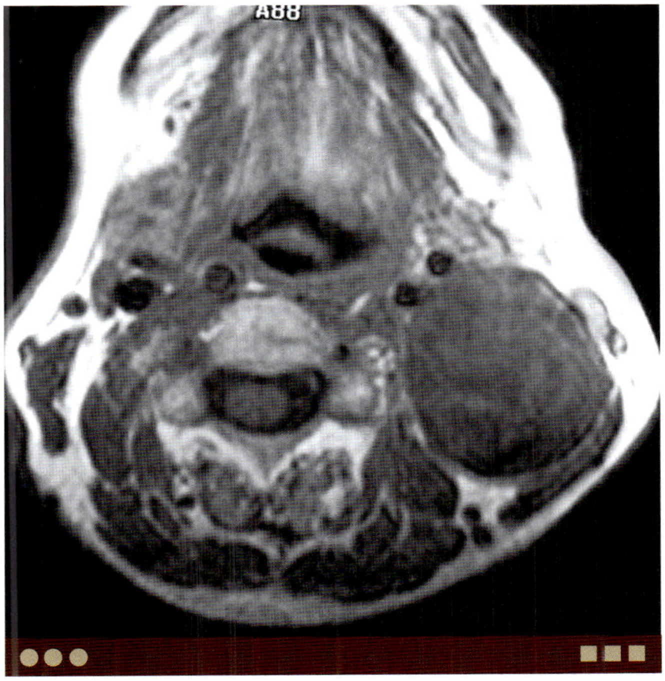

C. Internal carotid artery aneurysm, same patient as A. Axial T1W MR image demonstrates a round low-signal lesion posterolateral to the internal and external carotid arteries.

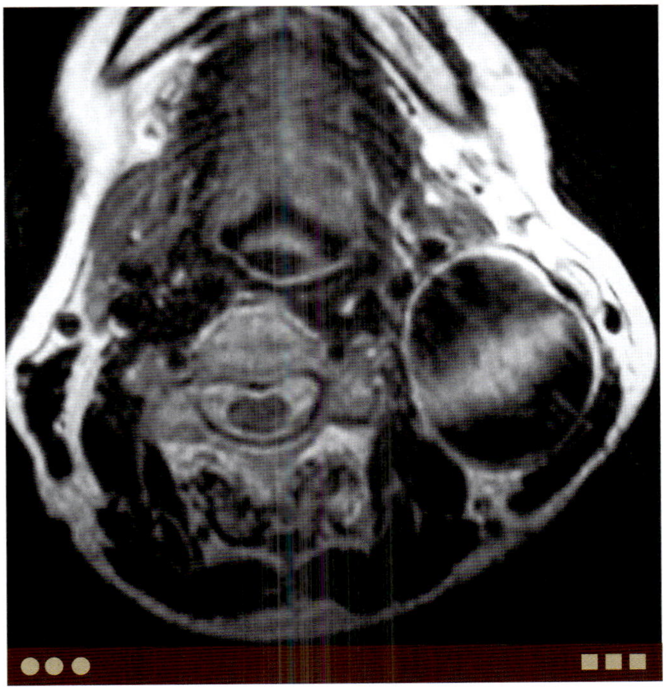

D. Internal carotid artery aneurysm, same patient as A. Axial T2W MR image demonstrates heterogeneous flow-voids in the lesion, with pulsation artifact.

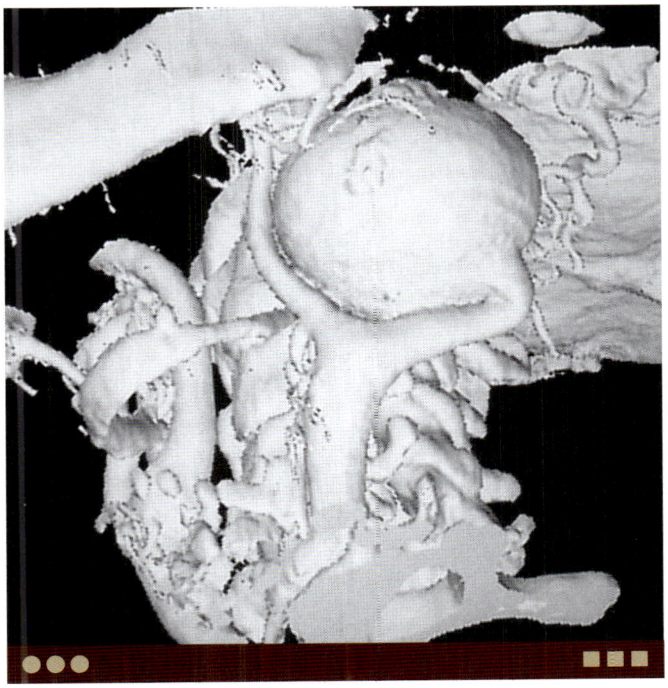

E. Internal carotid artery aneurysm, same patient as A. Surface rendered 3D CTA image demonstrates a round lesion contiguous to the internal carotid artery.

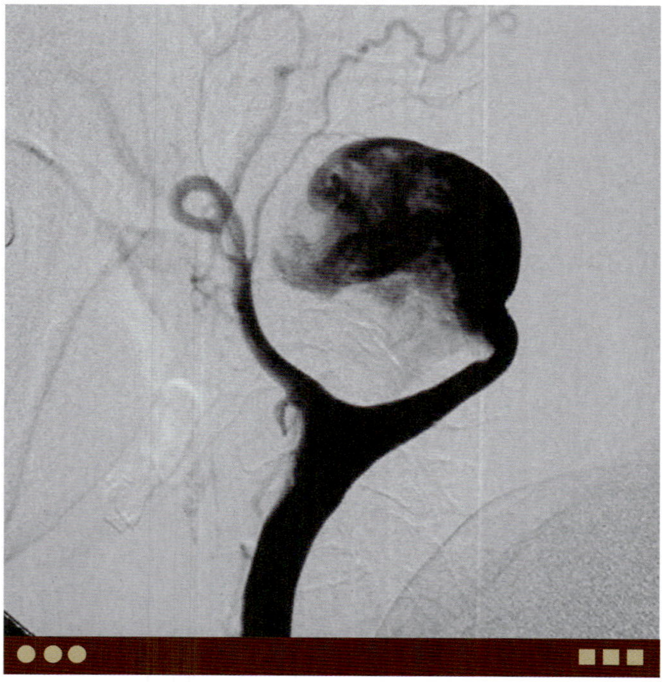

F. Internal carotid artery aneurysm, same patient as A. Common carotid arteriogram demonstrates contrast filling in the lesion.

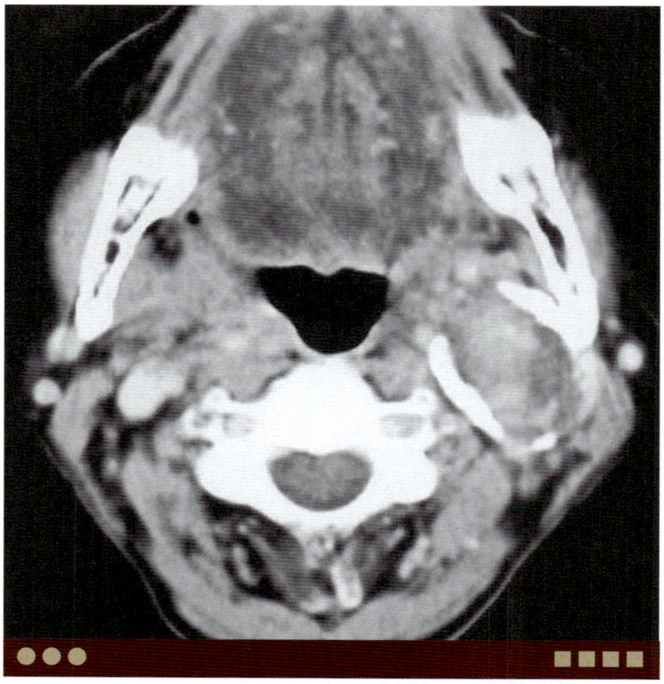

G. Partially thrombosed internal carotid artery aneurysm. Axial postcontrast CT demonstrates a heterogeneously enhancing lesion at the carotid bifurcation without normal appearing carotid arteries. Note dense calcification of the wall.

DIFFERENTIAL DIAGNOSIS IMAGES (H-J)

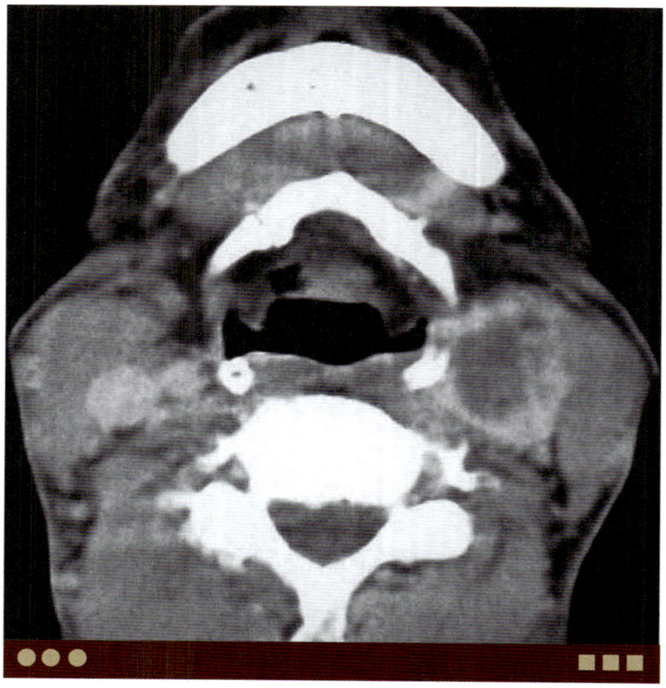

H. Common carotid artery pseudoaneurysm. Axial postcontrast CT demonstrates a partially thrombosed enhancing lesion near the carotid bifurcation. Note poorly defined heterogeneously enhancing wall.

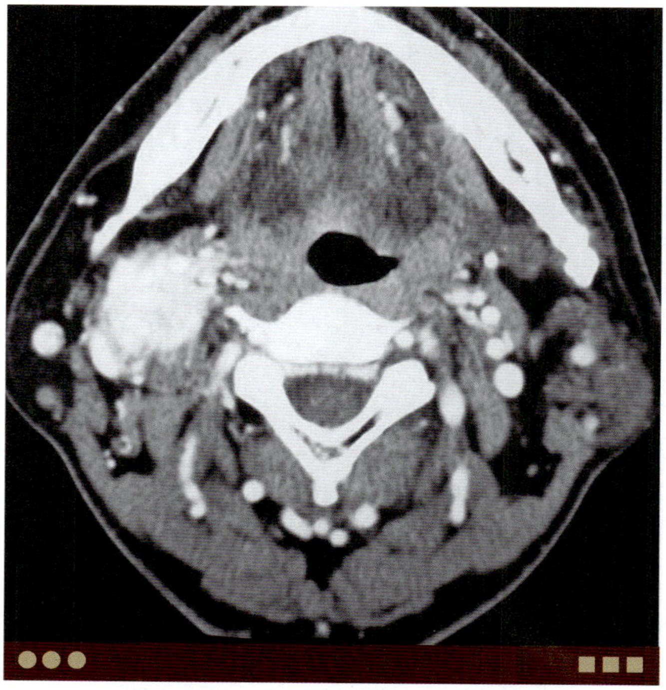

I. Paraganglioma (carotid body tumor). Axial postcontrast CT demonstrates an avidly enhancing tumor splaying and encasing the right internal and external carotid arteries.

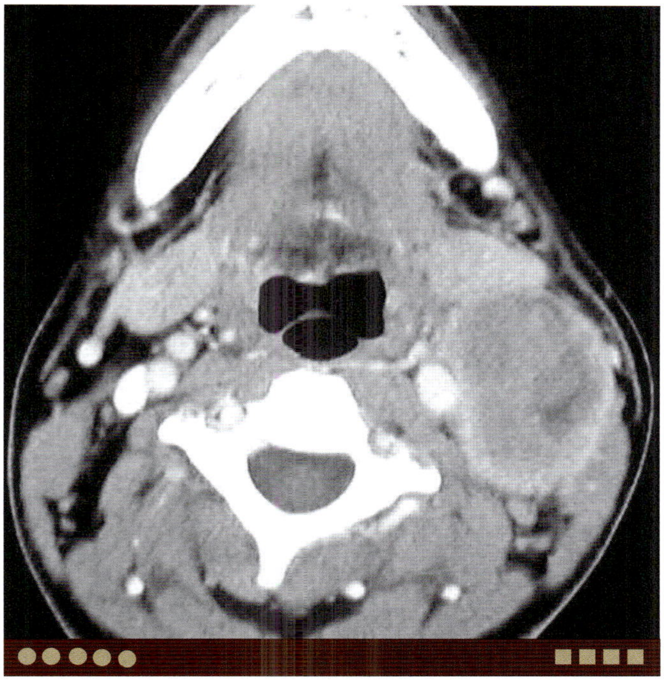

J. **Necrotic metastatic node**. Axial postcontrast CT demonstrates a heterogeneously enhancing lesion displacing the left carotid bifurcation.

Case 6–19 Retropharyngeal Carotid Artery/Medial Deviation of Carotid Artery

Osamu Sakai, Cory Siegel

PRESENTATION

Pulsatile pharyngeal mass.

FINDINGS

CT demonstrates an enhancing tubular structure running posterior to the posterior wall of the pharynx.

DIFFERENTIAL DIAGNOSIS

- Carotid artery aneurysm: This shows dilated caliber of the artery, often with calcification, not just tortuosity.
- Paraganglioma: This is seen as a very hypervascular mass with avid enhancement on CT and "salt-and-pepper" appearance on MRI.
- Castleman disease: This is a rare lymphoproliferative nodal disease that is usually very vascular.
- Retropharyngeal abscess or edema: Fluid density/signal is seen in the retropharyngeal space. Rim-enhancement suggests abscess formation.
- Prevertebral abscess: This condition is most commonly secondary to discitis/osteomyelitis, and often causes retropharyngeal edema. Evaluation for epidural abscess and cord compression is important.

COMMENTS

This is a 69-year-old man with pulsatile right neck mass.

Retropharyngeal internal or common carotid artery (ICA/CCA) is a common normal variant, often seen bilaterally. Atherosclerosis may contribute to this condition to some degree, however, this finding is considered to be an aberrancy.

Retropharyngeal ICA/CCA is usually asymptomatic and an incidental finding, however, patients may present with a sore throat, abnormal sensation, odynophagia, cervical pain, or pulsatile pharyngeal mass. Often a retropharyngeal ICA/CCA can easily be appreciated on exam.

Contrast-enhanced CT or MRI clearly demonstrates carotid arteries running posterior to the pharyngeal wall. However, on lateral neck radiograph or noncontrast-enhanced CT, it can be mistaken as thickening of the prevertebral soft tissue, which may be troublesome when cervical spine trauma or infection is clinically suspected. Of course, biopsy should never be recommended.

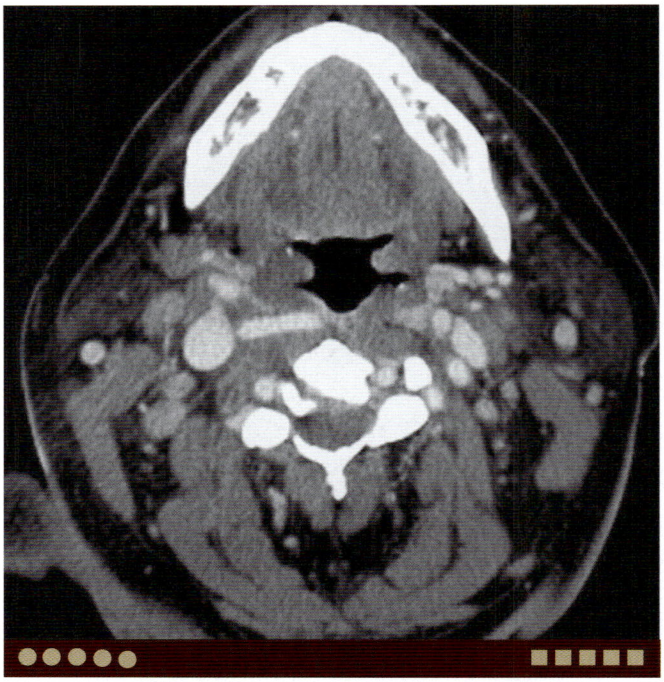

A. Retropharyngeal ICA. Axial postcontrast CT demonstrates a retropharyngeal course of the right ICA, transversely running at the oropharyngeal level. The left ICA is in normal location.

PEARLS

- **Retropharyngeal ICA/CCA is a common normal variant, often seen bilaterally.**
- **It is thought to be an aberrancy rather than elongation due to atherosclerotic disease or hypertension.**
- **It can be mistaken as thickening of the prevertebral soft tissue to suggest hematoma or infection on lateral neck radiograph or noncontrast-enhanced CT.**

ADDITIONAL IMAGES (B-G)

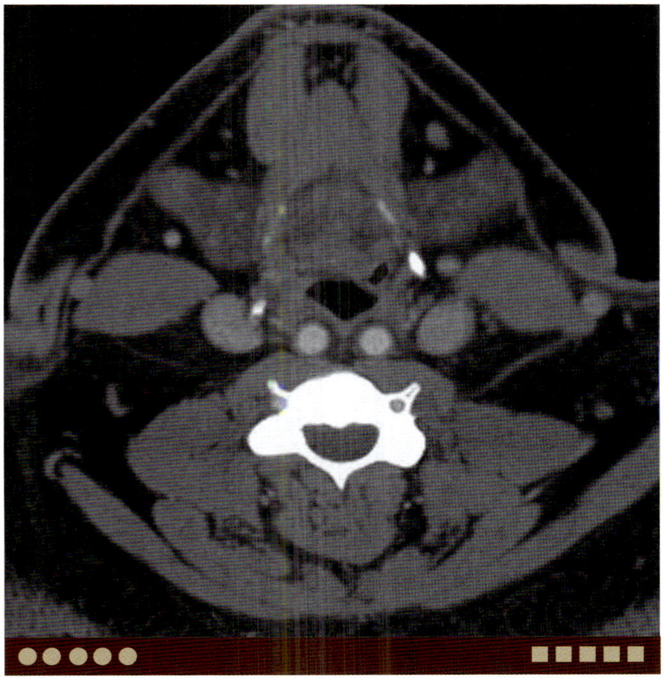

B. Retropharyngeal CCA. Axial postcontrast CT demonstrates bilateral CCAs in the retropharyngeal location, anteriorly displacing the posterior pharyngeal wall.

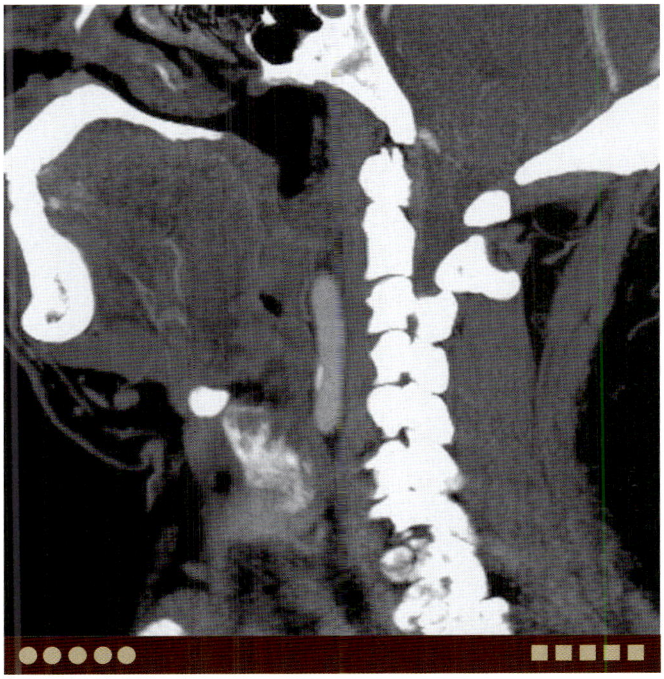

C. Retropharyngeal CCA, same patient as B. Sagittal postcontrast CT demonstrates the CCA posterior to the pharynx and anterior to the prevertebral muscle.

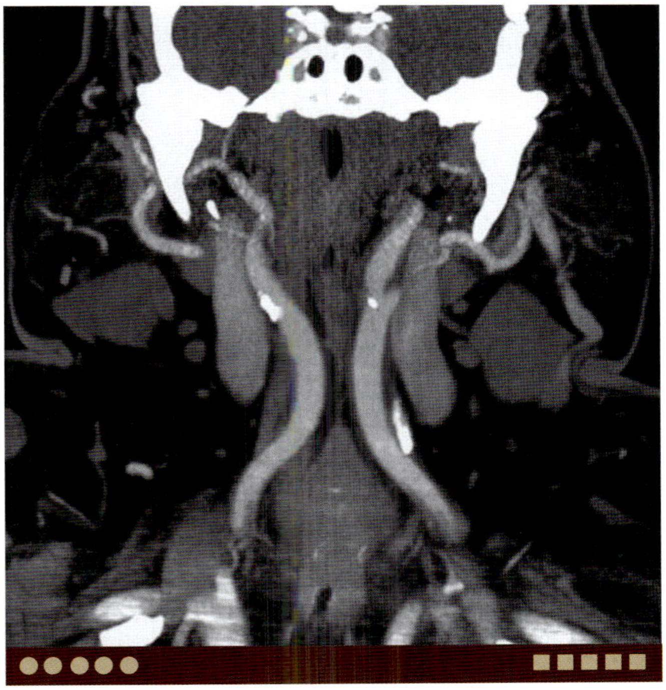

D. Retropharyngeal CCA, same patient as B. Coronal postcontrast CT demonstrates medially displaced CCAs.

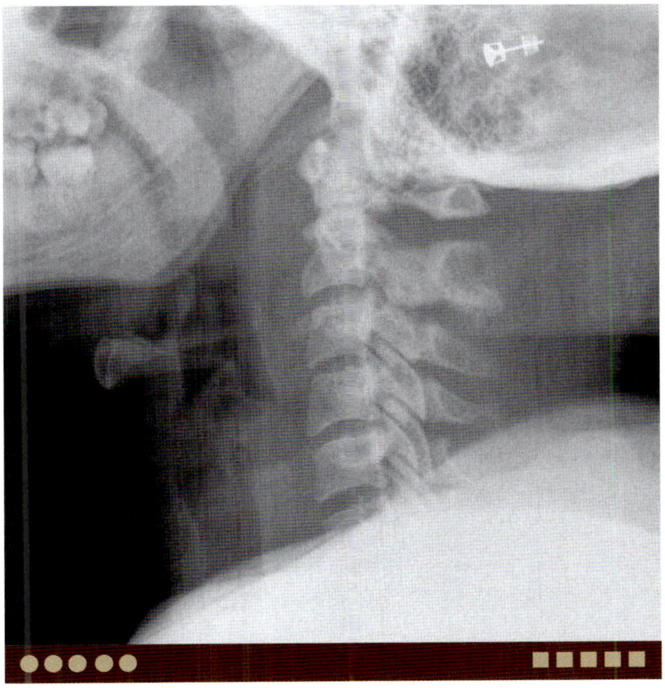

E. Retropharyngeal ICA in a patient status post motor vehicle collision. Lateral radiograph demonstrates thickened prevertebral soft tissue.

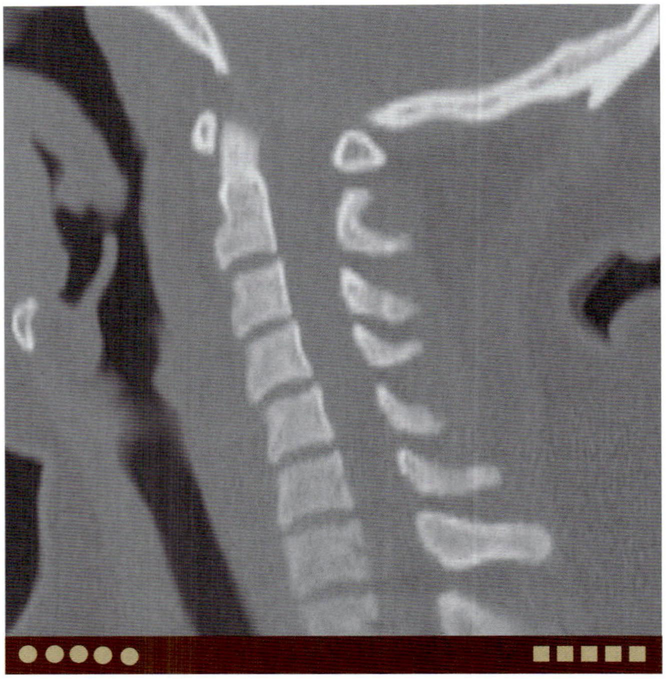

F. Retropharyngeal ICA in a patient status post motor vehicle collision, same patient as E. Sagittal bone window CT demonstrates thickened prevertebral soft tissue.

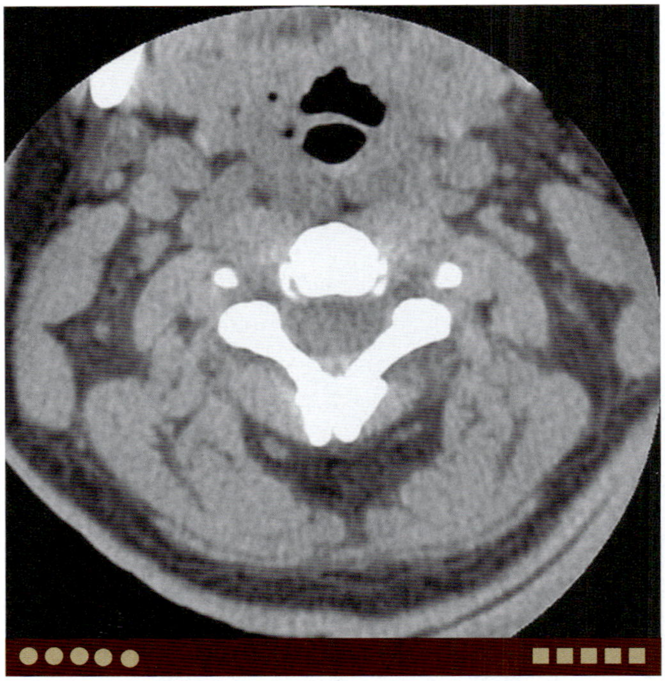

G. Retropharyngeal ICA in a patient status post motor vehicle collision, same patient as E. Axial soft tissue window CT demonstrates retropharyngeal ICAs. Note preserved fat density around the vessels.

DIFFERENTIAL DIAGNOSIS IMAGES (H-J)

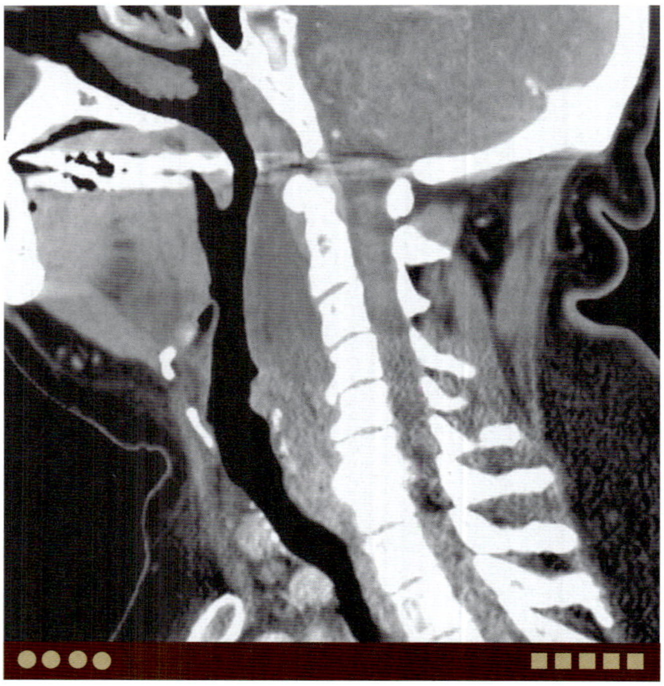

H. **Retropharyngeal edema**. Sagittal postcontrast soft tissue window CT demonstrates abnormal water density anterior to the prevertebral muscle without rim-enhancement.

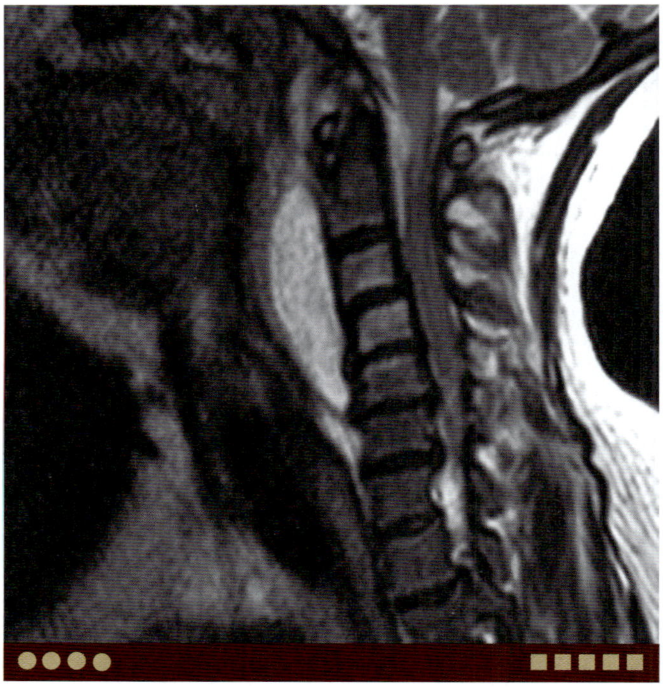

I. **Prevertebral abscess**. Sagittal T2W MR image demonstrates prevertebral fluid collection. Note epidural collection at C1 and C2 levels.

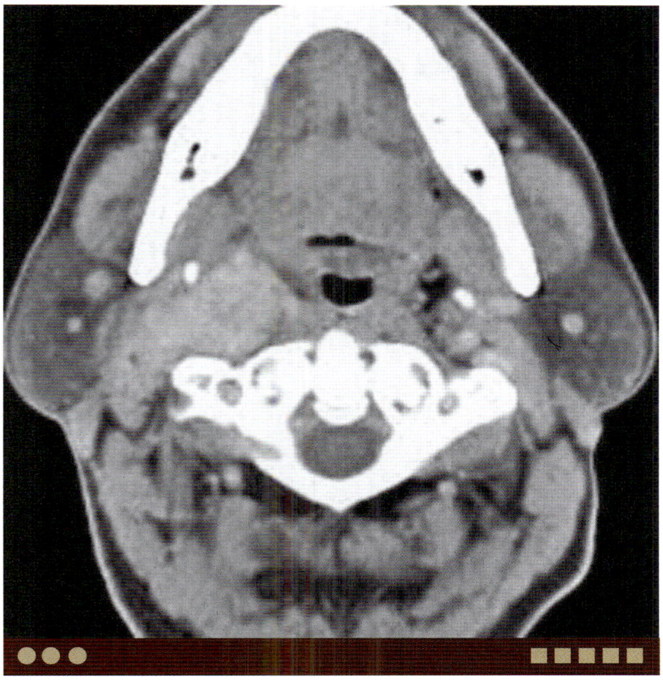

J. Glomus vagale. Axial postcontrast CT demonstrates an enhancing tumor in the right retrostyloid parapharyngeal space.

Case 6–20 Schwannoma—Vagus Nerve

Hiroki Kato, Osamu Sakai

PRESENTATION

Painless neck mass with vague symptoms of sore throat and dysphagia.

FINDINGS

CT and MRI demonstrate a well-demarcated lesion between the internal carotid artery and internal jugular vein, posterior to the vessels.

DIFFERENTIAL DIAGNOSIS

- Paraganglioma: This is a highly vascular tumor. Avid enhancement is seen on contrast-enhanced CT. "Salt-and-pepper" appearance is often seen on MRI.
- Neurofibroma: Neurofibroma associated with the vagus nerve is rare compared with schwannoma. Neurofibromas may be associated with neurofibromatosis, although a sporadic solitary neurofibroma is more common.
- Pleomorphic adenoma: This is the most common salivary gland tumor. Pleomorphic adenoma arising from the deep lobe of the parotid gland often extends into the parapharyngeal space through the stylomandibular tunnel and displaces the parapharyngeal space fat anteromedially.
- Lymphoma: Lymphoma demonstrates homogeneous density and signal similar to schwannoma, however it tends to demonstrate more lobulated appearance and involves multiple spaces without occluding vessels.

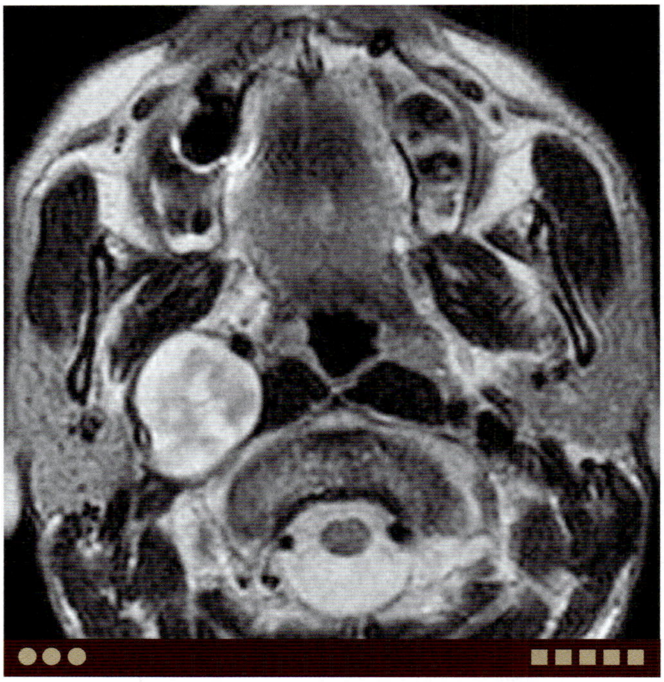

A. Vagus nerve schwannoma. Axial T2W MR image demonstrates a well-demarcated, slightly heterogeneous high-signal lesion, displacing the right ICA anteromedially and the IJV laterally.

COMMENTS

This is a 44-year-old man with slowly progressive dysphagia.

The vagus nerve runs between the internal or common carotid artery (ICA/CCA) and the internal jugular vein (IJV) at the posterior aspect of these vessels within the carotid sheath, although the carotid sheath is usually not completely formed in the suprahyoid neck. Therefore, vagus nerve schwannoma displaces the ICA/CCA anteromedially and the IJV laterally. On the other hand, a schwannoma from the sympathetic chain displaces the carotid vessels laterally because the sympathetic chain runs medial to the carotid vessels. Schwannomas in this region arise commonly from the vagus nerve, less commonly from the glossopharyngeal nerve or the superior sympathetic chain.

Imaging findings of vagus nerve schwannoma are similar to that of schwannomas in other locations; an ovoid or spindle-shaped, well-demarcated lesion with relatively homogeneous density or signal, although cystic or myxoid degeneration is not rare. Schwannoma does enhance after contrast, however, degree of enhancement is much less than that of paraganglioma on CT. This is very useful to differentiate schwannoma from paraganglioma. On MRI, schwannoma shows solid enhancement, while paraganglioma often demonstrates heterogeneous enhancement with "salt-and-pepper" appearance. On dynamic contrast-enhanced studies, schwannoma shows gradual enhancement while paraganglioma shows rapid enhancement and rapid wash-out.

PEARLS

- **Schwannoma from the vagus nerve displaces the ICA/CCA anteromedially and IJV laterally.**
- **Imaging findings are similar to that of schwannomas in other locations; an ovoid or spindle-shaped, well-demarcated lesion with relatively homogeneous density or signal, although cystic or myxoid degeneration is not rare.**
- **Contrast-enhanced CT and dynamic contrast-enhanced studies (CT or MRI) are helpful to differentiate it from paraganglioma.**

ADDITIONAL IMAGES (B-F)

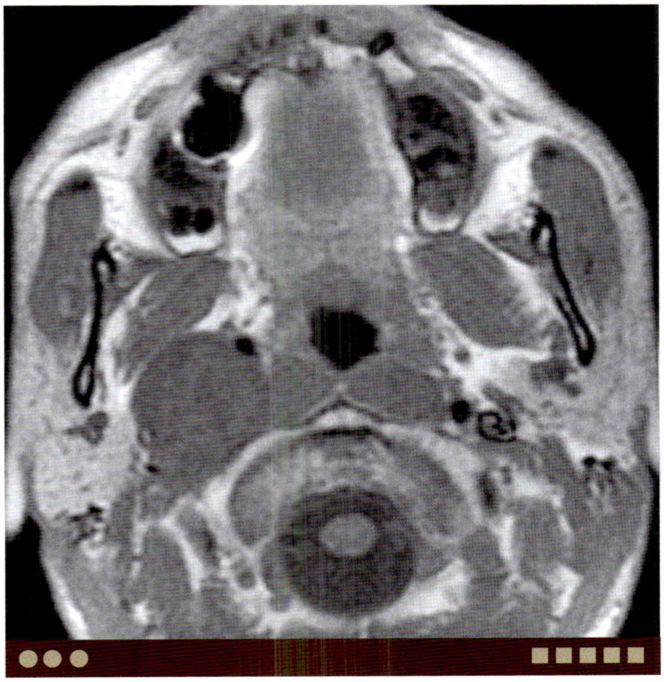

B. Vagus nerve schwannoma, same patient as A. Axial T1W image demonstrates homogeneous low-signal intensity.

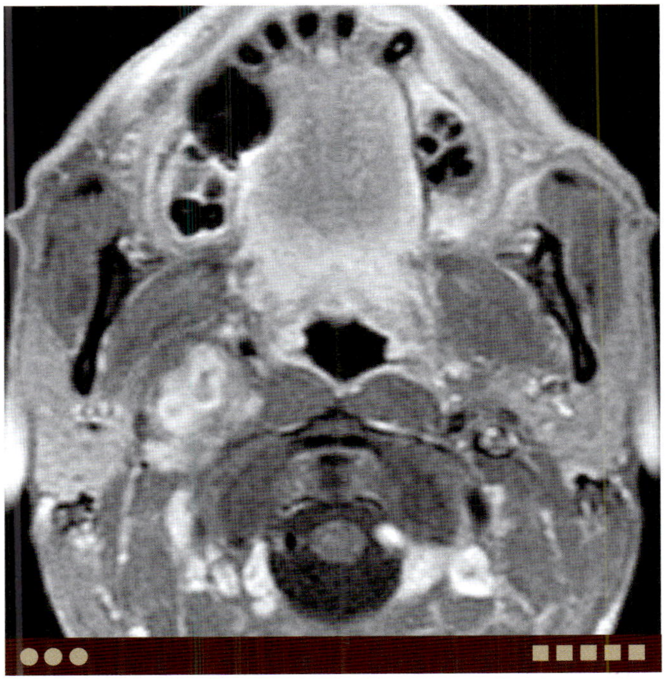

C. Vagus nerve schwannoma, same patient as A. Axial postcontrast fat-suppressed T1W image demonstrates slightly heterogeneous central enhancement.

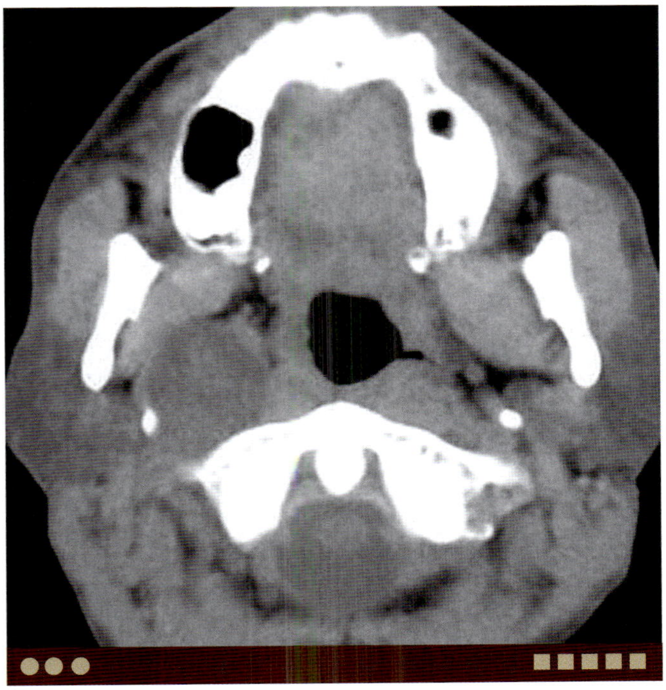

D. Vagus nerve schwannoma, same patient as A. Axial unenhanced CT demonstrates a homogeneous hypodense mass.

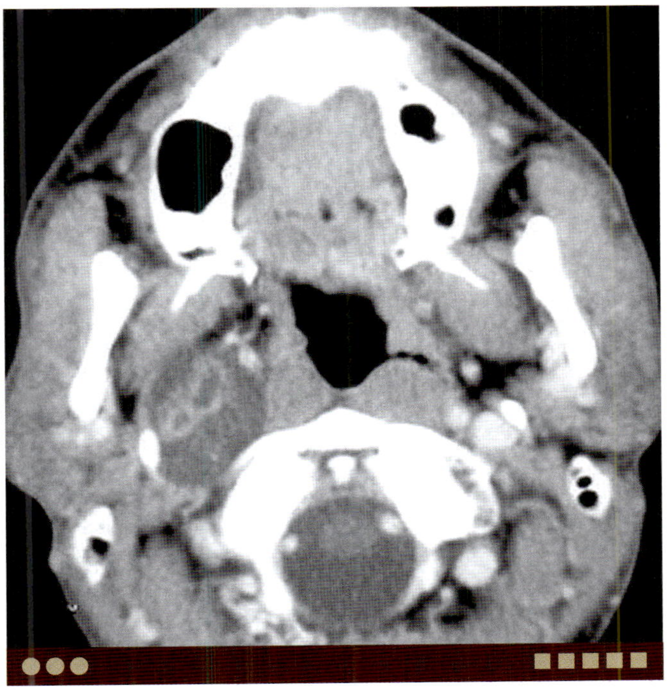

E. Vagus nerve schwannoma, same patient as A. Axial enhanced CT demonstrates mild central enhancement.

DIFFERENTIAL DIAGNOSIS IMAGES (G-J)

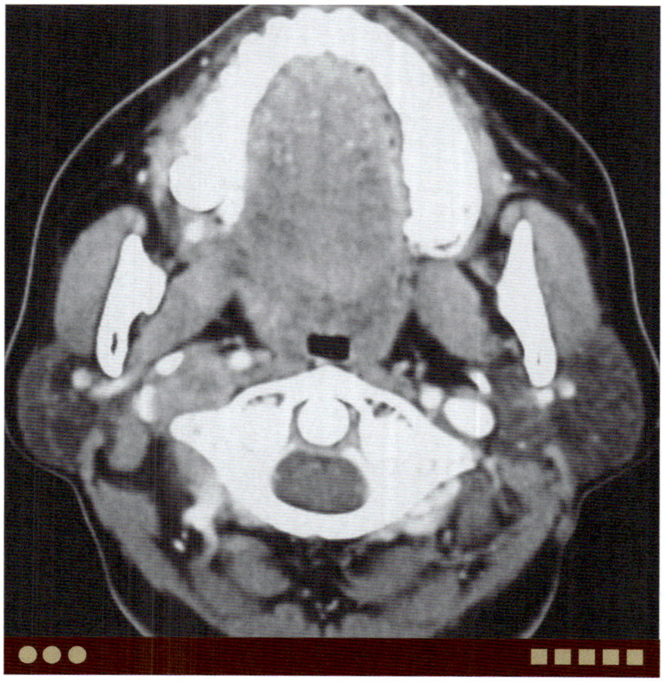

F. **Vagus nerve schwannoma** in a different patient. Axial enhanced CT demonstrates a heterogeneously enhancing lesion displacing the right ICA anteromedially, the IJV laterally and the styloid process anterolaterally.

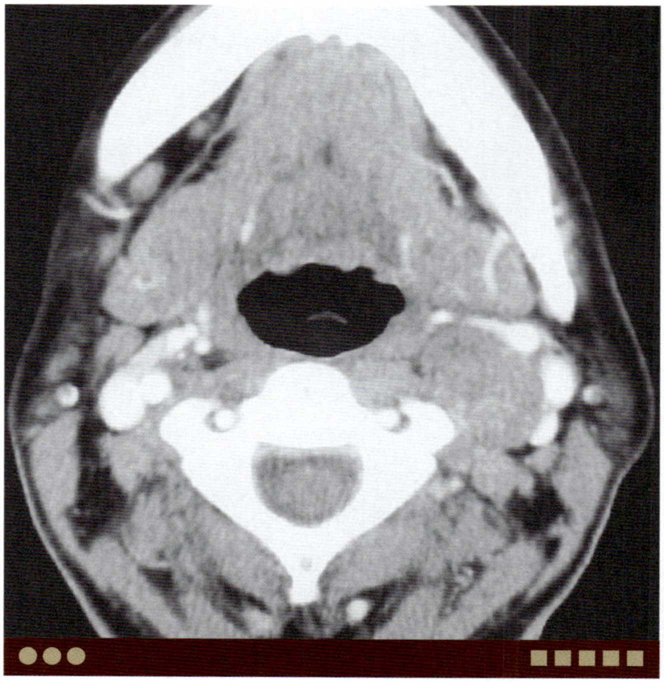

G. **Sympathetic trunk schwannoma**. Axial enhanced CT demonstrates a well-demarcated lesion displacing the left ICA and IJV laterally.

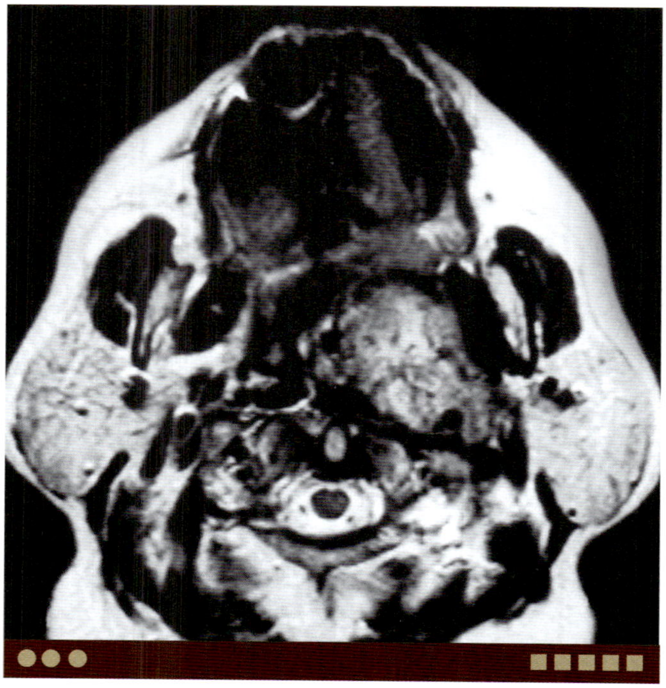

H. **Paraganglioma (glomus vagale)**. Axial T2W MR image demonstrates a large heterogeneous signal lesion displacing the ICA anteromedially. Note "salt-and-pepper" appearance within the lesion.

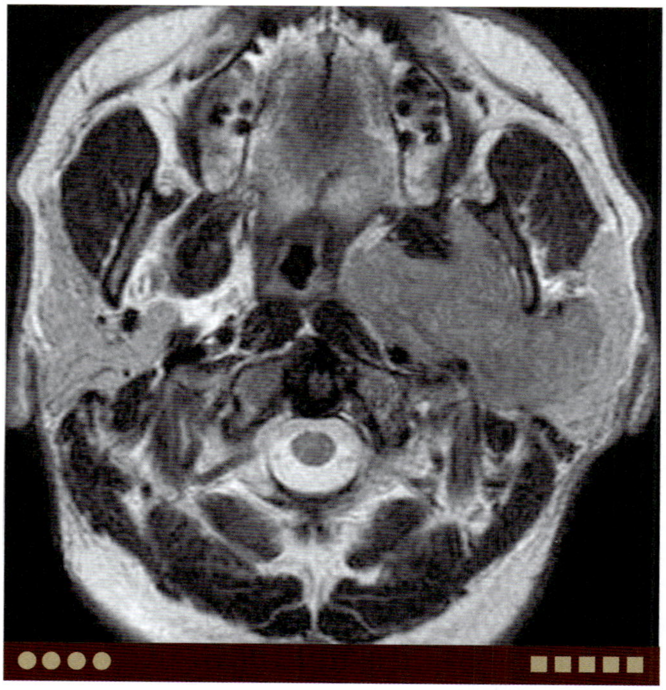

I. **Lymphoma**. Axial T2W MR image demonstrates a homogeneous signal mass involving the parotid, parapharyngeal, and masticator spaces, and displacing the ICA medially.

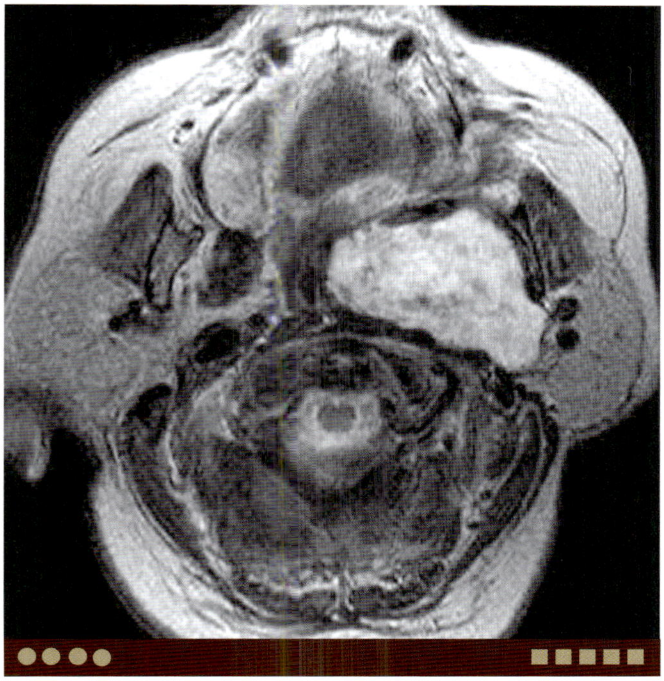

J. Pleomorphic adenoma from the deep lobe of the parotid gland. Axial T2W MR image demonstrates a high signal, slightly lobulated mass widening the stylomandibular tunnel and extending into the parapharyngeal space.

Case 6–21 Schwannoma—Sympathetic Trunk

Susmitha Reddy, Benjamin Ludwig, Osamu Sakai

PRESENTATION

Asymptomatic neck mass.

FINDINGS

CT demonstrates a well-demarcated soft tissue density mass displacing carotid vessels laterally with mild enhancement. MRI demonstrates intermediate-to-high T2 signal and relatively homogeneous enhancement.

DIFFERENTIAL DIAGNOSIS

- Neurofibroma: A tumor arising from the nerve sheath, which is often seen in patients with neurofibromatosis type I, although most neurofibromas are sporadic (90%). They are often difficult to differentiate from schwannomas by imaging alone.
- Paraganglioma: A highly vascular tumor, which demonstrates marked enhancement. The "salt-and-pepper" appearance on MRI is characteristic.
- Lymphoma: A neoplasm that demonstrates homogeneous density and signal similar to schwannoma; but tends to demonstrate a more lobulated appearance and involves multiple spaces without occluding vessels. Primary lymphoma in this region is rare.

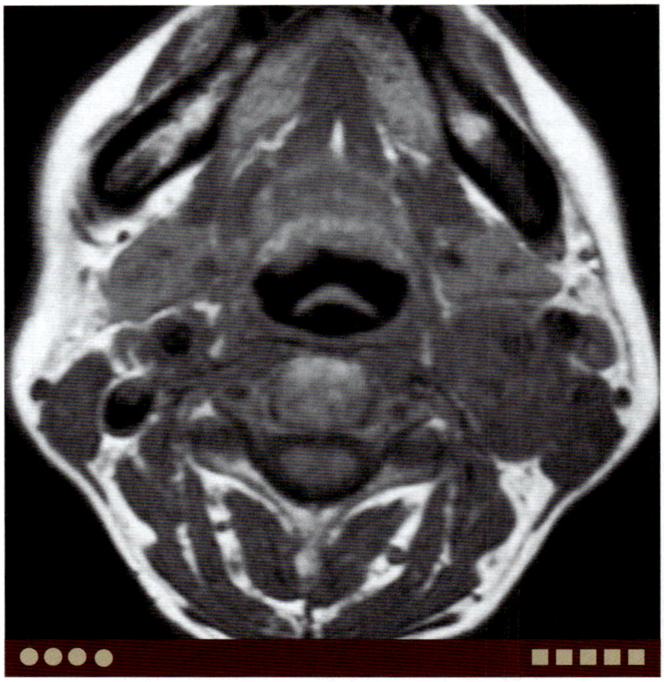

A. Schwannoma. Axial T1W image shows a hypointense mass displacing the left ICA anterolaterally.

COMMENTS

This is a 40-year-old woman with an asymptomatic left neck mass.

Schwannomas are encapsulated masses, which arise from the nerve sheath (perineural Schwann cells), and may involve any nerve in the body.

The sympathetic trunk is present in the medial portion of the retrostyloid parapharyngeal/carotid space, medial to the internal/common carotid arteries (ICA/CCA), and lateral to the lateral retropharyngeal space. The cervical sympathetic trunk is comprised of superior, middle and inferior cervical ganglia. The superior cervical ganglion (*ganglion cervicale superius*), the largest of the above three, is placed opposite the second and third cervical vertebrae and lies within the carotid sheath.

Schwannomas of the cervical sympathetic chain tend to push the ICA/CCA and internal jugular vein (IJV) anterolaterally as it courses medial to the ICA/CCA, whereas the schwannoma of the vagus nerve or other lower cranial nerves displace the ICA/CCA anteromedially as these nerves lie between the ICA and the IJV.

Imaging findings of schwannoma of the sympathetic plexus is similar to that of schwannomas in other locations.

On CT, schwannomas are typically spindle or ovoid-shaped circumscribed masses of soft tissue density. Mild enhancement is seen after contrast. On MRI, schwannomas demonstrate hypointensity on T1W and intermediate-to-high signal intensity on T2W images. Cystic degeneration may be present. Hetero- to homogenous enhancement is seen after contrast, which depends on the degree of cystic degeneration. In contrast to paragangliomas, no flow voids are present within schwannomas.

PEARLS

- **Schwannomas of the sympathetic trunk cause lateral displacement of the ICA/CCA and IJV, whereas schwannomas of the lower cranial nerves cause anteromedial displacement of the ICA/CCA.**
- **Imaging findings are similar to schwannomas in other locations.**

ADDITIONAL IMAGES (B-E)

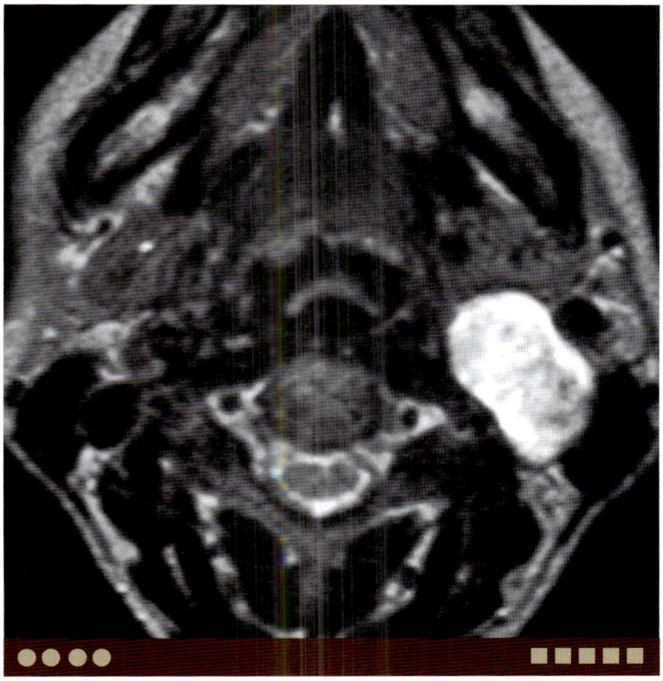

B. Schwannoma, same patient as A. Axial T2W image shows high-signal intensity lesion with heterogeneous signal areas.

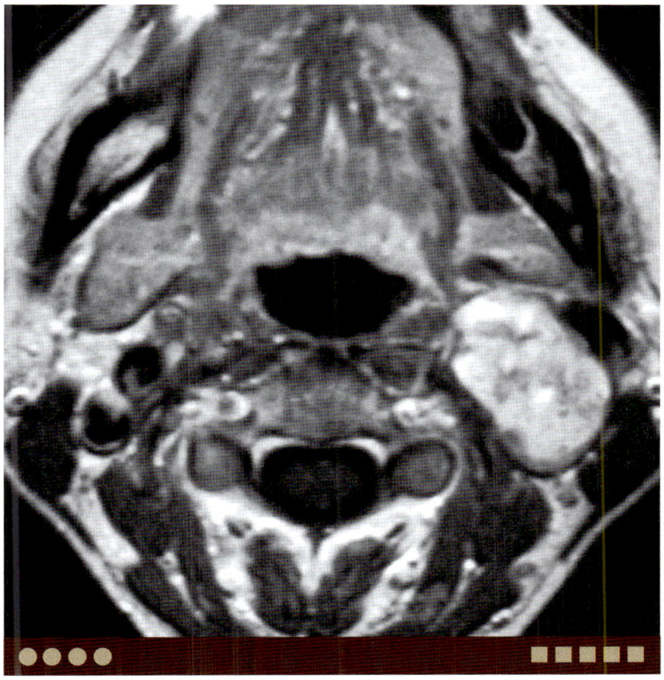

C. Schwannoma, same patient as A. Axial postcontrast T1W image shows enhancement of the lesion.

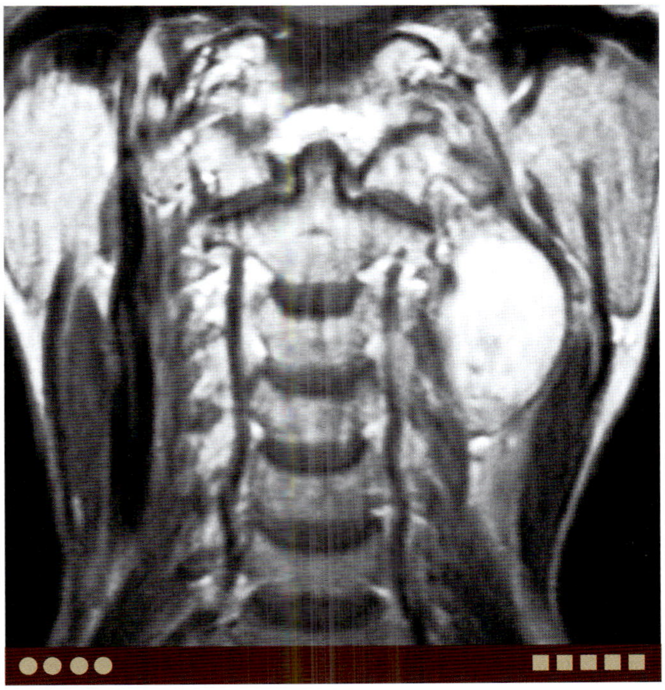

D. Schwannoma, same patient as A. Coronal postcontrast T1W image shows the enhancing lesion and its craniocaudal extension medial to the ICA.

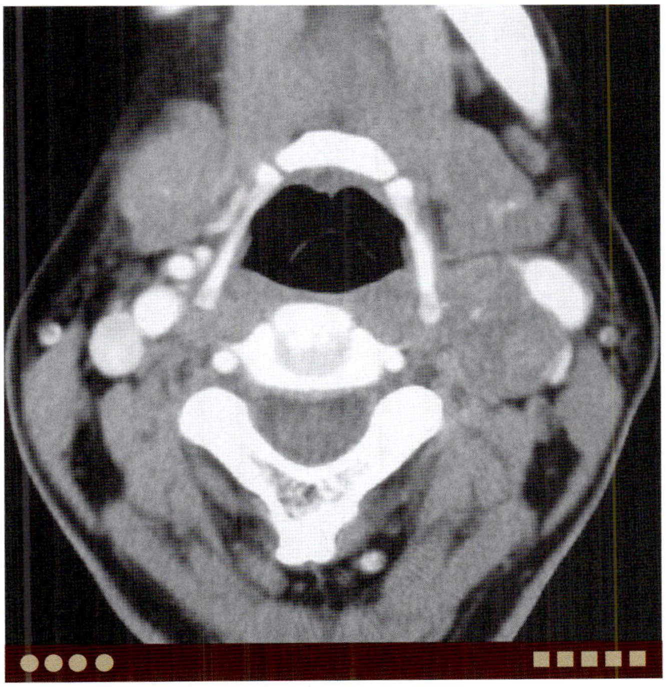

E. Schwannoma in a different patient. Axial postcontrast CT shows a well-demarcated lesion with mild enhancement displacing the left carotid bifurcation anterolaterally.

DIFFERENTIAL DIAGNOSIS IMAGES (F-I)

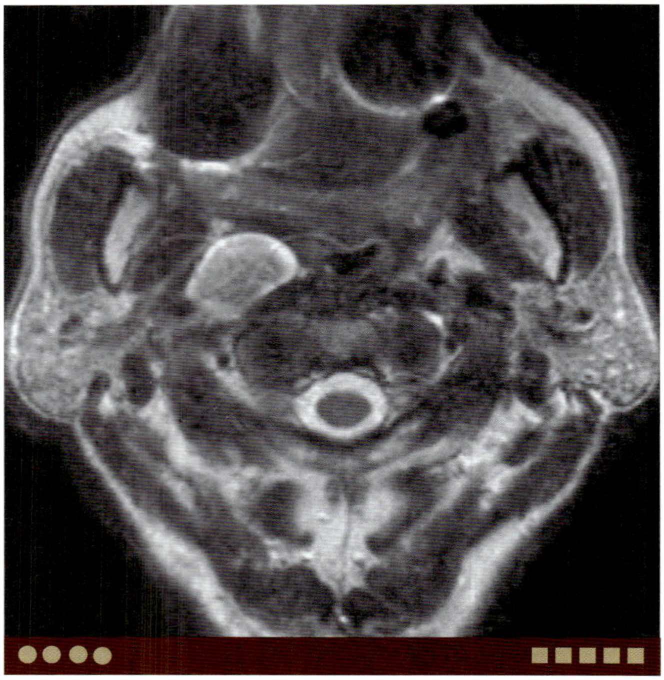

F. Neurofibroma. Axial T2W image demonstrates a high-signal lesion with central low signal.

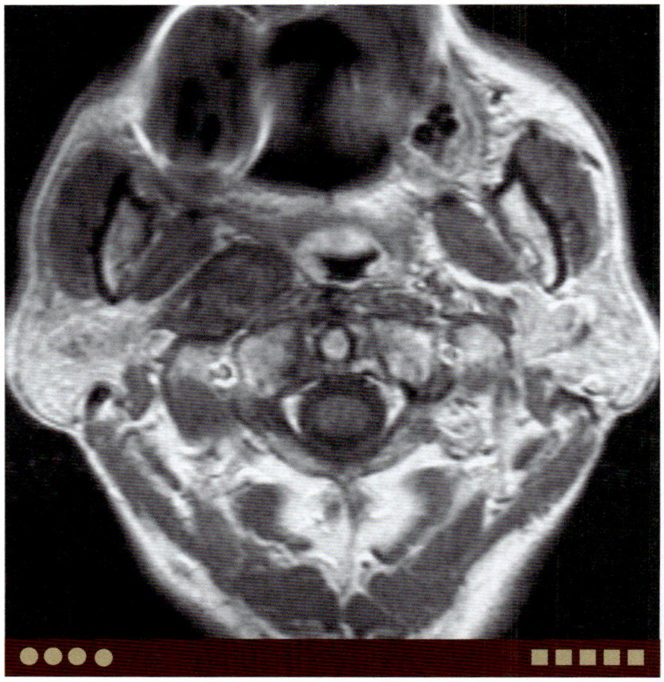

G. Neurofibroma, same patient as F. Axial postcontrast T1W image shows mild enhancement within the central portion of the lesion.

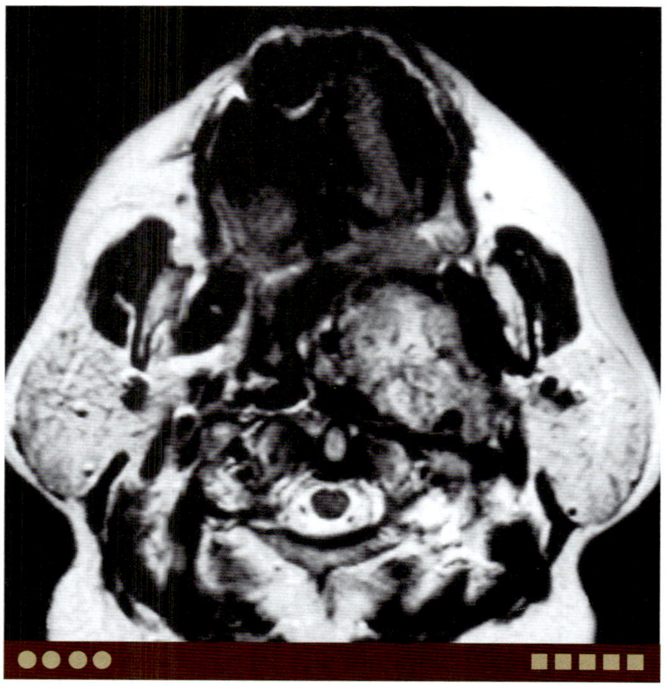

H. Paraganglioma (glomus vagale). Axial T2W MR image demonstrates a large heterogeneous signal lesion displacing the left ICA anteromedially. Note "salt-and-pepper" appearance within the lesion.

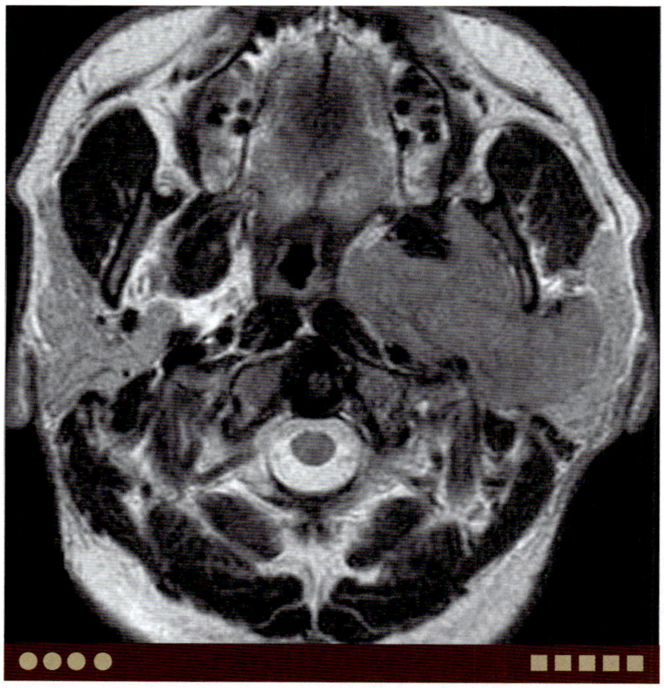

I. Lymphoma. Axial T2W MR image demonstrates a large, homogeneous, intermediate-signal lesion involving the left parapharyngeal, masticator, and parotid spaces.

Case 6–22 Prevertebral Abscess

Osamu Sakai, Benjamin Ludwig

PRESENTATION

Neck pain and fever.

FINDINGS

CT demonstrates prevertebral fluid and soft tissue thickening. MR images demonstrate fluid signal within the prevertebral space with peripheral enhancement. Similar findings are often present within the anterior epidural space.

DIFFERENTIAL DIAGNOSIS

- Retropharyngeal abscess: Typically result from infection of the upper respiratory tract, sinuses, or middle ear. Imaging demonstrates fluid confined to the retropharyngeal space with peripheral enhancement.
- Calcific tendinitis: A self-limited inflammatory reaction, secondary to hydroxyapatite deposition within the longus colli muscle tendon, which results in fluid within the prevertebral space. Associated findings include dystrophic calcifications within the longus colli tendon insertion.
- Prevertebral hematoma: This is secondary to trauma and usually the patient has clear history of injury.

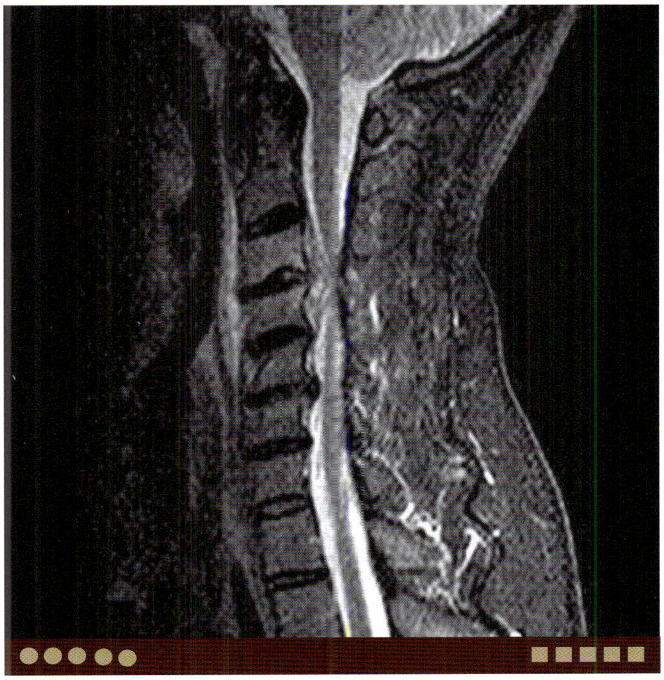

A. Prevertebral and epidural abscesses due to discitis/osteomyelitis. Sagittal fat-suppressed T2W image shows abnormal swelling and increased signal in the prevertebral and anterior epidural spaces. Note increased signal in C3 and C4 bodies and disc space suggesting discitis/osteomyelitis.

COMMENTS

This is a 41-year-old man with neck pain and fever.

The prevertebral space (PVS), also referred to as the paravertebral space, is encapsulated by the deep layer of the deep cervical fascia, and is located posterior to the retropharyngeal space (RPS) and danger space. The PVS extends from the skull base to the level of the coccyx and contents include the paravertebral muscles, vertebral bodies and their contents, thecal sac, and spinal cord.

Prevertebral abscesses most often occur secondary to discitis/osteomyelitis at adjacent cervical levels. Epidural extension of inflammation/abscess can be seen, which may result in cord compression and require emergent decompression. Differentiation from retropharyngeal abscess is important for patient management and surgical intervention, but may be difficult clinically. Imaging therefore plays a critical role in diagnosis and management of prevertebral abscesses by depicting compartmental anatomy, potential etiologies of prevertebral fluid, extent of inflammation, and the complication of epidural abscess with spinal cord compression.

MRI is the best modality to diagnose prevertebral pathologies and should be performed if prevertebral abscess is suspected. MRI findings include fluid signal within the PVS, which typically displaces the prevertebral fascia anteriorly, and demonstrates peripheral enhancement after contrast administration. Attention must be paid to the spine at this level to evaluate for associated findings of discitis/ osteomyelitis.

CT is complementary to MRI, and demonstrates obliteration of fat planes and peripherally enhancing fluid within the PVS. Initially, the retropharyngeal fat may be displaced anteriorly, but eventually inflammation extends into the RPS.

PEARLS

- **Prevertebral abscess is often secondary to discitis/osteomyelitis.**
- **Imaging can help differentiate prevertebral from retropharyngeal abscesses, which is often difficult clinically, and critical for subsequent treatment.**
- **Edema/inflammation within the retropharyngeal space is often seen secondary to prevertebral space infection.**

ADDITIONAL IMAGES (B-G)

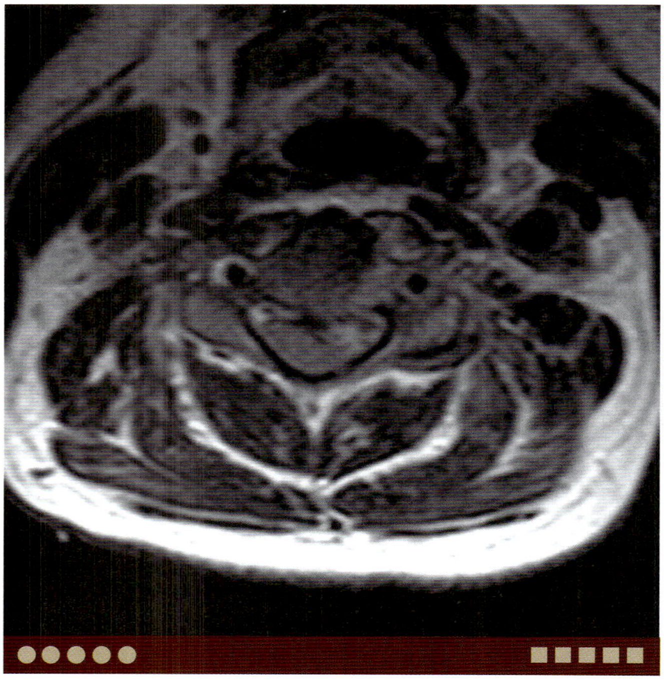

B. Prevertebral and epidural abscesses, same patient as A. Axial T2W image shows abnormal high signal in the PVS with heterogeneous high signal in the left longus colli muscle. Note fluid collection in the left anterior epidural space.

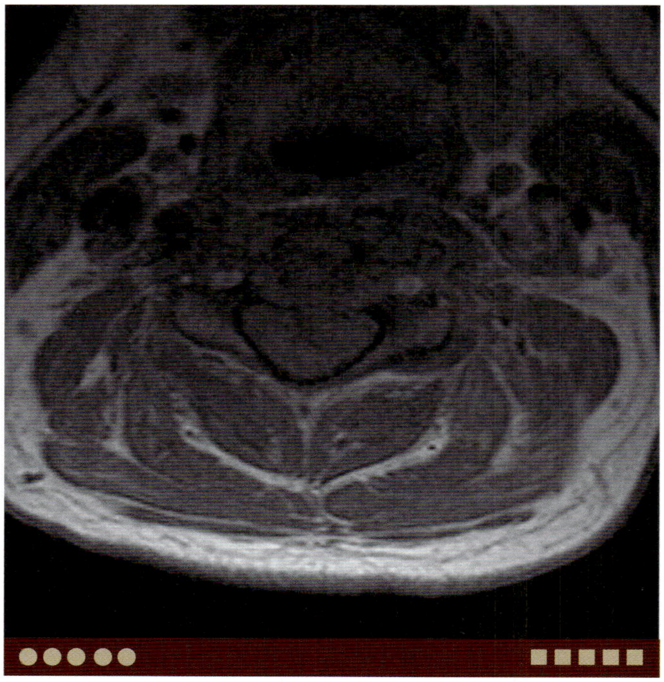

C. Prevertebral and epidural abscesses, same patient as A. Axial T1W image shows obscured fat signal in the PVS and anteriorly displaced but preserved high signal of the retropharyngeal fat.

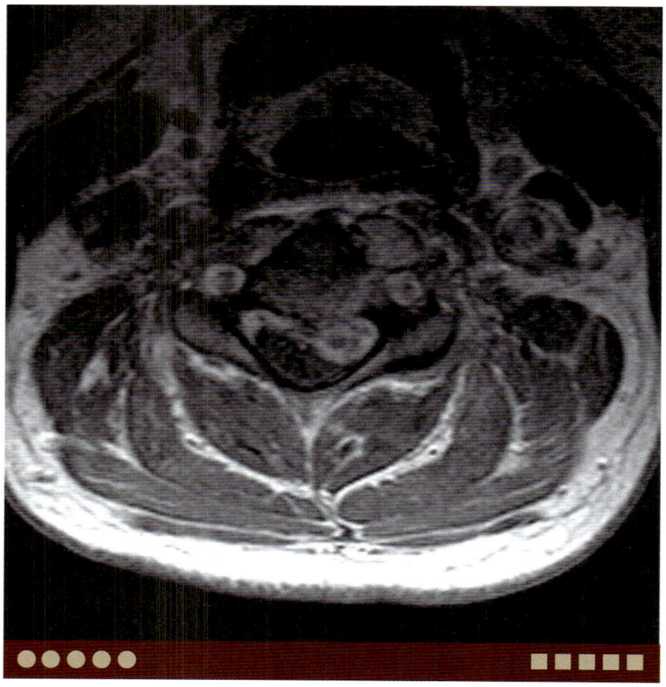

D. Prevertebral and epidural abscesses, same patient as A. Axial postcontrast T1W image shows abnormal enhancement of the PVS soft tissues, including the longus colli muscles. Note rim-enhancing fluid collection in the left anterior epidural space consistent with abscess.

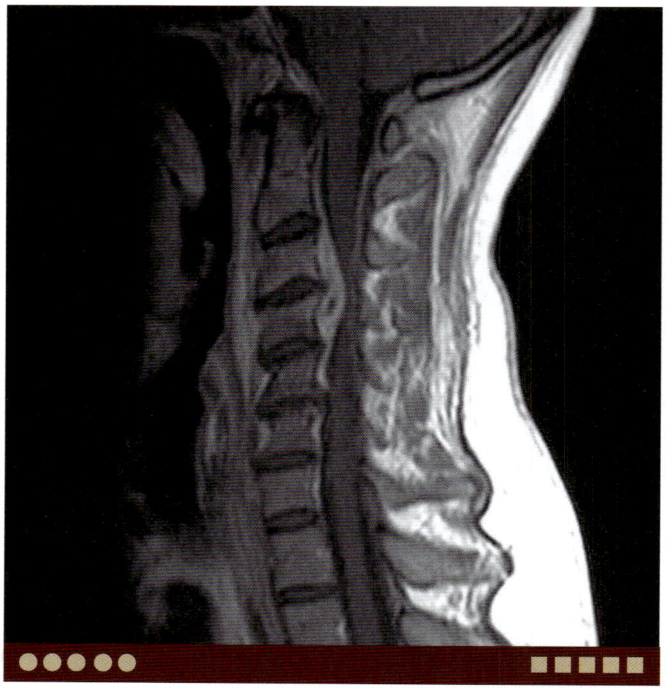

E. Prevertebral and epidural abscesses, same patient as A. Sagittal postcontrast T1W image shows abnormal enhancement in the prevertebral space and anterior epidural space Note small regions of fluid intensity within the epidural space, consistent with abscess.

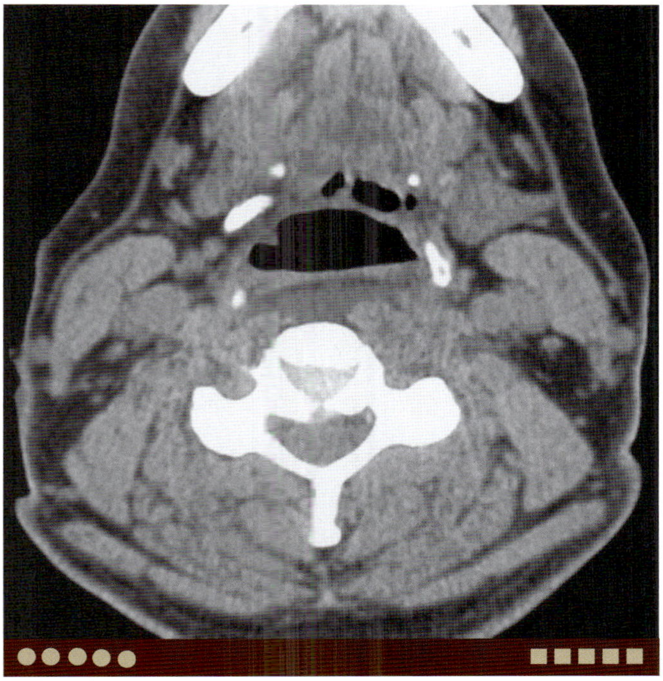

F. Prevertebral and epidural abscesses, same patient as A. Axial noncontrast CT shows fluid density and obliteration of fat density in the PVS. Note anteriorly displaced but preserved low density of the retropharyngeal fat. Increased density within the epidural space is less conspicuous compared to findings on MRI.

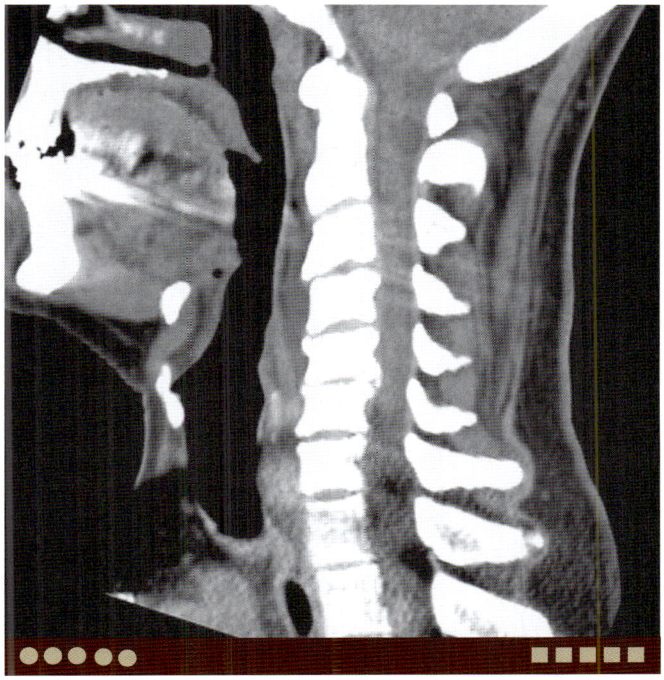

G. Prevertebral and epidural abscesses, same patient as A. Sagittal noncontrast CT shows abnormal fluid collection in the PVS, anterior to C3 to C5 bodies

DIFFERENTIAL DIAGNOSIS IMAGES (H-J)

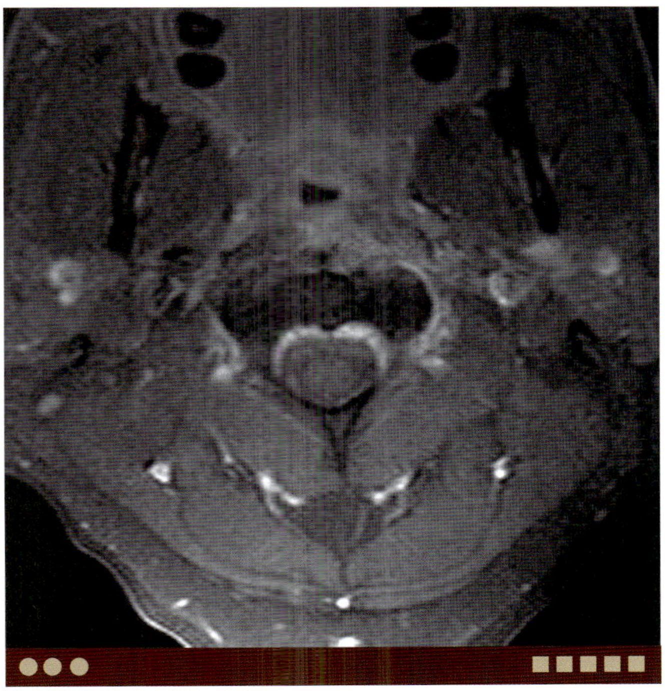

H. **Calcific tendinitis**. Axial postcontrast fat-suppressed T1W image at the C2 level shows swelling and enhancement of the longus colli muscles, left greater than right.

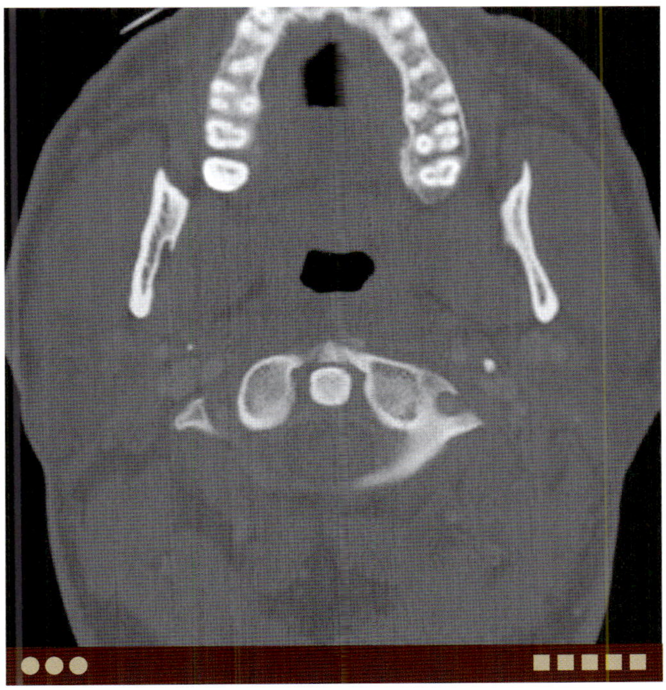

I. Calcific tendinitis, same patient as H. Axial CT in bone windows shows subtle calcification anterior to the anterior arch of the C1.

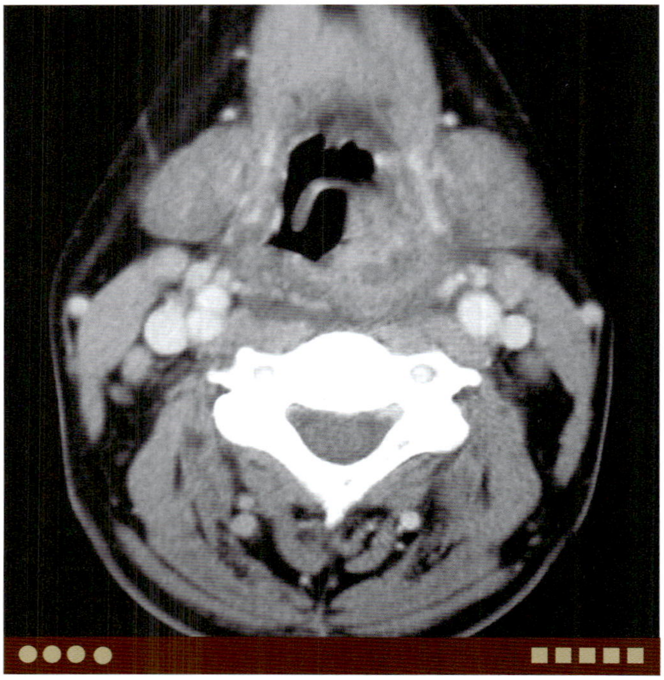

J. Retropharyngeal abscess. Axial postcontrast CT demonstrates rim-enhancing fluid collection centered in the left hypopharynx as well as fluid collection with mild rim-enhancement in the RPS.

Case 6–23 Eagle Syndrome

Brooke Devenney-Cakır, Osamu Sakai

PRESENTATION

Dysphagia and pain on rotation of the neck.

FINDINGS

Radiograph and CT demonstrate an elongated styloid process.

DIFFERENTIAL DIAGNOSIS

- Foreign body: Typically there is a history of foreign body ingestion. A fish or chicken bone may mimic the appearance of a calcified styloid process on radiographs. Foreign body can be easily differentiated on CT based on location, contour and density.
- Heterotopic ossification: This typically demonstrates more ill-defined density, not as organized and elongated as ossification/calcification of the stylohyoid ligament.

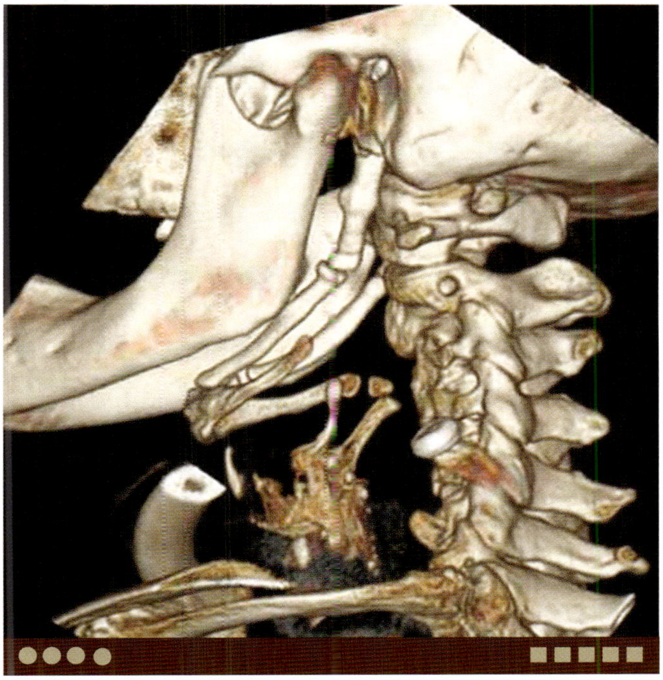

A. Eagle syndrome. Three-dimensional volume rendering reconstruction image from CT demonstrates ossified stylohyoid ligaments with articulations, extending from the skull base to the hyoid bilaterally.

COMMENTS

This is a 45-year-old male with neck pain and dysphagia.

Eagle syndrome is a constellation of symptoms which may include the sensation of a foreign body, hypersalivation, dysphagia, pain on rotation of the neck and extension of the tongue in the setting of an elongated styloid process or calcified/ossified stylohyoid ligament.

The normal length of the styloid process in an adult is about 2.5 cm whereas the styloid process in Eagle syndrome is greater than 3 cm. The presence of an elongated styloid process is not pathognomonic for Eagle syndrome because many patients with an elongated styloid process are asymptomatic (about 4% of the population) and only small percentages of this group are actually symptomatic.

There are several theories that have been proposed to explain the mechanism of symptoms: (1) fracture of the styloid process causing proliferation of granulation tissue, which causes pressure on the surrounding structures; (2) compression of adjacent nerves (cranial nerves V, VII, IX, and X) by elongated styloid process/ossified stylohyoid ligament; (3) degenerative and inflammatory changes in the tendinous portion of the stylohyoid insertion, called insertion tendonitis; (4) irritation of the pharyngeal mucosa by direct compression or post-tonsillectomy scarring; and (5) impingement of the carotid vessels, irritating the sympathetic nerves in the arterial sheath.

The diagnosis can be made by radiographs or CT. Physical examination may demonstrate a palpable styloid process in the tonsillar fossa and palpation of the tip may exacerbate the existing symptoms. CT provides precise relationship of an elongated styloid process or calcified/ossified stylohyoid ligament to surrounding soft tissue structures.

PEARLS

- **Eagle syndrome is a constellation of symptoms including the sensation of a foreign body, hypersalivation, dysphagia, facial and/or cervical spine pain in the setting of an elongated styloid process or calcified/ossified stylohyoid ligament.**
- **Normal adult styloid process is 2.5 cm, styloid process in Eagle syndrome is greater than 3 cm.**
- **Presence of an elongated styloid process is not pathognomonic for Eagle syndrome because it can be an incidental finding in an asymptomatic patient.**

ADDITIONAL IMAGES (B-G)

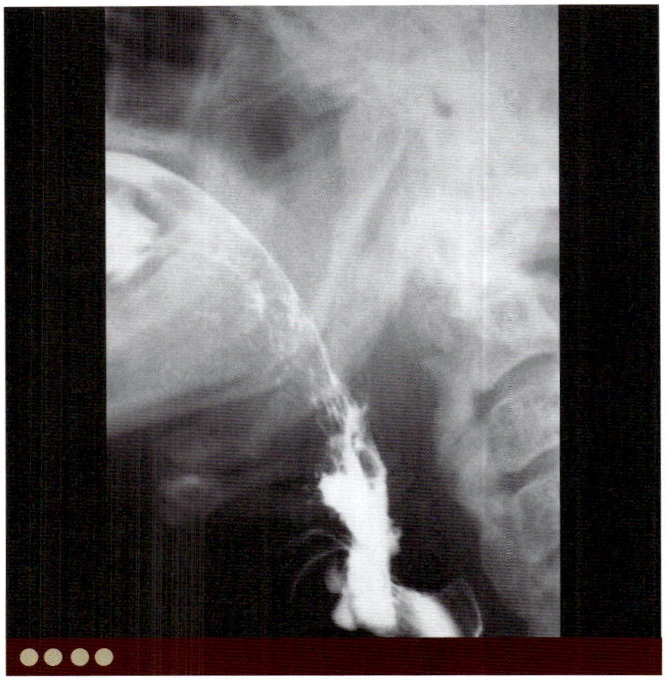

B. **Eagle syndrome** in a different patient. Barium swallow study demonstrates very thick ossified stylohyoid ligaments extending to the hyoid bilaterally.

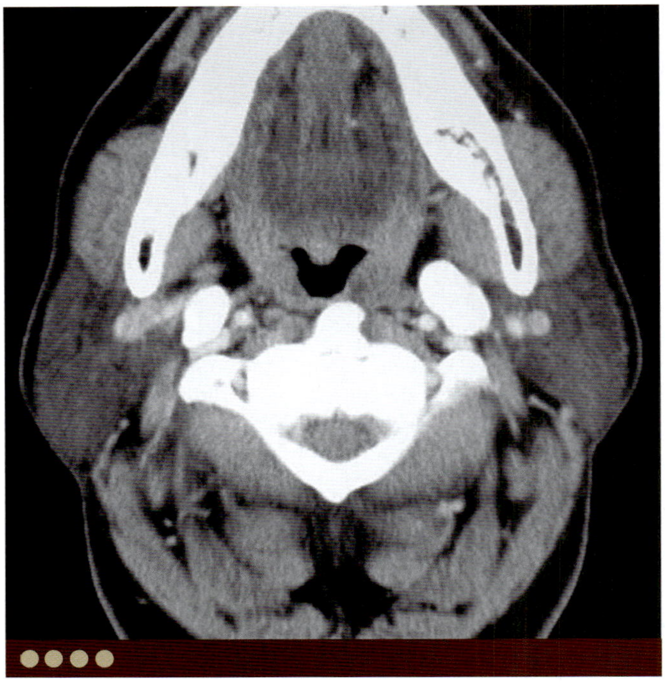

C. Eagle syndrome, same patient as B. Axial postcontrast CT demonstrates very thick ossified stylohyoid ligaments bilaterally.

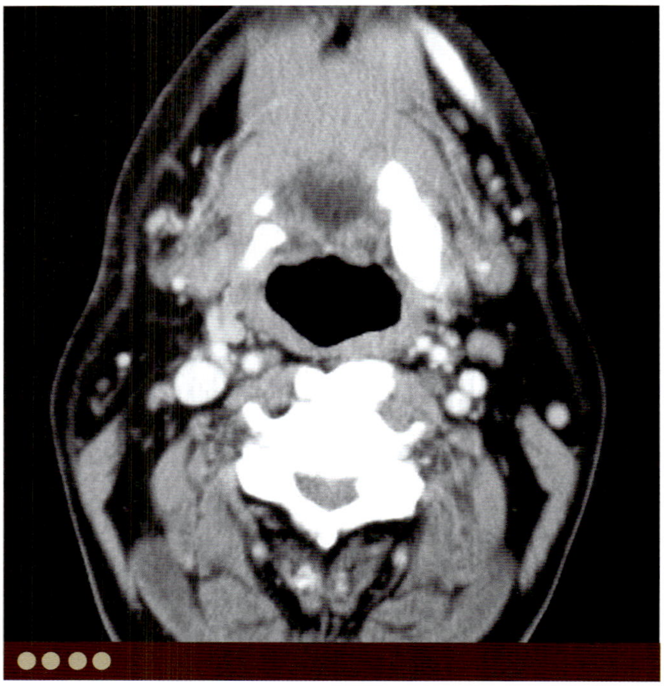

D. Eagle syndrome, same patient as B. Axial postcontrast CT at the hyoid level demonstrates thick ossified stylohyoid ligaments articulating with the hyoid.

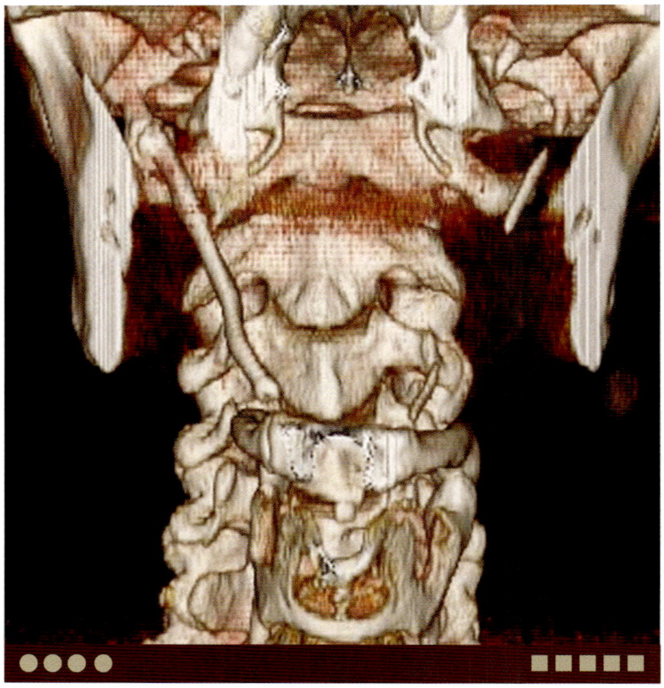

E. **Eagle syndrome** in a different patient. Three-dimensional volume rendering reconstruction image from CT demonstrates ossified stylohyoid ligaments, right longer than left.

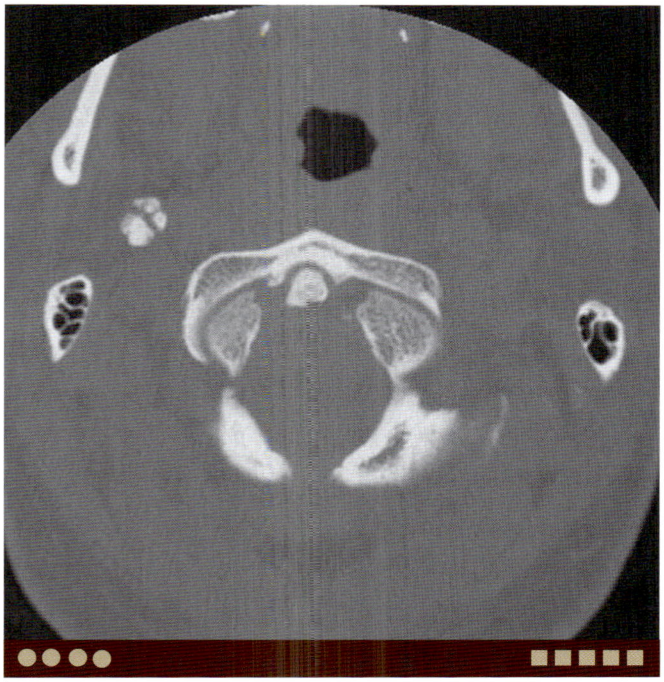

F. Eagle syndrome, same patient as E. Axial CT demonstrates thick ossified right stylohyoid ligament with osteoarthritic proliferative change.

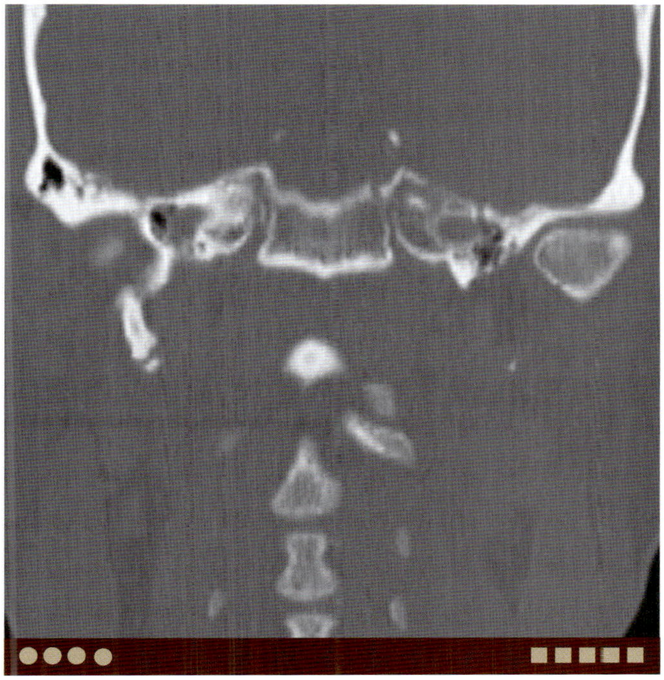

G. Eagle syndrome, same patient as E. Coronal CT demonstrates a thickened and elongated right styloid process.

DIFFERENTIAL DIAGNOSIS IMAGES (H-J)

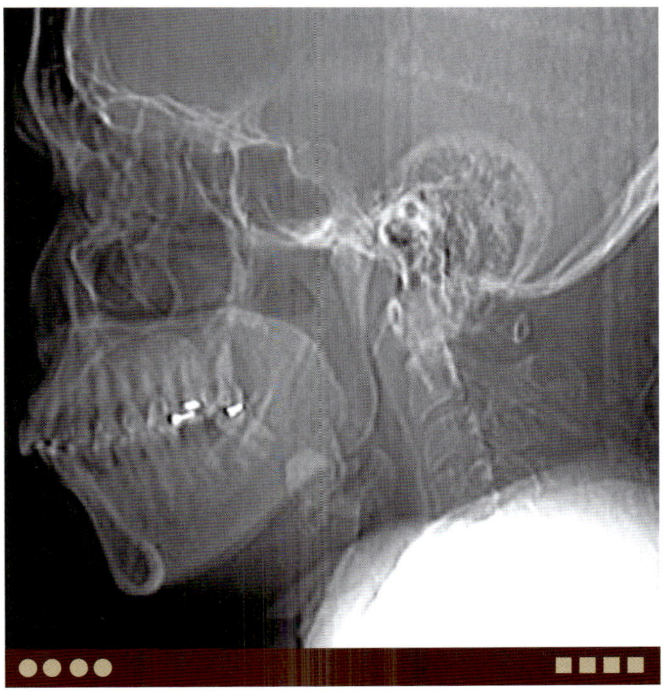

H. Sialolithiasis. Scout image of CT demonstrates slightly elongated round high density over the mandibular angle.

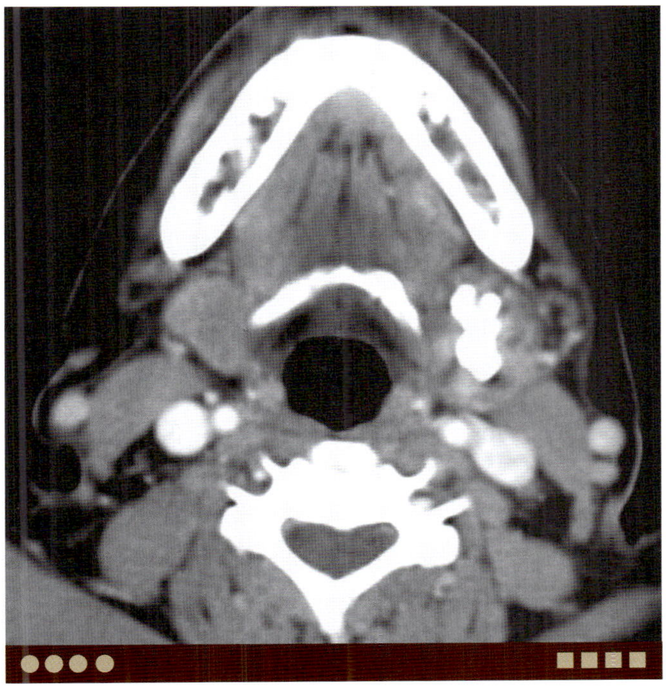

I. Sialolithiasis, same patient as H. Axial postcontrast CT demonstrates slightly lobulated dense calcification in the left submandibular gland, lateral to the hyoid.

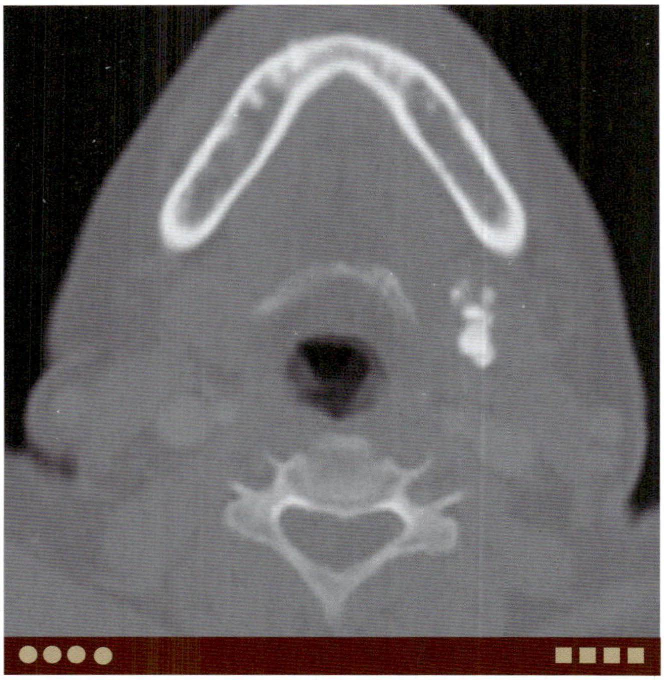

J. Sialolithiasis, same patient as H. Axial bone window CT demonstrates irregular-shaped calcifications, neither tubular nor corticated.

Case 6–24 Paraganglioma—Glomus Vagale

Brooke Devenney-Cakir, Osamu Sakai

PRESENTATION

Palpable neck mass, possible hoarseness.

FINDINGS

CT demonstrates an avidly enhancing mass below the skull base along the course of the vagus nerve, splaying the internal jugular vein and the internal carotid artery.

DIFFERENTIAL DIAGNOSIS

- Schwannoma: This occurs in similar locations, however enhancement on CT is less compared to paraganglioma. No flow-voids or "salt-and-pepper" appearance are seen on MRI.
- Castleman disease: This is a nodal disease and often very vascular. This usually displaces vessels rather than encasing them.
- Aneurysm: Normal carotid artery is usually missing with this condition; however, pseudoaneurysm may be seen with normal appearing carotid artery.
- Nodal metastasis: Metastases from renal dell carcinoma, hepatocellular carcinoma and thyroid cancer can be very vascular. These are usually multiple.

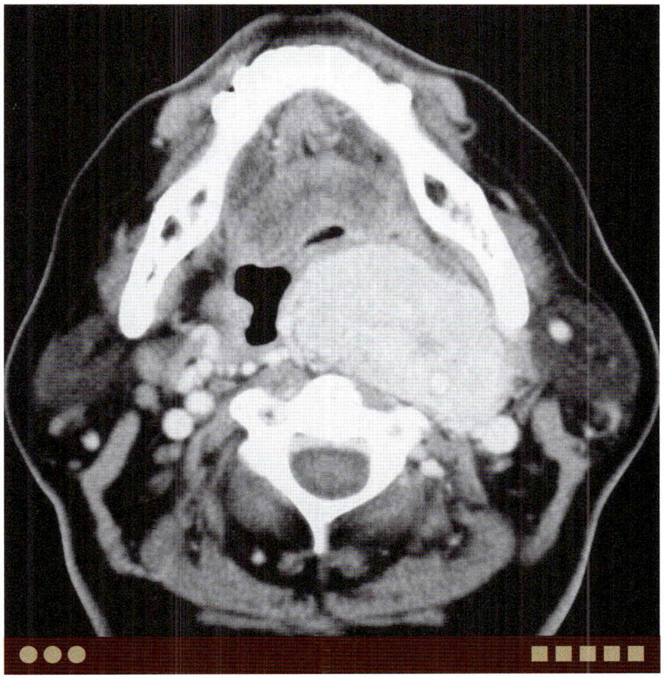

A. Glomus vagale. Axial CT demonstrates an avidly enhancing lesion encasing and displacing the left internal carotid artery anteromedially and internal jugular vein posterolaterally. The lesion also has mass effect on the airway.

COMMENTS

This is a 55-year-old woman with pulsatile left neck mass.

Paraganglioma is a benign tumor originated in the neural crest, and occurs anywhere between the skull base and aortic arch, along the carotid vessels. They are called differently based on locations; glomus jugulare at the skull base/jugular foramen, glomus vagale at the naso/oropharyngeal level, and carotid body tumor at the carotid bifurcation.

Paragangliomas are usually very hypervascular and demonstrate avid enhancement on CT. Vascularity is easily assessed by dynamic study. On MRI, characteristic "salt-and-pepper" appearance is seen corresponding to significantly increased vascularity on T2W images or postcontrast T1W images. Note due to prominent flow-voids the tumor may not demonstrate increased signal on postcontrast T1W images. Prior to surgical resection, embolization is often performed; however, catheter angiogram is not needed for diagnosis.

Glomus vagale tumors splay the internal jugular vein and internal carotid artery. In addition, this tumor often encases the internal carotid artery. It can be difficult to differentiate a large glomus vagale tumor from a glomus jugulare tumor. Typically glomus jugulare tumors arise from the jugular foramen and erode the bone prior to inferiorly extension to the neck. Glomus vagale tumors typically displace the internal jugular vein without erosion of the foramen. Schwannomas can also arise along the course of the carotid vessels, either from the lower cranial nerves (lateral to the carotid artery) or sympathetic trunk (medial to the carotid artery). However, they typically enhance less than paragangliomas on CT and should be easily differentiated. Further, "salt-and-pepper" appearance on MRI is not seen in schwannomas.

Similar to pheochromocytoma, paragangliomas can be bilateral, multiple, familial, and malignant. The entire neck should be evaluated for possible other lesions.

PEARLS

- **Paraganglioma occurs anywhere between the skull base and aortic arch in the neck, along the carotid vessels.**
- **Paraganglioma demonstrates avid enhancement on CT. Characteristic "salt-and-pepper" appearance is seen on T2W or postcontrast T1W MR images.**
- **Glomus vagale tumors splay the internal jugular vein and internal carotid artery, and encasement of the internal carotid artery can be seen.**
- **Paragangliomas can be bilateral, multiple, familial, and malignant.**

ADDITIONAL IMAGES (B-G)

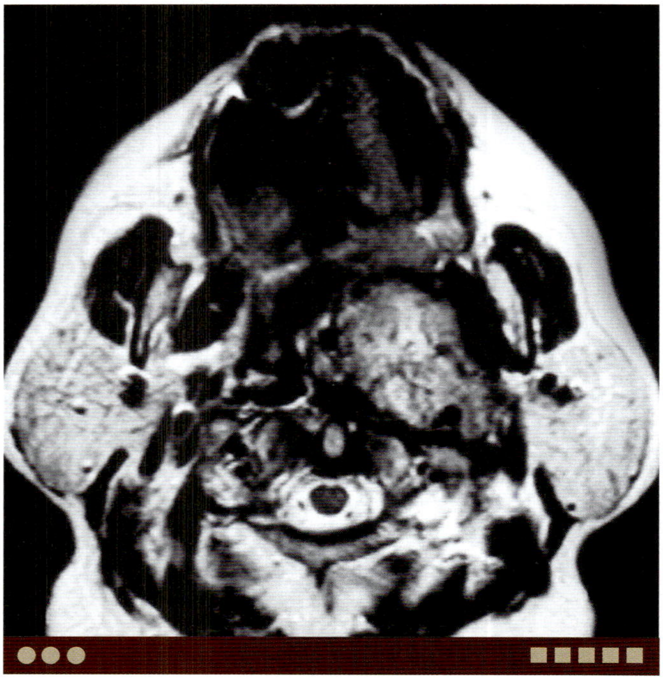

B. Glomus vagale, same patient as A. Axial T2W MR image demonstrates a hyperintense lesion with internal flow-voids, "salt-and-pepper" appearance.

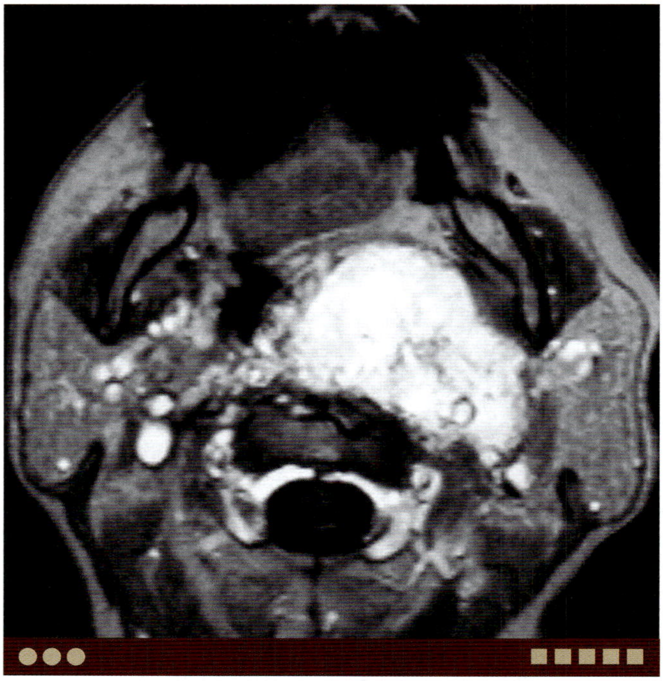

C. Glomus vagale, same patient as A. Axial dynamic contrast-enhanced T1W image (early phase) demonstrates avid enhancement of the lesion.

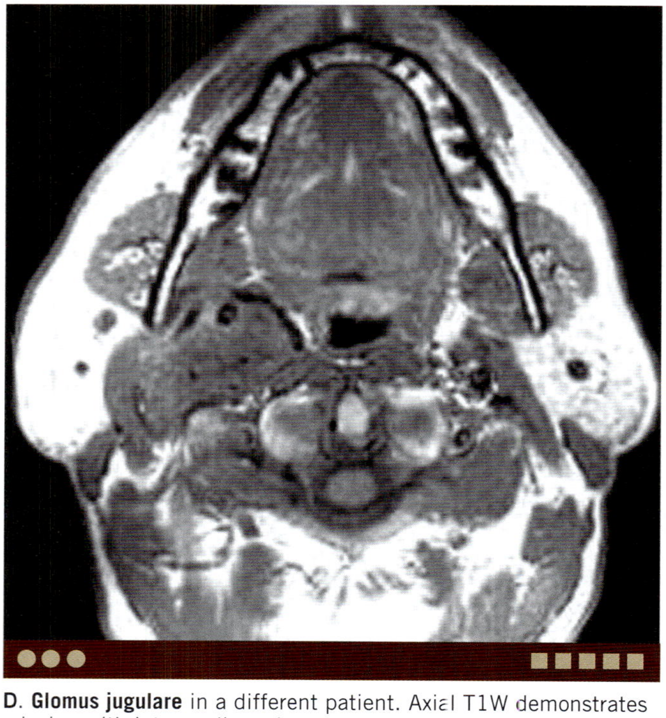

D. **Glomus jugulare** in a different patient. Axial T1W demonstrates a lesion with intermediate signal and internal flow-voids displacing the internal carotid artery and internal jugular vein anteriorly.

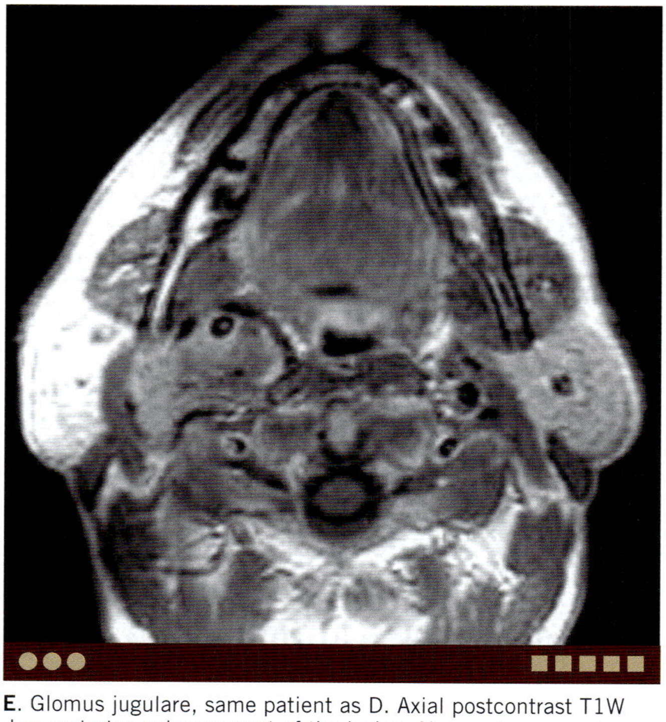

E. Glomus jugulare, same patient as D. Axial postcontrast T1W demonstrates enhancement of the lesion. Note enhancement on regular SE T1W may not be prominent.

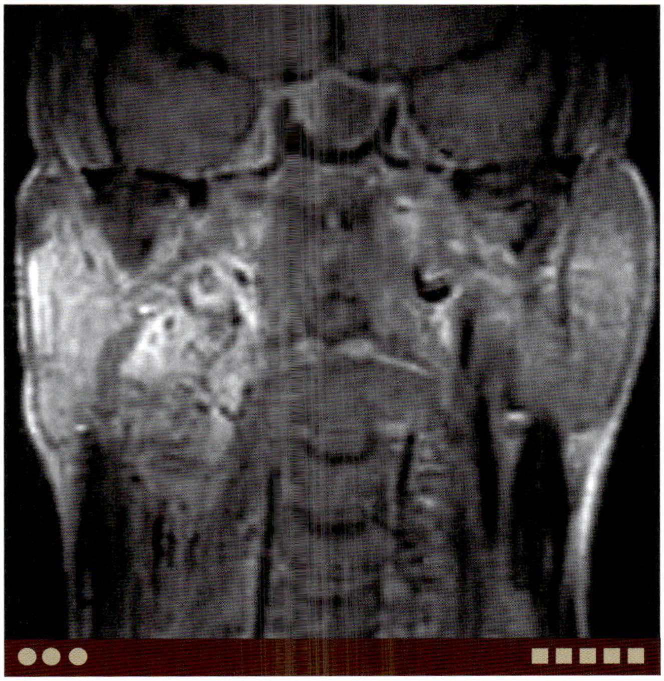

F. Glomus jugulare, same patient as D. Coronal postcontrast T1W demonstrates multiple flow-voids within the enhancing lesion.

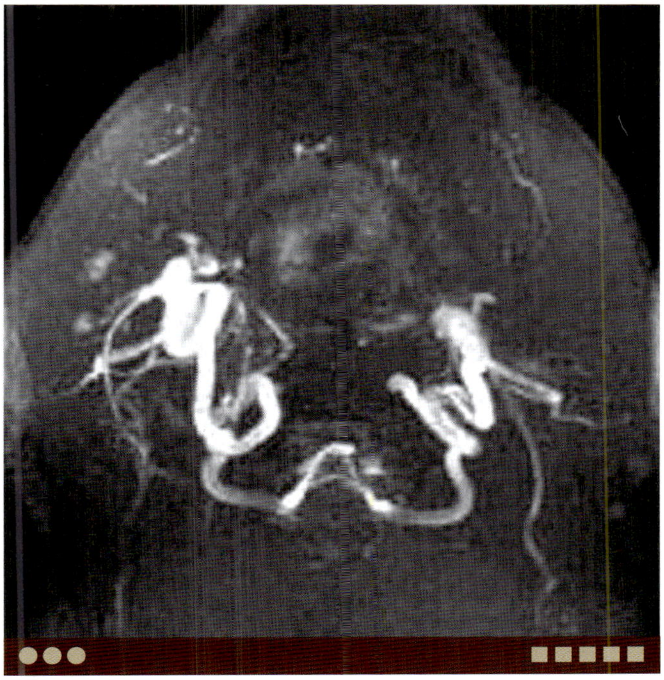

G. Glomus jugulare, same patient as D. Craniocaudal projection image of time-of-flight MRA MIP reconstruction demonstrates increased vascular supply to the lesion and anterior displacement of the right internal carotid artery. The tumor itself is hardly appreciated on time-of-flight MRA.

DIFFERENTIAL DIAGNOSIS IMAGES (H-J)

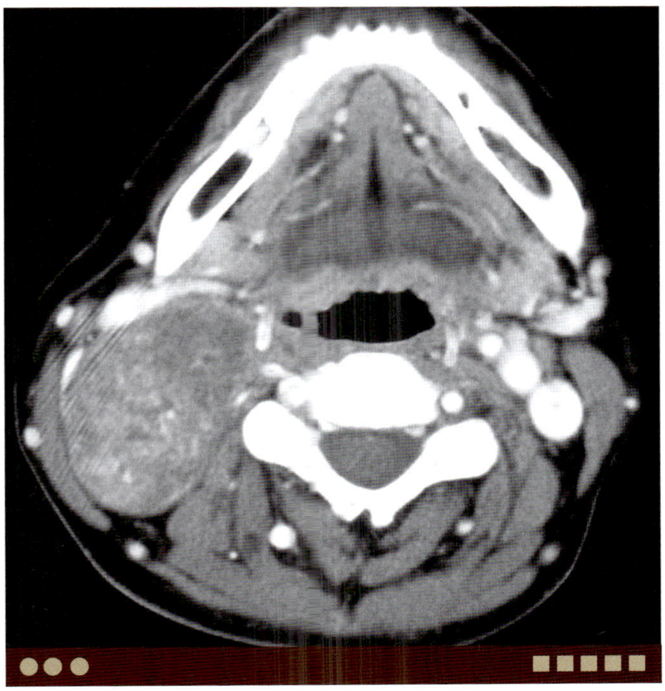

H. Schwannoma. Axial CT demonstrates a mildly enhancing tumor displacing the right carotid vessels without enactment.

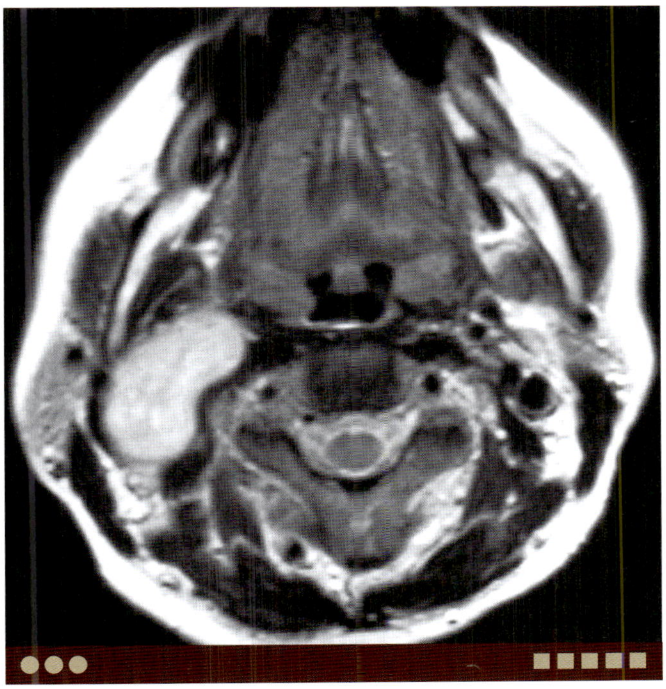

I. Schwannoma, same patient as H. Axial T2W MR image demonstrates a homogeneously hyperintense lesion without internal flow voids.

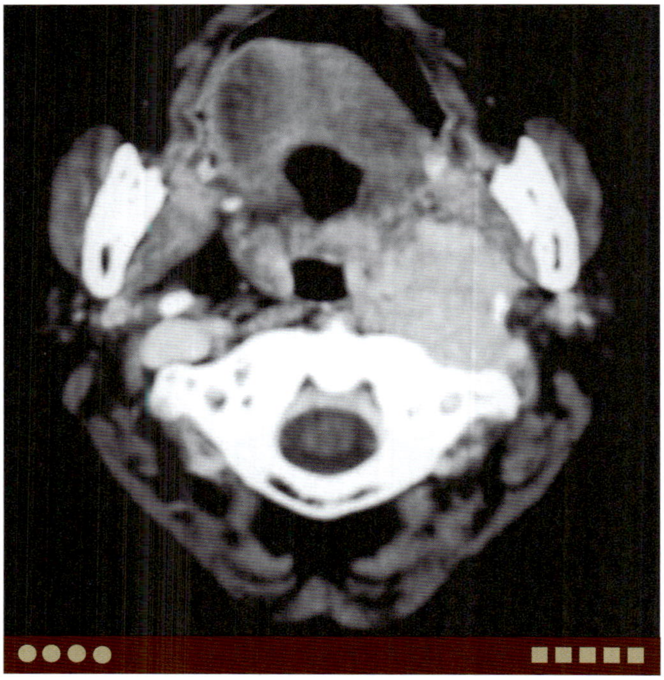

J. Metastasis from papillary thyroid carcinoma. Axial CT demonstrates a large, avidly enhancing metastatic left lateral retropharyngeal node.

Case 6–25 Calcific Tendinitis

Rohini Nadgir, Osamu Sakai

PRESENTATION

Gradual onset of neck pain and/or pain on swallowing following minor trauma.

FINDINGS

CT demonstrates prevertebral soft tissue thickening and edema with focal calcification at the level of C1 arch. MR images demonstrate edema within the retropharyngeal space and enlargement and edema within the longus colli muscles.

DIFFERENTIAL DIAGNOSIS

- Retropharyngeal abscess: This is usually due to infection through the pharynx or oral cavity. Infected fluid collection is seen in the retropharyngeal space with peripheral rim-enhancement on CT and MRI without calcification.
- Prevertebral abscess: This is infection and fluid collection in the prevertebral space typically occurring secondary to discitis/osteomyelitis at adjacent cervical levels. Epidural extension of inflammation can be seen. Prevertebral soft tissue calcification is not seen.

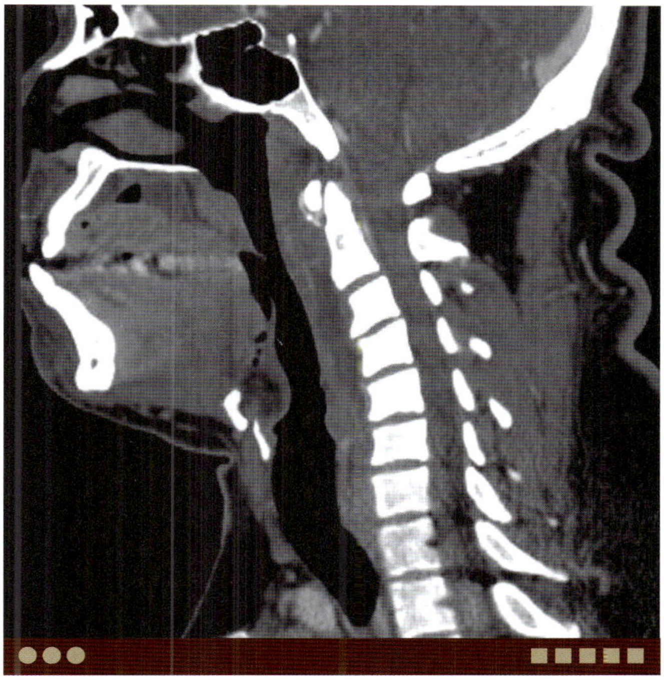

A. Calcific tendinitis. Sagittal contrast-enhanced CT demonstrates edema/fluid density without rim-enhancement in the retropharyngeal space. Note high density anterior to the anterior arch of the C1.

COMMENTS

Calcific tendinitis is a self-limited condition that can follow minor trauma (awkward neck positioning at time of awakening from sleep) presenting with gradual onset of neck pain and/or pain on swallowing. Associated low-grade fever and elevated white count may be present, which can raise clinical suspicion for retropharyngeal abscess, prompting additional imaging.

Although the precise pathophysiology is unknown, it is believed that calcium hydroxyapatite deposition within the longus colli muscle tendon results in an inflammatory foreign body reaction.

On imaging, calcific tendinitis can be distinguished from other differential considerations based on presence of classic calcium hydroxyapatite deposits just below the anterior arch of C1 level within the prevertebral muscles, best seen on CT, although these calcifications can be appreciable on cervical spine radiographs as well. These calcifications may resolve on follow-up imaging. On MRI, enlargement and edema of the longus colli muscles is seen with associated retropharyngeal space edema, typically extending to more inferior cervical levels. Peripheral rim-enhancement of the associated retropharyngeal fluid should not be seen. Marrow edema within C1 and C2 may be appreciable as well.

This condition is quite rare, but if diagnosed appropriately, more aggressive surgical management for the other clinically serious diagnostic considerations can be easily avoided. Treatment for calcific tendinitis, as opposed to the other diagnostic considerations, is supportive with analgesic medication and immobilization.

PEARLS

- **Calcific tendinitis is a self-limited condition that can follow minor trauma presenting with gradual onset of neck pain and pain on swallowing.**
- **Major diagnostic considerations include retropharyngeal versus prevertebral abscess.**
- **Calcific tendinitis can be distinguished from other differential considerations based on presence of classic dystrophic calcification within the prevertebral musculature best seen on CT.**
- **On MRI, edema within the retropharyngeal space and associated enlargement and edema within the longus colli muscles is seen.**

ADDITIONAL IMAGES (B-G)

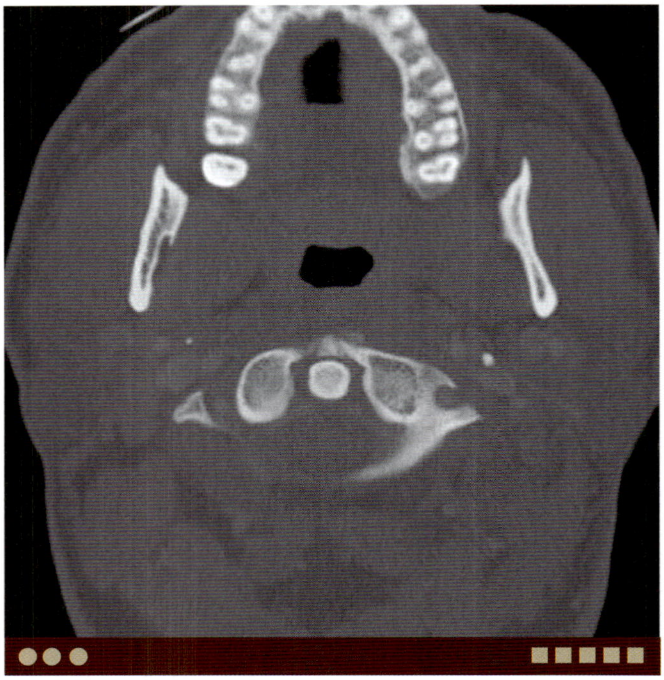

B. Calcific tendinitis, same patient as A. Axial bone window CT shows subtle calcification anterior to the anterior arch of the C1.

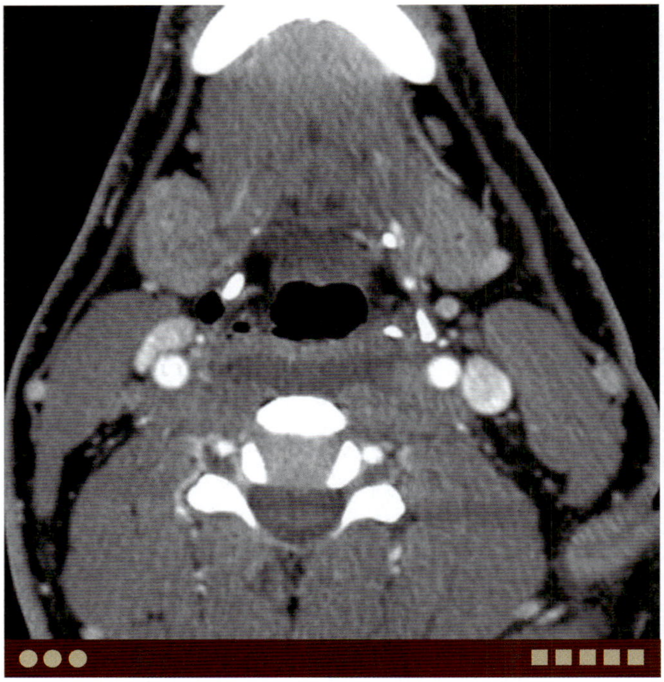

C. Calcific tendinitis, same patient as A. Axial postcontrast soft tissue window CT at C3 level shows edema/fluid density without rim-enhancement in the retropharyngeal space.

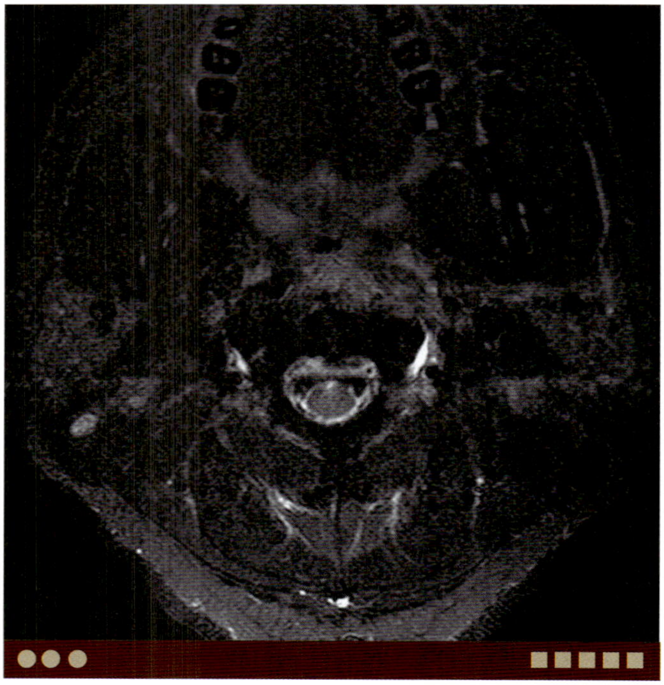

D. Calcific tendinitis, same patient as A. Axial fat-suppressed T2W image at C2 level shows increased signal and swelling of the longus colli muscles, left more than right.

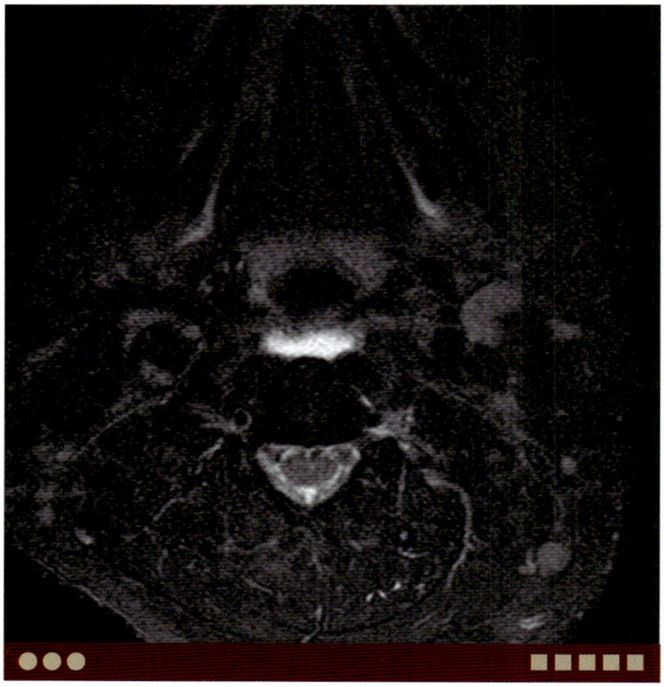

E. Calcific tendinitis, same patient as A. Axial fat-suppressed T2W image at C3 level shows retropharyngeal edema/fluid signal.

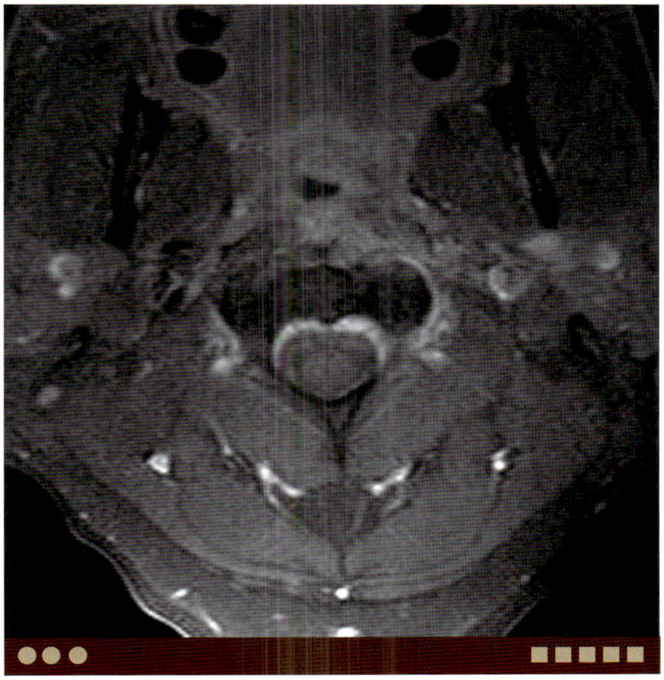

F. Calcific tendinitis, same patient as A. Axial postcontrast fat-suppressed T1W image at C2 level shows swelling and enhancement of the longus colli muscles, left more than right.

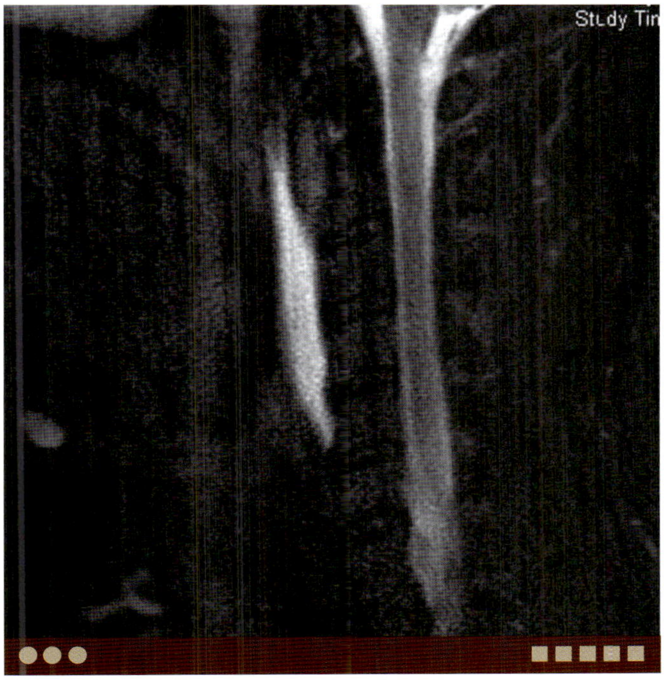

G. Calcific tendinitis, same patient as A. Sagittal fat-suppressed T2W image shows edema/fluid signal in the retropharyngeal space. There is no abnormal signal in the bone marrow or disc space to suggest discitis or osteomyelitis.

DIFFERENTIAL DIAGNOSIS IMAGES (H-J)

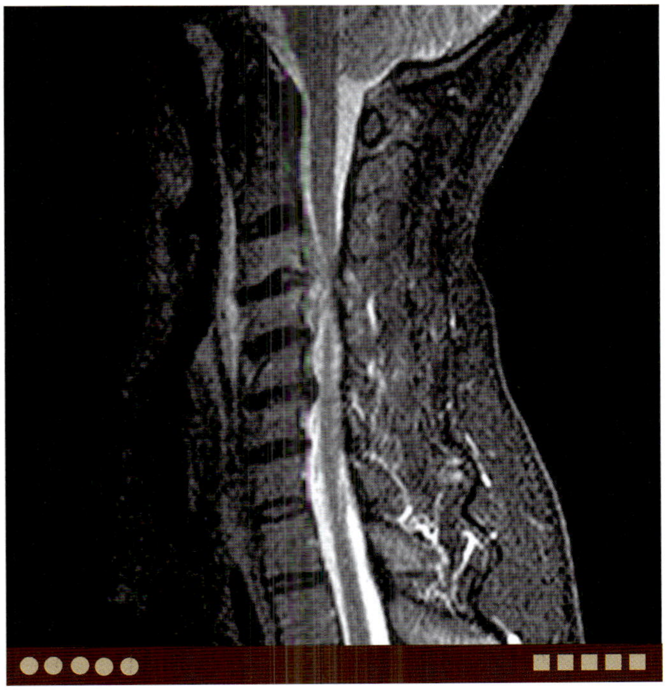

H. Discitis/osteomyelitis resulting in prevertebral and epidural abscess. Sagittal fat-suppressed T2W image shows increased signal in the bodies of C3 and C4 as well as the disc space. Note abnormal swelling and increased signal in the prevertebral space and anterior epidural space.

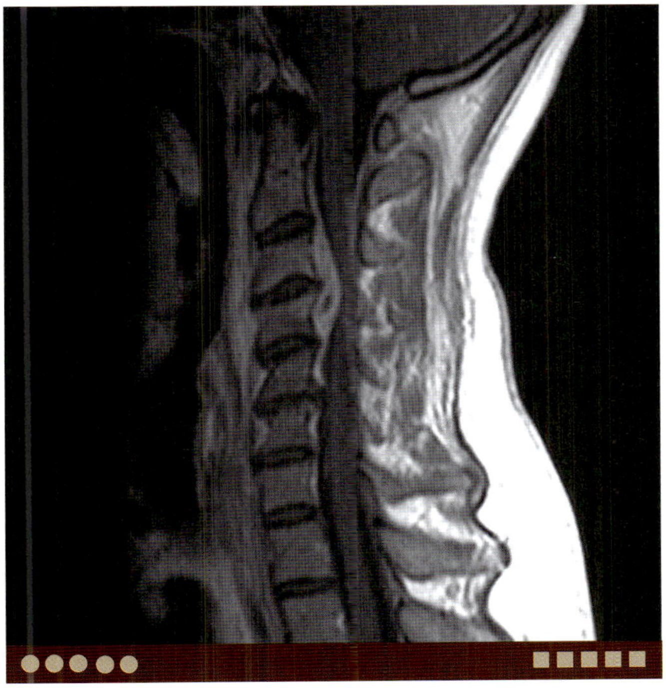

I. Discitis/osteomyelitis resulting in prevertebral and epidural abscess, same patient as H. Sagittal postcontrast T1W image shows abnormal enhancement in the prevertebral space and anterior epidural space with small nonenhancing areas consistent with abscess.

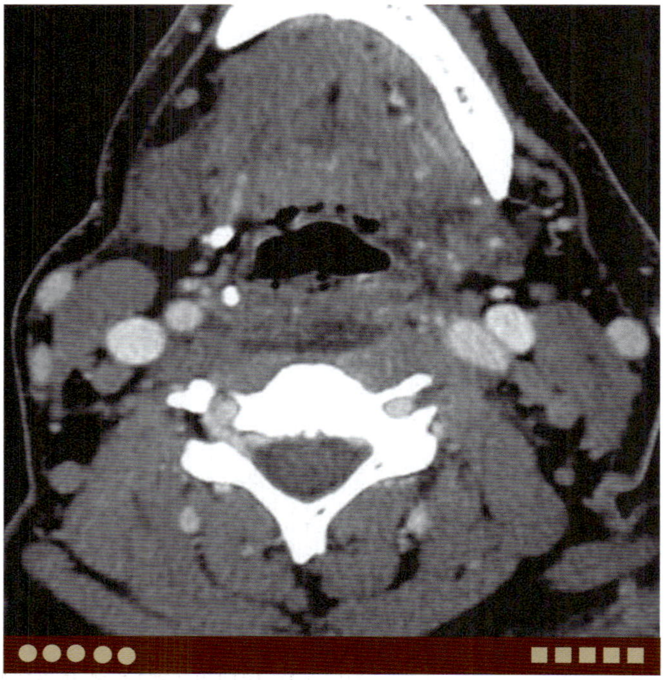

J. Retropharyngeal abscess. Axial postcontrast soft tissue window CT at C3 level shows fluid density with rim-enhancement in the retropharyngeal space.

Case 6–26 Relapsing Polychondritis

Hiroki Kato, Benjamin Ludwig, Osamu Sakai

PRESENTATION

Recurrent pain and swelling of the external ear.

FINDINGS

CT demonstrates increased attenuation and thickening of the auricles and tracheal walls.

DIFFERENTIAL DIAGNOSIS

- Tracheobronchopathia osteochondroplastica: A rare idiopathic disease characterized by formation of cartilaginous, osseous or mixed nodules in the tracheal and bronchial submucosa. CT demonstrates irregular thickening of the tracheal wall with small nodules and calcifications/ossification, which classically spares the posterior tracheal wall.
- Wegener's granulomatosis: A disease of unknown etiology characterized by necrotizing granulomatous vasculitis that can involve the upper and lower airways, lungs and kidneys. Tracheal involvement is characterized by concentric tracheal wall thickening, luminal narrowing, and calcifications associated with tracheal rings.
- Amyloidosis: A systemic disease characterized by progressive deposition of amyloid in the extracellular tissues. The larynx, pharynx and trachea are often involved. CT demonstrates nodular wall thickening and luminal narrowing of the airway, commonly with calcification.

COMMENTS

This is a 40-year-old woman with pain, redness, swelling, and tenderness involving both ears.

Relapsing polychondritis is a systemic, widespread, and destructive inflammatory disorder involving all types of cartilaginous structures, such as elastic cartilages of the ears and nose, hyaline cartilage of peripheral joints and tracheobronchial tree, and fibrocartilage. Further, relapsing polychondritis also involves other proteoglycan-rich structures, such as the eye, heart, blood vessels, and inner ear.

Clinically, the disease is characterized by recurrent episodes of painful inflammation, such as auricular chondritis, polyarthritis, nasal chondritis, ocular inflammation, and respiratory tract chondritis. Attacks tend to vary in severity, and last from days to weeks before resolving spontaneously.

The diagnosis of relapsing polychondrities is based on clinical symptoms, and about 25% of cases have coexistent diseases, usually autoimmune in nature. For example, systemic vasculitis (polyarteritis nodosa, Takayasu arteritis, giant cell arteritis, Wegener's granulomatosis), rheumatoid arthritis, Sjögren's syndrome, systemic lupus erythematosus, progressive systemic sclerosis, Reiter syndrome, Behcet disease, thyroid disease, ulcerative colitis, and paraneoplastic syndrome have been reported with relapsing polychondritis.

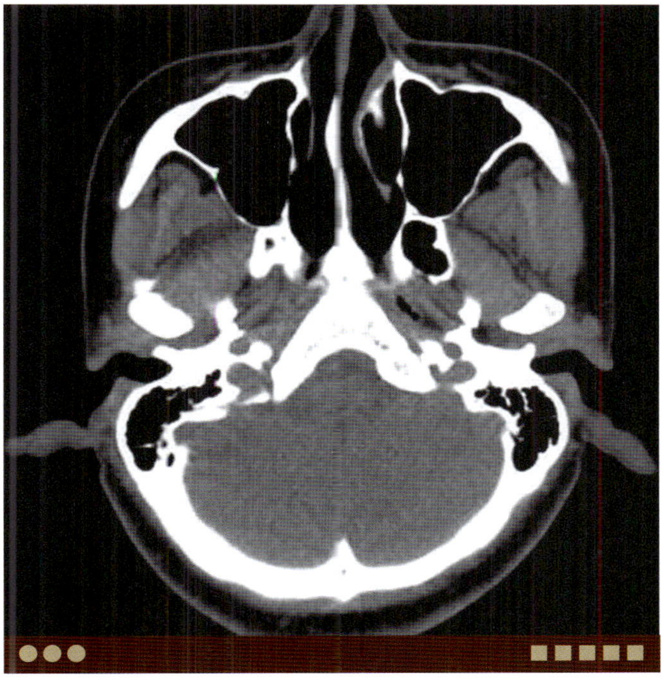

A. Relapsing polychondritis. Axial unenhanced CT demonstrates diffuse thickening of both auricles.

Imaging findings include increased attenuation and thickening of the auricles (a specific finding), as well as calcifications of the auricles, nasal cartilage collapse, and subglottic and tracheobronchial luminal narrowing, often with calcification. Increased attenuation and smooth thickening of tracheal and bronchial walls are the most common features of intrathoracic disease. As the condition affects hyaline cartilage in the trachea, the posterior tracheal wall is spared, similar to tracheobronchiopathia osteochondroblastica. The nature of airway wall thickening (smooth vs nodular) aids in differentiating the two entities.

PEARLS

- **Relapsing polychondritis is an uncommon, systemic disorder, which involves all types of cartilage, and most commonly affects the ears, nose, joints, and respiratory tract.**
- **The diagnosis of relapsing polychondritis is made based on clinical findings.**
- **Increased attenuation and smooth thickening of the auricles and the airway walls are common CT findings of relapsing polychondritis. With airway involvement, the posterior tracheal wall is spared.**

ADDITIONAL IMAGES (B-C)

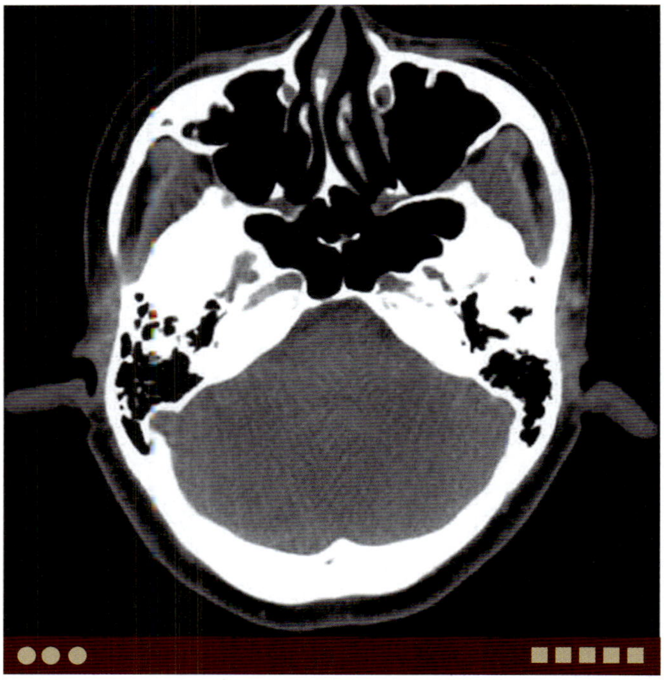

B. Relapsing polychondritis, same patient as A. Axial unenhanced CT demonstrates diffuse thickening of both auricles (higher level than A).

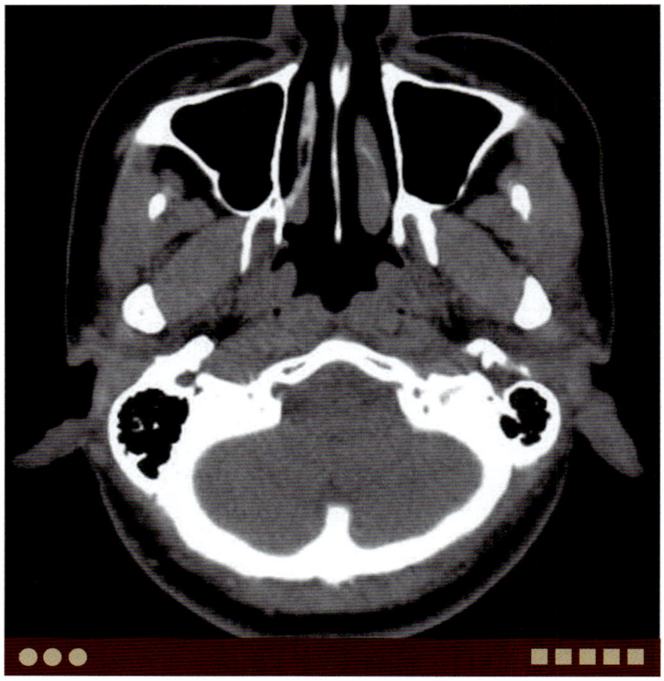

C. Relapsing polychondritis, same patient as A. Axial unenhanced CT demonstrates diffuse thickening of both auricles (lower level than A).

DIFFERENTIAL DIAGNOSIS IMAGES (D-I)

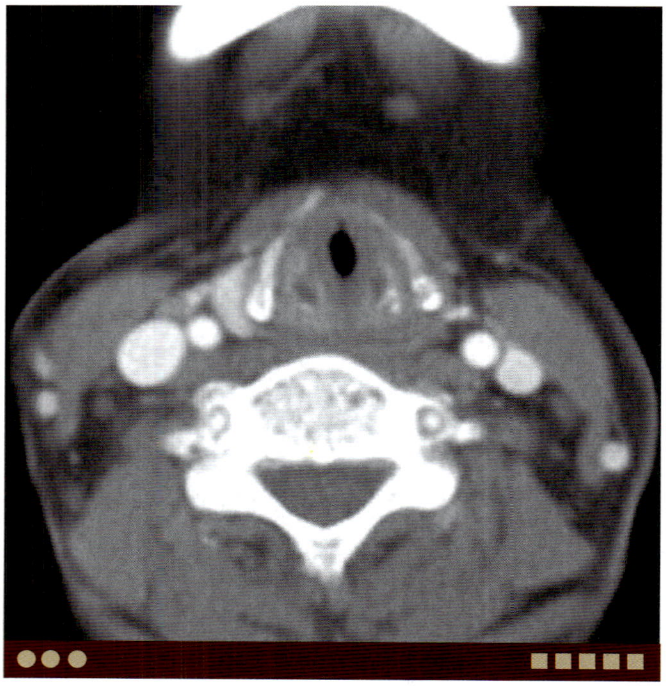

D. Amyloidosis. Axial contrast-enhanced CT demonstrates circumferential wall thickening of the subglottic larynx.

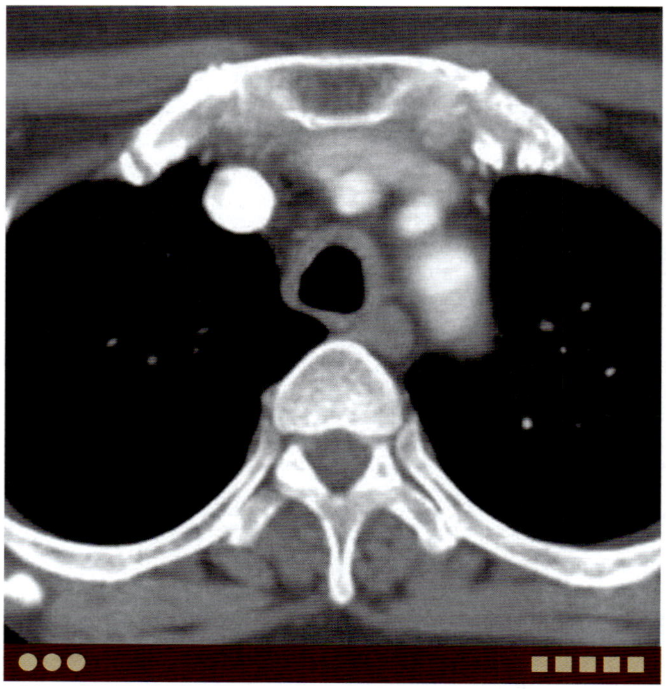

E. Amyloidosis, same patient as D. Axial contrast-enhanced CT demonstrates circumferential wall thickening of the trachea.

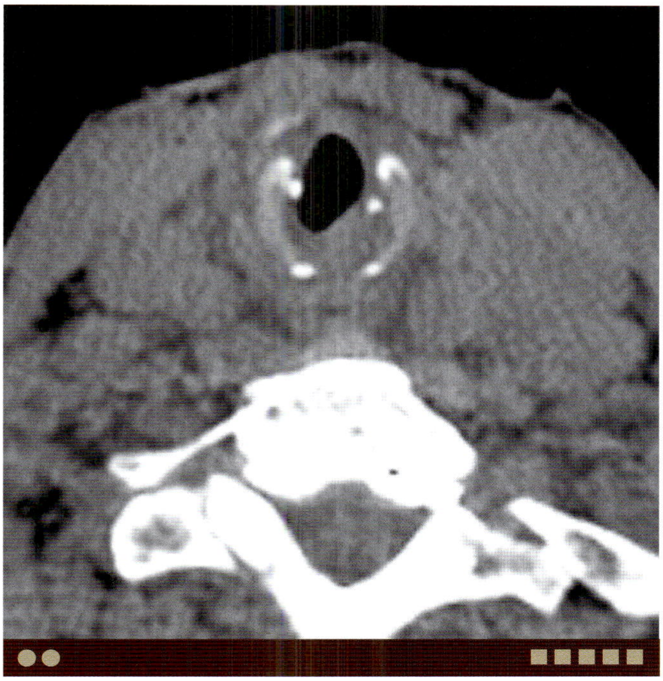

F. **Amyloidosis** in a different patient. Axial CT demonstrates slightly irregular concentric narrowing of the subglottic larynx. Note focal calcifications.

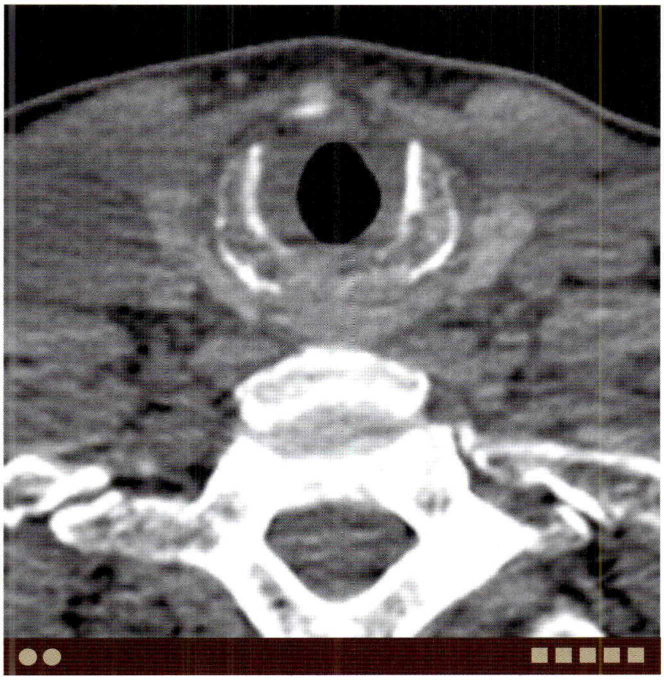

G. **Wegener's granulomatosis**. Axial CT demonstrates concentric soft tissue thickening in the subglottic larynx.

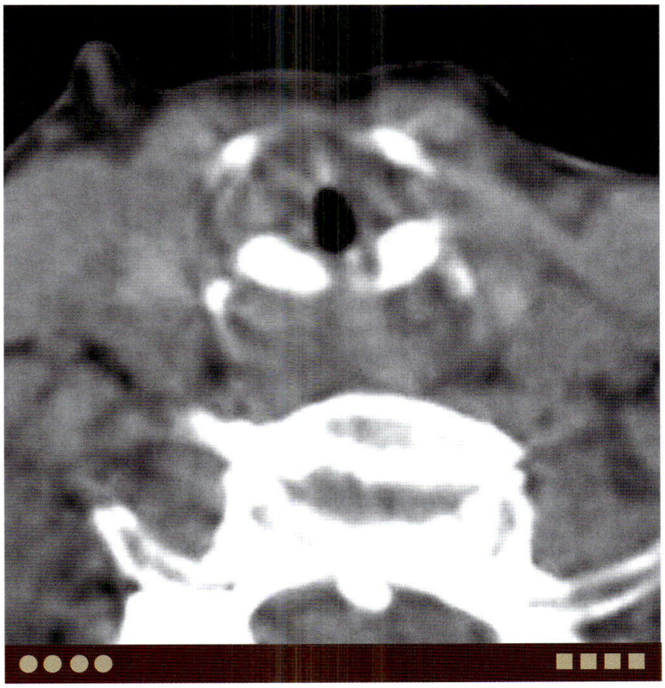

H. **Tracheobronchomalacia**. Axial CT demonstrates narrowing of the subglottic larynx.

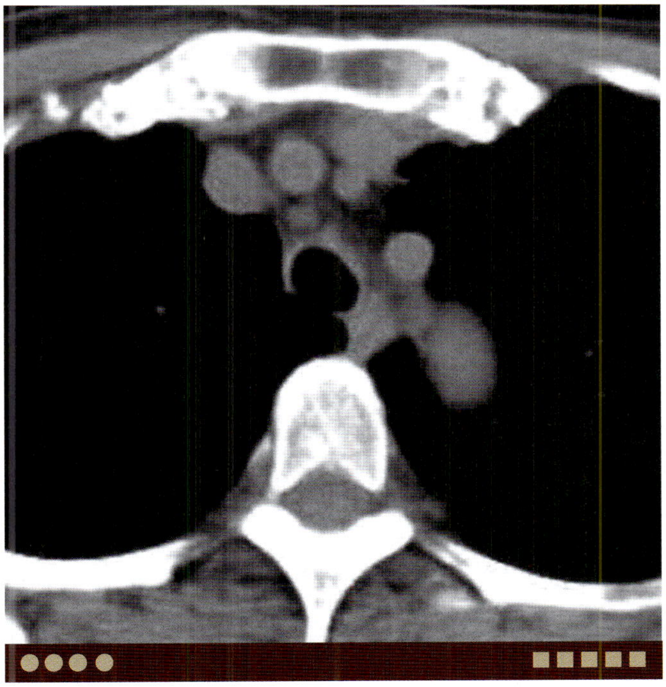

I. Tracheobronchomalacia, same patient as H. Axial CT demonstrates wall thickening of the cartilaginous segment of the trachea.

Case 6–27 Schwannoma at the Carotid Bifurcation

Osamu Sakai, Benjamin Ludwig, Susmitha Reddy

PRESENTATION

Non-pulsatile neck mass.

FINDINGS

CT demonstrates a mildly enhancing mass displacing and splaying the carotid bifurcation.

DIFFERENTIAL DIAGNOSIS

- Neurofibroma: A tumor arising from the nerve sheath, which is often seen in patients with neurofibromatosis type I, although most neurofibromas are sporadic (90%). They are often difficult to differentiate from schwannomas on imaging alone.
- Paraganglioma: This occurs in similar locations, but is a highly vascular tumor, which demonstrates marked enhancement. The "salt-and-pepper" appearance on MRI is characteristic.
- Castleman disease: This entity is a rare benign nodal lymphoproliferative disease. Enlarged nodes demonstrate marked, homogeneous enhancement.
- Nodal metastasis: Metastases are usually multiple and may be hypervascular. They are usually enlarged, with loss of normal nodal morphology, and heterogeneous in density or signal.

COMMENTS

This is a 41-year-old woman with non-pulsatile right neck mass.

Schwannomas are benign tumors arising from the Schwann cell, often seen in the cranial nerves (particularly sensory nerves), as well as the sympathetic trunk. They are usually painless masses which gradually increase in size; however, pain and cranial nerve impairment is not uncommon.

On CT, schwannomas are typically spindle or ovoid-shaped, well-demarcated masses of soft tissue density. Schwannomas associated with the vagus nerve displace the internal or common carotid artery anteromedially, while those associated with the sympathetic trunk displace the carotid artery anterolaterally. Schwannomas can arise near the carotid bifurcation and may demonstrate similar mass effect upon the vessels as carotid body tumors, however, vascular encasement is rare. Also, the degree of enhancement is significantly less in schwannomas compared to paragangliomas. Bone erosion/remodeling are commonly seen with paraspinal or skull base lesions.

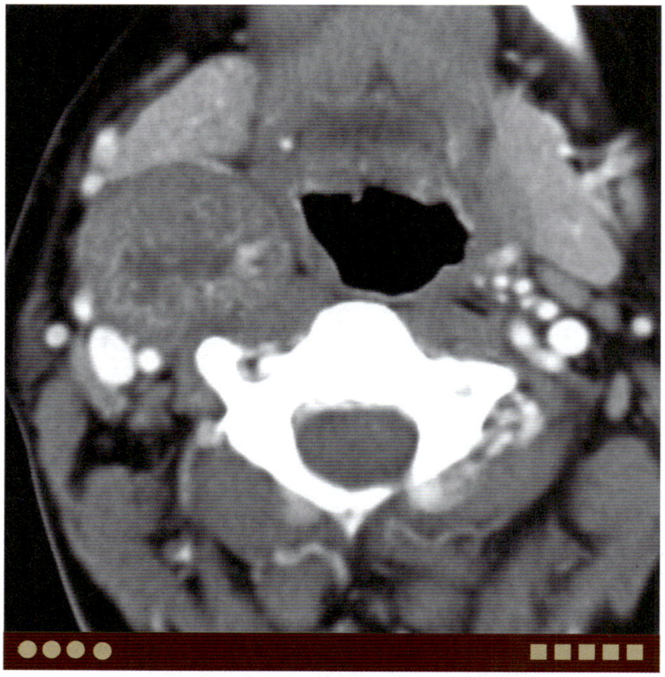

A. Schwannoma at the carotid bifurcation. Axial contrast-enhanced CT demonstrates a round, mildly enhancing mass with central cystic degeneration, anteromedial to the right carotid bifurcation.

On MRI, schwannomas demonstrate low signal on T1W images and intermediate signal on T2W images. Cystic degeneration is common as lesions increase in size. Fatty or hemorrhagic components may also be seen. Postcontrast images usually demonstrate relatively homogeneous enhancement without flow-voids.

PEARLS

- **Schwannomas are benign tumors arising from the Schwann cell, and are often seen in the cranial nerves (particularly sensory nerves), and the sympathetic trunk.**
- **Schwannomas are typically spindle or ovoid-shaped, well-demarcated masses of soft tissue density.**
- **Schwannomas demonstrate low signal on T1W and intermediate signal on T2W images, and relatively homogeneous enhancement. But cystic degeneration is also common.**
- **Schwannomas near the carotid bifurcation may splay the carotid bifurcation and mimic carotid body tumors.**

ADDITIONAL IMAGES (B-G)

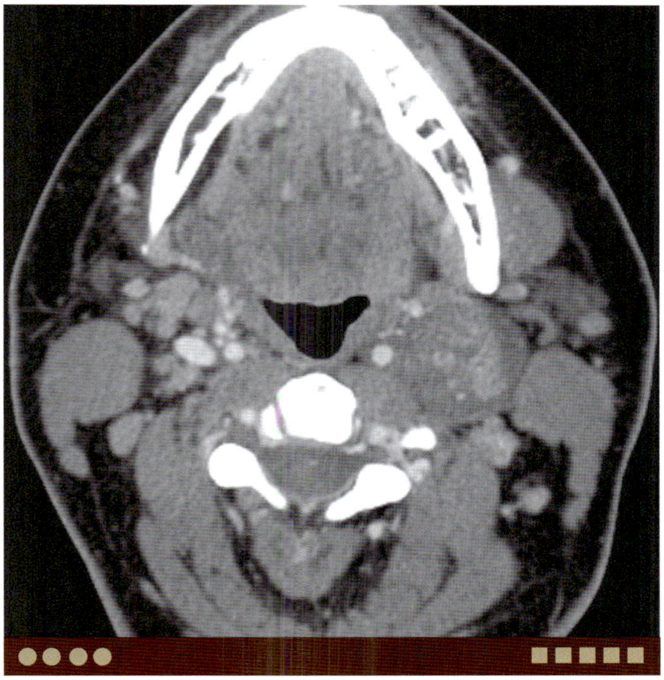

B. **Schwannoma** in a different patient. Axial contrast-enhanced CT demonstrates a round, heterogeneously enhancing mass, lateral to the left carotid bifurcation, likely arising from a lower cranial nerve.

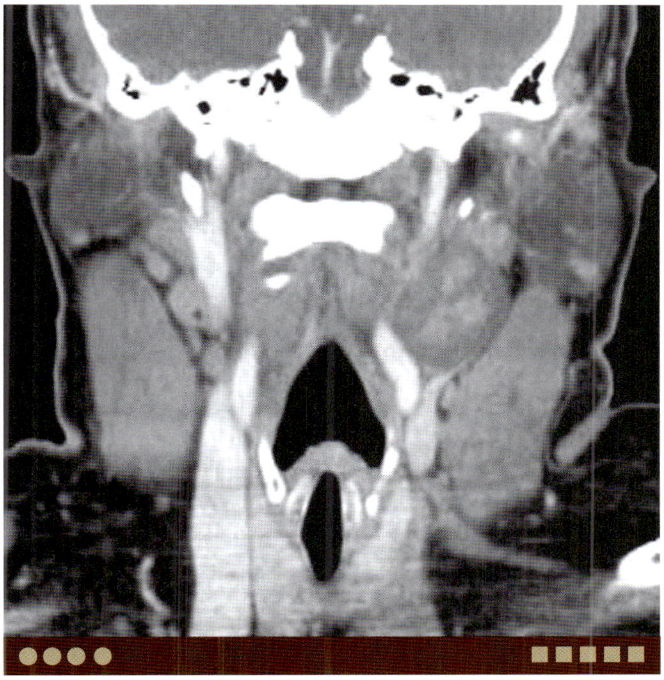

C. Schwannoma, same patient as B. Coronal contrast-enhanced CT demonstrates a round mass with enhancing foci, lateral to the left internal carotid artery.

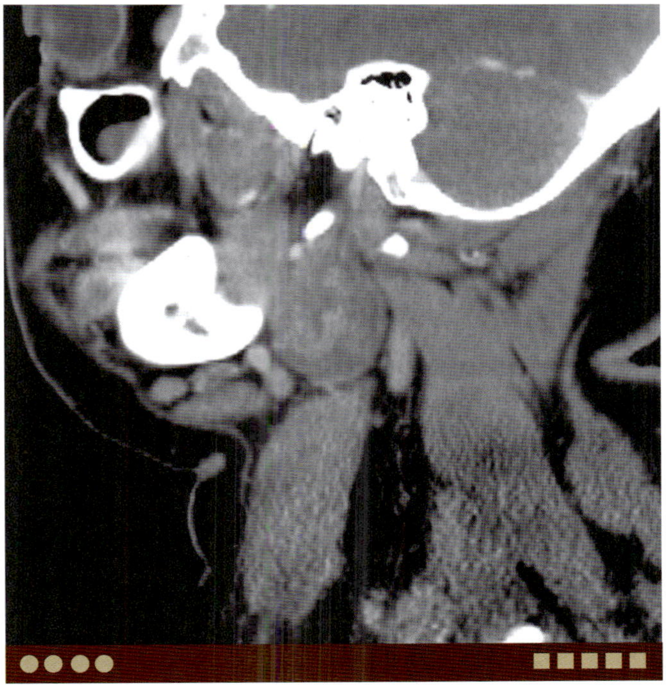

D. Schwannoma, same patient as B. Sagittal contrast-enhanced CT demonstrates a round mass with enhancing foci at the mandibular angle.

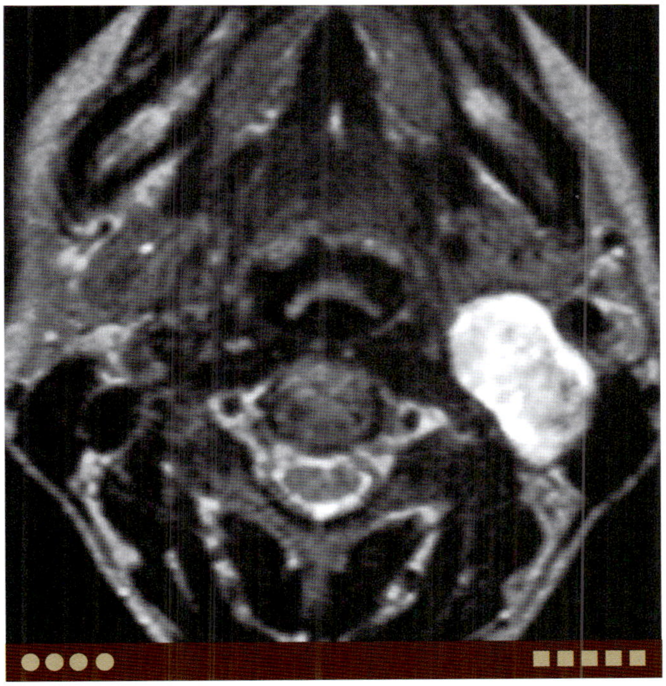

E. **Schwannoma** in a different patient. Axial T2W image demonstrates an ovoid-shaped, heterogeneously high-signal mass, medial to the left carotid bifurcation, likely arising from the sympathetic trunk.

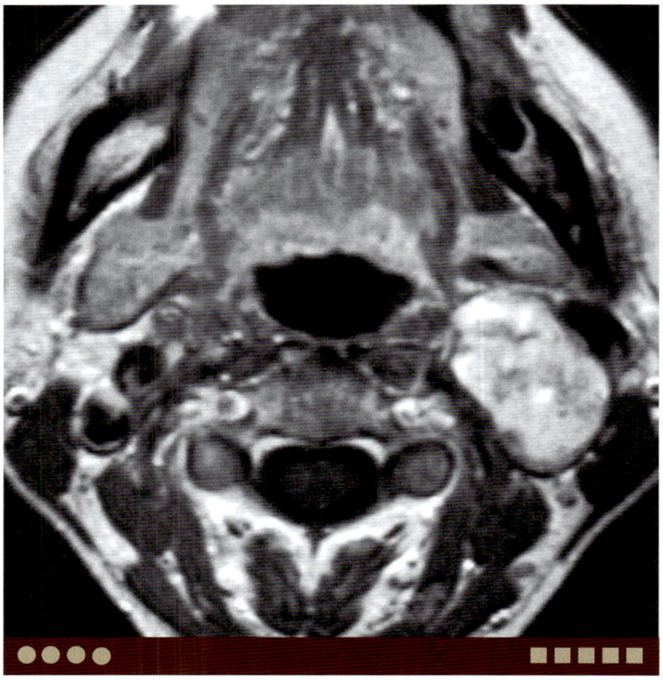

F. Schwannoma, same patient as E. Axial postcontrast T1W image demonstrates slightly heterogeneous enhancement of the lesion.

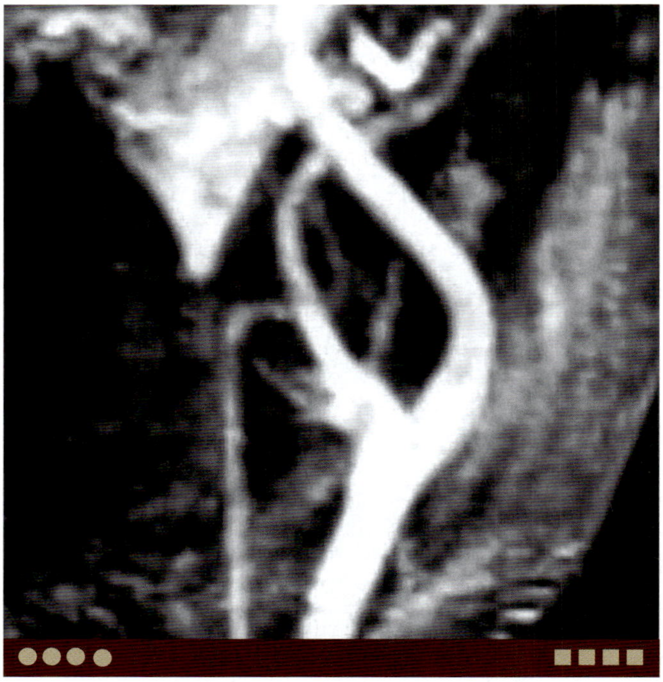

G. Schwannoma, same patient as E. Three-dimensional time-of-flight MRA MIP image shows splaying of the carotid bifurcation.

DIFFERENTIAL DIAGNOSIS IMAGES (H-J)

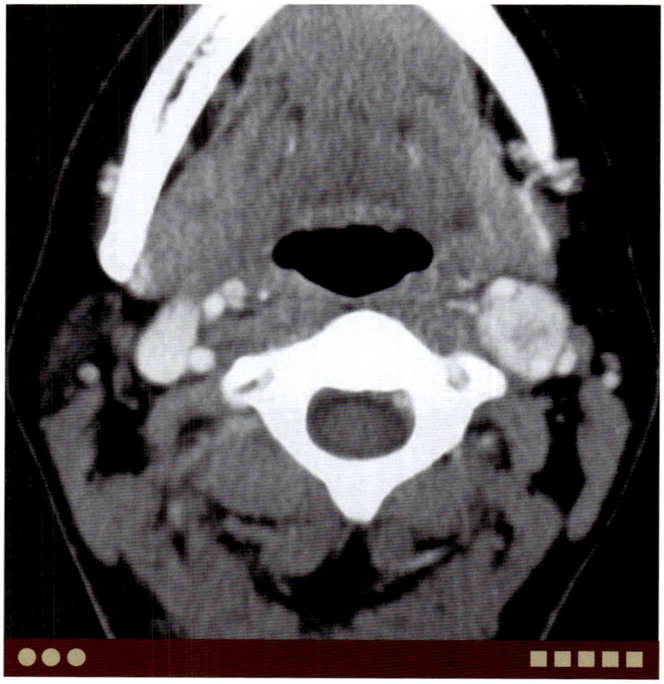

H. **Carotid body tumor**. Axial postcontrast CT demonstrates an avidly enhancing mass splaying the external and internal carotid arteries at the left carotid bifurcation.

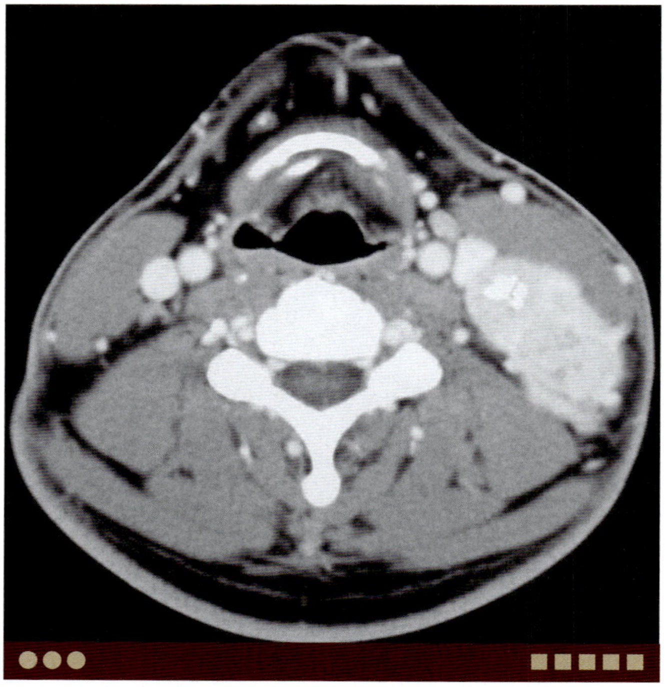

I. **Castleman disease**. Axial contrast-enhanced CT demonstrates an avidly enhancing lesion posterolateral to the left carotid vessels.

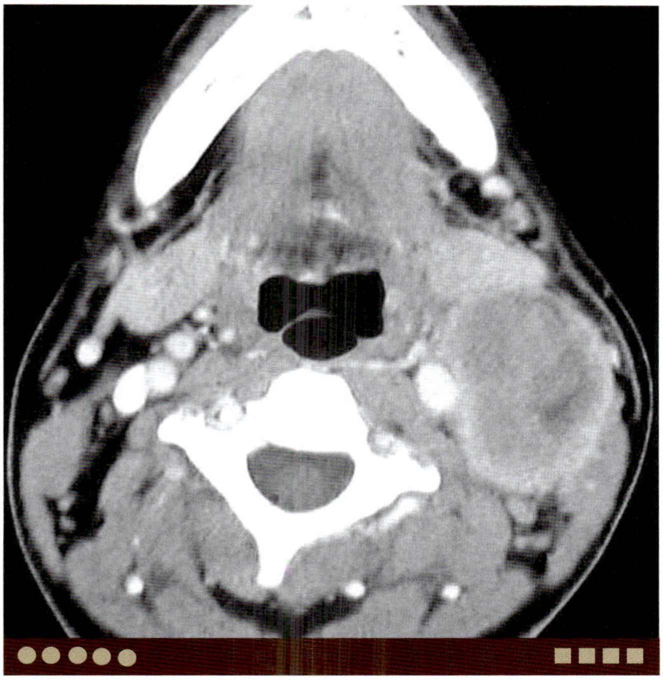

J. Metastatic node. Axial postcontrast CT demonstrates a heterogeneously enhancing lesion displacing the left carotid bifurcation medially.

Case 6–28 Kimura Disease

Akifumi Fujita, Benjamin Ludwig, Osamu Sakai

PRESENTATION

Unilateral cheek swelling with lymphadenopathy.

FINDINGS

CT and MRI demonstrate enhancing, infiltrative lesions within the subcutaneous tissues.

DIFFERENTIAL DIAGNOSIS

- Infection/inflammation: Infectious or inflammatory lesions in the subcutaneous soft tissue, such as cellulitis and phlegmon, may demonstrate an infiltrative appearance with associated cervical lymphadenopathy.
- Lymphoproliferative disorders and lymphoma: Lymphoproliferative disorders and lymphoma may occur in the subcutaneous soft tissue and salivary glands, and demonstrate an infiltrative appearance.
- Sarcoidosis: Sarcoidosis involves skin and other soft tissues. Orbital parotid, and nodal lesions are commonly seen in the head and neck.

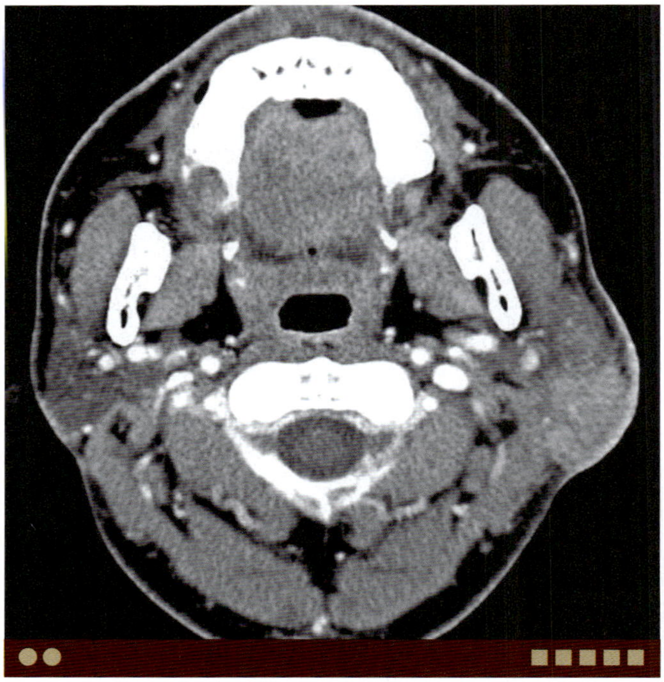

A. Kimura disease. Axial postcontrast CT demonstrates enlarged left parotid gland with an ill-defined enhancing mass infiltrating into the adjacent subcutaneous soft tissue.

COMMENTS

This is a 40-year-old man with left parotid and chin swelling.

Kimura disease is a benign chronic inflammatory disorder of unknown etiology which occurs most commonly in the head and neck. The disease is characterized by eosinophilic infiltration of lymphoid follicles, with associated peripheral eosinophilia, and elevated IgE. Kimura disease is more commonly seen in Japan and other Asian countries and affects mostly males in the second and third decades of life.

Kimura disease often occurs in the soft tissue near the salivary glands, most commonly in the parotid and submandibular regions. Nodal and salivary gland involvement is also common. Patients typically present with swelling, subcutaneous soft tissue masses, and asymmetric lymphadenopathy in the head and neck. These lesions are often painless and slowly enlarge over years.

CT and MR imaging findings of biopsy-proven Kimura disease have varied significantly. Described CT findings include subcutaneous lesions, enlarged nodes, and focal or infiltrative salivary gland lesions, all of which enhance after contrast administration. On MRI, lesions are hypointense on T1W and variably hyperintense on T2W images relative to salivary glands. Sonographic features include round, hypoechoic nodes with increased hilar vascularity within the submental, submandibular, and upper cervical nodal stations.

Given the diverse imaging features, Kimura disease should be considered when cervical lymphadenopathy and enhancing soft tissue or salivary gland lesions are encountered, particularly in young Asian males.

Currently, biopsy is used for diagnosis, in conjunction with peripheral eosinophilia and elevated IgE.

PEARLS

- **Kimura disease is a rare, idiopathic disease characterized by infiltrative soft tissue lesions, most common in the head and neck. Nodal and salivary gland involvement is also common.**
- **The disease is commonly seen in Japan and other Asian countries, most often in males in the second and third decades of life.**
- **CT, MRI, and ultrasound findings of Kimura disease vary widely. The diagnosis should be considered when one encounters subcutaneous lesions, lymphadenopathy, and salivary gland abnormalities in a young patient of Asian descent.**

ADDITIONAL IMAGES (B-G)

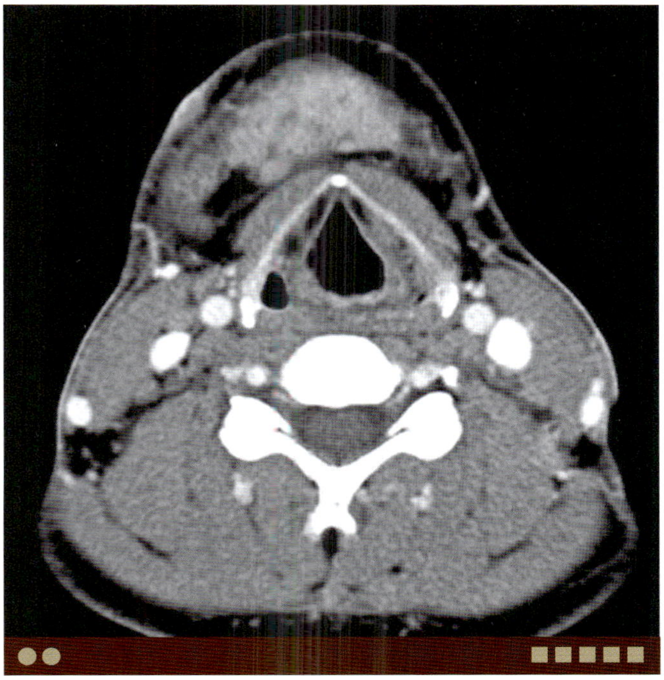

B. Kimura disease, same patient as A. Axial postcontrast CT demonstrates an ill-defined submental soft tissue mass with avid enhancement.

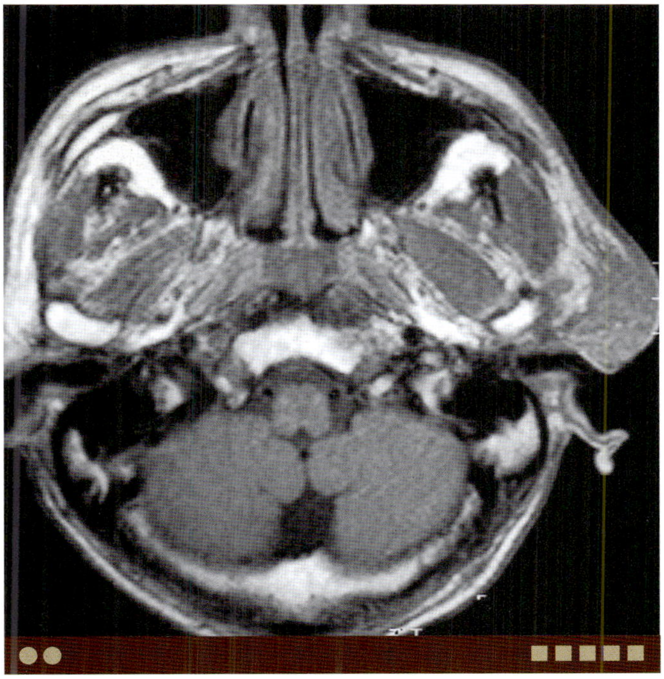

C. **Kimura disease** in a different patient. Axial T1W image demonstrates an ill-defined low-signal lesion in the subcutaneous soft tissue of the left parotid region.

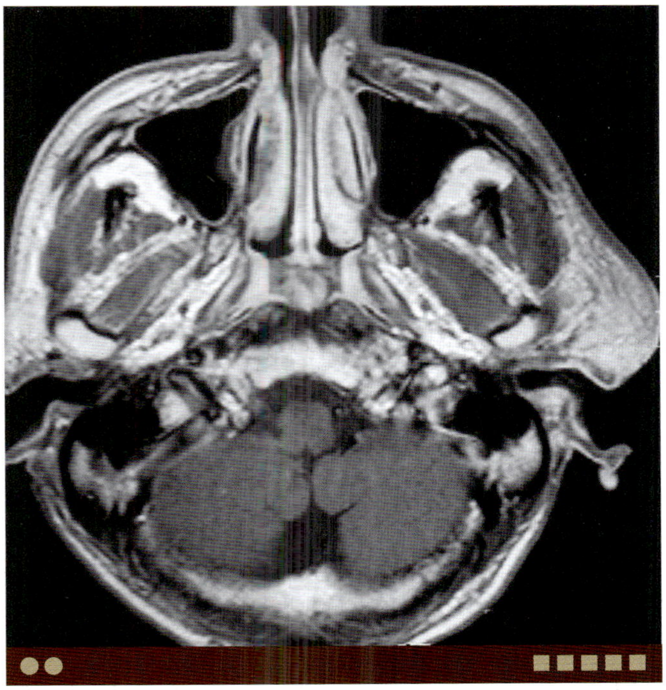

D. Kimura disease, same patient as C. Axial postcontrast T1W image demonstrates avid enhancement of the lesion.

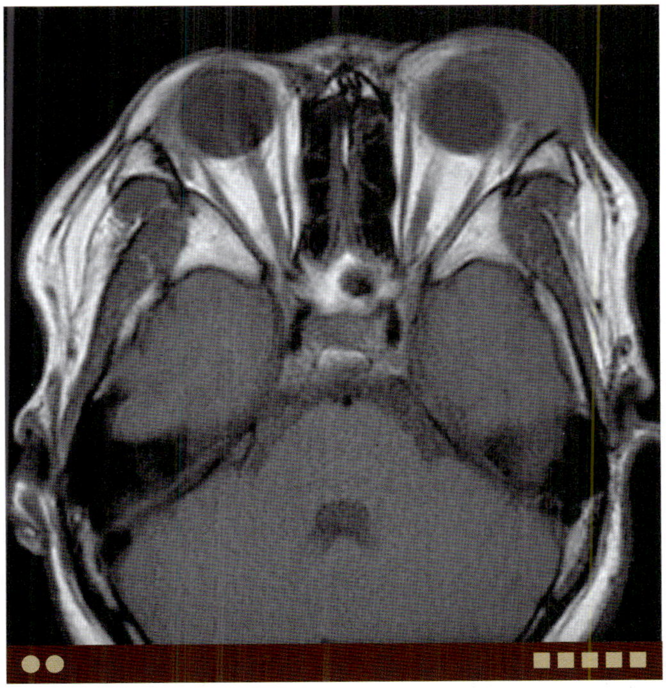

E. **Kimura disease** in a different patient. Axial T1W image demonstrates an ill-defined low-signal lesion in the left upper eyelid.

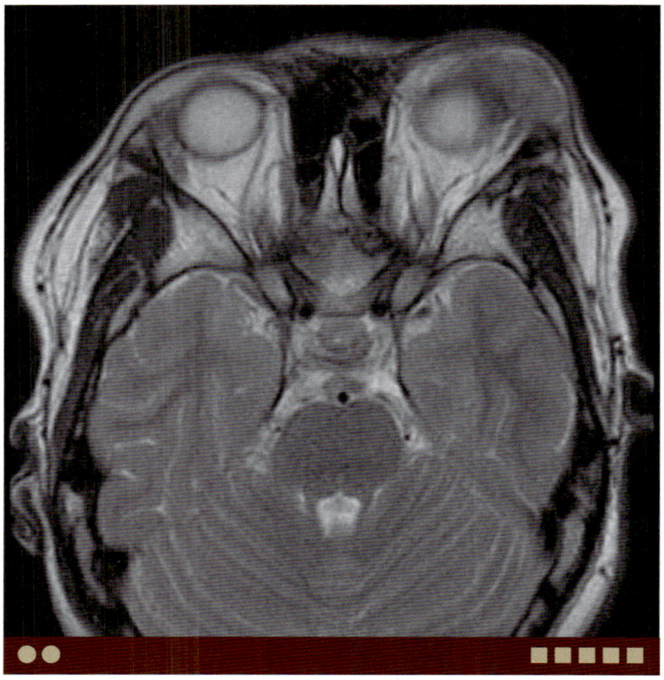

F. Kimura disease, same patient as E. Axial T2W image demonstrates intermediate-to-low signal of the les on.

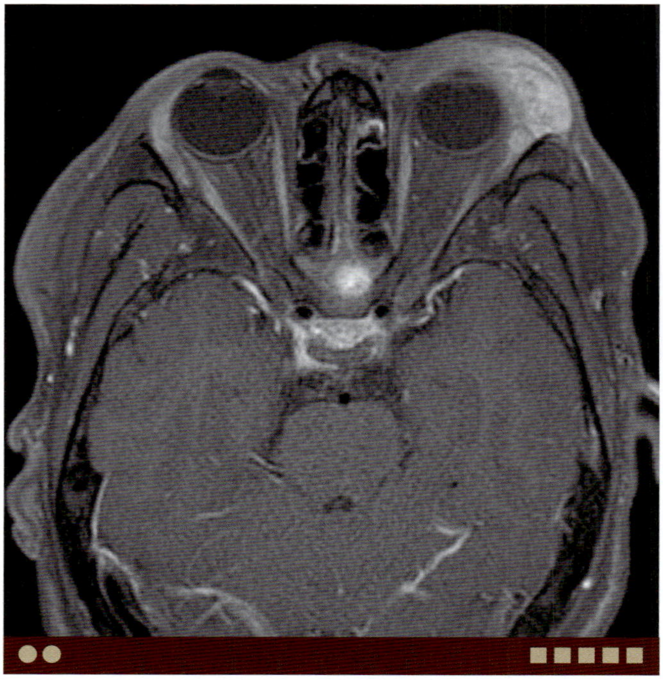

G. Kimura disease, same patient as E. Axial postcontrast fat-suppressed T1W image demonstrates avid enhancement of the lesion.

DIFFERENTIAL DIAGNOSIS IMAGES (H-J)

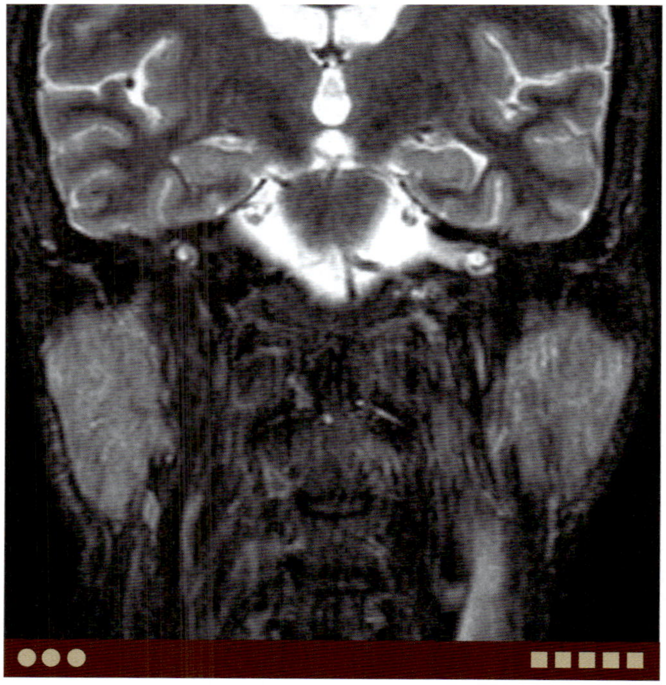

H. **Sarcoidosis**. Coronal STIR image demonstrates swelling of bilateral parotid glands with diffusely increased signal.

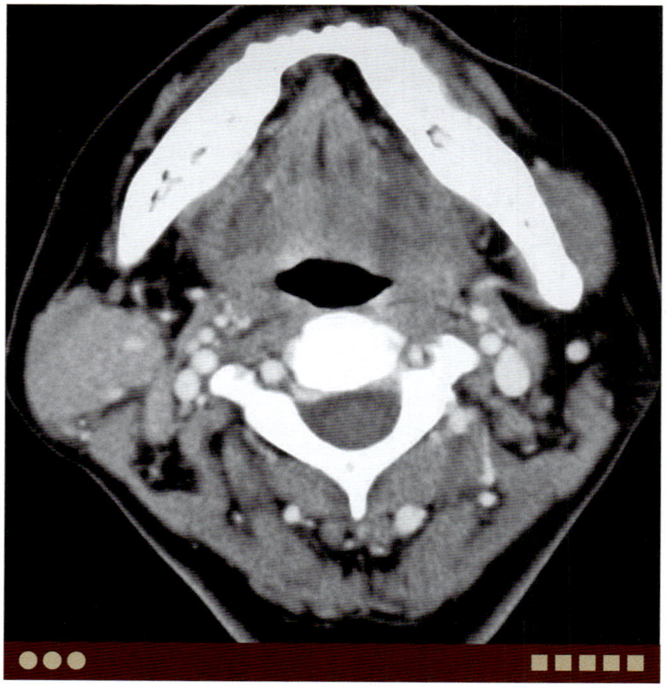

I. **Lymphoma arising from Sjögren's syndrome**. Axial contrast-enhanced CT demonstrates a homogeneously enhancing mass in the right parotid gland.

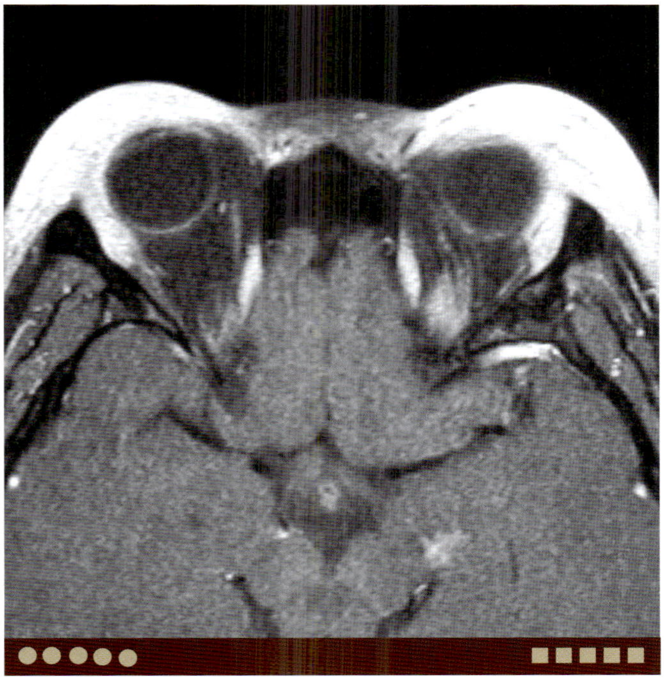

J. Idiopathic orbital inflammation. Axial contrast-enhanced fat-suppressed T1W image demonstrates marked swelling and enhancement of the periorbital soft tissues and lacrimal glands bilaterally.

Chapter 7

SALIVARY GLAND

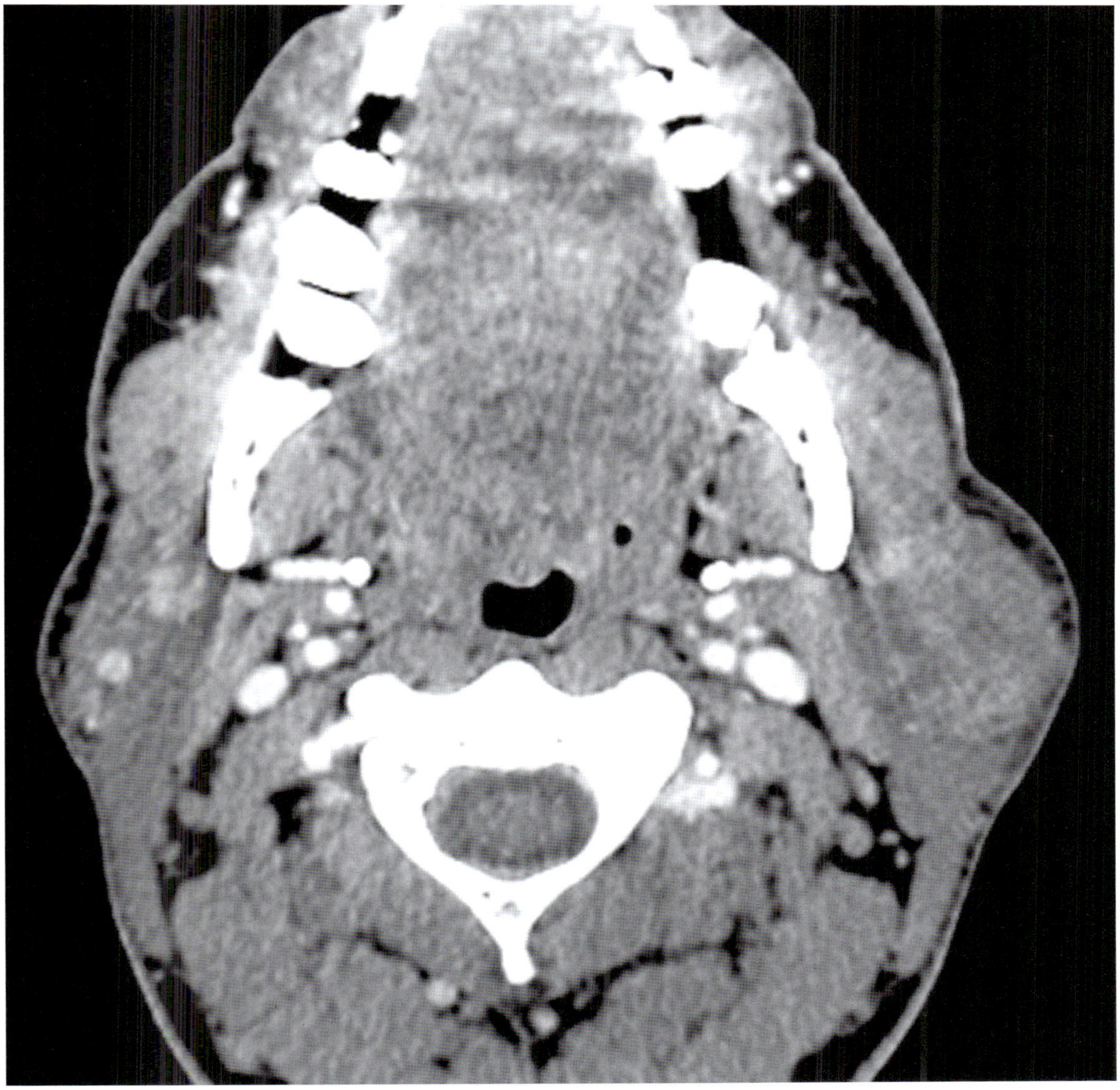

Case 7–1 Warthin's Tumor

Osamu Sakai, Asim Mian, Naoko Saito

PRESENTATION

Bilateral parotid swelling.

FINDINGS

CT and MRI demonstrate multiple masses in the bilateral parotid glands.

DIFFERENTIAL DIAGNOSIS

- Intra-/periparotid lymph nodes: Lymph nodes are usually located in the superficial lobe of the parotid gland and demonstrate similar density or signal to other nodes outside of the gland.
- Lymphoepithelial cysts (lesions) associated with HIV infection: This lesion demonstrates similar appearance to Warthin's tumor. The patient's HIV status should be determined. Cervical lymphadenopathy and nasopharyngeal lymphoid enlargement are often seen.
- Lymphoma: This is the most common malignancy which presents as multiple and bilateral lesions in the parotid glands. Cystic change is rare without treatment.
- Acinic cell carcinoma: This is the second most common malignant tumor which is presented as multiple and bilateral lesions in the parotid glands. This is, however, rare.

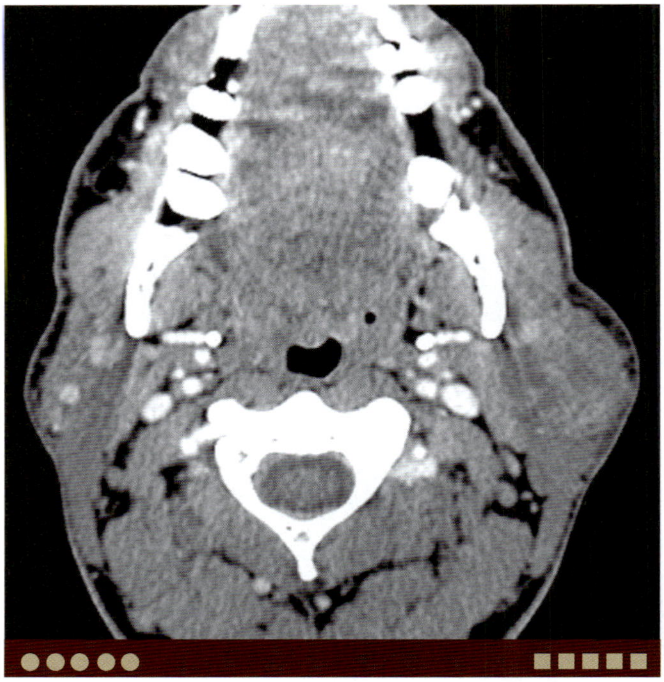

A. Warthin's tumor. Contrast-enhanced CT demonstrates a heterogeneously enhancing lesion in the left parotid gland. Note a small enhancing lesion is also present in the right parotid gland.

COMMENTS

This is a 65-year-old man with enlarged bilateral parotid glands.

Warthin's tumor, also known as benign papillary cystadenoma lymphomatosum, usually occurs in the parotid glands and occasionally in the submandibular glands. It is rare in the minor salivary gland in the oral cavity, although reported in the lip, palate and in the lacrimal gland. Contrary to pleomorphic adenoma which often occurs in women, Warthin's tumors usually occur in men, particularly older than 50 years old. It is often seen in the lower pole of the parotid gland. Patients often present with parotid swelling and pain. Bilaterality (>10%) and multiplicity are the unique features of this tumor.

Warthin's tumors often show proteinaceous or hemorrhagic cystic components and demonstrate increased density on CT. On MRI, cystic portions usually demonstrate high T2 signal, however, signal may be variable due to difference in protein concentration. Epithelial and lymphoid components demonstrate avid enhancement, which is rapid enhancement with rapid washout. This finding is helpful to differentiate it from pleomorphic adenoma and malignant tumors. Strong tracer accumulation on $^{99m}TcO^{4-}$ scintigraphy is also helpful to make a diagnosis.

Malignant transformation is uncommon, however, does occur. Increase in size, invasion to the adjacent structures and nodal metastasis have to be carefully evaluated.

PEARLS

- **Warthin's tumor is usually seen in elderly males.**
- **Warthin's tumor is often multiple and bilateral and tend to occur in the inferior portion of the parotid gland.**
- **Early enhancement and early washout is helpful to differentiate it from pleomorphic adenoma or malignant tumors.**

ADDITIONAL IMAGES (B-F)

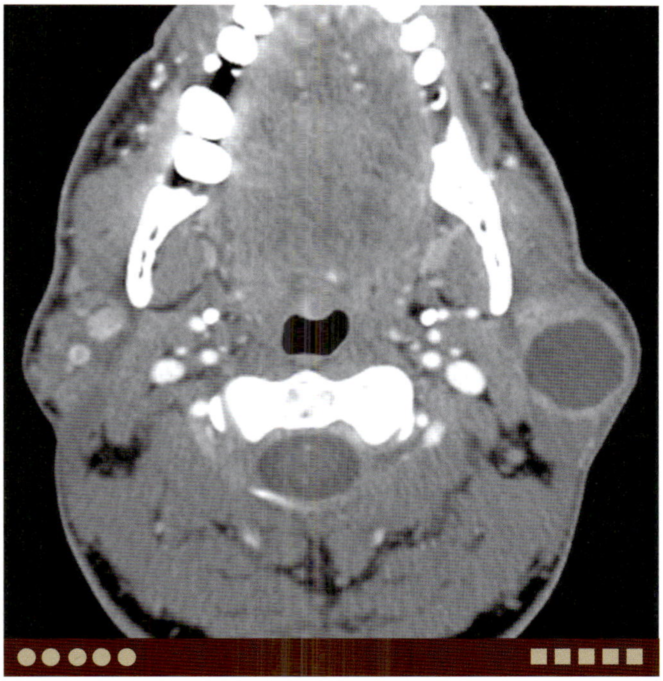

B. Warthin's tumor, same patient as A. Follow-up CT demonstrates a large cyst formation in the left parotid gland. The small enhancing lesion in the right parotid gland is stable.

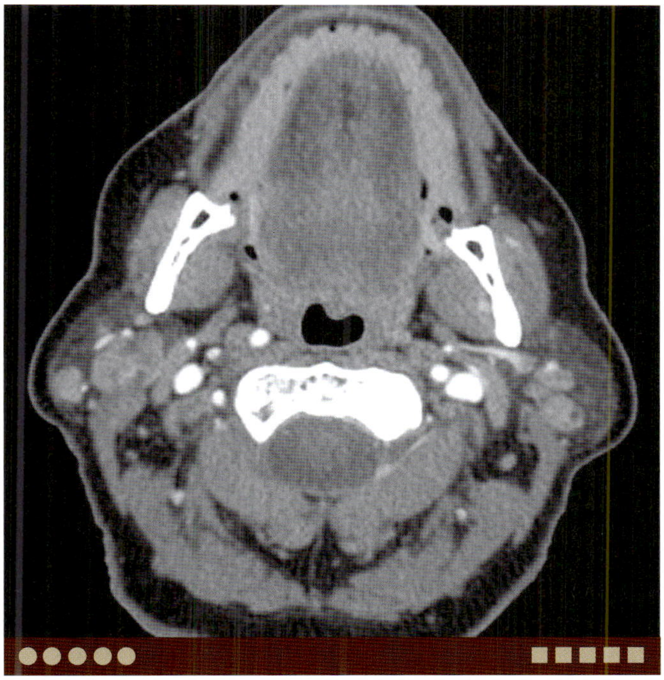

C. Warthin's tumor in a different patient. Axial contrast-enhanced CT demonstrates enhancing tumors in the inferior portion of the parotid gland bilaterally.

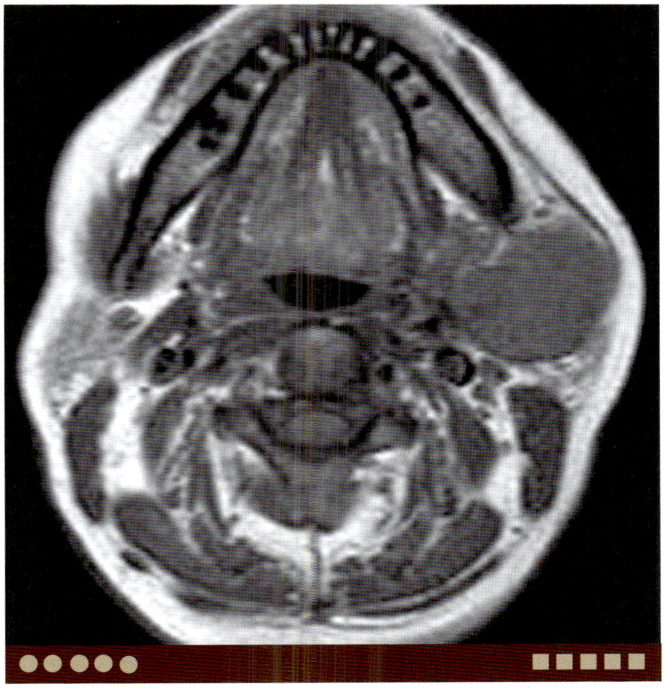

D. Warthin's tumor in a different patient. Axial T1W image demonstrates a large low-signal mass in the inferior portion of the left parotid gland.

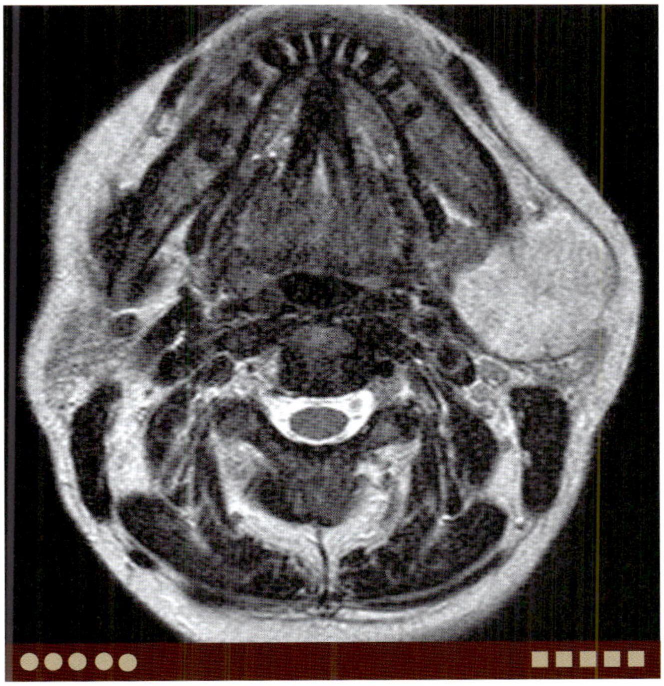

E. Warthin's tumor, same patient as D. Axial T2W image demonstrates relatively homogeneous, high signal in the lesion.

DIFFERENTIAL DIAGNOSIS IMAGES (G-I)

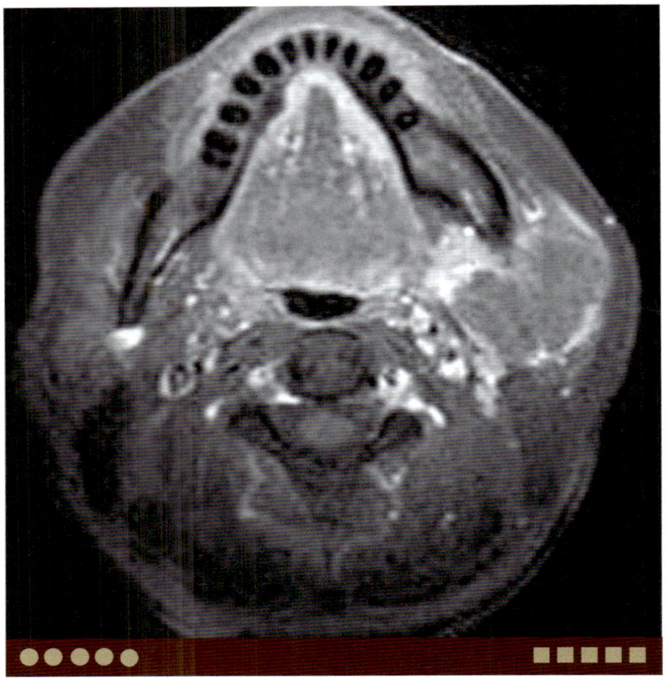

F. Warthin's tumor, same patient as D. Axial postcontrast fat-suppressed T1W image demonstrates peripheral enhancement in this cystic lesion.

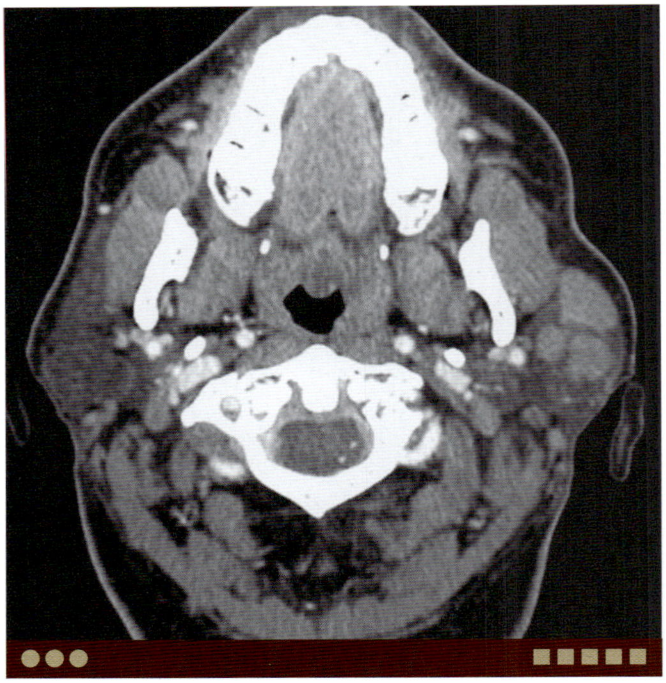

G. Lymphoma. Axial contrast-enhanced CT demonstrates multiple homogeneous density masses in the left parotid gland.

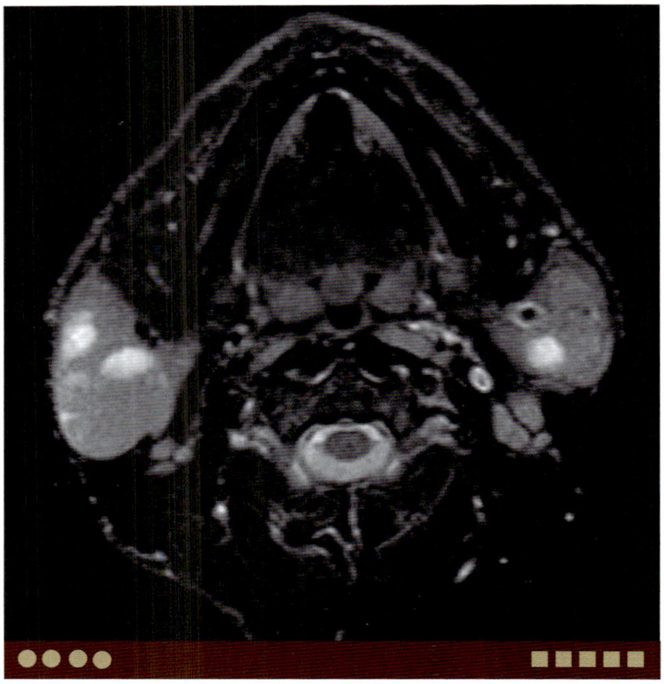

H. Lymphoepithelial lesions associated with HIV. Axial fat-suppressed T2W image demonstrates multiple high-signal lesions in the bilateral parotid glands. Note the cervical lymphadenopathy.

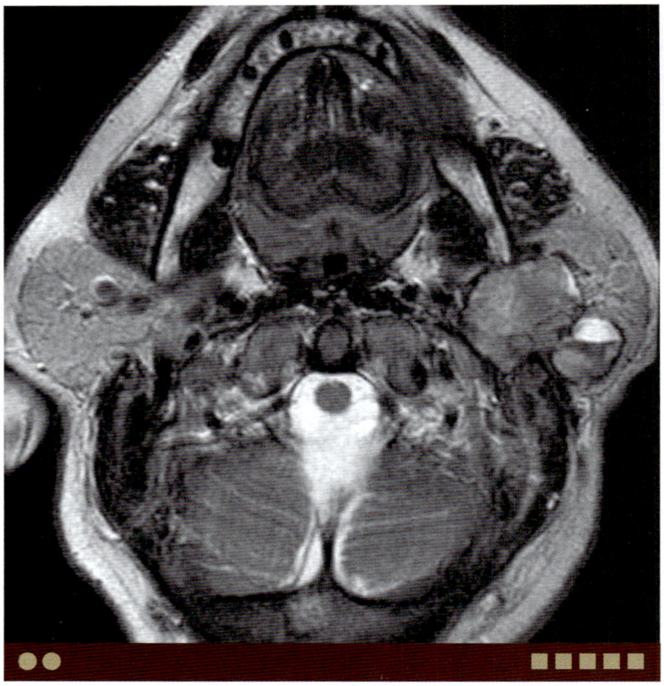

I. Acnic cell carcinoma. Axial T2W image demonstrates a heterogeneous intermediate-to-low signal tumor in the deep lobe of the left parotid gland. Note a partially cystic second lesion lateral to the main lesion.

Case 7–2 Pleomorphic Adenoma—Parotid Gland

Osamu Sakai, Naoko Saito, Asim Mian

PRESENTATION

Unilateral parotid swelling.

FINDINGS

CT and MRI demonstrate a well-circumscribed mass in the parotid gland.

DIFFERENTIAL DIAGNOSIS

- Warthin's tumor: This usually occurs in elderly men, most commonly in the inferior portion of the parotid glands. Lesions are often multiple and bilateral and can be cystic or solid.
- Mucoepidermoid carcinoma: This is the most common malignant parotid gland tumor. Regional cervical nodal metastasis is commonly seen. Low-grade tumor tends to have well-circumscribed margins.
- Lymphoma: Primary lymphoma of the parotid gland is rare. However, lymphoma is the most common malignancy which presents as multiple and bilateral lesions in the parotid glands. Cystic change is rare without treatment.
- Lymphoepithelial cysts (lesions) associated with HIV infection: This condition is usually multiple and bilateral, and may demonstrate similar appearance to Warthin's tumor. The patient's HIV status should be determined.

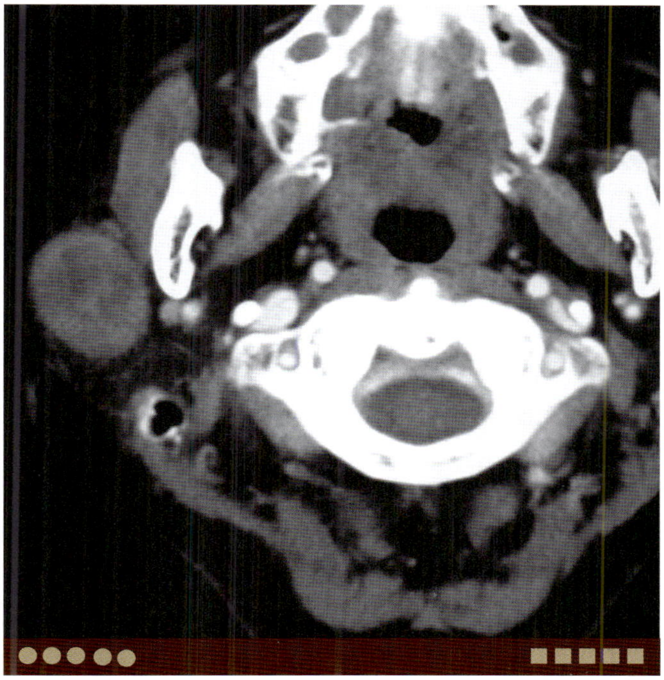

A. Pleomorphic adenoma. Axial contrast-enhanced CT demonstrates a well-circumscribed mass in the superficial lobe of the right parotid gland.

COMMENTS

This is a 45-year-old woman with right parotid mass.

Pleomorphic adenoma is the most common parotid tumor and represents about 70% to 80% of tumors arising in this region. This tumor is often seen in relatively young women, most commonly women in their forties and fifties. The majority of these tumors occur in the superficial lobe of the parotid gland; however, about 25% occur in the deep lobe. Histologically, this tumor demonstrates a mixture of epithelial and interstitial cells. It often has a thin capsule and smooth and well-demarcated margins with slight lobulation. This tumor demonstrates variable appearance from solid to almost totally cystic. Calcification is occasionally seen.

Typically pleomorphic adenoma demonstrates high signal on T2W image corresponding to myxoid degeneration or abundant glandular component. After contrast, the tumor demonstrates gradual enhancement. The delayed enhancement is helpful to differentiate from Warthin's tumor, which demonstrates quicker enhancement and washout. It is, however, difficult to differentiate pleomorphic adenomas from malignant tumors.

Rarely, carcinoma is accompanied with, or may arise from pleomorphic adenoma. Therefore, careful evaluation for invasion for the adjacent structures, perineural tumor spread and nodal metastasis is important.

The tumor arising from the deep lobe may extend medially into the parapharyngeal space through the stylomastoid tunnel, and seen as a parapharyngeal mass. Indeed, pleomorphic adenoma is the most common tumor in the parapharyngeal space.

PEARLS

- **Pleomorphic adenoma is the most common parotid tumor, often seen in women.**
- **Pleomorphic adenoma demonstrates delayed enhancement. This helps to differentiate it from Warthin's tumor.**
- **Pleomorphic adenoma is rarely malignant. However, careful evaluation for possible malignancy is important.**

ADDITIONAL IMAGES (B-G)

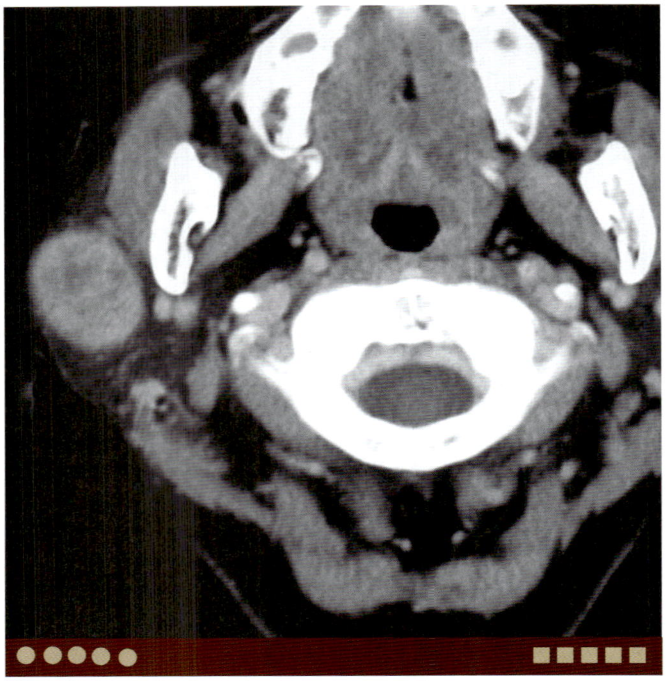

B. Pleomorphic adenoma, same patient as A. Axial delayed contrast enhanced CT demonstrates increased contrast enhancement of the lesion.

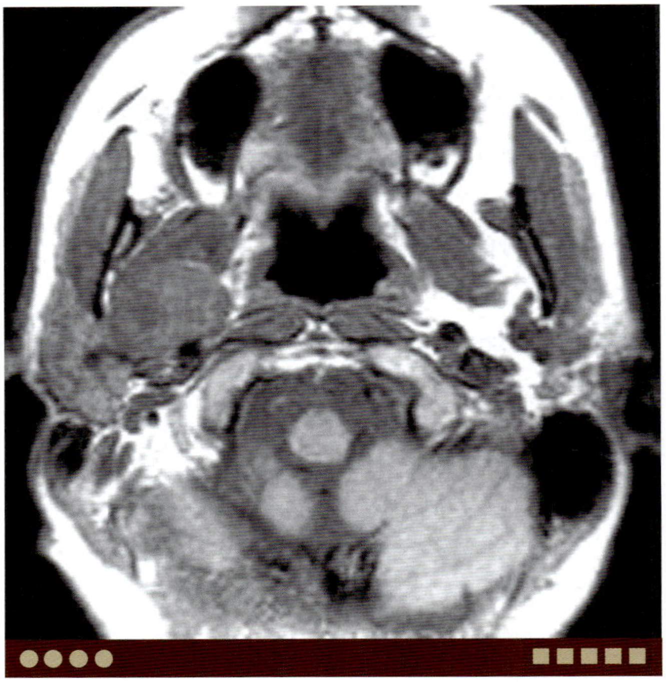

C. Pleomorphic adenoma in a different patient. Axial T1W image demonstrates a well-circumscribed low-signal mass in the deep lobe of the right parotid gland extending into the parapharyngeal space.

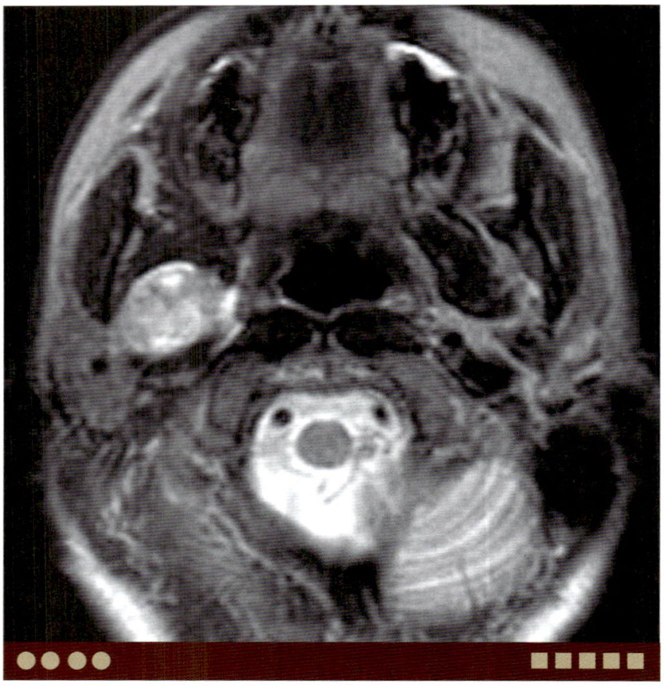

D. Pleomorphic adenoma, same patient as C. Axial T2W image demonstrates slightly heterogeneous high signals in the lesion.

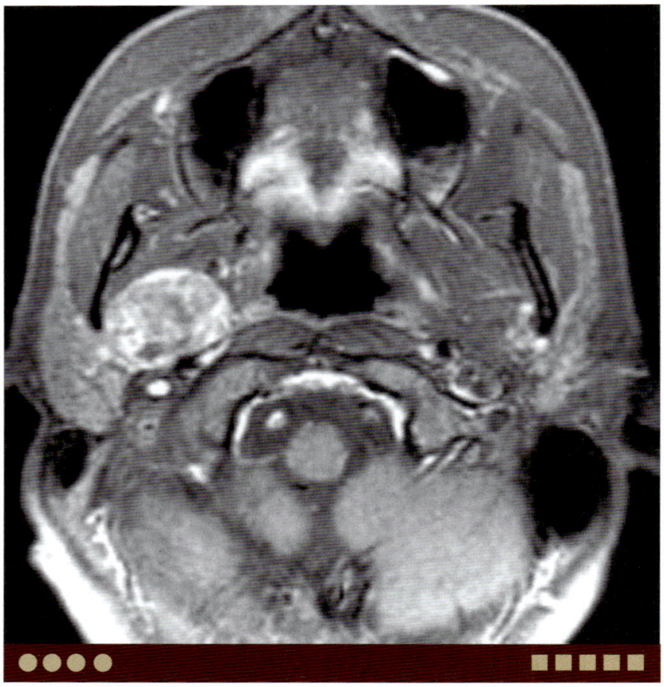

E. Pleomorphic adenoma, same patient as C. Axial postcontrast fat-suppressed T1W image demonstrates slight heterogeneous enhancement in the lesion.

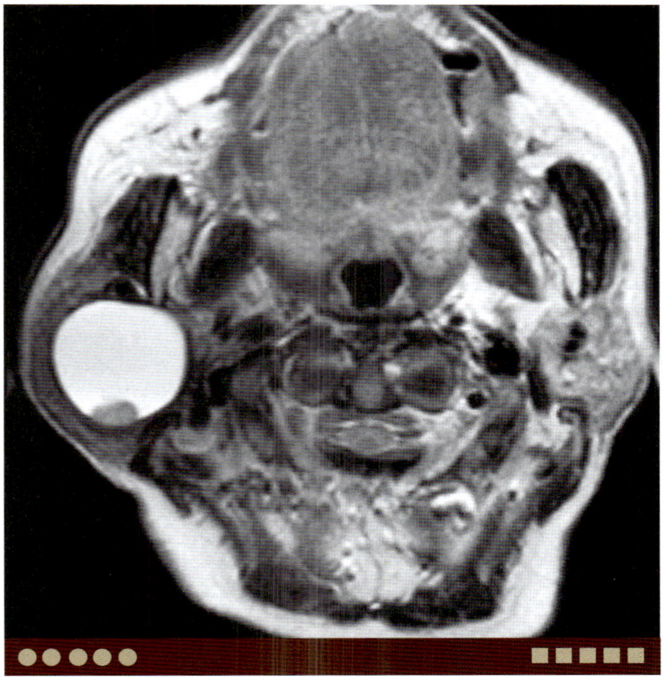

F. Pleomorphic adenoma in a different patient. Axial T2W image demonstrates a cystic lesion with a mural nodule in the right parotid gland.

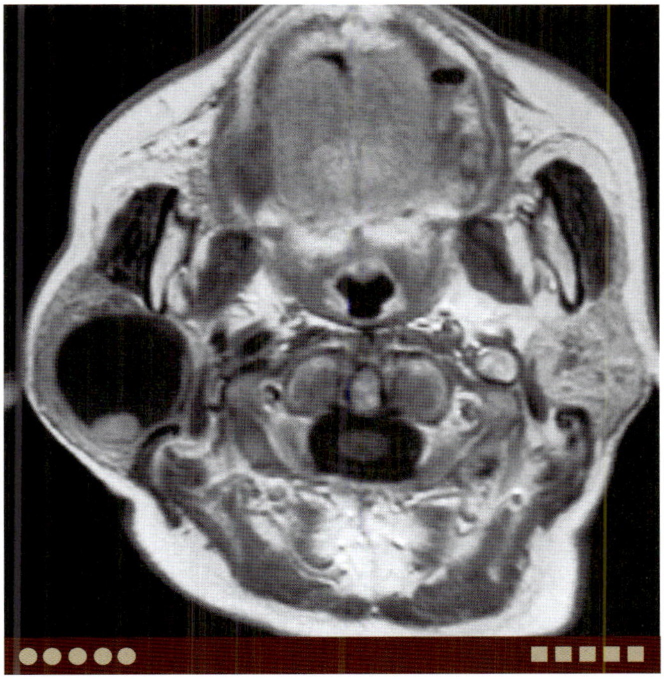

G. Pleomorphic adenoma, same patient as F. Axial postcontrast T1W image demonstrates slight enhancement in the mural nodule.

DIFFERENTIAL DIAGNOSIS IMAGES (H-J)

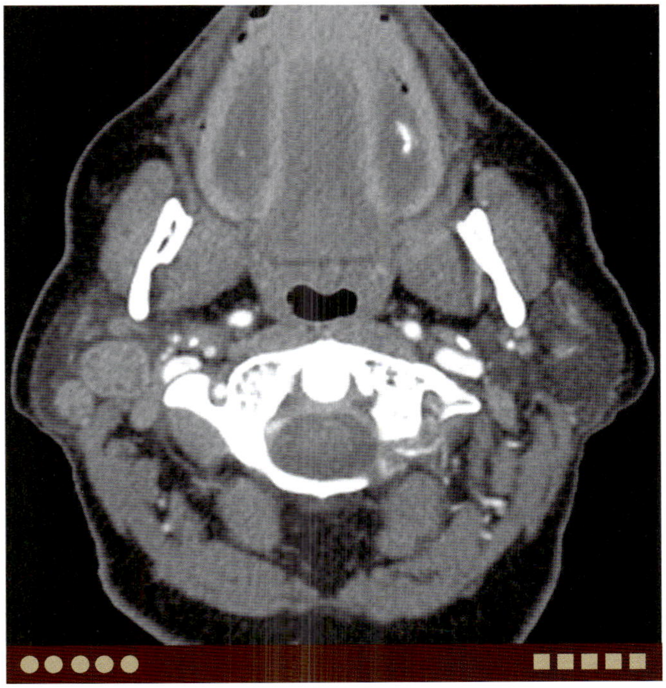

H. Warthin's tumor. Axial contrast-enhanced CT demonstrates two well-circumscribed enhancing masses in the inferior portion of the right parotid gland.

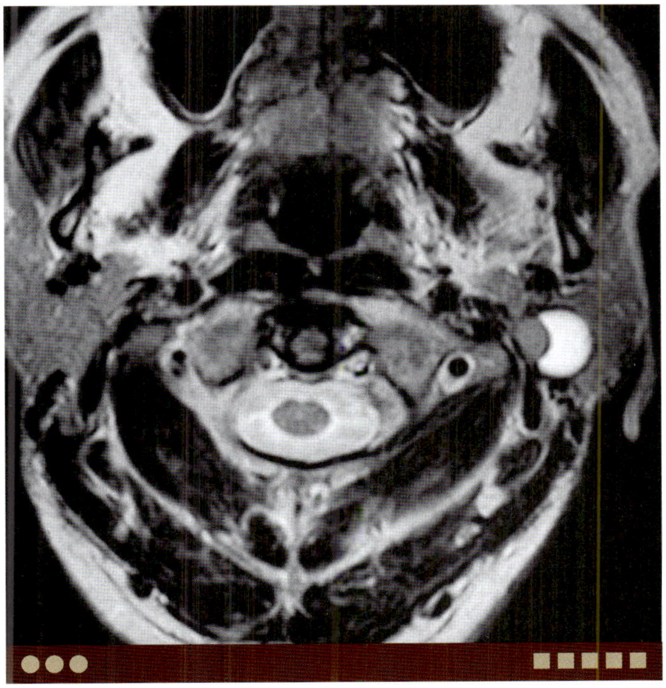

I. Basal cell adenoma. Axial T2W image demonstrates a cystic lesion with a mural nodule in the left parotid gland.

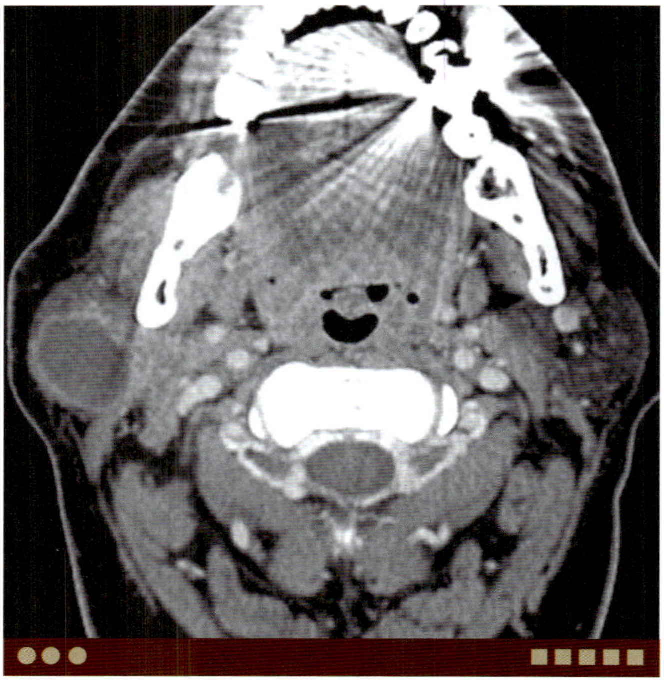

J. Mucoepidermoid carcinoma. Axial contrast-enhanced CT demonstrates a cystic tumor with irregular rim-enhancement in the right parotid gland.

Case 7–3 Adenoid Cystic Carcinoma—Submandibular Gland

Naoko Saito, Asim Mian, Osamu Sakai

PRESENTATION

Unilateral submandibular swelling.

FINDINGS

CT and MRI demonstrate a mass in the submandibular space.

DIFFERENTIAL DIAGNOSIS

- Mucoepidermoid carcinoma: This is the second most common malignant submandibular gland tumor. Low-grade tumor has a similar appearance to a benign tumor.
- Pleomorphic adenoma: This is the most common submandibular gland tumor. This tumor demonstrates a well-circumscribed mass. Dystrophic calcifications are sometimes seen and this finding helps to differentiate it from other tumors. It demonstrates delayed enhancement.
- Lymphatic malformation (lymphangioma): This is a congenital lymphatic malformation and often seen in infancy and childhood.

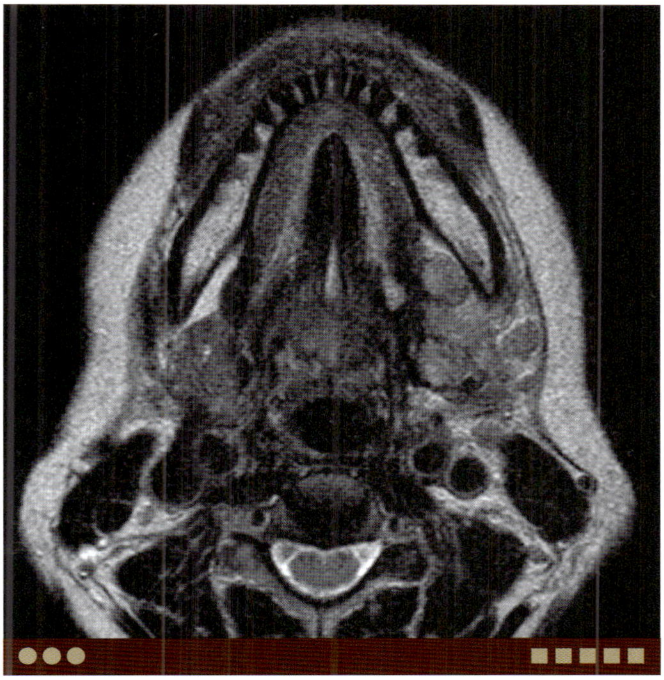

A. Adenoid cystic carcinoma. Axial T2W image demonstrates a lobulated/multinodular intermediate-signal lesion in the left submandibular space.

COMMENTS

This is a 38-year-old woman with a left submandibular mass.

Adenoid cystic carcinoma represents about 4% to 8% of all salivary gland tumors. They accounts for 2% to 6% of parotid gland tumors, 12% of submandibular gland tumors, 15% of sublingual gland tumors, 30% of minor salivary gland tumors, and 50% of lacrimal gland tumors. About 45% of the submandibular gland tumors are malignant and adenoid cystic carcinoma is the most common malignant tumor. This tumor is often seen in individuals in their forties and fifties and has a slight predilection for women.

Based on the WHO's classification system, adenoid cystic carcinomas are classified into three groups: tubular (well-differentiated or grade I), cribriform (moderately differentiated or grade II), and solid (poorly differentiated or grade III). The cribriform is the most common type, and the solid type is the least common. The solid type has the highest cellularity and poor prognosis.

On imaging, low-grade adenoid cystic carcinoma tends to have well-circumscribed margins while high-grade tumor shows infiltrating appearance. On T2W image, the high-grade tumor demonstrates low signal intensity corresponding to high cellularity. These findings may help to suggest higher grade tumor with poor prognosis.

Distant metastasis may occur 10 to 108 months (median 96) after initial diagnosis. Therefore, long-term follow-up is needed. Lung and bone are the most common sites of metastases; however, lymphatic spread is rare.

PEARLS

- **Adenoid cystic carcinoma is the most common malignant tumor in the submandibular gland.**
- **Adenoid cystic carcinomas are classified into three groups: tubular, cribriform, and solid. The solid type has the highest cellularity and poor prognosis.**
- **Low signal intensity on T2W image suggests solid type (high-grade) tumor.**

ADDITIONAL IMAGES (B-F)

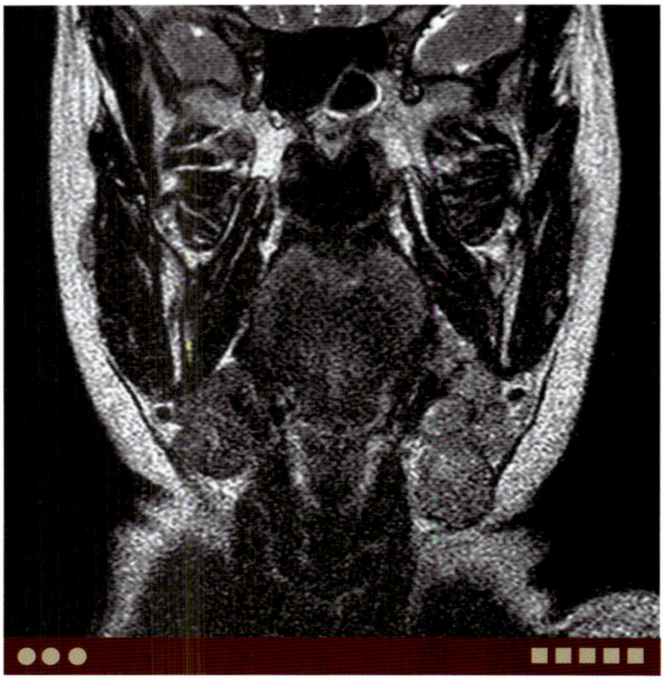

B. Adenoid cystic carcinoma, same patient as A. Ccronal T2W image demonstrates a lobulated, intermediate-signal lesion in the left submandibular space.

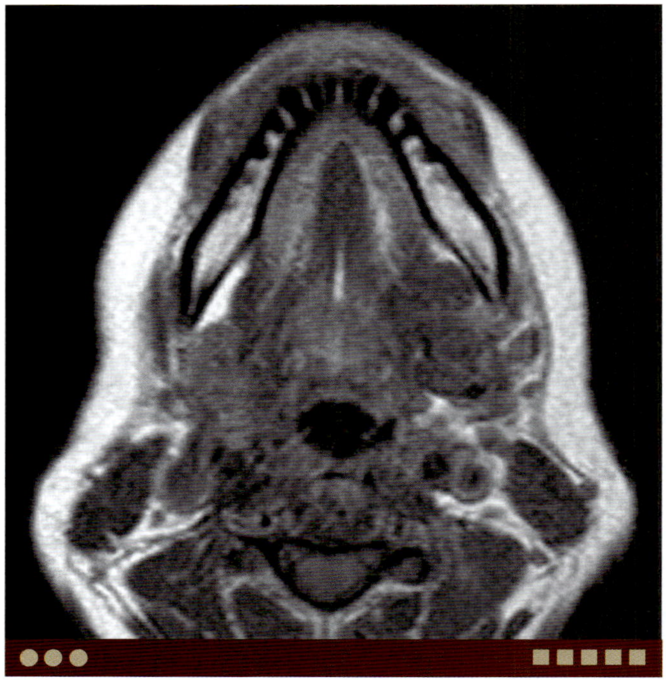

C. Adenoid cystic carcinoma, same patient as A. Axial T1W image demonstrates low signal in the lesion.

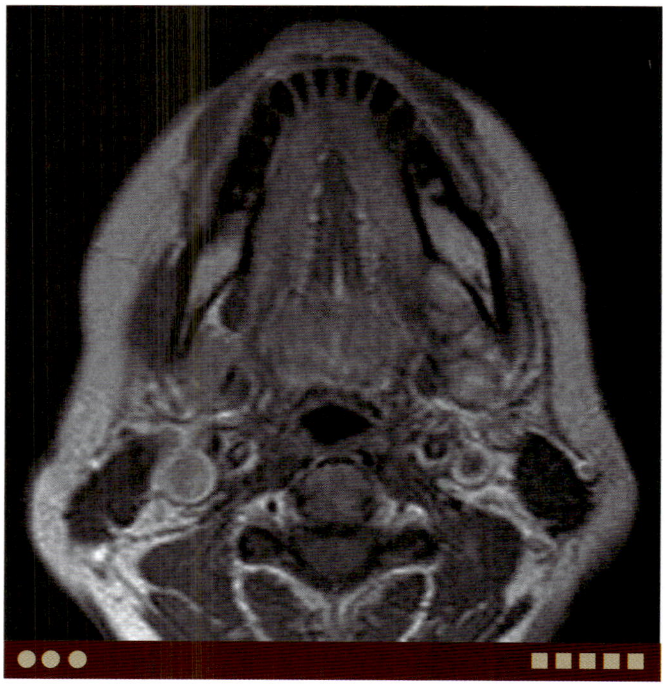

D. Adenoid cystic carcinoma, same patient as A. Axial postcontrast T1W image demonstrates enhancement of the lesion.

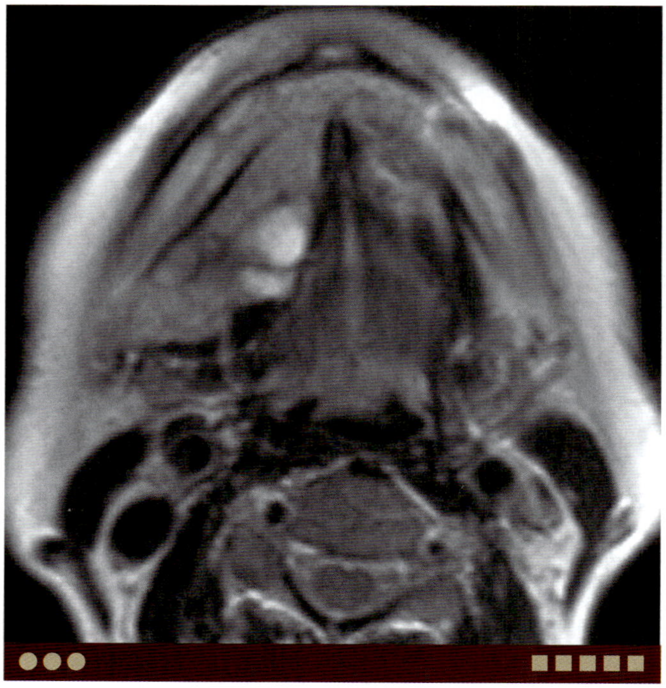

E. Sublingual adenoid cystic carcinoma in a different patient. Axial T2W image demonstrates a high-signal mass with cystic lesion in the right sublingual space.

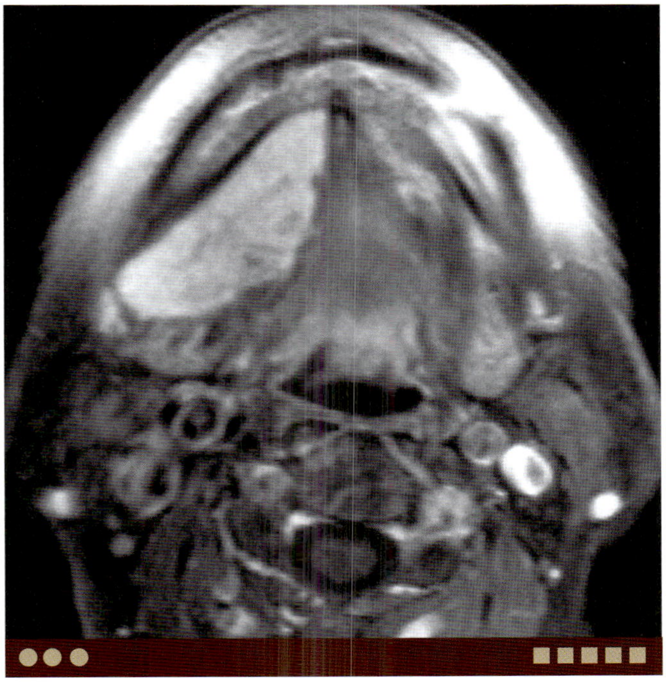

F. Sublingual adenoid cystic carcinoma, same patient as E. Axial postcontrast, fat-suppressed T1W image demonstrates slight heterogeneous enhancement in the lesion.

DIFFERENTIAL DIAGNOSIS IMAGES (G-I)

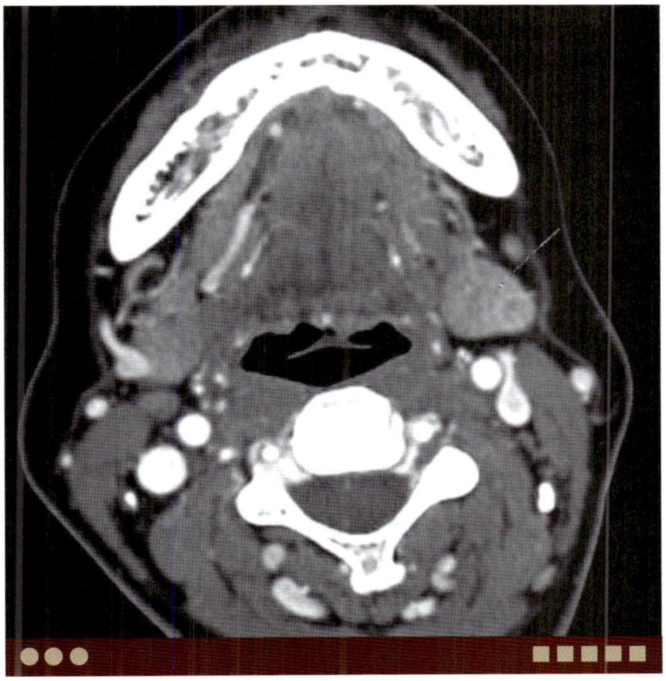

G. Mucoepidermoid carcinoma. Axial contrast-enhanced CT demonstrates a well-circumscribed lesion in the left submandibular gland (low-grade mucoepidermoid carcinoma).

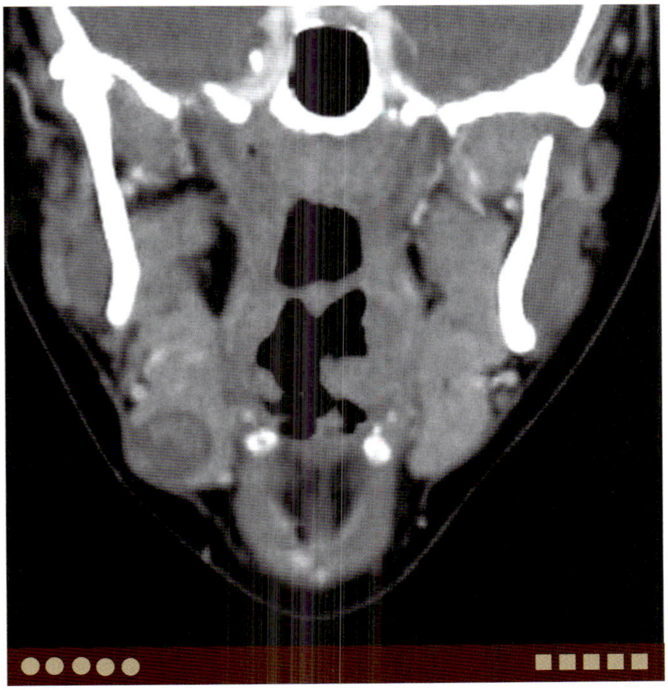

H. Pleomorphic adenoma. Coronal contrast-enhanced CT demonstrates a well-circumscribed and heterogeneously enhancing mass in the right submandibular gland.

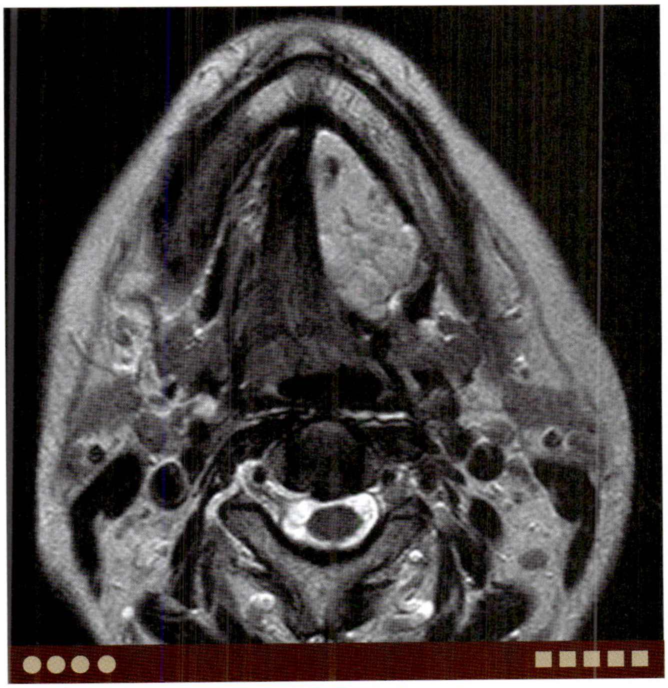

I. Lymphatic malformation of the sublingual space. Axial T2W image demonstrates a multicystic high-signal intensity mass in the left sublingual space.

Case 7–4 Acinic Cell Carcinoma

Naoko Saito, Asim Mian, Osamu Sakai

PRESENTATION

Parotid mass.

FINDINGS

CT and MRI demonstrate heterogeneous density/signal parotid tumors which may be bilateral or multiple.

DIFFERENTIAL DIAGNOSIS

- Warthin's tumor: This usually occurs in elderly men and are often multiple and bilateral. Lesions are commonly seen in the inferior portion of the parotid gland.
- Mucoepidermoid carcinoma: This is the most common malignant parotid gland tumor. Regional nodal metastasis is common. Low-grade tumors tend to show cystic appearance/high signal on T2W images.
- Pleomorphic adenoma: This tumor is the most common parotid tumor often seen in women in their forties and fifties. A solitary lesion with well-defined margins and variable internal signal is a common finding. Delayed enhancement is usually seen.
- Intra-/periparotid lymph nodes: Lymph nodes are usually located in the superficial lobe of the parotid gland and demonstrate similar density or signals to other nodes outside of the gland.

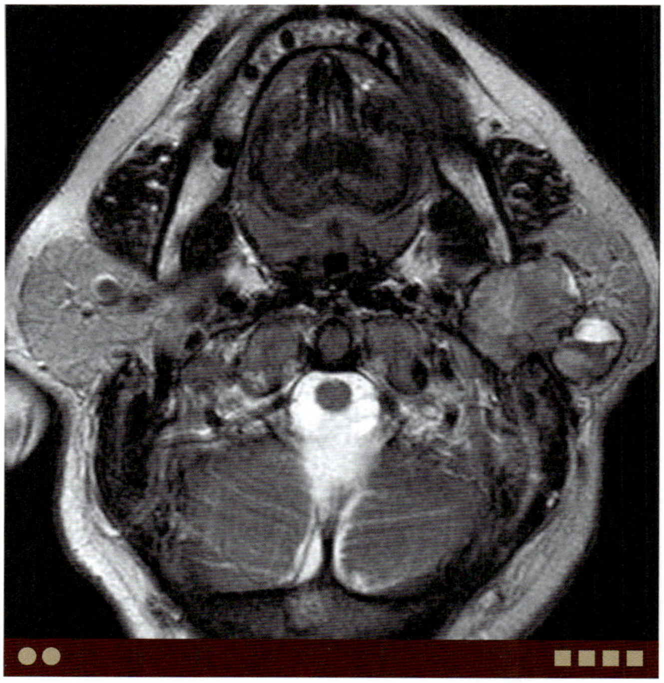

A. Acinic cell carcinoma. Axial T2W MR image demonstrates a heterogeneous intermediate-to-low signal tumor in the deep lobe of the left parotid gland. Note a partially cystic second lesion lateral to the main lesion.

COMMENTS

This is a 20-year-old woman with a left parotid mass.

Acinic cell carcinoma represents approximately 2% to 4% of all salivary gland tumors. About 90% of the tumors occur in the parotid gland with the minor salivary glands being the second most common site. This tumor is often seen in women in their forties and fifties. In children, this is the second most common malignant salivary gland tumor after mucoepidermoid carcinoma. Multiple or bilateral tumors may be present. Acinic cell carcinoma is the most frequent malignant epithelial tumor to present bilaterally.

Histologically, acinic cell carcinoma has four patterns: solid, microcystic, papillary-cystic, and follicular. A mixture of these patterns is common. Typically this tumor demonstrates a well-circumscribed mass and may be cystic; however, recurrent tumor may appear as a multinodular mass.

Acinic cell carcinoma often demonstrates nonspecific imaging features, therefore, it is difficult to differentiate from other parotid gland tumors. It often has a similar appearance to benign tumors. However, subtle invasive findings can be a clue to make a diagnosis of this malignant tumor. On T2W image, the tumor occasionally exhibits low signal corresponding to high cellularity, hemorrhage, fibrosis and calcification.

Although acinic cell carcinoma often has a benign appearance, lymphatic and hematogeneous metastases may occur. Lungs and bones are the most common metastatic sites. Large tumor size, deep lobe involvement, multinodular appearance, and metastasis predict poor prognosis.

PEARLS

- **Acinic cell carcinoma is sometimes multiple and bilateral in the parotid glands.**
- **Often acinic cell carcinoma demonstrates a well-circumscribed benign-appearing mass and may be cystic.**
- **Hemorrhage, fibrosis, and calcification are occasionally seen.**

ADDITIONAL IMAGES (B-G)

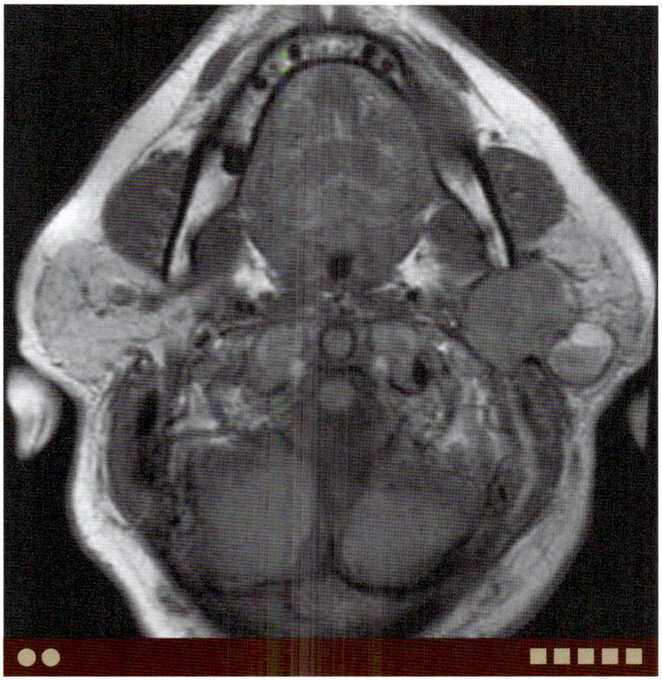

B. Acinic cell carcinoma, same patient as A. Axial T1W MR image demonstrates a low-to-intermediate signal tumor in the deep lobe of the left parotid gland. The second lesion shows high signal suggesting proteinaceous or hemorrhagic component.

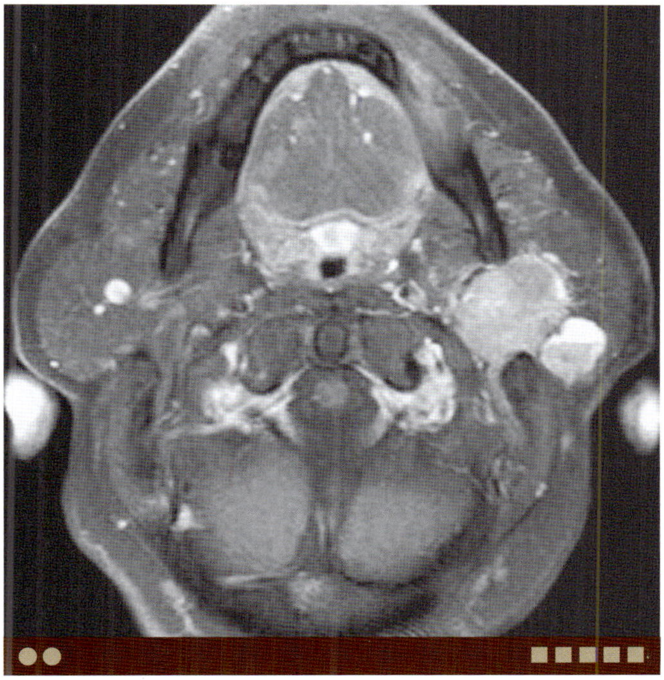

C. Acinic cell carcinoma, same patient as A. Axial postcontrast fat-suppressed T1W MR image demonstrates mild enhancement in the solid lesions. Abnormal enhancement in the left stylomastoid fat pad increases the possibility of facial nerve involvement.

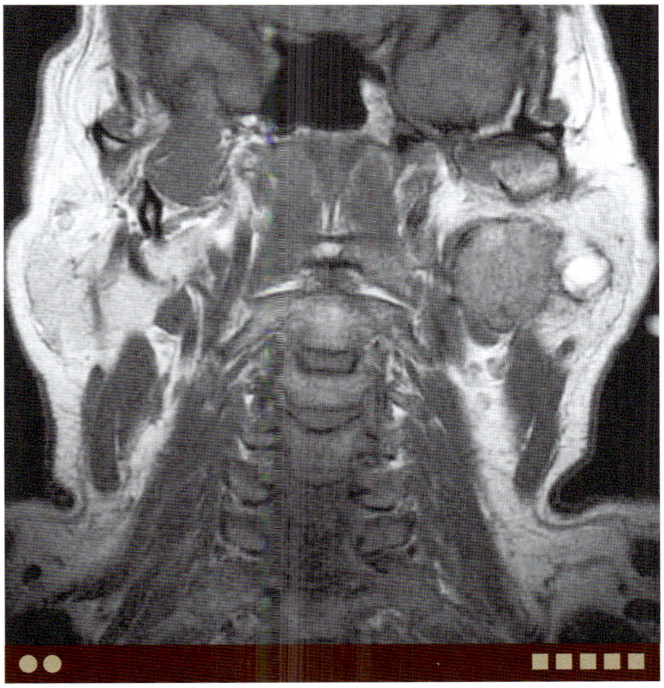

D. Acinic cell carcinoma, same patient as A. Coronal T1W MR image demonstrates the larger tumor in the deep lobe and the smaller second lesion in the superficial lobe of the left parotid gland.

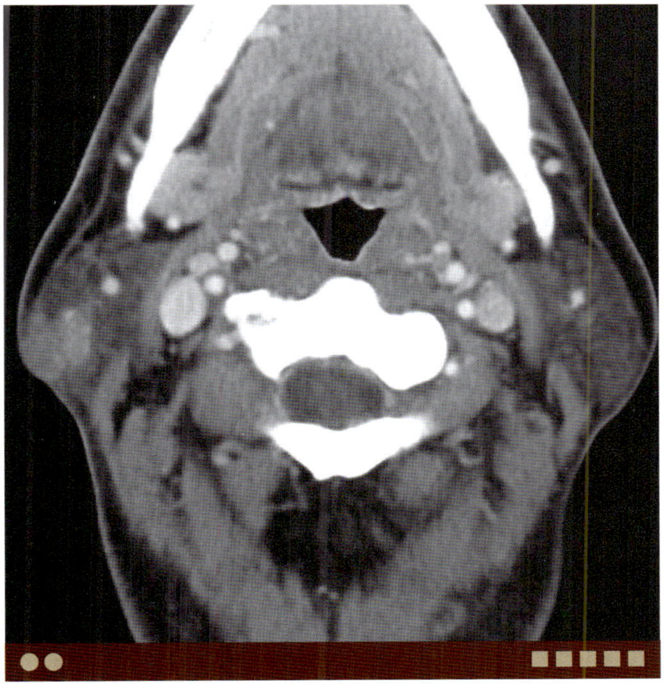

E. Acinic cell carcinoma in a different patient. Axial contrast-enhanced CT demonstrates lobulated mass in the superficial lobe of the right parotid gland. There is a slightly heterogeneous enhancement in the adjacent subcutaneous fat suggesting tumor invasion.

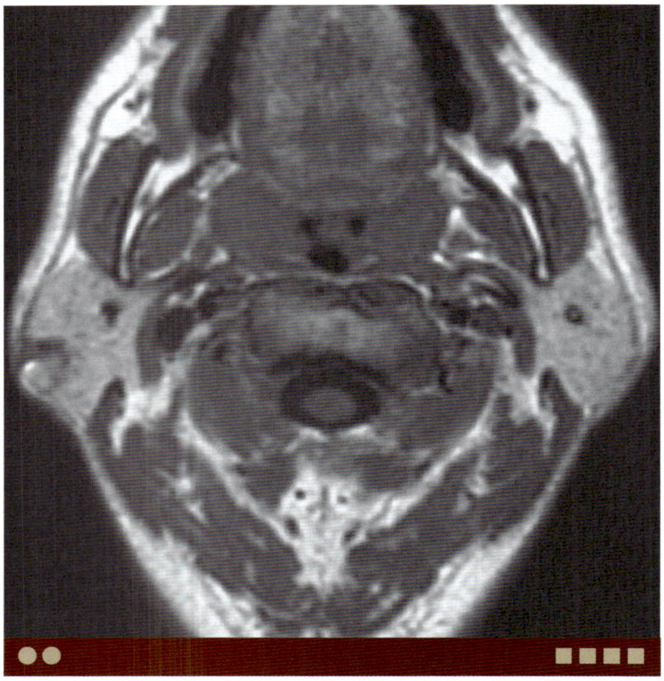

F. Acinic cell carcinoma, same patient as E. Axial T1W image demonstrates low-signal tumor with heterogeneous high signal which is suggestive of hemorrhage.

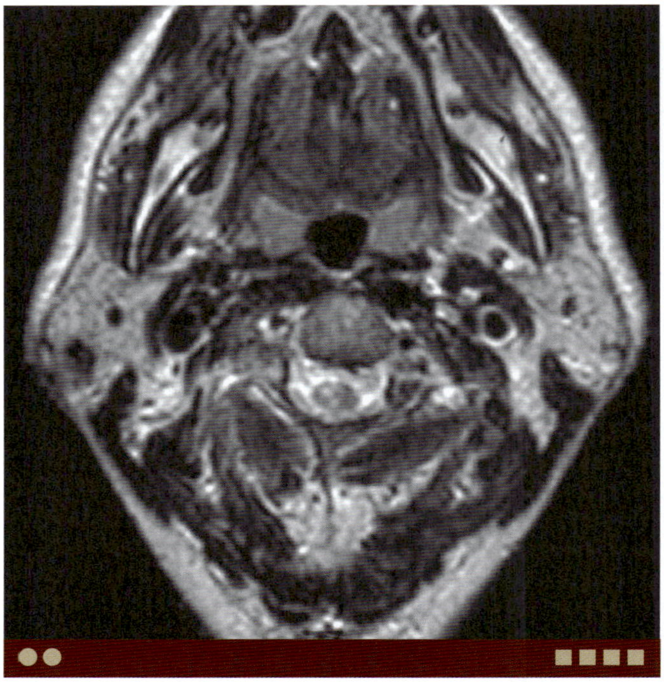

G. Acinic cell carcinoma, same patient as E. Axial T2W image demonstrates low signal in the lesion.

DIFFERENTIAL DIAGNOSIS IMAGES (H-J)

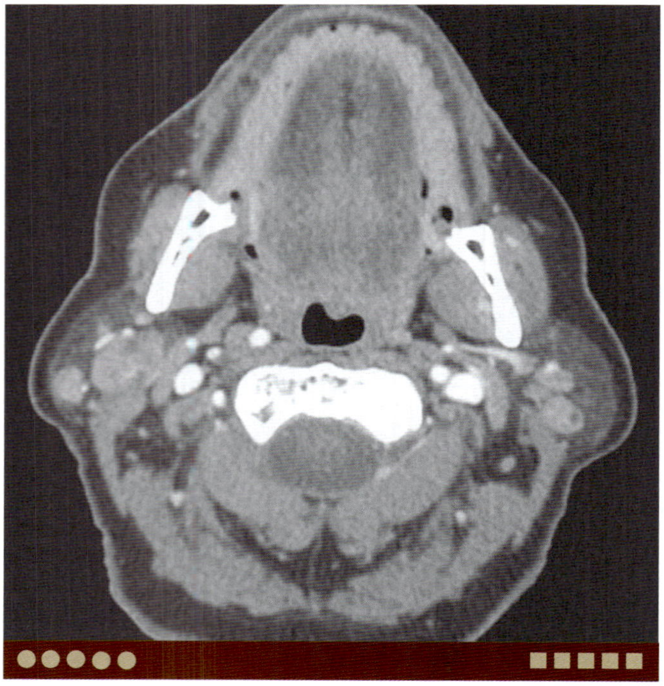

H. Warthin's tumor. Axial contrast-enhanced CT demonstrates multiple well-circumscribed masses in the bilateral parotid glands.

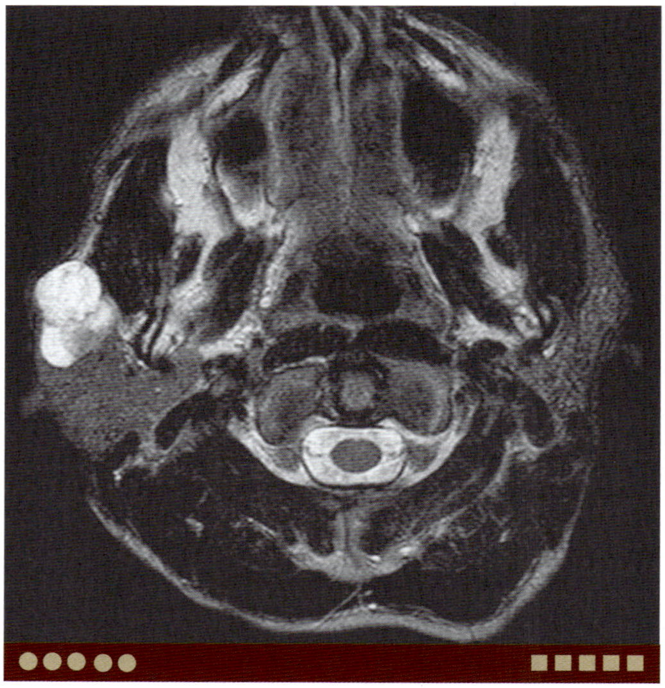

I. Pleomorphic adenoma. Axial T2W image demonstrates a well-circumscribed, lobulated, and multicystic high-signal tumor in the parotid gland.

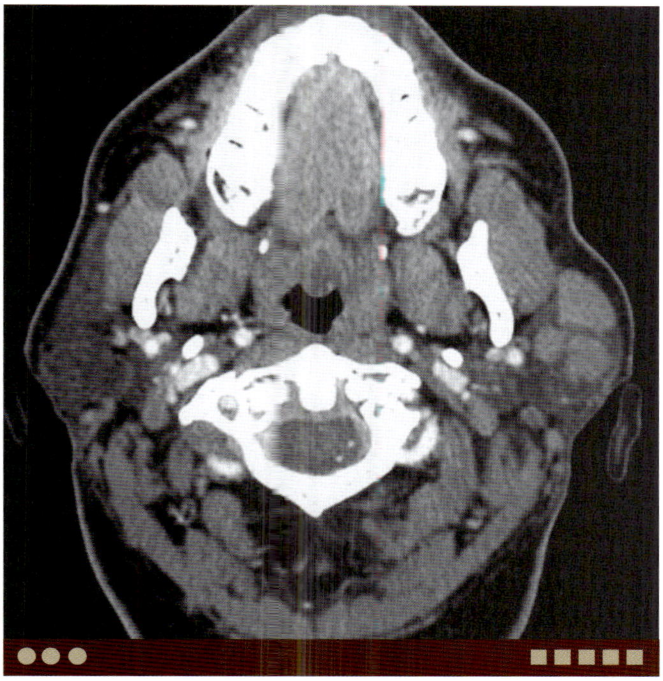

J. Lymphoma. Axial contrast-enhanced CT demonstrates multiple homogeneous-density masses in the left parotid gland. Identification of extraparotid nodal disease is helpful to suggest secondary lymphoma.

Case 7-5 Adenocarcinoma

Naoko Saito, Asim Mian, Osamu Sakai

PRESENTATION

Unilateral parotid mass.

FINDINGS

CT and MRI demonstrate a heterogeneously enhancing mass with irregular margins in the parotid gland.

DIFFERENTIAL DIAGNOSIS

- Mucoepidermoid carcinoma: This is the most common malignant parotid gland tumor. Regional cervical nodal metastasis is commonly seen.
- Adenoid cystic carcinoma: This is the second most common malignant tumor in the parotid gland. High-grade tumor (solid type) shows infiltrating appearance and low signal intensity on T2W image. This tumor has a high perineural invasion rate.
- Squamous cell carcinoma: Primary squamous cell carcinoma of the salivary gland is very rare. This tumor often has infiltrating appearance and intratumoral necrosis.

COMMENTS

This is a 49-year-old woman with a left parotid mass.

Adenocarcinoma consists about 9% of all salivary gland tumors. The majority of the tumors occur in the minor salivary glands and the parotid gland is the second most common site. This tumor is often seen in adults (20-70 years of age), and has no gender predominance. Patients often present with rapidly growing, painful parotid masses.

Histologically, adenocarcinomas are classified as grade I to III. Grade I tumors are characterized by mild pleomorphism with well-circumscribed margins. Grade III tumors are more solid and pleomorphic with infiltrating appearance and a poor clinical outcome. Grade II is classified between grades I and III.

Adenocarcinoma demonstrates nonspecific imaging features, therefore, it is difficult to differentiate from other primary parotid gland tumors. Low-grade tumors tend to have well-circumscribed margins while high-grade tumors often have infiltrating margins. On T2W image, the high-grade tumors demonstrate low signal intensity corresponding to high cellularity. Intratumoral necrosis is sometimes seen.

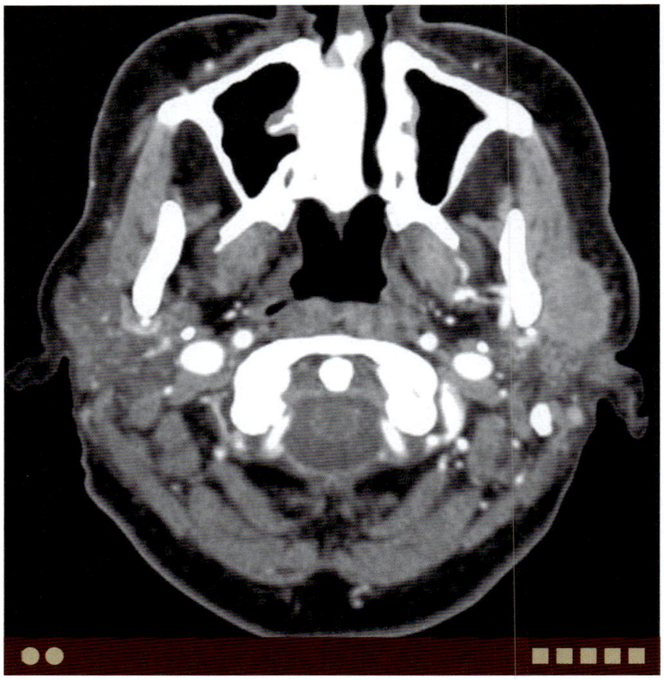

A. Adenocarcinoma. Axial contrast-enhanced CT demonstrates a heterogeneously enhancing tumor with irregular margins in the superficial lobe of the left parotid gland.

Carcinoma ex pleomorphic adenoma is a pleomorphic adenoma that has undergone malignant transformation, usually to adenocarcinoma. The patient usually has a long history (10-15 years) of pleomorphic adenoma that suddenly demonstrates rapid growth.

PEARLS

- **Painful parotid masses with rapid growth are the common clinical feature.**
- **Low-grade tumors tend to have well-circumscribed margins, while high-grade tumors often have infiltrating margins.**
- **Intratumoral necrosis is sometimes seen.**

ADDITIONAL IMAGES (B-G)

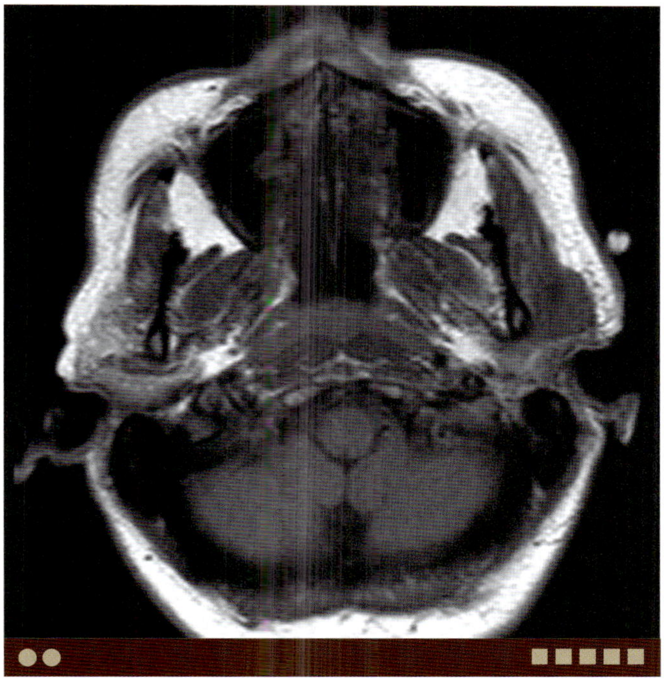

B. Adenocarcinoma, same patient as A. Axial T1W image demonstrates a heterogeneous low-signal lesion in the superficial lobe of the left parotid gland.

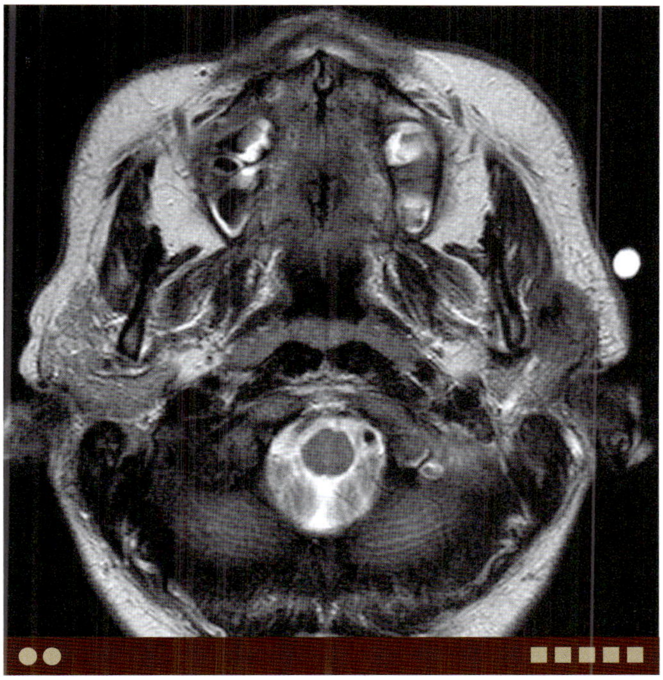

C. Adenocarcinoma, same patient as A. Axial T2W image demonstrates heterogeneously low signal in the lesion.

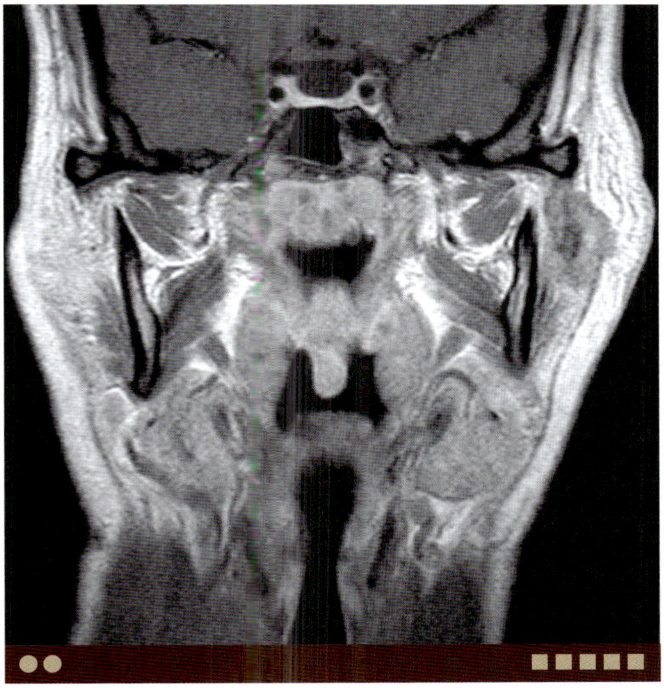

D. Adenocarcinoma, same patient as A. Coronal postcontrast T1W image demonstrates a heterogeneously enhancing tumor with irregular margins.

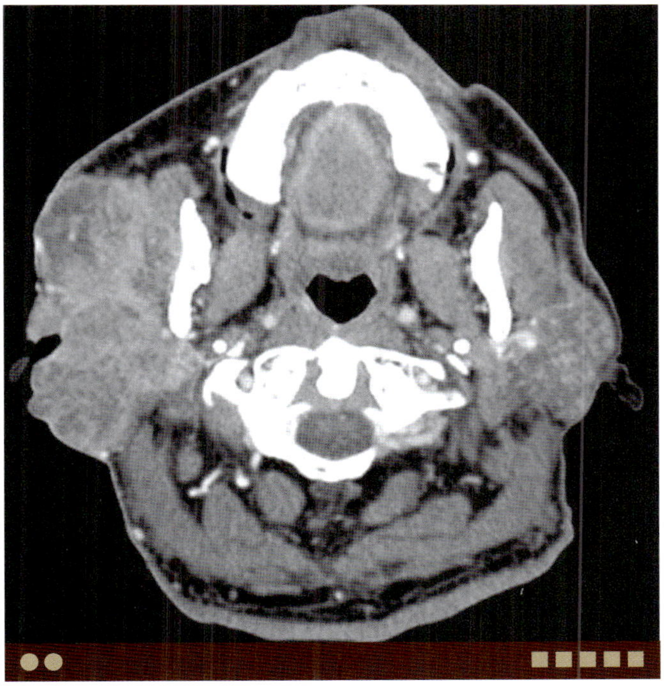

E. Adenocarcinoma in a different patient. Axial contrast-enhanced CT demonstrates a large, lobulated, heterogeneously enhancing tumor in the right parotid gland. The tumor invades the right masseter muscle and skin.

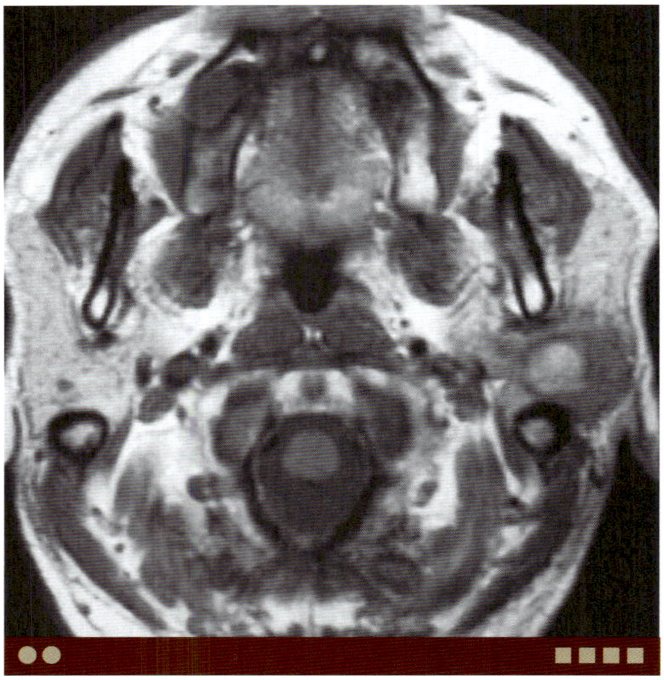

F. Carcinoma ex pleomorphic adenoma. Axial T1W image demonstrates a poorly circumscribed low-signal tumor with an area of high signal to suggest hemorrhage in the left parotid gland.

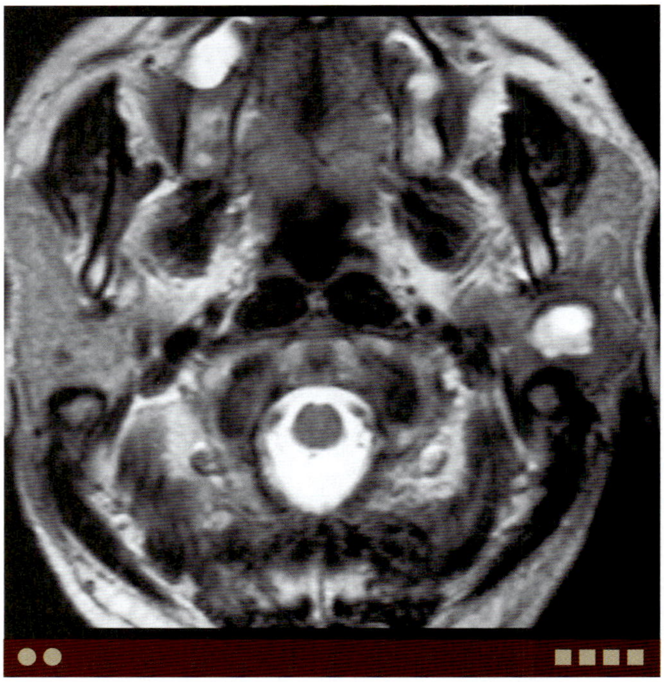

G. Carcinoma ex pleomorphic adenoma, same patient as F. Axial T2W image demonstrates ill-defined margins of the tumor. The central portion of the tumor shows heterogeneous high signal suggesting hemorrhage or necrosis.

DIFFERENTIAL DIAGNOSIS IMAGES (H-J)

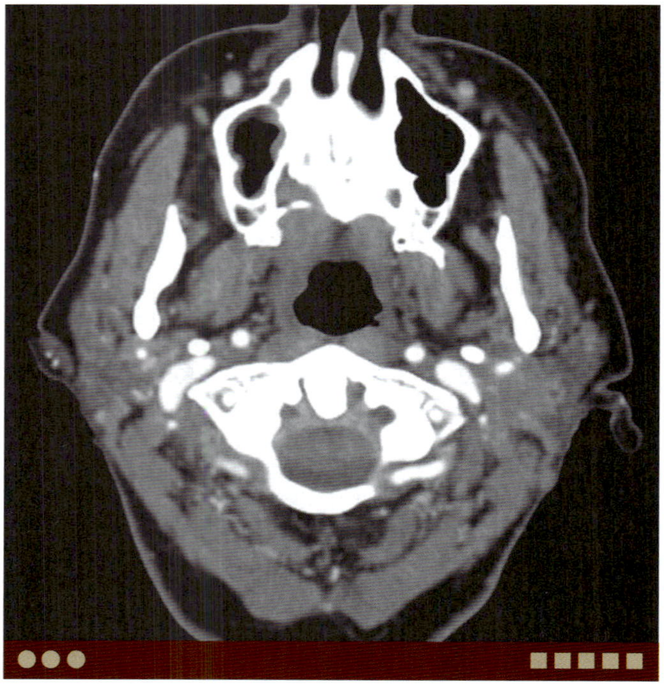

H. Adenoid cystic carcinoma (high grade). Axial contrast-enhanced CT demonstrates a poorly circumscribed tumor in the left parotid gland extending to the stylomastoid fat pad.

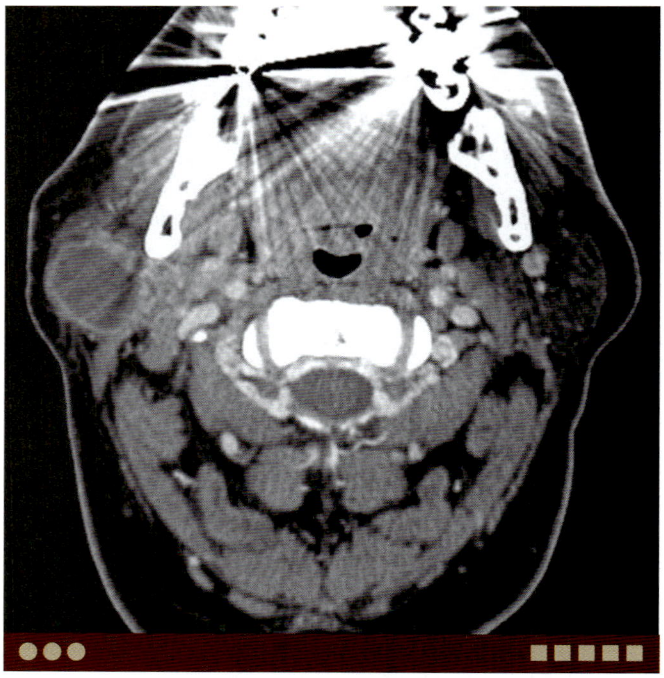

I. Mucoepidermoid carcinoma (high grade). Axial contrast-enhanced CT demonstrates a cystic mass with irregular rim-enhancement in the parotid gland. The lesion has infiltrative margins.

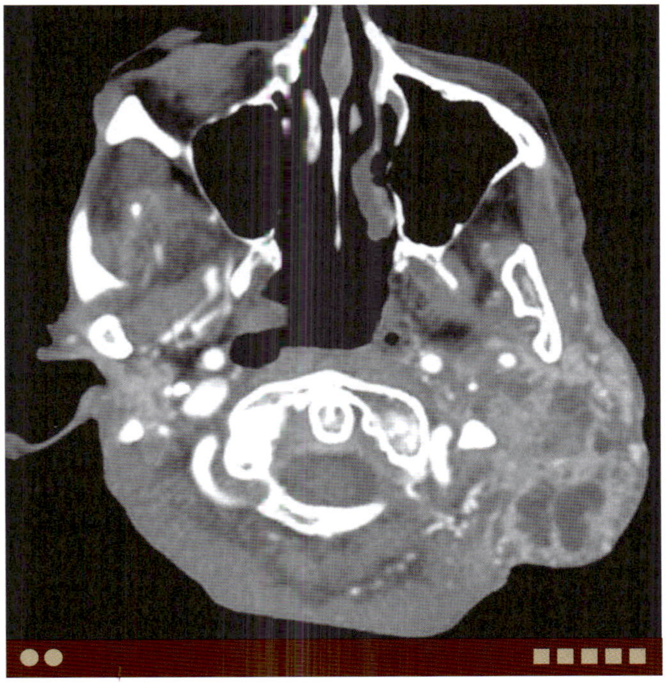

J. Squamous cell carcinoma. Axial contrast-enhanced CT demonstrates a large, poorly circumscribed, necrotic tumor in the left parotid gland. The tumor invades adjacent structures.

Case 7–6 Hemangioma

Naoko Saito, Asim Mian, Osamu Sakai

PRESENTATION

Unilateral parotid swelling.

FINDINGS

CT demonstrates enlargement of the parotid gland. Postcontrast images demonstrate avid enhancement.

DIFFERENTIAL DIAGNOSIS

- Lymphatic malformation (lymphangioma): This is one of the congenital low-flow vascular malformations. It demonstrates multiple intercommunicating cystic lesions with fluid–fluid levels, best seen on T2W images.
- Plexiform neurofibroma: This is pathognomonic for neurofibromatosis type I. The imaging finding may be very similar to vascular malformations and often involves more than one fascia-defined space. Mild enhancement is commonly seen after contrast.
- Parotitis: This is an acute infection of the parotid gland. Most bacterial infections occur unilaterally while viral infections usually occur bilaterally.

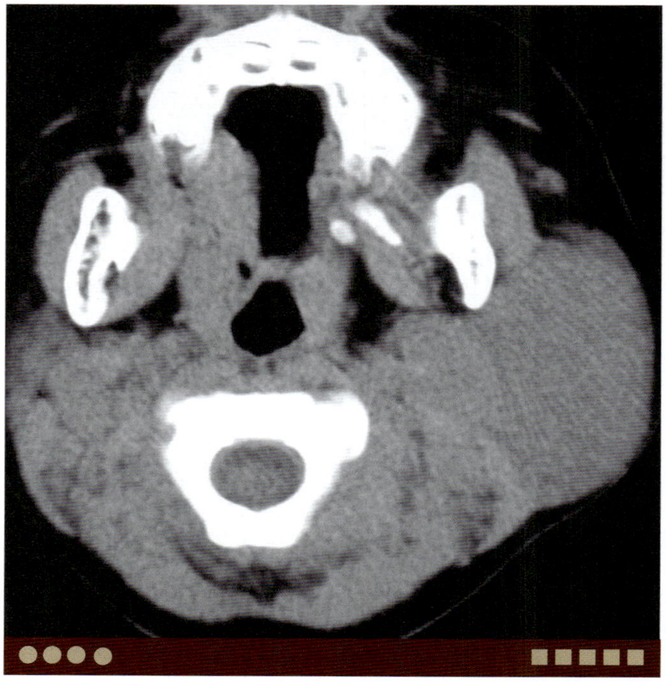

A. Hemangioma. Axial CT demonstrates a large, homogeneous, low-density lesion involving the entire left parotid gland.

COMMENTS

This is a 2-year-old boy with unilateral parotid swelling.

Hemangioma is the most common nonepithelial tumor of the salivary glands, furthermore, this is the most common salivary gland neoplasm in children. The majority of these lesions occur in parotid gland and involvement of submandibular gland is rare. Histologically, hemangiomas are classified into two types: capillary hemangioma and cavernous hemangioma.

Capillary hemangioma is composed of small capillary-sized vessels with plump endothelial cells. It represents 90% of parotid gland tumors in the first year of life and has a significant female predilection. Common clinical findings include unilateral, compressible, soft tissue mass with a bluish coloration in the overlying skin. Sometimes an associated hemangioma in the overlying skin is seen. Because most capillary hemangiomas regress spontaneously, surgery should be avoided and careful clinical follow-up is needed.

Cavernous hemangioma is composed of large, thin-walled vessels with flattened endothelial cells. It is often seen in older children and adults. Surgery is a treatment option because cavernous hemangioma does not regress spontaneously.

On CT, capillary hemangiomas tend to involve the entire parotid gland while cavernous hemangiomas usually demonstrate lobulated, enhancing masses. It may be seen to extend to the overlying skin. Very high signal on T2W image is a characteristic appearance. Postcontrast images usually demonstrate homogeneous enhancement.

PEARLS

- **Hemangioma is the most common salivary gland neoplasm in children.**
- **Capillary hemangioma is seen in the first year of life while cavernous hemangioma is seen in older children and adults.**
- **Capillary hemangiomas tend to involve the entire parotid gland while cavernous hemangiomas usually demonstrate lobulated, enhancing masses.**
- **Hemangioma demonstrates very high signal on T2W images.**

ADDITIONAL IMAGES (B-D)

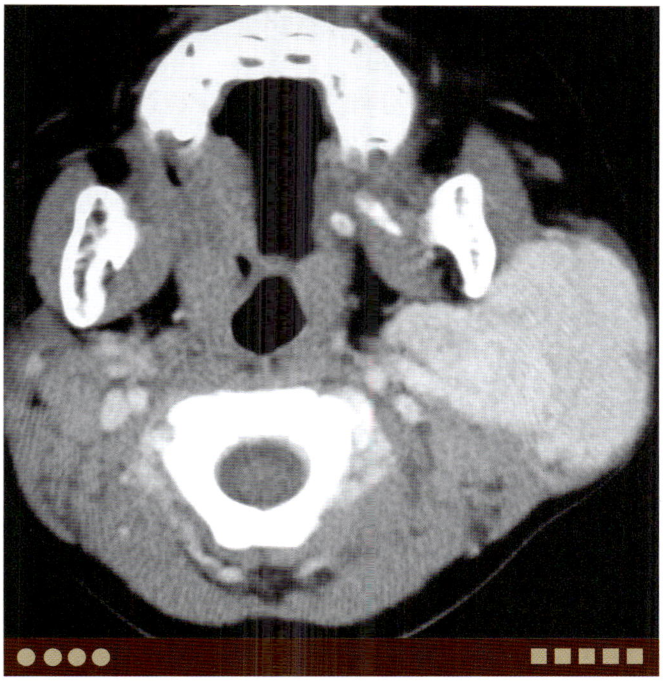

B. Hemangioma, same patient as A. Axial contrast-enhanced CT demonstrates strong, uniform enhancement within the lesion.

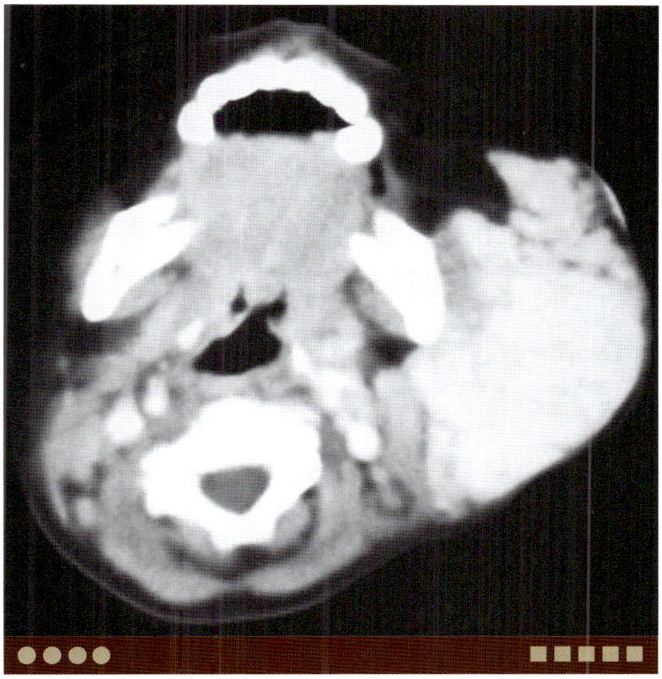

C. Hemangioma in a different patient (1-year-old infant). Axial contrast-enhanced CT demonstrates a large, avidly enhancing mass in the left parotid gland.

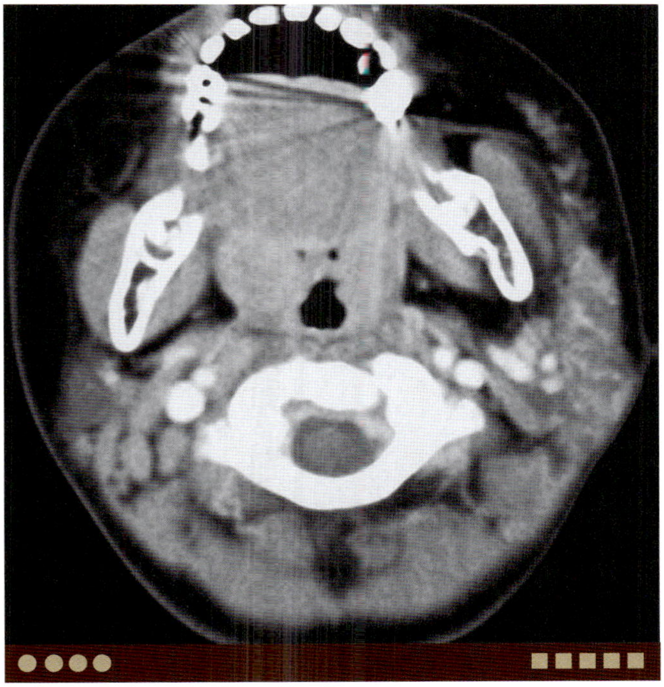

D. Hemangioma, same patient as C, at age 6. Axial contrast-enhanced CT demonstrates marked regression of the hemangioma.

DIFFERENTIAL DIAGNOSIS IMAGES (E-G)

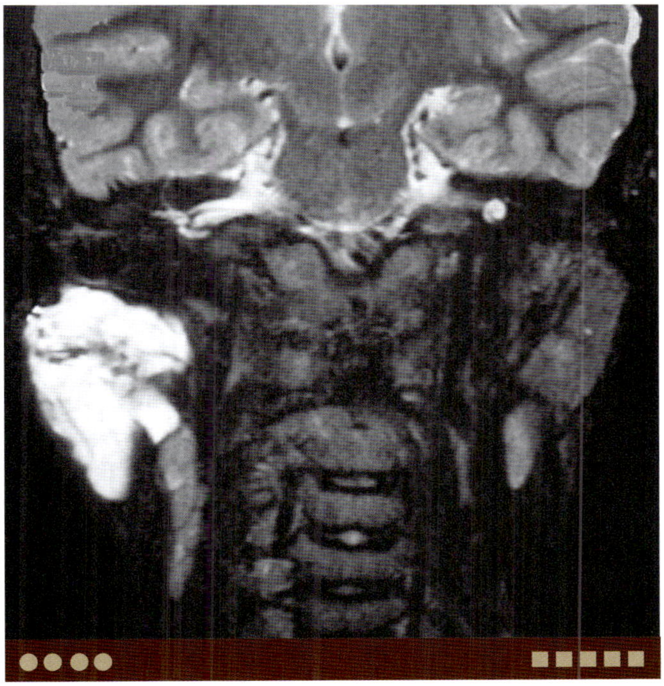

E. Lymphangioma. Coronal fat-suppressed T2W image demonstrates a lobulated, high-signal mass with septations in the right parotid gland. The lesion extends into the adjacent spaces.

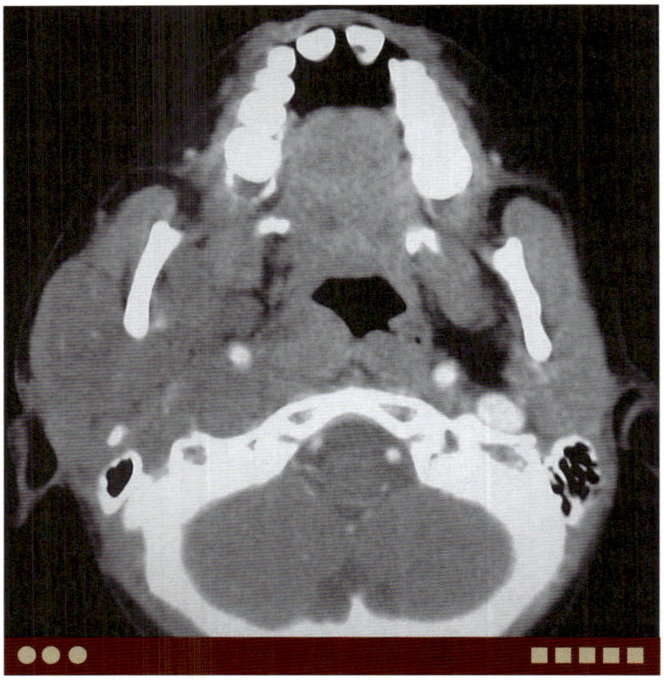

F. Plexiform neurofibroma. Axial contrast-enhanced CT demonstrates diffuse involvement of the right parotid gland by intermediate-density-lesion.

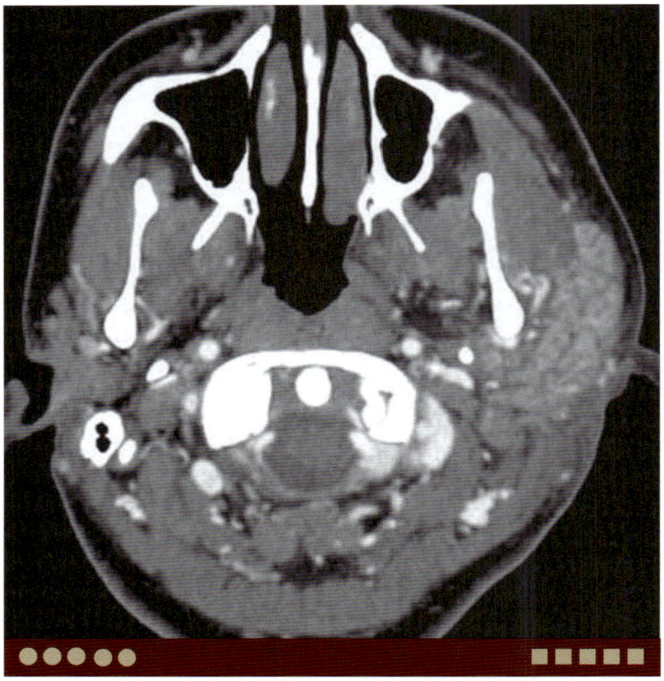

G. Acute parotitis. Axial contrast-enhanced CT demonstrates diffusely enlarged left parotid gland with enhancement. Fat stranding in the adjacent subcutaneous fat is noted.

Case 7–7 Lipoma

Naoko Saito, Asim Mian, Osamu Sakai

PRESENTATION

Parotid swelling.

FINDINGS

CT demonstrates a well-defined, fat density mass in the parotid gland.

DIFFERENTIAL DIAGNOSIS

- Liposarcoma: This tumor often demonstrates heterogeneous density or soft tissue component and infiltrative margins. Rapid increase in size and pain may be demonstrated.
- Fat deposition in the parotid gland: Fatty replacement can follow parenchymal atrophy from any causes including Sjögren's syndrome and infection. Overgrowth of fatty tissue in the parotid gland may result from diabetes mellitus or severe obesity.

COMMENTS

This is a 50-year-old woman with right parotid gland swelling.

Lipoma is a benign mesenchymal neoplasm composed of mature fat. Lipomas represent approximately about 1% of parotid gland tumors. They can arise either within the parotid gland or in the immediate periparotid region and usually it is impossible to distinguish the primary location. Radiologically, it is often difficult to detect the capsule; however, it is easily delineated from the adjacent structures.

Typically lipoma demonstrates well-defined, homogeneous, low density on CT and high signal on T1W MR images corresponding to mature fat. It sometimes demonstrates slightly heterogeneous intermediate signal on T2W image. On fat-suppressed image, significant signal loss is seen.

Rarely, lipomas show poorly defined margins, which are either infiltrating lipoma or occurring as a part of multiple systemic lipomatosis. Infiltrating lipoma may insinuate into the adjacent muscles and can cause hemorrhage and fibrotic changes. Multiple systemic lipomatosis causes diffuse fatty deposition throughout cervical regions. These lesions are not encapsulated.

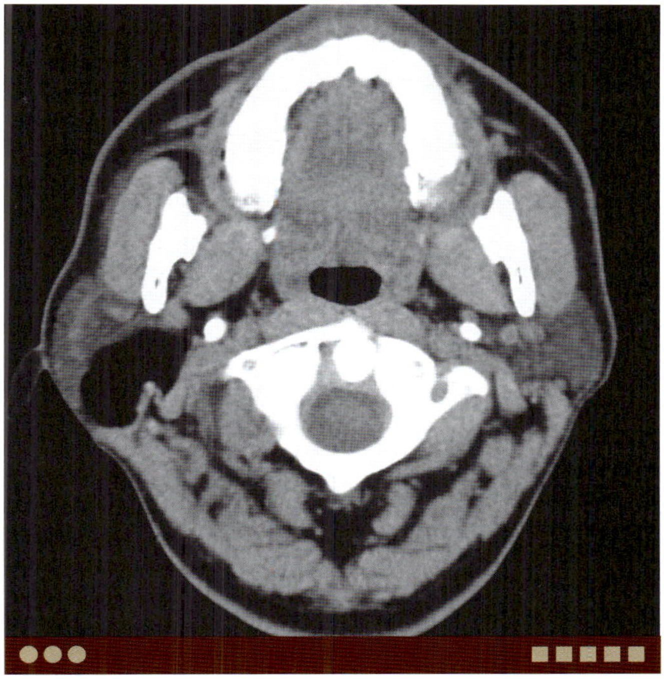

A. Lipoma. Axial CT demonstrates a well-defined, homogeneous, fat density mass in the parotid gland.

Differentiating from liposarcoma is important. Well-differentiated liposarcoma has similar appearance to the ordinary lipoma; however, there are several diagnostic clues. If a lipomatous mass shows a rapid increase in size or has an overall heterogeneously dense matrix, liposarcoma should be considered.

PEARLS

- **Lipoma consists about 1% of parotid gland tumors.**
- **Lipoma demonstrates well-defined, homogeneously low density on CT and high signal on T1W MR images corresponding to mature fat.**
- **Rapid increase in size or overall heterogeneously dense matrix in the lipomatous tumor suggests liposarcoma.**

ADDITIONAL IMAGES (B-D)

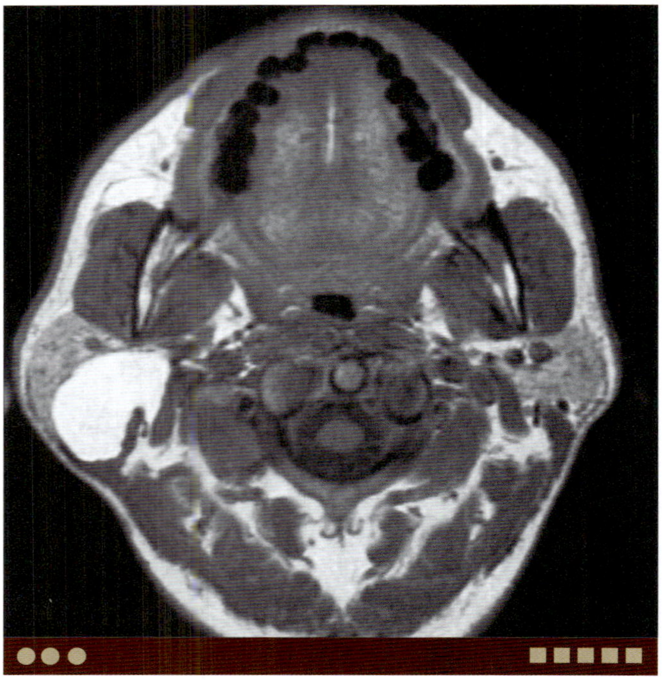

B. Lipoma, same patient as A. Axial T1W MR image demonstrates homogeneously high signal in the lesion.

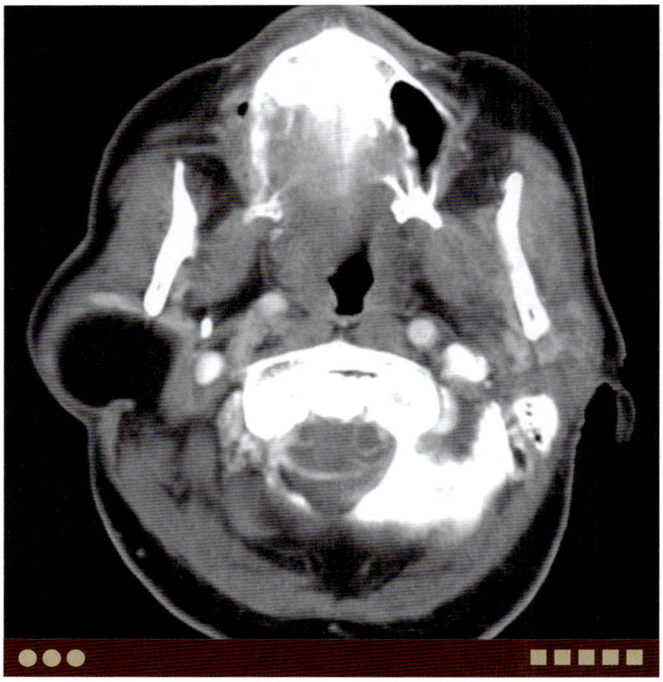

C. Lipoma in a different patient. Axial contrast-enhanced CT demonstrates a well-defined, fat density mass in the parotid gland. There is no enhancing area in the mass.

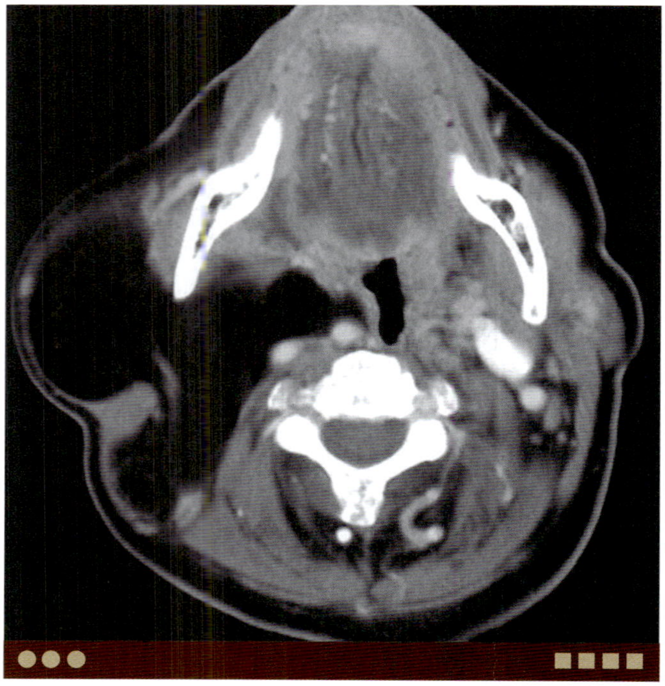

D. Lipoma, same patient as C. Axial contrast-enhanced CT demonstrates the lipomatous lesion also involves parapharyngeal and posterior cervical spaces.

DIFFERENTIAL DIAGNOSIS IMAGES (E-F)

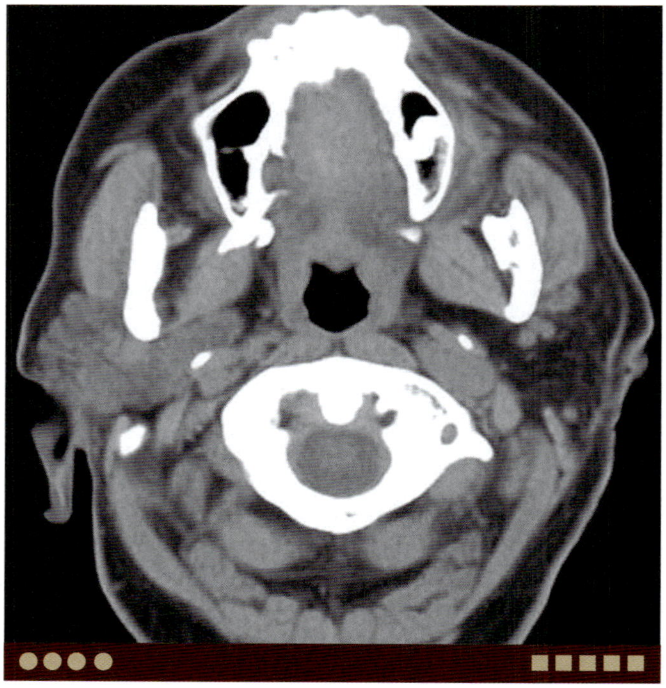

E. Fatty atrophy of the parotid gland. Axial noncontrast CT demonstrates fatty replacement in the left parotid gland. The gland is smaller compared with the right.

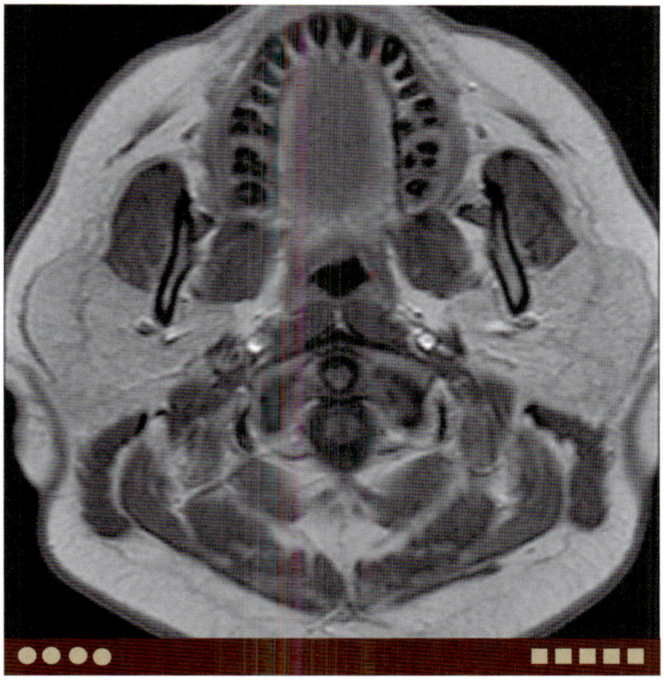

F. Diffuse fatty deposition. Axial T1W image demonstrates enlarged bilateral parotid glands with diffuse high signal.

Case 7-8 Lymphangioma—Parotid Gland

Naoko Saito, Asim Mian, Osamu Sakai

PRESENTATION

Unilateral parotid swelling.

FINDINGS

MRI demonstrates multiple intercommunicating cystic lesions in the parotid gland.

DIFFERENTIAL DIAGNOSIS

- Hemangioma: This is the most common salivary gland neoplasm in children. Very high signal is seen on T2W MR images like lymphangiomas, however, hemangiomas enhance after contrast.
- Branchial cleft cyst: The first branchial cleft cyst occurs close to or in the parotid gland.
- Pleomorphic adenoma: This tumor usually occurs in women in their forties and fifties. Gradual enhancement is a characteristic feature on contrast-enhanced imaging.

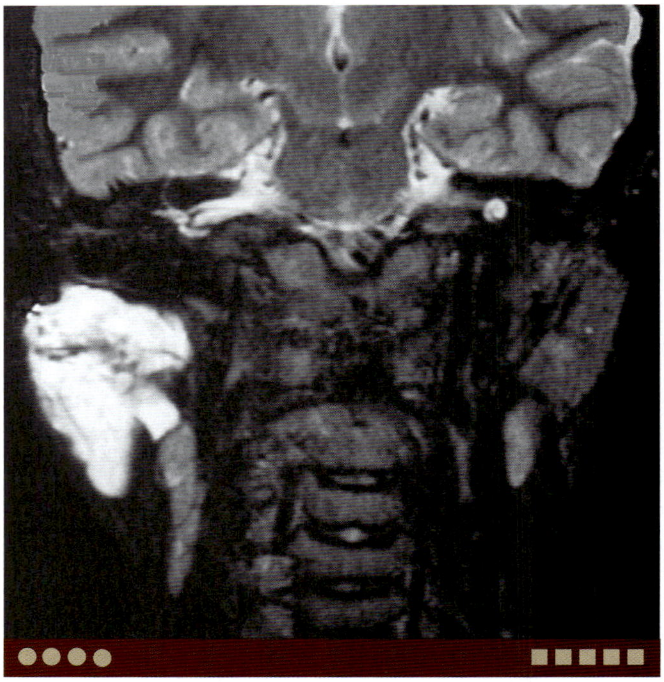

A. Lymphangioma. Coronal fat-suppressed T2W MR image demonstrates multi-lobulated, high-signal mass with septi in the right parotid gland. The lesion extends into the adjacent spaces.

COMMENTS

This is a 10-year-old boy with parotid swelling.

Lymphangiomas are congenital lymphatic malformations, one of the low-flow vascular malformations. They represent 5% to 6% of benign tumors in infancy and childhood and 80% to 90% of the patients are detected by the age of 2 years. The majority of these lesions occur in the head and neck, especially in the posterior triangle of the neck. They can involve the parotid and submandibular glands, muscles, and vessels.

Lymphangiomas are classified into three types: lymphangioma simplex, cavernous lymphangioma, and cystic lymphangioma (or cystic hygroma). In the head and neck, cystic lymphangiomas are the most common. These lesions can demonstrate from one cystic mass to multiple intercommunicating cystic masses.

Typically, lymphangioma demonstrates multiple intercommunicating cystic lesions with low signal on T1W image and high signal on T2W image. Within the cysts, fluid–fluid levels are often seen on T2W image reflecting hemorrhage or difference in protein or lipid concentration. On CT, these lesions are usually homogeneous low-density areas because the thin walls are not seen clearly. After contrast, enhancement of thin walls or septi may be seen. Thicker, solid-like enhancement suggests coexisting venous malformation (hemangioma) components. Further, infection may cause heterogeneous enhancement, often with inflammatory changes in the surrounding soft tissues.

Common clinical symptoms of lymphangioma in the parotid region include painless, soft mass and facial asymmetry. Sudden enlargement is often associated with infection or hemorrhage.

PEARLS

- **Eighty percent to 90% of lymphangiomas are diagnosed by the age of 2 years.**
- **Lymphangiomas often involve the adjacent tissues and spaces.**
- **Lymphangiomas demonstrate multiple intercommunicating cystic lesions with fluid–fluid levels, best seen on T2W MR images.**

ADDITIONAL IMAGES (B-F)

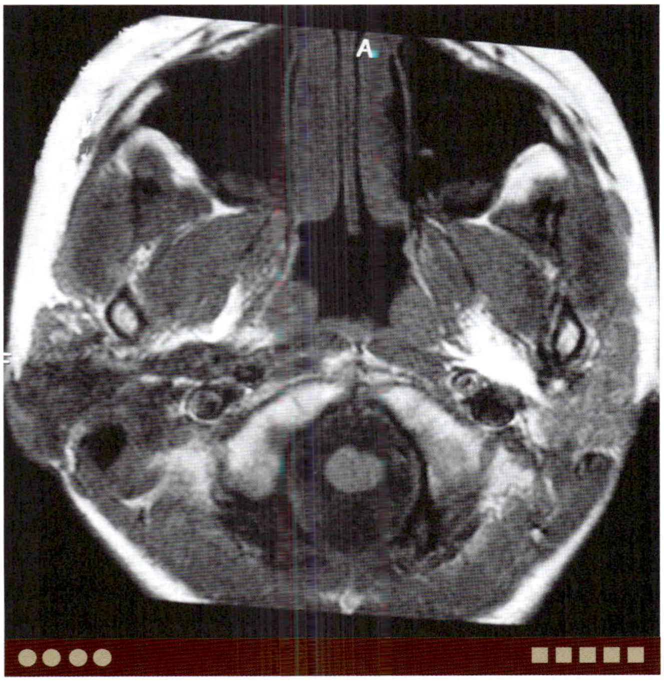

B. Lymphangioma, same patient as A. Axial T1W image demonstrates a low-signal mass in the posterior portion of the parotid gland.

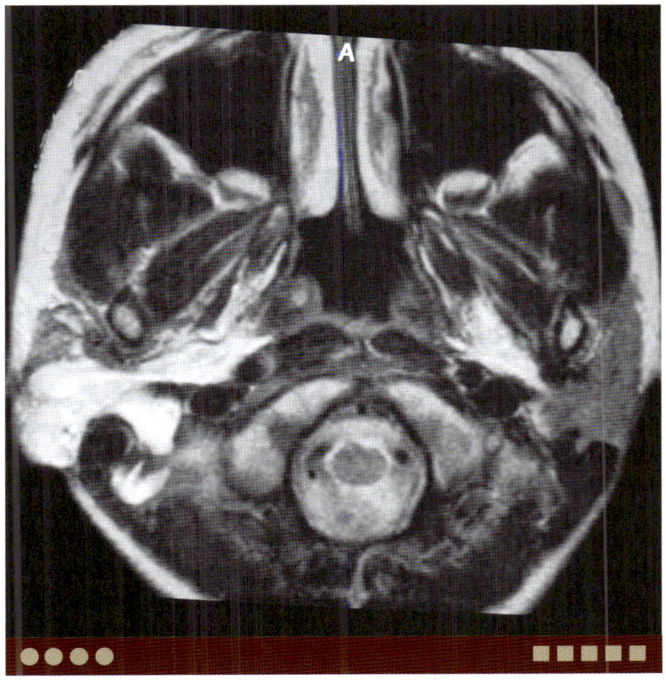

C. Lymphangioma, same patient as A. Axial T2W image demonstrates a high-signal mass extending into the parapharyngeal space.

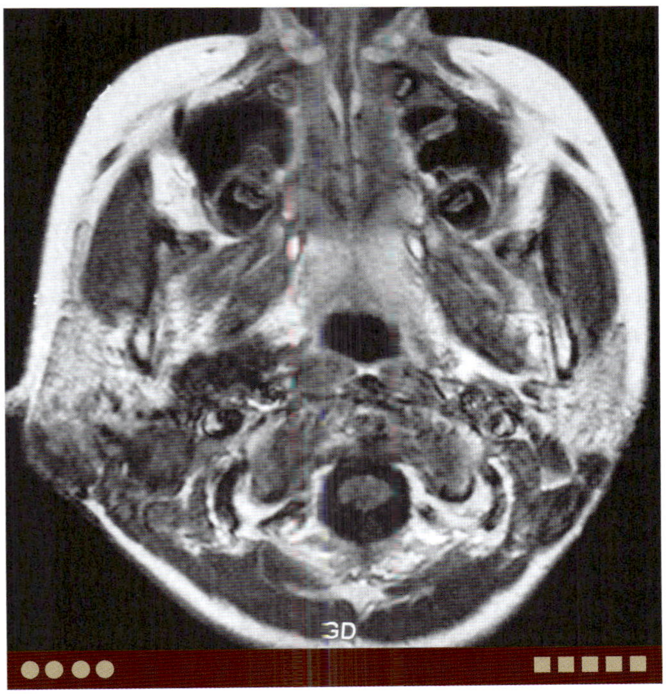

D. Lymphangioma, same patient as A. Axial contrast-enhanced T1W image demonstrates subtle enhancement of the cyst wall of the lesion without solid or thick enhancement.

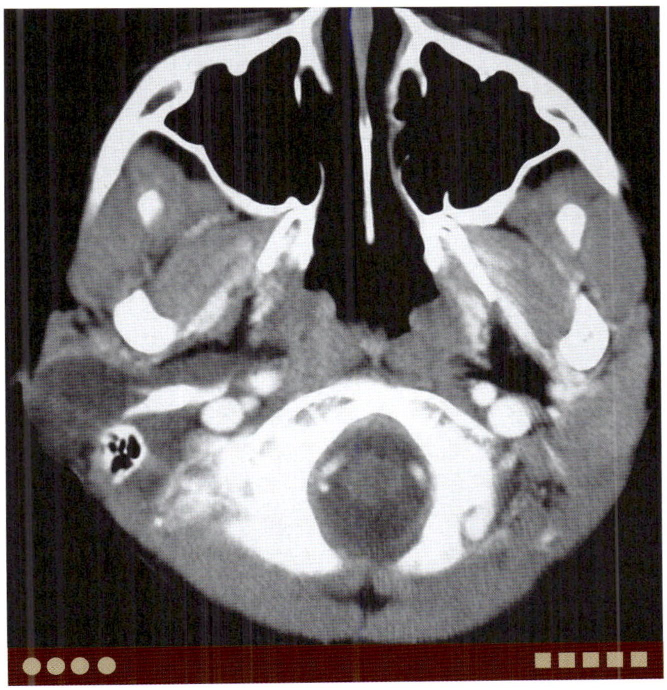

E. Lymphangioma, same patient as A. Axial contrast-enhanced CT demonstrates a low-density cystic-appearing lesion in the right parotid gland extending into the parapharyngeal space.

DIFFERENTIAL DIAGNOSIS IMAGES (G-H)

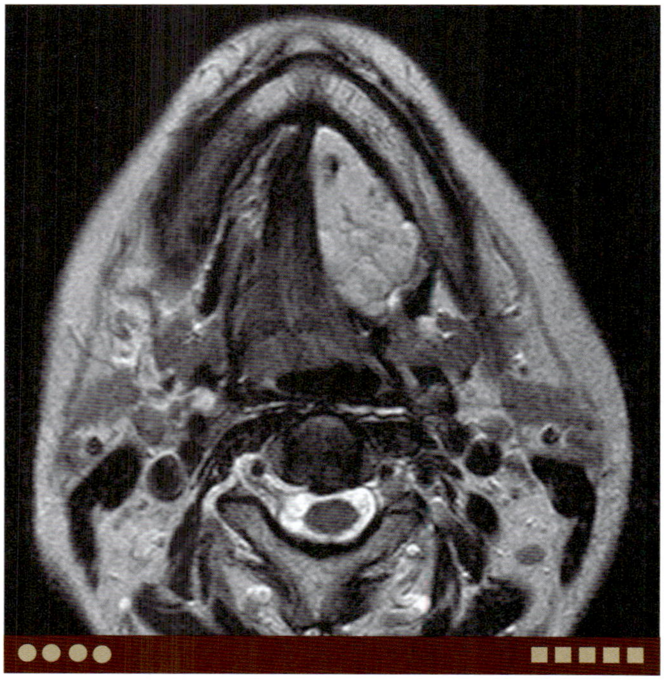

F. Lymphangioma of the sublingual space in a different patient. Axial T2W image demonstrates a multicystic high-signal lesion in the left sublingual space.

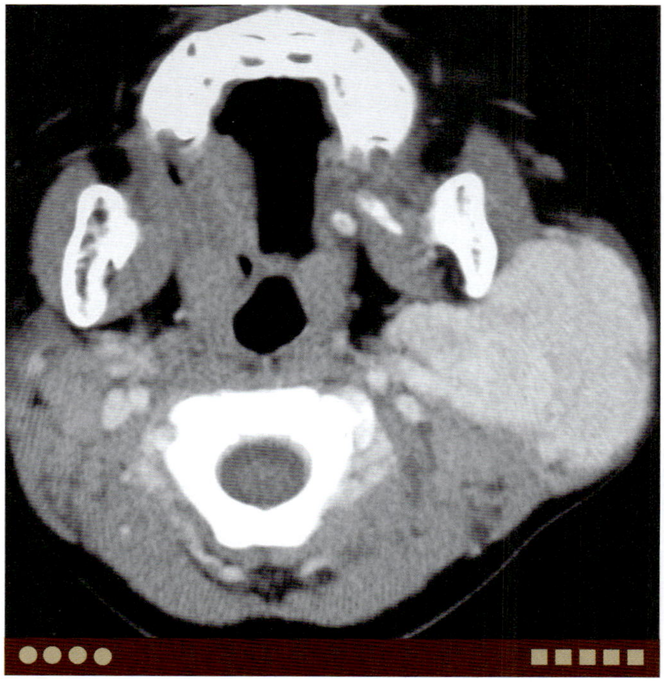

G. Hemangioma. Axial contrast-enhanced CT demonstrates a well-defined enhancing mass in the parotid gland.

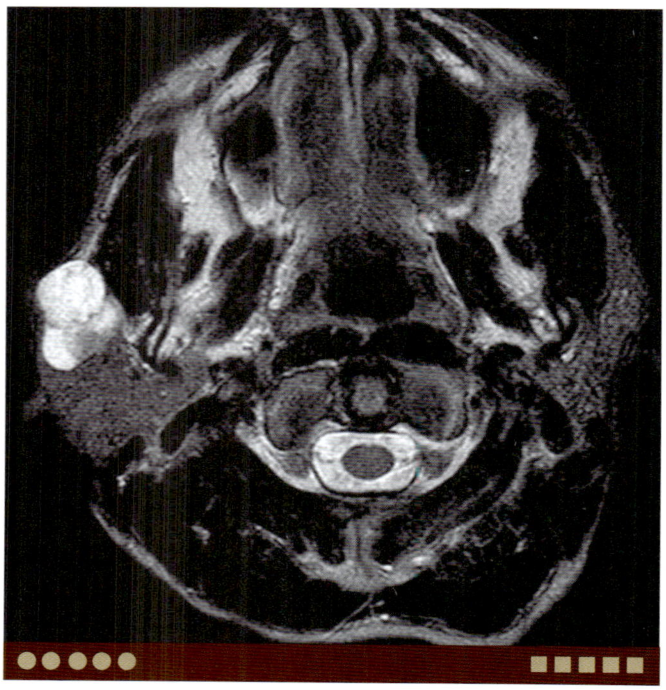

H. Pleomorphic adenoma. Axial T2W MR image demonstrates a well-defined, lobulated, and multicystic high-signal lesion in the parotid gland.

Case 7–9 Lymphoma—Parotid

Naoko Saito, Asim Mian, Osamu Sakai

PRESENTATION

Unilateral parotid swelling.

FINDINGS

CT demonstrates a well-circumscribed mass in the parotid gland.

DIFFERENTIAL DIAGNOSIS

- Warthin's tumor: This usually occurs in elderly men and often multiple and bilateral. Lesions are predominantly seen in the inferior portion of the parotid gland.
- Intra-/periparotid lymph nodes: Lymph nodes are usually multiple and small and located in the superficial lobe of the parotid gland and demonstrate similar density or signal to other nodes outside of the gland.
- Lymphoepithelial lesions associated with HIV infection: Lesions are usually multiple and bilateral, and solid and cystic. Sometimes they demonstrate similar appearance to Warthin's tumor. The patient's HIV status should be determined.

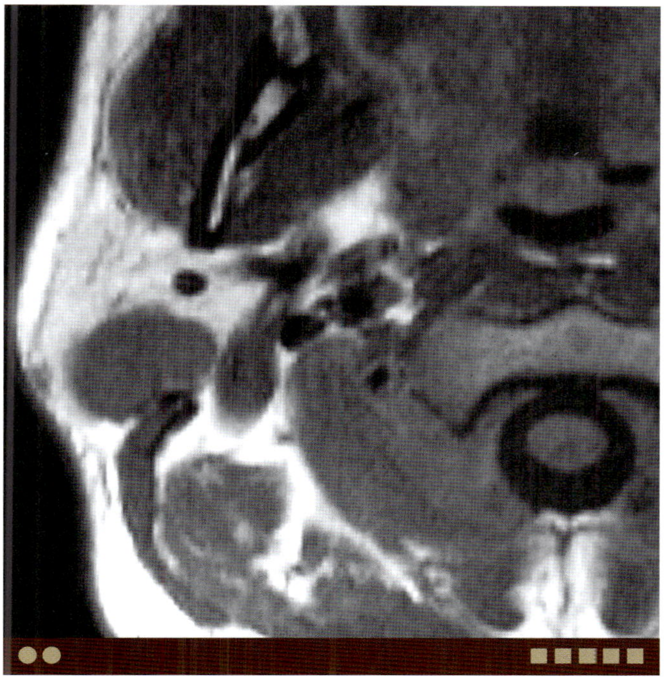

A. Primary lymphoma. Axial T1W image demonstrates a well-circumscribed, homogeneous low-signal mass in the posterior portion of the right parotid gland.

COMMENTS

This is a 40-year-old man with a unilateral parotid mass.

Lymphomas of the parotid gland are classified into two groups: primary lymphoma and secondary involvement due to systemic non-Hodgkin lymphoma.

Primary lymphoma of the salivary glands is very rare. About 80% of them occur in the parotid gland and are often seen in elderly people. These lymphomas are classified as mucosa-associated lymphoid tissue (MALT) lymphomas. The lesions can arise either in the intraparotid lymph node or parenchyma. Primary lymphoma has been reported to be accompanied with or arise from autoimmune disorders especially Sjögren's syndrome.

Secondary lymphoma in the parotid gland occurs in 1% to 8% of lymphomas and is most commonly seen with high-grade, diffuse large cell lymphoma. These lymphomas involve intraparotid lymph node as well as other cervical lymph nodes. Bilateral parotid gland involvement is sometimes seen. Identification of extraparotid nodal disease may be helpful in suggesting secondary lymphoma in the parotid gland.

On CT, lymphoma demonstrates a well-circumscribed homogeneous mass corresponding to enlarged intraparotid lymph node. In secondary lymphoma, multiple intraparotid masses with extraparotid lymphadenopathy are often seen. Typically, the mass demonstrates mild homogeneous enhancement, however, nodal necrosis may occur. On MRI, lymphoma demonstrates homogeneous intermediated intensity on all sequences. After contrast, lymphoma usually demonstrates mild homogeneous enhancement. If lymphoma involves the parenchyma, a diffuse infiltrative pattern with poorly defined margins or involvement of the entire gland is seen.

PEARLS

- **Primary lymphoma of the salivary glands is very rare.**
- **Lymphoma may be accompanied with or arise from autoimmune disease especially Sjögren's syndrome.**
- **In secondary lymphoma, multiple intraparotid lesions with adjacent extraparotid lymphadenopathy are often seen.**
- **Lymphoma demonstrates homogeneous intermediate signal on all MR imaging sequences.**

ADDITIONAL IMAGES (B-G)

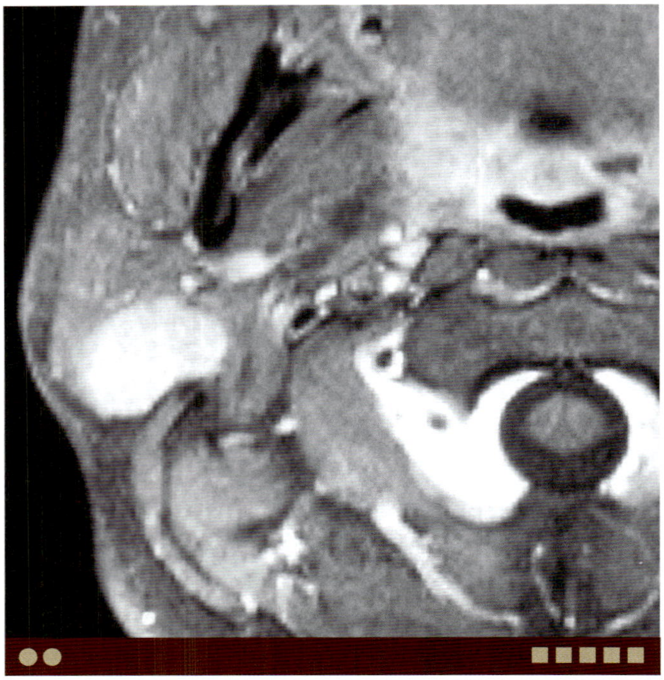

B. Primary lymphoma, same patient as A. Axial postcontrast fat-suppressed T1W image demonstrates homogeneous enhancement in the lesion.

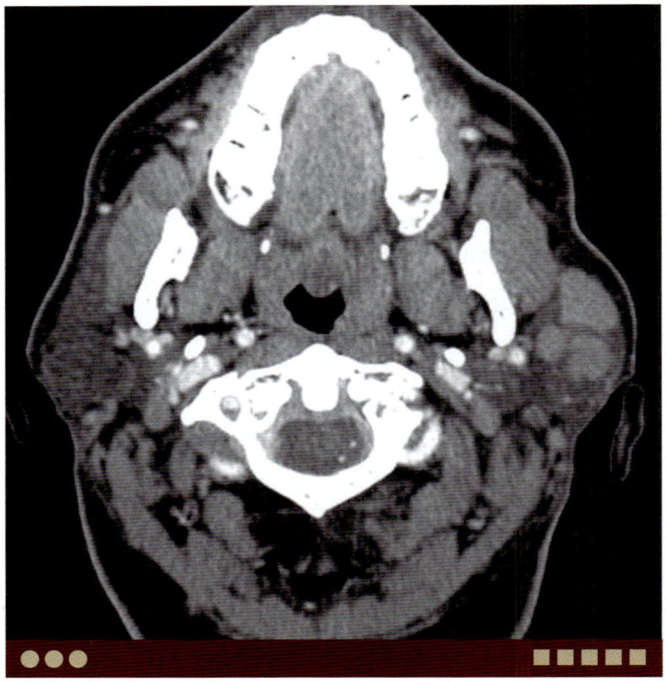

C. Secondary lymphoma. Axial contrast-enhanced CT demonstrates multiple masses with homogeneous enhancement in the left parotid gland.

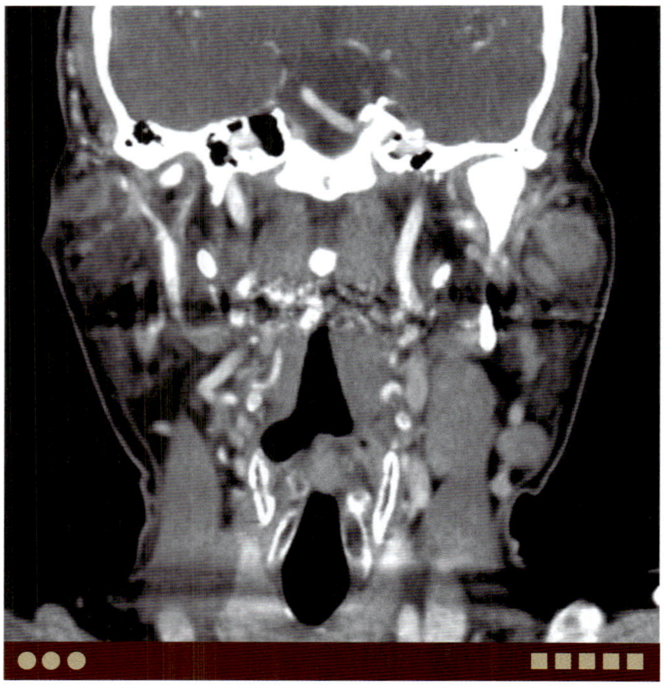

D. Secondary lymphoma, same patient as C. Coronal contrast-enhanced CT demonstrates multiple masses in the left parotid gland with cervical lymphadenopathy.

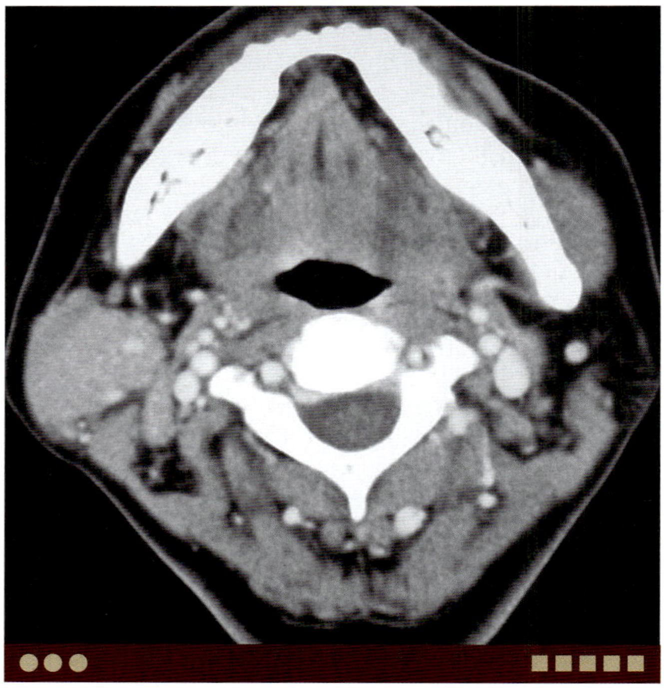

E. Lymphoma arising from Sjögren's syndrome. Axial contrast-enhanced CT demonstrates a homogeneously enhancing mass in the right parotid gland.

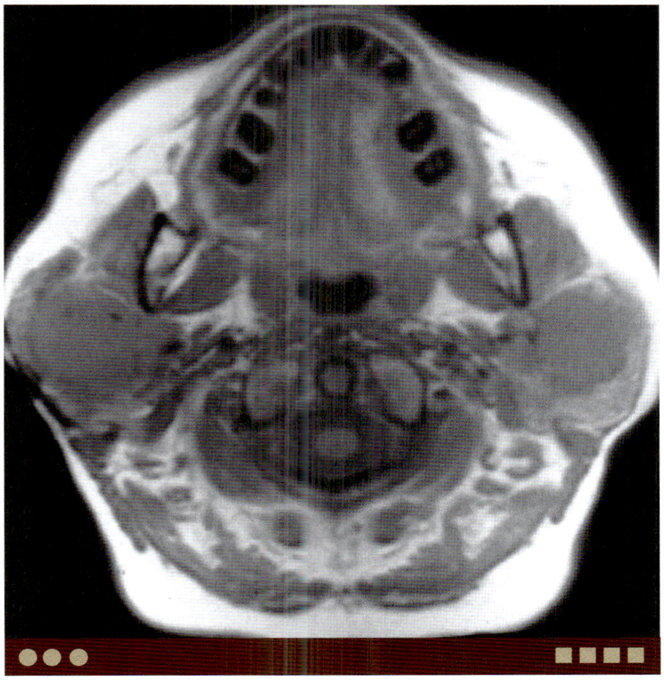

F. Lymphoma arising from Sjögren's syndrome in a different patient. Axial T1W image demonstrates homogeneous low-signal masses in the bilateral parotid gland.

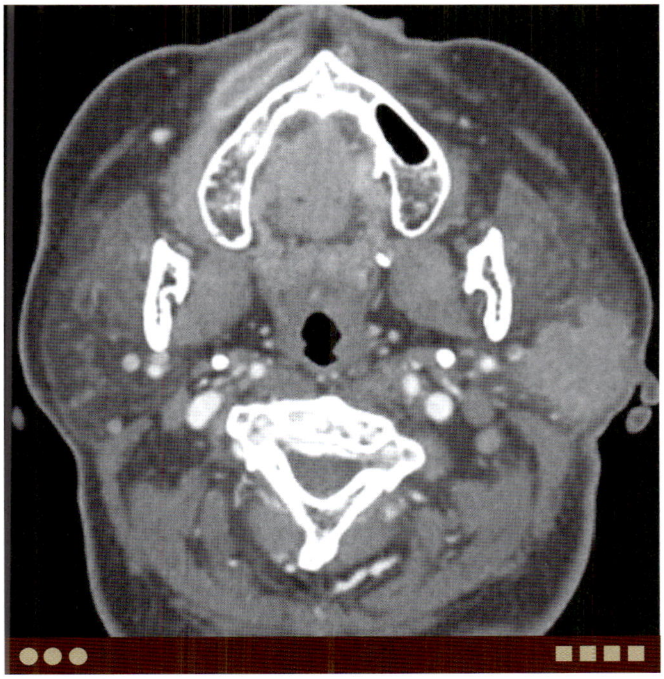

G. Hodgkin's lymphoma. Coronal contrast-enhanced CT demonstrates a homogeneous low-signal mass involving the left parotid gland.

DIFFERENTIAL DIAGNOSIS IMAGES (H-I)

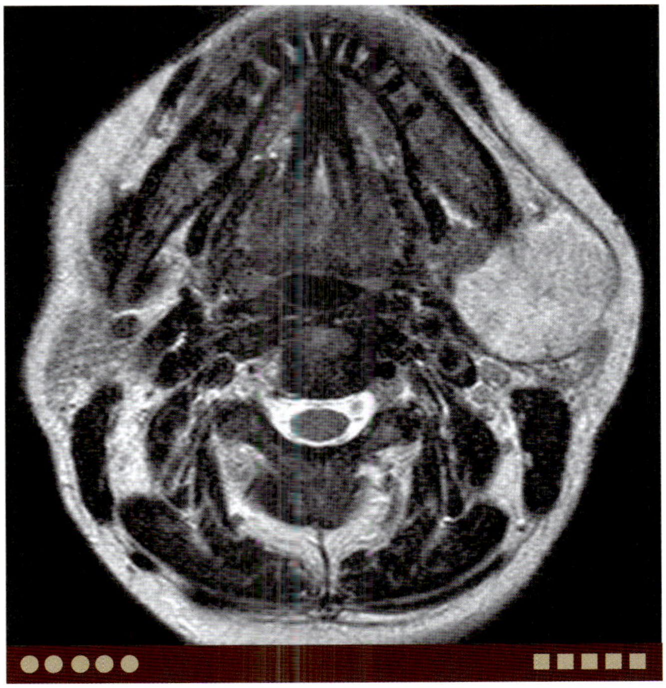

H. Warthin's tumor. Axial T2W image demonstrates a relatively homogeneous intermediate-to-high signal mass in the inferior portion of the parotid gland.

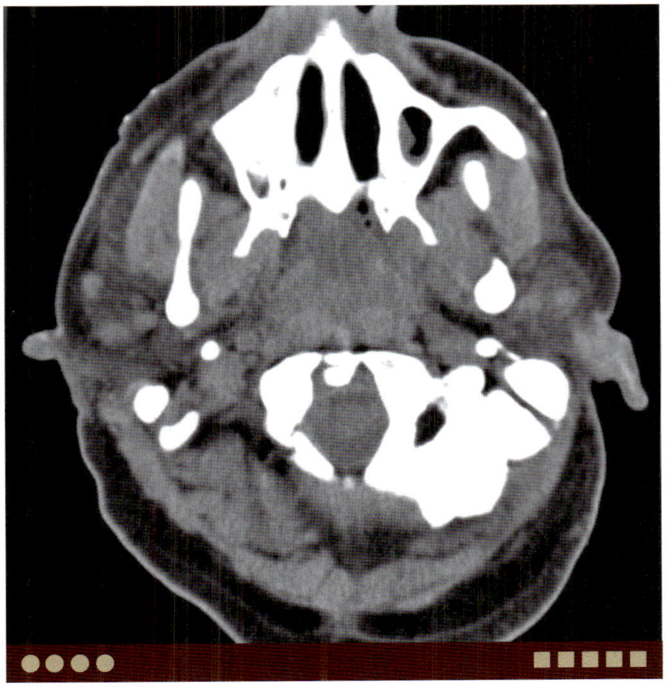

I. Lymphoepithelial lesions associated with HIV infection. Axial noncontrast CT demonstrates multiple nodular or cystic lesions in the bilateral parotid glands. Note enlarged adenoids.

Case 7–10 Sjögren's Syndrome

Akifumi Fujita, Naoko Saito, Asim Mian, Osamu Sakai

PRESENTATION

Bilateral parotid gland swelling and dry eye.

FINDINGS

CT shows bilateral parotid gland enlargement and heterogeneously increased density with punctuate calcification. MRI demonstrates diffuse multiple solid and cystic lesions in the bilateral parotid gland.

DIFFERENTIAL DIAGNOSIS

- Lymphoepithelial lesions associated with HIV: This condition shows mixed solid and cystic lesions within enlarged parotid glands, commonly associated with cervical lymphadenopathy and adenoid enlargement.
- Sarcoidosis: This is a systemic disease characterized by noncaseating granulomas. The parotid glands are affected in 10% to 30 % of patients. Multiple granulomas within bilateral enlarged parotid glands are sometimes seen.
- Warthin's tumor: This condition is occasionally multiple and bilateral. Tumor may be heterogeneous and may have cystic change.
- Lymphoma: Patients with Sjögren's syndrome have increased risk to develop lymphoma. This is the most common malignant tumor which presents as multiple and bilateral lesions in the parotid glands.

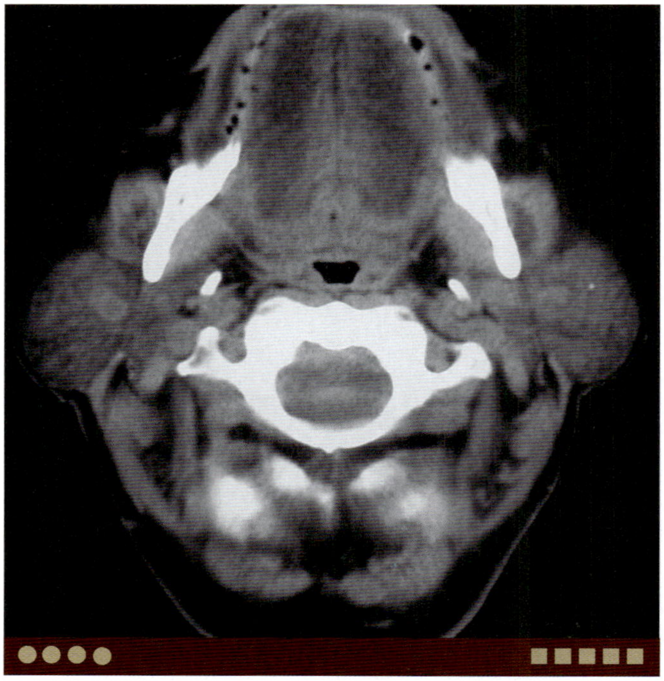

A. Sjögren's syndrome. Axial CT demonstrates enlarged bilateral parotid glands with slight fatty infiltration and heterogeneous density. A small calcification is noted.

COMMENTS

This is a 63-year-old man with increasing bilateral parotid swelling. He has a 20-year history of dry eye and Sjögren's syndrome was diagnosed recently.

Sjögren's syndrome is an autoimmune disorder of the exocrine glands that occurs either alone (*primary*) or with any of the connective tissue diseases (*secondary*). Secondary Sjögren's syndrome consists about 60% of all patients with Sjögren's syndrome and most of them have rheumatoid arthritis.

Xerostomia, keratoconjunctivitis sicca, and a connective tissue disease are the three major clinical presentations. Sjögren's syndrome is most commonly diagnosed in women in their forties and fifties; however, there is a slight male predominance in juvenile Sjögren's syndrome.

Histologically, it is characterized by periductal lymphocytic aggregates that extend into and destroy the salivary acinar parenchyma. Lymphoid infiltrate produces benign lymphoepithelial lesions. These show the same appearance as lymphoepithelial lesions associated with HIV. However, cervical lymphadenopathy and nasopharyngeal lymphoid enlargement are rare in Sjögren's syndrome.

In the early stages, CT and MRI are often negative. As the disease progresses, bilateral parotid enlargement and heterogeneously increased density becomes apparent. Punctate calcification may be present. Heterogeneous enhancement of the gland with solid and cystic parotid lesions is often seen. T1W MR images demonstrate a mixture of high and low signal in the parotid gland, representing fat deposition and inflammation of the gland respectively. T2W images show diffuse multiple high signal foci in the parotid gland. In the late stage, the glands become atrophic and fatty. Also, lymphoepithelial lesions develop, which demonstrate multiple bilateral well-circumscribed cystic lesions in the glands. MR sialography may be helpful to demonstrate punctuate, globular, cavitary, or destructive parotid distal ductal changes within the parotid gland.

There is a higher risk of lymphoma in patients with Sjögren's syndrome. Lymphomas developing in Sjögren's syndrome are classified as MALT (mucosa-associated lymphoid tissue) lymphomas.

PEARLS

- **CT demonstrates heterogeneous fatty and nodular density in enlarged parotid glands.**
- **MRI can demonstrate diffuse cystic and solid lesions in the parotid gland.**
- **Non-Hodgkin lymphoma may arise from Sjögren's syndrome.**

ADDITIONAL IMAGES (B-E)

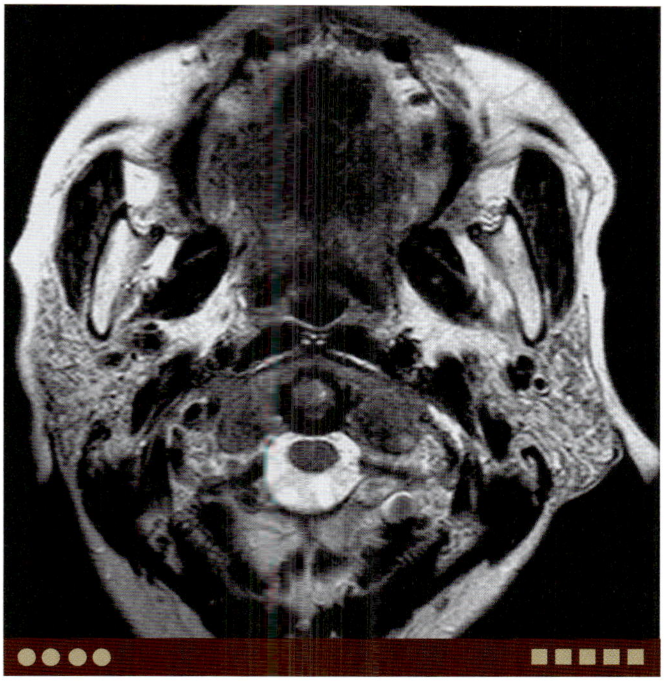

B. Sjögren's syndrome in a different patient. Axial T2W image demonstrates heterogeneous signal in the bilateral parotid glands.

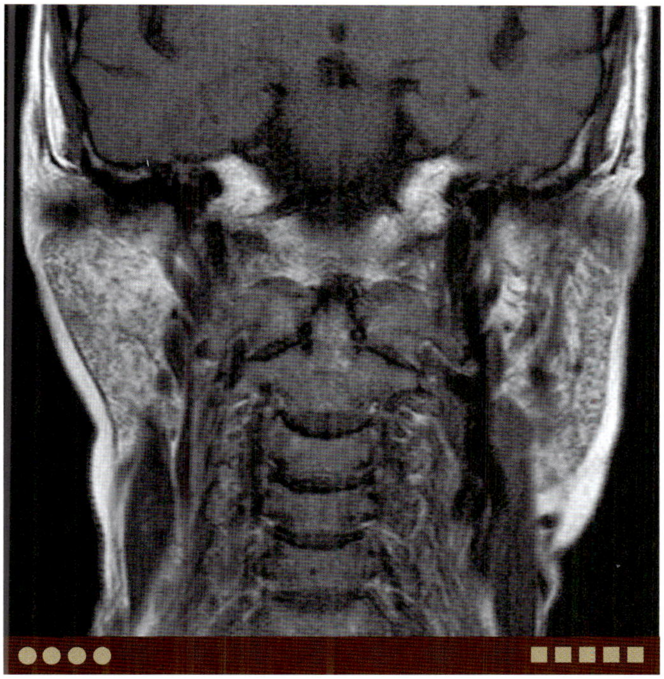

C. Sjögren's syndrome, same patient as B. Coronal T1W image demonstrates multiple small nodular lesions and diffuse fatty infiltration in the bilateral parotid glands.

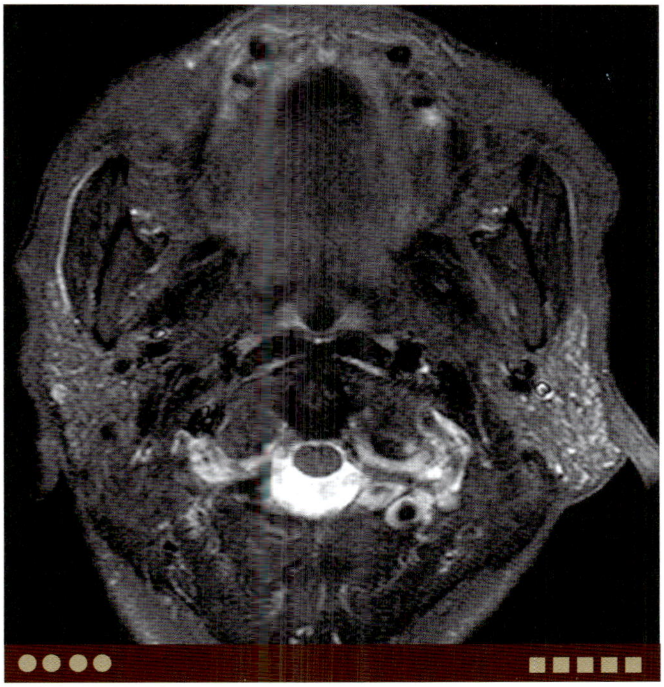

D. Sjögren's syndrome, same patient as B. Axial fat-suppressed T2W image demonstrates diffuse fatty glandular change and multiple small cystic lesions in the bilateral parotid glands.

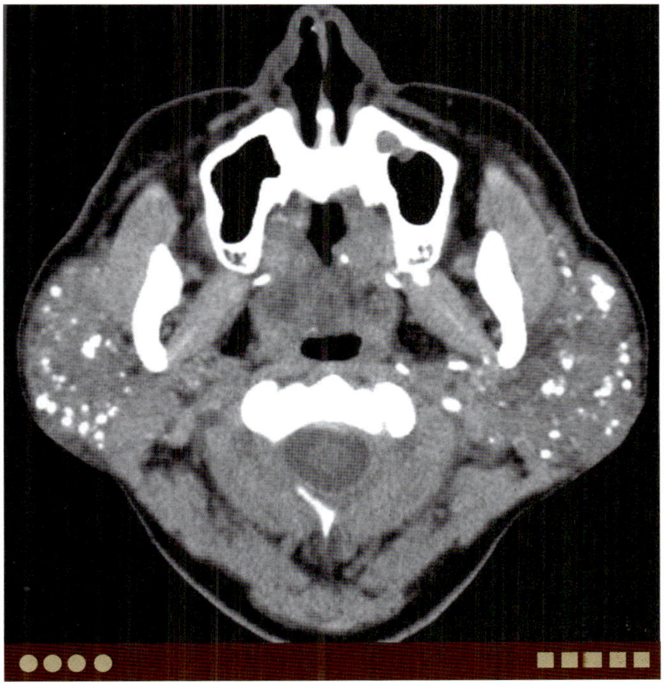

E. Sjögren's syndrome in a different patient. Axial CT demonstrates bilateral parotid swelling with increased nodular density and multiple punctuate calcification.

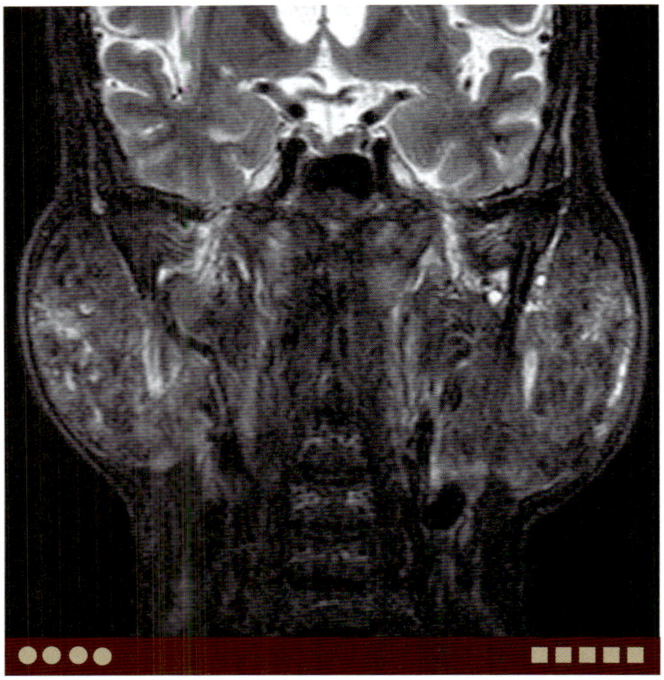

F. Sjögren's syndrome, same patient as E. Coronal STIR image demonstrates multiple high intensity foci in significantly enlarged parotid glands.

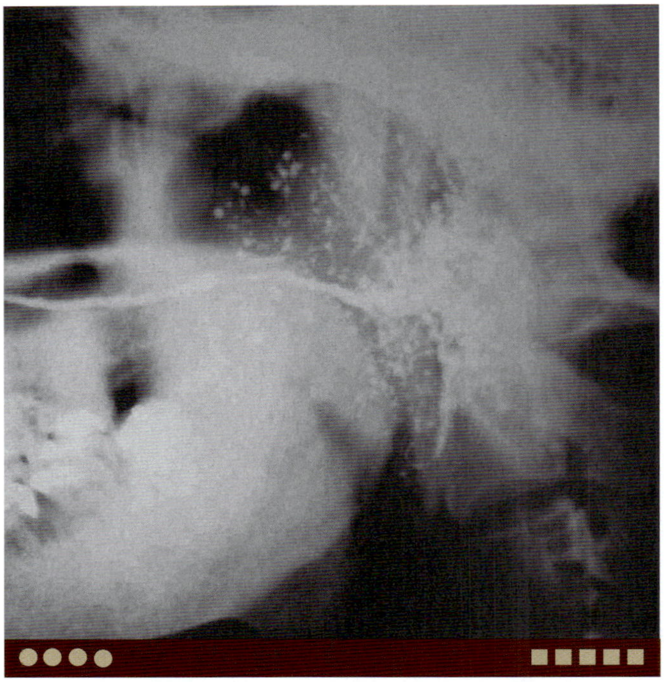

G. Sjögren's syndrome in a different patient. Parotid sialogram demonstrates multiple punctuate collections in the gland. This is a characteristic sialographic appearance which is referred as "apple-tree," "leafless fruit-laden–tree," or "mulberry-tree" appearance.

DIFFERENTIAL DIAGNOSIS IMAGES (H-J)

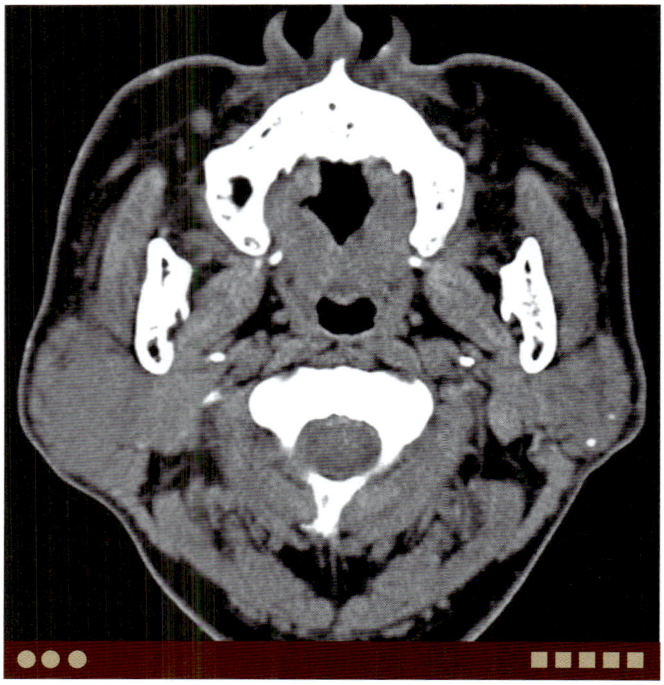

H. Lymphoma in Sjögren's syndrome. Axial noncontrast CT shows a homogeneous solid mass in the right parotid gland. Heterogeneous nodular density and punctuate calcification are noted in the left parotid gland.

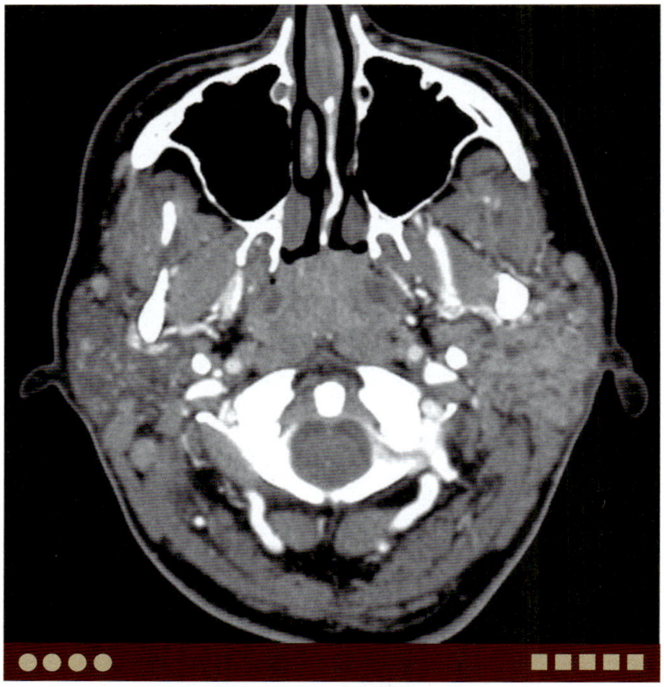

I. Lymphoepithelial lesions associated with HIV. Axial contrast-enhanced CT demonstrates multiple cystic and nodular lesions in the bilateral parotid glands. Note enlarged adenoids.

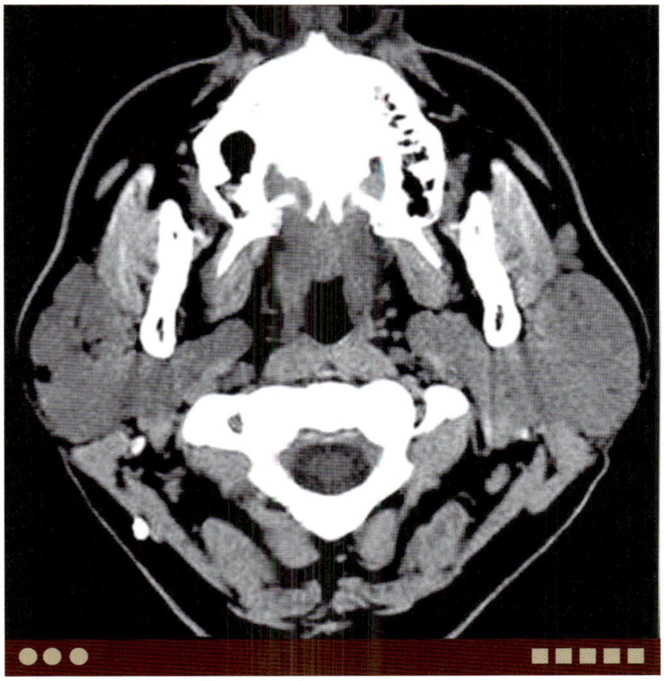

J. Sarcoidosis. Axial noncontrast CT demonstrates enlarged bilateral parotid glands.

Case 7-11 Kimura Disease

Misako Takeuchi, Akifumi Fujita, Asim Mian, Osamu Sakai

PRESENTATION

Swelling of the parotid gland with lymphadenopathy.

FINDINGS

MRI demonstrates an ill-defined lesion in the parotid gland and multiple enlarged cervical lymph nodes.

DIFFERENTIAL DIAGNOSIS

- Malignant salivary gland tumor: Malignant tumors tend to progress more rapidly than Kimura disease and facial nerve palsy is more common with malignant tumors.
- Lymphoma: Primary lymphoma of the parotid gland is rare. However, parotid glands are often involved secondary to systemic involvement.
- Sarcoidosis: This often demonstrates bilateral parotid glands swelling and enlargement of bilateral intra-/peri-parotid lymph nodes as well as cervical lymphadenopathy.
- Sjögren's syndrome: This condition usually shows multiple cystic and solid nodular lesions within enlarged parotid glands bilaterally. Fatty infiltration is commonly seen in the later stage of the disease The patient has increased risk of developing lymphoma.

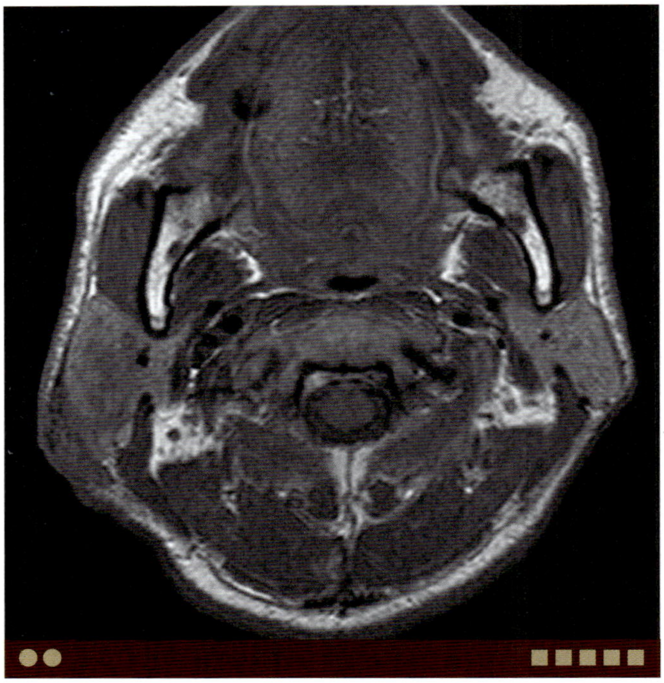

A. Kimura disease. Axial T1W image demonstrates an ill-defined low-signal lesion in the right parotid gland infiltrating beyond the capsule posteriorly.

COMMENTS

This is a 55-year-old man with right parotid swelling with lymphadenopathy.

Kimura disease is a benign chronic granulomatous disease of unknown etiology which occurs most commonly in the head and neck. This disease is characterized histopathologically by eosinophilic lymphfolliculoid granuloma, often with concomitant peripheral blood eosinophilia and elevated serum IgE. Kimura disease is more commonly seen in Japan and other Asian countries and affects mostly males from the second to fourth decade. Salivary lesions occur most commonly in the parotid and submandibular gland and uncommonly in the sublingual gland. Beyond head and neck regions, lesions often appear in axillary lymph nodes, inguinal lymph nodes and cubital subcutaneous soft tissues. Typical clinical presentation includes asymmetrical lymphadenopathy and subcutaneous soft tissue masses in the head and neck region. These lesions are painless, sometimes with itching of the surrounding skin and slowly progressive for years.

The differential diagnosis of Kimura disease includes angiolymphoid hyperplasia with eosinophilia, Hodgkin's disease, angioimmunoblastic T-cell lymphoma, Langerhans cell histiocytosis, florid follicular hyperplasia, Castleman disease, dermatopathic lymphadenopathy, Churg-Strauss syndrome, drug reaction, and parasitic lymphadenitis.

Enlarged lymph nodes are often oval shape without central necrosis. A salivary gland lesion tends to be ill-defined and often infiltrates beyond the capsule invading adjacent structures. On MRI, it shows various signal on T2W images depending on the degree of fibrosis. In the incipient period with less fibrosis it shows high signal, however, with advanced fibrosis it shows low signal. Postcontrast images demonstrate avid enhancement but with advanced fibrosis, it shows less enhancement. Avid enhancement is also seen in affected lymph nodes on postcontrast images.

PEARLS

- **Kimura disease demonstrates infiltrative lesions in the salivary glands and enlarged cervical lymph nodes. They show avid enhancement on postcontrast images.**
- **Avid enhancement of the lesion and affected nodes is often seen on postcontrast images.**
- **Kimura disease is important for the differential diagnosis of avidly enhancing lymph nodes, although it is difficult to be differentiated from other etiologies by imaging alone.**

ADDITIONAL IMAGES (B-E)

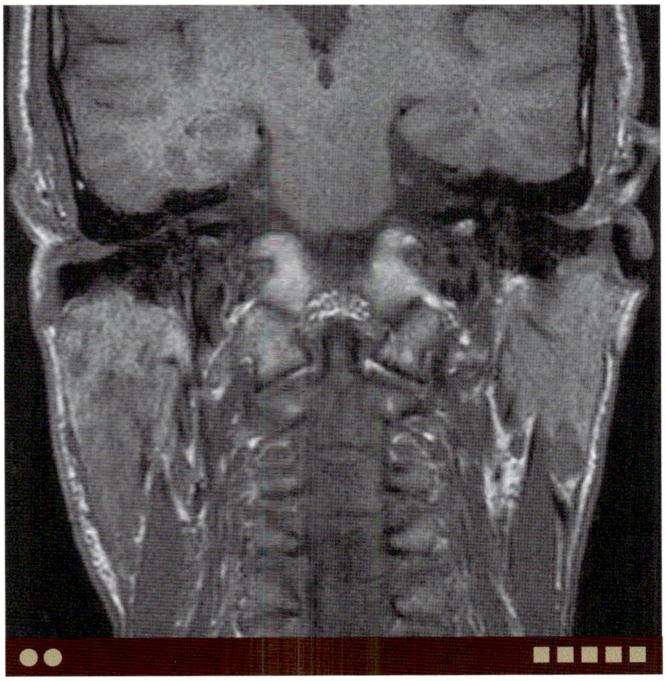

B. Kimura disease, same patient as A. Coronal T1W image demonstrates an ill-defined low-signal lesion in the right parotid gland and enlarged intra-/periparotid nodes are also seen bilaterally.

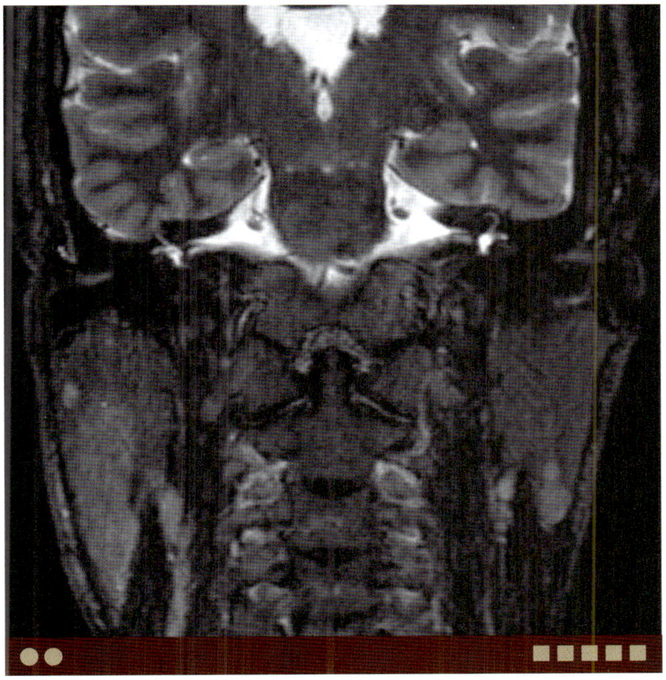

C. Kimura disease, same patient as A. Coronal STIR demonstrates an ill-defined high-signal lesion in the right parotid gland and enlarged intra-/periparotid nodes are also seen bilaterally.

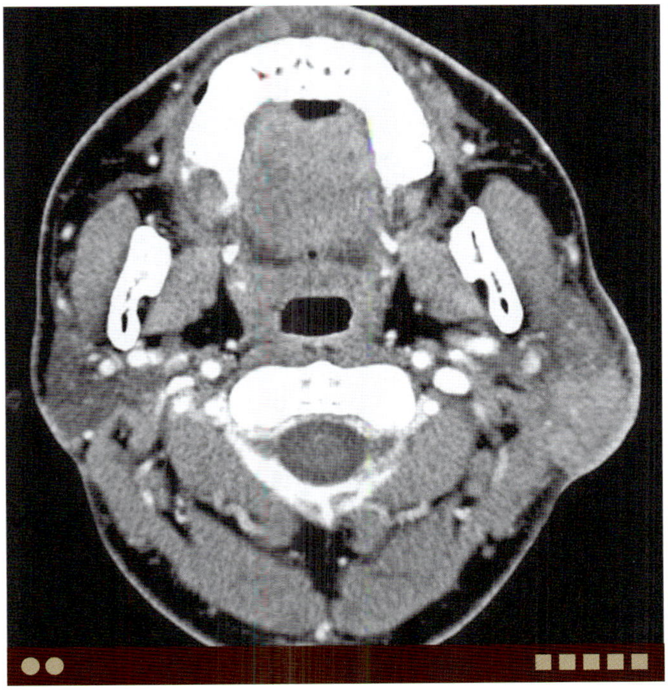

D. Kimura disease in a different patient. Axial postcontrast CT demonstrates enlarged left parotid gland with an ill-defined enhancing mass.

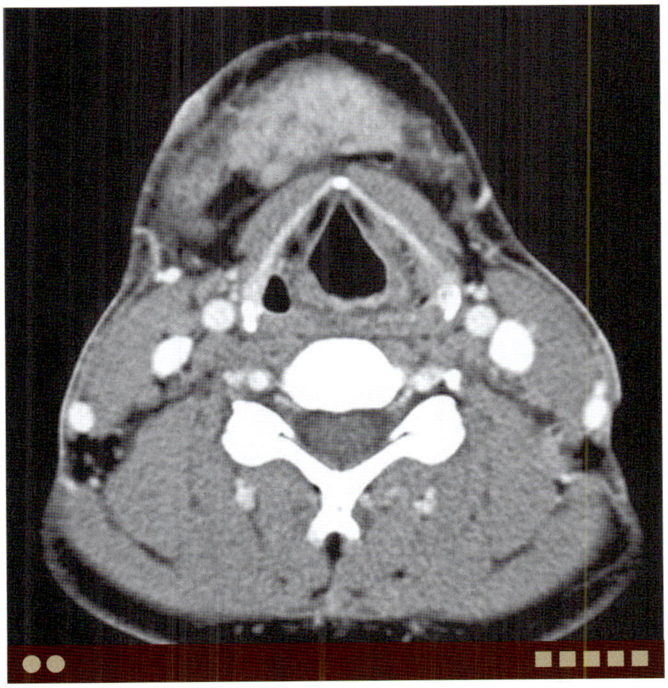

E. Kimura disease, same patient as D. Axial postcontrast CT demonstrates an ill-defined submental soft tissue mass with avid enhancement.

DIFFERENTIAL DIAGNOSIS IMAGES (F-I)

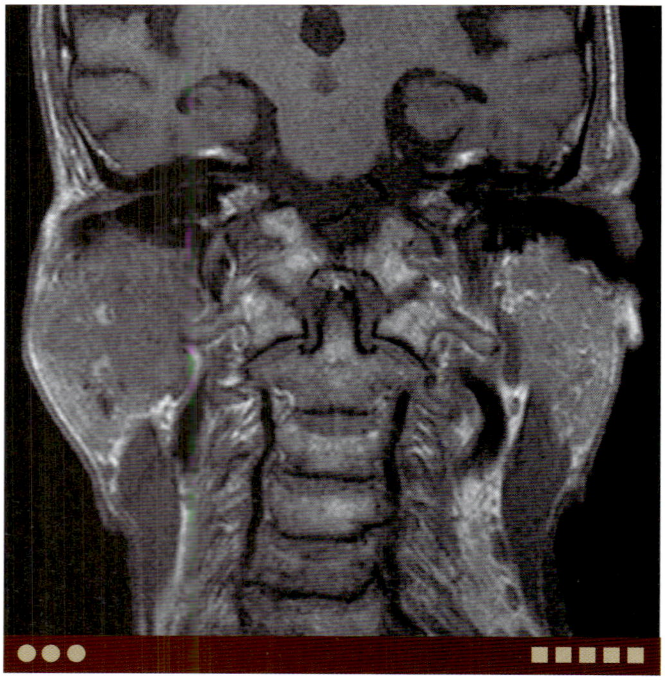

F. Salivary duct carcinoma. Coronal T1W image demonstrates an ill-defined low-signal mass in the right parotid gland.

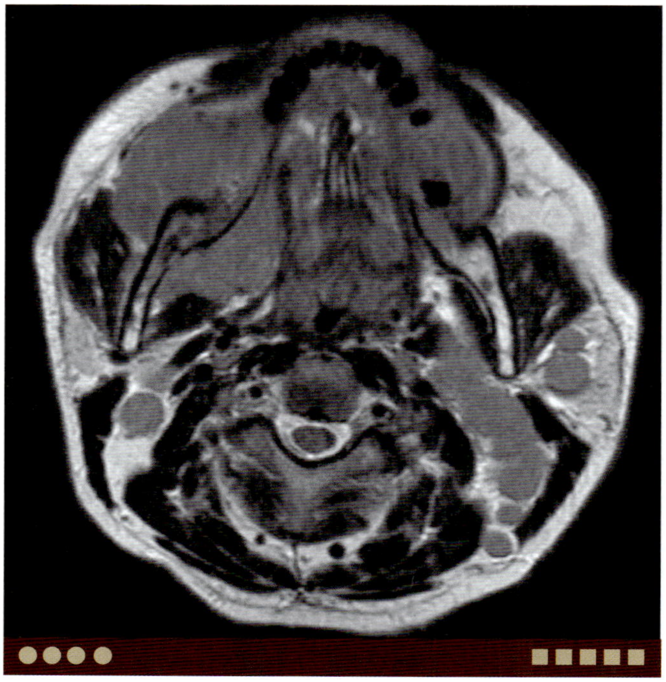

G. Lymphoma. Axial T2W image demonstrates multiple nonnecrotic enlarged nodes bilaterally with a large homogeneous signal mass involving the right mandible.

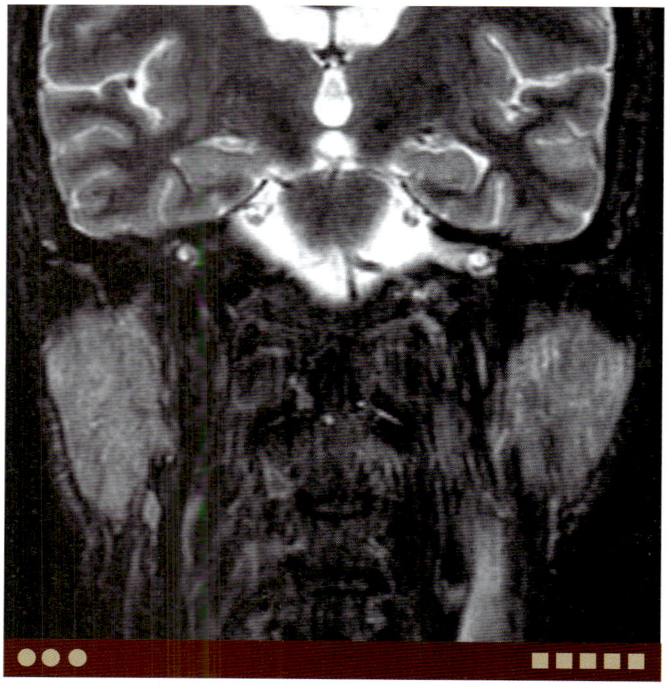

H. Sarcoidosis. Coronal STIR image demonstrates swelling of the bilateral parotid glands with diffusely increased signal.

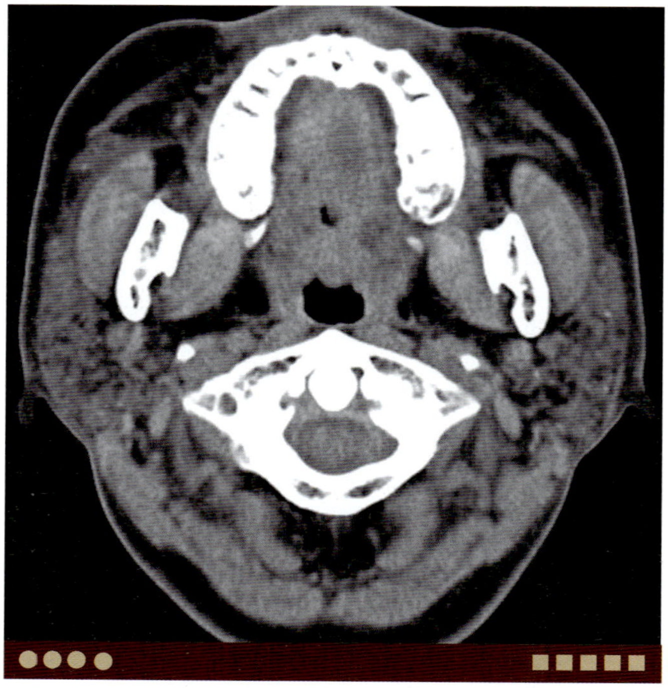

I. Sjögren's syndrome. Axial noncontrast CT demonstrates multiple nodular soft tissue densities in the bilateral parotid glands, demonstrating so-called salt-and-pepper appearance.

Case 7–12 Parotid Sarcoidosis

Shigeki Kijima, Akifumi Fujita, Asim Mian, Osamu Sakai

PRESENTATION

Diffuse bilateral parotid enlargement.

FINDINGS

MRI shows symmetrically enlarged parotid glands with increased signal on T2W and decreased signal on T1W images.

DIFFERENTIAL DIAGNOSIS

- Sjögren's syndrome: This condition shows variety of appearances based on each stage. Bilateral parotid swelling with multiple cystic and solid lesions may be seen. Punctuate calcification may be seen on CT.
- Lymphoma: This condition usually demonstrates multiple well-circumscribed homogeneous intraparotid masses with extraparotic lymphadenopathy.
- HIV-related benign lymphoepithelial lesion: This condition shows multiple cystic and solid masses with enlarged bilateral parotid grands associated with tonsillar hyperplasia and cervical reactive adenopathy.
- Warthin's tumor: This condition often demonstrates multiple masses, typically in the parotid tail, which can be unilateral or bilateral. This tumor usually occurs in men.

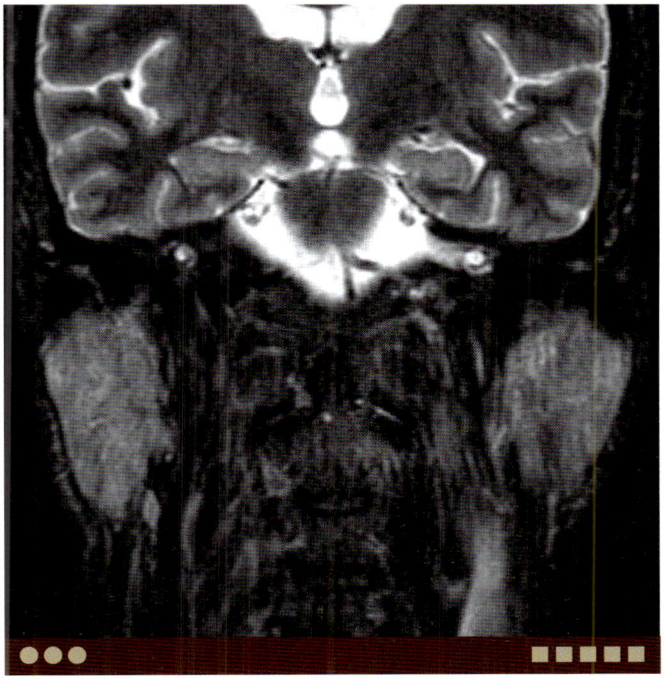

A. Sarcoidosis. Coronal STIR MR image shows symmetrically enlarged parotid glands with increased signal.

COMMENTS

This is a 55-year-old man with multiple nodules of the lower limbs. Bilateral parotid swelling is incidentally noted when he is hospitalized. Histopathological evaluation of the skin biopsy confirmed the diagnosis of sarcoidosis.

Sarcoidosis is a systemic disorder of unknown cause with a wide variety of clinical and radiological manifestations that is characterized by noncaseating granulomas with proliferation of epithelioid cells. Most patients are in the second to fourth decades of life. Diagnosis is usually made on the basis of these manifestations supported by histological findings.

Pulmonary involvement is reported in up to 90% of patients. Extrathoracic involvement can be an initial manifestation in one-half of symptomatic patients. Although skin and ocular lesions are common, the liver, spleen, lymph nodes, parotid glands, central nervous system (CNS), genitourinary system, muscles, and bones may also be involved.

Involvement of the parotid gland occurs in 6% of patients with sarcoidosis. It is commonly bilateral. The combination of fever, parotid gland enlargement, facial nerve palsy, and ocular involvement is designated as Heerfordt syndrome, which is usually a self-limiting process.

CT demonstrates swelling and multiple nodules in the bilateral parotid glands with enhancement. On MRI, affected parotid glands are typically enlarged, demonstrating increased signal intensity on T2W images and enhancement on postcontrast images. On Ga-67 citrate scintigraphy, simultaneous involvement of the parotid and lacrimal glands manifests as increased radiotracer accumulation bilaterally in these glands and normal accumulation in the nasopharynx, creating the appearance of a giant panda ("panda sign").

The clinical course and prognosis of sarcoidosis are highly variable, often correlating with the mode of onset. Corticosteroids are effectively used for treatment. Although some patients respond rapidly, others may require long-term therapy.

PEARLS

- **Sarcoidosis is a systemic disorder of unknown cause and parotid involvement is relatively rare.**
- **Bilateral parotid swelling with increased signal with T2W images and diffuse enhancement with postcontrast images are the common findings.**
- **Intraparotid and cervical lymphadenopathy is often associated.**

ADDITIONAL IMAGES (B-G)

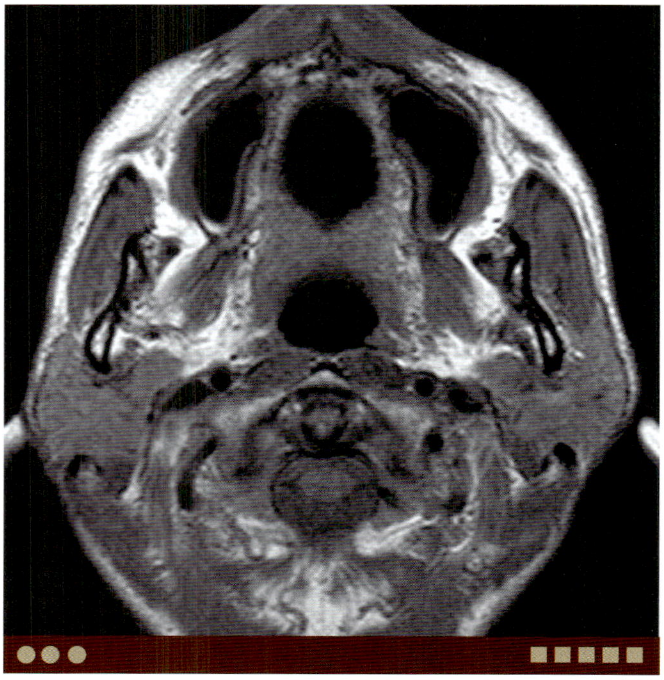

B. Sarcoidosis, same patient as A. Axial T1W image demonstrates bilateral parotid enlargement with decreased signal intensity.

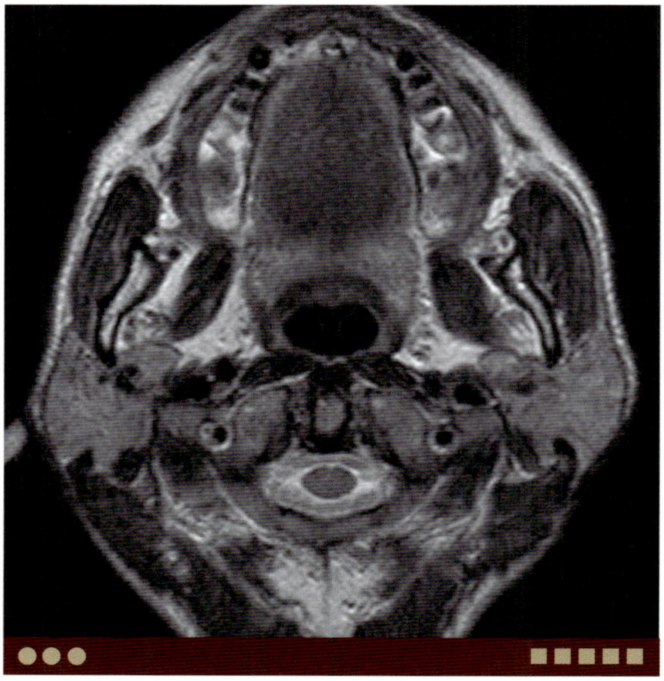

C. Sarcoidosis, same patient as A. Axial T2W image demonstrates bilateral parotid enlargement with increased signal. High intensity is also noted in the masticator and pterygoid muscle.

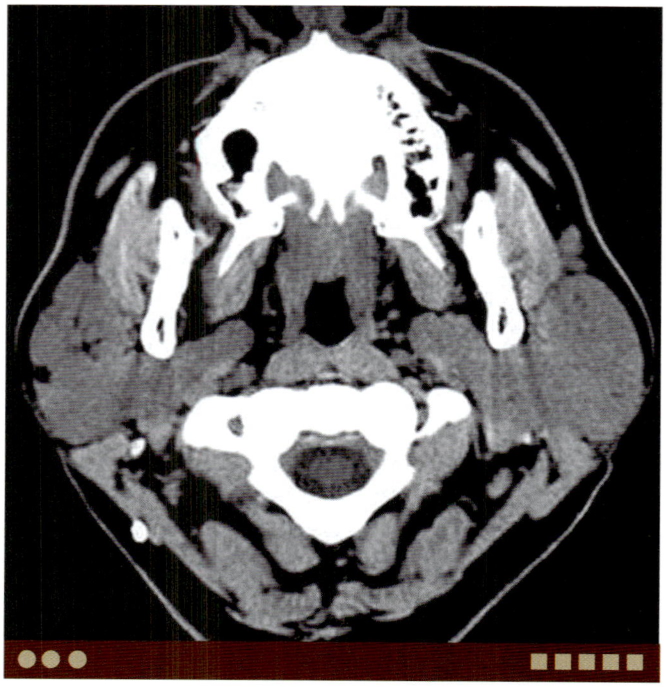

D. Sarcoidosis in a different patient. Axial CT demonstrates enlarged bilateral parotid glands.

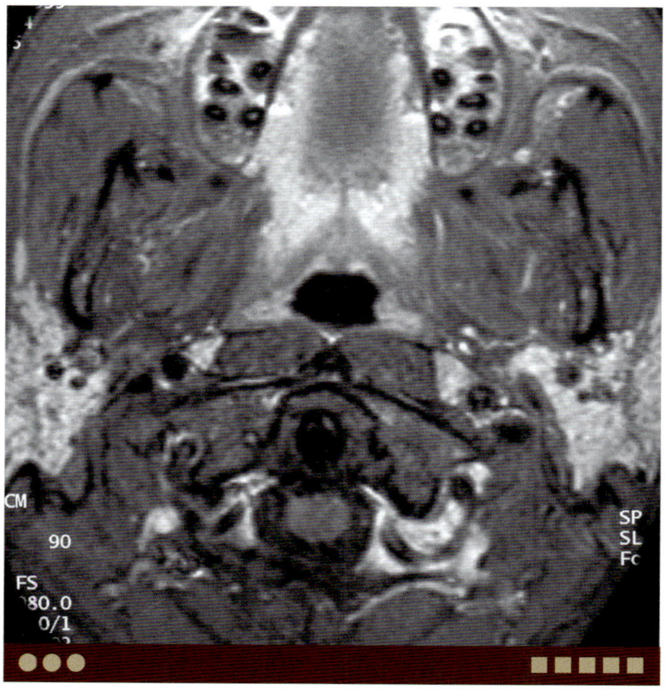

E. Sarcoidosis in a different patient. Axial postcontrast T1W MR image with fat-suppression shows diffuse enhancement of the parotid glands.

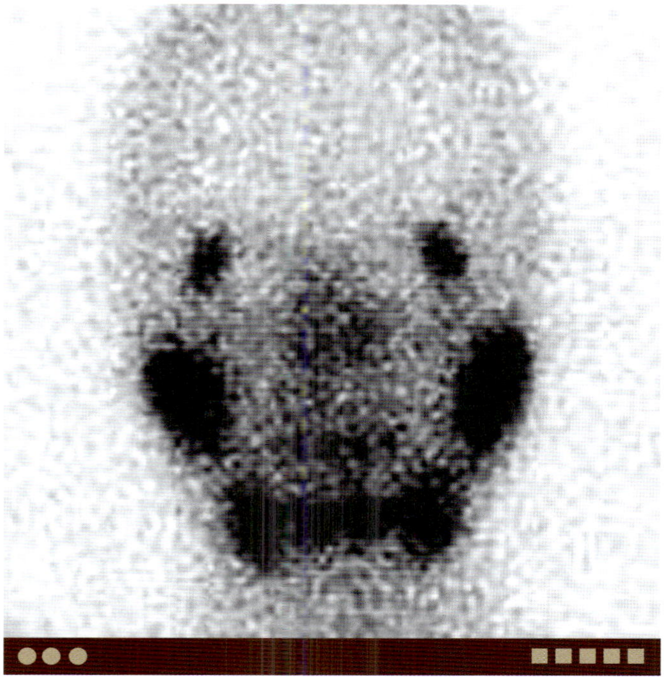

F. Sarcoidosis, same patient as E. Ga-67 scintigram demonstrates increased radiotracer accumulation in the lacrimal and parotid glands and normal accumulation in the nasopharynx, creating the appearance of a giant panda ("panda sign").

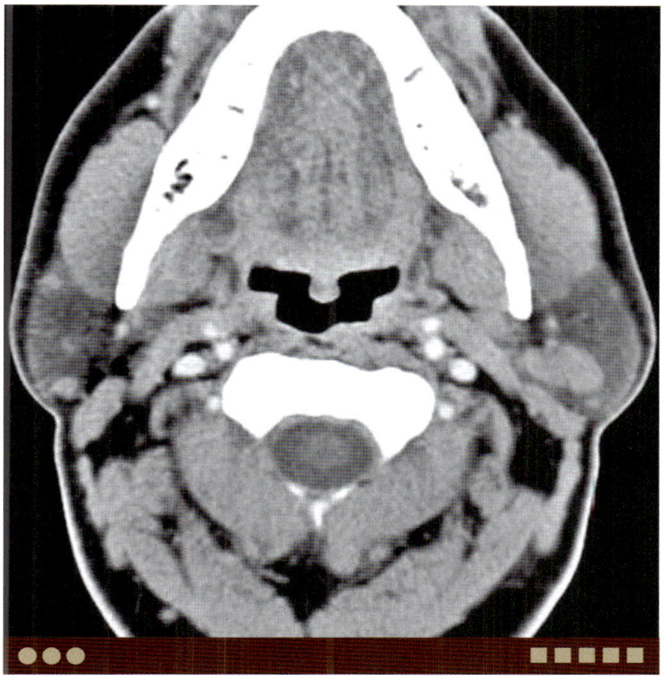

G. Sarcoidosis in a different patient. Axial postcontrast CT image demonstrates multiple nodules in the bilateral parotid glands.

DIFFERENTIAL DIAGNOSIS IMAGES (H-I)

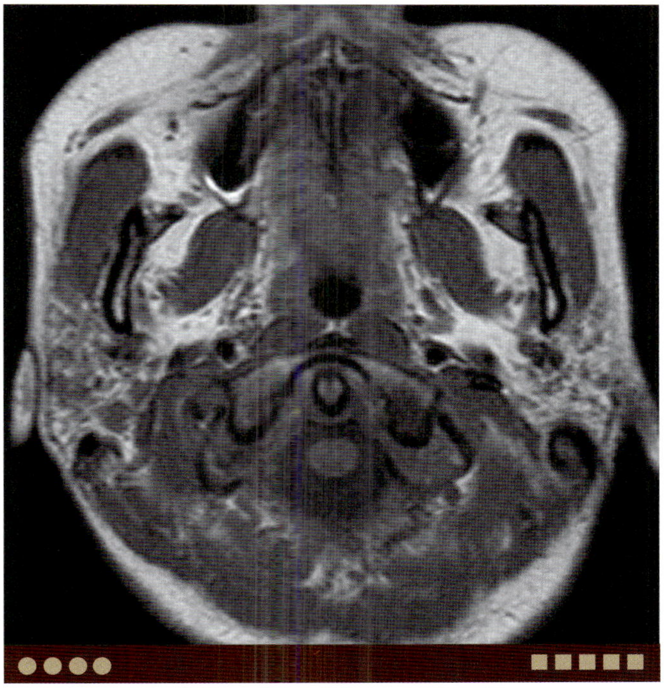

H. Sjögren's syndrome. Axial T1W image demonstrates heterogeneous fatty infiltration and nodular lesions in the bilateral parotid glands.

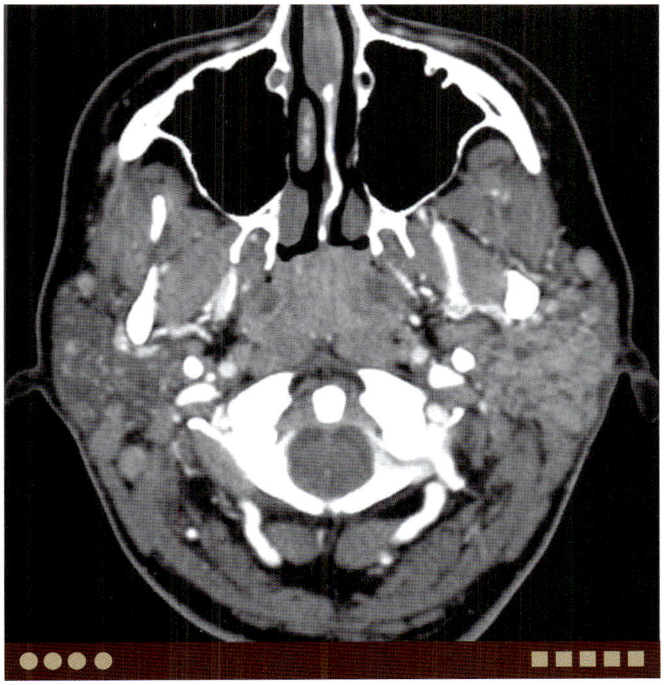

I. HIV-related benign lymphoepithelial lesion. Axial CT demonstrates multiple cystic and nodular lesions in the bilateral parotid glands. Note enlarged adenoids.

Case 7–13 Lymphoepithelial Lesions of the Parotid Gland Associated with HIV Positivity

Naoko Saito, Asim Mian, Osamu Sakai

PRESENTATION

Bilateral parotid swelling.

FINDINGS

CT and MRI demonstrate multiple cystic lesions in the bilateral parotid glands.

DIFFERENTIAL DIAGNOSIS

- Warthin's tumor: This usually occurs in elderly men and are often multiple and bilateral. Lesions are predominantly seen in the inferior portion of the parotid gland.
- Lymphoma: This is the most common malignant tumor which presents as multiple and bilateral lesions in the parotid glands. Cystic change is rare without treatment.
- Intra-/periparotid lymph nodes: Lymph nodes are usually multiple and small and located in the superficial lobe of the parotid gland and demonstrate similar density or signals to other nodes outside of the gland.
- Sjögren's syndrome: This usually occurs in women in their forties and fifties. Multiple small nodular and cystic lesions in enlarged parotid glands are commonly seen.

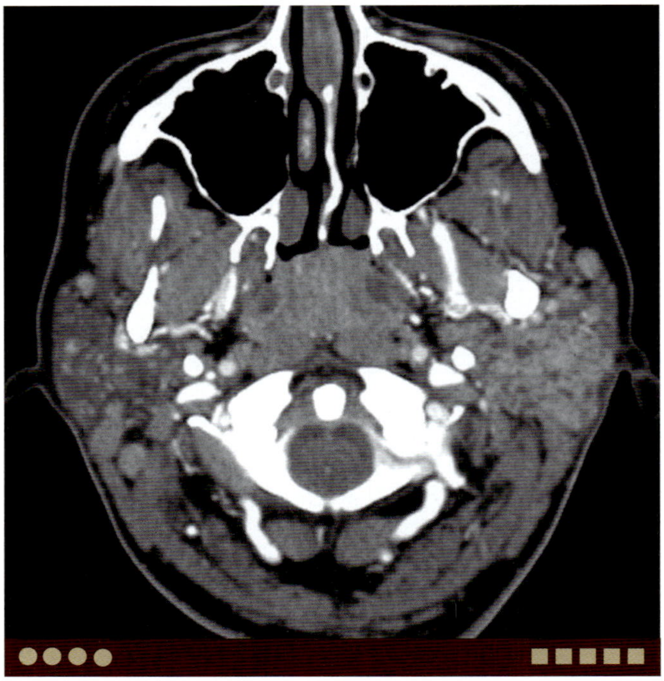

A. Lymphoepithelial lesions associated with HIV positivity. Axial contrast-enhanced CT demonstrates multiple cystic lesions in bilateral parotid glands. Enlarged nasopharyngeal adenoid tissue is also noted.

COMMENTS

This is a 56-year-old human immunodeficiency virus (HIV) positive man with bilateral parotid gland swelling.

The patients with HIV infection may develop lymphoepithelial lesions of the parotid gland. Cervical lymphadenopathy, nasopharyngeal lymphoid enlargement and lymphoepithelial lesions of the parotid gland are the three major head and neck imaging findings for HIV infection.

The term *lymphoepithelial cyst* had been used in the early literatures because of its characteristic multicystic appearance. Since cystic as well as solid intraparotid masses can occur, the term *lymphoepithelial lesion* has recently been used. However, this may be confusing because *benign lymphoepithelial lesion* has been used for histopathological changes from Sjögren's syndrome.

Lymphoepithelial lesions occur even in patients who do not develop full blown acquired immunodeficiency syndrome (AIDS). Therefore, it is important to consider HIV infection in case of the lymphoepithelial lesions of the parotid gland to initiate early intervention. Histologically, it appears cystic spaces lined by squamous epithelium accompanied by abundant lymphoid stroma. Two pathophysiologies are considered to cause lymphoepithelial lesions with HIV. One is HIV-related hyperplastic adenopathy of periparotid/intraparotid lymph nodes causing cystification of intranodal ducts. Another is basal cell hyperplasia of striated ducts and intense intraglandular lymphofollicular hyperplasia causing periductal obstruction and distal cyst formation.

Typically lymphoepithelial lesions demonstrate multiple bilateral well-circumscribed cystic and solid masses within enlarged parotid glands. It rarely occurs unilaterally. On CT, cystic lesions demonstrate low densities and solid lesions demonstrate slightly high densities with heterogeneous enhancement. On MRI, cystic lesions demonstrate low-to-intermediate signal on T1W images and high signal on T2W images and solid lesions demonstrate low-to-intermediate signal on T2W images.

PEARLS

- **Lymphoepithelial lesions of the parotid gland, cervical lymphadenopathy and nasopharyngeal lymphoid enlargement are the triad of head and neck imaging findings of HIV infection.**
- **Lymphoepithelial lesions demonstrate multiple bilateral well-circumscribed cystic and solid masses with enlarged parotid glands.**
- **Solid lesions demonstrate low-to-intermediate signal on T2W image and enhancement after contrast.**

ADDITIONAL IMAGES (B-F)

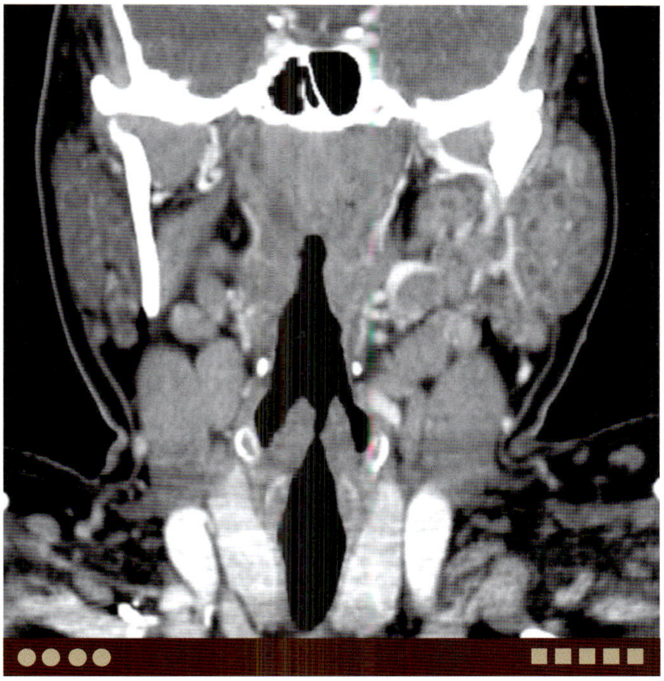

B. Lymphoepithelial lesions associated with HIV positivity, same patient as A. Coronal contrast-enhanced CT demonstrates multiple cystic lesions in bilateral parotid glands and cervical lymphadenopathy.

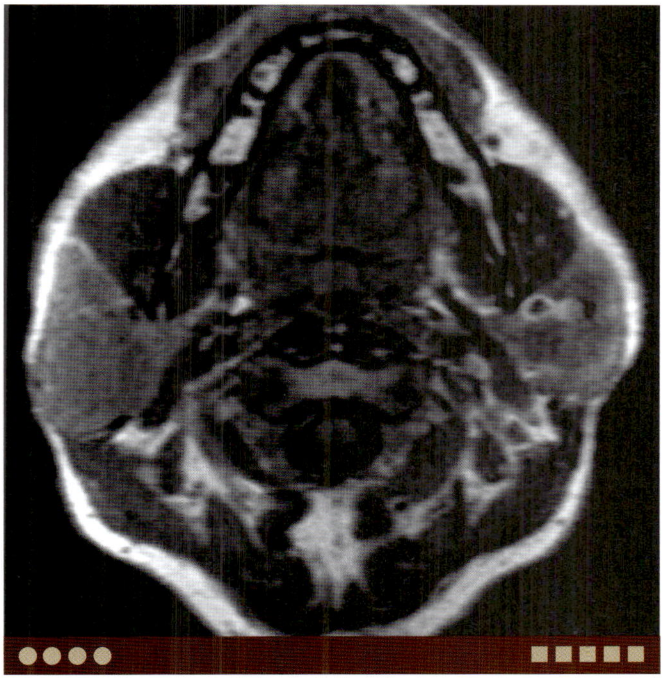

C. Lymphoepithelial lesions associated with HIV positivity in a different patient. Axial T1W image demonstrates multiple low-signal lesions in bilateral parotid glands.

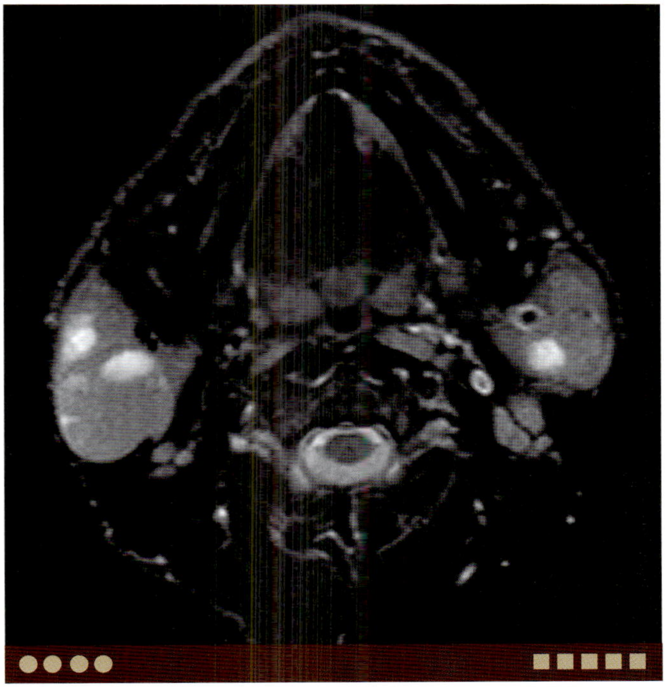

D. Lymphoepithelial lesions associated with HIV positivity, same patient as C. Axial fat-suppressed T2W image demonstrates multiple high-signal lesions in bilateral parotid glands and cervical lymphadenopathy.

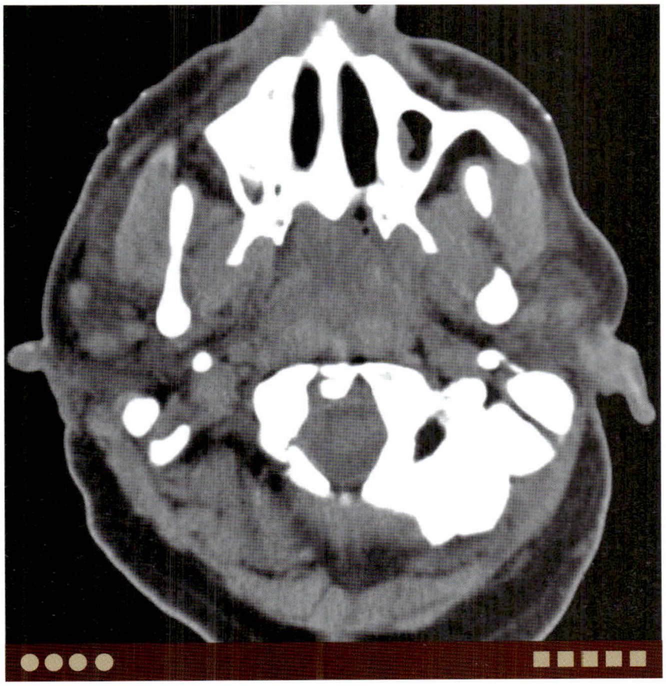

E. Lymphoepithelial lesions associated with HIV positivity in a different patient. Axial noncontrast-enhanced CT demonstrates multiple high-density lesions in bilateral parotid glands and enlarged adenoids.

DIFFERENTIAL DIAGNOSIS IMAGES (G-H)

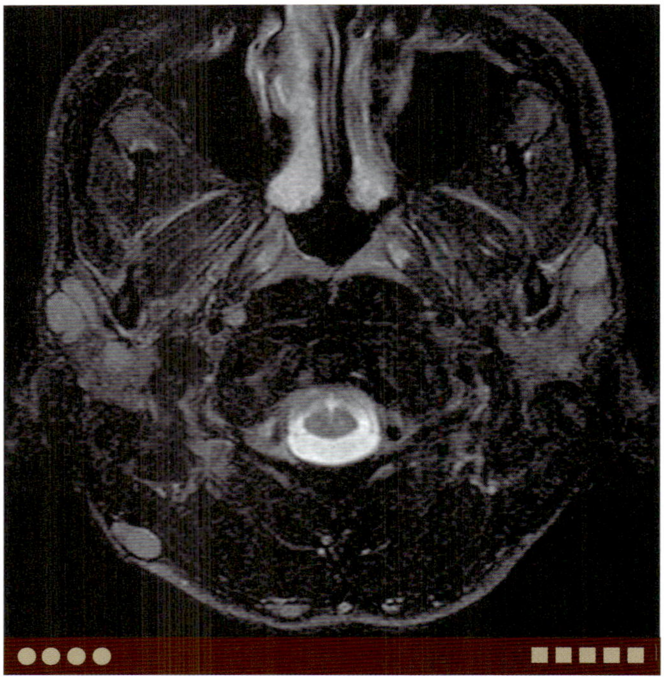

F. **Lymphoepithelial lesions associated with HIV positivity** in a different patient. Axial fat-suppressed T2W image demonstrates multiple high-signal intensity lesions in bilateral parotid glands as well as swelling of occipital lymph nodes.

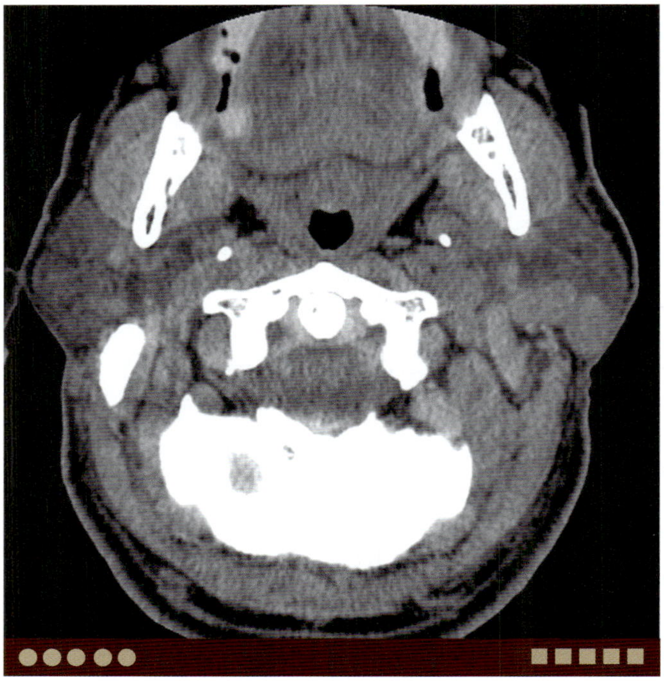

G. Warthin's tumor. Axial noncontrast CT demonstrates two soft tissue density masses in the left parotid gland.

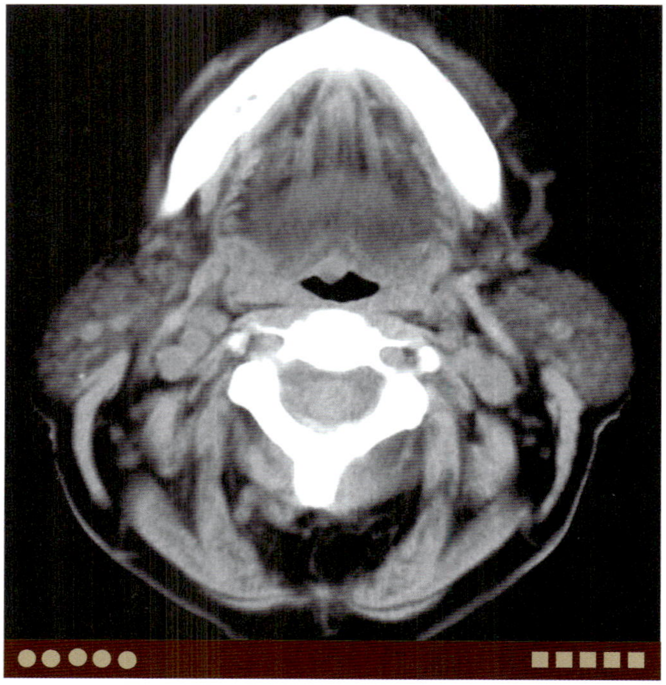

H. Sjögren's syndrome. Axial noncontrast CT demonstrates enlarged bilateral parotid glands with internal nodularity; multiple small low- and high-density areas.

Case 7–14 Epidermoid Cyst (Sebaceous Cyst, Atheroma)

Naoko Saito, Asim Mian, Osamu Sakai

PRESENTATION

Parotid mass.

FINDINGS

CT and MRI demonstrate a well-circumscribed cystic lesion in the subcutaneous tissue overlying the parotid gland.

DIFFERENTIAL DIAGNOSIS

- Parotid cyst: They are mainly divided into congenital cyst (e.g., branchial cleft cyst, lymphoepithelial cyst) and acquired cysts (e.g., ductal cyst, HIV-related parotid cyst). Usually there is no extension beyond the capsule of the parotid gland.
- Pleomorphic adenoma: This tumor is the most common parotid tumor, often seen in women in their forties and fifties. This tumor usually demonstrates delayed enhancement. Occasionally, lesions are almost entirely cystic.
- Warthin's tumor: This usually occurs in elderly men, and are often multiple and bilateral. Lesions are predominantly seen in the inferior portion of the parotid gland.

COMMENTS

This is a 46-year-old man with a left parotid mass.

Sometimes subcutaneous or skin lesions overlying salivary gland may present as a salivary gland mass clinically. There are many different terms describing the epidermal cyst: epidermoid cyst, epidermal inclusion cyst, sebaceous cyst, atheroma, trichilemmal cyst, and pilar cyst. Epidermoid cyst is the commonly used term among them.

Epidermoid cyst is the result of the proliferation of surface epidermoid cells within the dermis. There are three major causes of the lesions: (1) congenital sequestration of surface ectoderm, (2) occlusion of the pilosebaceous unit, and (3) implantation of epidermal cells into the dermis secondary to a penetrating injury and surgery. Epidermoid cyst has a thin squamous epithelial lining.

Epidermoid cysts can occur at any age, but they are usually identified in their thirties and forties. They often occur on the face, neck, back, and scrotum. Common clinical findings include slowly growing, painless mass, and discharge of cheesy, keratinous yellow-white material. Sudden enlargement and pain are often associated with infection.

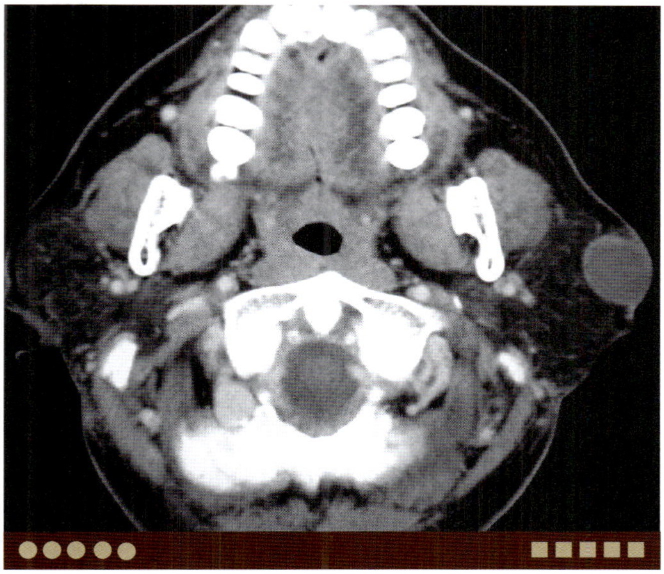

A. Epidermoid cyst. Axial contrast-enhanced CT demonstrates a well-circumscribed, low-density mass in the subcutaneous tissue overlying the left parotid gland. The mass attaches to the deep surface of the skin. There is a slight thickening of the adjacent skin.

Typically epidermoid cyst demonstrates a well-circumscribed mass with similar density and signal intensity of water. Occasionally, the lesion has slightly low density on CT and slightly high signal on T1W image, corresponding to keratin (protein) and cholesterol (lipid). The superficial margin of the lesion usually touches the deep skin line. Scattered calcifications are sometimes seen.

PEARLS

- **Epidermoid cysts can occur at any age, but they are usually identified in thirties and forties.**
- **Common clinical findings include slowly growing, painless mass, and discharge of cheesy, keratinous yellow-white material.**
- **Typically epidermoid cyst demonstrates a well-circumscribed mass with similar density and signal intensity to water.**

ADDITIONAL IMAGES (B-F)

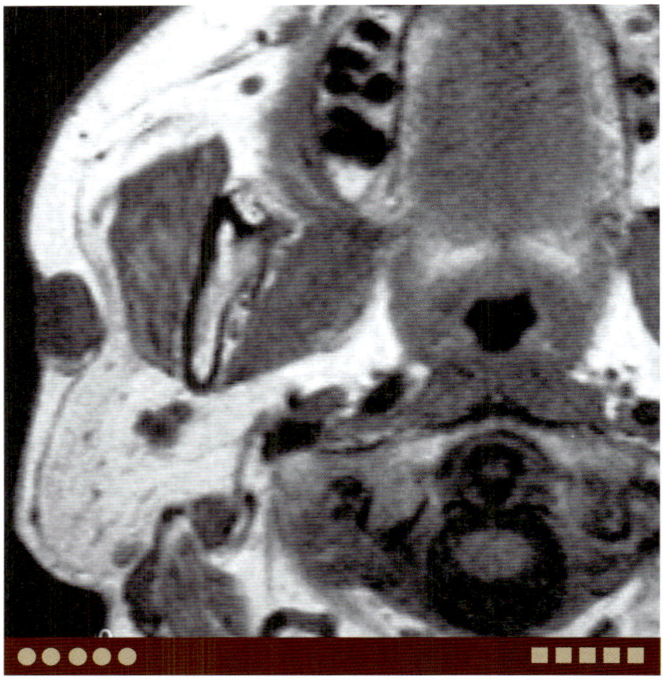

B. Epidermoid cyst in a different patient. Axial T1W image demonstrates a well-circumscribed, homogeneous, low-signal mass in the subcutaneous tissue overlying the right parotid gland. The mass abuts on the deep surface of the skin.

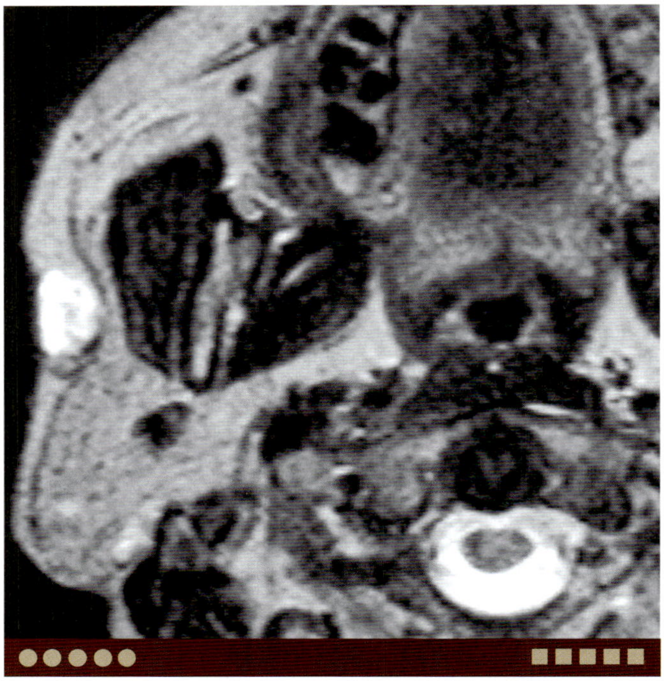

C. Epidermoid cyst, same patient as B. Axial T2W image demonstrates high signal in the lesion.

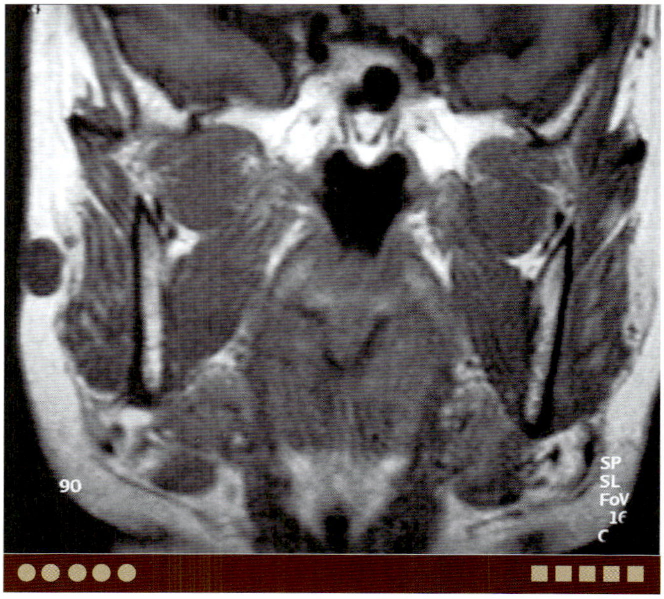

D. Epidermoid cyst, same patient as B. Coronal T1W image demonstrates a well-circumscribed, homogeneous, low-signal mass in the subcutaneous tissue overlying the right parotid gland attached to the deep surface of the skin.

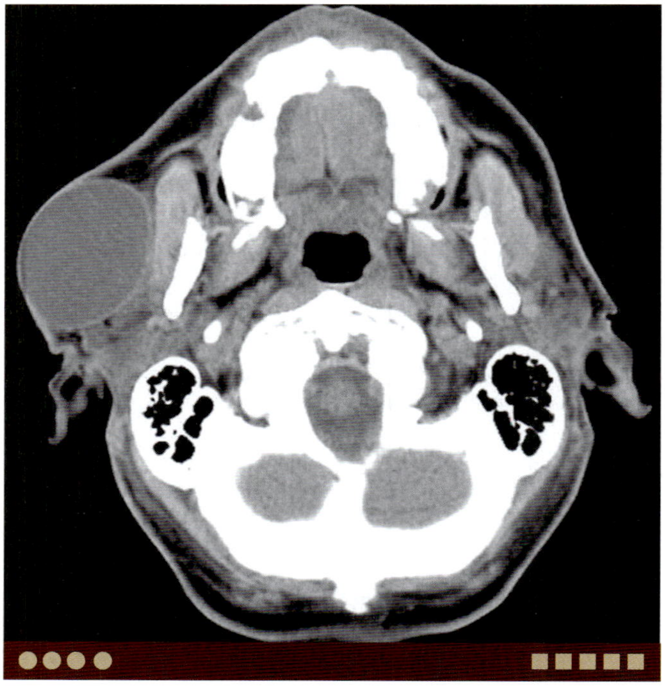

E. Epidermoid cyst in a different patient. Axial CT demonstrates a well-circumscribed, homogeneous, low-density mass over the parotid gland.

DIFFERENTIAL DIAGNOSIS IMAGES (G-H)

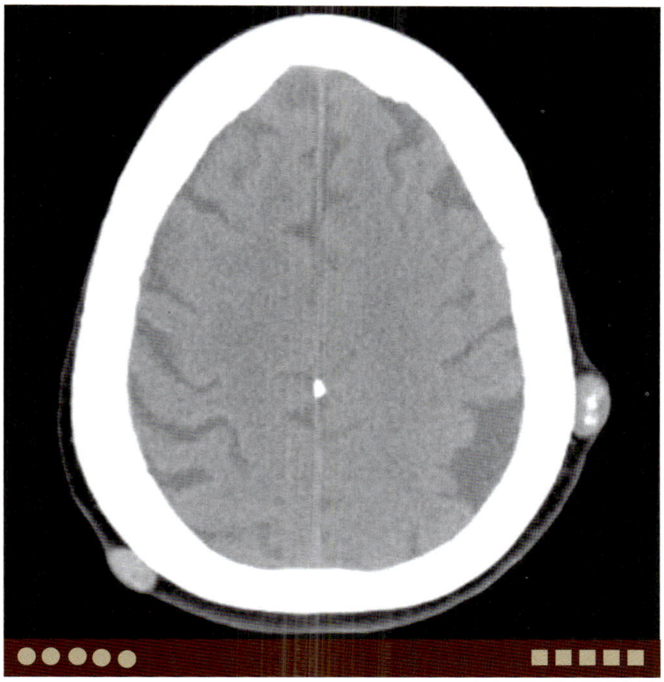

F. Epidermoid cyst in a different patient. Axial CT demonstrates well-circumscribed, dense, partially calcified subcutaneous lesions.

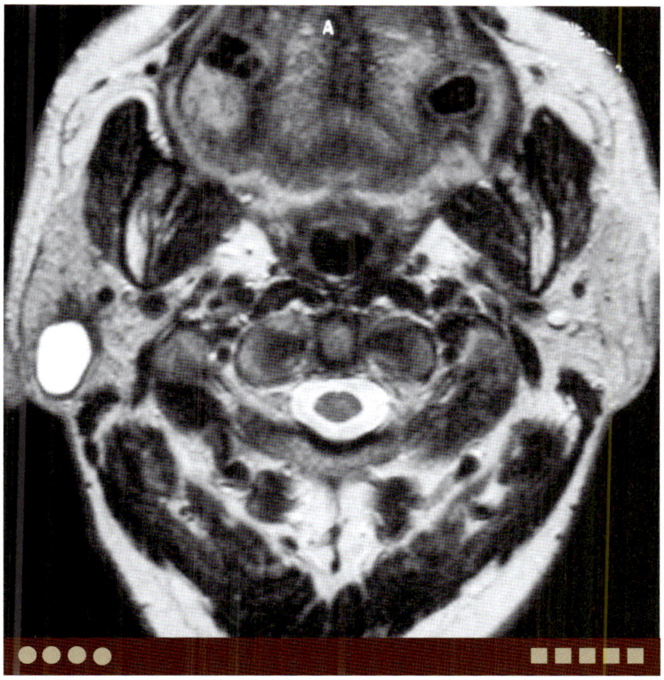

G. Acquired parotid cyst. Axial T2W image demonstrates a well-circumscribed high signal mass in the superficial lobe of the parotid gland. Postinflammatory fibrotic changes are seen anterior to the lesion.

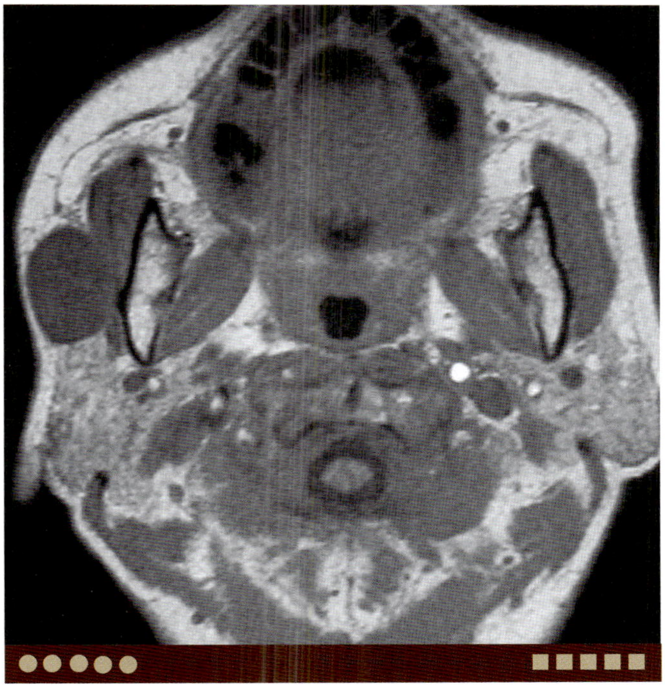

H. Pleomorphic adenoma. Axial T1W image demonstrates a well-circumscribed, homogeneous, low-signal cystic-appearing mass in the superficial lobe of the parotid gland.

Case 7-15 Basal Cell Adenocarcinoma

Naoko Saito, Asim Mian, Osamu Sakai

PRESENTATION

Unilateral parotid mass.

FINDINGS

Contrast-enhanced CT demonstrates a heterogeneously enhancing mass in the parotid gland.

DIFFERENTIAL DIAGNOSIS

- Basal cell adenoma: This is a rare benign salivary gland tumor. The typical imaging appearance is a well-defined mass with cystic component.
- Mucoepidermoid carcinoma: This is the most common malignant tumor in the parotid gland. Low-grade tumor tends to have well-circumscribed margins while high-grade tumor has infiltrating margins.
- Adenoid cystic carcinoma: This is the second most common malignant tumor in the parotid gland. High-grade tumor (solid type) shows infiltrating appearance and low signal on T2W image. This tumor has a high perineural invasion rate.
- Pleomorphic adenoma: This tumor is the most common parotid tumor, often seen in women in their forties and fifties. It demonstrates delayed enhancement.

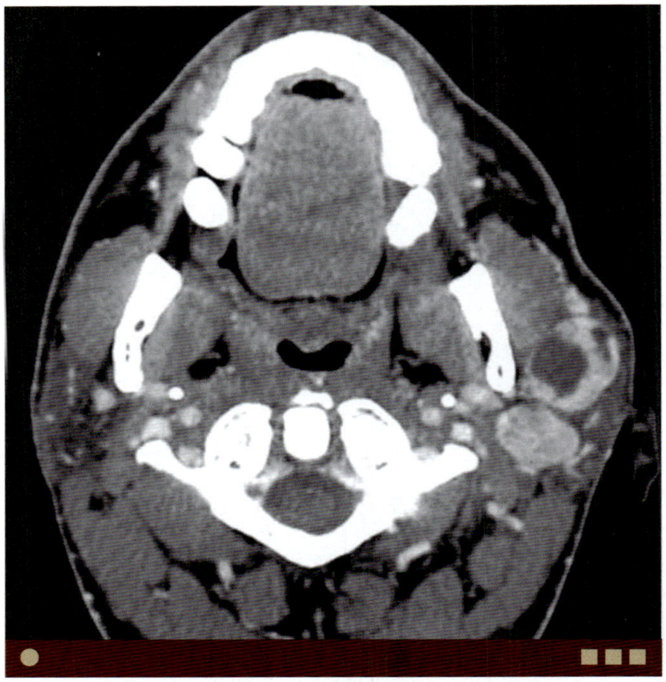

A. Basal cell adenocarcinoma. Axial contrast-enhanced CT demonstrates two well-circumscribed, heterogeneously enhancing masses in the left parotid gland. There are nonenhancing areas in the masses.

COMMENTS

This is a 40-year-old man with a left parotid mass.

Basal cell adenocarcinoma is a very rare tumor and accounts for less than 1% of major salivary gland tumors. About 90% of these tumors occur in the parotid gland. This tumor is often seen in individuals in their sixties, however, it may be found in a wide age range. This tumor is categorized as a malignant counterpart of basal cell adenoma. It may arise either de novo or via evolution from preexisting basal cell adenoma. The majority of the tumors arises de novo. While carcinoma ex pleomorphic adenoma occurs in the patients with a long history of pleomorphic adenoma, there is no relationship between malignant transformation and time. Although it is rare, bilaterality and multifocality of basal cell adenocarcinoma has been reported.

As basal cell adenomas, basal cell adenocarcinomas generally can be divided into four subtypes (solid, trabecular, tubular, and membranous) according to its predominant histological features. It has been suggested that the membranous type of basal cell adenoma has the highest risk for transforming into a basal cell adenocarcinoma. Basal cell adenocarcinoma is characterized by invasive and destructive morphologic growth in contrast to the noninvasive appearance of basal cell adenoma.

Basal cell adenocarcinoma demonstrates nonspecific imaging findings; therefore, it is difficult to differentiate from other malignant parotid gland tumors. The findings of infiltrative appearance and perineural invasion help to differentiate from basal cell adenoma.

Basal cell adenocarcinoma has a relatively high incidence of local recurrence, while regional lymph node and distant metastasis are rare.

PEARLS

- **Basal cell adenocarcinoma may arise either de novo or via evolution from preexisting basal cell adenoma. The majority of them arises de novo.**
- **Basal cell adenocarcinoma demonstrates nonspecific imaging findings of malignant salivary gland tumors. Infiltrative growth and perineural invasion help to differentiate from basal cell adenoma.**
- **Basal cell adenocarcinoma has a relatively high local recurrence rate.**

ADDITIONAL IMAGES (B-F)

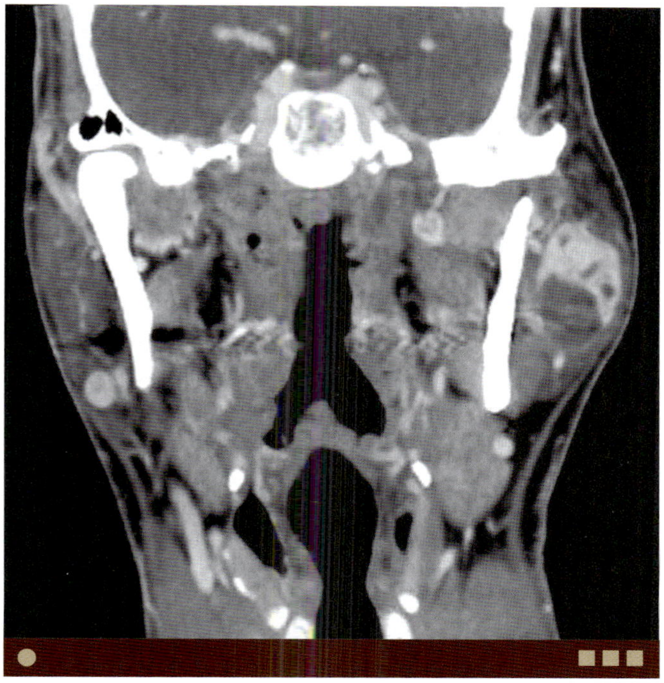

B. Basal cell adenocarcinoma, same patient as A. Coronal contrast-enhanced CT demonstrates a large enhancing tumor in the left parotid gland. Note a small round, well-circumscribed, slightly heterogeneously enhancing mass in the right parotid gland.

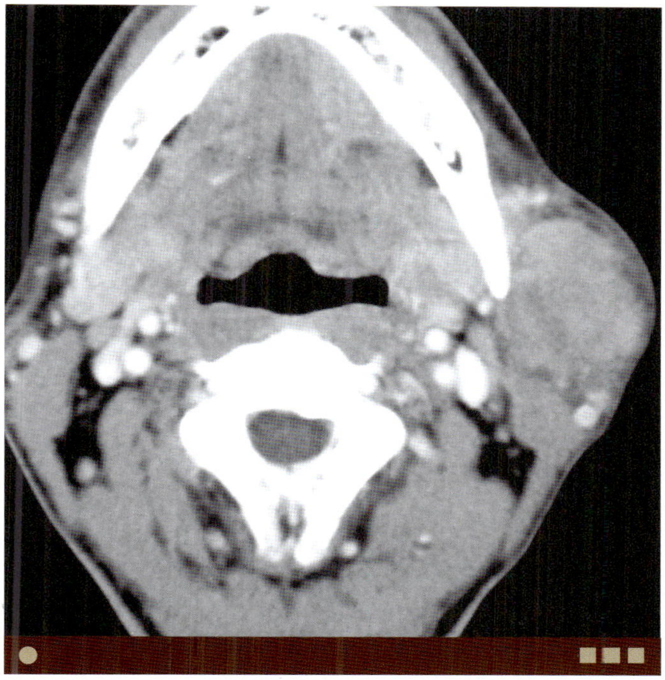

C. Basal cell adenocarcinoma in a different patient. Axial contrast-enhanced CT demonstrates a large poorly circumscribed, heterogeneously enhancing tumor in the left parotid gland.

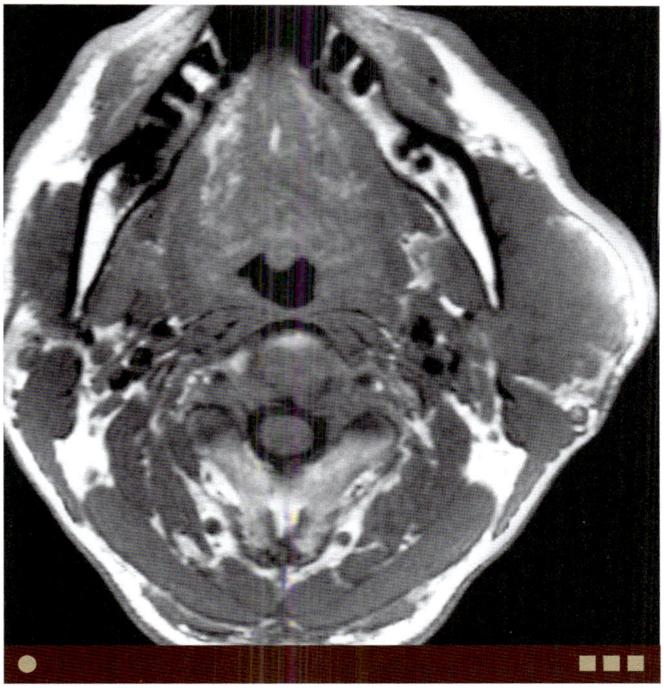

D. Basal cell adenocarcinoma, same patient as C. Axial T1W MR image demonstrates a large low-signal tumor with irregular margins in the left parotid gland.

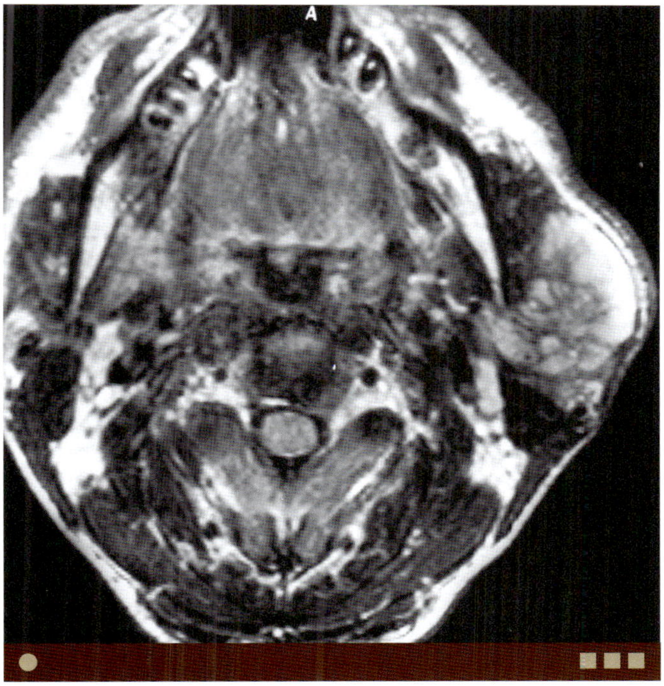

E. Basal cell adenocarcinoma, same patient as C. Axial T2W MR image demonstrates heterogeneous intermediate signal within the tumor.

DIFFERENTIAL DIAGNOSIS IMAGES (G-J)

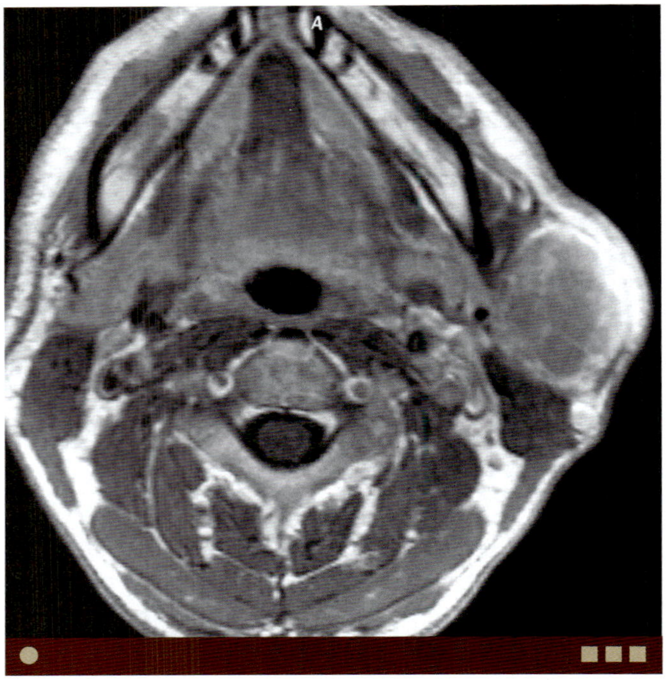

F. Basal cell adenocarcinoma, same patient as C. Coronal postcontrast T1W MR image demonstrates heterogeneous enhancement within the tumor.

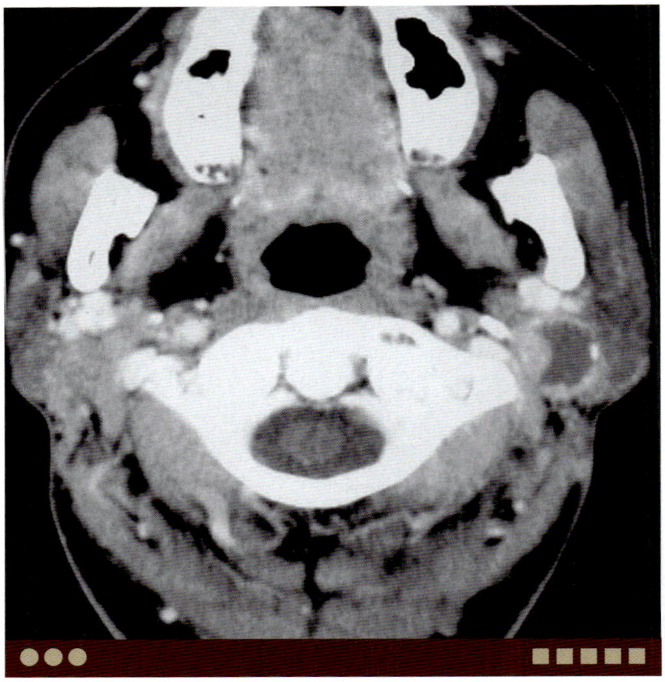

G. Basal cell adenoma. Axial contrast-enhanced CT demonstrates a cystic tumor with a mural nodule in the left parotid gland.

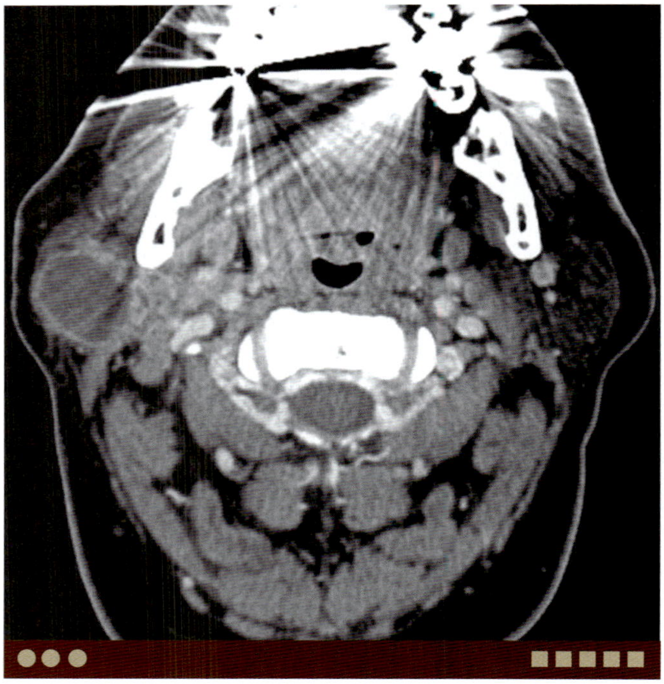

H. Mucoepidermoid carcinoma. Axial contrast-enhanced CT demonstrates a cystic-appearing tumor with mildly enhancing infiltrative margins in the right parotid gland.

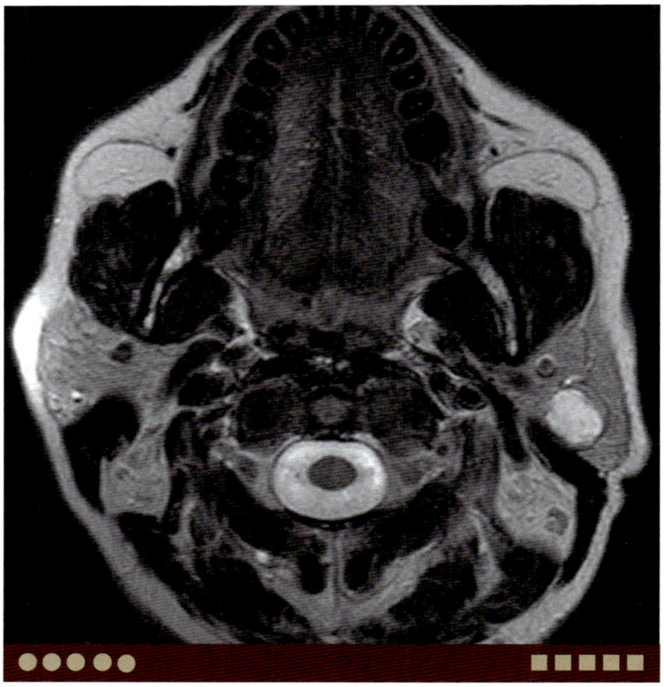

I. Pleomorphic adenoma. Axial T2W image demonstrates a well-circumscribed, slightly lobulated high-signal tumor in the parotid gland.

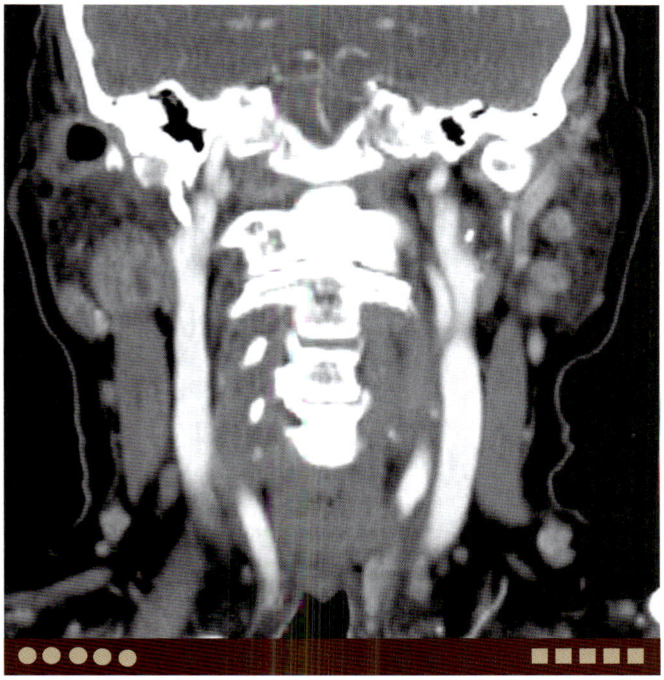

J. Warthin's tumor. Coronal contrast-enhanced CT demonstrates multiple well-circumscribed masses in the bilateral parotid glands.

Case 7–16 Oncocytoma

Naoko Saito, Asim Mian, Osamu Sakai

PRESENTATION

Bilateral parotid swelling.

FINDINGS

CT demonstrates multiple, well-demarcated, enhancing masses in the bilateral parotid glands.

DIFFERENTIAL DIAGNOSIS

- Warthin's tumor: This usually occurs in elderly men and are often multiple and bilateral. Lesions are commonly seen in the inferior portion of the parotid gland.
- Lymphoma: This is the most common malignant tumor which presents as multiple and bilateral lesions in the parotid glands. Cystic change is rare without treatment.
- Lymphoepithelial cysts (lesions) associated with HIV infection: This lesion demonstrates similar appearance to Warthin's tumor. The patient's HIV status should be determined. Cervical lymphadenopathy and nasopharyngeal lymphoid tissue enlargement are often seen.
- Acinic cell carcinoma: This is the second most common malignant tumor which presents as multiple and bilateral lesions in the parotid glands. This is, however, rare.

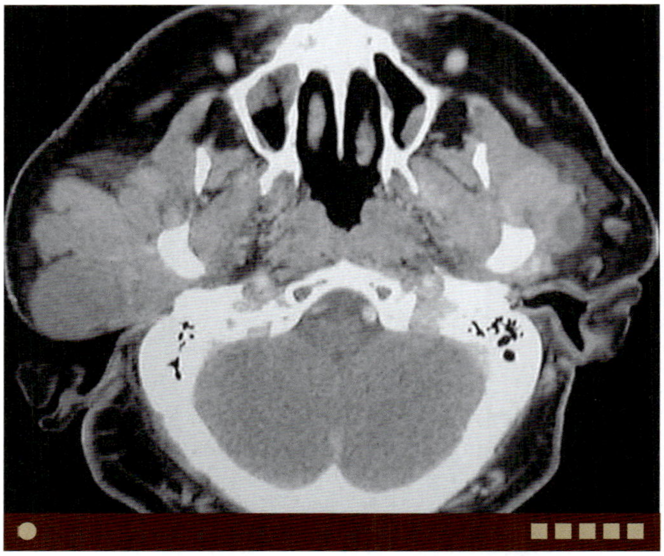

A. Oncocytoma. Axial contrast-enhanced CT demonstrates multiple solid masses in the bilateral parotid glands. Slightly heterogeneous enhancement is seen within the lesions.

COMMENTS

This is a 48-year-old woman with bilateral parotid swelling.

Oncocytoma is a rare epithelial benign tumor. Oncocytes are found in many types of tissue, including salivary glands, thyroid, pituitary gland, liver, kidneys, and gonads. The most dominant site for oncocytoma is the major salivary gland. The majority of them occur in the parotid glands, however, they account for 1% or less of all parotid gland tumors. Patients often present with painless parotid swelling. Bilaterality and multiplicity are sometimes present. Radiation exposure has been reported as one of the etiologic factors.

On imaging, oncocytomas demonstrate solitary or multiple solid masses with well-circumscribed margins. The imaging findings are nonspecific; therefore, it is difficult to differentiate from other benign and low-grade salivary gland tumors. On salivary scintigram, oncocytoma accumulates $^{99m}TcO^{4-}$, which is also a characteristic finding of Warthin's tumor.

Surgical excision usually affords cure, but recurrences due to a multifocal configuration or incomplete excision have been reported.

Oncocytic carcinoma, also referred to as malignant oncocytoma, arise in the salivary gland with most of these lesions occurring in the parotid gland. Invasive growth into adjacent tissues is a characteristic feature. They have high frequency of recurrence and metastasis.

PEARLS

- **Oncocytoma is a rare benign tumor and accounts for 1% or less of all parotid gland tumors.**
- **Bilaterality and multiplicity are sometimes present.**
- **Oncocytoma accumulates $^{99m}TcO^{4-}$ on salivary scintigram.**

ADDITIONAL IMAGES (B-C)

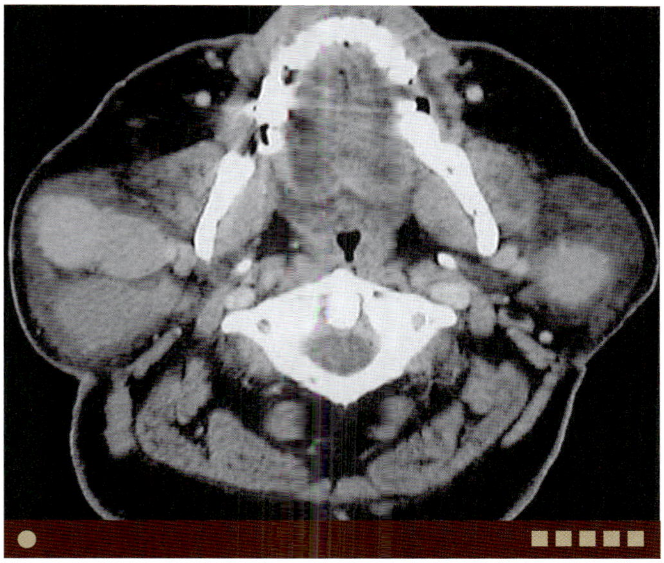

B. Oncocytoma, same patient as A. Axial contrast-enhanced CT at a slightly lower level demonstrates multiple homogeneously enhancing masses in the bilateral parotid glands.

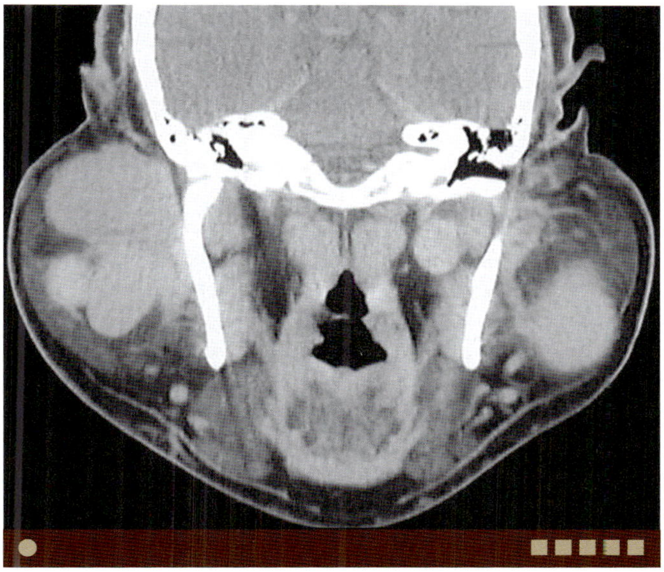

C. Oncocytoma, same patient as A. Coronal contrast-enhanced CT demonstrates multiple masses in the bilateral parotid glands. Adjacent normal parotid glands are slightly dense.

DIFFERENTIAL DIAGNOSES IMAGES (D-G)

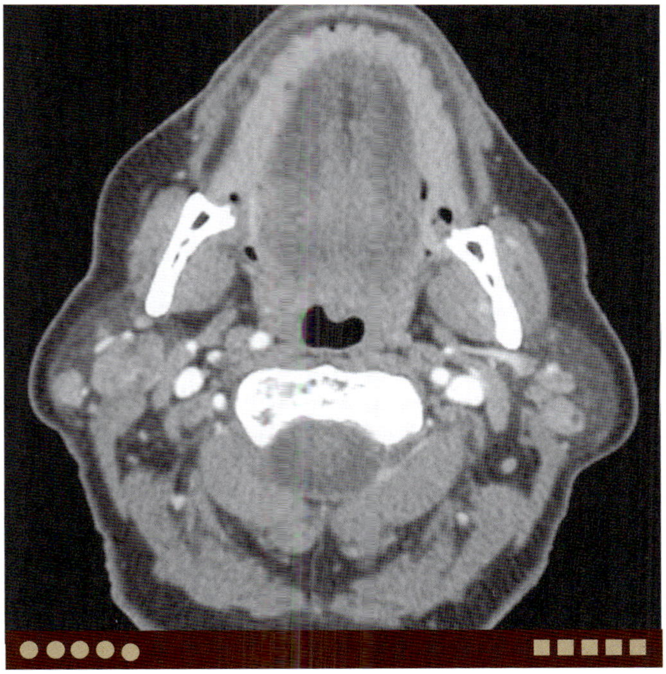

D. Warthin's tumor. Axial contrast-enhanced CT demonstrates multiple well-circumscribed masses in the bilateral parotid glands.

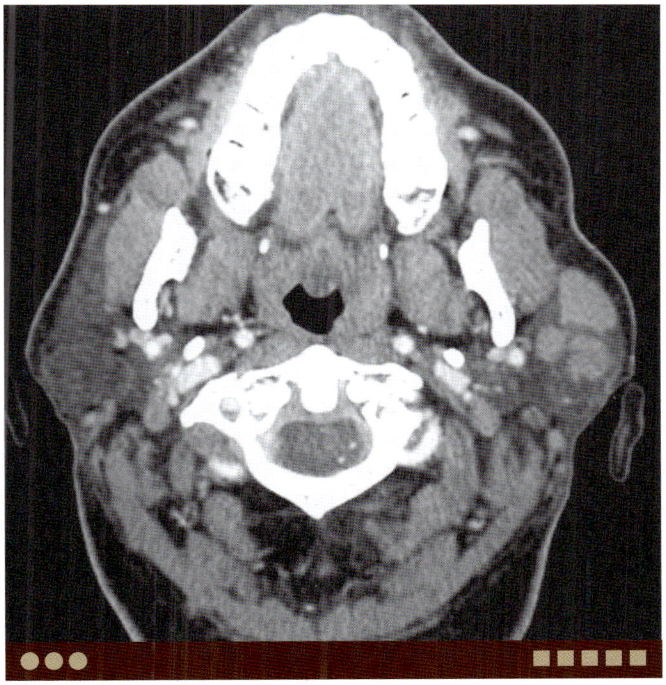

E. Secondary lymphoma. Axial contrast-enhanced CT demonstrates multiple masses with homogeneous enhancement in the left parotid gland. The identification of extraparotid nodal disease is helpful to suggest secondary lymphoma.

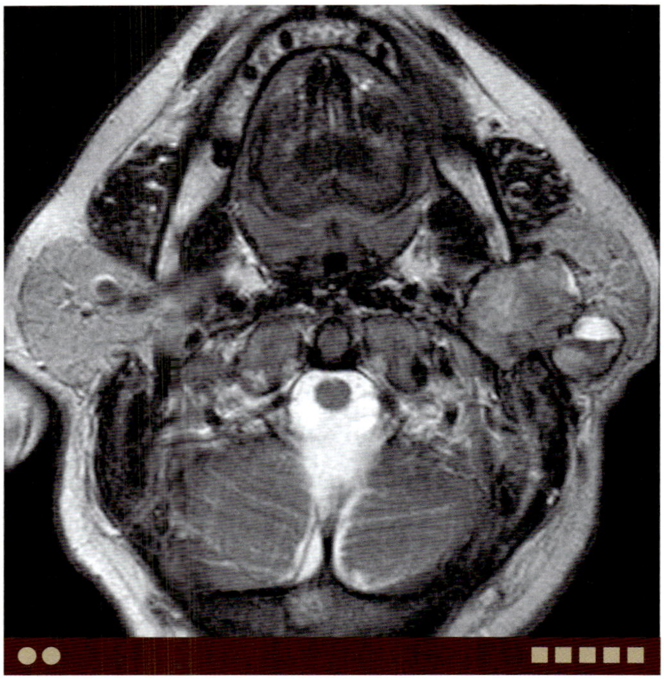

F. Acinic cell carcinoma. Axial T2W image demonstrates a heterogeneous intermediate-to-low signal tumor in the deep lobe of the left parotid gland. Note a partially cystic second lesion lateral to the main lesion.

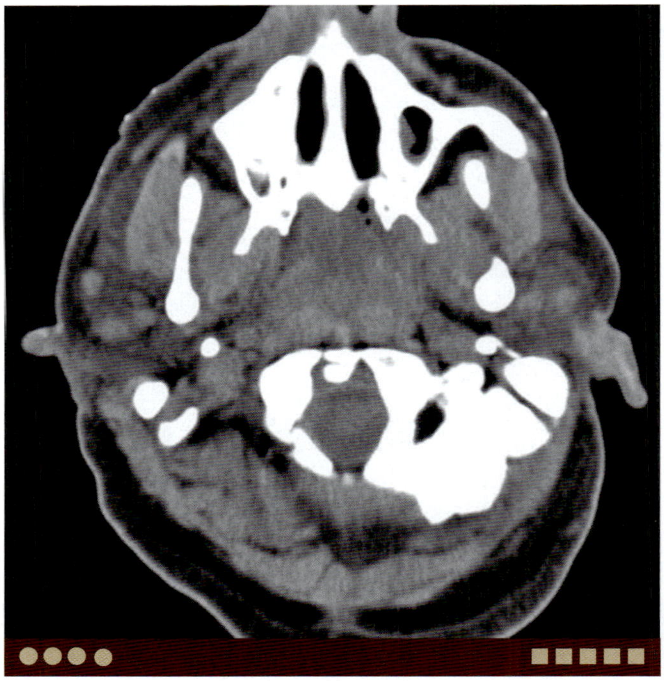

G. Lymphoepithelial lesions associated with HIV. Axial noncontrast CT demonstrates multiple high-density lesions in the bilateral parotid glands. Note enlargement of the nasopharyngeal lymphoid tissue.

Case 7–17 Adenoid Cystic Carcinoma—Parotid Gland

Naoko Saito, Asim Mian, Osamu Sakai

PRESENTATION

Facial pain.

FINDINGS

CT and MRI demonstrate a poorly circumscribed lesion showing low density on CT and low signal on both T1W and T2W images in the parotid gland.

DIFFERENTIAL DIAGNOSIS

- Mucoepidermoid carcinoma: This is the most common malignant parotid gland tumor. Regional nodal metastasis is commonly seen.
- Acinic cell carcinoma: This is a rare parotid gland tumor and can be multiple and bilateral. Hemorrhage, fibrosis and calcification are occasionally seen.
- Adenocarcinoma: This is a rare aggressive tumor with rapid growth. Imaging findings are nonspecific. Adenocarcinoma may arise from preexisting pleomorphic adenoma (carcinoma ex pleomorphic adenoma).

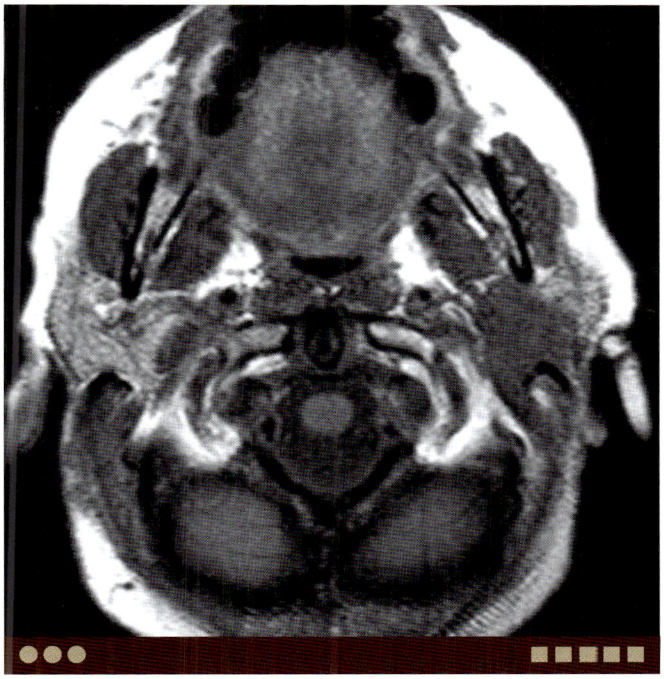

A. Adenoid cystic carcinoma. Axial T1W image demonstrates a poorly circumscribed low-signal tumor in the left parotid gland. The tumor extends to the stylomastoid foramen and obscures the normal fat pad, suggesting perineural tumor spread along the facial nerve.

COMMENTS

This is a 62-year-old woman with left facial pain.

Adenoid cystic carcinoma is the second most common malignant tumor in the parotid gland. This tumor is often seen in individuals in their forties and fifties with a slight predilection for women. It is rarely seen in children and adolescents younger than 20 years of age.

Histologically, adenoid cystic carcinoma is composed of ductal and abluminal myoepithelial cells. This tumor is rarely encapsulated and tends to extend along nerves, and "skip lesion" may be seen at considerable distances away from the main tumor mass.

Based on the WHO's classification system, adenoid cystic carcinomas are classified into three groups: tubular (well-differentiated or grade I), cribriform (moderately differentiated or grade II), and solid (poorly differentiated or grade III). The cribriform is the most common type and the solid type is the least common. The solid type has the highest cellularity and poor prognosis.

On imaging, low-grade adenoid cystic carcinoma tends to have well-circumscribed margins while high-grade tumor shows infiltrating appearance. High-grade tumor demonstrates low signal on T2W images corresponding to high cellularity. Therefore, low T2 signal suggests poor prognosis.

Adenoid cystic carcinoma has a high perineural tumor invasion rate. In the parotid gland, the tumor can spread along the facial nerve or via the auriculotemporal nerve to mandibular nerve (V3). Therefore, careful evaluation of the stylomastoid foramen and foramen ovale is important. Perineural tumor extension is probably best evaluated on precontrast T1W and postcontrast fat-suppressed T1W MR images. Fat suppression at the skull base may not be homogeneous, therefore, careful evaluation of the fat planes on precontrast T1W images is critical to diagnose perineural tumor extension.

Distant metastasis may occur 10 to 108 months (median, 96) after initial diagnosis. Therefore, long-term follow-up is needed. Hematogenous metastases to the lungs and bone are often seen, however, lymphatic spread is rare.

PEARLS

- **Adenoid cystic carcinomas are classified into three groups: tubular, cribriform, and solid. The solid type has the highest cellularity and poor prognosis.**
- **Low-signal intensity on T2W image suggests solid type (high-grade) tumor and poor prognosis.**
- **Adenoid cystic carcinoma has a high perineural invasion rate. In the parotid gland, the tumor can spread along the facial nerve or via the auriculotemporal nerve to the mandibular nerve (V3).**

ADDITIONAL IMAGES (B-F)

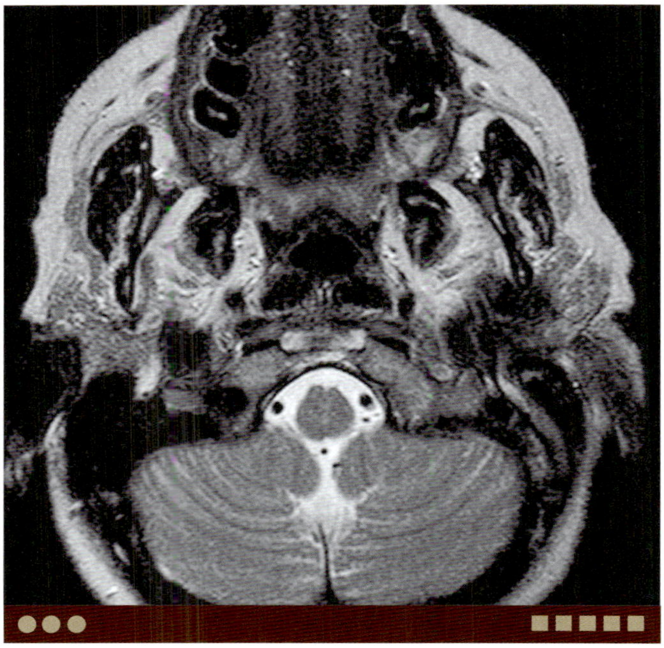

B. Adenoid cystic carcinoma, same patient as A. Axial T2W image demonstrates a low-signal tumor with infiltrating appearance. This low signal suggests a high-grade tumor.

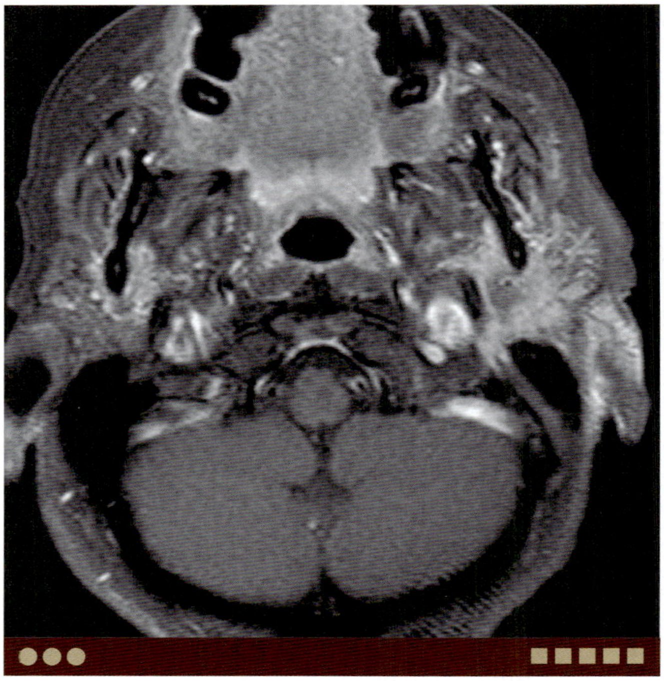

C. Adenoid cystic carcinoma, same patient as A. Axial postcontrast fat-suppressed T1W image demonstrates slight heterogeneous enhancement within the lesion. Abnormal enhancement is seen in the stylomastoid foramen to suggest perineural tumor invasion along the facial nerve.

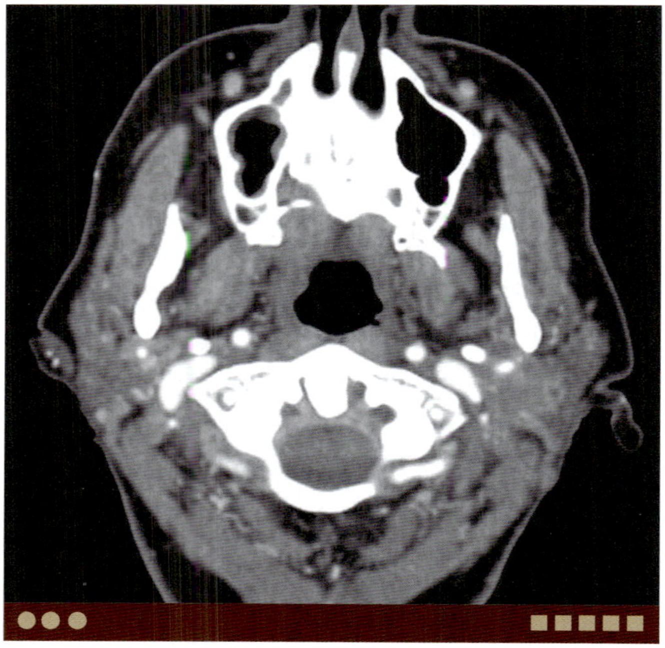

D. Adenoid cystic carcinoma, same patient as A. Axial contrast-enhanced CT demonstrates a poorly circumscribed enhancing tumor in the left parotid gland entering the stylomastoid foramen.

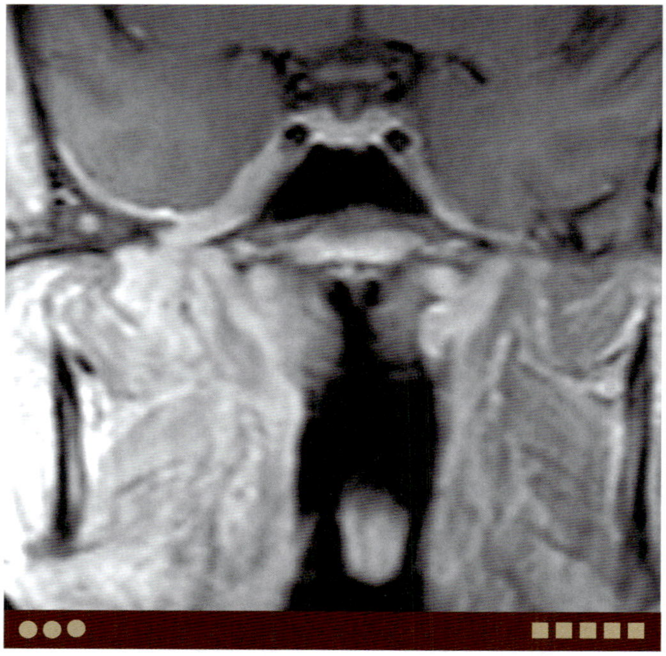

E. Adenoid cystic carcinoma (right parotid), perineural tumor spread in a different patient. Coronal postcontrast T1W image demonstrates thickening and enhancement of the right mandibular nerve (V3). The tumor extends intracranially via the foramen ovale and reaches the cavernous sinus. Note enhancement of right pterygoid and masseter muscles due to denervation myositis from injury of the V3.

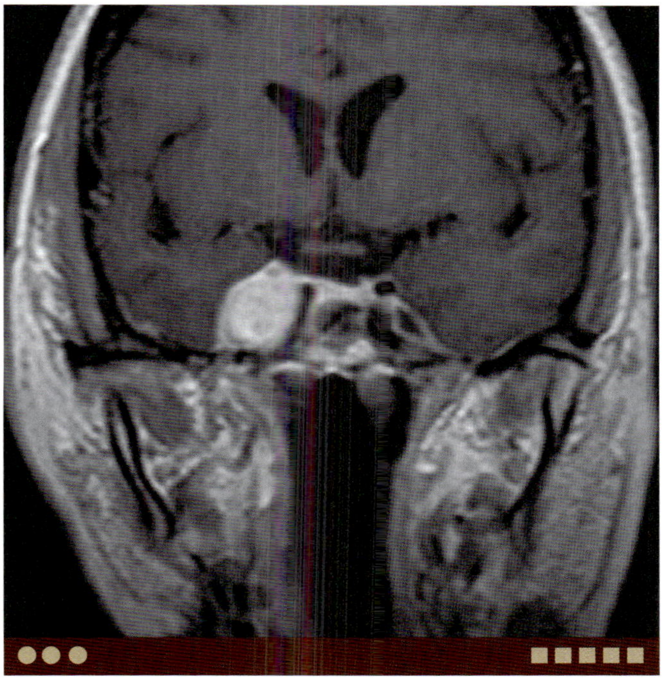

F. Adenoid cystic carcinoma (right parotid), skip perineural tumor spread in a different patient. Coronal postcontrast T1W image demonstrates an expansile enhancing tumor in the right paracavernous region without apparent mass below the skull base.

DIFFERENTIAL DIAGNOSIS IMAGES (G-I)

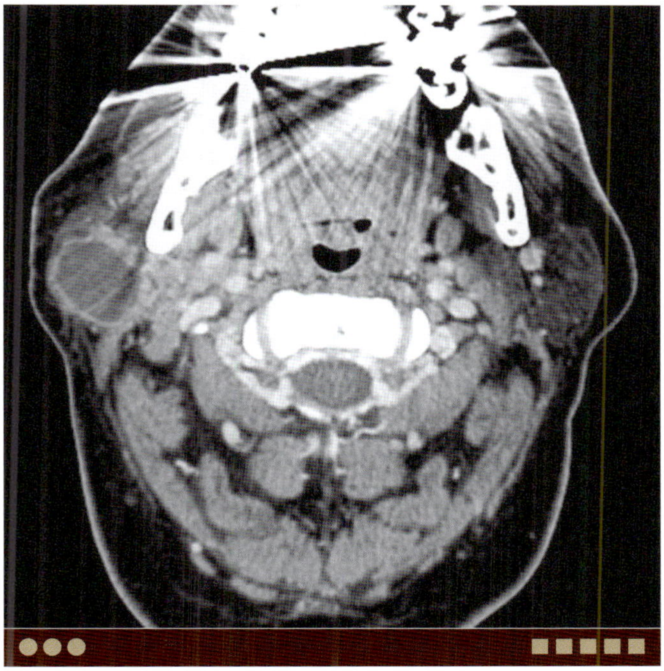

G. Mucoepidermoid carcinoma (high grade). Axial contrast-enhanced CT demonstrates a cystic-appearing tumor with rim-enhancement and infiltrative margins in the parotid gland.

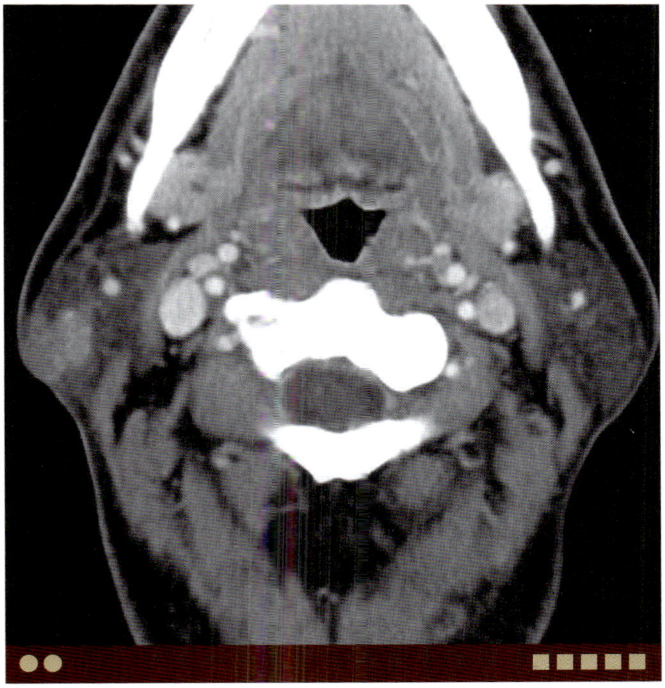

H. Acinic cell carcinoma. Axial contrast-enhanced CT demonstrates lobulated mass in the superficial lobe of the right parotid gland. There is tumor invasion into the subcutaneous fat and skin.

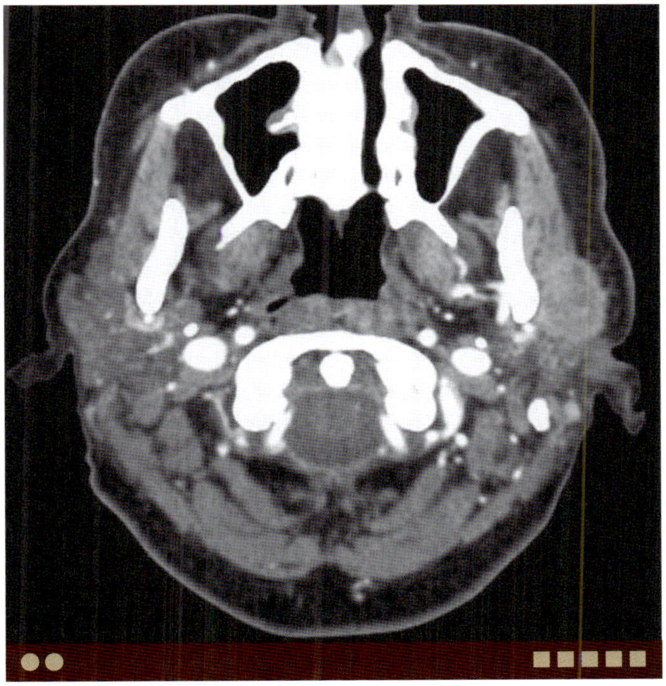

I. Adenocarcinoma. Axial contrast-enhanced CT demonstrates a heterogeneously enhancing tumor with irregular margins in the superficial lobe of the left parotid gland.

Case 7-18 Pleomorphic Adenoma—Submandibular Gland

Naoko Saito, Asim Mian, Osamu Sakai

PRESENTATION

Unilateral submandibular mass.

FINDINGS

CT and MRI demonstrate a well-circumscribed mass in the submandibular gland.

DIFFERENTIAL DIAGNOSIS

- Adenoid cystic carcinoma: This is the most common malignant submandibular gland tumor. High-grade tumor demonstrates low signal intensity on T2W image reflecting high cellularity.
- Mucoepidermoid carcinoma: This is the second most common malignant submandibular gland tumor. Low-grade tumor has a similar appearance to a benign tumor.

COMMENTS

This is a 25-year-old woman with right submandibular mass.

Pleomorphic adenoma is a benign tumor and the most common submandibular gland tumor, although about 50% of tumors arising in the submandibular gland are malignant. This tumor is often seen in relatively young women, most commonly women in their forties and fifties. Histologically, this tumor demonstrates a mixture of epithelial and interstitial cells. It often has a thin capsule and smooth and well-demarcated margins with slight lobulation. This tumor demonstrates variable appearance from solid to almost totally cystic. In the submandibular gland, the tumor tends to have a greater cystic component. Dystrophic calcifications are sometimes seen and this finding helps to differentiate from other tumors.

On imaging, pleomorphic adenoma has well-circumscribed margins. The large tumor tends to show a lobulated contour. Pleomorphic adenoma demonstrates slightly higher attenuation than surrounding parenchyma on CT. Calcification is occasionally seen. On MRI, typically the tumor demonstrates high signal on T2W images corresponding to myxoid degeneration or abundant glandular component. After contrast, the tumor demonstrates delayed enhancement.

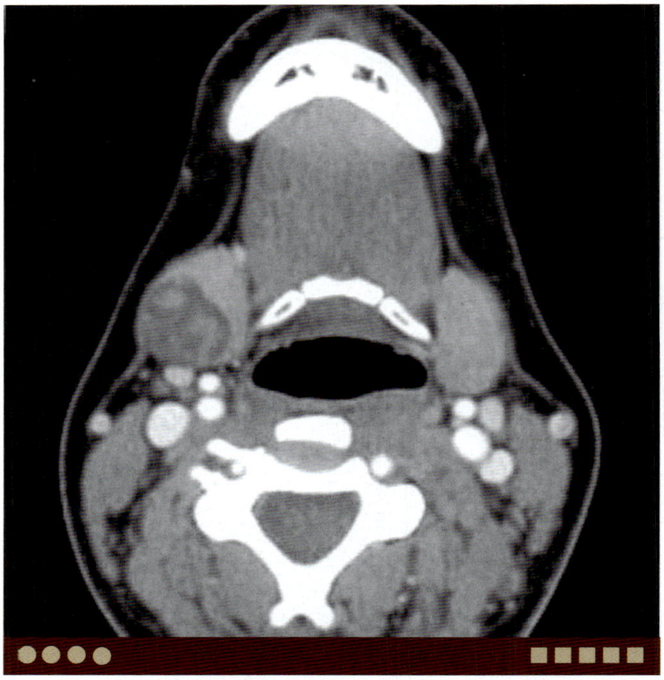

A. Pleomorphic adenoma. Axial contrast-enhanced CT demonstrates a well-circumscribed, heterogeneously enhancing mass in the right submandibular gland.

Rarely, carcinoma is accompanied with pleomorphic adenoma or carcinoma may arise from pleomorphic adenoma. Therefore, for careful evaluation for invasion of the adjacent structures, perineural tumor spread and nodal metastasis is important.

PEARLS

- **Pleomorphic adenoma is the most common submandibular gland tumor, although about 50% of tumors arising in the submandibular gland are malignant.**
- **Pleomorphic adenoma demonstrates delayed enhancement.**
- **Pleomorphic adenoma is rarely malignant. However, careful evaluation for possible malignancy is important.**

ADDITIONAL IMAGES (B–E)

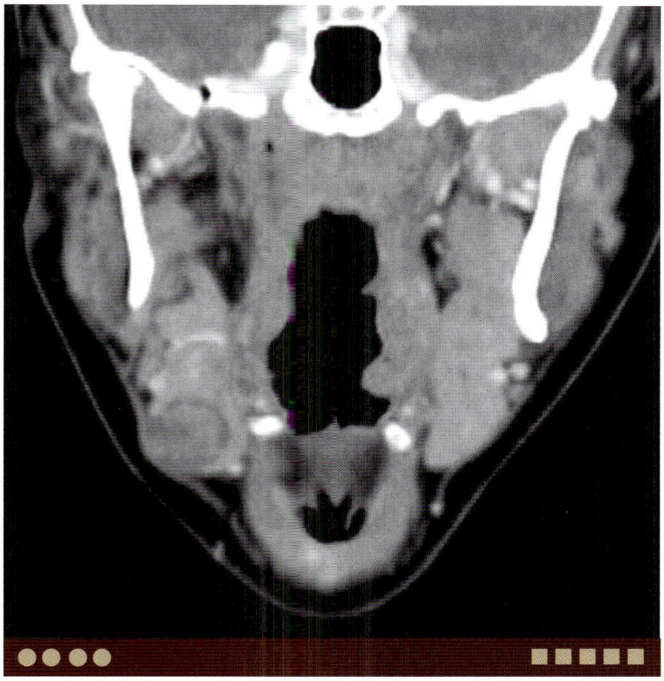

B. Pleomorphic adenoma, same patient as A. Coronal contrast-enhanced CT demonstrates a well-circumscribed, heterogeneously enhancing mass in the right submandibular gland.

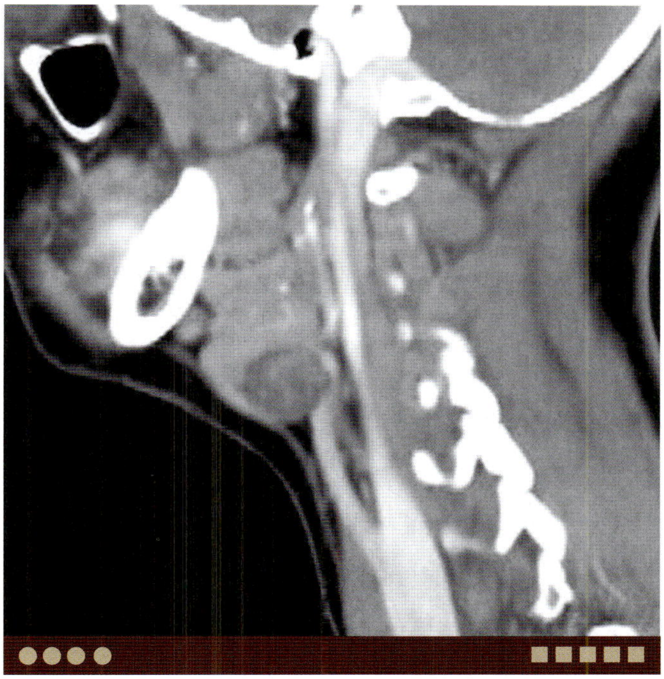

C. Pleomorphic adenoma, same patient as A. Sagittal contrast-enhanced CT demonstrates a well-circumscribed, heterogeneously enhancing mass in the submandibular gland.

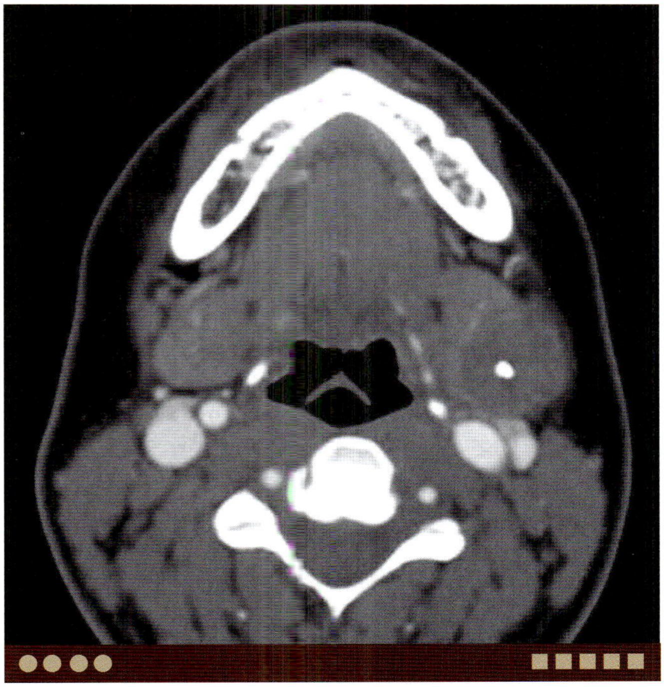

D. Pleomorphic adenoma in a different patient. Axial contrast-enhanced CT demonstrates a well-circumscribed, slightly enhancing mass in the left submandibular gland. There is a calcification within the mass.

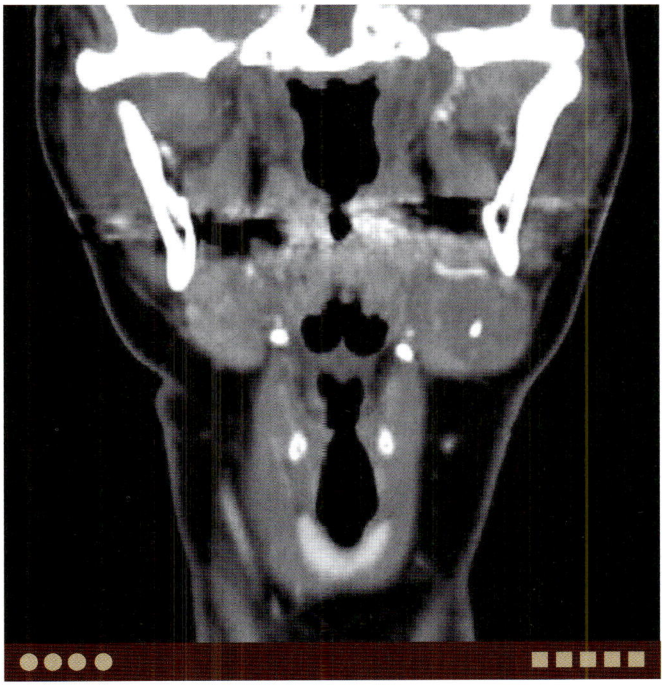

E. Pleomorphic adenoma, same patient as D. Coronal contrast-enhanced CT demonstrates a well-circumscribed, slightly enhancing mass with calcification in the left submandibular gland.

DIFFERENTIAL DIAGNOSIS IMAGES (F-H)

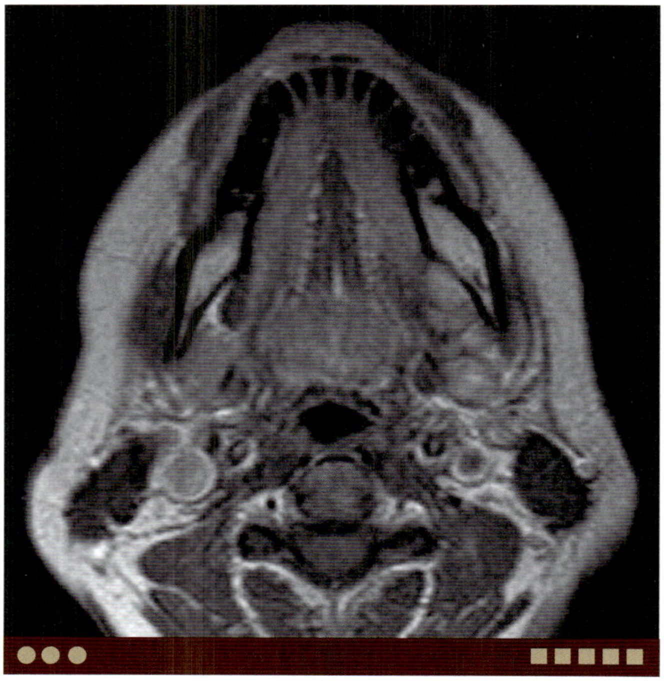

F. Adenoid cystic carcinoma. Axial postcontrast T1W image demonstrates an enhancing multicystic tumor in the left submandibular gland.

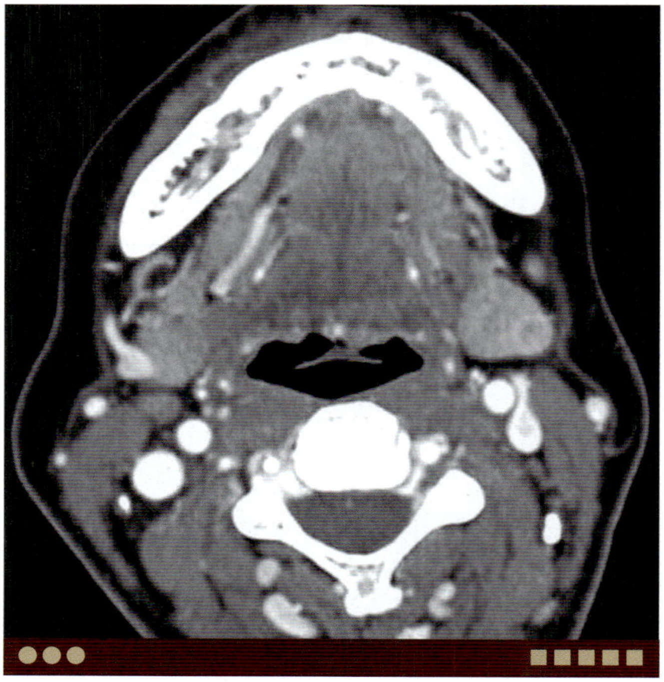

G. Mucoepidermoid carcinoma (low grade). Axial contrast-enhanced CT demonstrates a well-circumscribed, peripherally enhancing mass in the left submandibular gland.

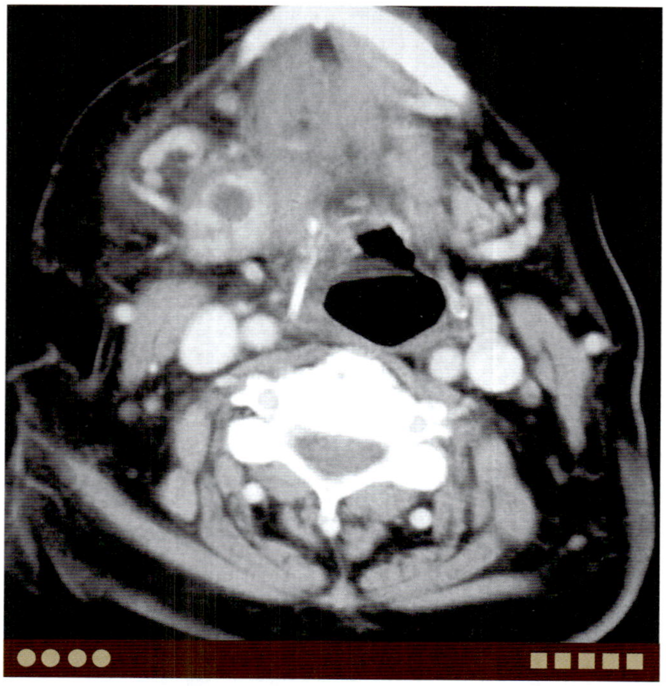

H. Submandibular gland abscess. Axial contrast-enhanced CT demonstrates a low-density area with rim-enhancement in the swollen right submandibular gland. There is adjacent fat stranding and thickening of platysma consistent with edema and inflammation.

Case 7–19 Mucoepidermoid Carcinoma—Submandibular Gland

Naoko Saito, Asim Mian, Osamu Sakai

PRESENTATION

Unilateral submandibular mass.

FINDINGS

CT demonstrates a heterogeneously enhancing tumor with internal low-density areas and poorly defined margins in the submandibular gland.

DIFFERENTIAL DIAGNOSIS

- Pleomorphic adenoma: This is the most common submandibular gland tumor. This tumor demonstrates well-circumscribed margins. Dystrophic calcifications are sometimes seen and this finding helps to differentiate from other tumors. Delayed enhancement is characteristic.
- Adenoid cystic carcinoma: This is the most common malignant submandibular gland tumor. High-grade tumor demonstrates low signal intensity on T2W image.
- Submandibular gland abscess: Fluid collection with rim-enhancement is seen surrounded by cellulitis and phlegmon.

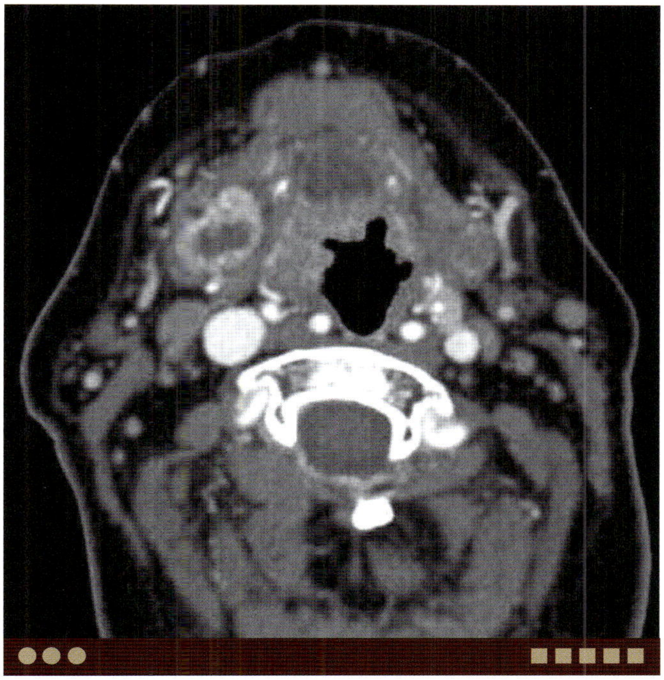

A. Mucoepidermoid carcinoma. Axial contrast-enhanced CT demonstrates a heterogeneous, peripherally enhancing tumor with poorly defined margins in the right submandibular gland.

COMMENTS

This is a 64-year-old woman with a right submandibular mass.

Mucoepidermoid carcinoma accounts for about 30% of malignant salivary gland tumors. It is the second most common malignant tumor in the submandibular gland. This tumor is often seen in individuals in their twenties and forties, however, it may be found at any age. Indeed, this tumor is the most common malignant salivary gland tumor in children and adolescents younger than 20 years of age.

Histologically, mucoepidermoid carcinoma is composed of varying proportions of epidermoid cells, mucus-secreting cells and cells intermediate between these cells. Based on the cell types, mucoepidermoid carcinomas are classified as low, intermediate, and high grade. Low-grade tumor is often characterized by prominent goblet cell component. On the other hand, high-grade tumor is characterized by necrosis with squamous cells. This tumor is rarely encapsulated but may appear well-circumscribed.

On imaging, low-grade mucoepidermoid carcinoma tends to have well-circumscribed margins, while high-grade tumor has infiltrating margins. Low-grade tumor tends to have a similar appearance to the benign tumor such as pleomorphic adenoma. High-grade tumors tend to show low signal on T2W images corresponding to high cellularity.

Intermediate- and high-grade tumors have high rate of recurrence and metastasis. Regional cervical lymph nodes are the most common metastatic sites. Distant metastasis is rare but it may involve the lungs, bones, and liver.

PEARLS

- **Mucoepidermoid carcinoma is the second most common malignant submandibular gland tumor.**
- **Low-grade mucoepidermoid carcinoma tends to have well-circumscribed margins, while high-grade tumor has infiltrating margins.**
- **Regional cervical lymph nodes are the most common sites for metastasis.**

ADDITIONAL IMAGES (B-E)

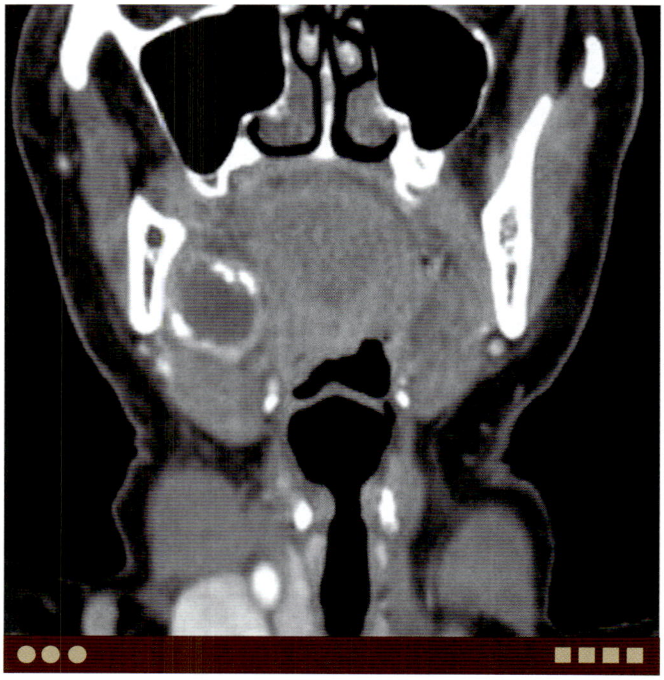

B. Mucoepidermoid carcinoma, same patient as A. Coronal contrast-enhanced CT demonstrates a peripherally enhancing cystic-appearing tumor with peripheral calcifications.

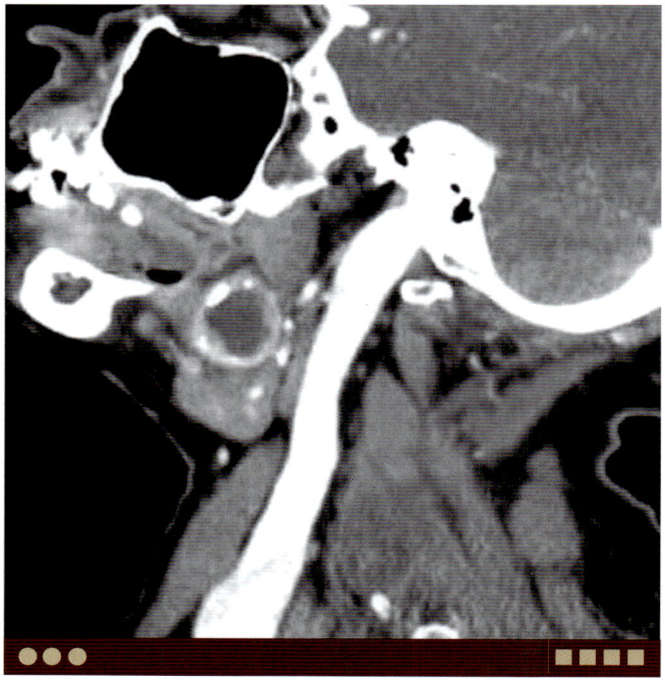

C. Mucoepidermoid carcinoma, same patient as A. Sagittal contrast-enhanced CT demonstrates a peripherally enhancing tumor with peripheral calcifications.

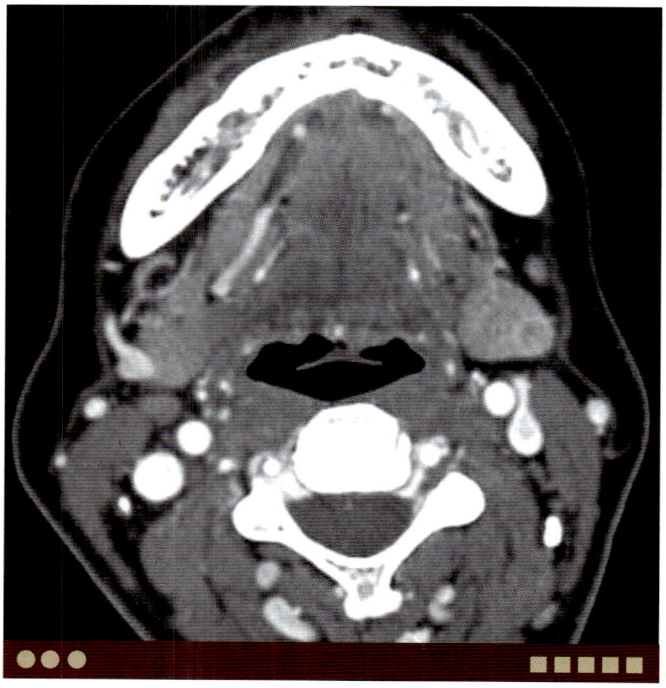

D. Low-grade mucoepidermoid carcinoma in a different patient. Axial contrast-enhanced CT demonstrates a well-circumscribed peripherally enhancing tumor in the superficial left submandibular gland.

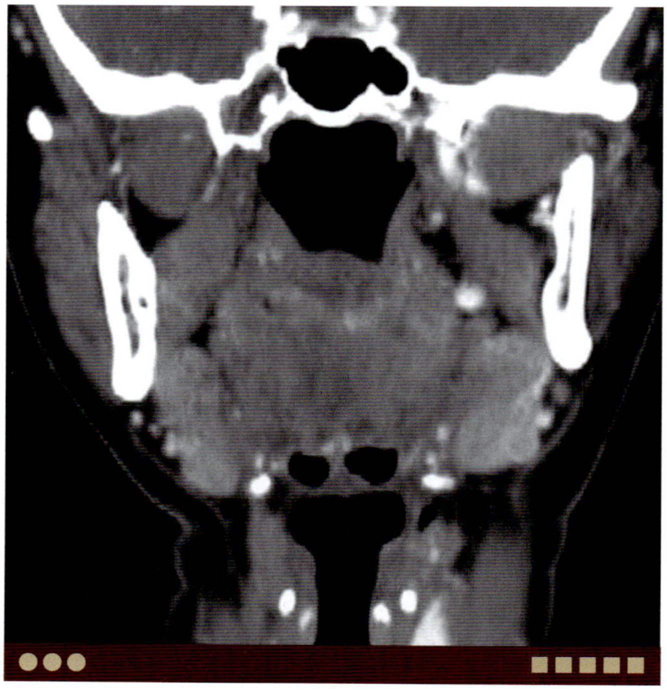

E. Low-grade mucoepidermoid carcinoma, same patient as D. Coronal contrast-enhanced CT demonstrates a well-circumscribed peripherally enhancing mass in the superficial left submandibular gland.

DIFFERENTIAL DIAGNOSIS IMAGES (F-H)

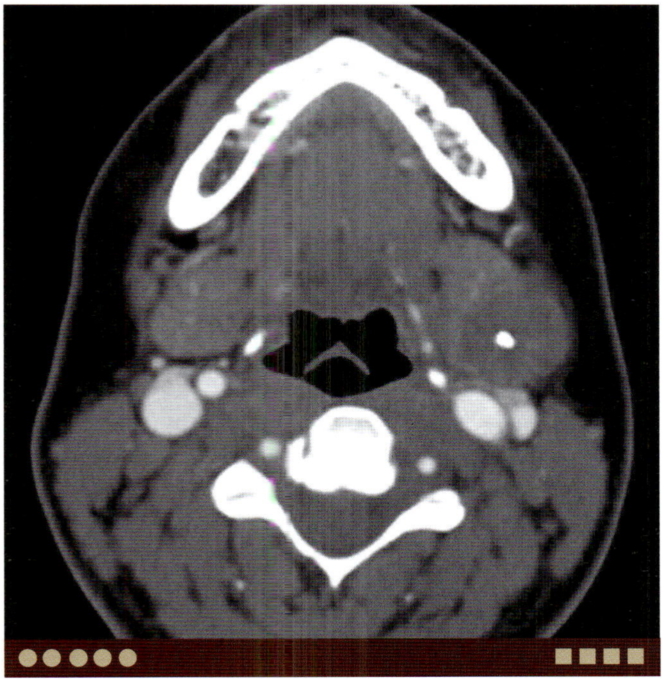

F. Pleomorphic adenoma. Axial contrast-enhanced CT demonstrates a well-circumscribed and slightly enhancing tumor in the left submandibular gland. There is a calcification within the mass, highly suggesting pleomorphic adenoma.

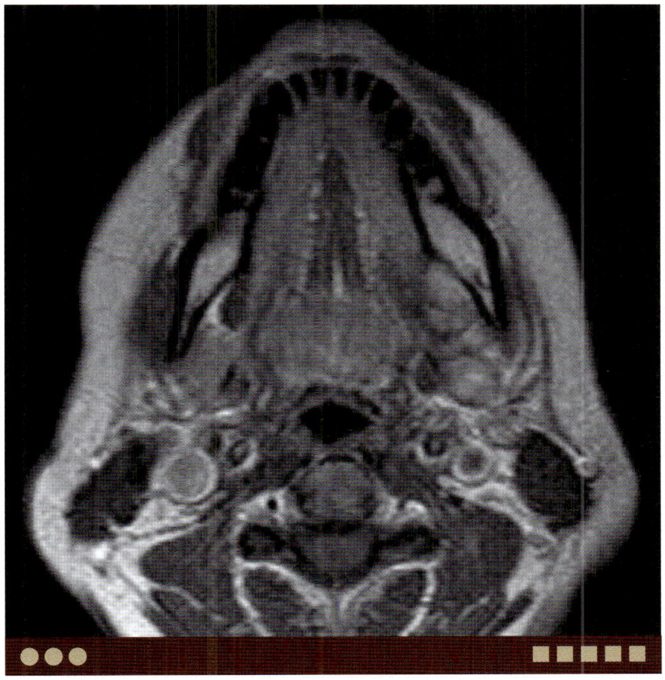

G. Adenoid cystic carcinoma. Axial postcontrast T1W image demonstrates an enhancing multicystic tumor in the left submandibular gland.

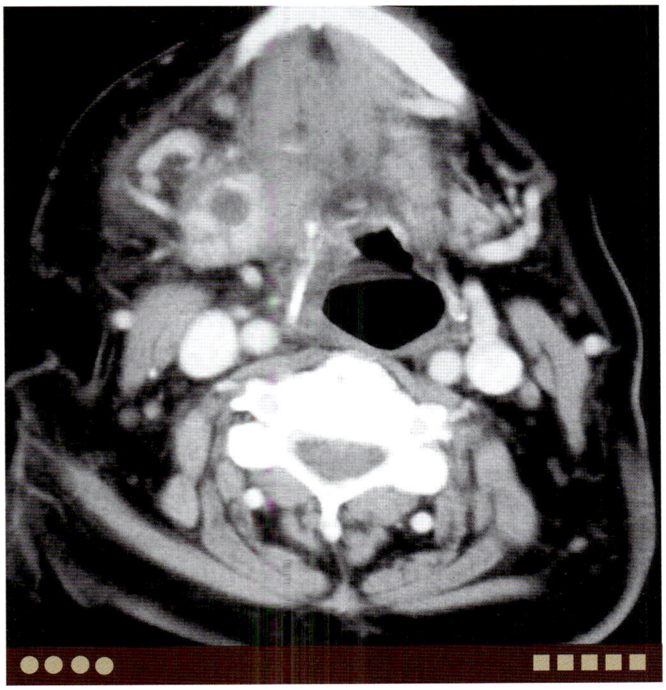

H. Submandibular gland abscess. Axial contrast-enhanced CT demonstrates a low-density area with rim-enhancement in the swollen right submandibular gland. There is adjacent fat stranding and thickening of platysma consistent with edema and inflammation.

Case 7–20 Mucoepidermoid Carcinoma—Parotid Gland

Naoko Saito, Asim Mian, Osamu Sakai

PRESENTATION

Unilateral parotid mass.

FINDINGS

Contrast-enhanced CT demonstrates a cystic mass with irregular rim-enhancement in the parotid gland.

DIFFERENTIAL DIAGNOSIS

- Adenoid cystic carcinoma: This is the second most common malignant tumor in the parotid gland after mucoepidermoid carcinoma. High-grade tumor (solid type) shows low signal on T2W image with an infiltrating appearance. This tumor has a high perineural invasion rate.
- Warthin's tumor: This usually occurs in elderly men, most commonly in the inferior portion of the parotid glands. Lesions are often multiple and bilateral and can be cystic or solid.
- Pleomorphic adenoma: This tumor is the most common parotid tumor, often seen in women in their forties and fifties. This tumor usually demonstrates delayed enhancement. Occasionally, lesions are almost entirely cystic.
- Adenocarcinoma: Adenocarcinoma arises as carcinoma ex pleomorphic adenoma from preexisting pleomorphic adenoma or de novo. Aggressive features are seen, however, imaging findings are nonspecific. Rapid growth is often seen.

COMMENTS

This is a 45-year-old man with right parotid mass.

Mucoepidermoid carcinoma accounts for about 30% of malignant salivary gland tumors. About half of the tumors occur in the major salivary gland and over 80% of them occur in the parotid gland. Mucoepidermoid carcinoma is the most common malignant parotid gland tumor. This tumor is often seen in individuals in their twenties and forties, however, it may be found at any age. Indeed, this tumor is the most common malignant salivary gland tumor in children and adolescents younger than 20 years of age. Radiation is an important etiologic factor and the latency periods may range from 7 to 32 years.

Histologically, mucoepidermoid carcinoma is composed of varying proportions of epidermoid cells, mucus-secreting cells, and cells intermediate between these cells. Based on the cell types, mucoepidermoid carcinomas are classified as low, intermediate, and high grade. Low-grade tumor is often characterized by prominent goblet cell component. On the other hand, high-grade tumor is characterized by necrosis with squamous cells. This tumor is rarely encapsulated but may appear well-circumscribed.

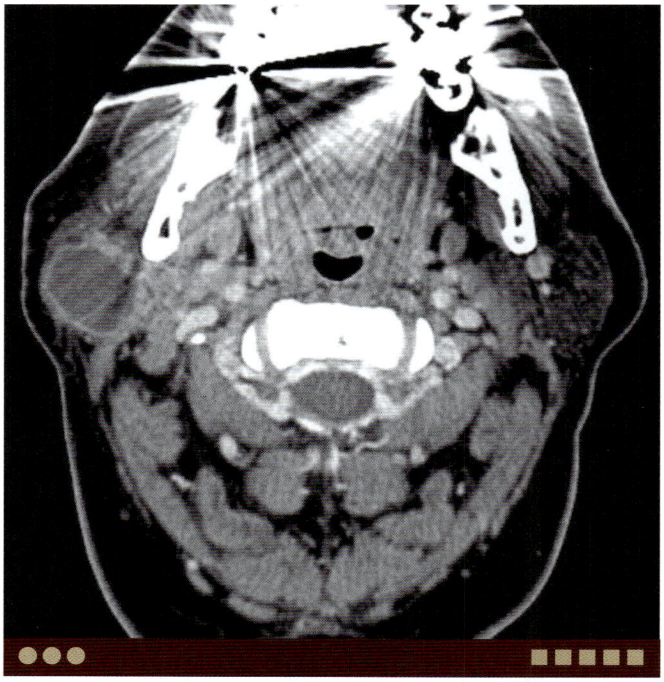

A. Mucoepidermoid carcinoma (high grade). Axial contrast-enhanced CT demonstrates a cystic tumor with irregular rim-enhancement in the right parotid gland.

On imaging, low-grade mucoepidermoid carcinoma tends to have well-circumscribed margins, similar to benign tumors, while high-grade tumor has infiltrating margins. Low-grade tumors have variable amount of serous and mucoid materials, therefore, they demonstrate low signal on T1W and high signal on T2W images. High-grade tumor demonstrates low signal on T2W images corresponding to high cellularity.

Intermediate and high-grade tumors have higher rates of recurrence and metastasis. Regional cervical lymph nodes are the most common sites for metastasis. Distant metastasis is rare but can involve the lungs, bones, and liver. High-grade mucoepidermoid carcinoma shows perineural invasion, therefore, careful evaluation of the stylomastoid foramen and foramen ovale is important.

PEARLS

- **Mucoepidermoid carcinoma is the most common malignant parotid gland tumor.**
- **Low-grade mucoepidermoid carcinoma tends to have well-circumscribed margins, while high-grade tumor has infiltrating margins.**
- **Regional cervical lymph nodes are the most common metastatic sites.**

ADDITIONAL IMAGES (B-F)

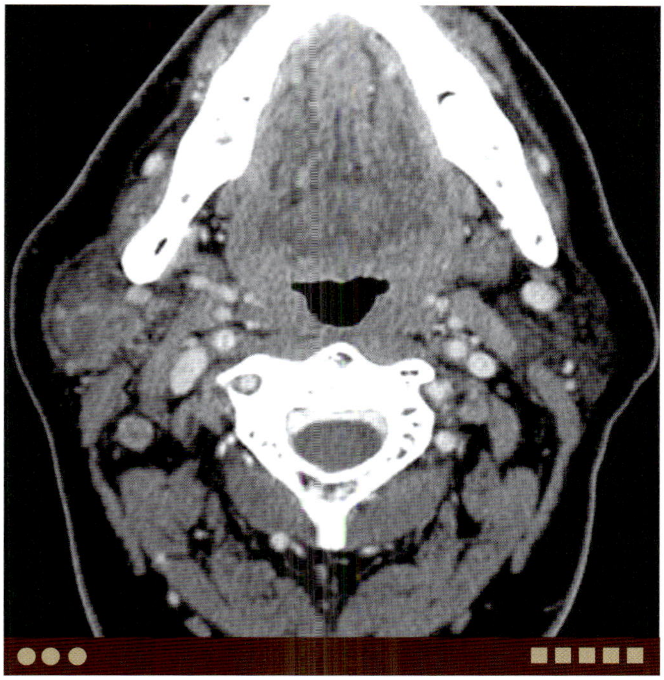

B. Mucoepidermoid carcinoma (high grade), same patient as A. Axial contrast-enhanced CT through the lower level shows the tumor to have infiltrative margins. Necrotic right level II node is noted, suggesting metastasis.

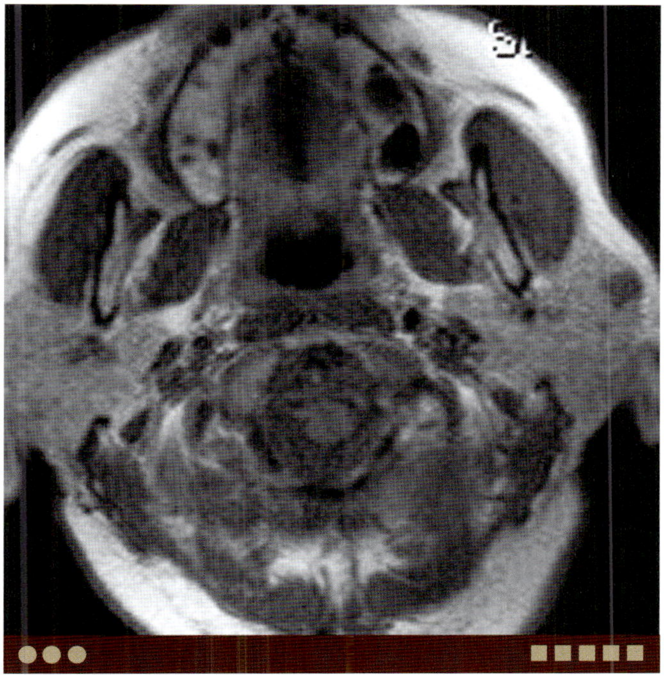

C. Mucoepidermoid carcinoma (low grade). Axial T1W image demonstrates a well-circumscribed low-signal intensity mass in the superficial lobe of the left parotid gland.

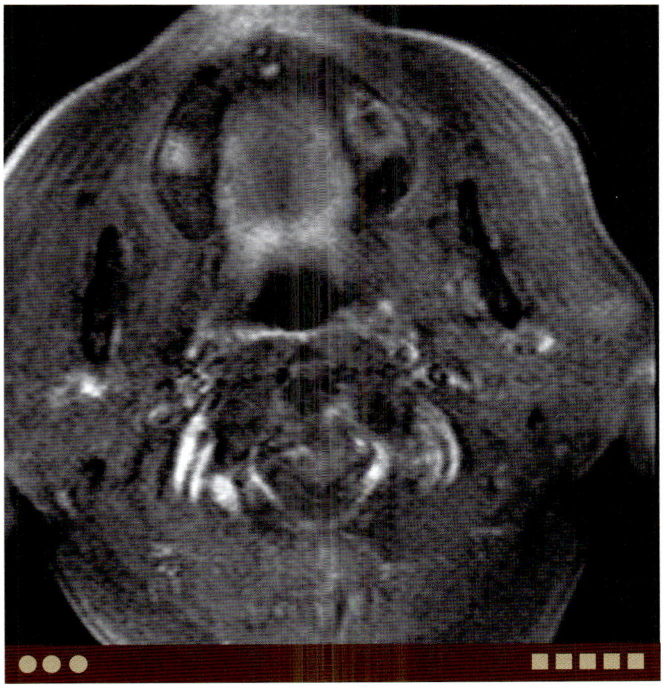

D. Mucoepidermoid carcinoma (low grade), same patient as C. Axial postcontrast, fat-suppressed T1W image demonstrates homogeneous enhancement in the lesion.

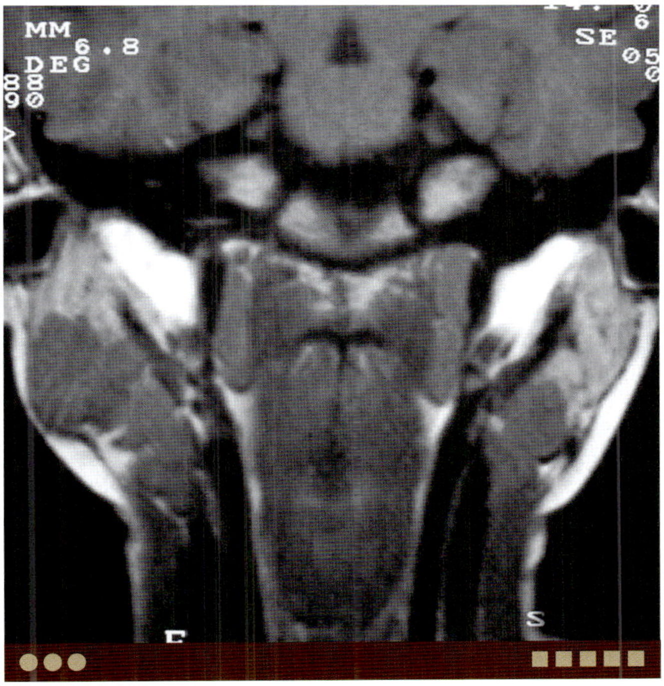

E. Mucoepidermoid carcinoma in a different patient (7-year-old boy). Coronal T1W image demonstrates a slightly lobulated low-signal tumor in the right parotid gland.

DIFFERENTIAL DIAGNOSIS IMAGES (G-J)

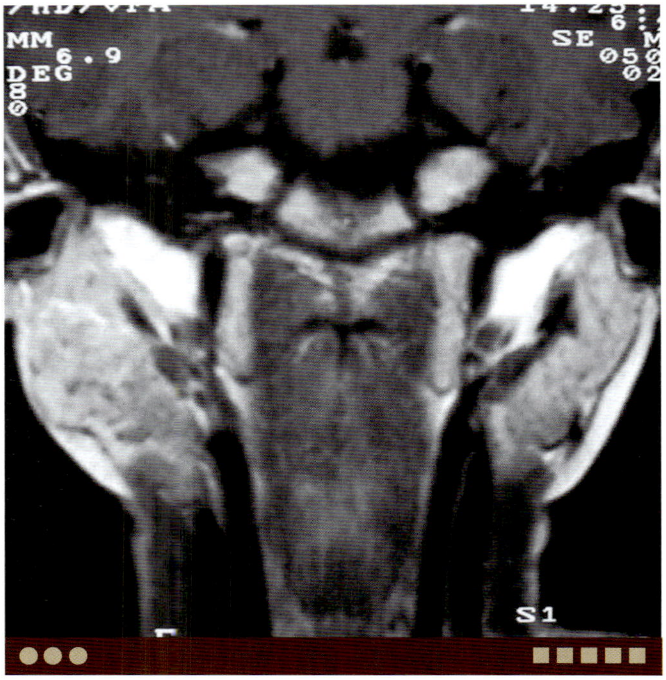

F. Mucoepidermoid carcinoma, same patient as E. Coronal post-contrast T1W image demonstrates homogeneous enhancement in the lesion.

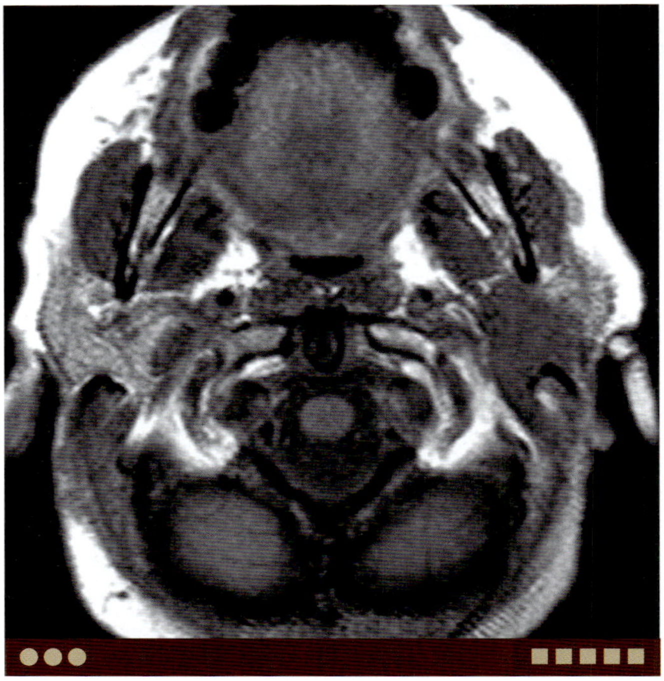

G. Adenoid cystic carcinoma. Axial T1W image demonstrates a poorly circumscribed low-signal tumor in the left parotid gland extending into the stylomastoid foramen.

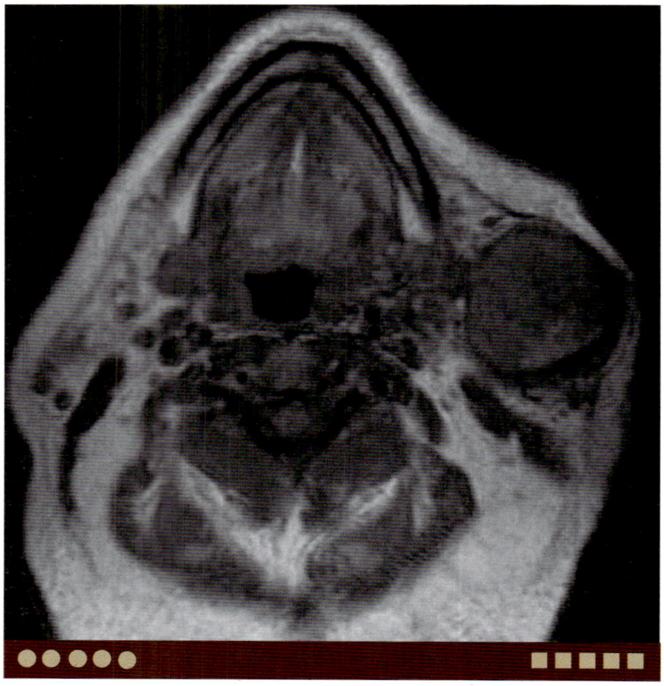

H. Warthin's tumor. Axial T1W image demonstrates a heterogeneous low-signal mass in the inferior portion of the left parotid gland. The lesion has heterogeneously high-signal areas corresponding to hemorrhage.

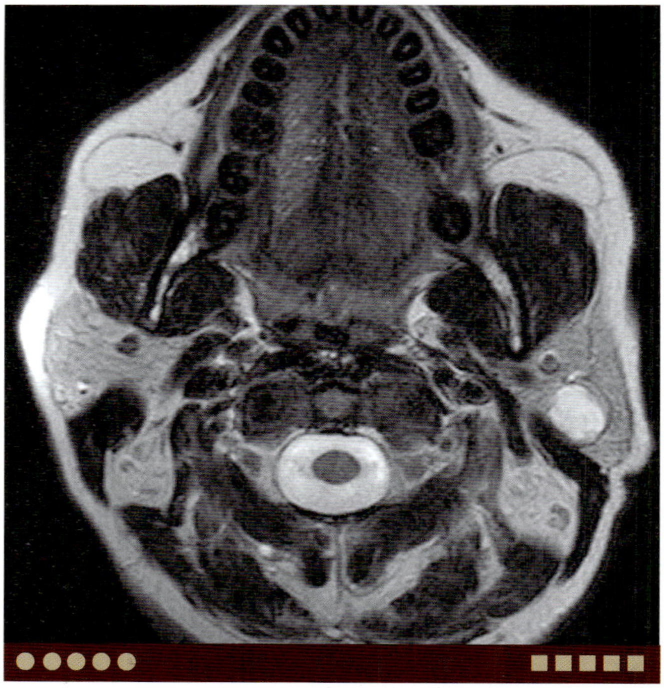

I. Pleomorphic adenoma. Axial T2W image demonstrates a well-circumscribed, slightly lobulated high-signal mass in the left parotid gland.

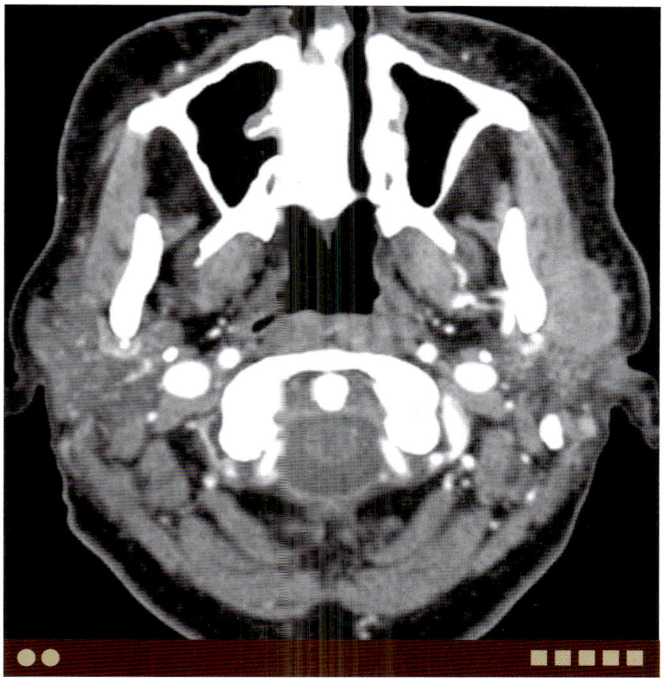

J. Adenocarcinoma. Axial contrast-enhanced CT demonstrates a heterogeneously enhancing tumor with irregular margins in the superficial lobe of the left parotid gland.

Case 7–21 Carcinoma Ex Pleomorphic Adenoma

Naoko Saito, Asim Mian, Osamu Sakai

PRESENTATION

Rapid increase in size of known pleomorphic adenoma.

FINDINGS

CT and MRI demonstrate a heterogeneous salivary gland tumor.

DIFFERENTIAL DIAGNOSIS

- Pleomorphic adenoma: Pleomorphic adenoma is the most common salivary gland tumor. It often shows heterogeneous low-to-intermediate signal on T1W and intermediate-to-high signal on T2W images with well-circumscribed margins.
- Mucoepidermoid carcinoma: Low-grade tumors often show cystic areas with well-delineated, smooth margins. High-grade tumors show heterogeneous low-to-intermediate signal on both T1W and T2W images with indistinct infiltrative margins.
- Adenoid cystic carcinoma: Like a mucoepidermoid carcinoma, adenoid cystic carcinoma shows either a benign (low-grade) or malignant (high-grade) appearance. Perineural tumor spread is common.

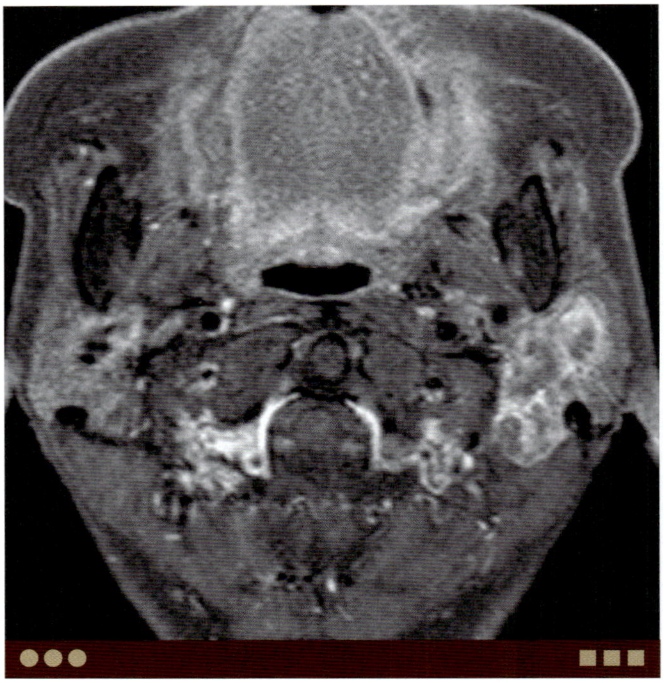

A. Carcinoma ex pleomorphic adenoma. Axial postcontrast fat-suppressed T1W image demonstrates a left parotid gland mass with heterogeneous enhancement and infiltrative margins.

COMMENTS

This is a 70-year-old woman who presented with a painless mass in the left parotid gland for 5 years with progressive left-sided facial palsy.

Malignant mixed salivary gland tumors should be divided into three different clinical and histological entities: (1) carcinoma ex pleomorphic adenoma, (2) carcinosarcoma, and (3) metastasizing pleomorphic adenoma. Carcinoma ex pleomorphic adenoma usually occurs in the major salivary glands, especially in the parotid gland. Malignant changes in pleomorphic adenoma are associated with a long duration, tumor recurrence, radiation therapy, advanced age, and tumor size. The patient presents with rapid growth of the known tumor, often with pain and facial nerve paralysis. Histological types of carcinomas occurring from pleomorphic adenomas are variable (e.g., undifferentiated carcinoma, adenocarcinoma, and squamous cell carcinoma).

Imaging findings of carcinomas ex pleomorphic adenomas are often nonspecific. However, they tend to have fairly low signal on both T1W and T2W images due to high cellularity. If carcinomas are localized within the capsule, well-delineated, smooth margins can be seen. However, focally or completely indistinct infiltrative margins can be seen once they extend beyond the capsule. Carcinoma ex pleomorphic adenoma often contains hemorrhage and necrotic tissue. CT and MRI demonstrate heterogeneous densities/signals and heterogeneous enhancement reflecting various pathologic conditions. Intratumoral hemorrhage shows high signal on T1W images. Calcification which is assumed from pleomorphic adenoma may be seen on CT. Cervical nodal metastasis with necrosis is often observed.

PEARLS

- **Carcinoma ex pleomorphic adenoma should be considered when patients present with rapid growth of known salivary gland tumors.**
- **Imaging findings of carcinoma ex pleomorphic adenoma are nonspecific, however, heterogeneous density or signal are often seen on CT and MRI, reflecting hemorrhage and necrosis.**
- **Carcinoma ex pleomorphic adenoma shows either smooth or infiltrative margins, depending on extension of the tumor.**

ADDITIONAL IMAGES (B-E)

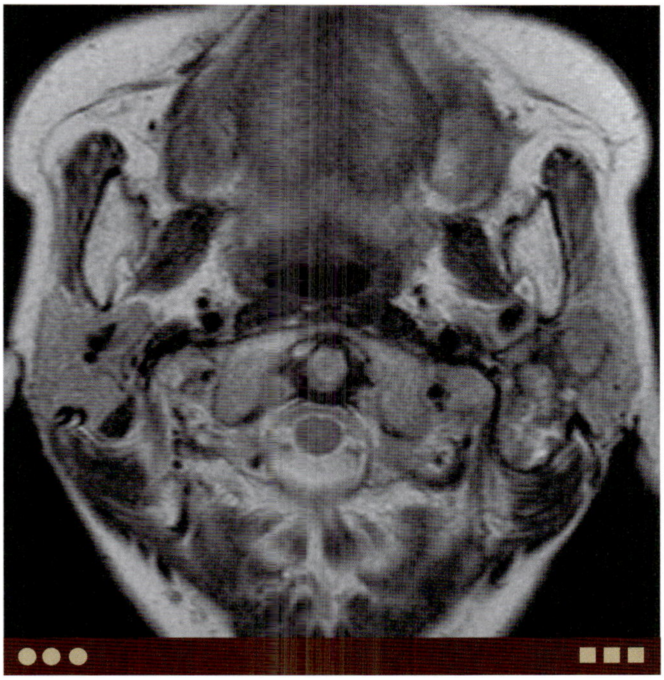

B. Carcinoma ex pleomorphic adenoma, same patient as A. Axial T2W image demonstrates heterogeneous low-to-high signal within the tumor.

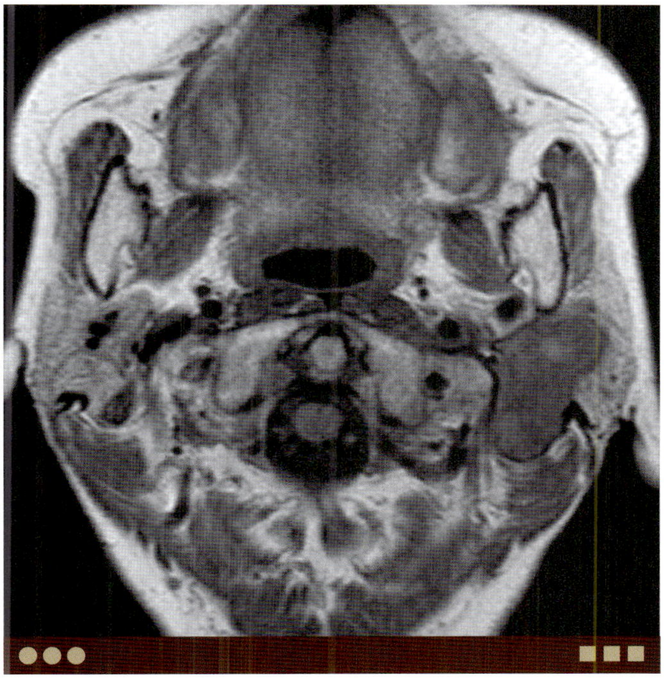

C. Carcinoma ex pleomorphic adenoma, same patient as A. Axial T1W image demonstrates focal high signal intensity in the tumor, reflecting intratumoral hemorrhage.

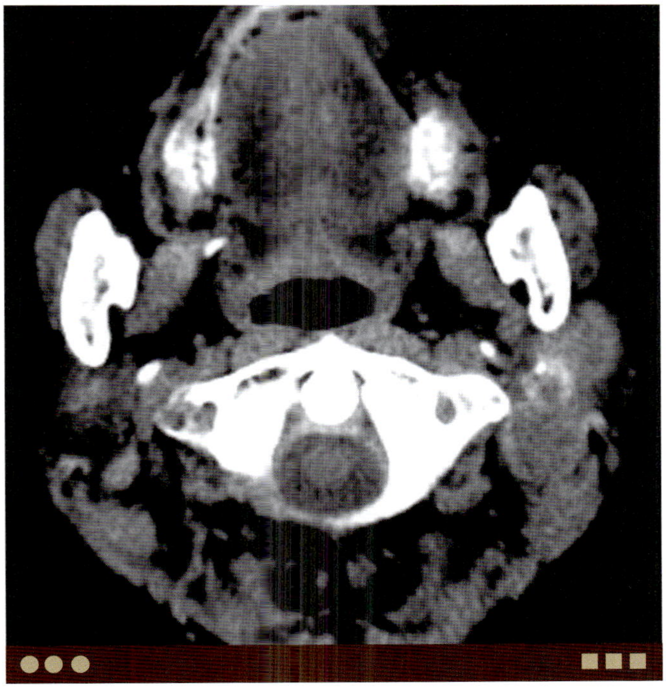

D. Carcinoma ex pleomorphic adenoma, same patient as A. Axial unenhanced CT demonstrates a left parotid gland tumor with calcification.

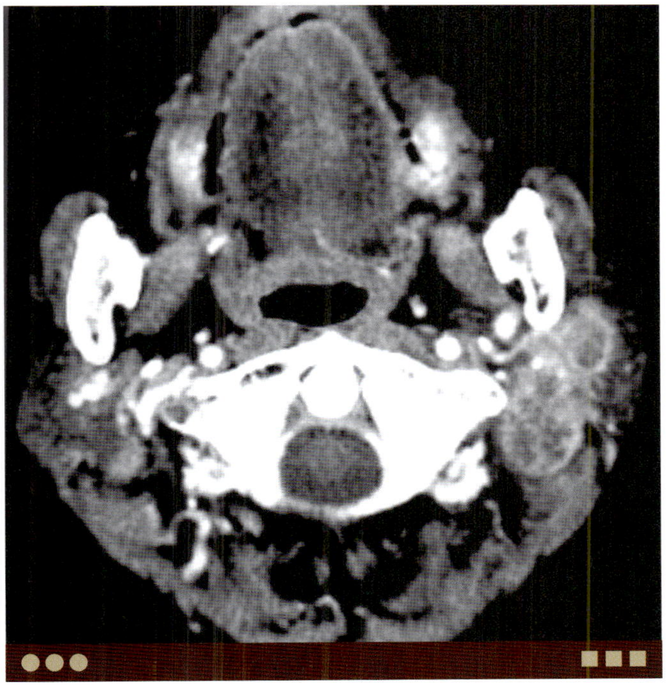

E. Carcinoma ex pleomorphic adenoma, same patient as A. Axial enhanced CT demonstrates heterogeneous enhancement in the tumor.

DIFFERENTIAL DIAGNOSIS IMAGES (F-G)

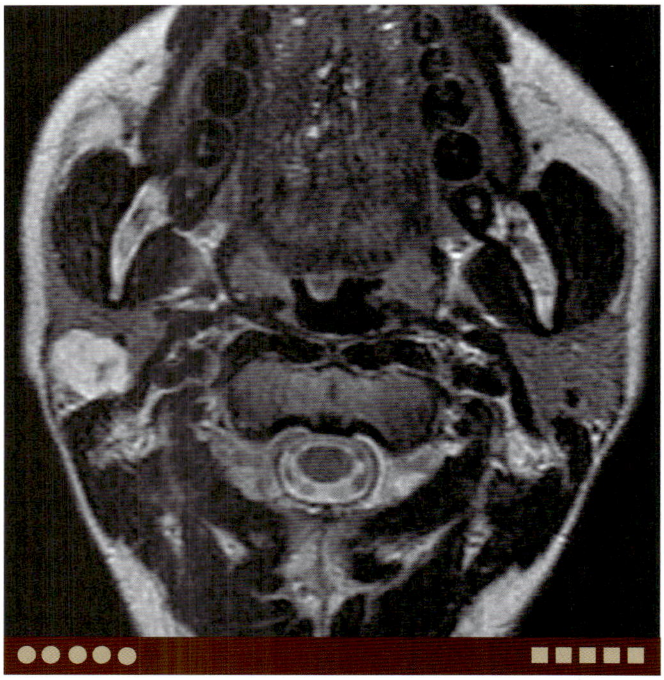

F. Pleomorphic adenoma. Axial T2W image demonstrates a right parotid gland tumor with homogeneous high signal intensity and slightly lobulated well-defined margin.

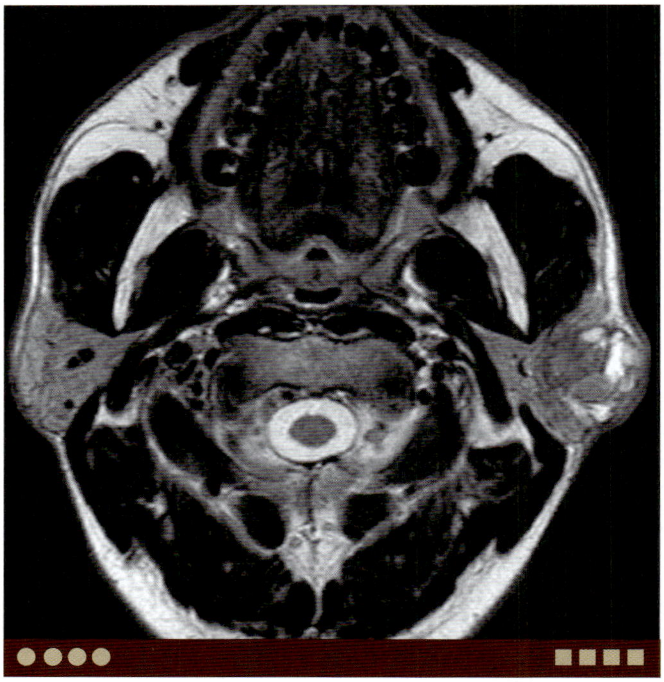

G. Mucoepidermoid carcinoma. Axial T2W image demonstrates a left parotid gland tumor with heterogeneous cystic components.

Case 7–22 Epithelial-Myoepithelial Carcinoma—Parotid

Hiroki Kato, Asim Mian, Osamu Sakai

PRESENTATION

Slowly enlarging mass within the parotid gland, associated with facial nerve pain and weakness.

FINDINGS

CT and MRI demonstrate a low-grade or benign-appearing parotid gland tumor.

DIFFERENTIAL DIAGNOSIS

- Pleomorphic adenoma: Pleomorphic adenoma is the most common salivary gland tumor. A small pleomorphic adenoma is fairly homogeneous and hyperintense on T2W images with hypointense capsules. However, large tumors often show heterogeneous signal. Total or subtotal cystic degeneration of benign pleomorphic adenomas is not common.
- Warthin's tumor: Warthin's tumors are composed of a lymphoid stroma and eosinophilic epithelial cells with cystic spaces. The cystic components filled with proteinaceous secretion vary from a few mm to 1-2 cm, and is recognized as high signal foci on T1W images.
- Mucoepidermoid carcinoma: Low-grade mucoepidermoid carcinomas are characterized by cysts containing mucin, which appear as high-intensity spots within the tumor on both T1WI and T2WI. Prominent cystic structures are the hallmark of low-grade mucoepidermoid carcinomas.
- Adenoid cystic carcinoma: Adenoid cystic carcinomas of the parotid gland tend to appear as benign, well-delineated tumors, while adenoid cystic carcinomas of the minor salivary gland usually have ill-defined margins.

COMMENTS

This is an 86-year-old woman presented with a painless mass in the left parotid gland for 3 months without facial nerve palsy.

Epithelial-myoepithelial carcinoma is a rare low-grade malignant salivary gland neoplasm defined by the World Health Organization (WHO) classification in 1991. Epithelial-myoepithelial carcinoma is rare and accounts for less than 1% of salivary gland tumors. It predominantly arises in the parotid gland; however, it has been described in the submandibular gland and in the minor salivary glands as well. The majority arises in patients in the seventh and eighth decades of life, with a female predominance. Although, they are thought to be of low-grade malignancy,

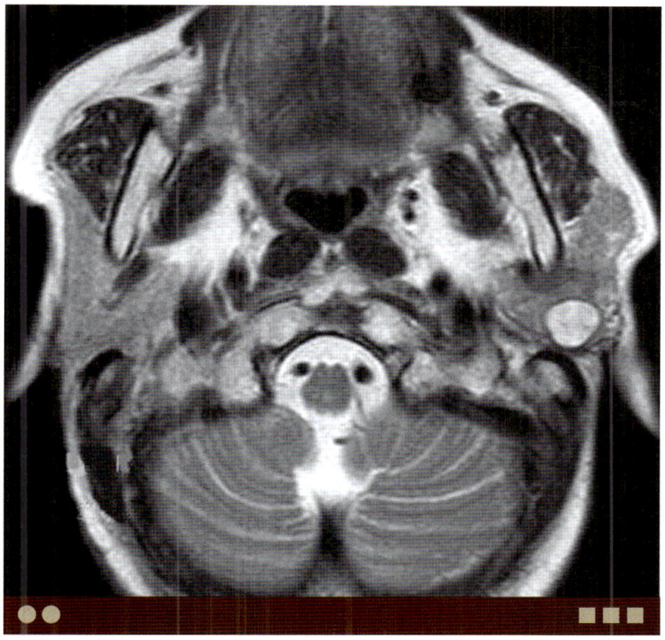

A. Epithelial-myoepithelial carcinoma. Axial T2W MR image demonstrates a well-demarcated, cystic-appearing high-signal lesion in the left parotid gland.

fatal courses are described due to their significant likelihood of local recurrence after resection. Regional nodal spread is seen, however, distant metastasis rarely occurs.

Imaging findings of epithelial-myoepithelial carcinoma are nonspecific, and it is very difficult to be differentiated from other more common parotid neoplasms by the imaging characteristics only. Epithelial-myoepithelial carcinoma is often seen as a low-grade, benign-appearing mass, which can be cystic. Therefore, it may be similar to Warthin's tumor.

The pathologic differential diagnosis includes clear cell carcinoma, mucoepidermoid carcinoma, acinic cell carcinoma, sebaceous carcinoma, and metastatic renal cell carcinoma.

PEARLS

- **Imaging findings of epithelial-myoepithelial carcinoma are nonspecific.**
- **Epithelial-myoepithelial carcinoma demonstrates a low-grade, benign-appearing mass.**
- **Epithelial-myoepithelial carcinoma may be cystic, and may be similar to Warthin's tumor.**

ADDITIONAL IMAGES (B-D)

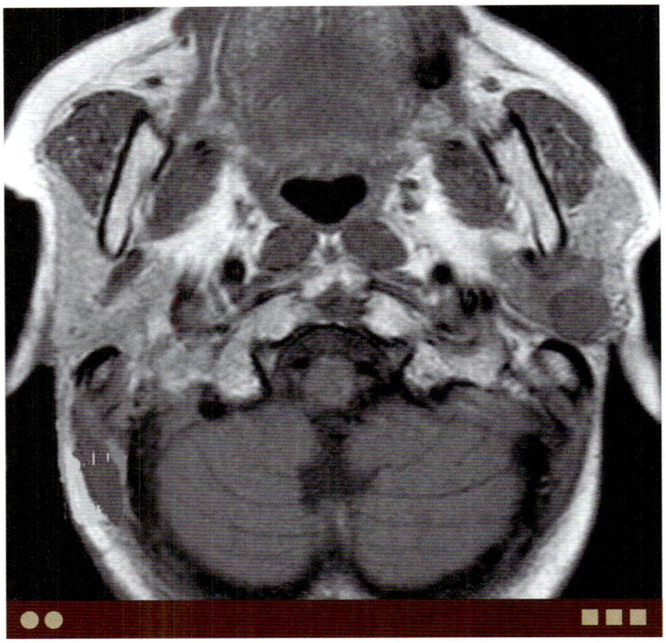

B. Epithelial-myoepithelial carcinoma, same patient as A. Axial T1W image demonstrates low signal.

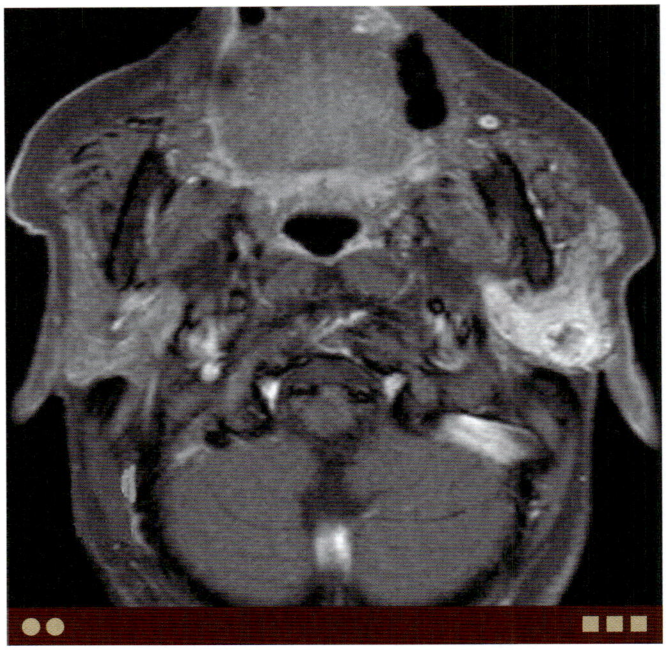

C. Epithelial-myoepithelial carcinoma, same patient as A. Axial postcontrast fat-suppressed T1W image demonstrates slightly heterogeneous peripheral enhancement.

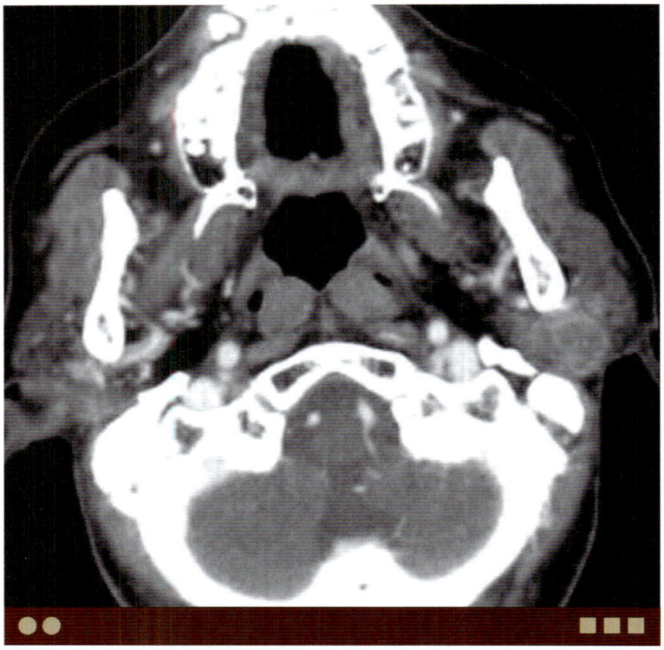

D. Epithelial-myoepithelial carcinoma, same patient as A. Axial enhanced CT demonstrates slightly heterogeneous peripheral enhancement.

DIFFERENTIAL DIAGNOSIS IMAGES (E-G)

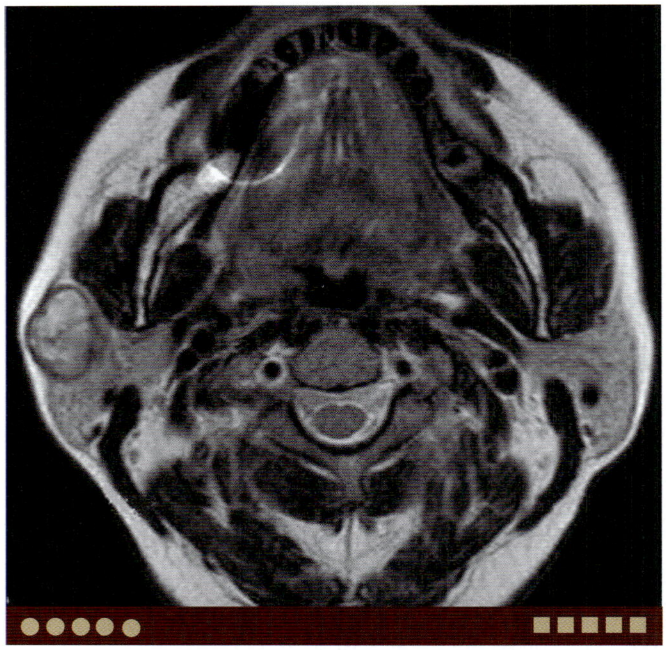

E. Pleomorphic adenoma. Axial T2W MR image demonstrates a slightly heterogeneous high-signal lesion with fibrous capsule in the right parotid gland.

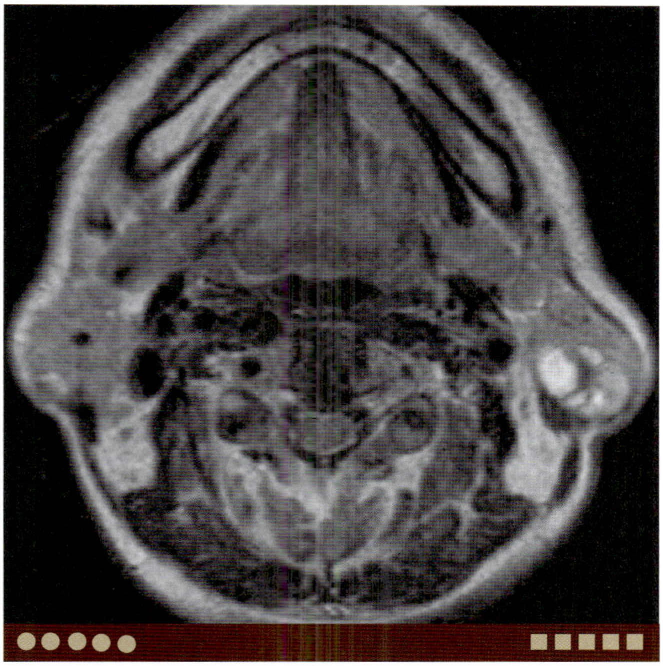

F. Warthin's tumor. Axial T2W MR image demonstrates a mass with multiple cystic components in the left parotid gland.

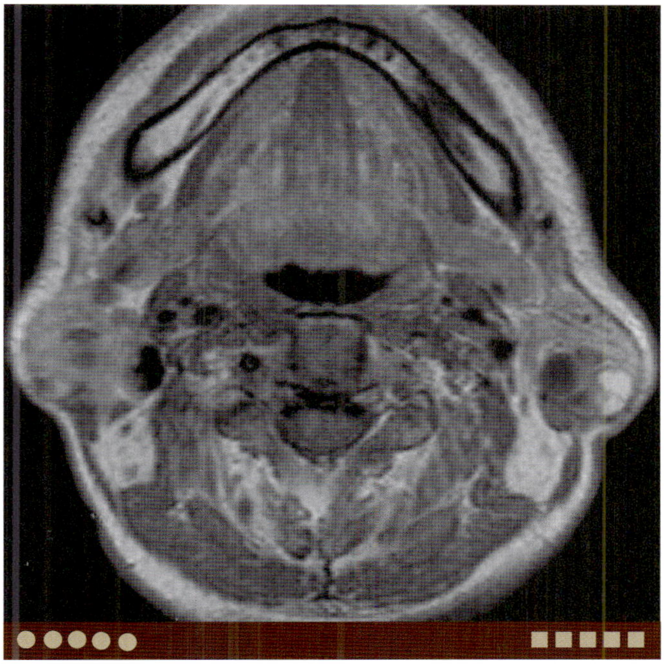

G. Warthin's tumor, same patient as F. Axial postcontrast T1W image demonstrates mild enhancement in the solid portion of the lesion. Multiple cystic portions show various signals reflecting difference in protein concentration.

Case 7-23 Schwannoma—Parotid (Facial Nerve)

Hiroki Kato, Asim Mian, Osamu Sakai

PRESENTATION

Palpable parotid mass with slowly progressing facial nerve paralysis.

FINDINGS

MRI demonstrates a smoothly demarcated, elongated lesion along the facial nerve.

DIFFERENTIAL DIAGNOSIS

- Pleomorphic adenoma: This is the most common parotid gland tumor and usually a single lesion. Imaging findings are often nonspecific; however, typical MR imaging findings include well-defined borders, lobulated contour and high T2 signal. Calcification may be seen.
- Warthin's tumor: This is the second most common benign tumor of the parotid gland after pleomorphic adenoma. It occurs largely in older men in the parotid gland or periparotid region, mostly involving the inferior pole of the gland. Multicentric lesions are seen more often seen with Warthin's tumor than any other salivary gland tumor.
- Hemangioma: Vascular/lymphatic tumor is the most common benign mesenchymal neoplasm. Hemangiomas in the parotid gland are usually cavernous type, although capillary hemangiomas of parotid gland have been reported. On MRI, marked T2 high signal and the presence of signal voids representing vessels and phleboliths are the hallmark features.
- Low-grade mucoepidermoid carcinoma, adenoid cystic carcinoma: Low-grade salivary gland malignant tumor often shows benign appearance.

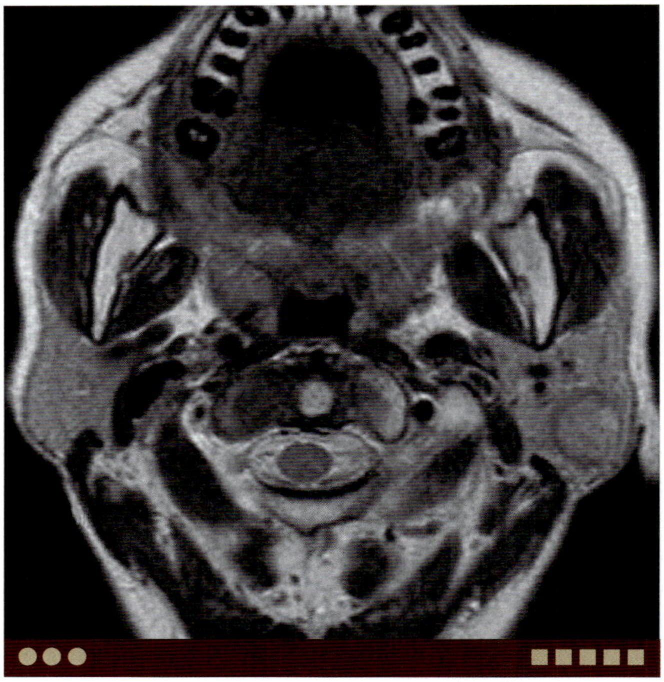

A. Schwannoma. Axial T2W MR image demonstrates a well-demarcated left parotid gland mass. Note low-signal fibrous capsule.

COMMENTS

This is a 57-year-old man with palpable left parotid mass.

Although approximately one-third of schwannomas occur in the head and neck, facial nerve schwannoma is rare. Facial nerve schwannoma may arise from any segments of the facial nerve, from the cerebellopontine angle to the peripheral branch in the parotid gland, but commonly seen in the genu and tympanic segment. Neurogenic tumors of the parotid gland are the second most common benign mesenchymal neoplasm after vascular/lymphatic tumors. Both schwannoma and neurofibroma occur in the parotid gland. There are no specific symptoms for facial nerve schwannoma, and diagnosis may be difficult. Therefore, facial nerve schwannomas in the parotid gland are frequently misdiagnosed preoperatively.

On CT and MRI, schwannomas are often seen as well-demarcated, fusiform masses. Frequently a low-signal intensity rim, reflecting fibrous capsule, is seen. They demonstrate intermediate signal on T1W and heterogeneous high signal on T2W images. The imaging findings of schwannomas reflect the pathological biphasic pattern with areas of high cellularity (Antoni type A) and less cellular areas where highly myxoid matrix predominates (Antoni type B). On dynamic contrast-enhanced study, schwannomas show delayed enhancement. On diffusion-weighted MR images, schwannomas show high ADC values. These imaging findings are similar to that of pleomorphic adenoma, which is the most common tumor in the parotid gland. However, multiplicity of facial nerve schwannoma (14%) may be helpful to make the diagnosis, because multiple pleomorphic adenomas are extremely rare. Meanwhile solitary neurofibroma affecting the major salivary gland is uncommon. Multiple neurofibromas and plexiform neurofibromas involving salivary glands are often seen associated with neurofibromatosis type I, von Recklinghausen's disease.

PEARLS

- **Schwannoma is the most common tumor associated with the facial nerve.**
- **Facial nerve schwannoma in the parotid gland is frequently misdiagnosed preoperatively.**
- **The differentiation of schwannoma and pleomorphic adenoma is often difficult. However, multiplicity of facial nerve schwannoma is helpful to make the diagnosis.**

ADDITIONAL IMAGES (B-E)

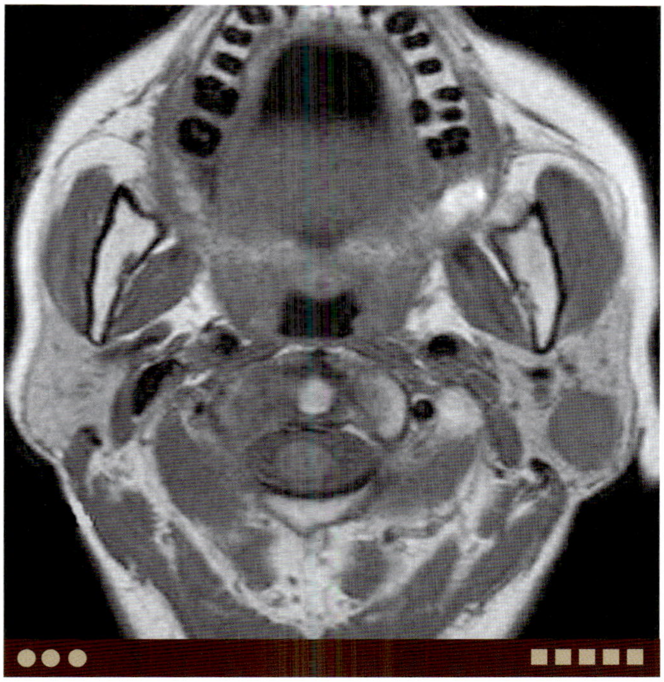

B. Schwannoma, same patient as A. Axial T1W image demonstrates low signal intensity.

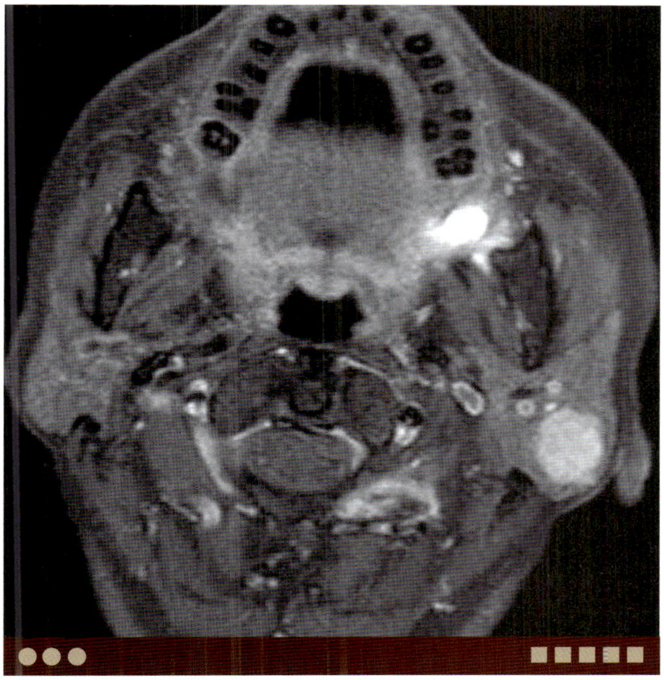

C. Schwannoma, same patient as A. Axial postcontrast fat-suppressed T1W image demonstrates homogeneous enhancement.

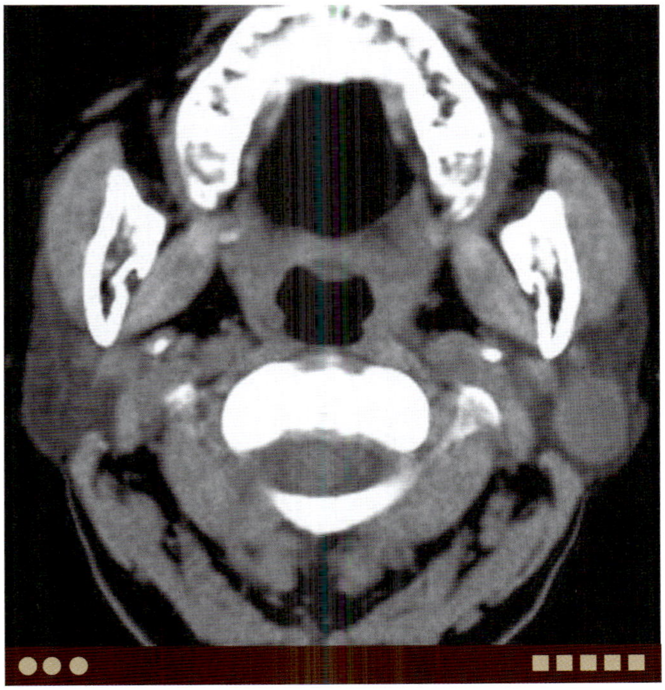

D. Schwannoma, same patient as A. Axial unenhanced CT demonstrates a homogeneous mass.

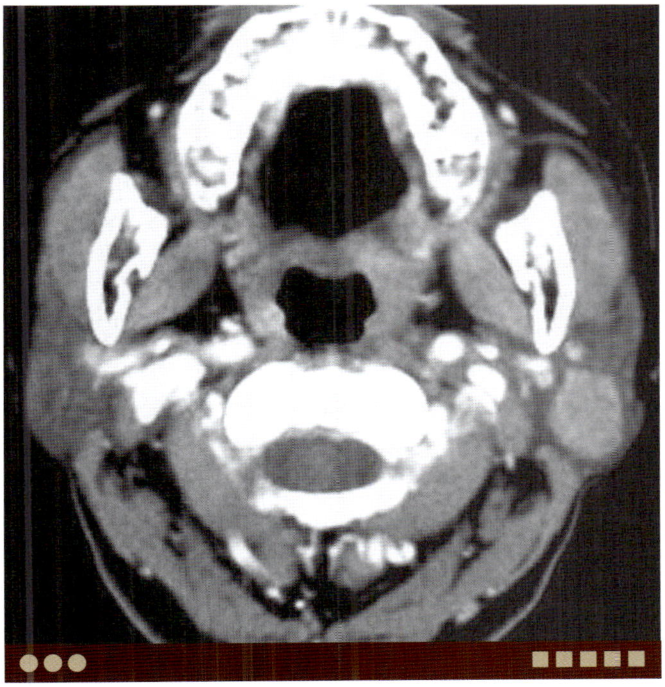

E. Schwannoma, same patient as A. Axial enhanced CT demonstrates homogeneous enhancement.

DIFFERENTIAL DIAGNOSIS IMAGES (F-G)

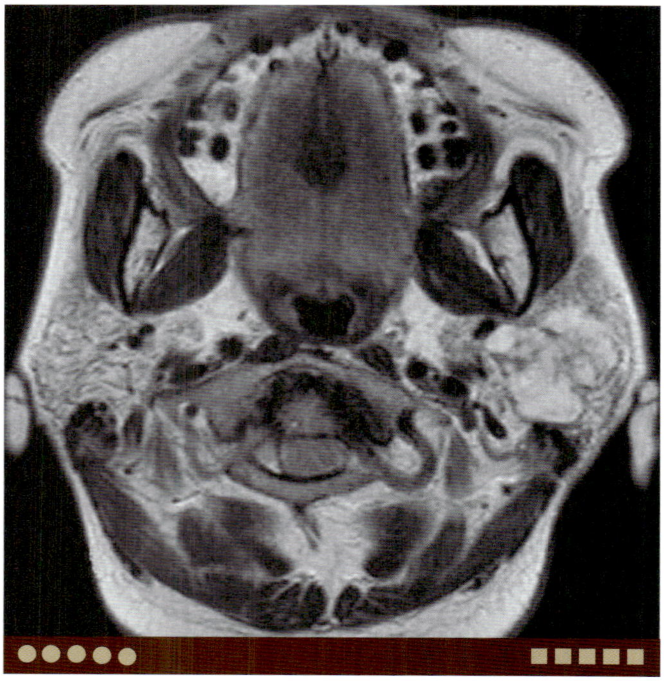

F. Pleomorphic adenoma. Axial T2W MR image demonstrates a lobulated, heterogeneous high-signal lesion in the left parotid gland.

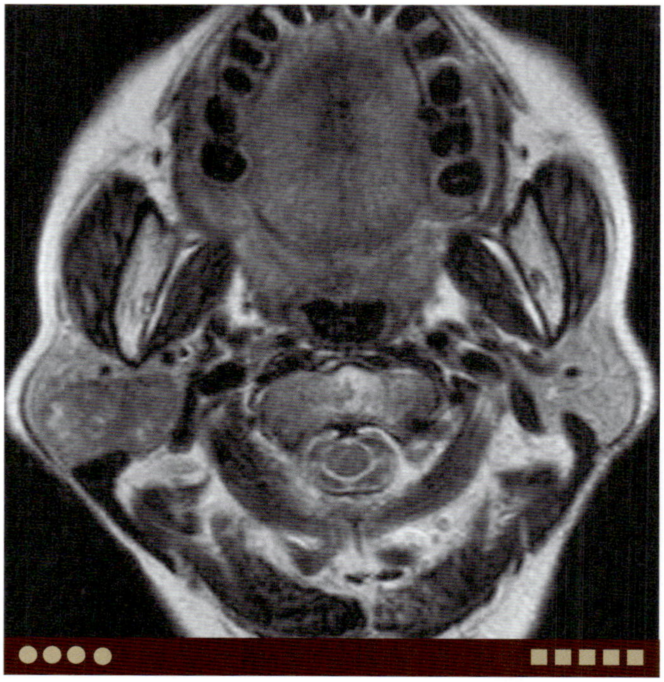

G. Warthin's tumor. Axial T2W MR image demonstrates a well-demarcated lesion with cystic components in the right parotid gland.

Case 7–24 Mumps Parotitis

Hiroki Kato, Asim Mian, Osamu Sakai

PRESENTATION

Swelling and pain of the salivary gland with fever.

FINDINGS

CT and MRI demonstrate enlarged salivary glands.

DIFFERENTIAL DIAGNOSIS

- Bacterial sialadenitis: Acute bacterial (suppurative) sialadenitis almost always involves the parotid gland. Heterogeneous enhancement is often seen on CT and MRI and a low-density area with peripheral enhancement suggests an abscess. Bacterial parotitis and parotid abscess are treated with antibiotics and surgical drainage if necessary.
- Sarcoidosis: Sarcoidosis is a systemic disease characterized by the formation of noncaseating granulomas in multiple organ systems. The parotid gland may be involved in up to 30% of patients.
- Sjögren's syndrome: Sjögren's syndrome is an autoimmune disorder characterized by inflammation and destruction of the exocrine glands, primarily the lacrimal and salivary glands.
- Lymphoma: Although rare primary lymphoma of the salivary glands most often involves the parotid gland and is classified as a mucosa-associated lymphoid tissue (MALT) lymphoma. Secondary lymphoma of the salivary glands is also rare but also most commonly involves the parotid gland.

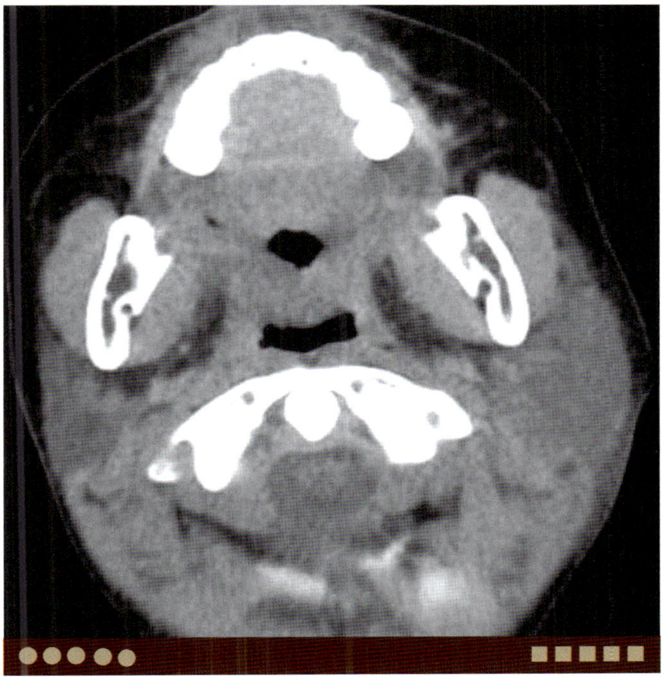

A. Mumps parotitis. Axial unenhanced CT demonstrates enlargement of the left parotid gland.

COMMENTS

This is a 5-year-old girl presenting with swelling and pain in the right parotid gland.

Mumps is by far the most common viral cause of parotitis in children, usually at the age of 5 to 14 years. Mumps is transmitted through airborne droplets from the coughs and sneezes of infected people. The virus that most commonly causes mumps is a paramyxovirus. The infection is more common during late winter and spring. Initially, patients are not very symptomatic but may have fever, loss of appetite, and headache. Swelling of the parotid glands usually starts on one side and then progresses to the other side rapidly.

Mumps is usually a mild illness; however, severe complications may be seen in a minority of cases. Encephalitis and meningitis occasionally occur. About 25% of male patients over age of 12 may develop inflammation of testicles (orchitis). Rarely, female patients may develop inflammation of ovaries (oophritis). Mumps also involves pancreas, thyroid and other areas of the body. Since there is no specific treatment for mumps, supportive treatment is applied.

In mumps parotitis, CT shows parotid gland enlargement with diffuse enhancement after intravenous administration of contrast material. MRI demonstrates an enlarged parotid gland that is hypointense on T1W and hyperintense on T2W images with enhancement.

PEARLS

- **Parotitis is the most common parotid disease in children and mumps is by far the most common viral cause of parotitis in children.**
- **Mumps parotitis is seen as parotid gland enlargement with diffuse enhancement on CT.**
- **Mumps parotitis shows hypointense on T1W and hyperintense on T2W images and enhancement in enlarged parotid glands.**

ADDITIONAL IMAGES (B-C)

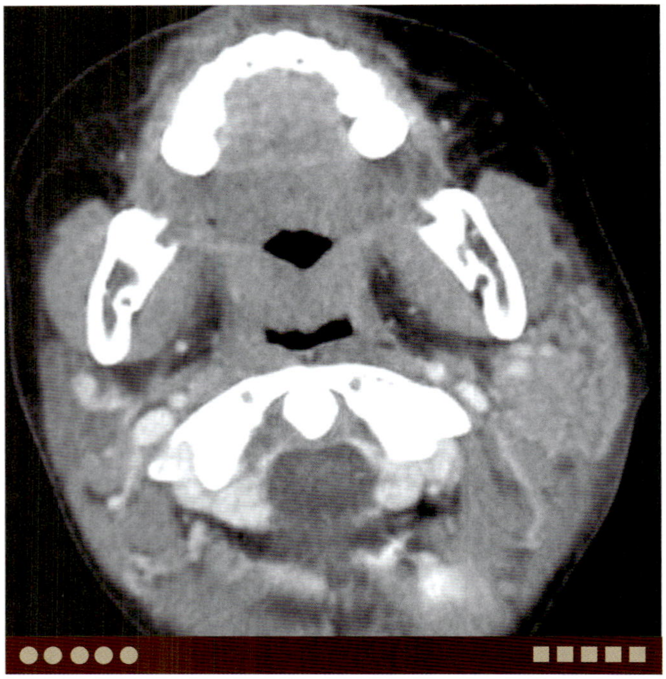

B. Mumps parotitis, same patient as A. Axial contrast-enhanced CT demonstrates diffuse enhancement in the enlarged gland with inflammatory change in the surrounding tissue.

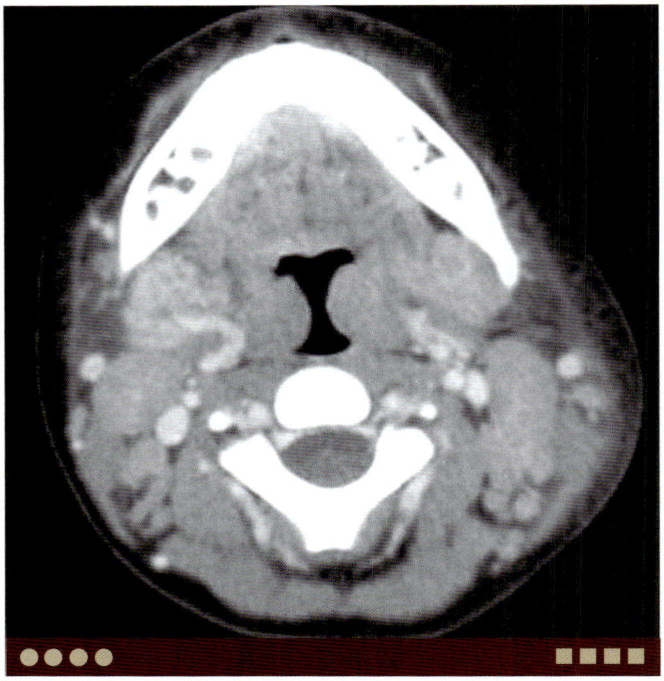

C. Mumps parotitis, same patient as A. Axial contrast-enhanced CT demonstrates enhancing reactive nodes bilaterally. Note inflammatory change in the left superficial soft tissue.

DIFFERENTIAL DIAGNOSIS IMAGES (D-G)

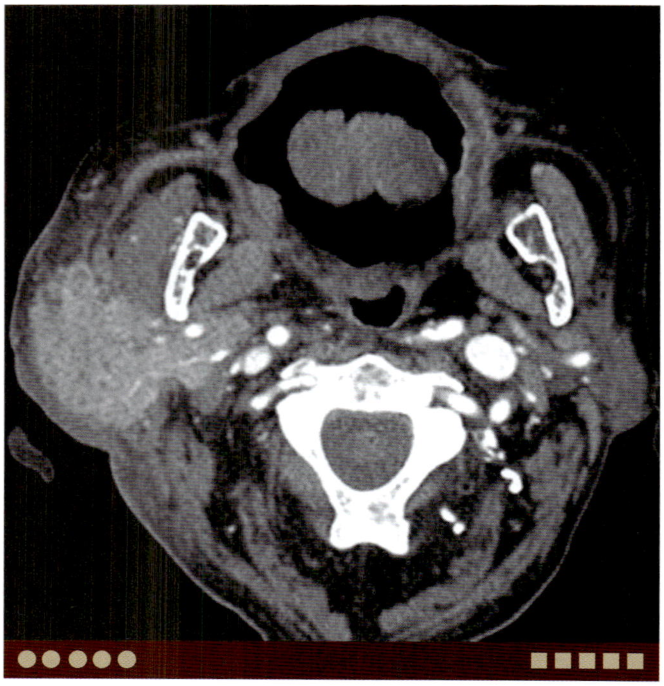

D. Pyogenic parotitis. Axial contrast-enhanced CT demonstrates right parotid gland swelling and heterogeneous enhancement. Note extensive inflammatory change in the superficial soft tissue.

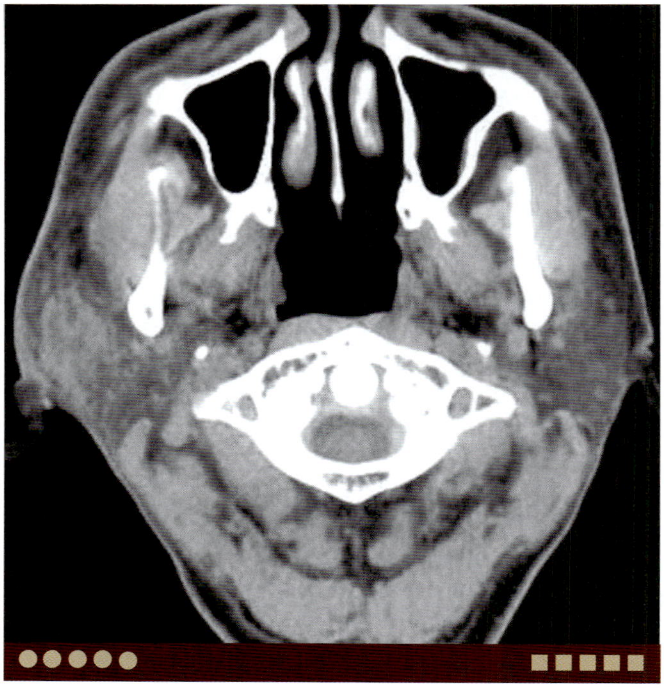

E. Parotitis due to sialolith. Axial unenhanced CT demonstrates right parotid gland swelling with internal heterogeneity.

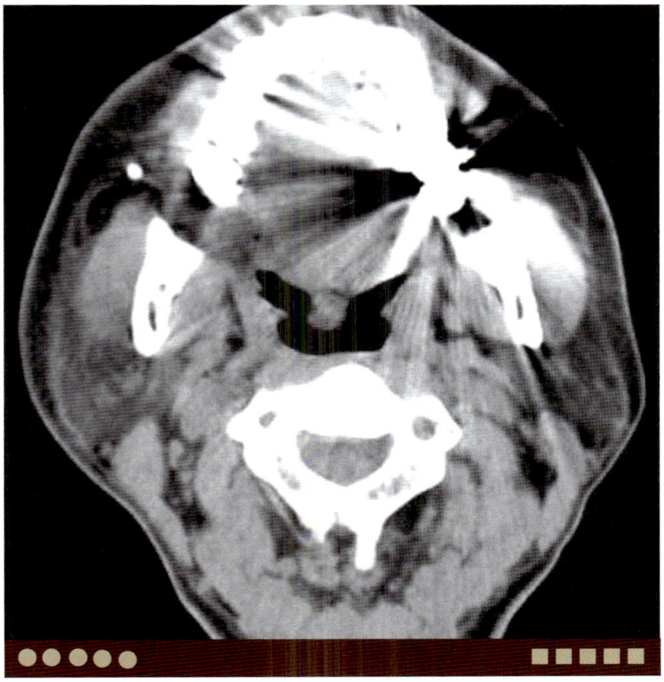

F. Parotitis due to sialolith, same patient as E. Axial unenhanced CT demonstrates a calcified sialolith in the right parotid duct.

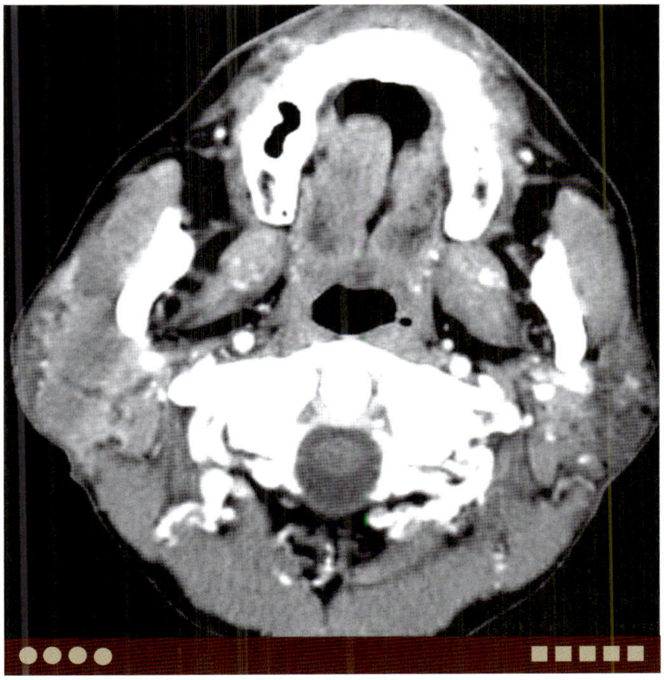

G. Follicular lymphoma. Axial contrast-enhanced CT demonstrates right parotid gland masses with homogenous enhancement.

Case 7–25 Primary Squamous Cell Carcinoma—Parotid

Hiroki Kato, Asim Mian, Osamu Sakai

PRESENTATION

Rapid growing mass within the parotid gland, associated with facial nerve paralysis.

FINDINGS

CT and MRI demonstrate an invasive tumor in the parotid gland.

DIFFERENTIAL DIAGNOSIS

- Metastatic parotid gland tumor: Cutaneous squamous cell carcinoma and malignant melanoma of the head and neck are likely to metastasize to the parotid gland. It is difficult to distinguish primary from metastatic parotid gland tumor.
- Mucoepidermoid carcinoma: High-grade mucoepidermoid carcinomas may have poorly defined and infiltrative margins. They have fewer cystic structures than the low-grade tumors.
- Adenoid cystic carcinoma: Adenoid cystic carcinomas with low signal on T2W images correspond to highly cellular tumors (solid subtype) with poor prognosis, while tumors with high T2 signal correspond to less cellular tumors (cribriform or tubular subtype) with better prognosis.

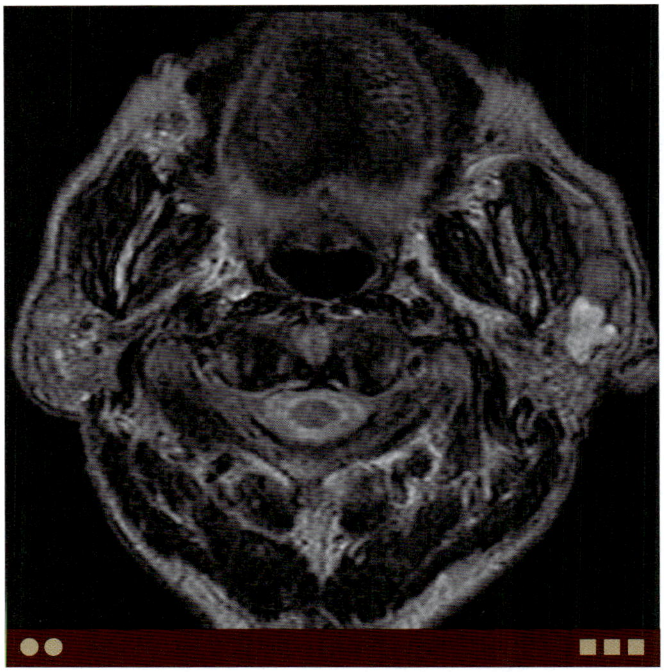

A. Primary SCCA of the parotid. Axial T2W MR image demonstrates a partially necrotic lesion in the left parotid gland.

COMMENTS

This is an 80-year-old man presented with a painful left parotid mass and facial nerve palsy.

Primary squamous cell carcinoma (SCCA) is uncommon in the parotid gland, and predominantly seen in men after the fifth decade. Association with previous irradiation has been described. This is aggressive malignancy with poor prognosis. Regional nodal metastasis is seen in 50% to 70% of patients.

To diagnose primary SCCA of the parotid gland, high-grade mucoepidermoid carcinoma and metastatic SCCA to the parotid gland must be excluded. Incidence of primary SCCA is much lower than metastasis to the parotid glands from scalp, face, auricular regions. Therefore, presence of such lesions suggests metastasis rather than primary parotid lesion. Primary submandibular SCCA is much less common than primary parotid SCCA. Rarely, SCCA occurs in the accessory parotid gland, parotid duct, sublingual gland, or minor salivary ducts.

Primary SCCA of the parotid gland demonstrates aggressive appearance; infiltrating and often necrotic. Like other high-grade malignancies, they tend to show heterogeneous low signal on T2W images corresponding to higher cellularity.

PEARLS

- **Primary SCCA of the parotid gland is rare. Metastatic SCCA to the parotid gland is more common.**
- **Primary SCCA of the parotid gland often demonstrates aggressive appearance such as infiltrative changes and intratumoral necrosis.**
- **Primary SCCA of the parotid gland tends to demonstrate low signal on T2W reflecting higher cellularity, which suggests poor outcome.**

ADDITIONAL IMAGES (B-E)

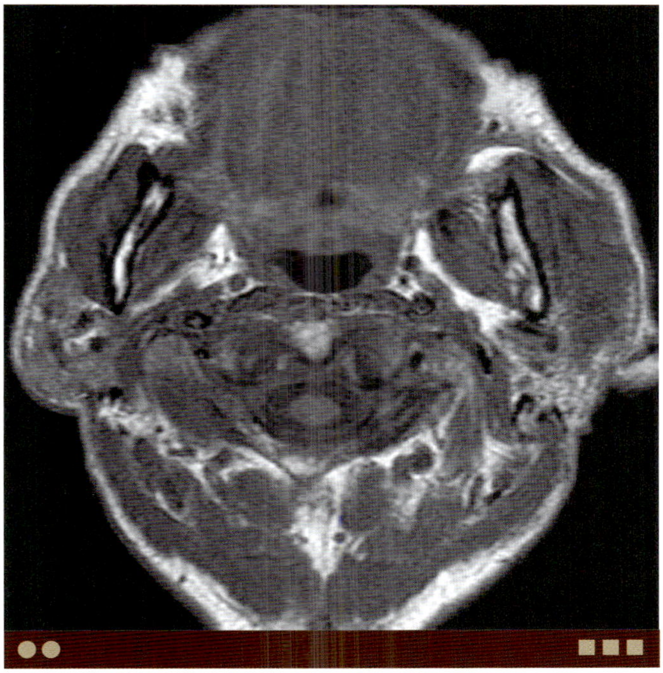

B. Primary SCCA of the parotid, same patient as A. Axial T1W image demonstrates an ill-defined low-signal lesion in the left parotid gland. Boundary between the tumor and the masseter muscle is poorly defined.

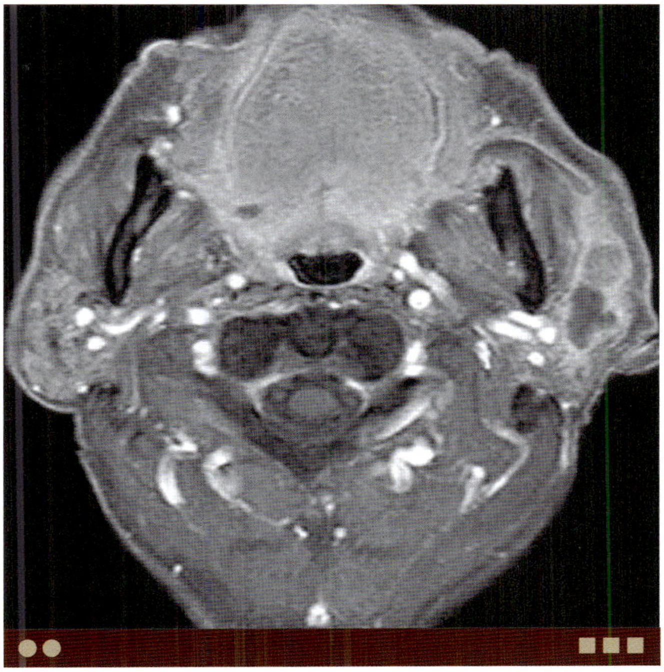

C. Primary SCCA of the parotid, same patient as A. Axial postcontrast fat-suppressed T1W image demonstrates heterogeneously enhancing tumor with necrotic components.

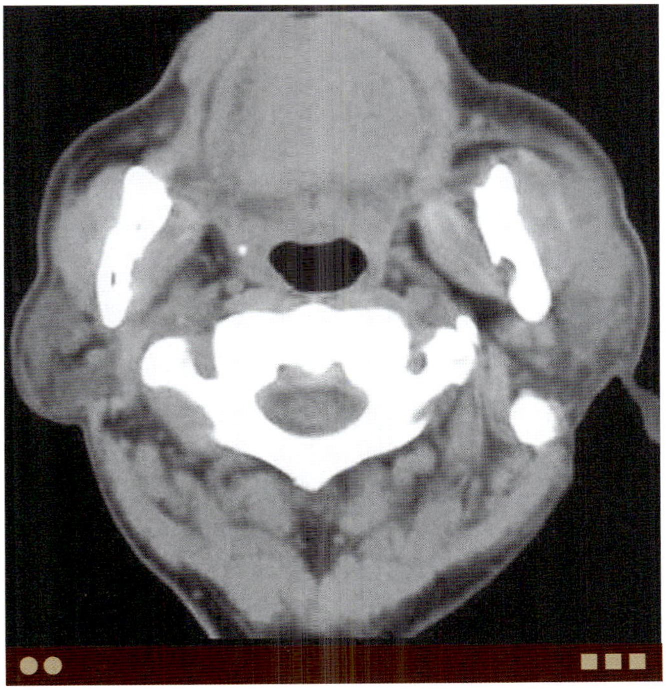

D. Primary SCCA of the parotid, same patient as A. Axial unenhanced CT demonstrates an infiltrative lesion in the left parotid gland.

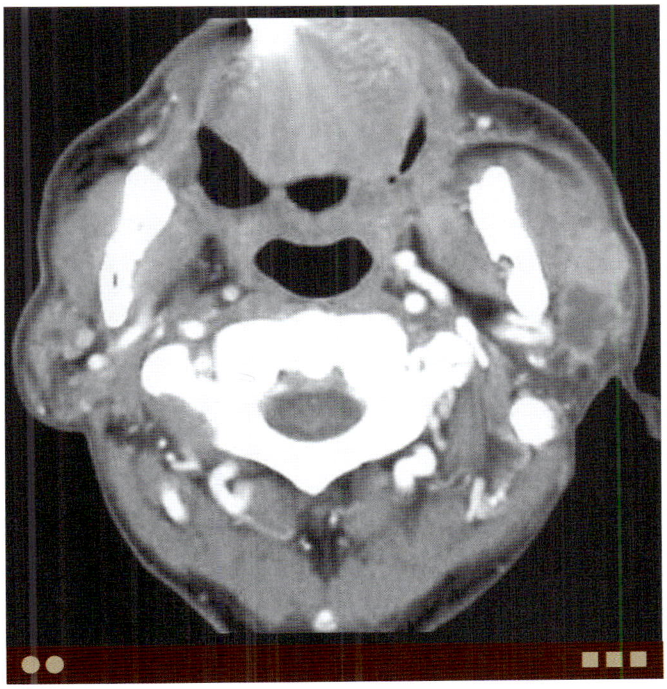

E. Primary SCCA of the parotid, same patient as A. Axial contrast-enhanced CT demonstrates heterogeneous enhancement with necrotic foci.

DIFFERENTIAL DIAGNOSIS IMAGES (F-I)

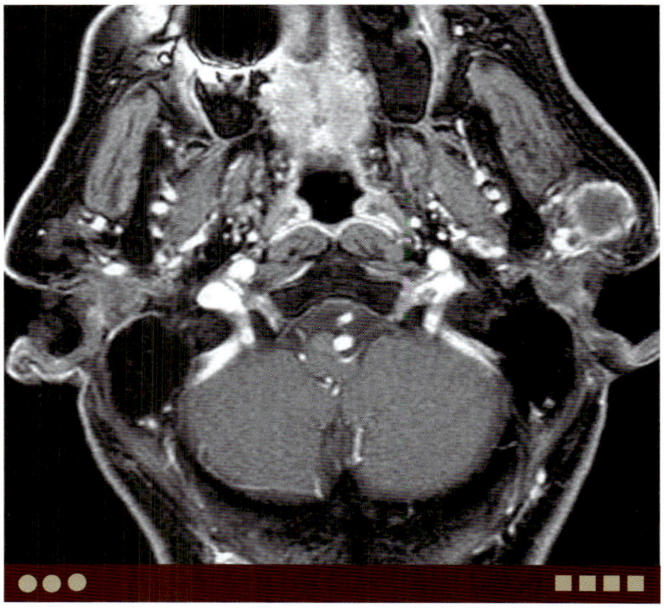

F. Parotid metastasis from cutaneous SCCA. Axial postcontrast fat-suppressed T1W MR image demonstrates a predominantly necrotic lesion with irregular rim-enhancement.

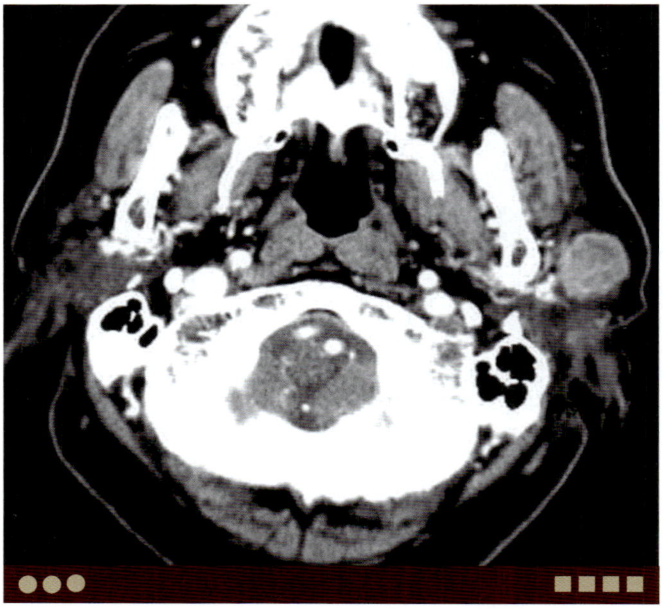

G. Parotid metastasis from cutaneous SCCA, same patient as F. Axial contrast-enhanced CT demonstrates a heterogeneously enhancing lesion in the left parotid.

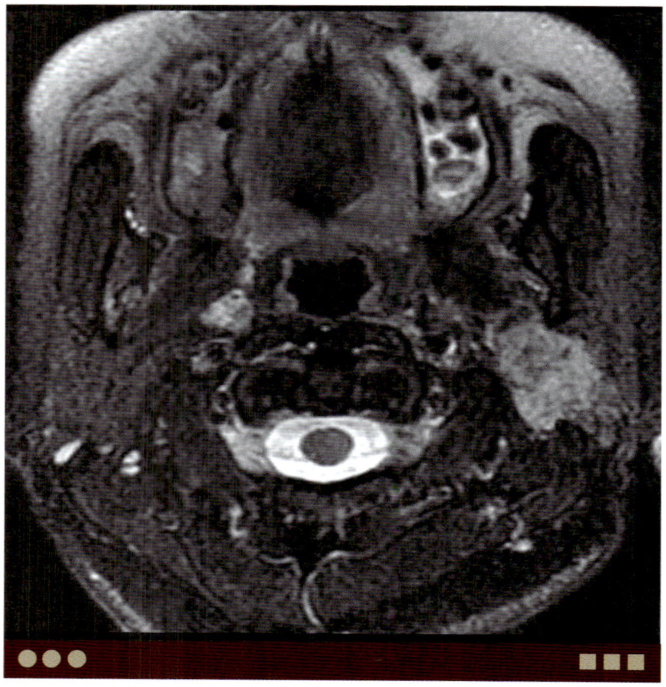

H. Parotid metastasis from cutaneous meibomian carcinoma. Axial postcontrast fat-suppressed T1W MR image demonstrates an infiltrating, enhancing lesion in the left parotid gland.

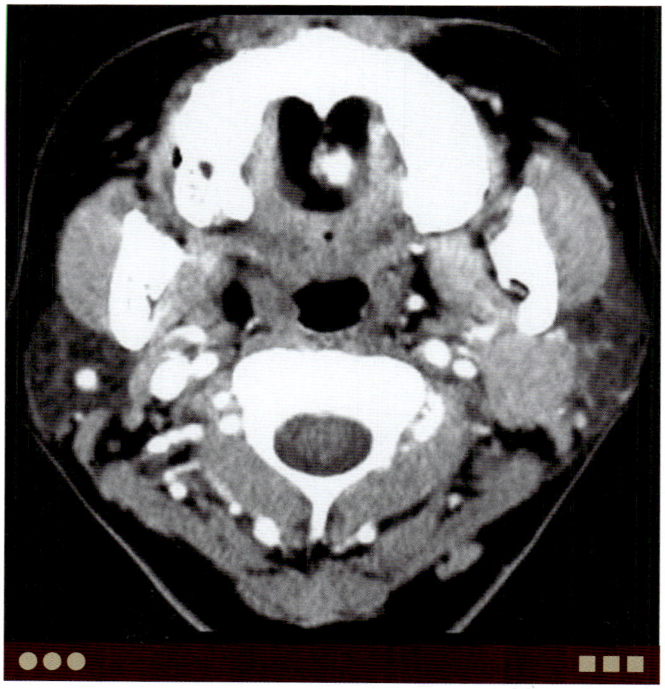

I. Parotid metastasis from cutaneous meibomian carcinoma, same patient as F. Axial contrast-enhanced CT demonstrates a heterogeneously enhancing lesion.

Case 7–26 Basal Cell Adenoma

Kevin Donahue, Osamu Sakai

PRESENTATION

A painless enlarging mass in the parotid region.

FINDINGS

CT and MRI demonstrate a well-demarcated cystic and solid parotid lesion with enhancing solid components.

DIFFERENTIAL DIAGNOSIS

- Basal cell adenocarcinoma: This is a malignant counterpart of basal cell adenoma and very rare, accounting for <1% of major salivary gland tumors. It may arise either de novo or via evolution from preexisting basal cell adenoma.
- Mucoepidermoid carcinoma: This is the most common malignant tumor in the parotid gland. Low-grade tumor tends to have well-circumscribed margins, while high-grade tumor has infiltrating margins.
- Adenoid cystic carcinoma: This is the second most common malignant tumor in the parotid gland. High-grade tumor (solid type) shows infiltrating appearance and low signal on T2W image. This tumor has a high perineural invasion rate.
- Pleomorphic adenoma: This tumor is the most common parotid tumor, often seen in women in forties and fifties. It demonstrates delayed enhancement.

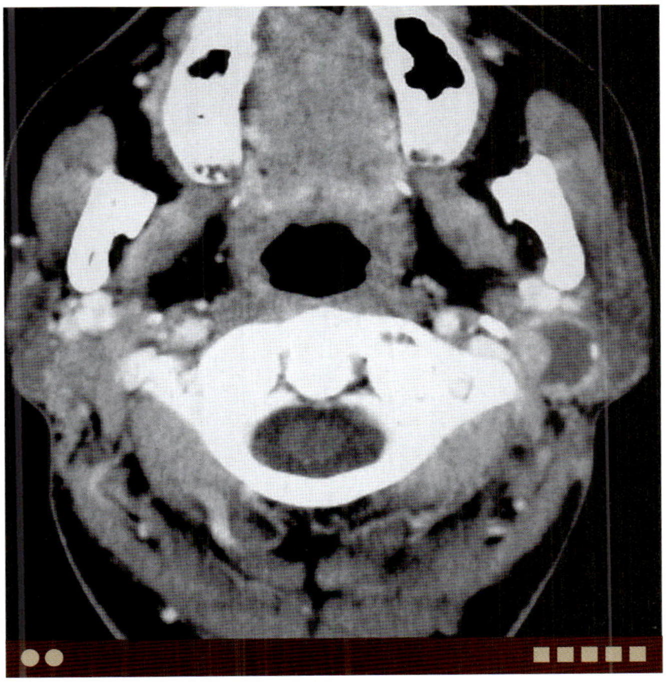

A. Basal cell adenoma. Axial contrast-enhanced CT demonstrates a cystic and solid lesion in the left parotid gland. The solid portions enhance relative to the remainder of the gland.

COMMENTS

This is a 39-year-old man with left parotid mass.

Basal cell adenoma is a rare benign epithelial tumor of the salivary gland that typically presents as a painless mass. Epithelial tumors are the most common form of salivary tumor accounting for greater than 85% of the total number of salivary tumors. Basal cell adenoma is an uncommon benign tumor representing 1% of the salivary epithelial tumors. Basal cell adenoma is more often seen in the superficial lobe and is more common in older patients.

Macroscopically, basal cell adenoma is generally a well rounded structure that frequently contains a cystic component. The tumor margins are typically smooth and well distinct. The solid portions of the tumor are relatively hyperattenuating to normal parotid tissue with brisk enhancement following administration of contrast. On MRI, the cystic portion is often hyperintense on both T1W and T2W images with enhancement of the solid portion following administration of contrast noted as well.

When diagnosing solitary cystic lesions of the parotid, basal cell adenoma must be considered, although this is rare. Other partially cystic solitary lesions include mucoepidermoid carcinoma, adenoid cystic carcinoma and pleomorphic adenoma. Warthin's tumors and lymphoepithelial lesions tend to be multiple and bilateral.

PEARLS

- **Basal cell adenoma is often seen as a cystic and solid parotid gland lesion with enhancement of the solid component.**
- **Basal cell adenoma is usually well circumscribed with smooth contour.**

ADDITIONAL IMAGES (B-G)

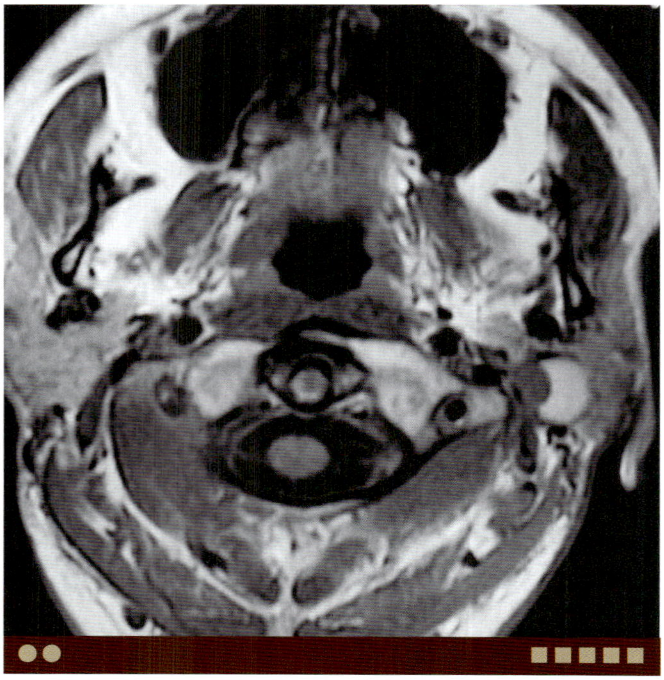

B. Basal cell adenoma, same patient as A. Axial T1W MR image demonstrates a hyperintense cystic component and a solid component hypointense to the remainder of the parotid gland.

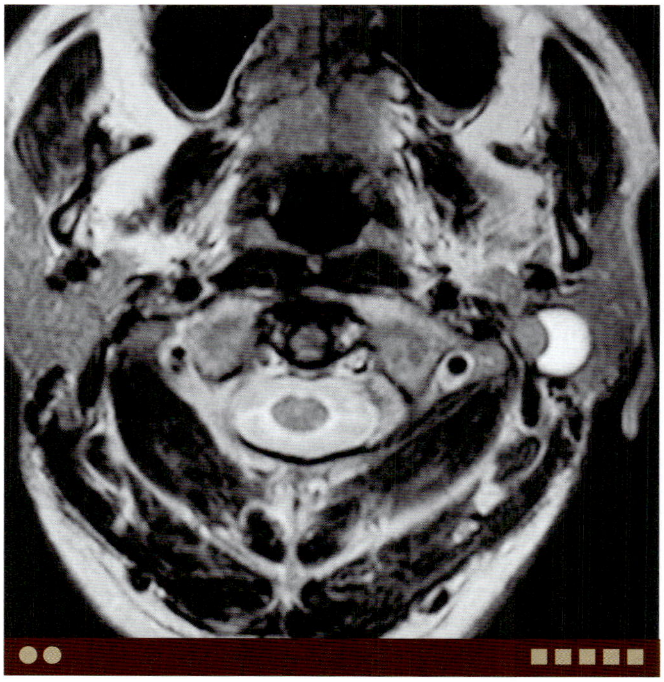

C. Basal cell adenoma, same patient as A. Axial T2W MR image demonstrates a well-circumscribed lesion in the left parotid lesion with hyperintense cystic component and intermediate signal solid component.

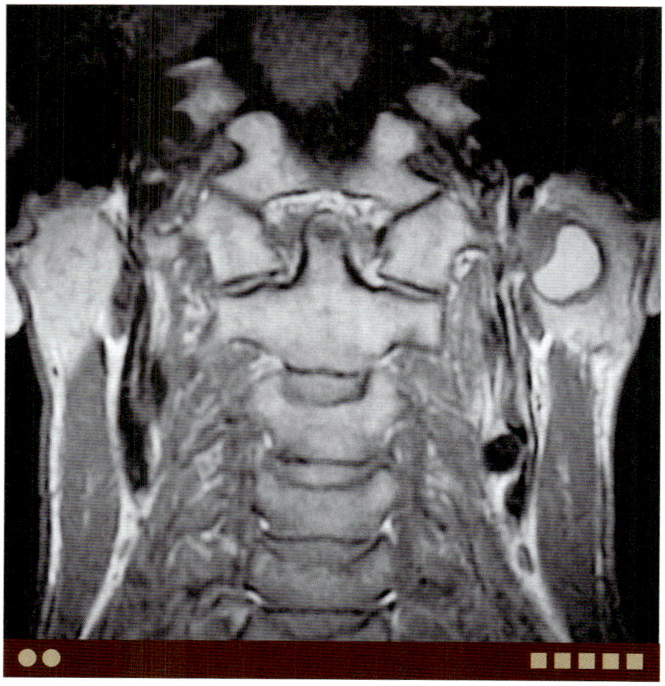

D. Basal cell adenoma, same patient as A. Coronal T1W MR image again demonstrates the well-circumscribed lesion in the left parotid gland. The cystic portion is hyperintense reflecting proteinaceous fluid, and solid portion is isointense relative to the parotid parenchyma

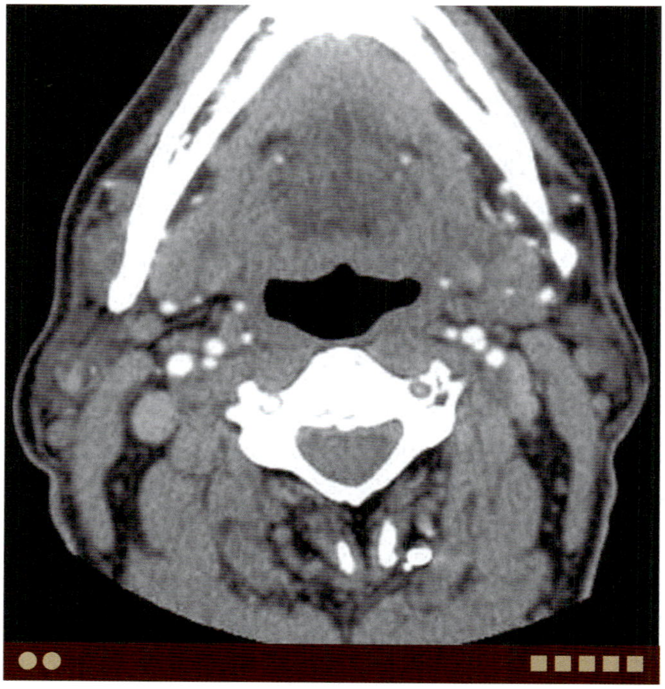

E. Basal cell adenoma in a different patient. Axial contrast-enhanced CT demonstrates a well-circumscribed partially cystic lesion with enhancing solid components in the right parotid gland.

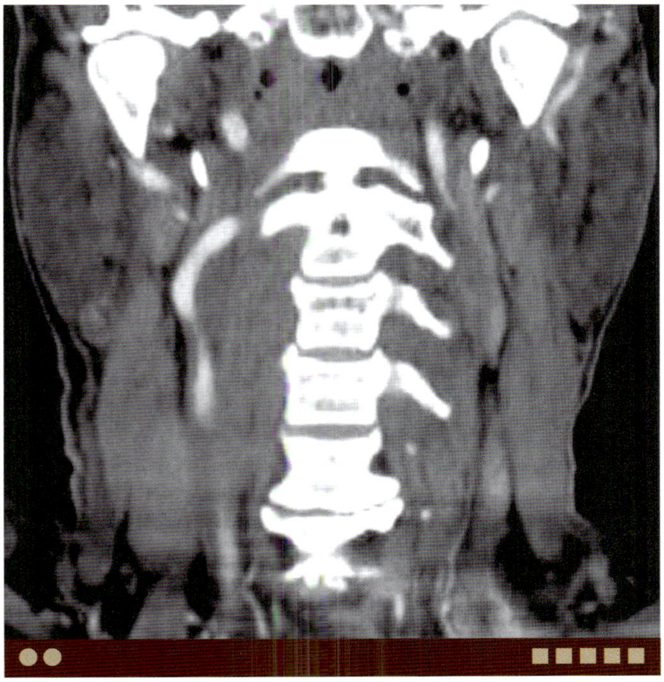

F. Basal cell adenoma, same patient as E. Coronal contrast-enhanced CT demonstrates a well-circumscribed cystic lesion with an enhancing nodule in the right parotid gland.

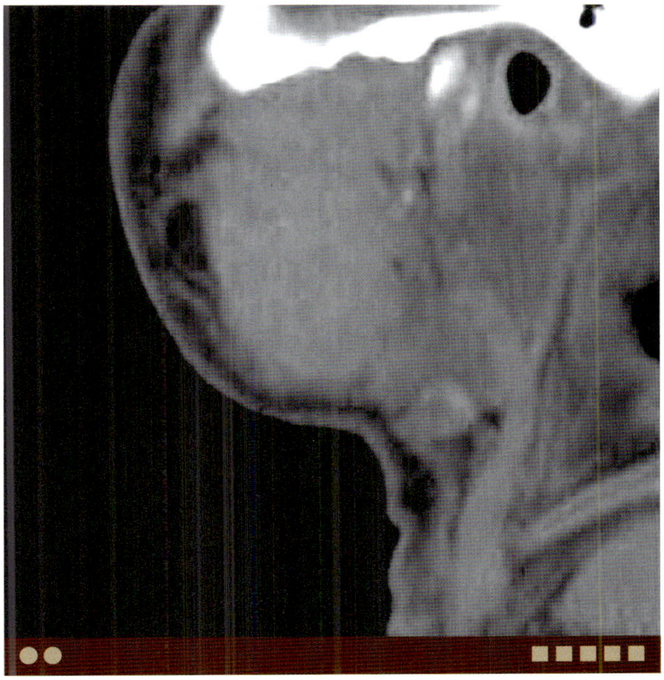

G. Basal cell adenoma, same patient as E. Sagittal contrast-enhanced CT demonstrates a peripherally enhancing cystic lesion with an enhancing nodule in the right parotid gland.

DIFFERENTIAL DIAGNOSIS IMAGES (H-J)

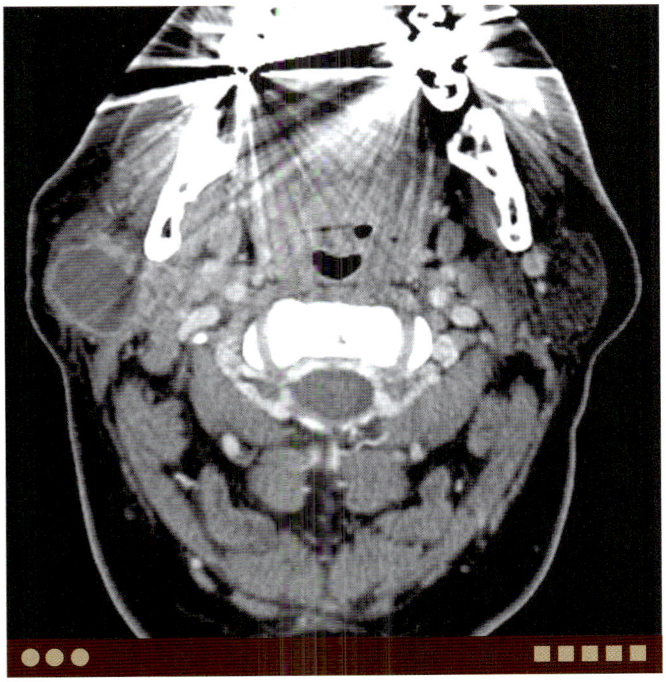

H. Mucoepidermoid carcinoma. Axial contrast-enhanced CT demonstrates a cystic-appearing tumor with mildly enhancing infiltrative margins in the right parotid gland.

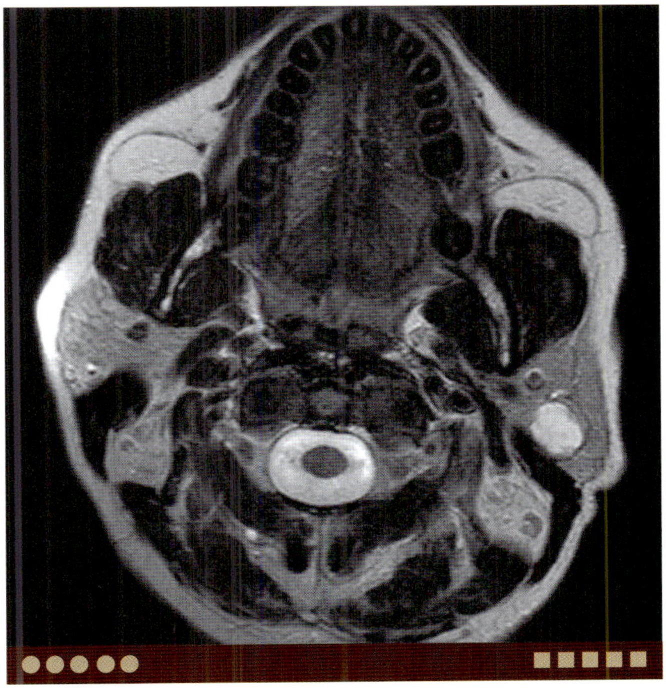

I. Pleomorphic adenoma. Axial T2W image demonstrates a well-circumscribed, slightly lobulated high-signal tumor in the left parotid gland.

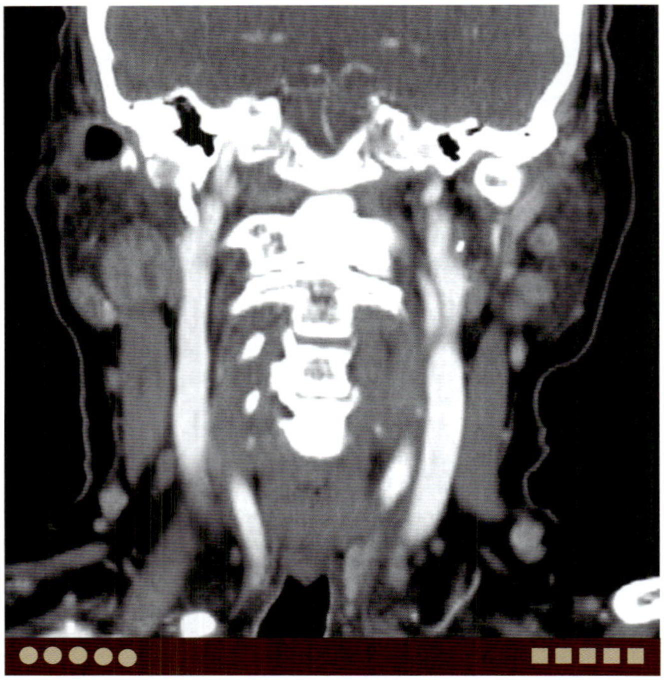

J. Warthin's tumor. Coronal contrast-enhanced CT demonstrates multiple well-circumscribed masses in the bilateral parotid glands.

Case 7–27 Disseminated Pleomorphic Adenoma

Rohini Nadgir, Osamu Sakai

PRESENTATION

Recurrent facial fullness in a patient with history of previously resected or biopsied pleomorphic adenoma.

FINDINGS

CT and MRI demonstrate multiple nodular cystic and solid masses in the parapharyngeal and submandibular spaces.

DIFFERENTIAL DIAGNOSIS

- Venous and venolymphatic malformations: These are slow-flow vascular malformations commonly seen in the head and neck. These lesions are multispacial, extending through multiple planes in the face and neck. Variable densities and signal are seen due to difference in flow and protein contents. Venous portions enhances after contrast. Presence of phlebolith suggests venous malformation.
- Hemangioma: This is the most common benign parotid tumor in children. Homogeneous enhancement and T2 high signal are usually seen. Spontaneous regression is often seen.
- Plexiform neurofibroma: Plexiform neurofibroma is another condition that can involve multiple fascia-defined spaces. Imaging findings may be similar to that of venolymphatic malformations.

COMMENTS

Pleomorphic adenomas, also known as benign mixed tumors, are by far the most common salivary gland tumors, particularly in the parotid gland. While classically described as well-defined T2 bright lesions with variable enhancement, there are no pathologically defining imaging features. Lesions can occasionally undergo cystic degeneration and may demonstrate associated calcifications.

Due to 15% chance of malignant transformation, surgical excision should be performed. Recurrence can occur due to incomplete resection or "spillage" at time of biopsy or surgery. For this reason, recurrent pleomorphic adenomas are typically multifocal in nature and can spread into deeper soft tissue planes of the head and neck.

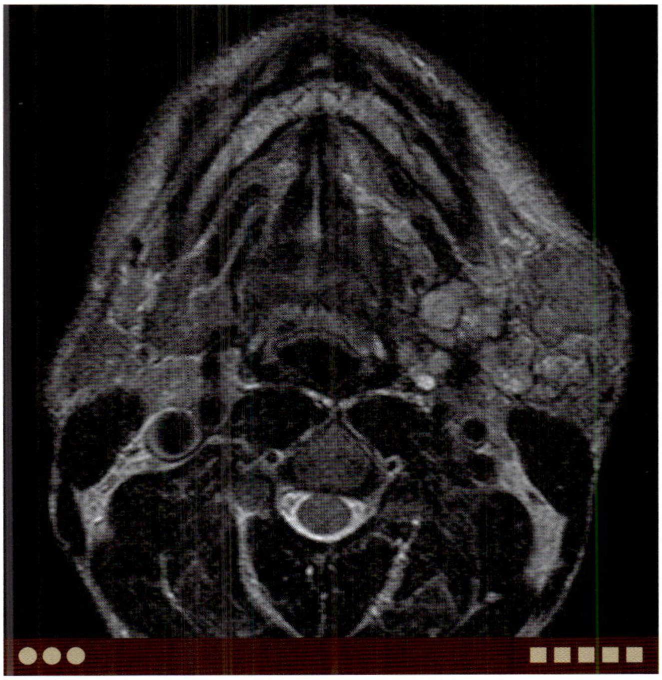

A. Disseminated pleomorphic adenoma. Axial T2W image demonstrates multiloculated lesions with variable signal intensity in the left submandibular space.

Disseminated pleomorphic adenoma is very difficult to surgically resect due to its multifocal nature, and therefore in such cases radiotherapy may be performed although its long-term efficacy remains unclear.

PEARLS

- **Pleomorphic adenomas are by far the most common salivary gland tumors, particularly in the parotid gland.**
- **Recurrence can occur due to incomplete resection or "spillage" at time of biopsy or surgery.**
- **Recurrent pleomorphic adenomas are typically multifocal in nature and can infiltrate into deeper soft tissue planes of the head and neck.**

ADDITIONAL IMAGES (B-D)

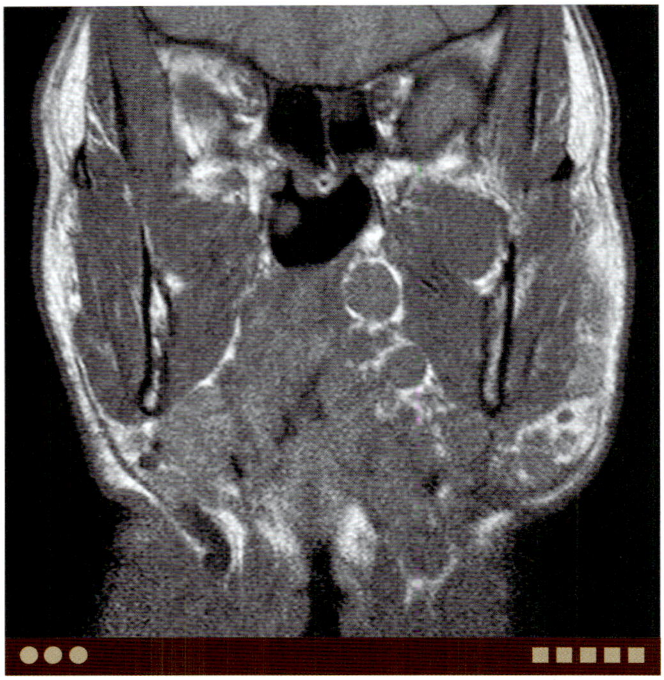

B. Disseminated pleomorphic adenoma, same patient as A. Coronal T1W image demonstrates numerous round lesions in the left parapharyngeal and submandibular spaces.

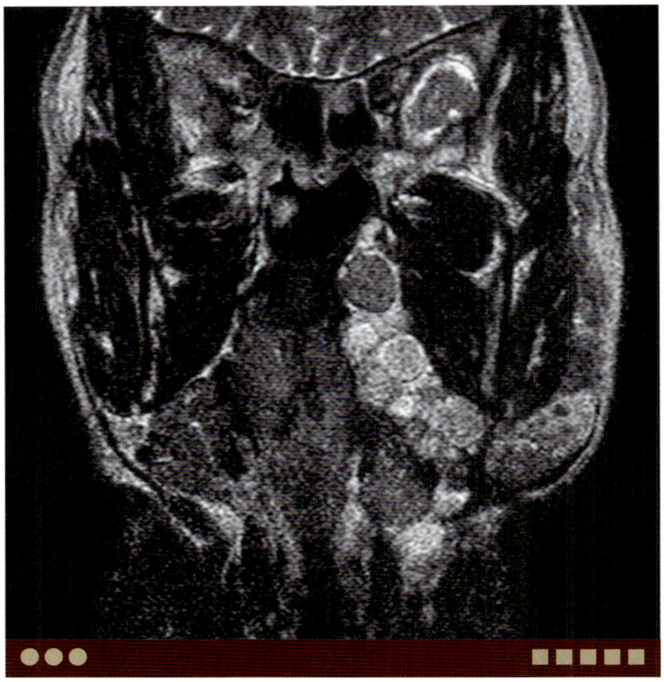

C. Disseminated pleomorphic adenoma, same patient as A. Coronal T2W image demonstrates the lesions in the left parapharyngeal and submandibular spaces showing variable signal intensities.

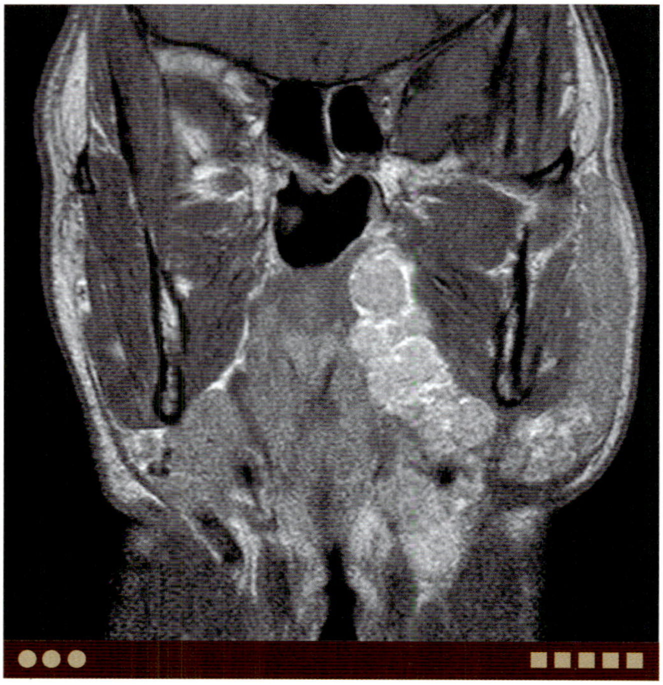

D. Disseminated pleomorphic adenoma, same patient as A. Coronal postcontrast T1W image demonstrates enhancement of the lesions.

DIFFERENTIAL DIAGNOSIS IMAGES (E-G)

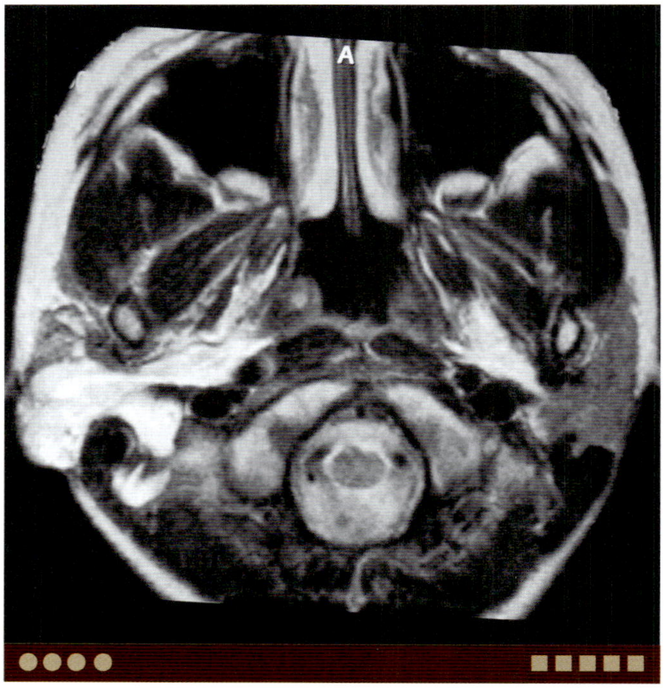

E. Lymphangioma. Axial T2W image demonstrates a high-signal mass in the right parotid region extending into the parapharyngeal space.

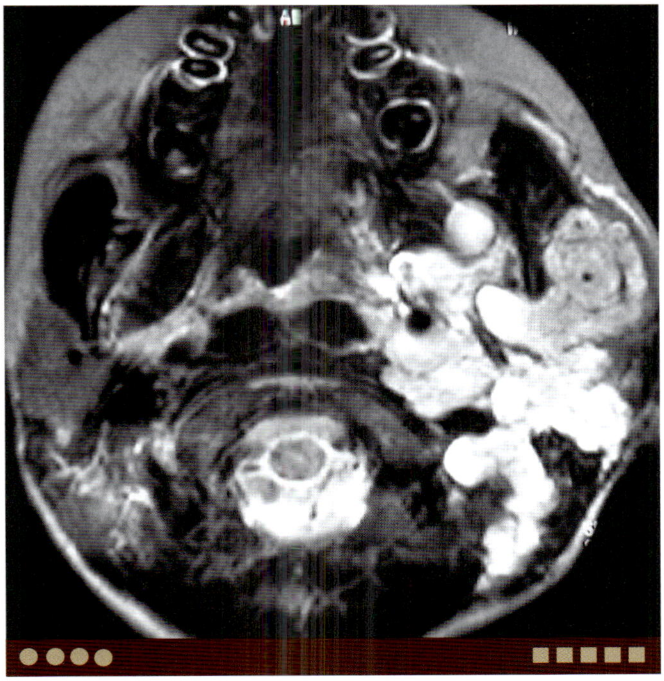

F. Plexiform neurofibroma. Axial T2W image demonstrates multiple lobulated high-signal lesions involving the left parotid, masticator, parapharyngeal, and paravertebral spaces.

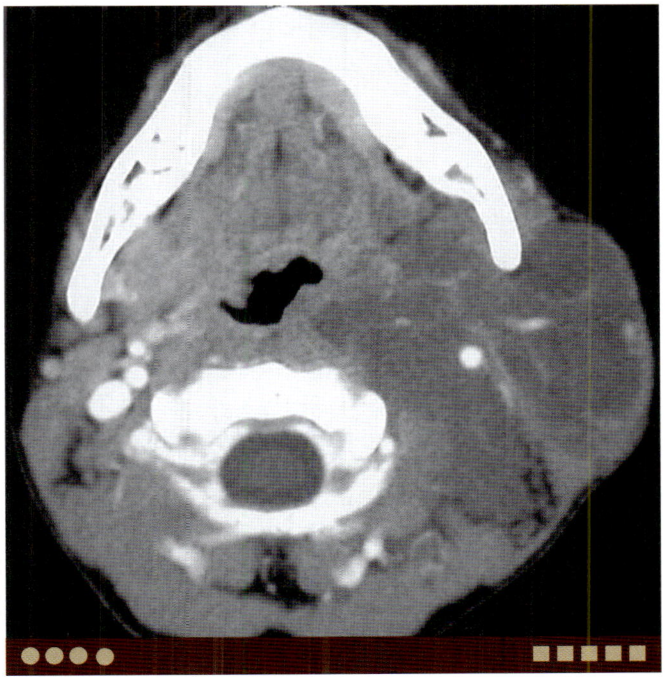

G. Plexiform neurofibroma in a different patient. Axial contrast-enhanced CT demonstrates a "multiloculated" low-density lesion involving the left parotid, masticator, parapharyngeal, and paravertebral spaces.

Case 7–28 Submandibular Sialolithiasis

Rohini Nadgir, Osamu Sakai

PRESENTATION

Painless firm submandibular mass.

FINDINGS

CT demonstrates a calculus obstructing of the submandibular duct and enlargement/inflammation of the submandibular gland.

DIFFERENTIAL DIAGNOSIS

- Submandibular ductal neoplasm: In absence of clearly identifiable obstructing calculus, enlargement of the submandibular duct and gland could be secondary to obstructing mass within the duct at the floor of mouth such as squamous cell carcinoma. Tumor may be too small to be visualized on imaging.
- Submandibular ductal stenosis: In absence of clearly identifiable obstructing calculus, narrowing or occlusion of the submandibular duct may be secondary to chronic inflammation related to diminished salivary flow/stasis or autoimmune etiologies such as Sjögren's syndrome and sarcoidosis. Drug-related, endocrine, and metabolic causes for ductal stenosis could also be considered.

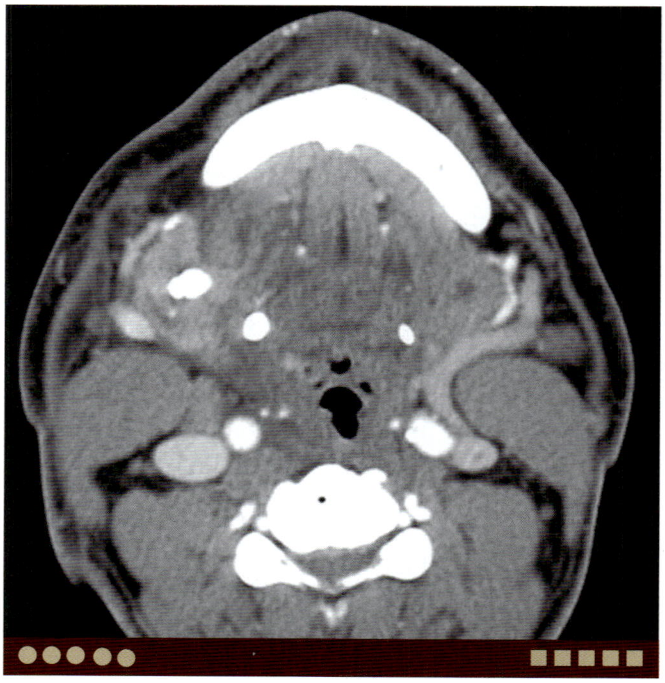

A. Sialolithiasis. Axial postcontrast CT shows a calculus within the swollen and hyperenhancing right submandibular gland.

COMMENTS

The submandibular duct is the most common salivary gland ductal system to be affected by sialolithiasis. This is because submandibular secretions tend to be thicker and more alkaline in nature than other salivary gland secretions, rendering them more prone to stone formation. Also, the dependent course of the submandibular duct within the floor of mouth allows for stasis and predisposes to stone formation.

If the submandibular gland is secondarily inflamed, patients present with unilateral painful submandibular swelling worsened with eating or gustatory stimulation. While smaller ductal calculi can be asymptomatic, larger calculi will obstruct and dilate the more proximal submandibular duct and the submandibular gland can become secondarily inflamed. Extremely large calculi can be formed occasionally in patients without severe symptoms. Clinically neoplasms can be suspected by slow growing firm masses due to sialolithiasis and chronic inflammation of the submandibular gland.

CT is ideal for identifying the calculus; on MRI calculi can be more easily missed. Inflamed ductal system will be dilated and margins can demonstrate enhancement. If the submandibular gland is also inflamed, the gland can be enlarged, relatively hyperenhancing, with adjacent fat stranding. Organized fluid collection within or adjacent to the gland and ductal system may also be seen. Chronic inflammation of the submandibular gland may demonstrate heterogeneous relatively low T2 signal, and it may be difficult to differentiate from malignancy.

PEARLS

- **The submandibular ductal system is the most common of the salivary gland ductal systems to be affected by sialolithiasis.**
- **Obstructed and inflamed ductal system will be dilated and margins can demonstrate enhancement. If the submandibular gland is also inflamed, the gland can be enlarged, relatively hyperenhancing, with adjacent fat stranding.**
- **CT is ideal for identifying the calculus; on MRI, calculi can be more easily missed.**
- **Chronic inflammation of the submandibular ductal system may mimic neoplasms clinically and radiologically.**

ADDITIONAL IMAGES (B–G)

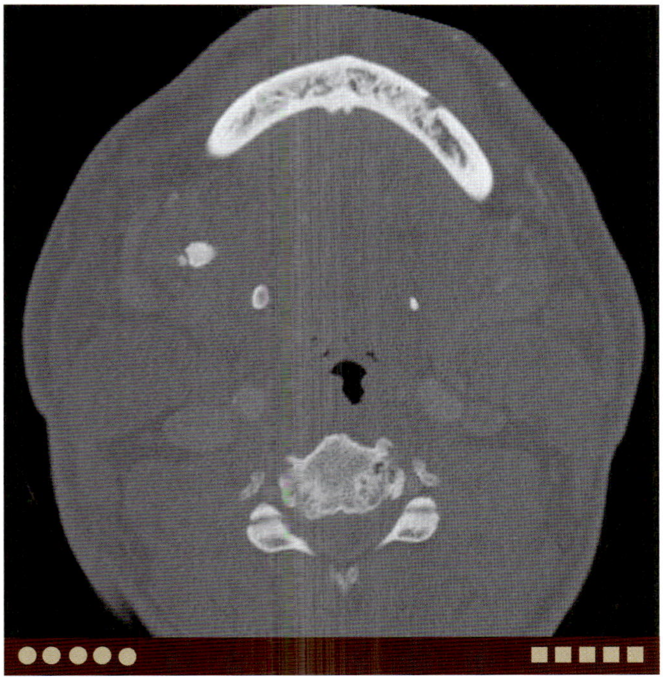

B. Sialolithiasis, same patient as A. Axial bone window CT confirms presence of calculi.

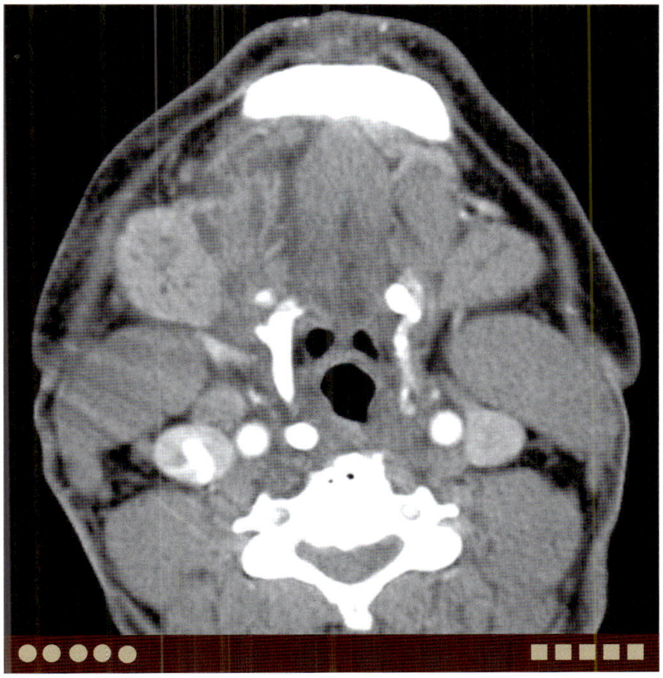

C. Sialolithiasis, same patient as A. Axial postcontrast CT at slightly lower level shows enlarged and hyperenhancing right submandibular gland. Note inflammatory change in the adjacent fat and thickening of the platysma muscle.

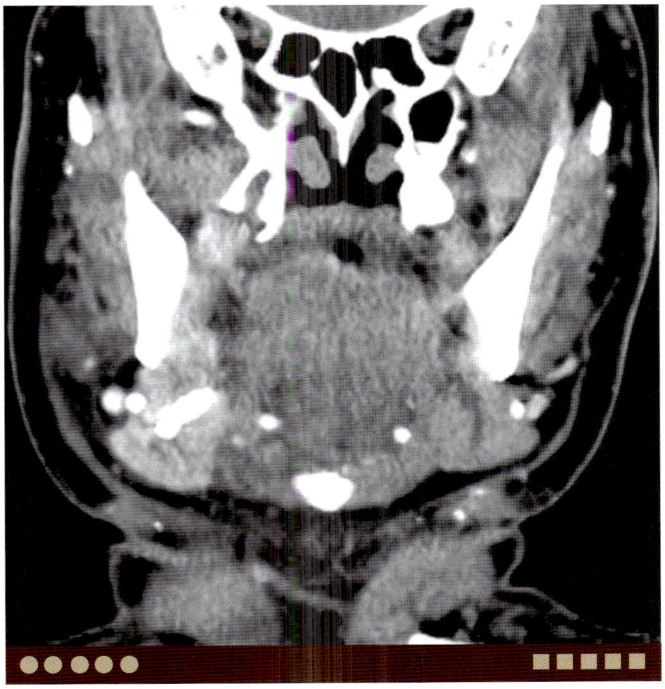

D. Sialolithiasis, same patient as A. Coronal postcontrast CT shows a calculus within the swollen and hyperenhancing right submandibular gland.

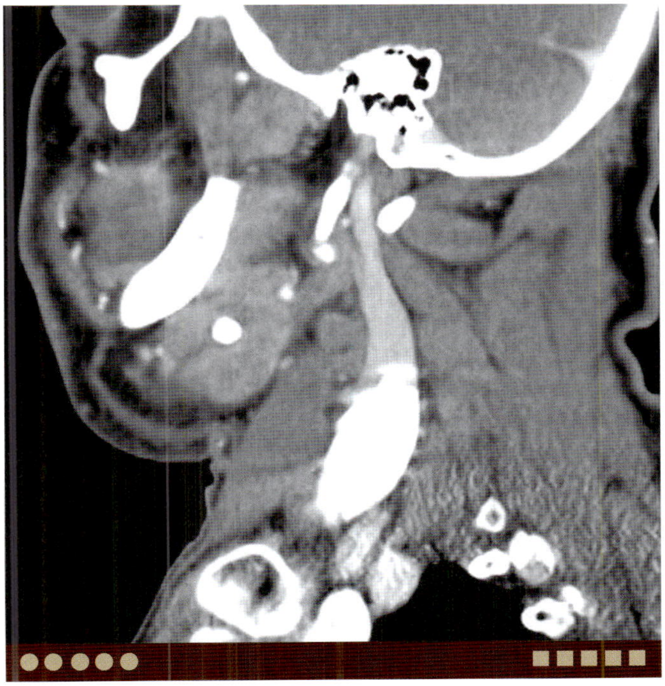

E. Sialolithiasis, same patient as A. Sagittal postcontrast CT shows a calculus within the swollen and hyperenhancing submandibular gland.

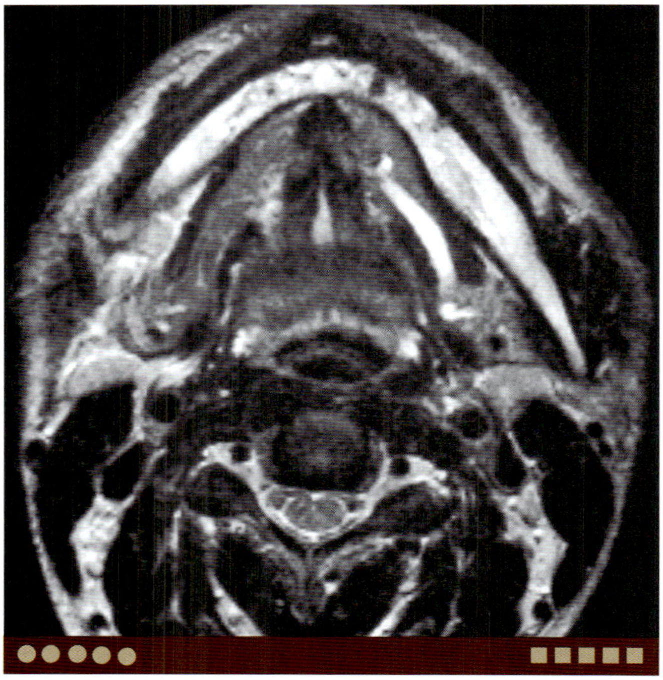

F. Sialolithiasis in a different patient. Axial T2W MR image shows a dilated left submandibular duct. A low-signal calculus obstructing the duct is seen.

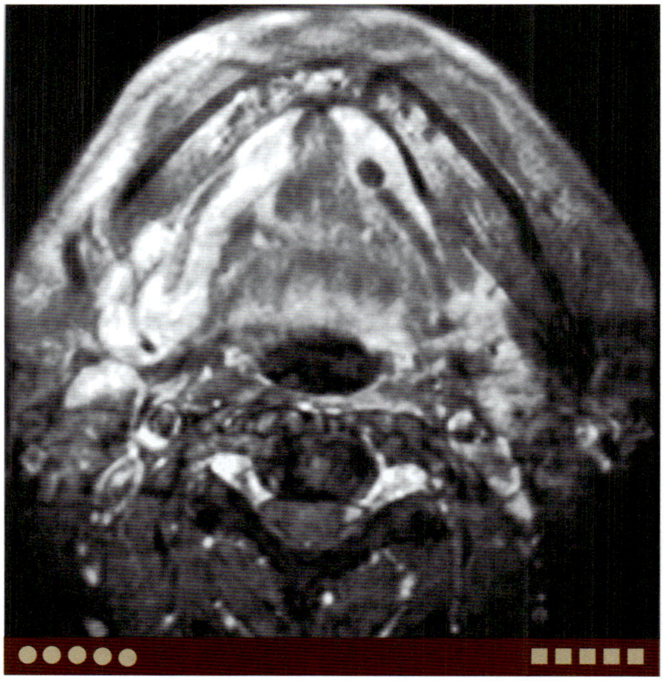

G. Sialolithiasis, same patient as F. Axial postcontrast fat-suppressed T1W MR image shows a dilated left submandibular duct. Note an ovoid-shaped calculus seen as signal-void.

DIFFERENTIAL DIAGNOSIS IMAGES (H-J)

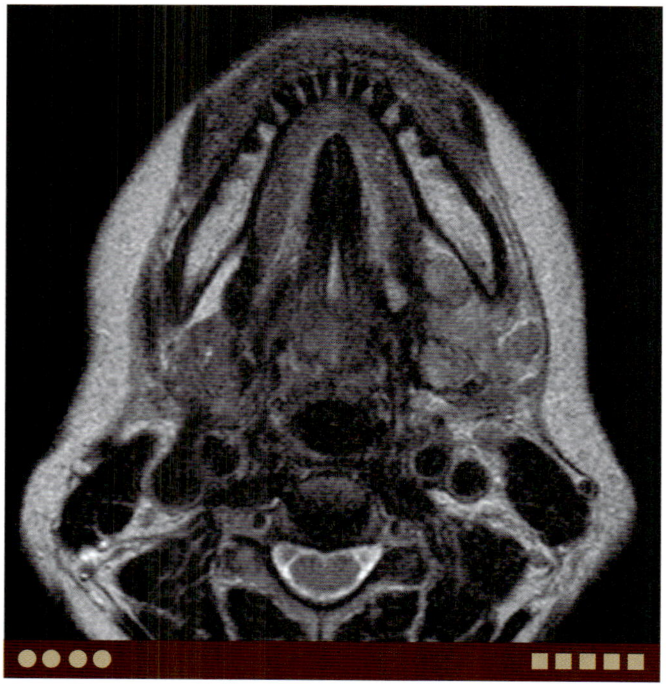

H. Adenoid cystic carcinoma. Axial T2W image demonstrates a lobulated/multinodular intermediate-signal lesion in the left submandibular space.

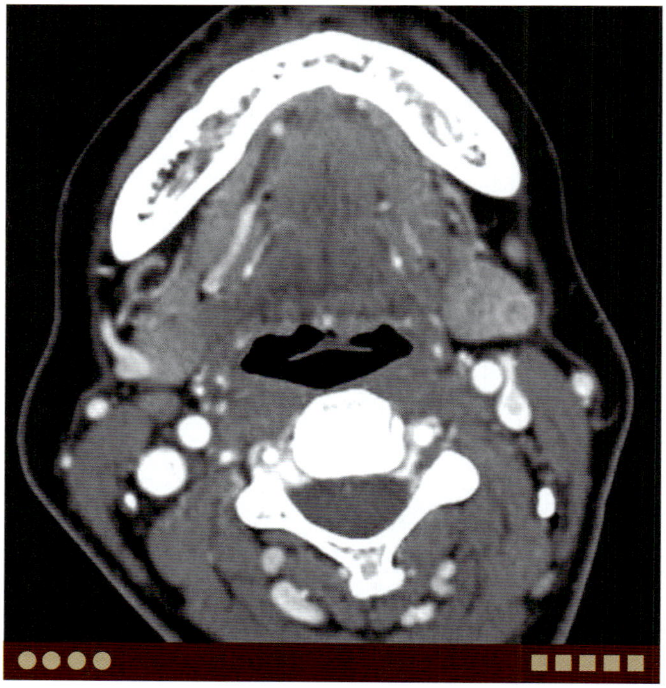

I. Mucoepidermoid carcinoma (low grade). Axial contrast-enhanced CT demonstrates a well-circumscribed cystic mass in the left submandibular gland.

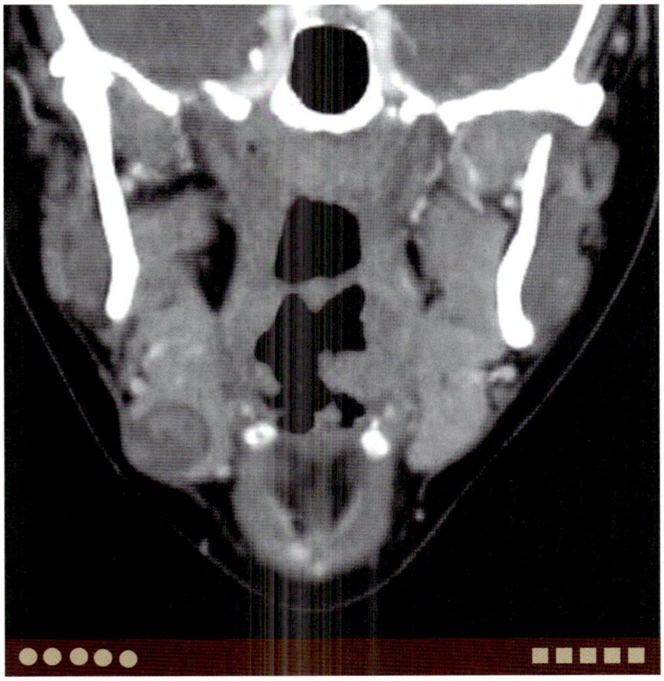

J. Pleomorphic adenoma. Coronal contrast-enhanced CT demonstrates a well-circumscribed, heterogeneously enhancing mass in the right submandibular gland.

Case 7–29 Acute Suppurative Parotitis

Benjamin Ludwig, Hiroki Kato, Osamu Sakai

PRESENTATION

Swelling, erythema, and tenderness anterior to the ear.

FINDINGS

CT demonstrates an enlarged, heterogeneous, enhancing parotid gland with inflammatory stranding within the subcutaneous tissues.

DIFFERENTIAL DIAGNOSIS

- Mumps parotitis: Mumps is by far the most common viral cause of parotitis in children, usually at the age of 5 to 14 years, and most commonly caused by paramyxovirus. Swelling of the parotid glands usually starts on one side and then progresses to the other side rapidly.
- Sjögren's syndrome: CT findings vary based on stage of disease, ranging from a normal gland to a honeycomb glandular appearance with solid and cystic lesions and calcifications, Sjögren's syndrome typically affects both parotids.
- Lymphoepithelial lesions associated with HIV positivity: CT demonstrates multiple cystic and solid lesions, which enlarge the parotids. Typically bilateral, with associated lymphoid hyperplasia and cervical adenopathy.
- Sialosis: Enlarged, dense parotid glands, without associated inflammatory stranding or lymphadenopathy. Typically presents with painless enlargement of the parotids.

COMMENTS

This is a 3-year-old boy with left preauricular swelling and pain.

Acute suppurative parotitis is most often unilateral, and results from ascending bacterial infection from the oral cavity. The parotid is preferentially affected given the large orifice of Stensen's duct within the oral cavity, susceptibility of the duct to oral trauma, and the less bacteriostatic nature of parotid secretions.

Acute parotitis may also result from viral etiologies. Patients are typically < 15, with prodromal symptoms and bilateral parotid pain and swelling. Other infectious and inflammatory etiologies including tuberculosis, cat scratch disease, and sarcoidosis result in parotitis.

In acute parotitis, ultrasound demonstrates a hypoechoic, heterogeneous, enlarged parotid with increased vascularity. Contrast-enhanced CT findings include an enlarged, heterogeneously enhancing parotid with inflammatory changes in the adjacent soft tissues. MRI demonstrates similar findings to CT. The T2 signal characteristics vary based on amount of edema (T2 hyperintense) versus cellular infiltration (T2 hypointense). Sialography is not performed in the acute setting, given risk of retrograde propagation of infection and duct rupture.

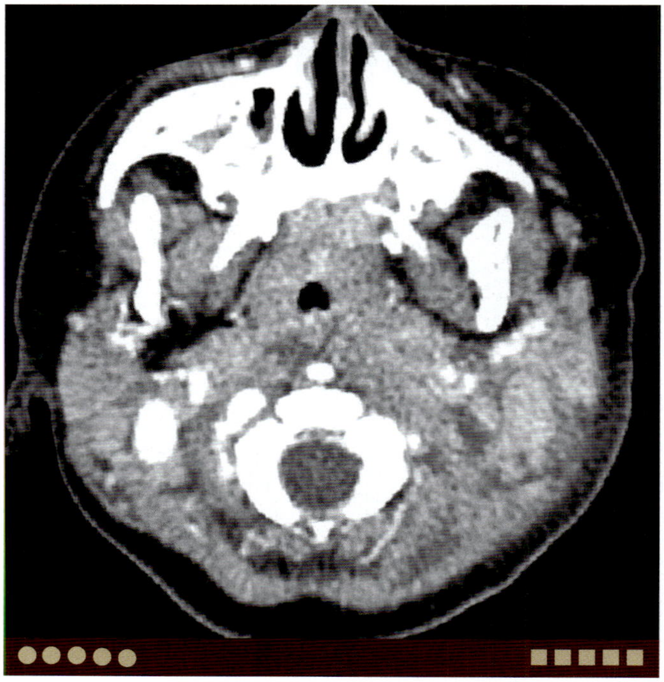

A. Supurative parotitis. Axial contrast-enhanced CT demonstrates left parotid enlargement and heterogeneous enhancement, with subcutaneous inflammatory stranding and enlarged lymph nodes.

Parotitis may also be secondary to sialolithiasis, and Stensen's duct should be carefully scrutinized. An obstructing sialolith results in proximal duct dilation, with duct wall enhancement. Intraglandular sialoliths result in sialadenitis less frequently.

Treatment includes rehydration, oral antibiotics, counseling on oral hygiene, and secretagogues. Complications include intraglandular abscess formation, which may extend into the deep spaces of the neck and thrombophlebitis of the retromandibular, facial, and internal jugular veins.

PEARLS

- **Acute suppurative parotitis is most often secondary to ascending bacterial infection from the oral cavity.**
- **Viral etiologies, autoimmune disease, and sialosis are typically bilateral processes.**
- **Calculus induced parotitis is also common, and it is imperative to scrutinize Stensen's duct to evaluate for sialolithiasis.**

ADDITIONAL IMAGES (B-C)

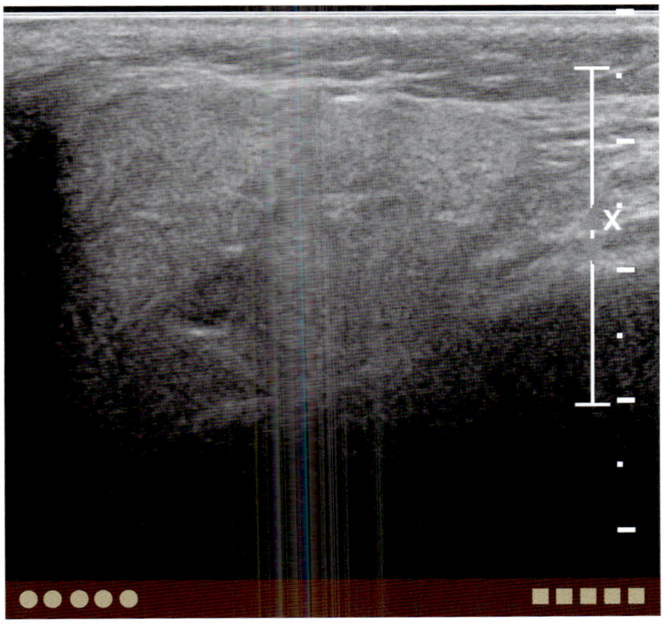

B. Supurative parotitis, same patient as A. Ultrasonography demonstrates asymmetric enlargement of the left parotid gland, which is heterogeneous in echotexture.

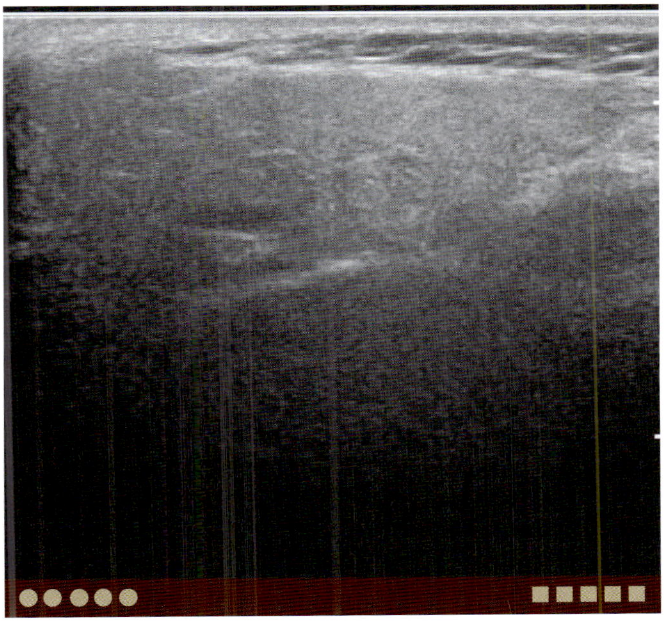

C. Normal right parotid gland, same patient as A. Ultrasonography demonstrates normal parotid gland with homogeneous echotexture.

DIFFERENTIAL DIAGNOSIS IMAGES (D-G)

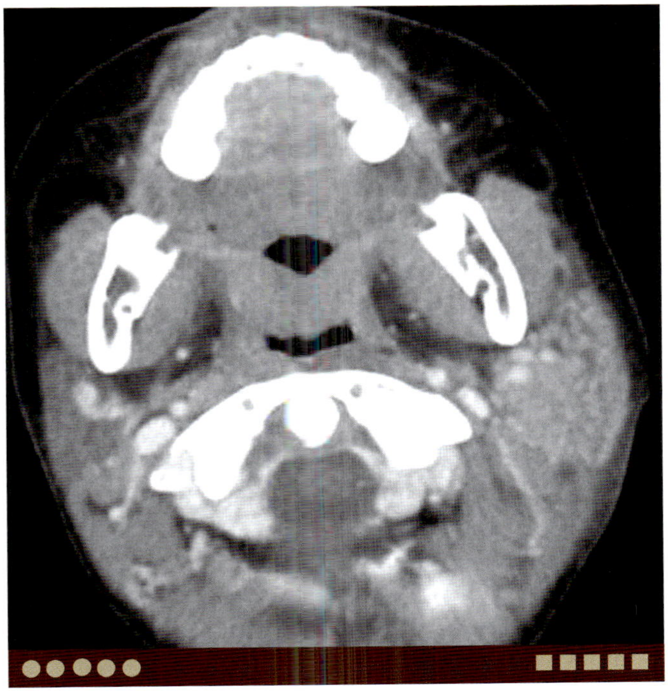

D. Mumps parotitis. Axial contrast-enhanced CT demonstrates diffuse enhancement in the enlarged gland with inflammatory change in the surrounding tissue.

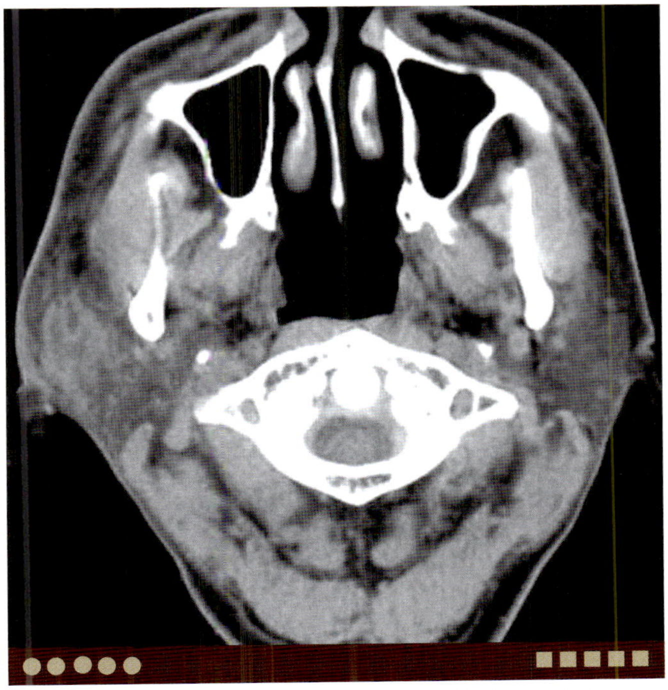

E. Parotitis due to sialolith. Axial unenhanced CT demonstrates right parotid gland swelling with internal heterogeneity.

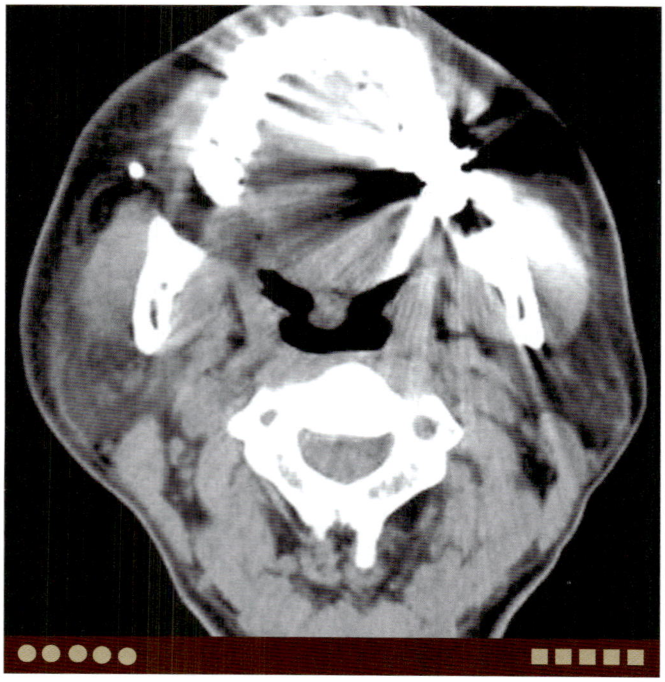

F. Parotitis due to sialolith, same patient as E. Axial unenhanced CT demonstrates a calcified sialolith in the right parotid duct.

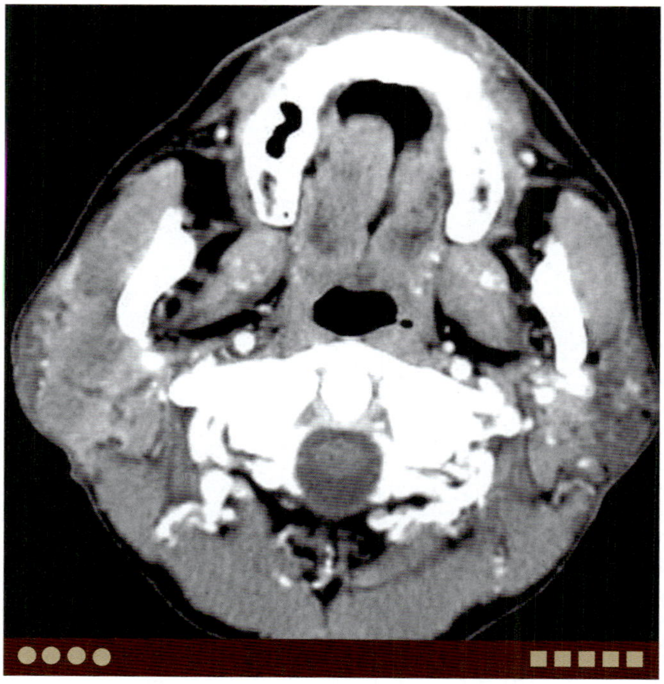

G. Follicular lymphoma. Axial contrast-enhanced CT demonstrates a right parotid gland mass with homogenous enhancement.

Case 7-30 Adenoid Cystic Carcinoma—Sublingual Gland

Akifumi Fujita, Margaret Chapman, Osamu Sakai

PRESENTATION

Swelling of the floor of mouth.

FINDINGS

CT and MRI show a mass in the sublingual gland.

DIFFERENTIAL DIAGNOSIS

- Pleomorphic adenoma: This lesion usually demonstrates a well-circumscribed high signal intensity mass on T2W images. However, it is difficult to differentiate from low-grade adenoid cystic carcinoma by imaging alone.
- Mucoepidermoid carcinoma: This cannot be differentiated from adenoid cystic carcinoma by CT or MR imaging.
- Lymphoma: This condition typically demonstrates a homogeneous mass lesion. Low signal intensity on T2W images and restricted diffusion reflect high cellularity.
- Schwannoma: This condition typically demonstrates an oval-shaped mass.
- Venous, venolymphatic and lymphatic malformation: This typically demonstrates high signal intensity on T2W images, however, imaging characteristics depend on vascular channel size. Enhancement is seen in the venous components. Presence of phleboliths is suggestive of venous malformation.

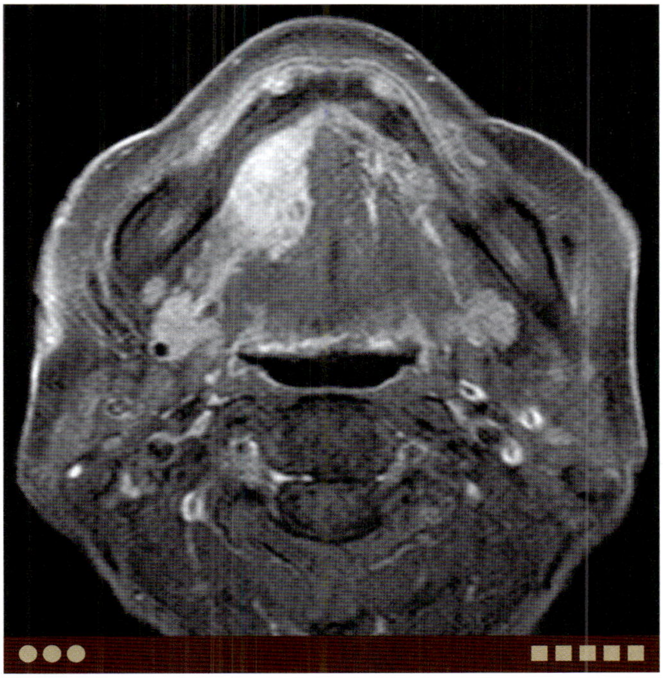

A. Adenoid cystic carcinoma. Axial postcontrast fat-suppressed T1W image demonstrates a well-circumscribed homogeneously enhancing mass of the right sublingual space.

COMMENTS

This is an 81-year-old woman with swelling of the floor of her mouth.

Adenoid cystic carcinoma is relatively rare in the parotid gland, comprising 2% to 6% of tumors in this location. However, it is more common in the submandibular and sublingual glands, comprising 12% and 15% of tumors arising in these glands, respectively. Further, it makes up about 30% of tumors in minor salivary glands with smaller glands tending to have a higher chance for malignancy. Eighty percent of parotid gland tumors are benign, however, 50% of submandibular gland tumors, and 70% to 80% of sublingual and minor salivary gland tumors are malignant. Therefore, malignancy has to be strongly suspected when diagnosing salivary gland tumors except those arising from the parotid gland.

Imaging findings of adenoid cystic carcinoma are often nonspecific. Signal intensity on T2W images reflects cellularity. It is suggested that low T2 signal is suggestive of higher cellularity and worse prognosis. Low-grade tumors are usually well-circumscribed and enhance homogeneously. High-grade tumors tend to be infiltrative with poorly defined margins.

Adenoid cystic carcinoma often presents with perineural tumor spread. It is important to cover the skull base and to evaluate the entire course of the nerve innervating the involved area. Skip perineural tumor spread can occasionally be seen.

It is always difficult to differentiate low-grade salivary gland tumors from benign tumors such as pleomorphic adenomas, schwannomas and venolymphatic malformations. Mucoepidermoid carcinoma and lymphoma are also important differential considerations.

PEARLS

- **More than half of tumors arising from the salivary gland, except the parotid gland, can be malignant.**
- **In adenoid cystic carcinoma, low T2 signal suggest higher cellularity and worse prognosis.**
- **Perineural tumor spread is often seen in adenoid cystic carcinoma. It is important to cover the skull base and to evaluate the entire course of the nerve innervating involved areas.**

ADDITIONAL IMAGES (B-D)

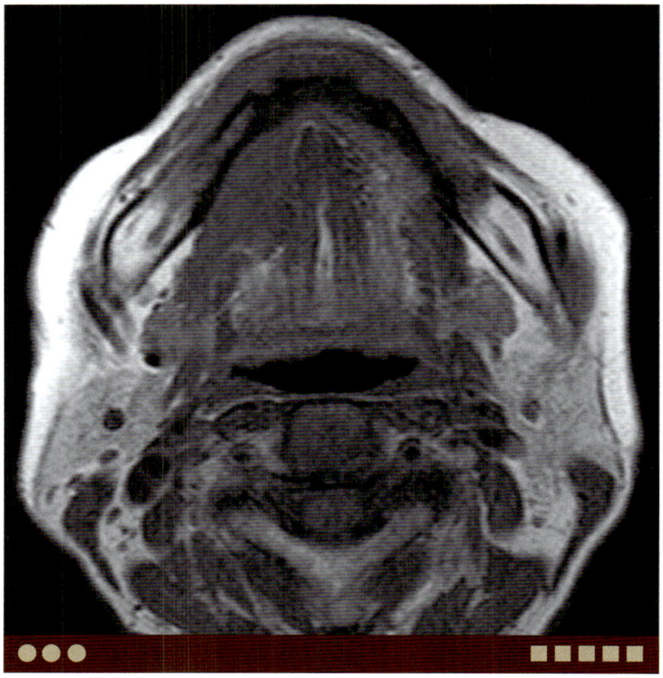

B. Adenoid cystic carcinoma, same patient as A. Axial T1W image demonstrates a homogeneous low-signal intensity mass.

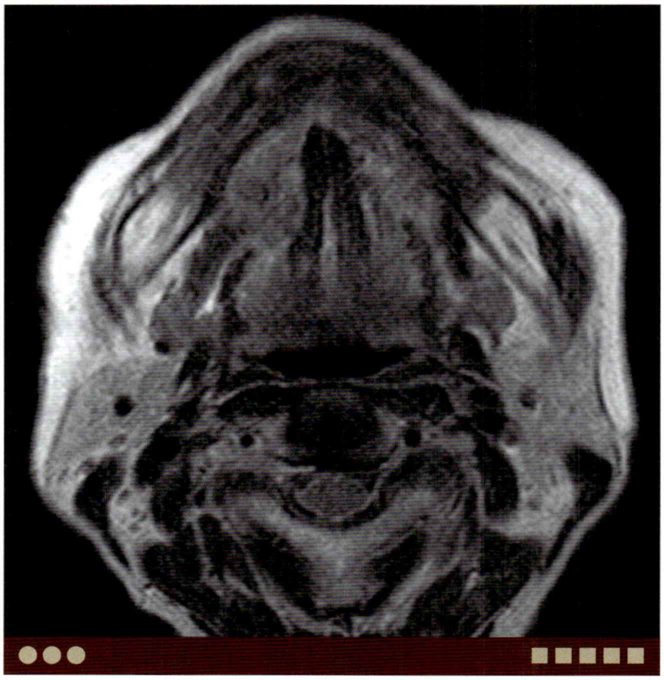

C. Adenoid cystic carcinoma, same patient as A. Axial T2W image demonstrates a heterogeneous low-signal intensity mass, suggestive of a high-grade malignant tumor.

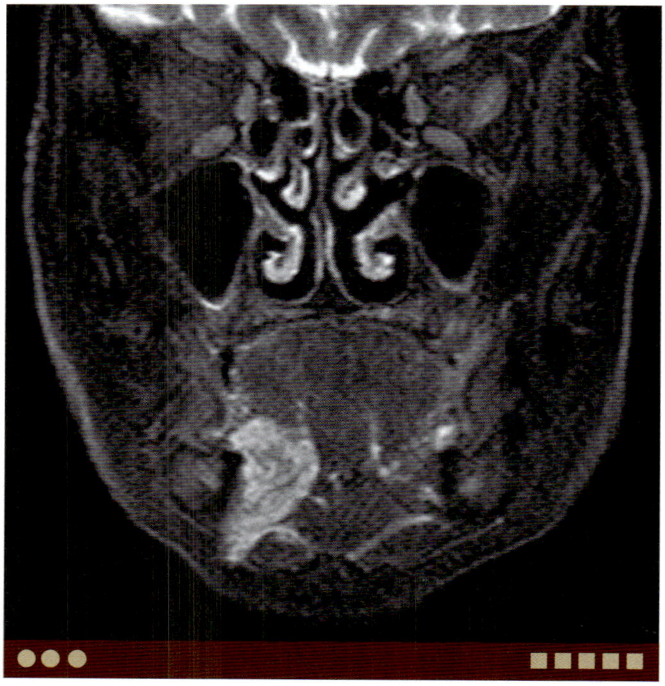

D. Adenoid cystic carcinoma, same patient as A. Coronal STIR image demonstrates infiltrative margin caudally, also suggestive of high-grade malignancy.

DIFFERENTIAL DIAGNOSIS IMAGES (E-G)

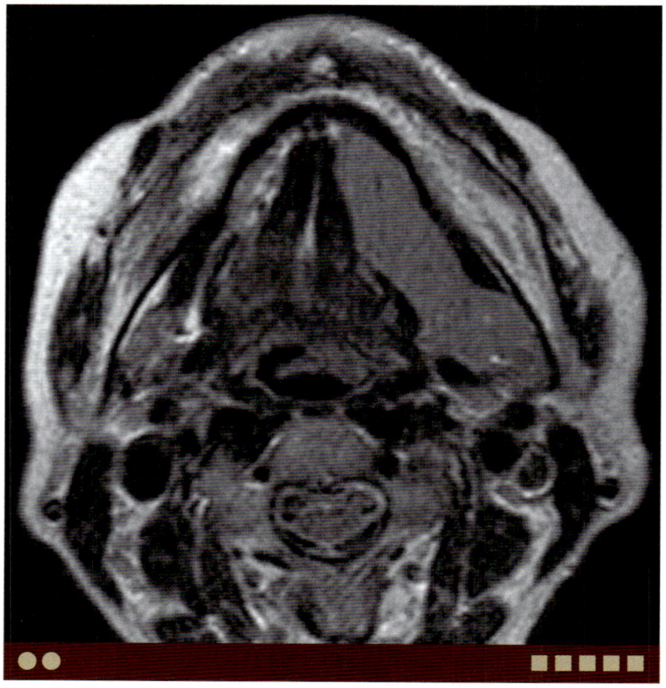

E. Lymphoma. Axial T2W image demonstrates a homogeneous intermediate-intensity mass of the left sublingual space infiltrating into the submandibular gland.

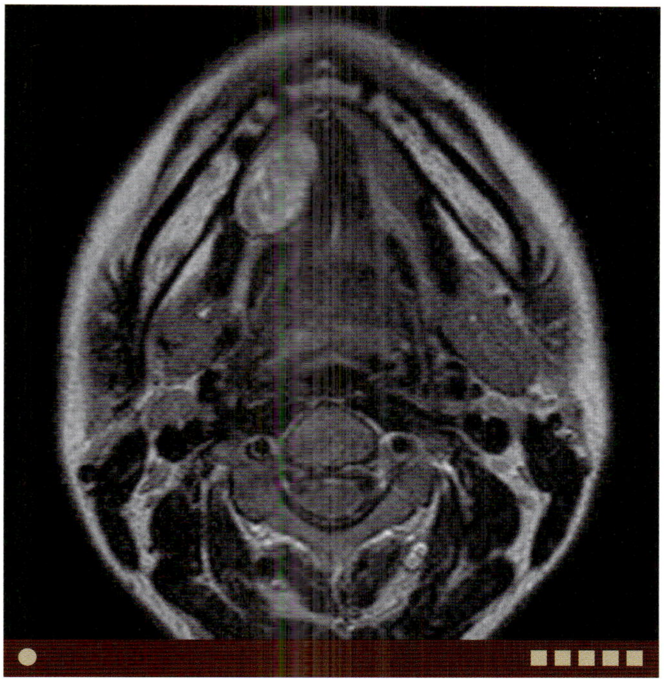

F. Schwannoma. Axial T2W image demonstrates a well-circumscribed oval mass of the right sublingual space. The normal sublingual gland is displaced anteriorly.

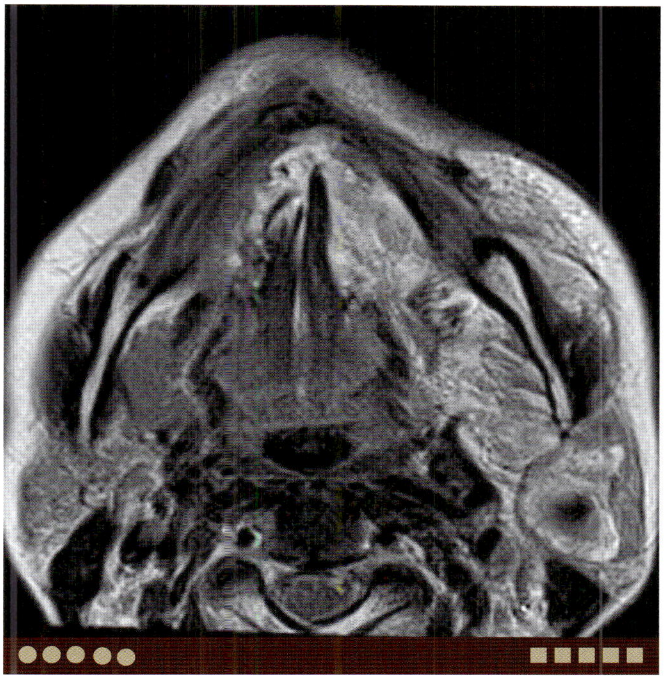

G. Venolymphatic malformation. Axial T2W image demonstrates a heterogeneous high-signal intensity mass-like lesion within the left sublingual space, submandibular space, masticator space, and parotid space. Multi-space involvement of the lesion suggests vascular malformation.

Chapter 8

ORAL CAVITY AND OROPHARYNX

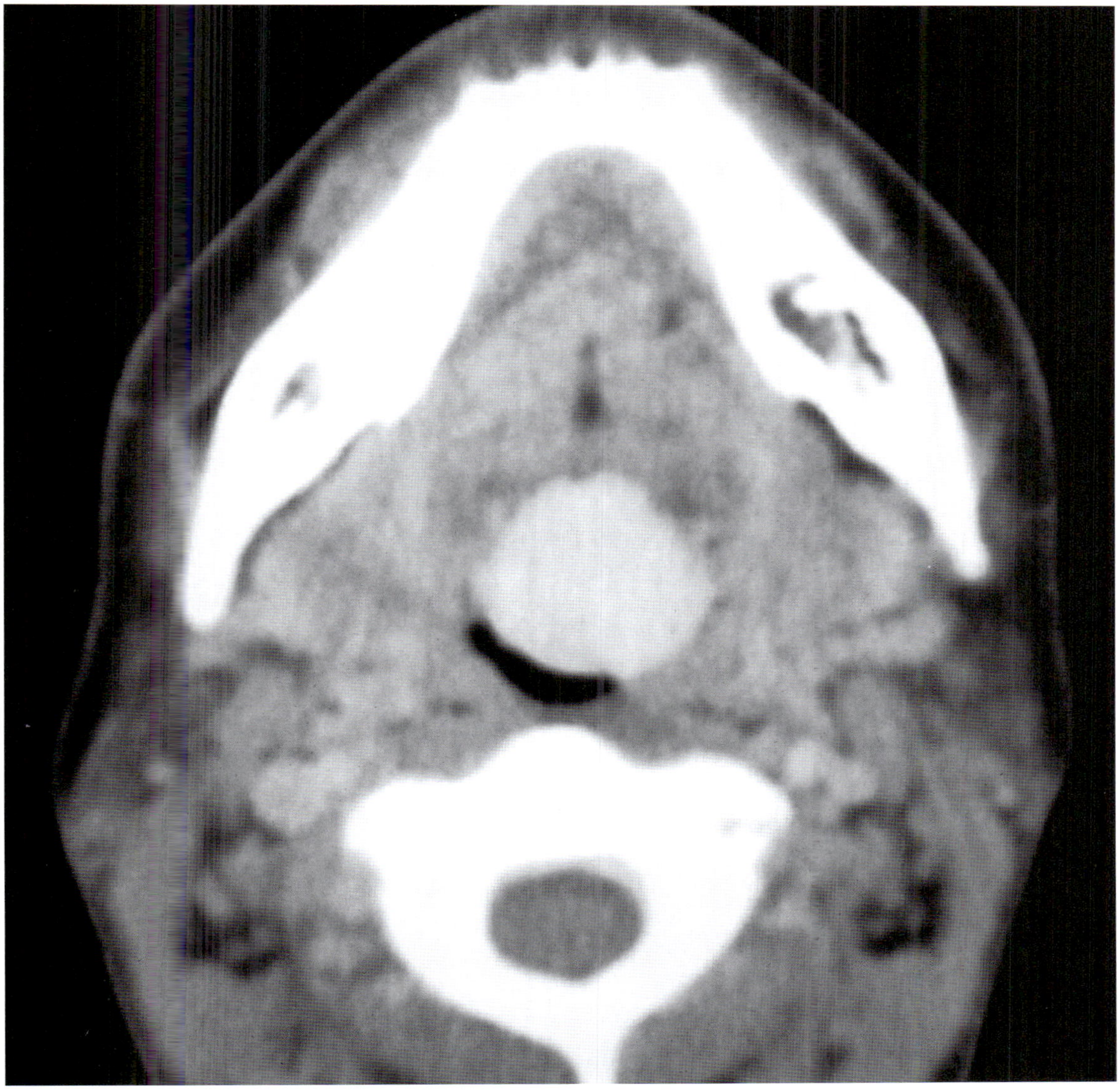

Case 8–1 Lingual Thyroid, Ectopic Thyroid

Osamu Sakai, Daniel Welier

PRESENTATION

Mass at the base of tongue.

FINDINGS

CT demonstrates a well-circumscribed, hyperdense mass at the base of tongue.

DIFFERENTIAL DIAGNOSIS

- Squamous sell carcinoma (SCCA): This is the most common tumor at the base of tongue. SCCA occasionally demonstrates avid enhancement, however, usually demonstrates more heterogeneous density/signal and enhancement with poorly defined margins.
- Lymphoma: Typically demonstrates a homogeneous infiltrative appearance with mild enhancement. Necrosis is not common.
- Lymphoid hyperplasia: This condition may be bulky, however, often preserves linear, septum-like striation without round, avid enhancement.
- Minor salivary gland tumors: Mucoepidermoid and adenoid cystic carcinomas can occur at the base of tongue, usually demonstrating more heterogeneous density/signal and ill-defined margins.

COMMENTS

This is a 34-year-old woman scanned for a mass at the base of tongue.

The thyroid gland descends from the foramen cecum at the base of tongue to the inferior neck through the thyroglossal duct. This process can be obstructed at any level. The lingual thyroid is a condition that results from early termination of this descent. This condition is often diagnosed in childhood, however, occasionally can be undiagnosed until middle age. In about 75% of patients, the lingual thyroid is the only functioning thyroid tissue, and about 70% of patients with lingual thyroid have hypothyroidism. Removal of this thyroid tissue results in hypothyroidism, and the patient will require hormonal supplementation for the rest of their life. Therefore, diagnosis of thyroid tissue in other location and evaluation of thyroid function is critical in patients with ectopic thyroid gland. Nuclear medicine studies with Tc-99m or I-123 are helpful for this assessment. On the other hand, a small amount of residual thyroid tissue may be seen along the course of the thyroglossal duct in patients with a normal thyroid gland, particularly with recent high-resolution imaging.

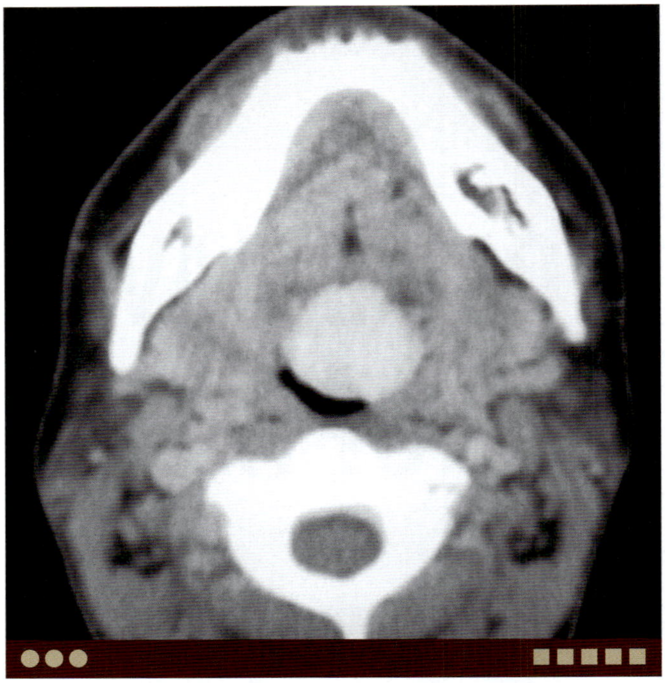

A. Lingual thyroid. Axial postcontrast CT demonstrates a well-demarcated, round, hyperdense mass at the base of tongue in midline.

Ectopic thyroid tissue demonstrates similar density/signal to the normal thyroid gland. Homogeneous high density and enhancement on CT is characteristic. On MRI, it demonstrates intermediate to slightly high signal on both T1W and T2W images. Neoplastic process must be suspected when heterogeneous density/signal or enhancement is noted because carcinomas, usually papillary carcinomas, can occur from the ectopic thyroid tissue. Other malignancies such as SCCA and minor salivary gland tumors may mimic ectopic thyroid as well.

PEARLS

- **Patients with lingual thyroid often do not have any other thyroid tissue, including a normal thyroid gland in expected location in the lower neck. Removal of this ectopic thyroid tissue results in hypothyroidism.**
- **This condition is often diagnosed in childhood; however, it can occasionally be left undiagnosed until middle age.**
- **Papillary carcinomas can occur from the ectopic thyroid tissue.**

ADDITIONAL IMAGES (B-E)

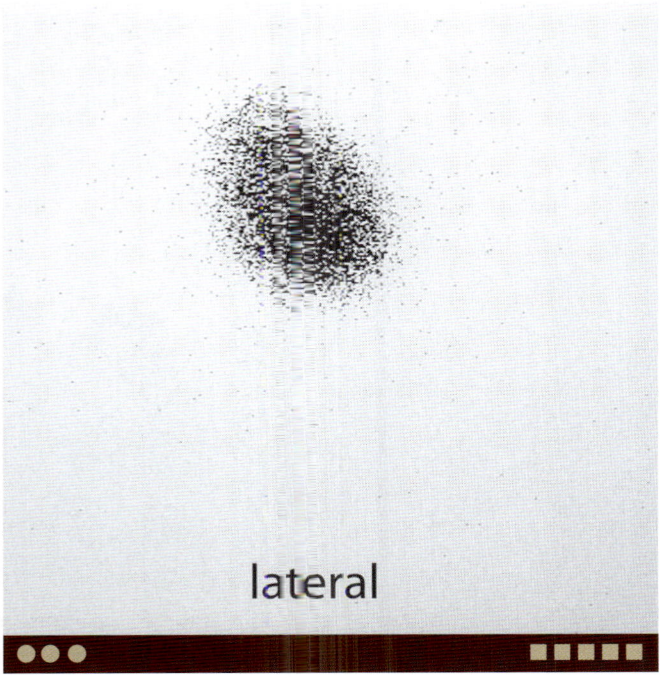

B. Lingual thyroid, same patient as A. I-123 scintigraphy demonstrates an area of increased uptake at the base of tongue without uptake in the lower neck.

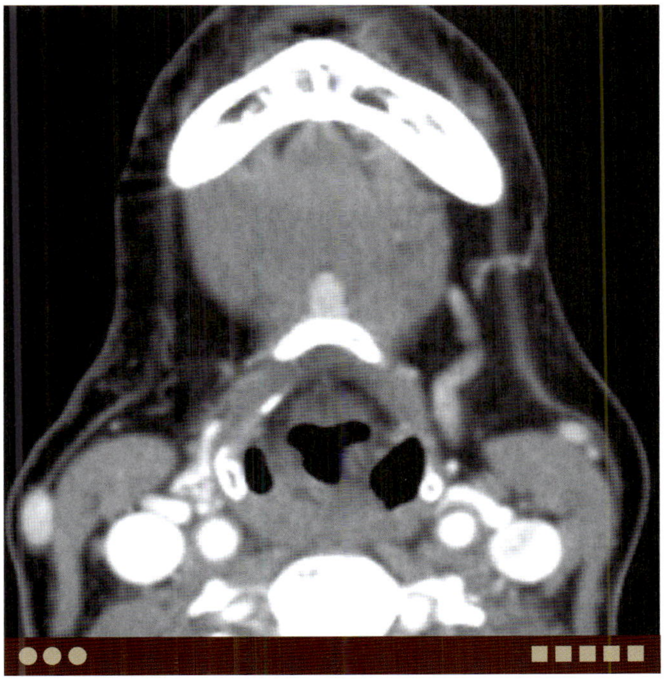

C. Ectopic thyroid in a different patient. Axial postcontrast CT demonstrates a small, round, hyperdense mass just above the hyoid bone in midline.

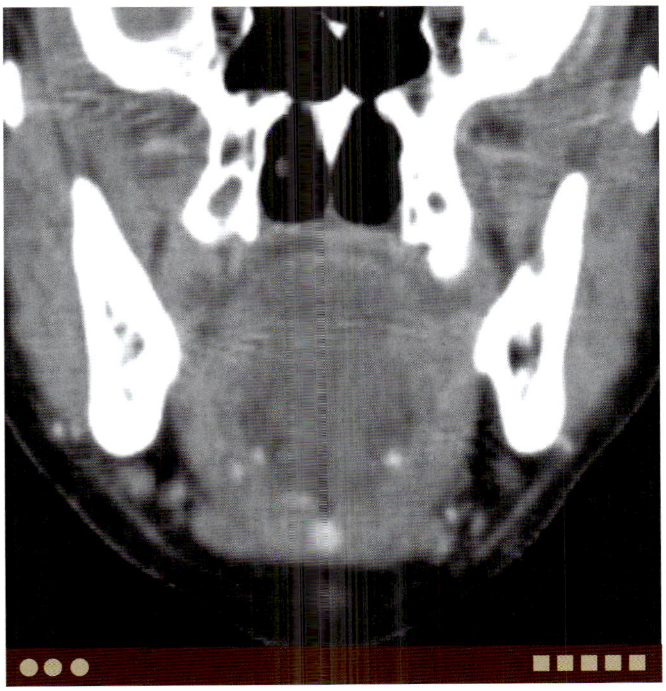

D. Ectopic thyroid, same patient as C. Coronal postcontrast CT demonstrates a small, round, hyperdense mass in the floor of mouth in midline.

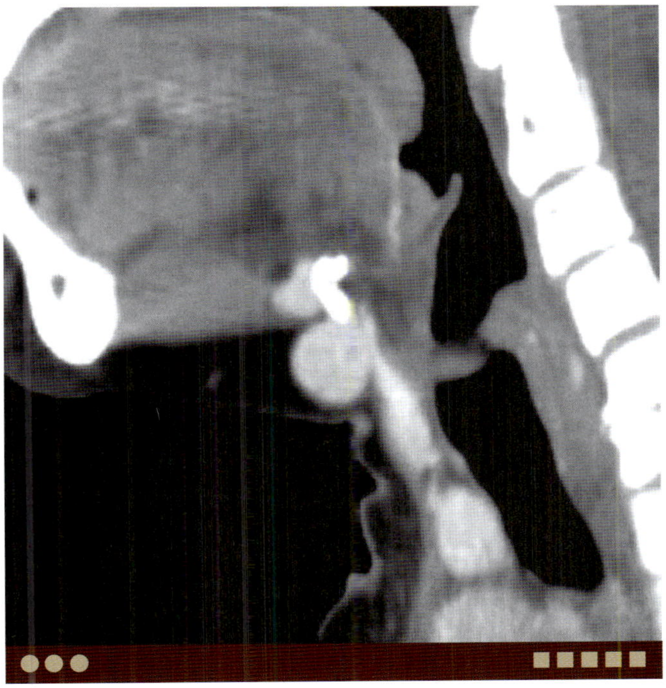

E. Ectopic thyroid, same patient as C. Sagittal postcontrast CT demonstrates multiple small, round hyperdense lesions along the course of the thyroglossal duct.

DIFFERENTIAL DIAGNOSIS IMAGES (F-H)

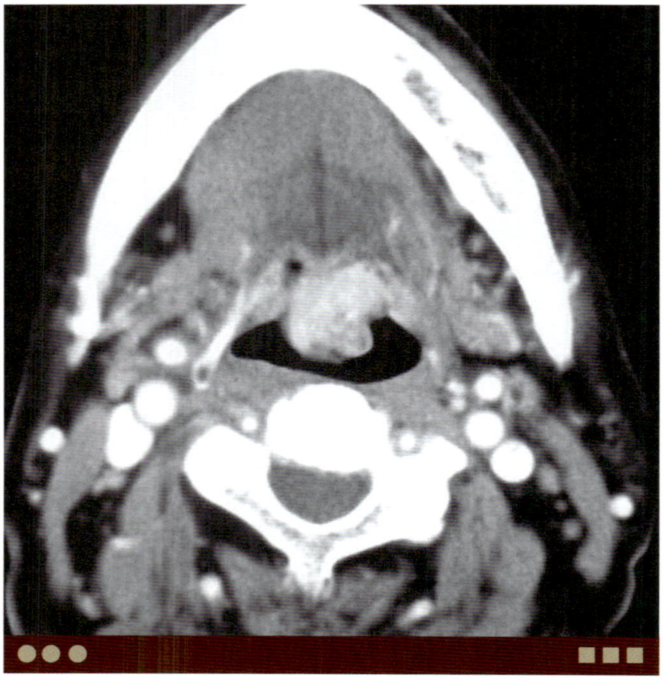

F. Mucoepidermoid carcinoma. Axial postcontrast CT demonstrates a heterogeneously enhancing, slightly irregular lesion at the base of tongue in midline.

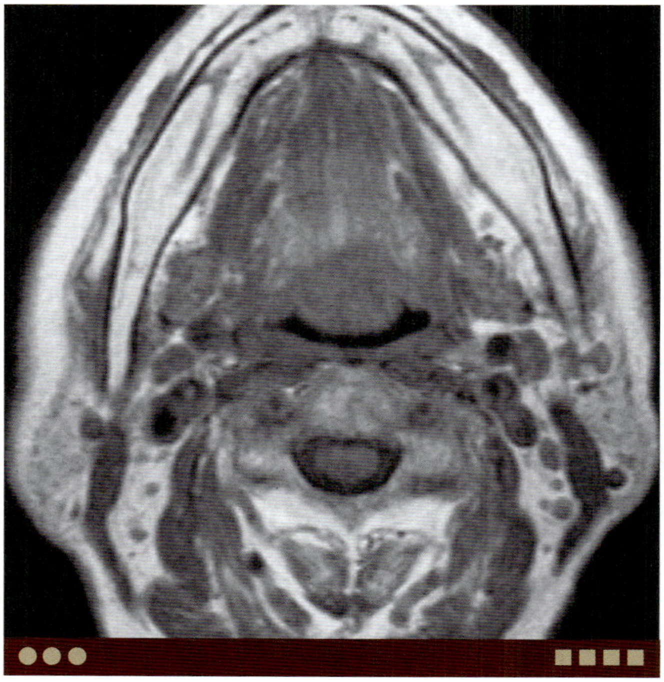

G. Mucoepidermoid carcinoma, same patient as F. Axial T1W MR image demonstrates a round, low-signal lesion at the base of tongue in midline.

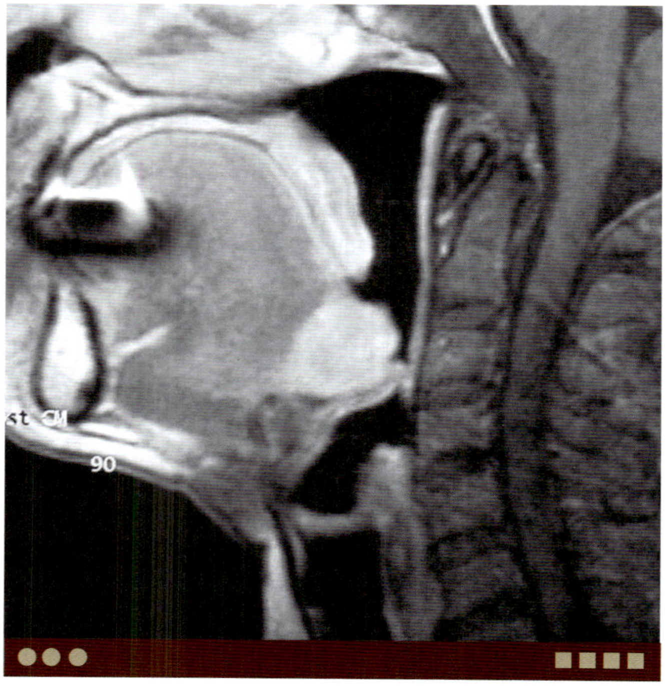

H. Mucoepidermoid carcinoma, same patient as F. Sagittal postcontrast T1W MR image demonstrates an avidly enhancing lesion at the base of tongue.

Case 8–2 Squamous Cell Carcinoma: Tongue

Osamu Sakai, Daniel Weber

PRESENTATION

Ulceration in the lateral tongue.

FINDINGS

CT demonstrates a heterogeneously enhancing lesion in the lateral tongue.

DIFFERENTIAL DIAGNOSIS

- Adenoid cystic carcinoma: Salivary gland tumor that often occurs in the sublingual gland and minor salivary glands and may involve the tongue. Perineural tumor spread is common.
- Mucoepidermoid carcinoma: Also a salivary gland tumor that often occurs in the sublingual gland and minor salivary glands and may involve the tongue. High-grade tumors tend to be solid and infiltrative.
- Lingual thyroid: Thyroid tissue located at the foramen cecum and seen as a well-demarcated, hyperdense lesion at the base of tongue on CT.

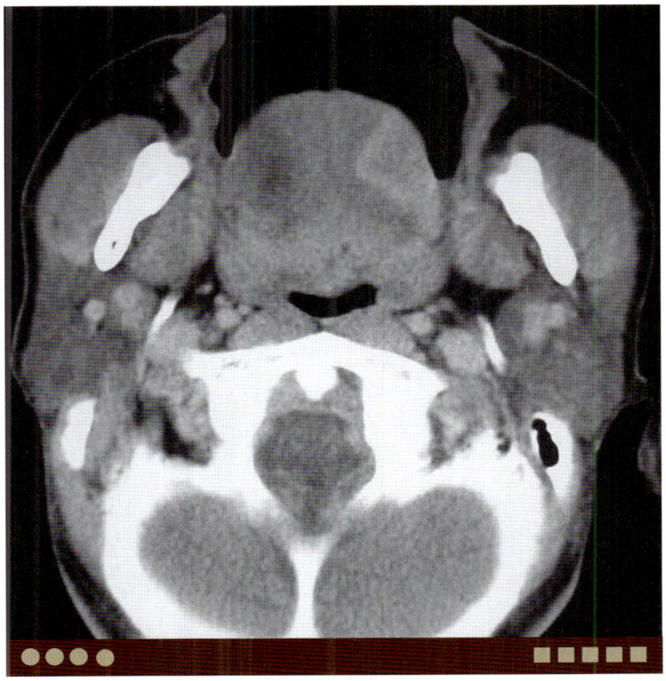

A. SCCA of the tongue. Axial postcontrast CT demonstrates a mildly enhancing, wedge-shaped tumor in the left lateral tongue.

COMMENTS

This is a 48-year-old man with ulceration in the left lateral tongue.

Squamous cell carcinoma (SCCA) is the most common malignancy occurring in the tongue accounting for more than 90% of malignancy in this region. Diagnosis of SCCA of the tongue is made by direct visualization and palpation, followed by biopsy. The role of imaging is to define the extent of the lesion and evaluate for possible nodal metastasis. Extension to the base of tongue, involvement of the sublingual nerve and vessels, involvement of the lingual raphe, contralateral extension, involvement of the oral floor, and invasion of the mandible should be carefully evaluated. SCCA in the tongue often occurs in the lateral aspect of the tongue. Therefore, axial and coronal planes should be basic scan planes, while the sagittal plane is helpful to evaluate for extension to the base of tongue. The tongue is composed of fatty musculature, therefore, tumors are often identified well on noncontrast T1W MR images. STIR images demonstrate tumors and surrounding inflammatory change as high signal. Tumor usually demonstrates rapid avid enhancement. Fat suppression is needed to evaluate for local extension of the tumor after contrast administration because the margin of the enhancing tumor can be obscured due to the fatty background. Contralateral nodal metastasis is common in patients with tongue cancer. Careful evaluation of the both sides of the neck is necessary, particularly in levels I and II.

PEARLS

- **Tumor is often identified well on precontrast T1W MR images due to fatty background.**
- **STIR and fat-suppressed postcontrast T1W images are also helpful to delineate the tumor extent.**
- **Axial and coronal are basic imaging planes, however, sagittal imaging is helpful to evaluate for extension to the base of tongue.**

ADDITIONAL IMAGES (B-G)

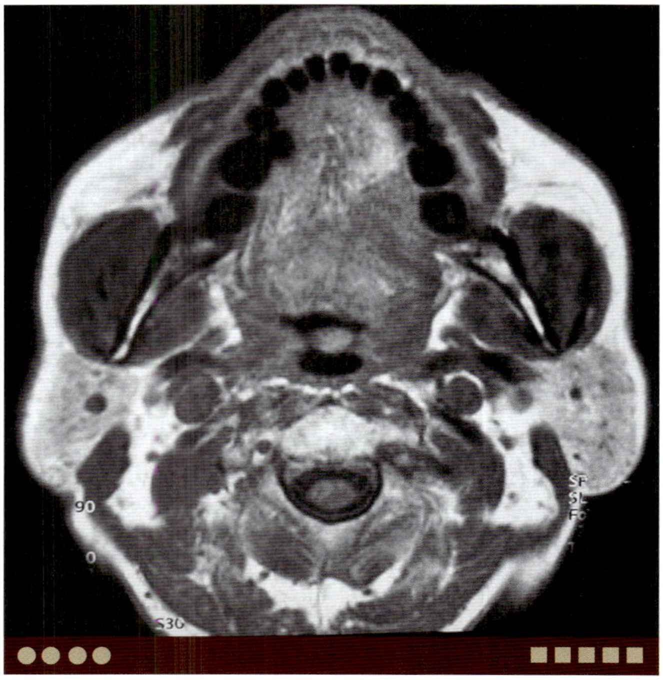

B. SCCA of the tongue, same patient as A. Axial T1W MR image demonstrates low signal in the tumor.

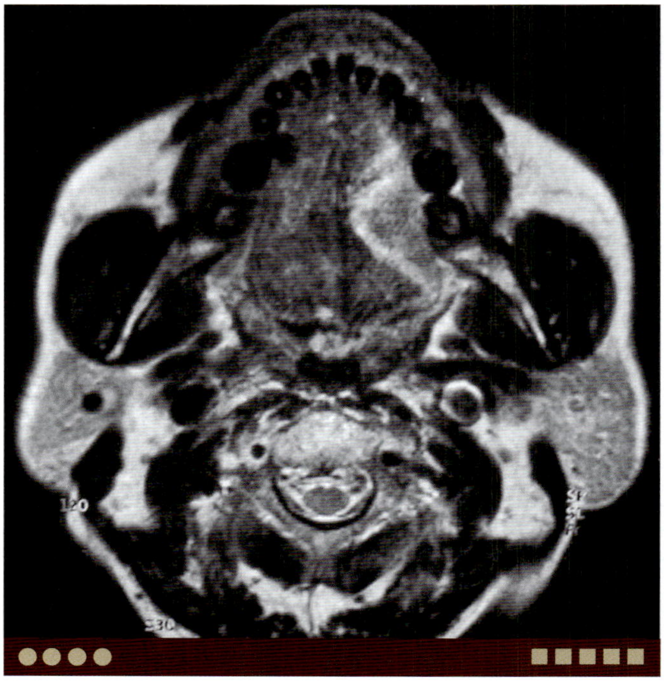

C. SCCA of the tongue, same patient as A. Axial T2W image demonstrates intermediate-to-high signal in the tumor.

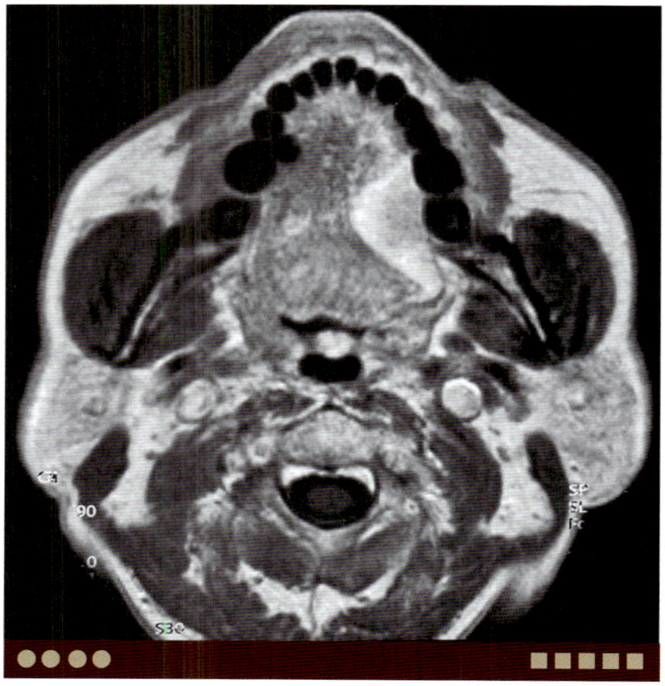

D. SCCA of the tongue, same patient as A. Axial postcontrast T1W image demonstrates enhancement of the tumor.

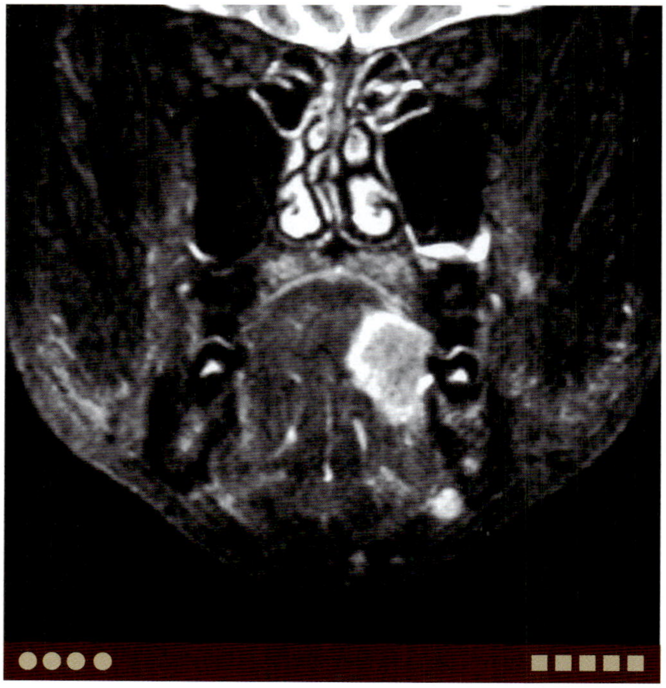

E. SCCA of the tongue, same patient as A. Coronal fat-suppressed T2W image demonstrates a well-demarcated, high-signal tumor in the left lateral tongue, abutting the genioglossus muscle, but not involving the lingual raphe.

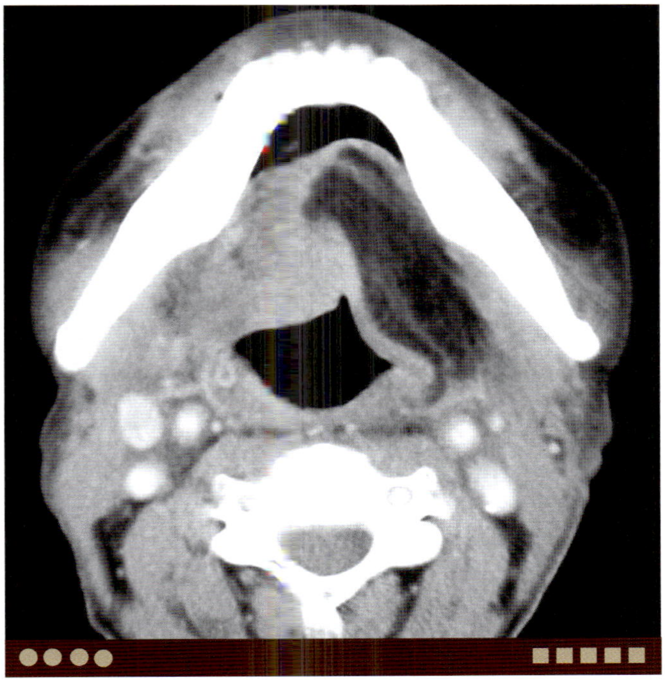

F. SCCA of the tongue, same patient as A, status-post hemiglossectomy and flap reconstruction. Axial postcontrast CT demonstrates fat density in the reconstructed left tongue.

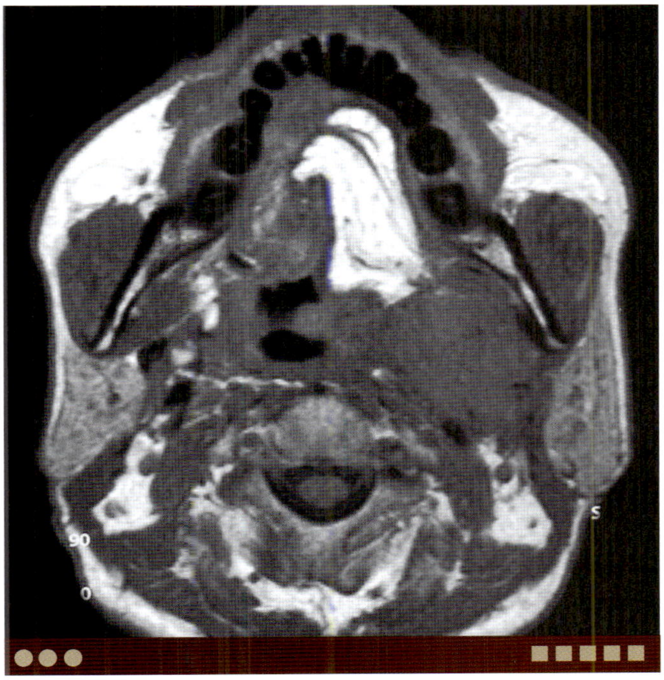

G. SCCA of the tongue, same patient as A, status-post hemiglossectomy and flap reconstruction. Axial T1W image demonstrates high signal from fatty tissue of the flap. Note a large low-signal mass posterior to the reconstruction site, compressing the left carotid vessels, consistent with recurrent tumor.

DIFFERENTIAL DIAGNOSIS IMAGES (H-J)

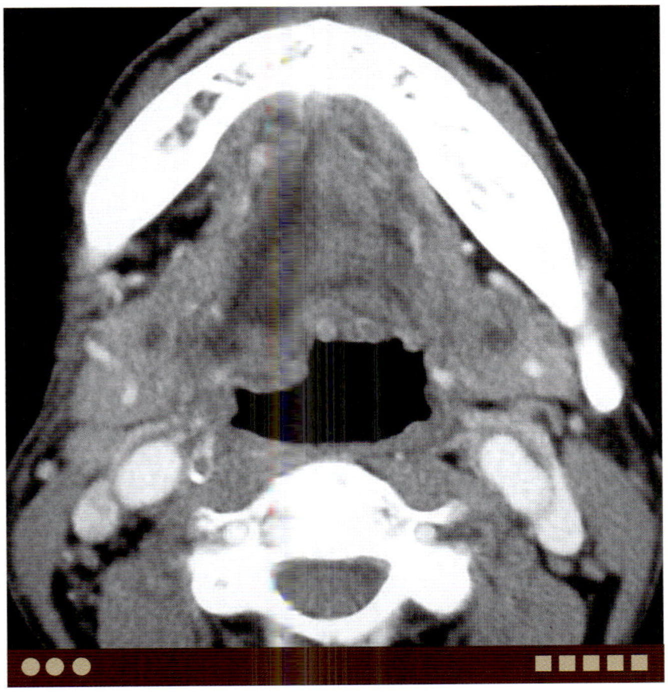

H. **Denervation myositis**. Axial postcontrast CT in a patient with nasopharyngeal carcinoma demonstrates decreased density and posterior protrusion of the right tongue consistent with subacute to chronic denervation myositic change due to hypoglossal nerve invasion.

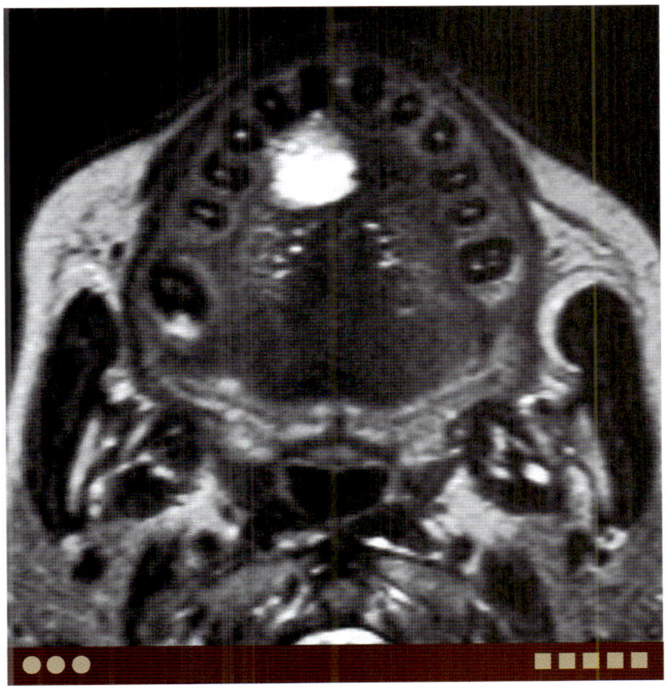

I. **Hemangioma**. Axial T2W image demonstrates a well-demarcated, very high-signal lesion in the anterior right tongue.

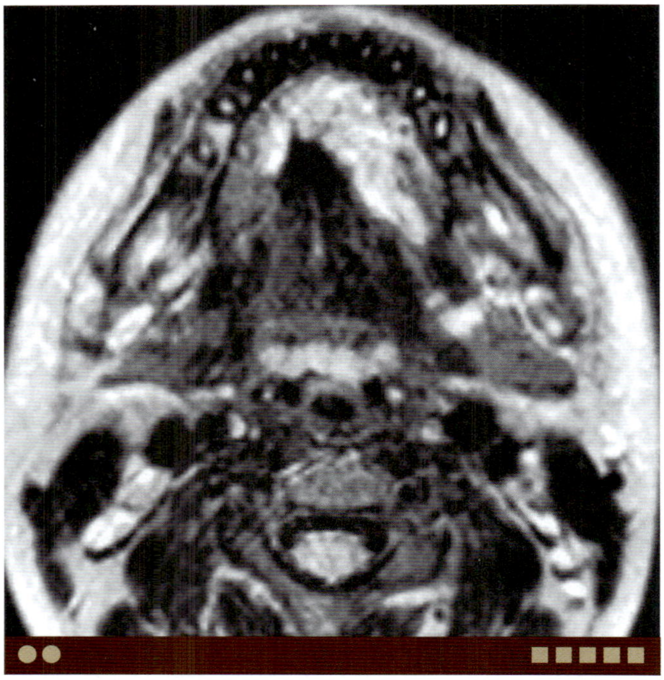

J. Neurofibroma. Axial T2W image demonstrates a slightly lobulated, high-signal lesion centered in the anterior left tongue crossing midline.

Case 8–3 Squamous Cell Carcinoma: Gingiva

Osamu Sakai, Daniel Weber

PRESENTATION

Gingival mass with ulceration.

FINDINGS

CT demonstrates an ill-defined lesion in the gingiva, often invading the mandible or maxilla.

DIFFERENTIAL DIAGNOSIS

- Mucoepidermoid carcinoma: This is a minor salivary gland tumor which may arise from the gingival mucosa. Occasionally, intraosseous primary mucoepidermoid carcinoma may occur.
- Leukemia: Gingival involvement by leukemic cell is occasionally seen, particularly in patients with acute myeloid leukemia.
- Lymphoma: Gingival lymphoma is rare. A gingival mass with cortex sparing marrow lesion is a characteristic imaging finding.
- Epulis fissuratum: Mucosal hyperplasia likely resulting from chronic low-grade trauma. This is well known to dentists, however, often unfamiliar to radiologists.
- Torus mandibularis: An exostosis that occurs at the lingual aspect of the anterior mandible; usually bilateral.

COMMENTS

This is a 70-year-old man with an anterior mandibular gingival mass.

Diagnosis of squamous cell carcinoma (SCCA) of the gingiva is made by direct visualization and followed by biopsy. Mucosal lesions are easily evaluated clinically. Therefore, the role of imaging is to define the extent of the lesion, particularly submucosal extension, and invasion into adjacent bone and neurovascular bundle. CT depicts subtle cortical destruction and is useful to evaluate for bony invasion. MRI is superior to evaluate for soft tissue lesions and bone marrow abnormality, while more clearly demonstrating tumor invasion and secondary inflammatory changes.

In the retromolar trigone, clinical evaluation is difficult and imaging has an important role in diagnosis of tumor extension. In cases with a large lesion, lesion identification may not be difficult; however, in certain instances, imaging findings may be very subtle and easily missed. These findings include subtle soft tissue density along the alveolus or posterolateral wall of the maxillary sinus, and subtle demineralization of the pterygoid plate or invasion of the insertion of the pterygoid muscles. Evaluation of the retroantral fat pad, fat in the pterygomaxillary fissure and pterygopalatine fossa is important. If the fat in these locations is involved, there is higher possibility of intracranial extension of the tumor by means of perineural tumor spread along the second branch of the trigeminal nerve (V2), reaching the paracavernous region and middle cranial fossa. In the mandible, evaluation of the fat anteromedial to the ramus, at the orifice of the mandibular canal, is important to diagnose perineural tumor spread along the third branch of the trigeminal nerve (V3).

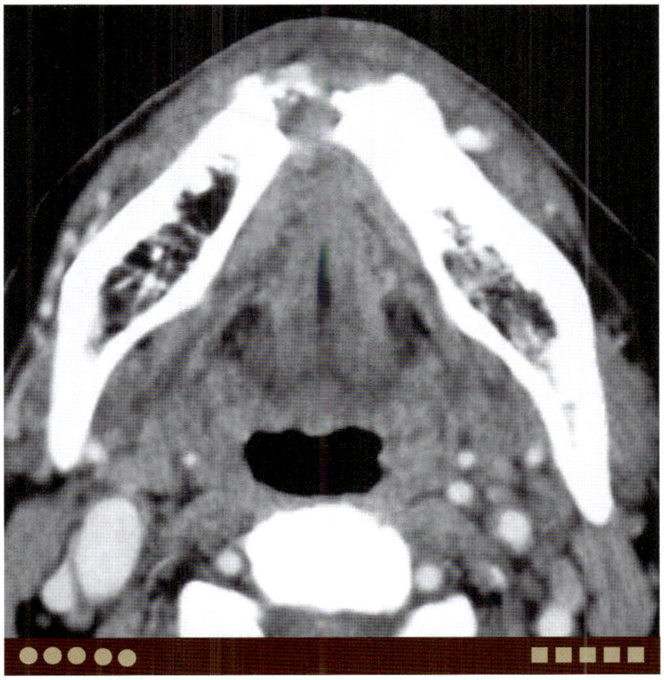

A. SCCA of the gingiva. Axial postcontrast CT demonstrates a heterogeneously enhancing lesion with destructive changes involving the anterior mandible.

PEARLS

- **SCCA is the most common malignancy involving the gingiva.**
- **CT is useful to evaluate for cortical destruction, and MRI is useful to evaluate for marrow involvement.**
- **Evaluation of the fat planes is important to diagnose perineural tumor spread.**

ADDITIONAL IMAGES (B-G)

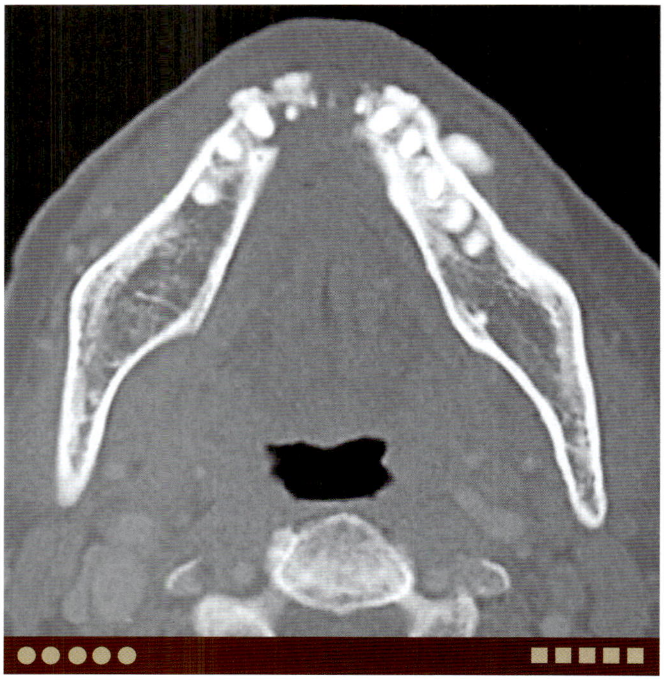

B. SCCA of the gingiva, same patient as A. Axial bone window CT more clearly demonstrates the bone destruction.

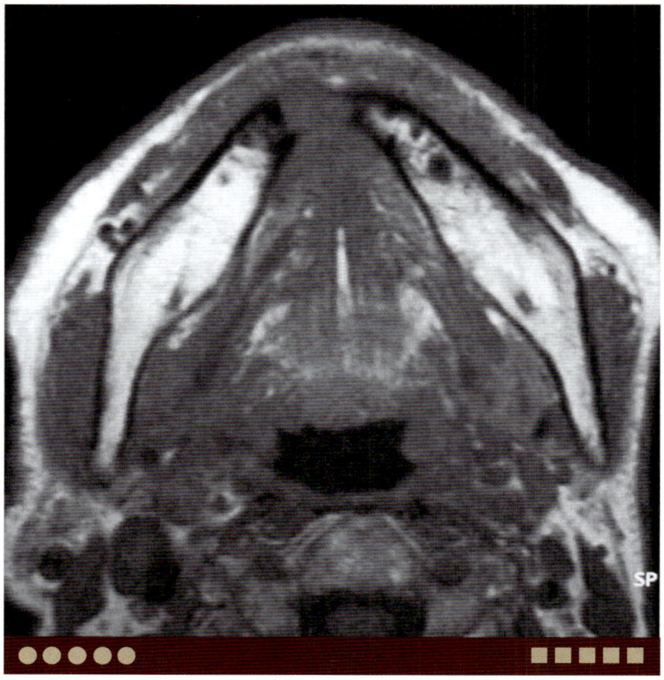

C. SCCA of the gingiva, same patient as A. Axial T1W MR demonstrates low signal in the tumor.

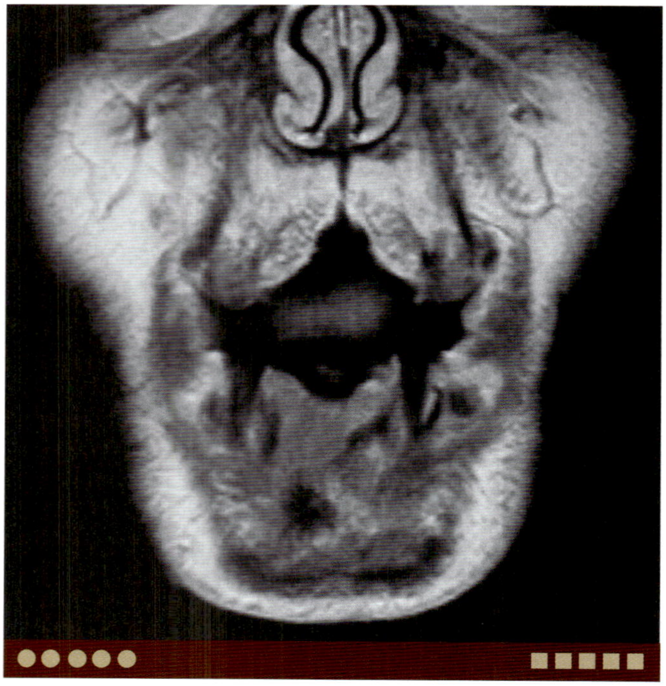

D. SCCA of the gingiva, same patient as A. Coronal postcontrast T1W MR demonstrates mild enhancement of the tumor invading the mandible.

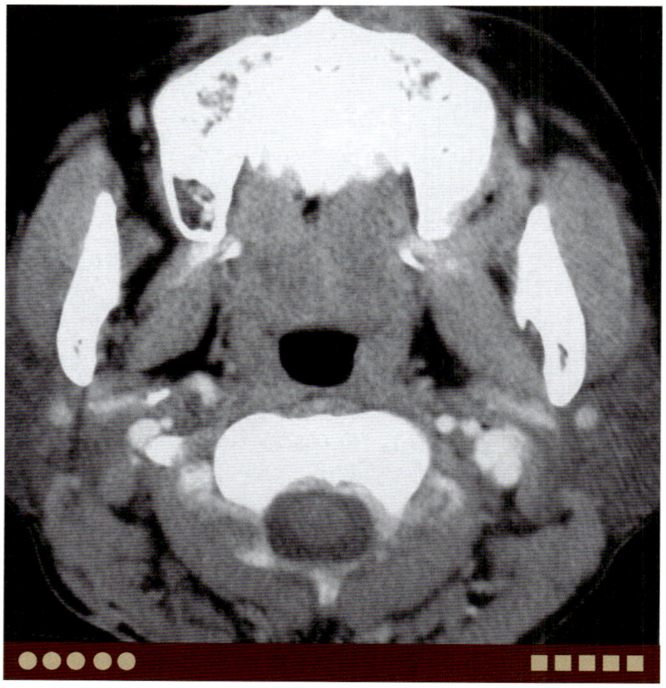

E. SCCA of the gingiva in a different patient. Axial postcontrast CT demonstrates subtle soft tissue density lateral to the maxilla on the left, obliterating the buccal fat. Note subtle cortical destruction and loss of normal fatty marrow compared with the right.

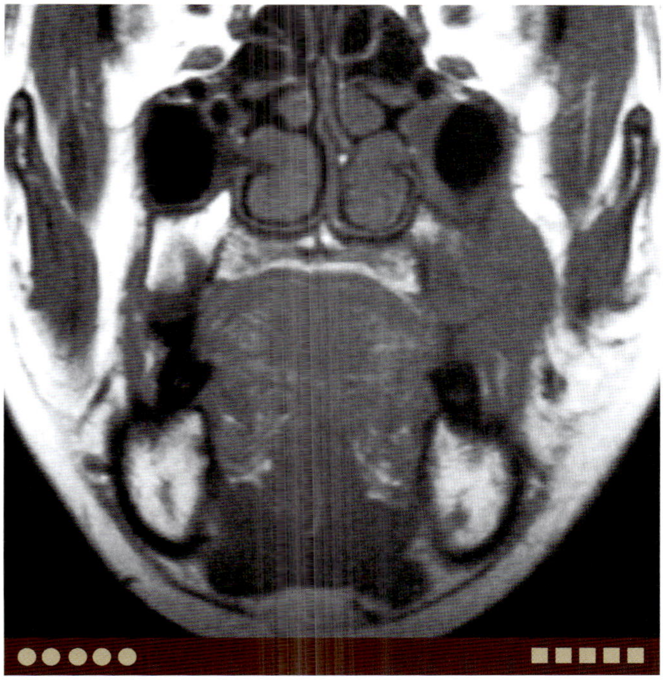

F. SCCA of the gingiva, same patient as E. Coronal T1W MR demonstrates a low-signal lesion involving the left maxillary alveolus and expanding into the buccal space.

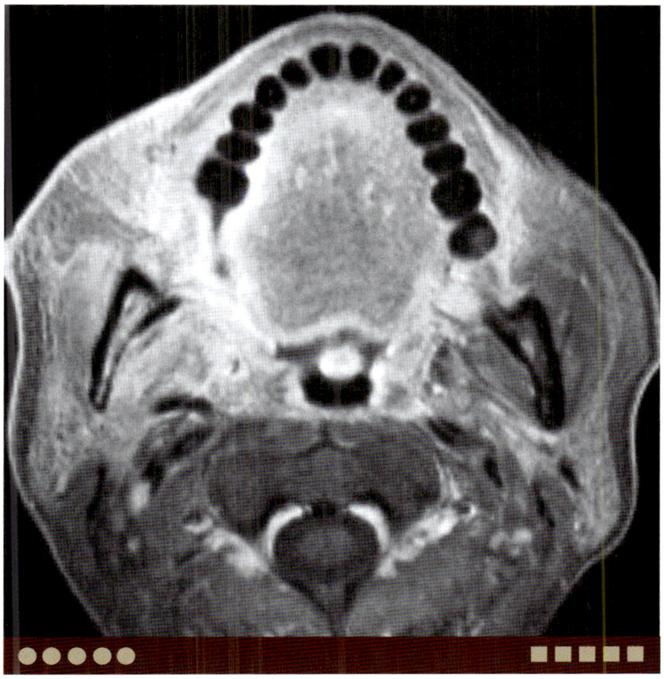

G. **SCCA of the gingiva** in a different patient. Axial postcontrast fat-suppressed T1W MR demonstrates heterogeneous enhancement in the right retromolar region. Note cortical destruction of the right mandibular ramus and bone marrow enhancement. There is also abnormal enhancement of right pterygoid and masseter muscles, consistent with a combination of direct invasion and denervation myositis due to V3 invasion.

DIFFERENTIAL DIAGNOSIS IMAGES (H-J)

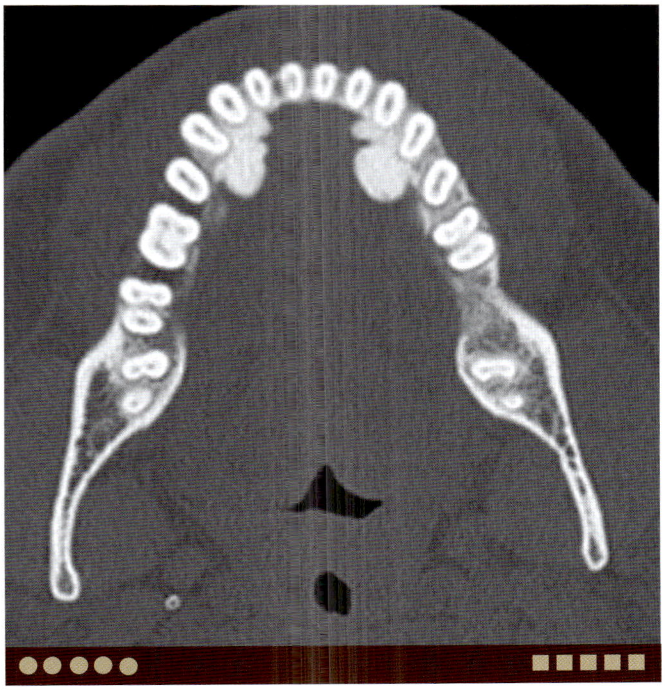

H. **Torus mandibularis**. Axial CT demonstrates nodular exostoses at the lingual aspect of the anterior mandible.

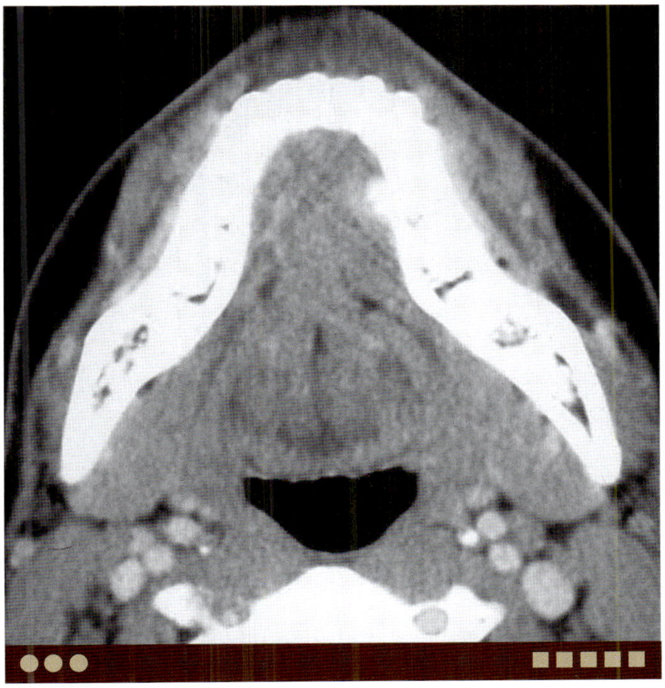

I. **Epulis fissuratum**. Axial postcontrast CT demonstrates a focal soft tissue mass with calcification at the lingual aspect of the left anterior mandible.

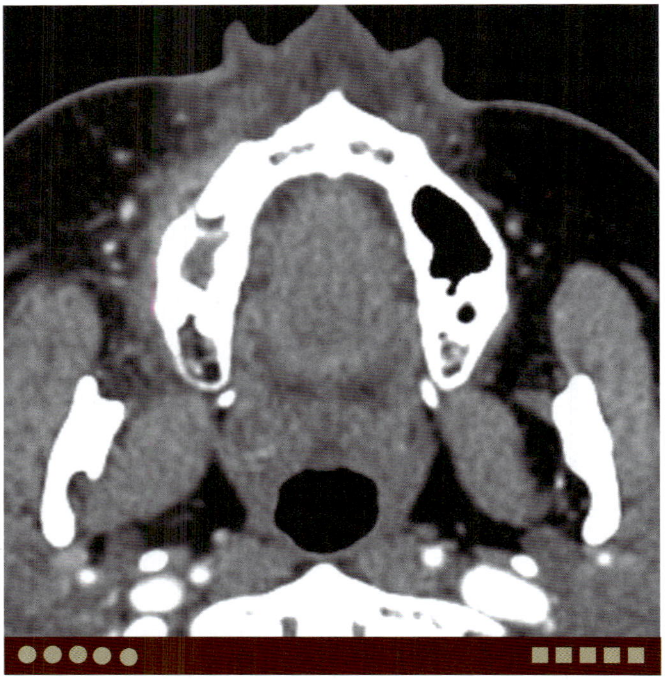

J. Periapical abscess. Axial postcontrast CT demonstrates a rim-enhancing lesion adjacent to the right maxilla. Note adjacent osteolytic lesion and opacification of the right maxillary sinus secondary to infection.

Case 8–4 Squamous Cell Carcinoma: Tonsil

Osamu Sakai, Daniel Weller

PRESENTATION

Tonsillar mass.

FINDINGS

CT and MRI demonstrate a mass arising from the palatine tonsil and necrotic lymph nodes.

DIFFERENTIAL DIAGNOSIS

- Lymphoid hyperplasia of the tonsils: Tonsillar prominence is common in children and young adults; typically bilateral and symmetric and often associated with prominent adenoids and cervical adenopathy. Enhancing septa are seen on contrast-enhanced CT and MR.
- Lymphoma: Second most common malignancy in the palatine tonsils. Lymphoma usually shows homogeneous density/signal with enlarged, non-necrotic lymph nodes.
- Pleomorphic adenoma: Typically a well-circumscribed mass arising from the minor salivary glands in the pharyngeal mucosa.
- Minor salivary gland cancers: Mucoepidermoid carcinoma and adenoid cystic carcinoma may arise in the tonsillar regions.

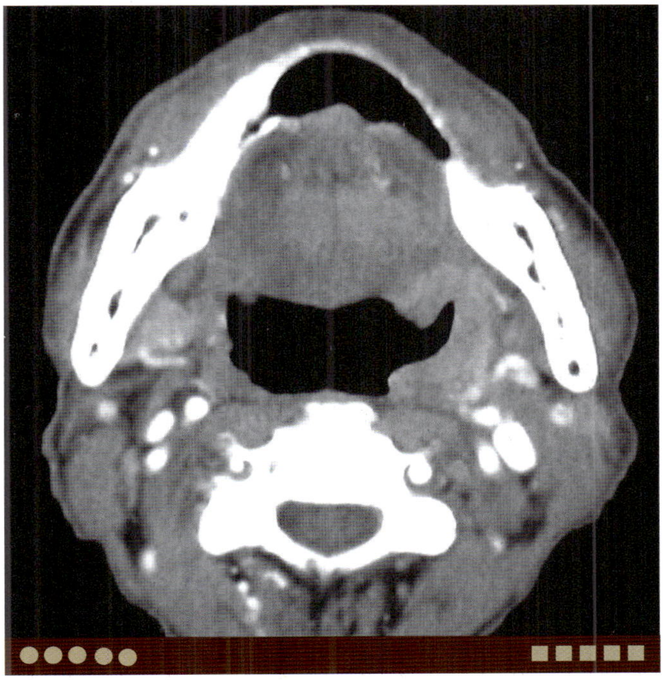

A. SCCA of the tonsil. Axial contrast-enhanced CT demonstrates a mildly enhancing lesion with large ulceration in the left palatine tonsil.

COMMENTS

This is a 70-year-old woman with left neck mass.

SCCA is the most common malignant tumor (>70%) arising in the tonsil, followed by lymphoma. Importantly, primary SCCA of the palatine tonsil can be small and patients may present with large metastatic nodes with unknown primary. These patients usually undergo panendoscopy and biopsy, and may undergo diagnostic tonsillectomy. Nasopharynx, base of tongue, and pyriform sinus are other common sites for SCCA of unknown primary. Smoking and alcohol abuse are common risk factors. In addition, human papilloma virus (HPV) has been shown to play an important role in developing SCCA in this region.

CT typically demonstrates a heterogeneously enhancing mass occupying the palatine tonsil, commonly with deep extension into the surrounding spaces. Associated nodal disease is often present at the time of diagnosis, typically with intranodal necrosis. Nodal metastasis is commonly seen in level II nodes and intra-/periparotid nodes. Inflammatory changes are often seen with nodal metastases, particularly in level II and peri-/intraparotid nodes, which can be misdiagnosed as parotid infection. MRI can provide more detailed information regarding diagnosis and lesion extension. Just like SCCA in other locations, tonsillar SCCA often demonstrates a heterogeneous signal mass with ulceration. However, occasionally the affected tonsil may show decreased T2 signal and volume, known as a "small and dark tonsil." Invasion beyond the pharyngeal constrictor muscles into the parapharyngeal space is often seen in advanced tumors.

PEARLS

- **SCCA is the most common malignant tumor arising in the tonsil, followed by lymphoma.**
- **The palatine tonsil is one of the common primary sites of SCCA with unknown primary.**
- **Tonsillar SCCA usually is seen as a heterogeneous density/signal mass with ulceration. However, the affected tonsil may show decreased T2 signal and volume.**

ADDITIONAL IMAGES (B-G)

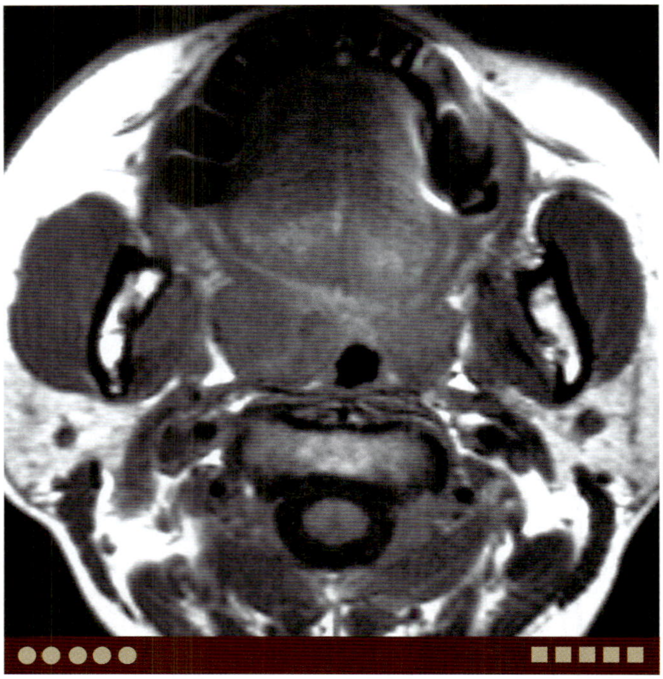

B. SCCA of the tonsil in a different patient. Axial T1W MR image demonstrates an enlarged right tonsil with preserved right parapharyngeal fat.

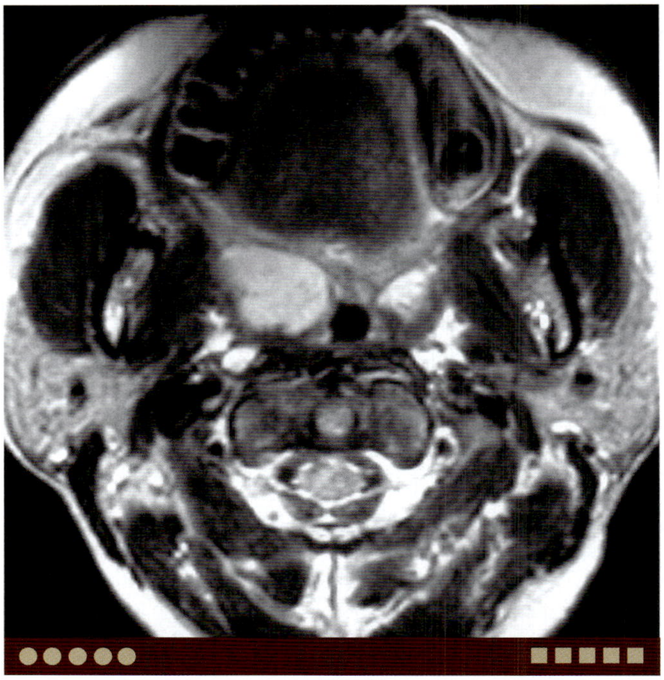

C. SCCA of the tonsil, same patient as B. Axial T2W image demonstrates an enlarged right tonsil showing high signal.

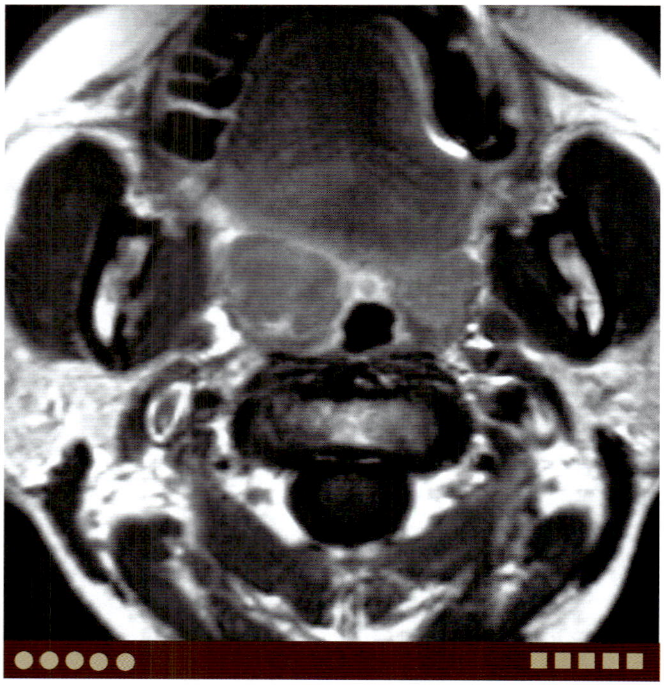

D. SCCA of the tonsil, same patient as B. Axial postcontrast T1W image demonstrates mild enhancement in the lesion.

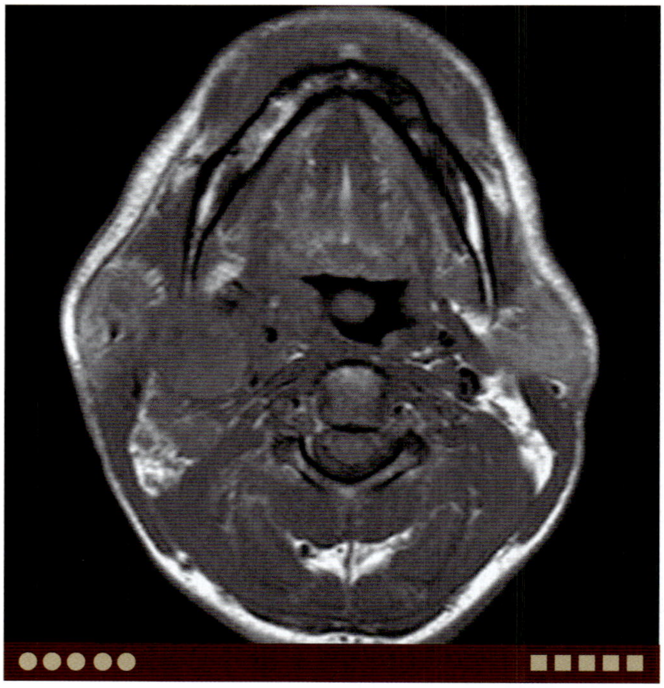

E. SCCA of the tonsil in a different patient. Axial T1W image demonstrates multiple metastatic right level II nodes displacing the carotid vessels and tonsil.

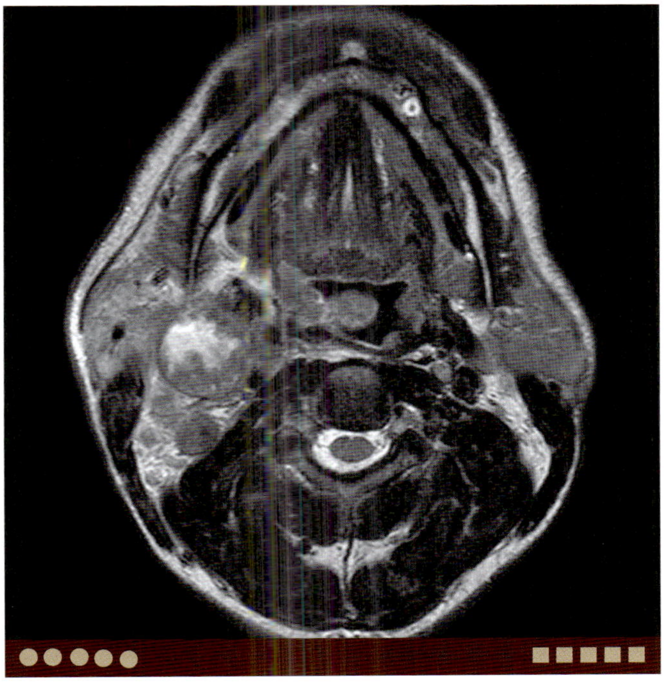

F. SCCA of the tonsil, same patient as E. Axial T2W image demonstrates multiple metastatic right level II nodes showing heterogeneous isointense to hyperintense signal. Note relatively small primary tumor in the right palatine tonsil.

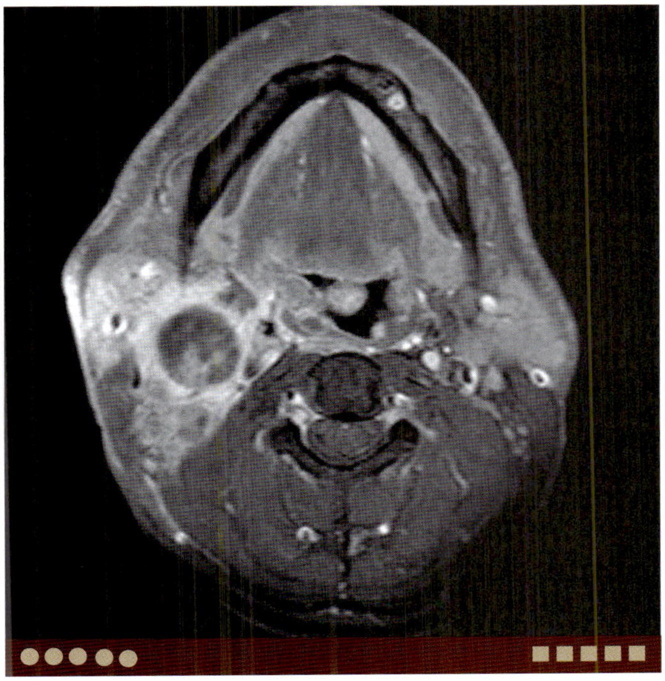

G. SCCA of the tonsil, same patient as E. Axial postcontrast fat-suppressed T1W image demonstrates heterogeneously enhancing nodal metastases with secondary inflammatory changes in the surrounding soft tissues. Ill-defined boundaries of nodes suggest extracapsular tumor spread. Note mildly enhancing small primary tumor in the right palatine tonsil.

DIFFERENTIAL DIAGNOSIS IMAGES (H-J)

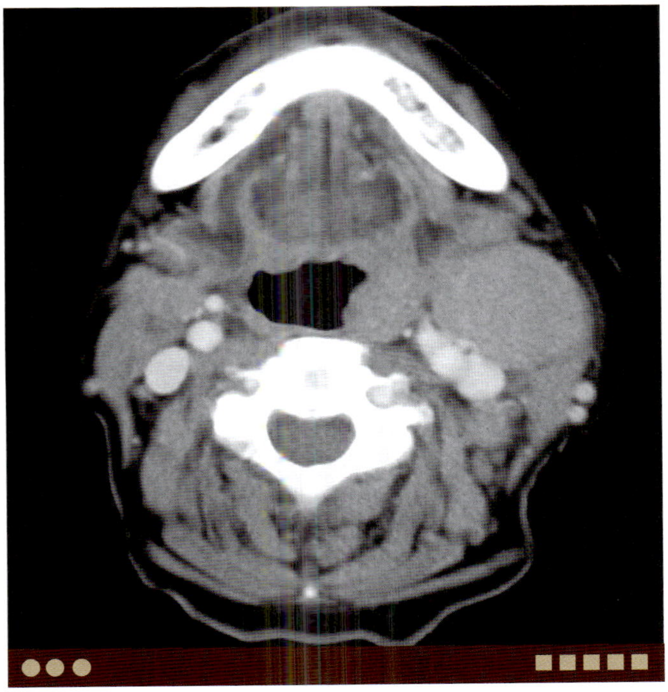

H. Lymphoma. Axial contrast-enhanced CT demonstrates a mildly enhancing lesion arising from the left palatine tonsil. Note large, mildly enhancing, non-necrotic left level II node.

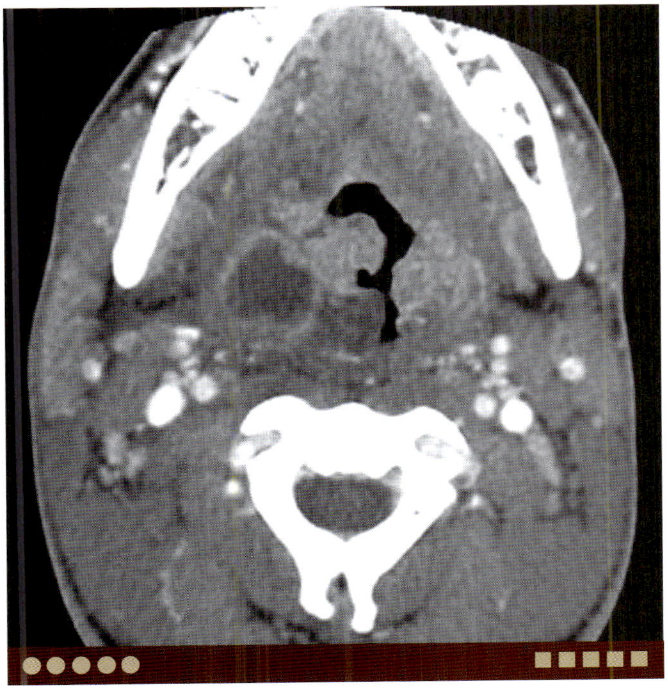

I. Peritonsillar abscess. Axial contrast-enhanced CT demonstrates a rim-enhancing fluid collection in the right peritonsillar region. The right palatine tonsil is displaced medially and there is narrowing the oropharyngeal lumen.

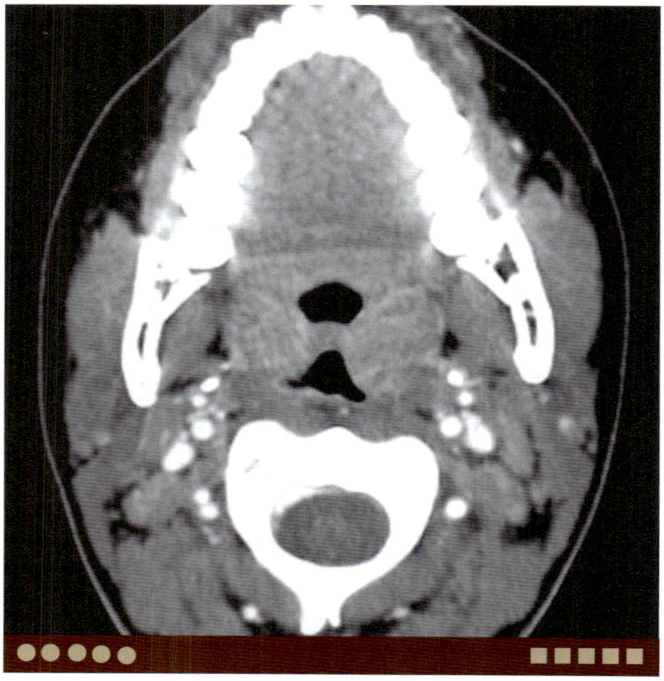

J. Tonsillitis. Axial contrast-enhanced CT demonstrates enlarged, enhancing tonsils bilaterally. Striation is seen; however, no apparent mass is noted in the tonsils.

Case 8–5 Hemangioma of the Tongue

Akifumi Fujita, Margaret Chapman, Osamu Sakai

PRESENTATION

Bluish-tinged soft mass in the tongue.

FINDINGS

MRI demonstrates a well-demarcated T2 high-signal intensity mass in the tongue

DIFFERENTIAL DIAGNOSIS

- Squamous cell carcinoma: This condition typically shows low-signal intensity on T2W images with heterogeneous enhancement following contrast administration. Ill-defined margins are often noted. This is usually differentiated from hemangiomas on clinical examination.
- Lymphoma: Often submucosal in location, this condition typically shows homogeneous signal on MRI, with lower-signal intensity on T2W images when compared to hemangiomas.
- Schwannoma: This condition may not be differentiated by imaging alone, although schwannomas usually show lower T2 signal than hemangiomas. Clinical findings usually help to differentiate these two entities.
- Venolymphatic malformation: This condition is typically less enhancing heterogeneous appearing with ill-defined margins.

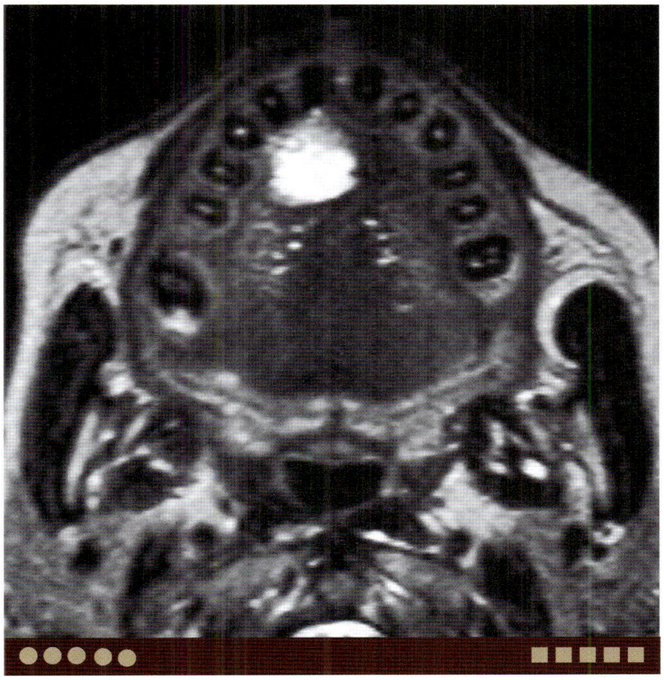

A. Hemangioma. Axial T2W image demonstrates a well-circumscribed homogeneous high-intensity mass of the right anterior tongue.

COMMENTS

This is a 45-year-old woman with a bluish-tinged soft tongue mass.

Hemangiomas are relatively common benign tumors of the tongue. They usually present as soft, bluish-tinged masses and are easily diagnosed clinically. Most hemangiomas are present at birth, but some may not manifest clinically until early childhood. They may regress spontaneously due to internal bleeding, thrombosis, or organization. However, adult presentation is not rare.

On CT and MRI, hemangiomas are seen as well-defined lesions with homogeneous density or signal, with very high-signal intensity on STIR or T2W images. Slow and sustained enhancement is characteristic after contrast administration. On imaging, hemangiomas may show similar findings to schwannomas; however clinical findings are usually different.

Angiography is not necessary for diagnosis, however, may be performed prior to sclerosis or resection to evaluate for possible high-flow components. When phleboliths are seen in the lesion, the vascular malformation is more likely to be venous rather than a hemangioma.

PEARLS

- **Hemangiomas are relatively common benign tumors of the tongue.**
- **They are well-marginated lesions demonstrating similar density to vessels on CT.**
- **High-signal intensity on STIR or T2W images is characteristic.**

ADDITIONAL IMAGES (B-D)

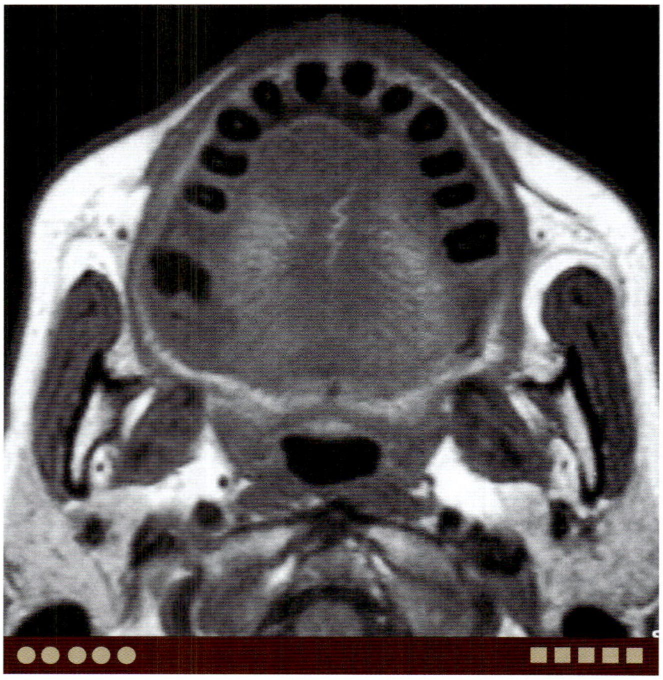

B. Hemangioma, same patient as A. Axial T1W image demonstrates a homogeneous intermediate-signal intensity mass.

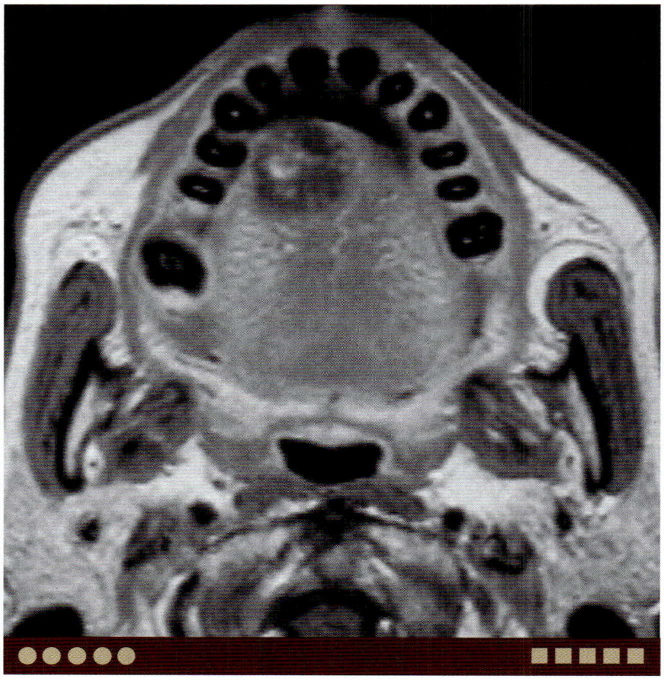

C. Hemangioma, same patient as A. Axial postcontrast T1W image demonstrates prominent partial enhancement of the tumor. Slow and sustained enhancement is characteristic.

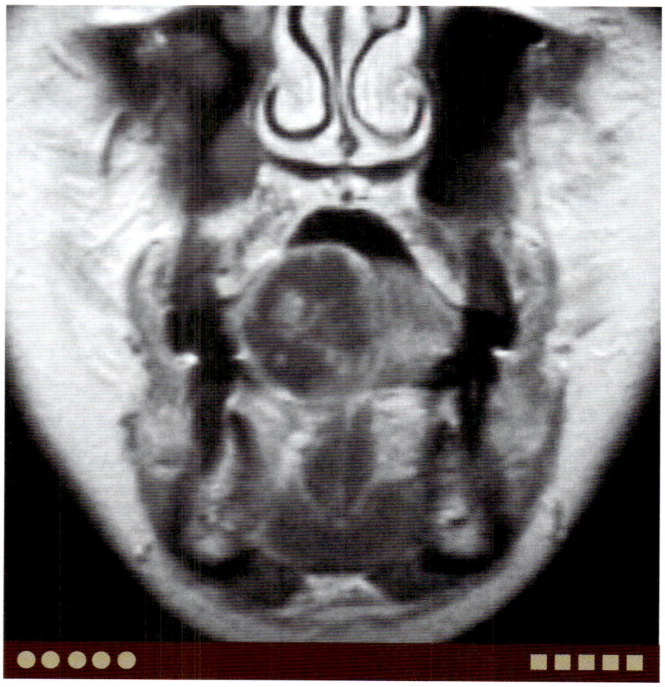

D. Hemangioma, same patient as A. Coronal postcontrast T1W image demonstrates sustained enhancement of the tumor.

DIFFERENTIAL DIAGNOSIS IMAGES (E-I)

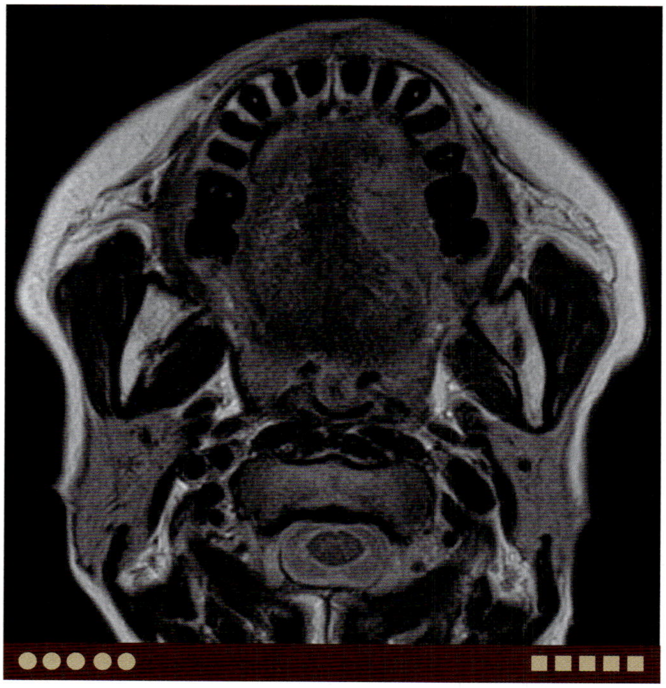

E. Squamous cell carcinoma. Axial T2W image demonstrates an ill-defined intermediate-signal intensity lesion of the left side of the tongue.

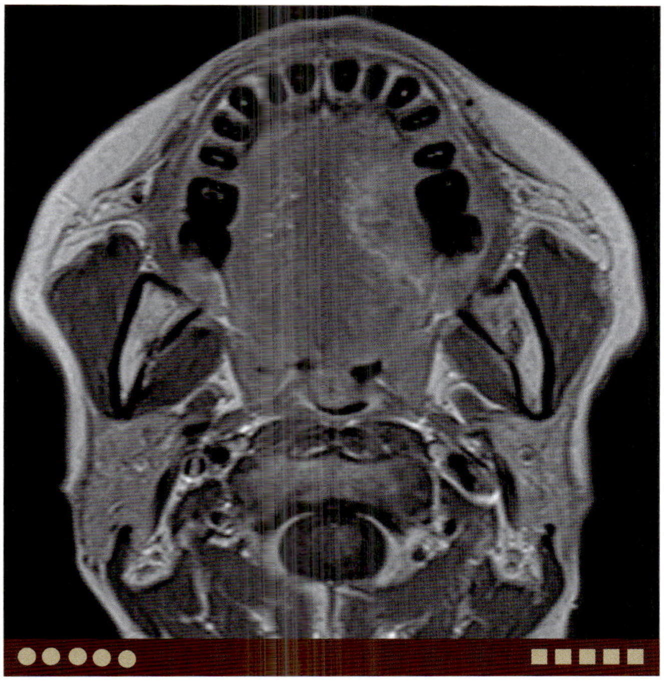

F. Squamous cell carcinoma, same patient as E. Axial contrast-enhanced T1W image demonstrates a heterogeneously enhancing tumor of the left tongue. Note the ill-defined margins of the tumor.

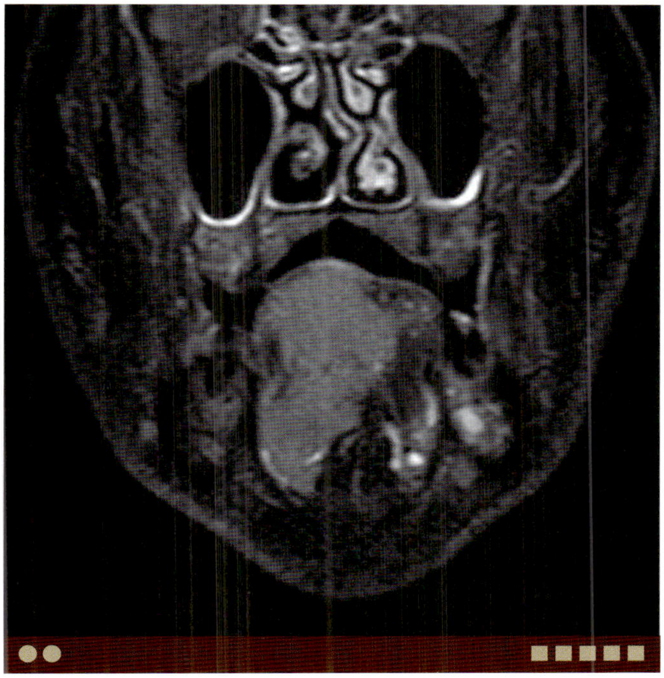

G. Lymphoma. Coronal STIR image demonstrates a homogeneous slightly high-signal intensity mass of the right tongue extending to the oral floor.

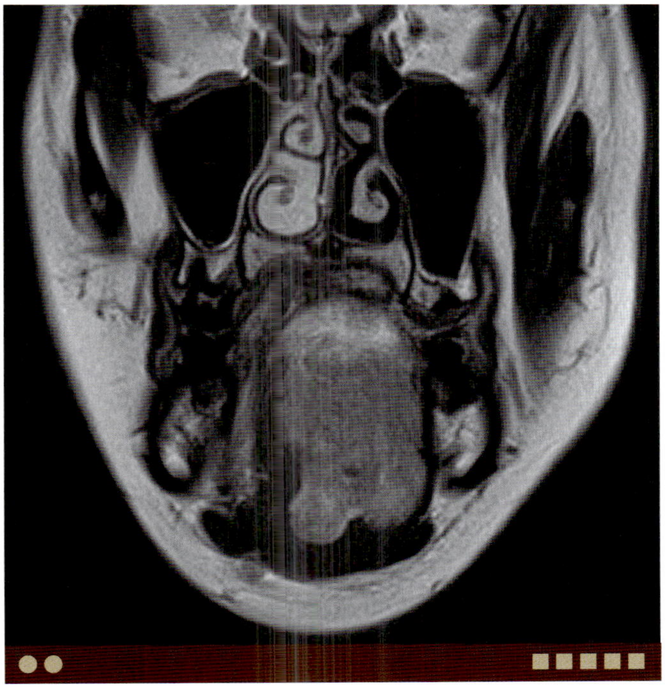

H. Schwannoma. Axial T2W image demonstrates a well-defined lobulated heterogeneous intermediate-to-high signal intensity mass of the left tongue and sublingual space.

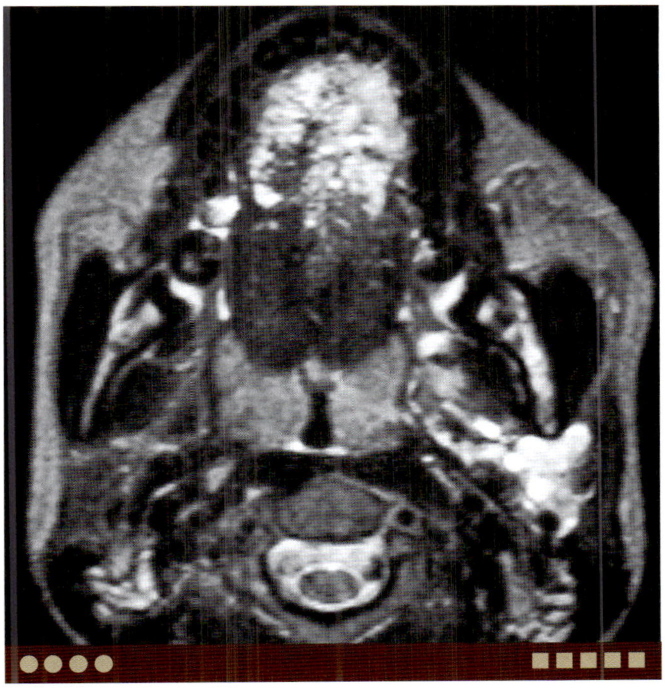

I. Venolymphatic malformation. Axial T2W image demonstrates a heterogeneous very high-signal intensity mass-like lesion of the anterior tongue. Note the ill-defined margins.

Case 8–6 Denervation of the Tongue

Akifumi Fujita, Margaret Chapman, Osamu Sakai

PRESENTATION

Tongue deviation.

FINDINGS

CT demonstrates decreased density of one side of the tongue.

DIFFERENTIAL DIAGNOSIS

- Recurrent or residual tumor: Posterior protrusion of the tongue caused by denervation may mimic recurrent or residual tumor. Denervation is usually differentiated clinically by the absence of mucosal abnormality and softness to palpation.
- Hemangioma: This is the most common benign tumor of the tongue. It usually demonstrates very high signal on T2W images.
- Proliferative myositis/cellulitis: Although uncommon, it is difficult to differentiate this condition from acute and subacute phases of denervation.

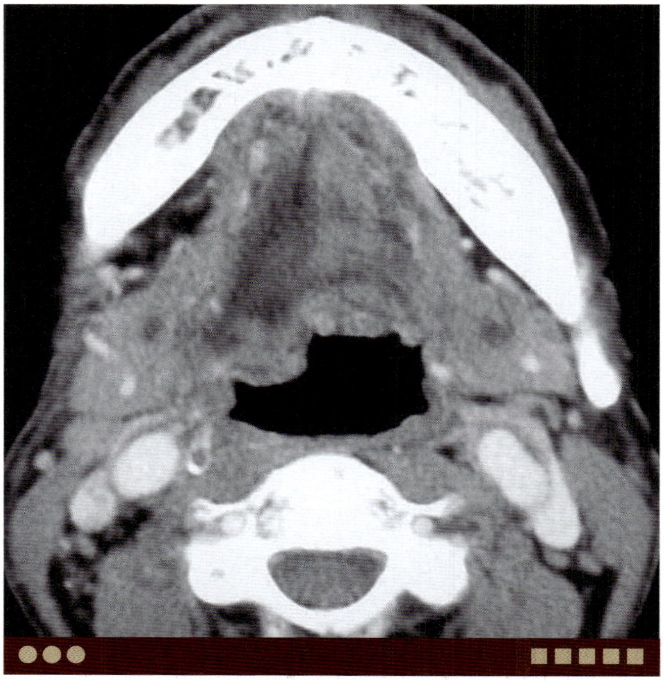

A. Denervation of the tongue (chronic phase). Axial contrast-enhanced CT demonstrates decreased density of the right side of the tongue. Note the posterior protrusion of the tongue.

COMMENTS

This is a 75-year-old man with nasopharyngeal carcinoma.

Denervation changes are seen after injury to the hypoglossal nerve by tumor invasion, trauma, or surgery. In the chronic state, volume loss and fatty changes are characteristic findings. However, in acute or subacute phases of denervation, the muscle demonstrates edema, inflammatory change, and increased volume (denervation myositis). Decrease in muscular tone results in posterior deviation of the tongue, with protrusion into the oropharyngeal lumen. This finding may mimic recurrent or residual tumor on imaging; however, this condition is easily differentiated clinically by the absence of mucosal abnormality and softness to palpation.

On CT and MRI, denervation changes of the tongue are seen in the area innervated by the hypoglossal nerve, typically unilaterally, with clear margination in midline. In the acute to subacute phase, the affected side demonstrates decreased density on CT, decreased T1 signal, increased T2/STIR signal, and strong enhancement after contrast administration. In the subacute to chronic phase, the affected muscle shows increased T1 signal, increased T2/STIR signal, and enhancement with fatty infiltration. Finally, in the chronic phase, decreased density on CT, increased T1 signal, and decreased signal on STIR without enhancement become apparent due to fatty change.

Denervation is an injury to the nerve proximal to the affected muscles; therefore, a search for the cause along the entire course of the nerve is essential. Careful history taking is important in understanding the underlying condition.

PEARLS

- **Injury to the hypoglossal nerve causes denervation changes of the ipsilateral half of the tongue.**
- **Increased T2/STIR signal with enhancement is seen in the acute to subacute phase of denervation myositis. Swelling and posterior protrusion of the tongue are often seen.**
- **Severe fatty infiltration and atrophy without contrast enhancement are seen in the chronic phase.**

ADDITIONAL IMAGES (B-F)

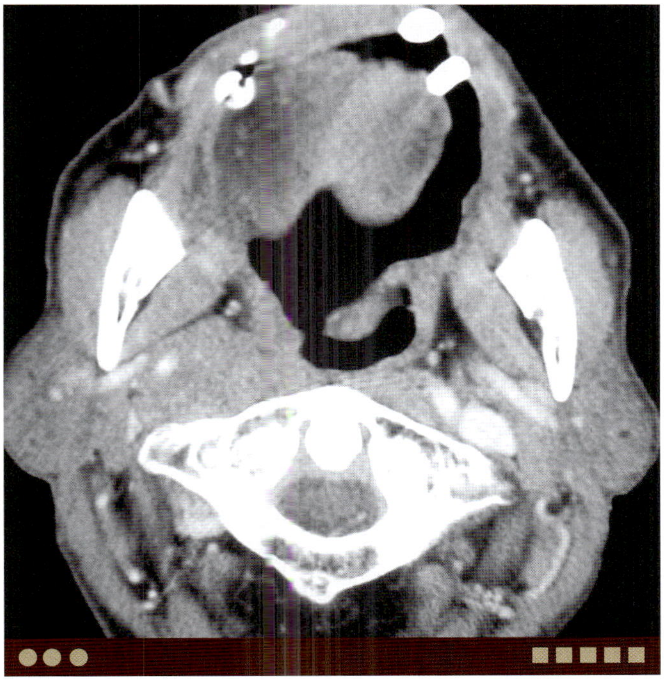

B. Denervation of the tongue (chronic phase), same patient as A. Axial CT demonstrates decreased density of the right side of the tongue. Swelling of the right nasopharynx is noted.

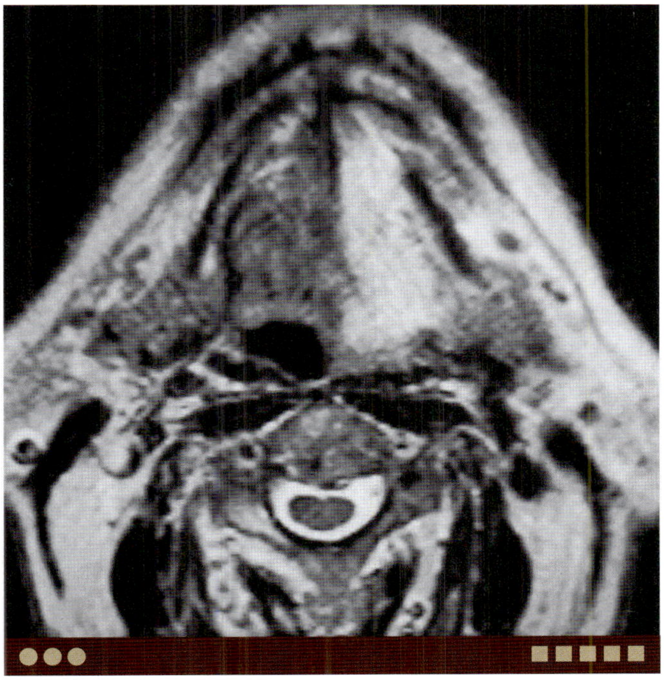

C. Denervation of the tongue (chronic phase) in a different patient. Axial T2W image demonstrates homogeneous high-signal of the left side of the tongue suggestive of fatty replacement due to invasion of the left hypoglossal nerve by nasopharyngeal carcinoma.

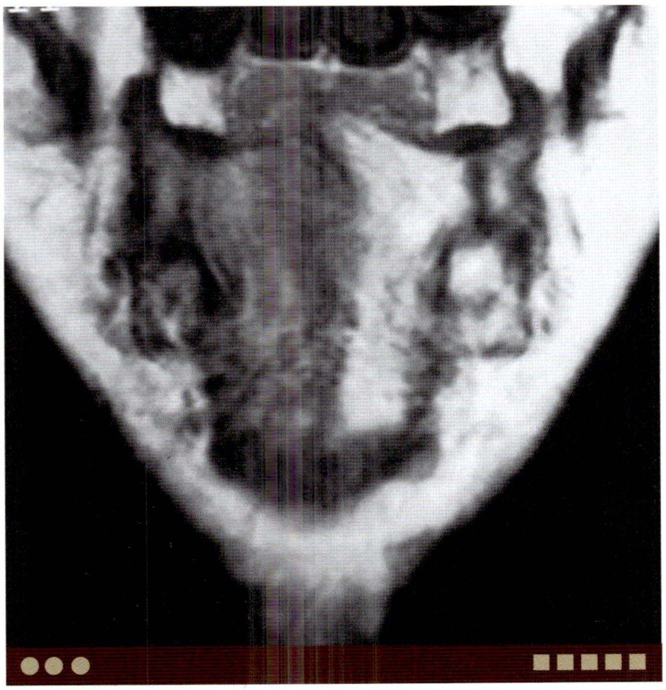

D. Denervation of the tongue (chronic phase), same patient as C. Coronal T1W image demonstrates decreased volume and homogeneous high signal of the left side of the tongue, consistent with fatty replacement secondary to chronic denervation.

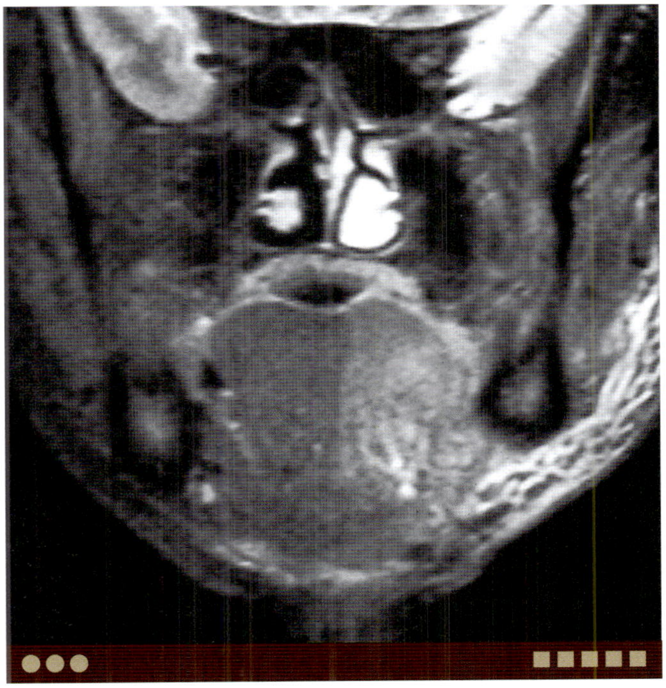

E. Denervation of the tongue (subacute phase) in a different patient. Coronal STIR image demonstrates swelling and high-signal intensity of the left side of the tongue consistent with subacute denervation secondary to left hypoglossal nerve invasion by submandibular gland adenoid cystic carcinoma.

DIFFERENTIAL DIAGNOSIS IMAGES (G-I)

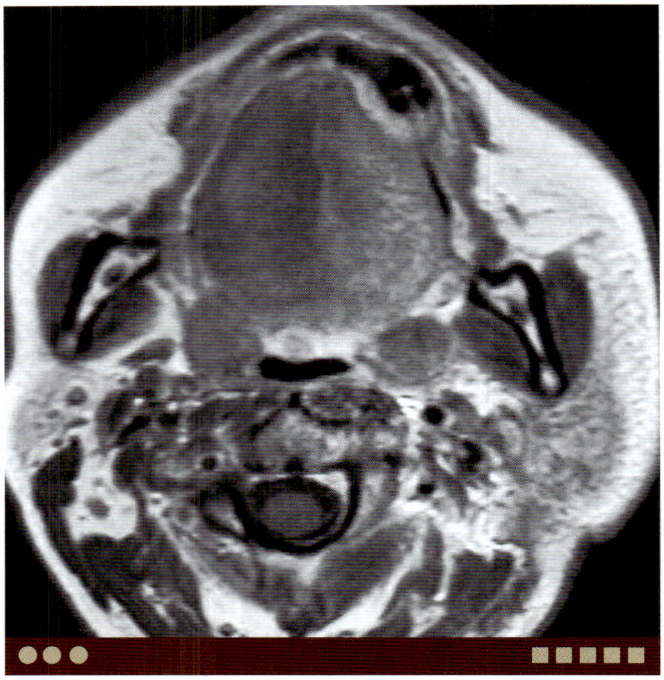

F. Denervation of the tongue (subacute phase), same patient as E. Axial T1W image demonstrates mild swelling of the left side of the tongue. High-signal intensity of the tongue suggests fatty infiltration.

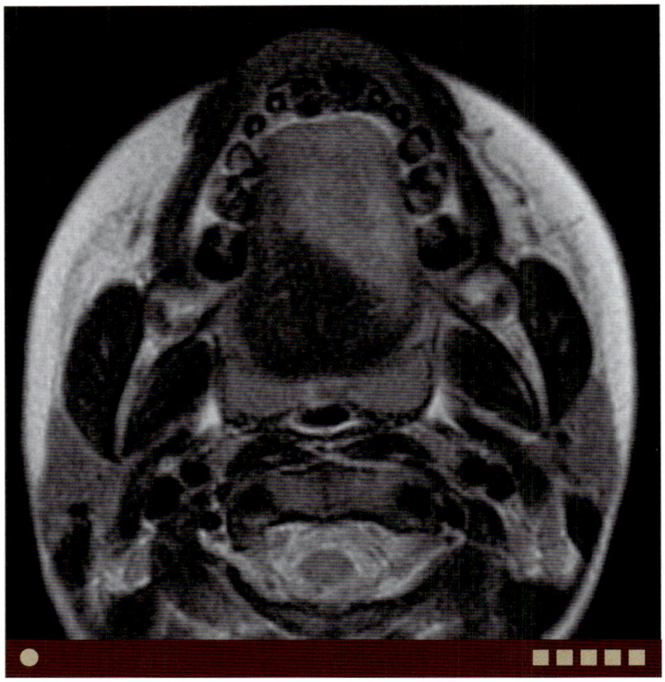

G. **Proliferative myositis**. Axial T2W image demonstrates high-signal intensity of the left side of the tongue. Patient presented with tongue swelling and pain.

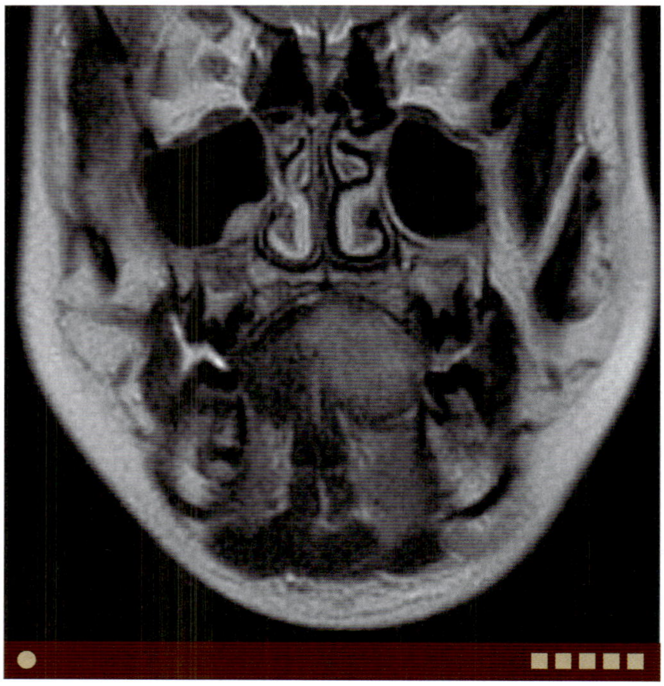

H. **Proliferative myositis**. Coronal T2W image demonstrates high-signal intensity of the left side of the tongue. Note contralateral infiltration of the inflammation. Patient was treated with antibiotics.

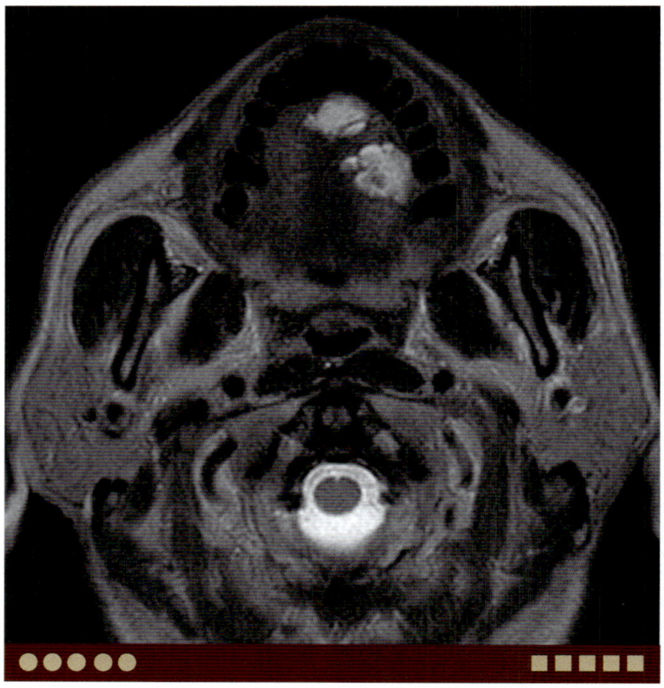

I. **Hemangioma**. Axial T2W image demonstrates multilobulated very high-signal intensity lesions in the left tongue without associated swelling or atrophy.

Case 8–7 Adenoid Cystic Carcinoma

Akifumi Fujita, Margaret Chapman, Osamu Sakai

PRESENTATION

Swelling of the sublingual space.

FINDINGS

CT and MRI show a mass within the sublingual gland.

DIFFERENTIAL DIAGNOSIS

- Pleomorphic adenoma: This usually demonstrates a well-circumscribed high-signal intensity mass on T2W images, but is difficult to differentiate from low-grade adenoid cystic carcinoma by imaging alone.
- Mucoepidermoid carcinoma: This cannot be differentiated by CT and MR imaging alone.
- Lymphoma: This condition typically demonstrates a homogeneous mass lesion. Low-signal intensity on T2W images and restricted diffusion on DWI reflects high cellularity.
- Schwannoma: This condition typically demonstrates an oval-shaped mass.
- Venolymphatic malformation: This lesion typically demonstrates high-signal intensity on T2W images; however, this finding depends on the vascular channel size. Phleboliths show round and oval signal-voids inside the lesion.

COMMENTS

This is an 81-year-old woman with swelling of the sublingual space.

Adenoid cystic carcinoma is a relatively rare entity in the parotid gland, representing only 2% to 6% of tumors. It is more common in the submandibular and sublingual glands, accounting for 12% and 15%, respectively of tumors arising in these glands. Further, it represents about 30% of tumors in minor salivary glands, with smaller glands having a higher chance of malignant tumors. 80% of parotid gland tumors are benign; however, 50% of submandibular gland tumors and 70% to 80% of sublingual and minor salivary gland tumors are malignant. Therefore, malignancy must be strongly suspected when diagnosing salivary gland tumors, with lowest suspicion for malignancy arising from lesions of the parotid gland.

Imaging findings of adenoid cystic carcinoma are often nonspecific. Signal intensity on T2W images reflects cellularity. It is suggested that low T2 signal represents higher cellularity and poor prognosis. Low-grade tumors are usually well-circumscribed and enhance homogeneously. High-grade tumors tend to be infiltrative with poorly defined margins.

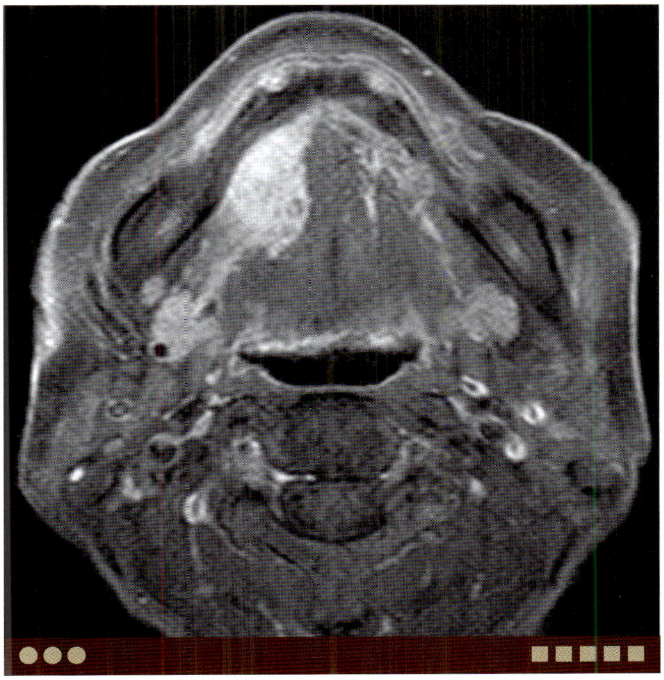

A. Adenoid cystic carcinoma. Axial postcontrast fat-suppressed T1W image demonstrates a well-circumscribed homogeneously enhancing mass of the right sublingual space.

Adenoid cystic carcinoma often presents with perineural tumor spread. It is important to thoroughly examine the skull base and the entire course of the nerve innervating the involved area. Skip perineural tumor spread is occasionally seen.

It is always difficult to differentiate low-grade salivary gland tumors from benign tumors such as pleomorphic adenomas, schwannomas, and venolymphatic malformations (hemangiomas). Lymphoma is also an important differential consideration on cross-sectional imaging.

PEARLS

- **More than half of tumors arising from the salivary glands can be malignant. As the potential for malignancy increases with lesions in smaller salivary glands, there is lower clinical suspicion for malignancy in parotid gland lesions.**
- **In adenoid cystic carcinoma, low T2 signal suggests higher cellularity and poor prognosis.**
- **Perineural tumor spread is often seen in adenoid cystic carcinoma. It is important to thoroughly examine the skull base and the entire course of the nerve innervating the involved area.**

ADDITIONAL IMAGES (B-D)

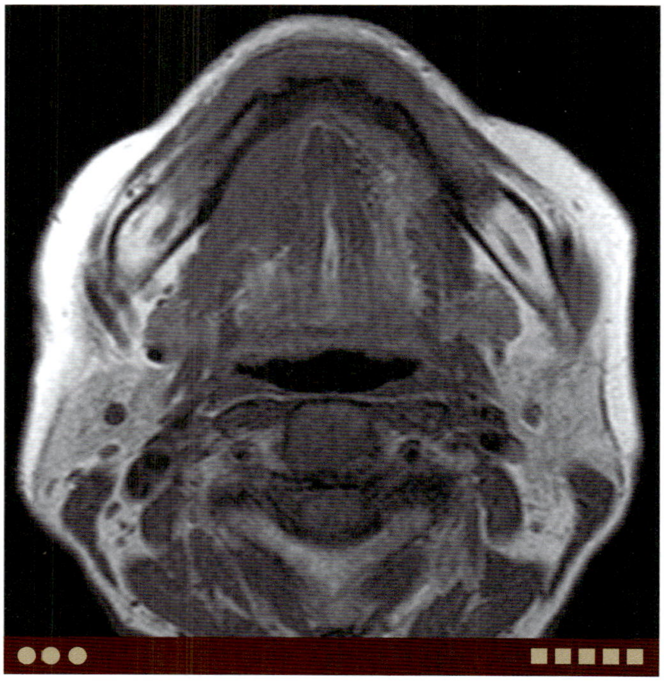

B. Adenoid cystic carcinoma, same patient as A. Axial T1W image demonstrates a homogeneous low-signal intensity mass in the right sublingual space.

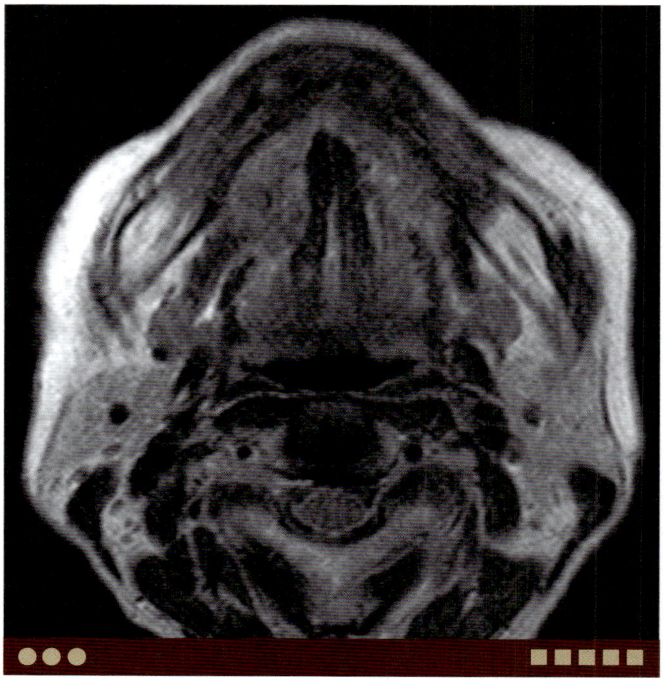

C. Adenoid cystic carcinoma, same patient as A. Axial T2W image demonstrates heterogeneous low-signal intensity of the mass, suggestive of a high-grade malignant tumor.

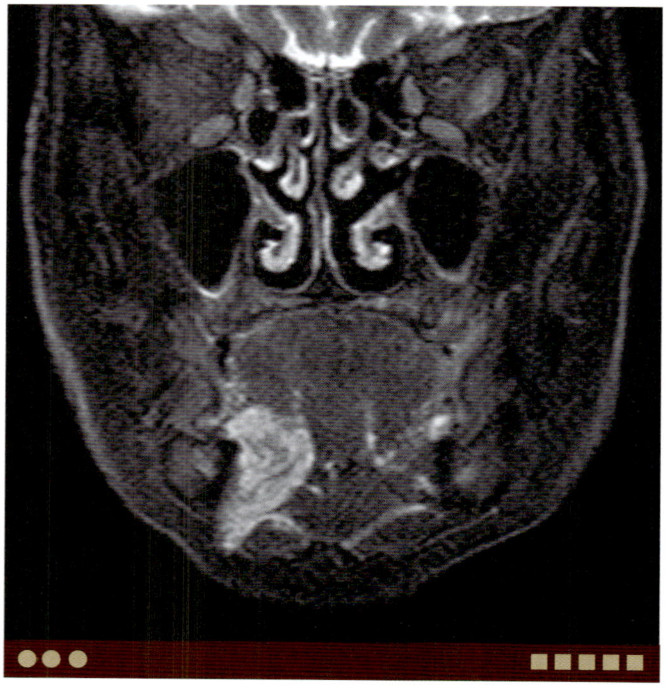

D. Adenoid cystic carcinoma, same patient as A. Coronal STIR image demonstrates an infiltrative margin caudally, also suggestive of a high-grade malignancy.

DIFFERENTIAL DIAGNOSIS IMAGES (E-G)

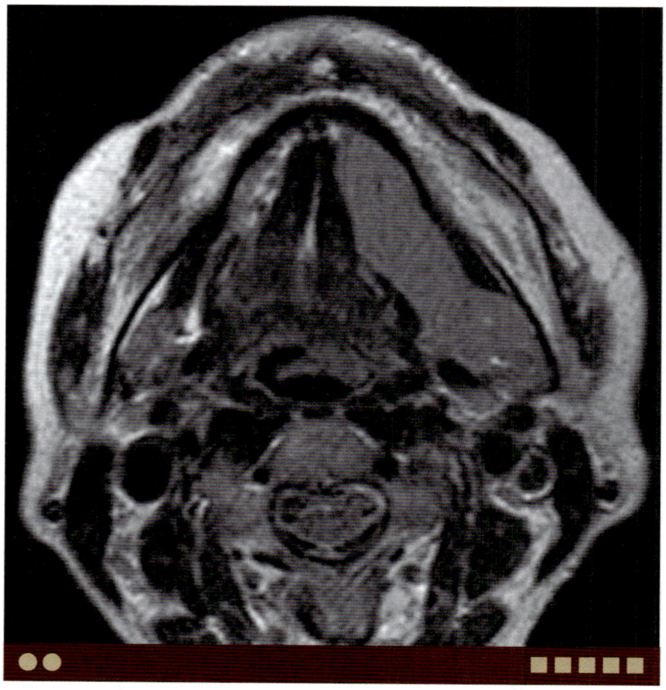

E. **Lymphoma**. Axial T2W image demonstrates a homogeneous intermediate-intensity lesion in the left sublingual space infiltrating into the submandibular gland.

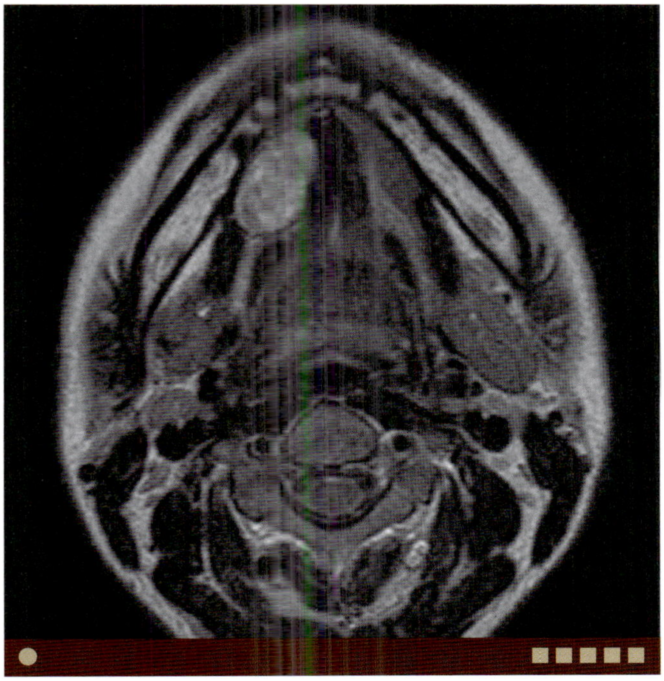

F. Schwannoma. Axial T2W image demonstrates a well-circumscribed oval mass in the right sublingual space. The normal sublingual gland is anteriorly displaced.

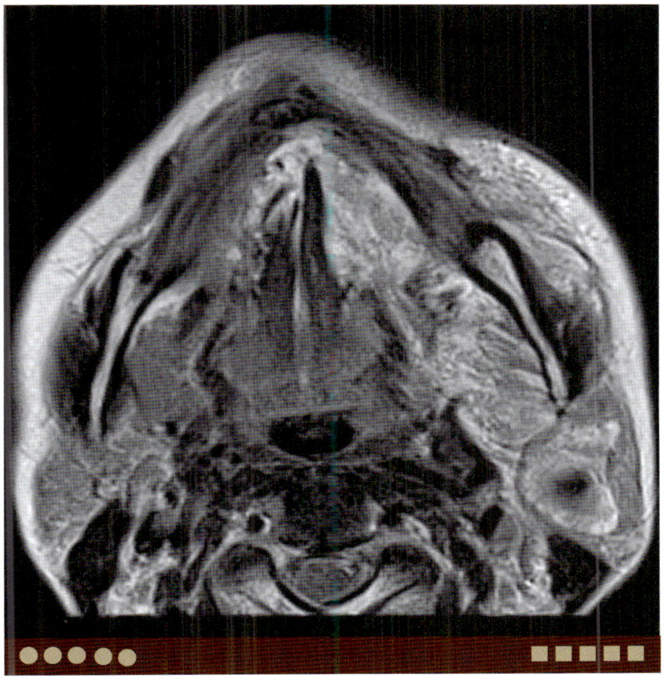

G. Venolymphatic malformation. Axial T2W image demonstrates a heterogeneous high-signal intensity mass-like lesion in the left sublingual space, extending into the submandibular, masticator, and parotid spaces. Multispace involvement of the lesion is suggestive of vascular malformation.

Case 8–8 Dermoid

Akifumi Fujita, Margaret Chapman, Osamu Sakai

PRESENTATION

Swelling of the floor of the mouth.

FINDINGS

CT demonstrates an ovoid cystic mass at the midline of the floor of the mouth.

DIFFERENTIAL DIAGNOSIS

- Epidermoid: This condition does not contain fat. It is often impossible to differentiate these lesions from non-fat-containing dermoids.
- Thyroglossal duct cyst: This occurs along the course of the thyroglossal duct. Suprahyoid lesions are difficult to differentiate from non–fat-containing dermoids and epidermoid cysts.
- Ranula: This condition usually occurs off-midline in the sublingual space. It occasionally extends to the submandibular space, so-called diving ranulas.
- Lymphatic malformation (lymphangioma): This condition typically occurs as a multiloculated, lobular cystic mass anywhere within the head and neck region, with preference in the posterior cervical triangle.

COMMENTS

This is a 4-month-old boy with swelling of the floor of the mouth.

Dermoids and epidermoids occur from aberrant migration of ectodermal tissues during development. They often grow slowly and are identified clinically as painless masses. Dermoids in the floor of the mouth may cause difficulty with swallowing or phonation. Most are diagnosed in childhood; however, presentation in adults is not rare.

In the floor of the mouth, dermoids can be divided into sublingual and submental types based on location. The sublingual region is the most common location, occurring here in 52% of cases, followed by submental (26%) and submandibular (6%) regions. For those cysts that lie above the mylohyoid muscle (sublingual), an intraoral approach to extracapsular excision is preferable. For lesions that lie inferior to the mylohyoid muscle (in the submental and submandibular regions), resection is usually via an external approach. Imaging is therefore extremely helpful for appropriate surgical planning. Dermoids can occur either at or just lateral to midline.

Dermoids have variable imaging characteristics due to complex contents, such as apocrine glands, sweat glands, sebaceous glands, and hair follicles. The lining is usually thicker and often calcifies. Sebaceous, lipid material in dermoids demonstrate similar density and signal intensity to fat on both CT and MRI. "Lipid-water levels," where

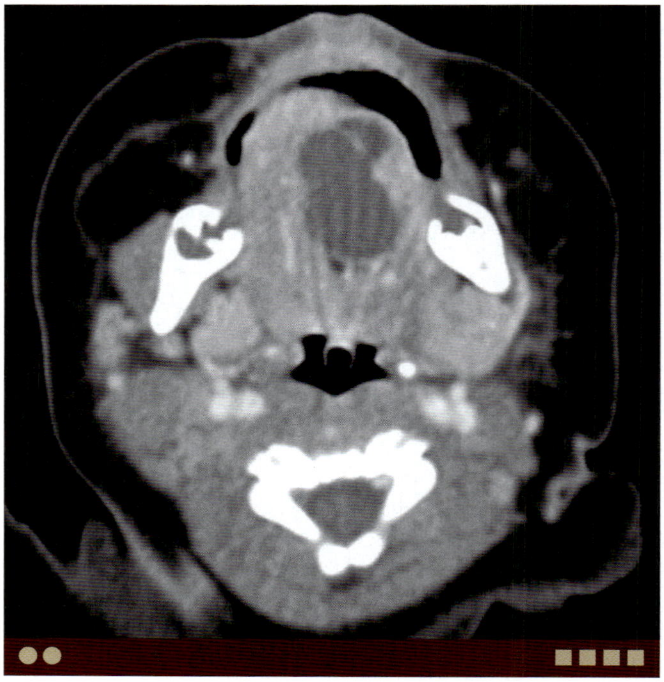

A. Dermoid. Axial contrast-enhanced CT demonstrates a cystic mass at the midline of the floor of the mouth. Fat is not obvious in this case.

lighter lipid material is visualized over proteinaceous debris, may be seen. Without apparent fat density or signal it is often difficult to differentiate dermoids from epidermoids radiologically. Pathology can misdiagnose dermoids as epidermoids due to failure to identify the dermal appendage structures from inadequate sampling or review.

Epidermoid cysts have a thin squamous cell lining and contain debris from desquamation of epithelial components, such as keratin, cholesterol, and some proteinaceous and lipid materials. They usually demonstrate water density, and occasionally slightly negative attenuation values on CT. They usually do not demonstrate very low density like true fat. On MRI, epidermoid cysts show slightly higher signal than water on T1W images and variable signal intensities on T2W images depending upon its contents. Calcification is rare.

PEARLS

- **Fat-containing cystic lesions of the sublingual, submental, and submandibular regions are diagnostic for dermoids.**
- **Fat in dermoids and fluid attenuation in epidermoids may differentiate the two, but it is impossible to differentiate these radiologically in the absence of fat.**
- **CT and MRI are extremely helpful in localizing the lesion in relationship to the mylohyoid muscle for surgical planning.**

ADDITIONAL IMAGES (B-C)

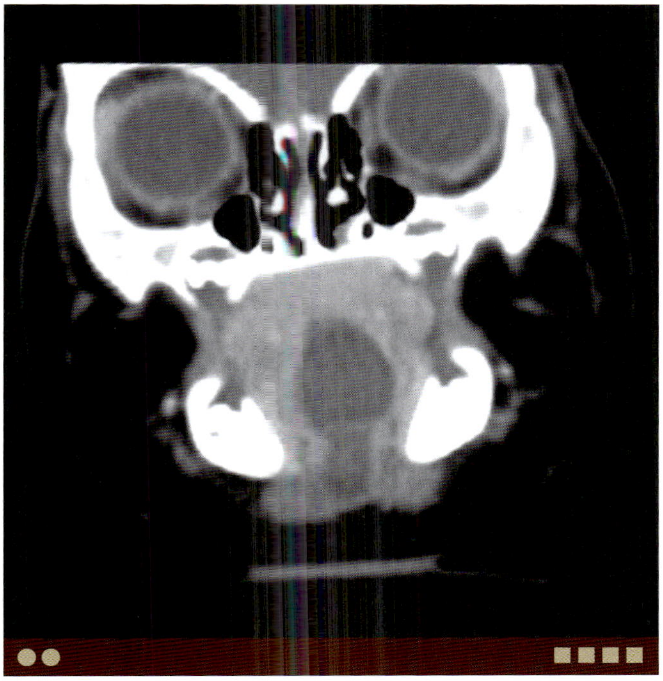

B. Dermoid, same patient as A. Coronal contrast-enhanced CT demonstrates a cystic mass at the midline of the sublingual space.

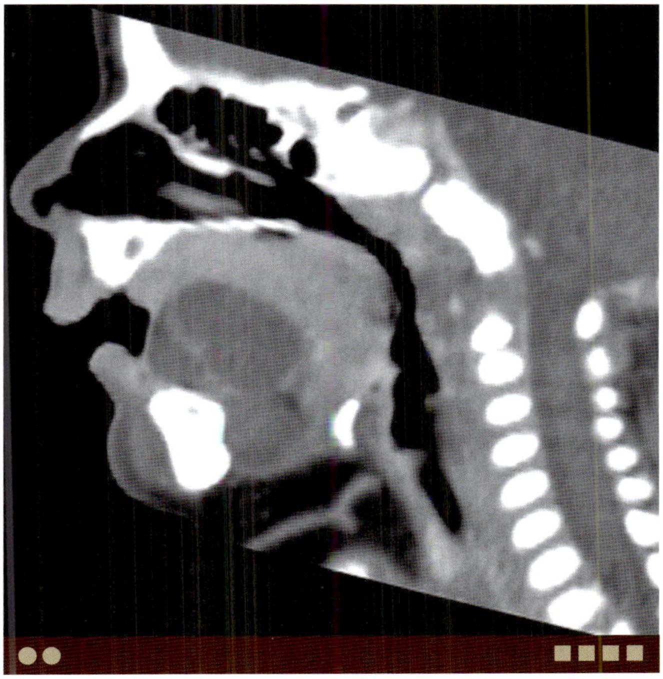

C. Dermoid, same patient as A. Sagittal contrast-enhanced CT demonstrates a cystic mass at the midline of the sublingual space. Note the fat density within postero-inferior part of the cystic lesion.

DIFFERENTIAL DIAGNOSIS IMAGES (D-I)

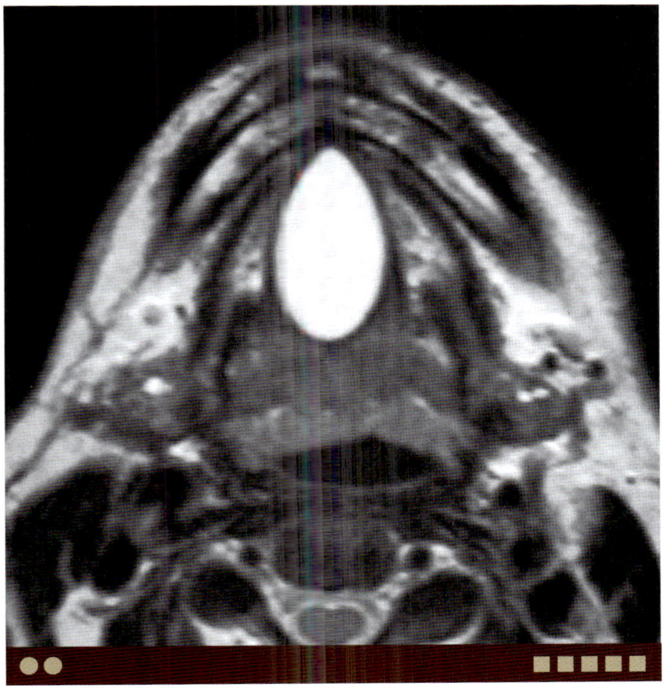

D. Epidermoid. Axial T2W image demonstrates a well-circumscribed high-signal cystic mass at the midline of the sublingual space.

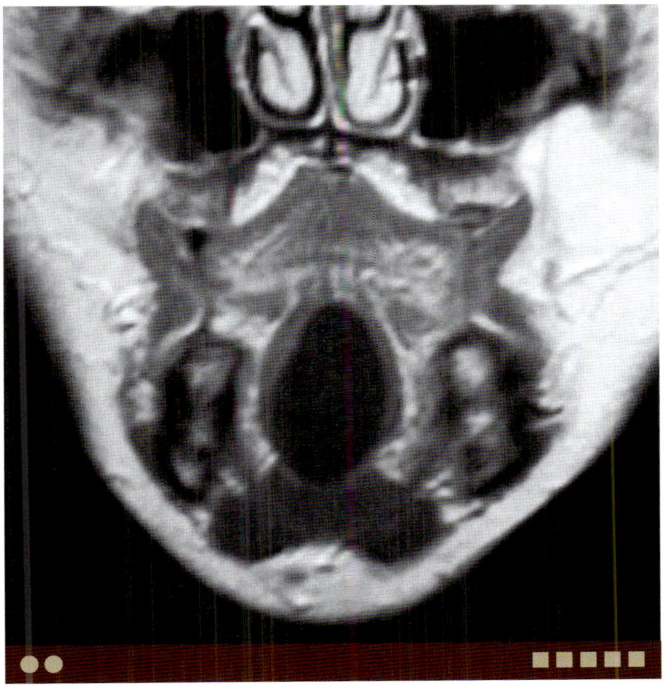

E. Epidermoid, same patient as D. Coronal contrast-enhanced T1W image demonstrates a homogeneous low-signal cystic mass within the sublingual region. There is no fat signal intensity.

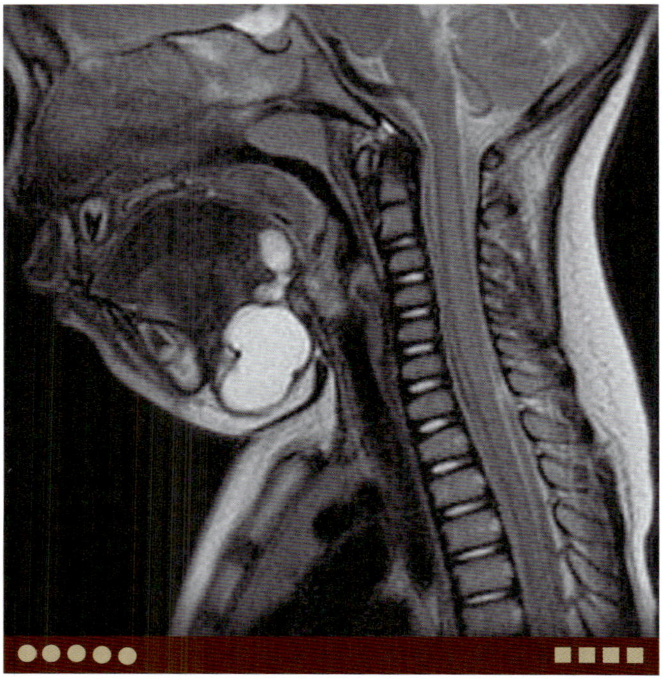

F. Thyroglossal duct cyst. Sagittal T2W image demonstrate a multilocula cystic mass at the midline of the sublingual space extending to the foramen cecum.

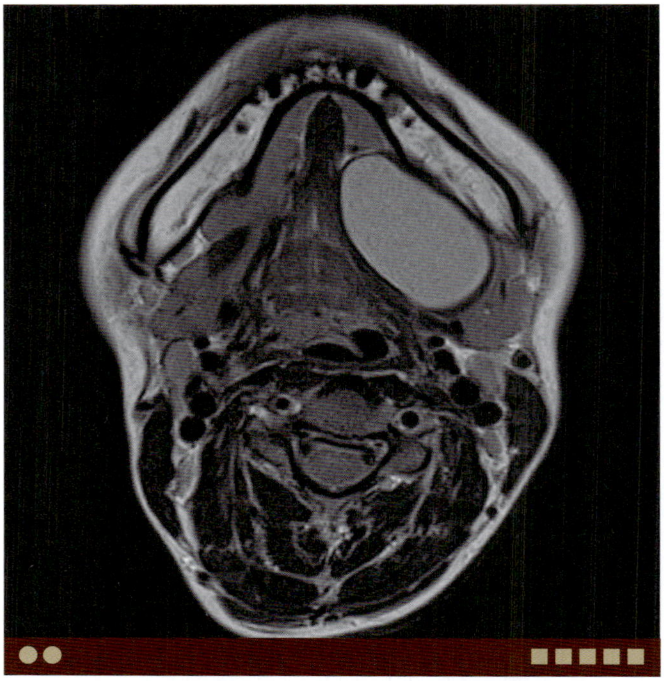

G. Epidermoid in a different patient. Axial T2W image demonstrates a well-circumscribed oval mass within the left sublingual space.

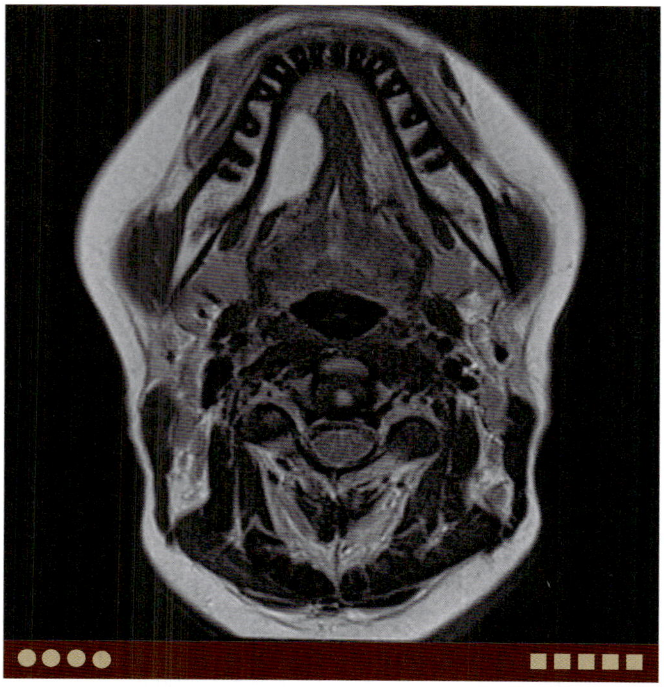

H. Ranula. Axial T2W image demonstrates a well-circumscribed cystic mass within the right sublingual space.

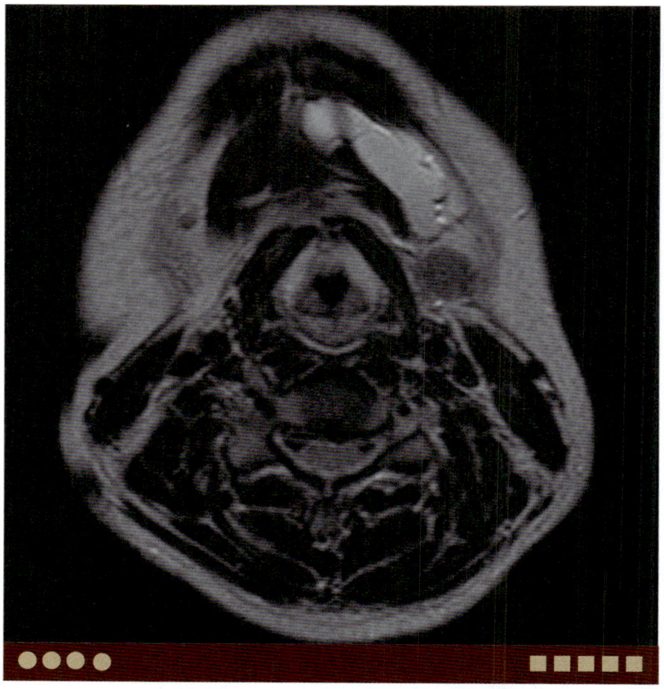

I. Lymphatic malformation. Axial T2W image demonstrates a lobular multiloculated cystic lesion within the left submandibular space.

Case 8–9 Ranula

Rohini Nadgir, Osamu Sakai

PRESENTATION

Painless swelling in sublingual region.

FINDINGS

CT and MRI demonstrate ovoid/elongated cystic lesions in the sublingual and/or submandibular spaces.

DIFFERENTIAL DIAGNOSIS

- Dermoid/epidermoid: These are congenital cystic lesions that contain epithelial elements and dermal appendages, typically midline or paramidline. The epithelial elements account for the cystic components, whereas the dermal appendages account for the fatty components. If fatty component is identified on imaging, the diagnosis is clear. Otherwise, differentiation between dermoid and epidermoid is difficult.
- Venolymphatic and lymphatic malformations: This condition is often seen in children or young adults. These lesions are multispatial, extending through multiple planes in the face and neck. Lesions can be T2 bright and heterogeneously enhancing. When nonenhancing, the lesion contents are more suggestive of lymphatic fluid (cystic hygroma) whereas any enhancing components are more suggestive of venous components.
- Abscess: Peripherally enhancing fluid collection indicates infected collection in the appropriate clinical setting.
- Necrotic sublingual lymph node: Necrosis within sublingual lymph node related to metastatic disease or infection can have a similar appearance, though this is not very common and is usually more rounded in configuration and located more posteriorly compared with ranula.

COMMENTS

A simple ranula is an epithelial-lined retention cyst related to the sublingual gland or minor salivary glands located within the sublingual space above the mylohyoid muscle, usually occurring as a consequence of prior trauma or inflammation. Such processes may cause stenosis or occlusion of the glandular ductal system, resulting in retention cyst formation. The cyst may enlarge and rupture into the sublingual space and with extension posteriorly into the submandibular space below the mylohyoid muscle (plunging or diving ranula) such that there is no longer clearly defined epithelial lining (pseudocyst).

On CT and MRI, ranulas are demonstrated as simple fluid-containing lesions centered in the sublingual/submandibular spaces without associated enhancing component. In the case of diving ranula, the bulk of the fluid collection is in the submandibular space, with smaller amount of fluid in the sublingual space, "tail sign." If the collection becomes infected, the lesion can demonstrate peripheral rim enhancement.

Because simple ranulas can be difficult to distinguish radiologically from epidermoid lesions and lymphatic malformation, biopsy is typically necessary prior to treatment.

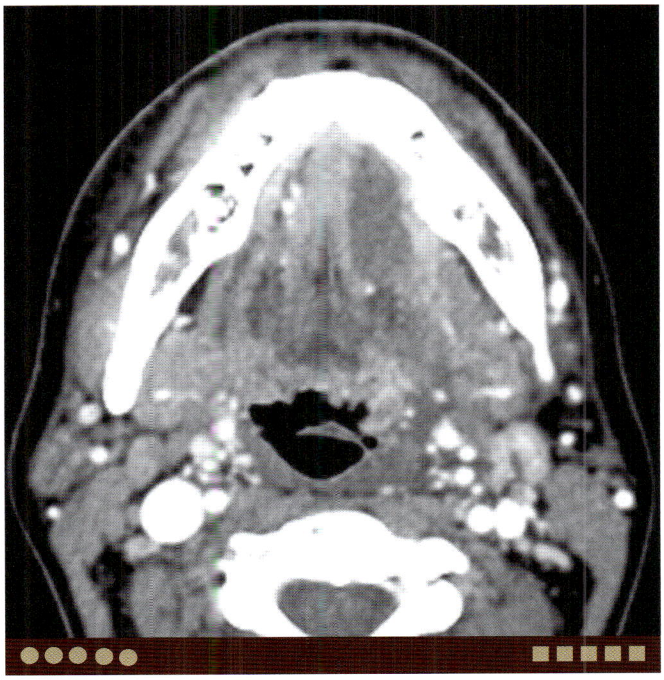

A. Ranula. Axial contrast-enhanced CT demonstrates a well-defined low-density lesion in the left sublingual space.

PEARLS

- **Simple ranula is an epithelial-lined retention cyst related to the sublingual gland located within the sublingual space above the mylohyoid muscle, usually a consequence of prior trauma or inflammation.**
- **Diving/plunging ranula is a pseudocyst extending below the mylohyoid muscle.**
- **On CT and MRI, ranulas are demonstrated as simple fluid-containing lesions centered in the sublingual/ submandibular spaces without associated enhancing component.**
- **Surgical resection of the sublingual gland and cyst provides the most definitive cure.**

If untreated, simple ranulas can rupture (diving ranula), and extend into deeper spaces of the head and neck. Occasionally ranulas can resolve on their own (typically in pediatric cases) although surgical resection of the sublingual gland and cyst provides the most definitive cure. It is important to define the extent of the lesion by imaging for surgical planning which may involve transoral versus open neck surgery. Sclerotheraphy is another treatment consideration.

ADDITIONAL IMAGES (B-G)

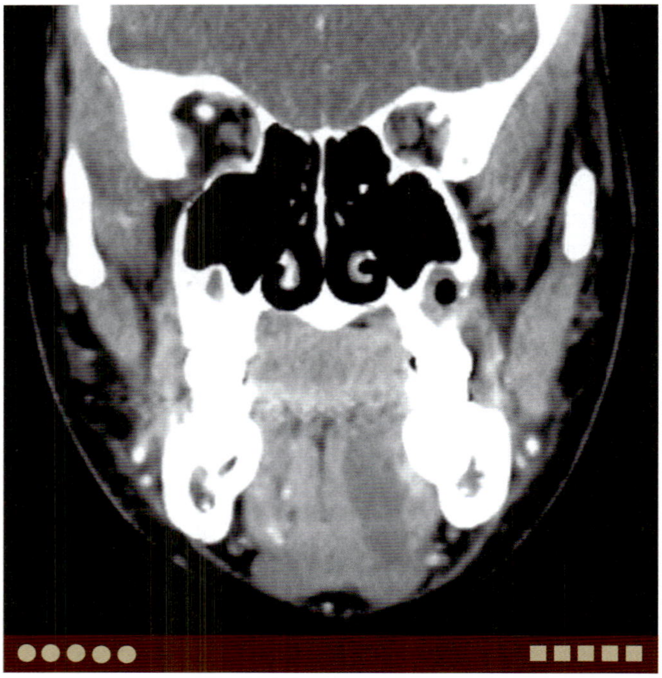

B. Ranula, same patient as A. Coronal contrast-enhanced CT demonstrates a cystic lesion in the left sublingual space, above the mylohyoid muscle.

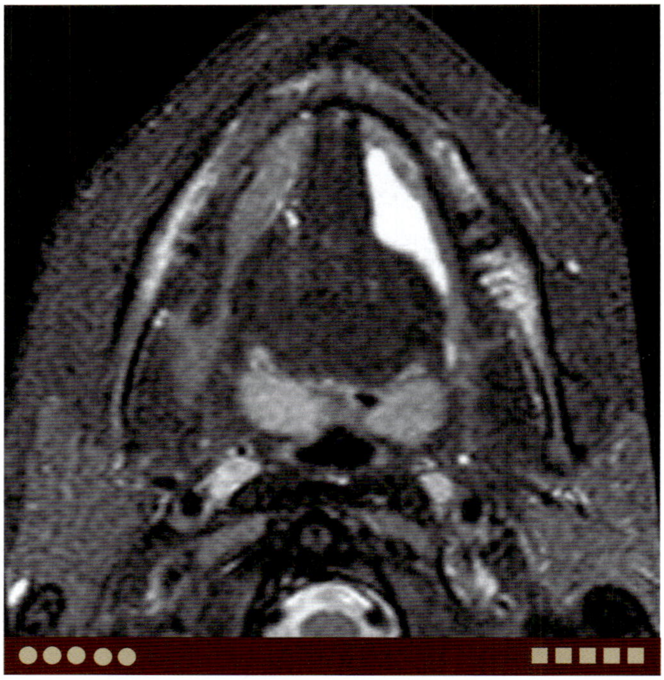

C. **Ranula** in a different patient. Axial fat-suppressed T2W image demonstrates a well-defined high-signal lesion in the left sublingual space.

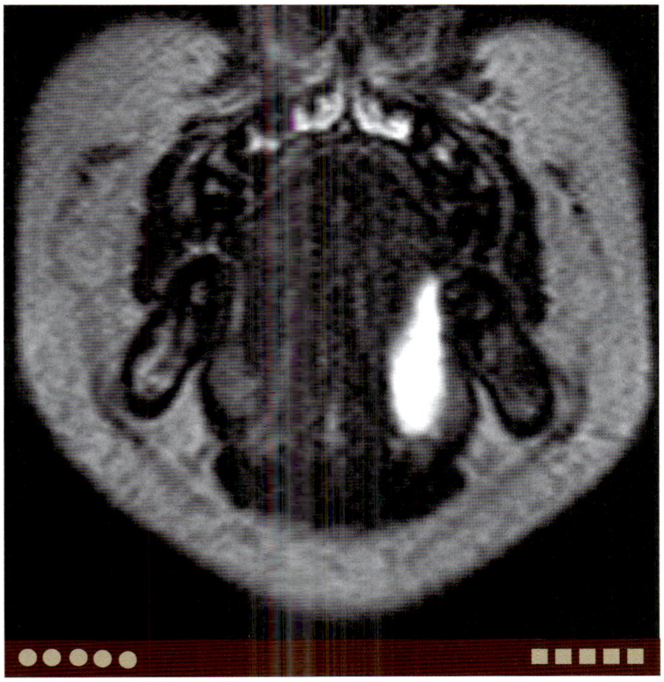

D. Ranula, same patient as C. Coronal T2W image demonstrates a well-defined high-signal lesion in the left sublingual space, above the mylohyoid muscle.

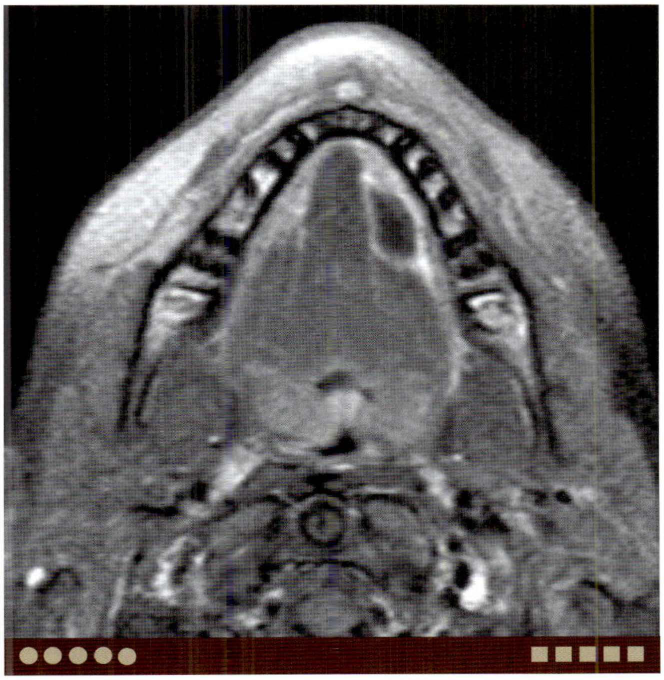

E. Ranula, same patient as C. Axial postcontrast fat-suppressed T1W image demonstrates a well-defined nonenhancing area in the left sublingual space.

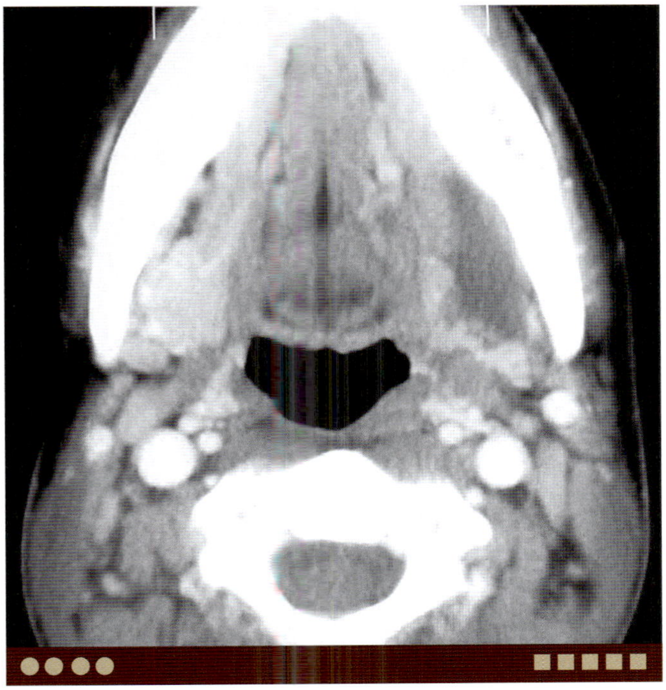

F. **Plunging/diving ranula**. Axial contrast-enhanced CT shows a low-density lesion along the lingual aspect of the left mandibular body.

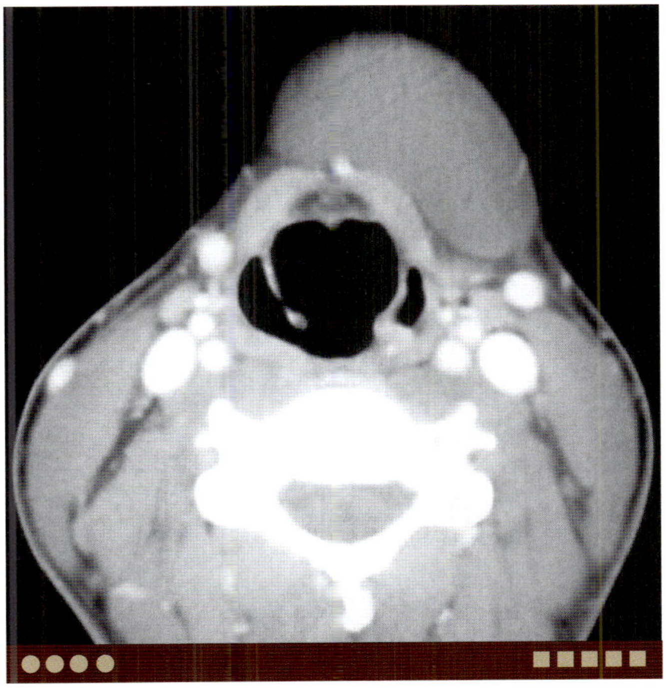

G. Plunging/diving ranula, same patient as F. Axial contrast-enhanced CT at the lower level shows a well-defined cystic lesion in the left anterior neck.

DIFFERENTIAL DIAGNOSIS IMAGES (H-J)

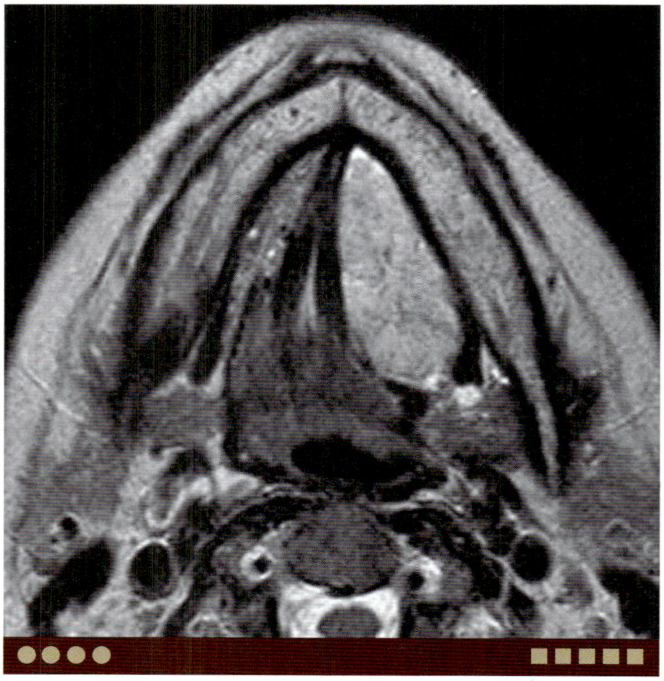

H. Lymphatic malformation. Axial T2W image shows an expansile high-signal lesion in the left sublingual space.

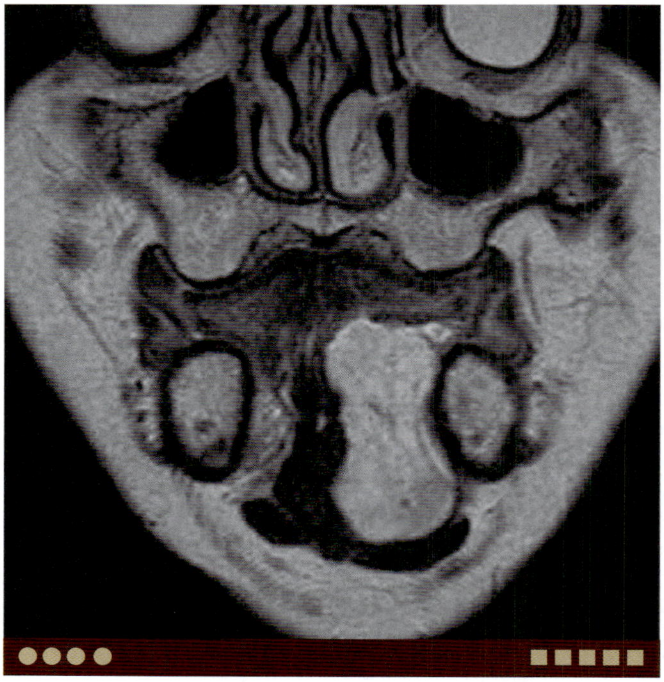

I. Lymphatic malformation, same patient as H. Coronal T2W image shows an expansile high-signal lesion in the left sublingual space, above the mylohyoid muscle.

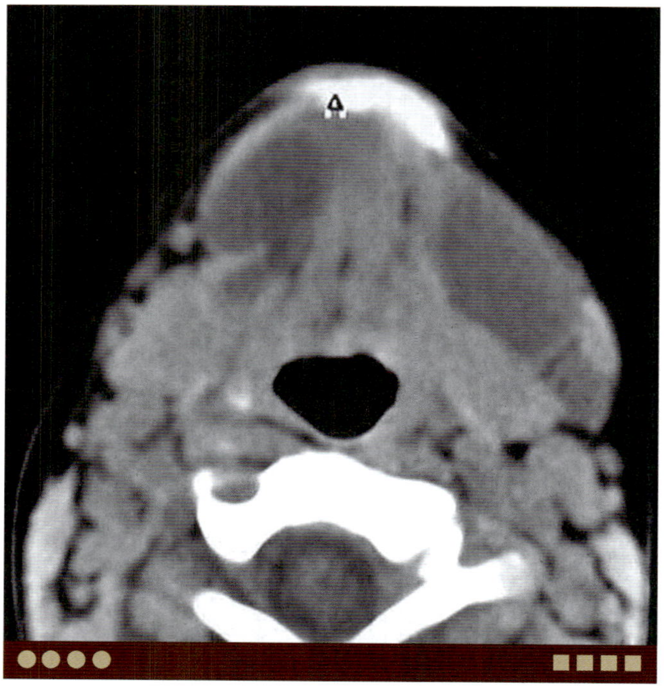

J. Lymphatic malformation in a different patient. Axial postcontrast CT shows multiloculated lesions in the bilateral submandibular spaces.

Case 8–10 Lymphoma—Tonsil

Brooke Devenney-Cakir, Osamu Sakai

PRESENTATION

Tonsillar mass.

FINDINGS

CT and MRI demonstrate a homogeneous density/signal mass arising from the palatine tonsil with enlarged lymph nodes without necrosis.

DIFFERENTIAL DIAGNOSIS

- Lymphoid hyperplasia of the tonsils: Tonsillar prominence is common in children and young adults, typically bilateral and symmetric and often associated with prominent adenoids and cervical adenopathy. Enhancing septa are seen on contrast-enhanced CT and MR.
- Squamous cell carcinoma (SCCA): SCCA is the most common malignancy in the oropharynx. The lesion is typically poorly circumscribed and heterogeneous in density, often with evidence of local invasion. Metastatic nodes often demonstrate intranodal necrosis.
- Pleomorphic adenoma: This lesion is typically a well-circumscribed mass arising from the minor salivary gland in the pharyngeal mucosa.

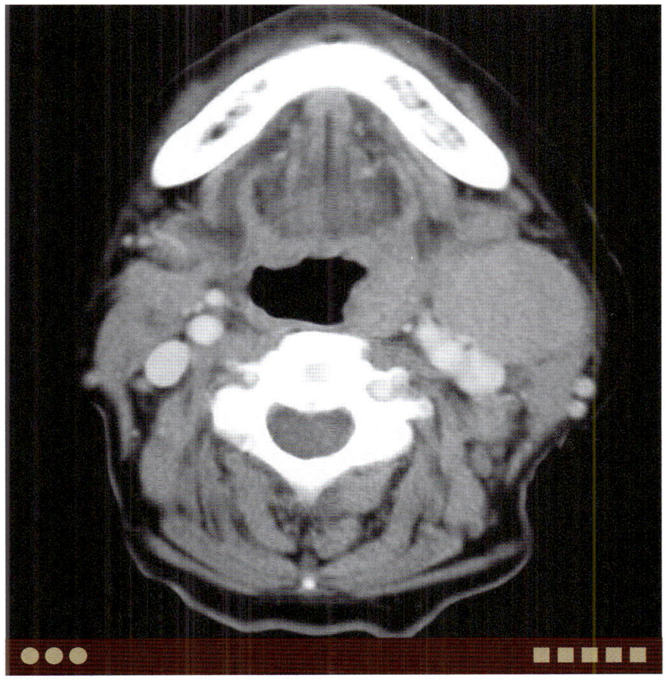

A. Lymphoma. Axial contrast-enhanced CT demonstrates a mildly enhancing tumor arising from the left palatine tonsil. Note a large mildly enhancing non-necrotic left level II node.

COMMENTS

This is a 70-year-old woman with left neck mass.

Tonsillar lymphomas are the second most common malignant tumors in this region following SCCA, although malignancy of the tonsils is not common accounting for approximately 0.5% of new malignancies in the United States every year. Lymphoma arising from the tonsil is usually non-Hodgkin lymphoma (NHL) B-cell type. Tonsillar lymphoma typically presents as a submucosal mass with asymmetrical enlargement of one tonsil. Unilateral lymphadenopathy is also often present.

Contrast-enhanced CT typically demonstrates a mildly enhancing tumor occupying the palatine tonsil commonly without deep extension into the surrounding spaces. Associated nodal disease is present in 50% of cases. The lymph nodes are typically large (>2 cm) and non-necrotic. Non-necrotic large nodes (>3 cm) are less likely to be SCCA and suggestive of lymphoma. Centrally necrotic lymph nodes can be seen in invasive NHL, especially in acquired immunodeficiency syndrome (AIDS) related.

MRI can provide additional details regarding diagnosis and possible extension of the lesion. T1W images typically demonstrate a large pharyngeal mucosal space mass, isointense to muscle. The signal characteristics of the lesion vary on T2W images depending on the cellularity of the lesion. Typically, the lesion is homogeneously hyperintense, while highly cellular lesions are generally less hyperintense. Postcontrast T1W images demonstrate mild homogeneous enhancement of the lesion. Presence of nonenhancing internal septa may be a finding to suggest benign lymphoid hyperplasia rather than lymphoma.

PEARLS

- **Lymphoma is the second most common malignant tumor in the tonsil following SCCA.**
- **Large non-necrotic nodes are commonly seen in lymphoma. However, intranodal necrosis can occur in invasive NHL, especially when it is AIDS related.**
- **Presence of nonenhancing internal septa may be a finding to suggest benign lymphoid hyperplasia rather than lymphoma.**

ADDITIONAL IMAGES (B-F)

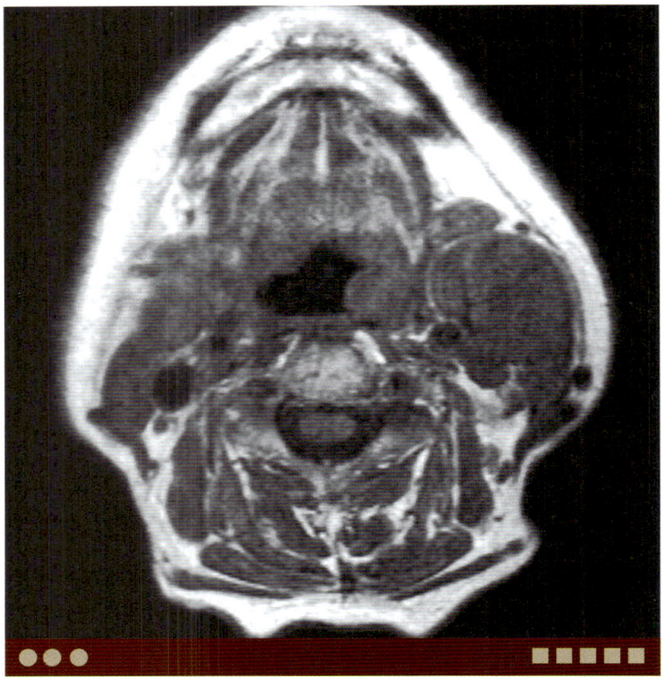

B. Lymphoma, same patient as A. Axial T1W image demonstrates a low-signal lesion in the left palatine tonsil. The large left level II node demonstrates homogeneously low signal.

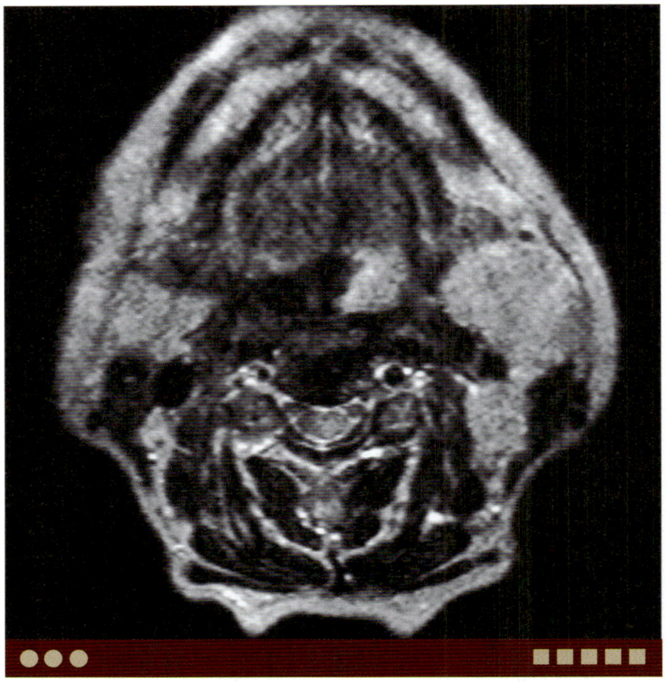

C. Lymphoma, same patient as A. Axial T2W image demonstrates a high-signal lesion in the left palatine tonsil. The large left level II node demonstrates homogeneously increased signal.

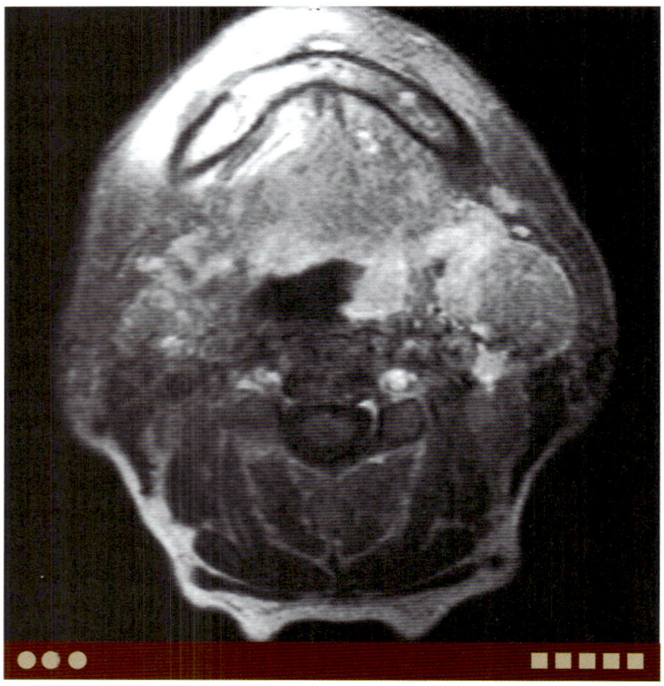

D. Lymphoma, same patient as A. Axial postcontrast fat-suppressed T1W image demonstrates mild homogeneous enhancement in the lesion. The node shows minimal enhancement.

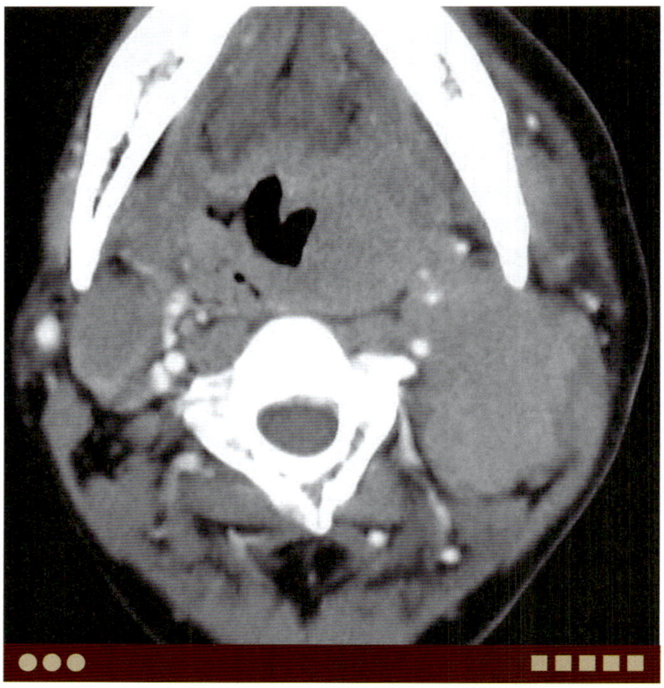

E. **Lymphoma** in a different patient. Axial contrast-enhanced CT demonstrates a mildly enhancing tumor in the left palatine tonsil. Large, mildly enhancing, non-necrotic level II nodes are seen bilaterally, left larger than right.

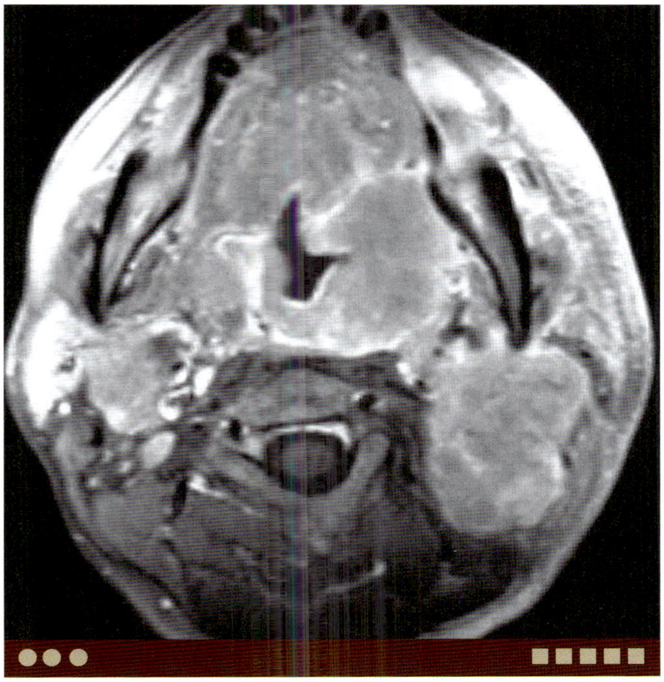

F. Lymphoma, same patient as E. Axial postcontrast fat-suppressed T1W image demonstrates mild homogeneous enhancement in the left tonsillar lesion as well as enlarged level II nodes. No necrosis is noted.

DIFFERENTIAL DIAGNOSIS IMAGES (G-J)

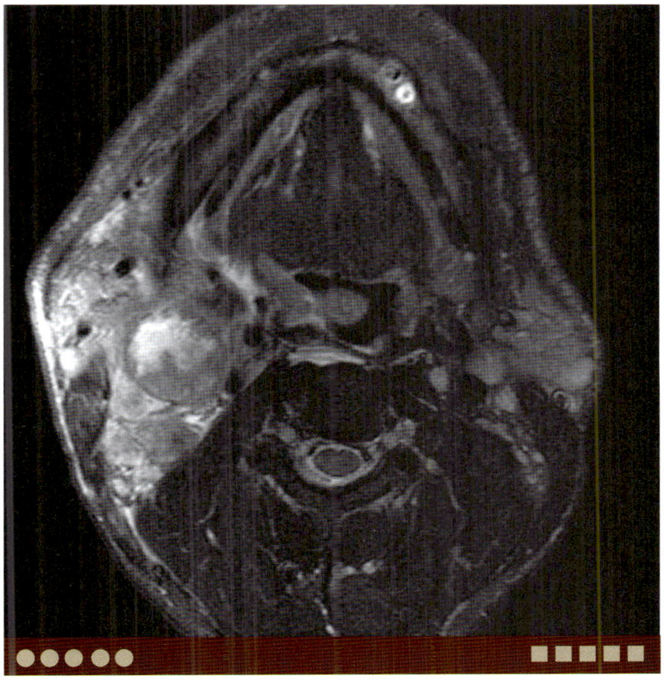

G. SCCA. Axial fat-suppressed T2W image demonstrates multiple metastatic nodes showing heterogeneous high signal. Ill-defined margins of nodes suggest extracapsular tumor spread. Note relatively small primary tumor in the right palatine tonsil.

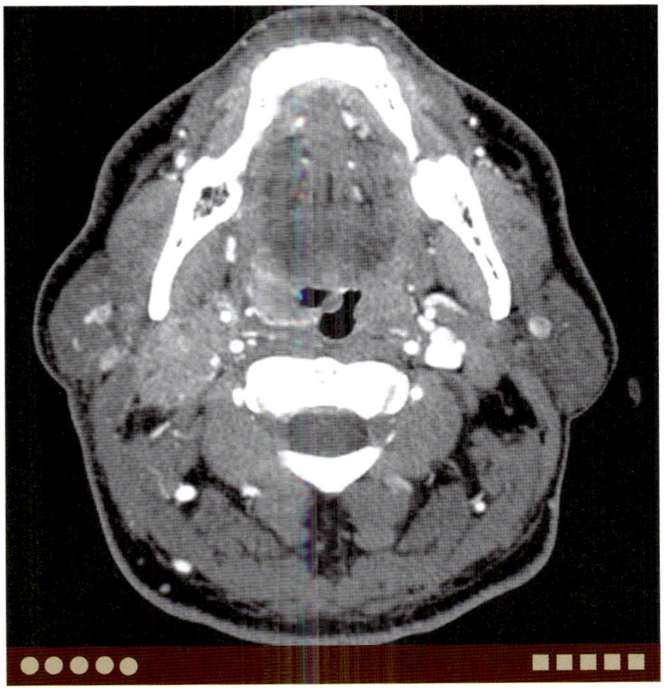

H. **SCCA** in a different patient. Axial contrast-enhanced CT demonstrates a heterogeneously enhancing lesion in the right tonsil. Note enhancing lymph nodes with poorly defined margins in the right level II consistent with nodal metastasis with extracapsular tumor extension.

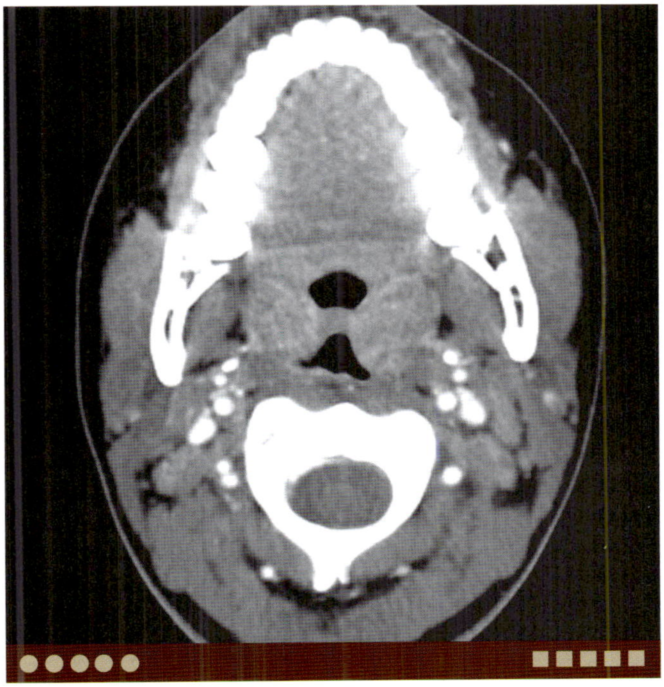

I. **Tonsillitis**. Axial contrast-enhanced CT demonstrates enhancing enlarged tonsils bilaterally. Striation is seen; however, no apparent mass is noted in the tonsils.

Case 8-11 Pleomorphic Adenoma—Palate

Brooke Devenney-Cakir, Csamu Sakai

PRESENTATION

A mass in the palate.

FINDINGS

CT and MRI demonstrate a well-circumscribed enhancing mass, arising from the palate, exerting some mass effect on the adjacent structure and bone erosion.

DIFFERENTIAL DIAGNOSIS

- Squamous cell carcinoma (SCCA): SCCA is the most common malignant tumor of the palate, and usually shows ill-defined, infiltrative margins and heterogeneous density/signal and enhancement.
- Adenoid cystic carcinoma: This is a malignant tumor arising from the minor salivary gland. High-grade tumors show higher cellularity and low signal on T2W images. Perineural tumor spread is common.
- Mucoepidermoid carcinoma: This is also a malignant tumor arising from the minor salivary gland. Low-grade tumors tend to be cystic and high-grade tumors tend to show more solid appearance.
- Lymphoma: This is a rare tumor in the palate but may demonstrate relatively well-circumscribed margins and homogeneous density/signal. Bone expansion or infiltration is more common than erosion.
- Torus palatinus: This is an exostosis arising from the hard palate.

COMMENTS

This is a 42-year-old woman with a mass in the palate.

Pleomorphic adenoma, also known as benign mixed tumor, is the most common benign tumor of the palate, although it is not very common. This lesion typically presents as a slowly growing submucosal mass visible on oral examination. Larger masses can prolapse into the airway, and untreated, can increase significantly to greater than 5 lbs. This lesion is most common between ages of 30 and 60 years with a 2:1 female predominance.

Pleomorphic adenoma of the palate typically is seen as a well-circumscribed mass, isodense to muscle on unenhanced CT. Contrast-enhanced CT typically demonstrates a mild, characteristically delayed enhancement. The lesion may be inhomogeneous if calcifications and/or cystic components are present. Benign-appearing bony remodeling may be noted when tumors are adjacent to the hard palate.

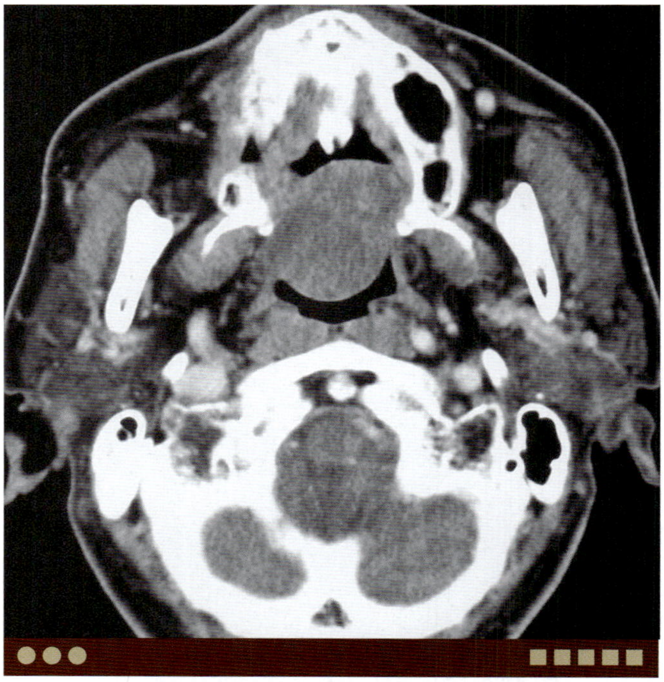

A. Pleomorphic adenoma of the palate. Axial postcontrast CT demonstrates a minimally enhancing, round mass in the soft palate, narrowing the airway.

On MRI, pleomorphic adenoma typically is isointense to muscle on T1W images. The lesion can have variable signal on T2W images but typically is hyperintense with respect to muscle. If calcifications are present, they will present as low or no signal. Contrast-enhanced T1W imaging most commonly demonstrate homogeneous enhancement, characteristically delayed enhancement.

PEARLS

- **Pleomorphic adenoma is the most common benign tumor of the palate.**
- **CT and MRI demonstrate a well-circumscribed mass, typically hyperintense to muscle.**
- **Calcification may be present. Benign-appearing bony remodeling may be noted when tumors are adjacent to the hard palate.**
- **Delayed enhancement is characteristic for pleomorphic adenoma.**

ADDITIONAL IMAGES (B–G)

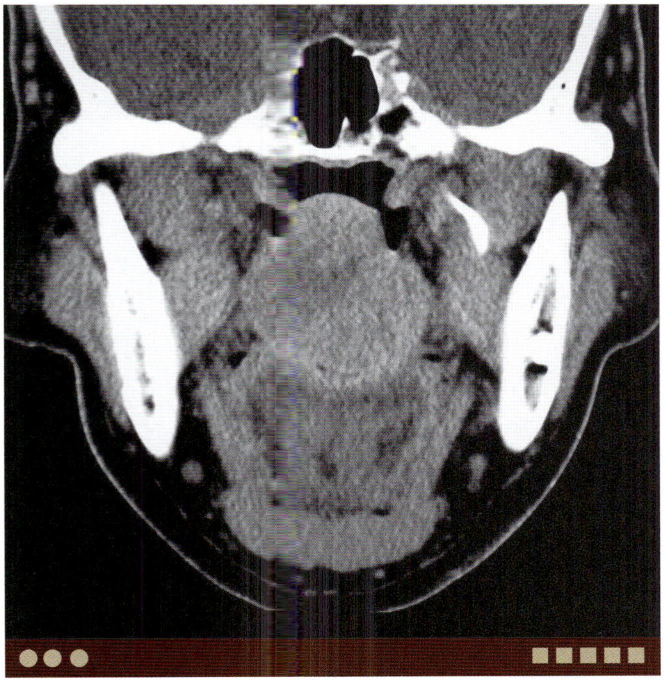

B. Pleomorphic adenoma, same patient as A. Coronal postcontrast CT (delayed phase) demonstrates increased enhancement of the tumor.

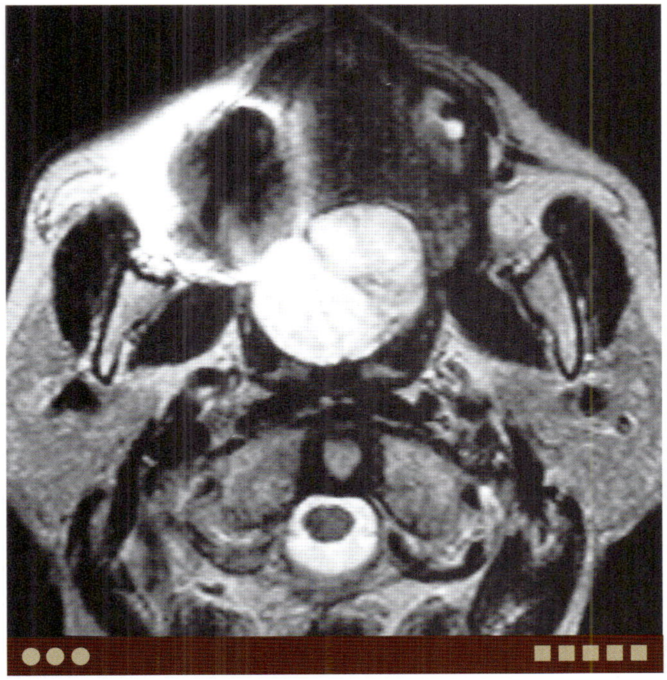

C. Pleomorphic adenoma, same patient as A. Axial T2W MR image demonstrates a well-demarcated, high-signal lesion with some internal septation.

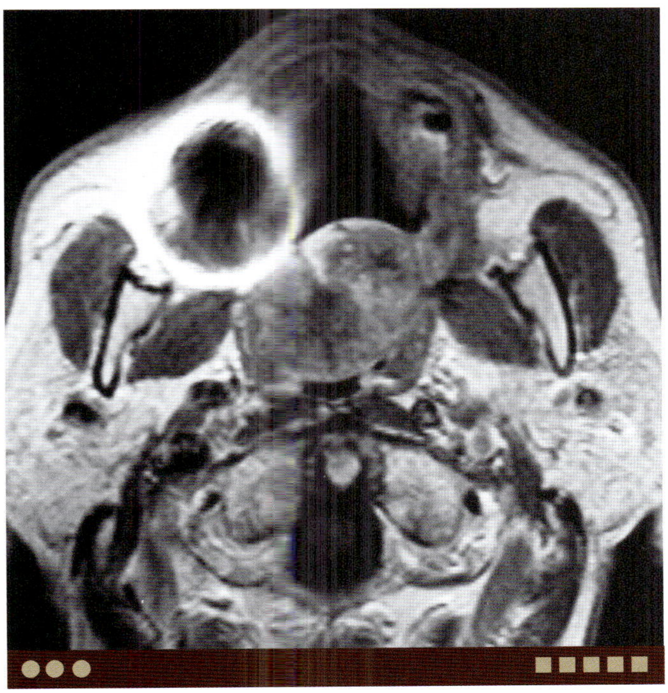

D. Pleomorphic adenoma, same patient as A. Axial postcontrast T1W MR image demonstrates slightly heterogeneous enhancement of the lesion.

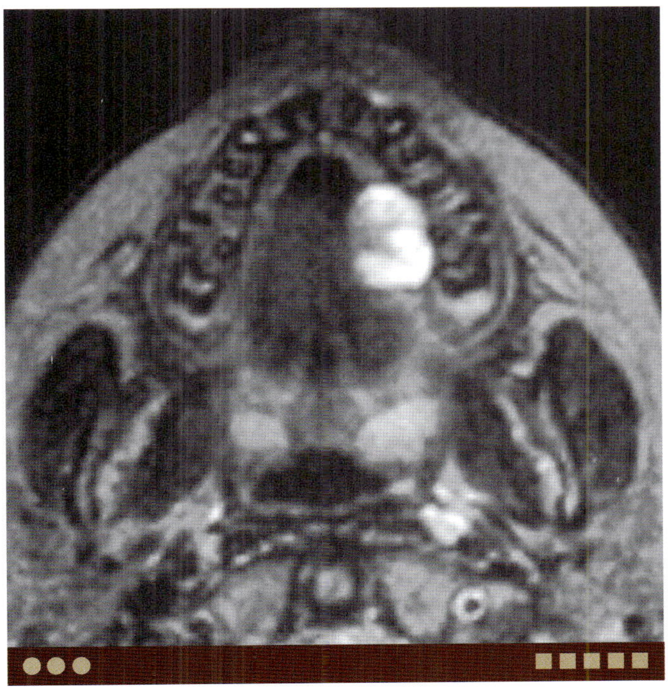

E. **Pleomorphic adenoma** in a different patient. Axial T2W MR image demonstrates a slightly lobulated, well-demarcated, high-signal lesion in the left hard palate.

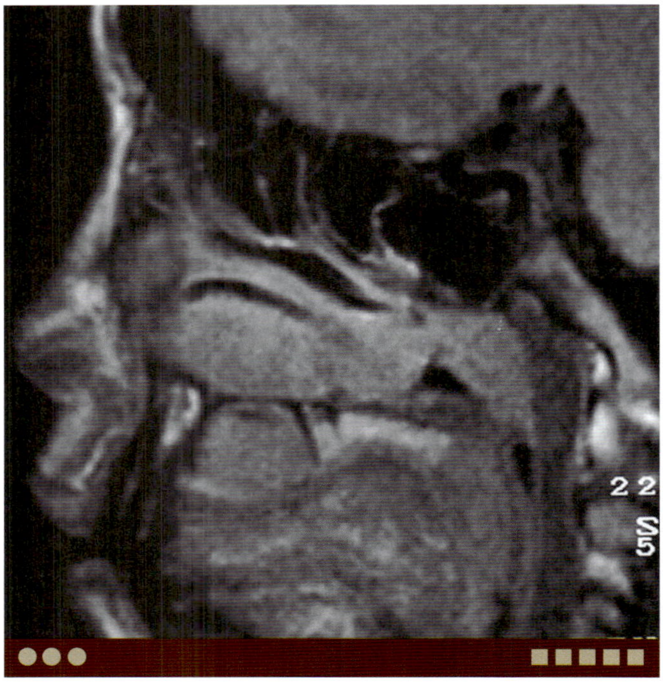

F. Pleomorphic adenoma, same patient as E. Sagittal T1W MR image demonstrates benign-appearing bony remodeling in the hard palate.

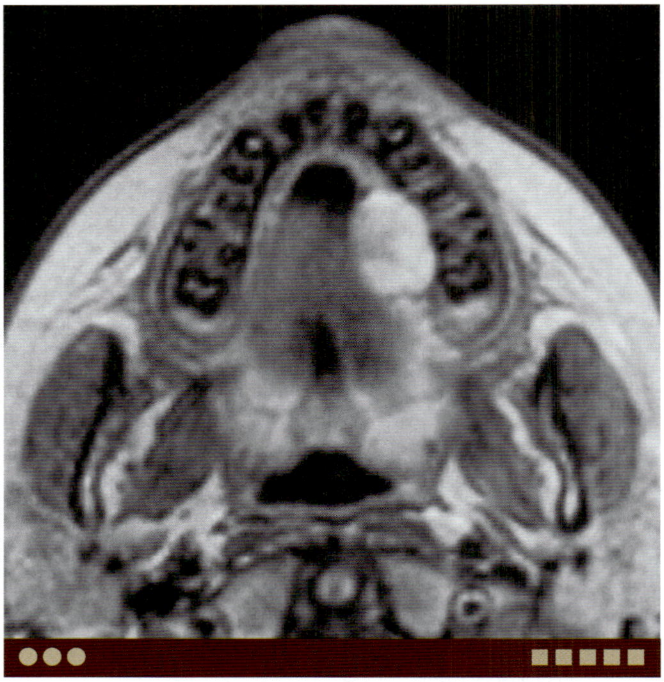

G. Pleomorphic adenoma, same patient as E. Axial postcontrast T1W MR image demonstrates homogeneous enhancement of the lesion.

DIFFERENTIAL DIAGNOSIS IMAGES (H-J)

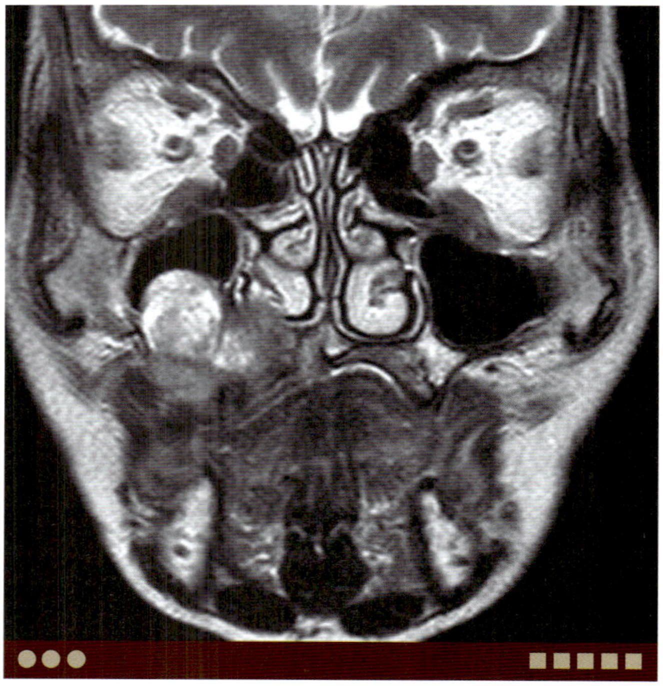

H. Adenoid cystic carcinoma. Coronal T2W MR image demonstrates a lobulated, heterogeneous high-signal lesion destructing the right hard palate and protruding into the right maxillary sinus.

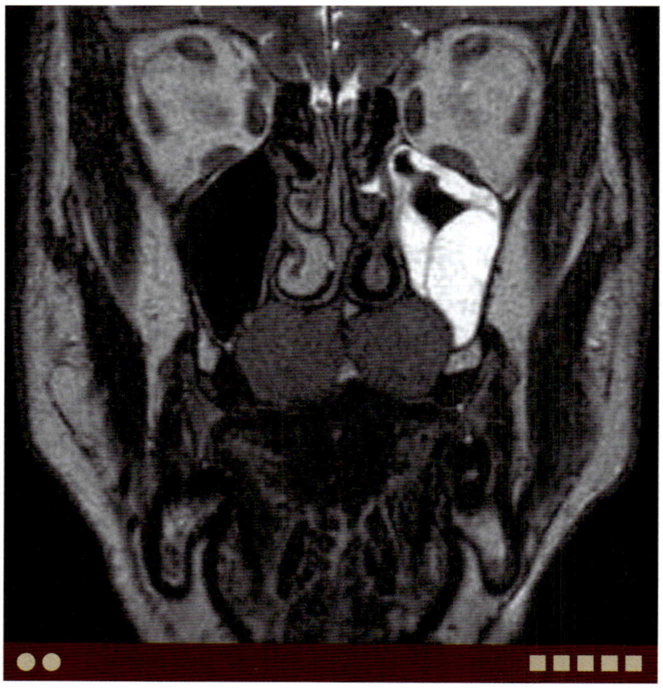

I. Lymphoma. Coronal T2W MR image demonstrates an expansile, homogeneous, intermediate-signal lesion in the hard palate.

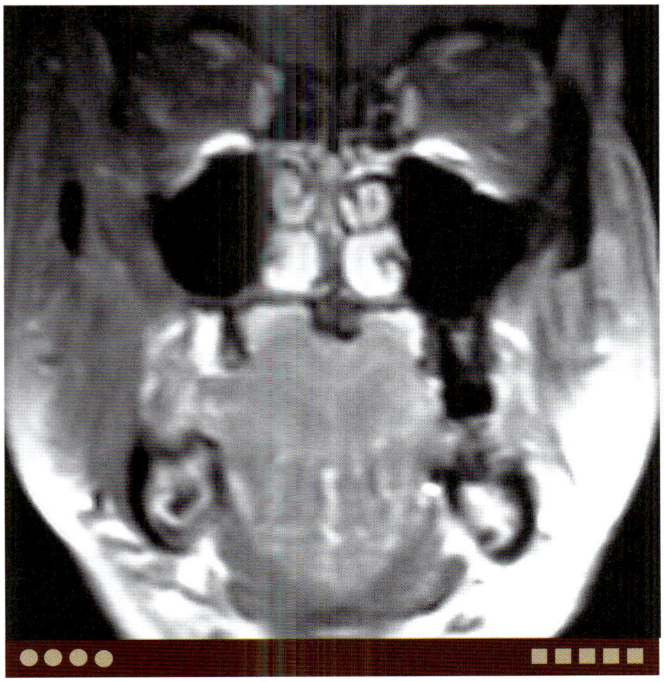

J. Torus palatinus. Coronal postcontrast fat-suppressed T1W MR image demonstrates an osseous protrusion in the hard plate in midline.

Case 8–12 Lymphoma—Palate

Brooke Devenney-Cakir, Osamu Sakai

PRESENTATION

A palatal mass.

FINDINGS

CT and MRI demonstrate an expansile homogeneous density/signal lesion in the palate.

DIFFERENTIAL DIAGNOSIS

- Squamous cell carcinoma (SCCA): SCCA is the most common malignant tumor of the palate, and usually shows ill-defined, infiltrative margins and heterogeneous density/signal and enhancement.
- Adenoid cystic carcinoma: This is a malignant tumor arising from the minor salivary gland. High-grade tumors show higher cellularity and low-signal on T2W images. Perineural tumor spread is common.
- Mucoepidermoid carcinoma: This is also a malignant tumor arising from the minor salivary gland. Low-grade tumors tend to be cystic and high-grade tumors tend to show more solid appearance.
- Pleomorphic adenoma: This is the most common benign tumor of the palate. Bone remodeling is often seen if it occurs near the hard palate.
- Torus palatinus: This is an exostosis arising from the hard palate.

COMMENTS

This is a 48-year-old man with a palatal mass.

Primary lymphoma of the palate is rare and represents a malignant neoplastic growth of lymphocytes or histiocytes. The most common malignancy of the palate is squamous cell carcinoma. Primary lymphoma of the palate occurs most commonly in patients older than 60 years but may be seen in younger patients, especially in the setting of AIDS. The tumor commonly arises from the junction of the hard and soft palates. Once the hard palate is affected it often shows expansile change.

Contrast-enhanced CT typically demonstrates a minimally enhancing homogeneous mass occupying the palate. MRI can provide additional details regarding diagnosis and possible extension of the lesion. On MRI lymphoma typically demonstrates homogeneously low signal on T1W and intermediate signal on T2W images, and homogeneous mild enhancement. Necrosis is rare without treatment. The T2W signal is similar to that of the oral mucosa, and significantly lower than sinonasal mucosa and retention cyst.

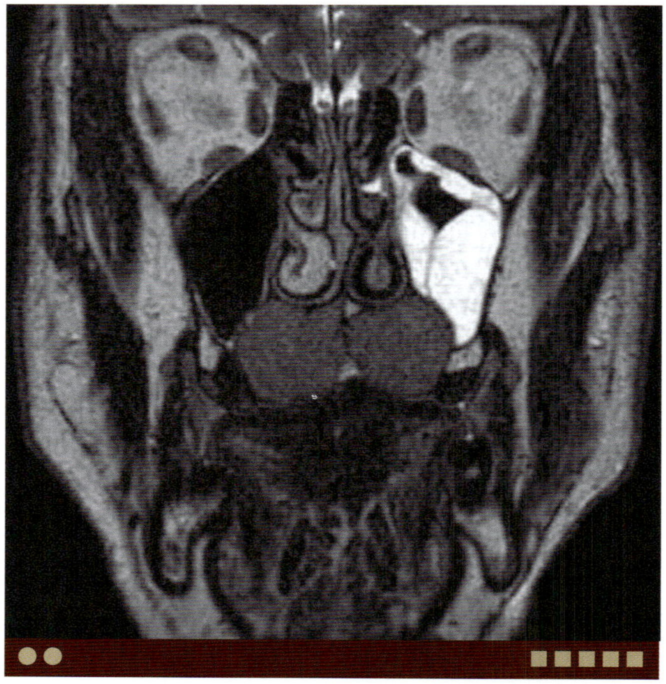

A. Lymphoma of the palate. Coronal T2W MR image demonstrates an expansile, homogeneous, intermediate-signal lesion in the hard palate.

PEARLS

- **Lymphomas involving the hard palate demonstrate expansile, homogeneous density/signal lesions with mild enhancement.**
- **SCCA is the most common malignancy arising from the palate. Minor salivary gland tumors such as adenoid cystic carcinoma and mucoepidermoid carcinoma also occur.**

ADDITIONAL IMAGES (B-G)

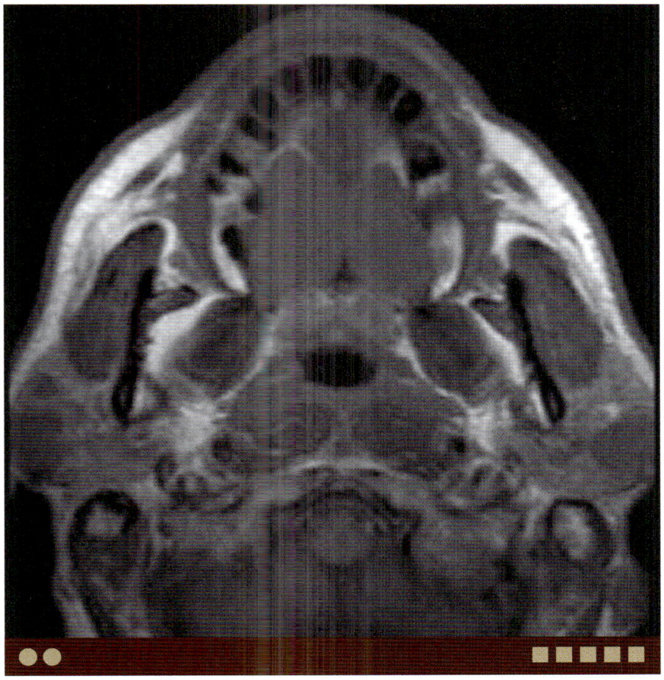

B. Lymphoma, same patient as A. Axial T1W MR image demonstrates a homogeneous, low-signal lesion in the hard palate.

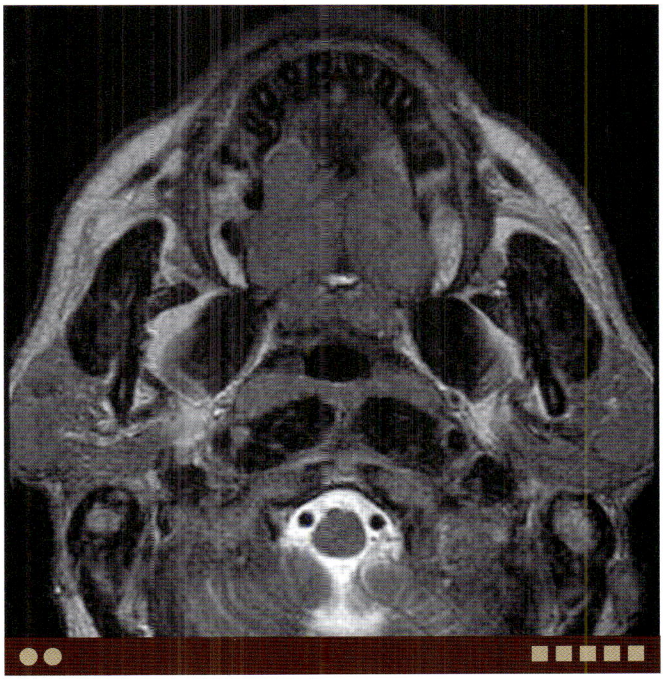

C. Lymphoma, same patient as A. Axial T2W MR image demonstrates a homogeneous, intermediate-signal lesion in the hard palate.

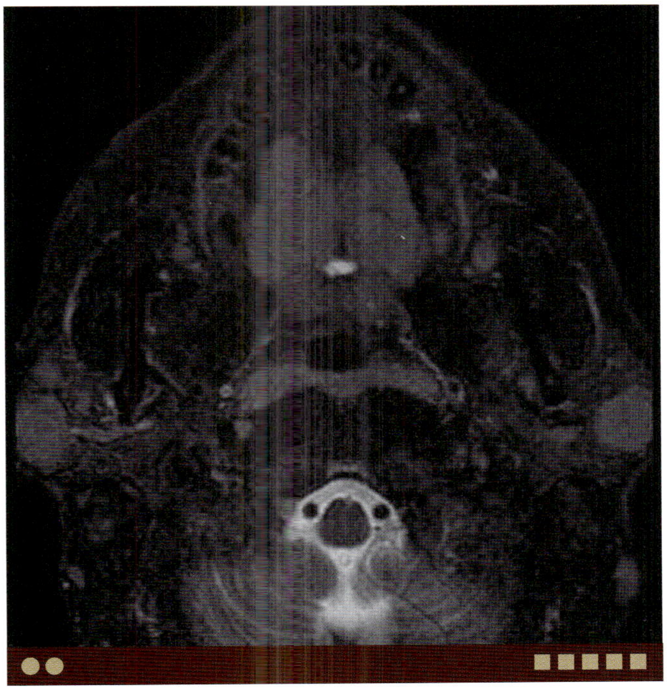

D. Lymphoma, same patient as A. Axial fat-suppressed T2W MR image demonstrates a homogeneous, intermediate-signal lesion in the hard palate.

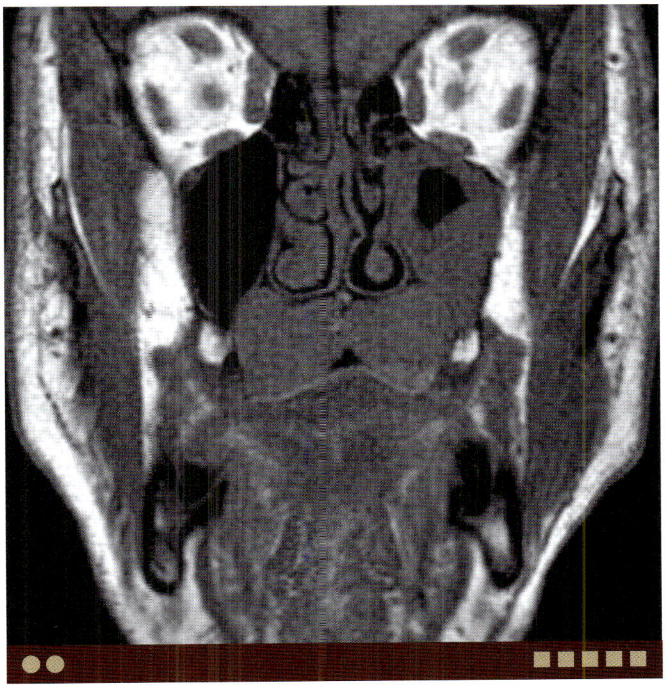

E. Lymphoma, same patient as A. Coronal T1W MR image demonstrates a homogeneous, low-signal lesion in the hard palate.

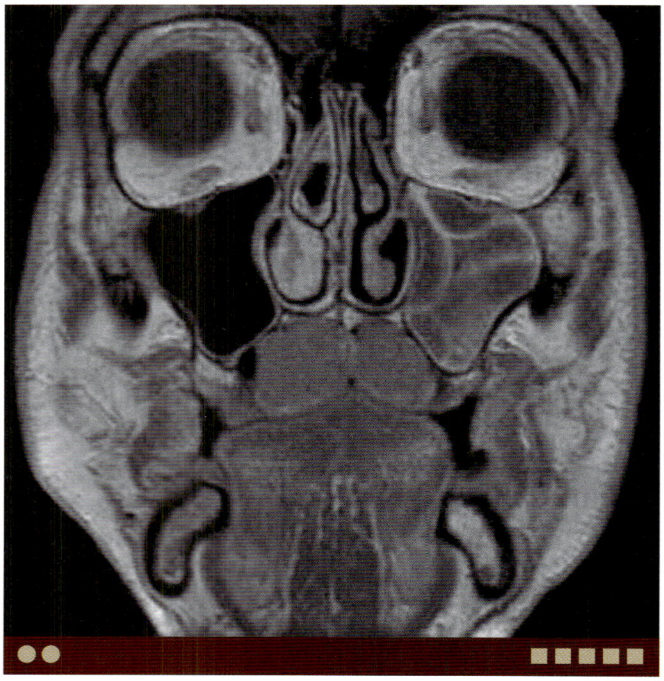

F. Lymphoma, same patient as A. Coronal postcontrast T1W MR image demonstrates mild, homogeneous enhancement of the lesion.

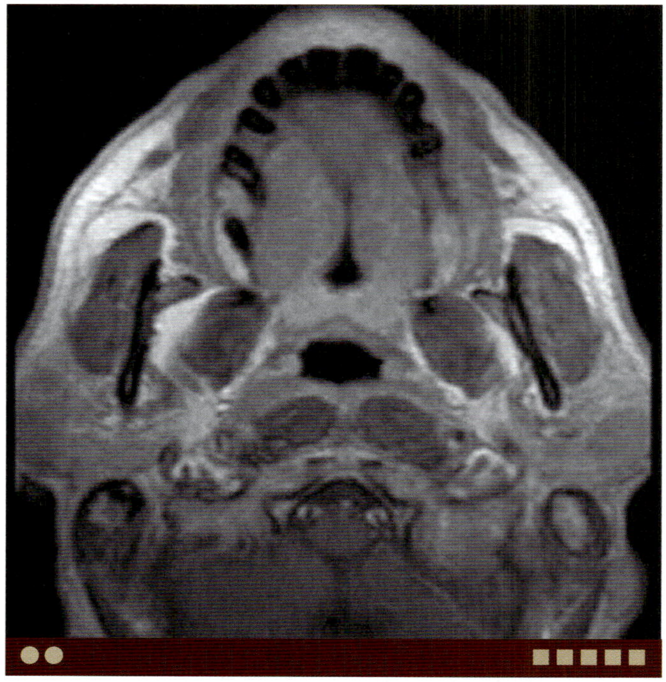

G. Lymphoma, same patient as A. Axial postcontrast T1W MR image demonstrates mild, homogeneous enhancement of the lesion.

DIFFERENTIAL DIAGNOSIS IMAGES (H-J)

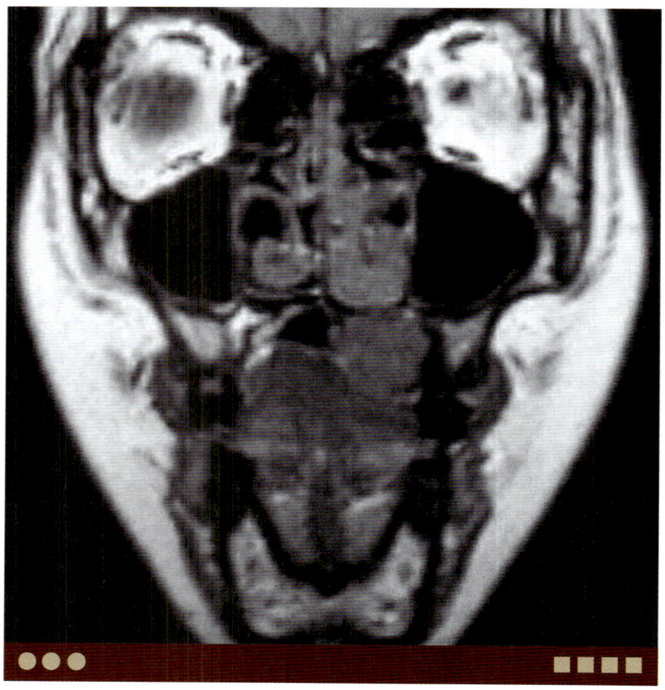

H. **Pleomorphic adenoma**. Coronal postcontrast T1W MR image demonstrates a homogeneously enhancing tumor in the left hard palate with bone remodeling/erosion.

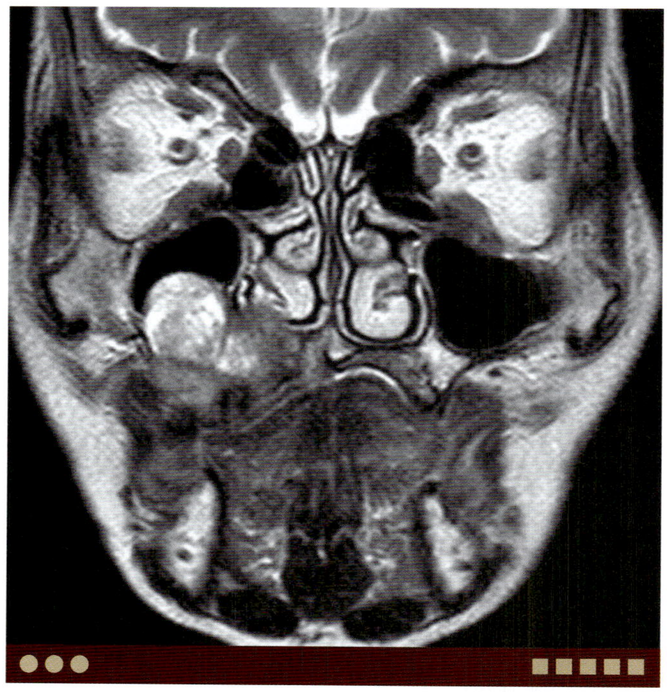

I. **Adenoid cystic carcinoma**. Coronal T2W MR image demonstrates a lobulated, heterogeneous high-signal lesion destructing the right hard palate and protruding into the right maxillary sinus.

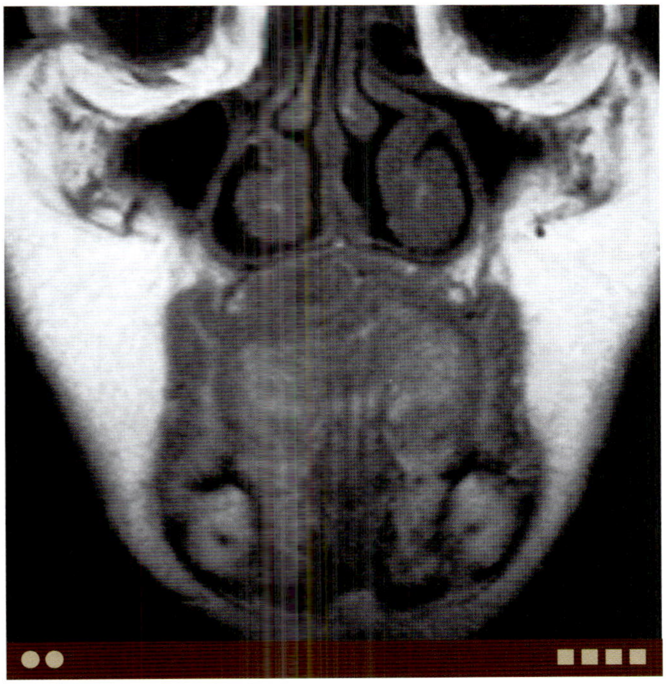

J. Melanoma. Coronal T1W MR image demonstrates an ovoid-shaped lesion tumor in the right palate with bone remodeling.

Case 8–13 Plexiform Neurofibroma—Neurofibromatosis Type I

Brooke Devenney-Cakir, Osamu Sakai

PRESENTATION

Sublingual fullness.

FINDINGS

Contrast-enhanced CT demonstrates an ill-defined hypoattenuating region in the sublingual region.

DIFFERENTIAL DIAGNOSIS

- Lymphatic malformation (lymphangioma): This condition will appear as an ill-defined low-density lesion on CT, extending into multiple fascia-defined spaces. This lesion will be homogeneously hyperintense on T2W MR images and may show no or subtle rim enhancement on postcontrast MR images. If more enhancement is seen, the lesion likely has a mixed venous component. No apparent enhancement is seen on CT.
- Venous malformation: This condition typically appears as a lobulated soft tissue lesion, isodense to muscle on CT with phleboliths and increased fat in the adjacent soft tissues. T2 high signal is characteristic. Contrast-enhanced CT and MRI typically show patchy delayed or homogeneous enhancement depending on lesion flow dynamics.
- Infantile hemangioma: This condition typically undergoes rapid growth during the first year of life. Contrast-enhanced MRI will show rapid, homogeneous, intense enhancement.
- Malignant peripheral nerve sheath tumor: This condition typically demonstrates a rapid increase in size, heterogeneous density/signal, and enhancement with invasive change to the adjacent structures.

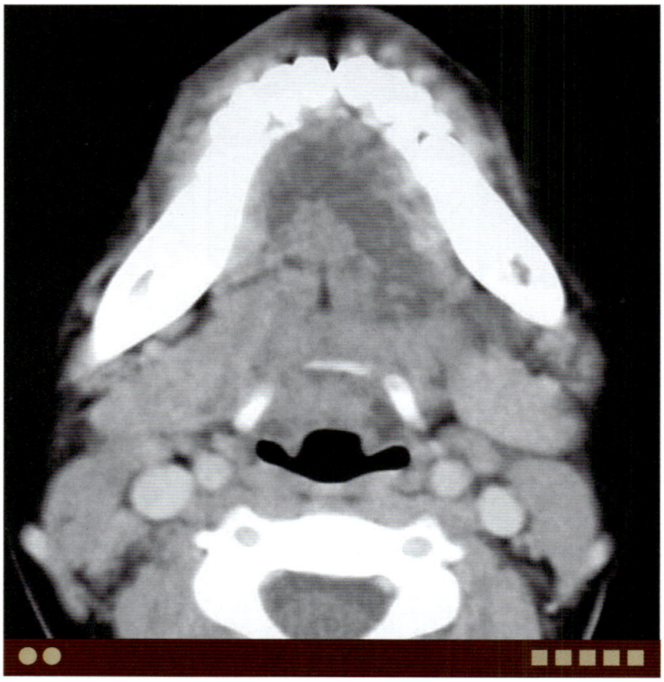

A. Plexiform neurofibroma. Axial postcontrast CT demonstrates an ill-defined hypoattenuating lesion in the left sublingual space, crossing the midline.

COMMENTS

This is an 11-year-old girl with known history of neurofibromatosis type I.

Neurofibromatosis type I (von Recklinghausen disease) is a common autosomal dominant condition occurring in 1:4000 individuals. The condition can include some of the following features: café-au-lait spots, axillary and inguinal freckling, lisch nodules, optic pathway gliomas, neurofibromas, and plexiform neurofibromas. A plexiform neurofibroma is a slow growing perineural tumor composed of Schwann cells, perineural cells, and fibroblasts and is virtually pathognomonic of type I neurofibromatosis. The tumor demonstrates an infiltrative growth pattern without regard to fascial boundaries. Plexiform neurofibromas can occur anywhere in the body; however, the first division of the trigeminal nerve, in the region of the orbital apex, is most often involved. Despite their common occurrence in the head and neck, only 4% to 7% are found in the oral cavity.

Neurofibromas are typically multifocal; thus imaging of the head and neck should be performed. Lesions occurring in nerves adjacent to the larynx and trachea must be identified as they may cause acute airway obstruction.

PEARLS

- **Plexiform neurofibromas are virtually pathognomonic of type I neurofibromatosis.**
- **CT typically demonstrates low attenuation even after contrast administration.**
- **Contrast-enhanced MRI will demonstrate an inhomogeneously enhancing, lobulated mass along the course of the involved peripheral nerve.**
- **Involvement of multiple fascia-defined spaces is often seen with plexiform neurofibroma.**

CT of plexiform neurofibromas typically demonstrates low attenuation even after contrast administration. The lesion may demonstrate a "target sign" because the central portion of the tumor will demonstrate minimal enhancement relative to the periphery. Neurofibromas are typically hyperintense on T2W MR images and can also show a "target sign" with central hypointensity and peripheral hyperintense signal due to high central collagen content. A "fascicular sign" can also be seen as multiple small irregular hypointense foci representing fascicular bundles and is typical of a benign lesion. Contrast-enhanced MRI will demonstrate an inhomogeneously enhancing, lobulated mass along the course of the involved peripheral nerve. Involvement of multiple fascia-defined spaces is often seen with plexiform neurofibroma.

ADDITIONAL IMAGES (B-D)

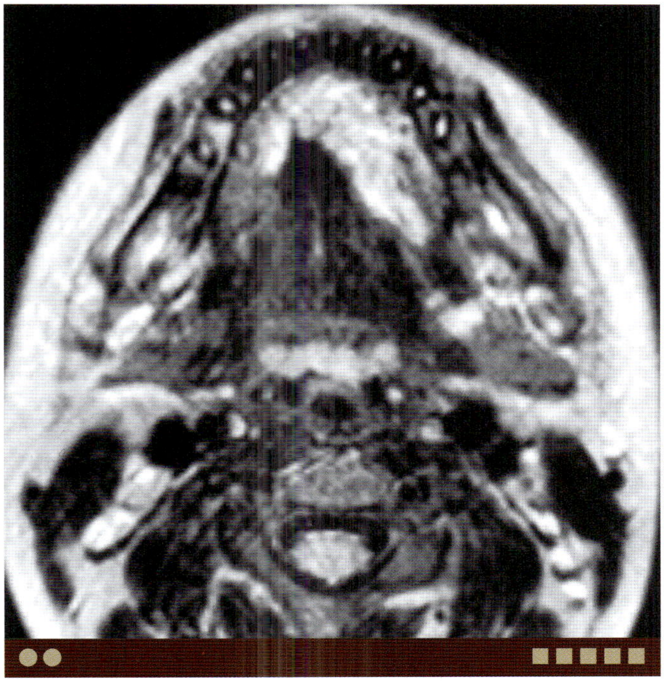

B. Plexiform neurofibroma, same patient as A. Axial T2W MR image demonstrates an ill-defined hyperintense lesion in the left sublingual space extending to the right. Focal regions of hypointensity may represent collagen or fascicular bundles.

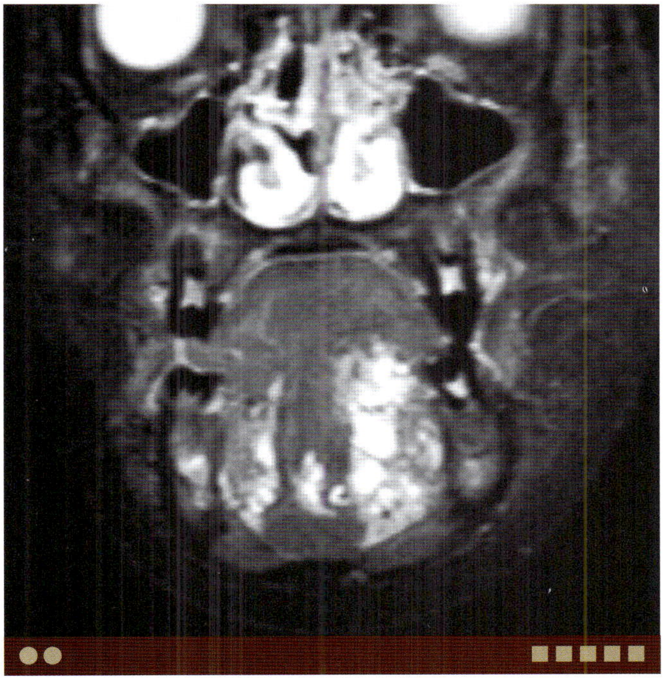

C. Plexiform neurofibroma, same patient as A. Coronal STIR MR image demonstrates inhomogeneously hyperintense sublingual lesion, left larger than right.

DIFFERENTIAL DIAGNOSIS IMAGES (E-G)

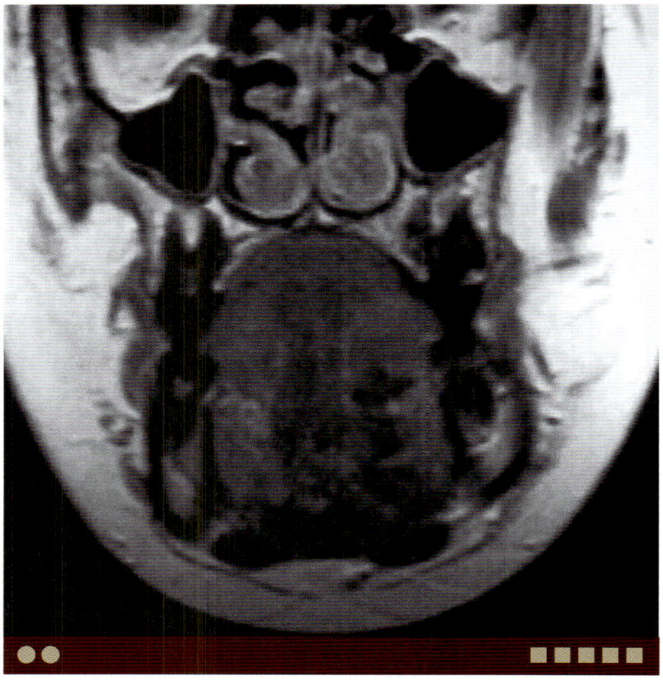

D. Plexiform neurofibroma, same patient as A. Coronal postcontrast T1W MR image demonstrates an inhomogeneously lobulated mildly enhancing lesion within the sublingual space.

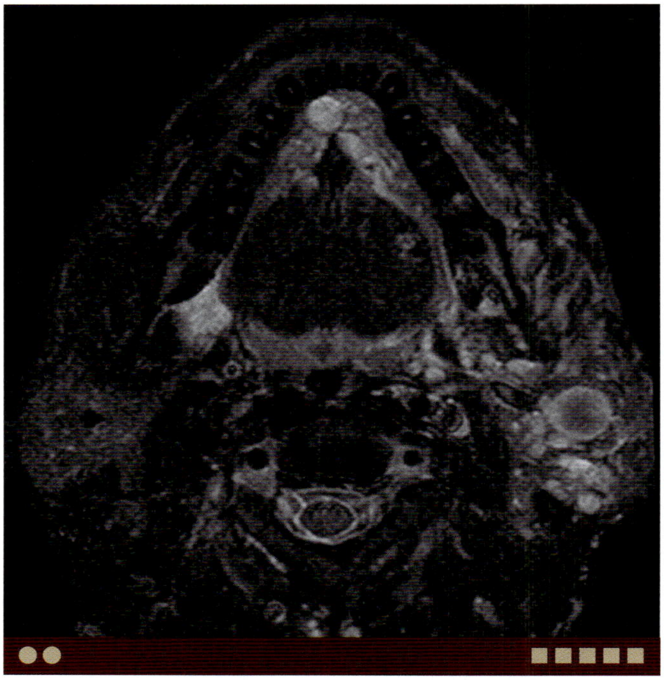

E. **Venolymphatic malformation**. Axial STIR MR image demonstrates a tubular, lobulated high-signal lesion in the sublingual space, left more than right. Note larger lesions involving the left masticator space and parotid gland.

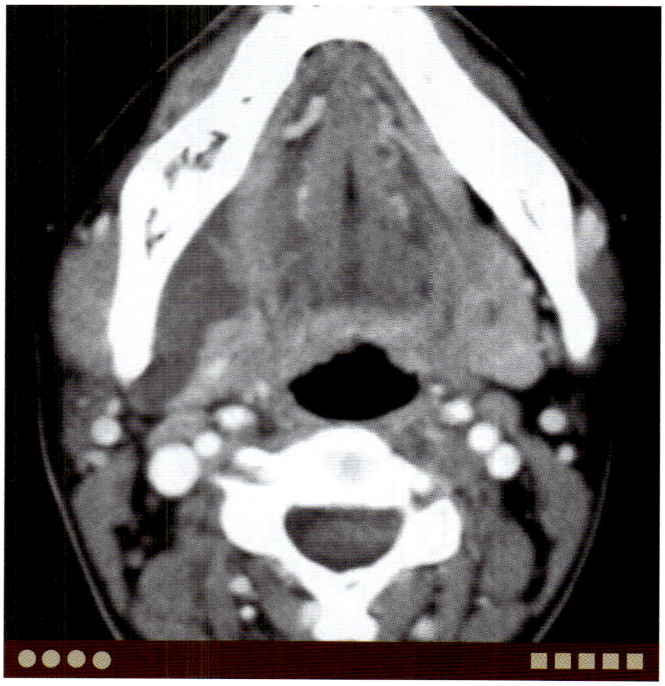

F. **Ranula**. Axial postcontrast CT demonstrates a well-defined water density lesion in the right submandibular space.

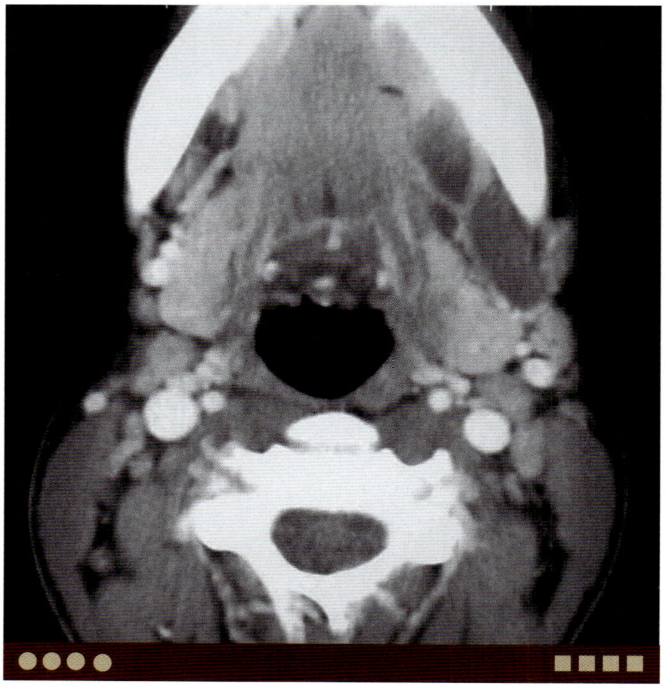

G. **Ranula** in a different patient. Axial postcontrast CT demonstrates a septated, well-defined water density lesion in the left submandibular space.

Case 8–14 Melanoma—Hard Palate

Brooke Devenney-Cakir, Osamu Sakai

PRESENTATION

Dark mass in the palate.

FINDINGS

CT demonstrates an avidly enhancing lesion in the mucosa of the oral cavity. T1W MR image demonstrates a hyperintense lesion.

DIFFERENTIAL DIAGNOSIS

- Squamous cell carcinoma (SCCA): SCCA is the most common malignancy in the oral cavity including the palate. CT demonstrates a heterogeneously enhancing lesion invading the adjacent bone, maxilla, or mandible.
- Mucoepidermoid carcinoma: This arises from the minor salivary gland of the oral cavity or oropharynx. High-grade lesions tend to show high cellularity while low-grade tumors tend demonstrate cystic appearance.
- Adenoid cystic carcinoma: This is also a minor salivary gland malignant tumor, commonly demonstrating perineural tumor spread. T2 low signal suggests high cellularity, high-grade, tumor, and poor outcome.

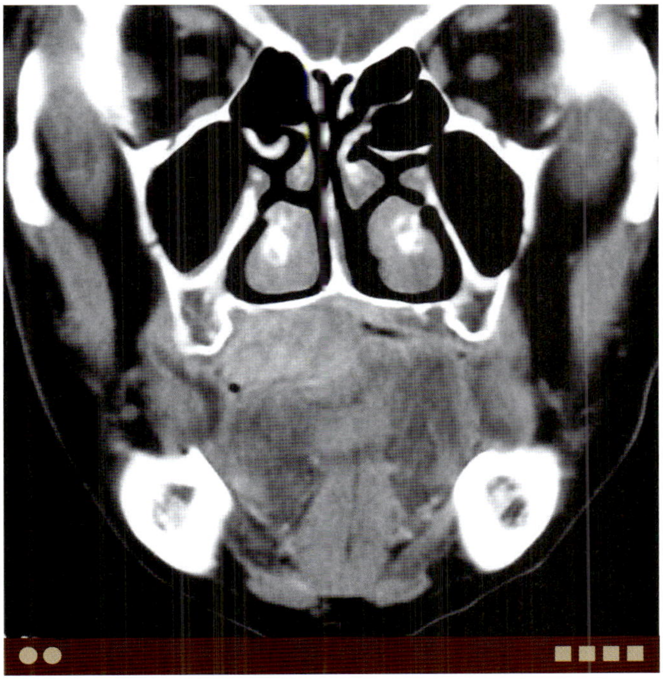

A. Melanoma. Coronal contrast-enhanced CT demonstrates a homogeneously enhancing ovoid tumor in the right palate.

COMMENTS

This is a 90-year-old woman with a dark palatal mass.

The incidence of malignant melanoma is increasing faster than any other human cancer with an increase in mortality rate second only to lung cancer. Melanoma accounts for 5% of all skin cancers but accounts for 65% of deaths. Twenty percent of melanomas occur in the head and neck. Malignant melanoma of the oral cavity is a rare condition, accounting for about 1% to 2% of all melanomas. Oral melanomas have extremely poor prognosis. The prognosis is closely related to tumor thickness and to the accompanying 50% prevalence of regional metastasis at presentation.

Given the rarity of oral melanoma in the general population, the risk factors are not clearly defined; however, possible etiologic factors include mechanical trauma, ill-fitting dentures, tobacco and alcohol use, and exposure to formaldehyde. However, in Japan, oral malignant melanoma is relatively common, with about 50% of cases occurring in the hard palate and the upper gingival.

Melanoma is highly vascular and often demonstrates avid enhancement on contrast-enhanced CT and MRI. Melanin has paramagnetic properties. Therefore, melanotic melanomas typically demonstrate a characteristic signal pattern—hyperintense on T1W and hypointense on T2W images. However, the signal pattern depends on degree of melanin concentration. "Amelanotic" melanoma shows nonspecific findings. Relatively homogeneous signal and avid enhancement, and bone erosion/remodeling are often seen.

PEARLS

- **Oral cavity melanoma is rare in the general population with a higher prevalence in Japan.**
- **Contrast-enhanced CT and MRI demonstrate avid enhancement.**
- **Melanotic melanomas have a characteristic intensity pattern appearing hyperintense on T1W and hypointense on T2W images.**

ADDITIONAL IMAGES (B-G)

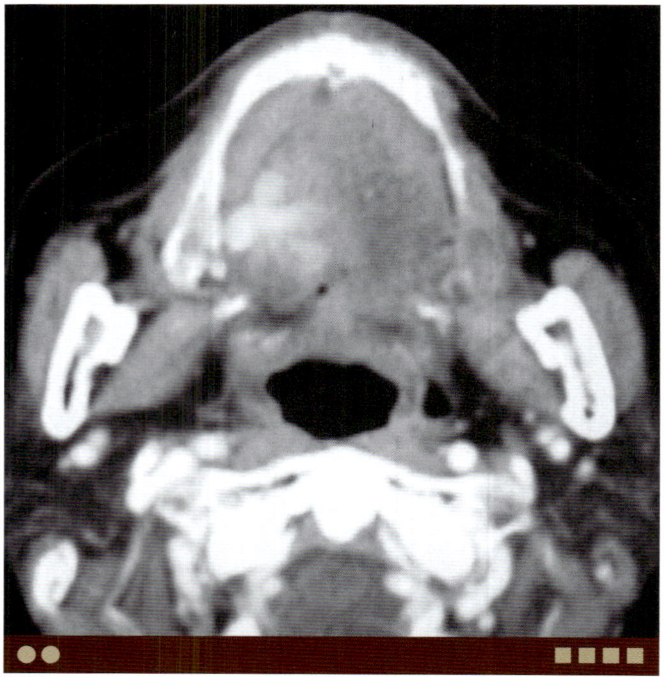

B. Melanoma, same patient as A. Axial contrast- enhanced CT demonstrates a slightly lobulated, avidly enhancing mass within the right aspect of the hard palate.

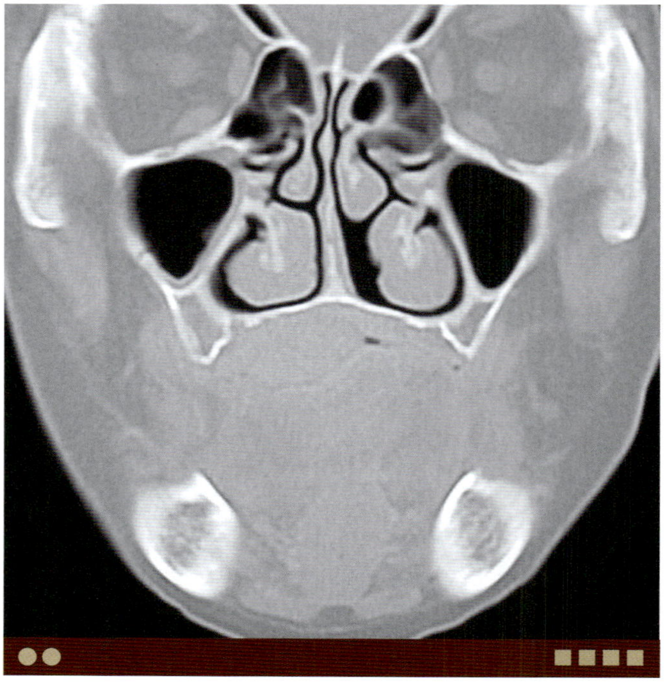

C. Melanoma, same patient as A. Coronal bone window CT demonstrates no bone destruction.

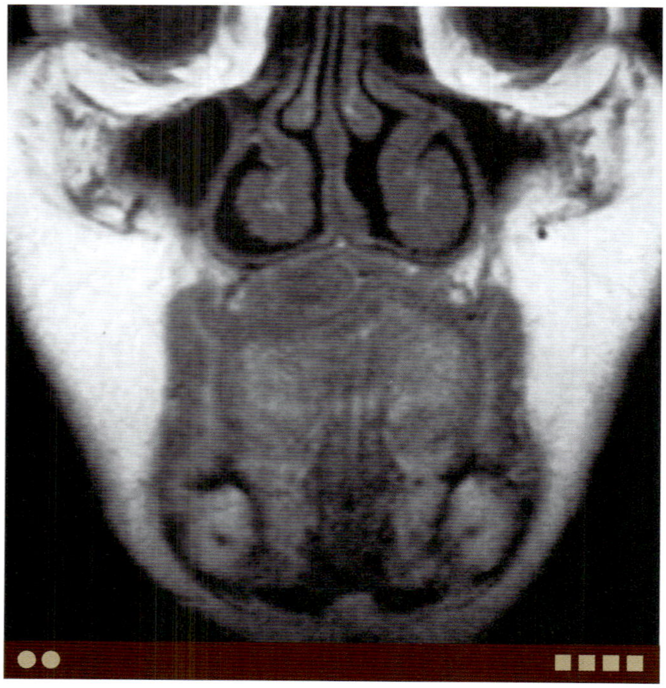

D. Melanoma, same patient as A. Coronal T1W image demonstrates a slightly heterogeneous isointense to slightly hyperintense lesion within right hard palate.

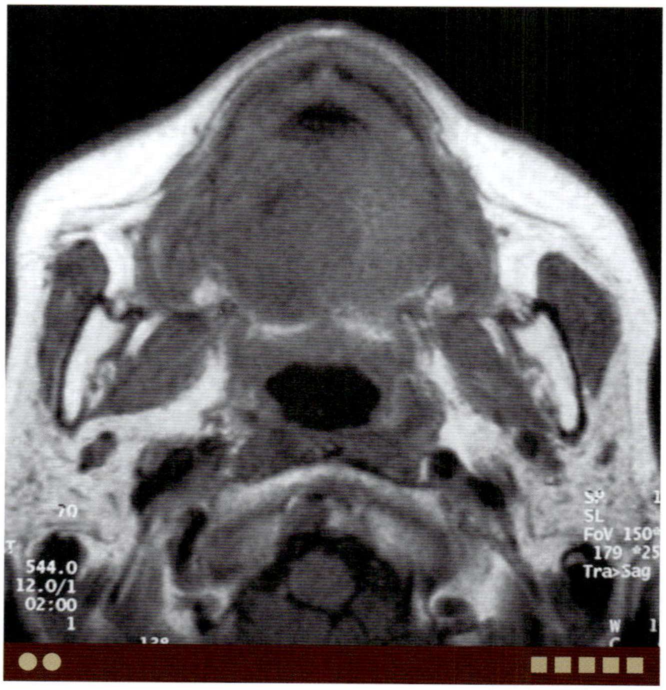

E. Melanoma, same patient as A. Axial T1W image demonstrates a low-signal lesion within right hard palate.

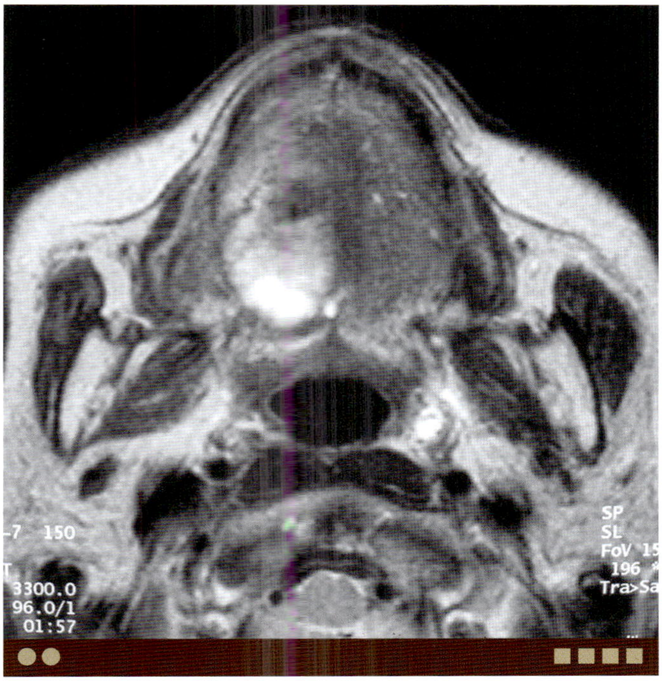

F. Melanoma, same patient as A. Axial T2W image demonstrates a slightly lobulated, high-signal lesion within right hard palate.

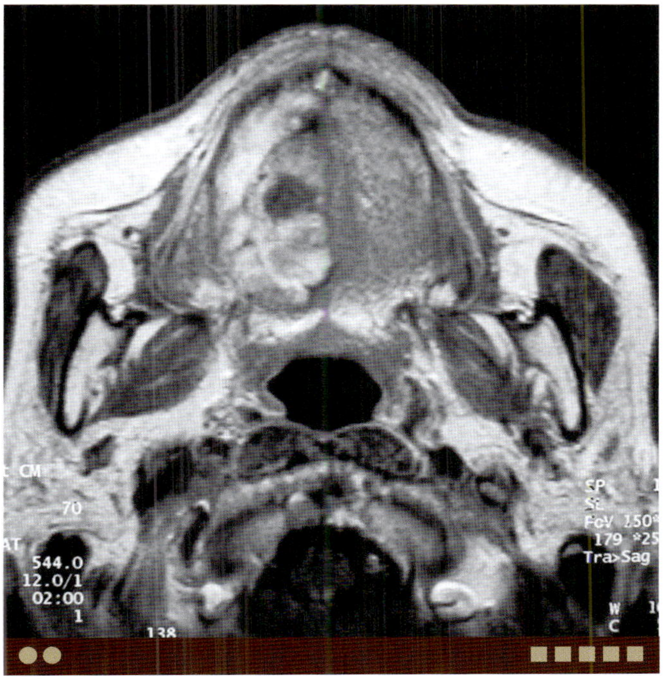

G. Melanoma, same patient as A. Axial postcontrast T1W image demonstrates a lobulated heterogeneously enhancing tumor within right hard palate.

DIFFERENTIAL DIAGNOSIS IMAGES (H-J)

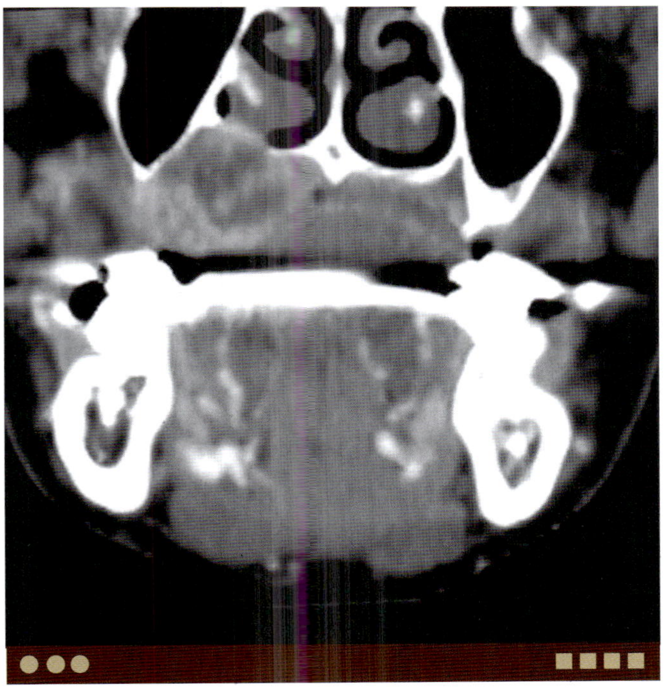

H. Adenoid cystic carcinoma. Coronal contrast-enhanced CT demonstrates a heterogeneously enhancing tumor in the right palate eroding the bone.

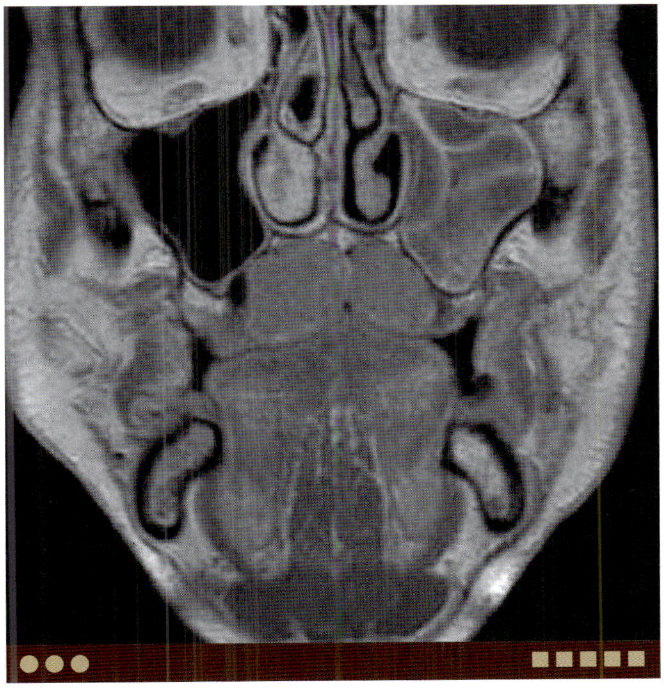

I. Lymphoma. Coronal postcontrast T1W MR image demonstrates homogeneously enhancing lesions expanding the hard palate bilaterally.

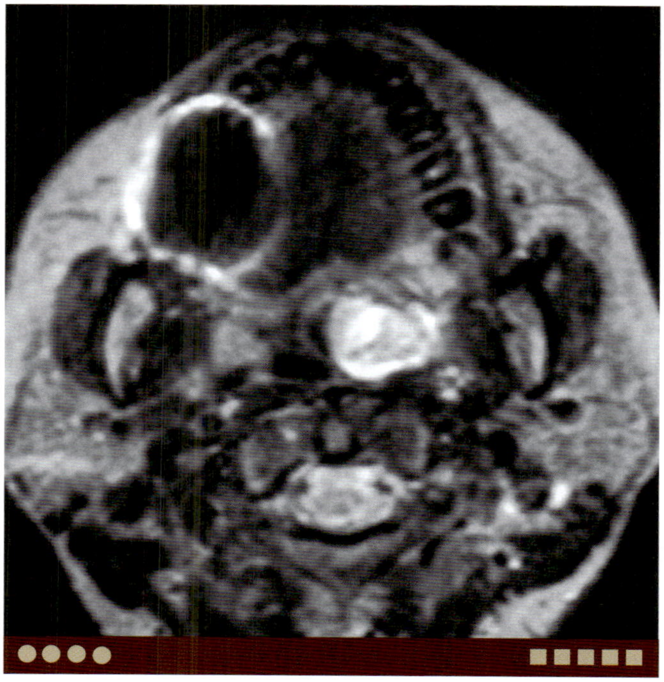

J. Pleomorphic adenoma. Axial T2W MR image demonstrates a slightly heterogeneous high-signal tumor in the left palate.

Case 8–15 Peritonsillar Abscess

Brooke Devenney-Cakir, Osamu Sakai

PRESENTATION

Fever, sore throat, and dysphagia.

FINDINGS

CT demonstrates a peripherally enhancing low-density lesion in the peritonsillar region causing mass effect on the adjacent airway.

DIFFERENTIAL DIAGNOSIS

- Tonsillar retention cyst: These patients are typically asymptomatic. There will not be adjacent soft tissue enhancement or edema. Focal calcifications can also be seen.
- Lymphoid hyperplasia of the tonsils: Tonsillar prominence is typically bilateral and symmetric, and typically associated with prominent adenoids and cervical adenopathy. Enhancing septa are seen on contrast-enhanced CT and MRI.
- Retropharyngeal abscess: This is abscess formation in the retropharyngeal space, typically accompanied by sepsis. Rim-enhancing fluid collection posterior to the pharynx and between the carotid arteries is seen.
- Tonsillar squamous cell carcinoma (SCCA): SCCA is typically poorly circumscribed with evidence of local invasion. SCCA with central necrosis and peripheral enhancement may mimic abscess.

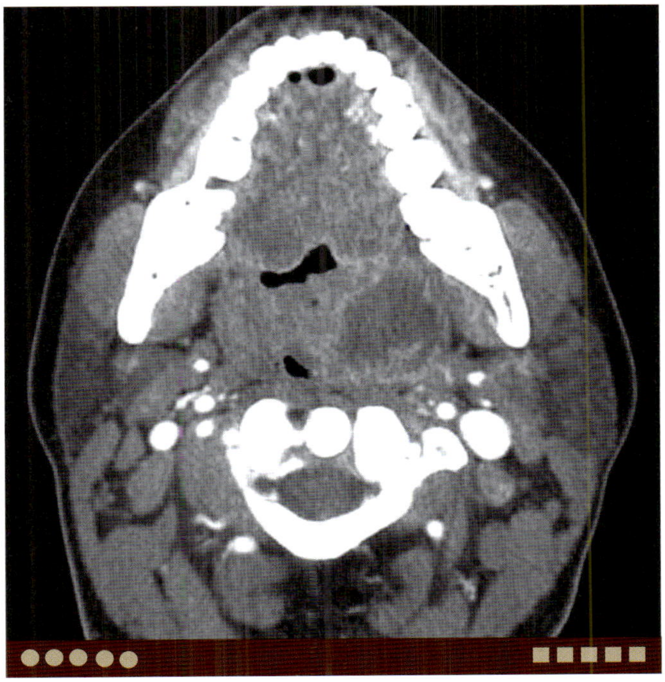

A. Peritonsillar abscess. Axial postcontrast CT demonstrates rim-enhancing fluid collection in the left peritonsillar region, lateral to the palatine tonsil. The parapharyngeal space fat is compressed.

COMMENTS

This is a 23-year-old woman with sore throat and fever.

Peritonsillar abscess is commonly seen in young adults, although it occurs at any age. It usually begins with acute tonsillitis manifested by tonsillar edema superficially and progresses into the deep soft tissues. Abscess formation can be seen within the tonsil or between the palatine tonsil and its capsule, usually at the superior pole. If left untreated, the tonsillar abscess may rupture into the pharyngeal airway or deep into the parapharyngeal and submandibular spaces. The most common organisms are beta-hemolytic *Streptococcus, Staphylococcus,* pneumococcus, and *Haemophilus.*

On CT, heterogeneous enhancement is seen in the peritonsillar soft tissue reflecting early infection, edema, and phlegmon development. This typically progresses onto abscess formation demonstrated on CT as a rim-enhancing fluid collection. Imaging is useful for diagnosis, presurgical localization of the peritonsillar abscess, and exclusion of trans-spatial abscess formation. MRI is not the first modality of choice; however, it is very useful to evaluate for abnormalities in the muscle and bone marrow.

PEARLS

- **Peritonsillar abscess is commonly seen in young adults, although it occurs at any age.**
- **Peritonsillar abscess is abscess formation between the palatine tonsil and its capsule, usually at the superior pole.**
- **CT is the modality of choice, and useful for diagnosis, presurgical localization of the abscess and exclusion of trans-spatial abscess formation.**

ADDITIONAL IMAGES (B-G)

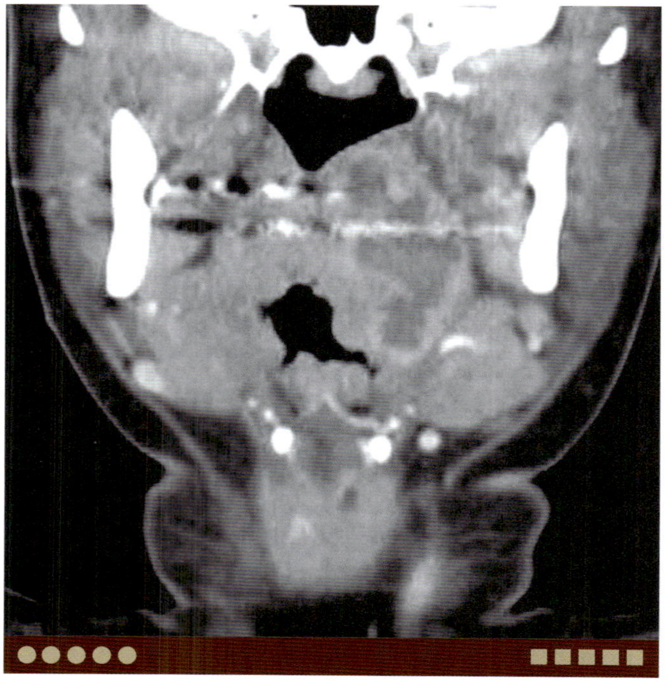

B. Peritonsillar abscess, same patient as A. Coronal postcontrast CT demonstrates craniocaudal extension of the slightly lobulated, rim-enhancing abscess, while bulging into the parapharyngeal space.

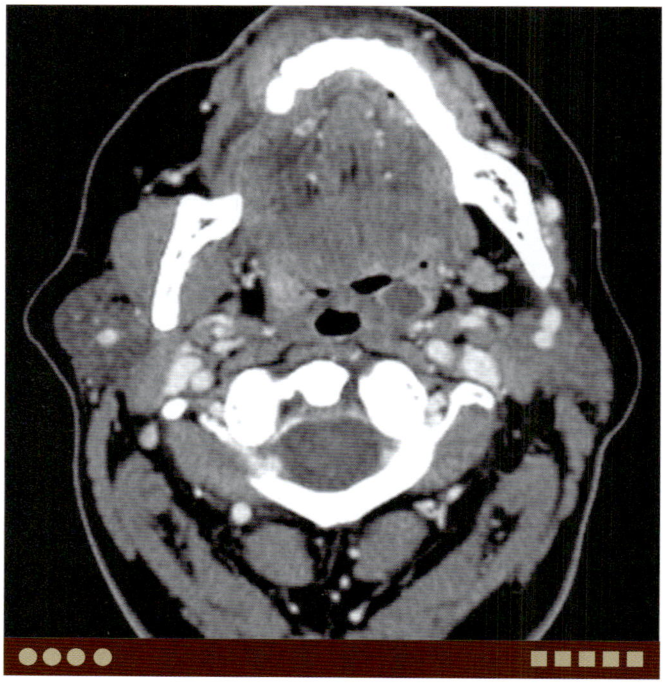

C. **Tonsillar abscess**. Axial postcontrast CT demonstrates a rim-enhancing fluid collection within the left palatine tonsil, close to the pharyngeal lumen.

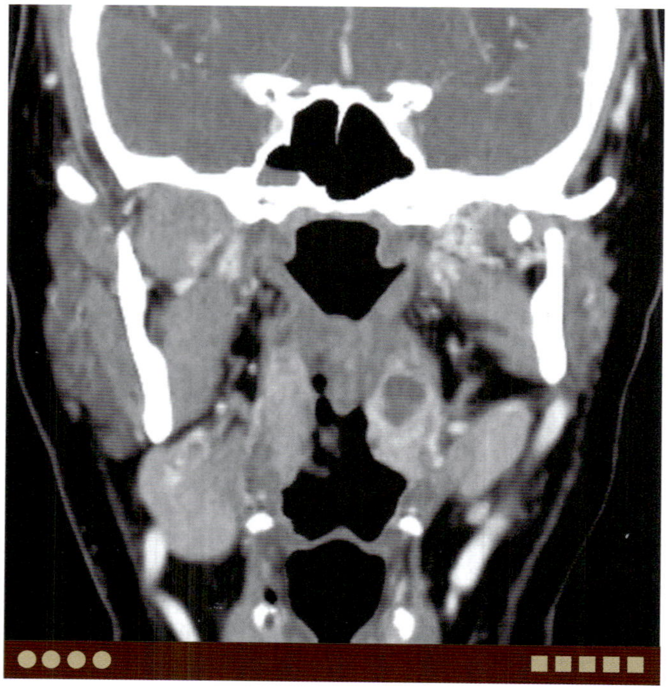

D. Tonsillar abscess, same patient as C. Coronal postcontrast CT demonstrates rim-enhancing fluid collection within the left palatine tonsil, close to the pharyngeal lumen.

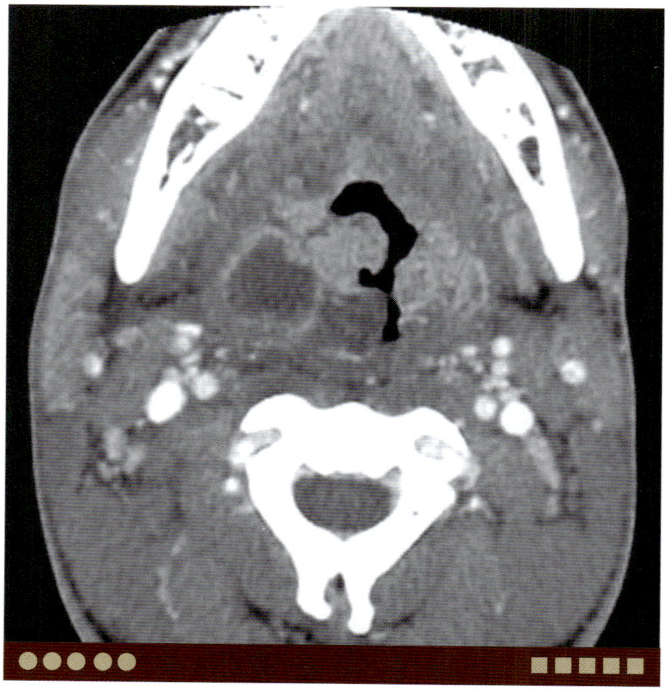

E. **Peritonsillar abscess** in a different patient. Axial postcontrast CT demonstrates a rim-enhancing fluid collection in the right peritonsillar region. The right palatine tonsil is displaced medially and narrowing the oropharyngeal lumen.

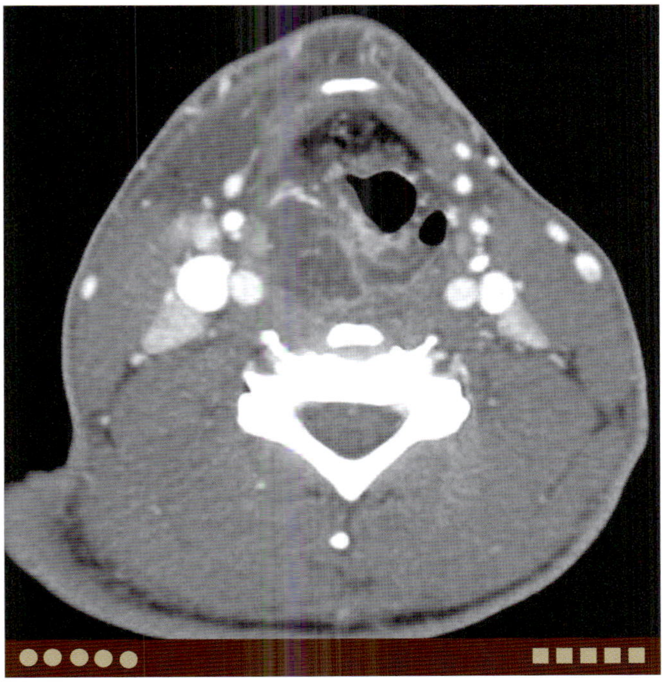

F. Peritonsillar abscess, same patient as E. Axial postcontrast CT demonstrates the abscess extending down to the level of pyriform sinus causing mass effect to the hypopharynx and supraglottic larynx. Note edema in the anterior neck superficially and enhancing level II nodes.

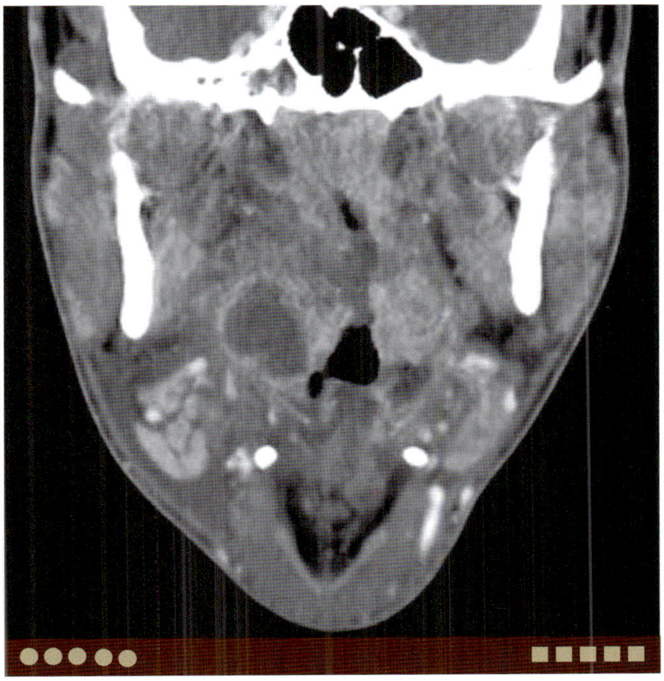

G. Peritonsillar abscess, same patient as E. Coronal postcontrast CT demonstrates the right peritonsillar abscess and edema in the right parapharyngeal and submandibular spaces.

DIFFERENTIAL DIAGNOSIS IMAGES (H-J)

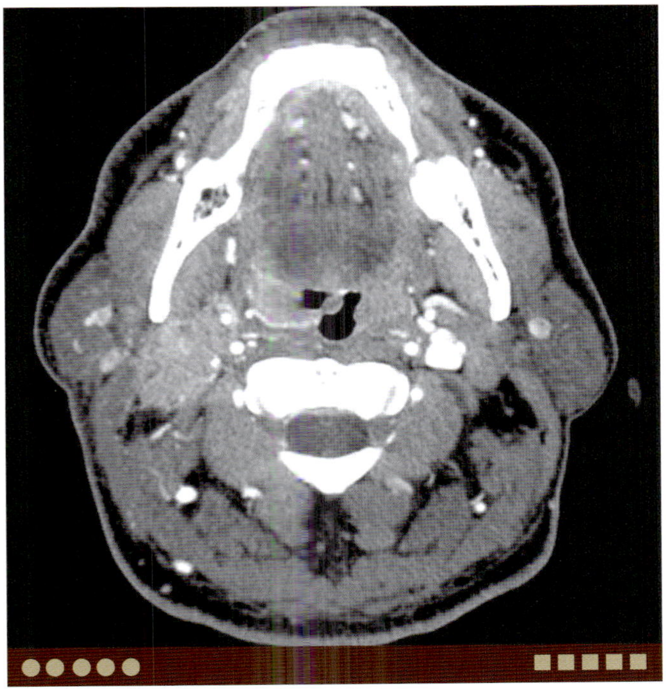

H. SCCA. Axial contrast-enhanced CT demonstrates a heterogeneously enhancing lesion in the right tonsil. Note enhancing right level II lymph nodes with poorly defined margins consistent with nodal metastasis with extracapsular tumor extension.

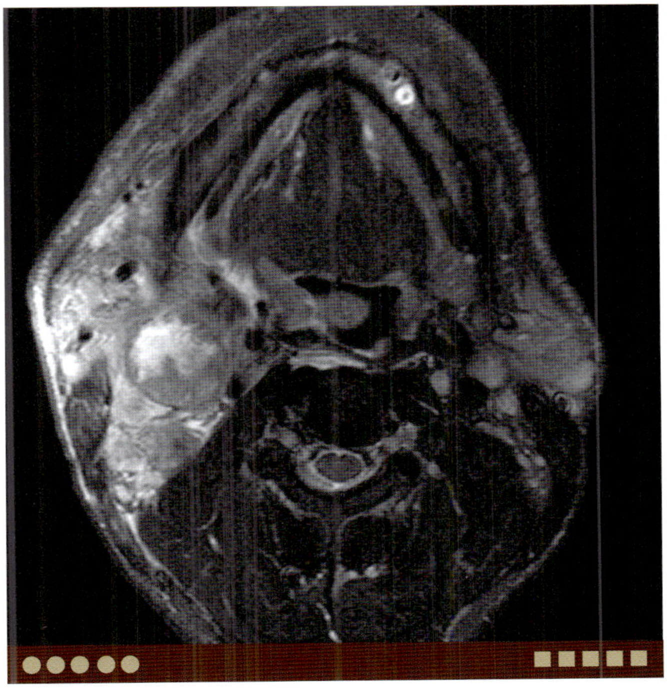

I. SCCA in a different patient. Axial fat-suppressed T2W image demonstrates a small intermediate lesion in the right palatine tonsil with poorly marginated large necrotic right level II nodes consistent with nodal metastasis with extracapsular tumor extension.

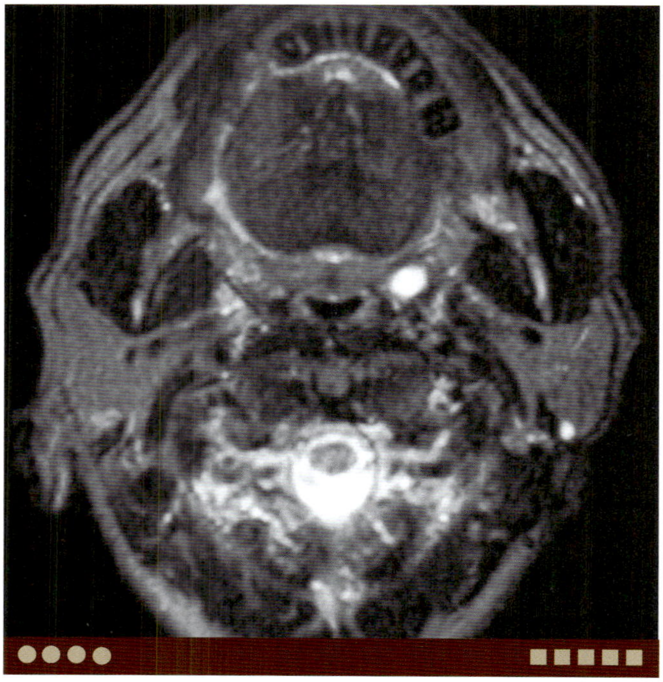

J. **Retention cyst**. Axial fat-suppressed T2W image demonstrates a cystic lesion in the left palatine tonsil without invasive findings.

Case 8–16 Lymphatic Malformation

Akifumi Fujita, Margaret Chapman, Osamu Sakai

PRESENTATION

Cheek swelling.

FINDINGS

CT and MR show a multilocular cystic mass with fluid–fluid levels within the submandibular region.

DIFFERENTIAL DIAGNOSIS

- Venous malformation: This condition also demonstrates high intensity on T2W images, however, enhances after contrast administration.
- Dermoid/epidermoid cyst: This condition is usually unilocular and often occurs in midline. Dermoid demonstrates fat density/signal intensity.
- Ranula: This condition usually occurs off-midline in the sublingual space. It occasionally extends to the submandibular space, so-called diving ranula.
- Thyroglossal duct cyst: This lesion is usually located at midline or slightly off-midline along the thyroglossal duct.
- Second branchial cleft cyst This lesion is usually unilocular and located posterior to the submandibular gland, anteromedial to the sternocleidomastoid muscle, and lateral to the carotid artery.

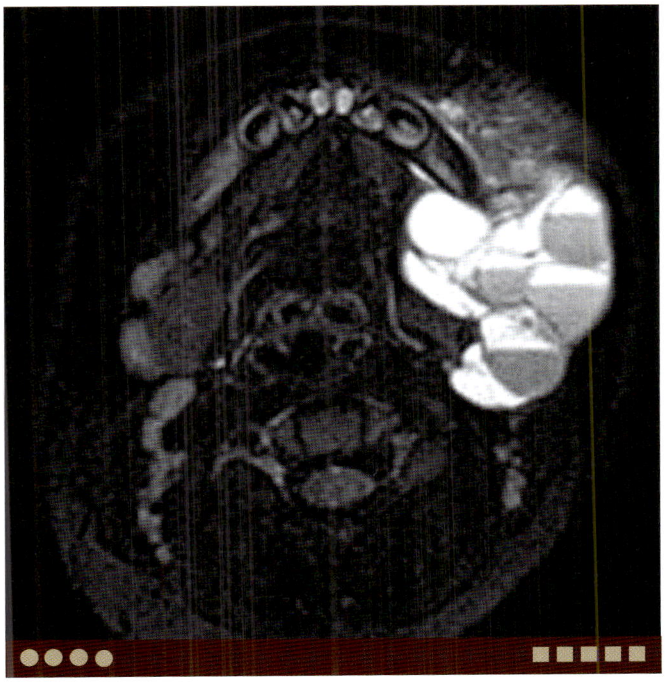

A. Lymphatic malformation. Axial STIR image demonstrates a multilocular cystic mass within the left submandibular region. Note the fluid–fluid level inside the mass.

COMMENTS

This is a 3-year-old girl with left cheek swelling after trauma.

Lymphatic malformations also known as lymphangiomas develop from congenital obstruction of lymphatic drainage. They can reside within vascular malformations and are considered to be a part of a spectrum of manifestations of the same pathologic process. These malformations tend to surround and infiltrate into normal anatomic structures. Approximately 75% of lymphatic malformations occur in the neck, generally in the posterior triangle, and 3% to 10% extend into the mediastinum. Spontaneous regression occurs in 6% of cases. Most often, lymphatic malformations are asymptomatic and manifest as painless masses. Ninety percent are detected by 2 years of age.

On CT and MRI, lymphatic malformations appear as multilocular, poorly circumscribed trans-spatial masses of fluid attenuation or signal intensity. After intravenous contrast material administration, there is usually no apparent central enhancement; however, the walls of septa may enhance, particularly if there is a history of surgery or infection. Occasionally, hemorrhagic areas and fluid–fluid levels can be seen. MRI is the most accurate technique for evaluating the extent of the lesion, the relationship of the lesion to neurovascular structures, and any associated venous malformations, factors that may be important for surgical planning.

PEARLS

- **Lymphatic malformations are considered to be a part of a spectrum of vascular manifestations of the same pathologic process.**
- **CT and MR images show multilocular masses of fluid attenuation/signal intensity.**

ADDITIONAL IMAGES (B-D)

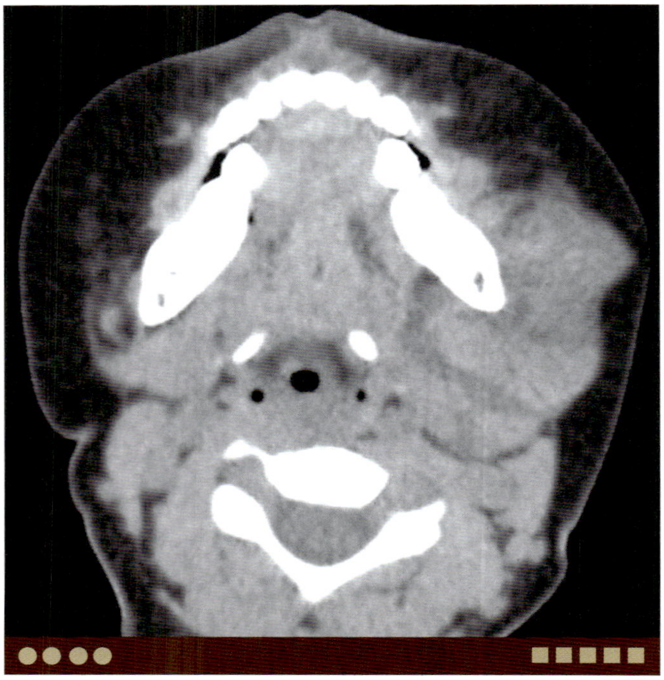

B. Lymphatic malformation, same patient as A. Axial CT demonstrates a multilocular cystic mass within the left submandibular region. Note the fluid–fluid level inside the mass and the dorsal high density suggestive of hemorrhage.

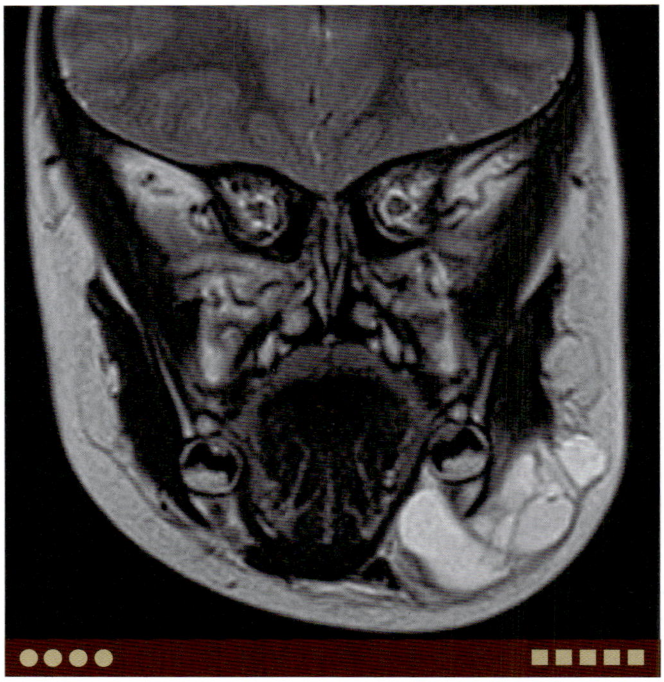

C. Lymphatic malformation, same patient as A. Coronal T2W image demonstrates a multilocular cystic mass within the left submandibular region.

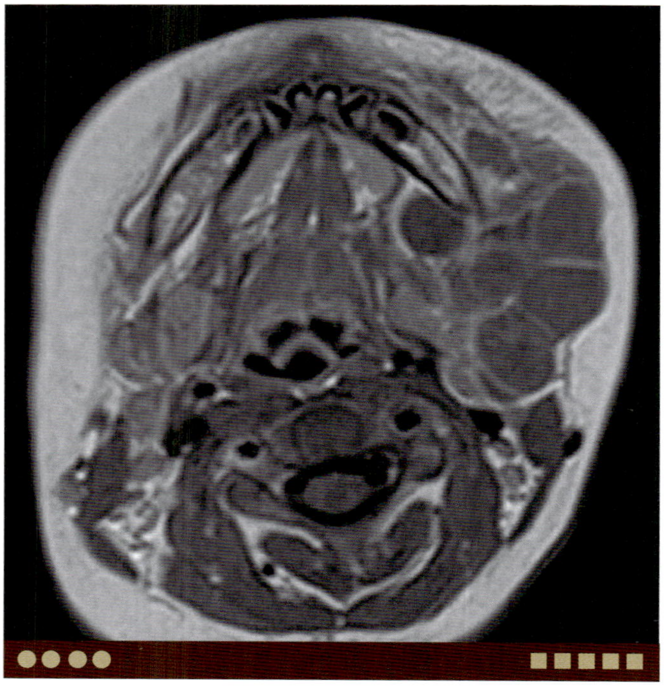

D. Lymphatic malformation, same patient as A. Axial postcontrast T1W image demonstrates a multilocular cystic mass within the left submandibular region with fluid–fluid level. Note the enhancing septa.

DIFFERENTIAL DIAGNOSIS IMAGES (E-J)

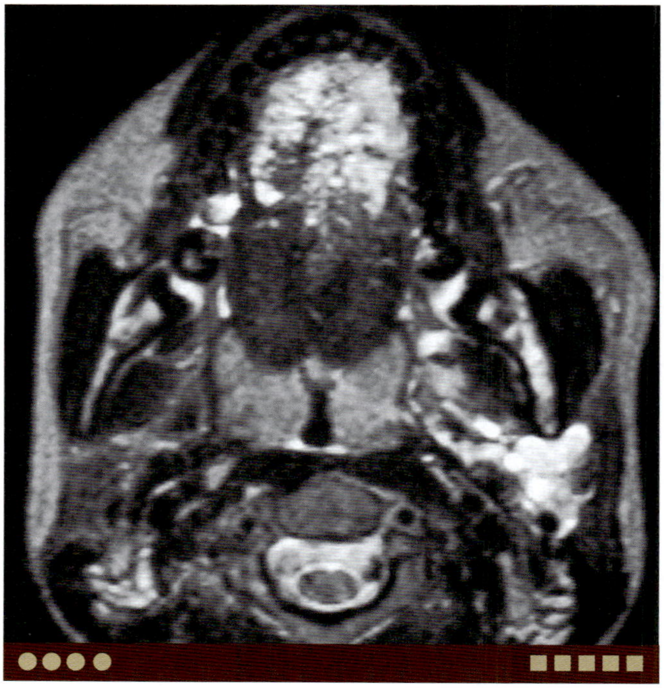

E. **Venolymphatic malformation**. Axial T2W image shows an ill-defined heterogeneous high-intensity lesion of the tongue. Left parapharyngeal and parotid lesions are also noted.

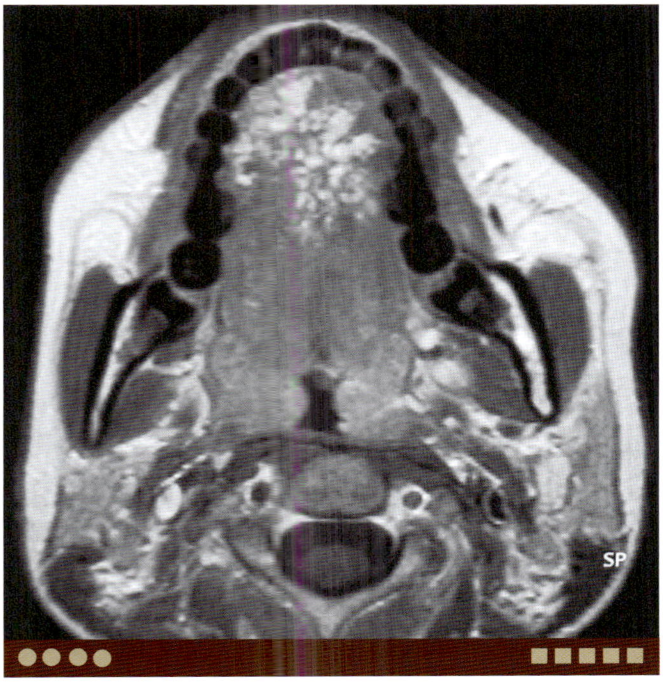

F. Venolymphatic malformation, same patient as E. Axial postcontrast T1W image shows heterogeneous enhancement of the tongue, left parapharyngeal space, and left parotid gland.

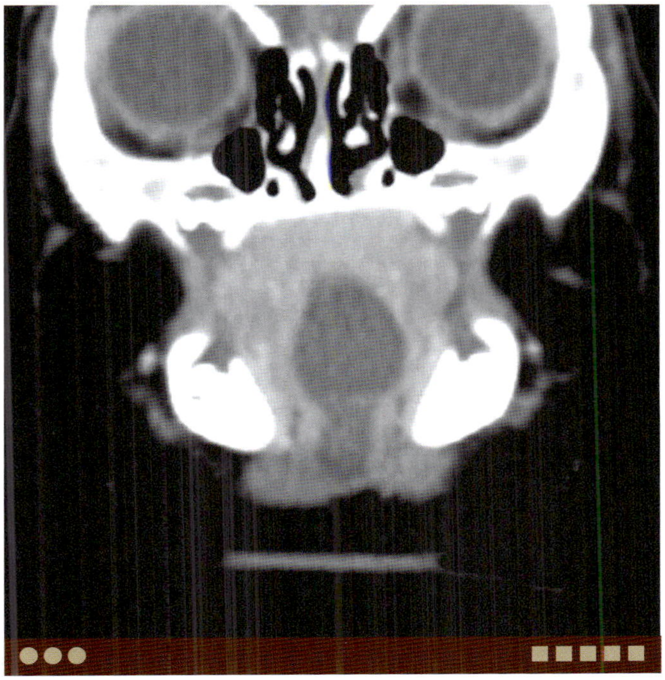

G. **Dermoid**. Coronal contrast-enhanced CT demonstrates a cystic mass at the midline of the sublingual space.

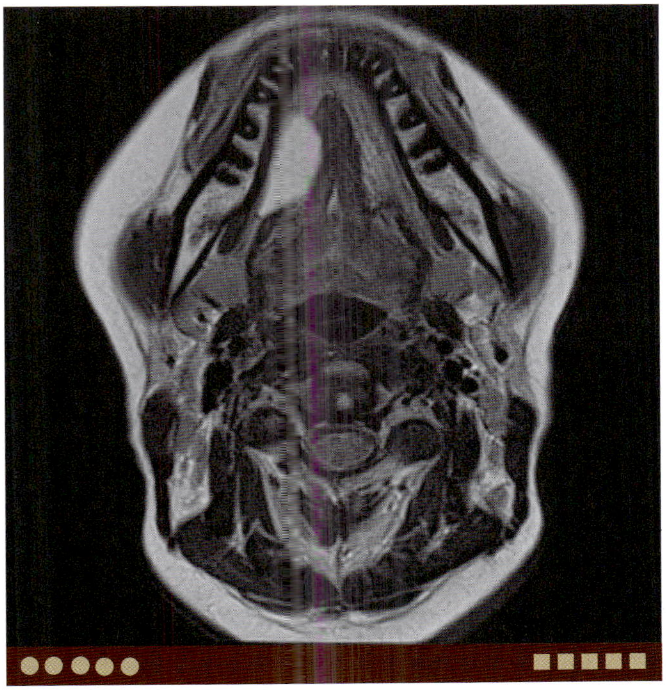

H. **Ranula**. Axial T2W image demonstrates a well-circumscribed cystic mass within the right sublingual space.

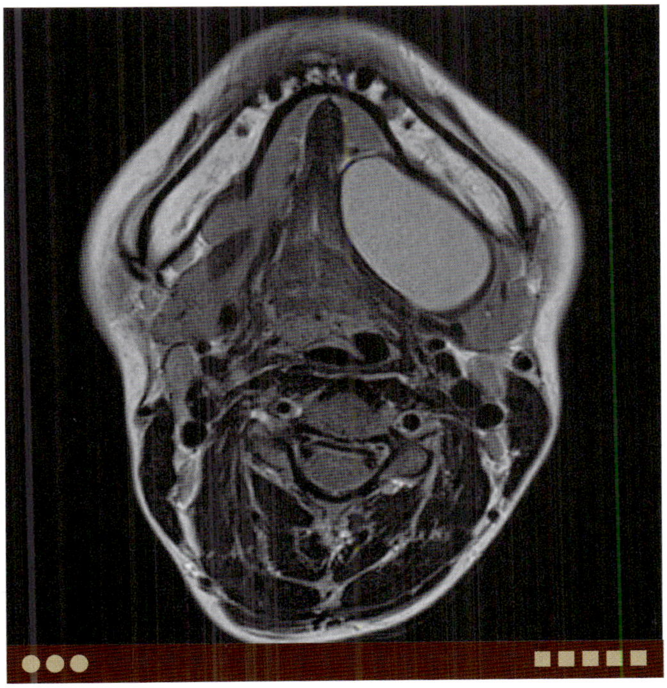

I. **Epidermoid**. Axial T2W image demonstrates a well-circumscribed high-signal intensity cystic mass in the left sublingual space.

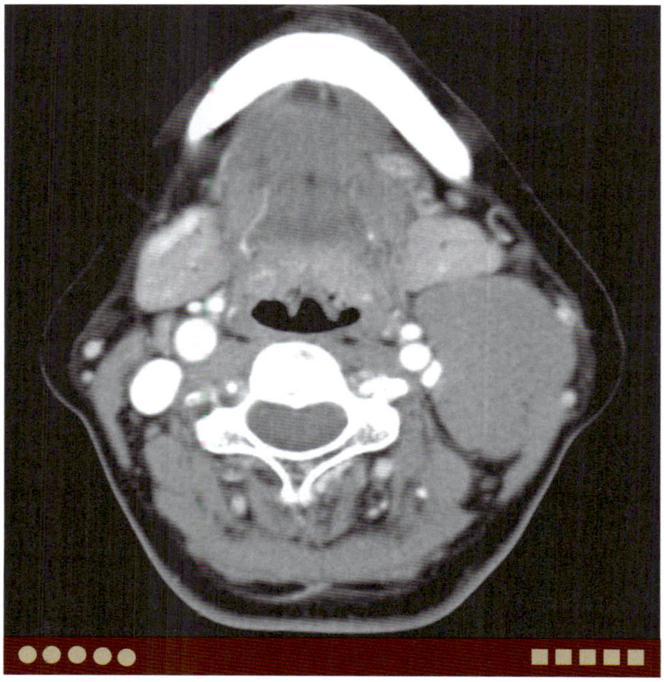

J. Second branchial cleft cyst. Axial postcontrast CT image demonstrates a unilocular cystic mass posterior to submandibular gland, anteromedial to sternocleidomastoid muscle, and lateral to the carotid artery.

Case 8–17 Arteriovenous Malformation (AVM)

Akifumi Fujita, Margaret Chapman, Osamu Sakai

PRESENTATION

Cheek swelling.

FINDINGS

CT and MR imaging demonstrate an enlarged vascular component within the buccal and masticator spaces.

DIFFERENTIAL DIAGNOSIS

- Venous malformation: This lesion usually demonstrates high-signal intensity on T2W images without flow-voids to suggest high-flow components and late phase enhancement after contrast administration. Presence of phlebolith suggests venous malformation.
- Lymphatic malformation: This lesion usually demonstrates multilocular masses of fluid attenuation/signal intensity. Postcontrast images show no apparent central enhancement; however, the walls or septa may enhance.

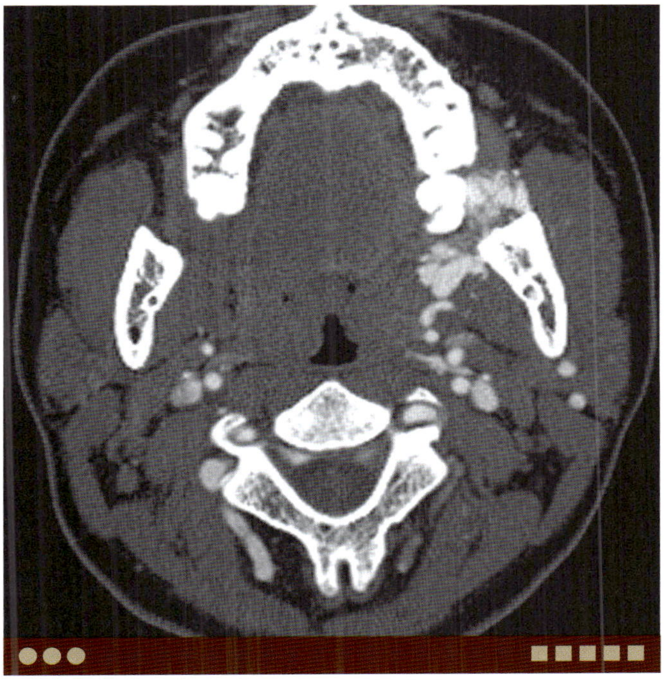

A. AVM. Axial postcontrast CT (CTA) demonstrates enlarged tortuous vascular components within the left buccal space.

COMMENTS

This is a 24-year-old woman with left cheek swelling.

AVMs are abnormal, direct communications between arteries and veins. They are usually high-flow malformations and thus fistulas are included in this category. The head and neck region is considered to be one of the more common sites for these malformations, including areas such as the tongue, lip, and cheek. Although AVMs are uncommon in the jaw, they may occur within the ramus and posterior mandibular body. Identification of an AVM in these locations is important as there is the potential for fatal hemorrhage after tooth extraction. AVMs are often treated conservatively, although surgical excision and embolization are possible.

Contrast-enhanced CT or CT angiography is very useful to demonstrate the enlarged and tortuous arteries and draining veins. It is extremely important to evaluate the lesion in bone windows to assess for osseous involvement. Demineralization and multiloculated cystic-appearing lesions may also be seen on radiographs.

On MRI, the enlarged arterial components appear as flow-voids on T1W and T2W images. Loss of normal high signal from fat in the mandible on T1W images suggests osseous involvement. Time-of-flight MRA may not be very useful, but dynamic contrast-enhanced MRA usually provides useful information regarding the extent of the lesion.

Catheter angiography is usually not necessary to make a diagnosis; however, it is useful to confirm the diagnosis and for treatment planning. These lesions typically do not show significant parenchymal staining on angiography.

PEARLS

- **AVMs are abnormal, direct communications between arteries and veins. They are usually high-flow lesions.**
- **MRI demonstrates the enlarged arterial components as flow-voids on T1W and T2W images.**
- **Catheter angiography is usually not necessary to make a diagnosis; however, it is useful to confirm the diagnosis and for treatment planning.**

ADDITIONAL IMAGES (B-F)

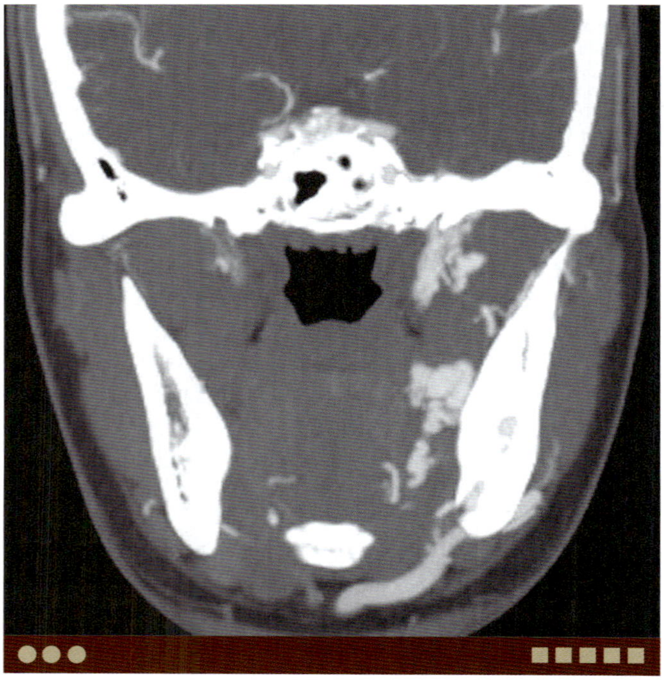

B. AVM, same patient as A. Coronal postcontrast CT (MIP) demonstrates enlarged tortuous vascular component within the left buccal, parapharyngeal, and masticator spaces. Note loss of normal fatty marrow in the left mandible.

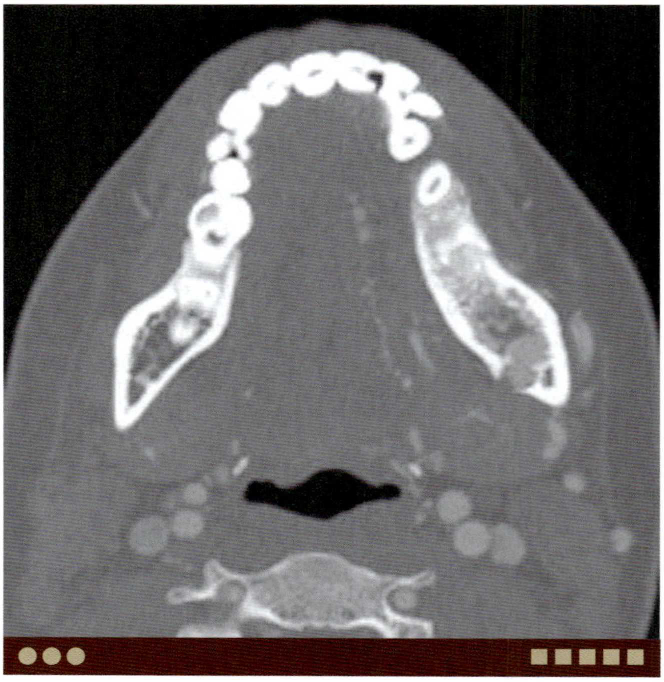

C. AVM, same patient as A. Axial postcontrast CT in bone windows demonstrates erosion of the mandible due to the enlarged vascular component inside.

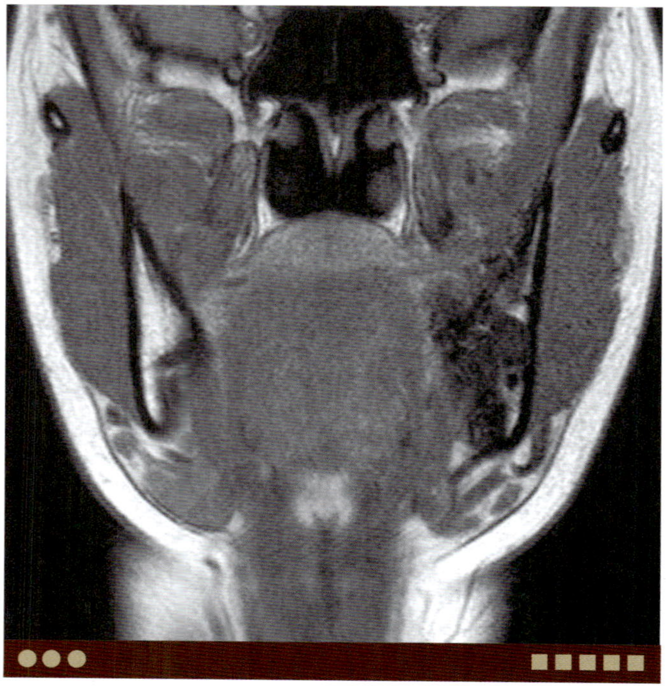

D. AVM, same patient as A. Coronal T1W image demonstrates loss of normal high signal from fatty marrow and signal-voids from high-flow vessels in the left mandible.

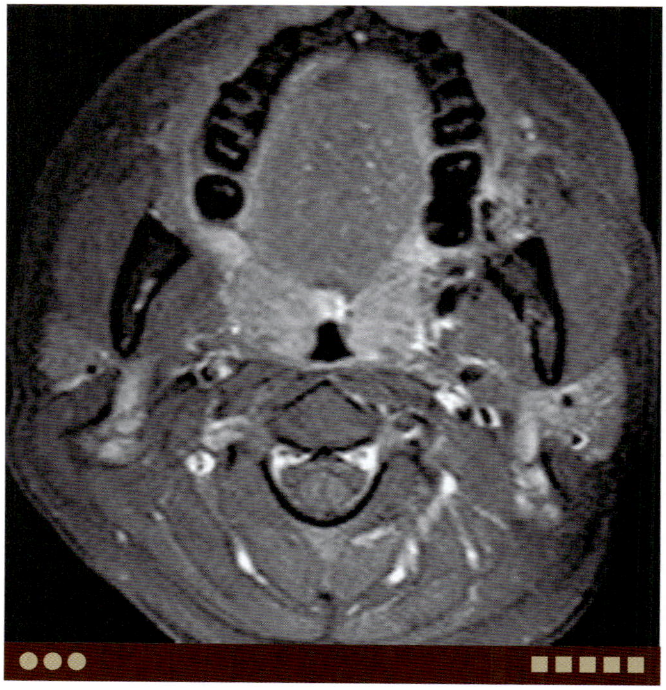

E. AVM, same patient as A. Axial postcontrast fat-suppressed T1W image demonstrates heterogeneous enhancement and flow-voids in the left buccal space.

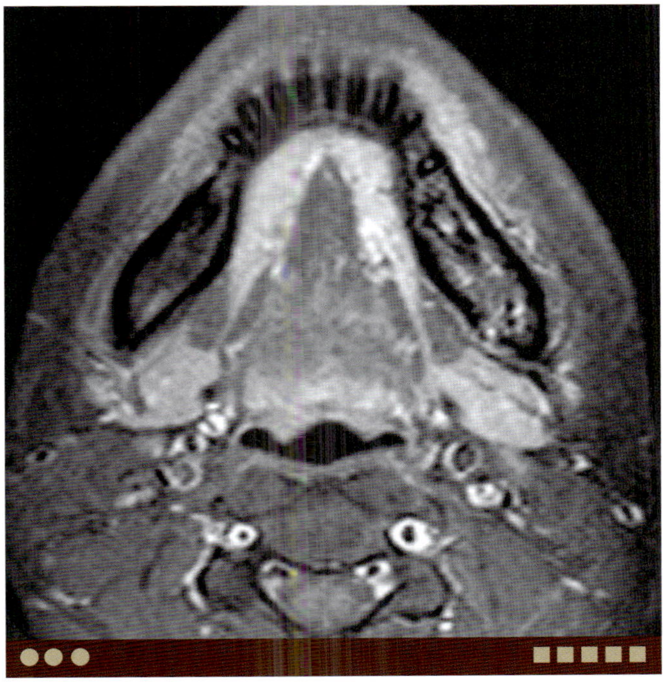

F. AVM, same patient as A. Axial postcontrast fat-suppressed T1W image also demonstrates flow-voids within the left mandible.

DIFFERENTIAL DIAGNOSIS IMAGES (G-J)

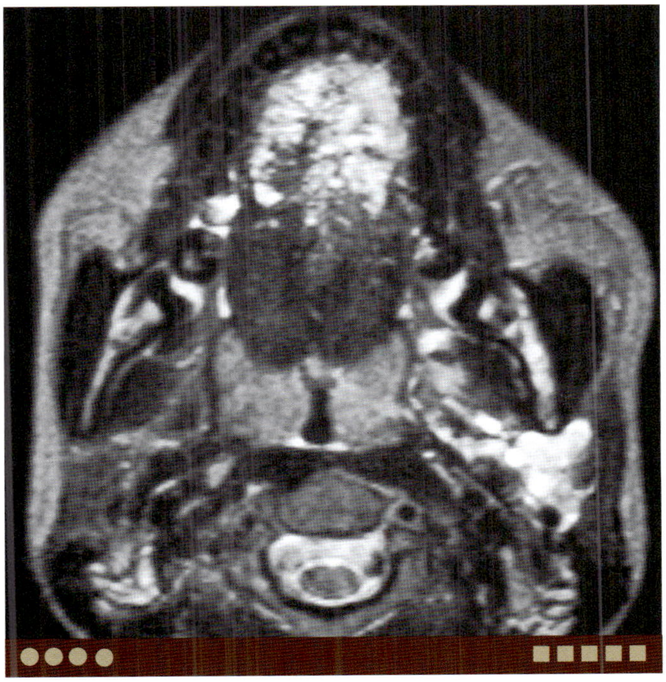

G. **Venolymphatic malformation**. Axial T2W image shows an ill-defined heterogeneous high-signal intensity lesion of the tongue. Left parapharyngeal and parotid lesions are also noted. Note no flow-voids in these lesions.

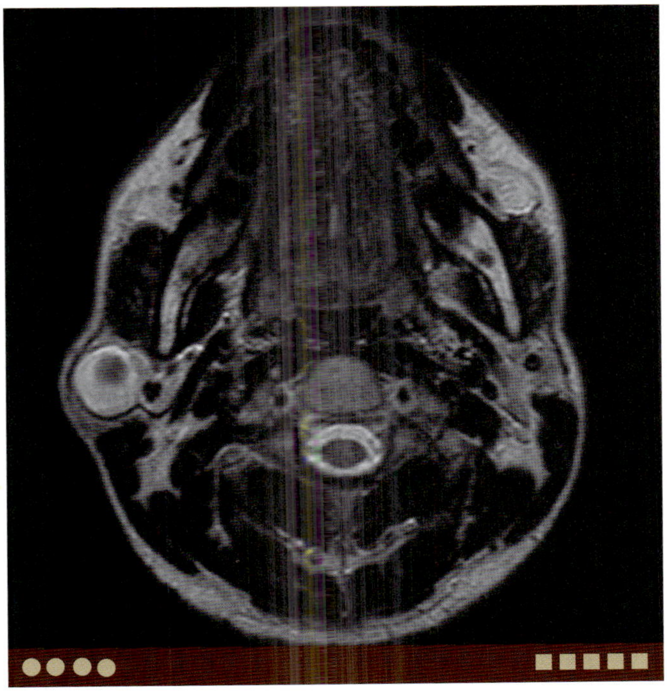

H. **Venolymphatic malformation** in a different patient. Axial T2W image demonstrates a high-signal intensity lesion within the right parotid space with internal signal-voids suggestive of phleboliths. No flow-voids are seen.

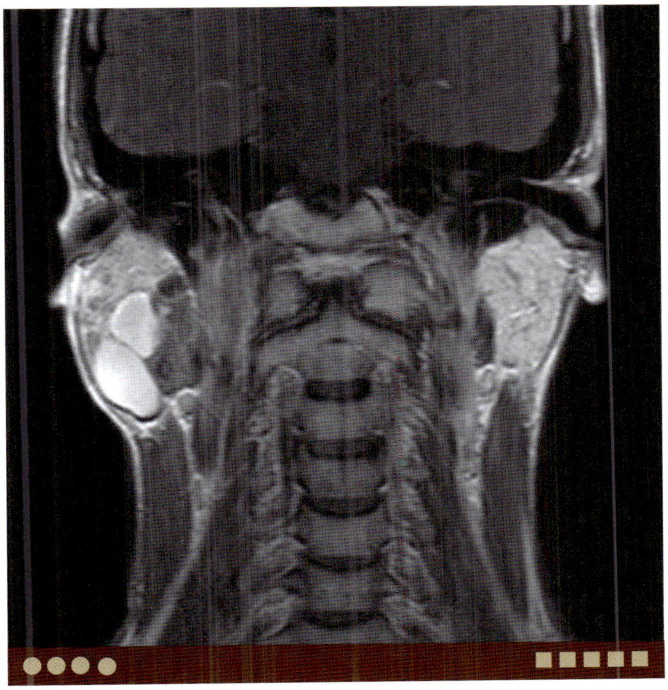

I. Venolymphatic malformation, same patient as H. Coronal post-contrast T1W image (late phase of dynamic study) demonstrates marked enhancement of the lesion within the right parotid space.

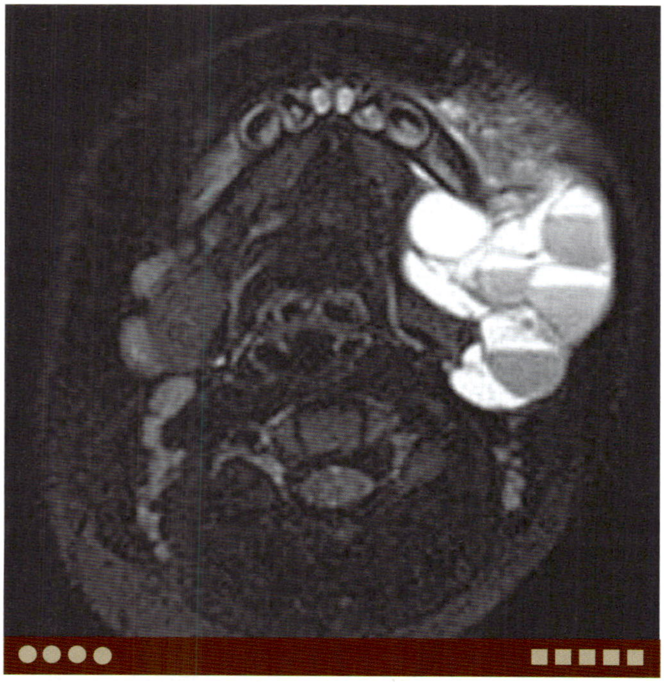

J. Lymphatic malformation. Axial STIR image demonstrates a multilocular cystic mass within the left submandibular region. Note the fluid–fluid level inside the mass without flow-voids.

Case 8–18 Mucoepidermoid Carcinoma—Palate

Hiroki Kato, Asim Mian, Osamu Sakai

PRESENTATION

Enlarging mass in the palate.

FINDINGS

CT and MRI demonstrate a benign- or malignant-appearing palatal lesion.

DIFFERENTIAL DIAGNOSIS

- Squamous cell carcinoma (SCCA): SCCA is the most common malignant tumor of the palate and usually shows ill-defined, infiltrative margins and heterogeneous density/signal and enhancement.
- Adenoid cystic carcinoma: Often a slow-growing, insidious disease with tendency to spread in a perineural fashion along the palatine branches of the maxillary division of the trigeminal nerve (V2).
- Pleomorphic adenoma: In the oropharynx/oral cavity, pleomorphic adenomas most commonly arise from the palate, followed by the upper lip and buccal mucosa. In the palate, they often cause remodeling/erosion of the adjacent bone.

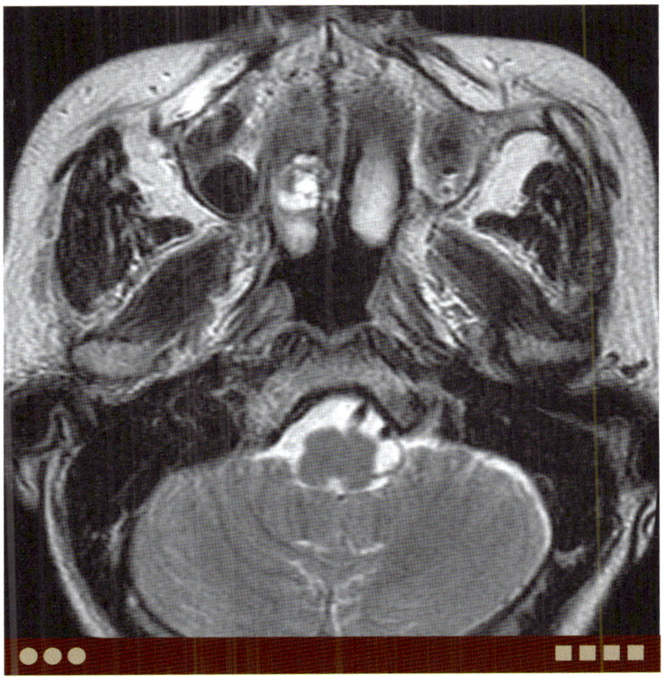

A. Mucoepidermoid carcinoma. Axial T2W MR image demonstrates a right palatal lesion with multicystic components suggesting a low-grade tumor.

COMMENTS

This is a 68-year-old woman presenting with a painless mass in the right palate.

Minor salivary gland cancers have their highest frequency in the posterior hard palate and soft palate. Mucoepidermoid carcinomas arise approximately 50% from the major salivary glands and 30% from the minor salivary glands. In the minor salivary glands, they most commonly arise from the palate; however, significant number of lesions may also be found in the retromolar region, floor of the mouth, lip, and tongue. Mucoepidermoid carcinoma is the most common malignant salivary gland neoplasm in children.

The histological pattern of mucoepidermoid carcinomas consists of a combination of squamous and mucous cells arranged in cords, sheets, or cystic configurations. They are classified as low-, intermediate-, and high-grade tumors. Low-grade mucoepidermoid carcinomas demonstrate smooth, "benign-appearing" margins and often have cystic areas containing mucin and occasionally with focal calcifications. They may have prominent cystic components and the cystic areas demonstrate high signal on both T1W and T2W images. Most areas of the tumors, except for the cystic components, show significantly low signal on T2W images, which may represent abundant fibrous tissue. Alternatively, high-grade mucoepidermoid carcinomas usually have poorly defined margins and may grossly infiltrate into the adjacent skin and soft tissues. High-grade mucoepidermoid carcinomas tend to be more solid with fewer cystic areas and are more homogeneous and often demonstrate intermediate-to-low signal on T2W images, reflecting their high cellularity.

PEARLS

- **Mucoepidermoid carcinoma is seen as a benign- or malignant-appearing mass.**
- **Low-grade mucoepidermoid carcinomas demonstrate smooth margins and are characterized by cystic components containing mucin.**
- **High-grade mucoepidermoid carcinomas tend to be more solid with fewer cystic areas and are more homogeneous, demonstrating low-to-intermediate signal on T2W images and have poorly defined margins.**

ADDITIONAL IMAGES (B-F)

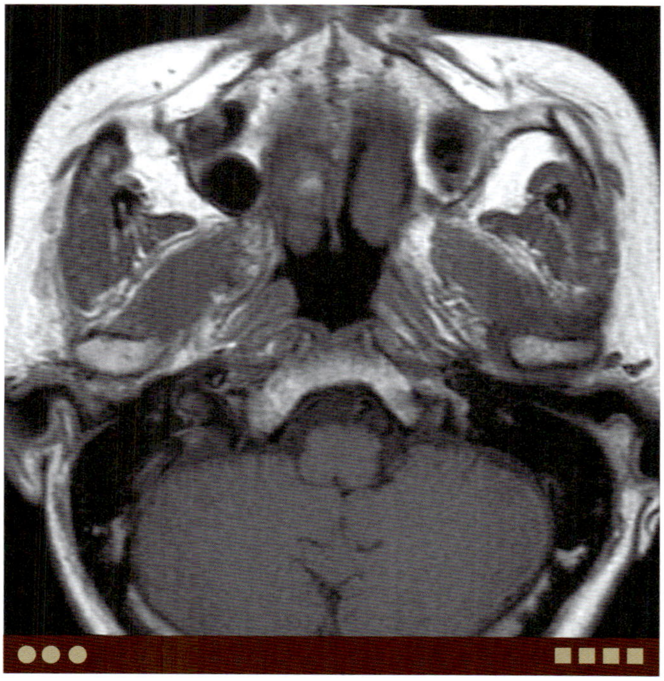

B. Mucoepidermoid carcinoma, same patient as A. Axial T1W image demonstrates a low-signal lesion with a focal high-signal area.

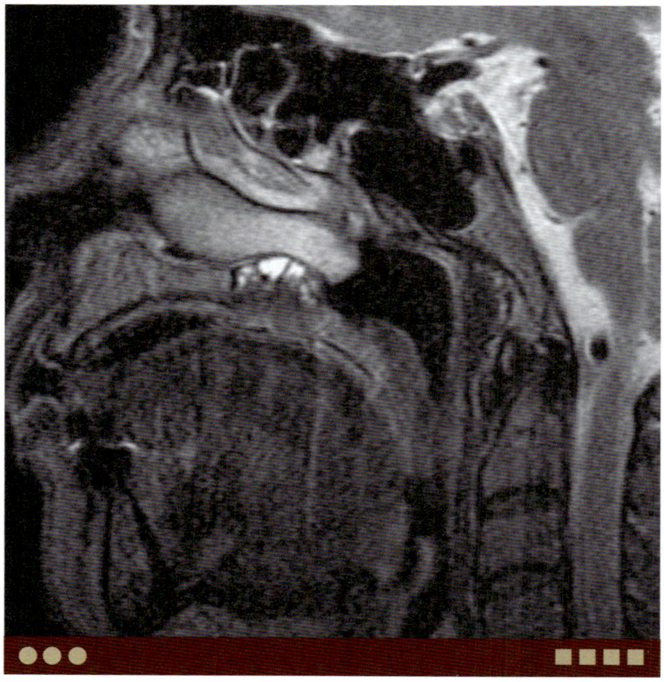

C. Mucoepidermoid carcinoma, same patient as A. Sagittal T2W image demonstrates a multicystic palatal lesion.

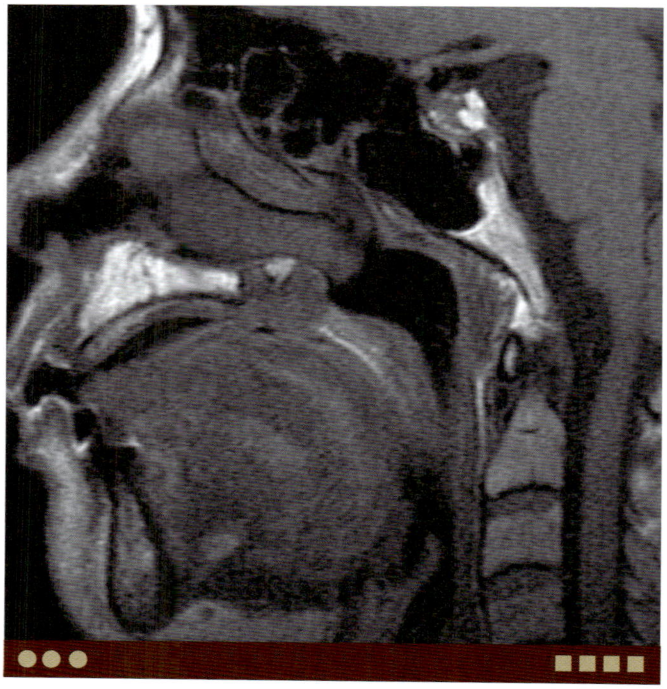

D. Mucoepidermoid carcinoma, same patient as A. Sagittal T1W image demonstrates a low-signal lesion with a focal high-signal area.

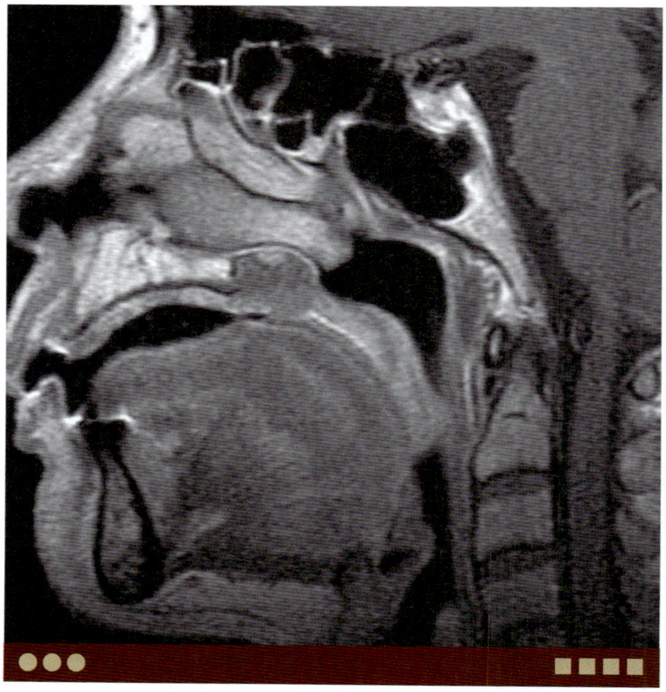

E. Mucoepidermoid carcinoma, same patient as A. Sagittal post-contrast T1W image demonstrates mottled enhancement.

DIFFERENTIAL DIAGNOSIS IMAGES (G-J)

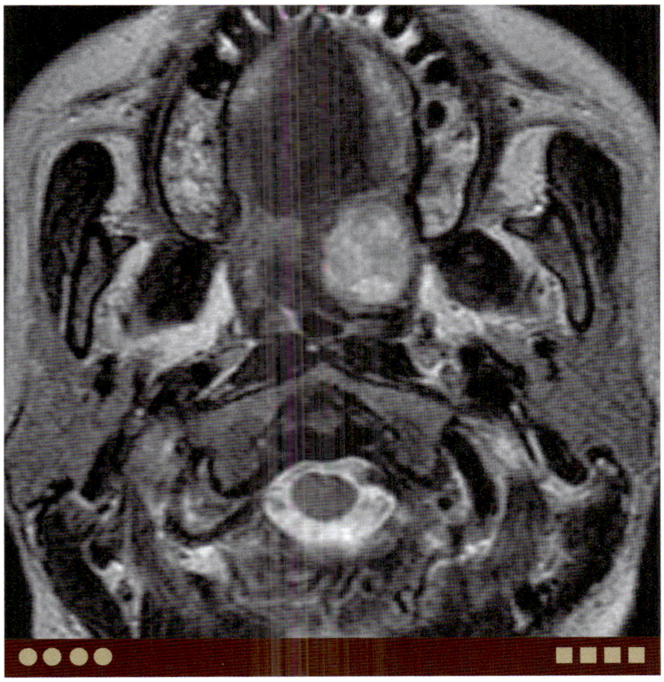

F. Pleomorphic adenoma. Axial T2W MR image demonstrates a well-demarcated left palatal lesion with heterogeneously high signal.

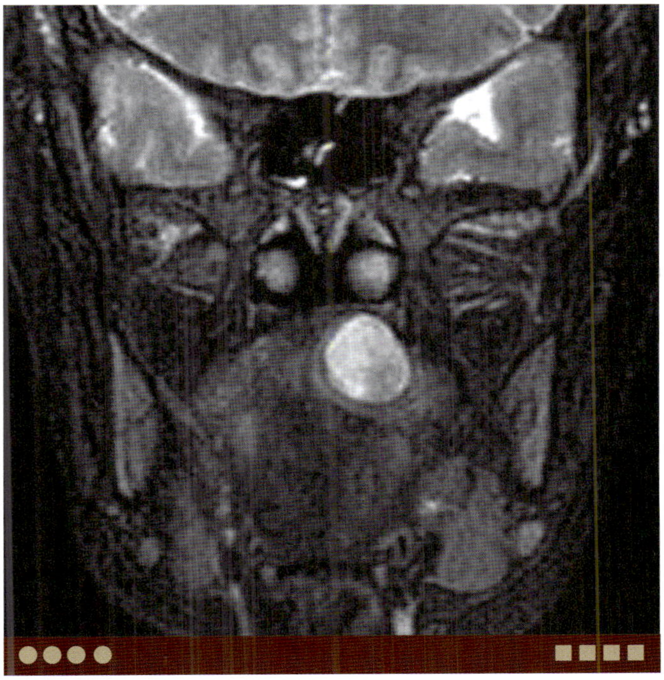

G. Pleomorphic adenoma, same patient as F. Coronal fat-suppressed T2W image demonstrates a well-delineated lesion with fibrous capsule.

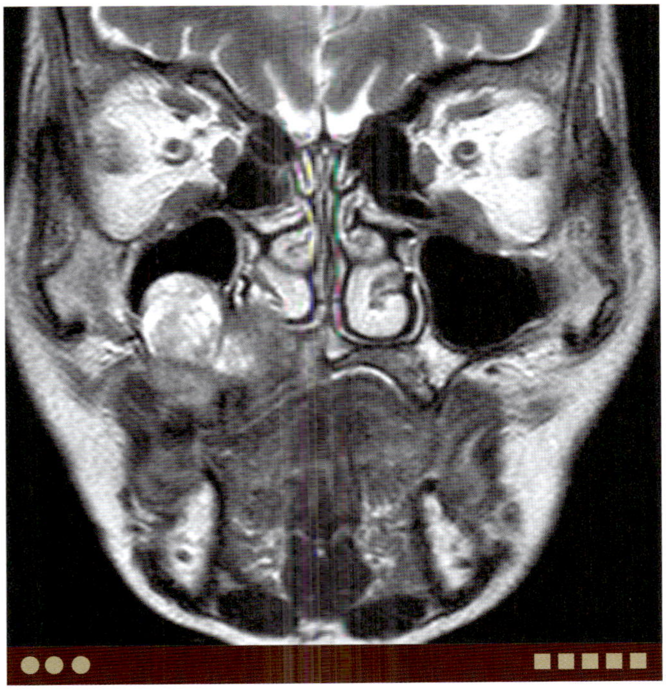

H. Adenoid cystic carcinoma. Coronal T2W MR image demonstrates a lobulated, heterogeneous high-signal lesion eroding the right hard palate and protruding into the right maxillary sinus.

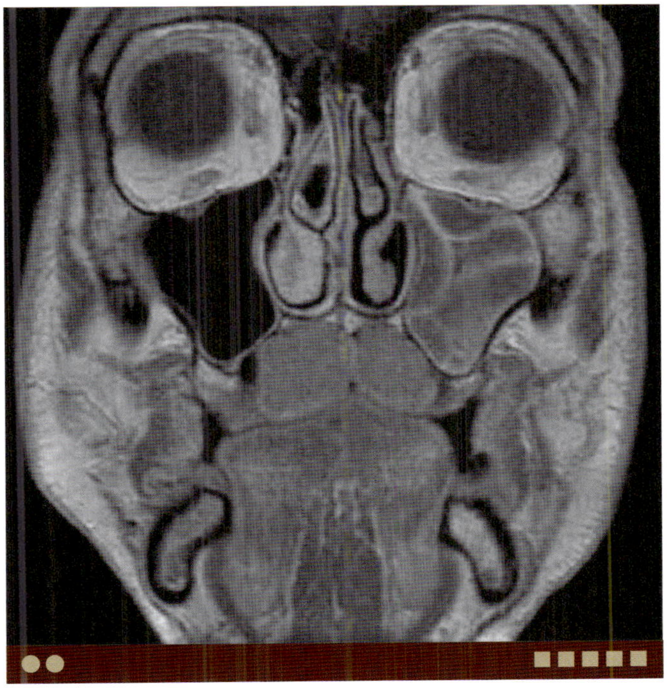

I. Lymphoma, same patient as A. Coronal postcontrast T1W MR image demonstrates mild, homogeneous enhancement of the lesion.

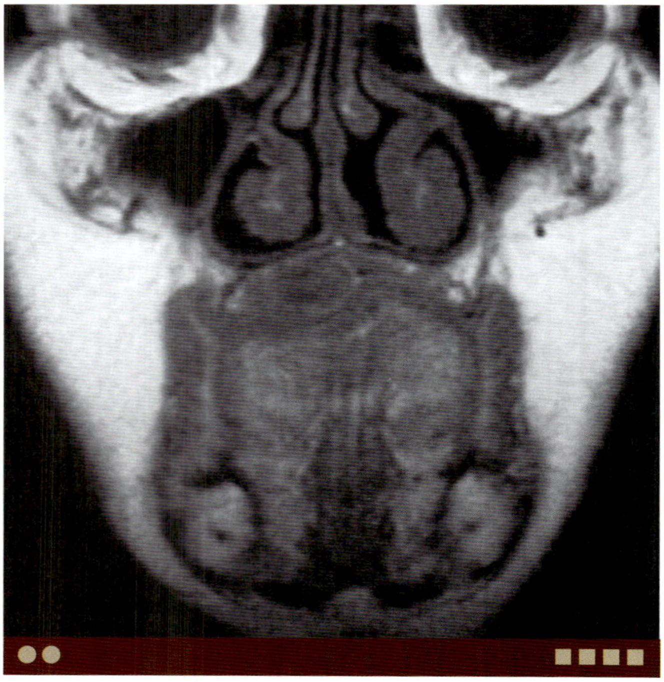

J. Melanoma. Coronal T1W MR image demonstrates an ovoid-shaped lesion in the right palate with bone remodeling.

Case 8–19 Hemangioma—Oropharynx

Hiroki Kato, Asim Mian, Osamu Sakai

PRESENTATION

A bluish mass in the oropharynx.

FINDINGS

CT and MRI demonstrate a well-defined, lobulated, enhancing lesion in the oropharynx.

DIFFERENTIAL DIAGNOSIS

- Squamous cell carcinoma (SCCA): SCCA is the most common malignant tumor of the oropharynx. Smoking and alcohol are important risk factors. They arise from the squamous epithelium of the mucosa of the soft palate, palatine and lingual tonsils, and pharyngeal walls.
- Lymphoma: Non-Hodgkin lymphoma is a common type of lymphoma in the oropharynx. Hodgkin lymphoma is rare in the pharynx. Homogeneous density/signal without necrosis is a common finding.
- Lingual thyroid: Lingual thyroid demonstrates high density on CT. If the thyroid anlage migration arrests, the thyroid tissue is seen at the base of tongue. In about 75% of the patients, the lingual thyroid is the only functioning thyroid tissue, and about 70% of patients with lingual thyroid have hypothyroidism.

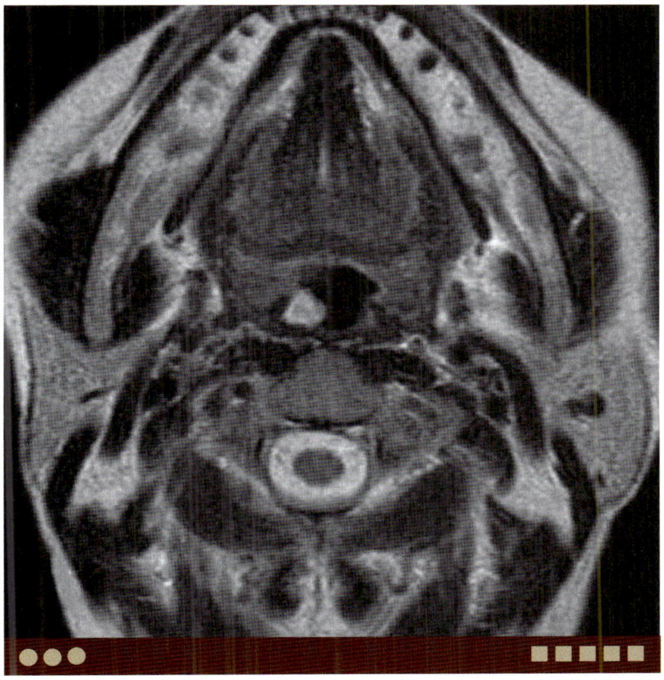

A. Hemangioma. Axial T2W image demonstrates a polypoid lesion with homogeneously high signal in the right oropharynx.

COMMENTS

This is a 59-year-old woman who presented with discomfort during swallowing.

Hemangiomas are the most common tumors in the head and neck among infants and children, accounting for approximately 7% of all benign soft tissue tumors. They typically present at birth, enlarge during the first year of life, and then often spontaneously involute by 5 years of age.

The classification for vascular lesions is based on their natural history as well as their cellular structure. Histopathologically, vascular lesions are categorized into two main groups: hemangiomas and vascular malformations. The vascular malformations are further classified as capillary, venous, arteriovenous, and lymphatic malformations depending on the predominant anomalous vascular channels. Alternatively, malformations can be categorized as either high-flow (arteriovenous) or low-flow (capillary, cavernous, venous) vascular lesions.

On CT and MRI, hemangiomas appear as well-defined, often lobulated, solid lesions. Hemangiomas tend to demonstrate similar density to the vasculature on CT. Enhancement, usually gradual, is seen after contrast. Presence of phlebolith is suggestive of venous malformation.

MRI is useful for characterizing and determining the extension of hemangiomas. Hemangiomas are isointense or slightly hyperintense to the muscle on T1W and markedly hyperintense on T2W images due to pooled blood. Contrast-enhanced MRI usually demonstrates avid enhancement with varying homogeneity. Presence of flow-voids suggests high-flow components. Combination of time-of-flight and dynamic contrast-enhanced MR angiography may be useful in distinguishing between high- and low-flow lesions. Arteriovenous shunts may be seen in high-flow lesion. It is important to distinguish between high- and low-flow lesions for therapeutic planning.

PEARLS

- **Hemangiomas are seen as well-defined, often lobulated, solid lesions on CT and MRI.**
- **Hemangiomas tend to demonstrate similar density to vessels on CT.**
- **Hemangiomas are isointense or slightly hyperintense to the muscle on T1W and markedly hyperintense on T2W image.**

ADDITIONAL IMAGES (B-D)

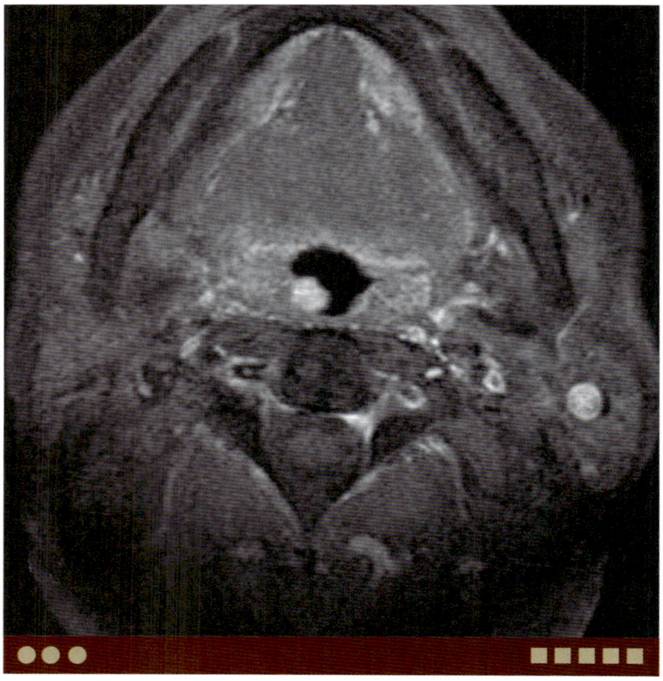

B. Hemangioma, same patient as A. Axial postcontrast fat-suppressed T1W image demonstrates homogeneous enhancement of the lesion.

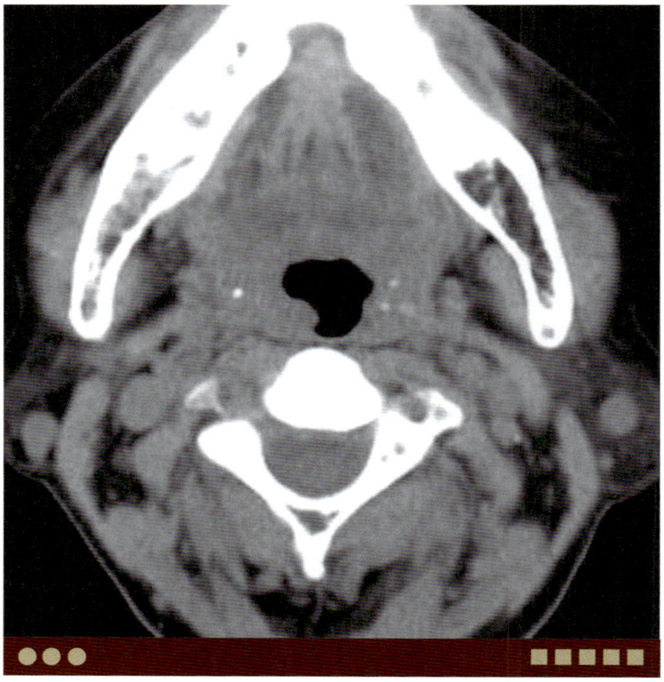

C. Hemangioma, same patient as A. Axial unenhanced CT demonstrates homogeneous soft tissue density in the lesion, isodense to the mucosa and muscle.

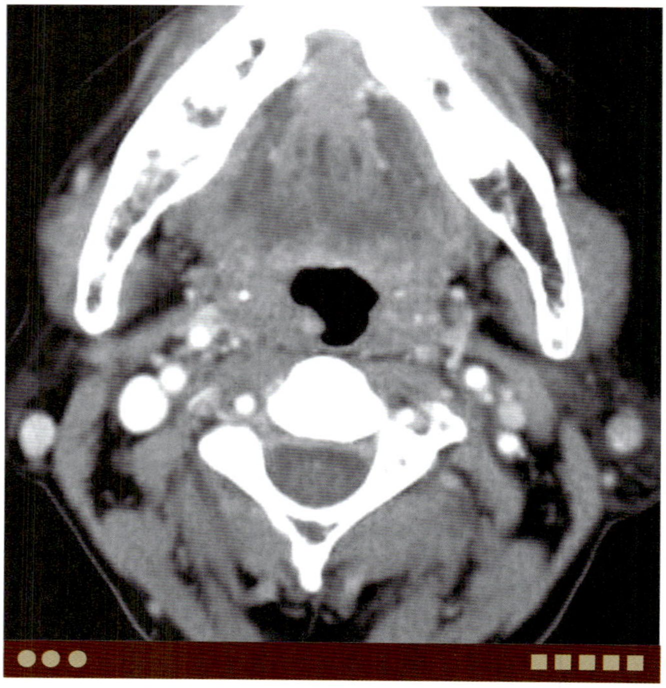

D. Hemangioma, same patient as A. Axial postcontrast CT demonstrates enhancement of the lesion.

DIFFERENTIAL DIAGNOSIS IMAGES (E-H)

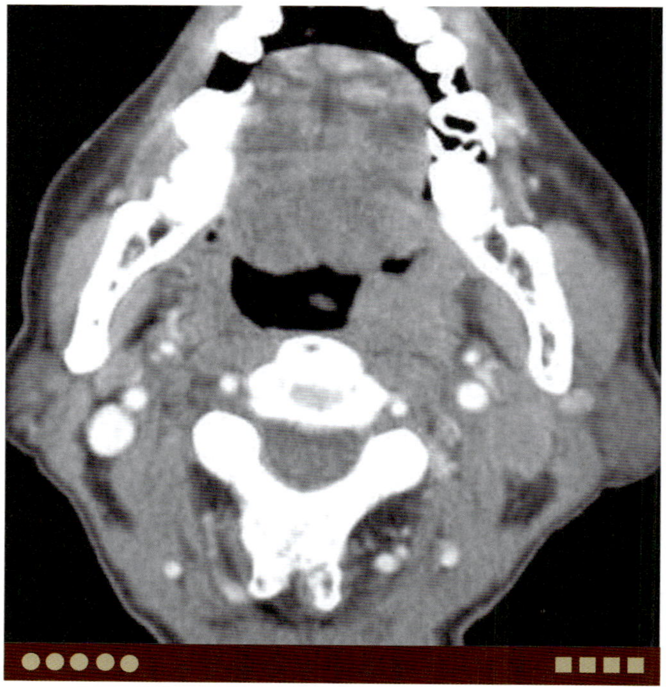

E. **SCCA**. Axial postcontrast CT demonstrates a mildly enhancing tumor in the left palatine tonsils. Left level II nodal metastasis is noted.

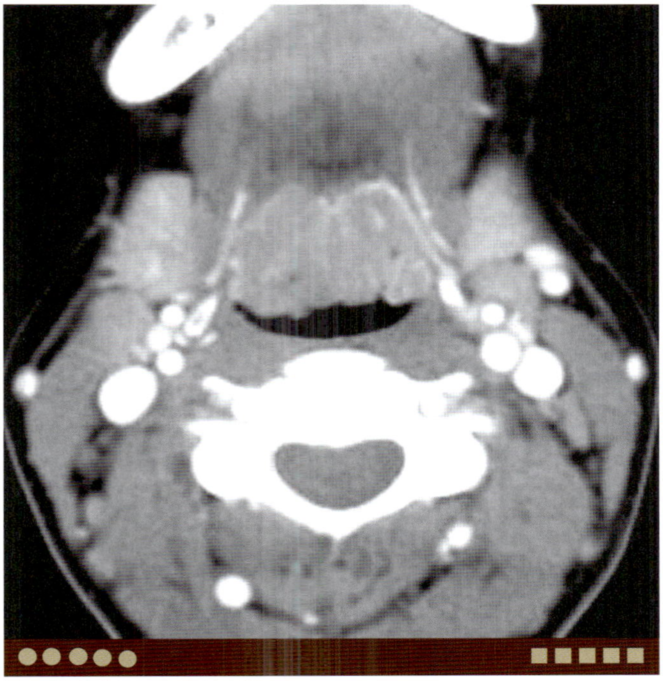

F. Lymphoma. Axial postcontrast CT demonstrates a relatively homogeneously enhancing tumor at the base of tongue.

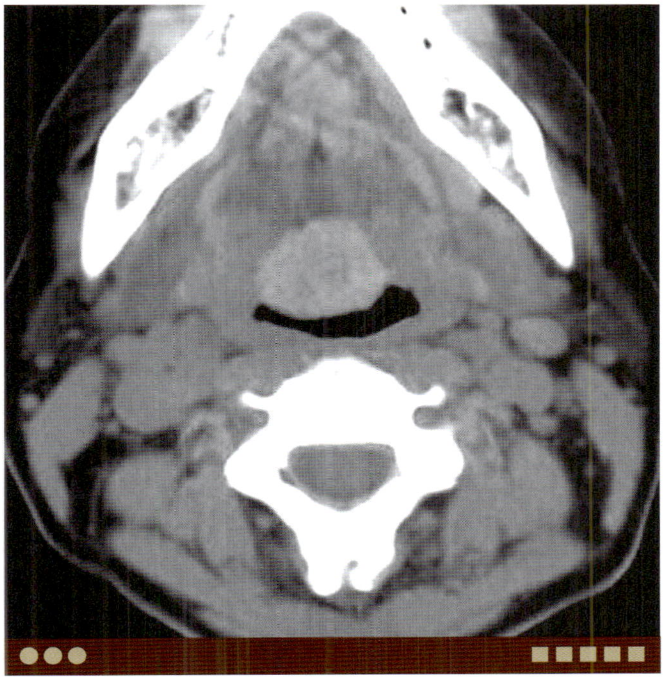

G. Lingual thyroid. Axial unenhanced CT demonstrates a hyperdense mass at the base of tongue.

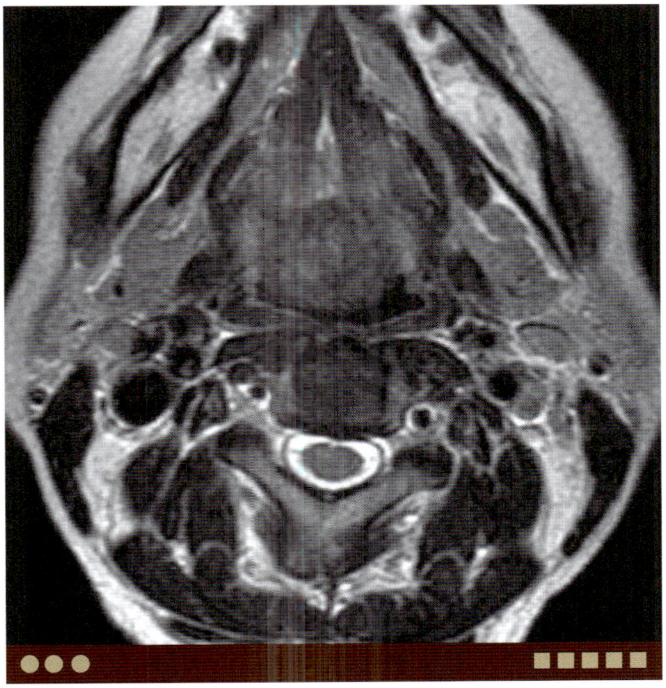

H. Lingual thyroid, same patient as G. Axial T2W image demonstrates a slightly heterogeneous hypointense mass at the base of tongue.

Case 8-20 Papilloma—Oropharynx

Hiroki Kato, Asim Mian, Osamu Sakai

PRESENTATION

Polypoid mass in the oropharynx.

FINDINGS

CT and MRI demonstrate a well-defined, polypoid lesion in the oropharynx.

DIFFERENTIAL DIAGNOSIS

- Squamous cell carcinoma (SCCA): Oropharyngeal SCCA shows an infiltrative growth pattern with moderate enhancement on CT and MRI. Large tumors often show heterogeneous appearance due to intratumoral necrosis, although small tumors may not be identified on images.
- Lymphoma: Lymphomas show usually homogeneous appearance both on CT and MRI. However, very large lesions may demonstrate heterogeneous appearance and hyperintense areas on T1W images, reflecting intratumoral hemorrhage.
- Tonsillitis/peritonsillar abscess: Acute infection of the tonsils can lead to tonsillitis and peritonsillar abscess, which is abscess formation within the potential space adjacent to the tonsils.

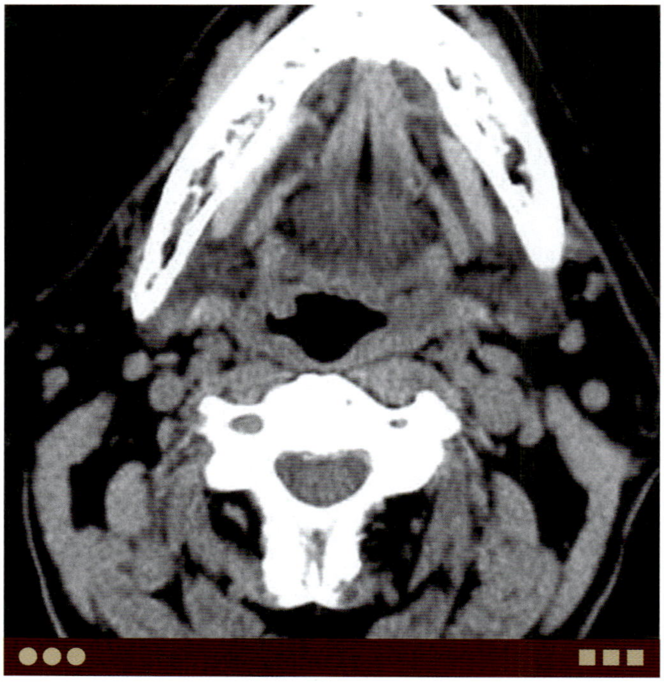

A. Papilloma. Axial unenhanced CT demonstrates a small polypoid lesion isodense to the mucosa in the right oropharynx.

COMMENTS

This is a 61-year-old man with an incidental polypoid lesion in the oropharynx.

Papillomas in the oral cavity and oropharynx are almost always squamous papilloma. This is the most common benign tumor, involving the larynx, trachea, and bronchi, and most of the lesions are thought to be associated with human papillomavirus (HPV). Squamous papillomas are exophytic, branching, pedunculated, or broad-based lesions, and consist of hyperplastic, well-differentiated squamous epithelium overlying central fibrovascular cores. Lesions may be multiple. They tend to recur after resection and may undergo malignant degeneration. They tend to be more aggressive in children, who frequently develop recurrent and progressive disease.

Squamous papilloma of the oral cavity and oropharynx occurs at any age, however, is often diagnosed in middle-age. Any oral surface may be affected, although lesions are usually found on lingual, labial, or buccal mucosa. Papillary and verruciform epithelial proliferations are common in the oral cavity and paraoral region. The typical presentation is a soft and pedunculated mass with numerous finger-like surface projections.

Radiological findings include nodular narrowing of the airway that may be either focal or diffuse. CT can demonstrate polypoid lesions, and is useful to assess size and shape of lesions and evaluate for possible invasive findings.

However, findings of papillomas are often nonspecific and it is difficult to differentiate them from other nonepithelial or mesenchymal tumors or early SCCA.

PEARLS

- **Papilloma is closely associated with HPV infection and occurs in the aerodigestive tract.**
- **Papilloma often shows a nonspecific polypoid lesion on CT and it is difficult to differentiate it from other benign nonepithelial or mesenchymal tumors, or early SCCA.**

ADDITIONAL IMAGE

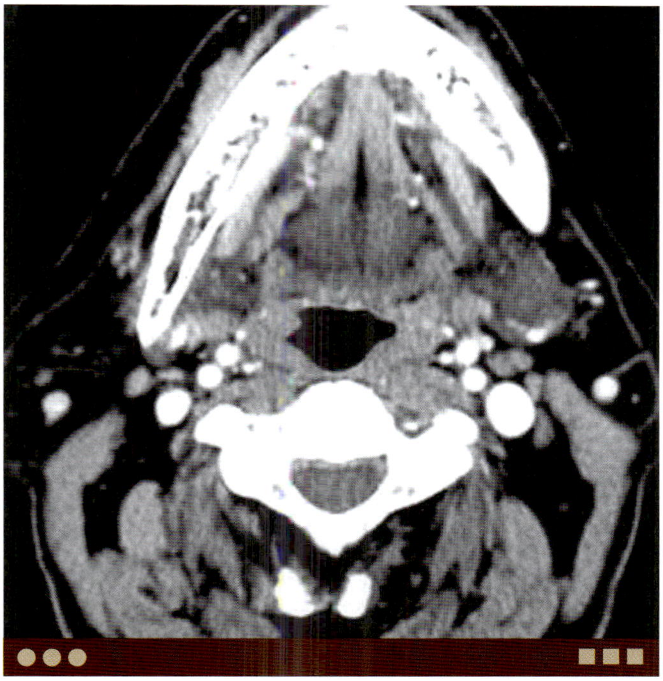

B. Papilloma, same patient as A. Axial contrast-enhanced CT demonstrates the polypoid lesion enhancing similar to the oropharyngeal wall.

DIFFERENTIAL DIAGNOSIS IMAGES (C-G)

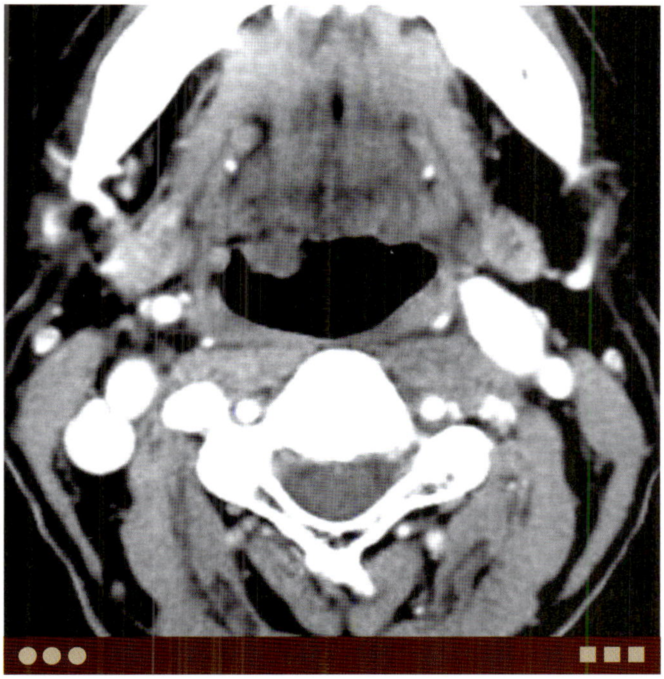

C. Hemangioma. Axial contrast-enhanced CT demonstrates an anterior oropharyngeal polypoid mass with minimal enhancement.

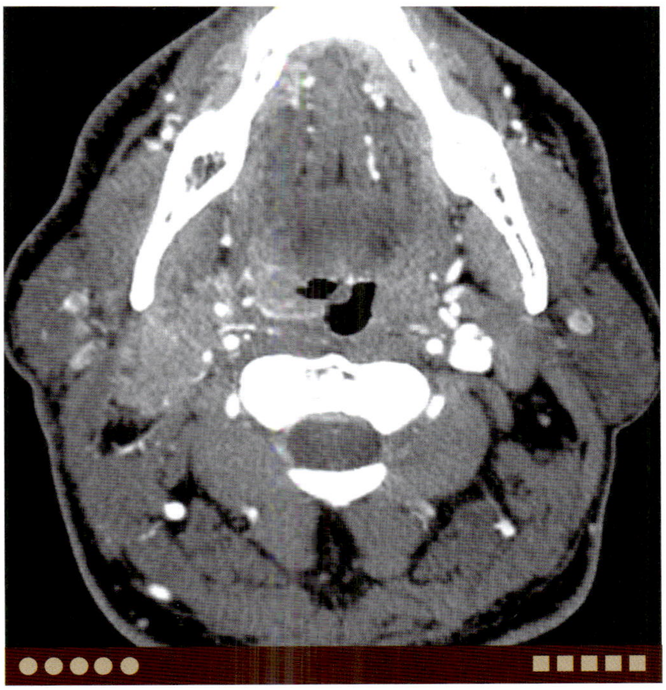

D. SCCA. Axial contrast-enhanced CT demonstrates a slightly exophytic enhancing tumor in the right tonsil. Note enhancing metastatic nodal disease at level II on the right.

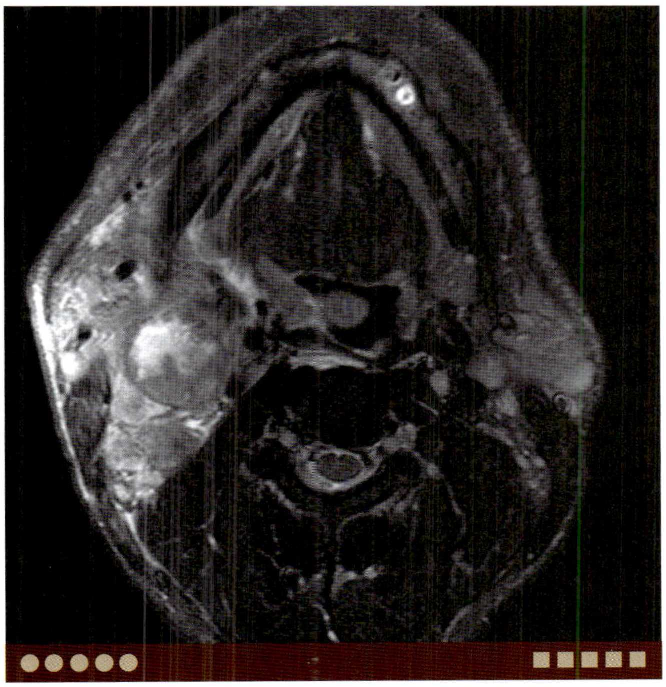

E. SCCA in a different patient. Axial T2W image demonstrates a small intermediate-signal tumor in the right tonsil with large metastatic nodes in the right level II involving the right parapharyngeal space.

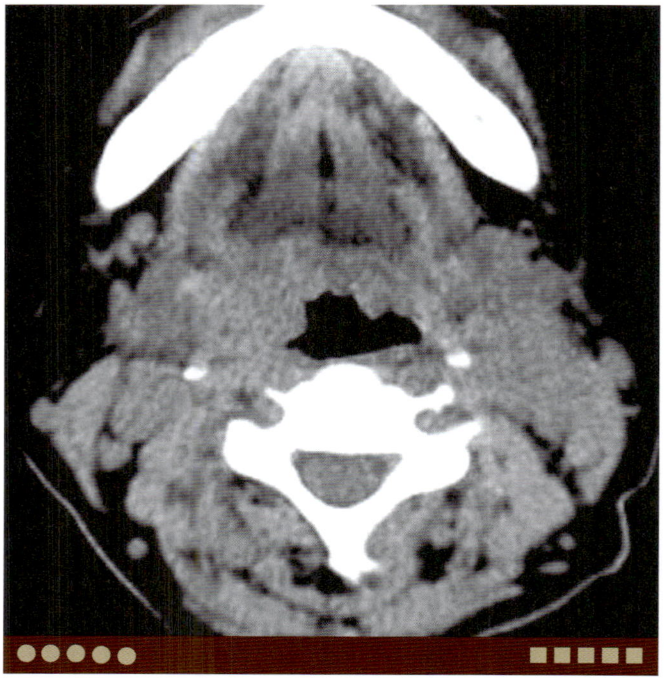

F. Diffuse large B-cell lymphoma. Axial unenhanced CT demonstrates a right oropharyngeal mass isodense to the muscle.

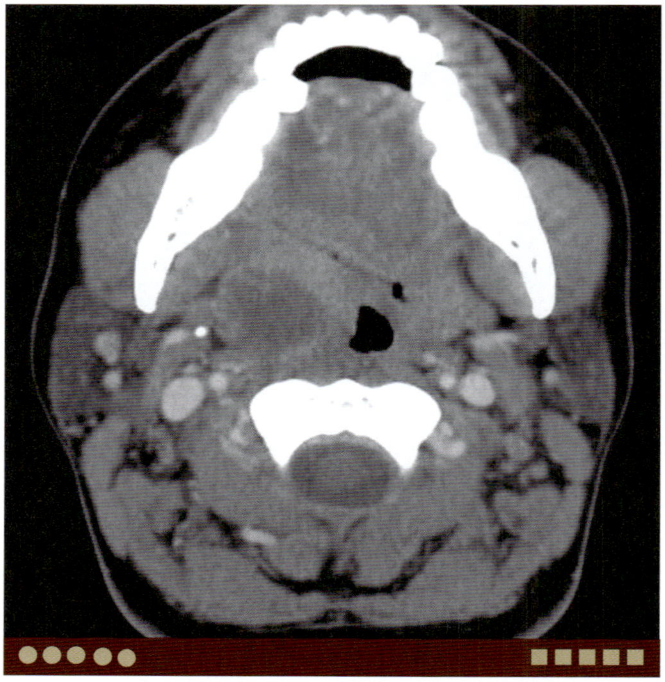

G. Peritonsillar abscess. Axial contrast-enhanced CT demonstrates a hypodense lesion with mild peripheral enhancement, lateral to the right palatine tonsil, which is displaced medially.

Case 8–21 Hemangioma—Palate

Hiroki Kato, Asim Mian, Osamu Sakai

PRESENTATION

Bluish mass in the palate.

FINDINGS

CT and MRI demonstrate a well-defined, lobulated, palatal mass with high T2 signal and enhancement.

DIFFERENTIAL DIAGNOSIS

- Pleomorphic adenoma: Pleomorphic adenoma is the most common benign neoplasm of the oral cavity in adults. Mixture of epithelial and fibromyxoid tissues with degenerative changes results in heterogeneous signal on T1W and T2W images and variable degree of enhancement.
- Adenoid cystic carcinoma: Adenoid cystic carcinomas originate from the minor salivary glands which can be found anywhere in the oral cavity. Low-grade tumors (cribriform or tubular subtype) show benign appearance with high signal on T2W images, while high-grade tumors demonstrates decreased T2 signal.
- Mucoepidermoid carcinoma: Low-grade tumors demonstrate benign appearance with prominent cystic components. The cystic areas containing mucin demonstrate high signal on both T1W and T2W images.
- Squamous cell carcinoma (SCCA): SCCA is the most common malignant tumor of the palate and shows an infiltrative growth pattern. Moderate enhancement is seen on CT and MRI. Larger tumors may be heterogeneous due to intratumoral necrosis.

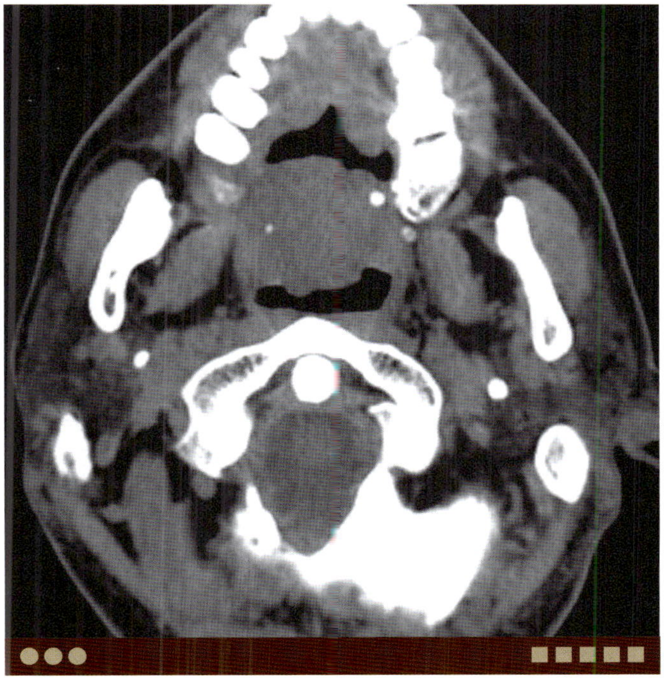

A. Hemangioma. Axial noncontrast-enhanced CT demonstrates a round, soft palatal mass with calcifications (phleboliths).

COMMENTS

This is a 42-year-old male who presented with a soft, painless mass in the soft palate.

Hemangioma of the palate is relatively rare, even though hemangiomas are relatively common in the head and neck. This is a benign condition; however, large lesions can cause airway compromise. Most hemangiomas in the oral cavity/oropharynx are likely developmental in origin and are composed of a mixture of hemangiomatous and lymphangiomatous elements. Recently, most hemangiomas have been renamed as venous malformations. The tongue and floor of mouth are the common sites in the oral cavity.

On CT, hemangiomas tend to demonstrate similar density to vessels. Presence of phlebolith strongly suggests venous malformation. MRI plays an important role in diagnosing, characterizing and determining the extent of the lesion. On T2W images, hemangioma are generally seen as a lobulated, markedly hyperintense mass that resembles a bunch of grapes. This appearance is due to cavernous or cystic vascular spaces containing stagnant blood. Fluid–fluid levels may also be seen within these spaces. Punctate or reticular hypointense areas may be present, representing fibrous tissue, flow-void, or calcification (phlebolith). These lesions usually demonstrate intermediate signal on T1W images. Occasionally, peripherally hyperintense areas reflecting fatty tissue are seen in the lesion on T1W images. Marked enhancement with varying homogeneity is seen after contrast.

PEARLS

- **Hemangiomas are seen as well-defined, lobulated, solid masses.**
- **Hemangiomas show markedly high signal on T2W and intermediate signal on T1W images. Sometimes peripheral T1 high signal reflecting fatty component is seen.**

ADDITIONAL IMAGES (B-C)

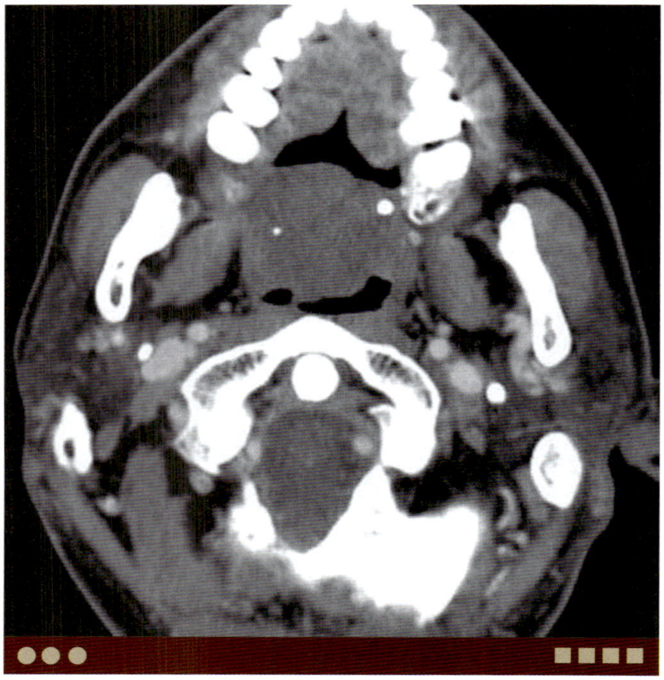

B. Hemangioma, same patient as A. Axial contrast-enhanced CT demonstrates minimal enhancement in the lesion.

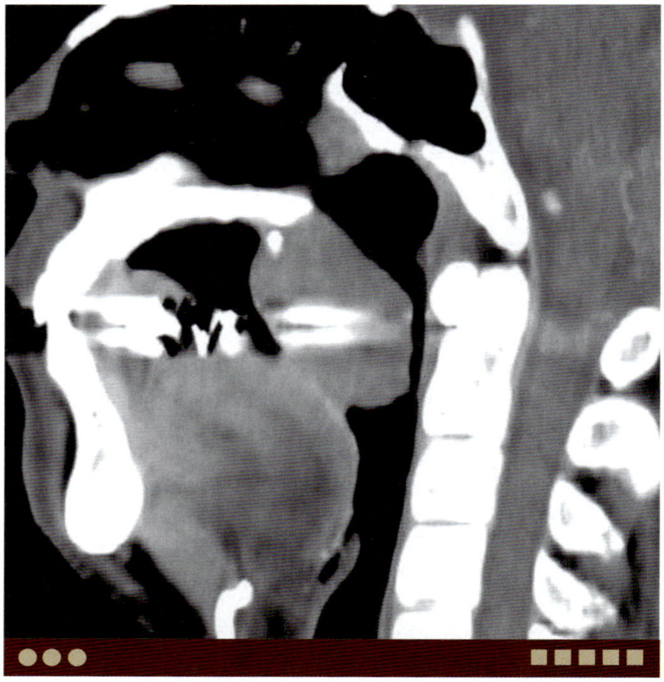

C. Hemangioma, same patient as A. Sagittal contrast-enhanced CT demonstrates a ovoid mass in the soft palate.

DIFFERENTIAL DIAGNOSIS IMAGES (D-H)

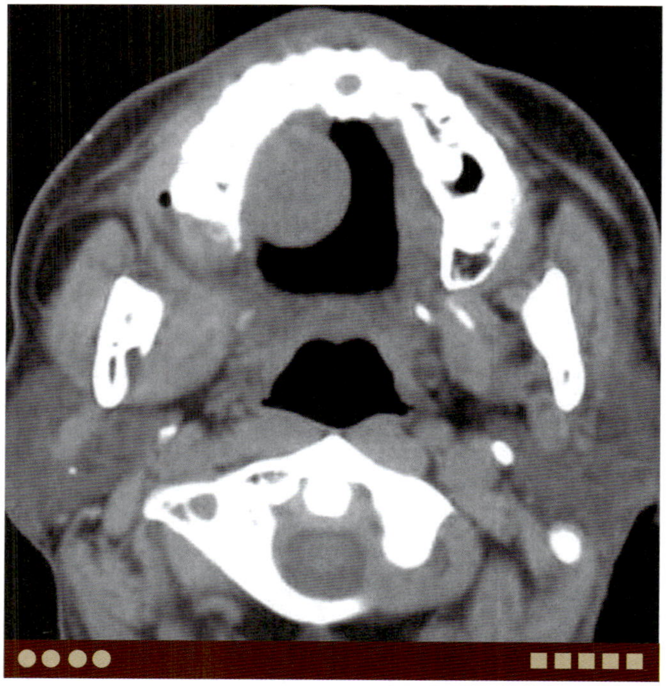

D. Pleomorphic adenoma. Axial unenhanced CT demonstrates a soft tissue density mass in the right soft palate.

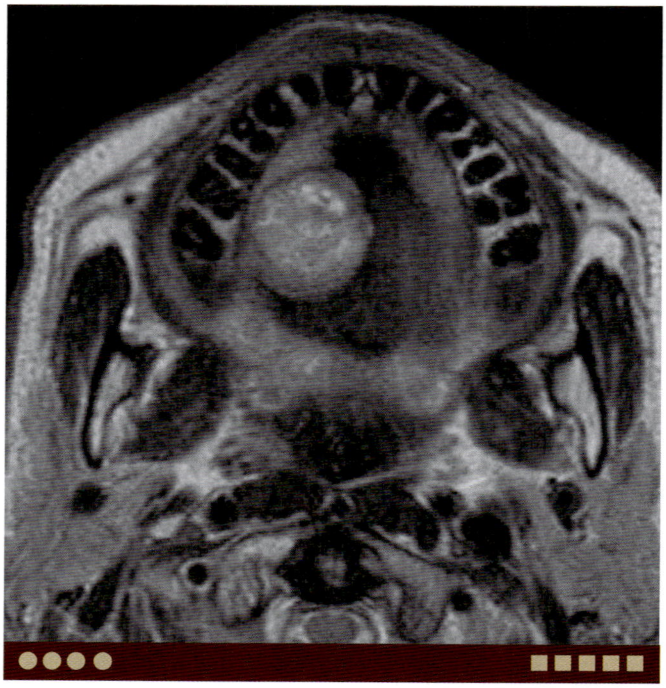

E. Pleomorphic adenoma, same patient as D. Axial T2W image demonstrates a well-defined, slightly heterogeneous, intermediate-to-high signal lesion.

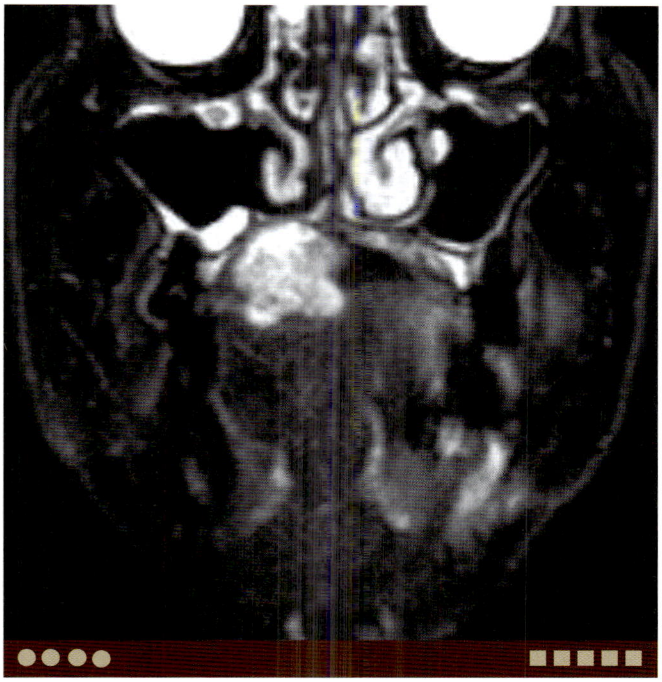

F. Pleomorphic adenoma, same patient as D. Coronal fat-suppressed T2W image demonstrates a lobulated lesion with heterogeneous high signal in the right palate.

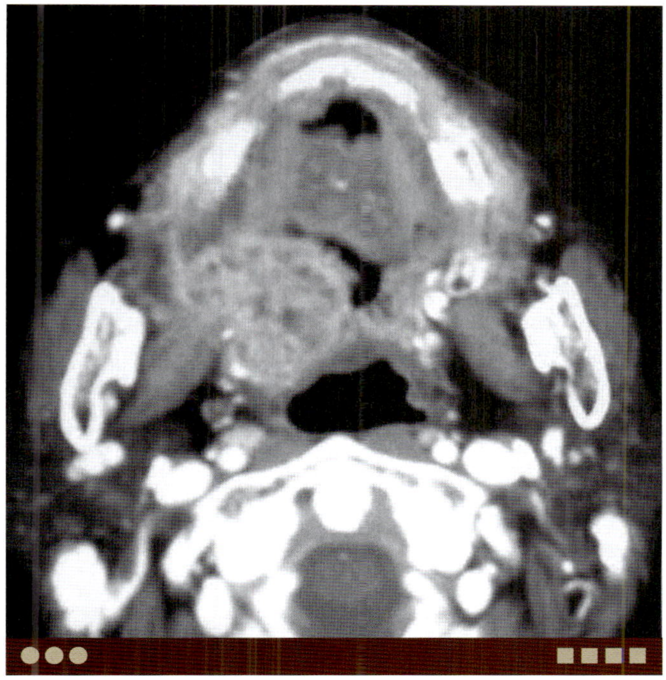

G. **Mucoepidermoid carcinoma**. Axial contrast-enhanced CT demonstrates a tumor with heterogeneous reticular enhancement in the right palate.

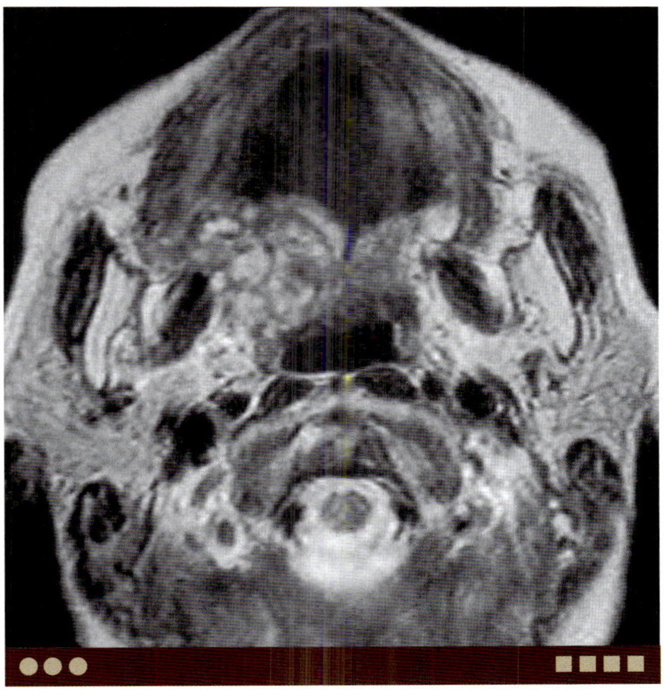

H. Mucoepidermoid carcinoma, same patient as G. Axial T2W image demonstrates multicystic components in the tumor.

Case 8–22 Thyroglossal Duct Cyst

Osamu Sakai, Akifumi Fujita, Asim Mian

PRESENTATION

Mass at the base of tongue.

FINDINGS

CT and MR demonstrate a cystic lesion at the base of the tongue.

DIFFERENTIAL DIAGNOSIS

- Lingual thyroid: Undescended/ectopic thyroid tissue demonstrates similar density to the normal thyroid gland on CT; homogeneous high density and enhancement. On MRI, it demonstrates intermediate to slightly high signal on both T1W and T2W images.
- Dermoid/epidermoid: Seen as a cystic mass at the midline of the floor of the mouth. Presence of fat suggests dermoid. Differentiation between dermoid and epidermoid is often difficult by imaging; however, the presence of fat strongly suggests a dermoid.
- Ranula: This condition usually occurs off-midline in the sublingual space. It occasionally extends to the submandibular space, so-called diving ranulas.
- Squamous sell carcinoma (SCCA): This is the most common tumor at the base of tongue, and usually demonstrates heterogeneous density/signal and enhancement with poorly defined margins.

COMMENTS

This is a 35-year-old woman with a mass at the base of tongue.

Thyroglossal duct cyst is a common congenital/developmental cystic lesion and usually located in the midline anterior neck. The thyroid gland descends from the foramen cecum at the base of tongue to the inferior neck through the thyroglossal duct. Thyroglossal duct cyst can occur along the thyroglossal duct, anywhere between the foramen cecum and thyroid, and most often seen around the level of the hyoid. The internal density or signal is similar to that of water. High density on CT is suggestive of residual or ectopic thyroid tissue, although increased density on CT or signal on T1W images may be seen with proteinaceous contents. Note in about 75% of patients with ectopic thyroid gland at the base of tongue, the lingual thyroid is the only functioning thyroid tissue. Therefore, diagnosis of thyroid tissue in other locations is critical in such patients.

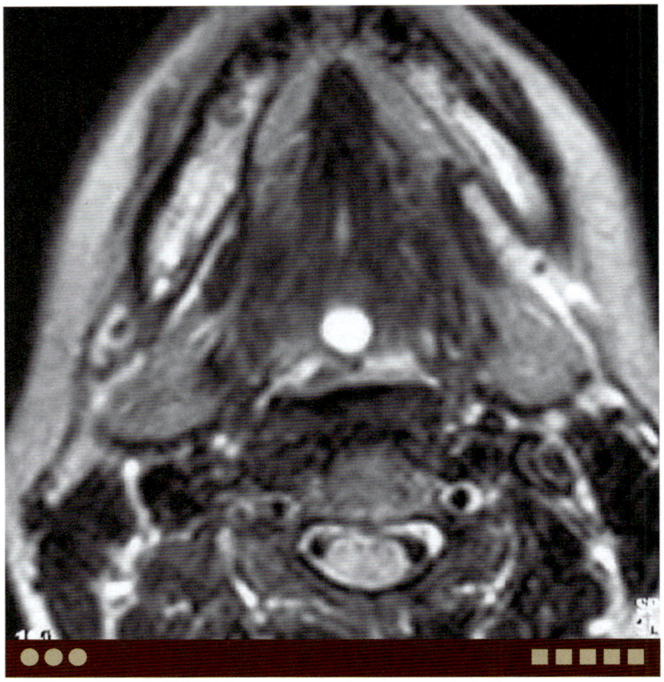

A. Thyroglossal duct cyst. Axial T2W MR image demonstrates a high-signal cystic lesion at the base of tongue in midline.

The differential diagnosis includes other cystic lesions, such as dermoid/epidermoid cysts, ranula, and minor salivary gland retention cyst. Solid lesions are more common at the base of tongue and should be ruled out first, including SCCA, lymphoma, minor salivary gland tumor, and thyroid cancer arising from the residual thyroid tissue, usually papillary carcinoma.

PEARLS

- **Thyroglossal duct cyst is a common congenital/developmental cystic lesion and occurs anywhere along the course of the thyroglossal duct, between the foramen cecum and thyroid.**
- **Residual thyroid tissue is occasionally seen in the cyst.**
- **Patients with lingual thyroid often do not have any other thyroid tissue. Removal of this ectopic thyroid tissue results in hypothyroidism.**

ADDITIONAL IMAGES (B-C)

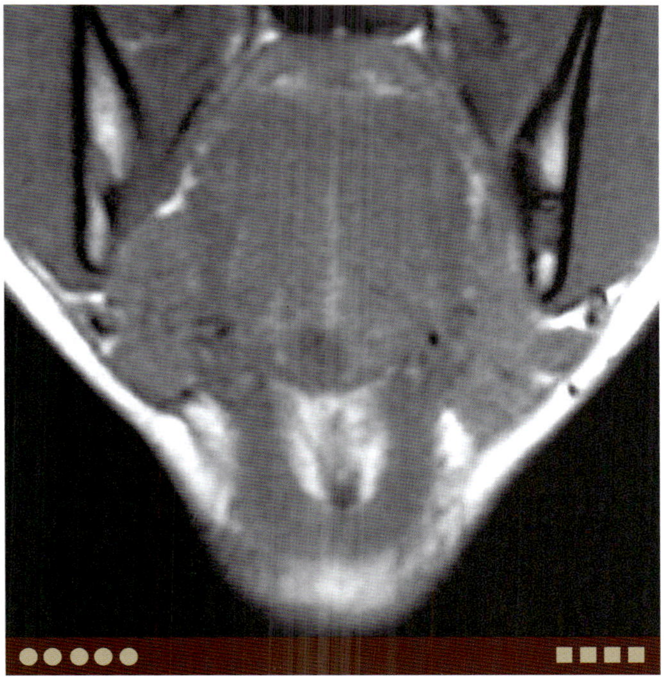

B. Thyroglossal duct cyst, same patient as A. Coronal T1W MR image demonstrates a low-signal cystic lesion at the midline of the base of tongue.

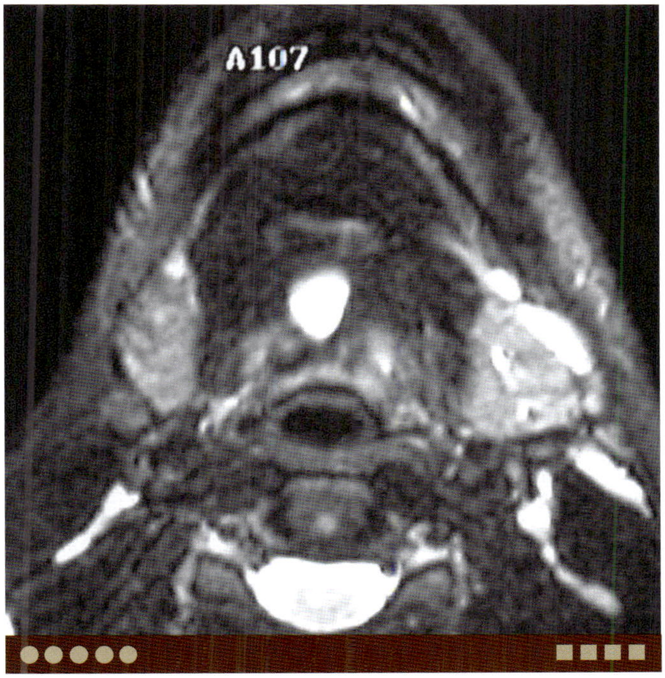

C. Thyroglossal duct cyst in a different patient. Axial STIR image shows a cystic lesion at the base of tongue in midline.

DIFFERENTIAL DIAGNOSIS IMAGES (D-H)

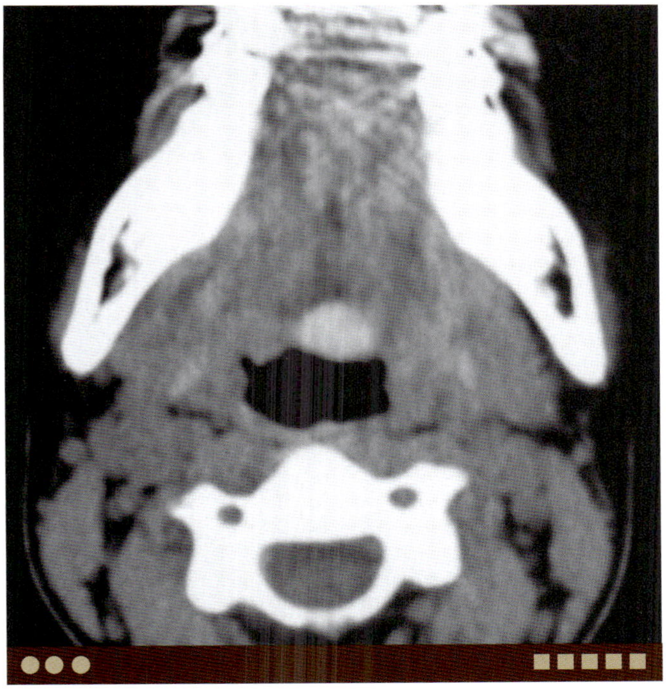

D. Lingual thyroid. Axial unenhanced CT demonstrates a well-demarcated, round, hyperdense mass at the midline of the base of tongue.

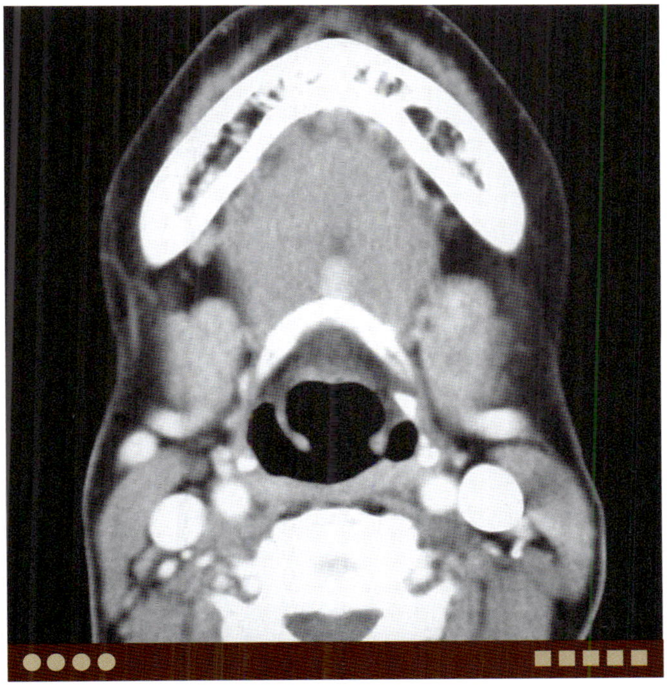

E. Residual/ectopic thyroid tissue. Axial contrast-enhanced CT shows a high-density nodular lesion in a midline location, anterior to the hyoid bone.

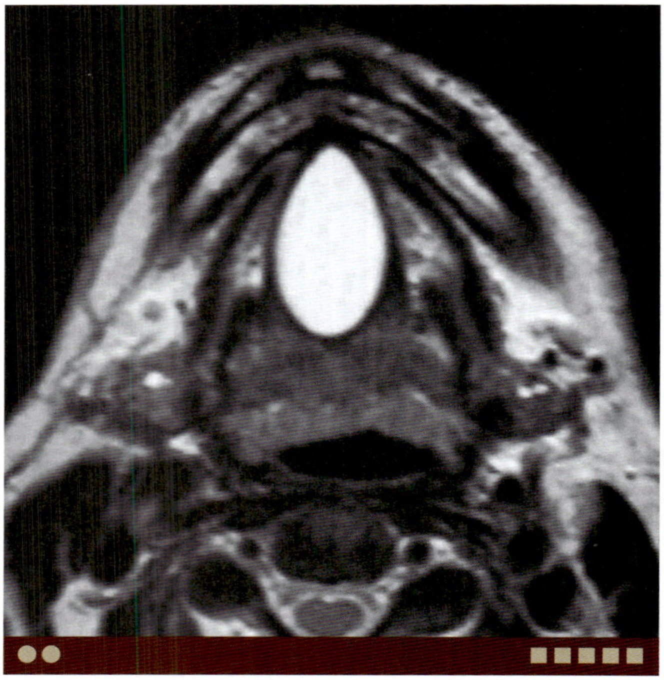

F. Epidermoid. Axial T2W image demonstrates a well-circumscribed, high-signal cystic mass at the midline of the sublingual space.

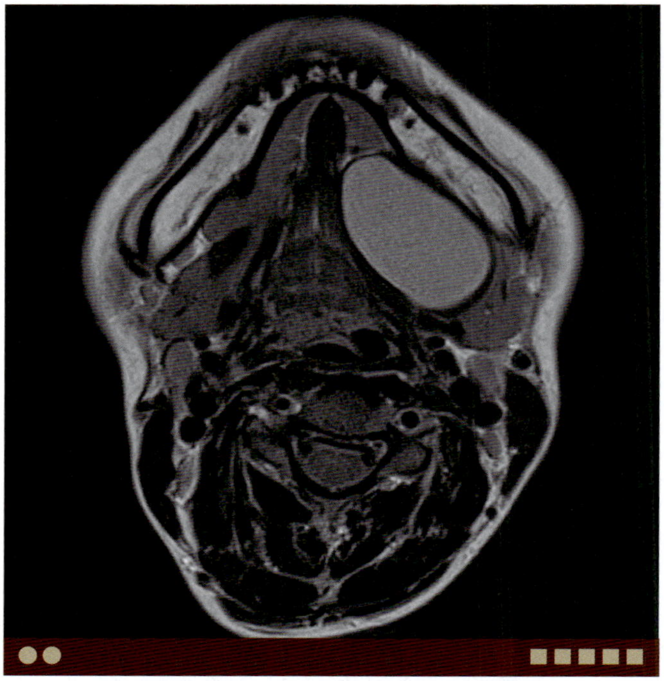

G. Epidermoid in a different patient. Axial T2W image demonstrates a well-circumscribed oval mass within the left sublingual space.

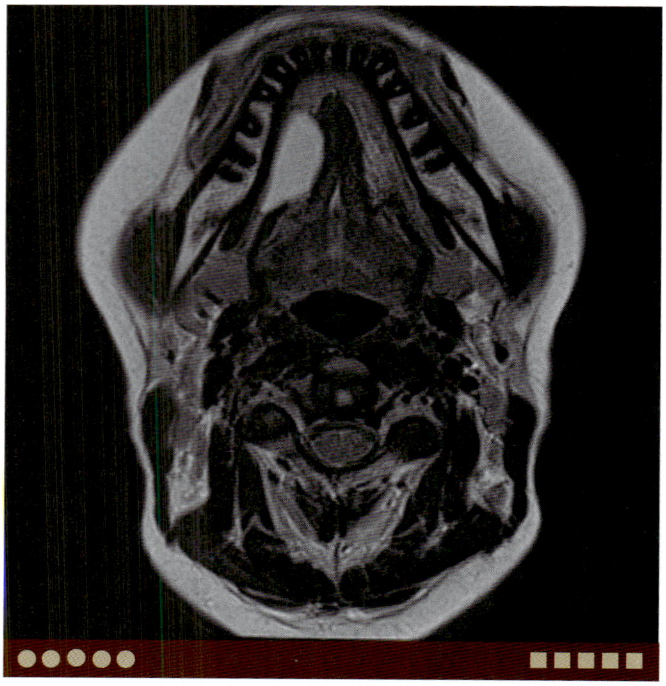

H. Ranula. Axial T2W image demonstrates a well-circumscribed cystic mass within the right sublingual space.

Chapter 9

JAW

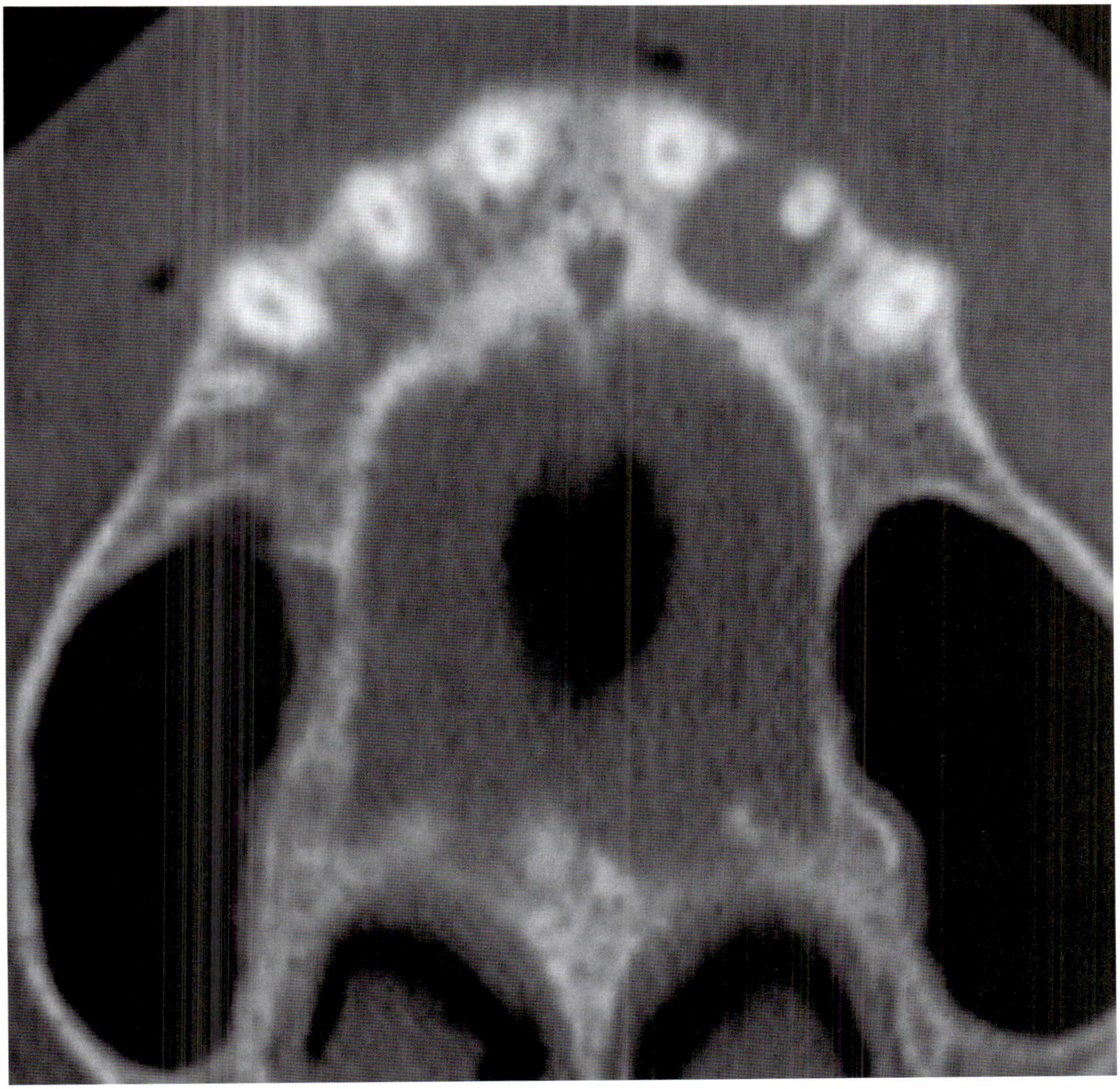

Case 9–1 Periapical (Radicular) Cyst

Osamu Sakai, Anita Gohel

PRESENTATION

Incidental finding.

FINDINGS

Computed tomography (CT) demonstrates a cystic lesion at the tooth root.

DIFFERENTIAL DIAGNOSIS

- Dentigerous (follicular) cyst: This is the most common developmental odontogenic cyst and lesion forms around the crown of an unerupted tooth.
- Early stage of periapical cemental dysplasia: This is usually seen in the mandibular anterior region in middle-aged black females. The associated teeth are vital.
- Nasopalatine duct cyst: This is a developmental cyst and one of the fissural cysts, which arises within the nasopalatine foramen or duct (incisive canal).

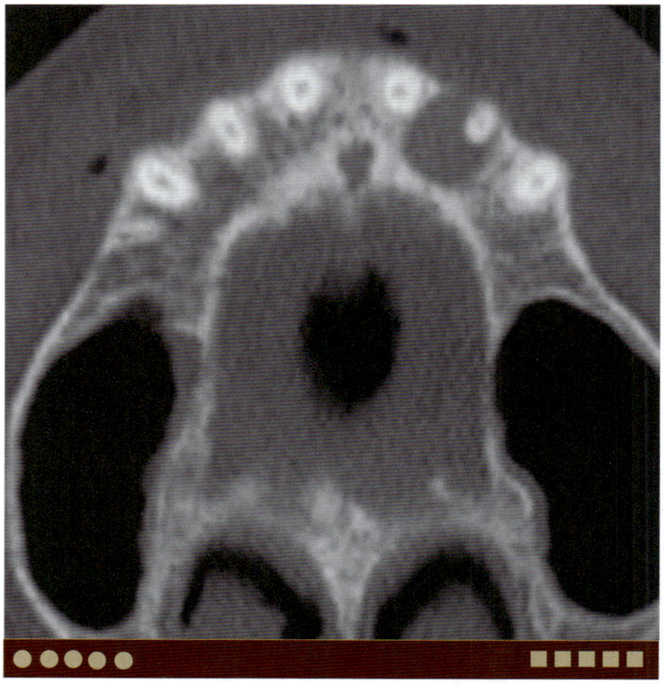

A. Periapical cyst. Axial CT demonstrates a round lucent lesion around the root of the lateral incisor.

COMMENTS

This is a 46-year-old man with focal maxillary swelling.

Periapical or radicular cyst is the most common odontogenic cyst and results from inflammation secondary to caries, trauma, or other conditions. The cyst lining is derived from the cell rests of Malassez. The peak prevalence of this asymptomatic cyst occurs between the third and sixth decades of life.

Typically, inflammatory products from a nonvital tooth spread to the apex (root) of the tooth, leading to secondary apical periodontitis, granuloma, or abscess or cyst formation. The cyst appears as a round or pear-shaped, well-defined radiolucent lesion with sclerotic borders. Dystrophic calcifications may be seen in long-standing cysts. Occasionally, it protrudes into the maxillary sinus, elevating the floor to cause "double floor sign." Most periapical cysts are less than 1 cm in diameter. It is important to note that imaging cannot always help distinguish a granuloma or abscess from a cyst. A periapical lucent lesion larger than 200 mm^3 is usually a periapical cyst. Periapical abscess may result in a fistula formation, followed by extraosseous abscess or infection. Evaluation of the tooth root is important in a patient with soft tissue inflammation around the mandible or maxilla.

Residual cyst is a generic term for any cyst that remains after extraction of the tooth. Therefore, most residual cysts are periapical cysts.

PEARLS

- **Periapical cyst is the most common odontogenic cyst, seen around the tooth root, containing the tooth root within the cyst.**
- **Periapical cyst is difficult to be differentiated from periapical granuloma or abscess; however, larger lesions tend to be periapical cysts.**

ADDITIONAL IMAGES (B-G)

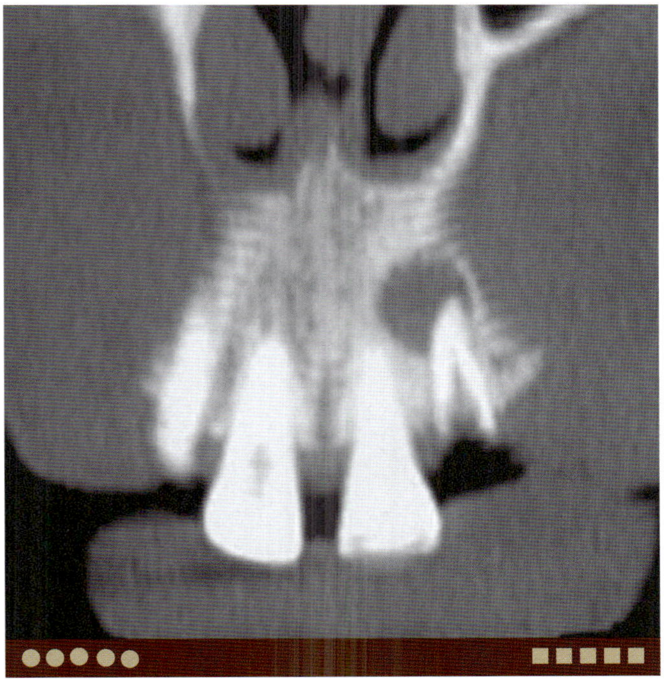

B. Periapical cyst, same patient as A. Coronal CT demonstrates a cyst around the root of the lateral incisor. Note a cavity in the crown of the tooth.

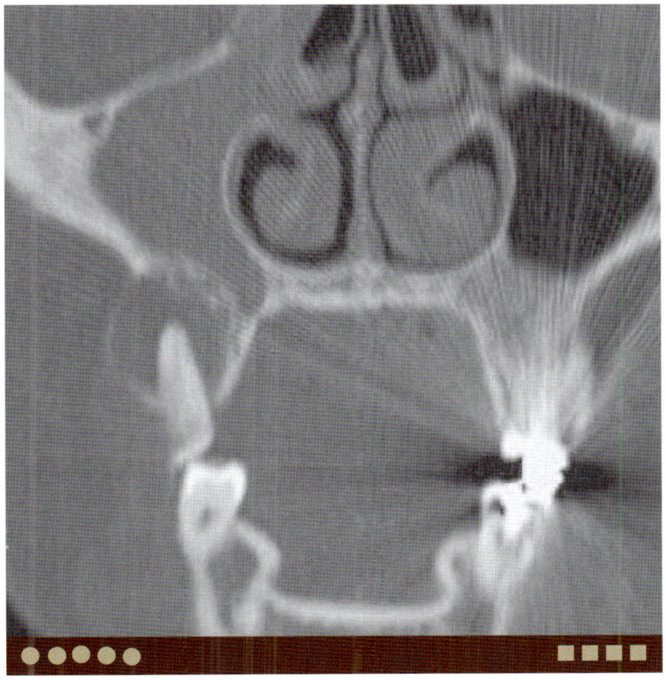

C. Periapical cyst in a different patient. Coronal CT demonstrates a cyst around the root of the premolar. Note irregularity of the superior cyst wall to suggest possible active inflammatory process and secondary inflammation in the maxillary sinus.

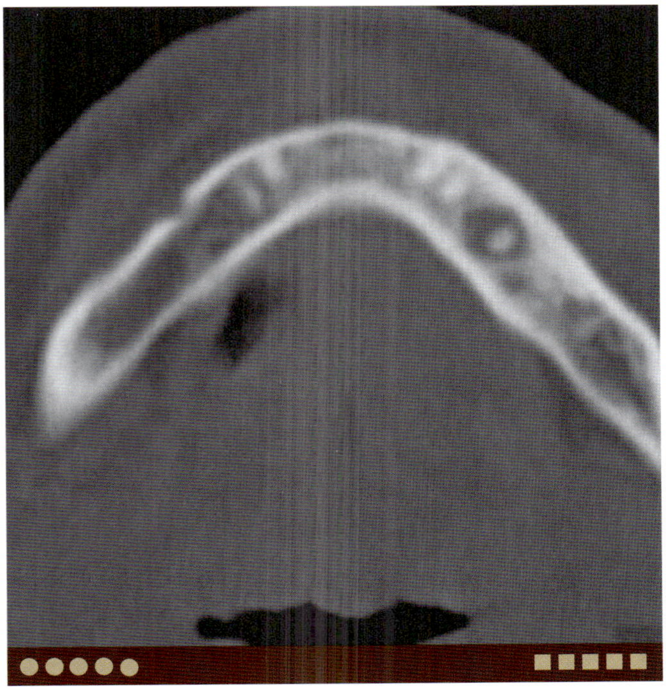

D. Periapical cyst in a different patient. Axial CT demonstrates an irregularly marginated lucent lesion around the root of the premolar with diffuse sclerotic change in the mandibular body, consistent with chronic inflammation.

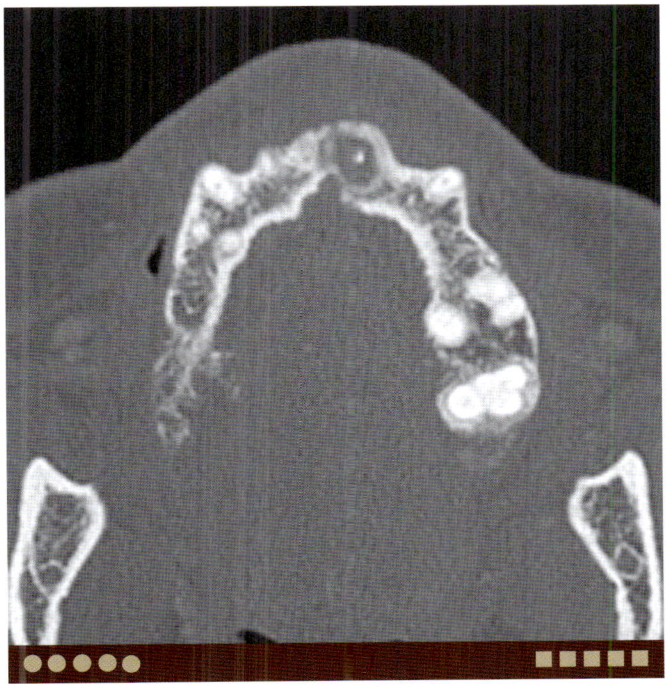

E. Periapical cyst in a different patient. Axial CT demonstrates a round lucent lesion around the root of the central incisor (tooth #9).

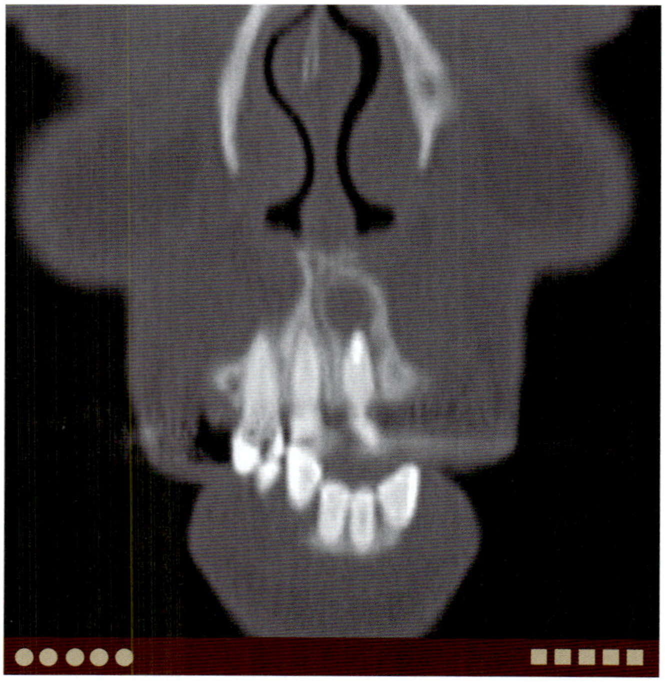

F. Periapical cyst, same patient as E. Coronal CT demonstrates a cyst around the tooth root. Note the tooth is status post root canal.

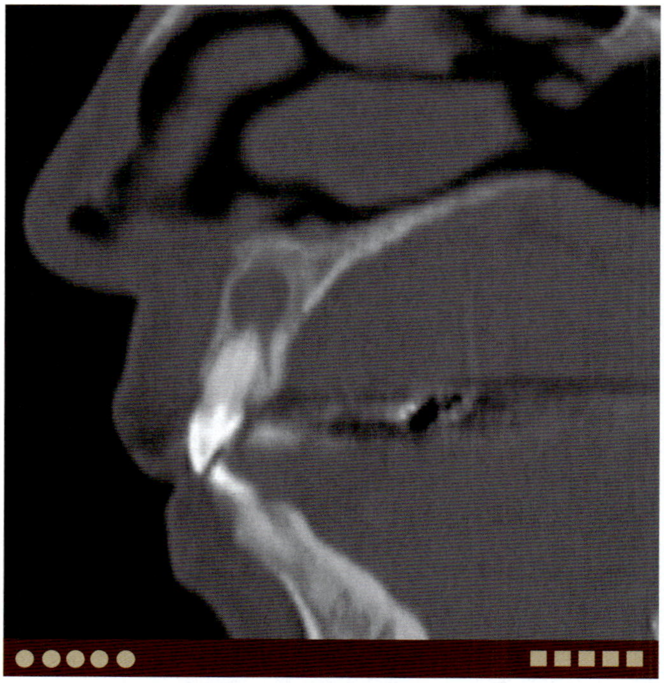

G. Periapical cyst, same patient as E. Sagittal CT demonstrates a cyst around the tooth root.

DIFFERENTIAL DIAGNOSIS IMAGES (H-J)

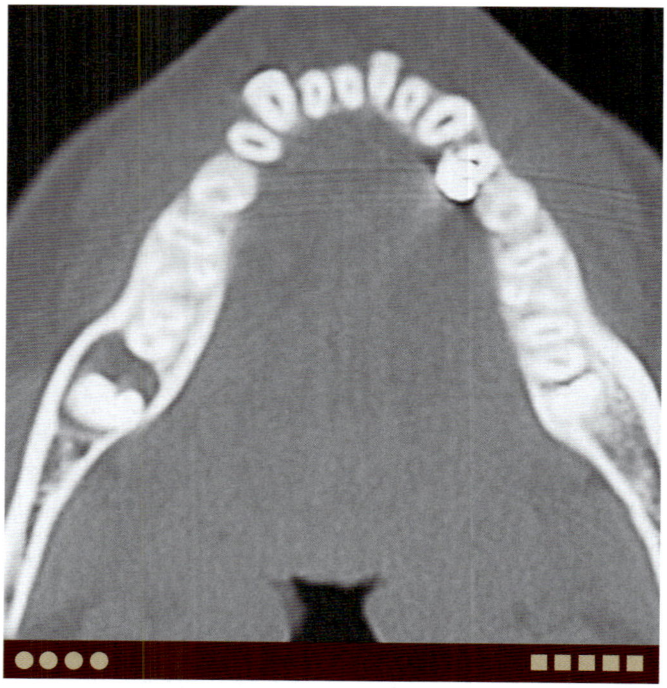

H. Dentigerous cyst. Axial CT demonstrates a lucent lesion around the molar. Note the crown is identified in the cyst.

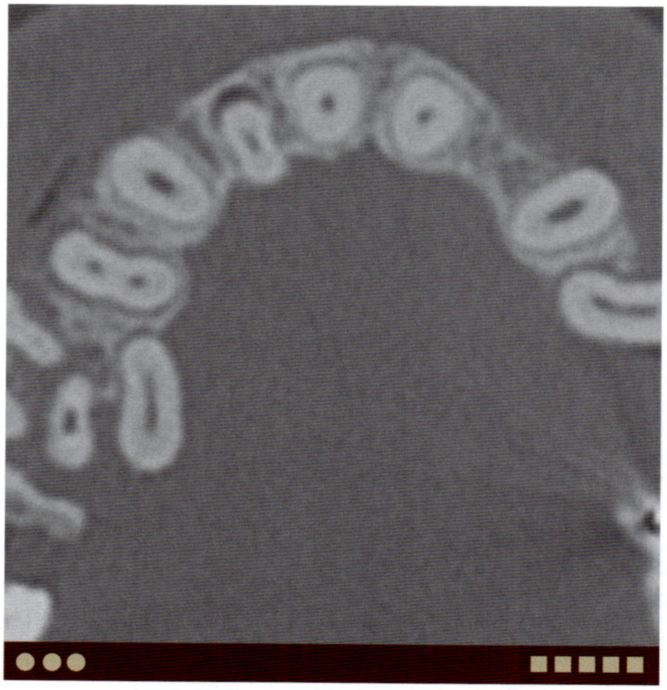

I. Tooth subluxation. Axial CT demonstrates lucency anterior to the right lateral incisor.

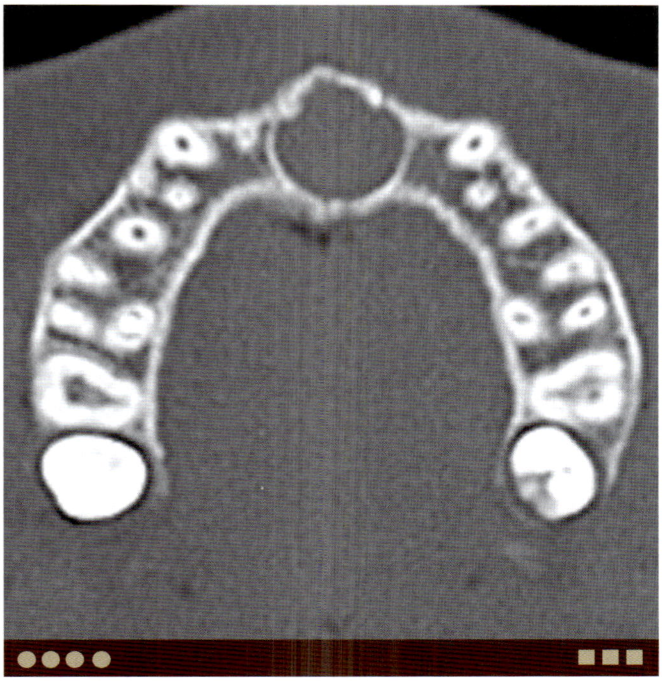

J. Nasopalatine duct cyst. Axial CT demonstrates a well-corticated cyst in the anterior maxilla in midline, separating the central incisors.

Case 9–2 Dentigerous (Follicular) Cyst

Osamu Sakai, Anita Gohel

PRESENTATION

An incidental lucent lesion in the mandible.

FINDINGS

CT demonstrates a cystic lesion containing the crown of the unerupted tooth.

DIFFERENTIAL DIAGNOSIS

- Hyperplastic follicle: Normal follicular space is less than 3 mm. If the follicular space is more than 6 mm, it is more likely a dentigerous cyst.
- Keratocystic odontogenic tumor: This may be seen around the crown of the teeth, but has a lesser tendency to expand or resorb teeth than dentigerous cyst.
- Ameloblastoma: This demonstrates significant expansile change with thinning/erosion of the cortex, and resorption and displacement of the adjacent tooth root.

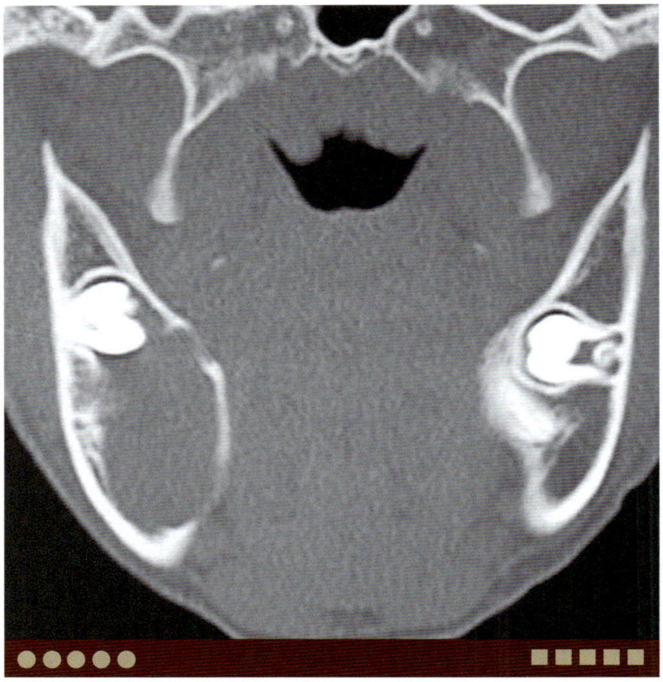

A. Dentigerous cyst. Coronal CT demonstrates an expansile cystic lesion containing the tooth crown in the posterior body of the mandible.

COMMENTS

This is a 17-year-old adolescent with an incidental lucent lesion in the mandible.

Dentigerous (follicular) cyst is the most common developmental odontogenic cyst. The lesion forms around the crown of an unerupted tooth, commonly the third molar, and is typically diagnosed in patients between 30 and 40 years of age. Fluid accumulates between the layers of reduced enamel epithelium or between the epithelium and the crown of the tooth.

Therefore, identifying the crown of a tooth projecting into the cystic cavity is pathognomonic.

The cyst appears radiologically as a well-demarcated radiolucent lesion attached at an acute angle to the cervical area of an unerupted tooth. The border of the lesion may be radiopaque.

A dentigerous cyst may become extremely large, often resorbing and displacing the roots of adjacent teeth and remodeling and expanding the mandible. However, the cortical bone is usually preserved. Cases of ameloblastic transformation of a dentigerous cyst in patients under 40 years have been reported.

PEARLS

- **Dentigerous cyst is the most common developmental odontogenic cyst.**
- **The lesion forms around the crown of an unerupted tooth, commonly the third molar.**
- **Mural ameloblastomas forming from the epithelial lining of the dentigerous cyst have been reported in patients less than 40 years of age.**

ADDITIONAL IMAGES (B-E)

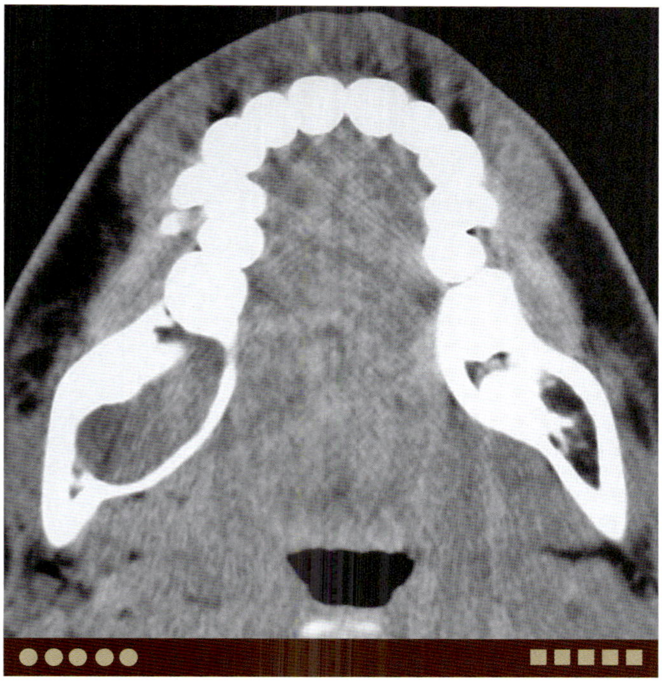

B. Dentigerous cyst, same patient as A. Axial soft tissue windowed CT demonstrates water density within the cyst. No extraosseous lesion is noted.

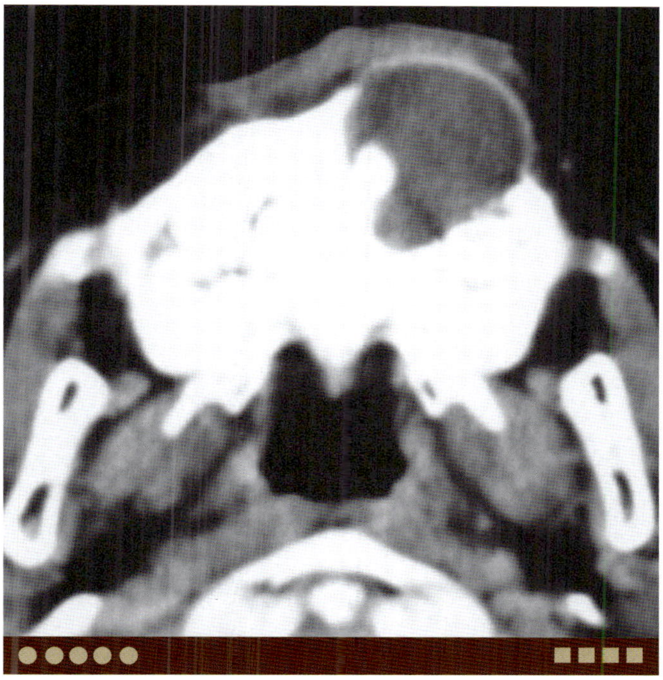

C. Dentigerous cyst in a different patient. Axial soft tissue windowed CT demonstrates an expansile cystic lesion in the anterior left maxilla.

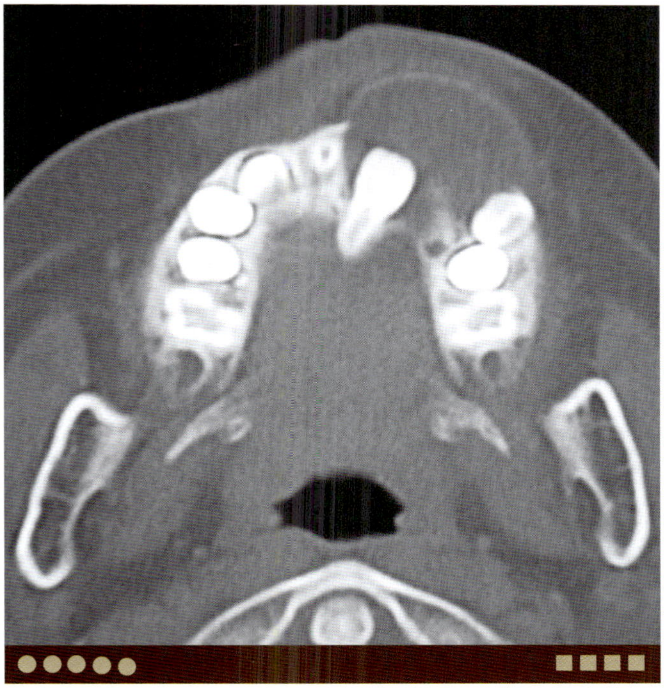

D. Dentigerous cyst, same patient as C. Axial bone-windowed CT demonstrates the tooth crown inside the cyst.

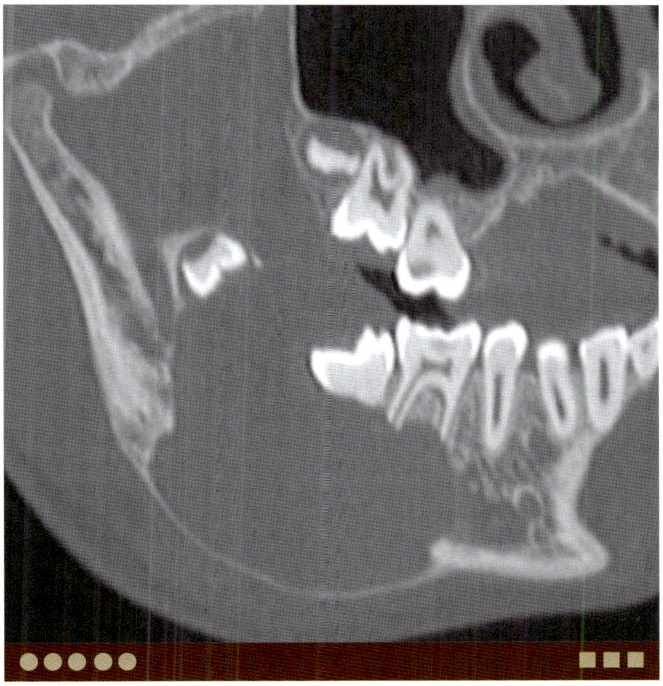

E. Dentigerous cyst in a different patient. Oblique-sagittal CT demonstrates an expansile cystic lesion in the posterior mandible containing the crown. Note significant thinning of the cortex of the mandible and resorption of tooth roots, atypical for dentigerous cyst.

DIFFERENTIAL DIAGNOSIS IMAGES (F-I)

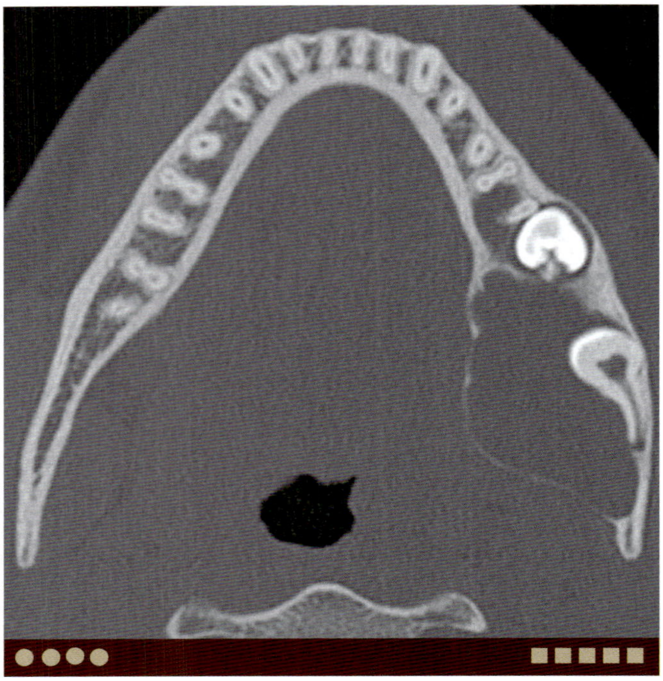

F. Ameloblastoma. Axial CT demonstrates an expansile cystic-appearing lesion in the posterior mandible containing the crown. Note significant thinning of the lingual cortex of the mandible.

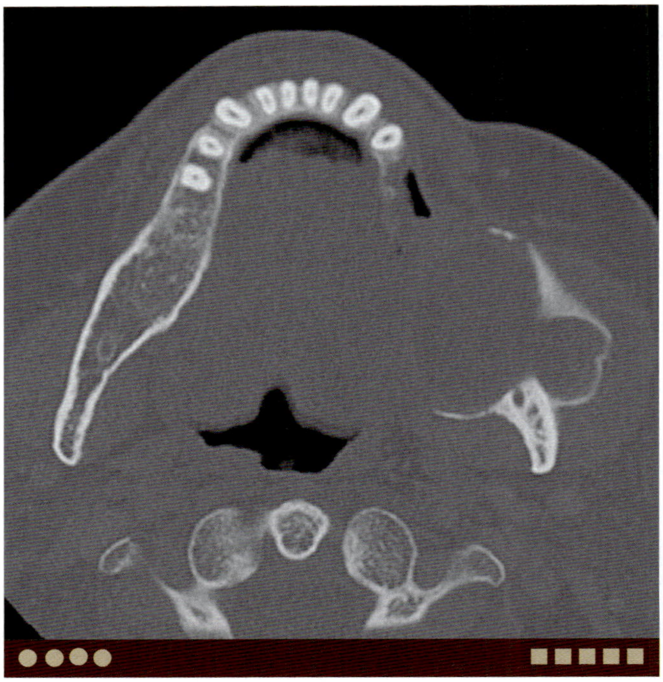

G. Ameloblastoma in a different patient. Axial CT demonstrates a lobulated, expansile lesion in the posterior body of the mandible extending to the ramus.

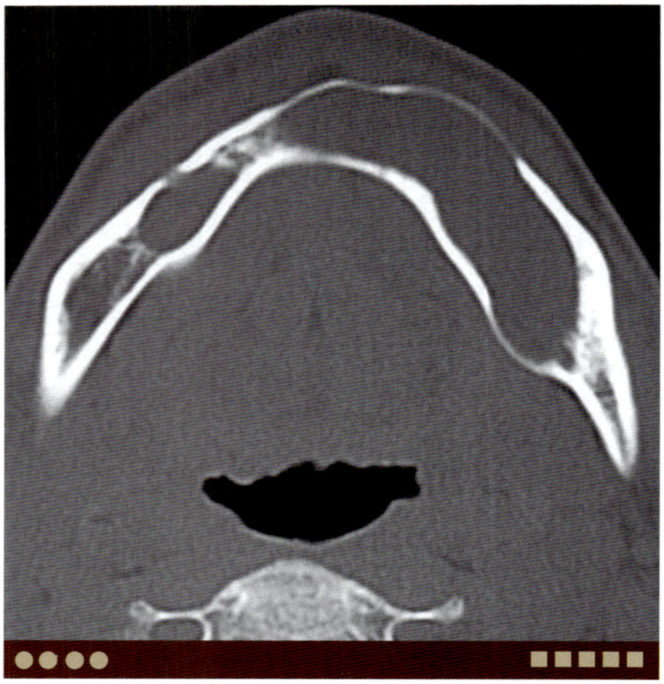

H. Keratocystic odontogenic tumor. Axial CT demonstrates a large cyst extending anteroposteriorly in the marrow cavity with wavy scalloping of the cortex without aggressive destruction.

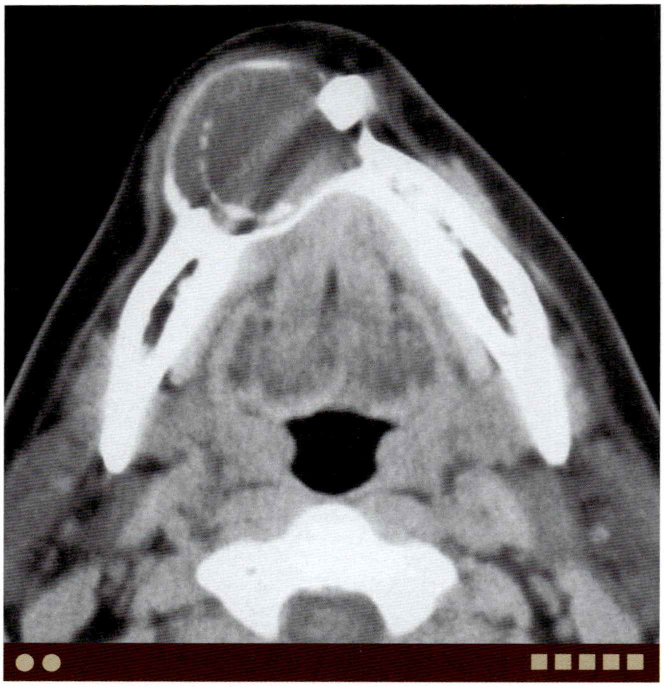

I. Adenomatoid odontogenic tumor. Axial soft tissue window CT demonstrates a cystic-appearing lesion containing a tooth crown as well as foci of calcification in the anterior body of the right mandible.

Case 9–3 Keratocystic Odontogenic Tumor

Osamu Sakai, Anita Gohel

PRESENTATION

Painless jaw swelling.

FINDINGS

CT demonstrates an elongated cystic lesion with smooth margins in the mandible.

DIFFERENTIAL DIAGNOSIS

- Radicular (periapical) cyst: This is the most common odontogenic cyst. The cyst forms around the root of the tooth.
- Dentigerous (follicular) cyst: This is the most common developmental odontogenic cyst and lesion forms around the crown of an unerupted tooth.
- Ameloblastoma: This is an odontogenic tumor and may form around the crown of an unerupted tooth.

COMMENTS

This is a 29-year-old man with swelling of the mandible.

Keratocystic odontogenic tumor (KCOT), formally termed as odontogenic keratocyst (OKC) is a benign, however, locally aggressive developmental odontogenic tumor, most commonly located in the body or ramus of the mandible. It arises from the dental lamina, which is found throughout the jaw and overlying alveolar mucosa and is lined by stratified keratinizing squamous epithelium. Therefore, the lesion can occur throughout periapical or primordial regions. KCOT can expand cortical bone and erode the cortex and has a high recurrence rate after resection. However, malignant transformation of KCOT is rare.

The lesion may be unilocular or multiloculated, often with daughter cysts that extend to the surrounding bone. Multiple KCOTs in a young patient should raise the possibility of basal cell nevus syndrome (Gorlin-Goltz syndrome). Associated findings with this autosomal dominant disorder include midface hypoplasia, frontal bossing and prognathism, mental retardation, calcification of the falx cerebri and dura, bifid ribs, and multiple basal cell carcinomas of the skin.

Typically, KCOT extends anteroposteriorly in the marrow cavity with wavy scalloping of the cortex. There may be an unerupted tooth in the lesion. On MRI, KCOT tends to show higher signal on T1W and lower signal on T2W images compared with dentigerous cyst and ameloblastoma.

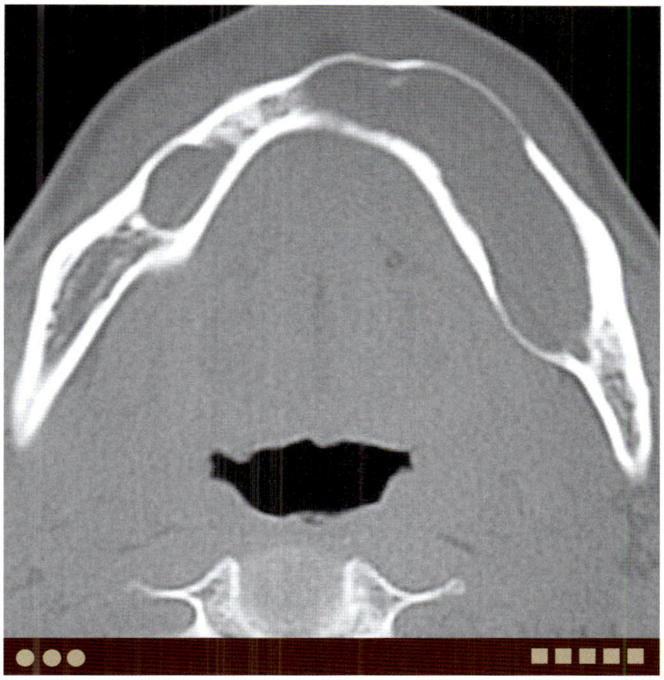

A. KCOT. Axial CT demonstrates a large cyst extending anteroposteriorly in the marrow cavity with wavy scalloping of the cortex without aggressive destruction. Note additional smaller lesion on the right.

PEARLS

- **KCOT is benign but locally aggressive, and has a high recurrence rate after resection.**
- **KCOT extends anteroposteriorly in the marrow cavity with wavy scalloping of the cortex.**
- **Multiple KCOTs in a young patient should raise the possibility of basal cell nevus syndrome (Gorlin-Goltz syndrome).**

ADDITIONAL IMAGES (B-F)

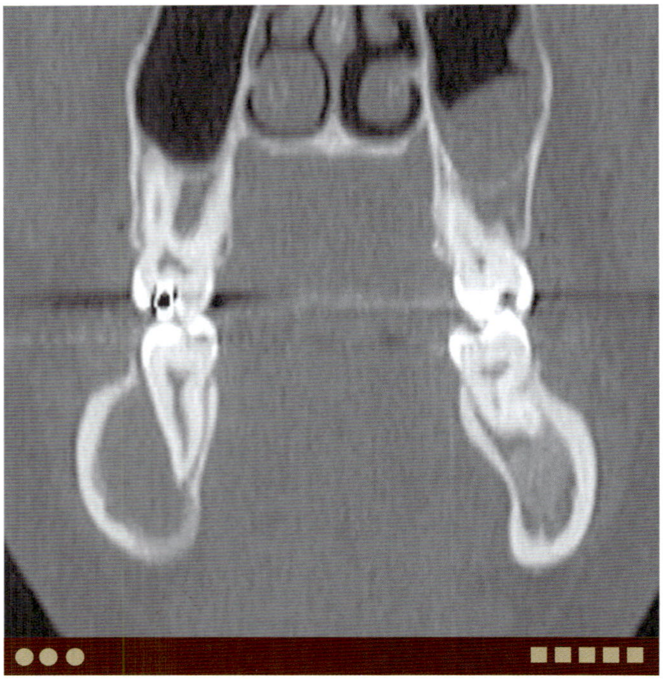

B. KCOT in a different patient. Coronal CT demonstrates an expansile cystic lesion in the right mandibular body with cortical thinning.

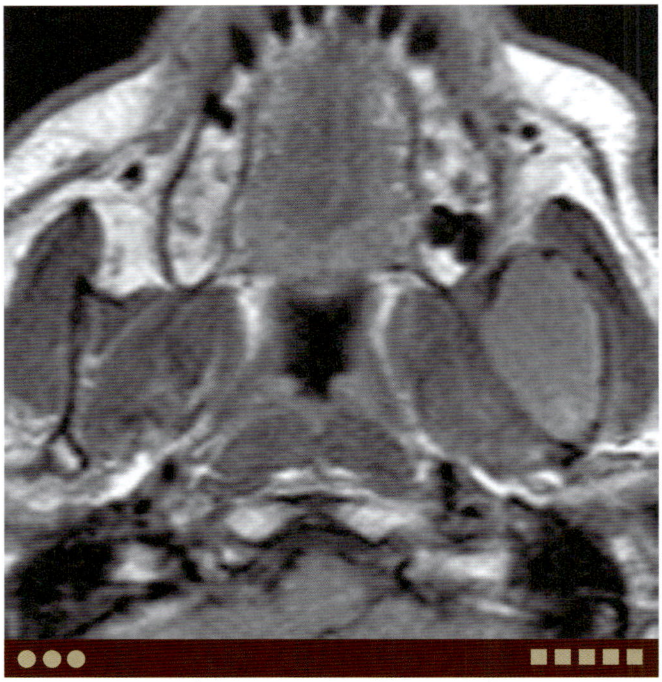

C. KCOT in a different patient. Axial T1W MR image shows an expansile cystic lesion in the mandibular ramus demonstrating intermediate-to-high signal.

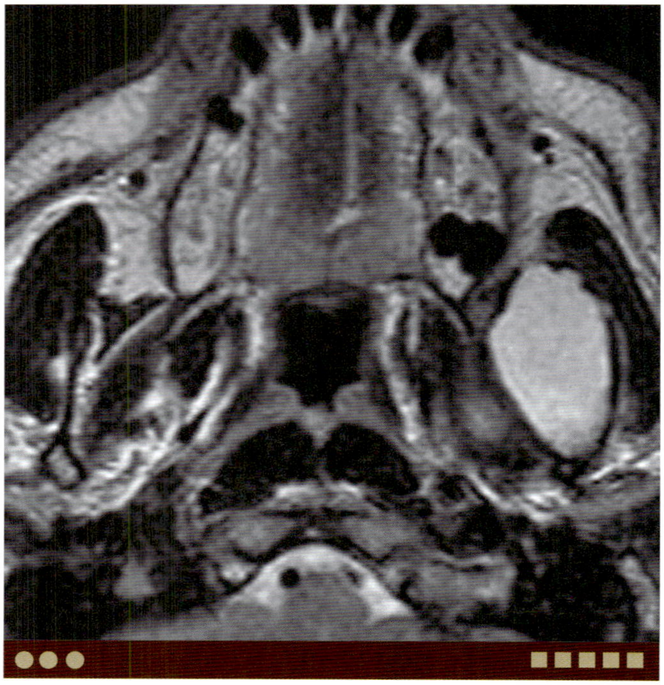

D. KCOT, same patient as C. Axial T2W MR image shows homogeneous high signal within the lesion.

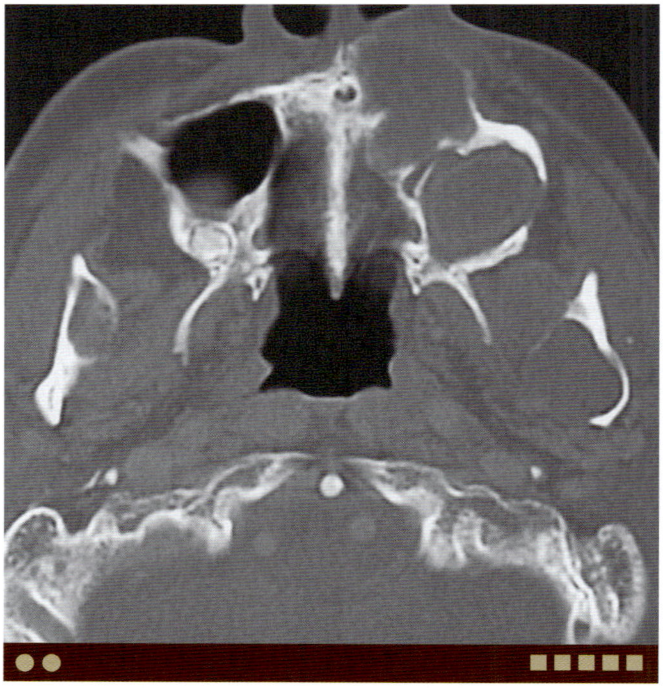

E. Basal cell nevus syndrome. Axial CT demonstrates multiple KCOTs in the maxilla as well as mandible.

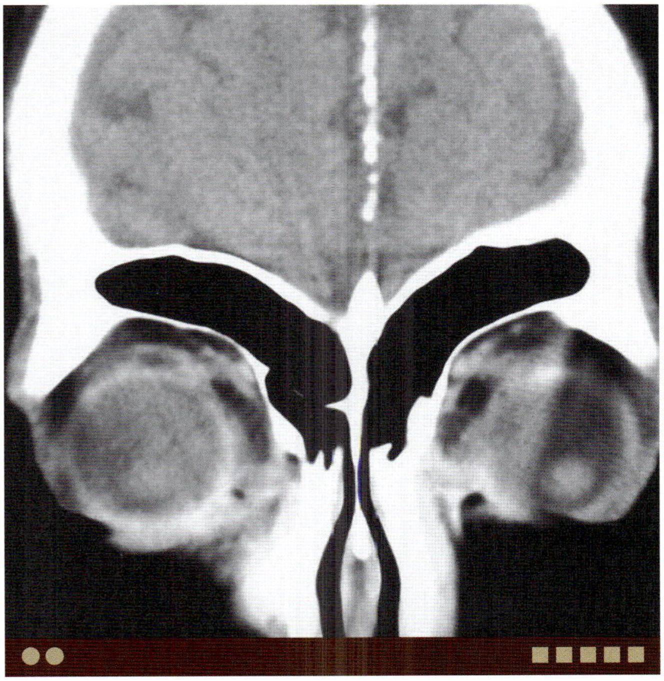

F. Basal cell nevus syndrome, same patient as E. Coronal CT demonstrates calcification of the falx.

DIFFERENTIAL DIAGNOSIS IMAGES (G-I)

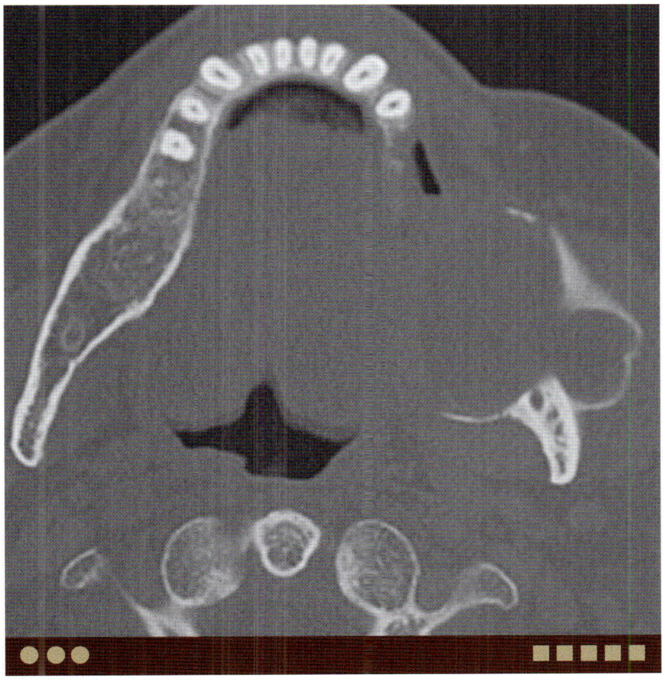

G. Ameloblastoma. Axial CT demonstrates a lobulated, expansile lesion in the posterior body of the left mandible extending to the ramus.

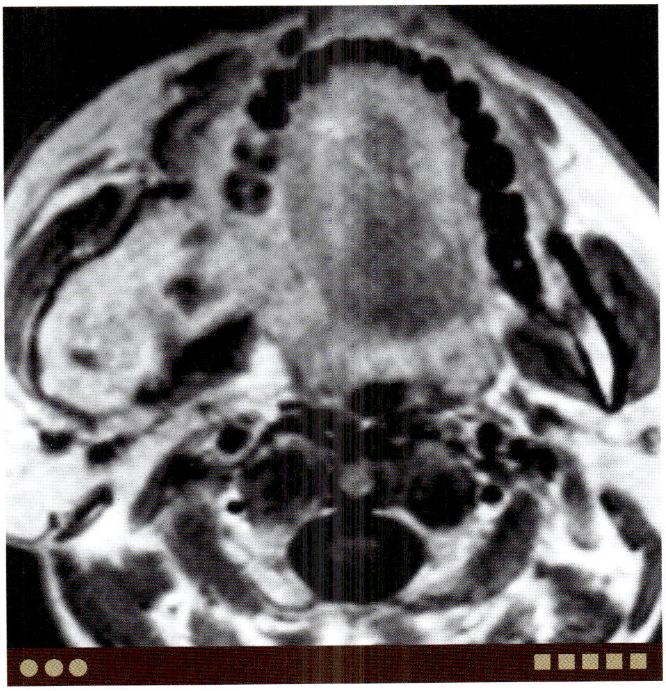

H. Ameloblastoma in a different patient. Axial postcontrast T1W image demonstrates a large enhancing lesion in the posterior body of the right mandible extending to the ramus.

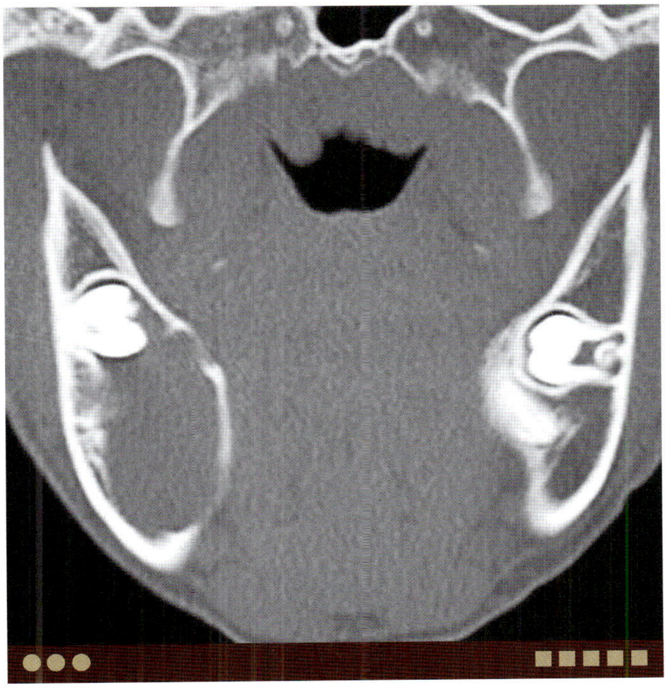

I. Dentigerous cyst. Coronal CT demonstrates an expansile lesion with an unerupted tooth in the posterior body of the right mandible.

Case 9-4 Ameloblastoma

Osamu Sakai, Anita Gohel

PRESENTATION

Painless jaw swelling.

FINDINGS

CT demonstrates an expansile cystic-appearing lesion in the posterior body of the mandible.

DIFFERENTIAL DIAGNOSIS

- Dentigerous (follicular) cyst: This is the most common developmental odontogenic cyst, which forms around the crown of an unerupted tooth.
- Keratocystic odontogenic tumor (previously called odontogenic keratocyst): This is a benign, however, locally aggressive developmental odontogenic tumor, most commonly located in the body or ramus of the mandible.
- Giant cell reparative cyst: This is a rare, benign, non-neoplastic lesion with a granulomatous appearance peculiarly affecting mandible and maxilla, and usually occurs in the second and third decades of life.
- Odontogenic myxoma: This is a rare, benign, locally invasive, multilocular neoplasm which is seen mainly in the mandible in the second and third decades of life.

COMMENTS

This is a 35-year-old man with painless jaw swelling.

Ameloblastoma is a benign epithelial odontogenic tumor arising from the enamel-forming cells of the odontogenic epithelium that have failed to regress during embryonic development. It usually diagnosed in twenties and thirties, about two-thirds are less than 40 years old without gender preference. It occurs in both the maxilla (20%) and mandible (80%), most commonly in the posterior body of the mandible, in the molar region. The expansile, radiolucent tumor can be unilocular or multilocular, with a characteristic "soap bubble–like" appearance, and unilocular lesions are more often seen in the maxilla. It is usually painless and the slow growth of the tumor can lead to significant expansion of the mandible.

Although multiple subtypes of ameloblastomas exist, most cannot be distinguished with radiology alone. Histopathologic analysis must provide the definitive subtype diagnosis of each lesion, with the exception of desmoplastic ameloblastoma. Distinguishing features of this subtype include multiple coarse internal calcifications with significant surrounding cortical destruction.

Typically, ameloblastoma demonstrates significant expansile change with thinning/erosion of the cortex, and resorption and displacement of the adjacent tooth root. CT findings of ameloblastoma include low-density cystic areas with scattered isodensity regions, representative of soft tissue components. Although ameloblastoma often shows similar findings to dentigerous (follicular) cyst and is difficult to be differentiated, it tends to have thick walls and solid component and shows more aggressive expansile change and cortical disruption. Extensive resorption of the roots of adjacent teeth is unique to ameloblastoma indicating aggressiveness. However, only histopathologic findings can help determine benignity and the absence of carcinomatous change. MRI better demonstrates thick walls and solid portions within the lesion better than CT, and is helpful to differentiate it from a dentigerous cyst.

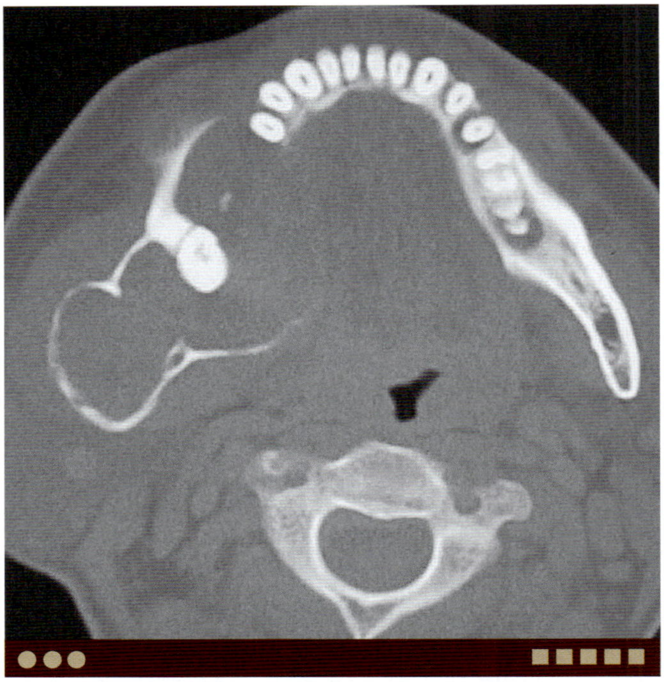

A. Ameloblastoma. Axial CT demonstrates a large, slightly lobulated, expansile lesion in the posterior body of the mandible extending to the ramus. Note displacement of the molar, significant erosion, and disruption of the cortex.

PEARLS

- **Ameloblastoma can be unilocular or multilocular and can demonstrate significant expansile change.**
- **Imaging findings of ameloblastoma may be similar to dentigerous cyst.**
- **Erosion of roots of adjacent teeth and disruption of the cortex indicates aggressiveness of the lesion and can be a clue to differentiate it from dentigerous cyst.**

ADDITIONAL IMAGES (B-G)

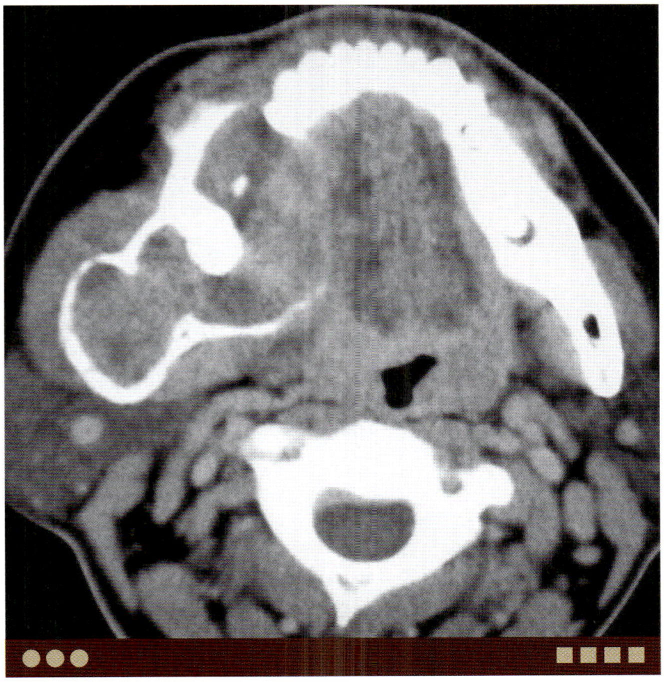

B. Ameloblastoma, same patient as A. Axial contrast-enhanced CT shows heterogeneous enhancement of the lesion.

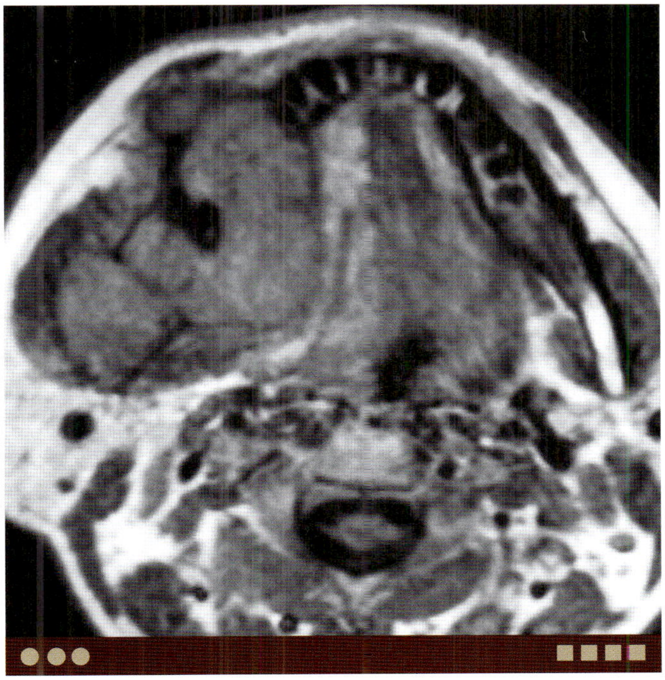

C. Ameloblastoma, same patient as A. Axial T1W MR image shows the lesion demonstrating heterogeneous intermediate signal.

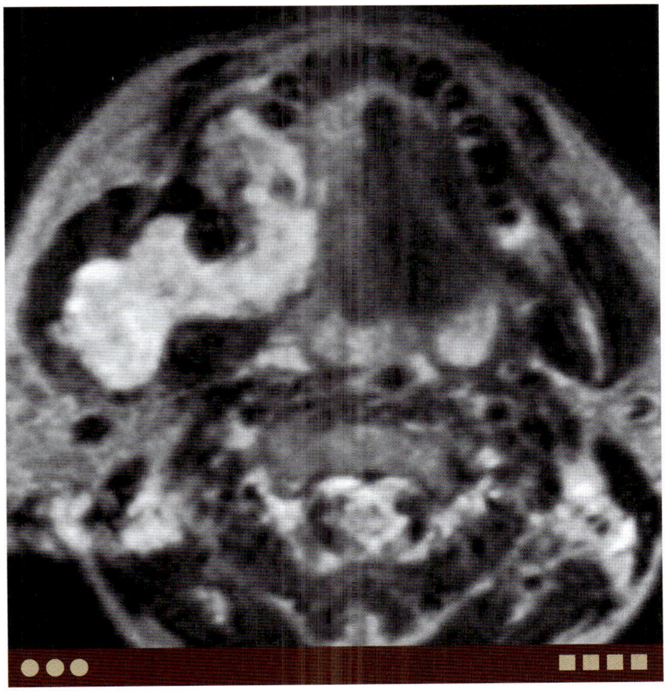

D. Ameloblastoma, same patient as A. Axial T2W MR image shows the lesion demonstrating heterogeneous high signal.

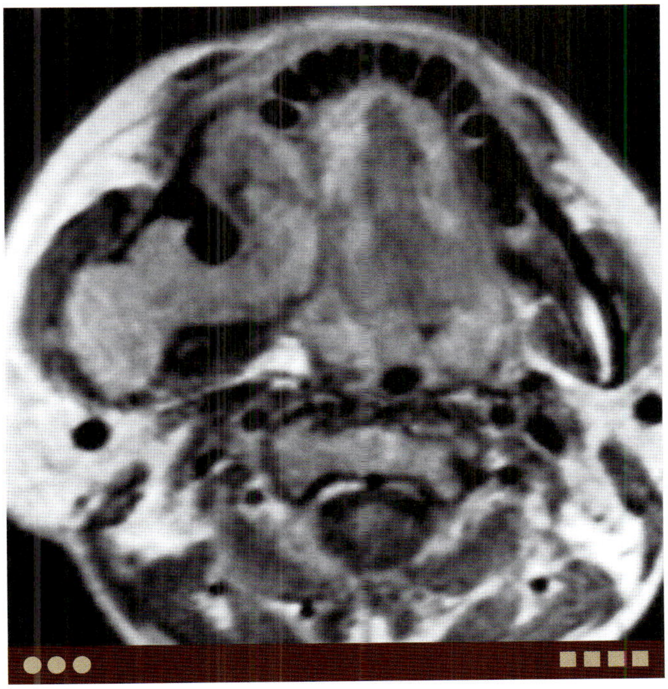

E. Ameloblastoma, same patient as A. Axial postcontrast T1W MR image shows heterogeneous enhancement of the lesion.

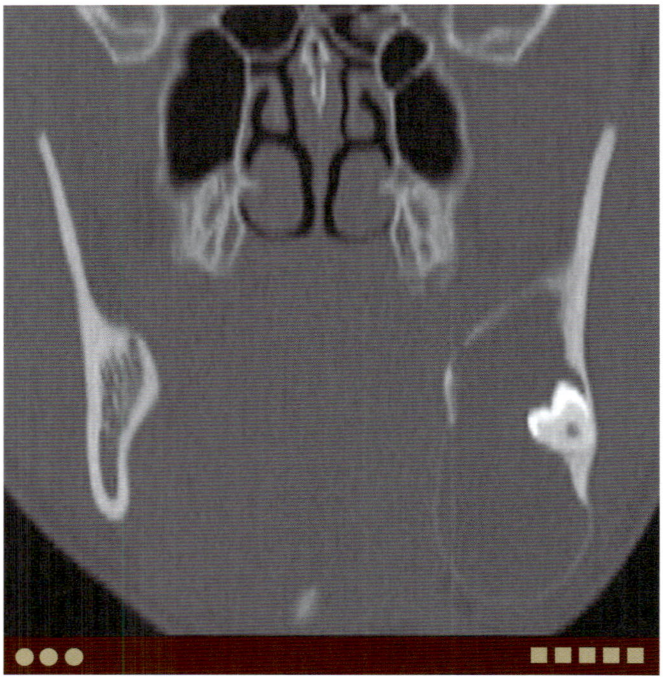

F. Ameloblastoma in a different patient. Coronal CT demonstrates a large, expansile lesion in the posterior body of the left mandible containing the crown.

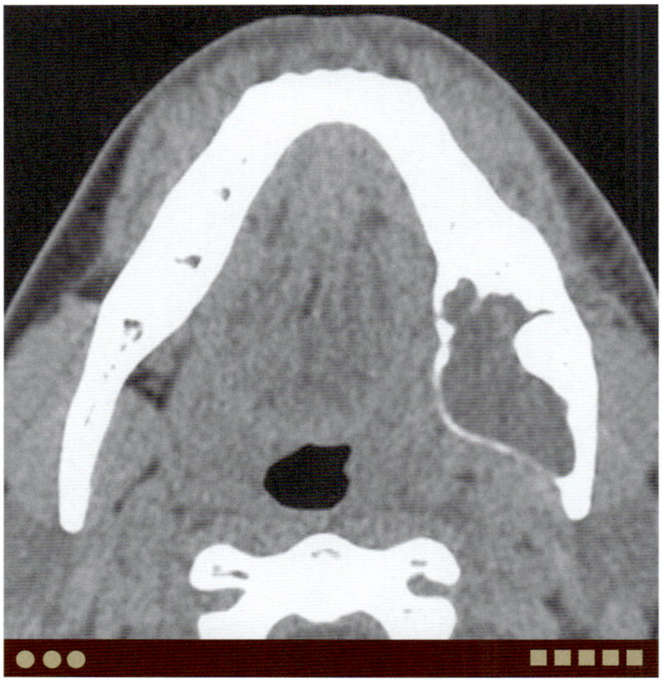

G. Ameloblastoma, same patient as F. Axial noncontrast soft tissue window CT shows water density of the lesion.

DIFFERENTIAL DIAGNOSIS IMAGES (H-J)

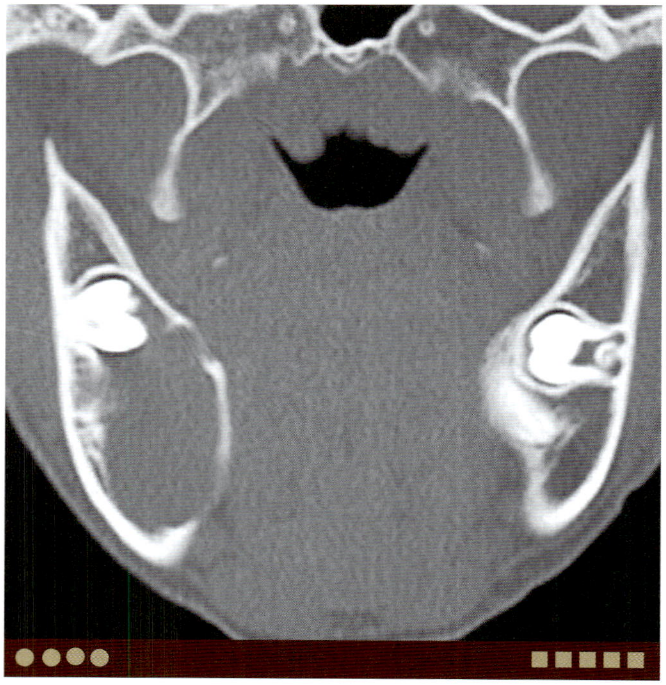

H. Dentigerous cyst. Coronal CT demonstrates an expansile lesion with an unerupted tooth in the posterior body of the right mandible.

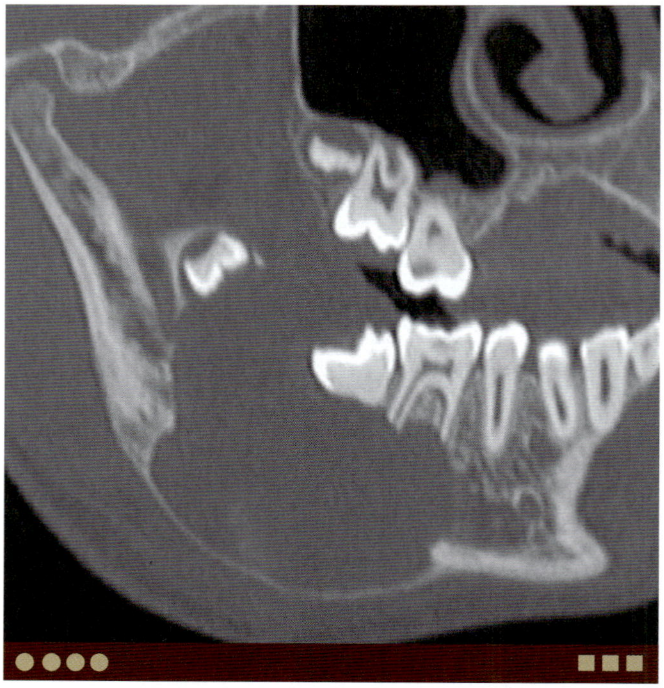

I. Dentigerous cyst in a different patient. Oblique-sagittal CT demonstrates an expansile cystic lesion in the posterior mandible containing the crown. Note significant thinning of the mandibular cortex of the mandible and resorption of tooth roots, atypical for dentigerous cyst.

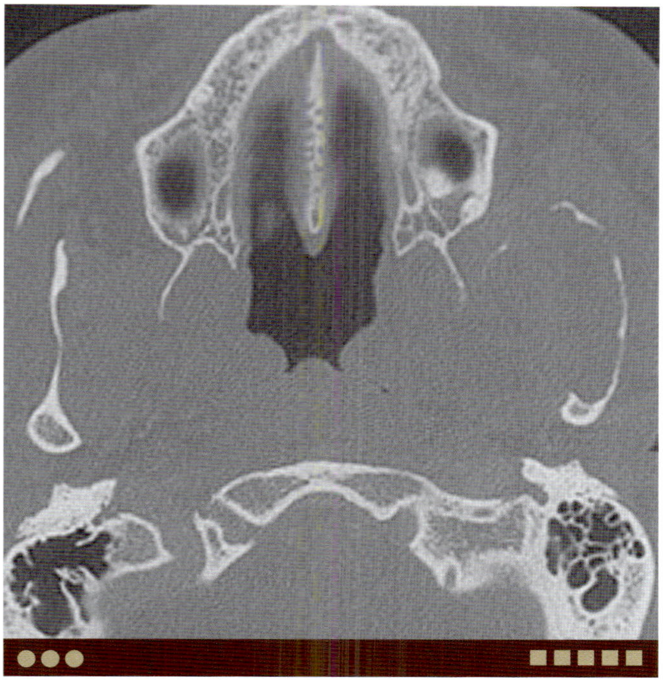

J. Keratocystic odontogenic tumor. Axial CT demonstrates an expansile lesion in the ramus of the left mandible with significant thinning of the cortex.

Case 9–5 Static Bone Cavity (Stafne Cyst)

Osamu Sakai, Anita Gohel

PRESENTATION

A lucent lesion noted in the panoramic radiograph at the dental checkup.

FINDINGS

CT demonstrates cortical bone defect in the lingual aspect of the angle of the mandible.

DIFFERENTIAL DIAGNOSIS

- Simple bone cyst: This often occurs in the body of the mandible and demonstrates cortical erosion/thinning but not cortical defect.
- Dentigerous (follicular) cyst: This is the most common developmental odontogenic cyst and contains a crown of an erupted tooth.
- Radicular (periapical) cyst: This is the most common odontogenic cyst containing a tooth root, and is not a cortical defect.
- Metastasis: Metastasis to the mandible is commonly seen in the posterior body, angle, or ramus.

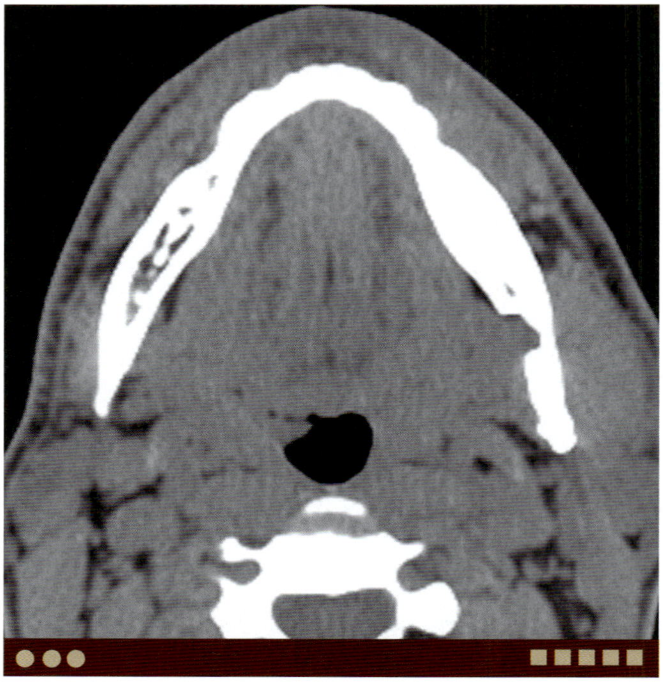

A. Static bone cavity. Axial soft tissue windowed CT demonstrates a lingual mandibular depression with heterogeneous density suggesting soft tissue and fatty tissue.

COMMENTS

This is a 36-year-old man with a "cystic" lesion in the mandibular angle incidentally found at the routine dental checkup.

Static bone cavity is also known as Stafne cyst or Stafne defect. However, this condition is not a cyst, actually it is a focal cortical bone defect in the lingual aspect of the angle or posterior body of the mandible, located below the mandibular canal. It is a lingual mandibular bone depression and is lined with an intact outer cortex.

It is believed to be a congenital/developmental lesion; however, the etiology is unknown and often incidentally discovered in the middle-aged patients. Classically it has been described that the submandibular gland tissue is seen in the defect; however, at least on imaging, often only fatty tissue filling the cavity is identified without soft tissue to suggest salivary gland.

On radiograph, it shows a cyst-like appearance with thick sclerotic wall in the posterior body or angle of the mandible. No more imaging is necessary; however, occasionally CT can be performed to rule out odontogenic or nonodontogenic cystic lesions. Static bone cavity is easily differentiated from odontogenic cysts by its location. CT demonstrates cortical defect in the lingual aspect of the mandibular angle, filled with fat with or without soft tissue density. MRI also demonstrates the lesion clearly although bony details are not provided.

PEARLS

- **Static bone cavity is also known as Stafne cyst. However, this condition is not a cyst, but a focal cortical bone defect.**
- **The location, the lingual aspect of the angle or posterior body of the mandible, below the mandibular canal, is unique enough to make the diagnosis and no further imaging is necessary.**
- **Classically it has been described that the submandibular gland tissue is seen in the defect; however, often only fatty tissue is identified in the cavity.**

ADDITIONAL IMAGES (B-F)

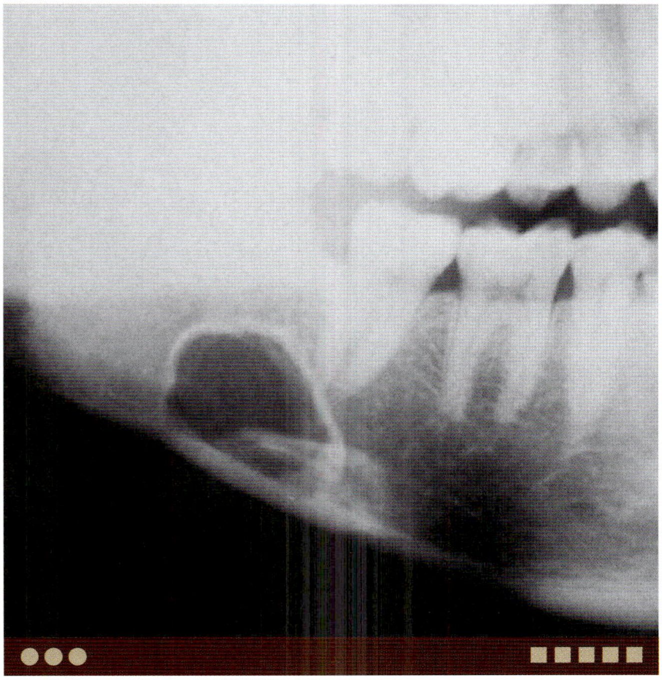

B. Static bone cavity in a different patient. Cropped panoramic radiograph reveals a well-defined, corticated radiolucency in the posterior body of the mandible.

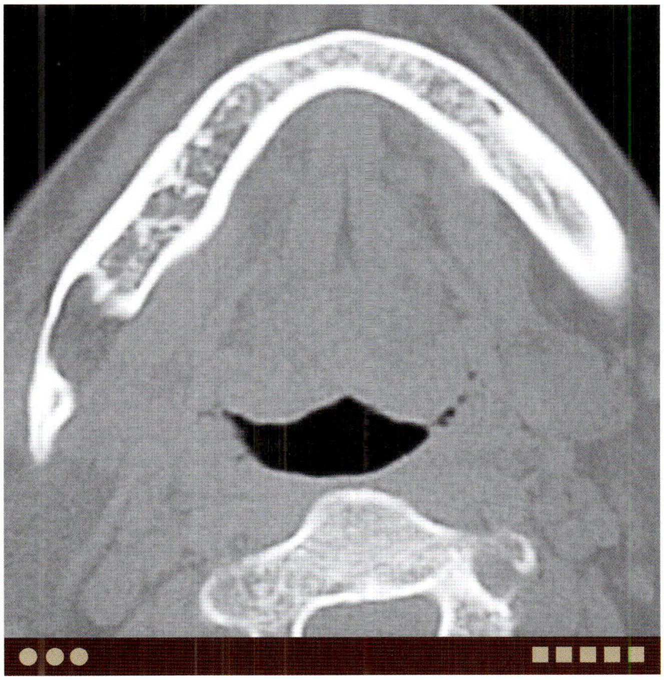

C. Static bone cavity, same patient as B. Axial CT demonstrates a well-defined lingual cortical defect in the posterior mandible

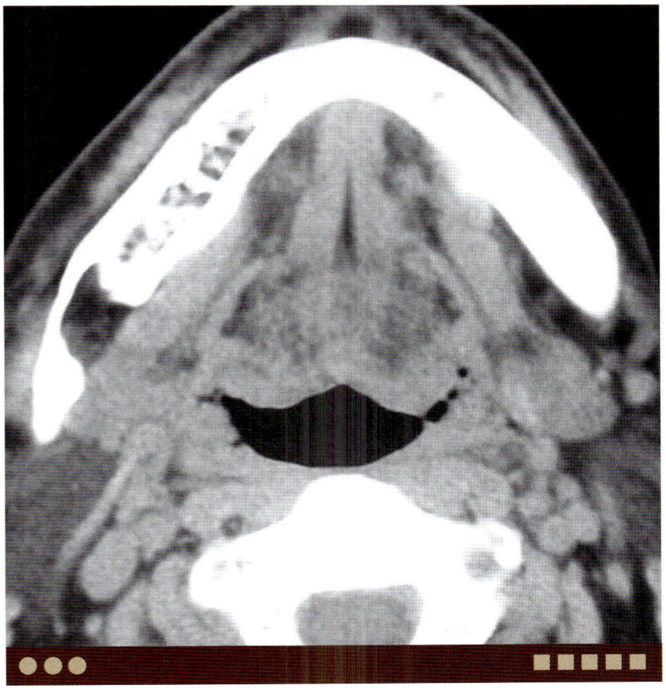

D. Static bone cavity, same patient as B. Axial soft tissue windowed CT reveals a lingual mandibular depression with slightly heterogeneous, predominantly fat density.

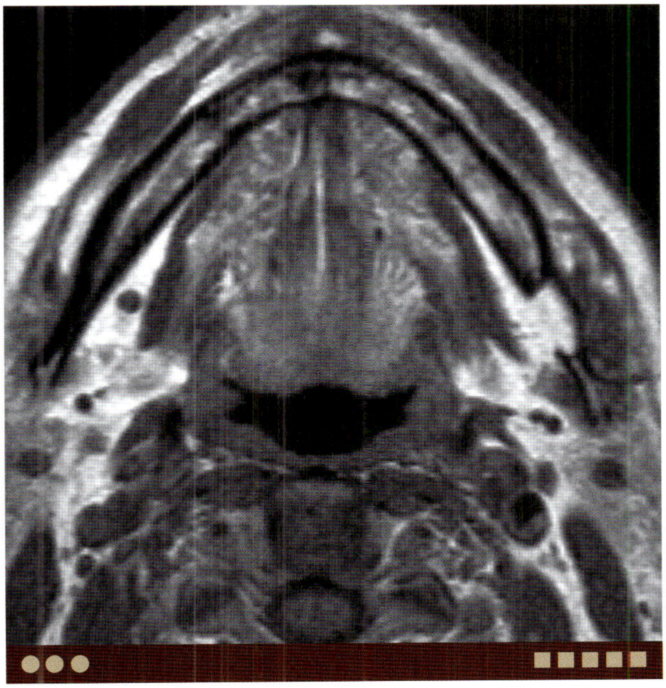

E. Static bone cavity in a different patient. Axial T1W MR image demonstrates a well-defined lingual cortical defect in the posterior left mandible filled with fat.

DIFFERENTIAL DIAGNOSIS IMAGES (G-I)

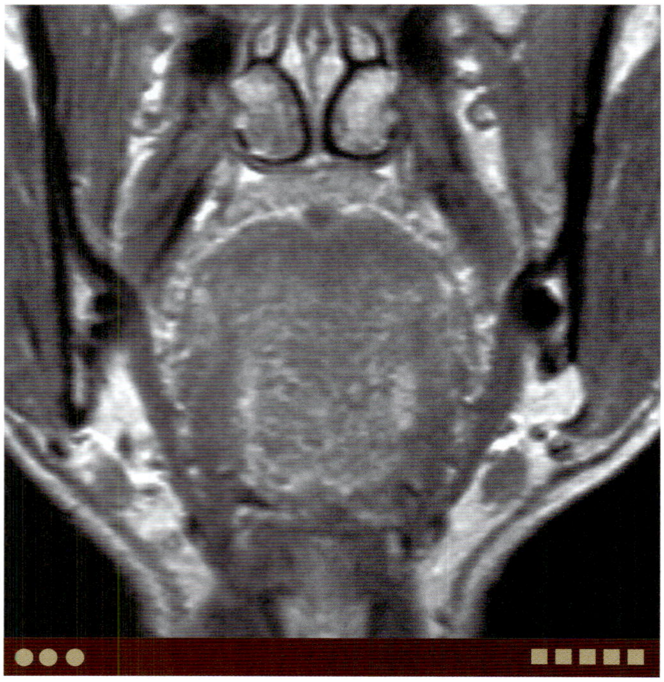

F. Static bone cavity, same patient as E. Coronal T1W MR image demonstrates a well-defined lingual cortical defect in the posterior left mandible filled with fat.

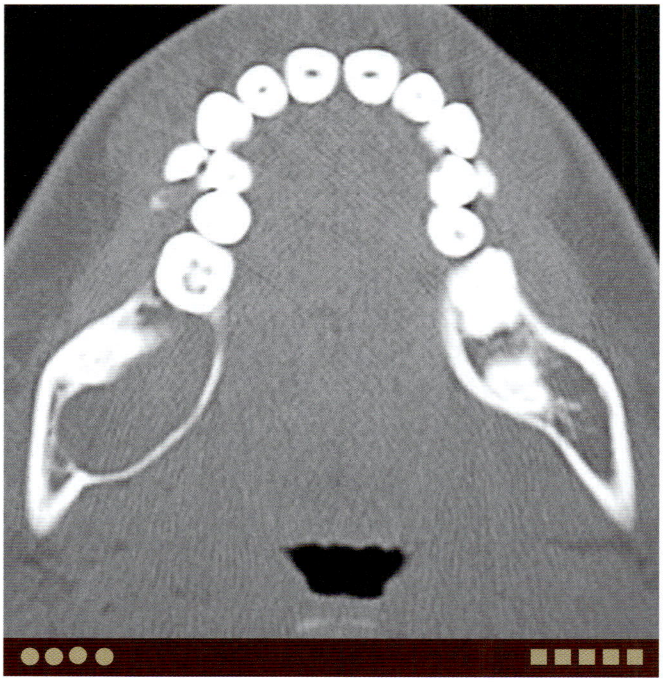

G. Dentigerous cyst. Axial CT demonstrates an expansile lesion with an unerupted tooth in the posterior body of the mandible.

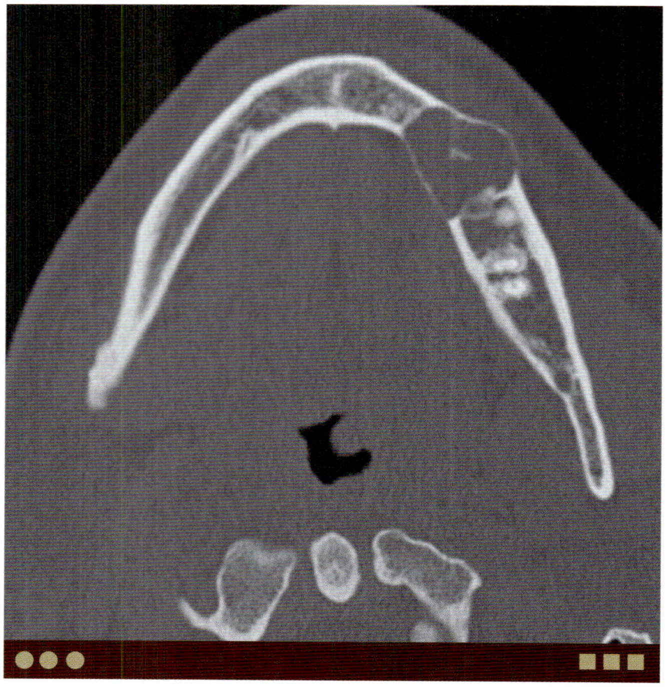

H. Simple bone cyst. Axial CT demonstrates a slightly expansile lesion in the anterior body of the left mandible with cortical thinning.

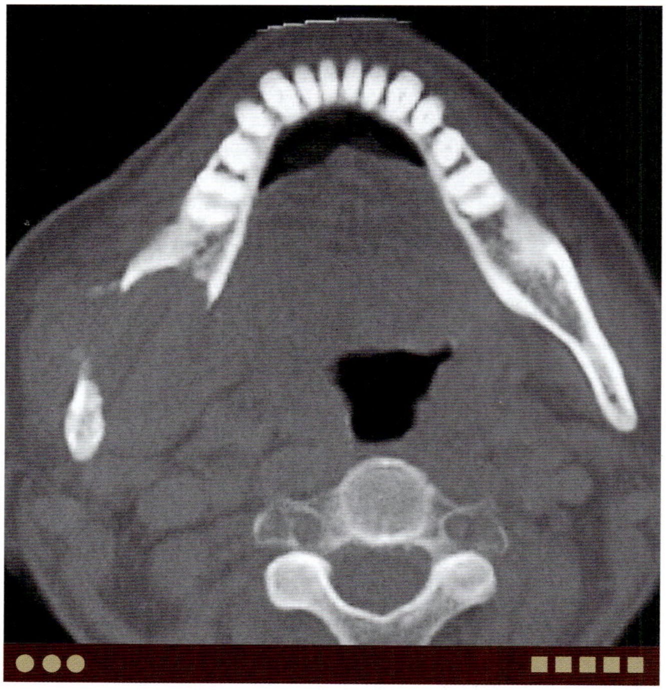

I. Metastasis from hepatocellular carcinoma. Axial CT demonstrates an expansile osteolytic lesion in the posterior body/angle of the right mandible.

Case 9–6 Nasoplatine Duct (Incisive Canal) Cyst

Osamu Sakai, Akifumi Fujita, Margaret Chapman

PRESENTATION

Incidental finding.

FINDINGS

CT demonstrates a well-marginated cystic lesion within the anterior hard palate at midline.

DIFFERENTIAL DIAGNOSIS

- Radicular (periapical) cyst: This contains a tooth root within the cystic cavity.
- Dentigerous (follicular) cyst: This contains a crown of a tooth within the cystic cavity.
- Nasoalveolar cyst: This lesion is also one of the fissural cysts, but is located slightly off-midline and involves the alveolus.
- Nasolabial cyst: This is also one of the fissural cysts, but is located more superficially, anteromedial to the maxilla with bony erosion.

COMMENTS

This is a 30-year-old man with a "cystic" lesion in the maxilla at midline incidentally found at a routine dental checkup.

The nasoplatine duct (NPD) or incisive canal is a round or heart-shaped osseous structure located in the anterior hard palate at midline that contains branches of the descending palatine and sphenopalatine arteries, the nasopalatine nerve, and mucus-secreting glands. It usually measures 5 mm in diameter and 5 mm in length. If its diameter exceeds 1 cm, it is called as a nasopalatine duct cyst (NPDC) or incisive canal cyst. This is one of the fissural cysts and the most common nonodontogenic cyst. Fissural cysts are named based on their location: nasopalatine duct cyst, nasolabial cyst, and nasoalveolar cyst. Globulomaxillary cyst is classified as an odontogenic cyst in a recent classification. NPDC is usually asymptomatic and found incidentally. With increasing size, it is clinically recognized as a submucosal mass. Rarely, it presents with infection or inflammation.

Median palatal cysts are rare fissural cysts that develop from epithelium entrapped at midline from the fusion of the lateral palatal shelves of the maxilla. Most "median palatal cysts" may represent posteriorly located nasopalatine duct cysts, because the NPD courses posteriorly and superiorly as it extends from the incisive canal to the nasal cavity.

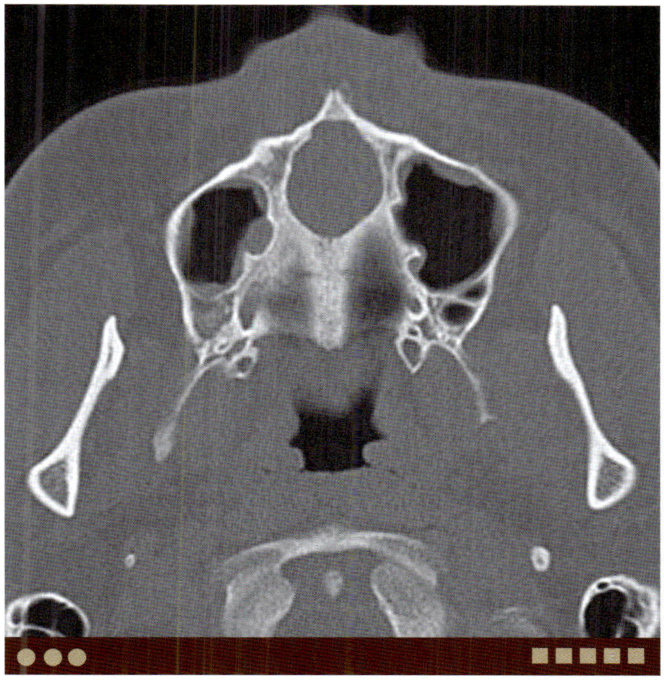

A. Nasopalatine duct cyst. Axial CT demonstrates an enlarged nasopalatine duct (incisive canal).

On imaging, NPDCs are seen as well-marginated expansile cystic lesions in the anterior hard palate at midline. Normal-appearing NPD is usually not identified. NPDCs separate the tooth roots; however, they do not contain them within their cystic cavity, an important distinguishing factor from most odontogenic cysts. On CT and MRI, NPDCs usually demonstrate homogeneous water density or signal. However, occasionally they contain proteinaceous fluid and show increased density and T1 signal.

PEARLS

- **NPDCs are common developmental cysts which occur in the anterior hard palate at midline.**
- **NPDCs displace the roots of the adjacent teeth.**
- **NPDCs typically demonstrate water density or signal, however, may exhibit increased density or T1 signal due to increased protein concentration.**
- **Median palatal cysts are rare fissural cysts arising from the hard palate, and are often confused with posteriorly located NPDCs.**

ADDITIONAL IMAGES (B-G)

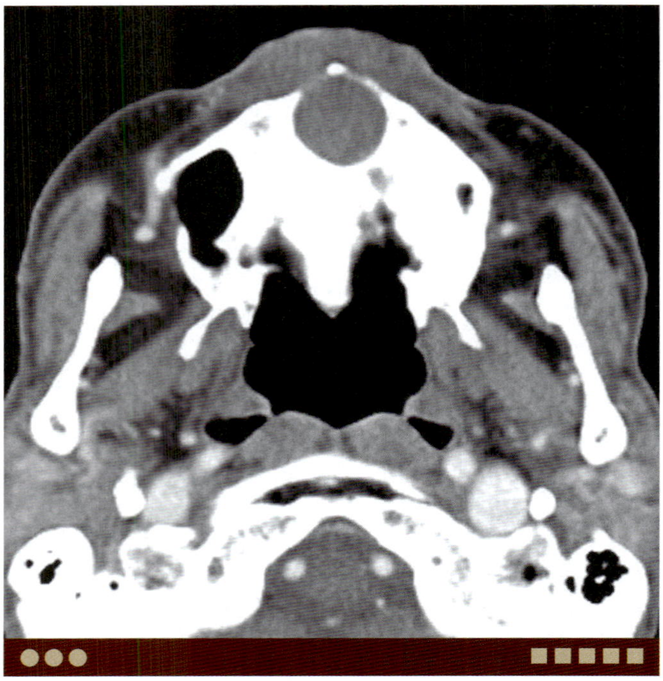

B. Nasopalatine duct cyst in a different patient. Axial soft tissue windowed CT demonstrates a homogeneous density cystic lesion in the anterior palate at midline.

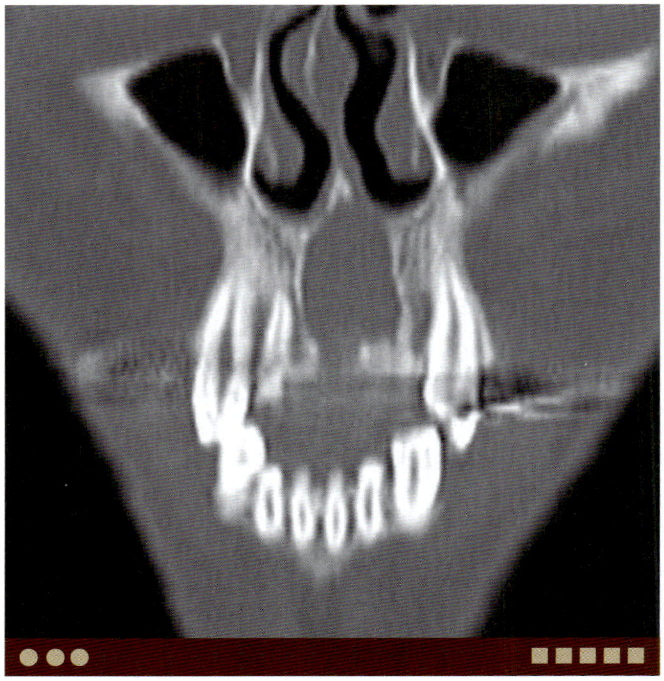

C. Nasopalatine duct cyst, same patient as B. Coronal bone windowed CT demonstrates an enlarged NPD separating the central incisors.

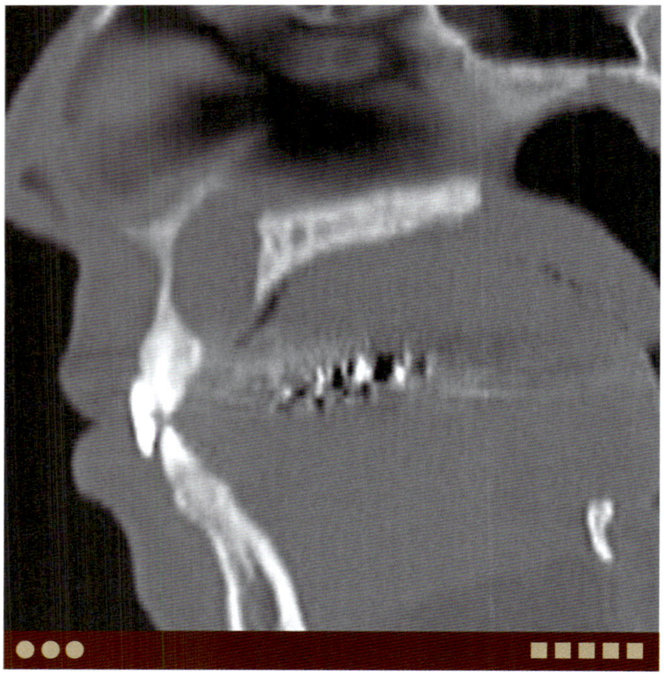

D. Nasopalatine duct cyst, same patient as B. Sagittal bone windowed CT demonstrates an enlarged NPD.

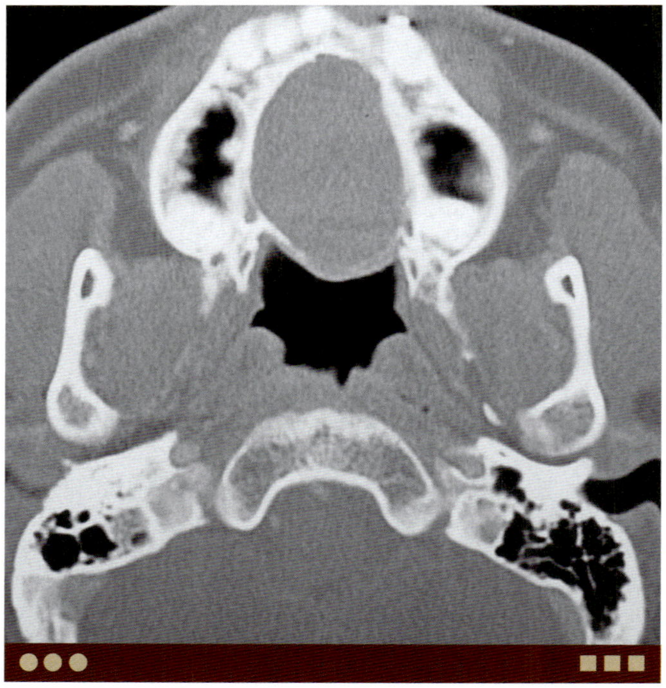

E. Median palatal cyst. Axial CT demonstrates a large cystic lesion in the palate.

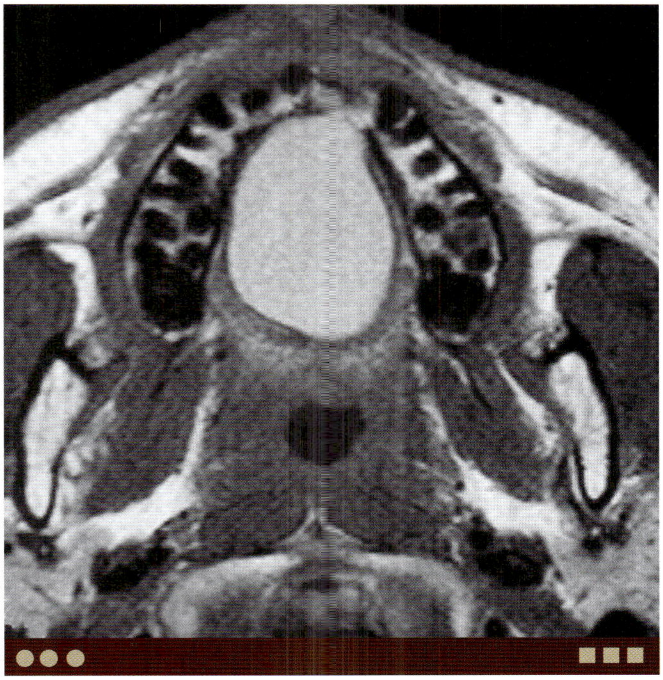

F. Median palatal cyst, same patient as E. Axial T1W MR image demonstrates a large high-signal cystic lesion in the palate at midline. The high T1 signal suggests proteinaceous content.

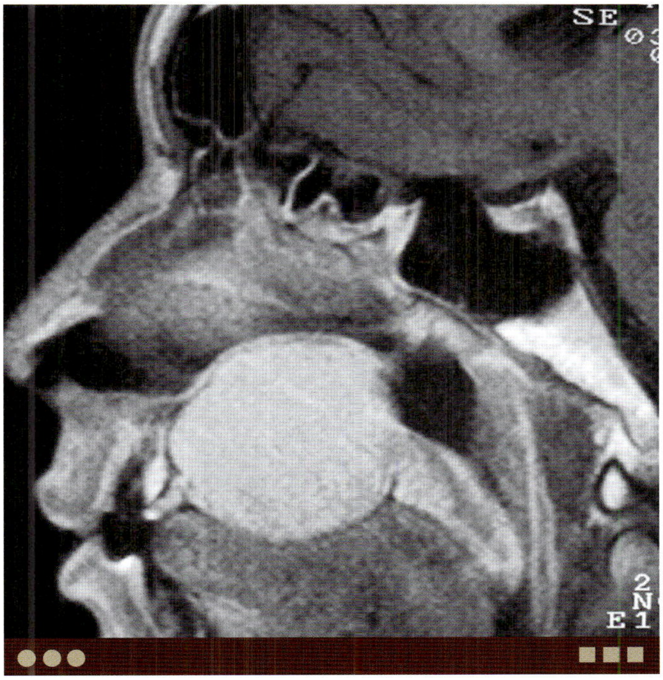

G. Median palatal cyst, same patient as E. Sagittal T1W MR image demonstrates a large high-signal intensity cystic lesion in the palate at midline.

DIFFERENTIAL DIAGNOSIS IMAGES (H-J)

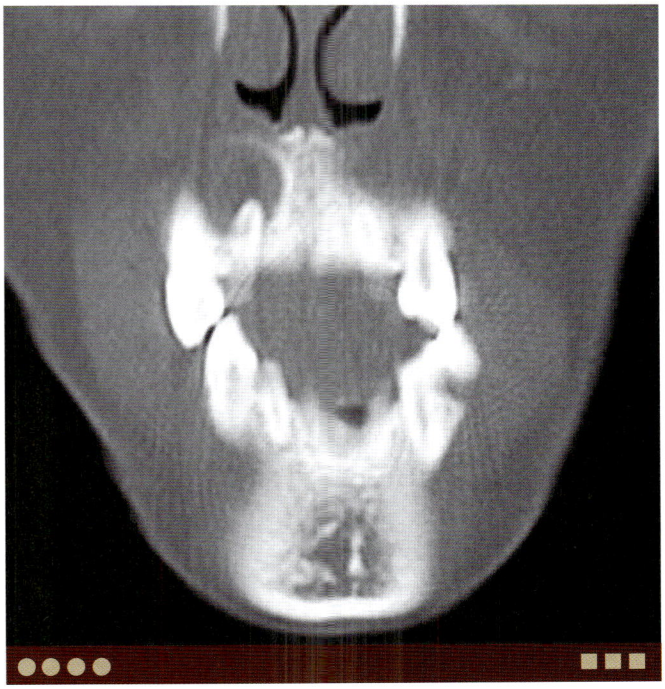

H. Radicular cyst. Coronal CT demonstrates a cystic lesion containing the root of the right maxillary central incisor.

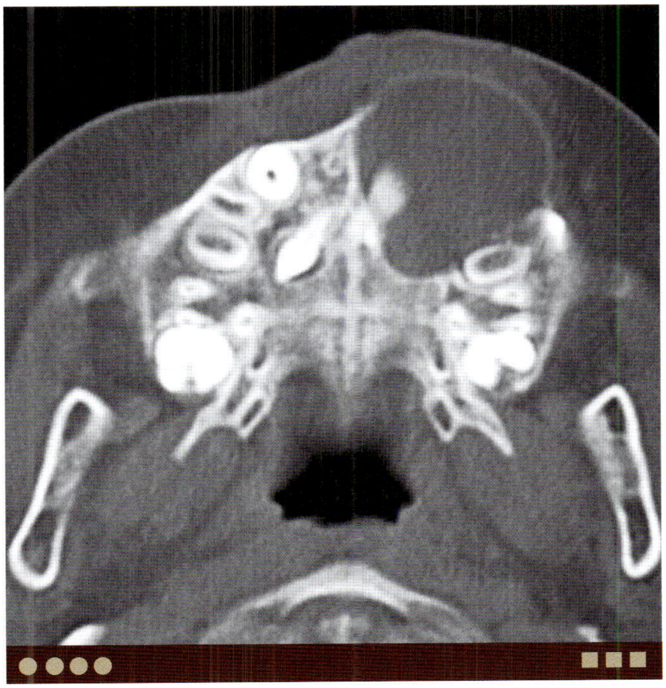

I. Dentigerous cyst. Axial CT demonstrates an expansile cystic lesion containing the crown of the tooth in the anterior left hard palate, not crossing midline.

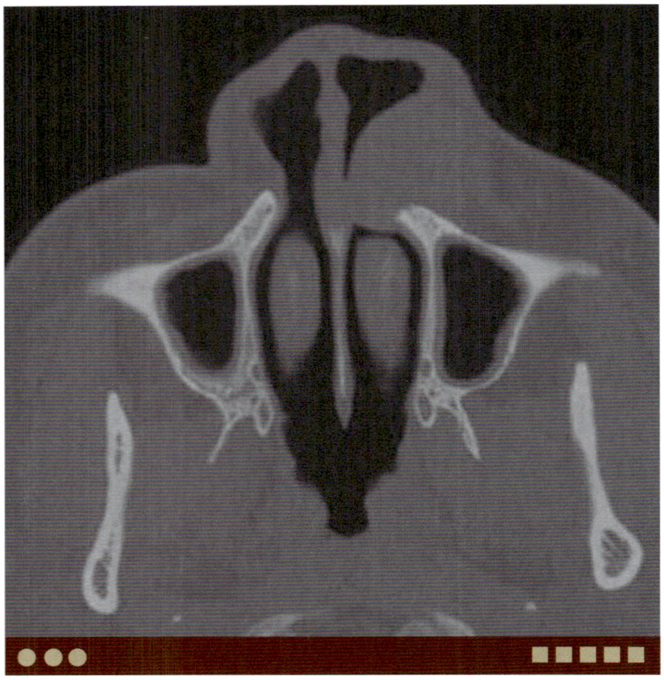

J. Nasoalveolar cyst. Axial bone windowed CT demonstrates a soft tissue density cystic lesion in the left nasal alar region with pressure erosion of the left maxilla.

Case 9–7 Osteomyelitis of the Jaw

Osamu Sakai, Daniel Weller

PRESENTATION

Jaw swelling and pain.

FINDINGS

CT demonstrates heterogeneous sclerotic changes in the mandible with loss of normal fatty marrow.

DIFFERENTIAL DIAGNOSIS

- Bisphosphonate-associated osteonecrosis of the jaw: This is a rare condition which occurs in patients on bisphosphonate therapy, particularly with intravenous administration.
- Osteoradionecrosis: This is a condition of radiation-induced bone necrosis, rare in patients who have received less than 60 Gy.
- Metastasis: This usually shows osteolytic change, most commonly seen in the posterior body and angle where abundant bone marrow is present.
- Osteosarcoma: This is a rare malignant tumor, and usually demonstrates osteoblastic changes with aggressive periosteal reaction.
- Fibrous dysplasia: Fibroosseous lesions demonstrating mixed density or ground-glass appearance without periosteal reaction or extraosseous soft tissue mass.

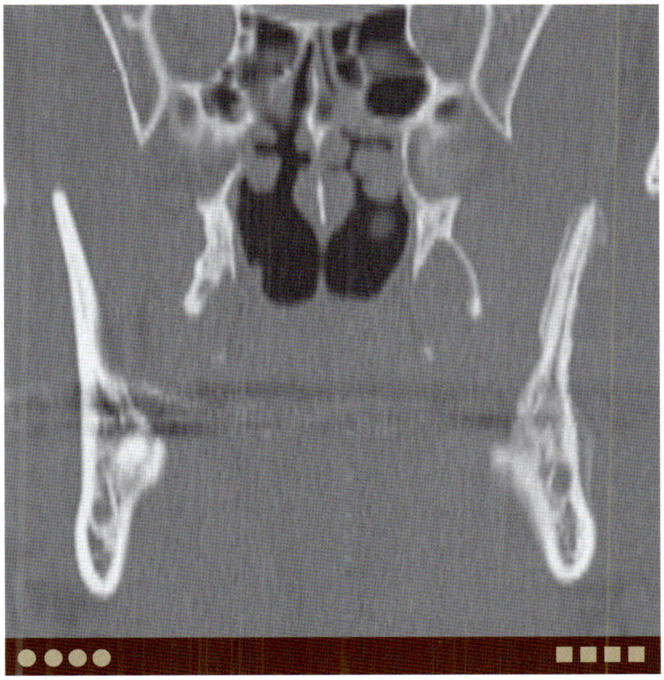

A. Acute osteomyelitis. Coronal CT demonstrates periosteal reaction in the left mandible, which shows mild sclerotic changes.

COMMENTS

This is a 65-year-old man with mandibular pain and swelling.

Osteomyelitis of the jaw is usually a polymicrobial disease, commonly from streptococci, *Bacteroides*, peptostreptococci, and others. Typical clinical presentations of acute osteomyelitis are fever, malaise, facial cellulitis, trismus, and significant leukocytosis. Chronic osteomyelitis may present with swelling, pain, purulence, and intraoral or extraoral draining fistulae.

Practically, CT demonstrates demineralization, osteolytic or destructive changes in the acute phase. With a chronic course, sclerotic changes occur. Similar to osteomyelitis in long bones, periosteal reaction/new bone formation is seen in the subacute phase of osteomyelitis. In chronic osteomyelitis, sclerotic change is a common imaging finding. Initially, the sclerosis is localized around the causative lesion, and later more diffuse sclerosis, occasionally involving the entire mandible, may occur.

MRI is very sensitive to marrow abnormality and useful to identify inflammation or infection of the mandible. However, findings are nonspecific, and evaluation is often limited by metallic artifacts from prior dental procedures. It should be noted that metallic artifact can be produced from dental bur fragments even without metallic hardware.

Sclerosing osteomyelitis or Garre osteomyelitis is a specific type of chronic osteomyelitis with prominent proliferative periostitis, usually seen in children or young adults. It usually starts with a focal mild infection, followed by extensive periosteal thickening and reactive bone formation that may extend through the entire mandible.

PEARLS

- **Acute osteomyelitis demonstrates demineralization or osteolytic changes.**
- **Sclerosis is a common finding for chronic osteomyelitis. Fistula or sequestrum can be seen.**
- **Prominent proliferative periostitis can be seen, particularly in children or young adults.**

ADDITIONAL IMAGES (B-F)

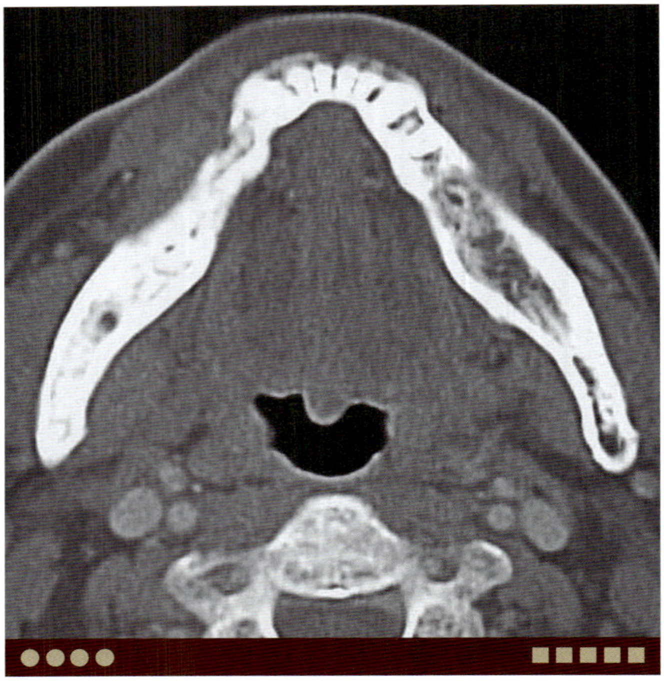

B. Chronic osteomyelitis in a different patient. Axial CT demonstrates diffuse sclerotic change in the right mandible.

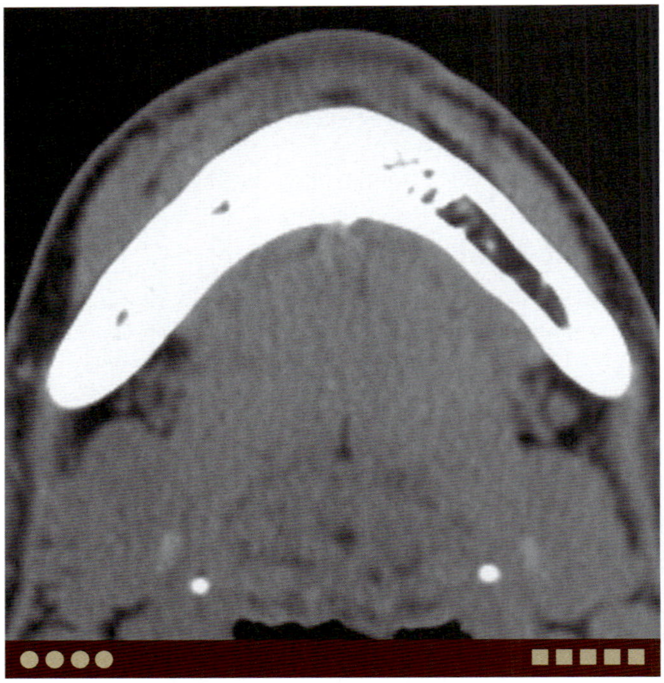

C. Chronic osteomyelitis in a different patient. Axial soft tissue windowed CT demonstrates loss of normal fatty marrow in the right mandible.

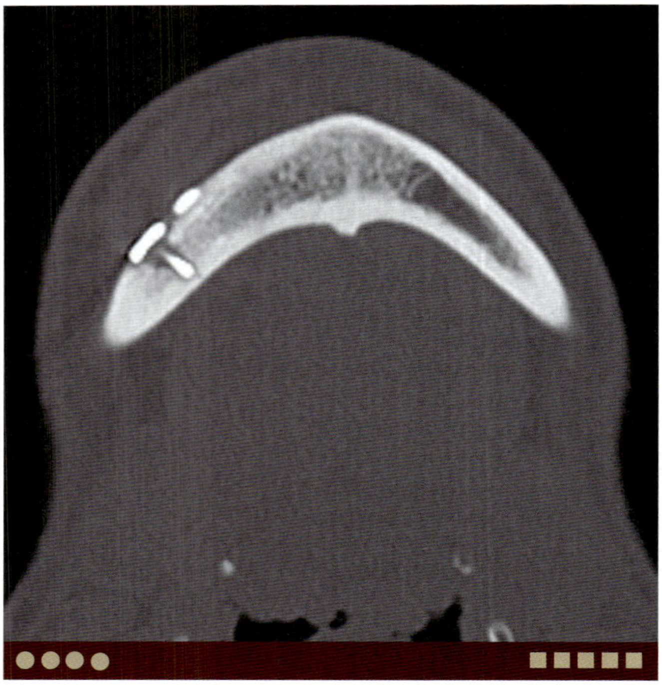

D. Chronic osteomyelitis, same patient as C. Axial CT demonstrates diffuse sclerotic changes in the right mandible. Note focal osteolysis around the infected screw.

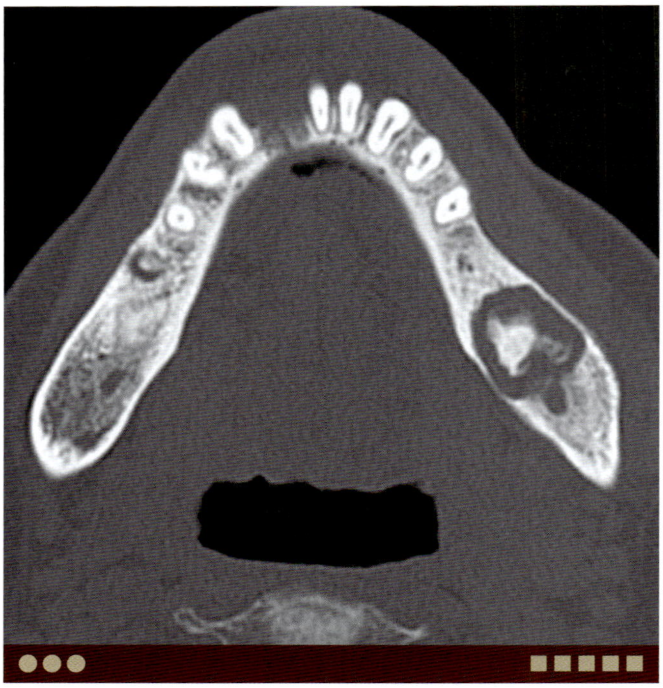

E. Chronic osteomyelitis in a different patient. Axial CT demonstrates a large osteolytic lesion with sequestrum in the left mandible. Note the entire mandible demonstrates diffuse sclerosis.

DIFFERENTIAL DIAGNOSIS IMAGES (G-I)

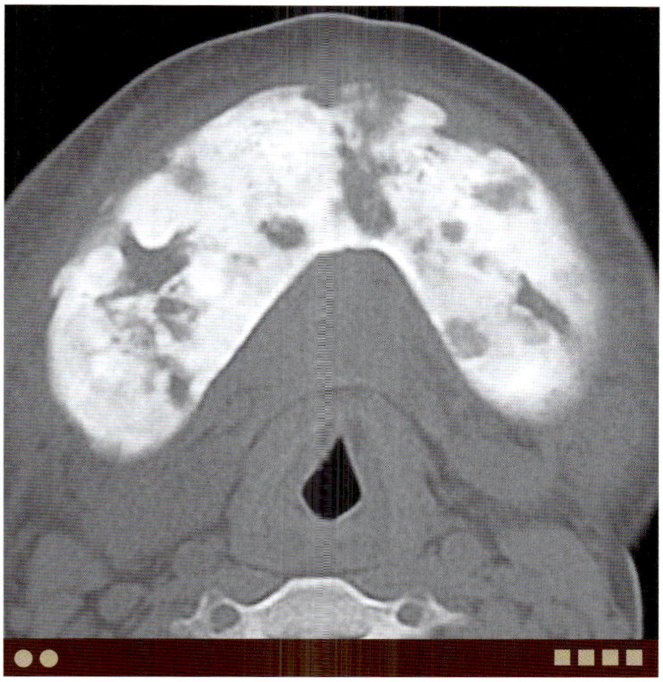

F. Sclerosing osteomyelitis. Axial CT demonstrates prominent proliferative changes with diffuse sclerosis and multiple osteolytic foci.

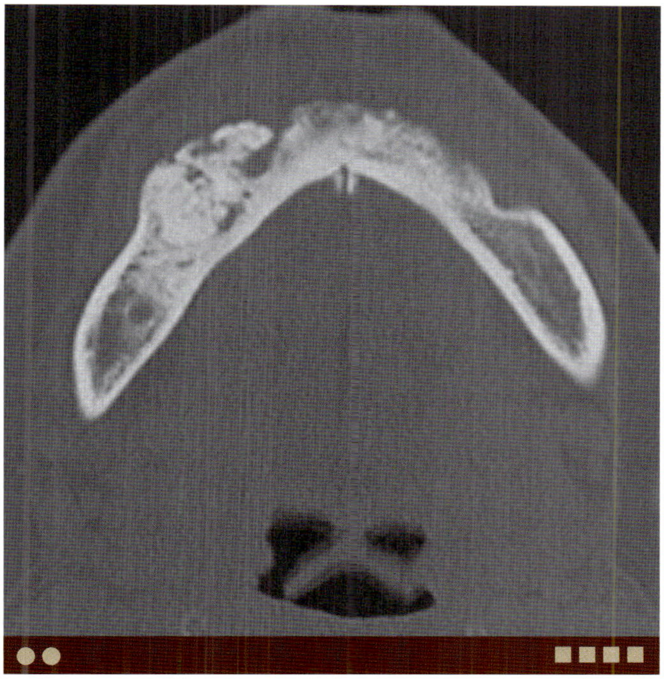

G. Bisphosphonate-associated osteonecrosis. Axial CT demonstrates sclerotic change and cortical destruction in the anterior body of the right mandible.

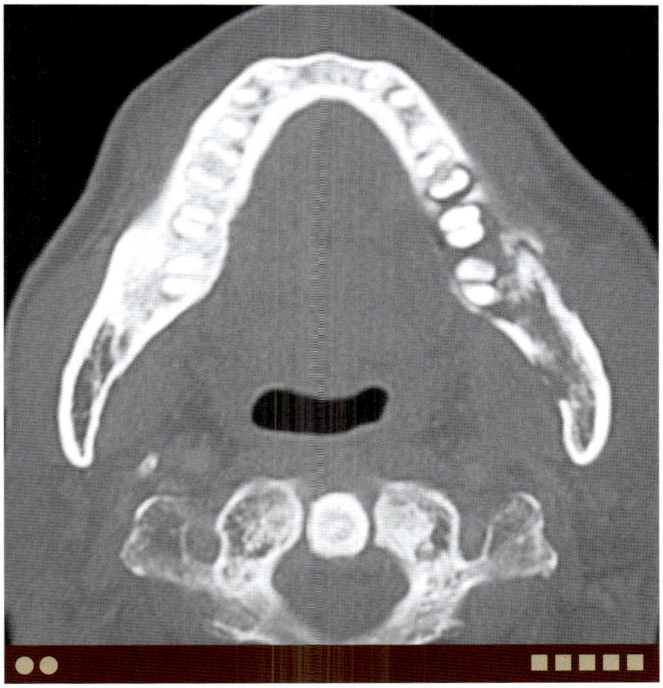

H. Osteoradionecrosis. Axial CT demonstrates diffuse demineralization and cortical destruction in the posterior body/ramus of the left mandible. Right mandible shows diffuse sclerotic changes consistent with osteitis.

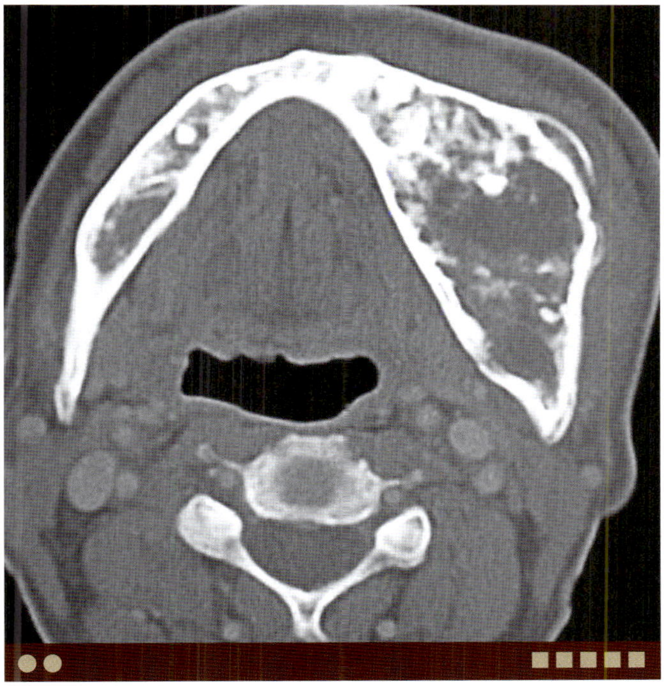

I. Fibrous dysplasia. Axial CT demonstrates a heterogeneously dense, expansile lesion in the left mandible, representing a mixture of sclerotic and cystic changes with preserved cortex.

Case 9–8 Renal Osteodystrophy, Hyperparathyroidism

Osamu Sakai, Anita Gohel

PRESENTATION

Diffuse swelling of the jaw in a patient on hemodialysis.

FINDINGS

CT demonstrates diffuse ground-grass density in the mandible.

DIFFERENTIAL DIAGNOSIS

- Chronic osteomyelitis: This condition demonstrates heterogeneous density; mixture of osteosclerotic and lytic changes, and occasionally shows expansion of the bone. Usually periodontal disease can be identified.
- Fibrous dysplasia: This condition often demonstrates a ground-grass appearance and resembles changes from hyperparathyroidism. However, it is usually more focal. Other fibroosseous lesions such as ossifying fibroma and Paget's disease may show similar findings.
- Paget's disease: This is a common disease of unknown etiology, usually seen in elderly people but unusual before age 40. Involvement of the skull and skull base is common, although any bones can be affected.

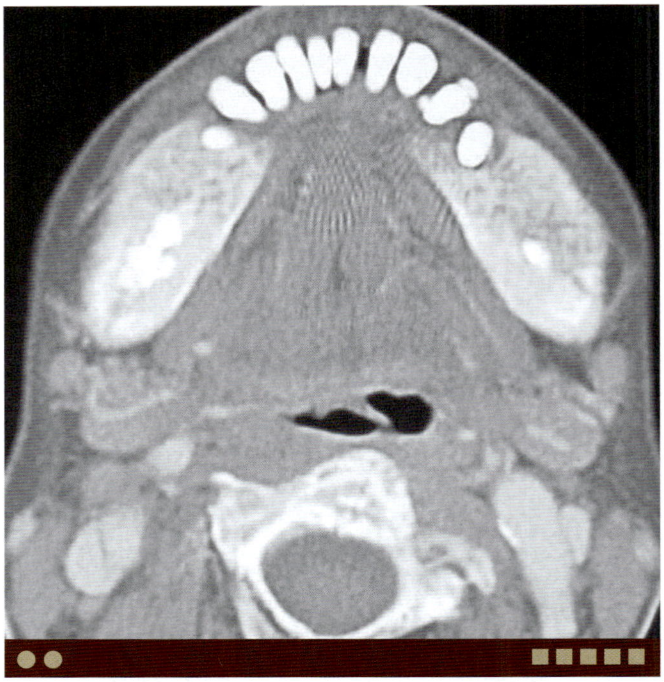

A. Renal osteodystrophy. Axial CT demonstrates expansile ground-grass density change in the body of the mandible.

COMMENTS

This is a 45-year-old woman on hemodialysis.

Chronic renal failure affects bone metabolism and two major types of condition are seen: high-turnover bone disease (increased bone resorption and formation) and low-turnover or aplastic bone disease (osteomalacia). Just like other bones, the maxilla and mandible are also affected by renal osteodystrophy as well as primary or secondary hyperparathyroidism. Generalized demineralization, subperiosteal resorption, bone cysts, and pathologic fractures are seen in these conditions, and radiographs demonstrate loss of the lamina dura, cortical thinning, coarsened trabecular pattern, and "salt-and-pepper"/ granular appearance of bone. The teeth stand out in distinction to the granular radiolucent bone.

Maxillofacial changes associated with hyperparathyroidism are not so emphasized although it is often present in various degrees in such patients. Historically, three forms have been described. The classic form is termed "osteitis fibrosa cystica," which is the result of mixed osteolytic and sclerotic change. Cortical thinning, coarsened trabecular patterns, osteolytic lesions, and "salt-and-pepper" appearance are seen. The second form mimics fibrous dysplasia, with a classic ground-glass pattern, however, which is more diffuse than true fibrous dysplasia and demonstrates poor corticomedullary distinction. The third form is "uremic leontiasis ossea." This rare form is characterized by significant hypertrophy of the jaws with serpiginous "tunneling" within the bone and impaired visualization of the cortex. This form is unique to renal osteodystrophy.

CT is the best modality to demonstrate findings associated with hyperparathyroidism in the maxillofacial bones, although loss of lamina dura and "salt-and-pepper" appearance are better seen with dental films and panoramic radiographs. Ground-grass appearance, sclerotic and osteolytic changes, and cyst formation are easily demonstrated by CT. However, these finding are nonspecific; therefore, clinical correlation is needed to make an appropriate diagnosis.

PEARLS

- **Maxillofacial changes associated with hyperparathyroidism are not rare.**
- **Three forms have been described: (1) "osteitis fibrosa cystica," (2) similar to true fibrous dysplasia, and (3) "uremic leontiasis ossea," which is unique to renal osteodystrophy.**
- **Findings may be similar to fibroosseous lesions, such as fibrous dysplasia, chronic osteomyelitis, and sclerotic metastasis. Clinical correlation is needed to make the diagnosis.**

ADDITIONAL IMAGES (B-F)

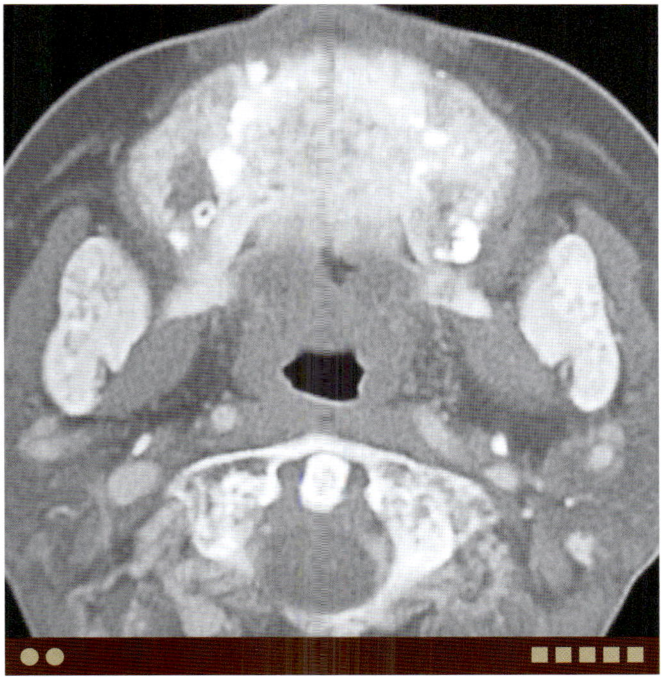

B. Renal osteodystrophy, same patient as A. Axial CT through the level of the hard palate demonstrates ground-glass density expansile changes in the hard palate, maxilla, and rami of the mandible.

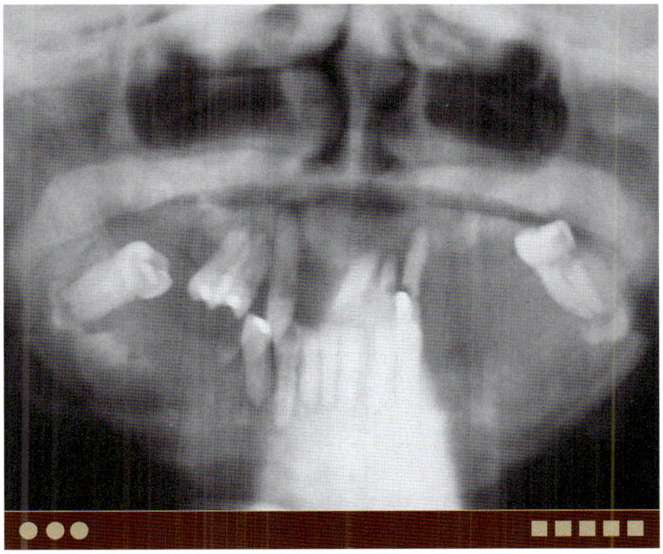

C. Renal osteodystrophy, same patient as A. Panoramic radiograph demonstrates diffuse osteomalacic changes in the maxilla and mandible. Note the missing lamina dura around the teeth. The teeth appear radiopaque in contrast to the granular radiolucent bone.

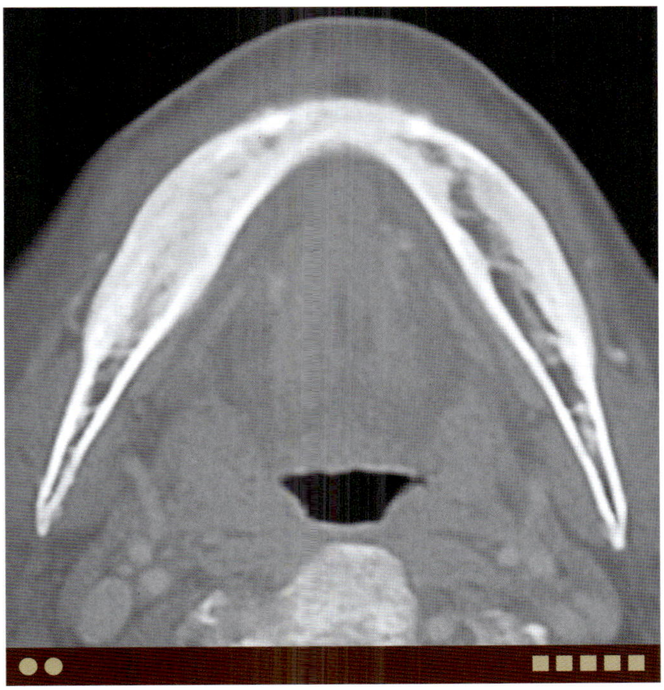

D. Renal osteodystrophy in a different patient. Axial CT demonstrates diffuse sclerotic changes in the mandible.

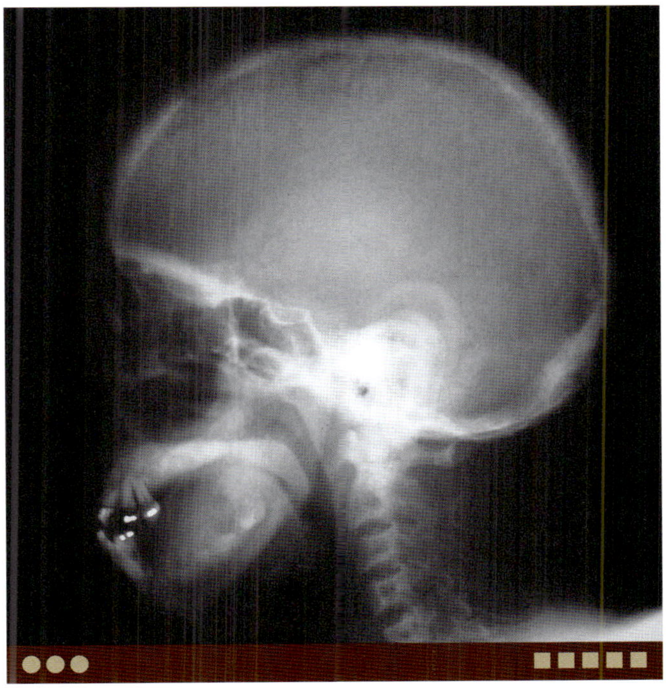

E. Renal osteodystrophy, same patients as D. Lateral radiograph of the skull demonstrates typical and "salt-and-pepper" appearance.

DIFFERENTIAL DIAGNOSIS IMAGES (G-I)

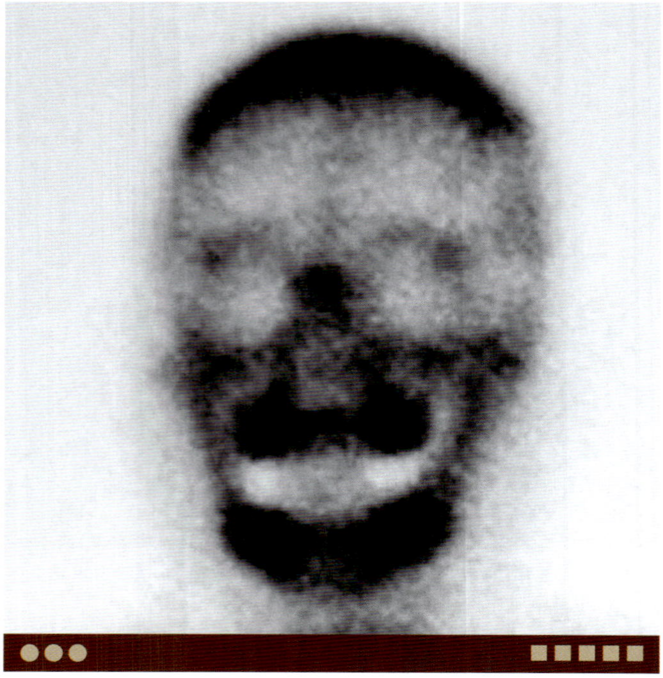

F. Renal osteodystrophy, same patients as D. Bone scan demonstrates increased uptake of the tracer in the maxilla and mandible as well as the vertex.

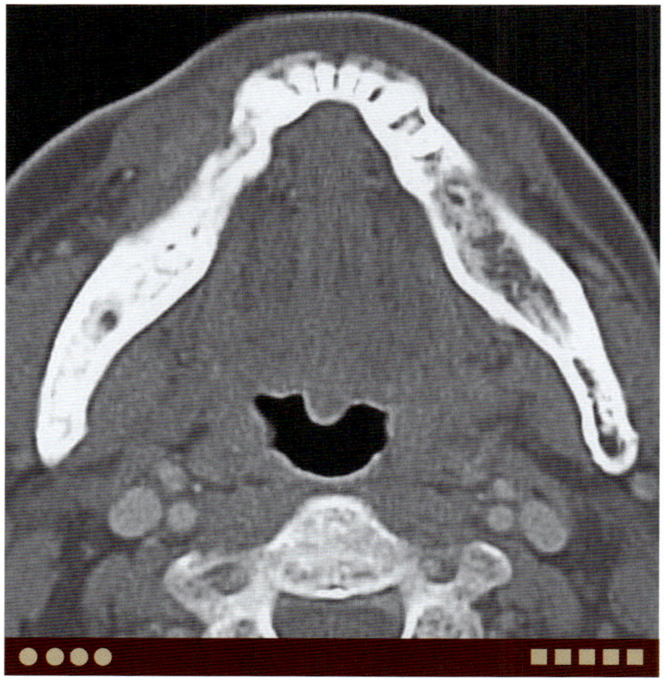

G. Chronic osteomyelitis. Axial CT demonstrates diffuse sclerosis in the right mandible. The left mandible is unremarkable.

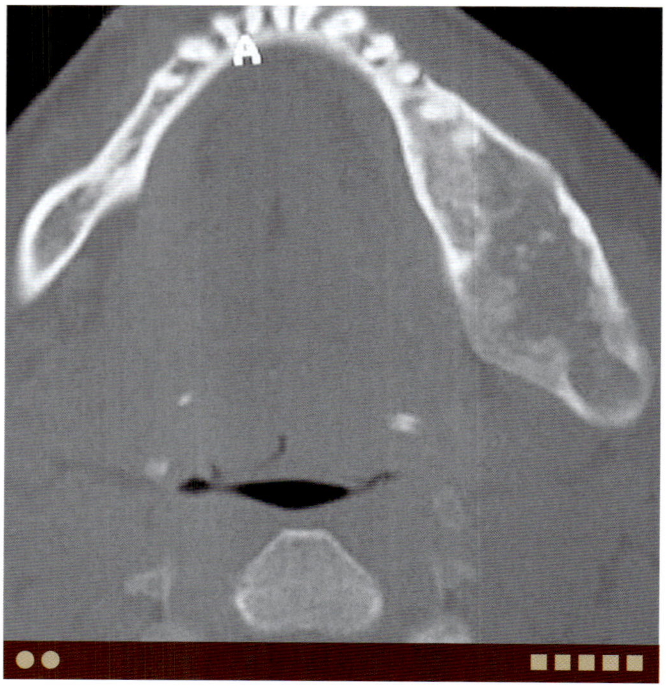

H. Fibrous dysplasia. Axial CT demonstrates a mixture of osteolytic and sclerotic change with expansion in the left mandibular body.

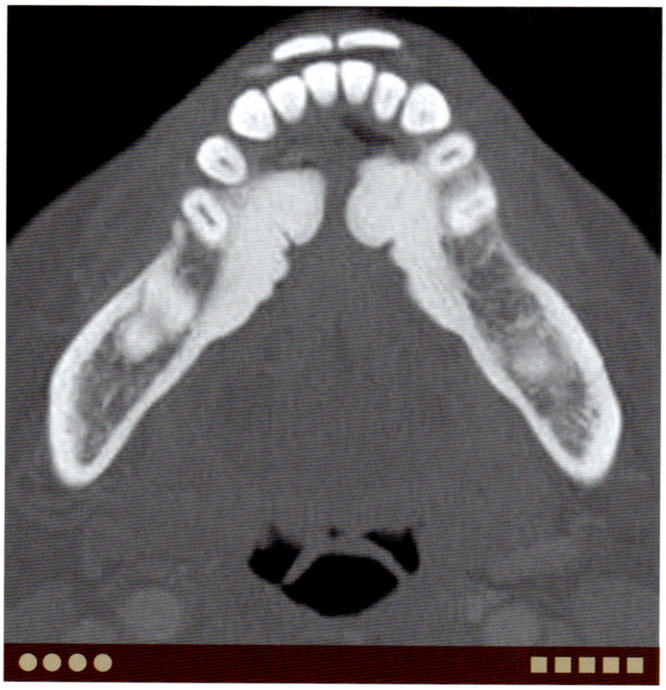

I. Torus mandibularis. Axial CT demonstrates exostoses along the lingual cortex of the anterior mandible bilaterally.

Case 9–9 Osteosarcoma

Osamu Sakai, Akifumi Fujita, Margaret Chapman

PRESENTATION

Jaw pain and swelling.

FINDINGS

CT demonstrates heterogeneous sclerotic changes with periosteal reaction in the mandible.

DIFFERENTIAL DIAGNOSIS

- Metastasis: This usually shows osteolytic change, most commonly seen in the posterior body and angle where abundant bone marrow is present.
- Chronic osteomyelitis: This condition demonstrates heterogeneous density with a mixture of osteosclerotic and lytic changes, and occasionally expansion of the bone. Usually periodontal disease can be identified.
- Bisphosphonate-associated osteonecrosis of the jaw: This is a rare condition which occurs in patients receiving bisphosphonate therapy, particularly by intravenous administration.
- Osteoradionecrosis: This is a condition of bone necrosis from radiation therapy, and is rare in patients who receive less than 60 Gy.
- Fibrous dysplasia: Fibroosseous lesions show mixed density or ground-glass appearance without periosteal reaction or extraosseous soft tissue mass formation.
- Epulis fissuratum: This condition demonstrates overgrowth of fibrous connective tissue in the mouth, with occasional calcification.
- Torus mandibularis: This is an exostosis which occurs along the lingual aspect of the anterior mandible.

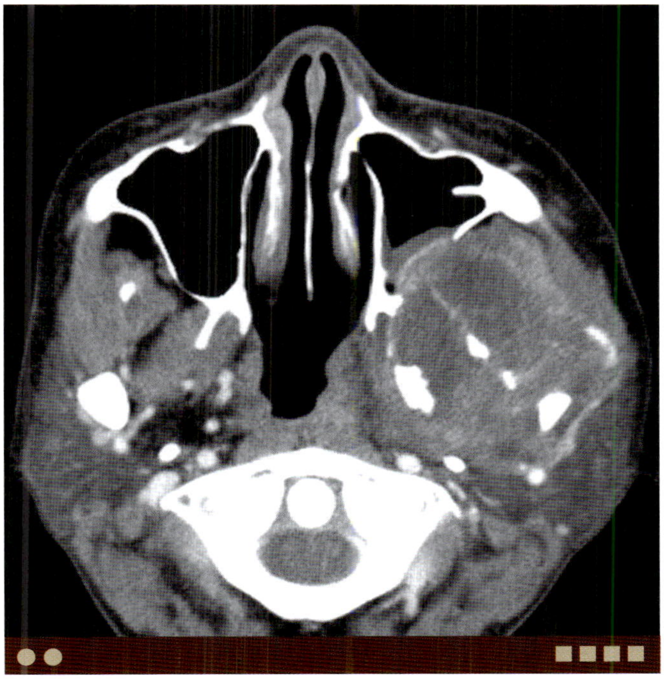

A. Osteosarcoma. Axial postcontrast CT demonstrates a heterogeneously enhancing tumor arising from the left mandibular ramus. Note intratumoral necrosis and foci of premature bones.

COMMENTS

This is a 41-year-old woman with jaw pain and swelling.

Osteosarcoma of the jaw accounts for approximately 6% to 9% of all osteosarcoma, and is more frequently seen in the mandible (maxilla:mandible = 1:1.6). It usually presents as swelling of the jaw and may take several months to establish a diagnosis. Osteosarcoma can be seen secondary to radiation therapy, Paget's disease, and fibrous dysplasia.

Histologically, osteosarcoma is subdivided into three types: osteoblastic, chondroblastic and low-grade types. It is similarly classified radiologically into three groups: osteoblastic (46%), osteolytic (31%), and mixed (23%) types.

Compared with classic osteosarcoma arising from the long bones, osteosarcoma of the mandible has several unique aspects. It generally occurs in older individuals (30-40 years) with less atypia, a longer interval before recurrence (20-29 months), and less metastasis. Low-grade, early-stage, or osteolytic lesions may demonstrate similar radiologic and histologic findings to benign conditions such as osteomyelitis, fibrous dysplasia, and granuloma.

CT demonstrates aggressive osteolytic and osteoblastic changes with periosteal reaction and extraosseous soft tissue mass formation. MRI better delineates the extent of bone marrow abnormality and extraosseous soft tissue involvement.

PEARLS

- **Osteosarcoma of the jaw occurs in an older population than "classic" osteosarcoma arising from the long bones.**
- **Osteosarcoma can be seen secondary to radiation therapy, Paget's disease, and fibrous dysplasia.**
- **Osteosarcoma of the jaw may demonstrate similar findings to benign conditions such as osteomyelitis, fibrous dysplasia, and granuloma.**

ADDITIONAL IMAGES (B-G)

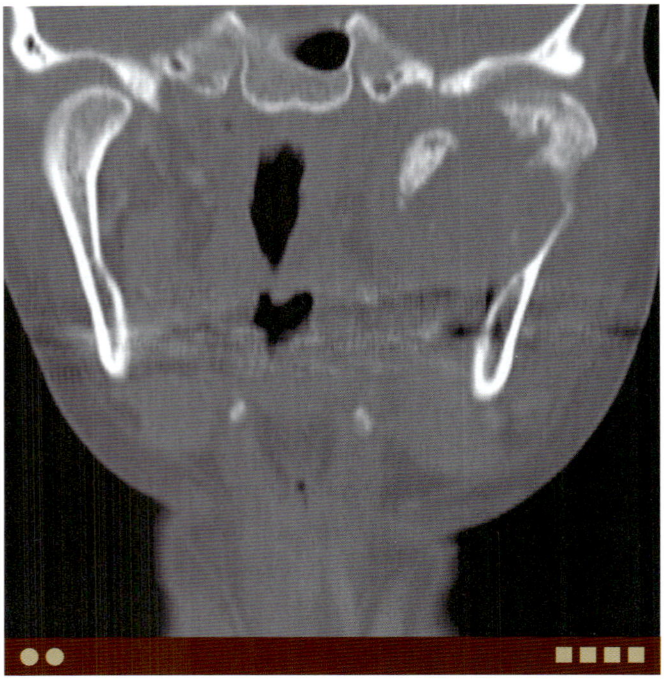

B. Osteosarcoma, same patient as A. Coronal bone window CT demonstrates bone destruction, sclerosis, and bone formation within the tumor.

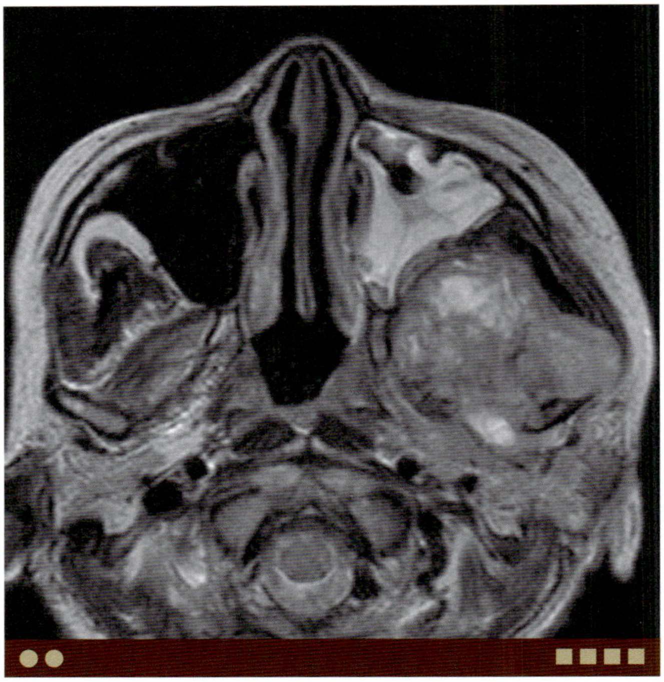

C. Osteosarcoma, same patient as A. Axial T2W MR image demonstrates a large heterogeneous intermediate-signal tumor arising from the left mandibular ramus.

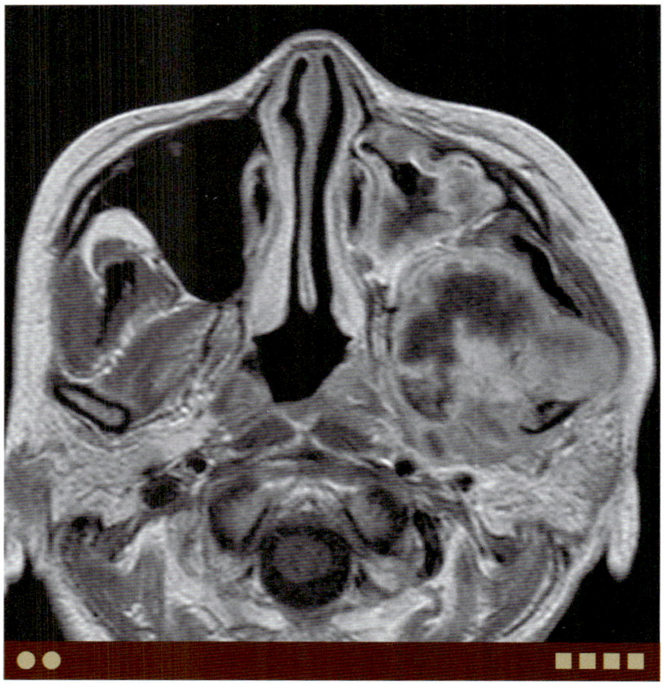

D. Osteosarcoma, same patient as A. Axia postcontrast T1W MR image demonstrates heterogeneous enhancement of the tumor. Note a large area of necrosis within the tumor.

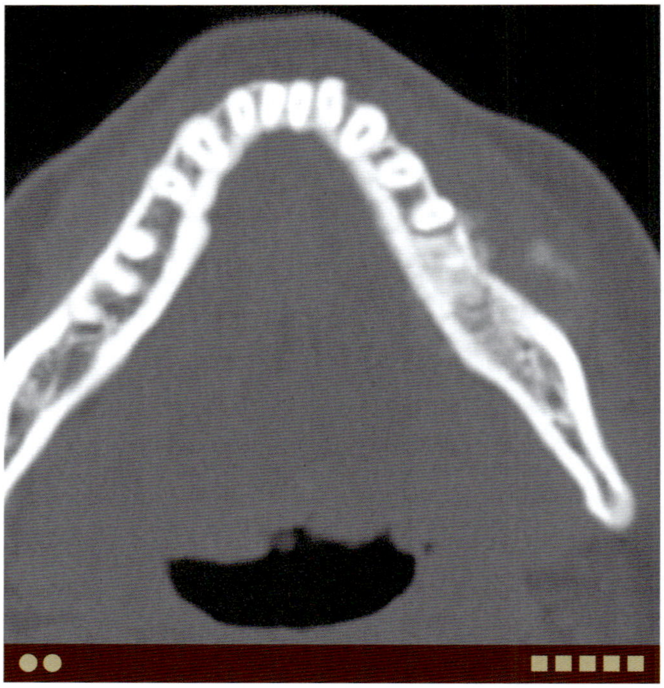

E. Osteosarcoma. Axial CT shows osteoblastic change in the body of the left mandible. Note the abnormal extraosseous soft tissue lesion with calcification/ossification along the buccal and lingual cortex.

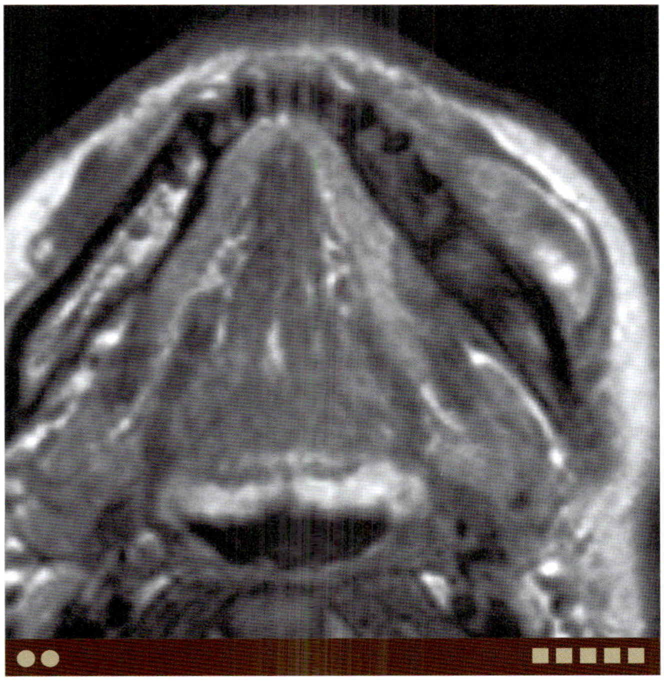

F. Osteosarcoma, same patient as E. Axial T2W MR image demonstrates heterogeneously decreased signal within the left mandibular body with extraosseous mass formation, buccal side larger than lingual side.

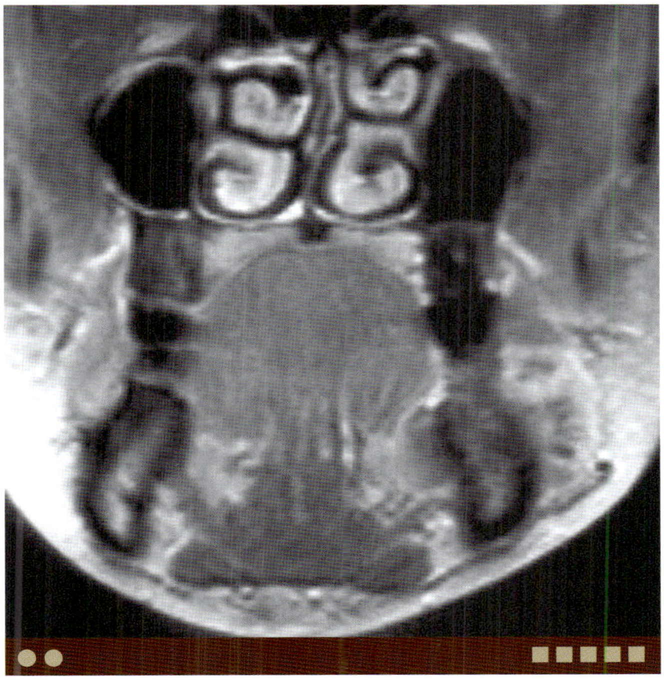

G. Osteosarcoma, same patient as E. Coronal postcontrast fat-suppressed T1W MR image demonstrates heterogeneous enhancement in the lesion.

DIFFERENTIAL DIAGNOSIS IMAGES (H-J)

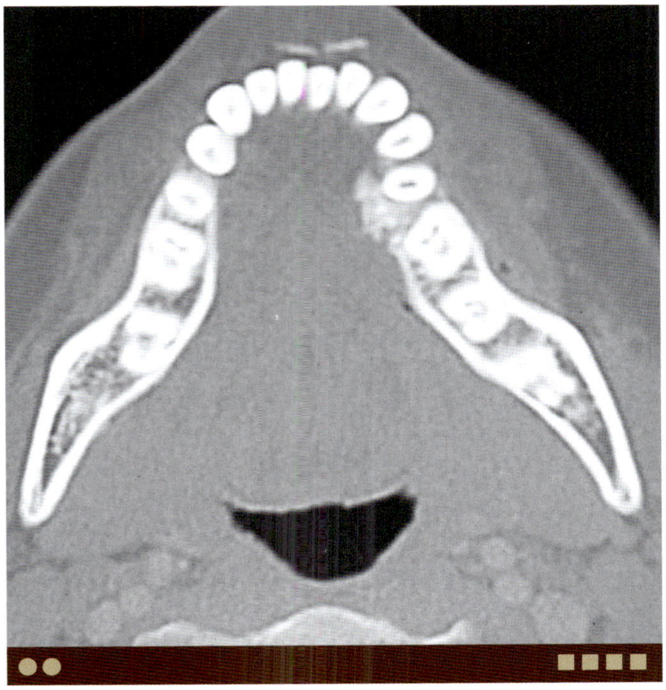

H. Epulis fissuratum. Axial CT demonstrates irregularly shaped calcification at the lingual aspect of the left mandible. This is less dense compared with a typical torus mandibularis.

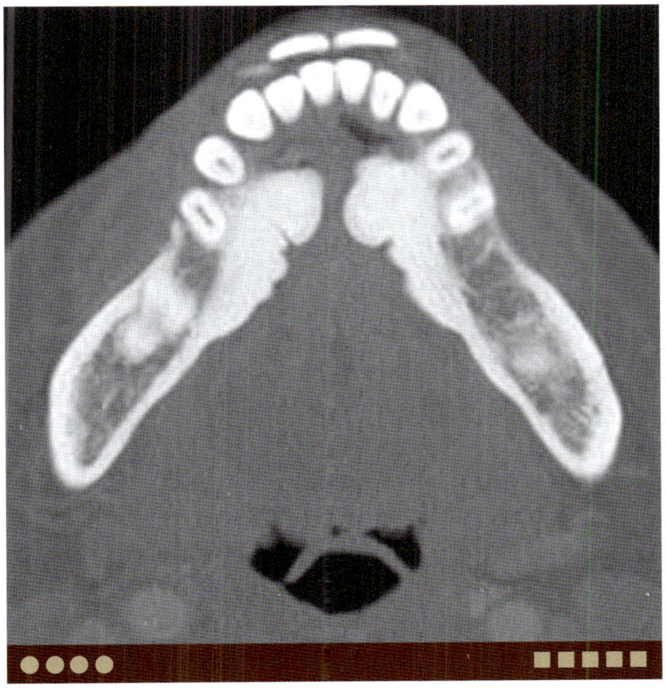

I. Torus mandibularis. Axial CT demonstrates lobulated, dense osseous proliferation along the lingual cortex of the mandible bilaterally.

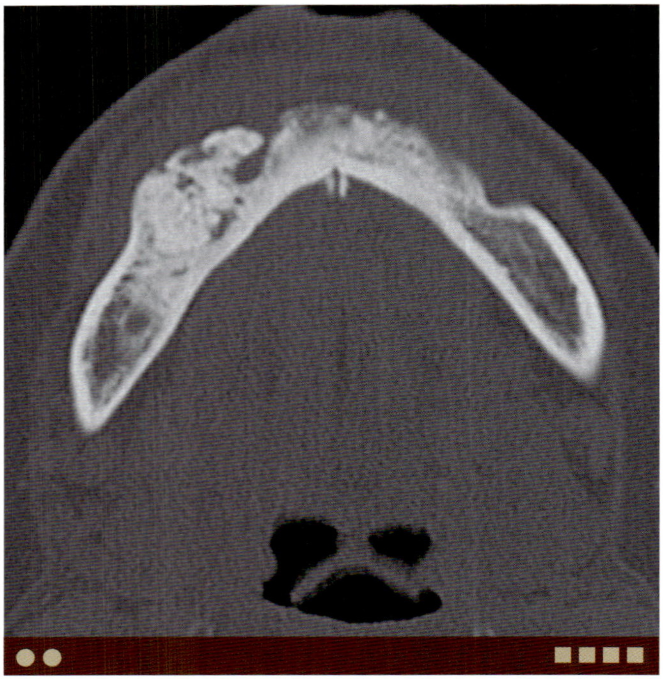

J. Bisphosphonate-associated osteonecrosis. Axial CT demonstrates sclerotic change and cortical destruction in the anterior body of the right mandible.

Case 9–10 Plasmacytoma/Multiple Myeloma

Osamu Sakai, Elisa Flower

PRESENTATION

Chin numbness.

FINDINGS

CT and MRI demonstrate a homogeneously enhancing expansile lesion in the mandible.

DIFFERENTIAL DIAGNOSIS

- Metastases: Metastases from vascular tumors such as thyroid cancer, renal cell carcinoma, and hepatocellular carcinoma show similar findings.
- Lymphoma: This may show less prominent osteolytic or expansile change compared with myeloma/plasmacytoma. However, extraosseous extension and perineural tumor spread is more often seen with lymphoma.
- Other "small round cell tumors": Any small round cell tumors show similar findings to myeloma/plasmacytoma on CT and MRI.

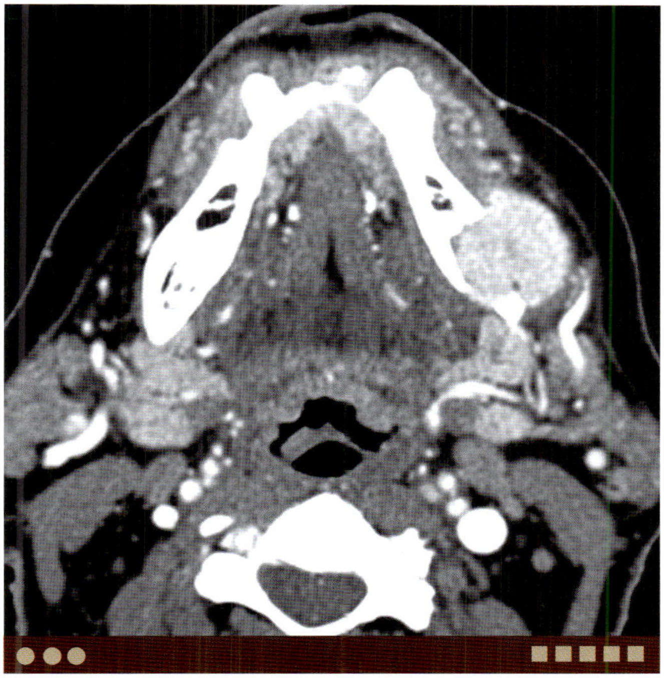

A. Plasmacytoma. Axial contrast-enhanced CT demonstrates an avidly enhancing expansile lesion in the left mandible.

COMMENTS

This is a 65-year-old woman with jaw swelling and pain.

Plasma cell tumor is a B-cell lymphoid neoplasm that involves the bone marrow as well as the soft tissues, and can be classified into multiple myeloma that involves multiple bones, solitary plasmacytoma that occurs in a single bone, and extramedullary plasmacytoma seen in the soft tissue. Histologically, they cannot be differentiated, and clinical presentation may be similar. If the tumor involves the mandible, "chin numbness" due to invasion of the inferior alveolar nerve is commonly noted.

CT usually demonstrates osteolytic change with expansile soft tissue mass formation. A narrow transition zone is typically seen, which is often termed as "punched-out," best seen in the skull. However, intraosseous lesion may be subtle, such as loss of trabeculation without cortical destruction. Similar to lymphoma, plasmacytoma/multiple myeloma demonstrates extraosseous extension without apparent cortical destruction. Therefore, careful evaluation of the adjacent soft tissue as well as the bone marrow is necessary. On CT and MRI the lesion usually demonstrates homogeneous density or signal intensity without necrosis, and avid homogeneous enhancement after administration of intravenous contrast. T1W images and short tau inversion recovery (STIR) images are very helpful to identify the lesion. T2W MR images usually demonstrate intermediate signal reflecting high cellularity of the lesion. Involvement of the nerve can be better assessed with postcontrast fat-suppressed T1W images, however, images may be degraded by inhomogeneous fat suppression; therefore, evaluation on precontrast and postcontrast non–fat-suppressed T1W images is crucial. Just like other parts of the body, metastases from vascular tumors such as renal cell carcinoma, thyroid cancer, and hepatocellular carcinoma may show similar findings.

PEARLS

- **Multiple myeloma/plasmacytoma of the mandible often presents with chin numbness.**
- **Classically, the tumor is seen as an expansile osteolytic lesion; however, the lesion is often subtle on images.**
- **T1W images and STIR images are very helpful to identify the lesion.**

ADDITIONAL IMAGES (B-G)

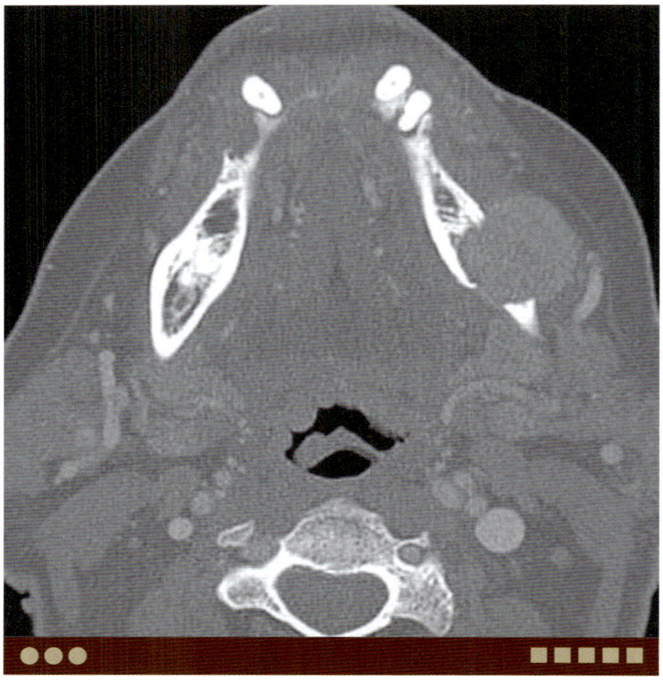

B. Plasmacytoma, same patient as A. Axial bone windowed CT demonstrates abrupt disruption of the buccal cortex of the left mandible as well as erosion of the lingual cortex.

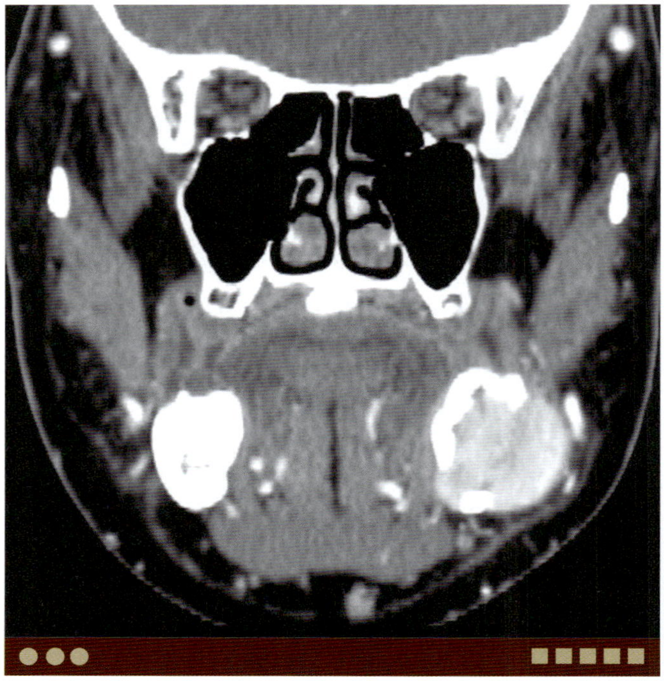

C. Plasmacytoma, same patient as A. Coronal contrast-enhanced CT demonstrates an avidly enhancing expansile lesion in the left mandible. There is mass effect to the adjacent structures without apparent invasion.

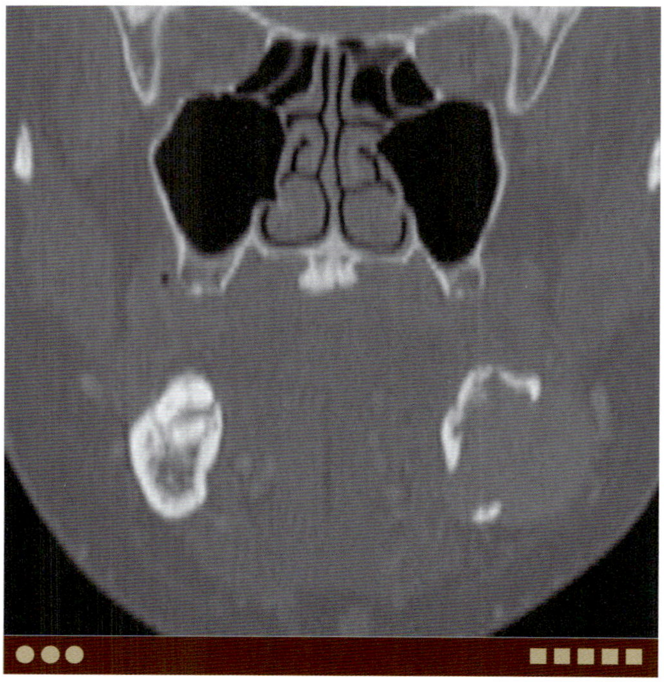

D. Plasmacytoma, same patient as A. Coronal bone window CT demonstrates destruction of the cortex of the left mandible by the expansile tumor.

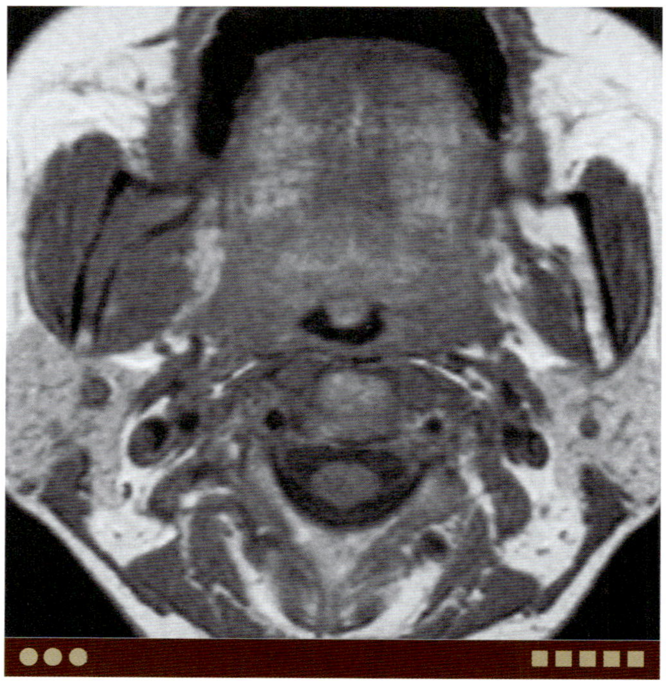

E. Multiple myeloma in a different patient. Axial T1W MR image demonstrates low-signal lesion in the ramus of the right mandible. Note loss of the signal-void from the bony cortex and very subtle soft tissue lesion along the cortex medially and laterally, representing extraosseous extension.

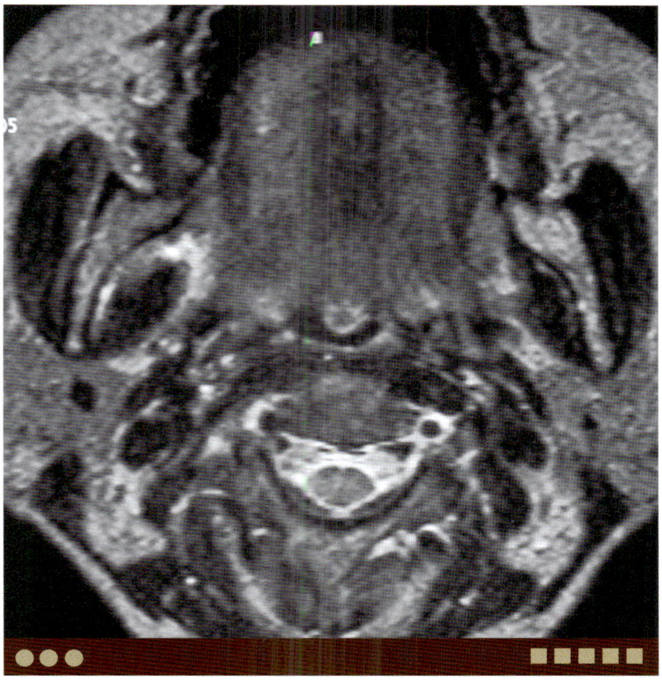

F. Multiple myeloma, same patient as E. Axial T2W MR image shows the lesion demonstrating intermediate signal, slightly lower than the normal marrow on the contralateral side, less obvious compared with T1W images. Extraosseous extension is again seen.

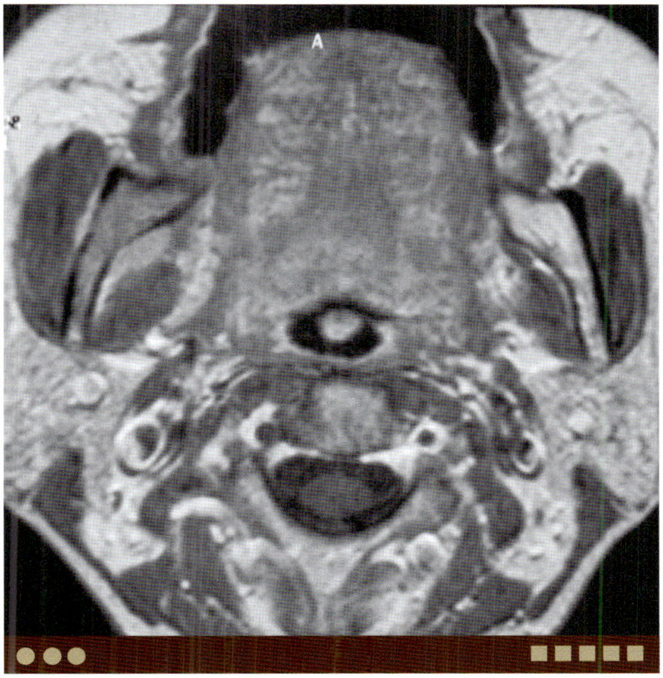

G. Multiple myeloma, same patient as E. Axial postcontrast non–fat-suppressed T1W MR image shows enhancement of the intraosseous lesion as well as the extraosseous lesion. Signal difference between the lesion and normal marrow or fat is less after contrast.

DIFFERENTIAL DIAGNOSIS IMAGES (H-J)

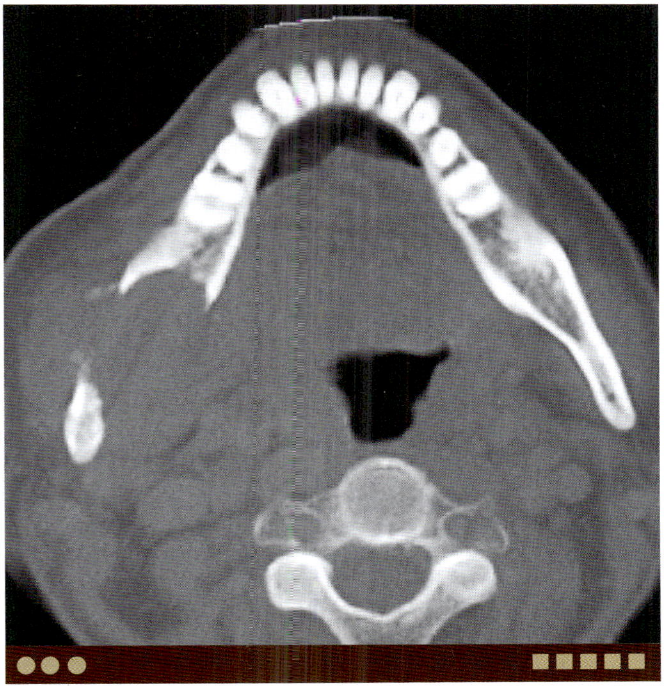

H. Metastasis, hepatocellular carcinoma. Axial bone windowed CT demonstrates abrupt disruption of the posterior body of the right mandible.

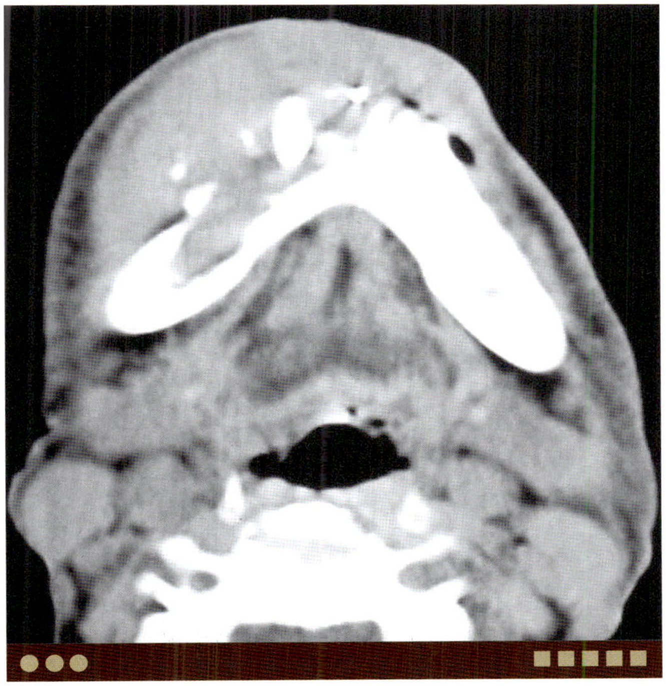

I. Metastasis, thyroid papillary carcinoma. Axial postcontrast CT demonstrates an avidly enhancing expansile lesion with a large extraosseous component in the body of the right mandible.

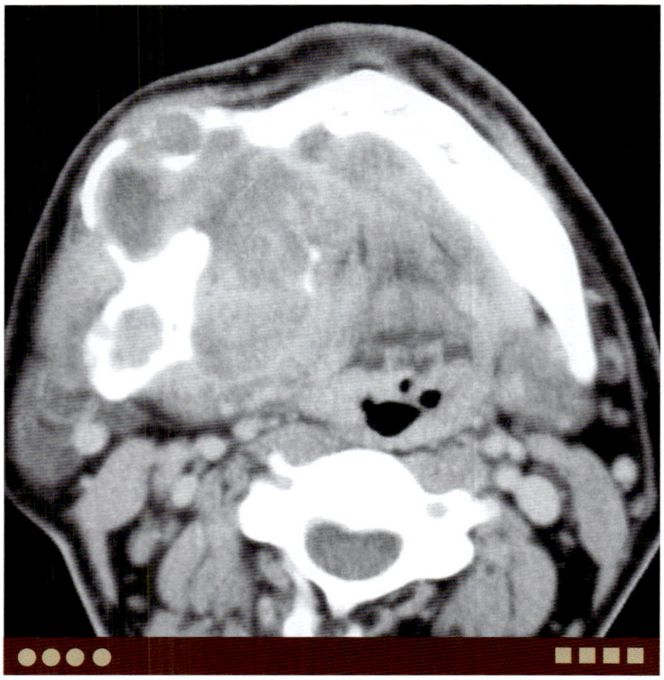

J. Ameloblastoma. Axial postcontrast CT shows a lobulated heterogeneously enhancing expansile lesion in the body of the right mandible.

Case 9–11 Metastatic Tumors

Osamu Sakai, Akifumi Fujita, Margaret Chapman

PRESENTATION

Jaw swelling.

FINDINGS

CT demonstrates an expansile-enhancing lesion in the mandible.

DIFFERENTIAL DIAGNOSIS

- Plasmacytoma/multiple myeloma: These are lymphoid tumors that demonstrate homogeneous-enhancing lesions.
- Lymphoma: This may show nonspecific osteolytic changes. Extraosseous extension and perineural tumor spread are commonly seen.
- Osteosarcoma: Osteosarcoma of the jaw accounts for about 6% to 9% of all osteosarcoma, and is most frequently seen in the mandible. A mixture of osteolytic and osteoblastic changes is commonly seen.

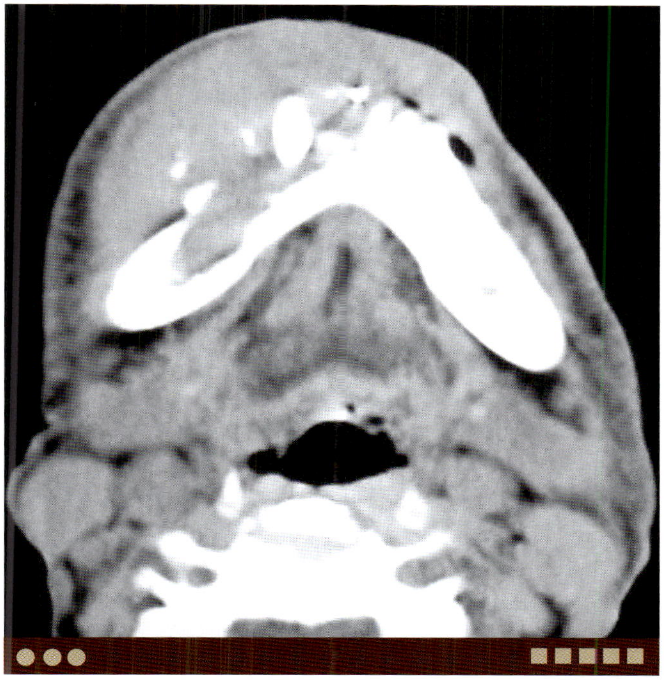

A. Metastasis from thyroid cancer. Axial contrast-enhanced CT demonstrates an enhancing expansile lesion with a large extraosseous component in the body of the right mandible.

COMMENTS

This is a 65-year-old woman with a history of thyroid cancer presenting with jaw swelling.

The mandible is susceptible to metastatic tumors because of its abundant bone marrow. Although metastatic disease can occur anywhere along the mandible, it is most commonly seen in the posterior body and angle where bone marrow is especially abundant. As in other parts of the skeletal system, most metastatic lesions are osteolytic and demonstrate nonspecific findings. Prostate cancer metastases, however, can be sclerotic while metastases from the thyroid, kidney, and liver are hypervascular and often expansile. Symptoms associated with metastatic disease include limited range of motion of the temporomandibular joint (TMJ) and pathologic fractures. Paresthesias of the chin and lower lip can be seen with involvement of the inferior alveolar nerve by metastatic tumors, multiple myeloma, or plasmacytoma.

CT easily demonstrates osteolytic or osteoblastic changes resulting from metastases. MRI is more useful in assessing bone marrow involvement and extraosseous extension of the metastatic lesions.

PEARLS

- **Metastatic tumors can occur anywhere within the jaw; however, they are most commonly seen in the posterior body or angle of the mandible.**
- **Most metastatic lesions are osteolytic and show nonspecific findings.**
- **Sclerotic or osteoblastic metastatic lesions can be seen in patients with prostate cancer.**

ADDITIONAL IMAGES (B-G)

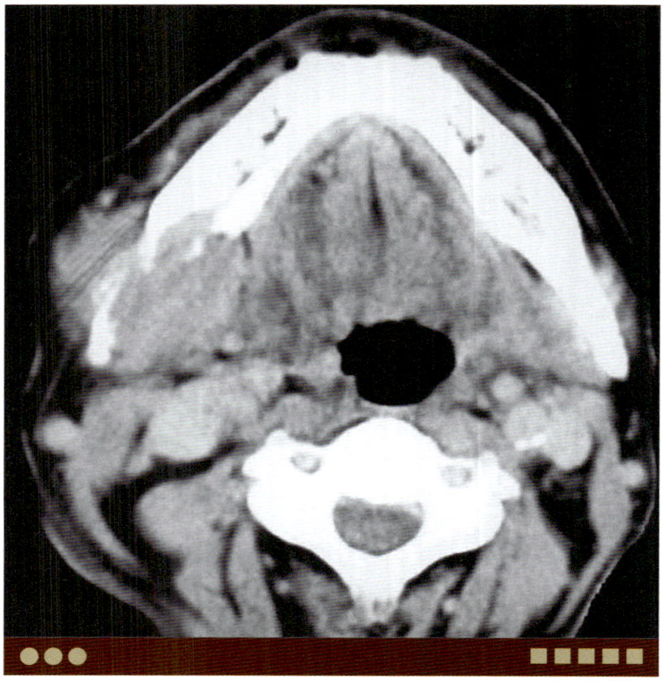

B. Metastasis from hepatocellular carcinoma. Axial contrast-enhanced CT demonstrates an enhancing expansile lesion in the posterior body/angle of the right mandible

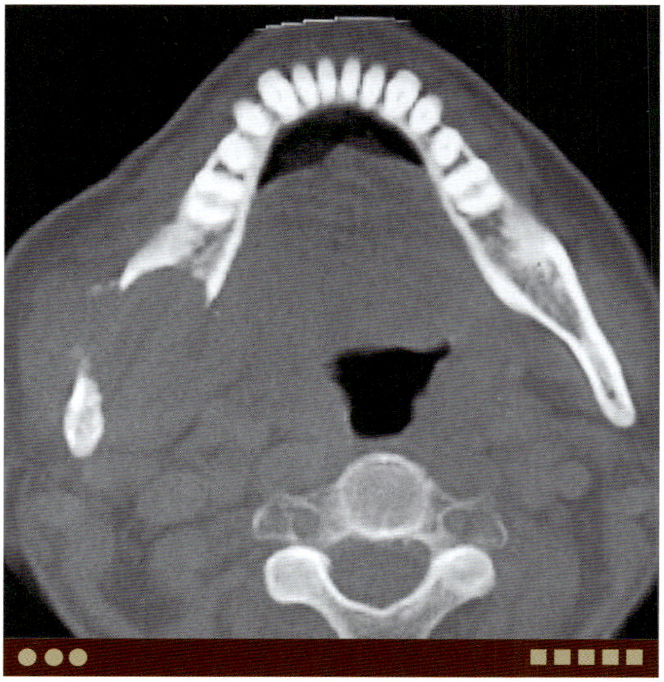

C. Metastasis from hepatocellular carcinoma, same patient as B. Axial bone window CT demonstrates an osteolytic lesion in the posterior body/angle of the right mandible.

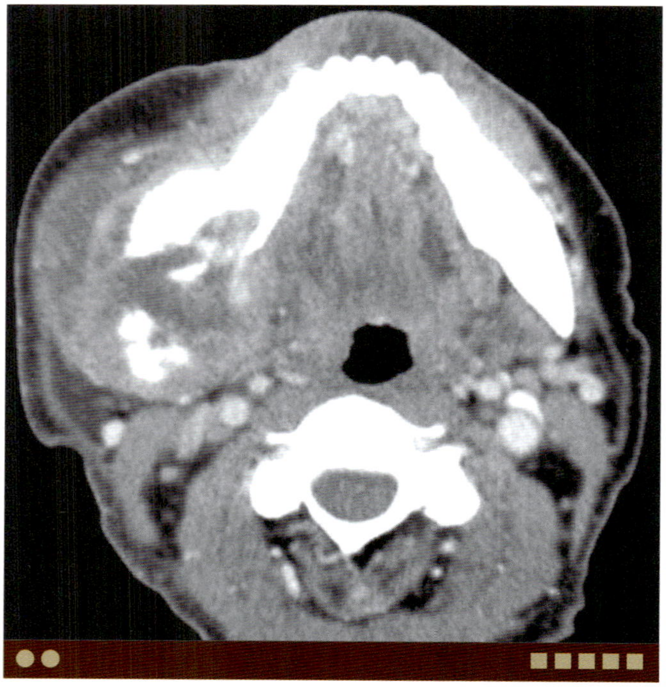

D. Metastasis from prostate cancer. Axial contrast-enhanced CT demonstrates a heterogeneously enhancing expansile lesion in the posterior body of the right mandible.

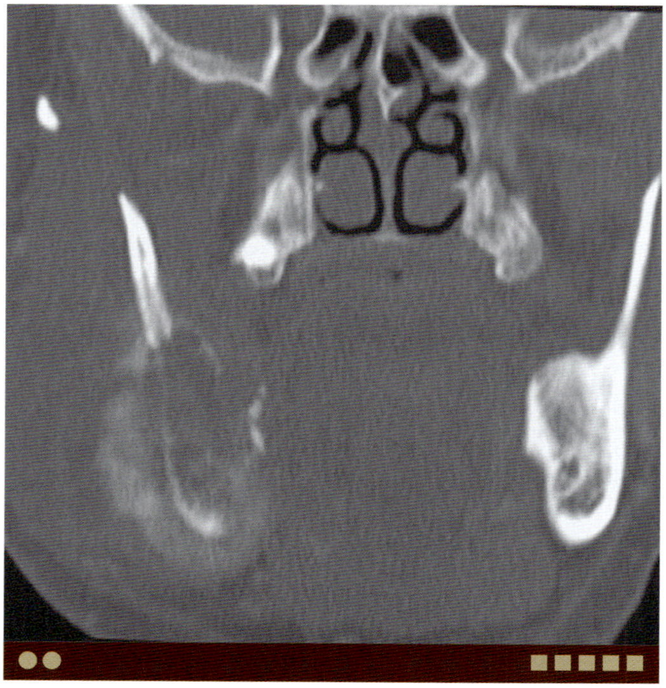

E. Metastasis from prostate cancer, same patient as D. Coronal bone window CT demonstrates prominent osteoblastic change of the lesion in the right mandible.

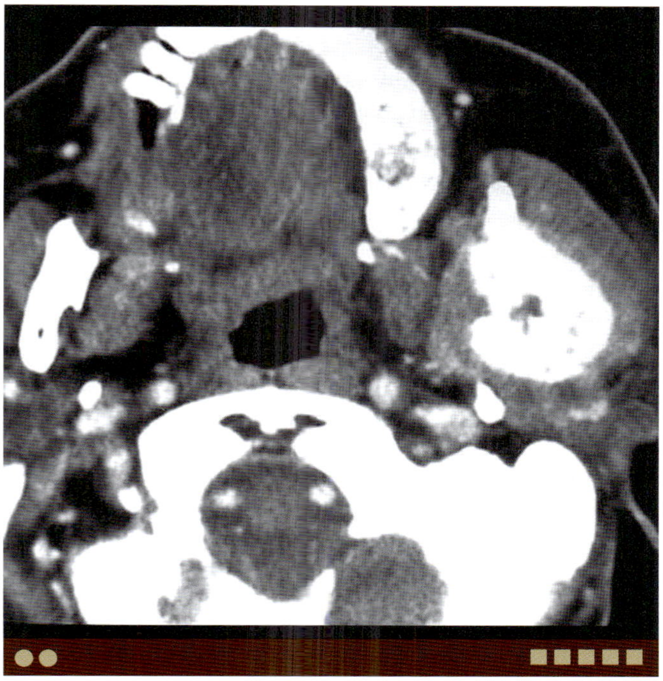

F. Metastasis from prostate cancer in a different patient. Axial contrast-enhanced CT demonstrates an expansile osteoblastic lesion in the ramus of the left mandible.

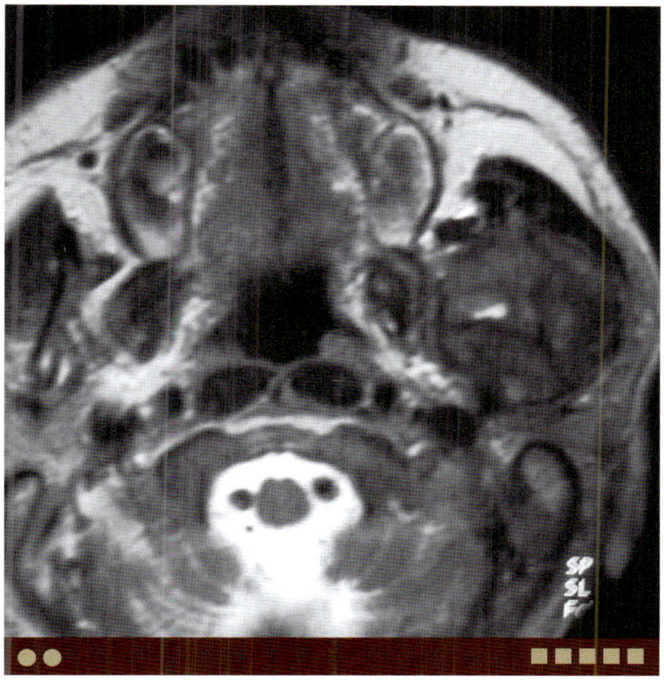

G. Metastasis from prostate cancer, same patient as F. Axial T2W MR image shows heterogeneous low signal in the lesion, consistent with osteoblastic metastasis

DIFFERENTIAL DIAGNOSIS IMAGES (H-J)

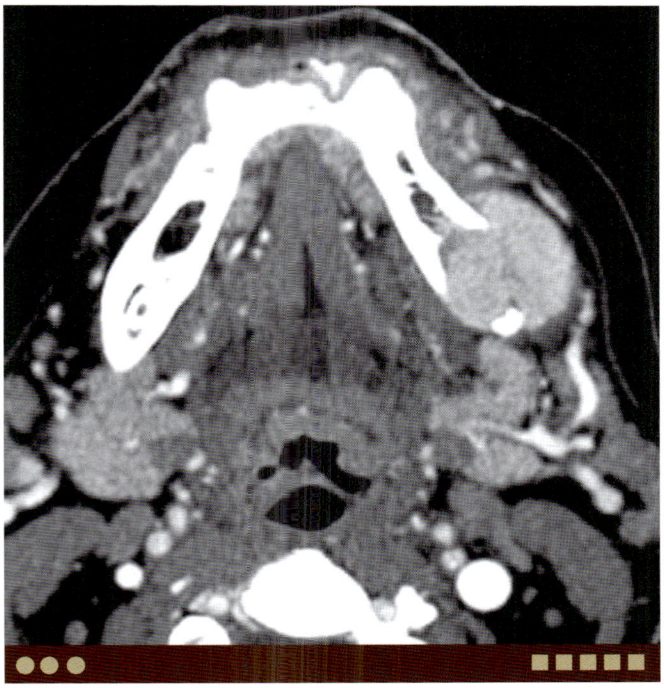

H. Plasmacytoma. Axial postcontrast CT shows an avidly enhancing expansile lesion in the posterior body of the left mandible.

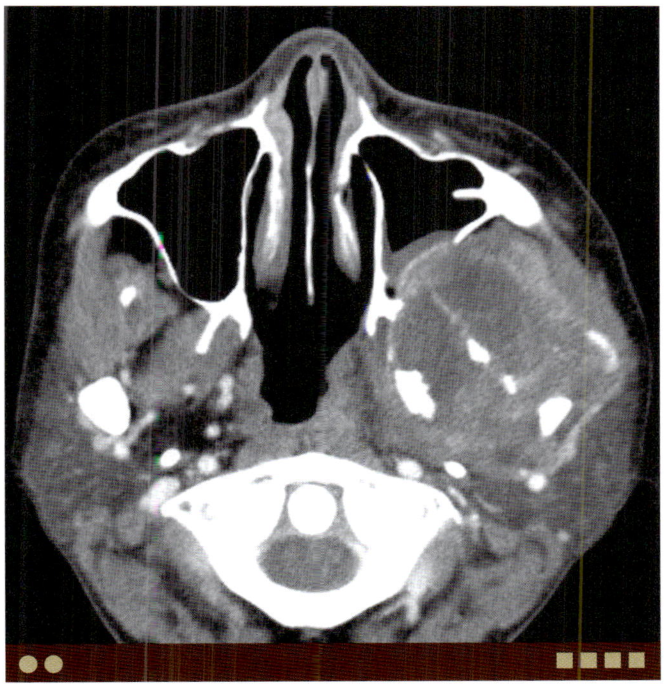

I. Osteosarcoma. Axial postcontrast CT demonstrates a heterogeneously enhancing tumor arising from the left mandibular ramus. Note intratumoral necrosis and foci of premature bones.

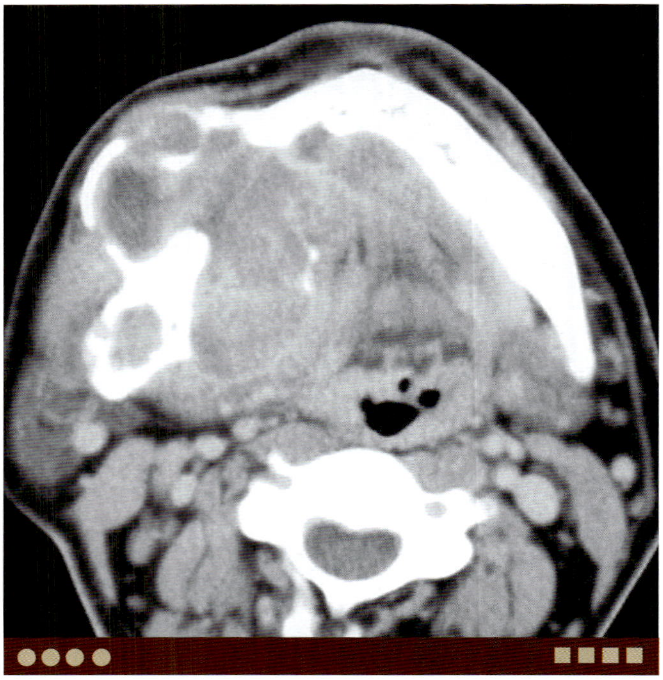

J. Ameloblastoma. Axial postcontrast CT shows a lobulated heterogeneously enhancing expansile lesion in the body of the right mandible.

Case 9–12 Bifid Mandibular Condyle

Osamu Sakai, Takashi Kaneda, Margaret Chapman

PRESENTATION

Temporomandibular joint (TMJ) pain.

FINDINGS

CT demonstrates a double-headed mandibular condyle.

DIFFERENTIAL DIAGNOSIS

- Osteoarthritis (OA): This is a common condition that demonstrates irregularity and sclerotic change of the mandibular condyle.
- Rheumatoid arthritis (RA): RA involves any joint including the TMJ.
- Osteochondroma: This is a rare tumor that, when found in the mandible, occurs exclusively within the condyle or coronoid process.

COMMENTS

This is a 74-year-old man with TMJ pain.

Bifid mandibular condyles (also know as double-headed mandibular condyles) are likely congenital/developmental anomalies, however, the etiology is not fully understood. Although rare, they are the most common condylar anomaly. Symptoms described with bifid condyles vary; however, in most instances patients are asymptomatic and this condition is most often diagnosed incidentally on panoramic radiograph. Bifid mandibular condyles usually have no clinical significance.

CT is an ideal imaging tool to evaluate the morphology of the condyle and to rule out other conditions including OA, RA, and other arthritides. Coronal imaging clearly demonstrates the characteristic double-headed mandibular condyle. On axial images, the bifid mandibular condyles may mimic deformities from OA changes due to partial volume averaging effects. However, with bifid mandibular condyles, there is preservation of the normal bony cortex, trabeculation, and marrow, which may be best seen on MRI.

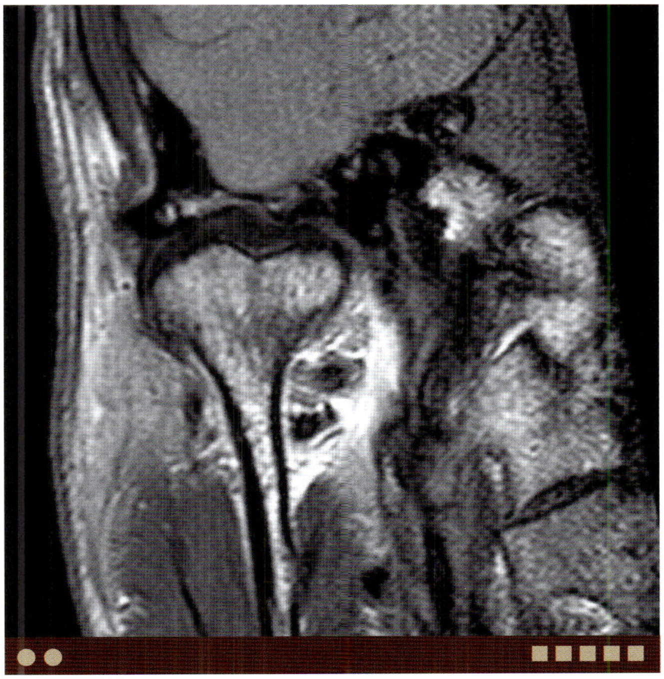

A. Bifid mandibular condyle. Coronal PDW MR image shows a bifid mandibular condyle. Note the normal marrow signal.

Treatment is conservative for symptomatic patients with TMJ disorders. Surgical treatment has been described in the literature for posttraumatic TMJ ankylosis in bifid condyles.

PEARLS

- **Although rare, bifid mandibular condyles are the most common anomaly of the mandibular condyle.**
- **They are often found incidentally, and usually there is no clinical significance.**
- **On axial images, imaging findings of this condition may be mistaken for changes resulting from OA.**

ADDITIONAL IMAGES (B-F)

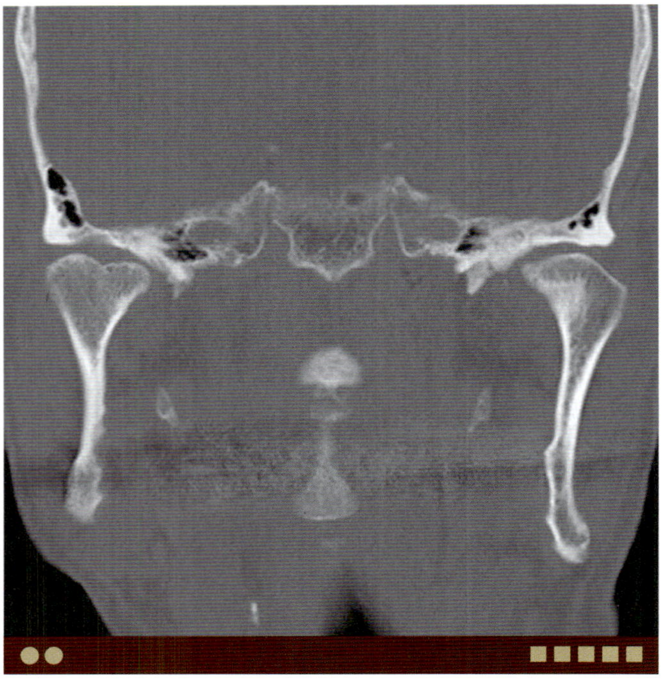

B. Bifid mandibular condyle, same patient as A. Coronal CT demonstrates a bifid right mandibular ccndyle, while the left condyle is normal in appearance.

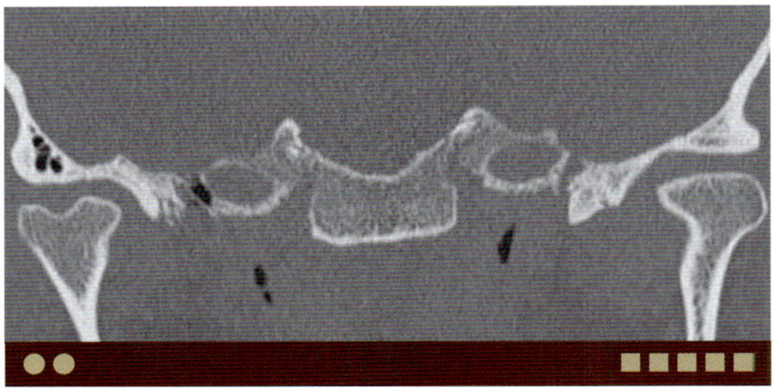

C. Bifid mandibular condyle in a different patient. Coronal CT demonstrates a right-sided bifid mandibular condyle. Note the preserved cortex, differentiating it from osteoarthritis and fracture.

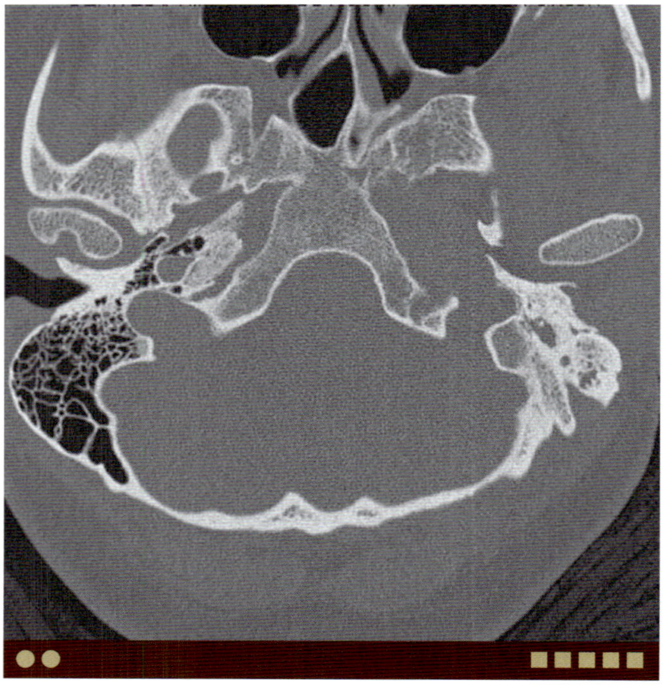

D. Bifid mandibular condyle, same patiert as C. Axial CT demonstrates a cleft in the right mandibular condyle. Again, the cortex is well preserved.

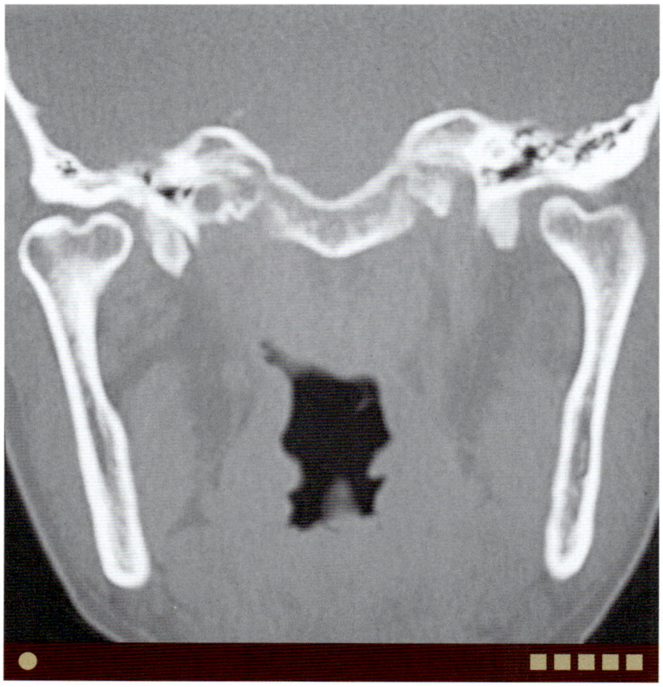

E. Bilateral bifid mandibular condyle. Coronal CT demonstrates bilateral bifid mandibular condyles.

DIFFERENTIAL DIAGNOSIS IMAGES (G-J)

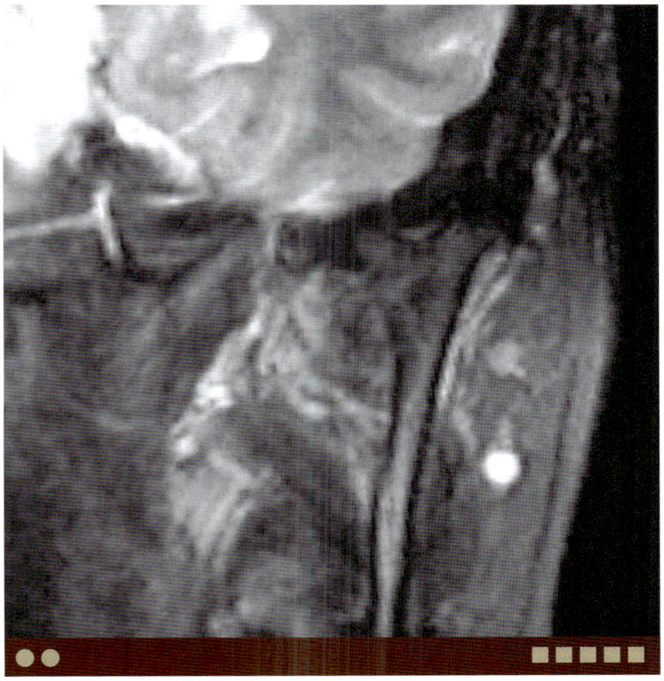

F. Bifid mandibular condyle in a different patient. Coronal T2W MR image shows a left-sided bifid mandibular condyle. Note the normal marrow signal.

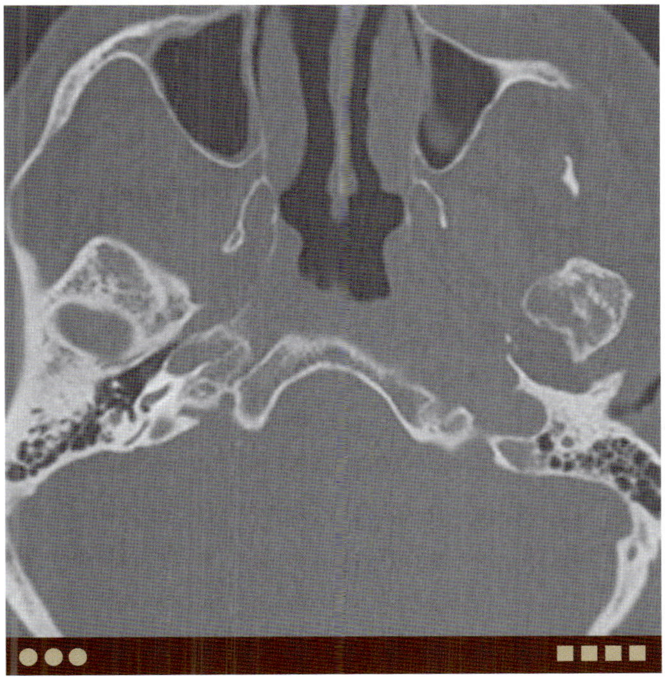

G. Healed fracture. Axial CT demonstrates deformity of the left mandibular condyle secondary to prior fracture.

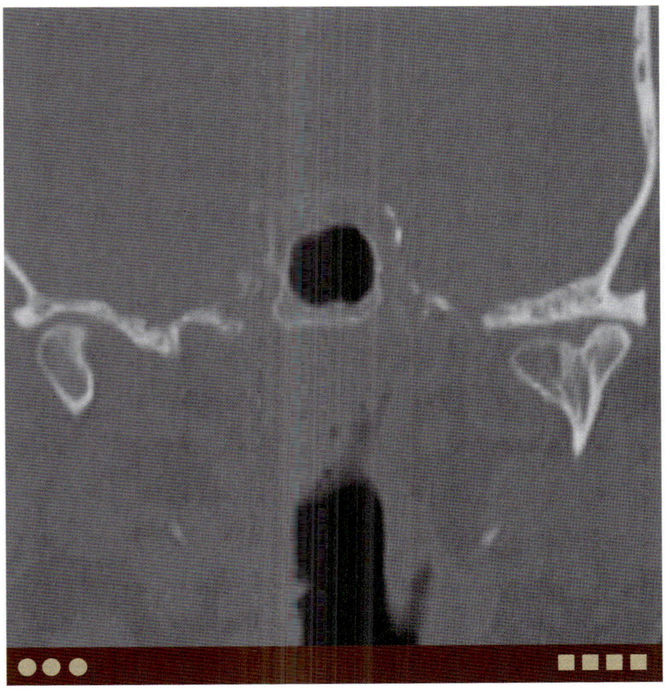

H. Healed fracture, same patient as G. Coronal CT demonstrates "bifid" left mandibular condyle resulting from prior fracture.

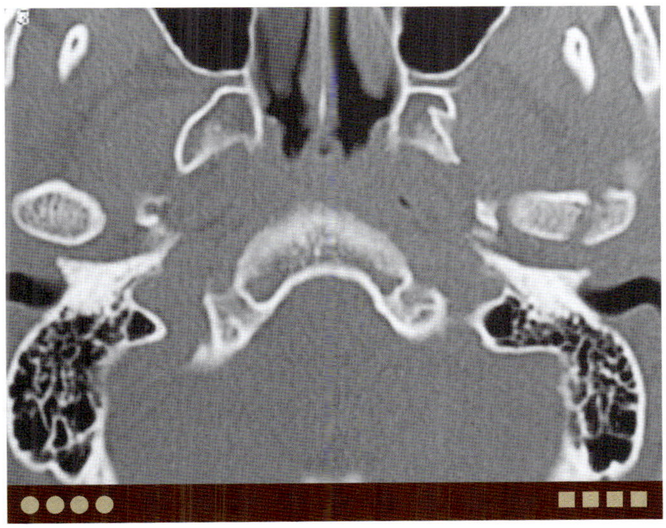

I. Fracture. Axial CT shows a fracture through the left mandibular condyle disrupting the cortex.

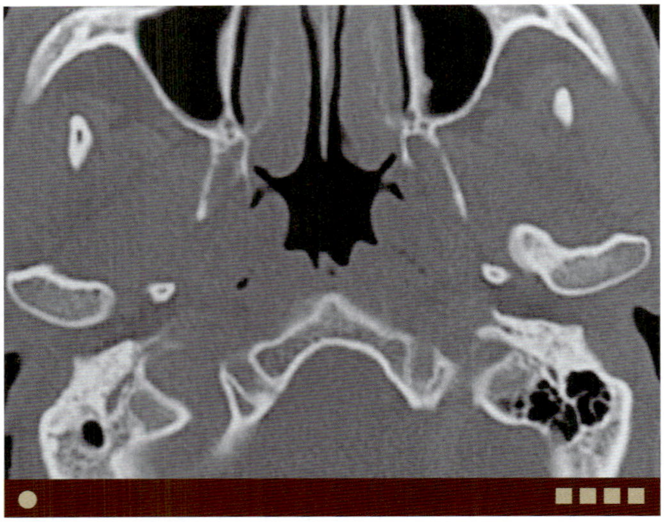

J. Osteochondroma. Axial CT shows an osteochondral lesion at the anteromedial aspect of the left mandibular condyle.

Case 9–13 Temporomandibular Joint Disorder

Osamu Sakai, Takashi Kaneda, Margaret Chapman

PRESENTATION

Temporomandibular joint (TMJ) pain and clicking.

FINDINGS

MRI demonstrates anterior dislocation of the disc.

DIFFERENTIAL DIAGNOSIS

- Osteoarthritis: This condition can be a sequela of temporomandibular joint disorder (TMJD) or trauma.
- Rheumatoid arthritis: Rheumatoid arthritis can be seen in the TMJ as well as in other parts of the body.
- Pseudogout: Calcium pyrophosphate dihydrate deposition is rare but can occur in the TMJ. Calcification is often seen.

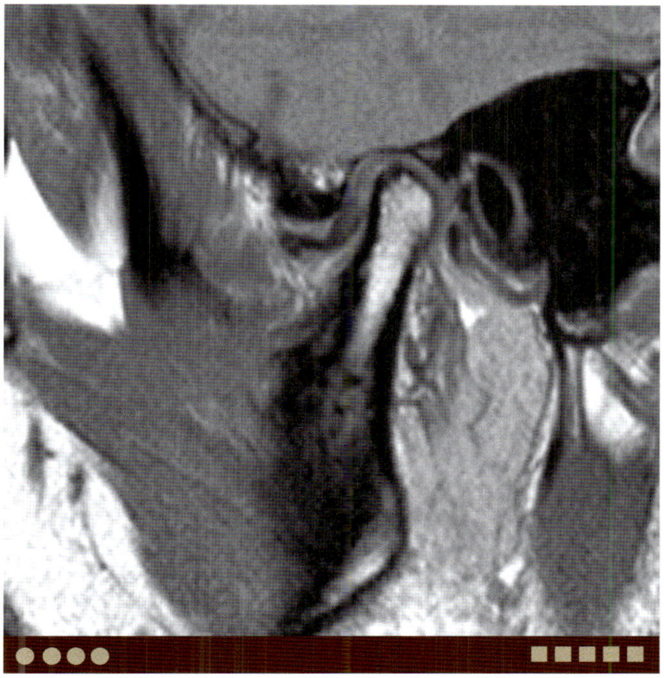

A. TMJD. Closed mouth oblique-sagittal PDW MR image demonstrates anterior dislocation of the disc.

COMMENTS

This is a 50-year-old woman with TMJ pain.

Temporomandibular joint disorder (TMJD) is a broad entity covering acute or chronic inflammation and dysfunction of the temporomandibular joint. The etiology of TMJ pain and dysfunction is unknown. Patients with this condition typically utilize multiple medical services, including dentistry, neurology, physical therapy, and psychology, as there are a variety of different treatment approaches.

TMJD is the most common TMJ condition referred for MRI. The role of MRI is to evaluate the joint morphologically and functionally, with special interest in imaging of the disc. As the disc is best seen on proton density-weighted (PDW) images, PDW oblique-sagittal imaging is the key sequence of TMJ MR. In addition, dynamic oblique-sagittal imaging with closed and open mouth views, and coronal imaging with T1W and T2W sequences should be performed to fully evaluate the joint. CT is helpful to evaluate bony cortex and trabeculae. The disc is also seen on CT, although MRI is the first-line modality to evaluate the disc and its associated pathology.

Normally the disc is seen as a bow tie-shaped low-signal structure between the mandibular condyle and glenoid fossa. The disc situates over the condyle, and normally the posterior band rests at the 12 o'clock position on the mandibular condyle. The tendinous insertion of the lateral pterygoid muscle is seen inferior to the anterior disc band.

Dislocation of the disc usually occurs anteriorly, and is often recaptured with opening of the mouth, usually associated with a "click." In more impaired conditions, there is no recapturing observed, and limited range of motion (decreased anterior translation and rotation of the condyle) is seen ("closed lock"). Medial dislocation is also often seen. Further, lateral or posterior dislocation is not rare.

Long-standing TMJD results in degeneration of the disc and osteoarthritis. Morphology of the condyle and glenoid fossa, as well as the disc, should be carefully evaluated. Osteosclerotic changes and joint effusions can be observed similar to findings seen in osteoarthritis of other joints. Further, the TMJ is susceptible to many conditions that affect other joints in the body, including other arthritides, trauma, dislocations, developmental anomalies, and neoplasms.

PEARLS

- **Normally the disc is seen as a bow tie-shaped structure between the mandibular condyle and glenoid fossa.**
- **Dislocation of the disc usually occurs anteriorly, and is often recaptured with opening of the mouth.**
- **Long-standing TMJD results in degeneration of the disc and osteoarthritis.**

ADDITIONAL IMAGES (B-H)

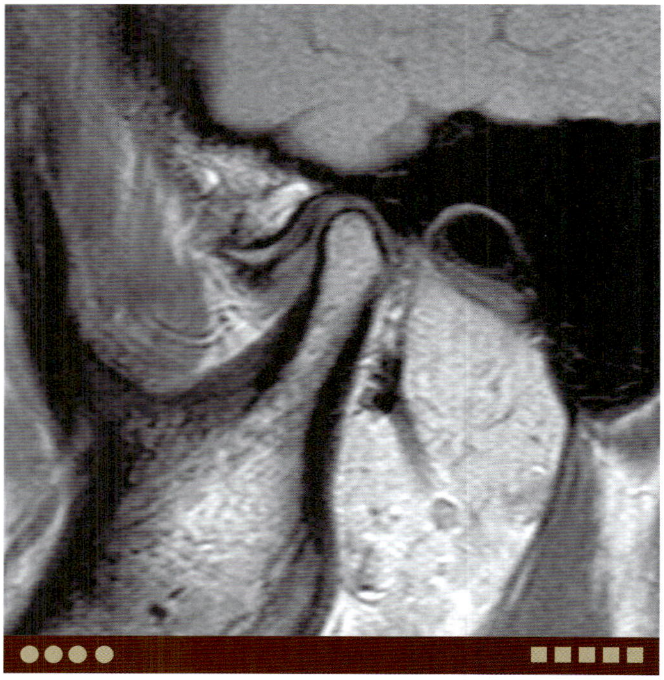

B. TMJD in a different patient. Closed mouth oblique-sagittal PDW MR image demonstrates anterior dislocation of the disc.

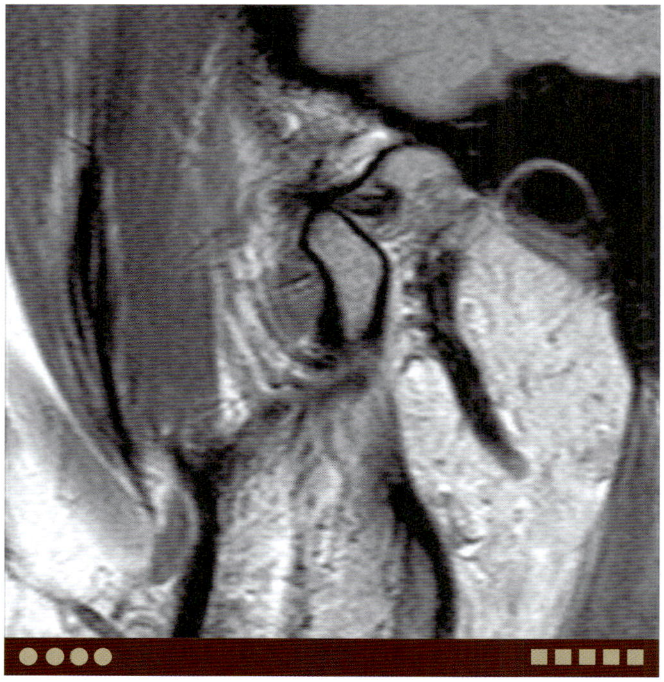

C. TMJD, same patient as B. Open mouth oblique-sagittal PDW MR image demonstrates anterior translation and rotation of the condyle and recapturing of the disc.

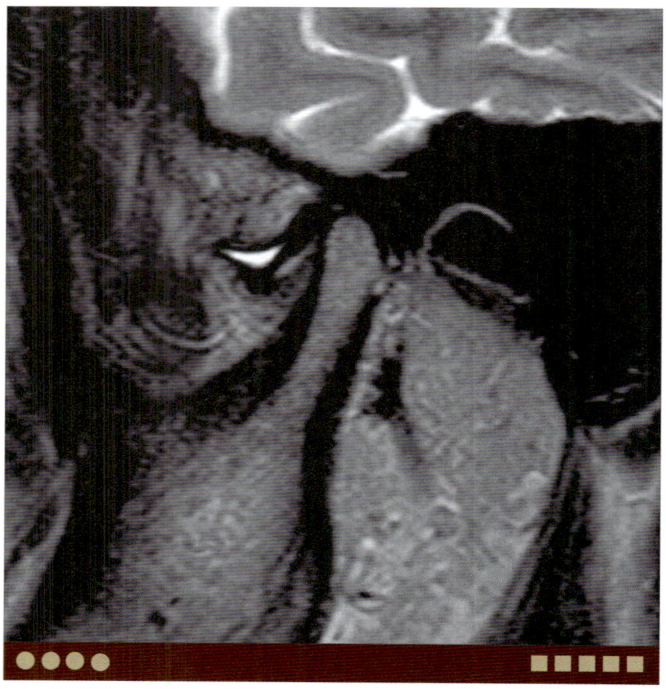

D. TMJD, same patient as B. Closed mouth oblique-sagittal T2W MR image demonstrates abnormal joint effusion and anteriorly dislocated disc.

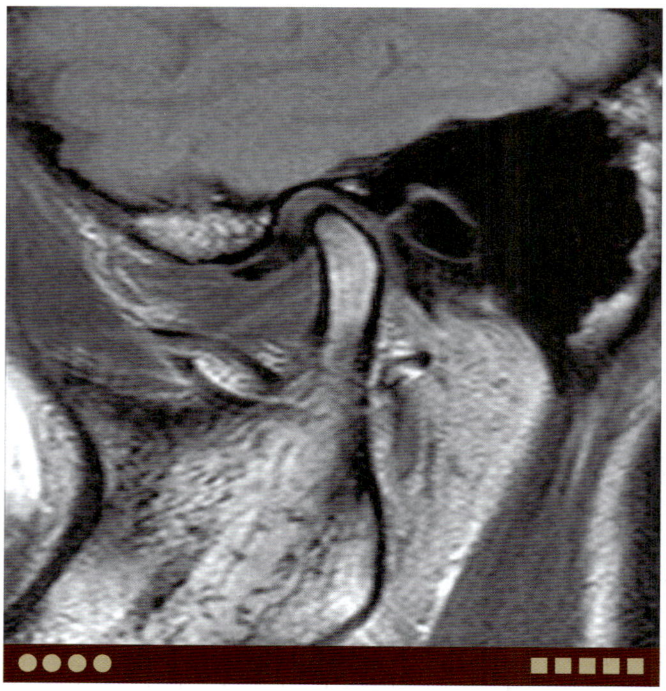

E. TMJD in a different patient. Closed mouth oblique-sagittal PDW MR image demonstrates anterior dislocation of the disc.

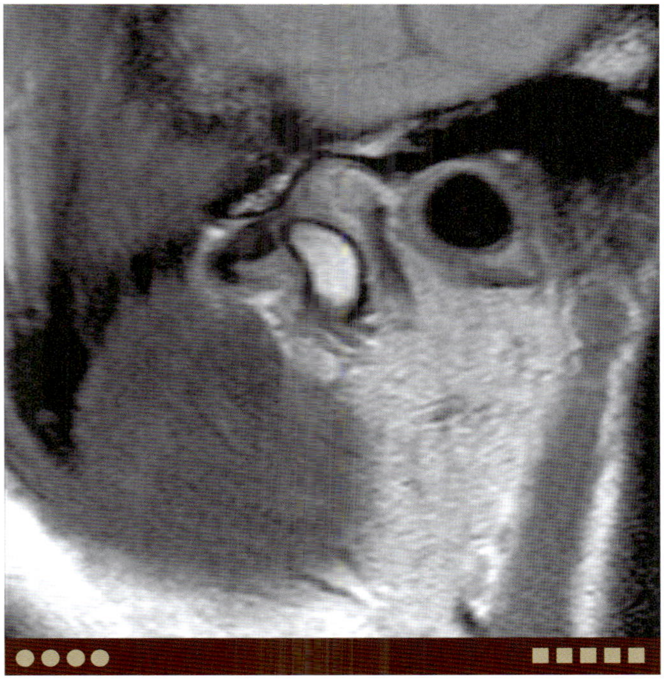

F. TMJD, same patient as E. Open mouth oblique-sagittal PDW MR image demonstrates slightly limited anterior translation and rotation of the condyle. No recapturing of the anteriorly dislocated disc is seen.

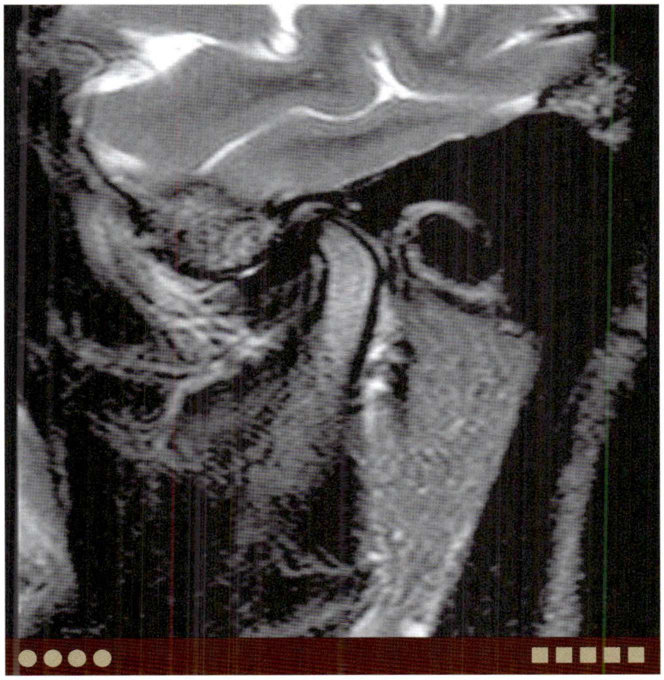

G. TMJD, same patient as E. Closed mouth oblique-sagittal T2W MR image demonstrates abnormal joint effusion and anteriorly dislocated disc.

DIFFERENTIAL DIAGNOSIS IMAGES (I-J)

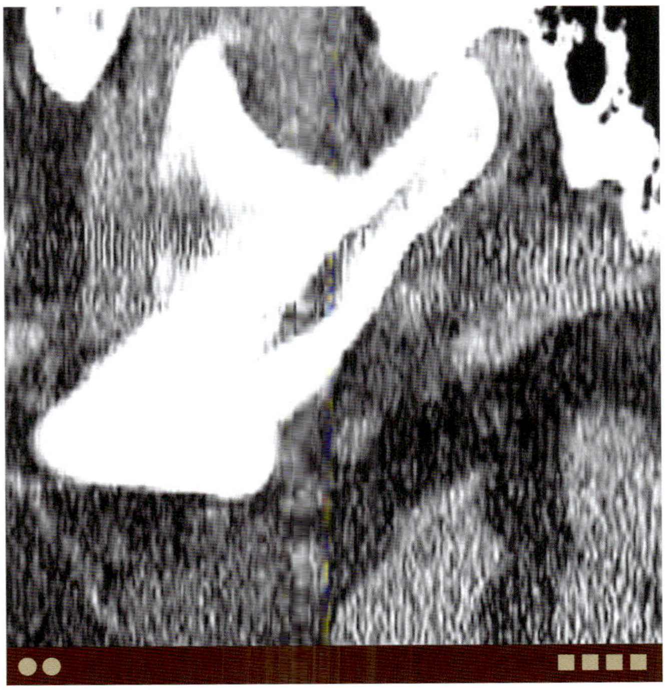

H. TMJD, posterior disc dislocation in a different patient. Closed mouth oblique-sagittal CT image demonstrates posterior dislocation of the disc. Note soft tissue density posterior to the condyle in the glenoid fossa.

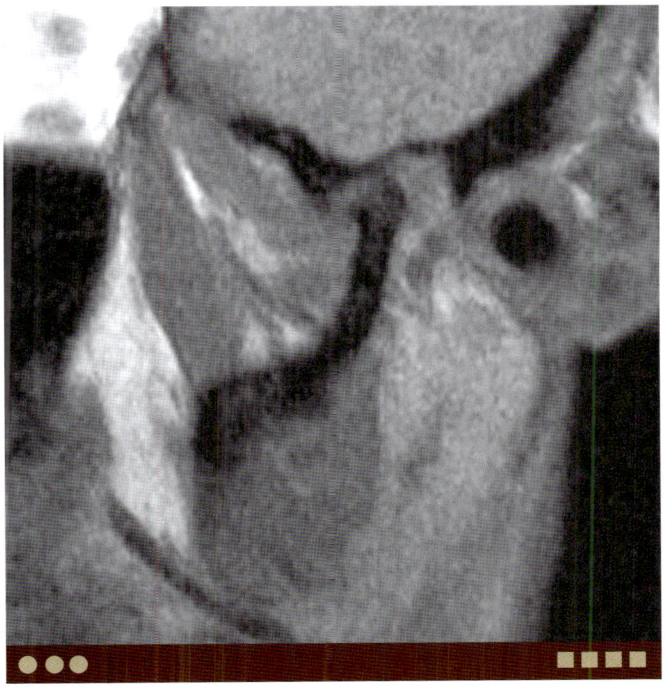

I. OA change from long-standing TMJD. Oblique-sagittal gradient-echo MR image demonstrates a thinned mandibular condyle with decreased marrow signal consistent with sclerosis. The disc is hardly appreciated.

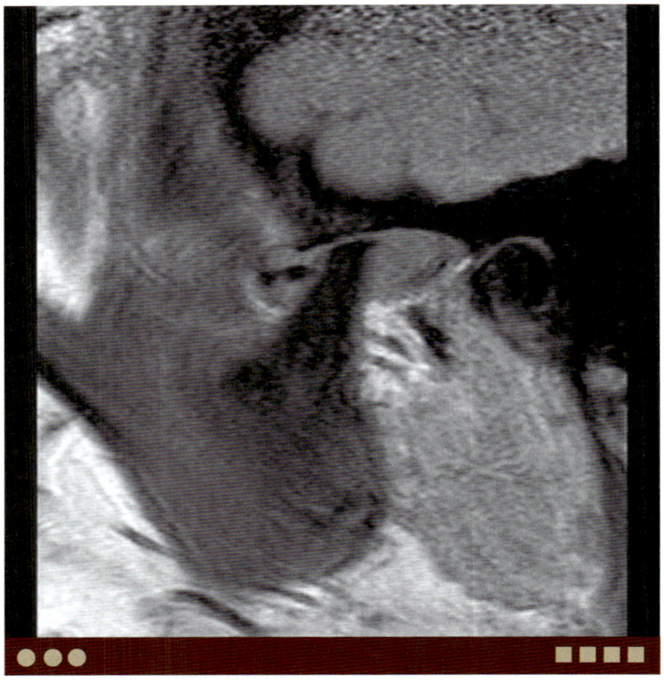

J. Rheumatoid arthritis. Closed mouth oblique-sagittal PDW MR image demonstrates thinned and deformed condyle and fullness of the joint capsule due to effusion and synovial proliferation. The disc is anteriorly dislocated.

Case 9–14 Rheumatoid Arthritis

Osamu Sakai, Takashi Kaneda, Margaret Chapman

PRESENTATION

TMJ pain.

FINDINGS

CT and MRI demonstrate arthritic changes in the temporomandibular joint (TMJ).

DIFFERENTIAL DIAGNOSIS

- Osteoarthritis: This is the most common cause of arthritic change in the TMJ and often represents sequela of TMJD or trauma.
- Pseudogout: Calcium pyrophosphate dihydrate deposition is rare, but can occur in the TMJ. Calcification is often seen.
- Suppurative arthritis: This condition usually demonstrates apparent inflammatory and infectious signs and symptoms clinically and radiologically.
- Synovial osteochondromatosis: This is usually seen in large joints, but it can be seen in the TMJ. Calcification or ossification is seen in the joint capsule.

COMMENTS

This is a 38-year-old woman with TMJ pain.

Rheumatoid arthritis (RA) is one of the autoimmune chronic inflammatory diseases that affects multiple tissues and organs, including the skin, blood vessels, heart, lungs, and muscles. RA most prominently involves synovial joints, where nonsuppurative proliferative synovitis often leads to destruction of cartilage and ankylosis. This is most commonly seen in small joints in the hands and feet; however, it occurs in the TMJ in greater than 20% of the patients affected with the disease.

CT and MRI findings of RA in the TMJ are usually nonspecific. Compared with osteoarthritis (OA), perforation of the disc is more commonly seen. Severe OA changes followed by ankylosis are seen in the late stages of RA. On MRI, abnormal enhancement is seen in the thickened synovia and fibrotic tissues.

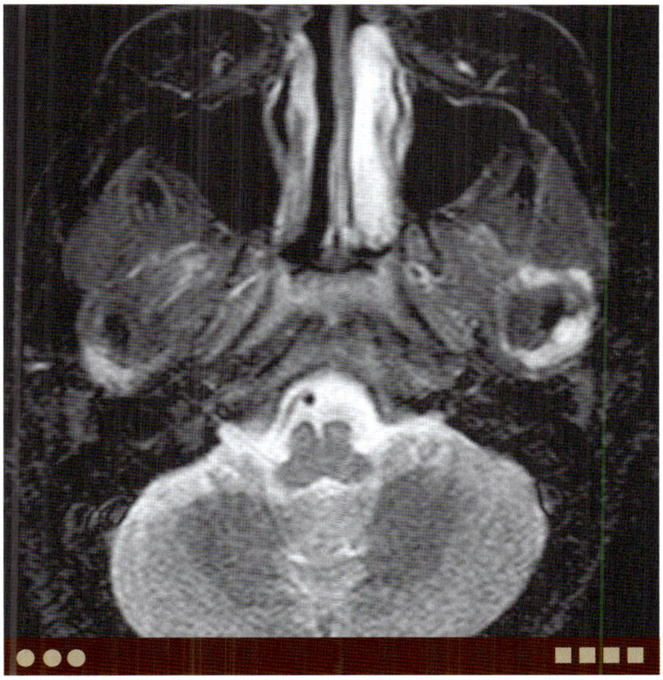

A. Rheumatoid arthritis. Axial STIR MR image demonstrates abnormal high signal in the bilateral TMJs, left worse than right.

In the head and neck, RA involvement of the atlantoaxial joint is well known; however, this condition can also affect the cricoarytenoid joint and TMJ. In addition, pachymeningeal enhancement is occasionally seen; therefore, careful evaluation of the intracranial structures and correlation with the history are important when interpreting TMJ imaging studies.

PEARLS

- **RA of the TMJ is not rare, and is seen in more than 20% of patients with RA.**
- **Findings of RA in the TMJ are similar to those in other joints.**
- **Intracranial involvement, such as pachymeningeal enhancement, can be seen in patients with RA.**

ADDITIONAL IMAGES (B-G)

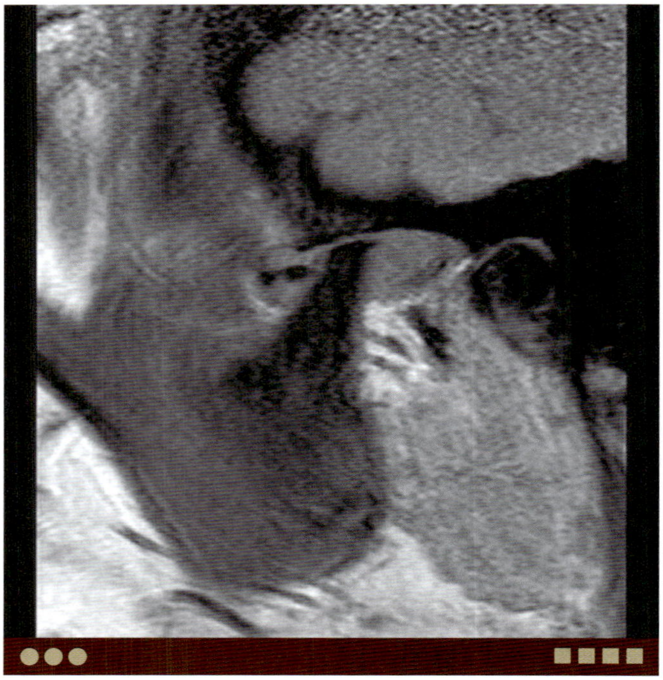

B. RA, same patient as A. Oblique-sagittal PDW MR image demonstrates a thinned and deformed condyle, anterior dislocation of the disc, joint effusion, and synovial proliferation.

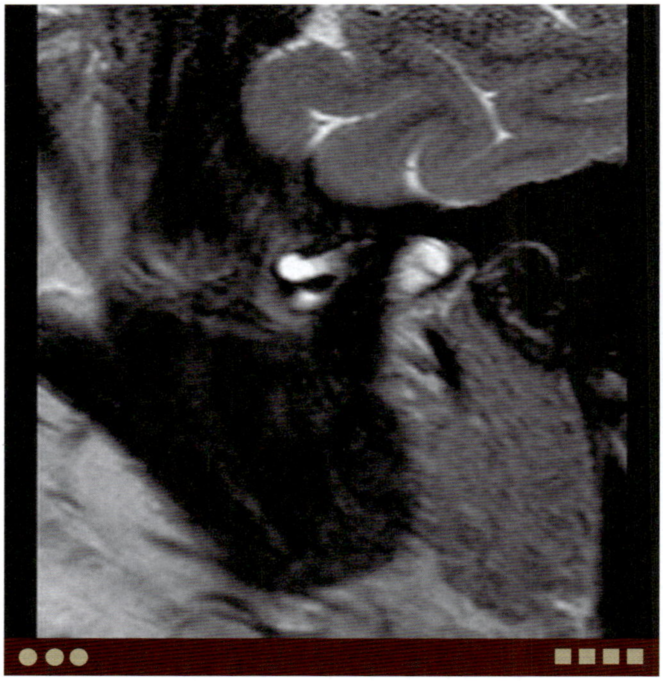

C. RA, same patient as A. Oblique-sagittal T2W MR image demonstrates high signal from the joint effusion and synovial proliferation.

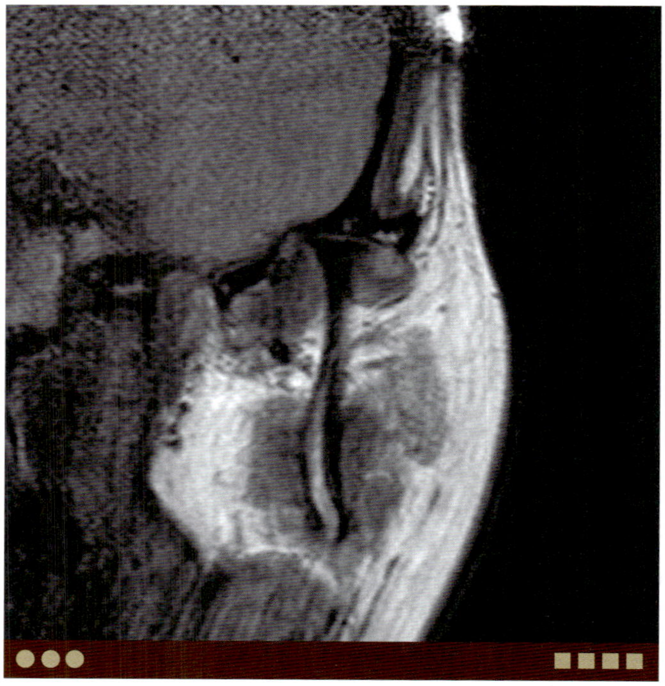

D. RA, same patient as A. Coronal PDW MR image demonstrates a thinned and deformed condyle and fullness of the joint capsule due to joint effusion and synovial proliferation.

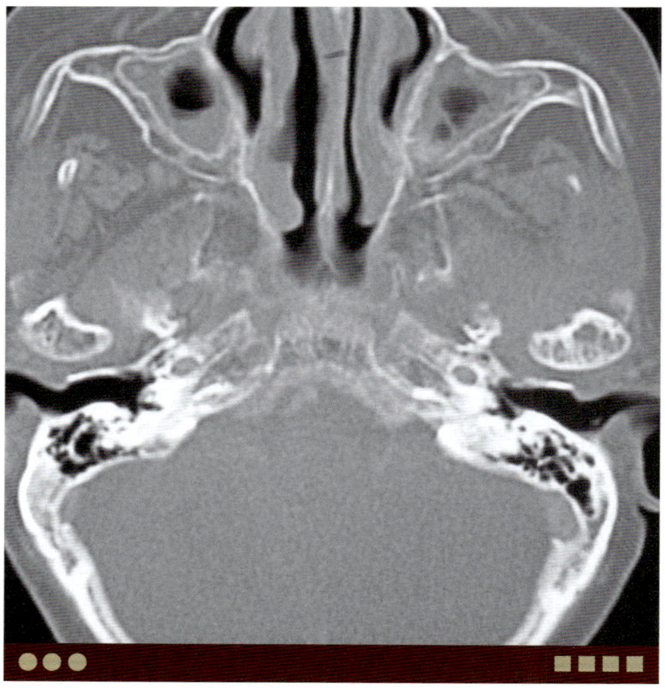

E. RA in a different patient. Axial CT demonstrates a mixture of sclerotic and lytic changes in the left mandibular condyle.

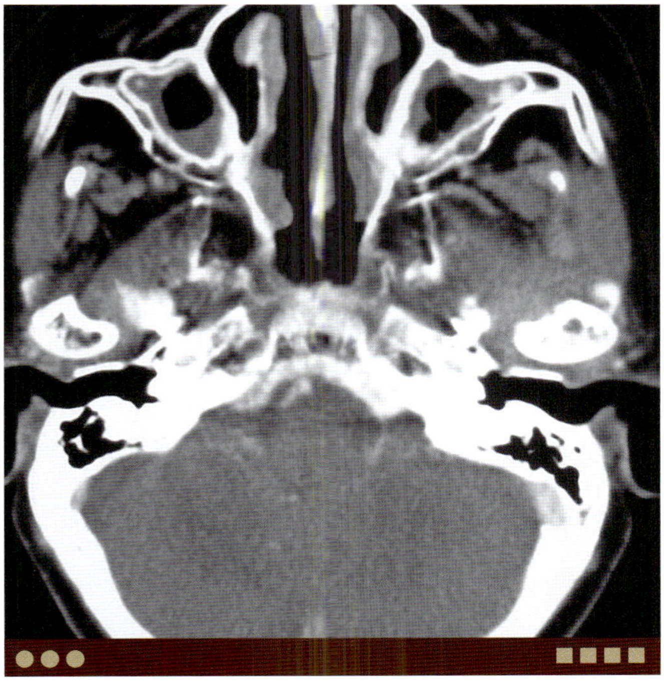

F. RA, same patient as E. Axial contrast-enhanced CT demonstrates abnormal soft tissue density around the left mandibular condyle obscuring the fat planes.

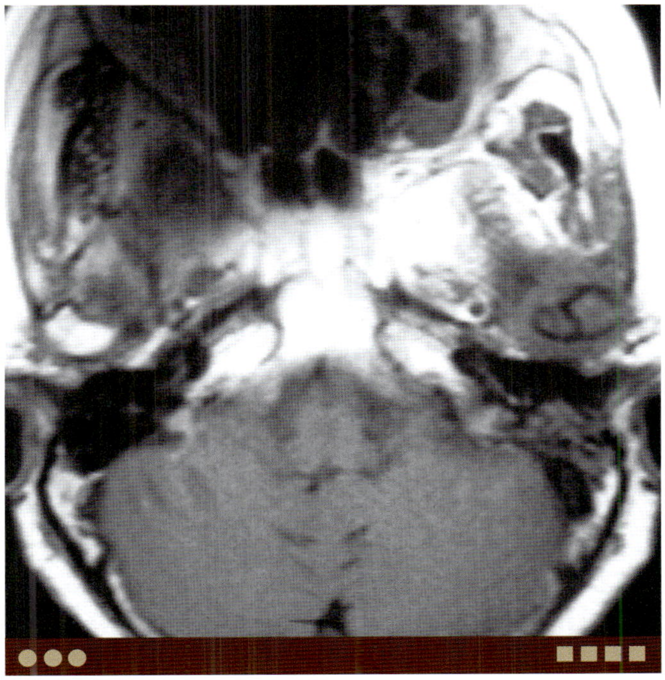

G. RA, same patient as E. Axial T1W MR image demonstrates abnormally decreased signal in the left mandibular condyle. Note abnormal intermediate signal around the condyle obscuring the fat planes consistent with synovial proliferation and fibrosis.

DIFFERENTIAL DIAGNOSIS IMAGES (H-J)

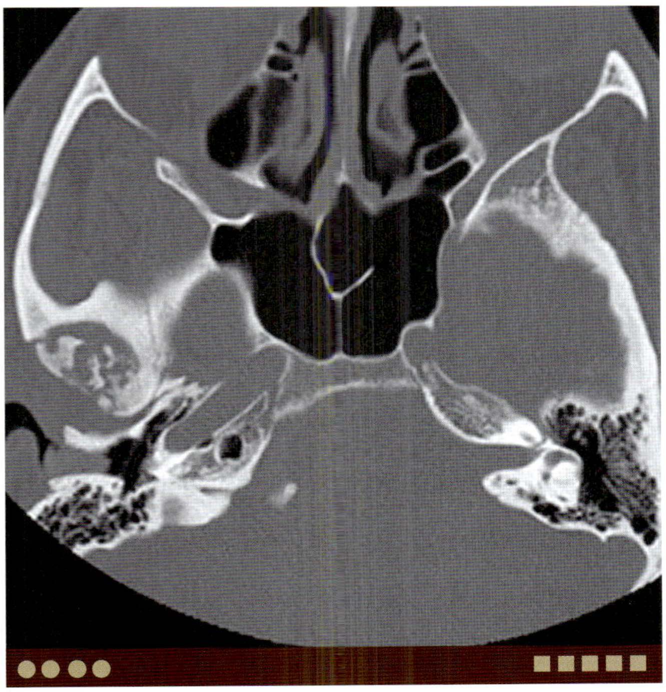

H. Osteoarthritis. Axial CT demonstrates a mixture of sclerotic and lytic changes in the right mandibular condyle.

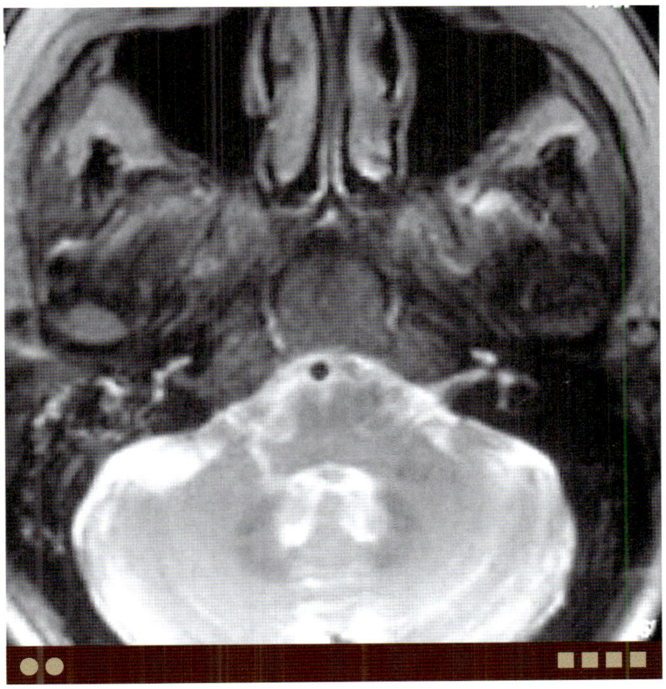

I. Pigmented villonodular synovitis. Axial T2W MR image demonstrates abnormally decreased signal in the left TMJ likely representing hemosiderin deposits.

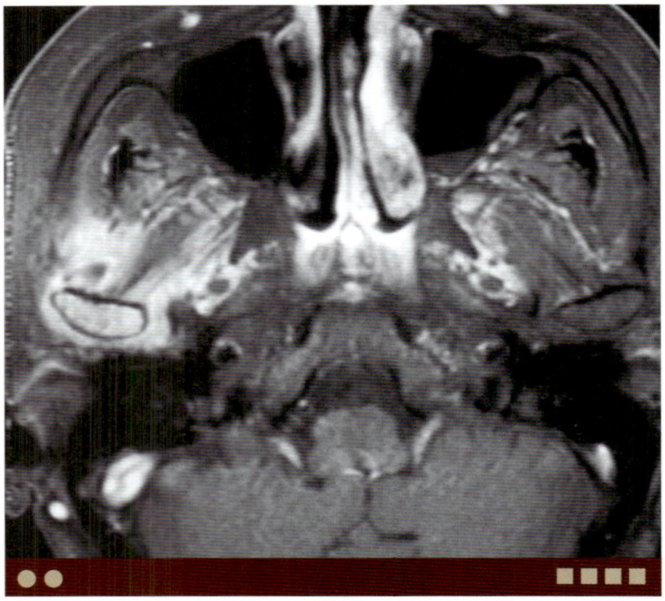

J. Septic arthritis. Axial postcontrast fat-suppressed T1W MR image demonstrates avid enhancement in the right TMJ, including the condyle and periarticular soft tissues. A small nonenhancing area indicates joint effusion.

Case 9–15 Synovial Chondromatosis

Osamu Sakai, Daniel Welier

PRESENTATION

TMJ swelling.

FINDINGS

CT demonstrates multiple high-density nodular lesions in the expanded joint capsule of the TMJ.

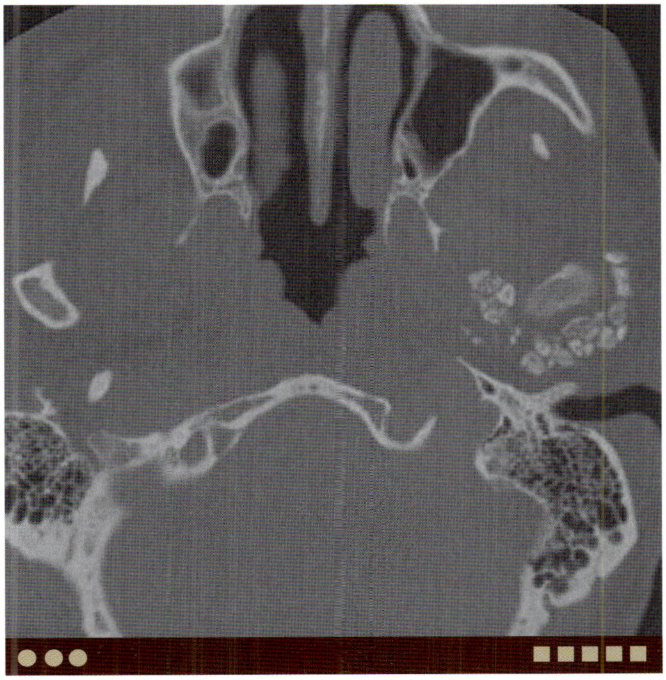

A. Synovial chondromatosis. Axial CT demonstrates multiple ossified fragments with smooth margins in the left TMJ. Note some are well corticated and contain central low density consistent with bone marrow.

DIFFERENTIAL DIAGNOSIS

- Osteoarthritis: This condition is the most common arthritic change in the TMJ and usually a sequela of TMJD or trauma.
- Calcium pyrophosphate dihydrate deposition (CPPD, pseudogout): This condition is rare in the TMJ, but occurs as seen in other joints.
- Tumoral calcinosis: This is an uncommon condition characterized by periarticular soft tissue hyperplasia and calcification.
- Chondromyxoid fibroma: This is a rare tumor which can occur in the temporal bone
- Pigmented villonodular synovitis: Decreased signal on T2W MR images is seen in the TMJ due to hemosiderin deposits. Calcification is not seen.

COMMENTS

This is a 41-year-old woman with preauricular swelling.

Synovial chondromatosis is a benign condition characterized by synovial membrane proliferation and metaplasia. This condition is also termed synovial osteochondromatosis. Synovial chondromatosis often occurs in large joints such as the knee, shoulder, and hip; however, it can be seen in the TMJ. Nodular proliferation and metaplasia of the synovial lining may break off into the joint. Within the joint, the fragments are nourished by synovial fluid, and can grow, calcify, and ossify. The fragments may vary in size from several millimeter to several centimeter. The calcified or ossified fragments may be embedded in the synovium or free in the joint capsule. Expansion of the joint capsule is often seen.

CT can easily depict calcified or ossified fragments. Joint calcification may be seen in other conditions such as pseudogout (CPPD) and chondrosarcoma. However, calcification or ossification in synovial chondromatosis usually has smooth margins, and occasionally bone marrow can be identified inside of the fragments, which is helpful to make the diagnosis. Irregularity of the joint surface and sclerosis or hyperostosis of the glenoid fossa and mandibular condyle are often seen.

MRI can better delineate expanded joint capsules and the extent of the lesion, although calcification or ossification is not well seen on MRI. High T1 signal from the marrow in the ossified fragment can be observed. Joint effusion is better demonstrated on MRI. The fragments are seen as filling defects in the expanded joint space on T2W or postcontrast T1W images.

PEARLS

- **Synovial chondromatosis is a benign condition characterized by synovial proliferation and metaplasia.**
- **CT can easily depict calcified or ossified fragments with smooth margins.**
- **High T1 signal from the marrow in the ossified fragment can be observed on MRI, and the fragments can be seen as filling defects in the expanded joint space on T2W or postcontrast T1W images.**

ADDITIONAL IMAGES (B-G)

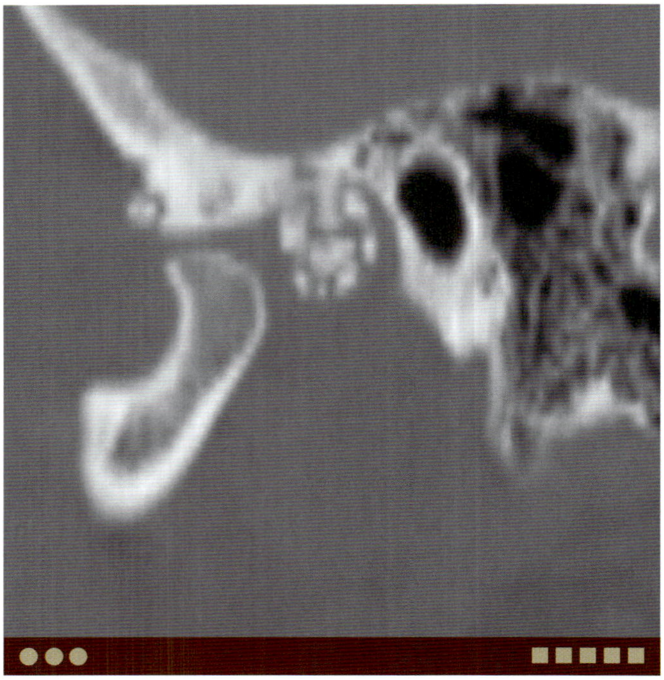

B. Synovial chondromatosis, same patient as A. Sagittal CT demonstrates multiple ossified fragments in the glenoid fossa.

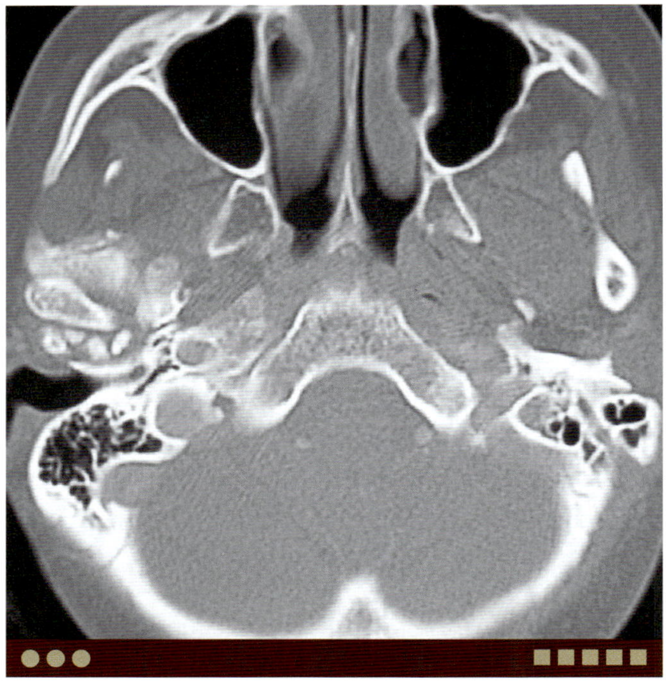

C. Synovial chondromatosis in a different patient. Axial CT demonstrates multiple ossified fragments with smooth margins in the right TMJ. Note some are well corticated and contain central low density consistent with bone marrow.

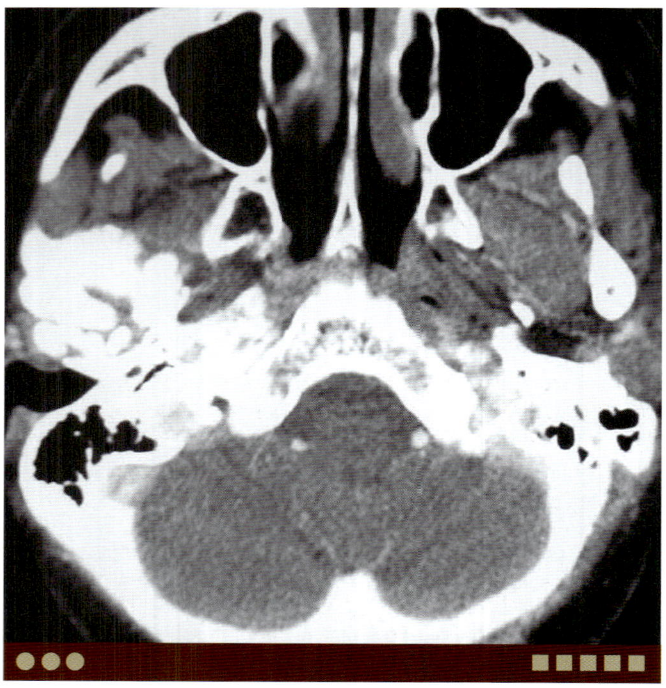

D. Synovial chondromatosis, same patient as C. Axial contrast-enhanced soft tissue windowed CT demonstrates calcified or ossified fragments in the right TMJ.

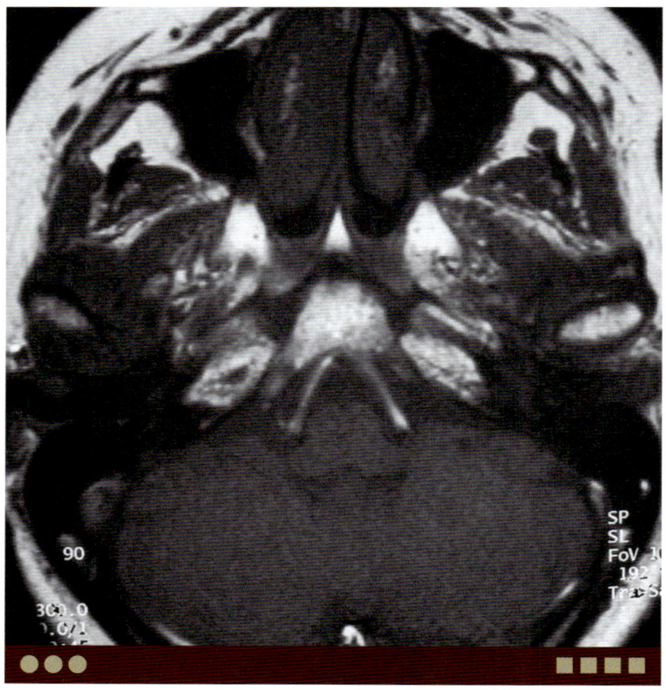

E. Synovial chondromatosis, same patient as C. Axial T1W MR image demonstrates expanded joint capsule containing low-signal foci representing calcified or ossified fragments. Note some fragments demonstrate high signal from the bone marrow.

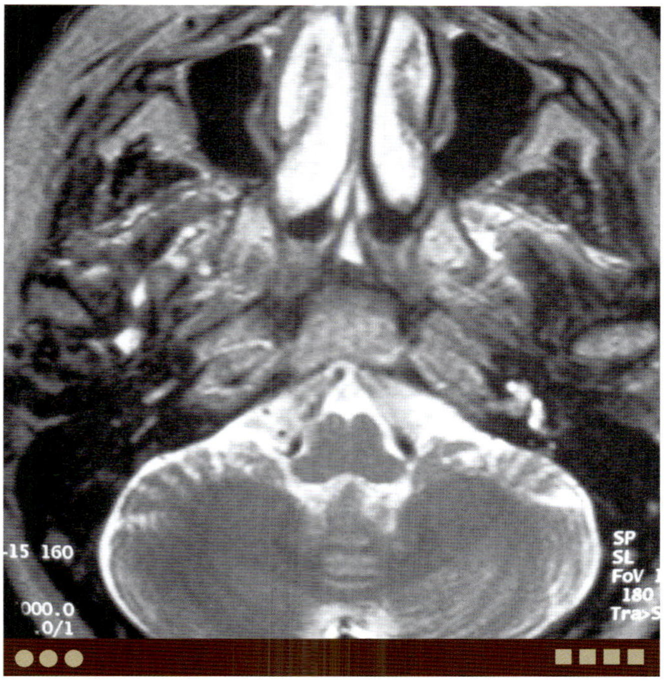

F. Synovial chondromatosis, same patient as C. Axial T2W MR image demonstrates the expanded joint capsule showing foci of heterogeneous signal; low signal from the fragments and high signal from joint effusion.

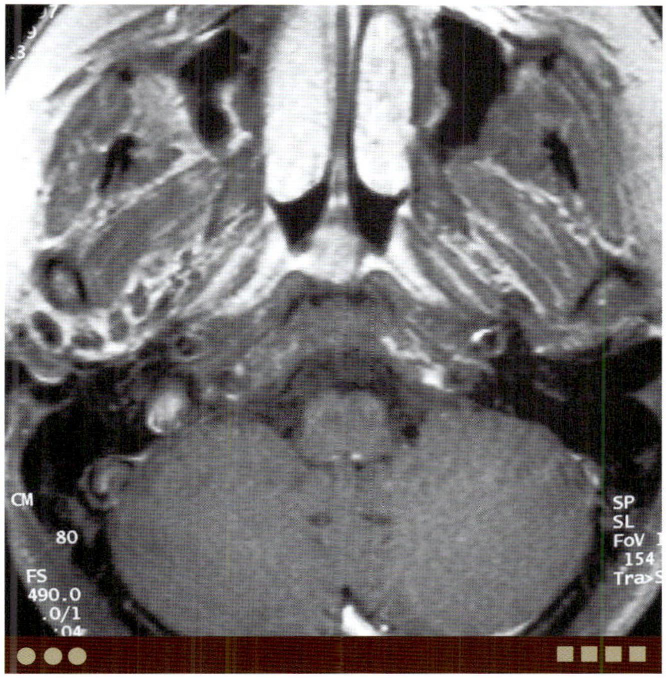

G. Synovial chondromatosis, same patient as C. Axial postcontrast fat-suppressed T1W MR image demonstrates enhancement of the synovium in the expanded joint capsule with multiple signal-voids from the fragments.

DIFFERENTIAL DIAGNOSIS IMAGES (H-J)

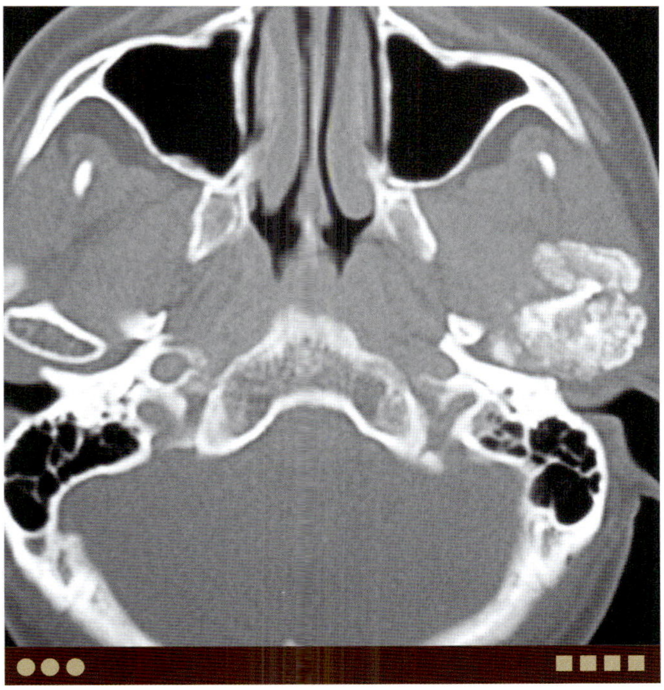

H. CPPD. Axial CT demonstrates amorphous calcification in the left TMJ and deformity of the mandibular condyle.

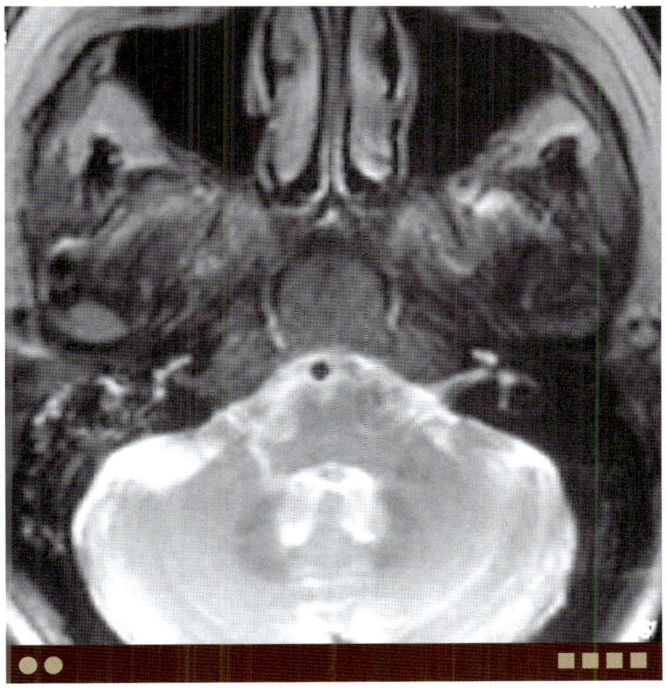

I. Pigmented villonodular synovitis. Axial T2W MR image demonstrates decreased signal in the left TMJ due to hemosiderin deposits.

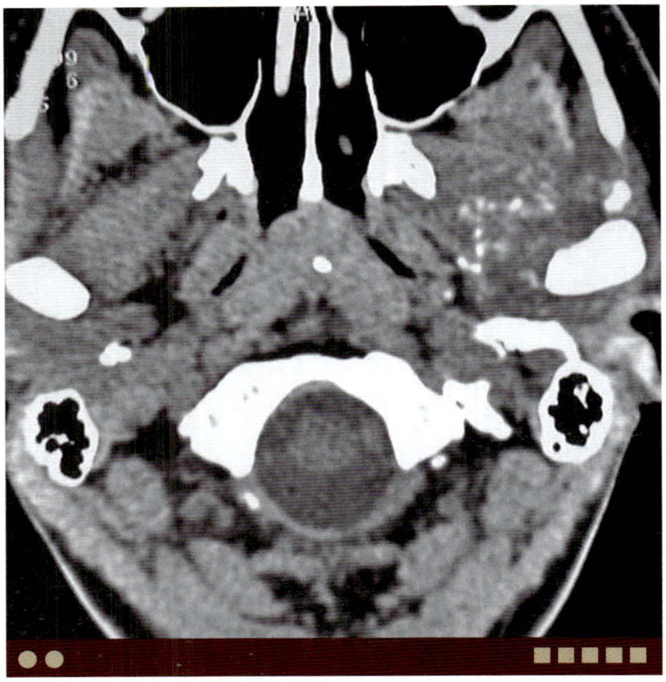

J. Chondromyxoid fibroma. Axial CT demonstrates heterogeneous soft tissue densities with multifocal calcifications around the left mandibular condyle.

Case 9–16 Calcium Pyrophosphate Dihydrate Deposition (Pseudogout)

Osamu Sakai, Andrew Akman

PRESENTATION

TMJ swelling and pain.

FINDINGS

CT demonstrates amorphous calcification in the joint capsule of the TMJ.

DIFFERENTIAL DIAGNOSIS

- Synovial chondromatosis: This is a benign condition characterized by synovial membrane proliferation and metaplasia. Calcified or ossified fragments are seen in the joint capsule.
- Osteoarthritis: This condition is the most common type of arthritic change in the TMJ and a sequela of TMJD or trauma.
- Pigmented villonodular synovitis: This condition is characterized by decreased signal on T2W MR images in the TMJ secondary to hemosiderin deposition. Calcification is not visualized.

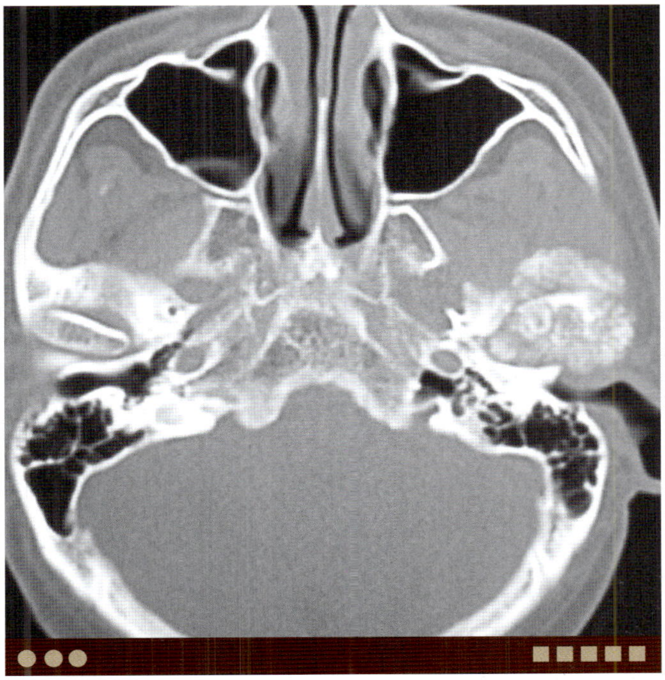

A. CPPD. Axial CT demonstrates amorphous calcification in the region of the left TMJ. The mandibular condyle shows cystic or osteolytic lesions and is not well identified.

COMMENTS

This is a 41-year-old man with preauricular swelling.

Calcium pyrophosphate dihydrate deposition (CPPD), "pseudogout" is characterized by the accumulation of calcium pyrophosphate dihydrate crystals in intra-articular and periarticular soft tissues, and occasionally affects the temporomandibular joint (TMJ) and temporal bone, causing pain, swelling, trismus, and hearing loss.

CPPD is characterized by the presence of crystal deposits that demonstrate positive birefringence under polarized light and typically have blunt/squared ends, whereas the crystals of uric acid in gout are needle shaped and demonstrate negative birefringence with polarized light.

CPPD can be divided into two groups: common/diffuse and tumoral. The former usually affects larger joints and often follows trauma, surgery, or ischemic heart disease, and the later affects smaller joints such as the TMJ, cervical spine, and hand.

CT is the best modality to identify and characterize joint calcification in the TMJ. However, diagnosis of CPPD is challenging because symptoms and imaging findings are not very characteristic and occasionally may mimic chondrosarcoma. Radiographs of the wrist or knee and laboratory findings may help make the diagnosis.

PEARLS

- **CPPD in the TMJ is not very rare.**
- **CT can easily depict intra- or periarticular calcification.**
- **CPPD has two groups: common/diffuse and tumoral. The tumoral type affects the TMJ as well as cervical spine and hand.**

ADDITIONAL IMAGES (B-F)

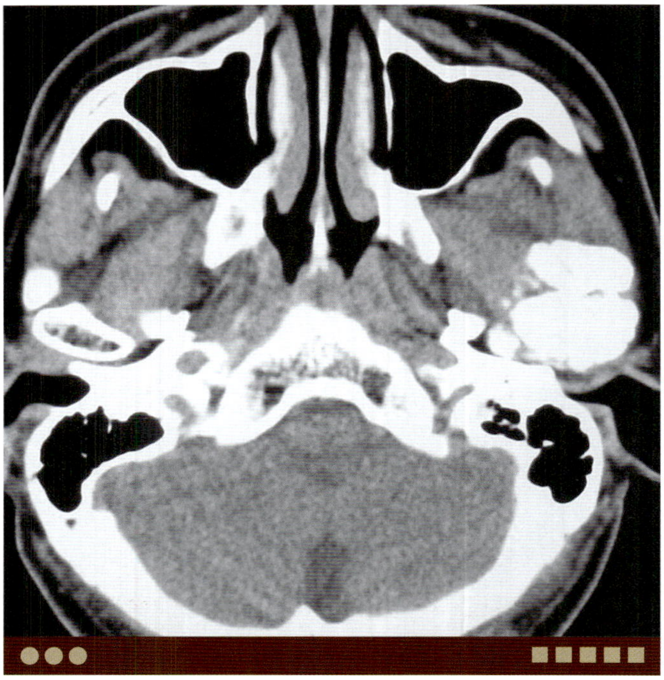

B. CPPD, same patient as A. Axial noncontrast-enhanced soft tissue windowed CT better demonstrates the extent of the lesion.

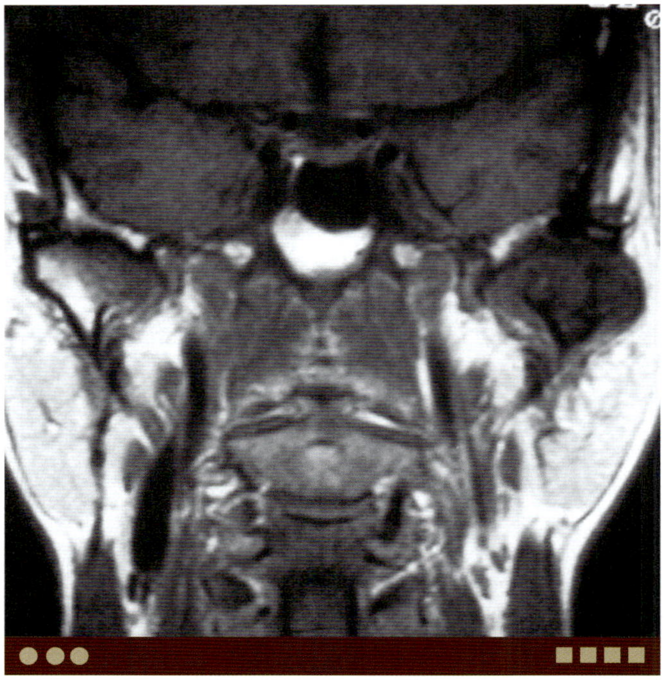

C. CPPD, same patient as A. Coronal T1W MR image demonstrates an expanded joint capsule filled with heterogeneous low-signal materials. Note loss of the normal high signal from the fatty marrow in the mandibular condyle.

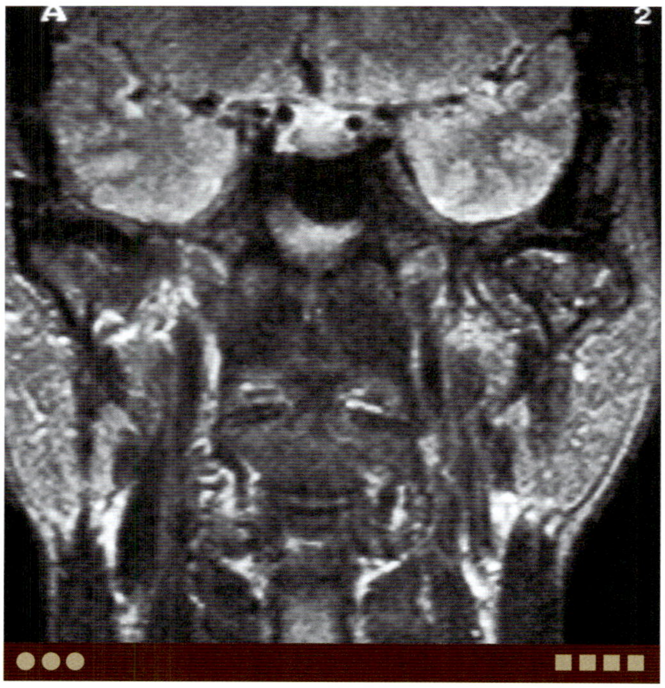

D. CPPD, same patient as A. Axial T2W MR image demonstrates heterogeneous signals in the mandibular condyle and expanded joint capsule filled with heterogeneous low-signal materials.

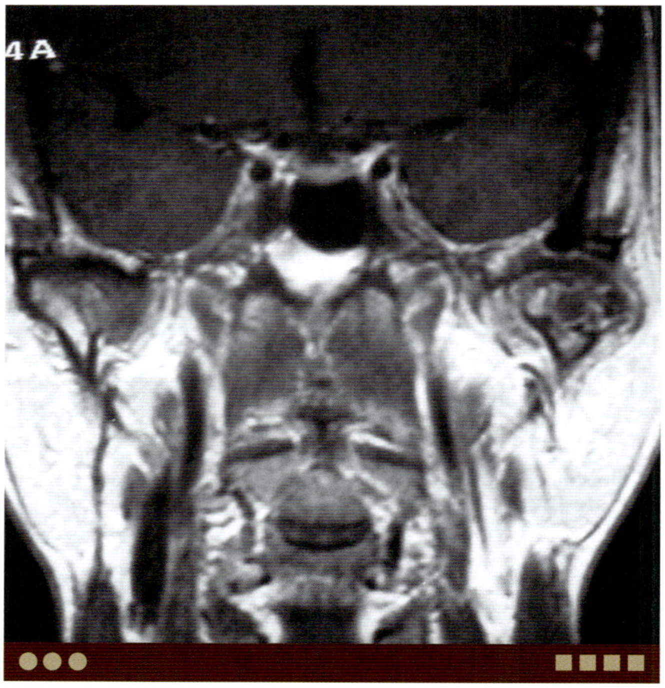

E. CPPD, same patient as A. Axial postcontrast T1W MR image demonstrates heterogeneous enhancement of the thickened synovium. Cystic degenerative changes of the mandibular condyle are better delineated by enhancing cyst walls.

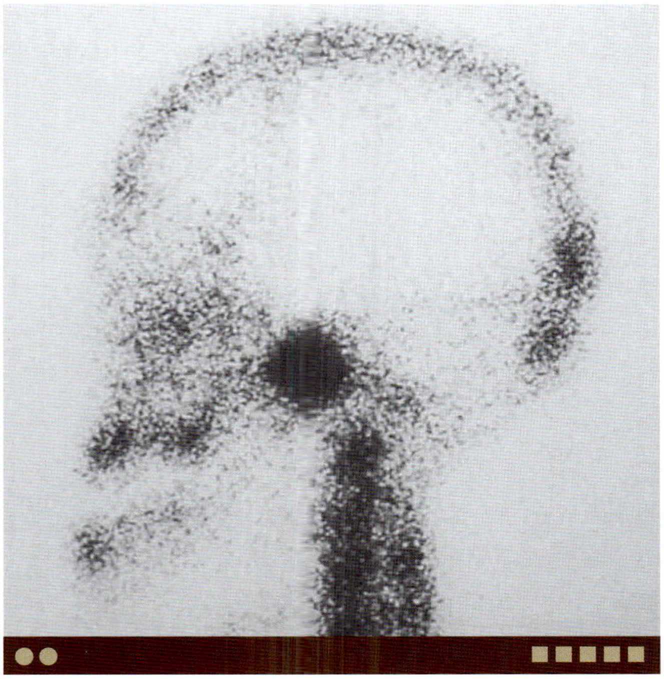

F. CPPD, same patient as A. Bone scan demonstrates increased uptake in the TMJ.

DIFFERENTIAL DIAGNOSIS IMAGES (G-H)

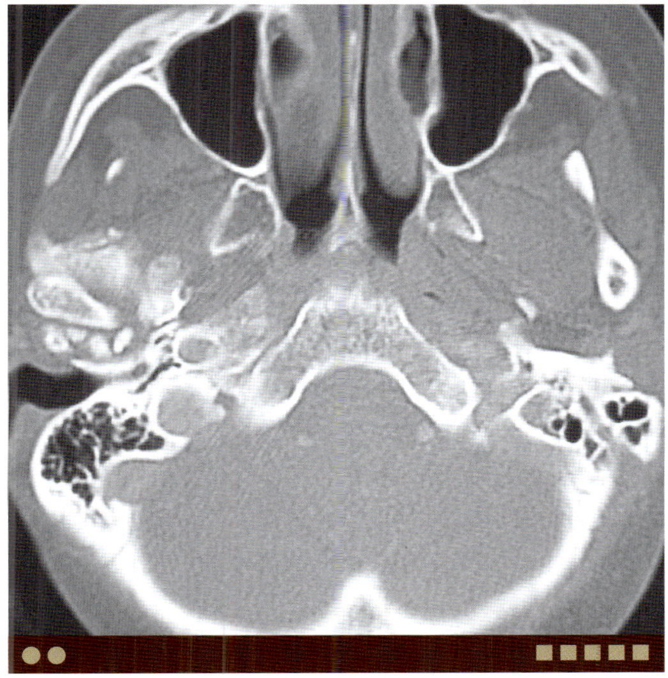

G. Synovial chondromatosis. Axial CT demonstrates multiple calcified/ossified bodies with smooth margins.

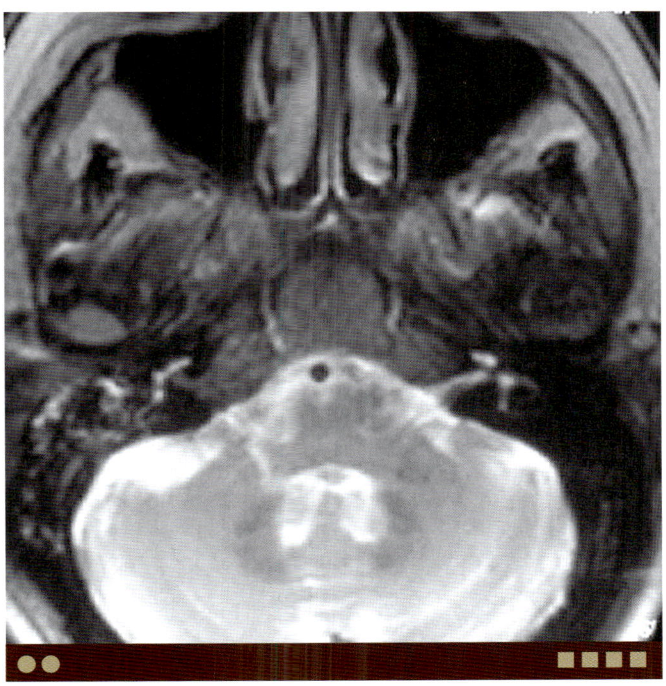

H. Pigmented villonodular synovitis. Axial T2W MR image demonstrates decreased signal in the left TMJ due to hemosiderin deposits.

Case 9–17 Torus Palatinus

Osamu Sakai, Margaret Chapman

PRESENTATION

Bump in the hard palate.

FINDINGS

CT demonstrates an osseous protrusion in the hard palate at midline.

DIFFERENTIAL DIAGNOSIS

- Pleomorphic adenoma: This is the most common benign tumor in the hard palate. Bony erosion may be seen.
- Schwannoma: This condition may show findings similar to pleomorphic adenoma. Smooth bone remodeling or erosion is commonly seen.
- Squamous cell carcinoma: This is the most common malignant tumor in the palate. Normal fat just below the greater palatine foramen should be confirmed on every case to exclude perineural tumor spread.

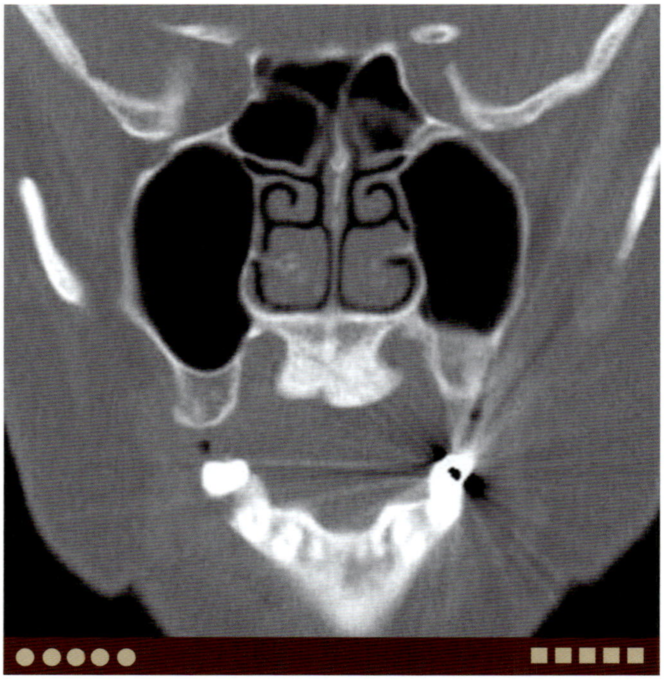

A. Torus palatinus. Coronal CT demonstrates a slightly lobulated, dense osseous protrusion of the hard palate.

COMMENTS

This is a 44-year-old woman who underwent CT for sinusitis.

Torus palatinus is an exostosis (focal bony growth) of the palate in midline, often demonstrating a lobulated appearance. It is usually less than 2 cm in diameter; however, larger sizes can be seen. It is considered a developmental anomaly, although it does not present until adult life. Patients are usually middle-aged women, with lesions seen more commonly among the Asian population.

Torus palatinus usually has no clinical significance and there is no need for treatment. However, this condition may complicate the fabrication of dentures, and surgery may be performed. Ulceration or burning of the overlying mucosa is often seen.

Exostosis is also often seen in the mandible (torus mandibularis) and maxillary alveolus without clinical significance.

On CT, the osseous protrusion is clearly seen on coronal and sagittal planes, while the lobulated appearance may be better demonstrated on axial images. MRI may demonstrate high signal on T1W images from the bone marrow in the center of the torus palatinus.

PEARLS

- **Torus palatinus is a focal osseous proliferation of the hard palate at midline.**
- **There is usually no clinical significance; however, this condition may complicate the fabrication of dentures.**
- **CT clearly demonstrates a well-corticated osseous protrusion. MRI may show bone marrow in addition to the signal-void from the dense bone.**

ADDITIONAL IMAGES (B-E)

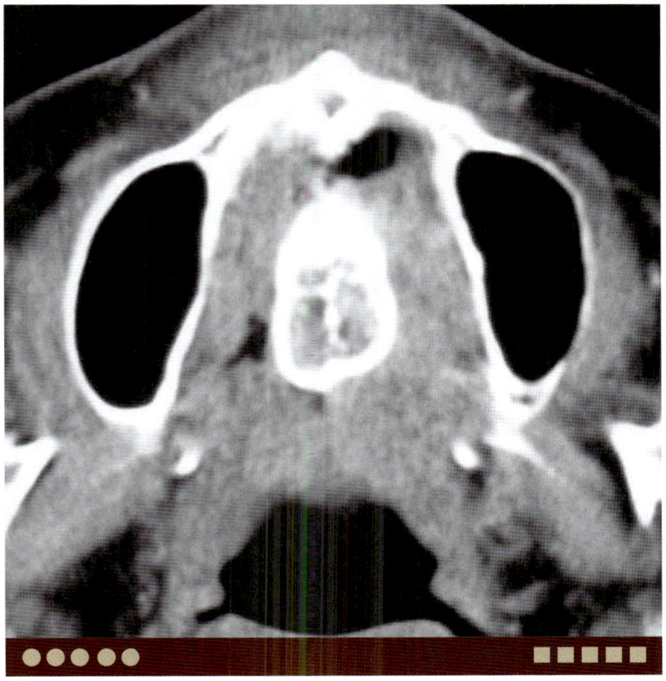

B. Torus palatinus in a different patient. Axial CT demonstrates an osseous protrusion of the hard palate with internal trabeculation and marrow density.

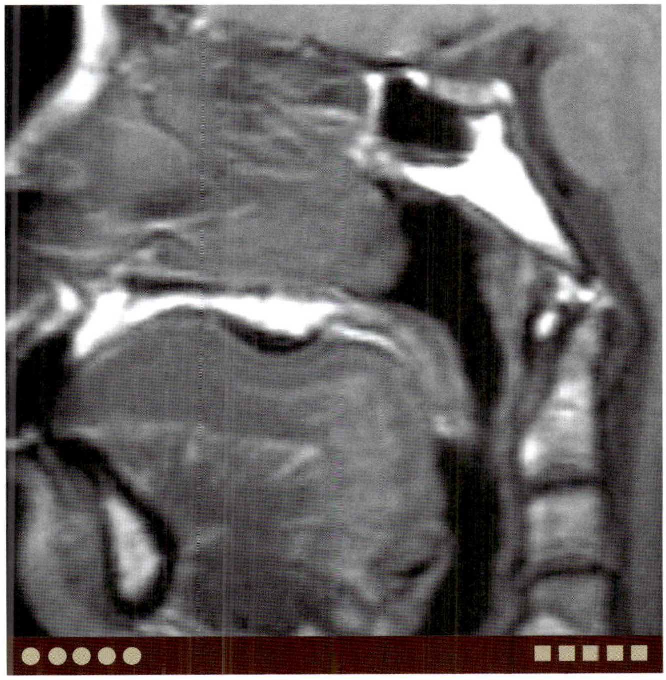

C. Torus palatinus in a different patient. Sagittal T1W MR image demonstrates proliferation of the cortex and thickened marrow in the hard palate.

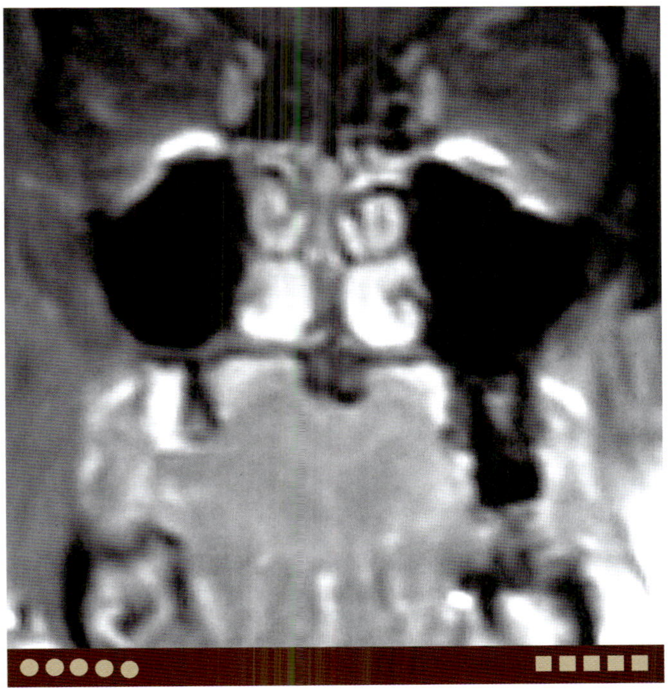

D. Torus palatinus in a different patient. Coronal postcontrast fat-suppressed T1W MR image demonstrates midline protrusion of the hard palate. Note normal marrow signal in the torus.

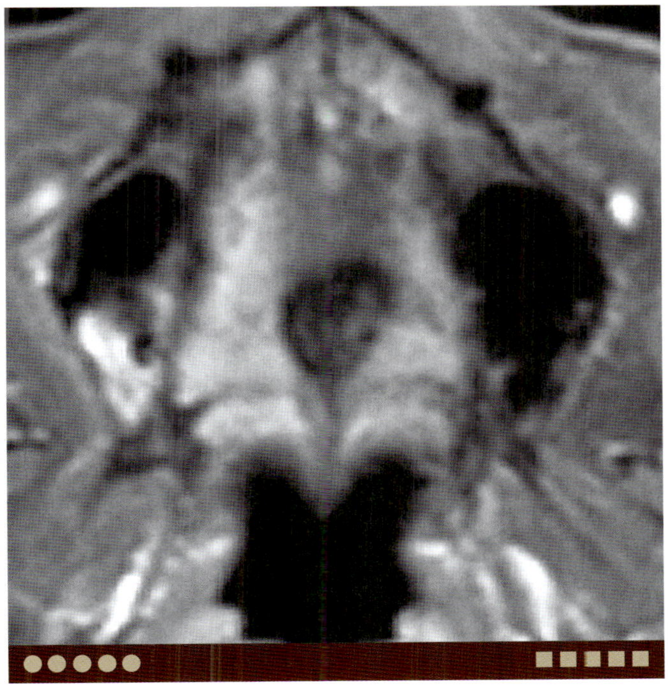

E. Torus palatinus same patient as D. Axial postcontrast fat-suppressed T1W MR image demonstrates a well-corticated osseous protrusion with normal marrow.

DIFFERENTIAL DIAGNOSIS IMAGES (F-H)

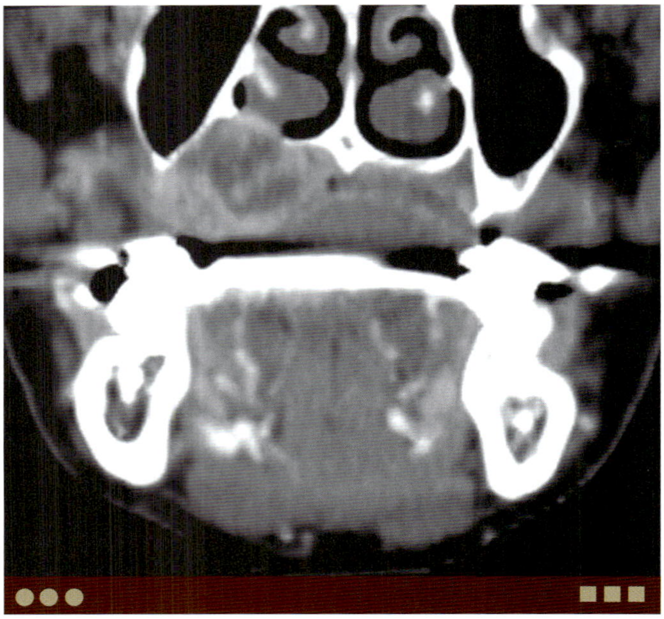

F. Adenoid cystic carcinoma. Coronal contrast-enhanced CT demonstrates a rounded heterogeneously enhancing lesion in the right palate eroding the adjacent bone. Involvement of the greater palatine foramen raises the possibility of perineural tumor spread.

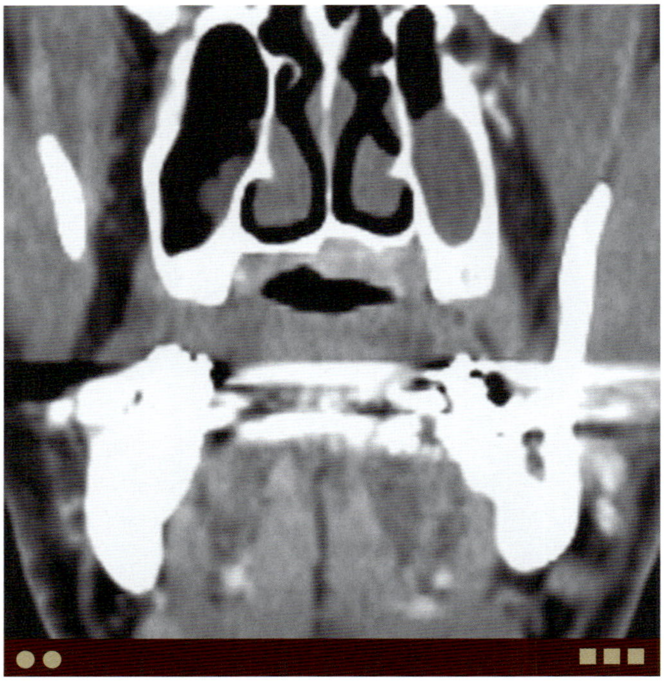

G. Adenocarcinoma. Coronal contrast-enhanced CT demonstrates a small heterogeneously enhancing lesion in the left palate eroding the bone.

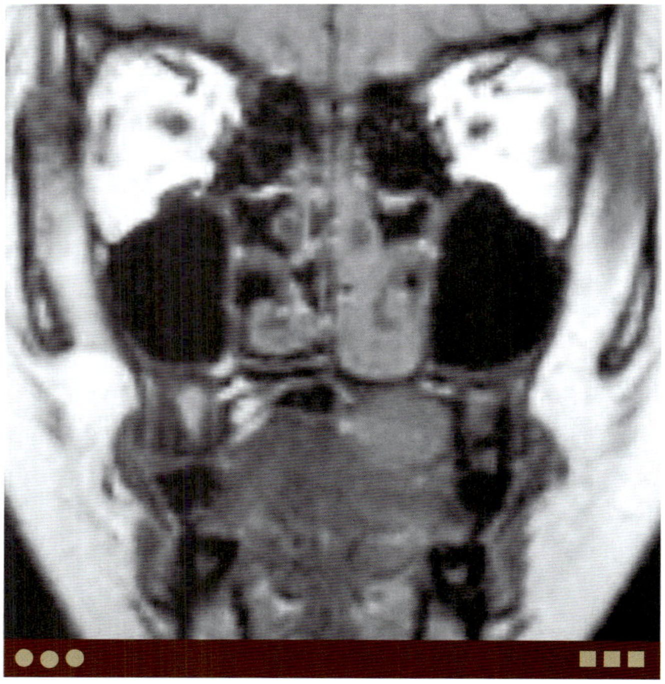

H. Pleomorphic adenoma. Coronal postcontrast T1W MR image demonstrates a round-enhancing tumor eroding the left hard palate.

Case 9–18 Fibrous Dysplasia

Osamu Sakai, Margaret Chapman

PRESENTATION

Asymmetric jaw swelling.

FINDINGS

CT demonstrates an expansile ground-grass density osseous lesion within the mandible and/or maxilla.

DIFFERENTIAL DIAGNOSIS

- Ossifying fibroma: This is a benign fibroosseous lesion composed of lamellar bone with prominent osteoblastic rimming in dense fibrous stroma. This demonstrates nearly identical radiological findings to fibrous dysplasia.
- Chronic osteomyelitis: This condition demonstrates heterogeneous density on CT, including a mixture of osteosclerotic and lytic changes, and occasionally expansion of the bone. Usually periodontal disease can be identified.
- Paget's disease: This is a common disease of unknown etiology. This is usually seen in elderly individuals, and is unusual in patients under age 40. Involvement of the skull and skull base is common, although any bone can be affected.

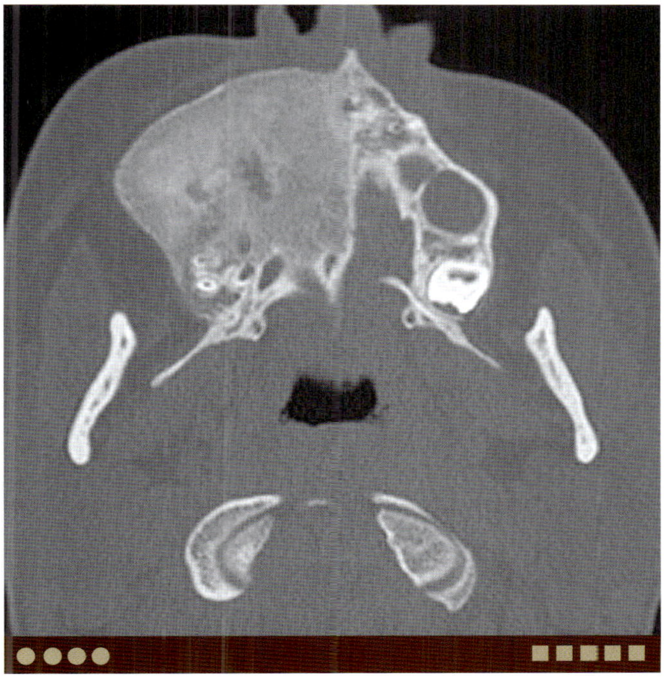

A. Fibrous dysplasia. Axial CT demonstrates an expansile ground-grass lesion in the right maxilla.

COMMENTS

This is a 65-year-old man with an asymmetric jaw.

Fibrous dysplasia can occur anywhere in the body, and is often seen in the maxillofacial bones and skull base. This condition can present at any age but is often diagnosed before 20 years. Fibrous dysplasia can be subdivided into three types: monostotic, polyostotic, and McCune-Albright syndrome. Lesions are usually unilateral. When found in the head and neck, this condition often involves contiguous bones on the same side; however, skull and skull base lesions often cross midline. Ipsilateral lesions in the maxilla and mandible are often seen although they are not contiguous.

Because of similar radiographic findings, cherubism has been described as a subtype of fibrous dysplasia that specifically involves the mandible and maxilla. However, recent genetic analysis has shown these to be separate entities.

On CT, a ground-grass appearance is thought to be a typical finding; however, cystic change is also commonly seen. Radiologically, fibrous dysplasia may be difficult to differentiate from other benign fibroosseous lesions. Narrowing of osseous canals and foramina is seen due to bone expansion and occasionally results in cranial nerve impairment.

On MRI, fibrous dysplasia demonstrates low signal on T1W images and variable signal on T2W images, depending on the degree of fibrotic or osseous changes. "Fresh" fibrotic change demonstrates high signal on T2W images and avid enhancement after contrast.

Malignant tumors, such as osteosarcoma, fibrosarcoma, chondrosarcoma, and malignant fibrohistiocytoma may rarely occur from fibrous dysplasia, particularly in patients with the polyostotic form, McCune-Albright syndrome.

PEARLS

- **Fibrous dysplasia is a common benign fibroosseous lesion.**
- **It is usually unilateral and involves contiguous bones. Ipsilateral maxillary and mandibular lesions are also often seen, although these are not contiguous.**
- **A ground-grass appearance is a typical finding of fibrous dysplasia; however, cystic change is also common.**

ADDITIONAL IMAGES (B-F)

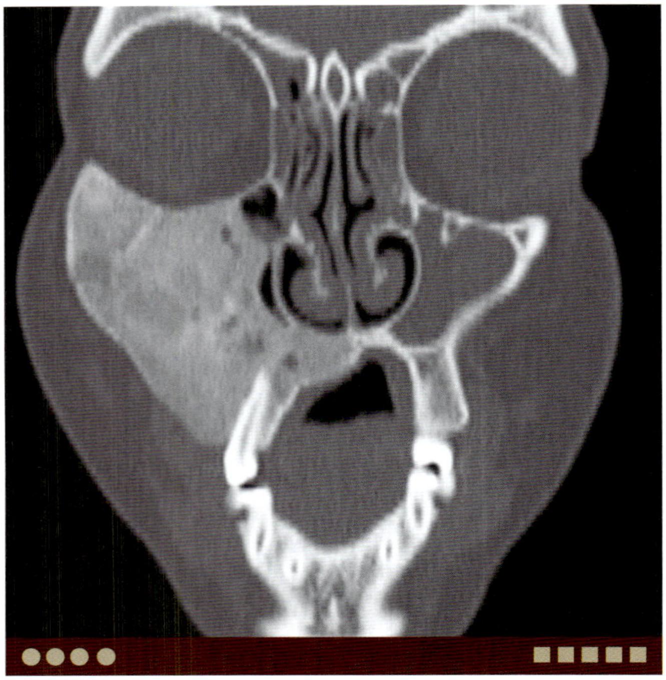

B. Fibrous dysplasia, same patient as A. Coronal CT demonstrates an expansile ground-grass-appearing lesion in the right maxilla extending to the alveolar ridge and palate.

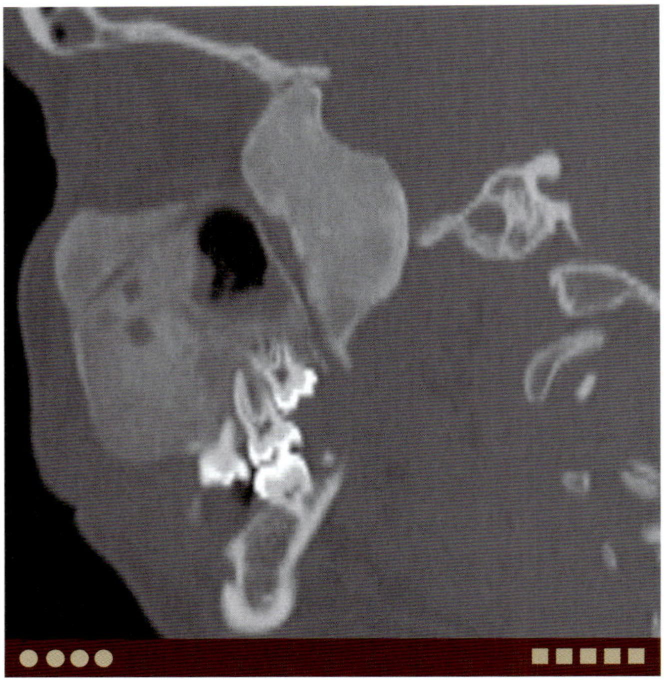

C. Fibrous dysplasia, same patient as A. Sagittal CT demonstrates expansile ground-grass maxillary and pterygoid lesions. Note narrowed maxillary sinus and involvement of the infraorbital groove and pterygopalatine fossa.

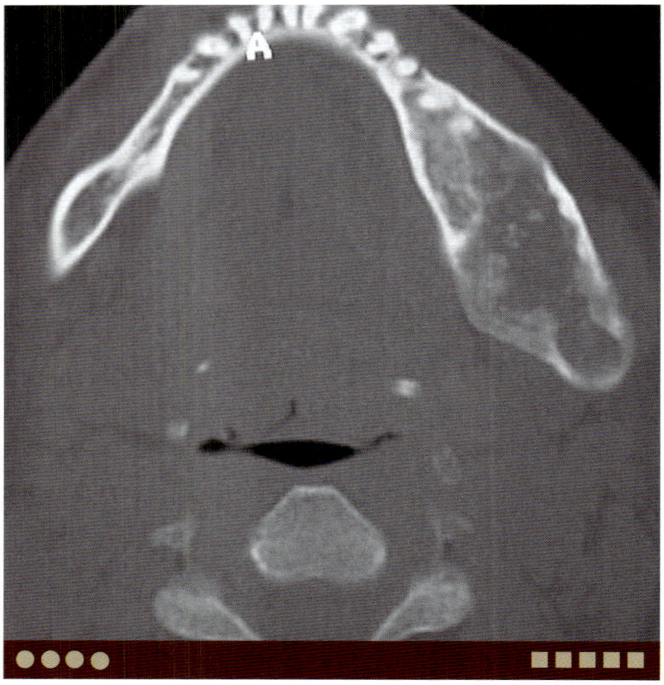

D. Fibrous dysplasia in a different patient. Axial CT demonstrates an expansile ground-grass and cystic-appearing lesion in the posterior body of the left mandible.

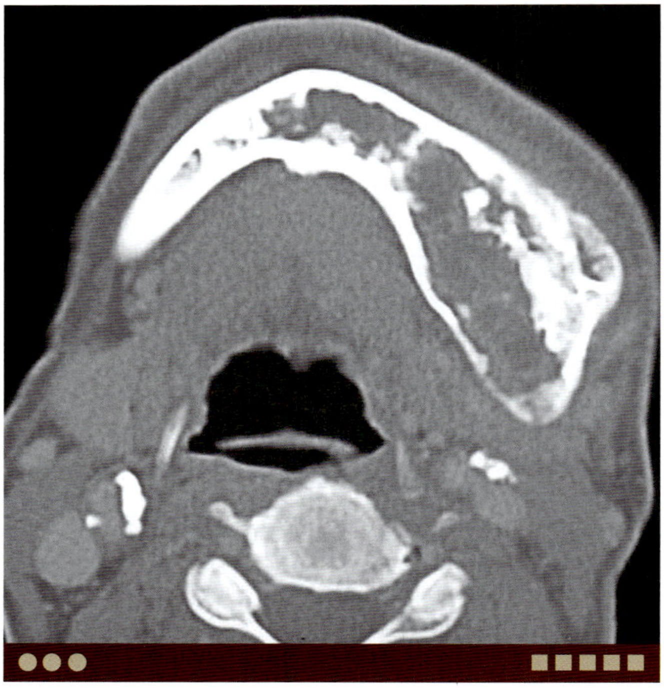

E. Fibrous dysplasia in a different patient. Axial CT demonstrates an expansile lesion with coarse internal calcifications in the left mandible.

DIFFERENTIAL DIAGNOSIS IMAGES (G-J)

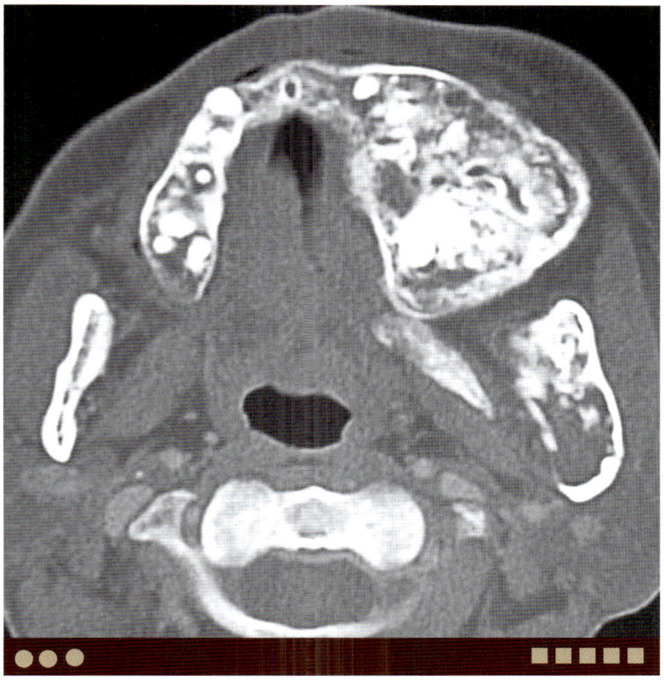

F. Fibrous dysplasia, same patient as E. Axial CT through the maxilla demonstrates lesions in both the maxilla and mandible on the same side.

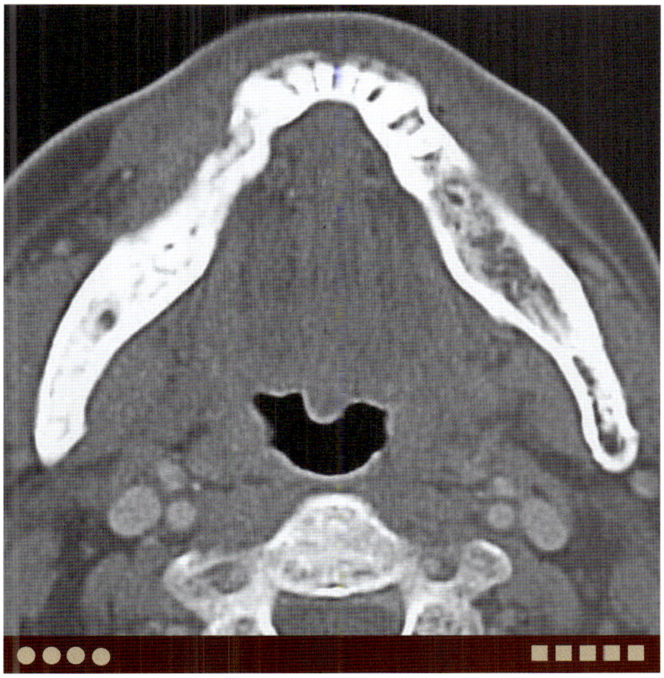

G. Chronic osteomyelitis. Axial CT demonstrates diffuse sclerotic changes in the right mandibular body.

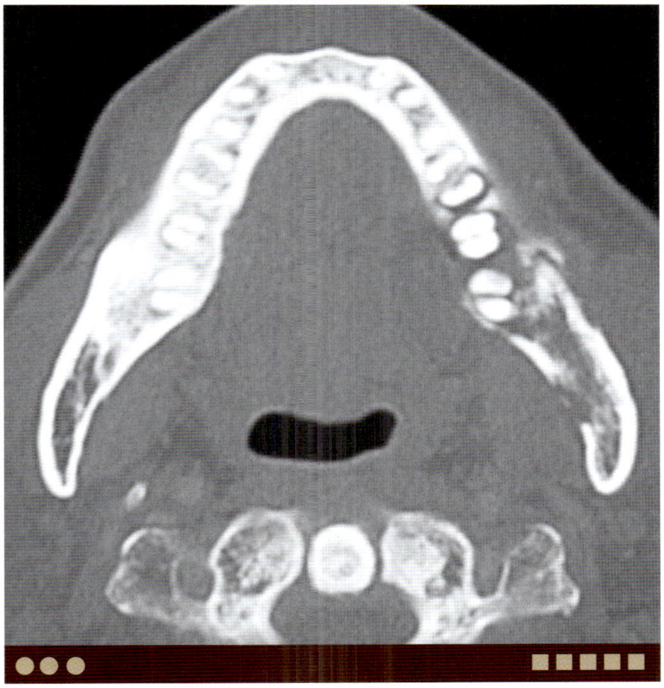

H. Osteoradionecrosis. Axial CT demonstrates diffuse demineralization and cortical destruction in the posterior body/ramus of the left mandible. There is diffuse sclerotic change consistent with osteitis identified in the right mandible.

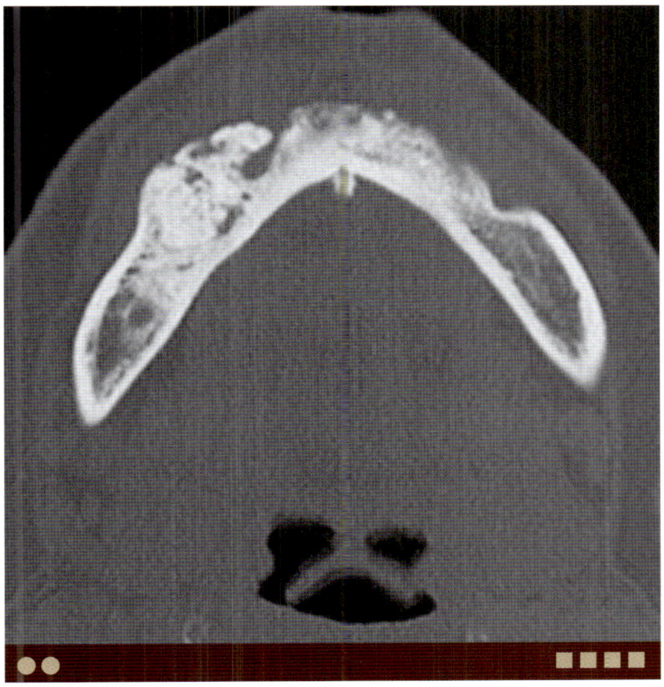

I. Bisphosphonate-associated osteonecrosis. Axial CT demonstrates sclerotic changes in the anterior mandible, right greater than left, and foci of osteolysis. Buccal cortical destruction is noted.

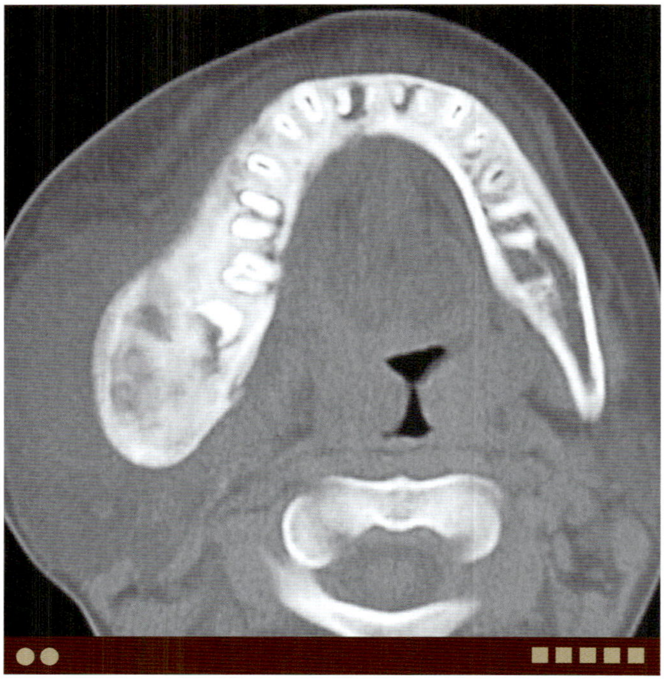

J. Sclerosing osteomyelitis. Axial CT demonstrates expansile change of the right mandible with a mixture of sclerosis and osteolysis.

Case 9–19 Nasoalveolar (Nasolabial) Cyst

Osamu Sakai, Margaret Chapman

PRESENTATION

Lip swelling.

FINDINGS

CT demonstrates a well-marginated cystic lesion at the root of the nose with erosion of the maxilla.

DIFFERENTIAL DIAGNOSIS

- Radicular (periapical) cyst: This lesion contains a tooth root within the cystic cavity.
- Dentigerous cyst: This lesion contains a crown of the tooth within the cystic cavity.
- Nasopalatine duct cyst: This is located within the nasopalatine foramen or canal and causes expansion of these structures.
- Dermoid/epidermoid cyst: This lesion may occur in the subdermal layer on the face. If focal or diffuse fat density or signal is present on CT and MR images, the diagnosis of dermoid can be made.

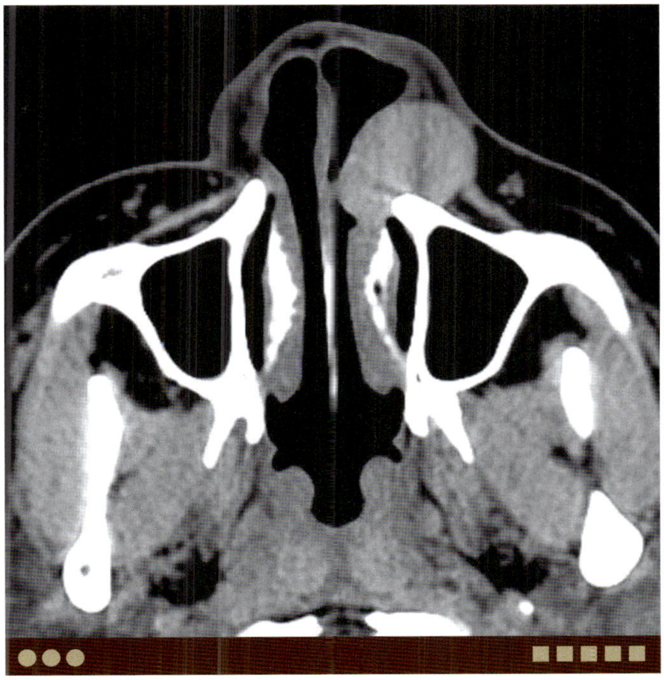

A. Nasoalveolar cyst. Axial CT shows a round soft tissue density lesion in the left nasal alar region.

COMMENTS

This is a 44-year-old man with swelling of the left nasal ala.

Nasoalveolar cysts, also known as nasolabial cysts or Klestadt cyst, are rare nonodontogenic cysts that arise in the nasal alar region. They are usually smooth, cystic lesions located between the upper lip and nasal aperture that are easily identified by clinical examination and by imaging. These lesions are more common in women than men (3:1), and are occasionally bilateral (about 10%). Although they are usually asymptomatic, they may cause protrusion of the upper lip, elevation of the nasal ala, and effacement of the nasolabial fold. Rapid increase in size and infection may occur.

Controversy exists surrounding the etiology of nasoalveolar cysts, with both congenital and acquired mechanisms being postulated. Most investigators support the idea that the development of this lesion is analogous to fissural cysts, and that embryonic nasal epithelium is trapped between the merging maxillary process and the medial and lateral nasal processes. Nasoalveolar cysts are lined by respiratory epithelium, although squamous metaplasia may be seen in infected lesions.

Typically, CT demonstrates a smooth water density cystic lesion in the nasal alar region, anteromedial to the maxilla. Pressure erosion of the underlying bone is commonly seen. With an increase in protein concentration within the cyst due to mucinous secretion, hemorrhage, or infection, the cyst shows increased density on CT and increased T1 and decreased T2 signal on MRI.

PEARLS

- **Nasoalveolar cysts arise in the nasal alar region and are most likely developmental cysts, although the etiology is controversial.**
- **CT demonstrates a smooth cystic lesion in the nasal alar region, anteromedial to the maxilla, often associated with pressure erosion of the underlying bone.**
- **Increased protein concentration within the cyst results in increased density on CT, and increased T1 and decreased T2 signal on MRI.**

ADDITIONAL IMAGES (B-E)

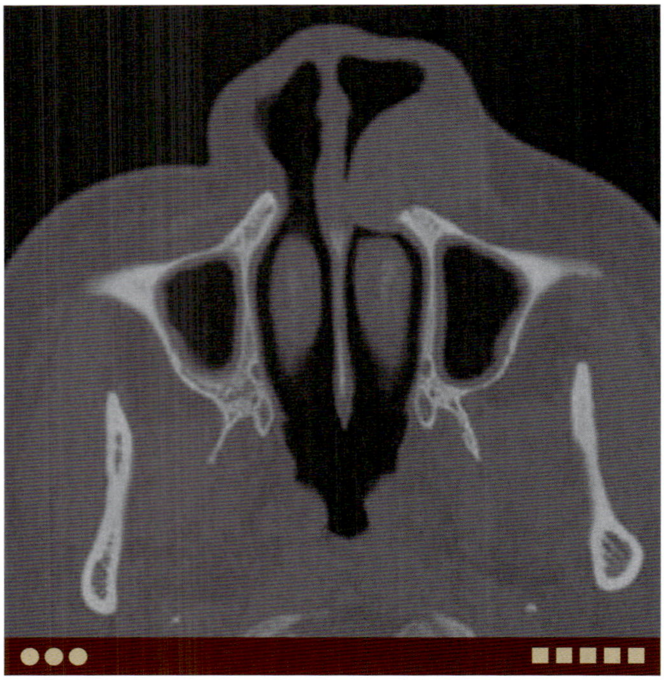

B. Nasoalveolar cyst, same patient as A. Axial bone window CT demonstrates pressure erosion of the maxi la.

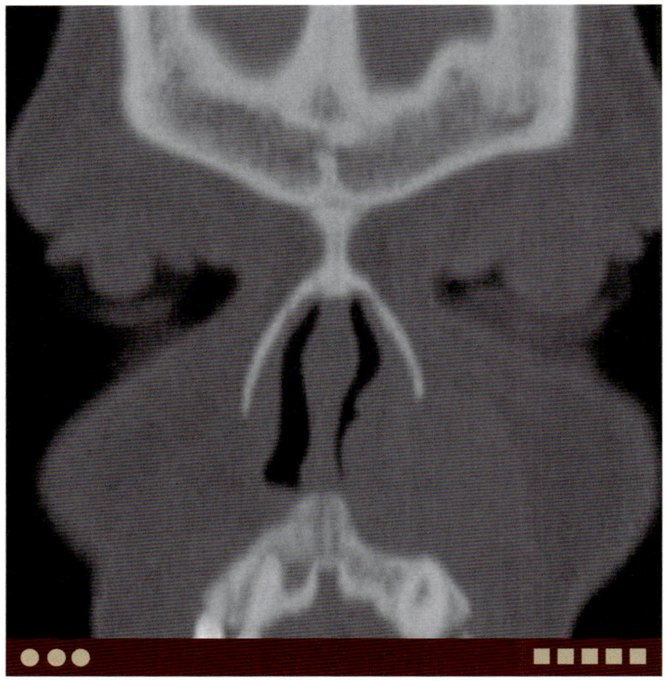

C. Nasoalveolar cyst, same patient as A. Coronal bone window CT demonstrates pressure erosion/remodeling of the underlying maxilla.

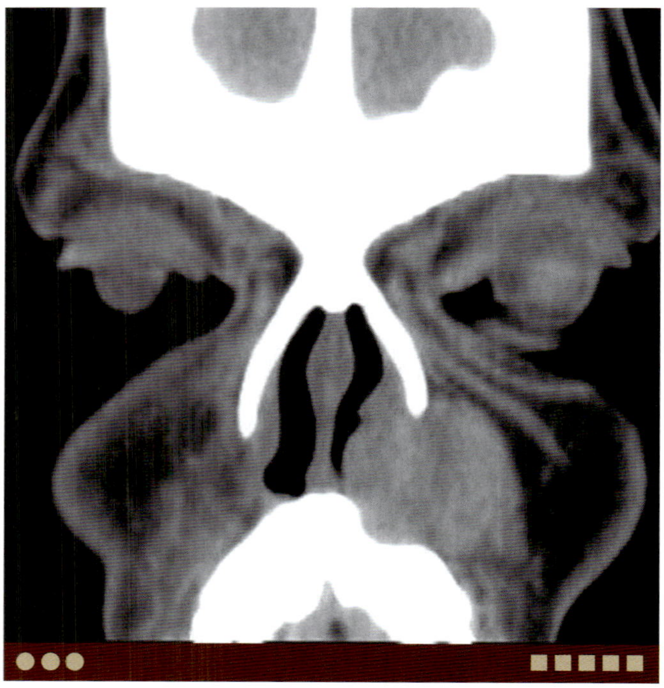

D. Nasoalveolar cyst, same patient as A. Coronal soft tissue window CT demonstrates a round soft tissue density lesion in the left nasal alar region.

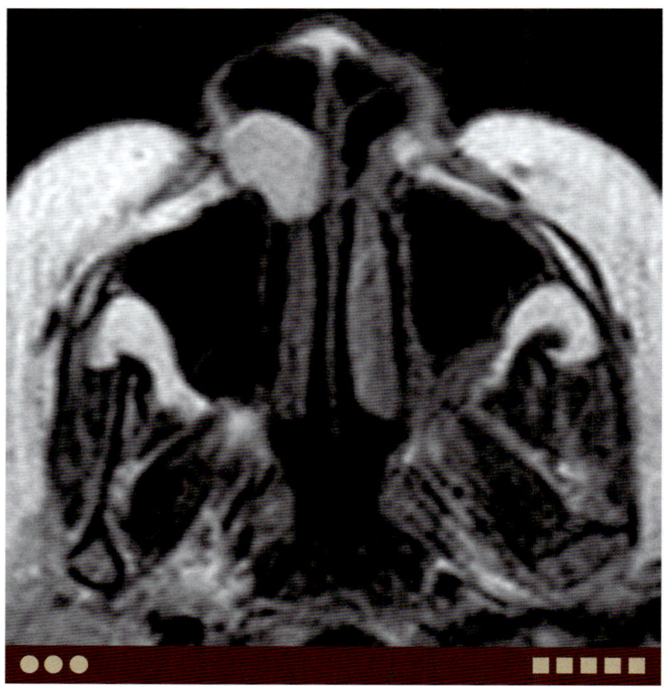

E. Nasoalveolar cyst in a different patient. Axial FLAIR MR image demonstrates a high-signal lesion suggesting proteinaceous contents.

DIFFERENTIAL DIAGNOSIS IMAGES (F-H)

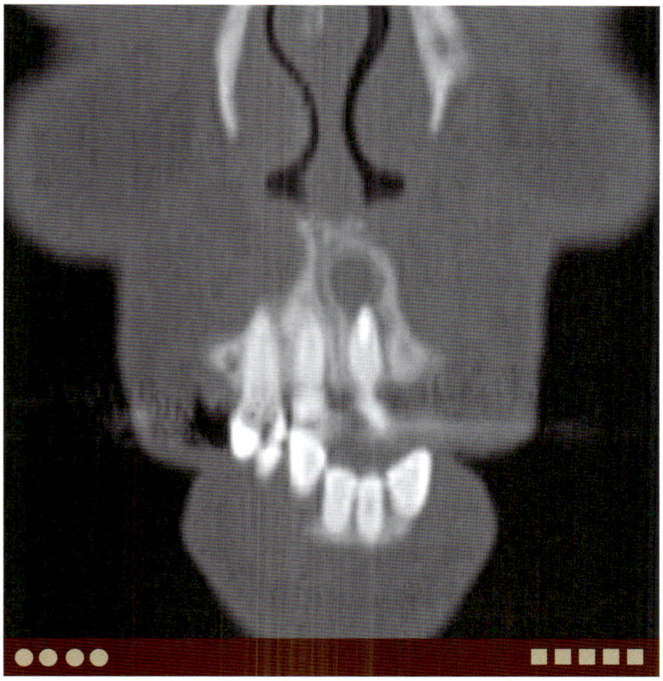

F. Radicular cyst. Coronal CT demonstrates a cystic lesion adjacent to the root of tooth #9 (left maxillary central incisor). Note the tooth is status post root canal.

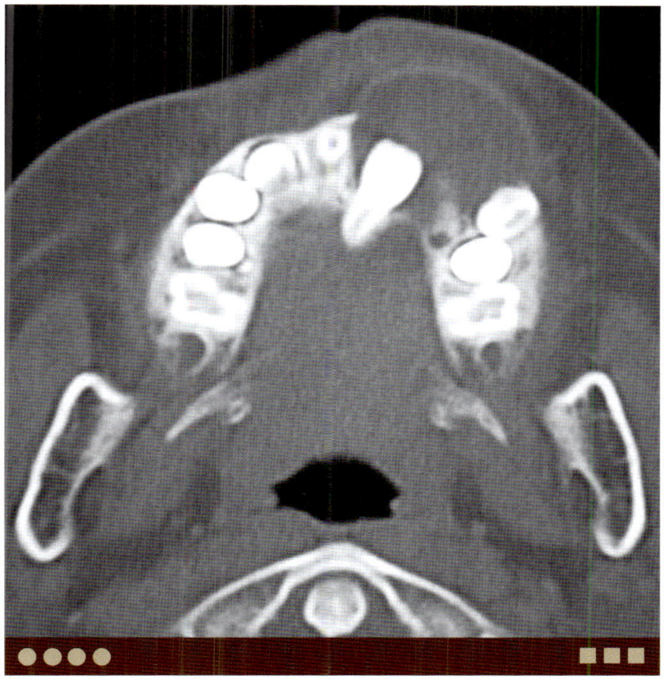

G. Dentigerous cyst. Axial CT demonstrates an expansile lesion containing the crown of an erupted tooth.

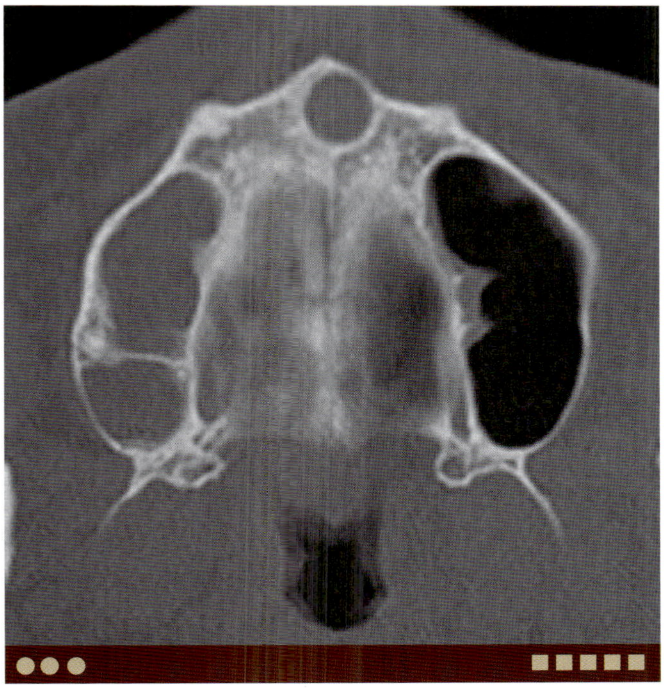

H. Nasopalatine duct (incisive canal). Axial CT demonstrates a slightly prominent, but less than 1 cm in diameter, nasopalatine duct (incisive canal).

Case 9–20 Odontoma

Osamu Sakai, Margaret Chapman

PRESENTATION

Incidental finding of toothlike structures.

FINDINGS

CT demonstrates dysplastic toothlike structures within the mandible or maxilla.

DIFFERENTIAL DIAGNOSIS

- Cemento-osseous dysplasia: This condition presents as a more ill-defined focal sclerotic lesion. Its density is much less than that of enamel.
- Chronic inflammation/infection: This condition causes focal or diffuse sclerotic change around the tooth.
- Ameloblastic fibroma, ameloblastic fibrodentinoma, and ameloblastic fibro-odontoma: These tumors typically appear as well defined, usually multiloculated, pericoronal radiolucent lesions, with odontogenic ectomesenchyme with or without hard tissue formation.
- Ossifying fibroma: This is a well-defined lesion with a thin, radiolucent line representing a fibrous capsule. The internal architecture is mixed radiolucent-radiopaque depending on the amount and form of the calcified materials. The density is lower than that of odontoma.

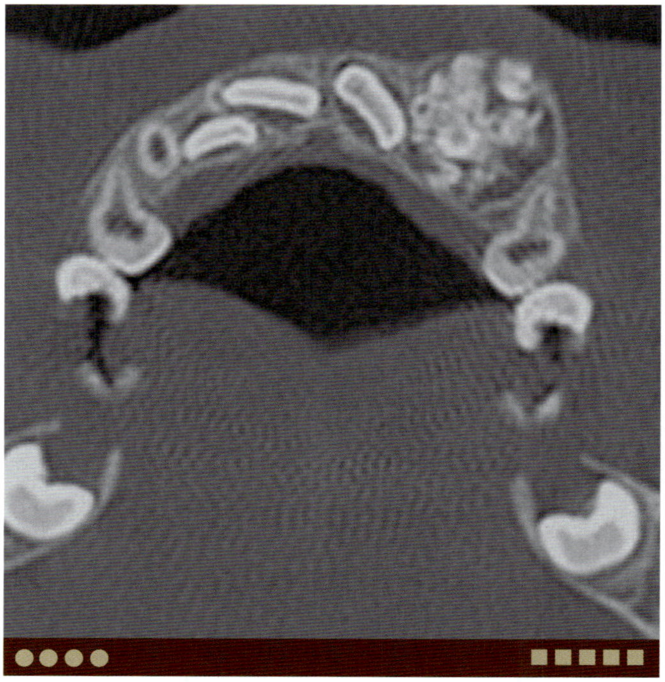

A. Odontoma, complex type. Axial CT demonstrates a slightly expansile lesion with multiple masses of dental tissue. Note the mass effect upon adjacent teeth.

COMMENTS

This is a 5-year-old girl with a maxillary mass.

Odontoma is by far the most common odontogenic tumor (actually a "hamartoma") accounting for about 70% of all cases. The lesion consists of various tooth components, such as dentin and enamel. About half of odontomas are associated with an impacted tooth, and most are diagnosed by 20 years of age; however they may develop before or after eruption of the tooth. Odontoma is initially radiolucent; however, it evolves to contain small calcifications. Eventually, the tumor forms a radiopaque mass with a lucent rim.

Odontomas are subdivided into compound and complex types, depending on their composition when compared with normal teeth. The compound type of odontoma has radiographically identifiable tooth components (abortive teeth), whereas the complex type contains multiple masses of dental tissue with amorphous calcifications. Odontomas can cause impaction or resorption of adjacent teeth.

PEARLS

- **Odontoma is by far the most common odontogenic tumor, and is actually a "hamartoma."**
- **Odontomas are subdivided into compound and complex types depending on their composition when compared with normal teeth.**
- **Odontomas can cause impaction or resorption of adjacent teeth.**

ADDITIONAL IMAGES (B-E)

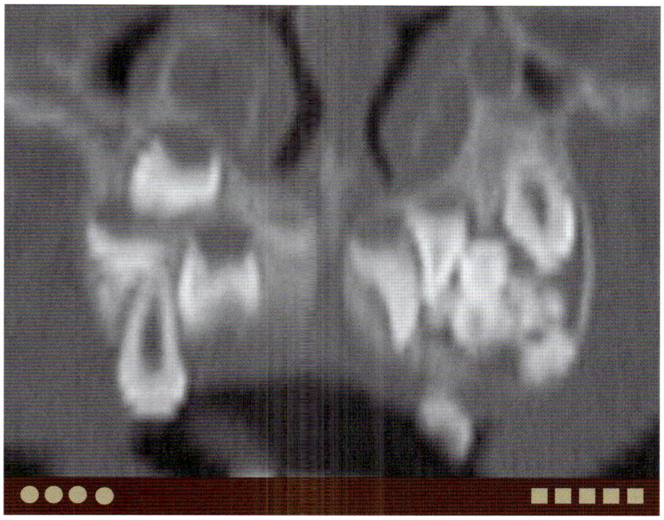

B. Odontoma, complex type, same patient as A. Coronal CT also demonstrates multiple dysplastic tooth elements within the lesion.

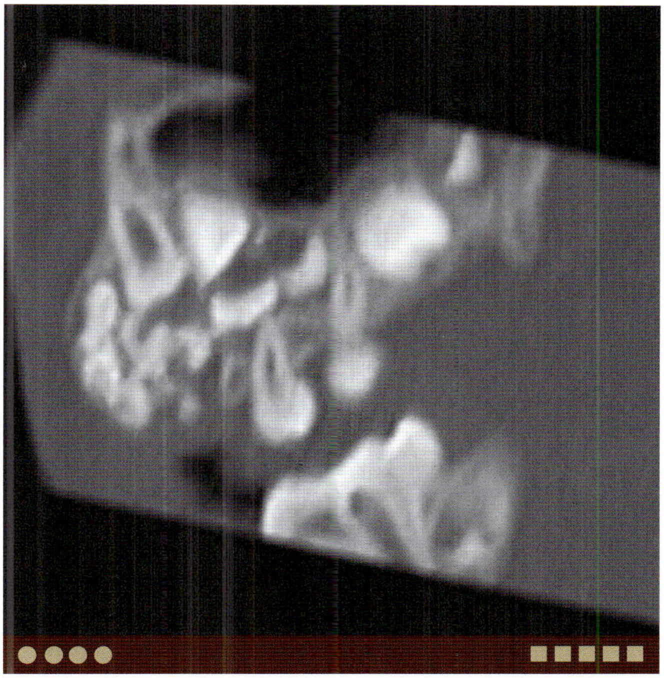

C. Odontoma, complex type, same patient as A. Sagittal CT also demonstrates multiple dysplastic tooth elements within the lesion.

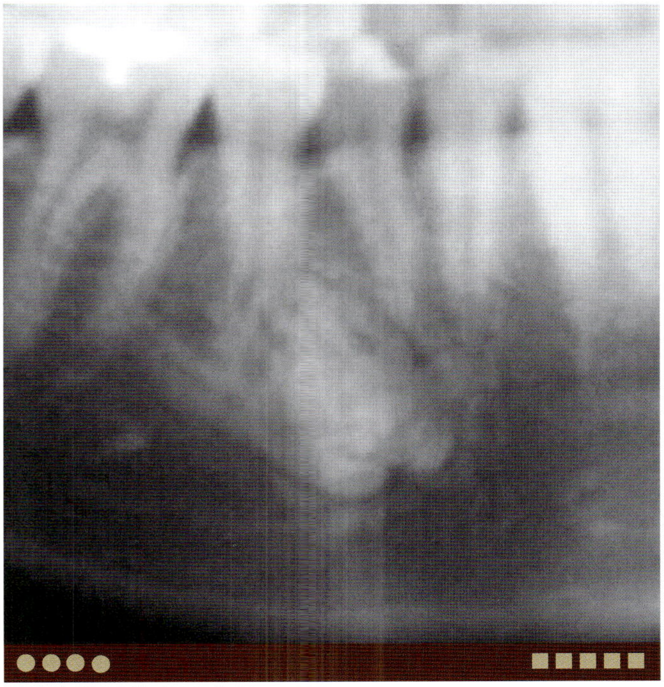

D. Odontoma, compound type. Magnified view of a panoramic radiograph demonstrates mature dental elements surrounded by a lucent rim, displacing and eroding the adjacent teeth roots.

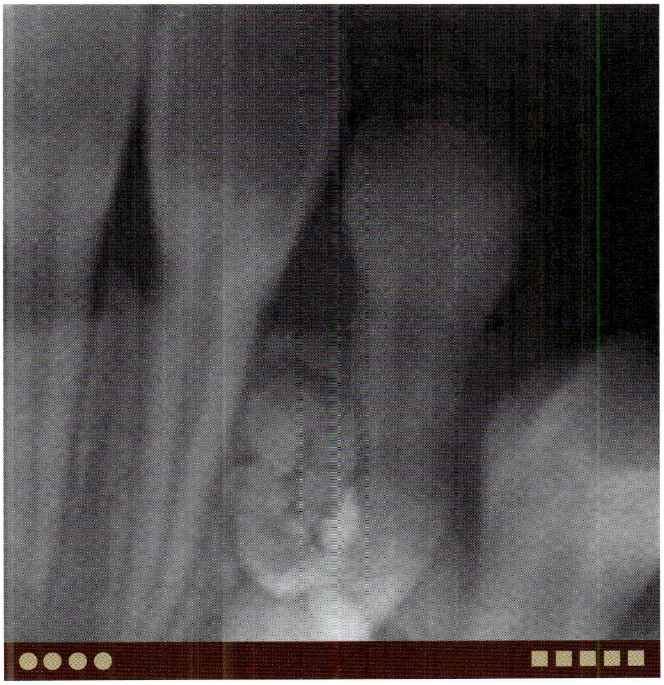

E. Odontoma, compound type in a different patient. Magnified view of a panoramic radiograph demonstrates mature dental elements surrounded by a lucent rim, displacing and eroding the adjacent teeth roots.

DIFFERENTIAL DIAGNOSIS IMAGES (G-I)

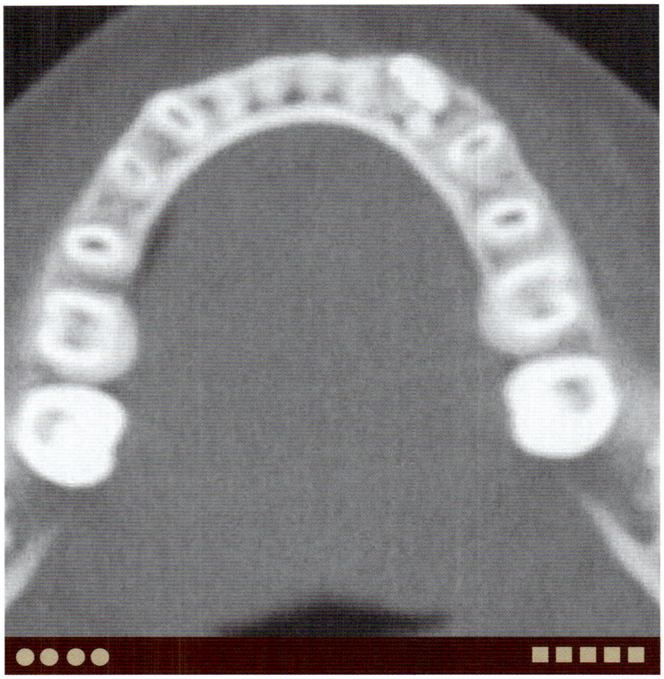

F. Odontoma, compound type, same patient as E. Axial CT demonstrates dysplastic tooth elements in the anterior left mandible.

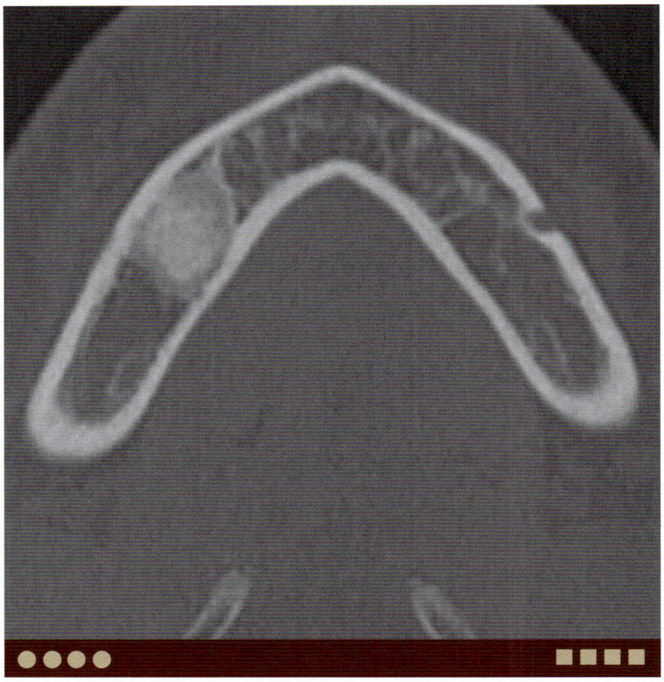

G. Cemento-osseous dysplasia. Axial CT demonstrates a focal sclerotic lesion with ill-defined margin in the right mandible.

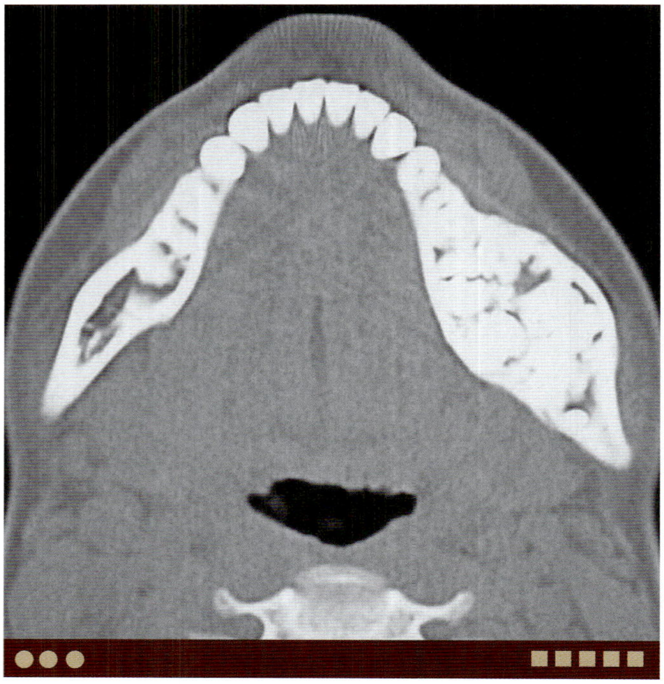

H. Ameloblastic fibroma. Axial CT demonstrates a slightly expansile lesion with high-density material in the posterior body of the left mandible.

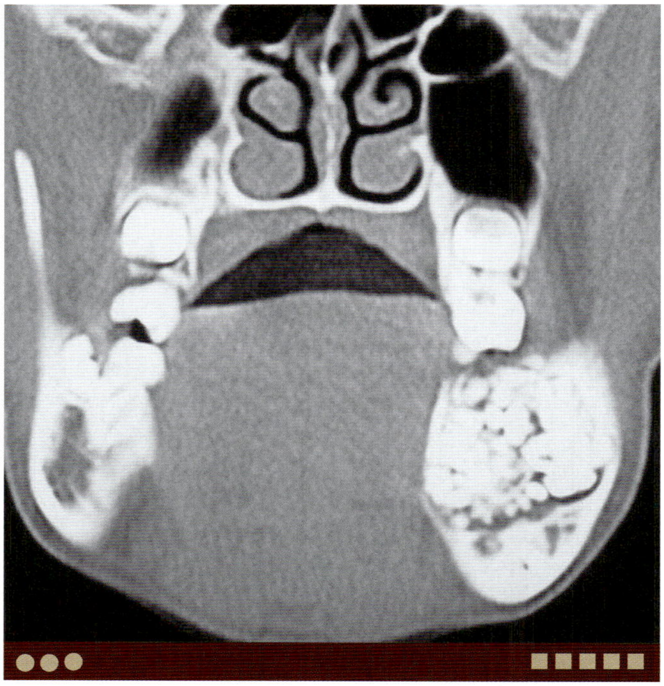

I. Ameloblastic fibroma, same patient as G. Coronal CT demonstrates a slightly expansile lesion with high-density material in the left mandible.

Case 9–21 Osteoarthritis

Osamu Sakai, Daniel Weller

PRESENTATION

TMJ pain.

FINDINGS

CT and MRI demonstrate degenerative changes, including sclerosis and spur formation in the temporomandibular joint.

DIFFERENTIAL DIAGNOSIS

- Rheumatoid arthritis: This condition is not uncommon in the TMJ in patients with rheumatoid arthritis. Findings are often nonspecific; however, enhancement of proliferated synovium is seen after contrast administration.
- Pseudogout: Calcium pyrophosphate dihydrate deposition is rare, but occurs in the TMJ and shows degenerative changes.
- Suppurative arthritis: This condition usually demonstrates apparent inflammatory and infectious pictures clinically and radiologically.

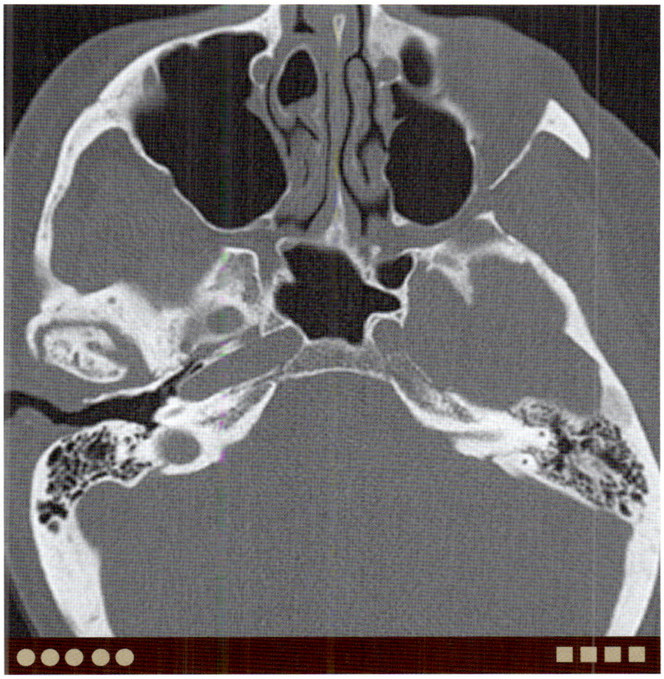

A. OA. Axial CT demonstrates sclerosis and cystic changes of the condyle. A large spur is seen anteriorly.

COMMENTS

This is a 72-year-old man with bilateral TMJ pain.

Osteoarthritis (OA) is the most common arthritis in the TMJ. OA can be seen as a resultant of long-term internal derangement or trauma. Any arthritis can develop secondary OA. Just like OA in other joints, OA in the TMJ also causes joint space narrowing, sclerotic change, spur formation, subcortical cysts, as well as degeneration of the disc. Thinning and deformity of the condyle is often seen in advanced OA, and ankylosis and pseudoarthrosis are seen in the late stage, particularly after trauma.

CT is the best modality to evaluate osseous structures, while MRI can better evaluate the disc, other soft tissue structures as well as bone marrow. Sclerotic change, spur formation, subcortical cysts, and deformity of the condyle are clearly visualized on CT, particularly with multiplanar reformats. MRI better demonstrates marrow signal change, joint effusion, and disc disease. Loss of T1 hyperintensity from normal fatty marrow is typically seen in OA secondary to edema or sclerosis.

Imaging is important to direct appropriate therapy for every patient, and to exclude more serious underlying conditions. It is important to note that the marrow of the condyle is susceptible to metastatic disease.

PEARLS

- **OA is common in the TMJ as well as other joints.**
- **Joint space narrowing, sclerotic change, spur formation, subcortical cysts, as well as degeneration of the disc are seen in OA of the TMJ.**
- **CT is the best modality to evaluate osseous structures, while MRI can better evaluate the disc, bone marrow, and other soft tissue structures.**

ADDITIONAL IMAGES (B-E)

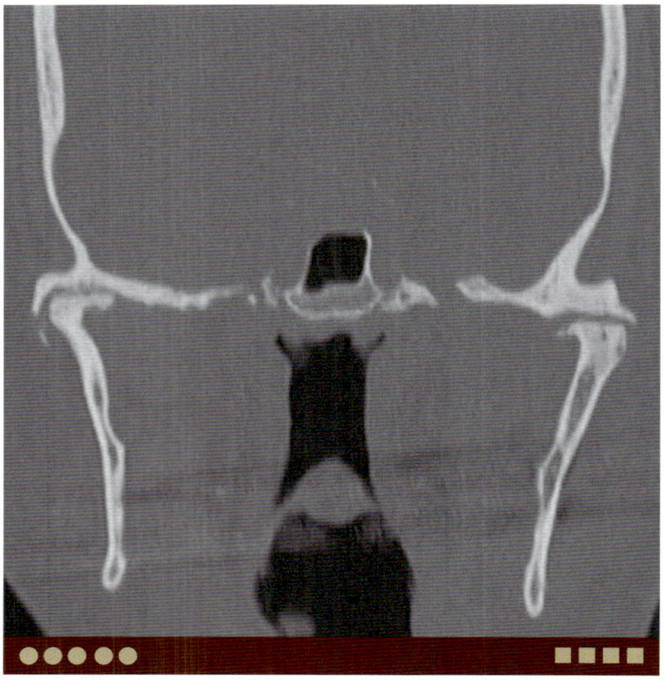

B. OA, same patient as A. Coronal CT demonstrates joint space narrowing and flattening of the condyles bilaterally. Spur formation is seen at the medial aspect of the condyles.

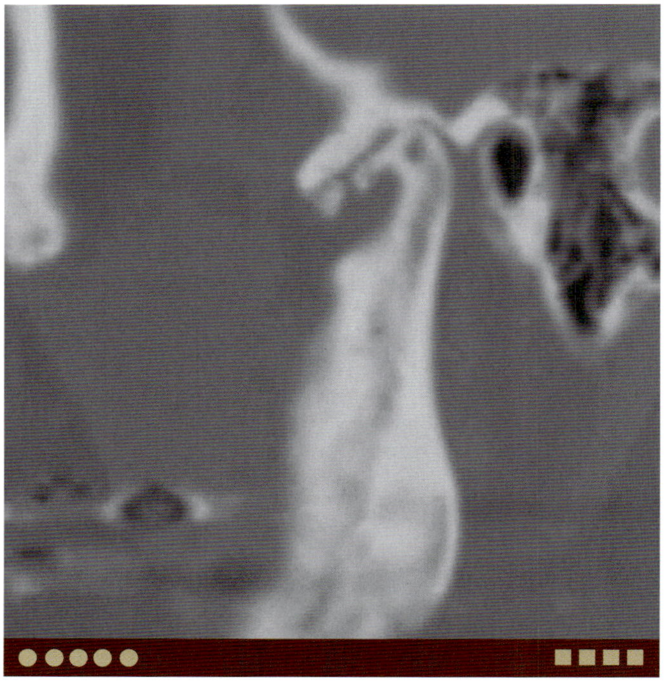

C. OA, same patient as A. Sagittal CT demonstrates joint space narrowing and thinning of the condyle with subcortical cyst and anterior spur formation.

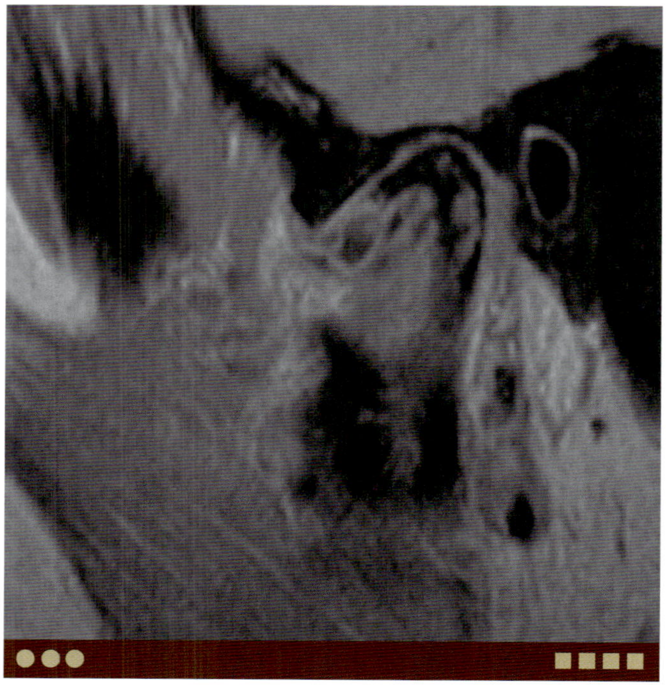

D. OA, same patient as A. Oblique-sagittal proton density-weighted MR image demonstrates joint space narrowing, thinning, and sclerotic change of the condyle. Normal disc is not identified.

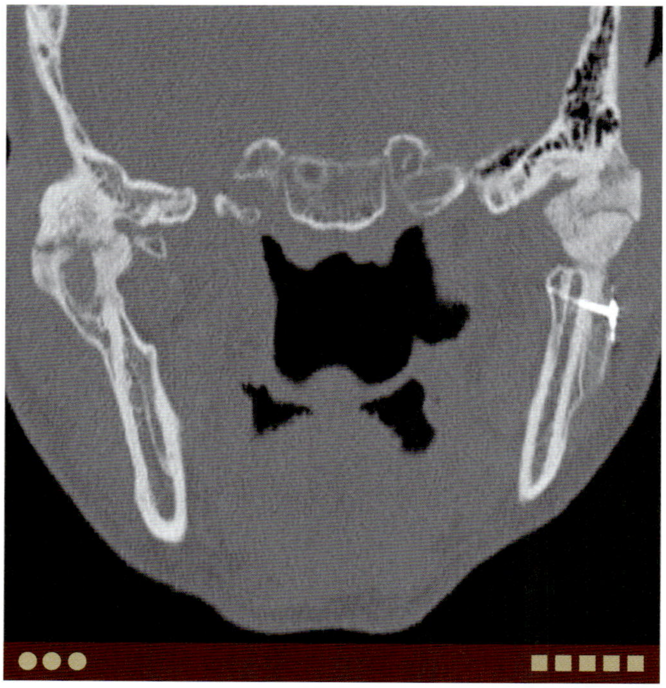

E. OA, ankylosis and pseudoarthrosis after traumatic injury. Coronal CT demonstrates significant hypertrophic degenerative changes in the TMJs bilaterally. Note ankylosis and pseudoarthrosis bilaterally.

DIFFERENTIAL DIAGNOSIS IMAGES (F-I)

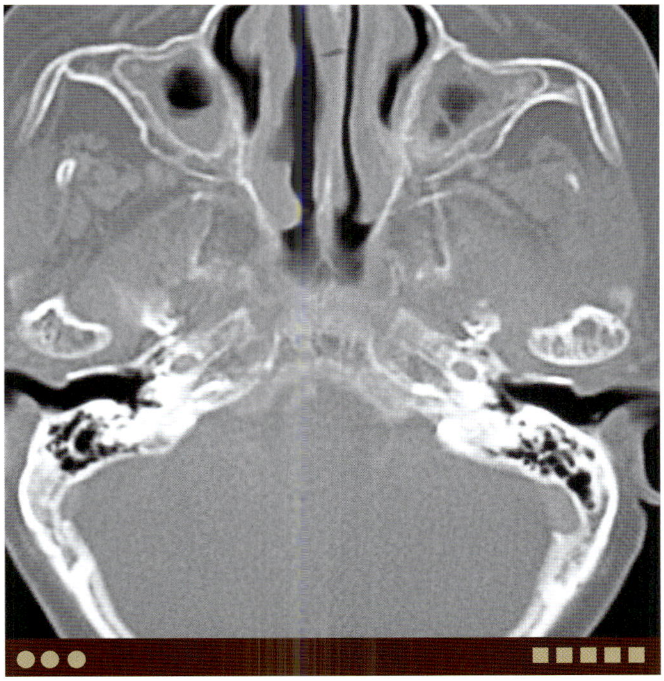

F. Rheumatoid arthritis. Axial CT demonstrates a mixture of sclerotic and lytic changes in the left mandibular condyle.

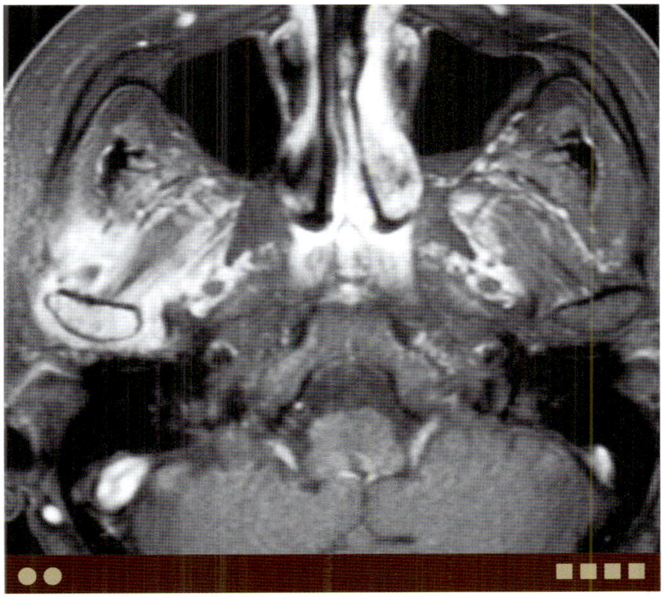

G. Septic arthritis. Axial postcontrast fat-suppressed T1W MR image demonstrates avid enhancement in the right TMJ, including the condyle and periarticular soft tissues. A small nonenhancing area within the joint indicates effusion.

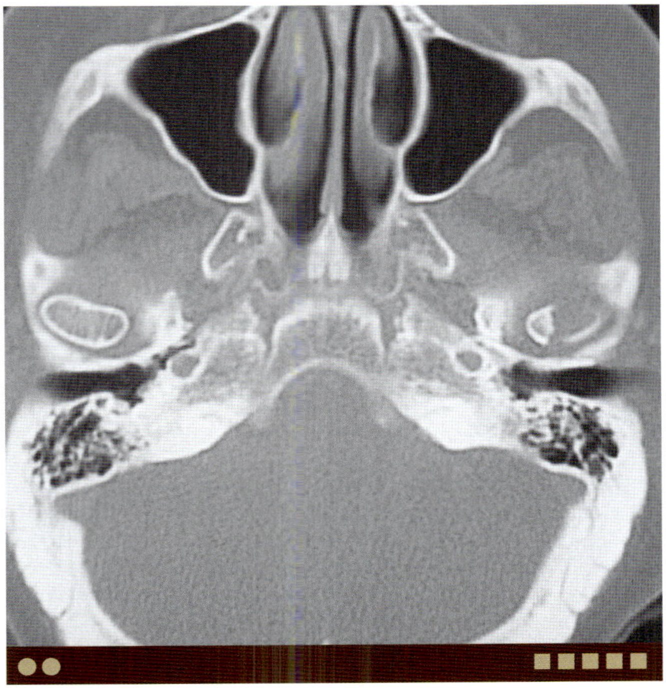

H. Metastasis from thyroid cancer. Axial CT demonstrates osteolytic change in the left mandibular condyle.

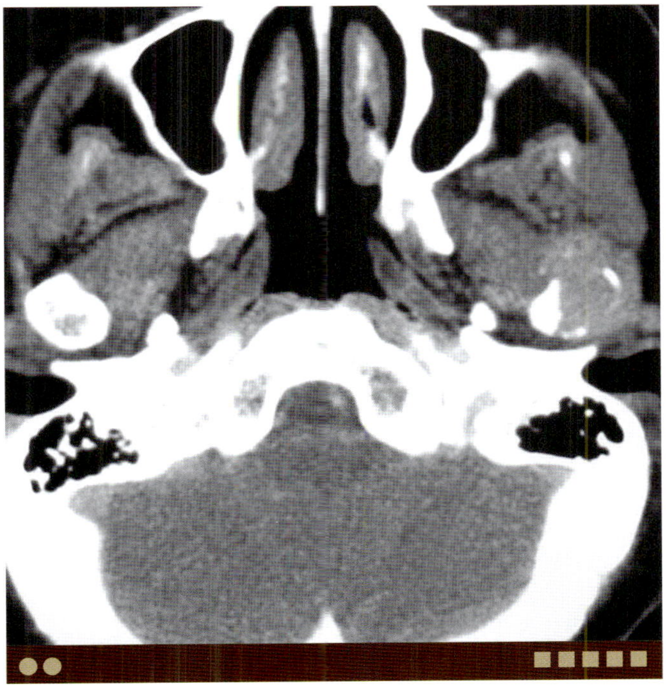

I. Metastasis from thyroid cancer, same patient as H. Axial contrast-enhanced soft tissue windowed CT demonstrates an expansile, mildly enhancing lesion in the left mandibular condyle.

Case 9–22 Bisphosphonate-Associated Osteonecrosis

Osamu Sakai, Margaret Chapman

PRESENTATION

Pain, ulcer, and deformity of the mandible.

FINDINGS

CT demonstrates permeative and destructive changes in a patient with a history of bisphosphonate treatment.

DIFFERENTIAL DIAGNOSIS

- Chronic osteomyelitis: This condition demonstrates heterogeneous bone density with a mixture of sclerotic and lytic changes, with or without periosteal reaction, and occasionally expansion of the bone. Periodontal disease is often identified.
- Osteoradionecrosis: This condition represents bone necrosis following radiation therapy, and is rare in patients receiving less than 60 Gy.
- Paget's disease: This is a common disease of unknown etiology, usually seen in elderly patients, but unusual before age 40. Involvement of the skull and skull base is common, although any bone can be affected.
- Metastasis: This usually shows osteolytic change, most commonly seen in the posterior body and angle where abundant bone marrow is present. However, sclerotic metastasis can be seen with prostate and breast cancers.

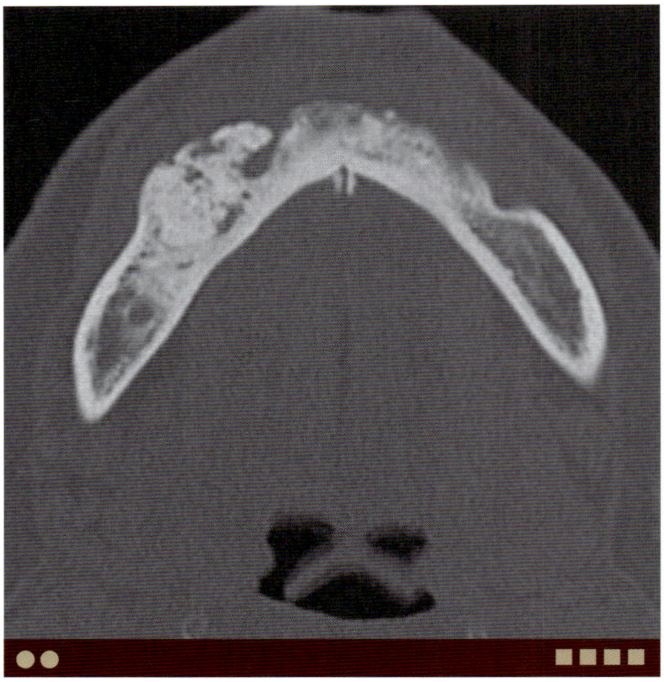

A. BON. Axial CT demonstrates sclerotic changes in the anterior mandible, right greater than left, with foci of osteolysis. Buccal cortical destruction is noted.

COMMENTS

This is a 79-year-old woman with breast cancer on chronic bisphosphonate therapy.

Bisphosphonate-associated osteonecrosis (BON) of the jaw has become more clinically apparent since 2003, and is particularly associated with the use of zolendronic acid and pamidronate. Many cases have a reported association with dental procedures such as tooth extraction; however, BON may occur spontaneously in patients taking bisphosphonates. The risk for developing BON appears to be much higher for cancer patients on intravenous bisphosphonate therapy than for those receiving oral treatment. The clinical differential diagnosis of BON should include neuralgia-inducing cavitary osteonecrosis (NICO). Unlike patients with BON, patients with NICO present with atypical facial pain or trigeminal neuralgia, which often has been present for years.

Imaging findings are often nonspecific. Osteosclerosis is seen in the majority of patients with BON to a variable extent. Less frequently, osteolysis, periosteal reaction, sequestra, fistula formation, and soft tissue swelling are seen, likely associated with infection. The radiologic differential diagnosis for BON includes chronic sclerosing osteomyelitis, osteoradionecrosis, metastasis, myeloma, and Paget's disease. Careful clinical correlation is needed to differentiate from these conditions.

PEARLS

- **Spontaneous bone necrosis of the jaw occurs in patients treated with bisphosphonates.**
- **Findings are nonspecific; however, sclerotic change is seen in the majority of patients. Osteolysis, periapical lucencies, periosteal reaction, sequestra, and fistula formation are also seen.**

ADDITIONAL IMAGE

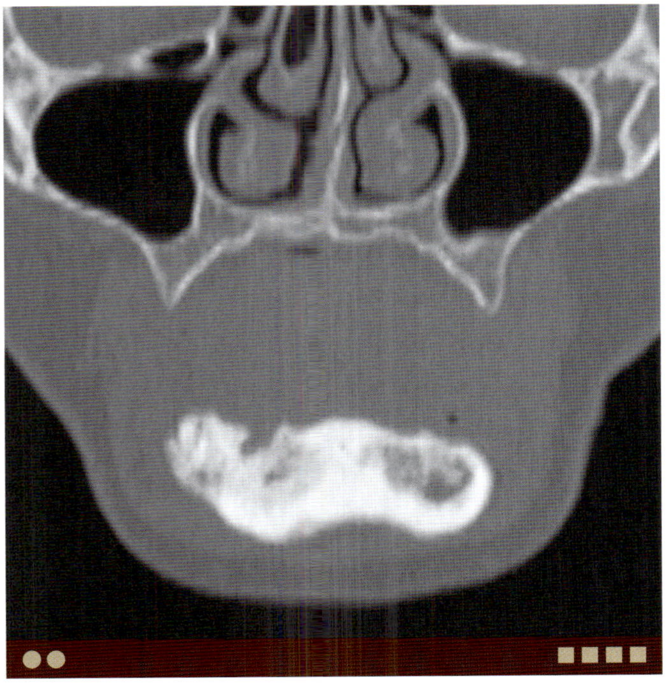

B. BON, same patient as A. Coronal CT demonstrates sclerotic changes and cortical destruction of the right anterior mandible.

DIFFERENTIAL DIAGNOSIS IMAGES (C-F)

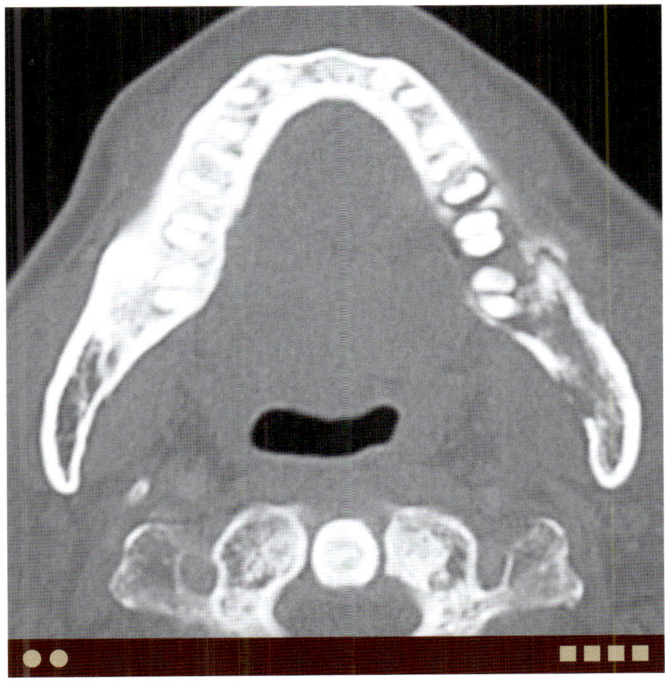

C. Osteoradionecrosis. Axial CT demonstrates permeative osteolytic change in the posterior body and ramus of the left mandible. The right mandible shows sclerotic change consistent with osteitis.

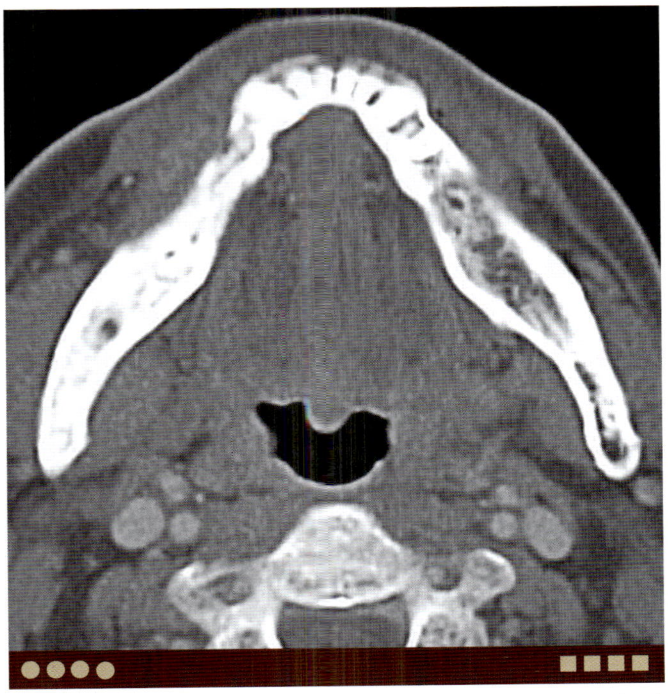

D. Chronic osteomyelitis. Axial CT demonstrates diffuse sclerosis of the right mandible.

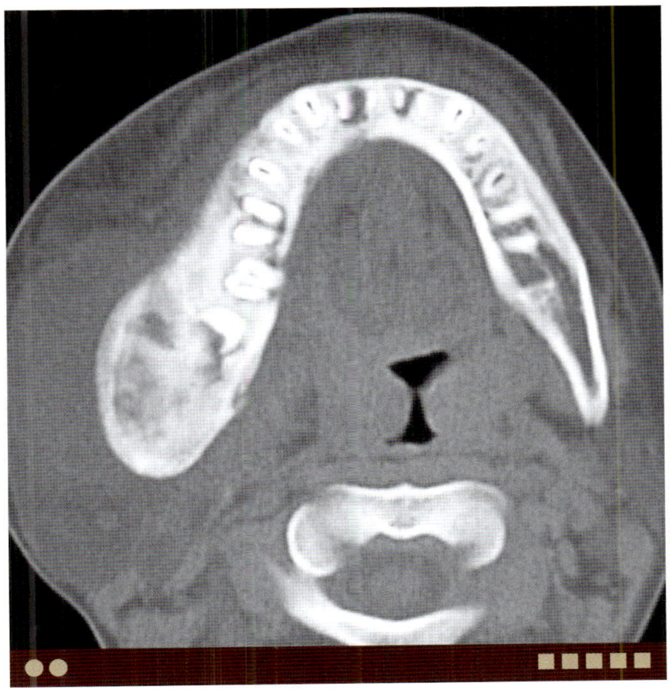

E. Sclerosing osteomyelitis. Axial CT demonstrates expansile change of the right mandible with a mixture of sclerosis and osteolysis.

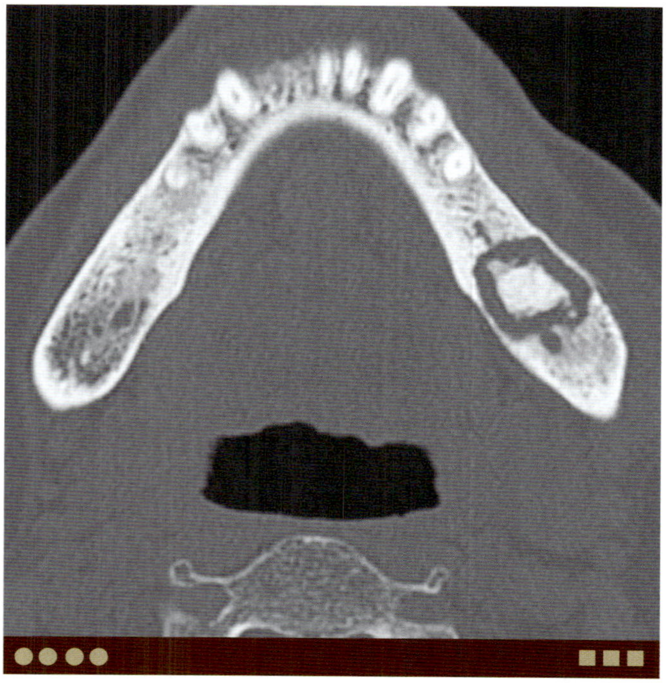

F. Chronic osteomyelitis. Axial CT demonstrates an area of osteolysis with sequestrum in the left mandibular body.

Case 9–23 Osteoradionecrosis

Osamu Sakai, Daniel Weller

PRESENTATION

Pain, ulceration, and deformity of the mandible.

FINDINGS

CT demonstrates permeative and destructive changes in a patient treated with radiotherapy for floor of mouth cancer.

DIFFERENTIAL DIAGNOSIS

- Chronic osteomyelitis: This condition demonstrates heterogeneous bone density; mixture of sclerotic and lytic changes, with or without periosteal reaction, and occasionally shows expansion of the bone. Periodontal disease is usually identified.
- Bisphosphonate-associated osteonecrosis of the jaw: This is a rare condition that occurs in patients with history of bisphosphonate therapy, particularly with intravenous administration.
- Metastasis: This usually shows osteolytic change, most commonly seen in the posterior body and angle of the mandible, where abundant bone marrow is present.
- Osteosarcoma: This is a rare malignant tumor, usually demonstrating osteoblastic changes with aggressive periosteal reaction.
- Epulis fissuratum: This is a condition of an overgrowth of fibrous connective tissue in the mouth, and rarely calcifies.

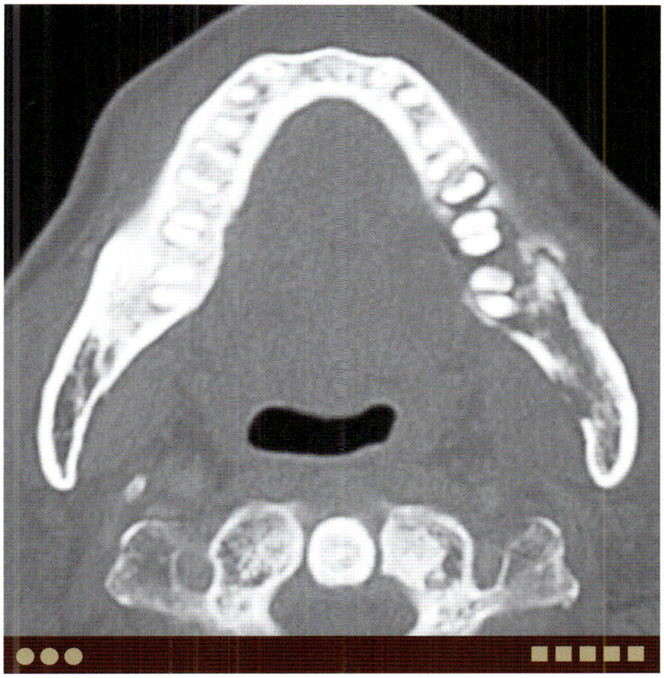

A. Osteoradionecrosis. Axial CT demonstrates diffuse demineralization and cortical destruction in the posterior body/ramus of the left mandible. Right mandible shows diffuse sclerotic changes consistent with osteitis

COMMENTS

This is a 69-year-old man with history of radiotherapy for oropharyngeal carcinoma.

Osteoradionecrosis is a condition of bone necrosis from prior radiation therapy. This occurs rarely in patients who received less than 60 Gy. This condition develops following radiation injury when the bone reparative capacity within the field is insufficient to conquer the injury. The incidence of osteoradionecrosis has decreased recently due to newer radiation protocols such as 3D conformational radiation therapy, intensity-modulated radiotherapy, preventive measures prior to radiotherapy, and dental hygiene during radiotherapy.

Three grades of this condition are recognized:

Grade I: exposure of alveolar bone

Grade II: no response to hyperbaric oxygen therapy requiring sequestrectomy/saucerization

Grade III: full-thickness involvement and/or pathological fracture

Imaging findings are nonspecific; however, mixture of osteolysis and osteosclerosis is often noted with destructive changes. Pathological fracture can be seen.

PEARLS

- **Osteoradionecrosis is a condition of bone necrosis from prior radiation therapy.**
- **Findings are nonspecific; however, mixture of osteolysis and osteosclerosis is often noted with destructive changes. Pathological fracture can be seen.**

ADDITIONAL IMAGES (B-D)

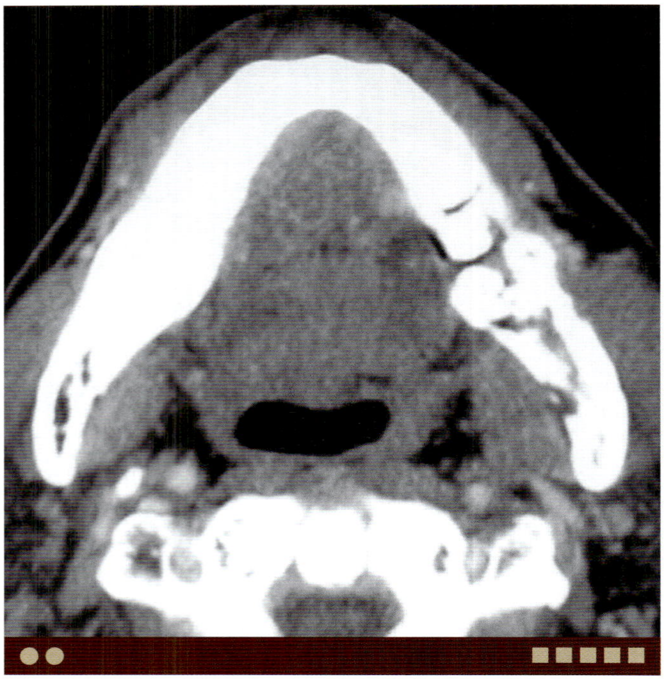

B. Osteoradionecrosis, same patient as A. Axial postcontrast soft tissue windowed CT demonstrates loss of normal fatty marrow in the left mandible and swelling of the left masseter and pterygoid muscles.

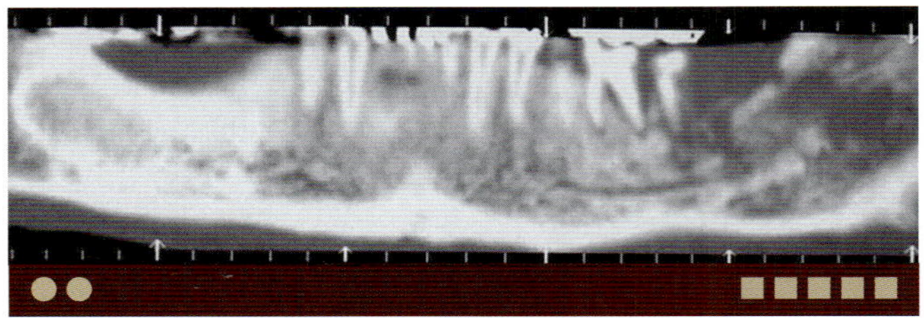

C. Osteoradionecrosis, same patient as A. Panoramic reconstruction of CT demonstrates permeative changes in the posterior body/angle of the left mandible.

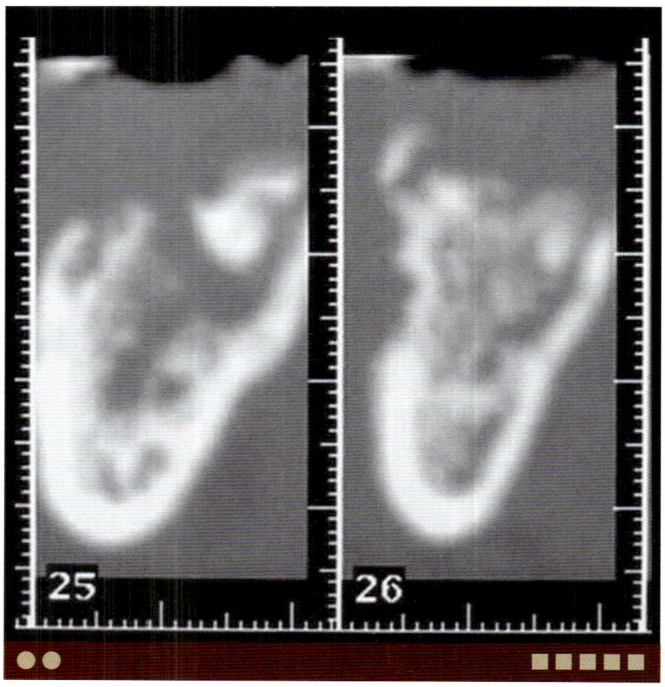

D. Osteoradionecrosis, same patient as A. Coronal reconstructions of CT through the posterior body of the left mandible demonstrate diffuse demineralization and cortical destruction.

DIFFERENTIAL DIAGNOSIS IMAGES (E-G)

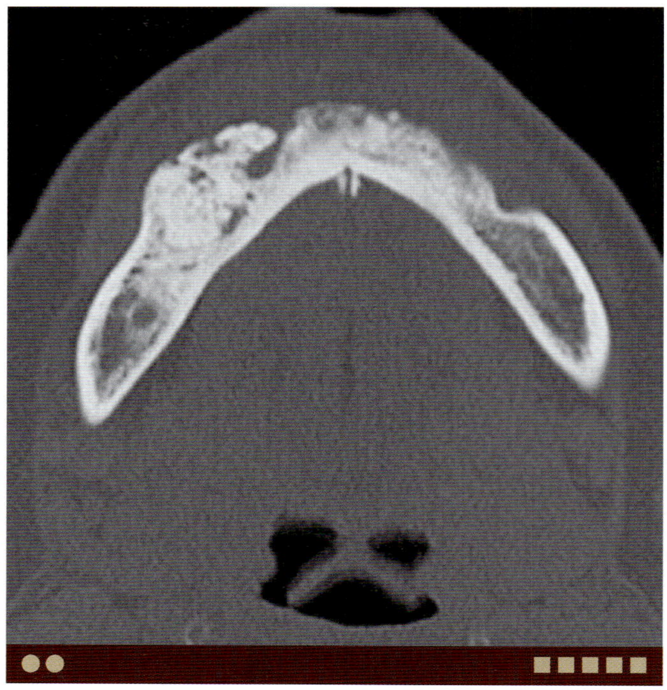

E. Bisphosphonate-associated osteonecrosis. Axial CT demonstrates mixture of sclerosis and osteolysis in the anterior mandible, more pronounced on the right side.

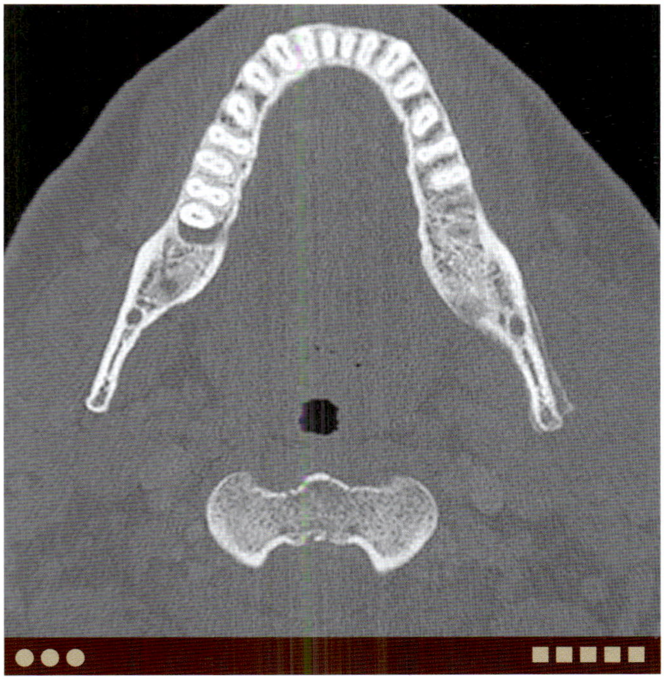

F. Chronic osteomyelitis. Axial CT demonstrates sclerotic changes in the posterior body of the left mandible. Note periosteal reaction in the left ramus and swelling of the left masseter muscle.

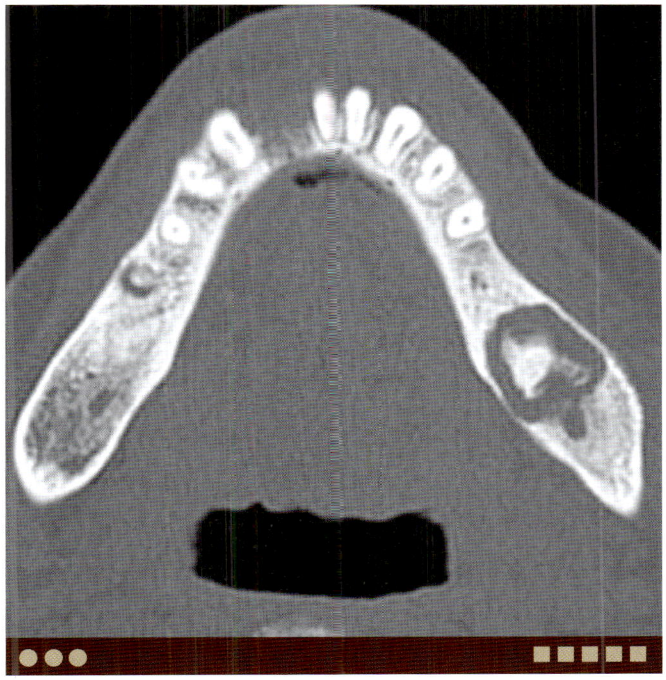

G. Chronic osteomyelitis. Axial CT demonstrates diffuse sclerotic changes of the mandible. Sequestrum is noted in the left mandible surrounded by an osteolytic lesion.

Case 9–24 Periapical Abscess

Osamu Sakai, Margaret Chapman

PRESENTATION

Jaw pain and swelling.

FINDINGS

CT demonstrates a cystic lesion at the tooth root.

DIFFERENTIAL DIAGNOSIS

- Periapical granuloma and cyst: Periapical abscess, granuloma, and cyst represent different phases of the same pathological process and may be difficult to distinguish from each other radiographically.
- Dentigerous cyst: This lesion represents the most common developmental odontogenic cyst, demonstrating a cyst around the crown of an unerupted tooth. Infection may cause more complicated imaging findings, such as a thickened wall.
- Nasopalatine duct cyst: This is a fissural cyst that arises from the nasopalatine duct (incisive canal) during development. It may become symptomatic secondary to infection.
- Squamous cell carcinoma (SCCA) SCCA is the most common malignancy of the oral cavity. Occasionally, patients present with symptoms similar to infection.

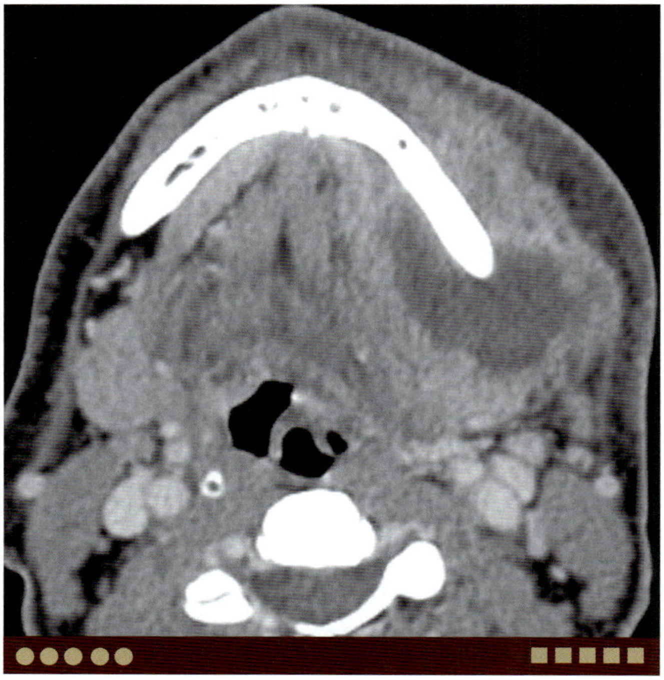

A. Periapical abscess. Axial contrast-enhanced CT demonstrates a soft tissue abscess around the left mandibular angle, surrounded by a larger area of cellulitis.

COMMENTS

This is a 43-year-old woman with left jaw swelling and pain.

Odontogenic infection is one of the major causes of maxillofacial infection that requires imaging. Identifying periapical lucency is the key to the appropriate diagnosis and management in affected patients. Periodontitis-related lesions account for the majority of periapical lucencies. Caries formation leading to erosion of the enamel and dentin can lead to an acute or chronic infection of the pulp. Apical periodontitis occurs when the infection spreads down the root and through the apical foramen, resulting in an acute immune response characterized by the recruitment of neutrophils, resultant vascular congestion, and periodontal ligament edema. The inflammatory reaction progresses with neutrophils causing localized tissue destruction and recruitment of osteoclasts and odontoclasts which cause bone and root resorption, respectively.

These findings are seen as a lucent area surrounding the tooth root. Periapical infection/inflammation can present as an acute or chronic process. Periapical abscess, granuloma, and cyst represent different phases of the same pathologic process and are difficult to distinguish from each other radiographically, although ill-defined borders suggest an acute process, and sharply defined borders suggest a chronic process.

This condition may result in "odontogenic" sinusitis and extraosseous abscess around the mandible or maxilla. Therefore, careful evaluation for dental disease, such as periapical lucency and caries, is essential for patient management to identify the primary source of infection in patients with maxillofacial infection. In patients with a soft tissue abscess around the jaw, a fistula extending from the periapical lucency to the abscess is often identified on CT.

PEARLS

- **Odontogenic infection is one of the major causes of maxillofacial infection that require imaging.**
- **Identifying periapical lucency is the key to the appropriate diagnosis and management in such patients.**
- **A fistula is often identified on CT in patients with a soft tissue abscess around the jaw.**

ADDITIONAL IMAGES (B-G)

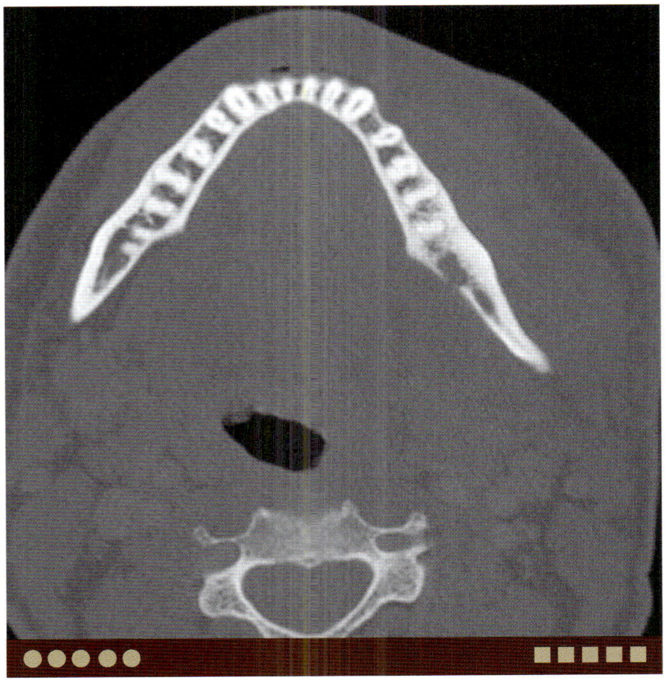

B. Periapical abscess, same patient as A. Axial bone window CT demonstrates a focal lucency with destruction of the lingual cortex in the molar region consistent with periapical abscess and fistula, the cause of the soft tissue abscess.

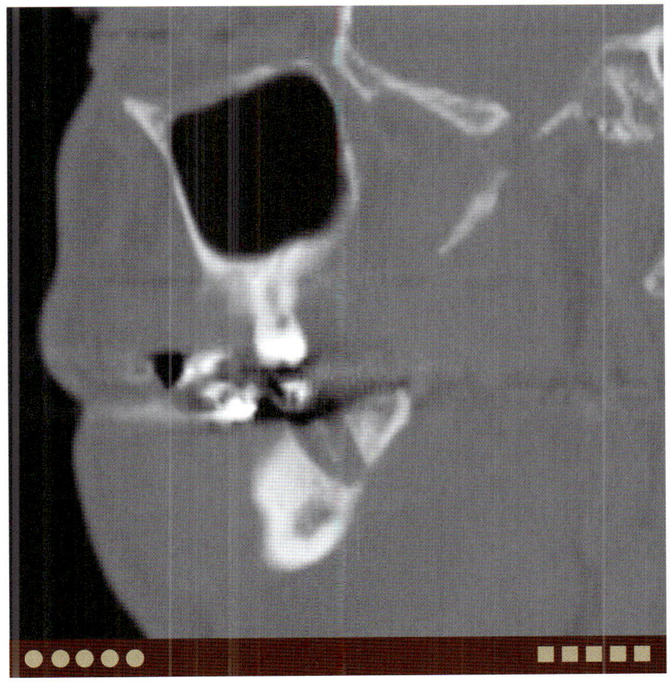

C. Periapical abscess, same patient as A. Sagittal bone window CT clearly demonstrates periodontal lucency and cortical disruption.

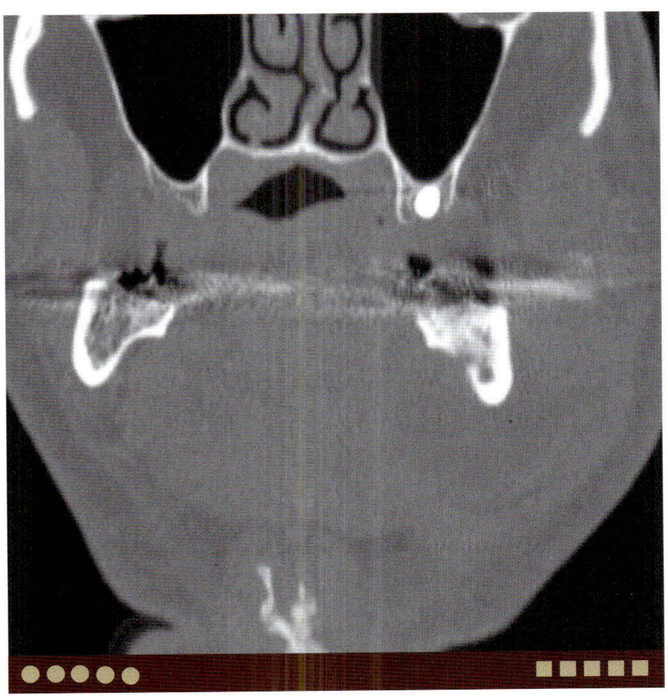

D. Periapical abscess, same patient as A. Coronal bone window CT demonstrates lingual cortical disruption and sclerotic change of the left mandible.

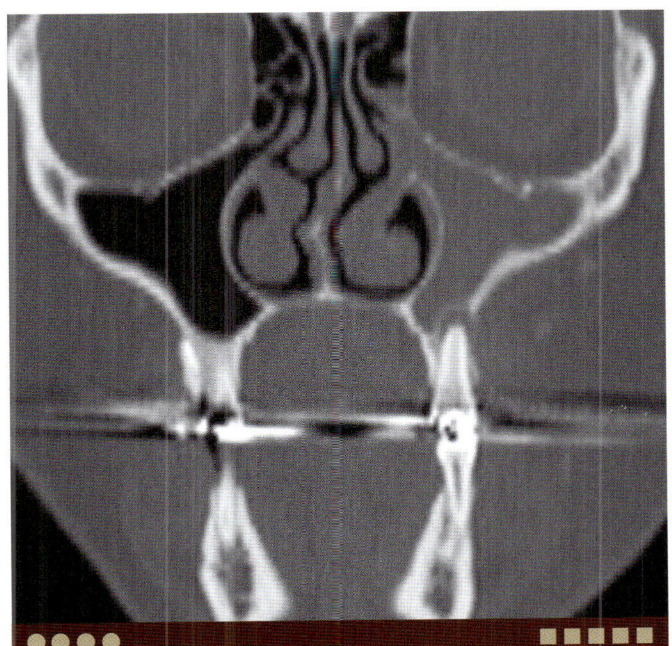

E. Periapical abscess in a different patient presenting with sinusitis and cheek pain. Coronal CT demonstrates complete opacification of the left maxillary sinus. Note a small periapical cyst focally elevating the floor of the maxillary sinus.

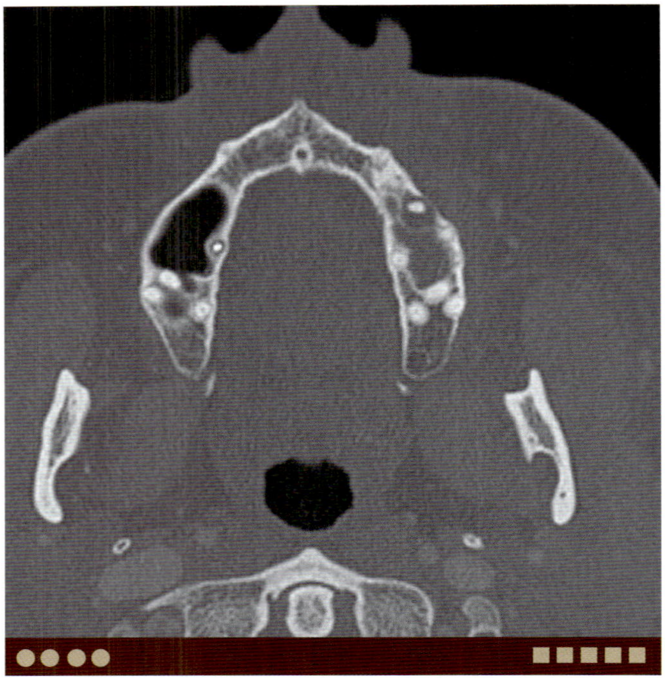

F. Periapical abscess, same patient as E. Axial CT demonstrates a lucent lesion around the tooth root. Note buccal cortical thinning.

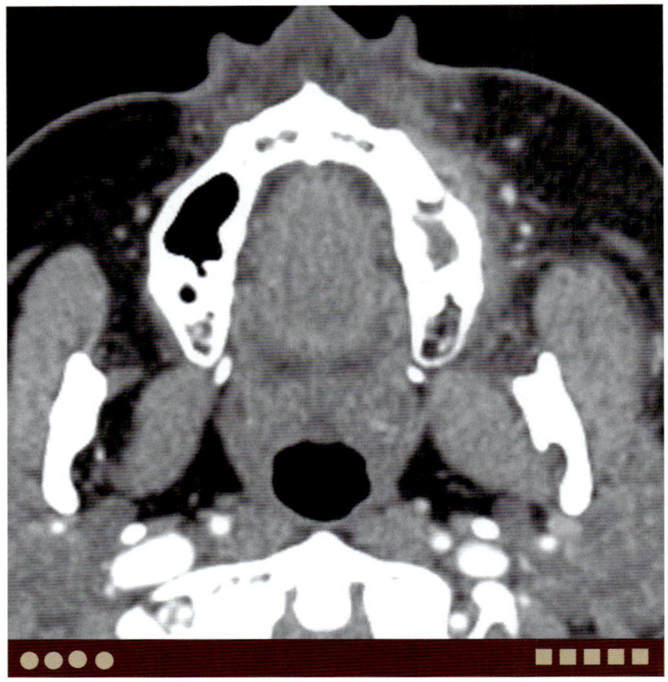

G. Periapical abscess, same patient as E. Axial contrast-enhanced soft tissue window CT demonstrates a small abscess adjacent to the periapical lucent lesion.

DIFFERENTIAL DIAGNOSIS IMAGES (H-I)

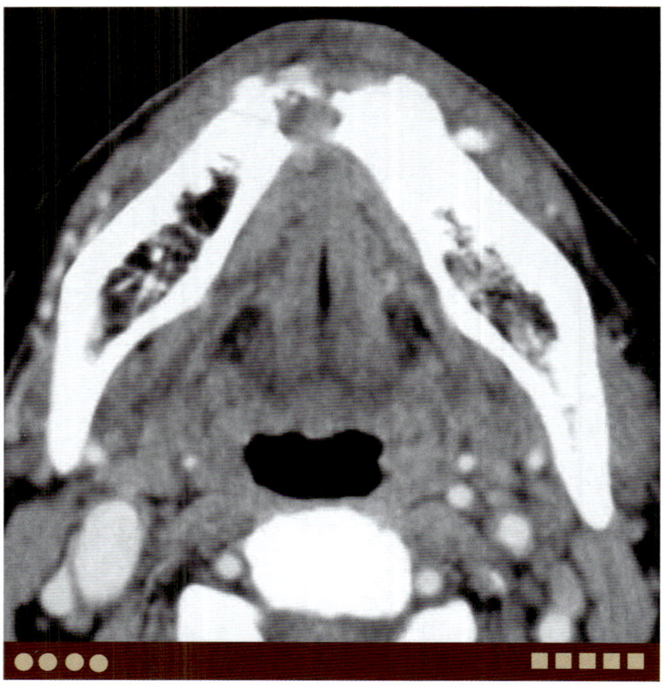

H. SCCA. Axial contrast-enhanced CT demonstrates disruption of the mandible at the symphysis with soft tissue density.

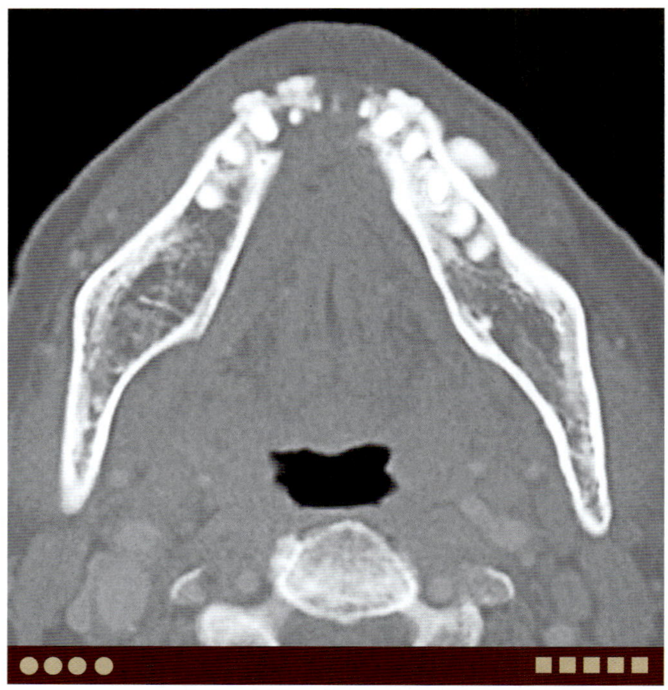

I. SCCA, same patient as H. Axial bone window CT clearly demonstrates bone destruction at the mandibular symphysis.

Case 9–25 Pigmented Villonodular Synovitis

Osamu Sakai, Daniel Welie.

PRESENTATION

Temporomandibular joint (TMJ) pain.

FINDINGS

T2W MR images demonstrate arthritic changes with decreased signal in the TMJ.

DIFFERENTIAL DIAGNOSIS

- Osteoarthritis: This condition is the most common arthritic change in the TMJ, usually a sequela of TMJD or trauma.
- Pseudogout: Calcium pyrophosphate dihydrate deposition is rare, but can occur in the TMJ. Calcification is often seen.
- Rheumatoid arthritis (RA): TMJ involvement is not uncommon in patients RA, seen in more than 20% of patients.
- Synovial osteochondromatosis: This is often seen in a large joint, however, can be seen in the TMJ. Multiple calcified or ossified fragments are seen in the joint.

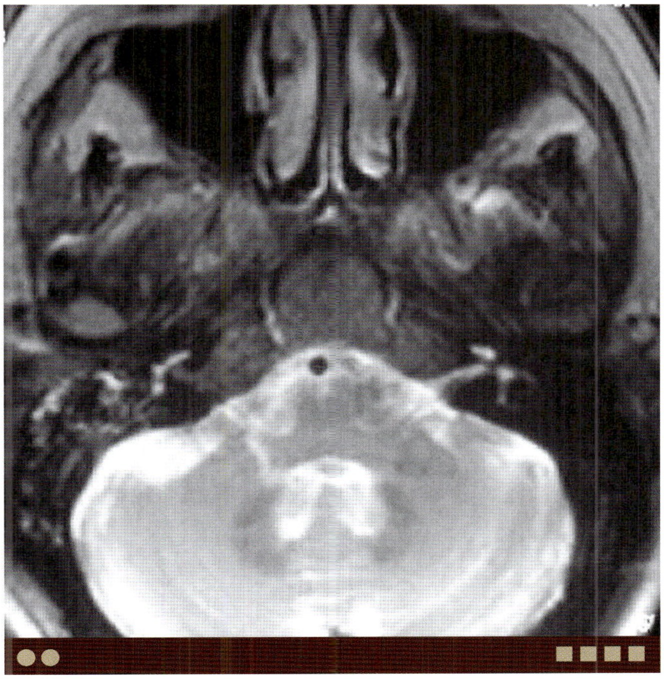

A. PVNS. Axial T2W MR image demonstrates markedly decreased signal in and around the left mandibular condyle.

COMMENTS

This is a 57-year-old man with TMJ pain.

Pigmented villonodular synovitis (PVNS) is a rare proliferative disorder affecting the synovium. It is often seen in the second and third decades of life as a slowly growing, non-tender swelling of the joint. It is almost exclusively a monarticular lesion and most often seen in large joints, such as knee, hip, shoulder, ankle, and wrist. However, any synovial joint can be affected. Involvement of the TMJ is very rare; however, it can be associated with destruction of the mandibular condyle and invasion of the infratemporal fossa.

CT demonstrates erosion or destruction of the mandibular condyle and abnormal soft tissue which expands the joint capsule. Calcification is not seen. MRI is very useful in diagnosing PVNS. The lesion usually demonstrates heterogeneously decreased T2 signal with blooming corresponding to abundant hemosiderin deposits, which is very characteristic for this condition. However, signal can be very variable depending on the degree of hemosiderin deposition and other factors. An area of high T2 signal corresponding to a loculated cyst of joint fluid is often seen. Further, increased T1 signal from lipid in foamy macrophages may be seen.

PVNS is very vascular, and preoperative embolization may be performed. However, evaluation of vascularity is difficult by conventional MRI

PEARLS

- **PVNS is a rare proliferative disorder affecting the synovium and can be seen in the TMJ.**
- **Decreased signal on T2W MR images corresponding to hemosiderin deposits is characteristic.**
- **PVNS is locally aggressive, and bony erosion or destruction is often seen. The lesion may show extracapsular extension and invade the infratemporal fossa.**

ADDITIONAL IMAGES (B-C)

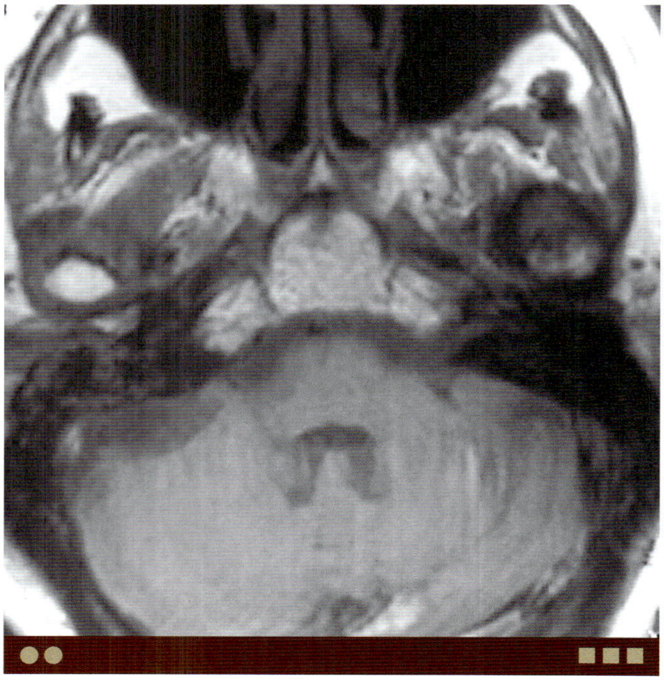

B. PVNS, same patient as A. Axial T1W MR image demonstrates heterogeneously decreased signal in and around the left mandibular condyle.

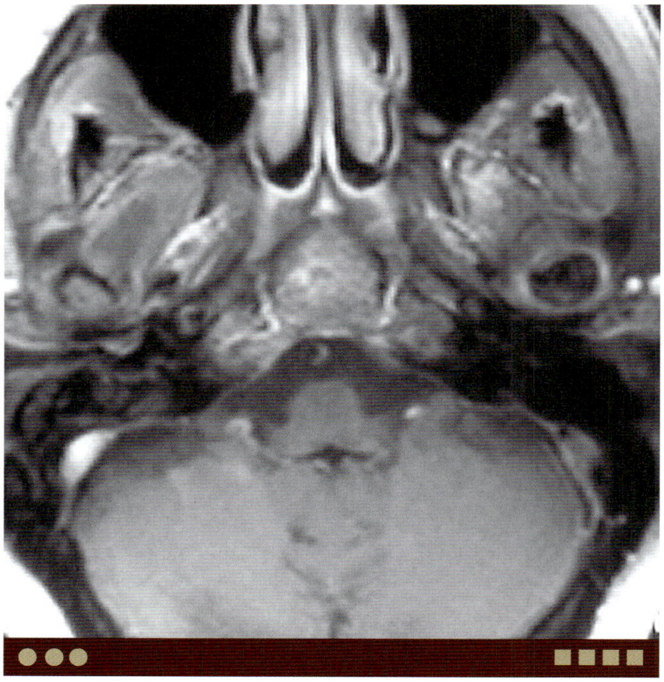

C. PVNS, same patient as A. Axial postcontrast fat-suppressed T1W MR image demonstrates enhancement around the left mandibular condyle.

DIFFERENTIAL DIAGNOSIS IMAGES (D-G)

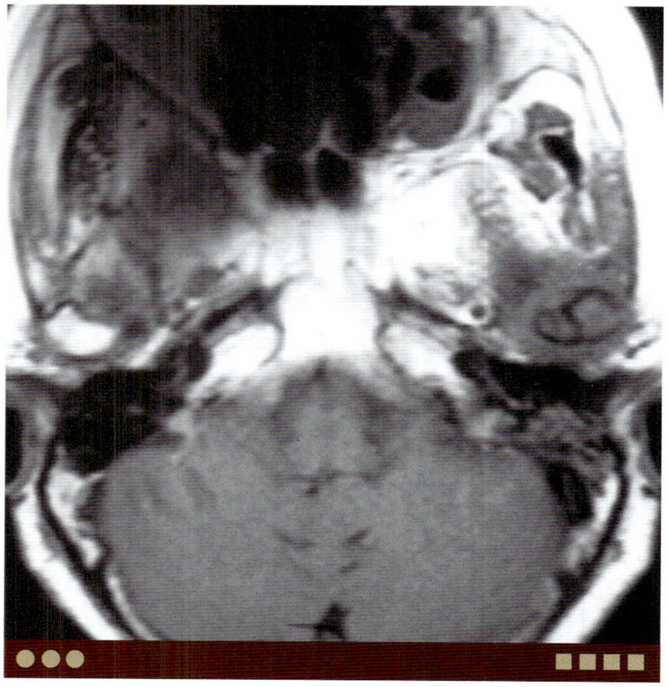

D. Rheumatoid arthritis. Axial T1W MR image demonstrates abnormally decreased signal in and around the left mandibular condyle consistent with synovial proliferation and fibrosis.

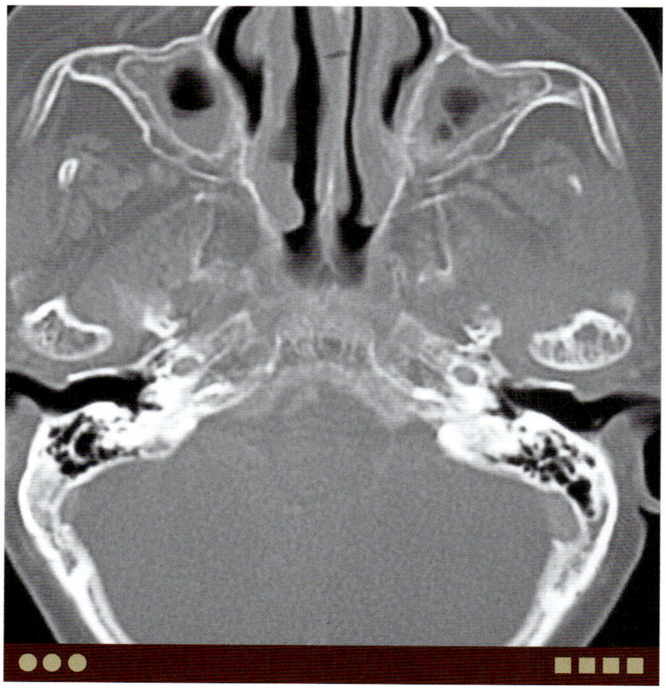

E. Rheumatoid arthritis, same patient as D. Axial CT demonstrates mixture of sclerotic and lytic changes of the left mandibular condyle.

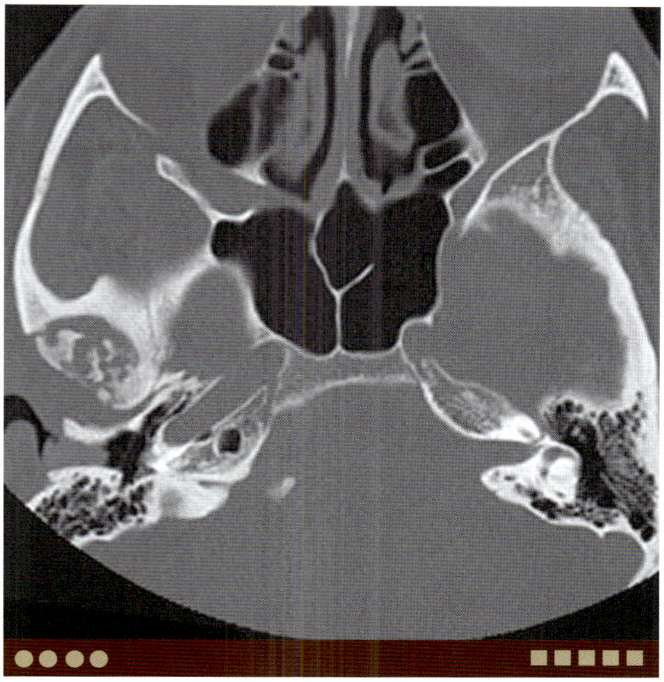

F. Osteoarthritis. Axial CT demonstrates mixture of sclerotic and lytic changes in the right mandibular condyle.

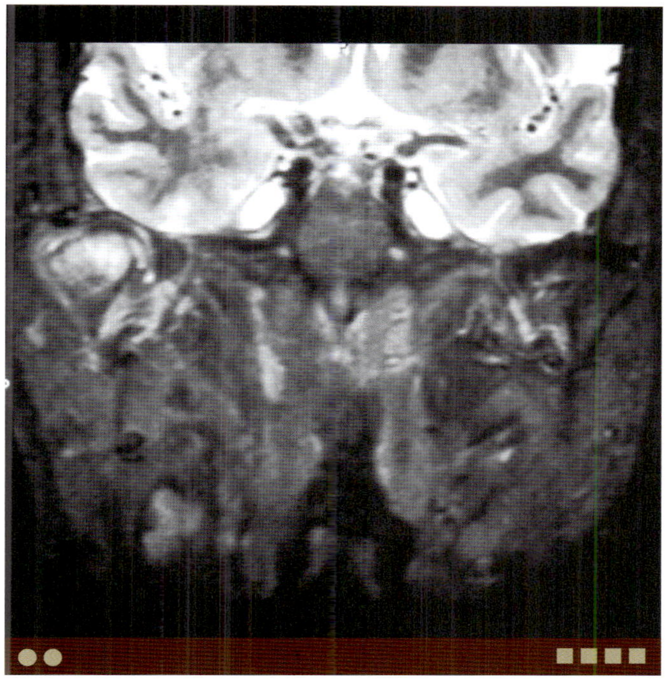

G. Septic arthritis. Coronal STIR image demonstrates abnormal high signal in the right mandibular condyle with joint effusion.

Case 9–26 Torus Mandibularis

Osamu Sakai, Margaret Chapman

PRESENTATION

Bump along the lingual surface of the mandible.

FINDINGS

CT demonstrates dense osseous protrusions along the lingual aspect of the anterior mandible.

DIFFERENTIAL DIAGNOSIS

- Epulis fissuratum: This condition represents overgrowth of fibrous connective tissue in the mouth that rarely calcifies.
- Osteosarcoma: This condition shows more aggressive osteoblastic and osteolytic changes with periosteal reaction. Compared with classic osteosarcoma arising from the long bones, osteosarcoma of the mandible is seen in an older age group.
- Chronic osteomyelitis: This condition may demonstrate either diffusely increased or heterogeneous density, a mixture of osteosclerotic and lytic changes, and occasionally expansion of the bone. Usually periodontal disease is also present.
- Fibrous dysplasia: Fibroosseous lesions show mixed density or ground-glass appearance without periosteal reaction or extraosseous soft tissue mass.

COMMENTS

This is a 47-year-old woman who underwent a CT evaluation for "bumps" in her gum.

Torus mandibularis is a lobulated or nodular focal bony growth of the mandible that is usually bilateral and located along the lingual aspect of the anterior mandible. This condition is different from torus palatinus (exostosis of the hard palate) in that it is less common and more likely to be acquired, rather than congenital/developmental. Torus mandibularis may be more commonly seen in males. There is no clinical significance, although affected individuals may be more susceptible to trauma and ulceration of the overlying mucosa.

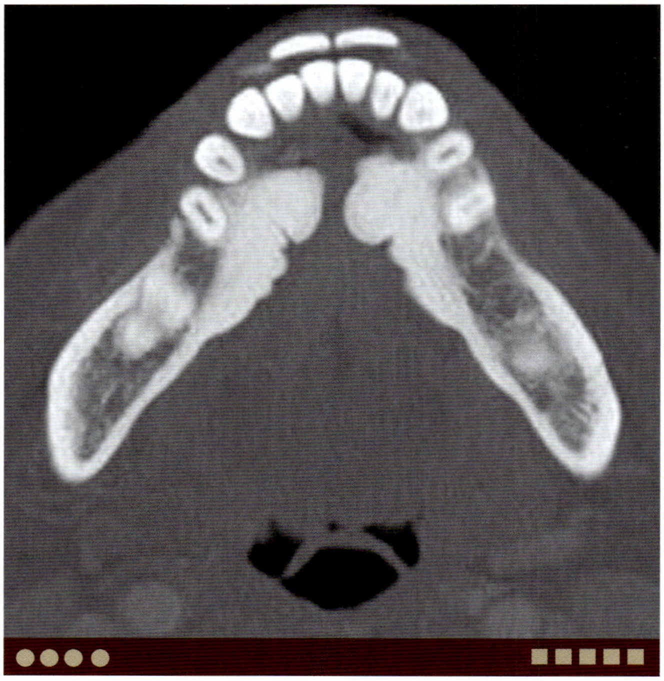

A. Torus mandibularis. Axial CT demonstrates lobulated, dense osseous proliferation along the lingual cortex of the mandible bilaterally.

Similar osseous protrusions are also seen in the maxillary alveolus (alveolar exostosis), more commonly in the buccal (buccal exostosis) than lingual side.

CT will clearly demonstrate the dense osseous protrusions. These exostoses are seen as signal-voids on MRI.

PEARLS

- **Torus mandibularis is focal bony growth of the mandible along the lingual aspect of the anterior mandible, and is usually bilateral.**
- **There is no associated clinical significance; however, affected patients may be more susceptible to trauma and ulceration of the overlying mucosa.**
- **CT clearly demonstrates the dense osseous protrusions. These exostoses are seen as signal-voids on MRI.**

ADDITIONAL IMAGES (B-D)

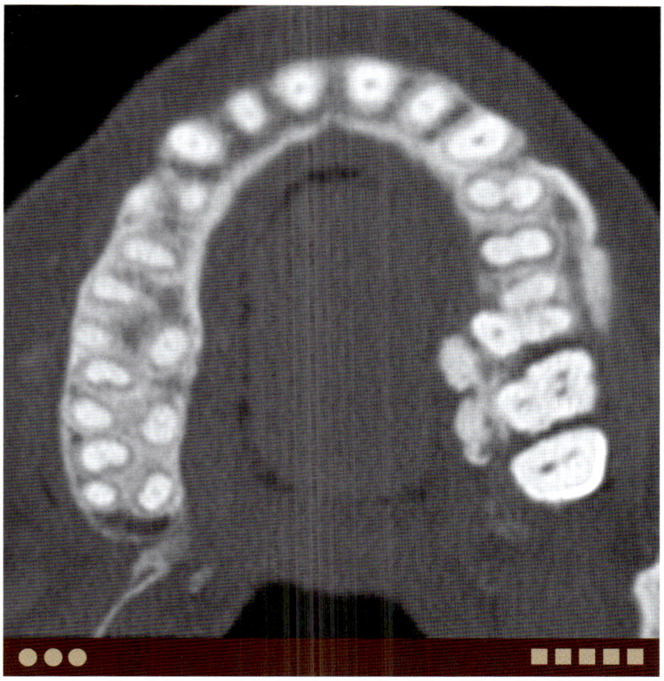

B. Alveolar exostosis. Axial CT demonstrates osseous protrusions along the buccal and lingual cortex of the left maxilla.

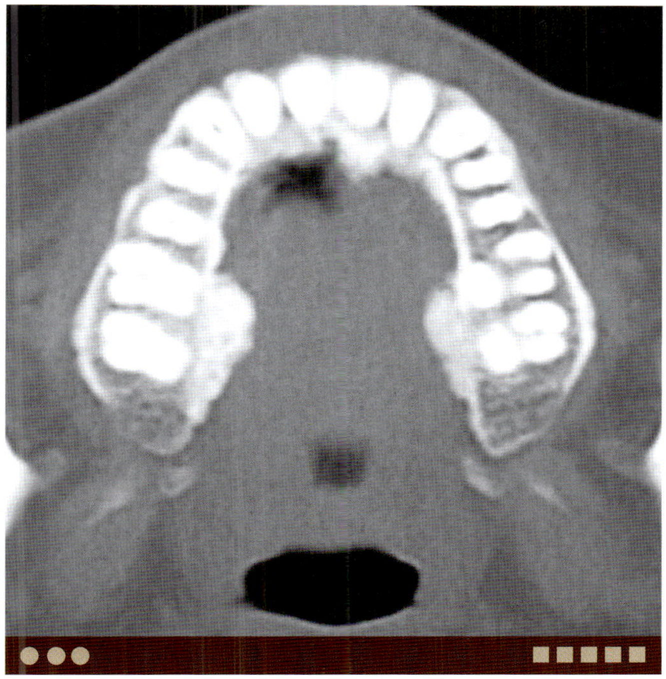

C. Alveolar exostosis in a different patient. Axial CT demonstrates osseous protrusions along the lingual cortex of the maxilla bilaterally.

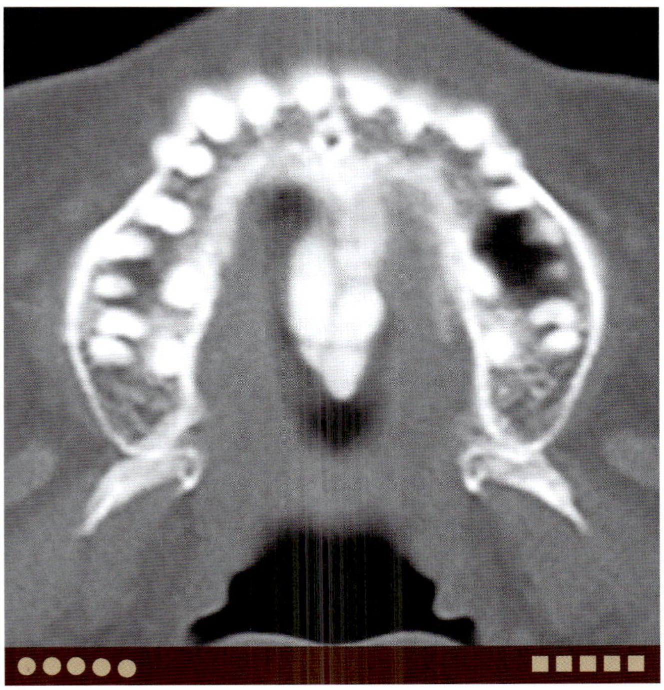

D. Torus palatinus. Axial CT demonstrates lobulated osseous protrusions in the hard palate in midline.

DIFFERENTIAL DIAGNOSIS IMAGES (E-G)

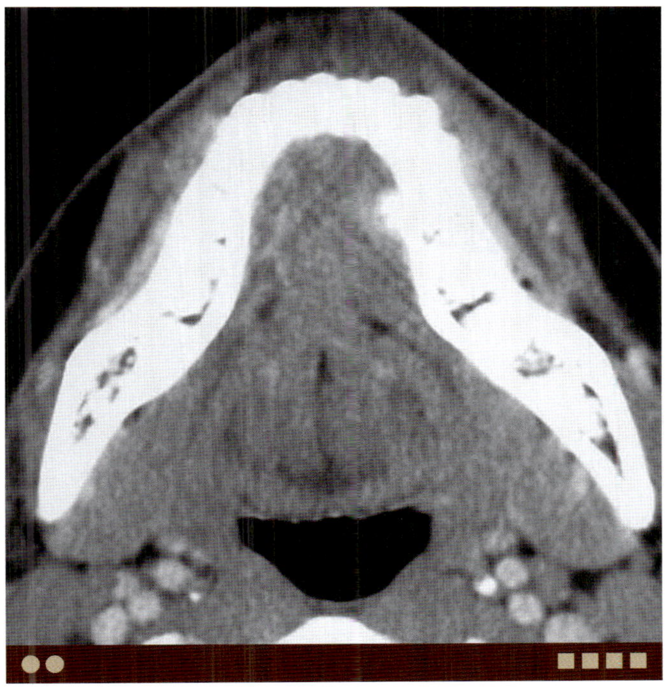

E. Epulis fissuratum. Axial contrast-enhanced CT demonstrates a high-density lesion of the lingual aspect of the left mandible.

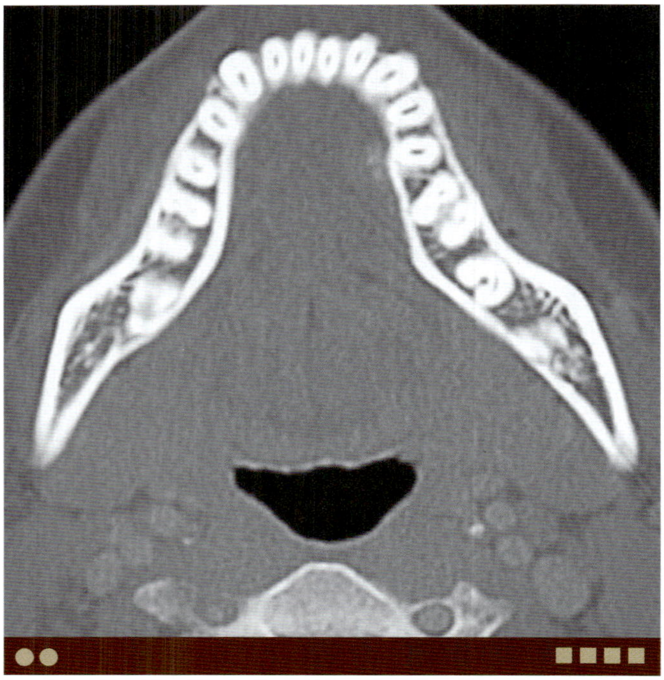

F. Epulis fissuratum, same patient as E. Axial bone windowed CT shows faint calcification.

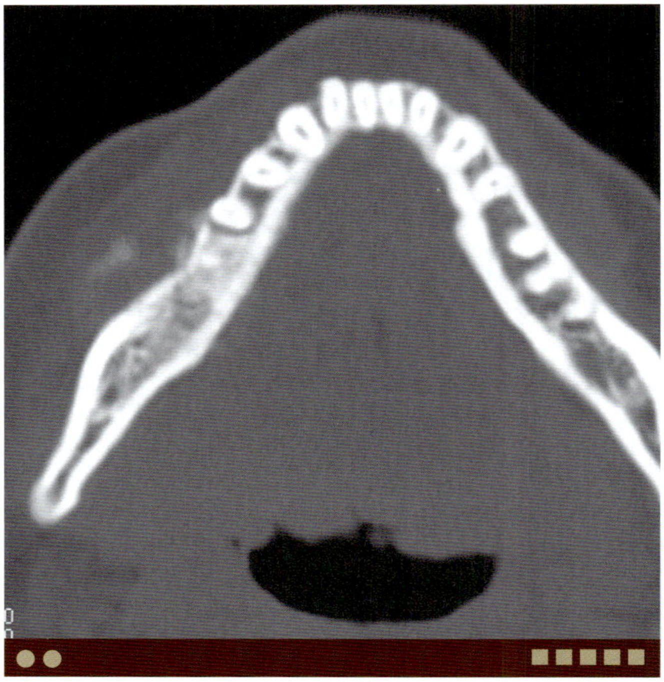

G. Osteosarcoma. Axial CT shows osteoblastic change in the body of the right mandible. Note the abnormal extraosseous soft tissue lesion with calcification/ossification along the buccal and lingual cortex.

Case 9–27 Osteoblastoma

Hiroki Kato, Margaret Chapman, Osamu Sakai

PRESENTATION

Occasional pain, tenderness, and discomfort of the jaw.

FINDINGS

CT demonstrates an osteolytic lesion with a sclerotic rim.

DIFFERENTIAL DIAGNOSIS

- Osteomyelitis: Osteomyelitis of the mandible is classified into osteolytic, mixed, sclerosing, sequestrum, and irregular trabeculation patterns. Acute osteomyelitis tends to be osteolytic.
- Fibrous dysplasia: Classically, this condition is seen as an expansile ground-glass density lesion on radiograph and CT. Other appearances such as homogeneously increased density and cystic changes are also often seen.
- Osteosarcoma: Osteosarcoma is rare but does occur in the jaw. Some osteoblastomas are locally aggressive and have atypical histopathologic features, and are often difficult to differentiate from low-grade osteosarcoma.

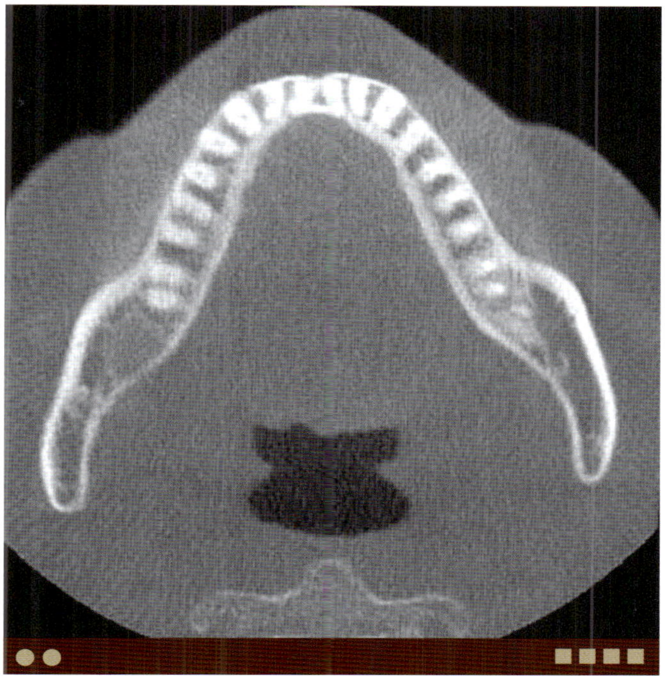

A. Osteoblastoma. Axial unenhanced CT demonstrates an osteolytic lesion with a slightly sclerotic rim within the posterior body of the right mandible.

COMMENTS

This is a 46-year-old man presenting with pain and tenderness of the right mandible.

Osteoblastoma is a rare benign tumor accounting for less than 1% of all bone tumors and approximately 3.5% of benign bone tumors. It usually arises in young patients and develops in the long bones and posterior elements of the spine. It can also be seen within the posterior mandible but is rare in this location, comprising less than 5% of all osteoblastomas. Occasionally patients complain of pain, tenderness, and discomfort associated with the lesion. The time from onset of symptoms to diagnosis is typically several months because it is a rare entity and radiographic studies are often negative early in the course of the disease.

Osteoblastoma is characterized by interconnecting trabeculae of woven bone and is rimmed by prominent osteoblasts. Radiographs demonstrate either osteolytic or osteoblastic changes, and reactive sclerosis is a common feature. On CT, osteoblastoma is typically seen as an osteolytic lesion with a sclerotic rim; however, they can be predominantly osteolytic with little matrix mineralization. On MRI, they are often hypointense on T1W images and hyperintense on T2W images, and enhance after contrast administration. Depending on the degree of tumor matrix mineralization or sclerosis, T2W images may show areas of hypointensity.

Osteoblastomas are highly vascular and locally aggressive, and require complete resection.

PEARLS

- **Osteoblastoma often arises in the long bones and posterior elements of the spine, and rarely within the posterior mandible.**
- **CT typically demonstrates an osteolytic lesion with an osteosclerotic rim.**
- **Osteoblastoma typically demonstrates low signal on T1W and variable signal on T2W images, depending on the degree of mineralization/sclerosis, and enhancement following contrast administration.**

ADDITIONAL IMAGES (B-E)

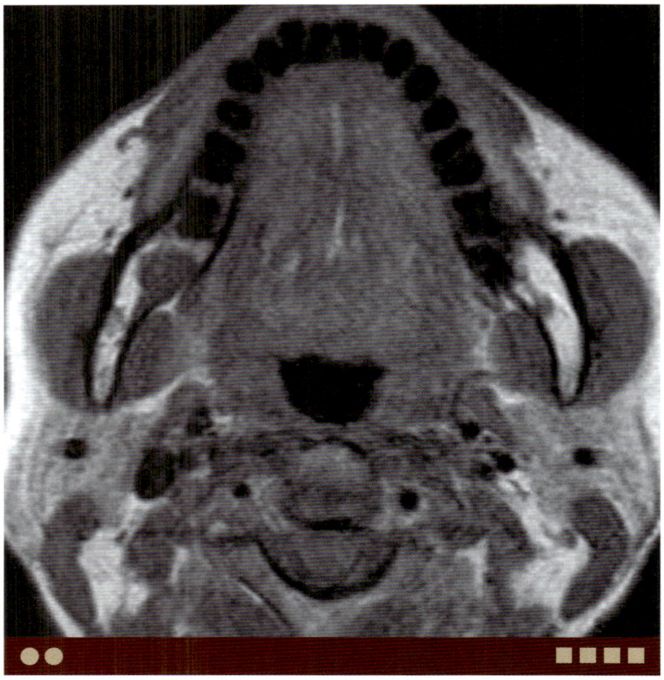

B. Osteoblastoma, same patient as A. Axial T1W image demonstrates low signal in the tumor.

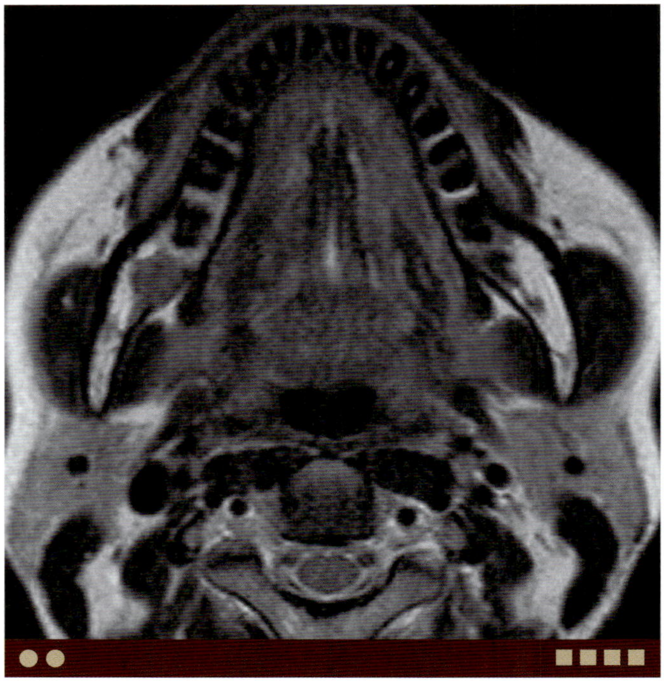

C. Osteoblastoma, same patient as A. Axial T2W image demonstrates an intermediate-signal tumor in the right mandible.

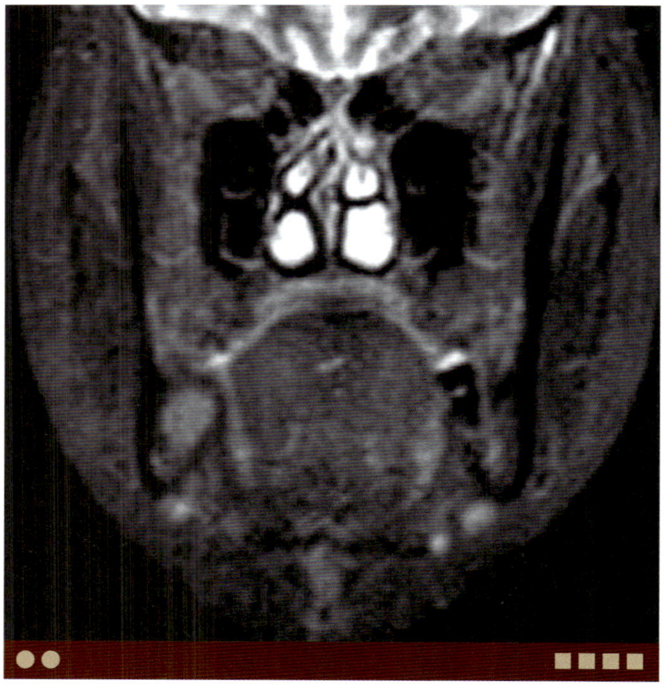

D. Osteoblastoma, same patient as A. Coronal fat-suppressed T2W image demonstrates high signal in the tumor.

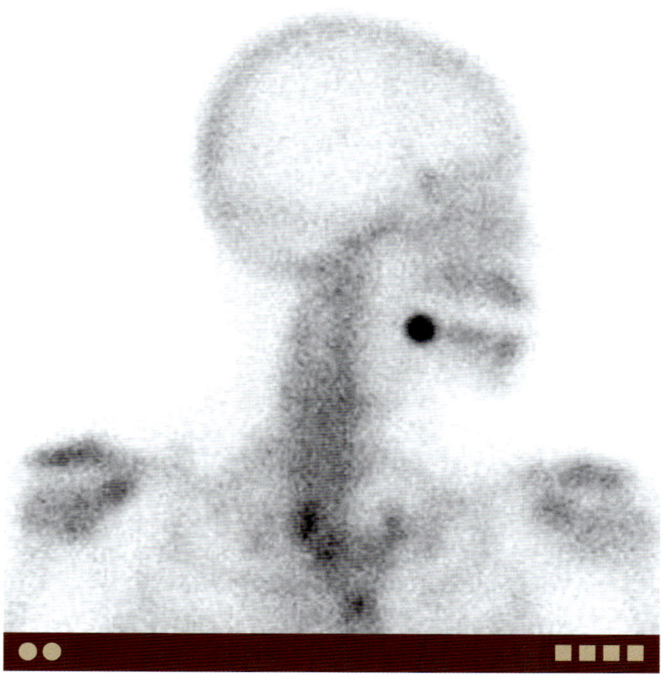

E. Osteoblastoma, same patient as A. 99mTc-MDP scintigraphy demonstrates marked uptake in the tumor.

DIFFERENTIAL DIAGNOSIS IMAGES (F-H)

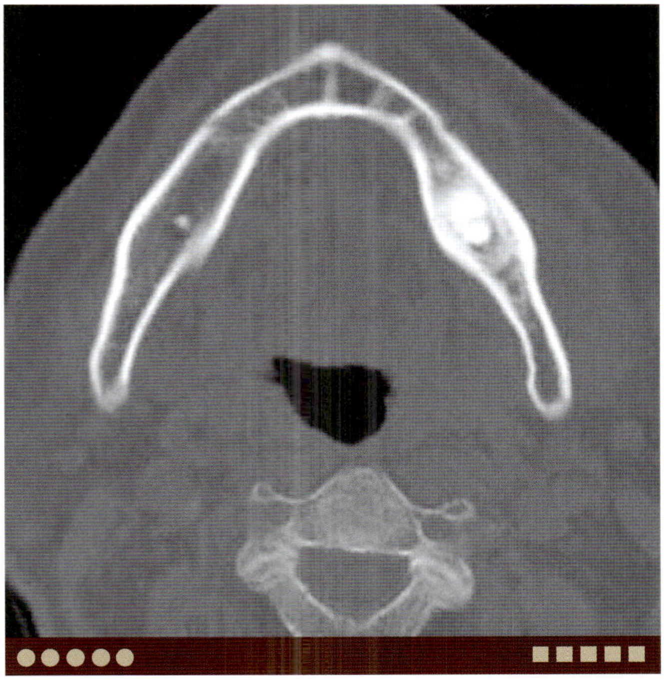

F. Chronic osteomyelitis. Axial unenhanced CT demonstrates focal osteosclerosis within the left mandible.

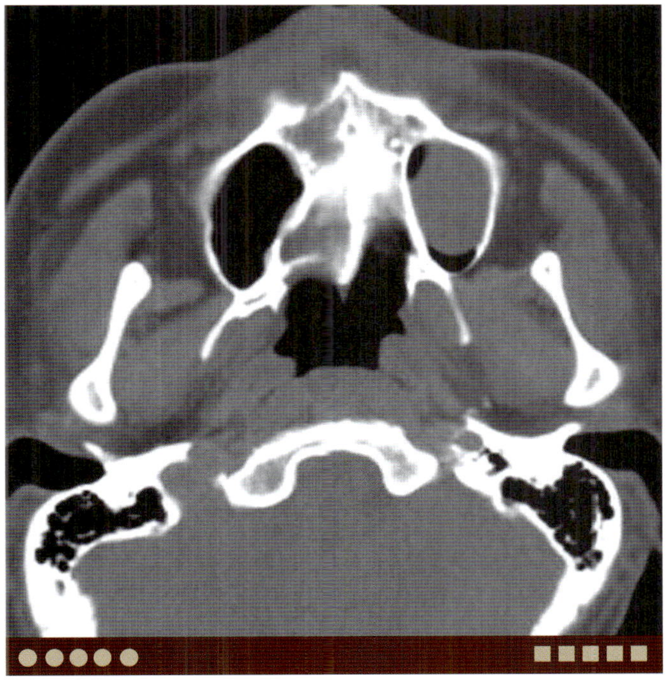

G. Acute osteomyelitis. Axial unenhanced CT demonstrates an osteolytic region in the anterior right maxilla.

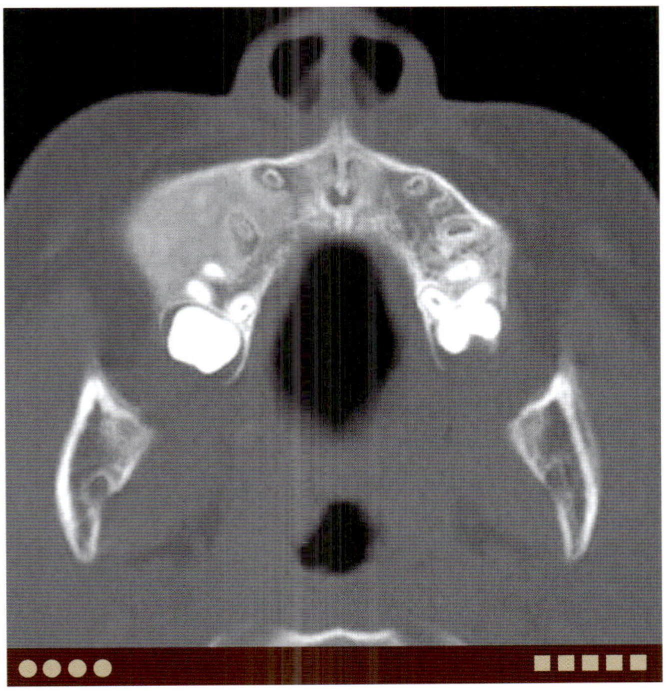

H. Fibrous dysplasia. Axial unenhanced CT demonstrates an expansile ground-glass density lesion within the right maxilla.

Case 9–28 Osteochondroma: Mandibular Condyle

Hiroki Kato, Margaret Chapman, Osamu Sakai

PRESENTATION

Mandibular asymmetry.

FINDINGS

CT and MRI demonstrate an exophytic bone lesion with cortical and marrow continuity with the underlying bone.

DIFFERENTIAL DIAGNOSIS

- Bifid condyle: This is a double-headed mandibular condyle, likely representing a congenital/developmental anomaly. Although rare, this is the most common anomaly of the condyle.
- Prior fracture and degenerative changes: Healed fractures and degenerative change may show deformity of the condyle and exophytic osseous proliferation.
- Osteoma: Osteoma is a benign lesion resulting from the continuous formation of both compact and cancellous bone. Osteomas are often seen in the mandibular body. If multiple, Gardner syndrome should be considered.
- Osteoblastoma: Osteoblastoma is rare in the maxillofacial region. It has a pleomorphic histologic appearance, with a well-vascularized, osteoblastic, connective tissue stroma in which benign giant cells may be present.
- Chondroma: This is a benign tumor composed of mature cartilage. Chondroid tumors of the jaws are rare.
- Chondroblastoma: This is a rare tumor in the jaw, which demonstrates proliferating chondroblasts on histologic examination.

COMMENTS

This is a 50-year-old woman presenting with discomfort in the right temporomandibular joint.

Osteochondroma is one of the most common benign tumors of bone, representing approximately 35% to 50% of all benign tumors and 8% to 15% of all primary bone tumors. They rarely arise in the cranial and maxillofacial bones, because these bones develop by intramembranous ossification. Almost all mandibular osteochondromas arise from the condyle or coronoid process.

Osteochondromas of the mandibular condyle are usually diagnosed in older patients (average age 40 years). They are found most often on the medial aspect of the mandibular condyle, followed by the anterior, and rarely the lateral or superior aspects of the bone. The growth of osteochondromas is usually slow and causes ipsilateral vertical displacement and elongation of the mandible, and an

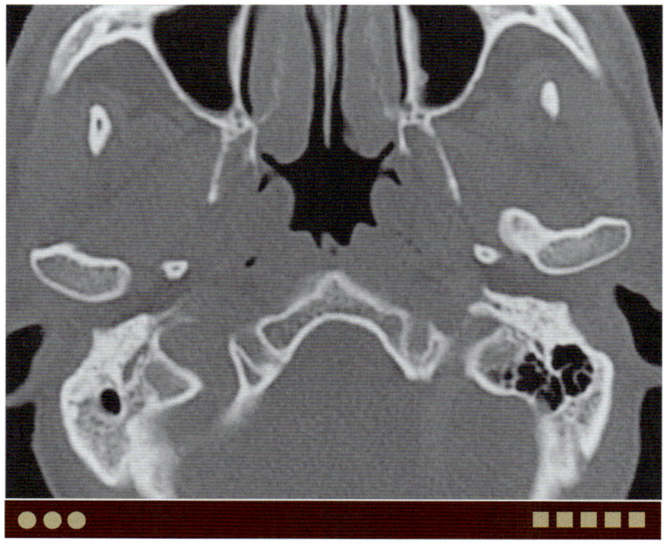

A. Osteochondroma. Axial unenhanced CT demonstrates an exophytic bone lesion in the anteromedial aspect of the left mandibular condyle.

increase in the vertical height of the condyle, neck, ramus, and mandibular body on the affected side. This typically results in vertical elongation of the affected side of the face, and progressively increasing mandibular asymmetry. Clinical symptoms may include malocclusion, disc displacement, loss of condylar function, and rarely pain.

Radiographically, osteochondroma is composed of cortical and medullary bone protruding from and continuous with the underlying bone. CT with 3D and multiplanar reconstructions demonstrates cortical and marrow continuity of the lesion and parent bone. MRI is useful in evaluating the relationship between the lesion and surrounding structures and to assess for the hyaline cartilage cap.

PEARLS

- **Almost all mandibular osteochondromas arise from the condyle or coronoid process.**
- **Radiograph and CT demonstrate an exophytic bone lesion with cortical and marrow continuity to the underlying bone.**
- **MRI is useful in evaluating the relationship between the lesion and surrounding structures and to assess for the hyaline cartilage cap.**

ADDITIONAL IMAGES (B-G)

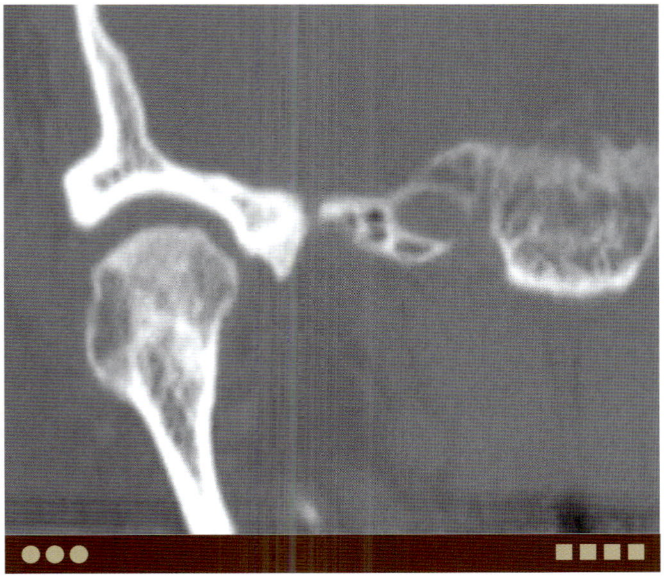

B. Osteochondroma in a different patient. Coronal unenhanced CT demonstrates a slightly exophytic lesion in the lateral aspect of the right mandibular condyle.

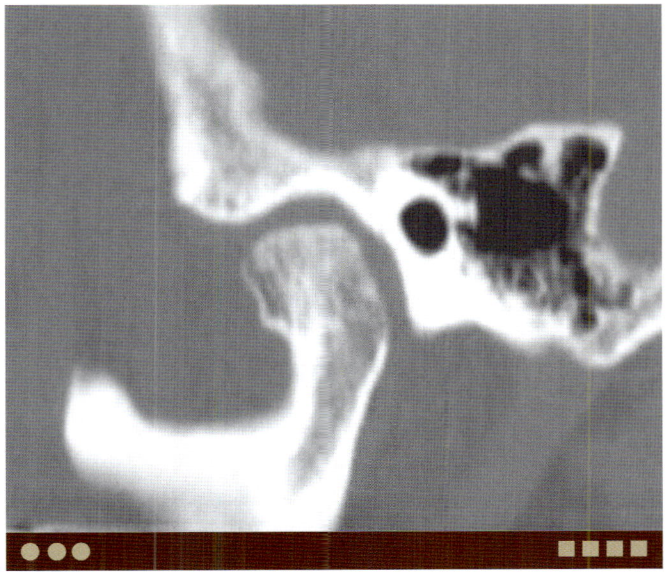

C. Osteochondroma, same patient as B. Sagittal unenhanced CT demonstrates the lesion in the anterior aspect of the condyle.

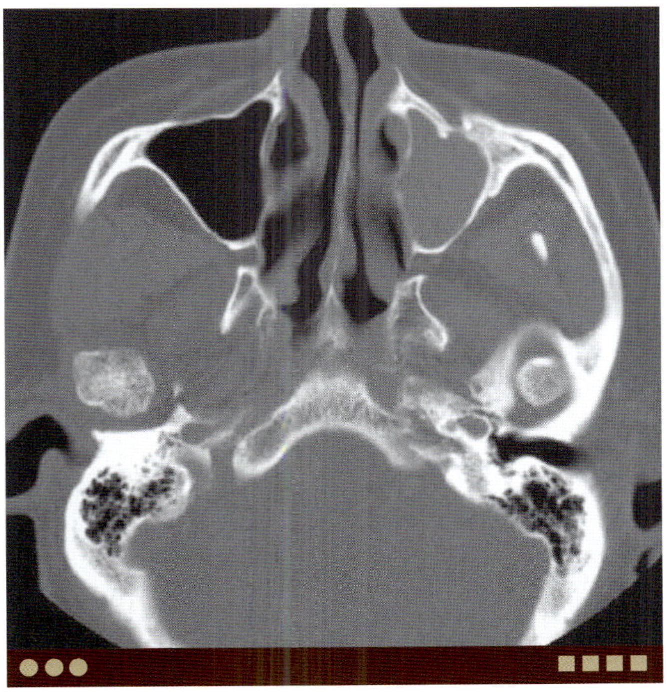

D. Osteochondroma, same patient as B. Axial unenhanced CT demonstrates a slightly exophytic lesion in the right mandibular condyle.

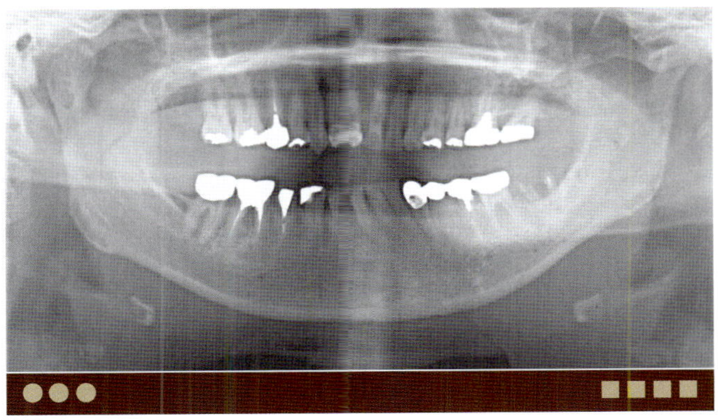

E. Osteochondroma, same patient as B. Panoramic radiograph demonstrates a lesion with mixed density in the right mandibular condyle.

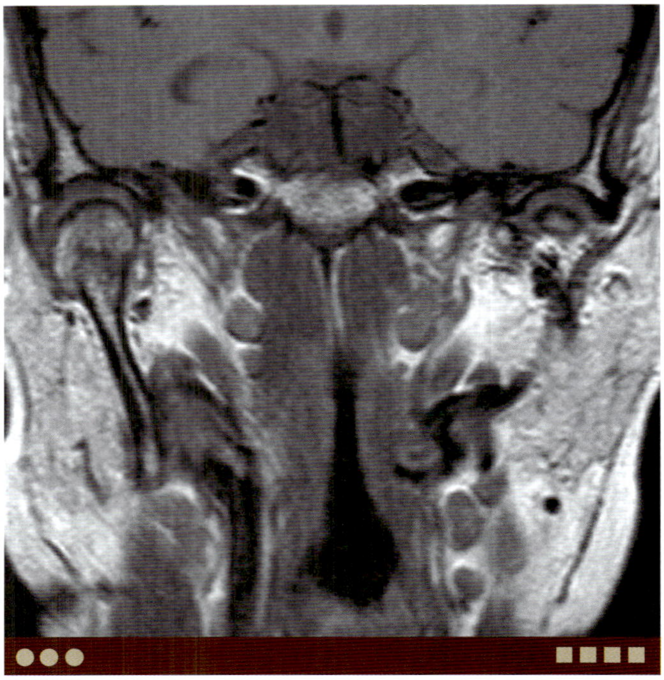

F. Osteochondroma, same patient as B. Coronal PDW image demonstrates the continuity of the lesion and the underlying bone.

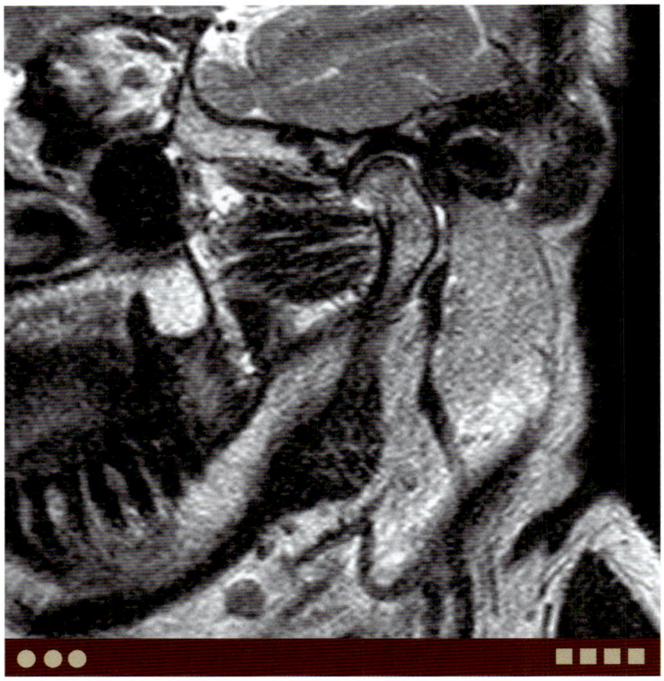

G. Osteochondroma, same patient as B. Sagittal T2W image demonstrates no cartilage cap.

DIFFERENTIAL DIAGNOSIS IMAGES (H-J)

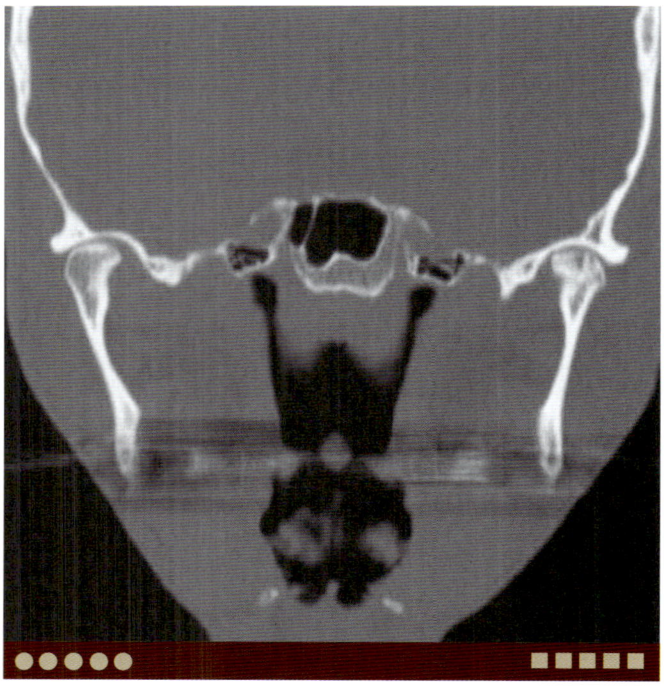

H. Degenerative joint disease. Coronal unenhanced CT demonstrates sclerotic change and subcortical cysts in the left mandibular condyle.

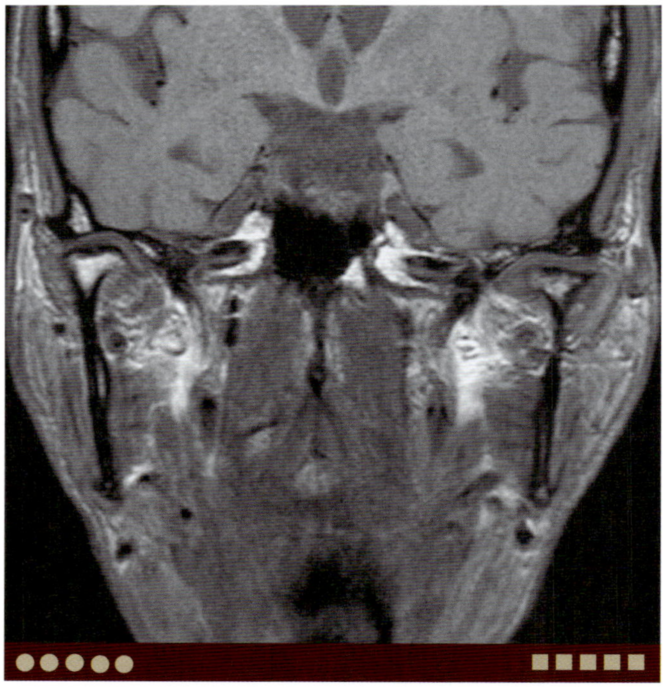

I. Degenerative joint disease in a different patient. Coronal PDW MR image demonstrates a deformity of the left mandibular condyle.

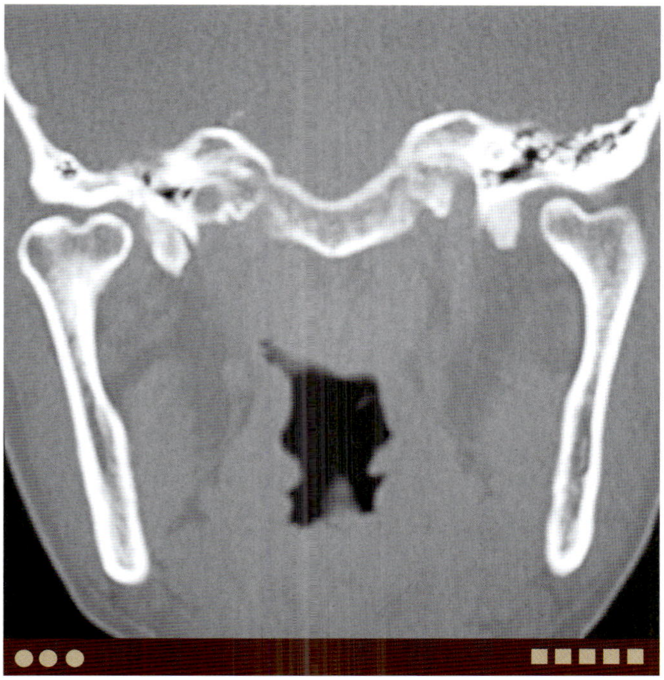

J. Bifid condyle. Coronal unenhanced CT demonstrates double-headed condyles bilaterally.

Case 9–29 Adenomatoid Odontogenic Tumor

Osamu Sakai, Andrew Akman

PRESENTATION

Jaw swelling.

FINDINGS

CT demonstrates a cystic lesion containing calcification between the incisors of the maxilla or mandible.

DIFFERENTIAL DIAGNOSIS

- Dentigerous (follicular) cyst: This is the most common developmental odontogenic cystic lesion, commonly found in the molar regions.
- Ameloblastoma: This lesion demonstrates similar findings to a dentigerous cyst, is commonly found in the molar regions, and typically shows a multilocular or soap-bubble appearance. However, these lesions may also occur in the anterior mandible or maxilla and can be unilocular.
- Radicular (periapical) cyst: These lesions form around the tooth roots and are the most common odontogenic cystic lesions.
- Keratocystic odontogenic tumor (previously called odontogenic keratocyst): This is a benign, however, locally aggressive developmental odontogenic tumor, most commonly located in the body or ramus of the mandible.
- Nasopalatine duct cyst: This is a developmental cyst and one of the fissural cysts which arises from the nasopalatine duct (incisive canal). This lesion does not contain a tooth.

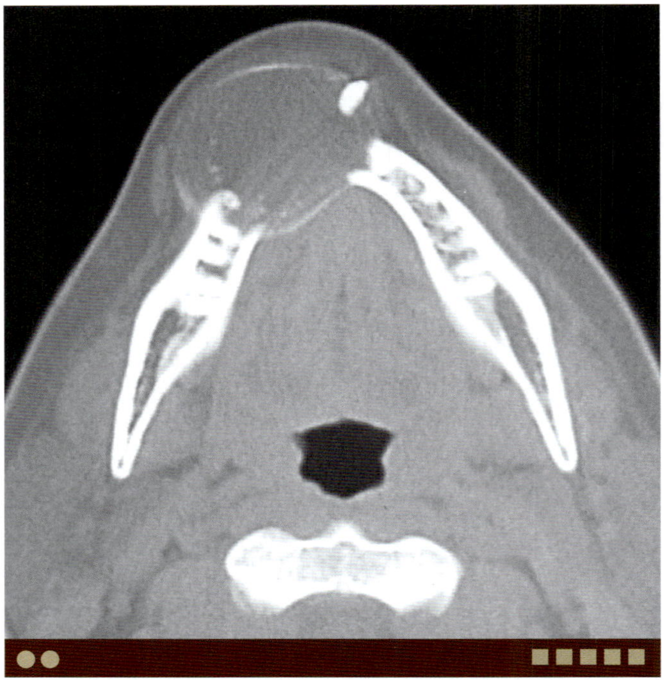

A. Adenomatoid odontogenic tumor. Axial CT demonstrates an expansile cystic lesion within the anterior mandible containing an unerupted tooth and calcifications.

COMMENTS

This is a 13-year-old boy with swelling of the mandible.

Adenomatoid odontogenic tumor (AOT) is a rare tumor that has odontogenic epithelium with mature, fibrous stroma without odontogenic ectomesenchyme. It is typically diagnosed in female patients in the second decade of life and often found in the maxilla (70%). An AOT most commonly appears as a well-demarcated radiolucent lesion containing varying amounts of punctate calcifications and causing expansion of the involved bone. The lesion can displace or prevent the eruption of teeth. In about 75% of cases, it is associated with an unerupted tooth. If attached to teeth, AOTs are found more apically on the root than dentigerous cysts.

AOT is often remembered as the "two-thirds tumor," (1) two-thirds appear in the second and third decades, (2) two-thirds involve females, (3) two-thirds occur in the anterior maxilla, and (4) two-thirds are associated with an unerupted tooth (usually the cuspid). This is a rare tumor; however, the characteristic imaging findings along with appropriate patient demographics can help to narrow the differential diagnosis.

CT clearly demonstrates an expansile cystic-appearing lesion in the anterior maxilla or mandible, with internal calcification, often involving an unerupted tooth.

PEARLS

- **AOT is a rare tumor that has odontogenic epithelium with mature, fibrous stroma without odontogenic ectomesenchyme.**
- **AOT is the "two-thirds tumor," (1) second and third decades, (2) female, (3) anterior maxilla, and (4) unerupted tooth.**
- **AOT is rare, however, can be easily diagnosed by the characteristic imaging findings and appropriate patient demographics.**

ADDITIONAL IMAGES (B-C)

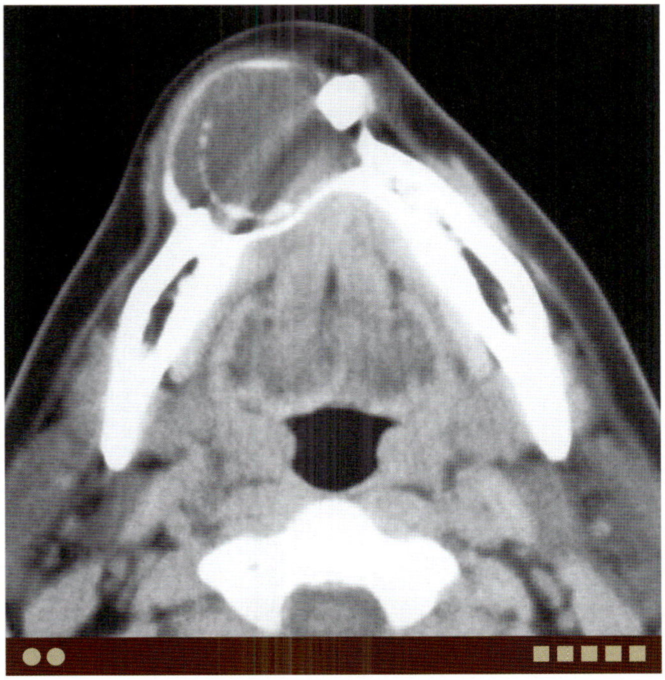

B. AOT, same patient as A. Axial CT with soft tissue window demonstrates the lesion showing internal water density with calcifications. An unerupted tooth is located peripherally.

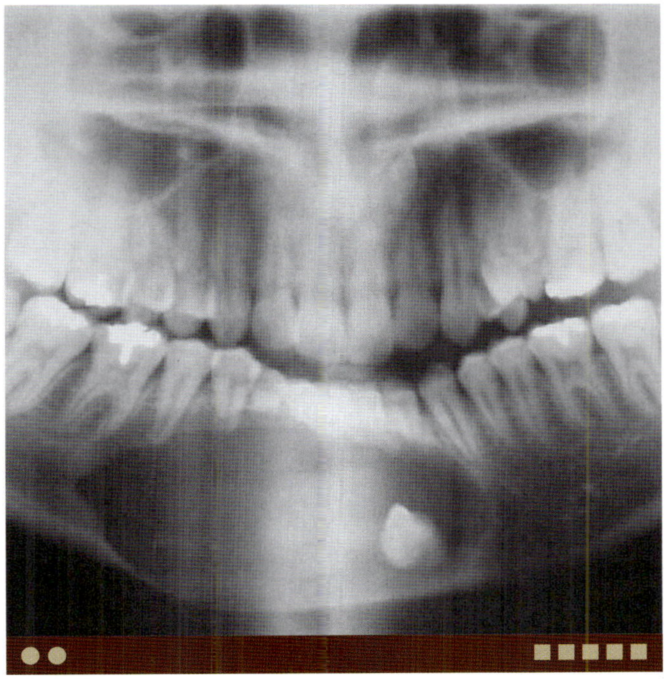

C. AOT, same patient as A. Panoramic radiograph demonstrates the lesion displacing and eroding adjacent teeth roots.

DIFFERENTIAL DIAGNOSIS IMAGES (D-H)

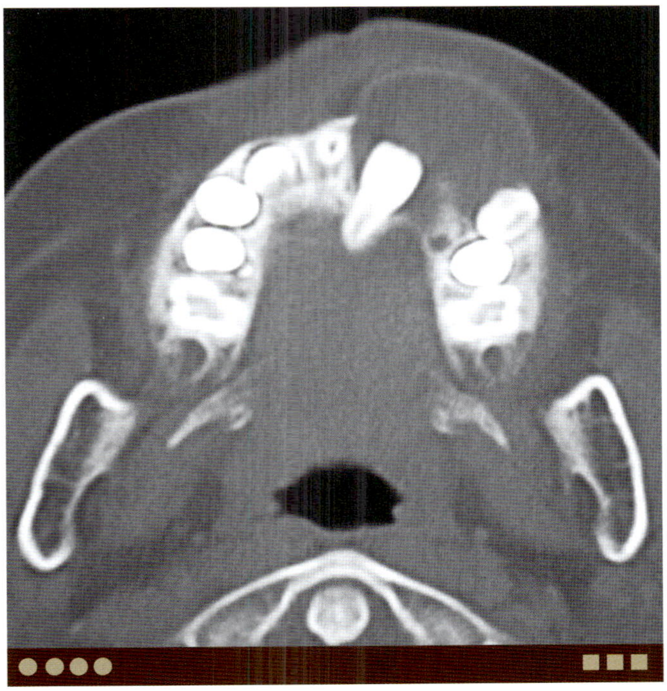

D. Dentigerous cyst. Axial CT demonstrates an expansile cystic lesion that contains the crown of an unerupted tooth in the anterior left maxilla.

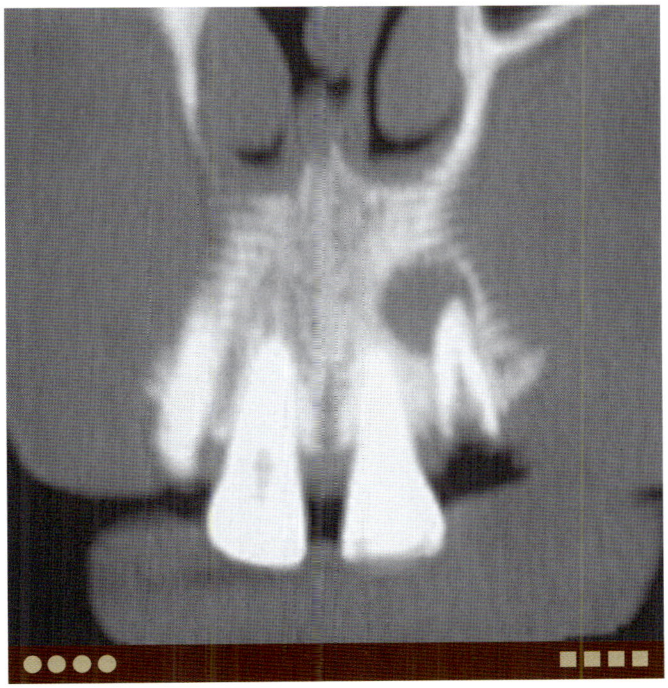

E. Periapical cyst. Coronal CT demonstrates a cystic lesion around the root of a tooth with a cavity.

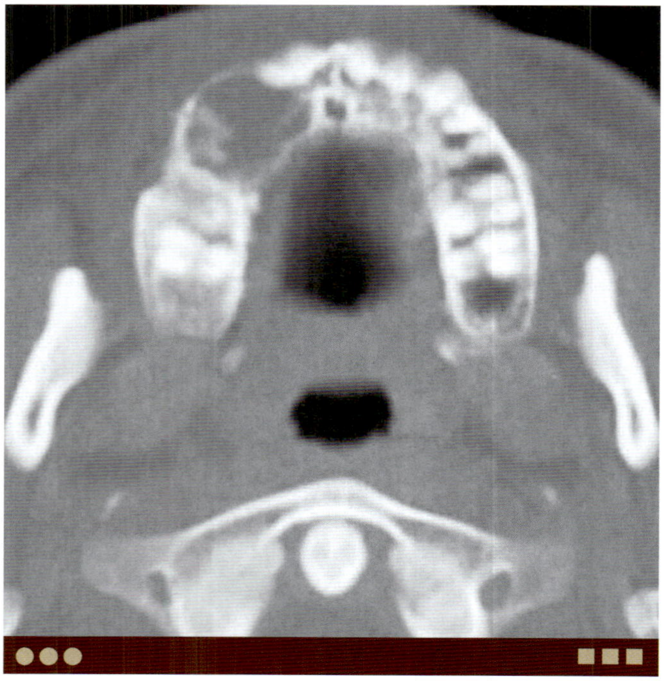

F. Ameloblastoma. Axial CT demonstrates a slightly expansile cystic-appearing lesion with some internal calcification in the anterior maxilla.

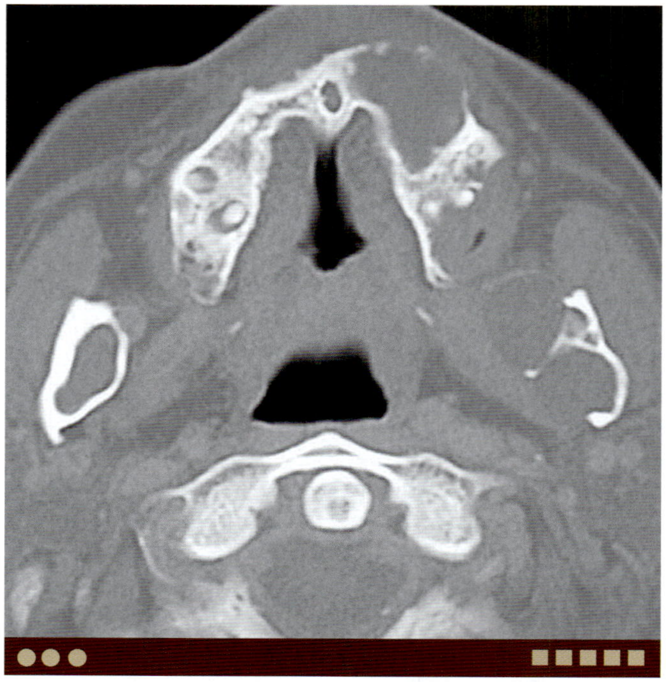

G. Keratocystic odontogenic tumor. Axial CT demonstrates a cystic lesion in the anterior maxilla. Note other cystic lesions involving bilateral mandibular rami.

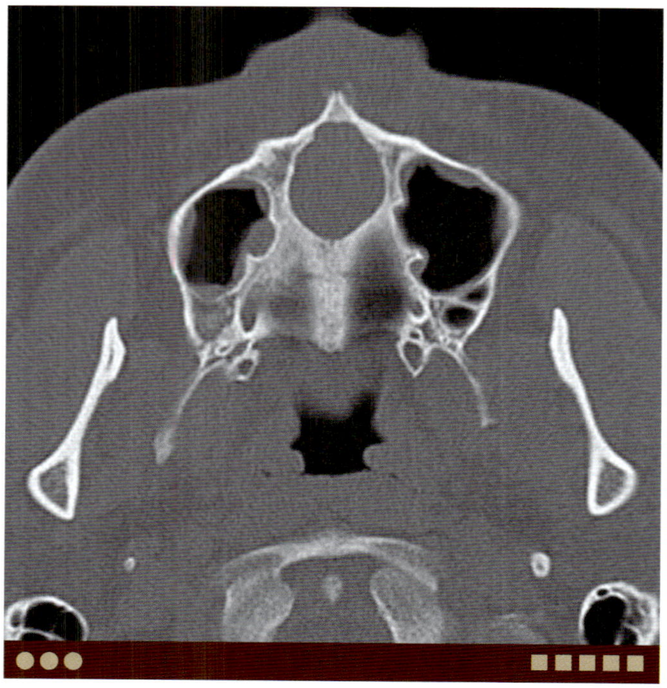

H. Nasopalatine duct cyst. Axial CT demonstrates an enlarged nasopalatine duct (incisive canal). The lesion does not contain a tooth.

Case 9–30 Cemento-Osseous Dysplasias

Anita Gohel, Osamu Sakai

PRESENTATION

Jaw swelling.

FINDINGS

CT demonstrates a lucent or ground-glass lesion surrounding the apices of teeth.

DIFFERENTIAL DIAGNOSIS

- Radicular (periapical) cyst: This is the most common odontogenic cyst and the lesion forms around the root of the tooth.
- Benign cementoblastoma: This is an odontogenic tumor seen usually at the apices of mandibular posterior teeth.
- Chronic osteomyelitis: The late stage of cemento-osseous dysplasia may resemble osteomyelitis with sequestrum formation.

COMMENTS

This is a 29-year-old woman who underwent CT after trauma.

Cemento-osseous dysplasias are a group of dysplasias which include periapical and florid cemento-osseous dysplasias. They typically occur in a middle-aged black female and usually are discovered as incidental findings. Sometimes these lesions can become quite large and cause expansion. The associated teeth are vital.

Periapical cemental dysplasia (PCD) usually is seen in the periapical region of the anterior mandible. Florid cemento-osseous dysplasia is a more extensive form of PCD. The lesions are usually bilateral. The lesions may be multifocal and in the early stage they are radiolucent. Dysplastic cemento-osseous tissue fills these radiolucent lesions and lesions show mixed density, and during later stages they may appear radiopaque. Large lesions can cause displacement of the mandibular canal and the maxillary sinus floor.

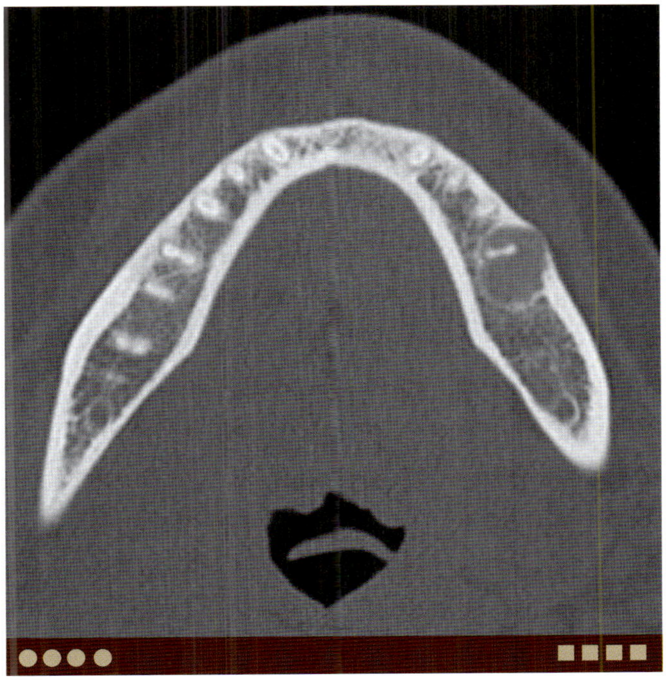

A. Cemento-osseous dysplasia. Axial CT demonstrates a radiolucent lesion causing expansion and thinning of the buccal cortical plate.

PEARLS

- **Cemento-osseous dysplasia is usually seen as an incidental finding in middle-aged black females.**
- **The lesions are often multifocal, bilateral, and may be radiolucent, mixed density, or radiopaque.**
- **Simple bone cysts may form with these lesions.**

ADDITIONAL IMAGES (B-F)

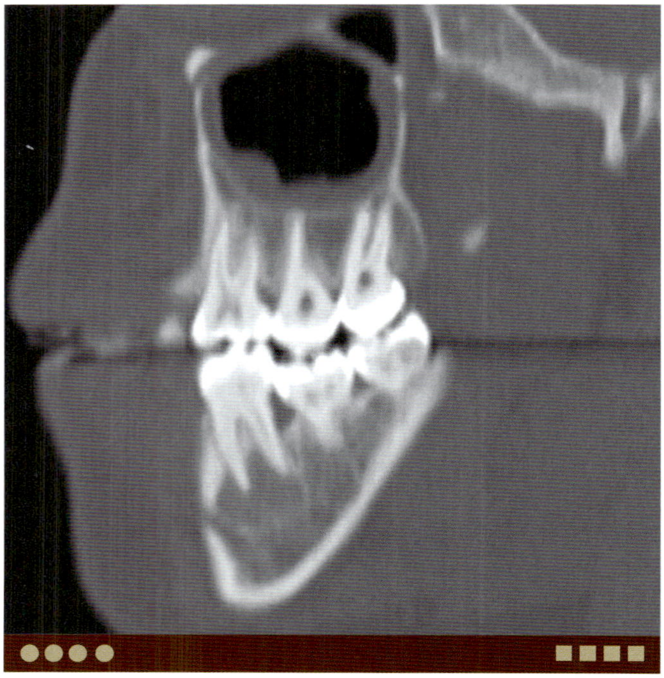

B. Cemento-osseous dysplasia, same patient as A. Sagittal CT demonstrates the lesion at the apices of the molar teeth.

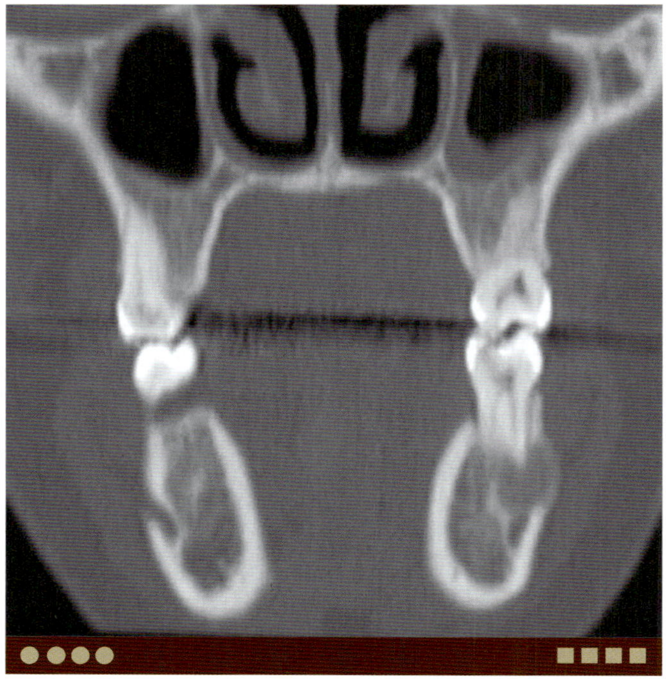

C. Cemento-osseous dysplasia, same patient as A. Coronal CT demonstrates the lesion causing expansion and thinning of the buccal cortical plate.

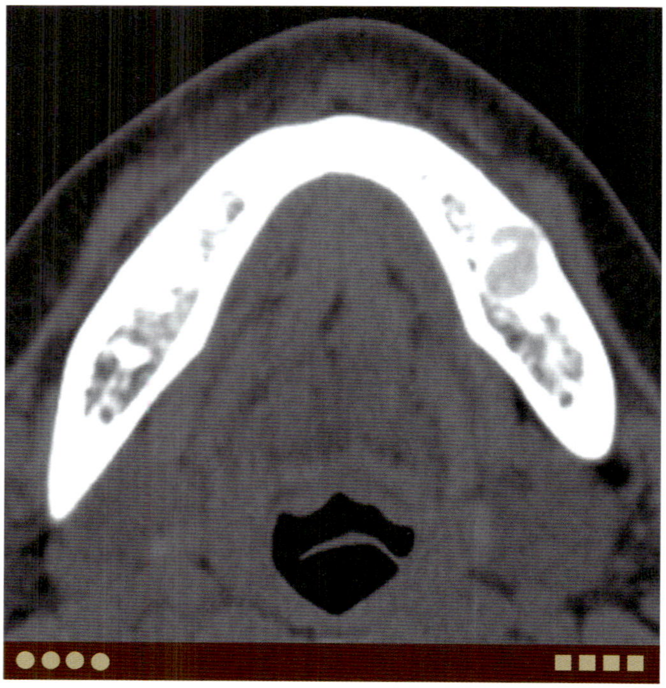

D. Cemento-osseous dysplasia, same patient as A. Axial soft tissue window CT demonstrates a slightly expansile lesion with ground-glass density.

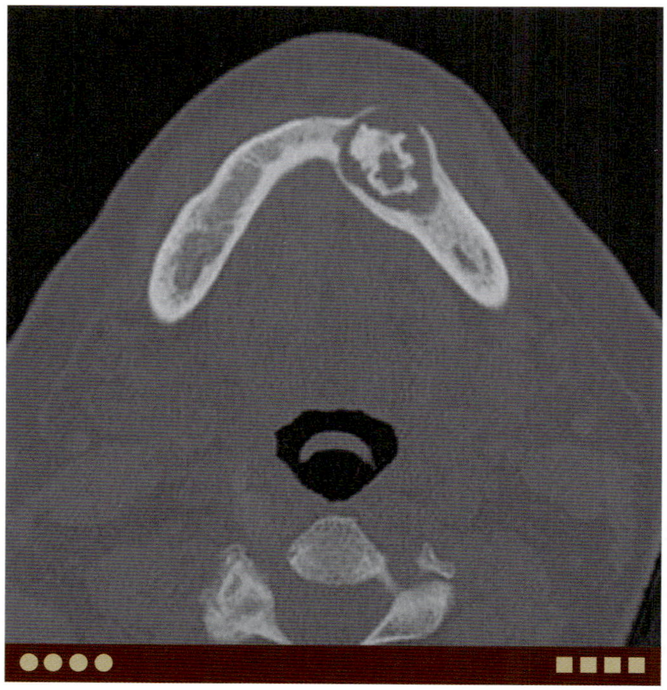

E. Cemento-osseous dysplasia, late phase. Axial CT demonstrates an expansile lucent lesion thinning the buccal cortex with internal radiodense foci.

DIFFERENTIAL DIAGNOSIS IMAGES (G-H)

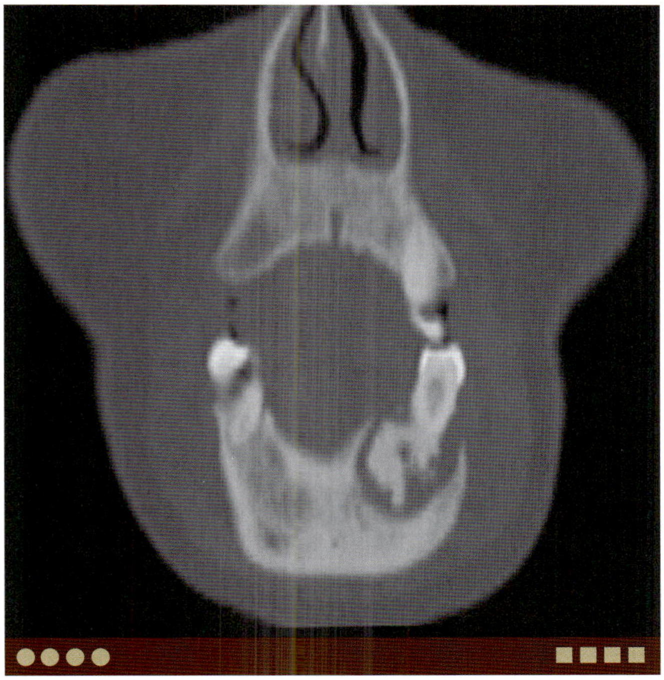

F. Cemento-osseous dysplasia, late phase, same patient as E. Coronal CT demonstrates a vital associated tooth.

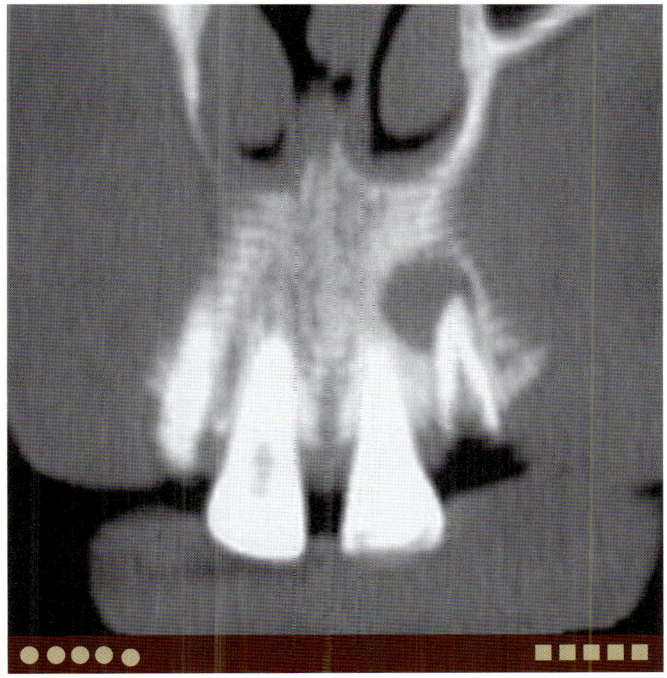

G. Radicular (periapical) cyst. Coronal CT demonstrates a cyst around the root of the lateral incisor. Note a cavity in the crown of the tooth.

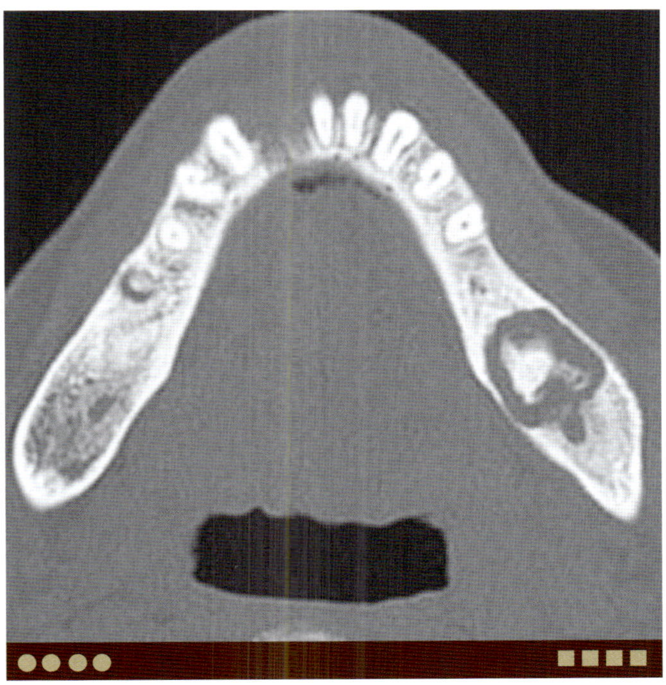

H. Chronic osteomyelitis. Axial CT demonstrates a large osteolytic lesion with sequestrum in the left mandible. Note the entire mandible demonstrates diffuse sclerosis.

Case 9–31 Central Giant Cell Lesion (Granuloma)

Anita Gohel, Osamu Sakai

PRESENTATION

Jaw swelling.

FINDINGS

CT demonstrates an expansile lesion in the anterior mandible.

DIFFERENTIAL DIAGNOSIS

- Ameloblastoma: This is an odontogenic tumor seen more in the posterior mandibular region and has well-defined coarse trabeculation within the lesion.
- Odontogenic myxoma: This is an odontogenic tumor usually seen in the premolar and molar region of the mandible.
- Aneurismal bone cyst: This is also a reactive lesion seen more often in posterior mandible and causes considerable expansion.
- Brown tumors of hyperparathyroidism: These can appear radiologically and histologically identical to central giant cell lesion. However, the patient's age and laboratory test results should easily help distinguish between these two entities.

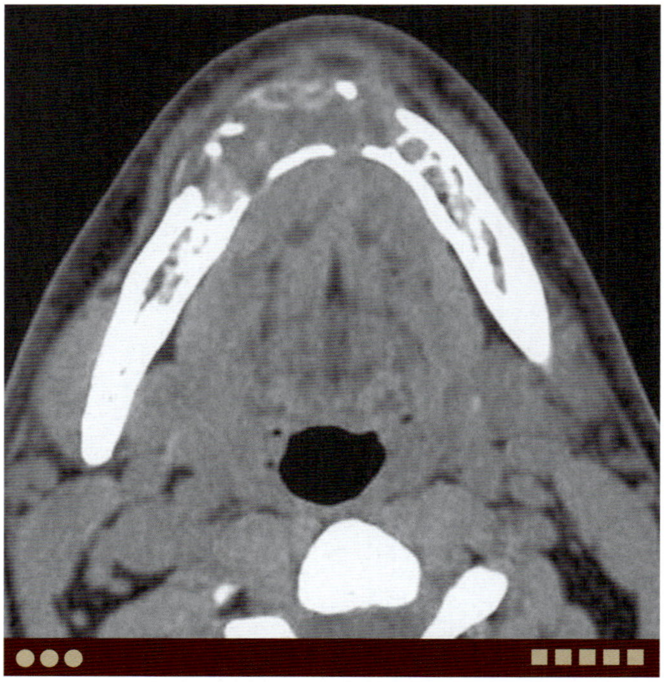

A. CGCL. Axial precontrast CT with soft tissue window demonstrates a soft tissue density lesion with small foci of calcifications destructing the anterior mandible. The lesion crosses the midline.

COMMENTS

This is a 33-year-old man with swelling of the mandible.

Central giant cell lesion (granuloma) (CGCL), as known as giant cell reparative granulomas, is a single lesion in a spectrum of altered vascular and reactive responses within bone. This is most frequently seen in patients in the second and third decades of life with female predominance. The majority of these lesions are found in the anterior mandible. Initially, CGCL manifests as a small, unilocular radiolucent lesion that can mimic an odontogenic cyst. With development, however, the lesion becomes multilocular, exhibiting a honeycomb appearance. These lesions can cross the midline in the mandible. The lesions are expansile and may have a multilocular appearance. Ill-defined, thin trabeculations which run at right angles to the periphery are frequently seen. There may be thinning of the cortex. They can cause displacement and resorption of teeth.

PEARLS

- **CGCL is usually seen in individuals less than 30 years of age.**
- **CGCLs are seen more in the anterior mandibular region.**
- **CGCLs may have faint mineralization within the lesions.**

ADDITIONAL IMAGES (B-E)

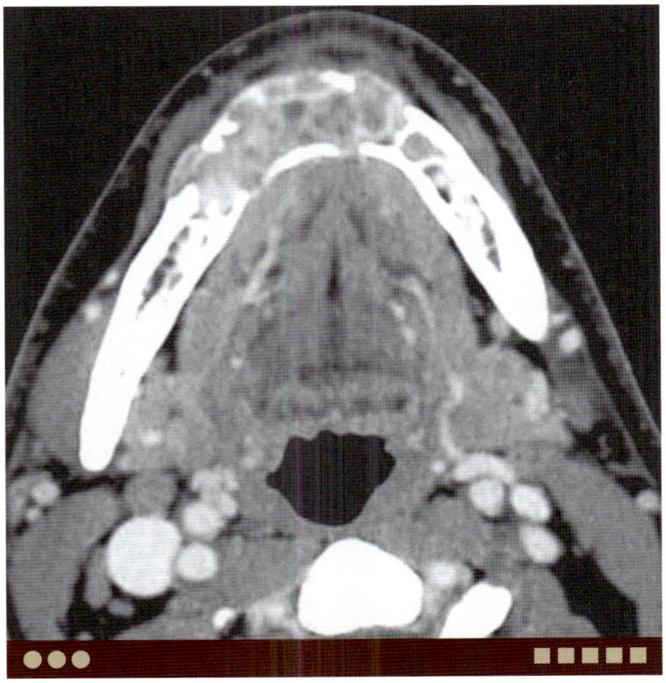

B. CGCL, same patient as A. Axial postcontract CT shows avid, heterogeneous enhancement of the lesion.

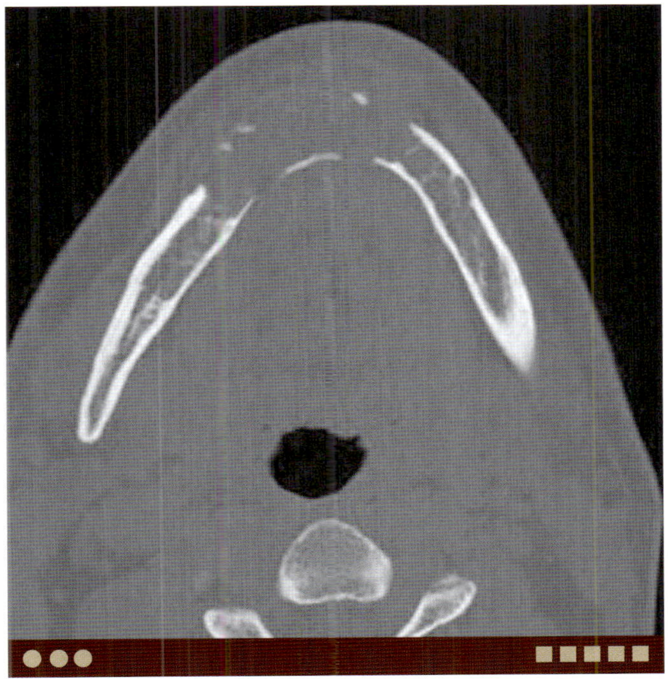

C. CGCL, same patient as A. Axial CT with bone window demonstrates an expansile osteolytic lesion with cortical erosion/thinning and small foci of calcification.

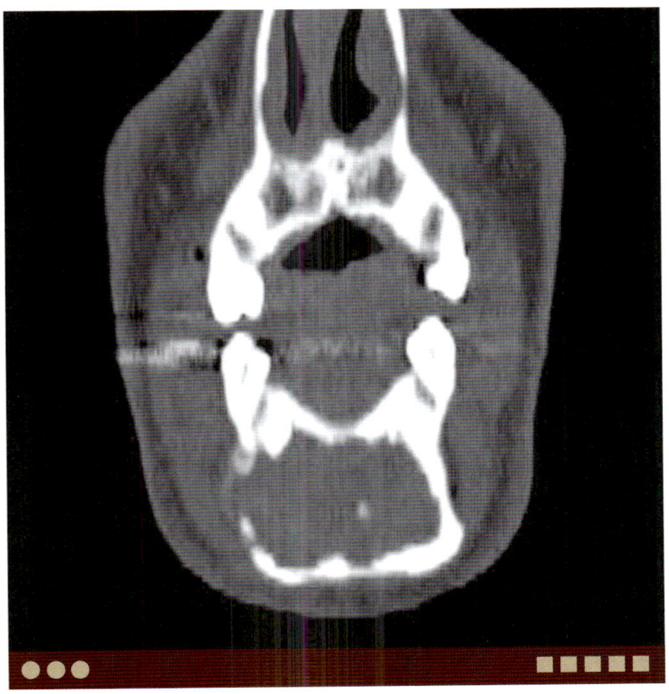

D. CGCL, same patient as A. Coronal precontrast CT with soft tissue window demonstrates an expansile, soft tissue density lesion with small foci of calcification in the anterior mandible.

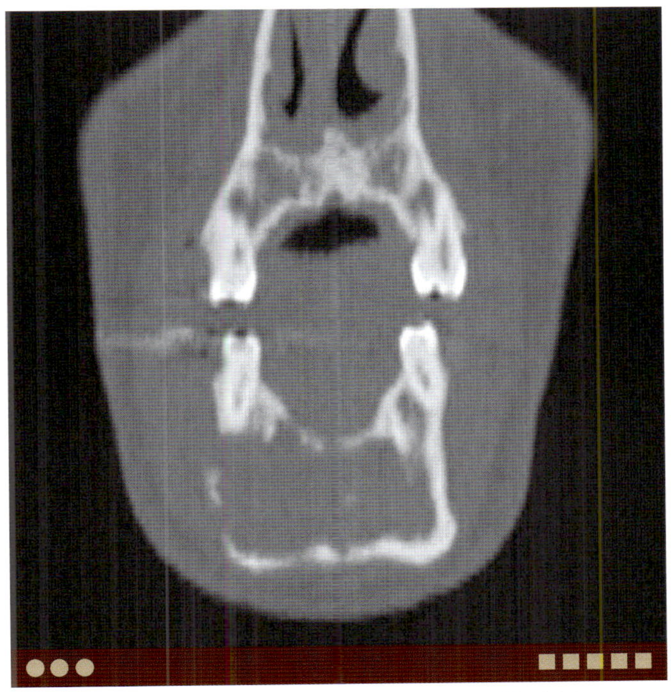

E. CGCL, same patient as A. Coronal precontrast CT with bone window demonstrates an expansile lesion with cortical erosion and small foci of calcification in the anterior mandible.

DIFFERENTIAL DIAGNOSIS IMAGES (F-H)

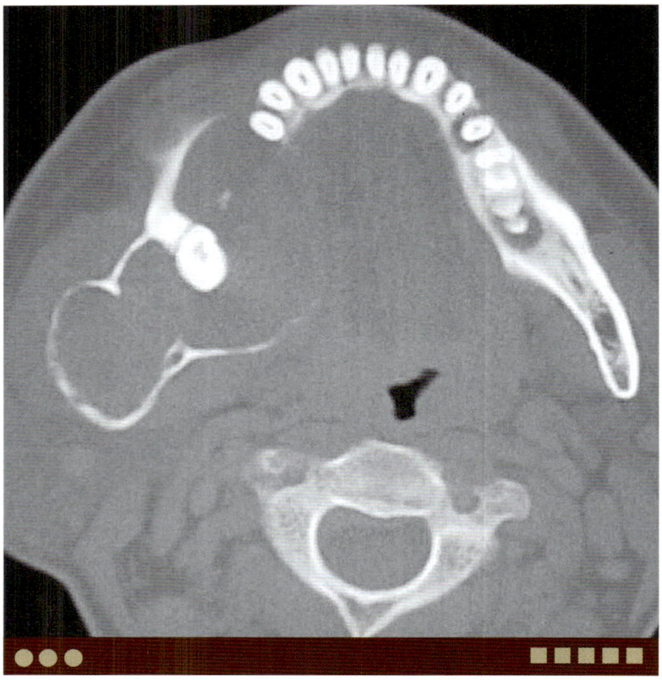

F. Ameloblastoma. Axial CT demonstrates a large, slightly lobulated, expansile lesion in the posterior body of the mandible extending to the ramus. Note displacement of the molar, significant erosion, and disruption of the cortex.

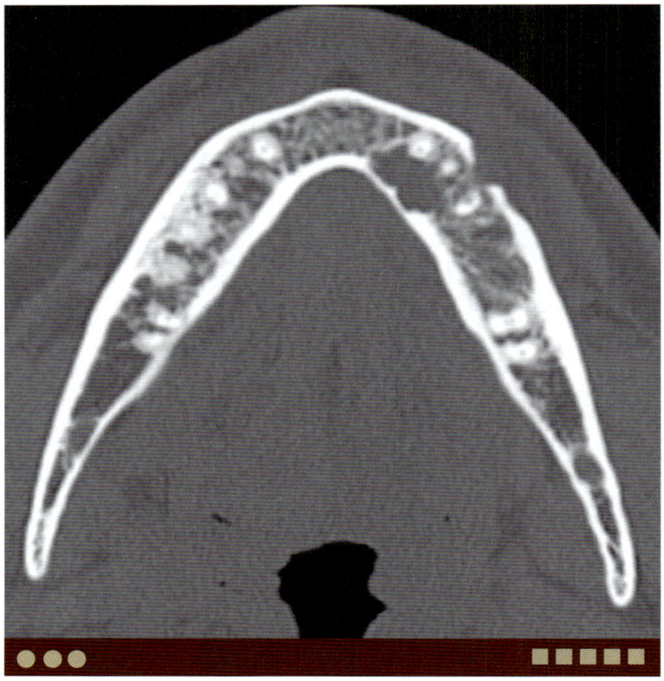

G. Odontogenic myxoma. Axial CT scan reveals a lesion in the mandible causing thinning of the lingual cortical plate.

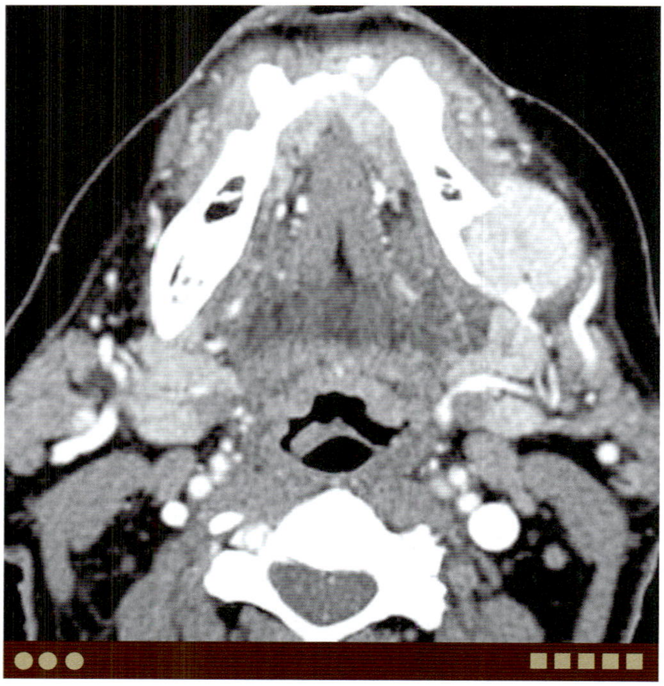

H. Plasmacytoma. Axial contrast-enhanced CT demonstrates an avidly enhancing expansile lesion in the left mandible. This tumor usually occurs in older patients.

Case 9–32 Odontogenic Myxoma

Anita Gohel, Akifumi Fujita, Osamu Sakai

PRESENTATION

Jaw swelling.

FINDINGS

CT demonstrates an expansile lesion in the mandible.

DIFFERENTIAL DIAGNOSIS

- Ameloblastoma: This is a benign epithelial odontogenic tumor arising from the enamel-forming cells of the odontogenic epithelium, and may form around the crown of an unerupted tooth.
- Dentigerous (follicular) cyst: This is the most common developmental odontogenic cyst and lesion forms around the crown of an unerupted tooth.
- Radicular (periapical) cyst: This is the most common odontogenic cyst and the lesion forms around the root of the tooth.

COMMENTS

This is a 48-year-old man with swelling of the mandible.

Odontogenic myxoma (myxofibroma) is a rare benign odontogenic mesodermal tumor usually in the tooth-bearing areas of the jaw. It is usually seen in patients between the age of second and sixth decades of life with a slight female predilection. It is locally aggressive and can cause extensive bony destruction and extends into the surrounding structures. They are usually expansile and can displace and loosen teeth. Root resorption is rare. They may appear multilocular and can occur around the crown of an impacted tooth. The treatment of choice is surgical excision; however, they have a high recurrence rate (around 25%).

Odontogenic myxoma is often clinically and radiographically indistinguishable from ameloblastoma, appearing as a multiloculated radiolucent lesion with internal osseous trabeculae. This rare tumor typically manifests in the second or third decade of life.

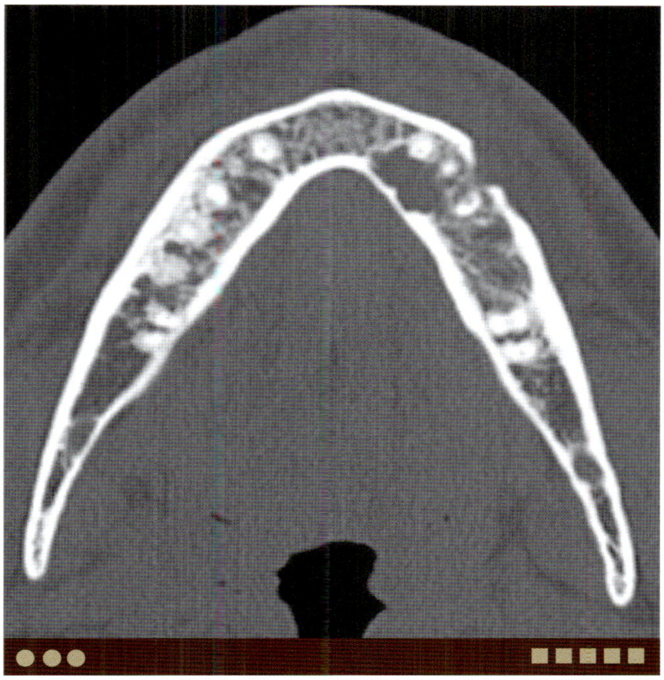

A. Odontogenic myxoma. Axial bone window CT reveals a lesion in the left anterior mandible causing thinning of the lingual cortical plate.

PEARLS

- **Odontogenic myxomas are usually seen in patients over second and sixth decades of life.**
- **They may occur pericoronally around an impacted tooth.**
- **They may have fine septations within the lesions and can cause displacement and loosening of the teeth.**

ADDITIONAL IMAGES (B-G)

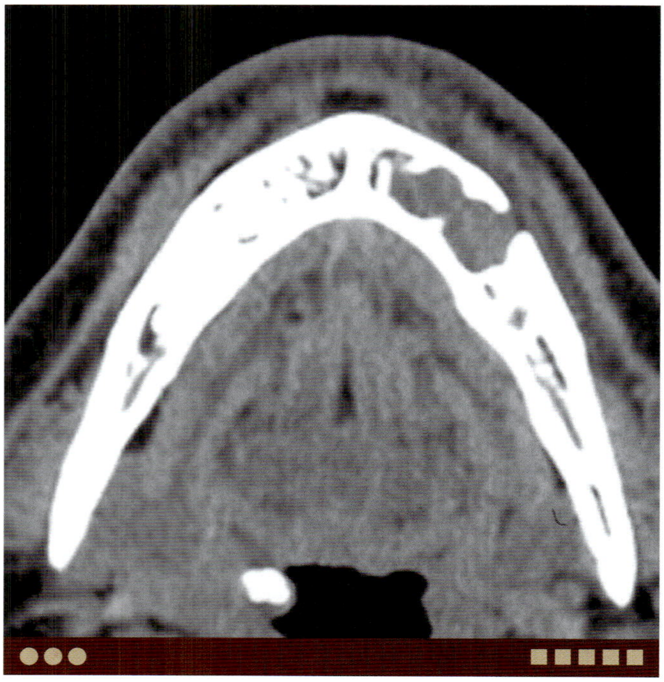

B. Odontogenic myxoma, same patient as A. Axial soft tissue window CT shows a lesion with soft tissue attenuation and scalloping border.

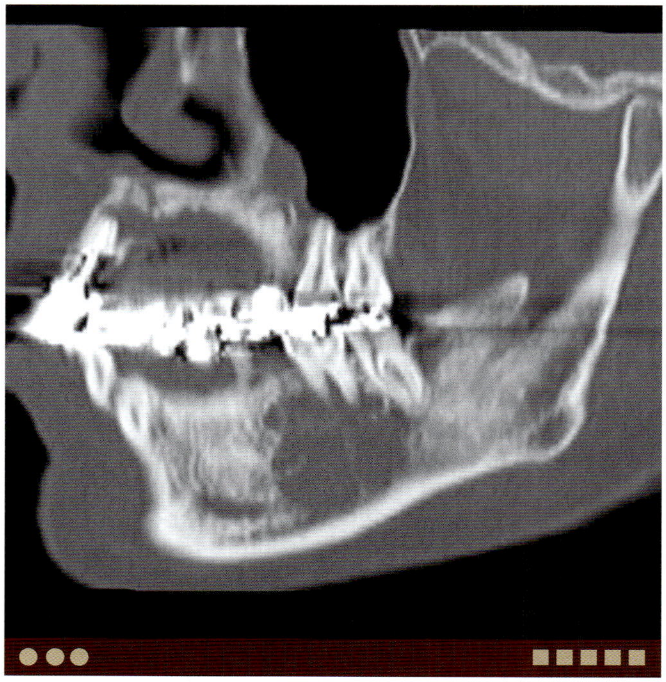

C. Odontogenic myxoma in a different patient. Sagittal bone window CT demonstrates a lucent lesion with slight lobulation in the mandibular body.

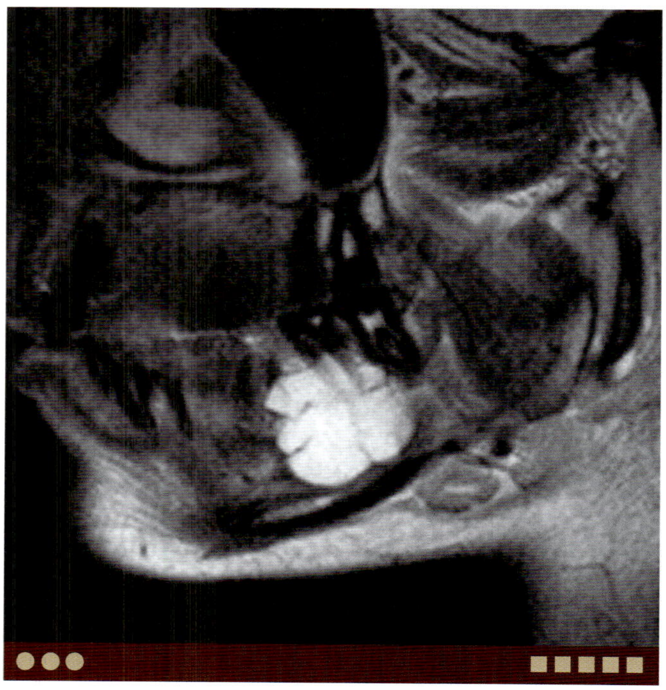

D. Odontogenic myxoma, same patient as C. Sagittal T2W MR image demonstrates a slightly lobulated high-signal lesion.

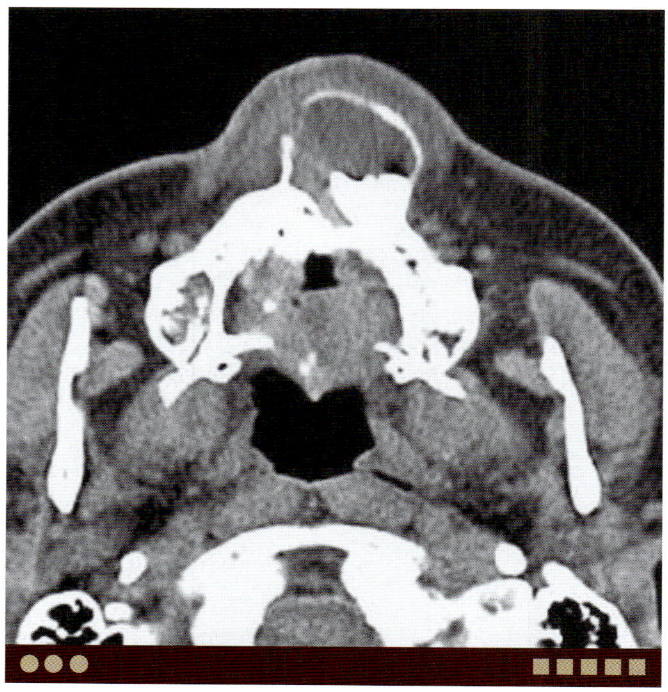

E. Odontogenic myxoma in a different patient. Axial soft tissue window CT shows an expansile lesion with a crown in the anterior maxilla.

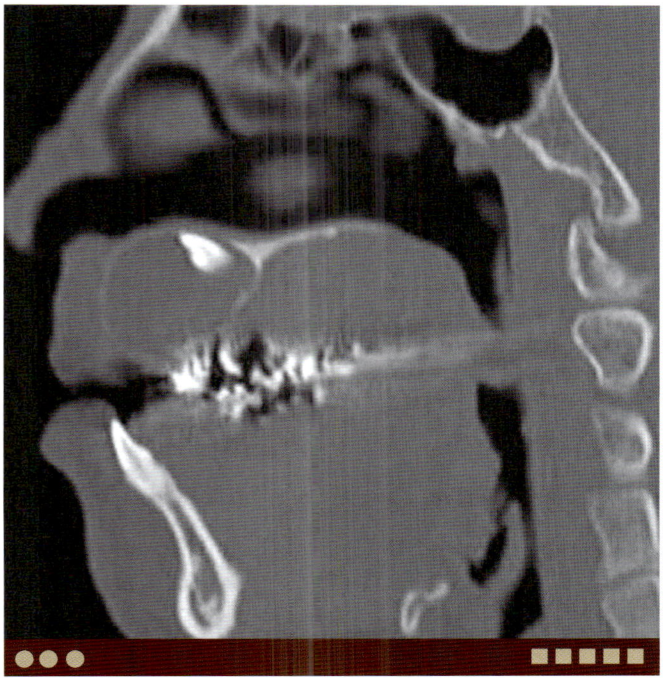

F. Odontogenic myxoma, same patient as E. Sagittal bone window CT shows an expansile lesion containing a tooth.

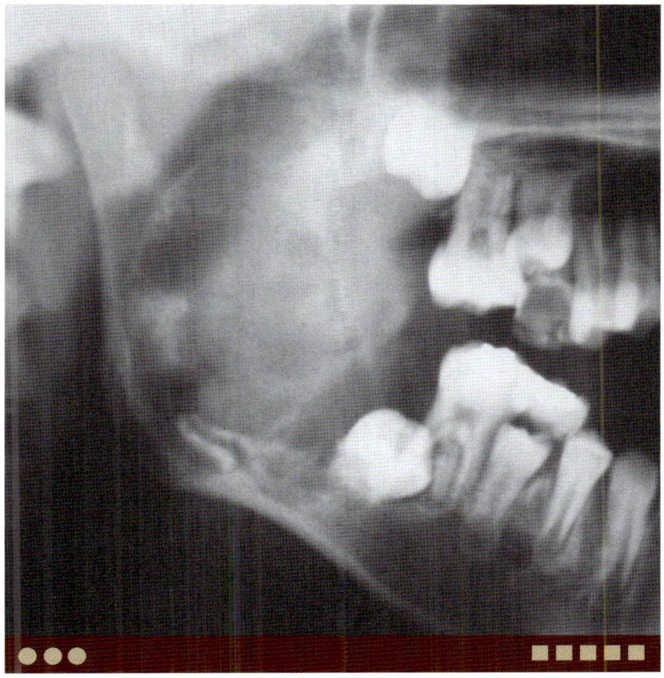

G. Odontogenic myxoma in a different patient. Magnified view of panoramic tomogram shows an expansile lesion in the posterior body/angle of the mandible.

DIFFERENTIAL DIAGNOSIS IMAGES (H-J)

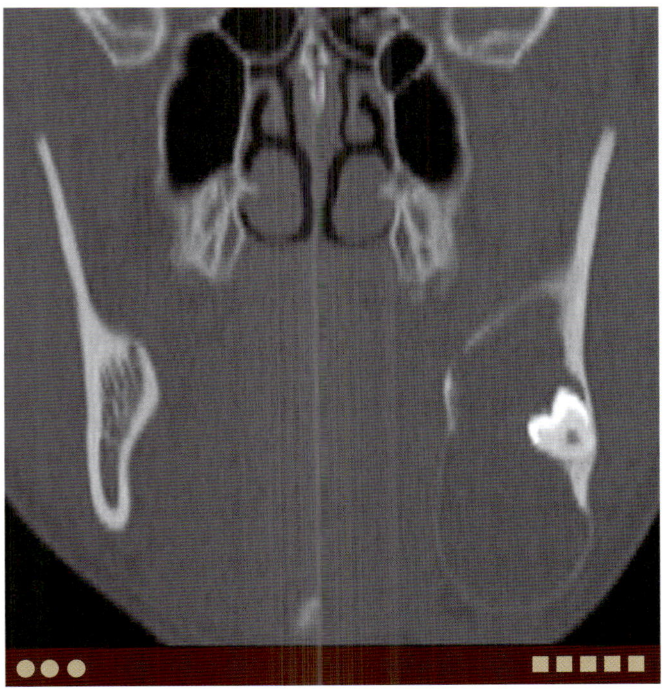

H. Ameloblastoma. Coronal bone window CT demonstrates a large, expansile lesion in the posterior body of the left mandible containing the crown.

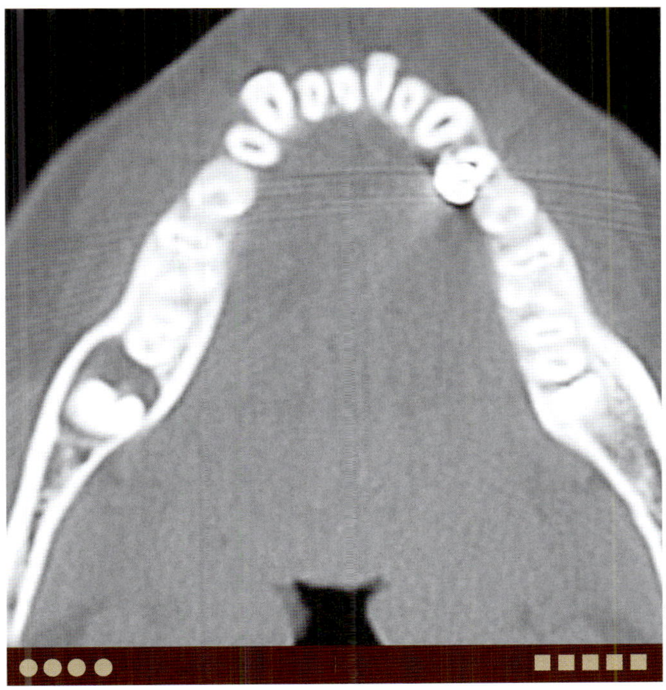

I. Dentigerous cyst. Axial bone window CT demonstrates a lucent lesion around the molar. Note the crown is identified in the cyst.

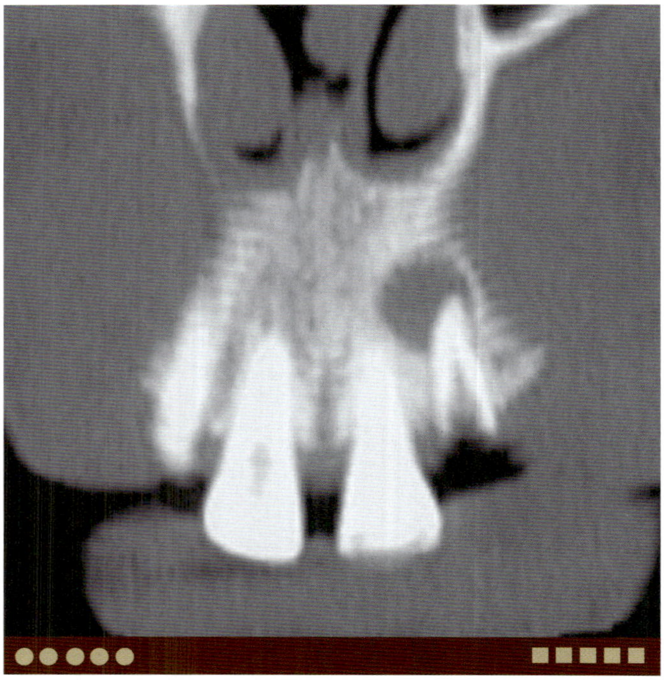

J. Periapical cyst. Coronal bone window CT demonstrates a cyst around the root of the lateral incisor. Note a cavity in the crown of the tooth.

Case 9–33 Simple Bone Cyst

Osamu Sakai, Andrew Akman, Anita Gohel

PRESENTATION

An incidental lucent lesion in the mandible.

FINDINGS

CT shows a large cystic-appearing lesion in the mandible involving and scalloping between multiple teeth roots.

DIFFERENTIAL DIAGNOSIS

- Keratocystic odontogenic tumor: This may be found around the crown of an impacted tooth, and cause expansion, displacement, and root resorption.
- Ameloblastoma: This demonstrates significant expansile change with thinning/erosion of the cortex, and resorption and displacement of the adjacent teeth.

COMMENTS

This is a 19-year-old man with a cystic lesion identified on dental radiograph.

Simple bone cysts are also known as traumatic, solitary, or hemorrhagic bone cysts. These lesions are not true cysts, but rather unilocular bony cavities filled with clear fluid, sanguineous fluid, or air. They are thought to result from trauma, which leads to intramedullary hemorrhage and subsequent resorption, although the exact mechanism is not known. They usually occur in the first two decades of life. They can also be seen in older patients within the lesions of cemento-osseous dysplasia.

These pseudocysts are most commonly located in the marrow space of the posterior mandible and appear slightly irregular with poorly defined borders. Classically these lesions are noted to "scallop" between the roots of adjacent teeth and are associated with cortical thinning. There should be no evidence of root resorption or tooth displacement. In addition, the mandibular cortex may be thinned secondary to osseous expansion. These lesions are often asymptomatic and may eventually resolve.

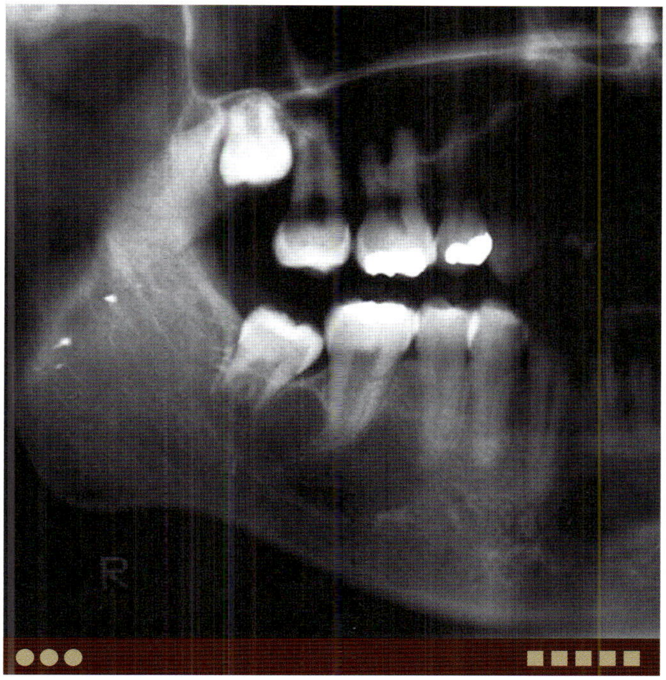

A. Simple bone cyst. Cone-downed view of panoramic radiograph demonstrates a cystic lesion without root resorption in the posterior body of the mandible.

PEARLS

- **Simple bone cysts are also known as traumatic, simple, or hemorrhagic bone cysts.**
- **Simple bone cysts are thought to result from trauma, which leads to intramedullary hemorrhage and subsequent resorption.**
- **There should be no root resorption or tooth displacement, but the cortex may be thinned.**

ADDITIONAL IMAGES (B-D)

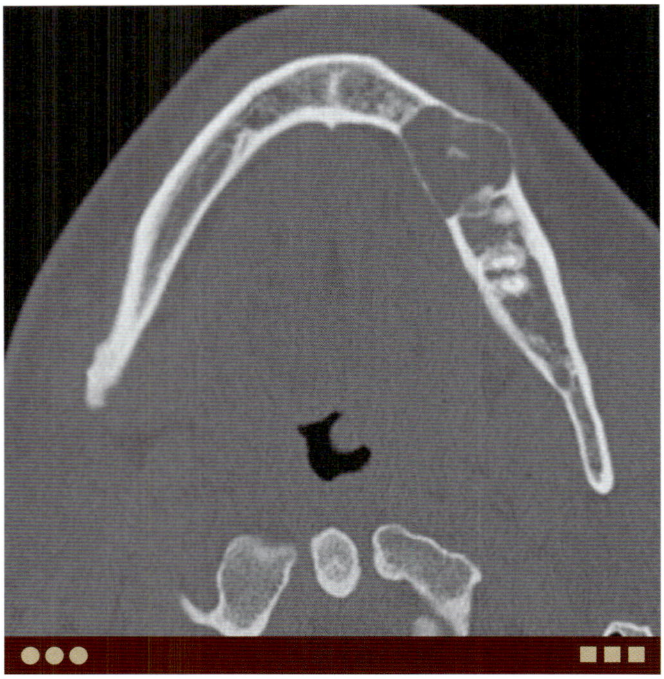

B. Simple bone cyst in a different patient. Axial CT demonstrates an expansile cystic lesion thinning the buccal and lingual cortex of the anterior mandible.

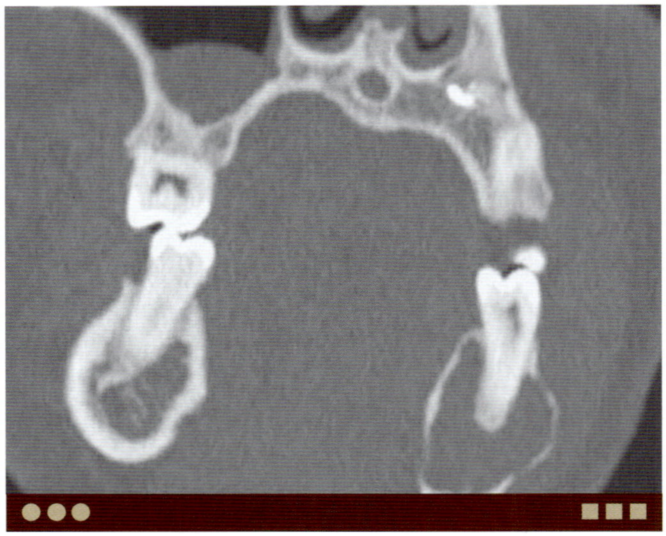

C. Simple bone cyst, same patient as B. Coronal CT demonstrates an expansile cystic lesion thinning the buccal and lingual cortex of the mandible. Note the intact tooth within the lesion.

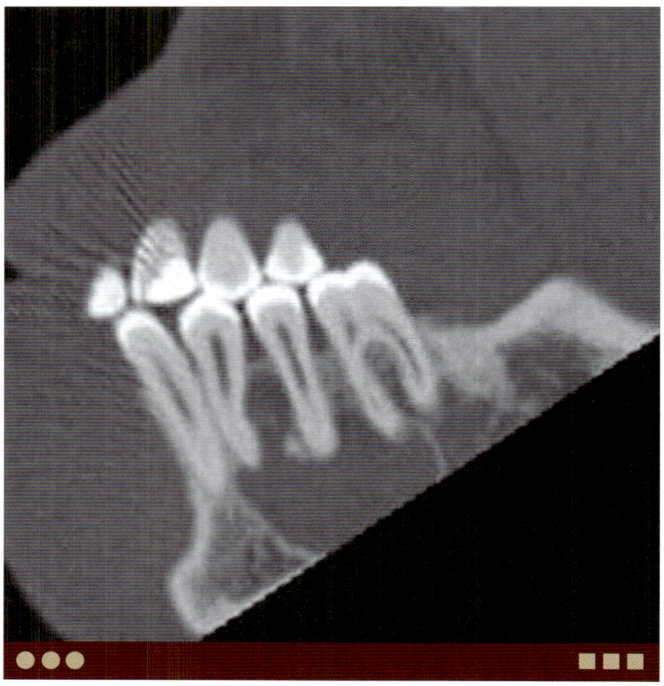

D. Simple bone cyst, same patient as B. Sagittal CT demonstrates a cystic lesion. There is no erosion or resorption of tooth roots within the lesion. The lesion appears to scallop between the roots without causing any significant displacement.

DIFFERENTIAL DIAGNOSIS IMAGES (E-G)

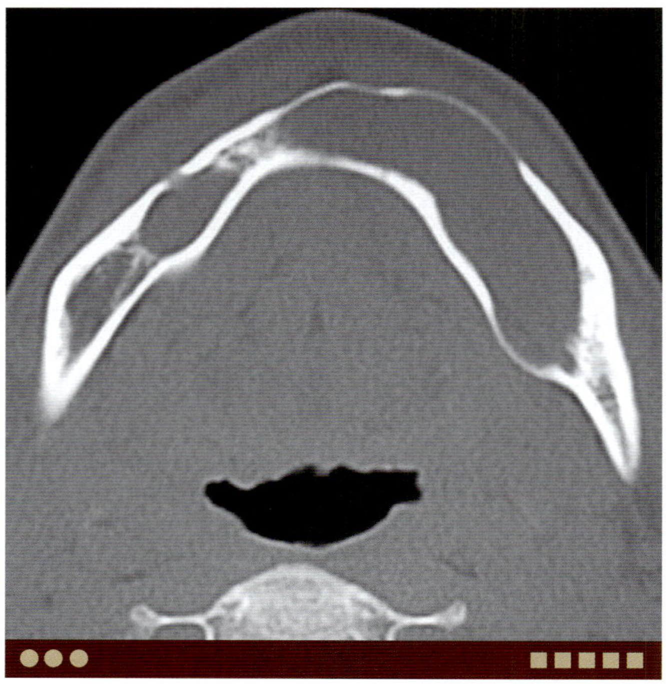

E. Keratocystic odontogenic tumor. Axial CT demonstrates a large cyst inside the marrow cavity of the anterior mandible with wavy scalloping cortical margin, causing expansion and thinning of the cortical boundaries.

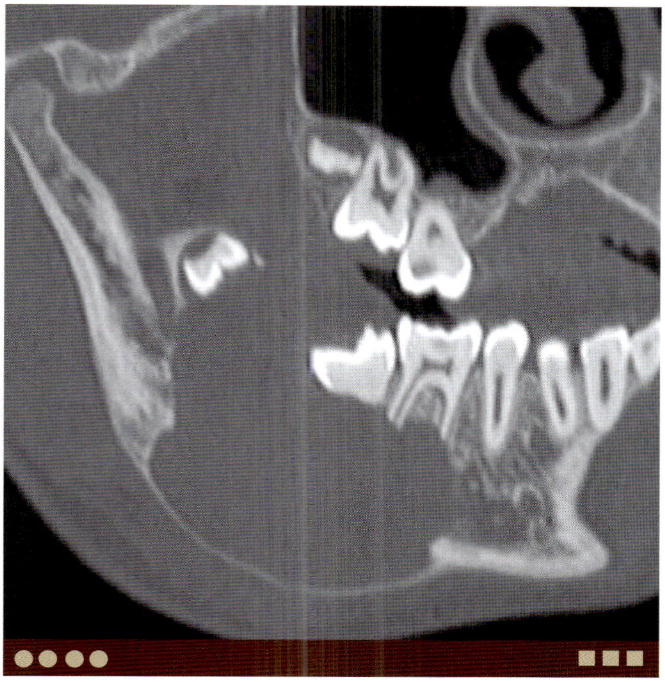

F. Dentigerous cyst. Oblique-sagittal CT demonstrates an expansile cystic lesion in the posterior mandible containing the crown of the third molar. Note the displacement of teeth, significant thinning of the mandibular cortex, and resorption of the associated roots, findings atypical for a dentigerous cyst.

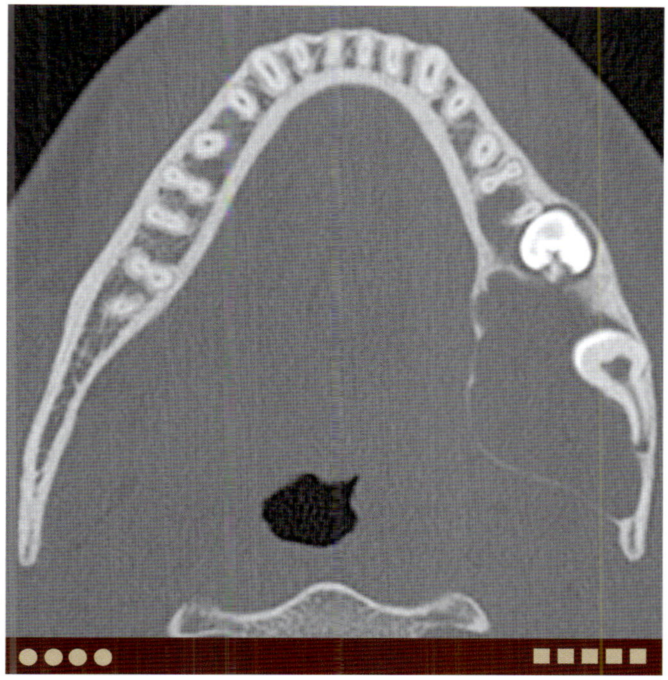

G. Ameloblastoma. Axial CT demonstrates an expansile cystic-appearing lesion in the posterior mandible containing the crown. Note the significant thinning of the lingual cortex of the mandible with expansion and displacement of teeth.

Chapter 10

LARYNX AND HYPOPHARYNX

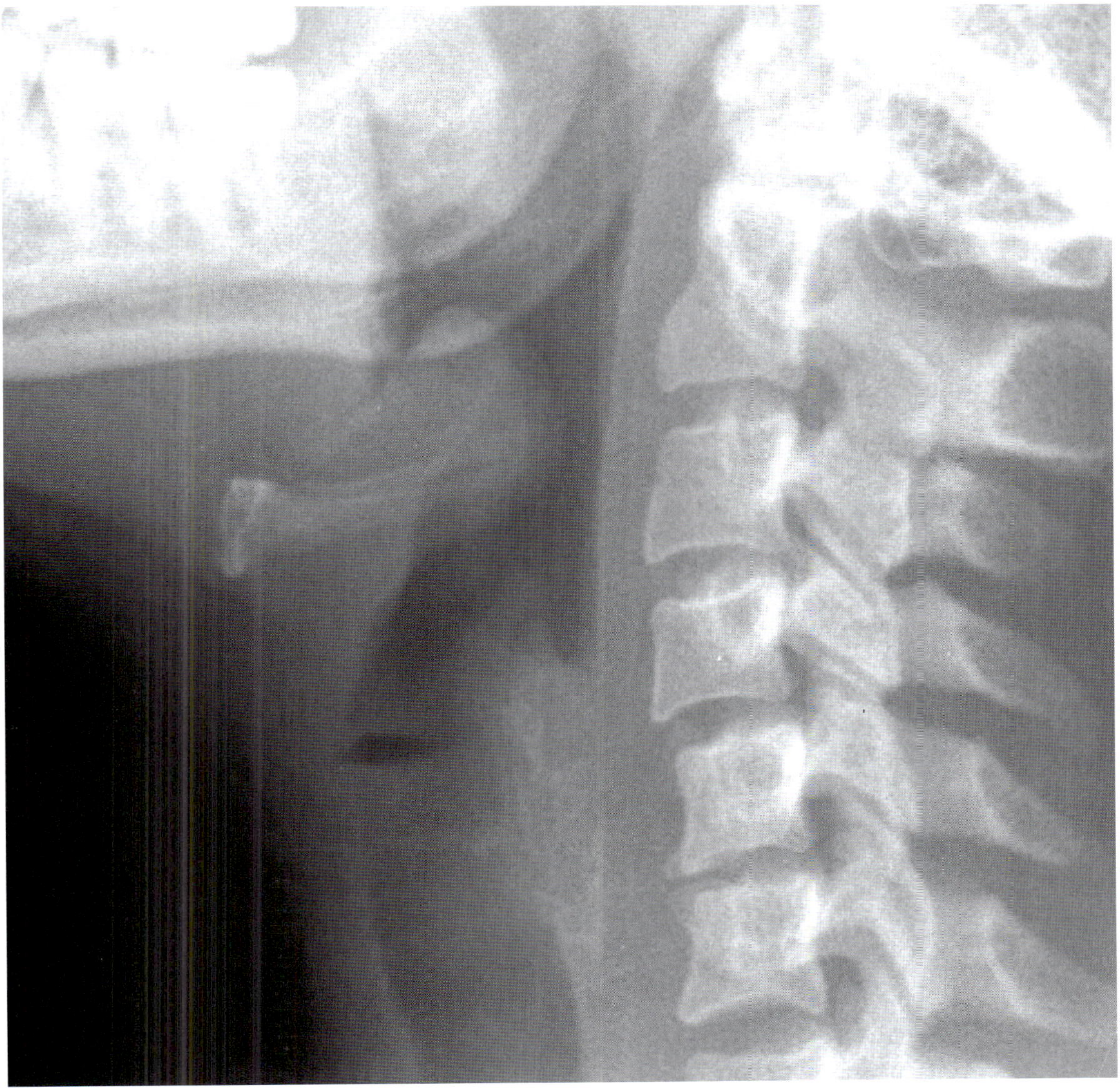

Case 10–1 Acute Epiglottitis/Supraglottitis

Osamu Sakai, Benjamin Ludwig

PRESENTATION

Fever, sore throat, drooling, respiratory distress, and posturing with neck extension.

FINDINGS

Lateral soft tissue neck radiograph demonstrates a thickened epiglottis and aryepiglottic folds. CT Neck with contrast demonstrates a thickened epiglottis.

DIFFERENTIAL DIAGNOSIS

- Angioedema: Results in rapid swelling/edema of the mucosa and submucosa. Although often mediated by allergies or complement (C1) deficiency, medications including angiotensin-converting enzyme (ACE) inhibitors are well-known causes of this condition.
- Omega epiglottis: This condition is often seen in patients with laryngomalacia, as a result of the tightly curled epiglottis, in the shape of the Greek letter omega when viewed during laryngoscopy. This finding may also be seen when the epiglottis is imaged in an oblique manner.
- Postradiation change: Thickening of the epiglottis is often seen after radiation. This should be easily differentiated from acute epiglottitis by the history and symptoms, and related findings within the soft tissues, including reticulation within the subcutaneous fat and platysmal thickening.
- Amyloidosis: Extracellular deposition of abnormal proteins results in a thickened epiglottis, sometimes with calcification.
- Caustic injury: Thermal or chemical irritation of the oropharynx, epiglottis, and upper gastrointestinal tract results in mucosal edema, resulting in a thickened epiglottis.

COMMENTS

This is an 18 year-old woman with sore throat, hoarse voice, and difficulty swallowing.

Acute epiglottitis/supraglottitis is a true emergency and one of the most serious conditions of the larynx given the potential for airway compromise. Fever, sore throat, drooling, posturing with neck extension, and respiratory distress are common clinical symptoms. If untreated, rapid respiratory decompensation follows.

Historically, epiglottitis occurs in children, with *Haemophilus influenzae* as the most common etiology.

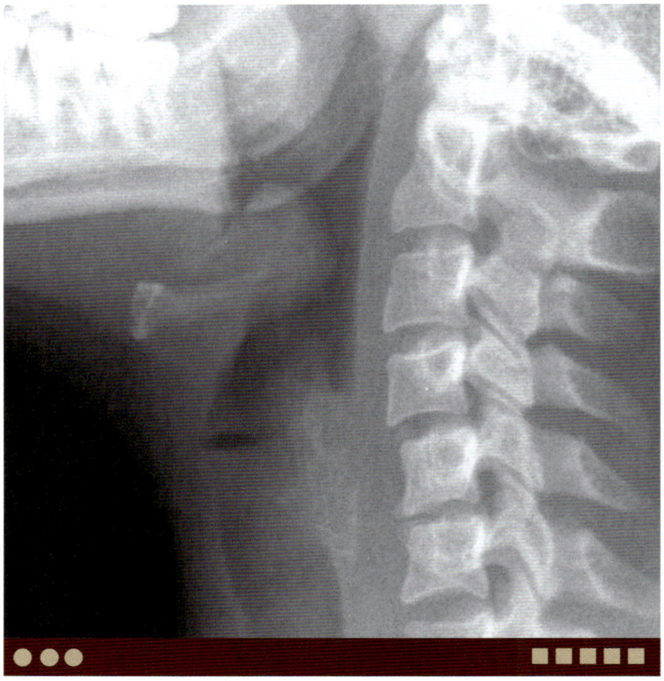

A. Epiglottitis. Lateral radiograph demonstrates a thickened, bulbous epiglottis.

Patients are typically slightly older than the typical age distribution for laryngotracheobronchitis (croup), with the most common ages ranging from 1 to 5 years. Given routine *H. influenzae* vaccination in children, the incidence has decreased markedly in the pediatric population. Recent literature suggests that epiglottitis is now more common in adults and may even affect those previously immunized against *H. influenzae*.

As epiglottitis is a clinical diagnosis, imaging should not delay bronchoscopy or securing an airway. If the patient's condition permits, an upright, lateral neck radiograph is the

PEARLS

- **Acute epiglottitis is a true emergency and one of the most serious conditions of the larynx.**
- **With high clinical suspicion for epiglottitis, the patient's clinical condition and airway management take precedent over imaging.**
- **Upright, lateral neck radiograph is the imaging modality of choice, and demonstrates a swollen epiglottis, resulting in the classic "thumb sign" and thickening of the aryepiglottic folds.**

imaging modality of choice in suspected epiglottitis. An edematous epiglottis results in the classic radiographic "thumb sign," with the additional finding of aryepiglottic fold thickening.

CT is not necessary and not recommended in the acute setting, as supine positioning is avoided in the potentially unstable patient. CT, however, may be performed in patients with unsuspected epiglottitis and reveal significantly thickened epiglottis and aryepiglottic folds. CT may also evaluate additional causes of epiglottic/aryepiglottic fold thickening, including caustic ingestion, laryngeal edema (angioedema), foreign body, hemorrhage, epiglottic cyst, amyloidosis, and postradiation edema/fibrosis.

ADDITIONAL IMAGES (B-E)

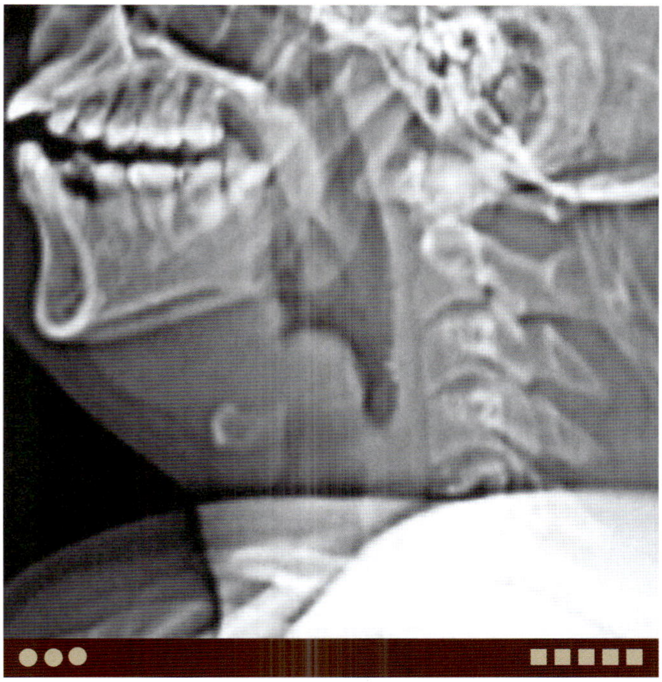

B. Epiglottitis in a different patient. Lateral scout image of CT demonstrates thickened epiglottis.

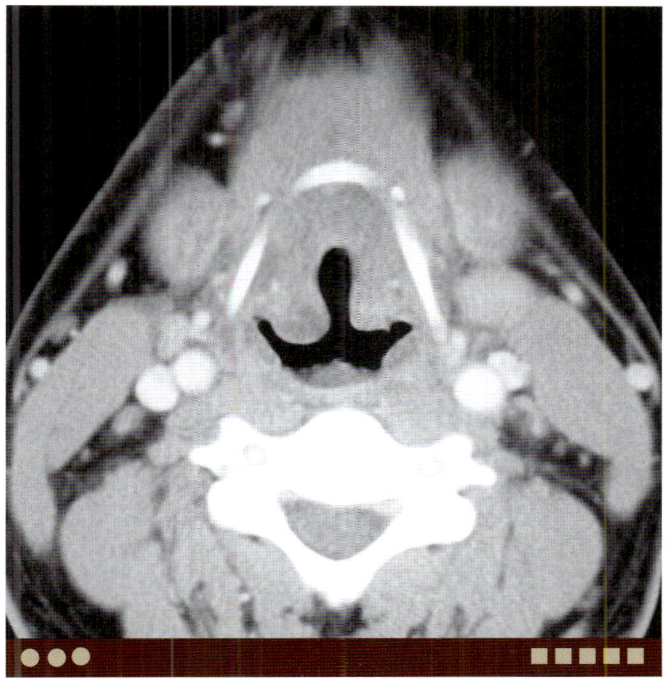

C. Epiglottitis, same patient as B. Axial contrast-enhanced CT demonstrates thickened aryepiglottic folds.

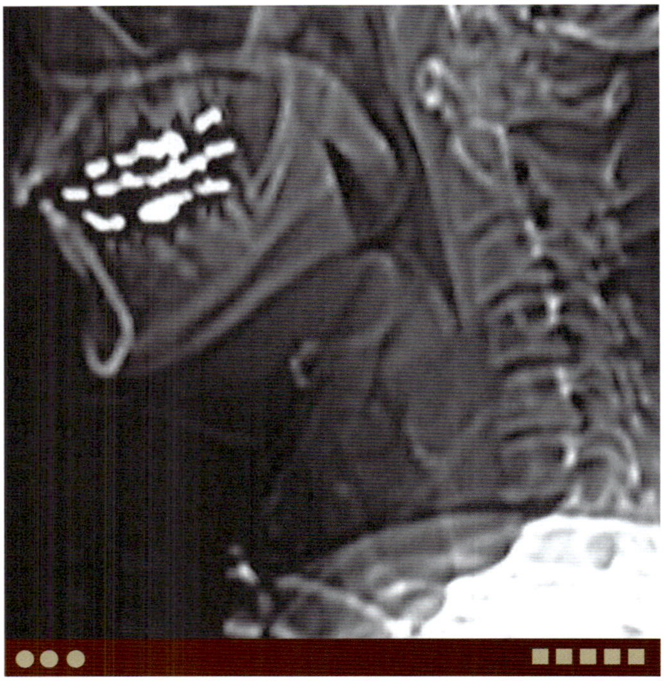

D. Epiglottitis in a different patient. Lateral scout image of CT demonstrates significantly thickened epiglottis.

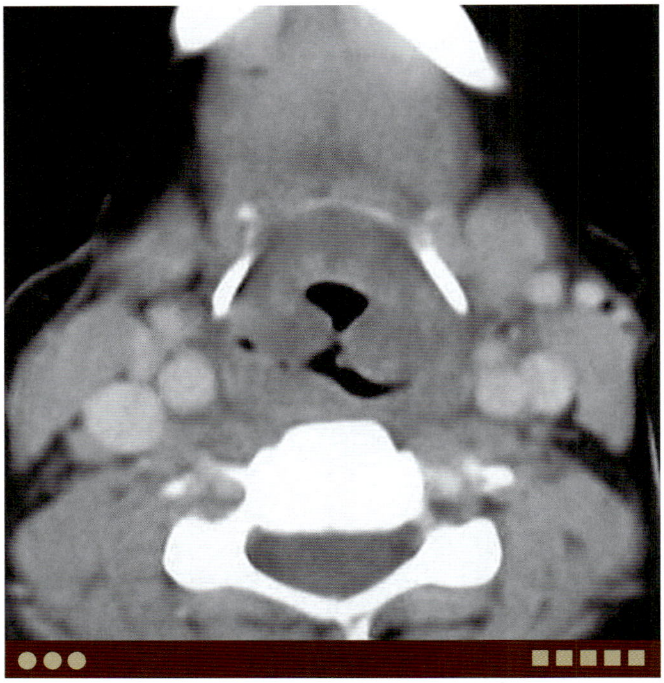

E. Epiglottitis, same patient as D. Axial contrast-enhanced CT demonstrates thickened aryepiglottic fold.

DIFFERENTIAL DIAGNOSIS IMAGES (F-H)

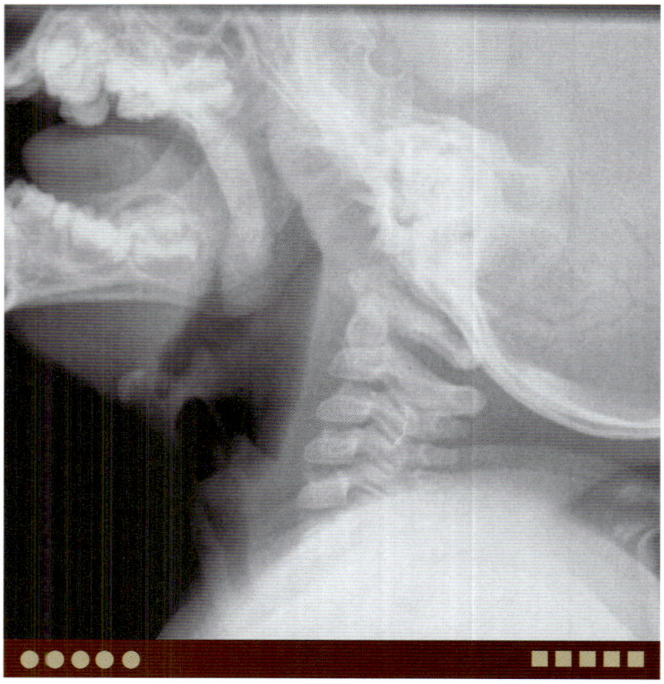

F. Croup (laryngotracheobronchitis). Lateral radiograph demonstrates subglottic narrowing and overdistension of the hypopharynx.

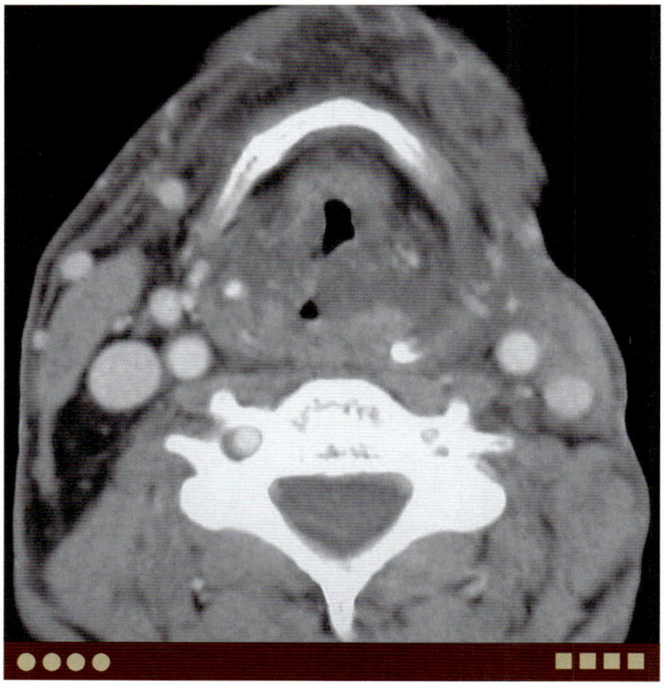

G. Postradiation laryngeal edema. Axial contrast-enhanced CT shows a thickened epiglottis demonstrating heterogeneous density. Note edematous changes in the subcutaneous fat in the anterior neck, and changes from left-sided neck dissection.

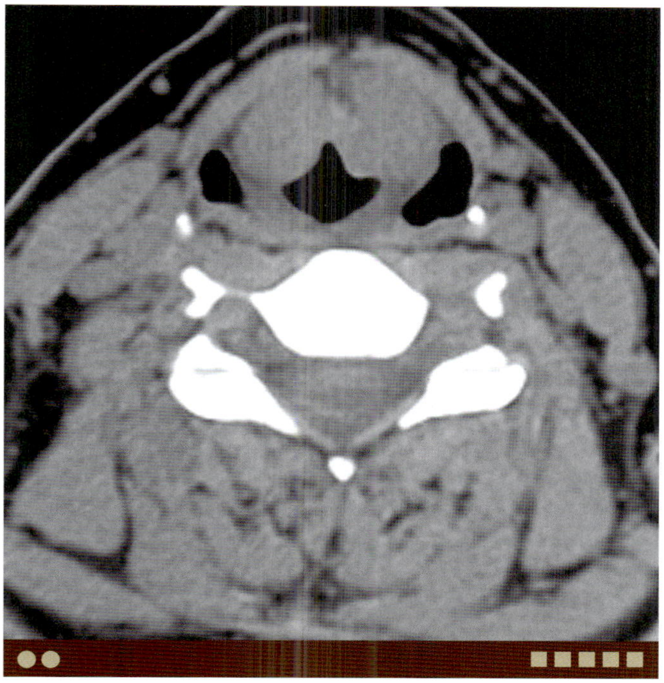

H. Amyloidosis. Axial noncontrast CT demonstrates homogeneous density lesions in the aryepiglottic folds.

Case 10–2 Laryngeal Edema (Angioedema)

Osamu Sakai, Jimmy Wang

PRESENTATION

Hoarseness and dyspnea.

FINDINGS

CT demonstrates edema in the soft tissues of the larynx narrowing the airway.

DIFFERENTIAL DIAGNOSIS

- Acute epiglottitis: This is most commonly caused by *H. influenzae* infection. Fever and sore throat is a common presentation.
- Omega epiglottis: This condition is often seen in patients with laryngomalacia. The shortened aryepiglottic folds cause the epiglottis to be furled.
- Postradiation change: Thickening of the epiglottis and other laryngeal tissues is often seen after radiation. This should be easily differentiated from acute epiglottitis by the history and symptoms.
- Amyloidosis: This condition may cause diffusely thickened epiglottis and other laryngeal tissues, sometimes with calcification.

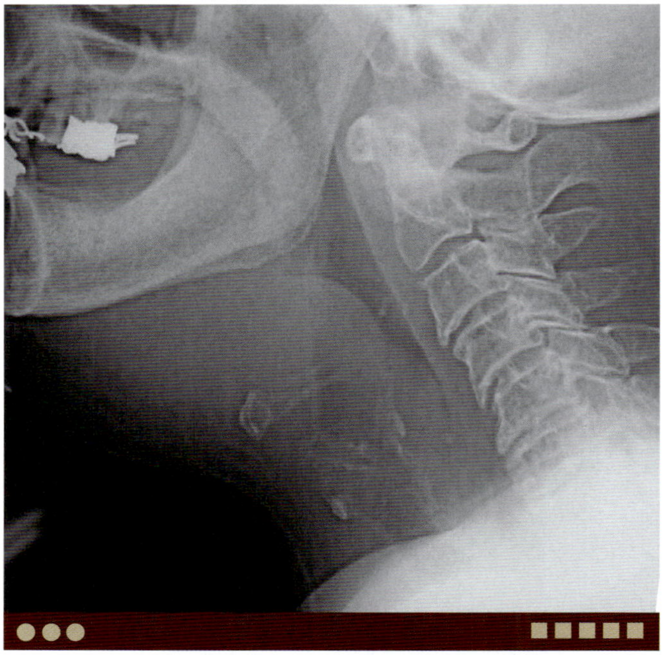

A. Laryngeal edema. Lateral radiograph demonstrates significant thickening of the supraglottic soft tissues.

COMMENTS

This is a 66-year-old man with hoarseness and dyspnea.

Laryngeal edema, angioedema, is diagnosed clinically and requires emergent treatment without imaging. This condition is rapid swelling/edema of the skin, mucosa, and submucosal tissues, mediated by an allergic reaction. ACE inhibitors are well-known cause of this condition. There are several causes of laryngeal edema: (1) hereditary angioedema, (2) acquired angioedema, (3) angioedema associated with allergic reactions, often associated with urticaria, (4) angioedema secondary to medications, and (5) idiopathic angioedema.

If imaging is performed, edema and soft tissue swelling of the larynx, narrowing the airway are seen. Similar findings can also be seen during or after radiation therapy for head and neck cancers, which may persist for a long time. Therefore, clinical findings and appropriate history are important for diagnosis and patient management.

PEARLS

- **Laryngeal edema, angioedema, is diagnosed clinically and requires emergent treatment.**
- **Diffuse swelling of the mucosa and submucosal tissues are seen in the larynx, narrowing the airway.**

ADDITIONAL IMAGES (B-C)

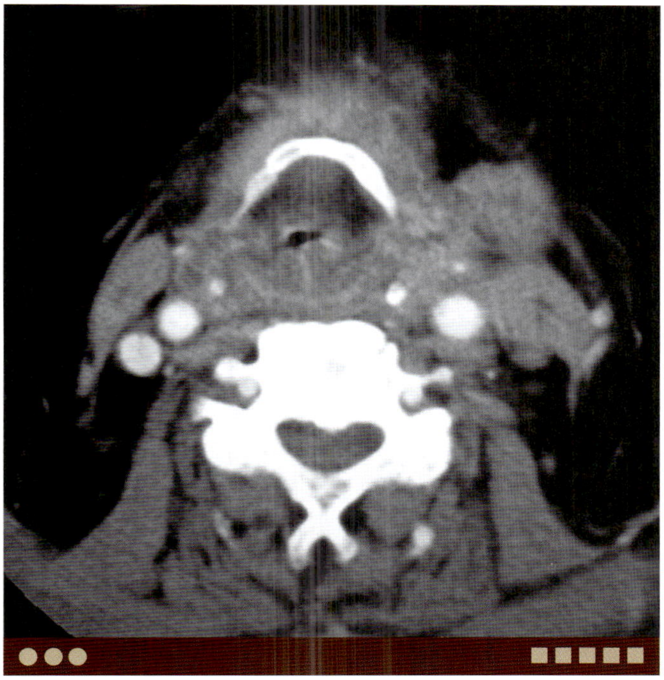

B. Laryngeal edema, same patient as A. Axial postcontrast CT demonstrates thickening of the submucosal tissues in the supraglottic larynx narrowing the airway.

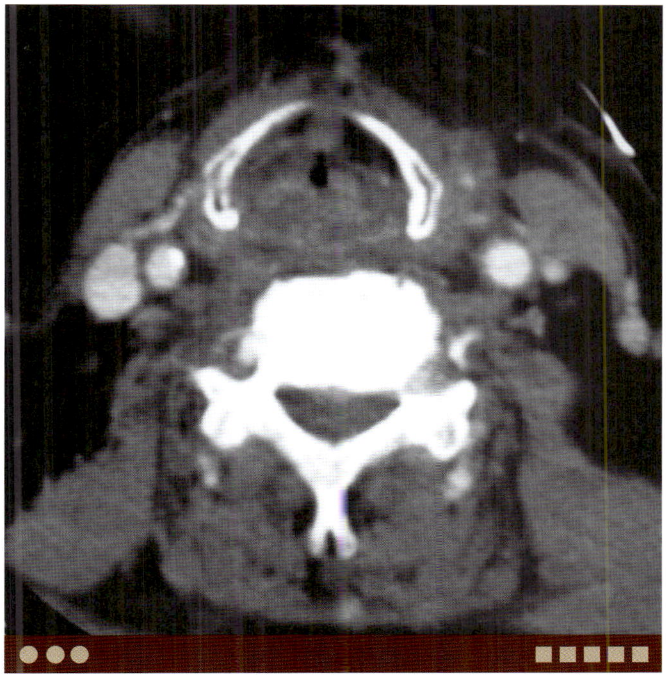

C. Laryngeal edema, same patient as A. Axial postcontrast CT demonstrates thickening of the submucosal tissues in the glottic larynx narrowing the airway.

DIFFERENTIAL DIAGNOSIS IMAGES (D-G)

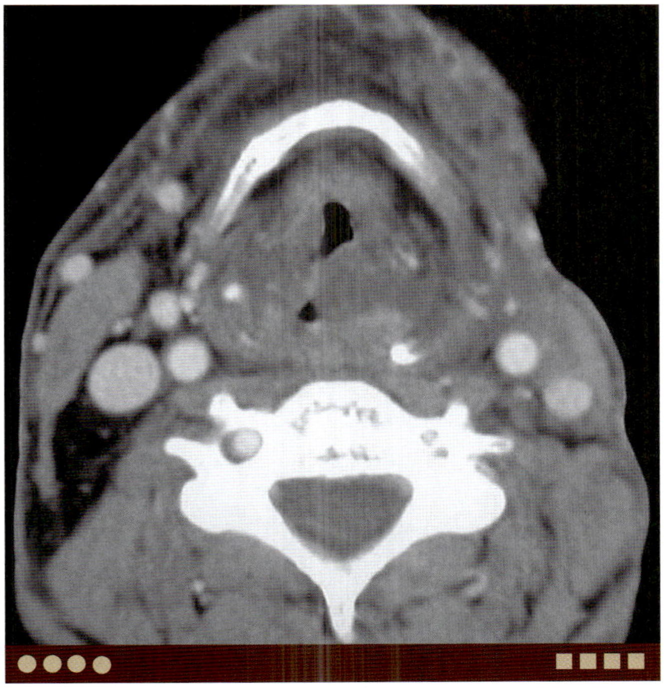

D. Postradiation laryngeal edema. Axial postcontrast CT demonstrates a thickened epiglottis demonstrating heterogeneous density. Note edematous changes in the subcutaneous fat in the anterior neck and changes from left-sided neck dissection.

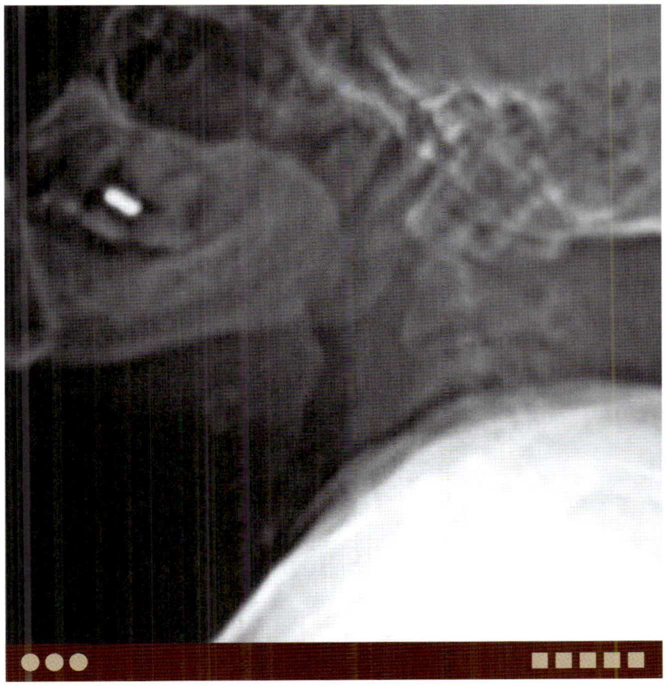

E. Retropharyngeal edema. Lateral scout view of CT demonstrates retropharyngeal/prevertebral soft tissue thickening.

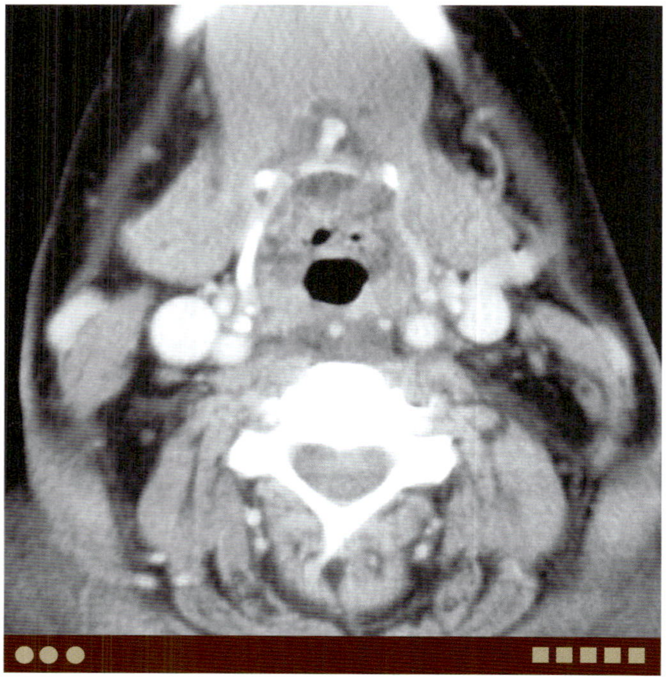

F. Retropharyngeal edema, same patient as E. Axial postcontrast CT demonstrates edema and thickening of the retropharyngeal space. The airway is preserved.

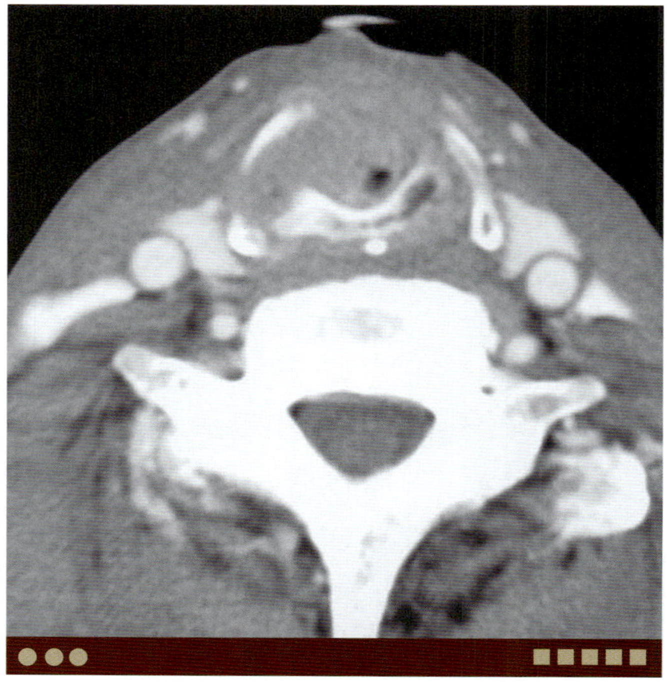

G. Squamous cell carcinoma. Axial postcontrast CT demonstrates a heterogeneously enhancing soft tissue mass lesion narrowing the laryngeal lumen. Note invasion and destruction of the anterior portion of the thyroid lamina and right cricoid cartilage.

Case 10–3 Laryngocele, Saccular Cyst

Osamu Sakai, Jimmy Wang

PRESENTATION

Incidental finding; sometimes dysphasia and dyspnea.

FINDINGS

CT demonstrates air density or fluid-filled cyst in the lateral supraglottic larynx.

DIFFERENTIAL DIAGNOSIS

- Vallecular cyst: This is a retention cyst in the vallecula.
- Thyroglossal cyst: This is a congenital/developmental cyst and located in the midline around the hyoid level.
- Squamous cell carcinoma (SCCA): SCCA is the most common malignant tumor of the larynx. Further, laryngoceles may be secondary to obstruction of the laryngeal ventricle by SCCA.
- Schwannoma: This is a rare tumor, however, important for the differential diagnosis of submucosal tumors in the larynx. This often arises in the supraglottic larynx.

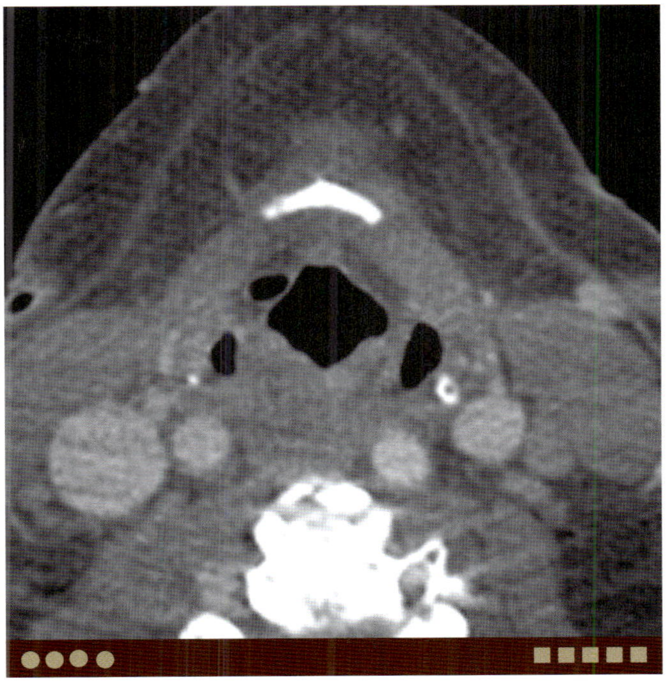

A. Laryngocele. Axial CT demonstrates a small air density in the right supraglottic fat.

COMMENTS

This is a 58-year-old man with hoarseness.

A laryngocele is an air-filled, saccular dilatation of the laryngeal ventricular appendix. If it is filled with fluid, it is called a saccular cyst. Laryngoceles are often seen in glassblowers due to continual forced expiration producing elevated pressures in the larynx, and also seen in people with chronic obstructive airway disease. It is often asymptomatic; however, occasionally it causes dysphasia and dyspnea. The symptom varies depending on its location and size.

Sometimes, laryngoceles protrudes laterally between the hyoid and thyroid cartilage, lateral to the thyrohyoid membrane; this is called an external laryngocele. The ones confined medial to the thyrohyoid membrane is called an internal laryngocele. If the lesion is seen in both sides of the thyrohyoid membrane, it is called a mixed laryngocele. However, based on the mechanism, there is no pure external laryngocele.

There is no clinical significance in laryngocele itself. However, laryngoceles may be due to obstruction of the laryngeal ventricle by a small glottic cancer. Therefore, when a laryngocele is identified on images, careful radiological and clinical evaluation for glottic cancer is needed.

PEARLS

- **Laryngocele is an air-filled, saccular dilatation of the laryngeal ventricular appendix.**
- **If it is fluid filled, it is called as a saccular cyst.**
- **Laryngocele may be due to a small glottic cancer obstructing the laryngeal ventricle.**

ADDITIONAL IMAGES (B-D)

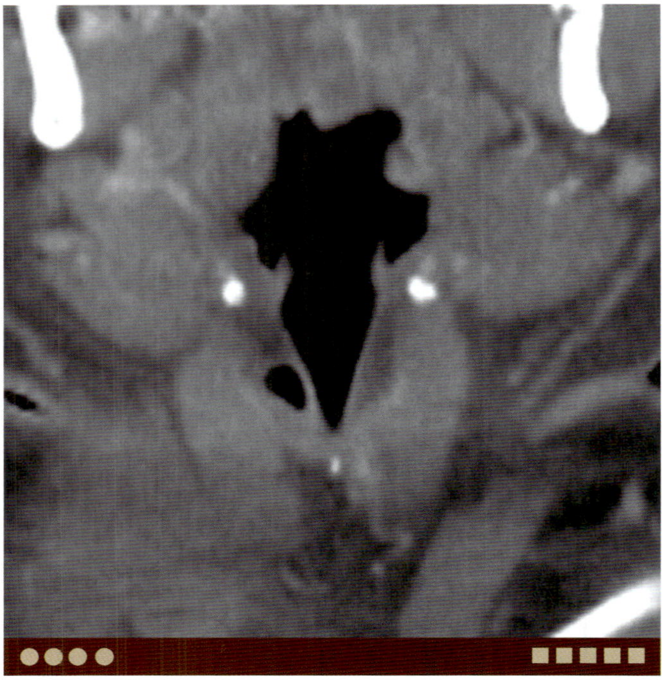

B. Laryngocele, same patient as A. Coronal CT demonstrates craniocaudally elongated air density in the right supraglottic fat.

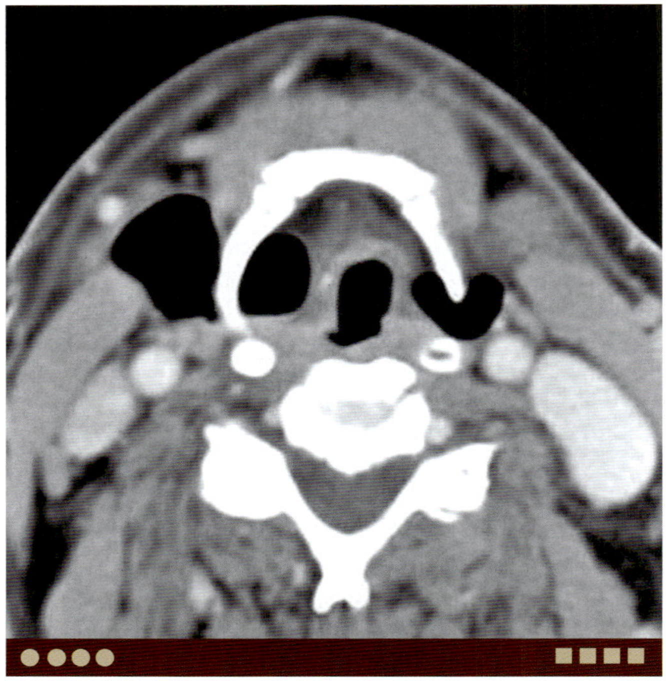

C. Bilateral laryngoceles in a different patient. Axial CT demonstrates a larger "external" component of laryngocele on the right.

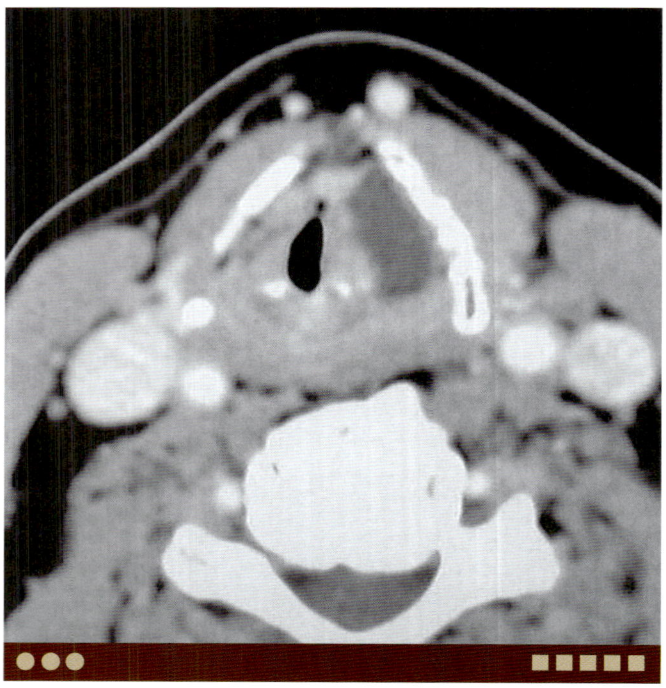

D. Saccular cyst. Axial postcontrast CT demonstrates a fluid-filled lesion in the left paraglottic space.

DIFFERENTIAL DIAGNOSIS IMAGES (E-G)

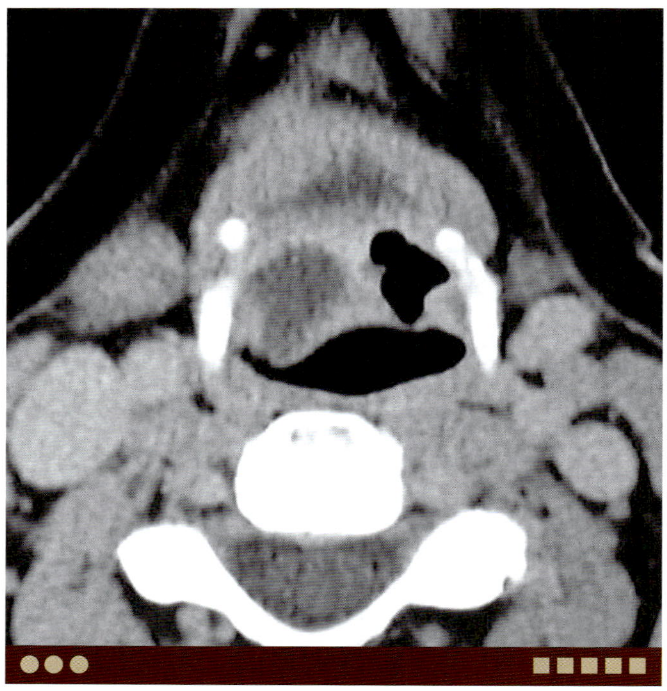

E. Vallecular cyst. Axial postcontrast CT demonstrates a fluid-filled lesion in the right valleculla.

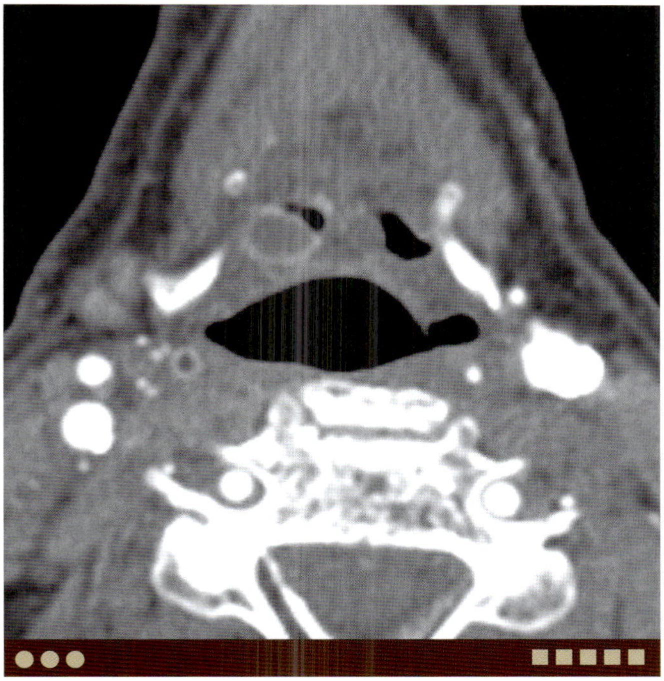

F. Vallecular cyst in a different patient. Axial postcontrast CT demonstrates a rim-enhancing fluid-filled lesion in the right vallecula.

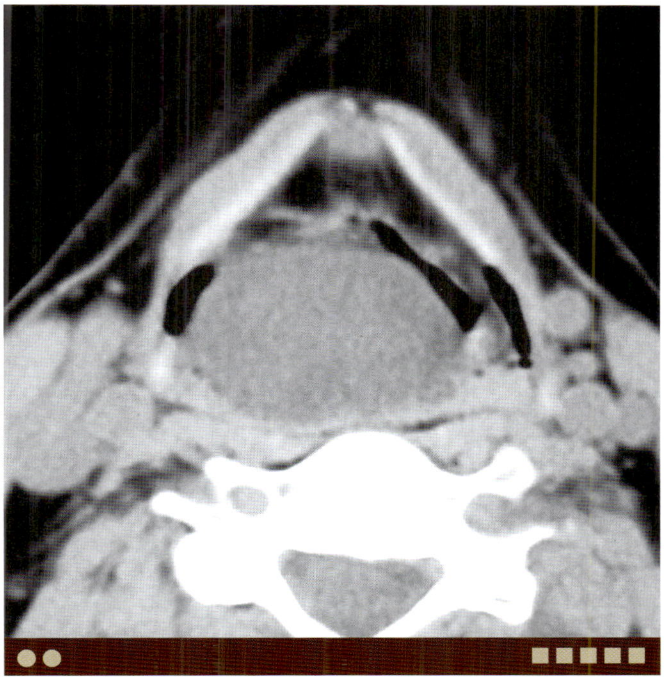

G. Schwannoma. Axial noncontrast CT demonstrates a homogeneous low-density lesion in the supraglottic larynx.

Case 10–4 Hypopharyngeal Squamous Cell Carcinoma

Osamu Sakai, Jimmy Wang

PRESENTATION

Ear pain.

FINDINGS

CT demonstrates an ill-defined heterogeneous density lesion in the pyriform sinus.

DIFFERENTIAL DIAGNOSIS

- Lymphoma: This usually demonstrates more homogeneous density or signal compared with squamous cell carcinoma (SCCA).
- Adenoid cystic carcinoma: This is a relatively rare tumor arising from the minor salivary gland. Imaging findings can be similar to SCCA and indistinguishable.
- Amyloidosis: This demonstrates nodular mucosal thickening or submucosal mass often with calcification.

COMMENTS

This is a 63-year-old man with left ear pain.

The tip of the pyriform sinus is one of the blind spots for the ENT clinician. Lesions deep in the pyriform sinus are often difficult to detect clinically. Therefore, imaging plays an important role in diagnosing such lesions. Patients with hypopharyngeal SCCA often present with a neck mass, which is a nodal metastasis, or ear pain (referred pain associated with the glossopharyngeal nerve) without known primary lesion. The pyriform sinus is one of the primary sites for nodal metastasis from unknown primary with nasopharynx, tonsils, and base of tongue being the other areas. These anatomical sites must be carefully evaluated radiologically as well as clinically. At the time of diagnosis of hypopharyngeal carcinoma, nodal metastasis is already present in about 75% of cases, and 15% are bilateral. Five to fifteen percent of patients with hypopharyngeal carcinoma have a second primary lesion; therefore, the entire aerodigestive tract should be carefully evaluated.

On imaging, it is important to confirm symmetry of the hypopharynx. Even very subtle asymmetry may suggest underlying tumor in an appropriate clinical setting such as nodal metastasis or ear pain. The lesion is often mainly submucosal without apparent mucosal abnormality.

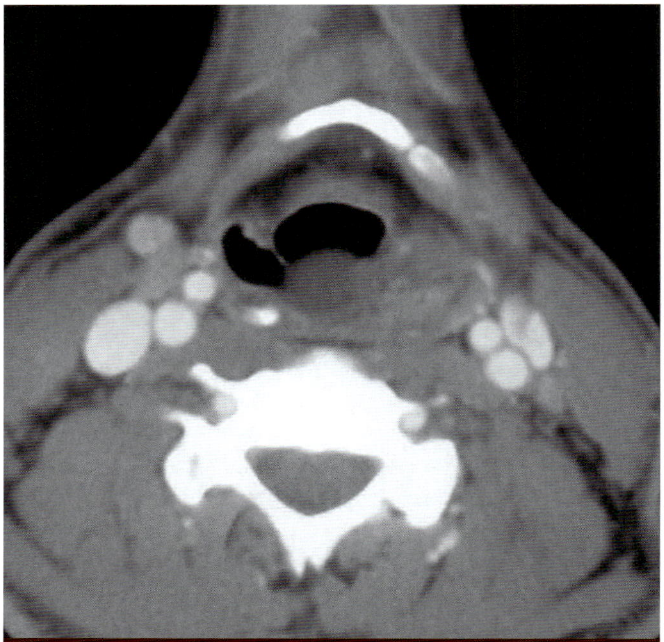

A. Hypopharyngeal SCCA. Axial CT demonstrates a heterogeneously enhancing tumor occupying the left pyriform sinus. Note tumor extension to the paraglottic fat.

It is often difficult to diagnose the primary site in tumors involving the medial aspect of the pyriform sinus and aryepiglottic fold, hypopharyngeal versus supraglottic laryngeal carcinomas. However, laryngeal extension of hypopharyngeal carcinoma is more common than hypopharyngeal extension of supraglottic laryngeal carcinomas.

PEARLS

- **The hypopharynx is one of the primary sites for cervical nodal metastasis from unknown primary site.**
- **The tip of the pyriform sinus is a blind spot for the clinician. Therefore, imaging plays an important role.**
- **Otalgia, ear pain, is a common presentation for hypopharyngeal tumors.**

ADDITIONAL IMAGES (B-E)

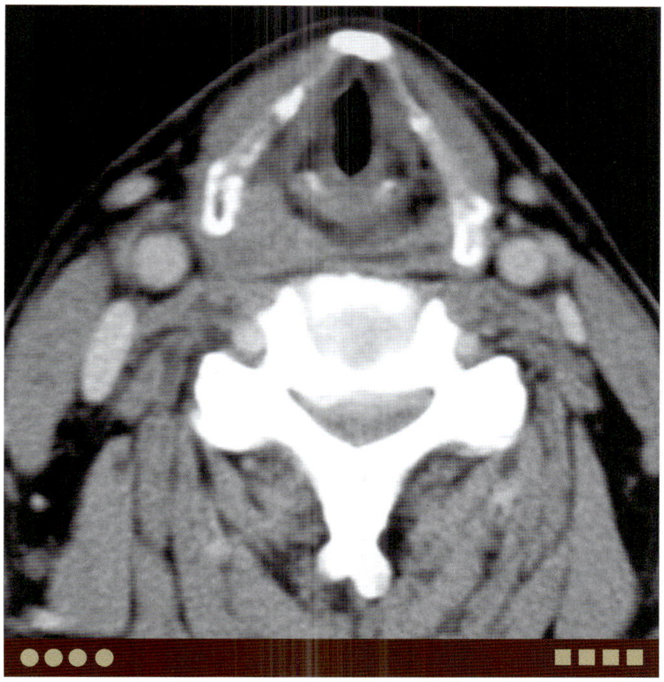

B. Hypopharyngeal SCCA in a different patient. Axial CT demonstrates asymmetry in the right hypopharyngeal soft tissue, posterolateral to the right arytenoid cartilage.

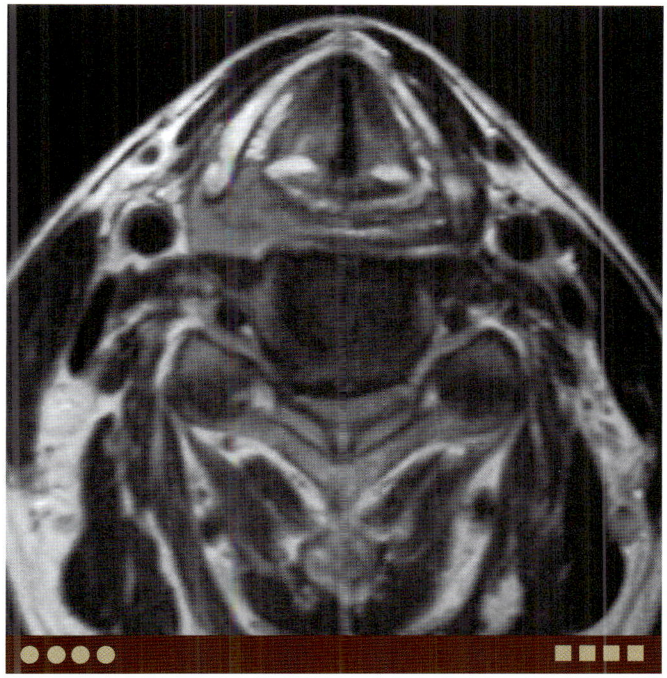

C. Hypopharyngeal SCCA, same patient as B. Axial T2W MR image demonstrates a lesion demonstrating slightly increased signal, posterolateral to the right arytenoid cartilage. This is SCCA arising from the tip of the right pyriform sinus.

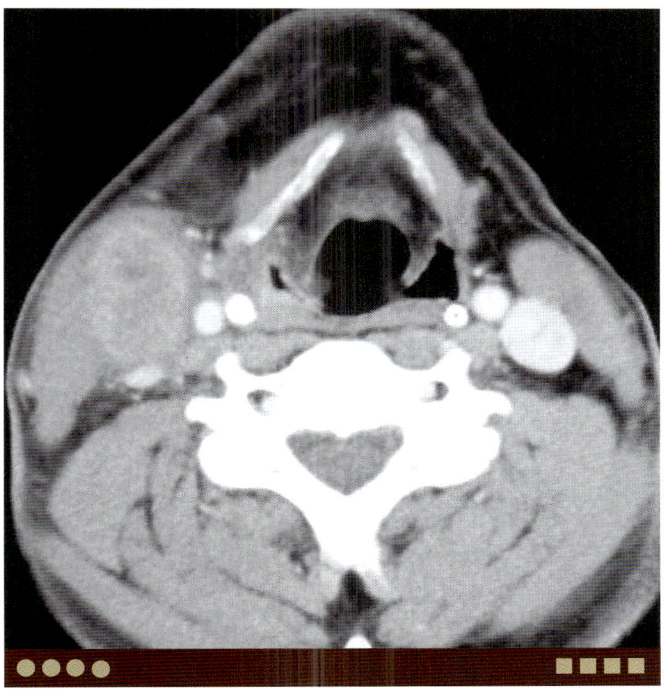

D. Hypopharyngeal SCCA in a different patient. Axial CT demonstrates heterogeneously enhancing deformed right pyriform sinus. Note a heterogeneously enhancing enlarged node in the right level III with ill-defined margins, representing extracapsular tumor spread.

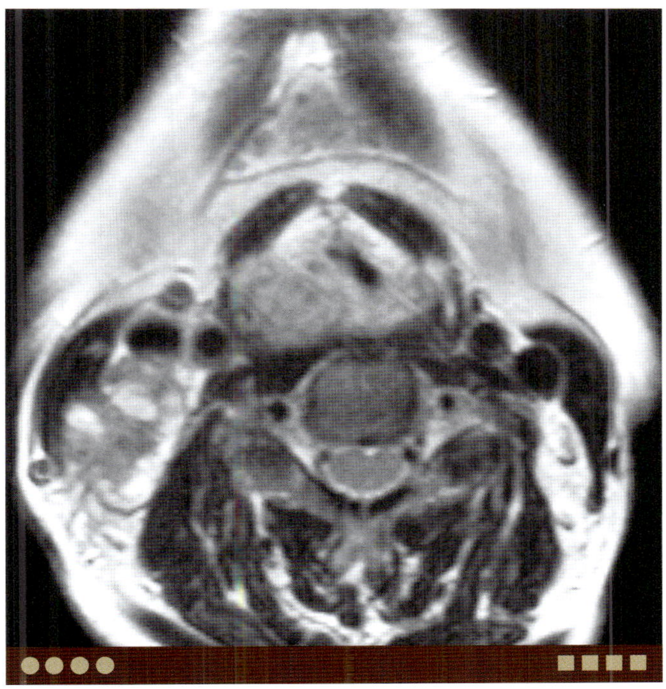

E. Hypopharyngeal SCCA in a different patient. Axial T2W image demonstrates a submucosal lesion in the right pyriform sinus with necrotic right level III nodes.

DIFFERENTIAL DIAGNOSIS IMAGES (F-G)

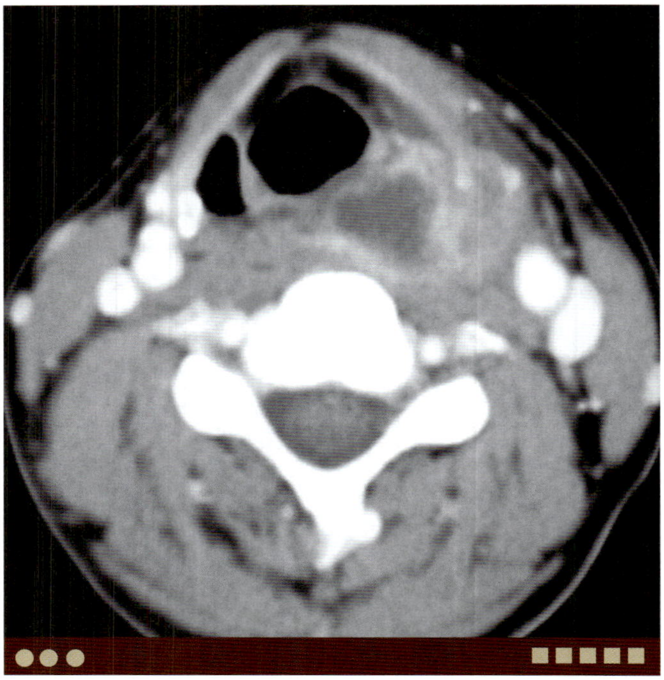

F. Pyriform sinus fistula, developmental anomaly. A heterogeneous rim-enhancing lesion centered in the left pyriform sinus. Lower slices demonstrate abscess in the left lobe of the thyroid (not shown).

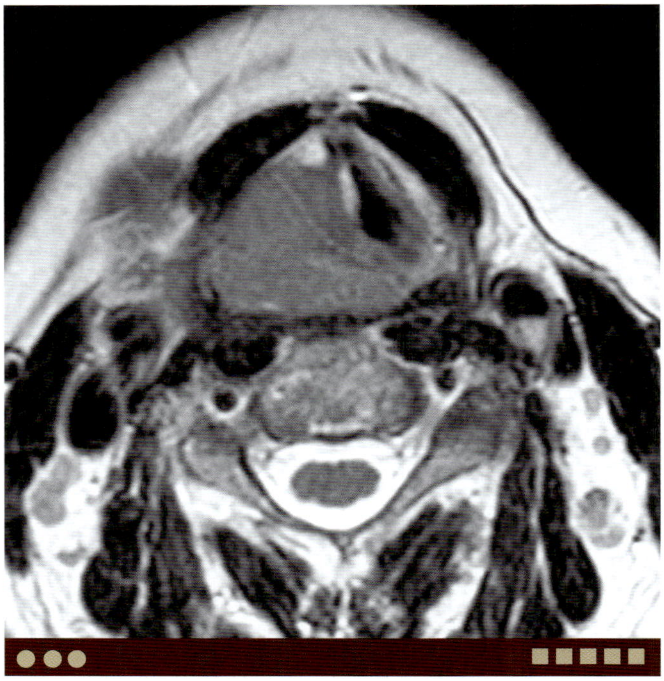

G. Lymphoma. Axial T2W image shows a homogeneous intermediate-signal lesion involving the right paraglottic space and displacing the cord medially.

Case 10–5 Chondrosarcoma

Osamu Sakai, Jimmy Wang

PRESENTATION

Lump in the neck and hoarseness.

FINDINGS

CT demonstrates a well-demarcated mass with stippled calcification in the laryngeal cartilage.

DIFFERENTIAL DIAGNOSIS

- Chondroma: This is a benign tumor without aggressive features, such as soft tissue density and invasion into the adjacent structures.
- Cartilage invasion by tumors arising from adjacent structures: Squamous cell carcinoma invades the laryngeal cartilage. The paraglottic fat invasion by tumor raises the possibility of cartilage involvement. Thyroid cancers invade the cartilage from the lateral cortex.
- Metastasis: The laryngeal cartilage contains marrow and can have metastasis. This usually shows heterogeneous soft tissue density, not fat density. Splaying of the medial and lateral cortex of the cartilage suggests the lesion is growing from within the marrow, while invasion by tumors arising from adjacent structures destroys the cartilage from outside.

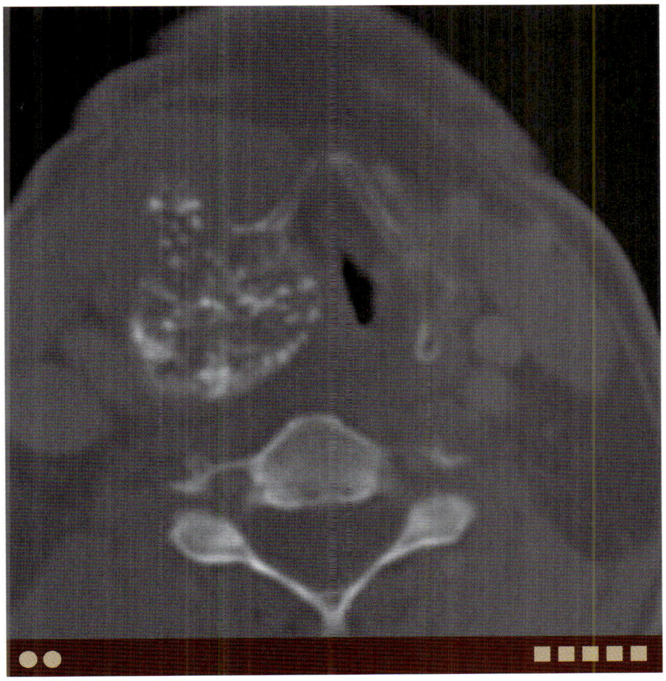

A. Chondrosarcoma. Axial CT demonstrates coarse or stippled calcification in the focally expanded lesion in the thyroid lamina.

COMMENTS

This is a 38-year-old man with hoarseness.

Chondrosarcomas are rare tumors accounting for less than 1% of all laryngeal tumors, and usually occur in the fourth to sixth decades of life with male-to-female predominance, 5:1 to 10:1. In the larynx, they typically originate in the hyaline cartilage, most commonly in the cricoid cartilage (approximately 70% of cases), followed by the thyroid cartilage. The symptoms depend on the location of the tumor. Endolaryngeal and subglottic growth causes dyspnea as the airway is progressively narrowed, whereas extralaryngeal growth, originating in the posterior cricoid, can produce dysphagia. Limited laryngeal mobility causes hoarseness. Thyroid cartilage lesions are likely to produce a painless neck mass.

Laryngeal chondrosarcoma is relatively low grade, both in clinical aggressiveness and histologic findings, unlike other head and neck chondrosarcomas. Often, they can be successfully controlled with local excision. Rarely, however, an additional aggressive and rapidly fatal malignant mesenchymal component may develop within the lesion (dedifferentiation).

On CT, coarse or stippled calcification within the tumor is the characteristic finding for chondrosarcoma, as seen in other chondroid lesions. Diagnosis of tumor extension is important to determine the type and feasibility of conservative surgery.

MRI has superior contrast resolution of the tumor and contiguous tissues and useful to determine tumor extension to the adjacent soft tissues. Typically, chondrosarcoma shows high signal on T2W images with multiple signal-voids from calcification or ossification.

PEARLS

- **Laryngeal chondrosarcoma is a rare tumor of the larynx.**
- **Laryngeal chondrosarcoma demonstrates coarse or stippled calcification on CT and high signal on T2W MR images.**

ADDITIONAL IMAGES (B-F)

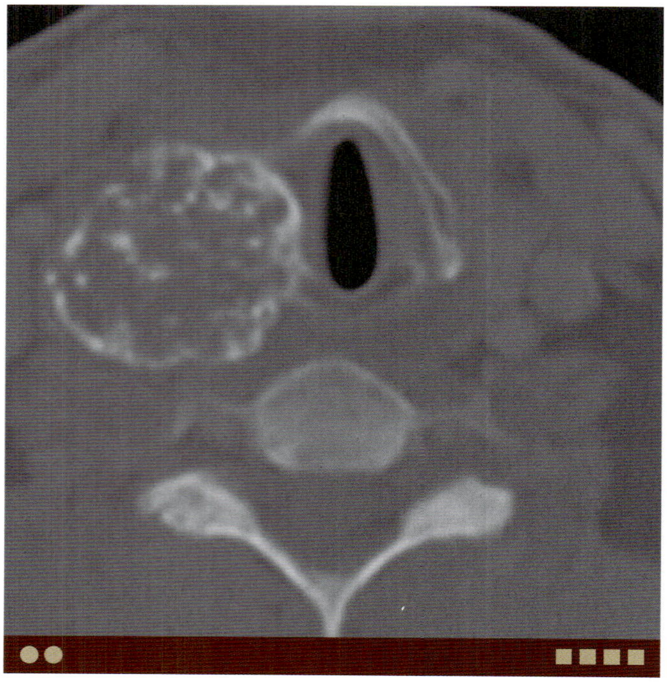

B. Chondrosarcoma, same patient as A. Axial CT through the lower level demonstrates an expansile mass arising from the right thyroid cartilage.

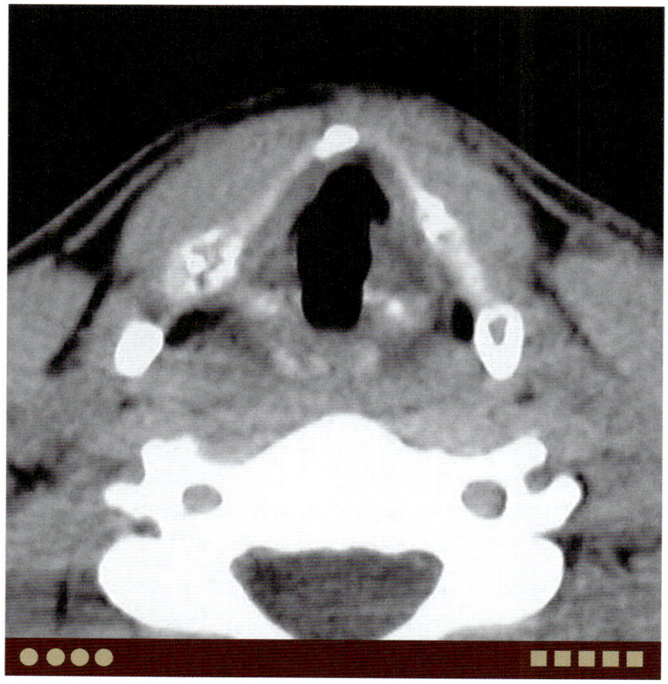

C. Chondroma. Axial CT (soft tissue window) demonstrates a focal thickening of the right thyroid lamina with coarse or stippled calcification.

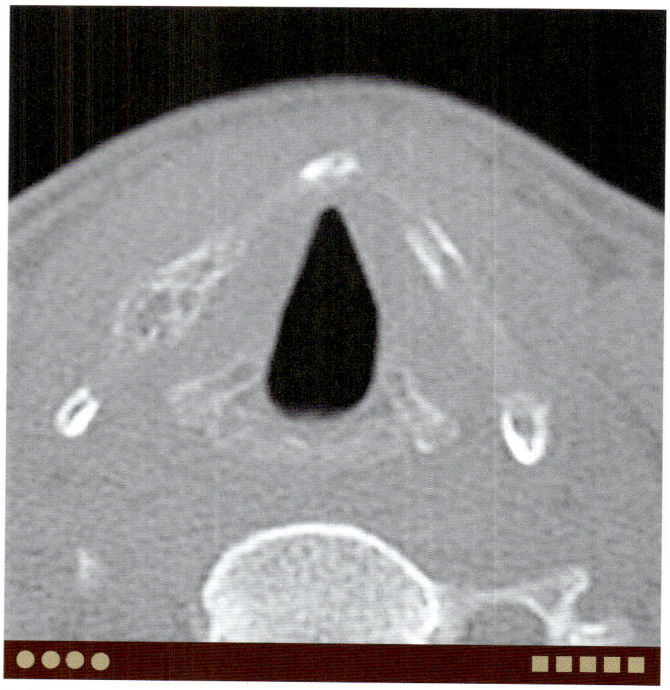

D. Chondroma, same patient as C. Axial CT (bone window) demonstrates a focal thickening of the right thyroid lamina with coarse or stippled calcification.

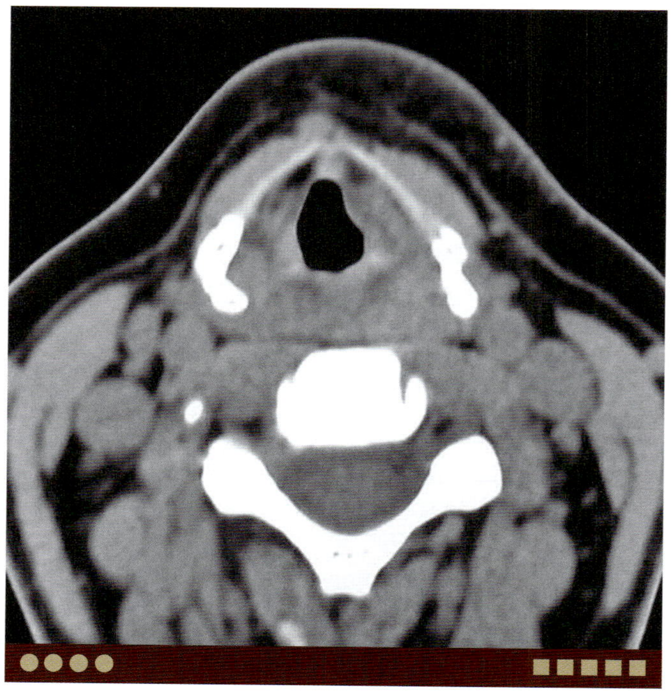

E. Healed fractures. Axial CT (soft tissue window) demonstrates deformity of the thyroid lamina bilaterally.

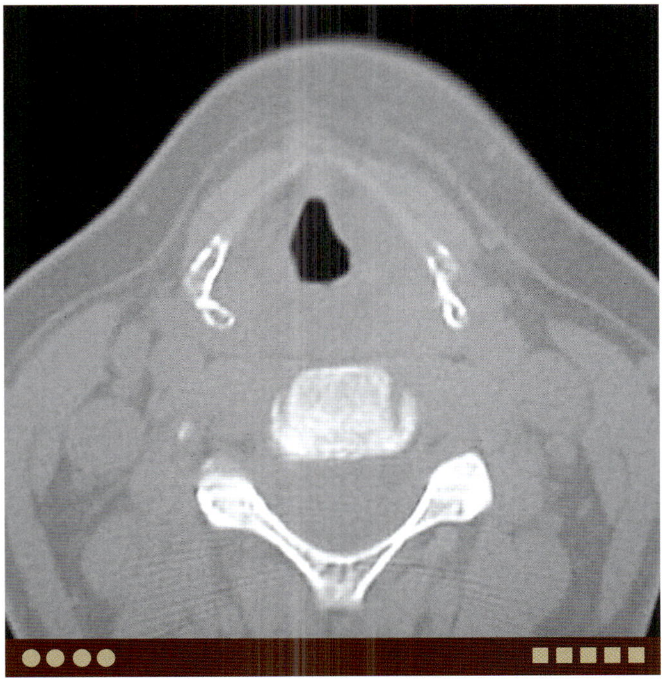

F. Healed fractures, same patient as E. Axial CT (bone window) demonstrates deformity of the thyroid lamina bilaterally.

DIFFERENTIAL DIAGNOSIS IMAGE

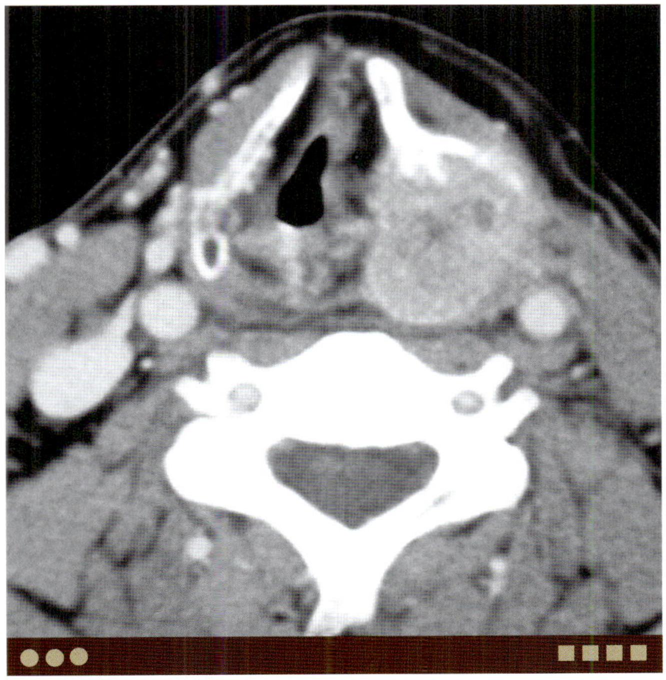

G. Metastasis. Axial postcontrast CT demonstrates a heterogeneously enhancing tumor spraying the medial and lateral cortex of the left thyroid lamina.

Case 10-6 Laryngeal Carcinoma, Supraglottic

Osamu Sakai, Jimmy Wang

PRESENTATION

Hoarseness.

FINDINGS

CT demonstrates a tumor in the supraglottic larynx, above the level of the true vocal cord.

DIFFERENTIAL DIAGNOSIS

- Adenoid cystic carcinoma: This is rare in the larynx. The imaging findings are similar to SCCA and often indistinguishable.
- Lymphoma: This usually demonstrates homogeneous density/signal and mild enhancement.
- Amyloidosis: This demonstrates nodular or diffuse mucosal soft tissue thickening or submucosal mass, often with calcification.
- Schwannoma: This is a rare tumor in the larynx, however, important for the differential diagnosis of submucosal tumors in the larynx. This often arises in the supraglottic larynx.

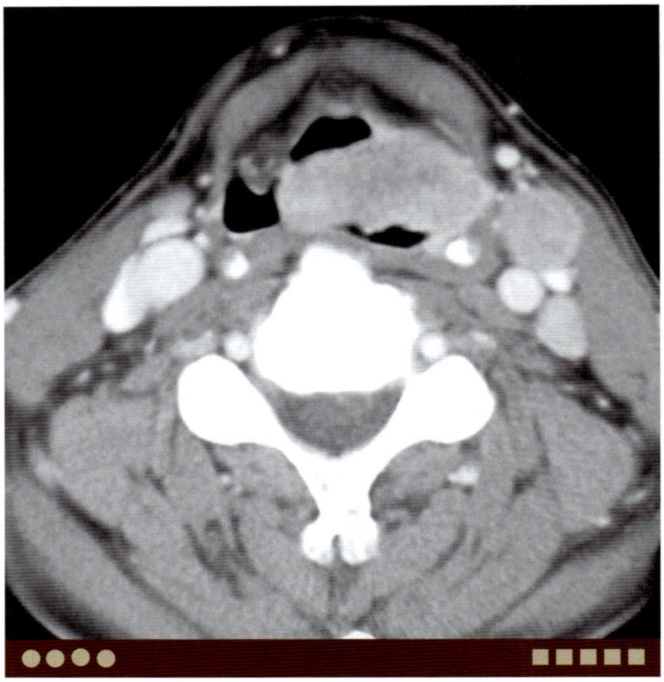

A. Supraglottic SCCA. Axial CT demonstrates a heterogeneously enhancing tumor involving the left aryepiglottic fold. Note enhancing left level III metastatic nodes.

COMMENTS

This is a 50-year-old man with hoarseness and difficulty swallowing.

The supraglottic larynx contains structures above the true vocal cord, such as the false cords, laryngeal ventricles, aryepiglottic folds, and epiglottis. The supraglottic larynx has abundant lymphatics; therefore, contralateral nodal metastasis often occurs in patients with supraglottic tumors.

The supraglottic larynx contains a large amount of fatty tissue, which is clearly seen as low density on CT and high signal on T1W MR images. The preepiglottic and paraglottic spaces are important areas when diagnosing laryngeal tumors. Once tumors extend into the preepiglottic fat, the risk of nodal metastasis will significantly increase. Also, this is a clinically blind spot; therefore, imaging plays an important role. Tumor extension into the paraglottic space increases the risk of cartilage involvement because there is no definite fascial barrier. If there is preserved low density on CT or high signal on T1W MR images within the cartilage, tumor invasion to the cartilage is virtually excluded, while other density or signal patterns may be due to tumor invasion or edema secondary to tumors. Cartilage invasion will be further discussed later in a separate section.

PEARLS

- **The supraglottic larynx has abundant lymphatics; therefore, contralateral nodal metastasis often occurs in patients with supraglottic tumors.**
- **The supraglottic larynx contains a large amount of fatty tissue, which is clearly seen as low density on CT and high signal on T1W MR images. Abnormal soft tissue density or signal in this area raises the possibility of tumor extension.**

ADDITIONAL IMAGES (B-D)

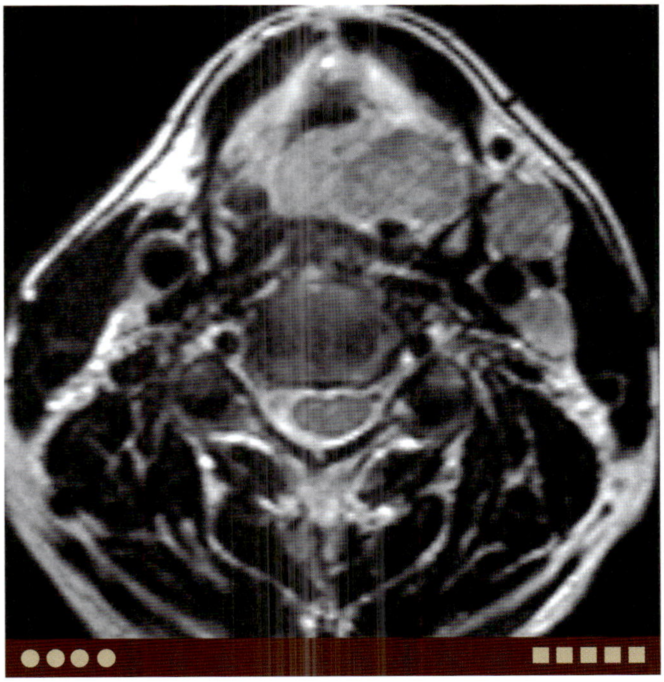

B. Supraglottic SCCA, same patient as A. Axial T2W MR image shows the lesion demonstrating heterogeneous intermediate-to-high signal. The metastatic left level III nodes demonstrate similar signal to the primary lesion.

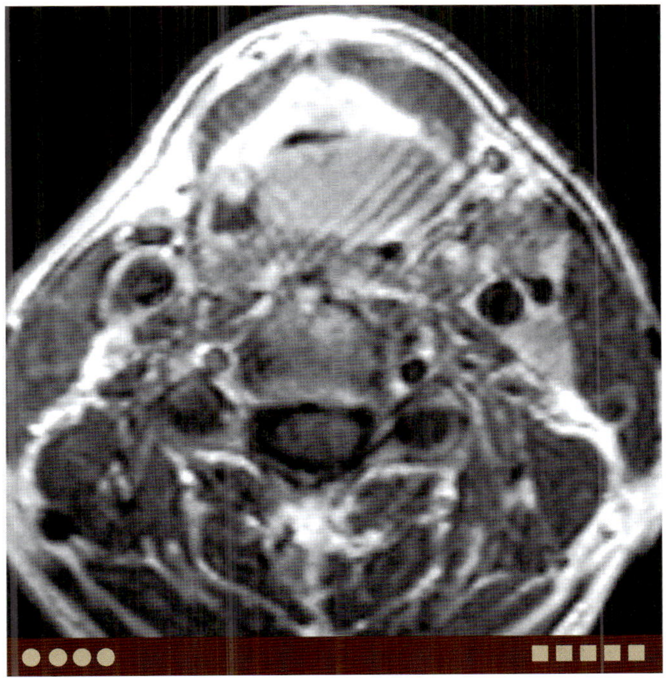

C. Supraglottic SCCA, same patient as A. Axial postcontrast T1W MR image demonstrates heterogeneous enhancement in the primary lesion as well as metastatic nodes.

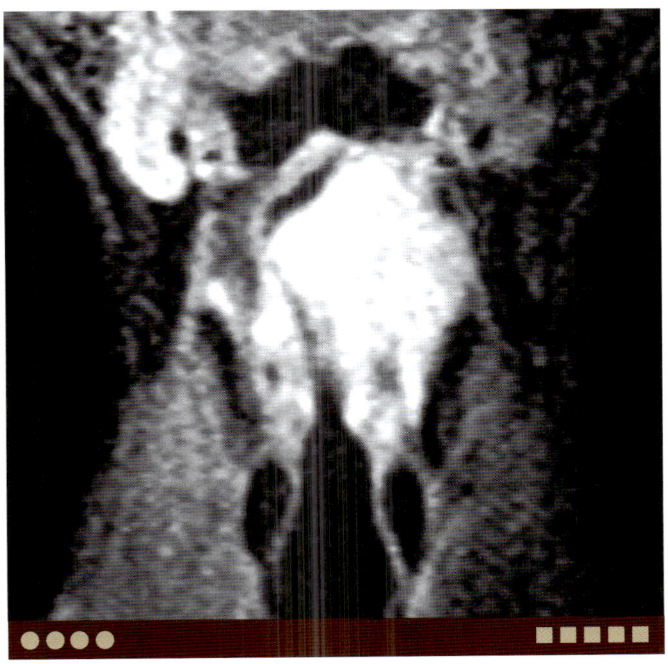

D. Supraglottic SCCA, same patient as A. Coronal postcontrast fat-suppressed T1W image demonstrates heterogeneous enhancement of the lesion. Note the extent of the tumor from the level of the epiglottis to the true vocal cord. Note left thyroid lamina preserves normal low T1 fat-suppressed signal.

DIFFERENTIAL DIAGNOSIS IMAGES (E-H)

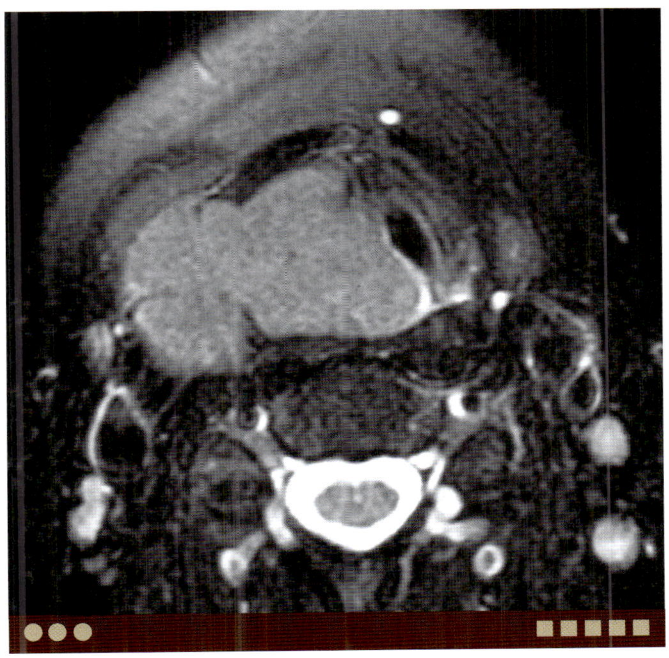

E. Lymphoma. Axial T2W image shows an intermediate-signal lesion involving the right aryepiglottic fold with lateral extension. Note homogeneous signal of the lesion without necrosis.

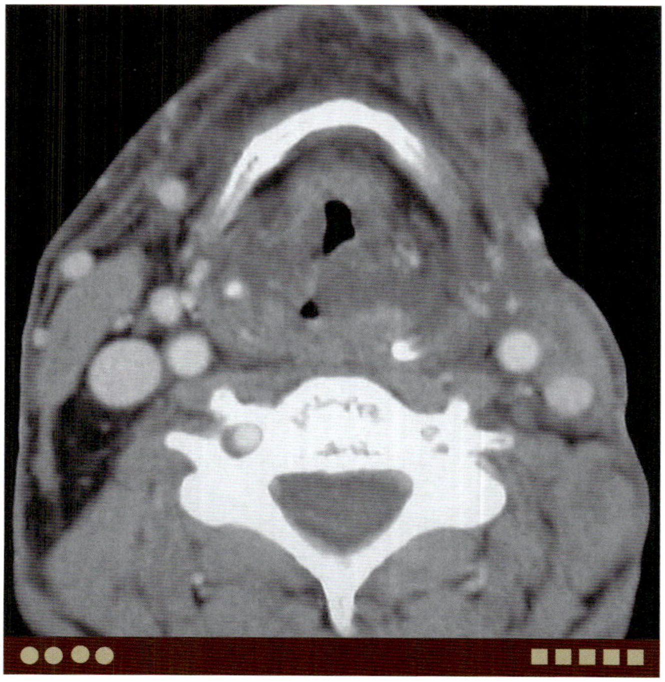

F. Postradiation edema and fibrosis. Axial postcontrast CT demonstrates diffuse swelling and heterogeneous density of the supraglottic soft tissues as well as subcutaneous fat.

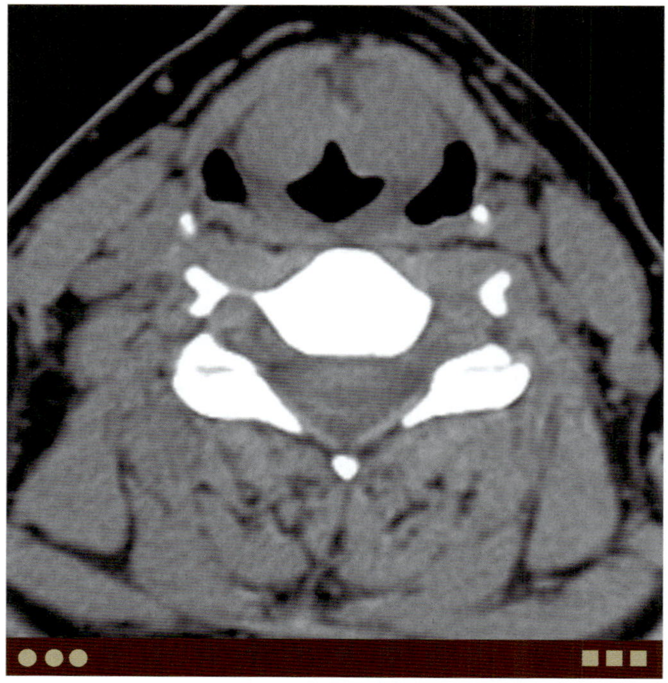

G. Amyloidosis. Axial CT demonstrates homogeneous density lesions involving the aryepiglottic folds.

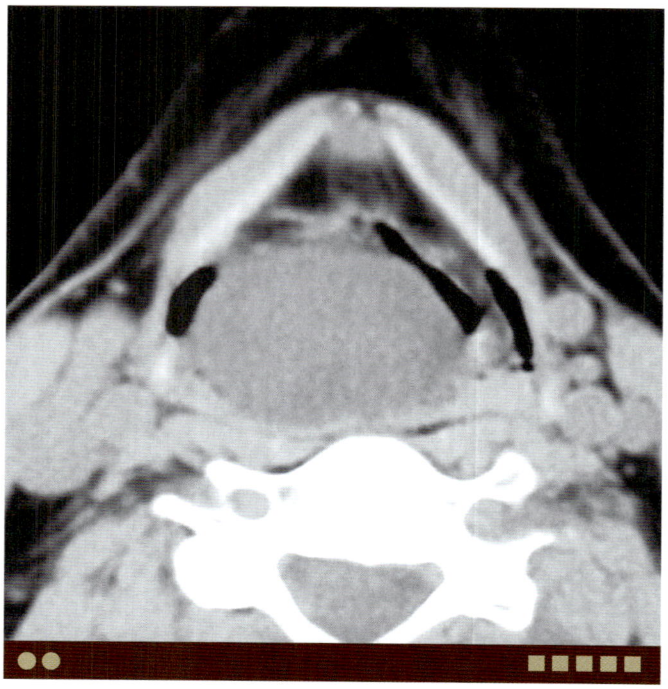

H. Schwannoma. Axial noncontrast CT demonstrates a homogeneous low-density lesion in the supraglottic larynx.

Case 10–7 Laryngeal Carcinoma, Glottic

Osamu Sakai, Jimmy Wang

PRESENTATION

Hoarseness.

FINDINGS

CT and MRI demonstrate a mass involving the true vocal cord.

DIFFERENTIAL DIAGNOSIS

- Adenoid cystic carcinoma: This is rare in the larynx. The imaging findings are similar to SCCA and often indistinguishable.
- Lymphoma: This usually demonstrates homogeneous density/signal and mild enhancement.
- Amyloidosis: This demonstrates nodular or diffuse mucosal thickening or submucosal mass often with calcification.
- Rhabdomyoma and rhabdomyosarcoma: These are rare submucosal tumors. Rhabdomyosarcoma tends to demonstrate more aggressive features.

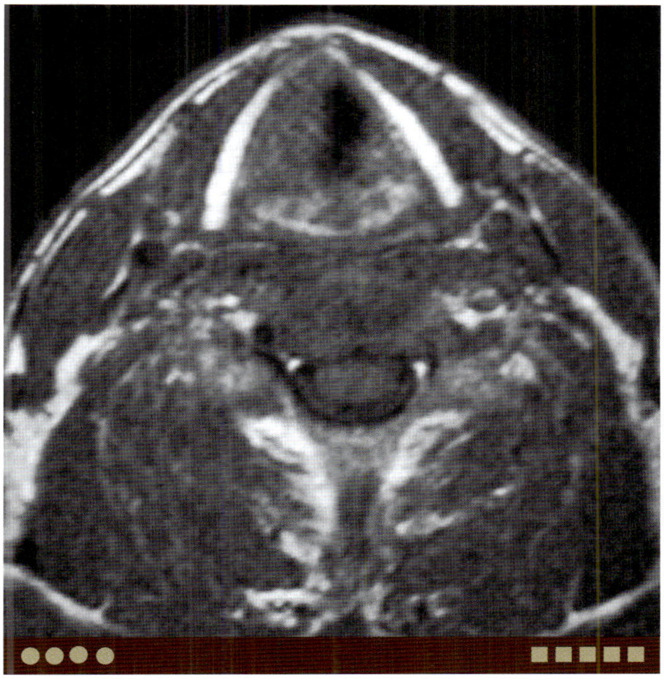

A. Glottic SCCA. Axial T1W MR image demonstrates thickening of the right vocal cord.

COMMENTS

This is a 75-year-old man with hoarseness.

Glottic squamous cell carcinoma (SCCA) is the most common laryngeal cancer, confined within the glottis, the true vocal cord. The glottic larynx contains few lymphatics. Therefore, nodal metastasis is not common early, which usually occurs after tumor extension to the supraglottis or subglottis. Glottic and subglottic tumors usually have ipsilateral nodal metastasis. If the tumor extends to the anterior commissure and anterior subglottis, metastasis to the middle and lower anterior cervical nodes, the Delphian node, and levels VI and VII nodes may occur. If the tumor extends to the supraglottic larynx, contralateral nodal metastasis occurs more frequently.

The main role of imaging in evaluation of laryngeal cancers is to provide precise information regarding local extension of the tumor. This is helpful for selecting suitable treatment options. Extension to the preepiglottic and paraglottic space is very important because it increases the risk of nodal metastasis and cartilage invasion. Abnormal soft tissue density in the preepiglottic and paraglottic spaces in the glottic and supraglottic larynx is a strong indicator for tumor extension to these spaces. In addition, any soft tissue density medial to the cricoid in the subglottic larynx is a strong indicator for subglottic tumor extension.

If there is preserved fat with low density on CT or high signal on T1W MR images within the adjacent cartilage, tumor invasion into the cartilage is virtually excluded. Other cartilage densities or signal patterns may be due to tumor invasion or edema secondary to tumors. Cartilage invasion will be further discussed later in a separate section.

PEARLS

- **Glottic carcinoma is confined within the glottis, the vocal cord.**
- **The glottic larynx contains few lymphatics. Therefore, nodal metastasis is not common, which usually occurs after tumor extension to the supraglottis or subglottis.**
- **Abnormal soft tissue density in the preepiglottic and paraglottic spaces in the glottic and supraglottic larynx is a strong indicator for tumor extension to these spaces.**

ADDITIONAL IMAGES (B-D)

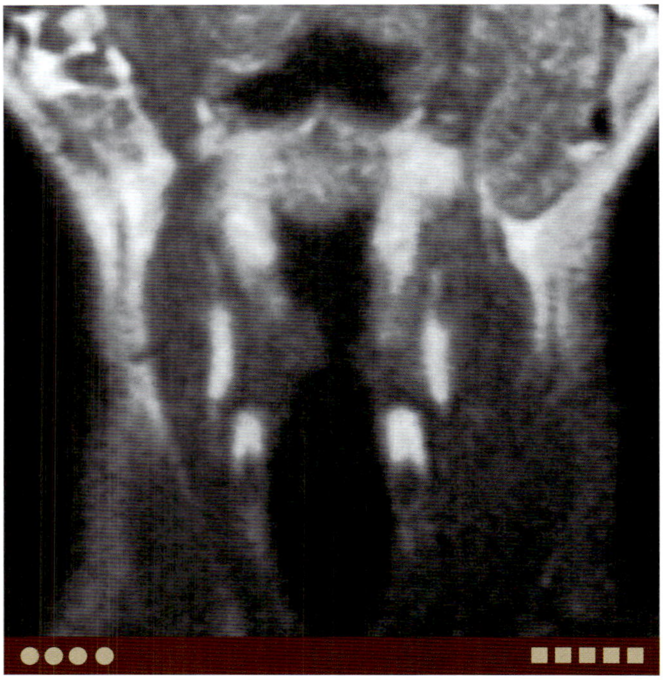

B. Glottic SCCA, same patient as A. Coronal T1W image demonstrates nodular thickening of the right vocal cord.

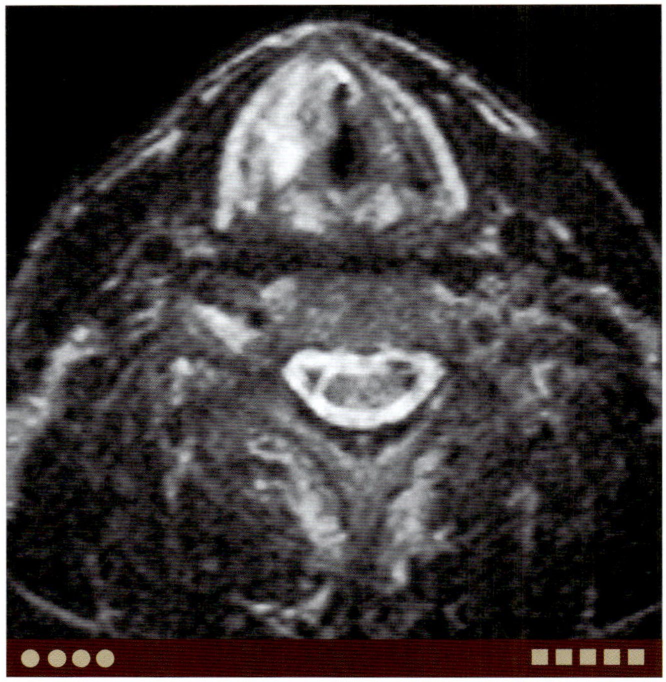

C. Glottic SCCA, same patient as A. Axial T2W image shows the right vocal cord lesion demonstrating heterogeneous high signal.

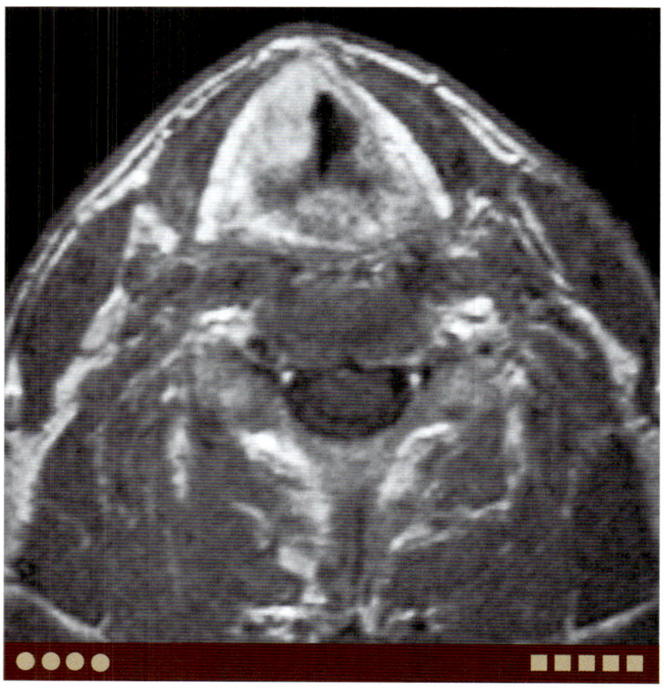

D. Glottic SCCA, same patient as A. Axial postcontrast T1W image shows the right vocal cord lesion demonstrating heterogeneous enhancement.

DIFFERENTIAL DIAGNOSIS IMAGES (E-G)

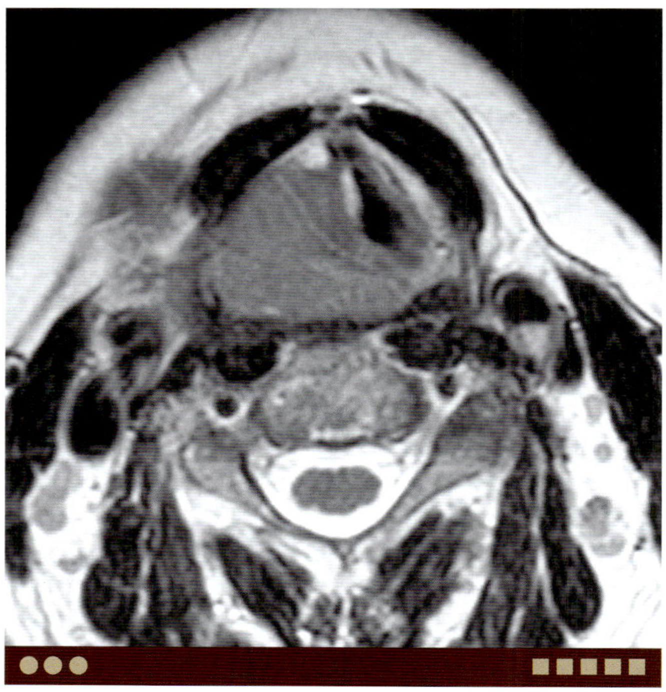

E. Lymphoma. Axial T2W image shows a homogeneous intermediate-signal lesion involving the right paraglottic space and displacing the cord medially.

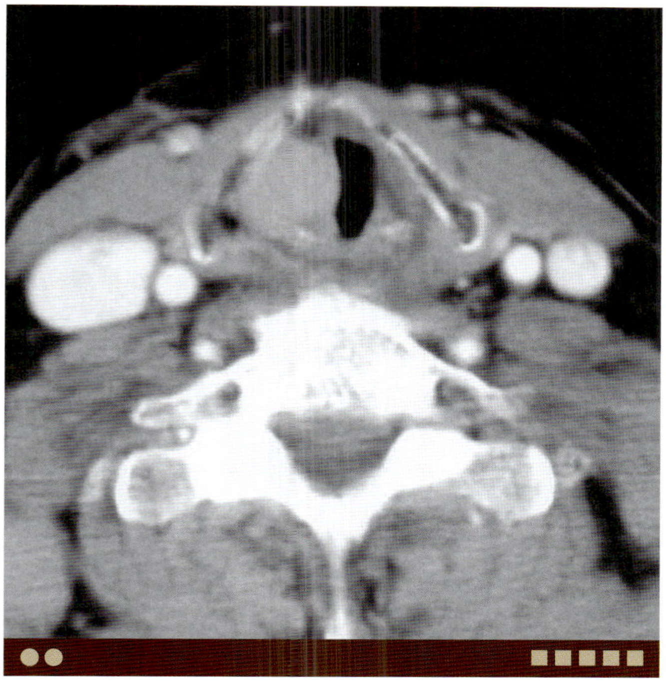

F. Rhabdomyoma. Axial postcontrast CT demonstrates a homogeneously enhancing lesion in the right cord.

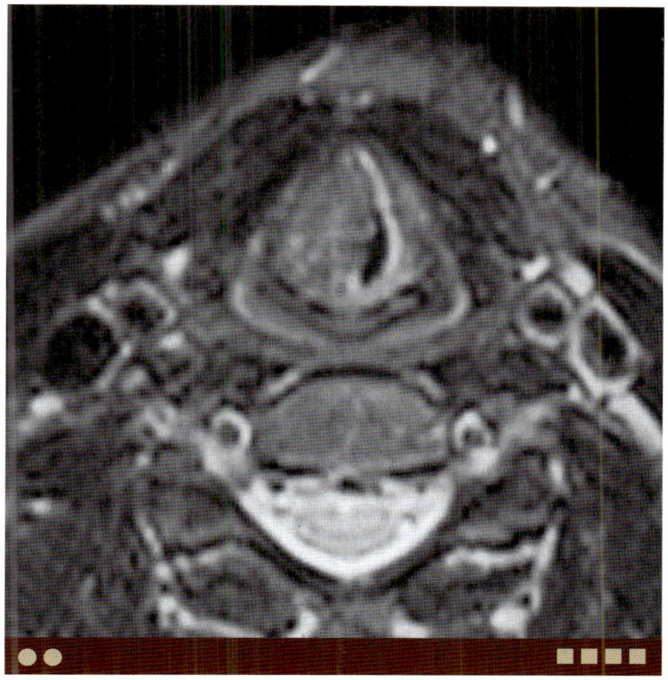

G. Granular cell tumor. Axial T2W image shows a slightly heterogeneous intermediate-signal lesion involving the right cord.

Case 10–8 Laryngeal Carcinoma, Subglottic

Osamu Sakai, Jimmy Wang

PRESENTATION

Hoarseness and stridor.

FINDINGS

CT demonstrates a mass involving the subglottis.

DIFFERENTIAL DIAGNOSIS

- Adenoid cystic carcinoma: This is rare in the larynx. The imaging findings are similar to SCCA and often indistinguishable.
- Lymphoma: This usually demonstrates homogeneous density/signal and mild enhancement.
- Amyloidosis: This demonstrates nodular mucosal soft tissue thickening or submucosal mass often with calcification.
- Rhabdomyoma and rhabdomyosarcoma: These are rare submucosal tumors. Rhabdomyosarcoma tends to demonstrate more aggressive features.

COMMENTS

This is a 78-year-old man with hoarseness and stridor.

Subglottic carcinoma is difficult to visualize clinically. Therefore, imaging is important to identify the lesion as well as to define its extent because inferior extent is important for surgical and radiation therapy planning. On imaging, no tissue should be seen medial to the cricoid cartilage ring. Presence of soft tissue in this location is a strong indicator for mass lesion. This is a very important finding, particularly when the lesion is symmetric, because it may be missed if asymmetry is searched to diagnose a subglottic lesion. Subglottic extension should be evaluated for in every patient with glottic or supraglottic SCCA because presence of subglottic involvement dramatically changes treatment options. Subglottic extension is often submucosal and difficult to evaluate clinically.

Glottic and subglottic tumors usually have ipsilateral nodal metastasis. If the tumor extends to the anterior commissure and anterior subglottis, metastasis to the middle and lower anterior cervical nodes, the Delphian node, and levels VI and VII nodes may occur. If the tumor extends to the supraglottic larynx, contralateral nodal metastasis occurs more frequently.

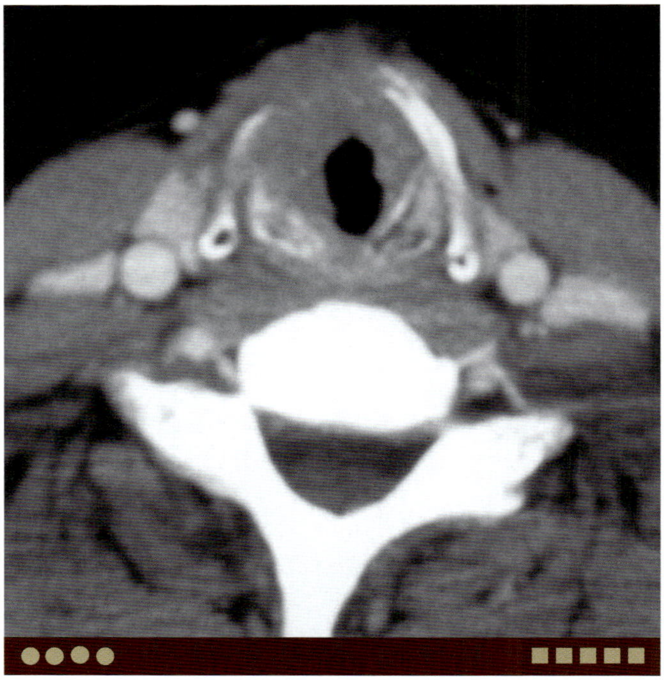

A. Subglottic SCCA. Axial contrast-enhanced CT demonstrates irregular thickening of the mucosa medial to the cricoid ring, right more than left, and anterior more than posterior. Note erosion/destruction and sclerosis of the right cricoid cartilage, consistent with cartilage invasion.

The subglottic larynx can be involved by various other neoplastic, infectious and inflammatory conditions. Evaluation of the trachea and bronchi is also necessary for diagnosis and appropriate patient management.

PEARLS

- **In the subglottic larynx, no soft tissue should be identified medial to the cricoid ring.**
- **Subglottic and transglottic extension should be evaluated for in every patient with glottic or supraglottic SCCA, because presence of subglottic involvement dramatically changes treatment options.**

ADDITIONAL IMAGES (B-E)

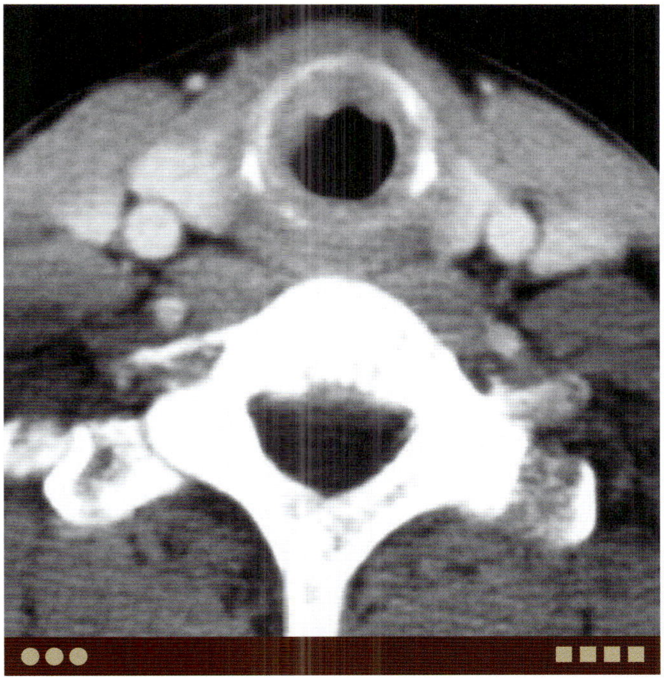

B. Subglottic SCCA, same patient as A. Axial contrast-enhanced CT through a lower level demonstrates concentric thickening of the mucosa medial to the tracheal ring, tumor extension.

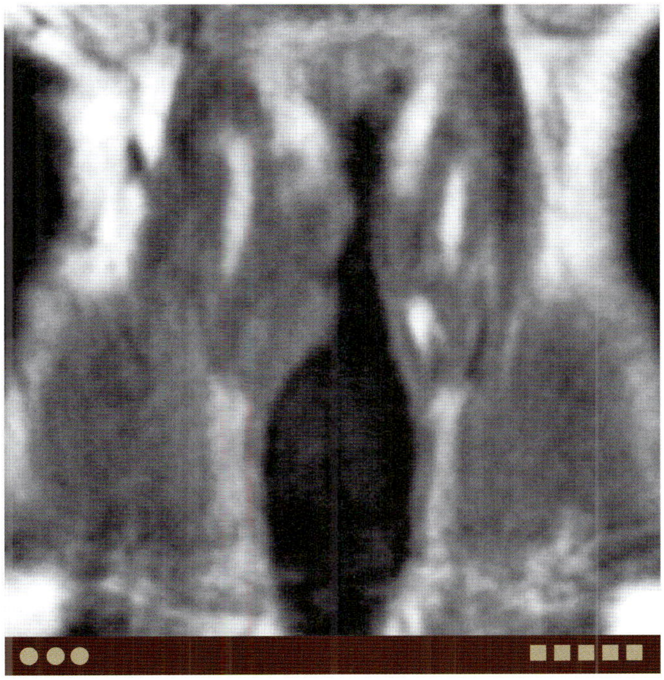

C. Subglottic SCCA, same patient as A. Coronal T1W MR image shows a low-signal lesion in the right subglottic larynx. Note loss of high signal in the right cricoid cartilage consistent with cartilage invasion.

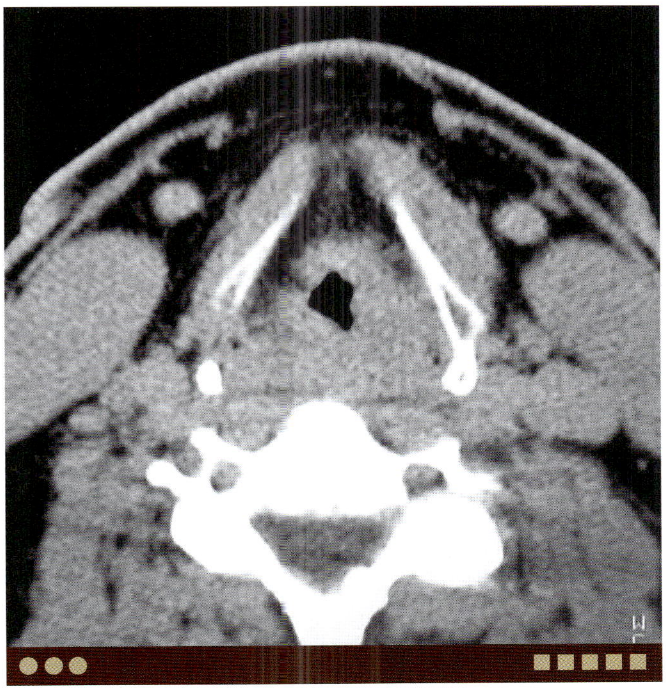

D. Transglottic tumor extension. Axial noncontrast CT through the supraglottic larynx demonstrates asymmetric soft tissue thickening on the left with obliteration of the paraglottic fat.

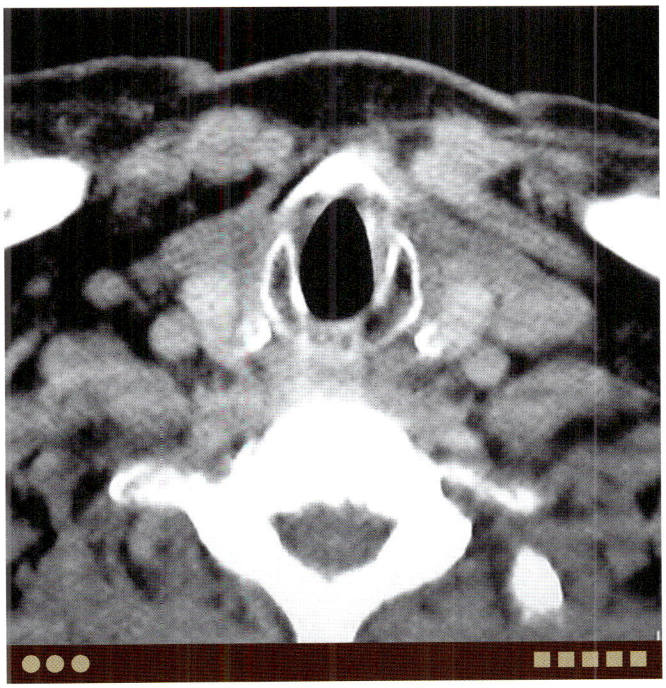

E. Transglottic tumor extension, same patient as D. Axial noncontrast CT through the subglottic larynx demonstrates very slight asymmetric soft tissue density on the left suggesting subglottic tumor extension.

DIFFERENTIAL DIAGNOSIS IMAGES (F-G)

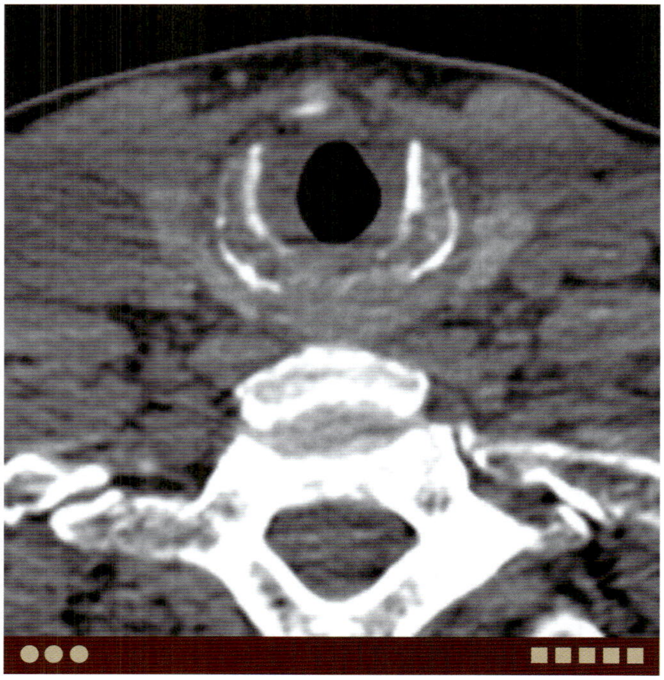

F. Wegener's granulomatosis. Axial noncontrast CT through the subglottic larynx demonstrates concentric thickening of the mucosa medial to the cricoid ring.

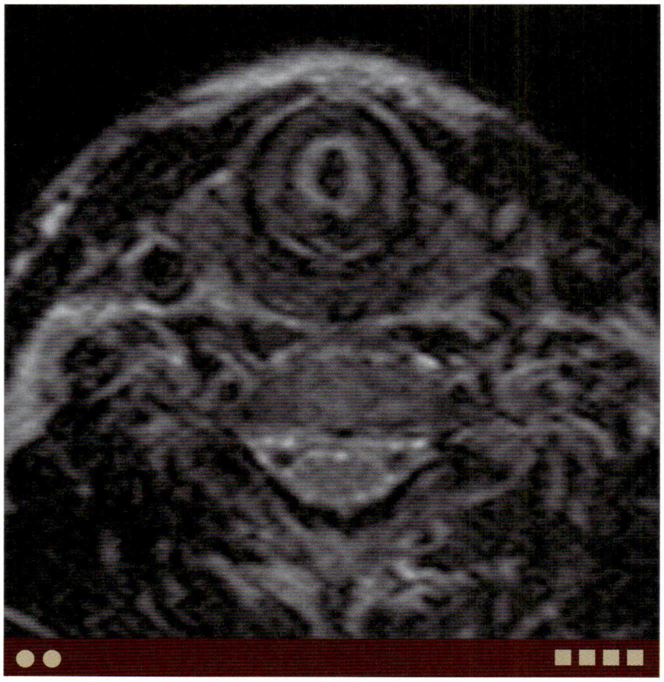

G. Amyloidosis. Axial T2W MR image shows concentric thickening of the submucosa medial to the cricoid ring.

Case 10–9 Laryngeal Carcinoma, Cartilage Invasion

Osamu Sakai, Jimmy Wang

PRESENTATION

Hoarseness.

FINDINGS

CT demonstrates erosion/destruction of the laryngeal cartilage.

DIFFERENTIAL DIAGNOSIS

- Lymphoma: Just like in other sites this tends to demonstrate homogeneous density/signal and enhancement. Necrosis without treatment is rare.
- Adenoid cystic carcinoma: This is the most common minor salivary gland tumor; however, in the larynx, minor salivary gland tumors rarely occur and constitute less than 1% of laryngeal tumors.
- Metastasis: The laryngeal cartilage contains marrow and can have metastasis. This usually shows heterogeneous soft tissue density, not fat density. Splaying of the medial and lateral cortex of the cartilage suggests the lesion is growing in the marrow, while invasion by tumors arising from adjacent structures destroys the cartilage from outside.

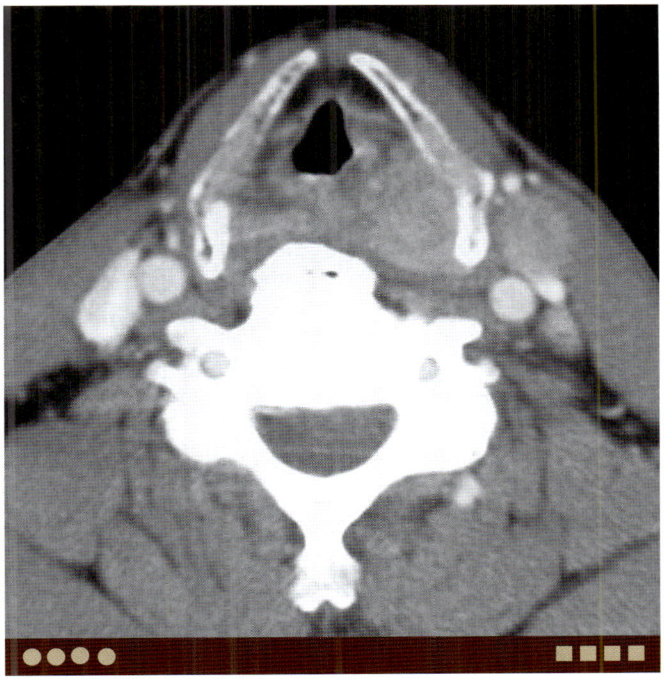

A. SCCA, cartilage invasion. Axial CT demonstrates a tumor in the left supraglottic larynx invading into the paraglottic fat and contacting the thyroid lamina. No apparent erosion or destruction is noted; however, slight sclerosis is noted. Note left level III nodal metastases.

COMMENTS

This is a 65-year-old man with hoarseness.

Cartilage invasion is considered to be a significant prognostic indicator. This previously has been a contraindication for partial laryngectomy or radiation therapy; however, this concept has been questioned and treatment options have been changed recently.

Diagnosis of cartilage invasion is often difficult both with CT and MRI. MRI is believed to be more sensitive. However, CT is much easier to acquire and cortical erosion and gross destruction, particularly transcartilaginous invasion (extralaryngeal tumor extension), is easily demonstrated on CT, while MRI suffers from motion artifacts from swallowing and breathing.

If the fat is preserved in ossified cartilage containing fatty marrow, we can rule out tumor invasion. Therefore, low density on CT and high signal on T1W MR images are reassuring findings. If the region is low signal on both T1W and T2W images, this area is considered as nonossified cartilage. If the region is low signal on T1W and high signal on T2W images, it is considered as abnormal, tumor versus edema due to inflammatory response to the adjacent tumor.

Sclerotic changes in the cartilage may suggest microscopic tumor invasion because SCCA is known to stimulate osteoblast activity; however, this is not very reliable sign. Heterogeneous and asymmetric ossification or calcification of the cartilage is very common in the normal population.

PEARLS

- **Preserved fat planes, such as preepiglottic and paraglottic fat, strongly suggest that the tumor does not reach those areas.**
- **No soft tissue should be identified medial to the cricoid ring in the subglottic larynx.**
- **Preserved fat density or signal is the only reliable finding for intact cartilage when evaluating for possible cartilage tumor invasion.**

ADDITIONAL IMAGES (B-F)

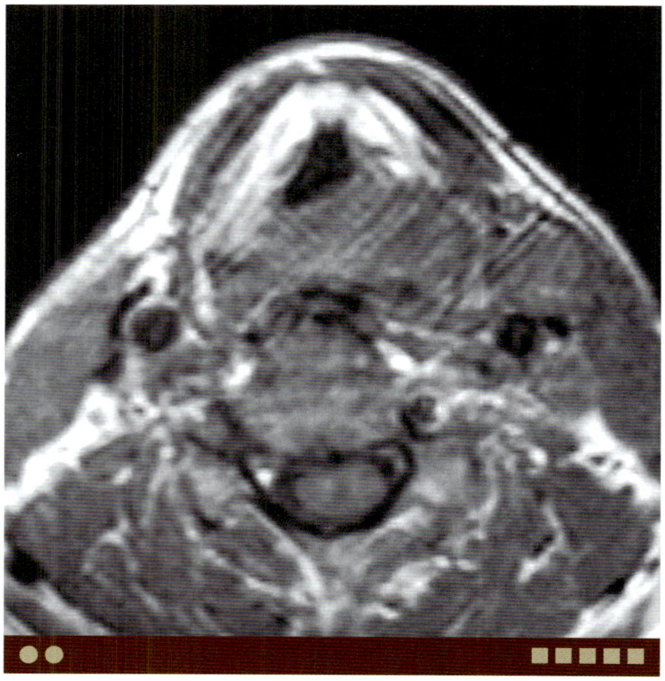

B. SCCA, cartilage invasion, same patient as A. Axial T1W MR image demonstrates decreased signal in the thyroid lamina contacted by the tumor, suggesting edema or tumor infiltration, or partial volume averaging. Note significant motion artifact degrading the image.

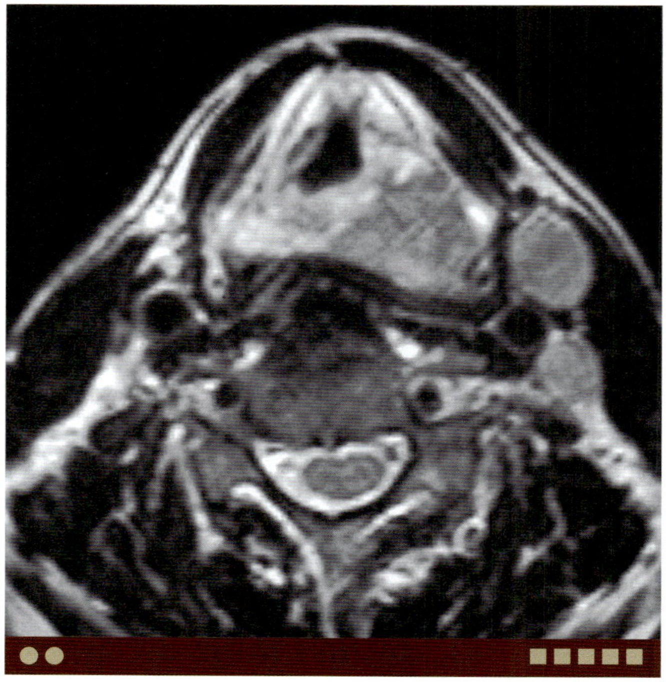

C. SCCA, cartilage invasion, same patient as A. Axial T2W image shows the region demonstrating high signal, similar to the rest of marrow, suggesting intact marrow space; however, microinvasion cannot be excluded. Note left level III nodal metastases.

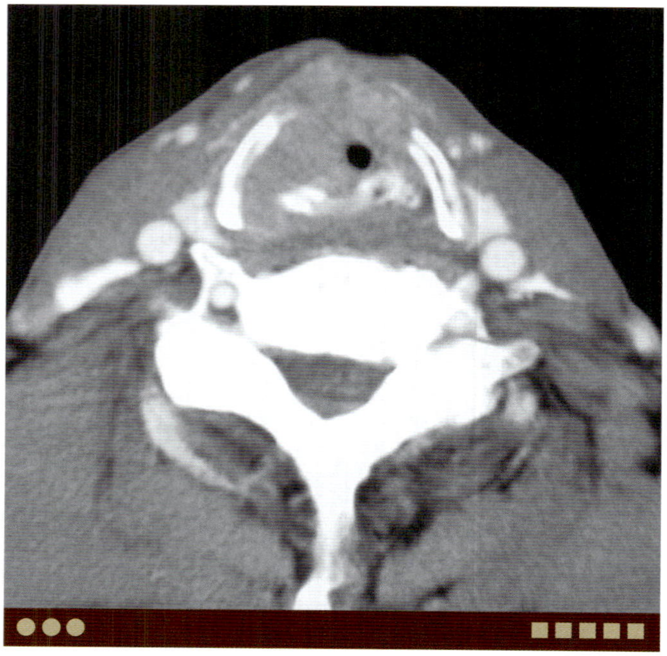

D. Gross cartilage invasion, transcartilaginous extension (thyroid cartilage). Axial postcontrast CT demonstrates a heterogeneously enhancing tumor destructing the thyroid lamina anteriorly and bilaterally, left more than right. Note enhancing tumor outside of the cartilage. Erosion and sclerosis are also seen in the right cricoid.

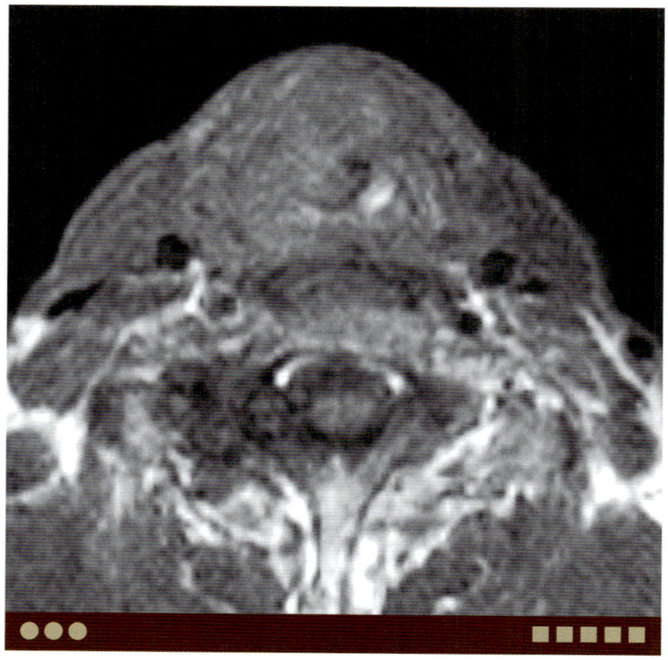

E. Transcartilaginous extension, same patient as D. Axial precontrast T1W image shows the tumor invading through thyroid lamina bilaterally. Loss of high signal from the fatty marrow is also seen in the right cricoid consistent with tumor invasion.

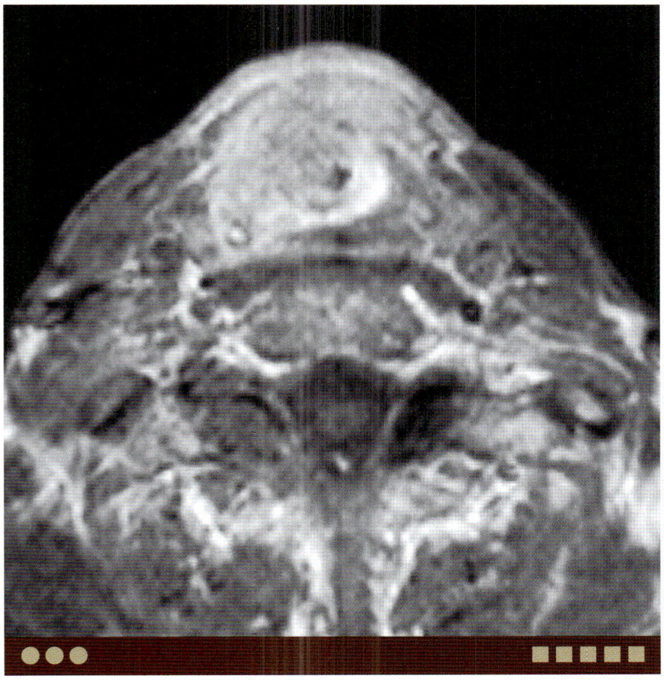

F. Transcartilaginous extension, same patient as D. Axial postcontrast T1W image shows the tumor demonstrating heterogeneous enhancement, extending to the superficial soft tissues through the thyroid cartilage.

DIFFERENTIAL DIAGNOSIS IMAGES (G-H)

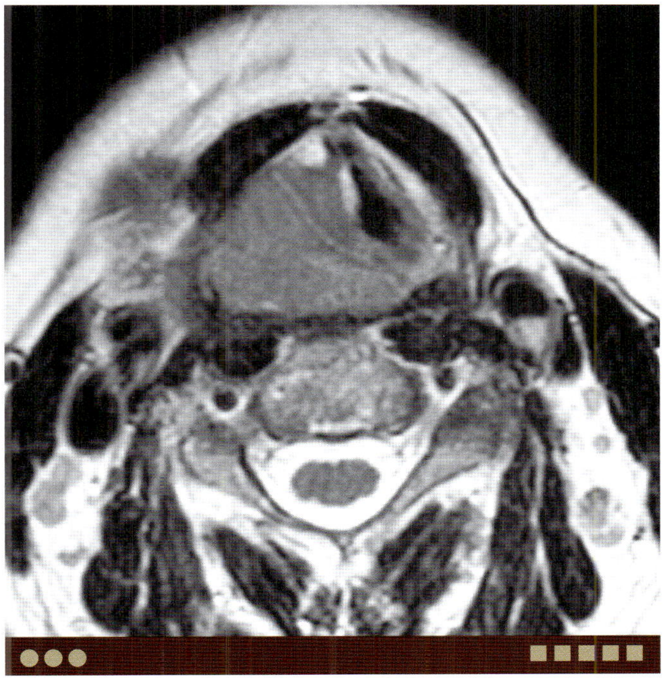

G. Lymphoma. Axial T2W image demonstrates a homogeneous intermediate-signal lesion centered in the right supraglottic/glottic larynx involving the right thyroid lamina, which also demonstrates intermediate signal.

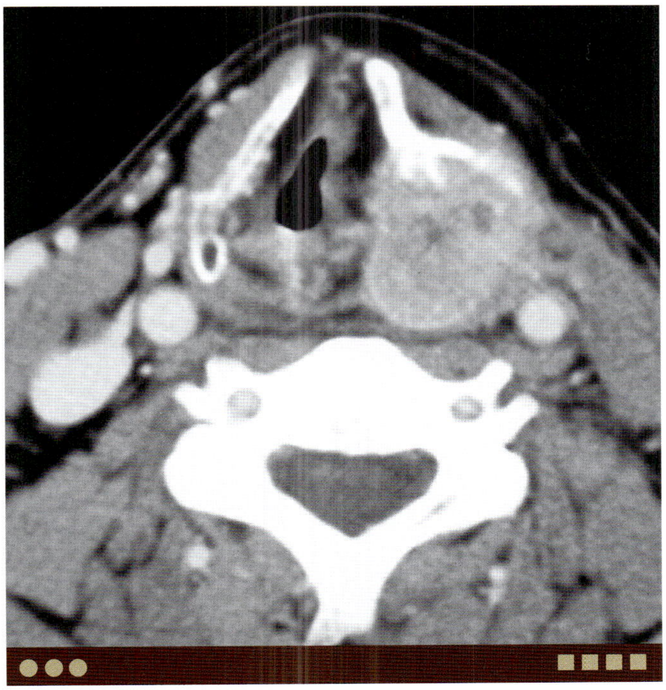

H. Metastasis. Axial postcontrast CT demonstrates a heterogeneously enhancing tumor spraying the medial and lateral cortex of the left thyroid lamina.

Case 10–10 Lymphoma

Osamu Sakai, Jimmy Wang

PRESENTATION

Hoarseness.

FINDINGS

CT and MRI demonstrate a homogeneous density/signal mass involving the larynx and hypopharynx.

DIFFERENTIAL DIAGNOSIS

- Squamous cell carcinoma (SCCA): This usually demonstrates heterogeneous density/signal and variable enhancement.
- Adenoid cystic carcinoma: This is rare. The imaging finding is similar to SCCA and often indistinguishable.
- Rhabdomyoma and rhabdomyosarcoma: These are rare submucosal tumors. Rhabdomyosarcoma tends to demonstrate more aggressive features.
- Amyloidosis: This demonstrates nodular mucosal thickening or submucosal mass, often with calcification.

COMMENTS

This is a 49-year-old man with hoarseness.

Primary laryngeal lymphomas are very rare, and laryngeal involvement is often seen as a part of systemic disease. Laryngeal lymphomas usually have large submucosal components centered in the supraglottic larynx. Then tumors extend into the glottis, with less frequent spread to the subglottis, laryngeal cartilage, and strap muscles. Contiguous lesions to the base of tongue or palatine tonsils are often seen. These are often diffuse large B-cell lymphomas or mucosa-associated lymphoid tissue (MALT) lymphomas.

Similar to lymphomas in other locations, they demonstrate homogeneous density similar to muscle on CT without necrosis. Signal on MRI is also homogeneous. Necrosis before treatment is rare. Mild enhancement is usually seen after contrast.

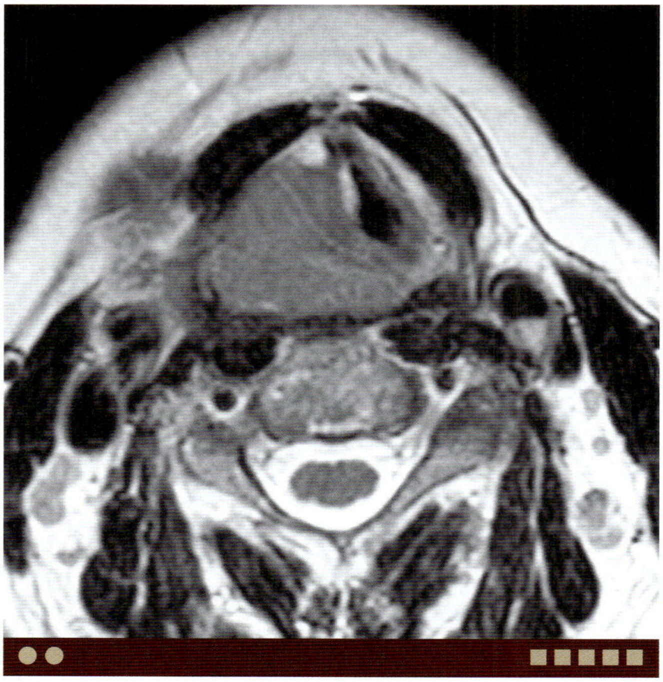

A. Lymphoma. Axial T2W MR image demonstrates homogeneous intermediate-signal lesion centered in the right paraglottic space in the supraglottis and glottis. The vocal cord is deviated to the left.

PEARLS

- **Primary laryngeal lymphomas are very rare.**
- **Laryngeal lymphomas usually have large submucosal components centered in the supraglottis.**
- **Laryngeal lymphomas demonstrate homogeneous density/signal, and necrosis before treatment is rare.**

ADDITIONAL IMAGES (B-D)

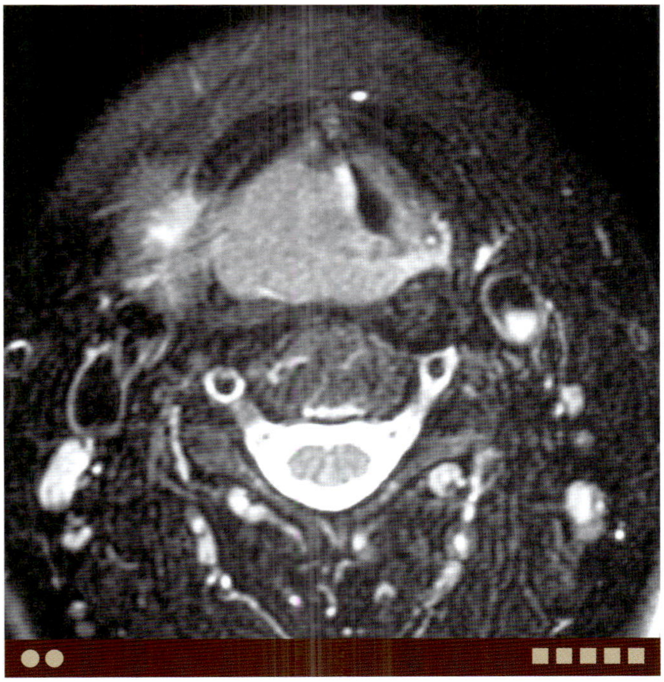

B. Lymphoma, same patient as A. Axial STIR image shows the lesion demonstrating homogeneous intermediate-to-high signal. Note extralaryngeal extension on the right.

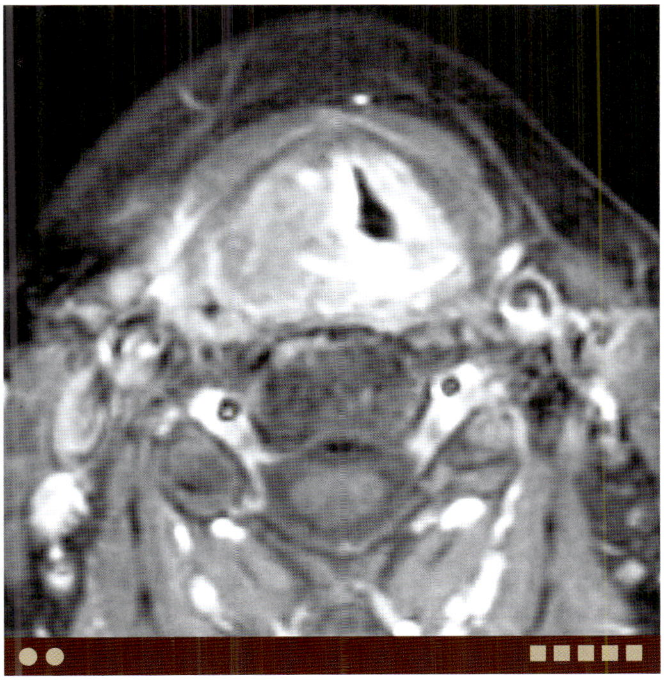

C. Lymphoma, same patient as A. Axial postcontrast fat-suppressed T1W image shows mild enhancement of the lesion.

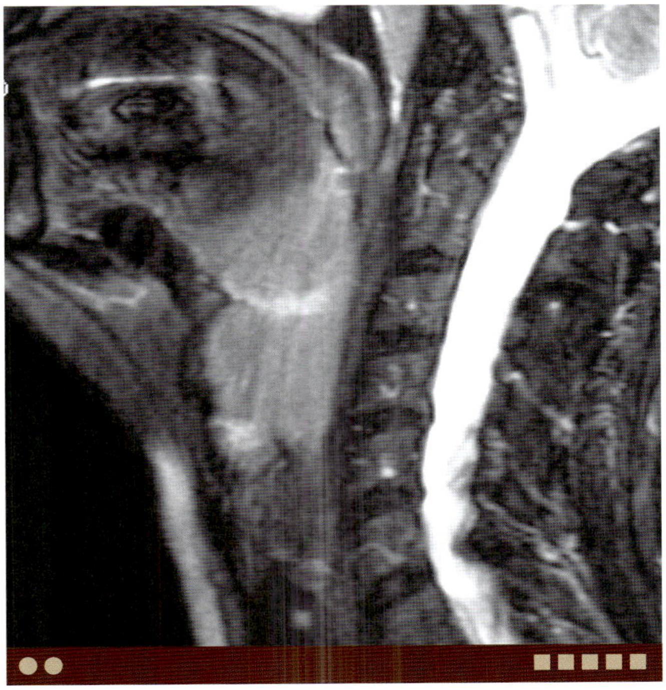

D. Lymphoma, same patient as A. Sagittal STIR image shows contiguous lesions to the base of tongue.

DIFFERENTIAL DIAGNOSIS IMAGES (E-H)

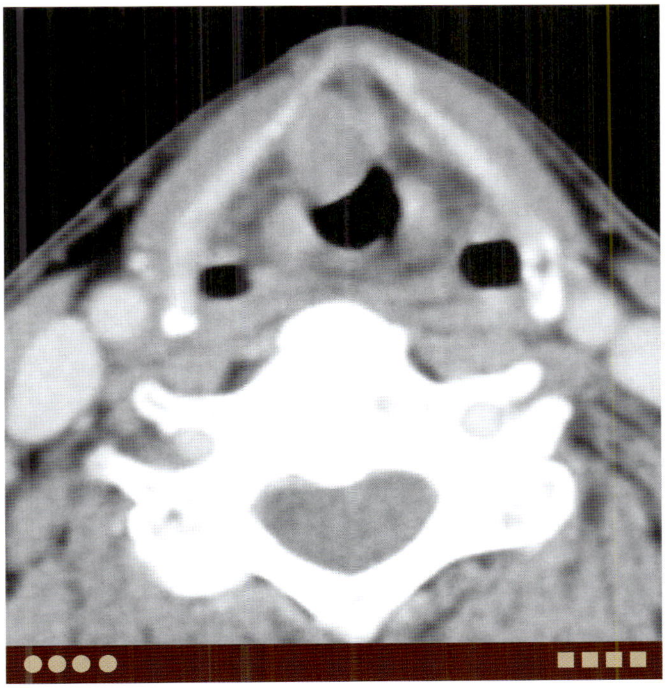

E. Squamous cell carcinoma. Axial contrast-enhanced CT shows a round lesion in the right supraglottic larynx.

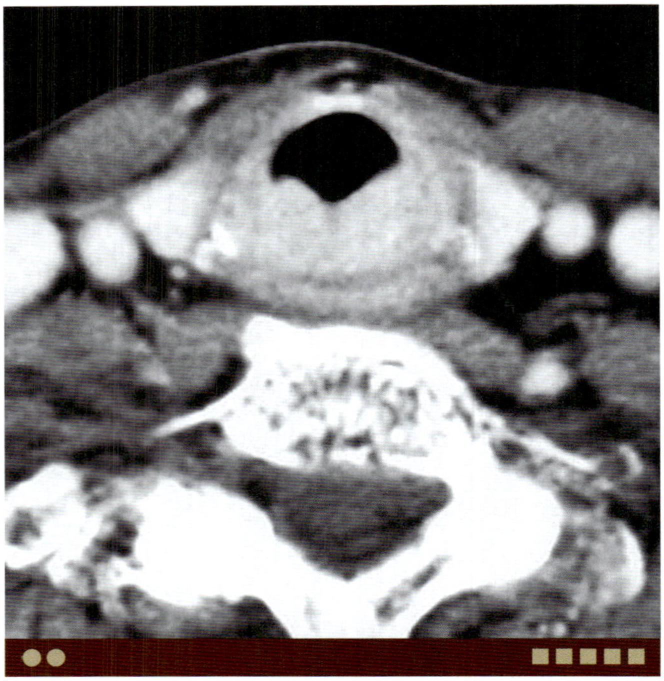

F. Plasmacytoma. Axial contrast-enhancec CT shows a homogeneously enhancing tumor in the posterior subglottis.

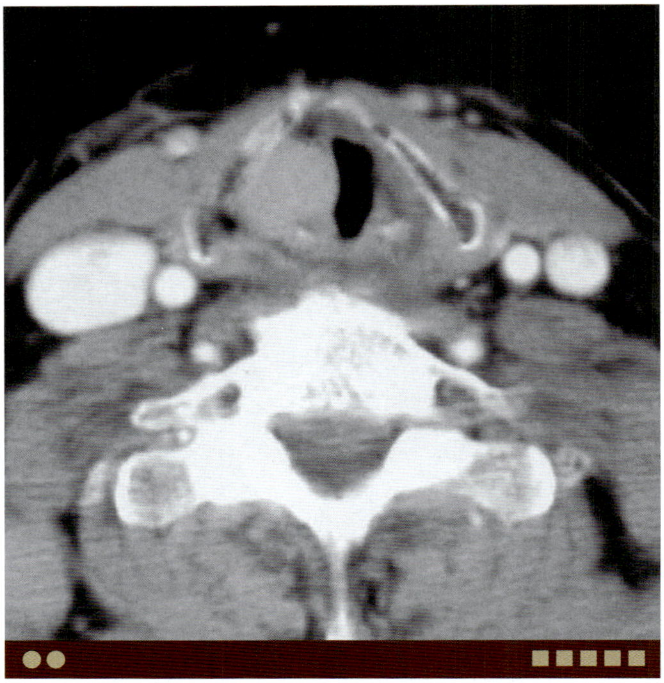

G. Rhabdomyoma. Axial contrast-enhanced CT demonstrates a homogeneously enhancing lesion in the right cord.

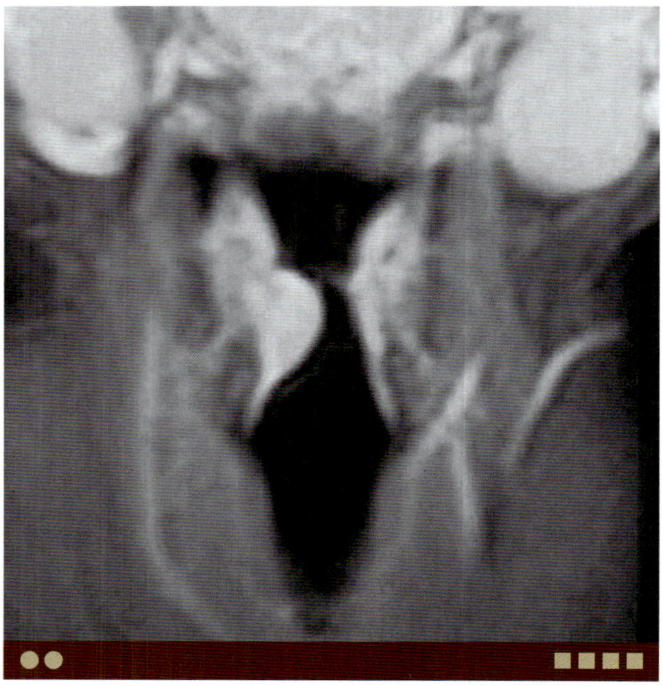

H. Granular cell tumor. Coronal postcontrast fat-suppressed T1W MR image shows a homogeneously enhancing lesion involving the right cord.

Case 10–11 Amyloidosis

Osamu Sakai, Akira Murakami

PRESENTATION

Hoarseness.

FINDINGS

CT and MRI demonstrate irregular thickening of the vocal cord.

DIFFERENTIAL DIAGNOSIS

- Squamous cell carcinoma: This is the most common malignancy and usually demonstrates heterogeneous density/signal and variable enhancement.
- Wegener's granulomatosis: This condition occurs anywhere in the aerodigestive tract and causes concentric narrowing of the lumen or nodular masses.
- Chondrosarcoma: This is the most common primary malignant tumor of the laryngeal cartilage and demonstrates internal calcification and local invasion.
- Extramedullary plasmacytoma: This is a B-cell tumor which can be found in the upper respiratory tract, and is often a coexistent lesion; localized amyloidosis is found in 15% of cases of extramedullary plasmacytoma.

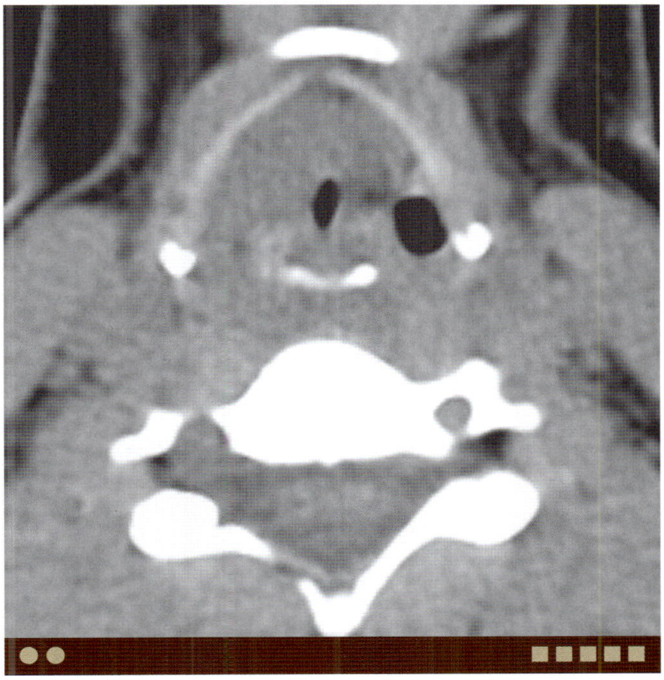

A. Amyloidosis. Axial noncontrast CT demonstrates thickening of the aryepiglottic folds, right more than left, and abnormal soft tissue density in the right paraglottic fat.

COMMENTS

This is a 55-year-old woman with hoarseness.

Amyloidosis is a rare disorder of deposition of abnormal amount of proteins in various organs. Clinically, amyloidosis can be categorized into either systemic or localized disease. About 10% to 15% are localized, which is rare and relatively benign condition. In the head and neck, most amyloidomas are secondary to the localized form. The lesions are most often the result of abnormal immunoglobulin light chains which are deposited locally by a clone of plasma cells. The resulting insoluble fibrillar proteins produce the characteristic apple-green birefringence under polarized light microscopy, which is seen in all amyloid deposits.

Although amyloidosis is seen anywhere in the aerodigestive tract, the larynx is the most common site; vocal cords and ventricles are commonly affected. Presenting symptoms include hoarseness, cough, and sensation of fullness. Stridor and dyspnea may be seen in patients with extensive involvement in the larynx or trachea. Presence of amyloid can be confirmed histologically by the characteristic Congo red staining under polarized light microscopy, through immunohistochemical stains, or by electron microscopic findings.

Amyloid deposits can be diffuse submucosal deposit or focal nodular deposit. On CT, it usually demonstrates soft tissue density with or without calcification. On MRI, amyloidomas show low signal on T1W, and low-to-intermediate signal on T2W images, with little-to-no enhancement.

Macroglossia and lymphadenopathy are both characteristics more typical of systemic amyloid disease. Further clinical assessment is needed in these cases to assess further organ system involvement.

PEARLS

- **Head and neck amyloidosis is most commonly seen in the larynx; however, it can occur anywhere in the entire aerodigestive tract.**
- **Amyloid deposits can be diffuse submucosal deposit or focal nodular deposit. Calcification is common.**
- **Amyloidoma shows low signal on T1W and T2W MR images, and no or minimal enhancement.**

ADDITIONAL IMAGES (B-D)

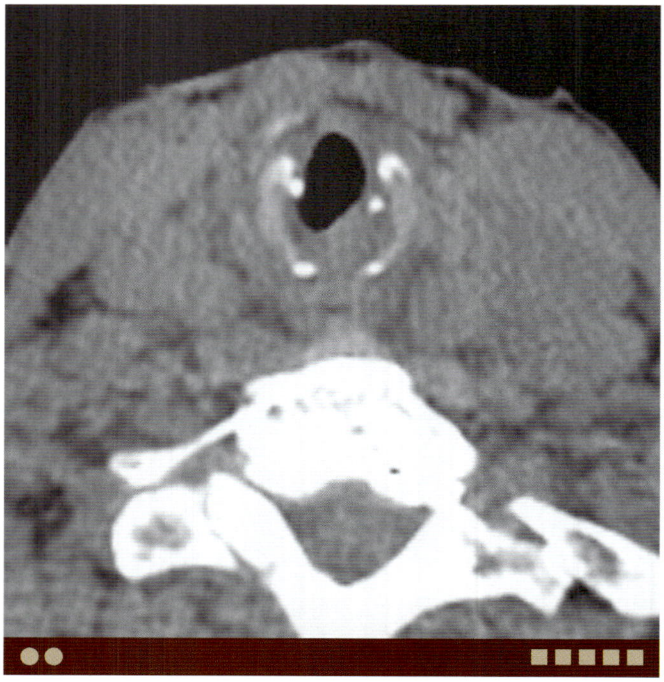

B. Amyloidosis in a different patient. Axial CT demonstrates slightly irregular concentric narrowing of the subglottis. Note focal calcifications.

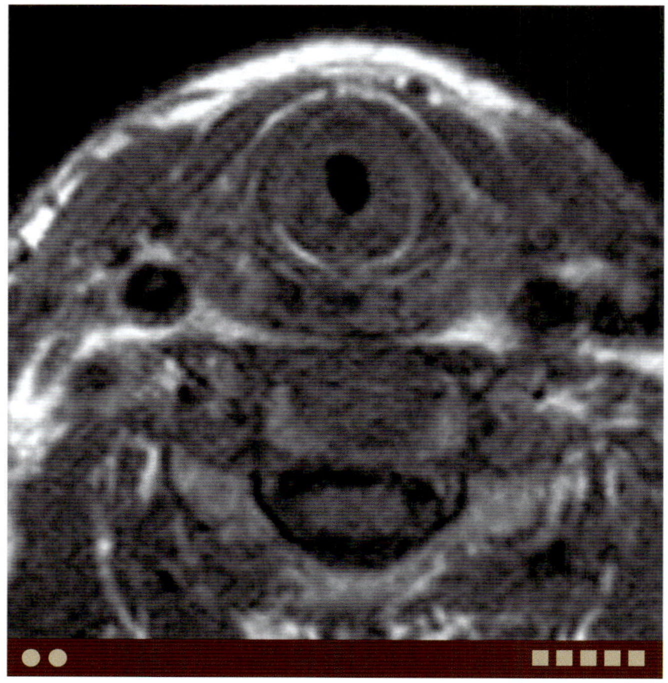

C. Amyloidosis in a different patient. Axial T1W MR image shows circumferential narrowing of the subg ottis due to submucosal amyloid deposit.

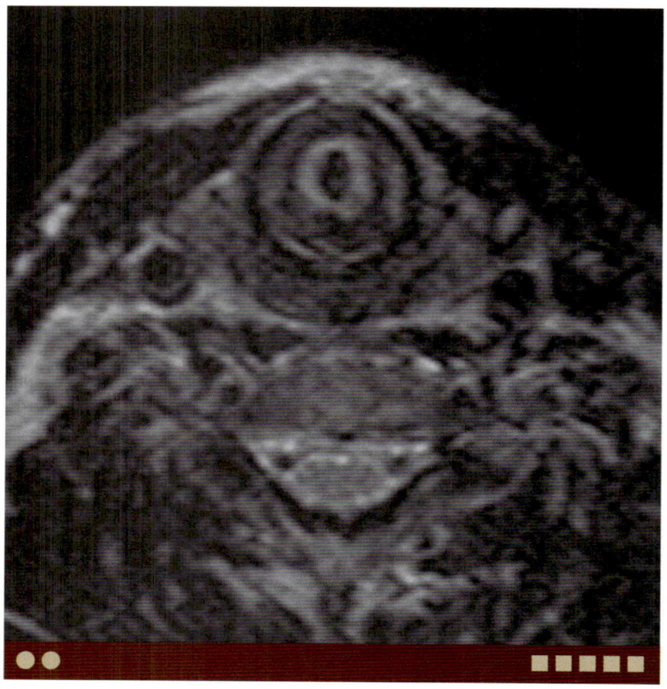

D. Amyloidosis, same patient as C. Axial T2W MR image shows circumferential narrowing of the subglottis due to submucosal amyloid deposit. Note iso-to-low signal of the lesion.

DIFFERENTIAL DIAGNOSIS IMAGES (E-H)

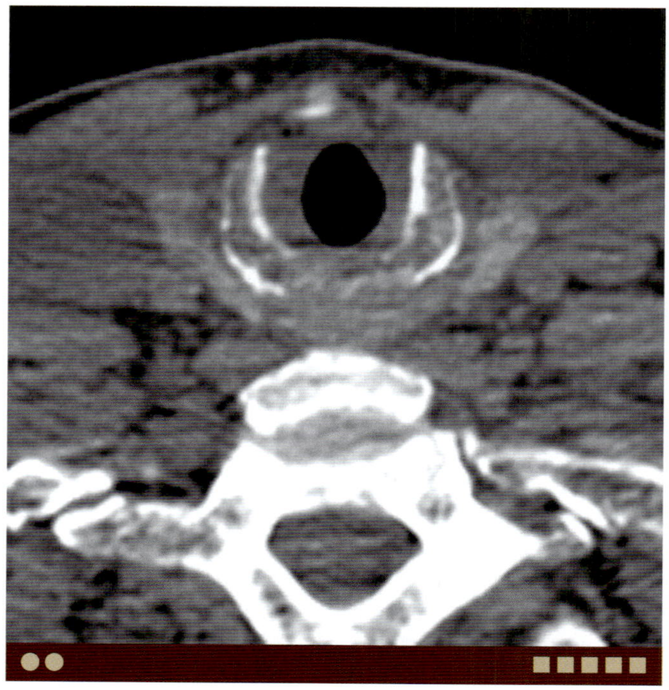

E. Wegener's granulomatosis. Axial noncontrast CT demonstrates slightly irregular circumferential soft tissue thickening in the subglottis, very similar to amyloidosis.

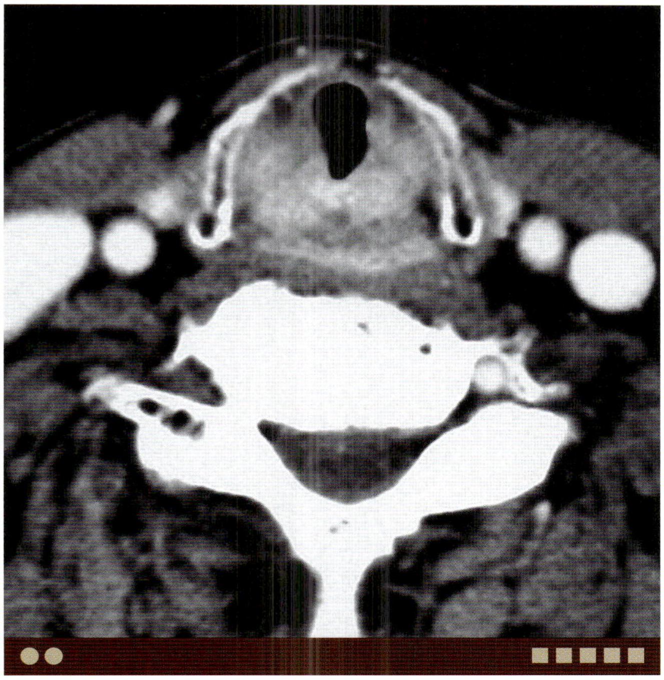

F. Plasmacytoma. Axial postcontrast CT shows a homogeneously enhancing tumor in the posterior glottis and subglottis.

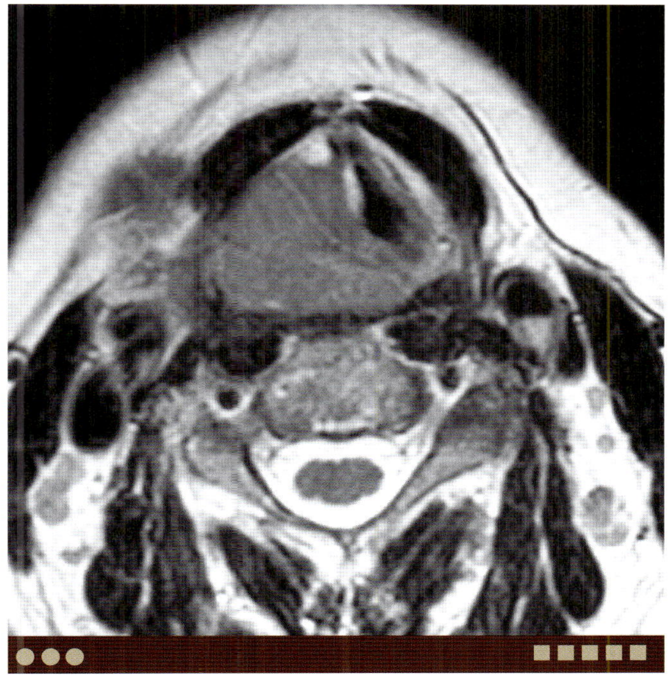

G. Lymphoma. Axial T2W MR image shows homogeneous intermediate-signal lesion centered in the right paraglottic space.

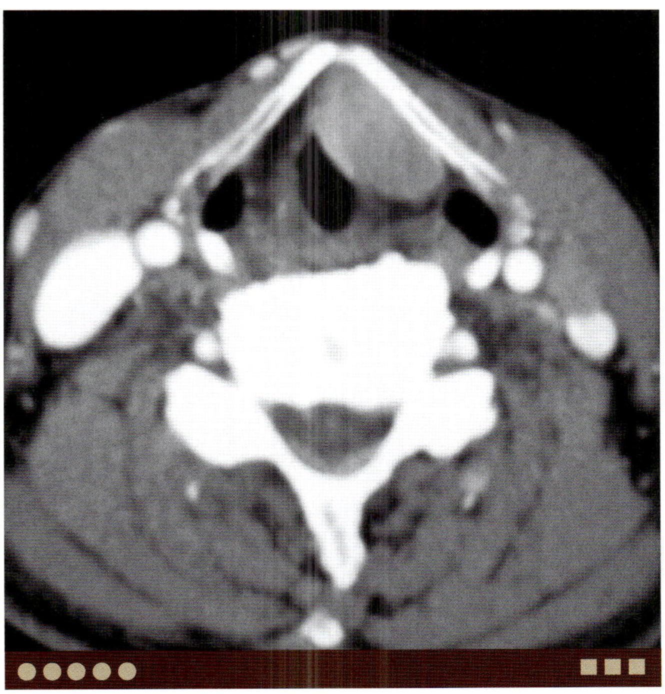

H. Squamous cell carcinoma. Axial postcontrast CT shows an enhancing tumor in the left supraglottic larynx.

Case 10–12 Laryngeal and Tracheal Papillomatosis

Osamu Sakai, Jimmy Wang

PRESENTATION

Hoarseness.

FINDINGS

CT demonstrates multiple nodular lesions in the larynx and trachea.

DIFFERENTIAL DIAGNOSIS

- Vocal cord polyp: This develops mainly from overuse of the voice and is seen in the true vocal cord.
- Squamous cell carcinoma (SCCA): SCCA can be polypoid in appearance and human papilloma virus (HPV) infection can cause SCCA as well as papillomas.
- Amyloidosis: This condition causes amyloid deposits in the submucosa with or without calcification.

COMMENTS

This is a 35-year-old man with hoarseness.

Laryngeal papillomatosis is a rare condition caused by HPV infection (types 6 and 11) in the larynx and other areas of the respiratory tract. It causes multiple tumors, papillomas, to develop over time. These can recur frequently and may require repetitive surgeries, and rarely can progress to squamous cell carcinomas. Without treatment, it is potentially fatal as uncontrolled growths can obstruct the airway.

Laryngeal and tracheal papillomatosis is usually diagnosed in the pediatric population; two-thirds of cases are diagnosed in patients under 4 years old. Clinically, it usually presents with hoarseness. Usually, it is localized in the larynx; however, dissemination to the trachea and bronchi are not uncommon. Typically, it will be less prominent after adolescence; fewer than 1% of cases result in airway dissemination and pulmonary parenchymal disease.

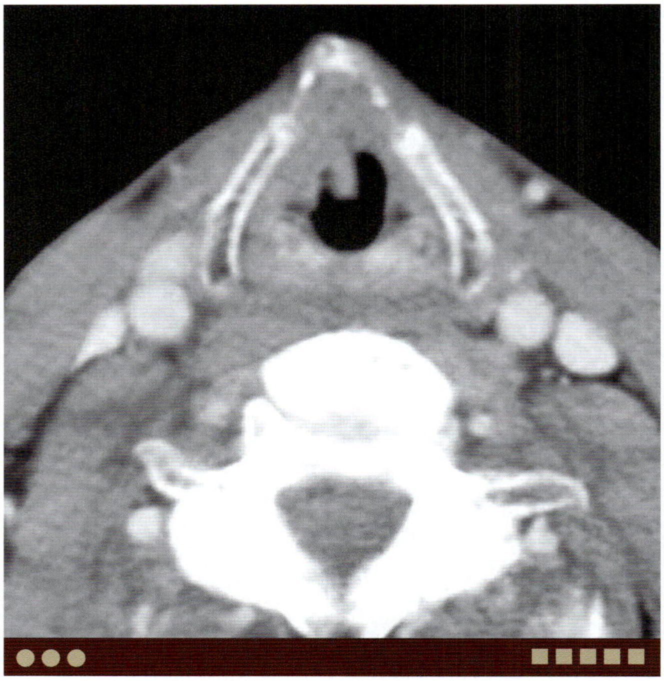

A. Laryngeal papillomatosis. Axial contrast-enhanced CT demonstrates a polypoid lesion in the anterior portion of the right vocal cord.

Histologically, it is papillary, cauliflower-like proliferation of the squamous epithelium. Endoscopic resection often using carbon dioxide laser is the mainstay of treatment.

PEARLS

- **Laryngeal and tracheal papillomatosis is caused by human papilloma virus (types 6 and 11).**
- **Laryngeal and tracheal papillomatosis is usually diagnosed in the pediatric population.**
- **Usually, it is localized in the larynx; however, dissemination to the trachea and bronchi are rare (<1%).**

ADDITIONAL IMAGES (B–E)

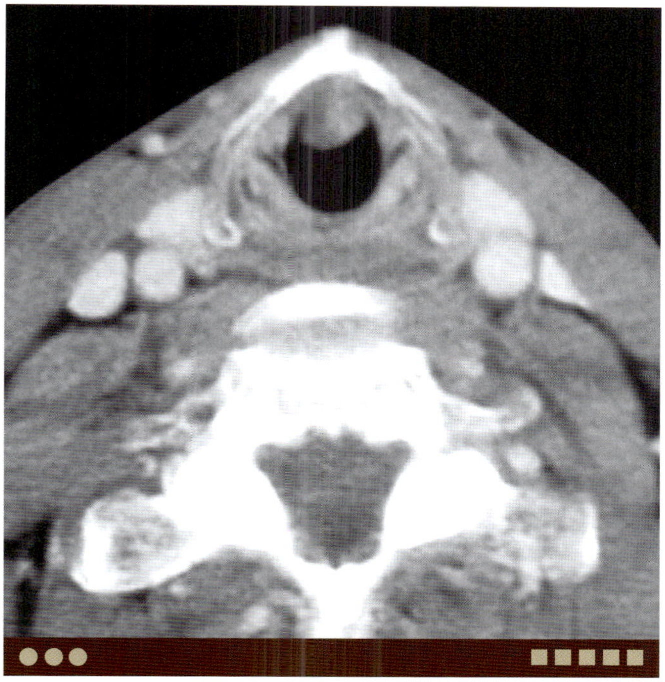

B. Laryngeal papillomatosis, same patient as A. Axial contrast-enhanced CT through the subglottic larynx demonstrates a round polypoid lesion anteriorly.

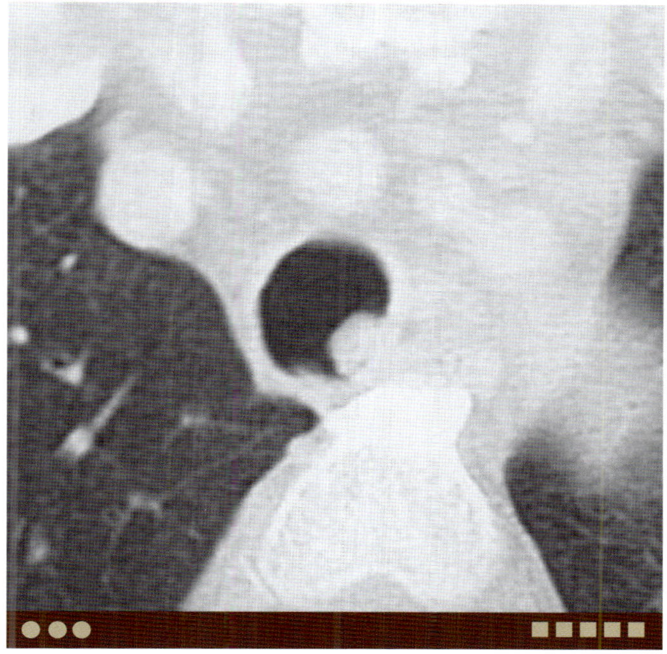

C. Laryngeal papillomatosis, same patient as A. Axial CT through the trachea demonstrates a polypoid lesion

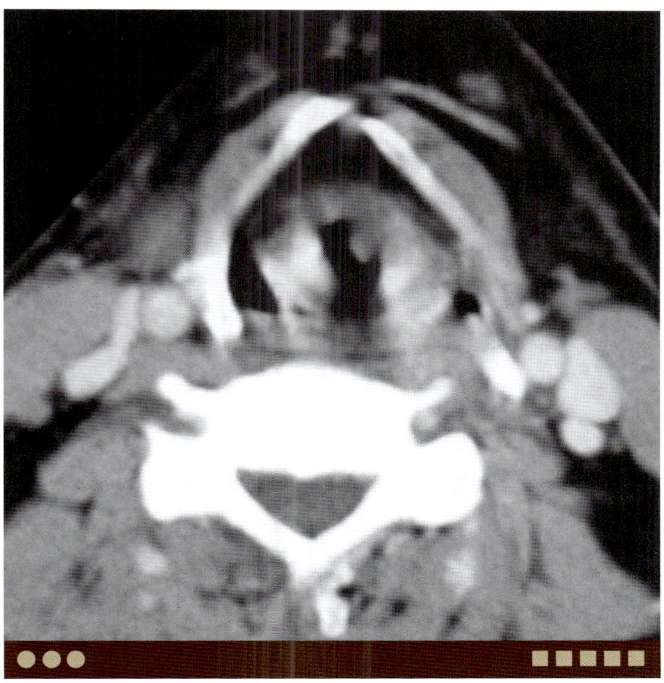

D. Laryngeal papillomatosis in a different patient. Axial contrast-enhanced CT through the supraglottic larynx demonstrates diffuse thickening of the aryepiglottic folds and a polypoid lesion on the left.

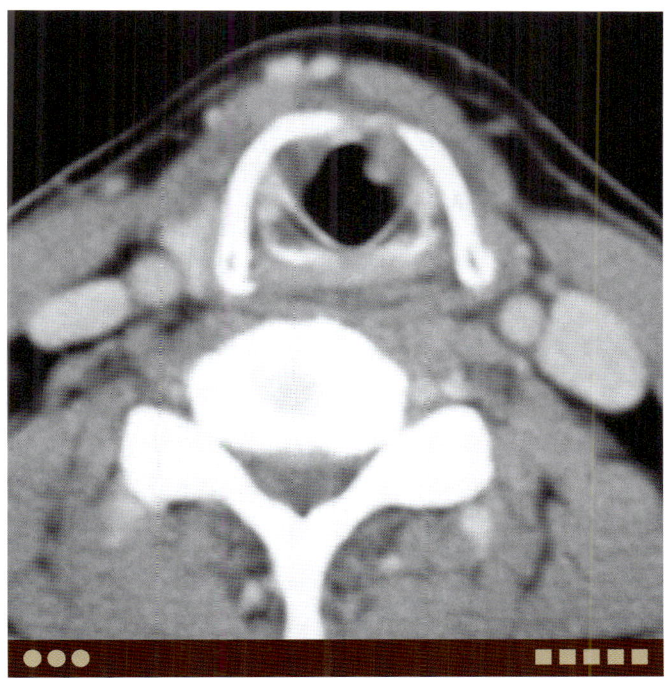

E. Laryngeal papillomatosis, same patient as D. Axial contrast-enhanced CT through the subglottic larynx demonstrates a polypoid lesion on the left.

DIFFERENTIAL DIAGNOSIS IMAGES (F-G)

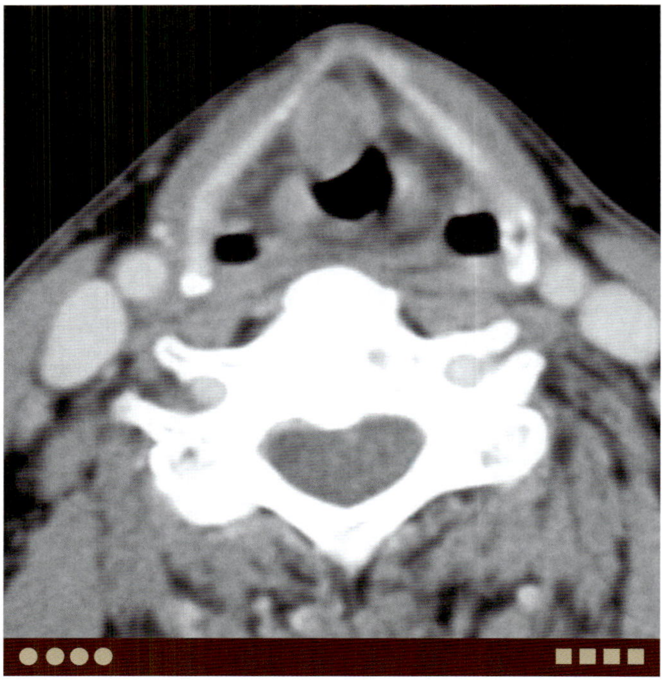

F. Squamous cell carcinoma. Axial contrast-enhanced CT through the supraglottic larynx demonstrates a nodular lesion anteriorly and on the right.

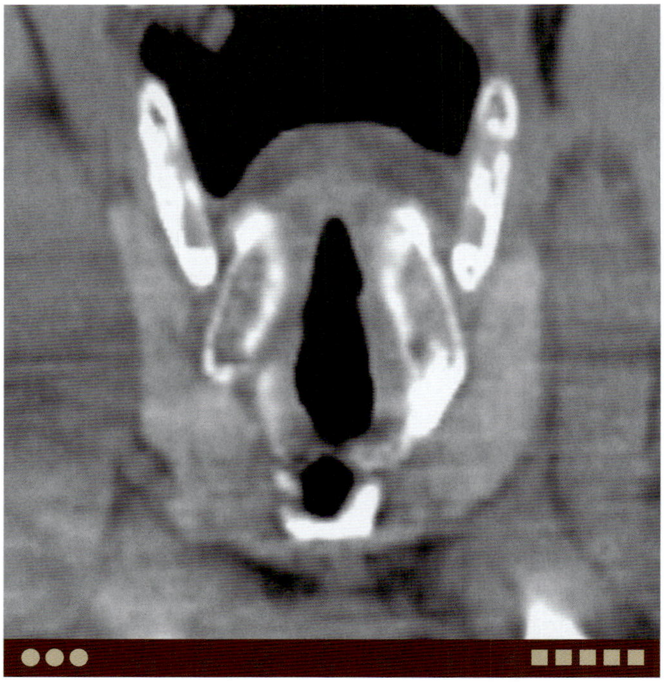

G. Wegener's granulomatosis. Coronal noncontrast CT through the larynx demonstrates diffuse mucosal thickening of the subglottis and upper trachea and nodular lesions in the upper trachea.

Case 10–13 Laryngeal Schwannoma

Osamu Sakai, Jimmy Wang

PRESENTATION

Hoarseness.

FINDINGS

CT demonstrates a well-demarcated soft tissue density mass in the larynx.

DIFFERENTIAL DIAGNOSIS

- Squamous cell carcinoma: This is the most common malignancy and can be seen as a submucosal tumor.
- Lymphoma: This often demonstrates a large homogeneous density/signal mass in the supraglottic larynx.
- Hemangioma: This is rare condition, often seen in children, in the subglottic region. This demonstrates very high signal on T2W MR images.
- Retention cyst: This is often seen in the vallecula or supraglottis.
- Saccular cyst: This water-filled laryngocele may mimic a solid mass.

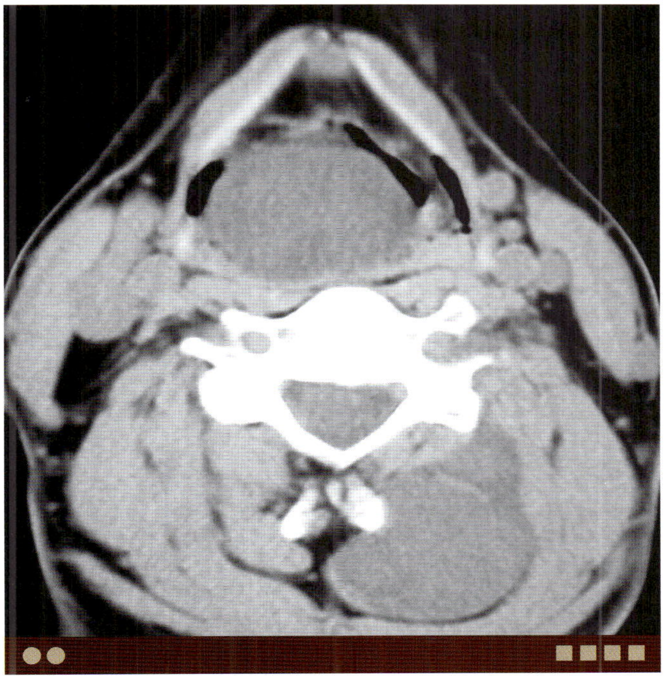

A. Schwannoma. Axial CT demonstrates a tumor in the supraglottic larynx, demonstrating homogeneous low density. Note another lesion in the left posterior paraspinal muscles demonstrating similar density.

COMMENTS

This is a 38-year-old man with hoarseness.

Neurogenic tumors such as schwannoma and neurofibroma are rare in the larynx. Laryngeal schwannoma usually grows very slowly and is often diagnosed between 50 and 60 years old with female predominance. The symptom varies depending on its location and size, such as pain, dysphagia, dyspnea, dysphonia, and hoarseness. Most schwannomas arise in the supraglottic larynx, and involve the false cord, aryepiglottic fold, and epiglottis, from the superior laryngeal nerve. This is a rare tumor, however, important for the differential diagnosis of submucosal tumors in the larynx.

On CT, it demonstrates relatively homogeneous soft tissue density with mild enhancement. Calcification is rarely seen. On MRI, it usually demonstrates low signal on T1W and intermediate-to-high signal on T2W images. Relatively homogeneous enhancement is seen after contrast.

PEARLS

- **Laryngeal schwannoma is a rare submucosal tumor of the larynx.**
- **Laryngeal schwannoma demonstrates soft tissue density on CT, low signal on T1W, and intermediate-to-high signal on T2W images and relatively homogeneous enhancement.**

ADDITIONAL IMAGES (B-D)

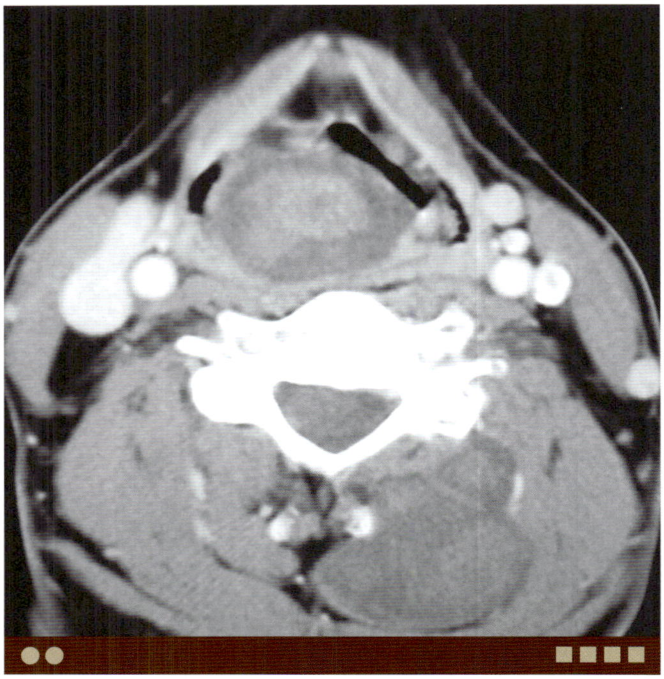

B. Schwannoma, same patient as A. Axial postcontrast CT demonstrates mild enhancement in the tumors.

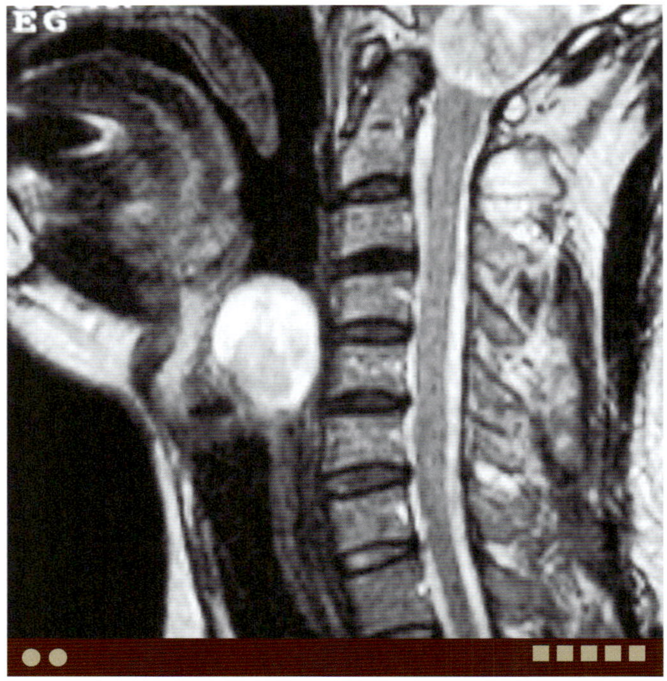

C. Schwannoma, same patient as A. Sagittal T2W image shows the lesion in the supraglottic larynx demonstrating high signals. Note a heterogeneously high-signal lesion at the foramen magnum, another schwannoma.

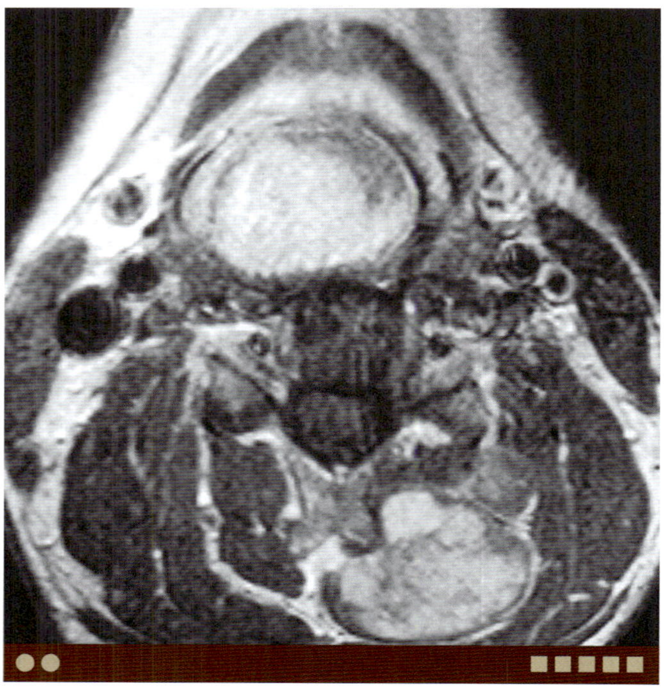

D. Schwannoma, same patient as A. Axial postcontrast T1W image shows slightly heterogeneous enhancement of the tumors.

DIFFERENTIAL DIAGNOSIS IMAGES (E-H)

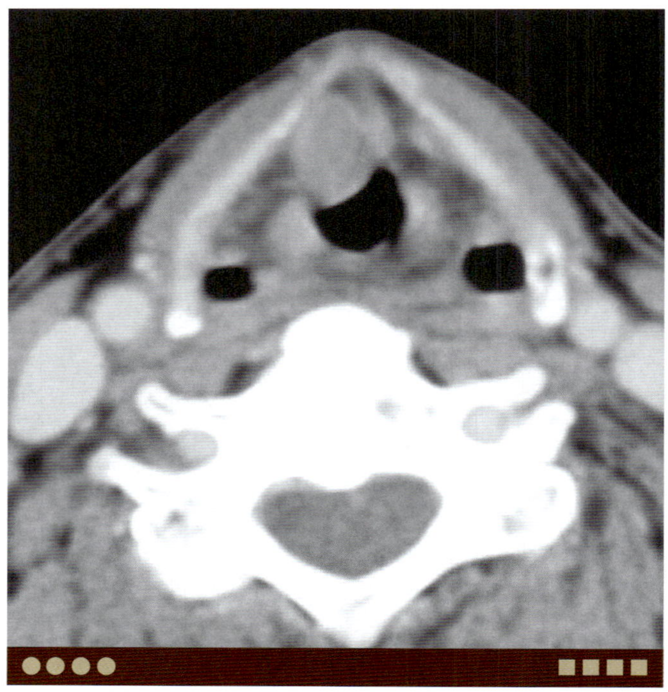

E. Squamous cell carcinoma. Axial contrast-enhanced CT shows a round lesion in the right supraglottic larynx.

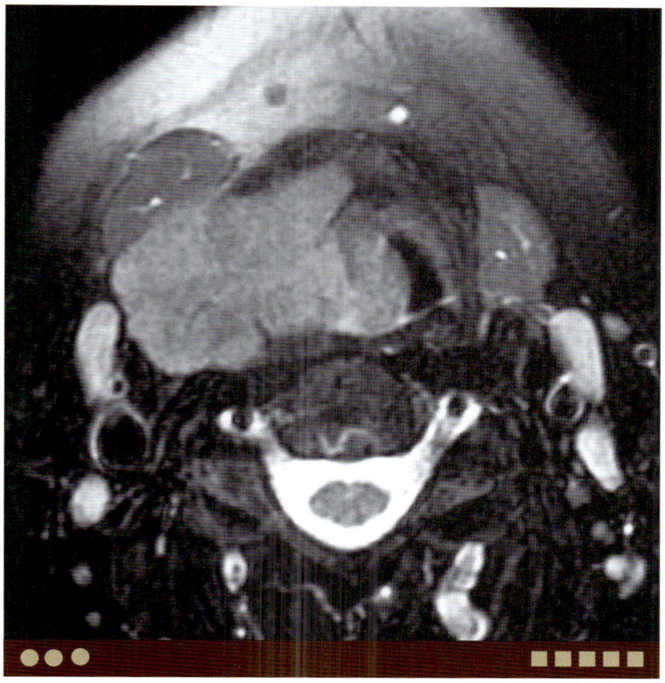

F. Lymphoma. Axial STIR image demonstrates a lobulated, homogeneous intermediate-signal lesion centered in the right supraglottic larynx.

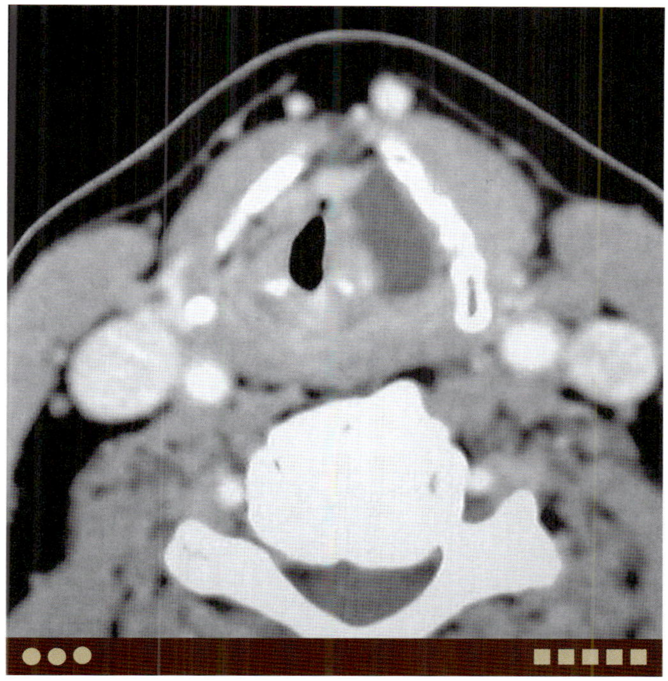

G. Saccular cyst. Axial CT demonstrates a fluid-filled lesion in the left paraglottic space.

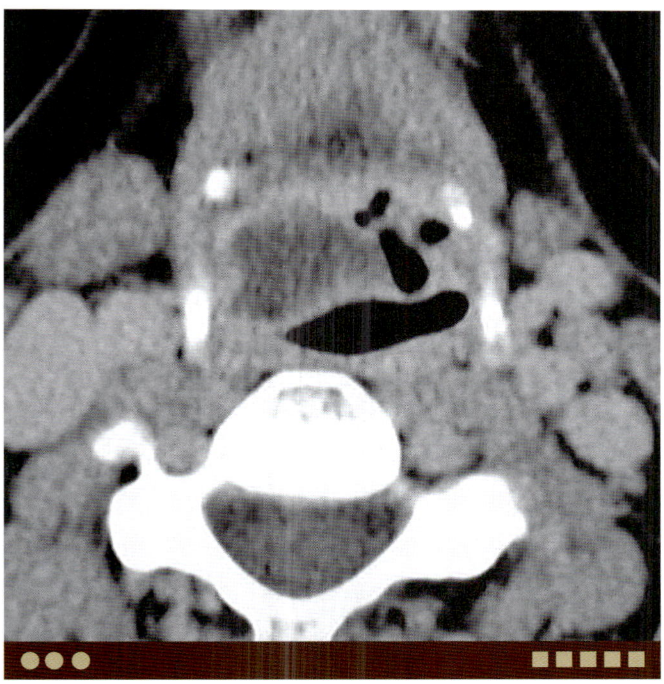

H. Vallecular cyst. Axial CT shows a water density lesion in the right vallecula.

Case 10–14 Recurrent Laryngeal Nerve Palsy

Osamu Sakai, Jimmy Wang

PRESENTATION

Hoarseness.

FINDINGS

CT demonstrates dilated laryngeal ventricle.

DIFFERENTIAL DIAGNOSIS

- Patient positioning: Slight asymmetry of the larynx may be seen secondary to patient positioning and scan plane.

COMMENTS

This is a 65-year-old man with hoarseness.

Recurrent laryngeal nerve palsy (vocal cord paralysis) is diagnosed clinically, and the role of imaging is to identify the causative lesion, not to make the diagnosis. It is important to cover the entire course of the vagus nerve and recurrent laryngeal nerve from the skull base to the aortic arch. The vagus nerve exits from the jugular foramen with glossopharyngeal and spinal accessory nerves as well as the internal jugular vein. Below the hyoid, the vagus nerve is the only cranial nerve that runs within the carotid sheath. The recurrent laryngeal nerve is a branch of the vagus nerve. Usually, the left nerve goes to the level of aorticopulmonary window and the right nerve goes to the level of subclavian artery, and then the nerves ascend to innervate the laryngeal muscles. It used to be difficult to obtain thin sections covering a wide field of view, but now with multidetector computed tomography (MDCT) thin slices are easily obtained in a short period of time with less motion artifacts. Multiplanar reformations, particularly coronal images, are helpful to evaluate the larynx as well.

Evaluation of the larynx itself may not be important in cases of known vocal cord paralysis, because it is directly visualized and evaluated by the otolaryngologist. However, familiarity with images findings of recurrent laryngeal nerve palsy is important for unknown vocal cord paralysis cases. These findings are (1) widening of the pyriform sinus, (2) dilatation of the laryngeal ventricle, (3) atrophy of the thyroarytenoid muscle (vocal cord), (4) medial deviation and rotation of the arytenoid cartilage, and (5) atrophy of the posterior cricoarytenoid muscle. On MRI, denervation myositic change, increased T2 signal, and abnormal enhancement of the affected muscles may be seen in acute/subacute phase of denervation.

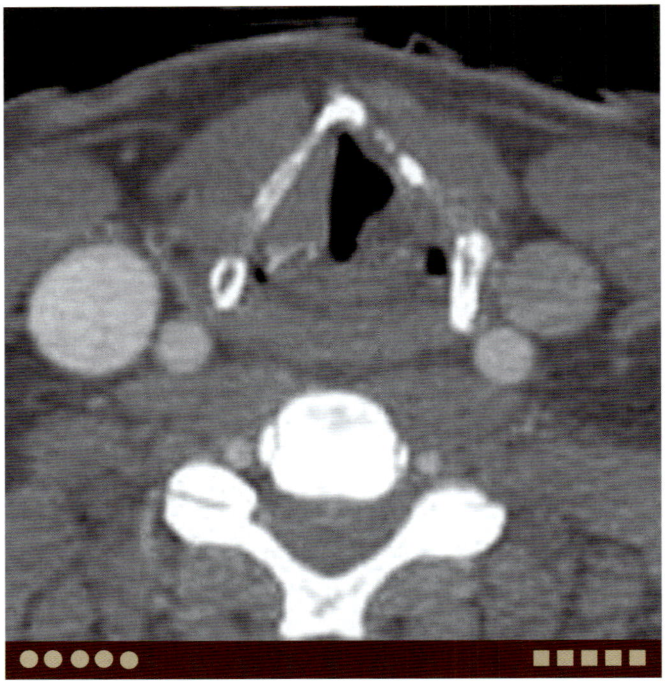

A. Recurrent laryngeal nerve palsy. Axial CT demonstrates atrophy of the left cord and widening of the left laryngeal ventricle.

PEARLS

- **To evaluate the cause of recurrent laryngeal nerve palsy, it is important to cover the entire course of the vagus nerve and recurrent laryngeal nerve from the skull base to the aortic arch.**
- **Imaging findings of recurrent laryngeal nerve palsy are widening of the pyriform sinus, dilatation of the laryngeal ventricle, atrophy of the thyroarytenoid muscle, medial deviation and rotation of the arytenoid cartilage, and atrophy of the posterior cricoarytenoid muscle.**

ADDITIONAL IMAGES (B-F)

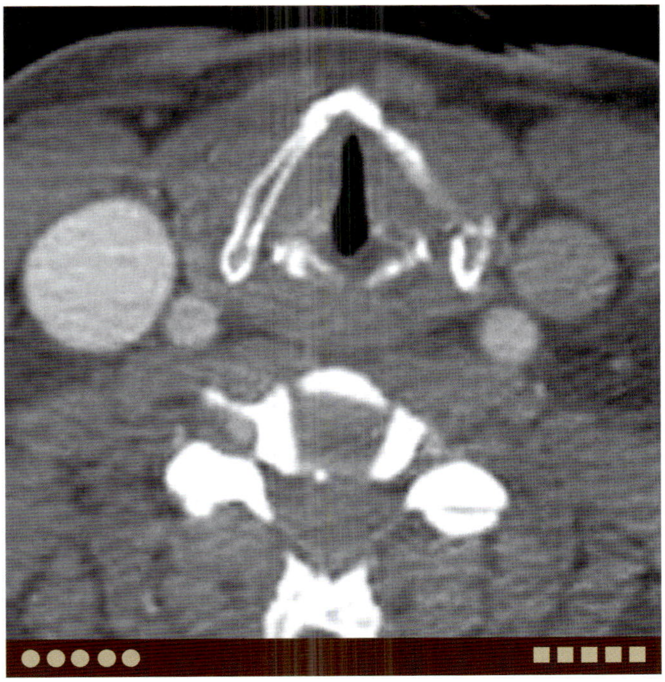

B. Recurrent laryngeal nerve palsy, same patient as A. Axial CT through the arytenoid demonstrates atrophy of the left posterior cricoarytenoid muscle.

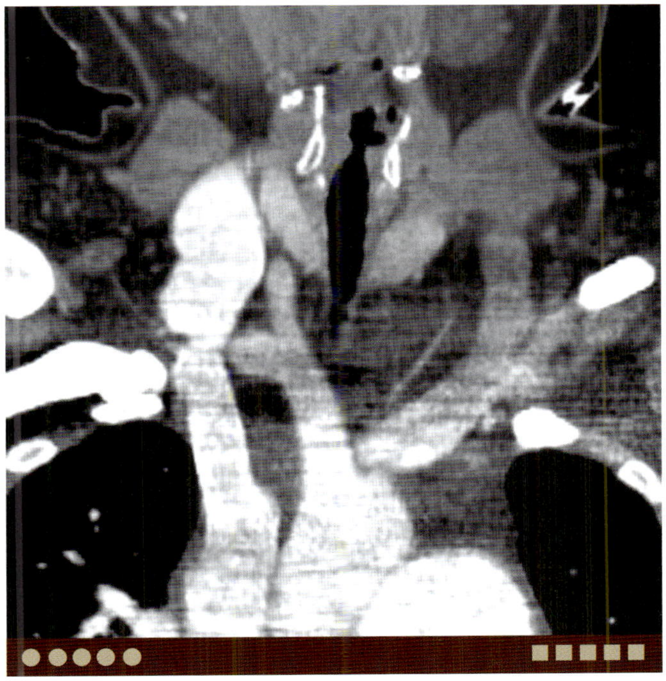

C. Recurrent laryngeal nerve palsy, same patient as A. Coronal CT demonstrates atrophy of the left cord and widening of the left laryngeal ventricle. Note an enlarged pulmonary artery.

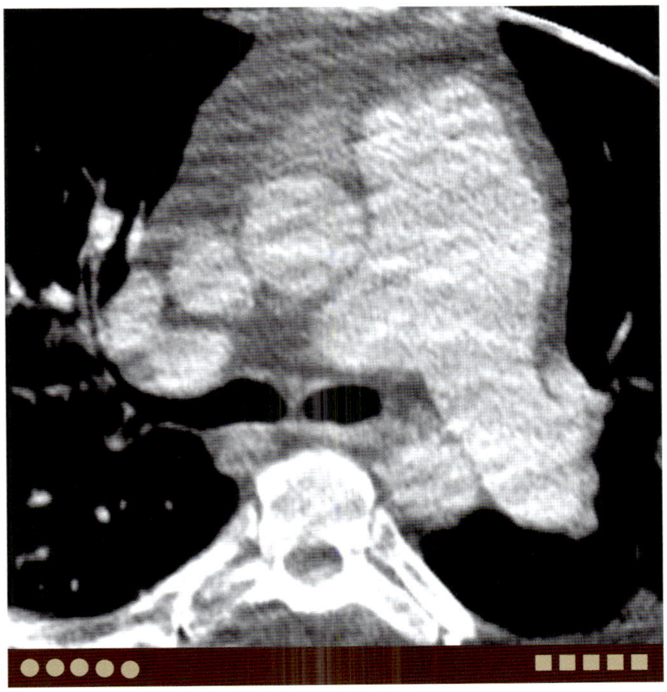

D. Recurrent laryngeal nerve palsy, same patient as A. Axial CT through the aorticopulmonary window demonstrates significantly enlarged pulmonary artery, which can cause left-sided recurrent laryngeal nerve palsy (Ortner's syndrome).

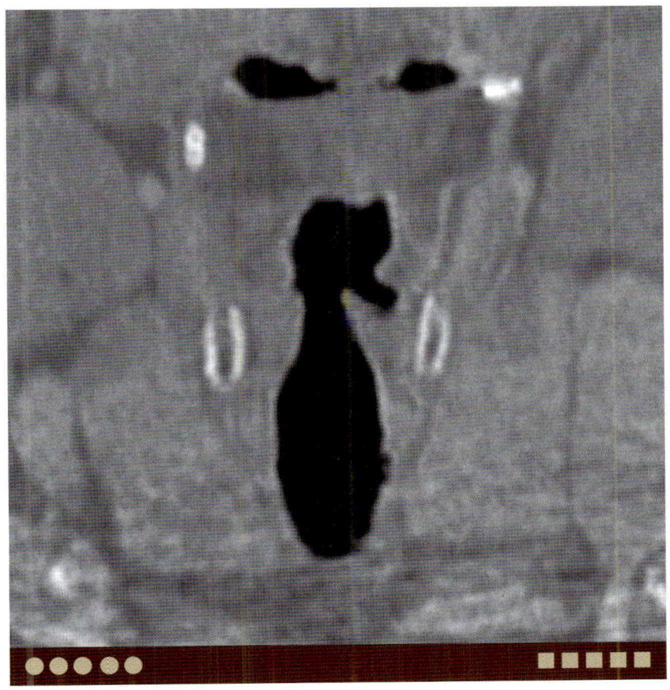

E. Recurrent laryngeal nerve palsy in a different patient. Coronal CT demonstrates atrophy and medial deviation of the left cord and widening of the left laryngeal ventricle.

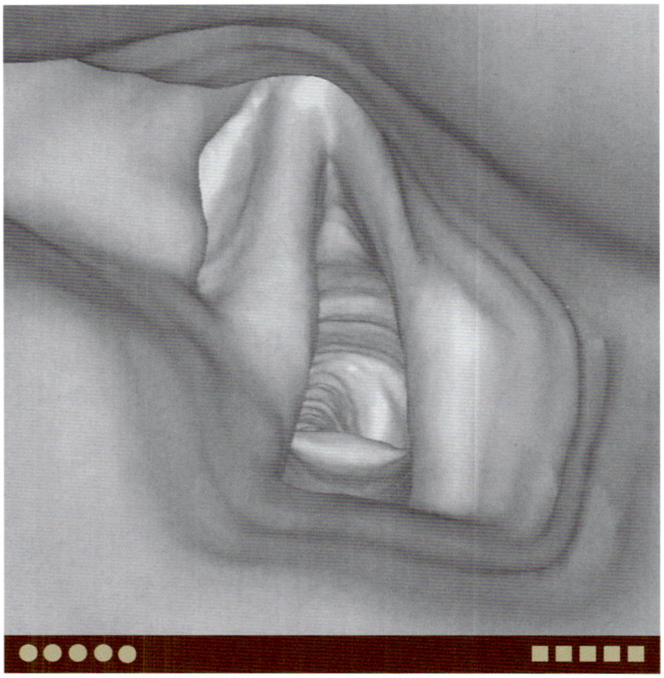

F. Recurrent laryngeal nerve palsy, same patient as E. 3D reconstruction, "virtual endoscopy" image view from supraglottic larynx demonstrates dilated left laryngeal ventricle and left cord atrophy.

Case 10–15 Granular Cell Tumor

Osamu Sakai, Jimmy Wang

PRESENTATION

Hoarseness.

FINDINGS

MRI demonstrates a homogeneously enhancing tumor in the glottis.

DIFFERENTIAL DIAGNOSIS

- Squamous cell carcinoma (SCCA): SCCA is the most common malignant tumor in the larynx. It usually demonstrates heterogeneous density/signal and invasive appearance; however, occasionally it shows homogeneous density/signal and is well circumscribed.
- Lymphoma: This laryngeal presentation usually demonstrates a submucosal, homogeneous, relatively low-signal lesion on T2W images.
- Rhabdomyoma and rhabdomyosarcoma: These are rare submucosal tumors. Rhabdomyosarcoma tends to demonstrate more aggressive features.
- Amyloidosis: This is a rare deposition disorder of abnormal amount of proteins and demonstrates nodular soft tissue thickening or a submucosal mass, often with calcification.

COMMENTS

This is a 55-year-old woman with hoarseness.

Granular cell tumor (GCT), also known as Abrikossoff tumor, is usually a benign, slowly growing neoplasm. In 1926, Abrikossoff called these tumors myoblastomas because he thought the tumor was of skeletal muscle origin; however, currently GCTs are generally accepted to be of neurogenic origin. GCTs can occur in any part of the body, and can be single or multiple; however, about half of all GCTs occur in the head and neck and most commonly in the tongue. It has female predominance, is more common in black population, and often presents between the third and sixth decades of life. More than half of GCTs of the larynx involve the true cord, particularly posterior cord and arytenoid regions, however, other parts of the larynx can be involved. GCTs in the pediatric population are rare, but often involve the anterior and subglottic regions in contrast to adults.

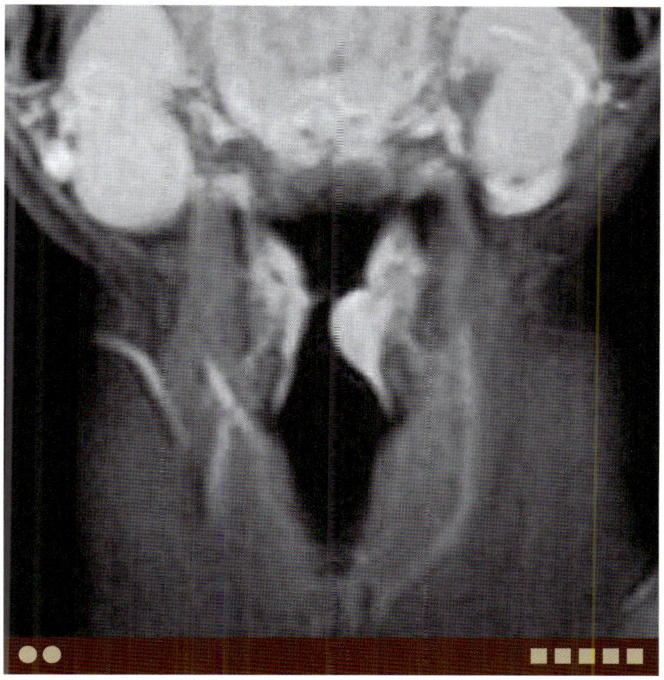

A. Granular cell tumor. Coronal postcontrast fat-suppressed T1W MR image demonstrates a homogeneously enhancing tumor in the left vocal cord.

On CT, GCTs are seen as a solid lesion with relatively homogeneous enhancement. On MRI, they tend to show slightly hypointense signal on T1W, heterogeneously increased signal on T2W images, and relatively homogeneous enhancement. However, imaging findings of GCTs are often nonspecific, and often difficult to differentiate from SCCA radiologically.

PEARLS

- **GCT is a rare laryngeal tumor, often involves the true cord.**
- **GCTs show relatively homogeneous enhancement on CT.**
- **GCTs show slightly hypointense signal on T1W, heterogeneously increased signal on T2W images, and homogeneous enhancement on MRI.**

ADDITIONAL IMAGES (B-F)

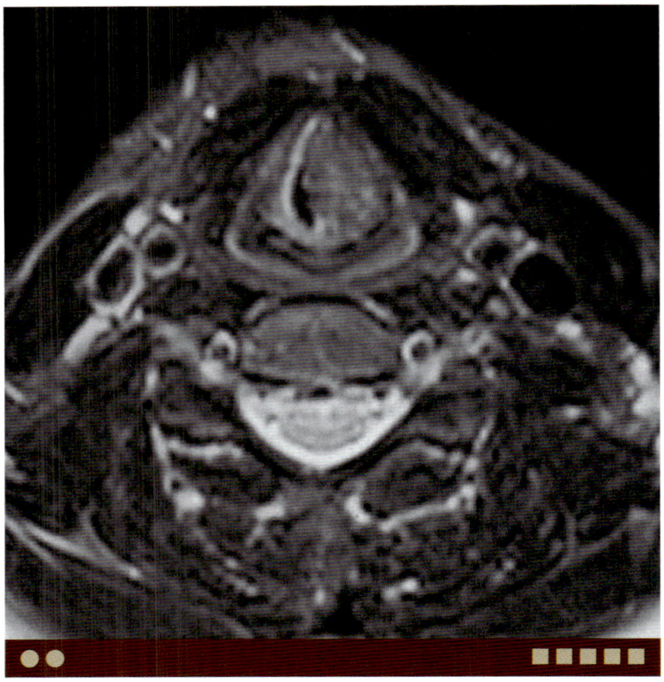

B. GCT, same patient as A. Axial T2W image shows slightly heterogeneous increased signal of the lesion.

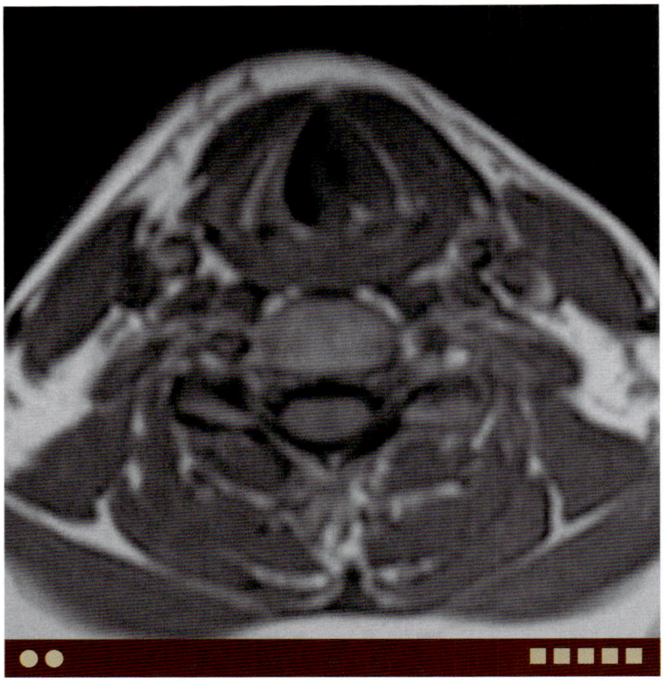

C. GCT, same patient as A. Axial T1W image shows low signal of the lesion.

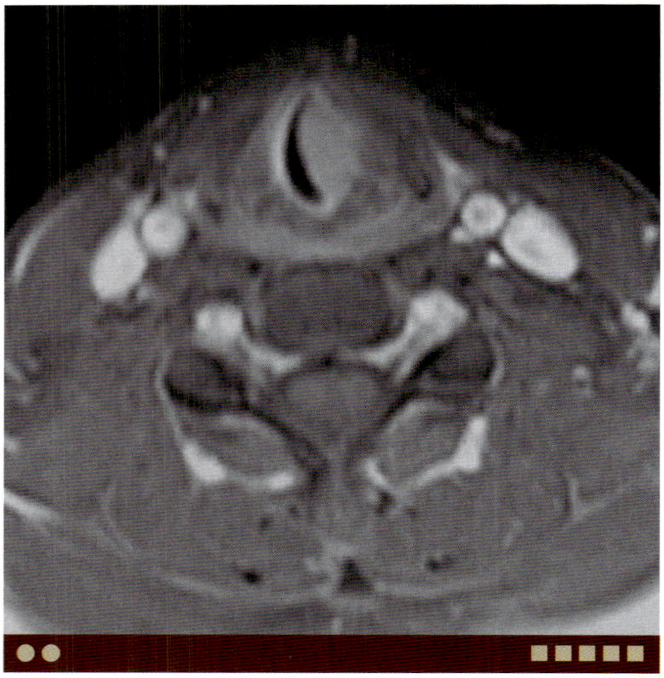

D. GCT, same patient as A. Axial postcontrast fat-suppressed T1W image shows homogeneous enhancement of the lesion.

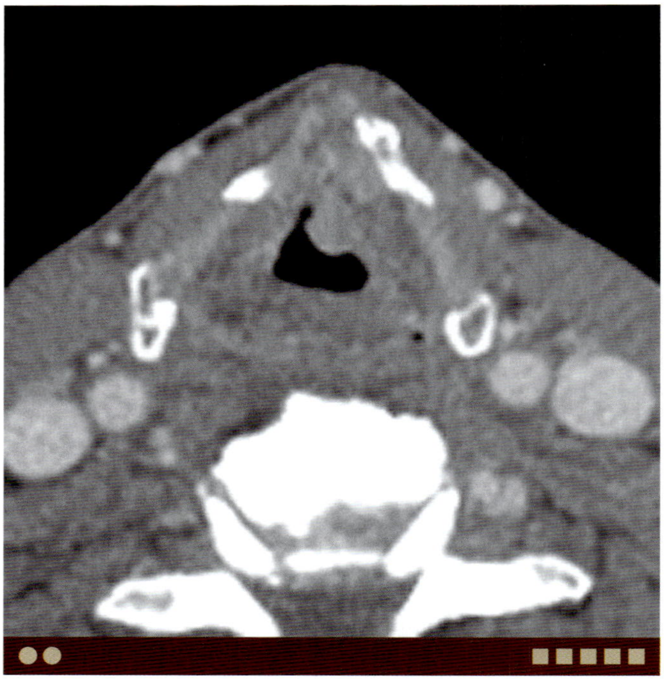

E. GCT in a different patient. Axial contrast-enhanced CT shows a homogeneously enhancing lesion in the left supraglottic larynx.

DIFFERENTIAL DIAGNOSIS IMAGES (G-I)

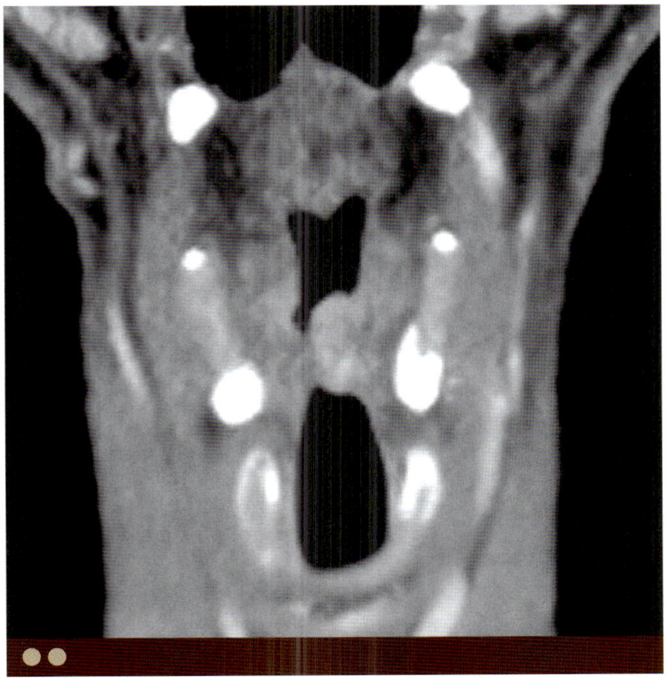

F. GCT, same patient as E. Coronal contrast-enhanced CT shows a homogeneously enhancing lesion seen in the left supraglottis and glottis.

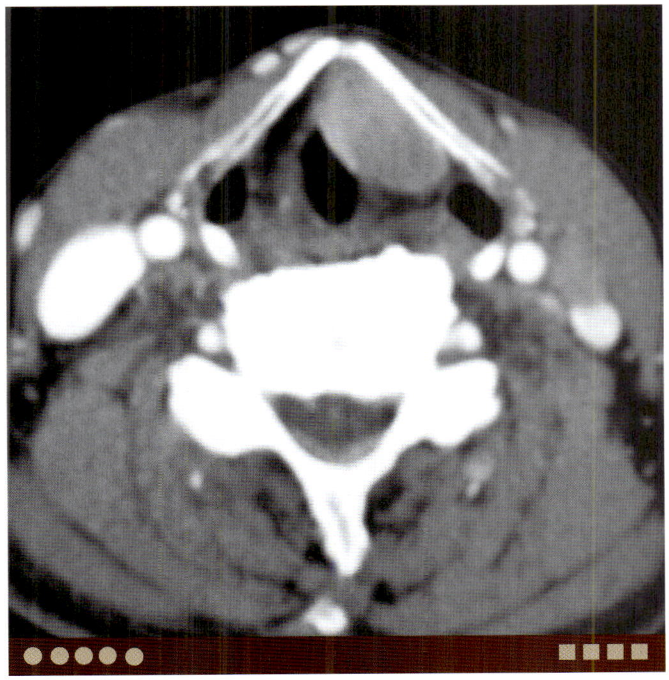

G. Squamous cell carcinoma. Axial contrast-enhanced CT shows a round lesion in the left supraglottic larynx

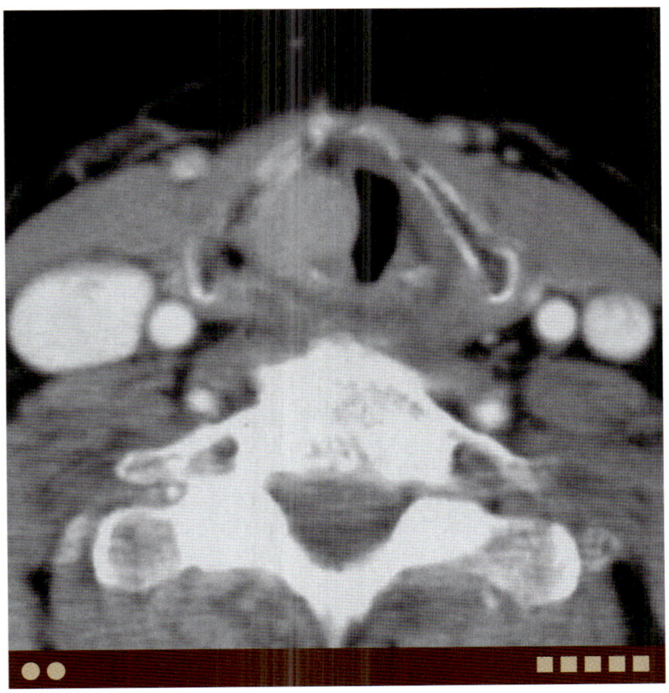

H. Rhabdomyoma. Axial contrast-enhanced CT demonstrates a homogeneously enhancing lesion in the right cord.

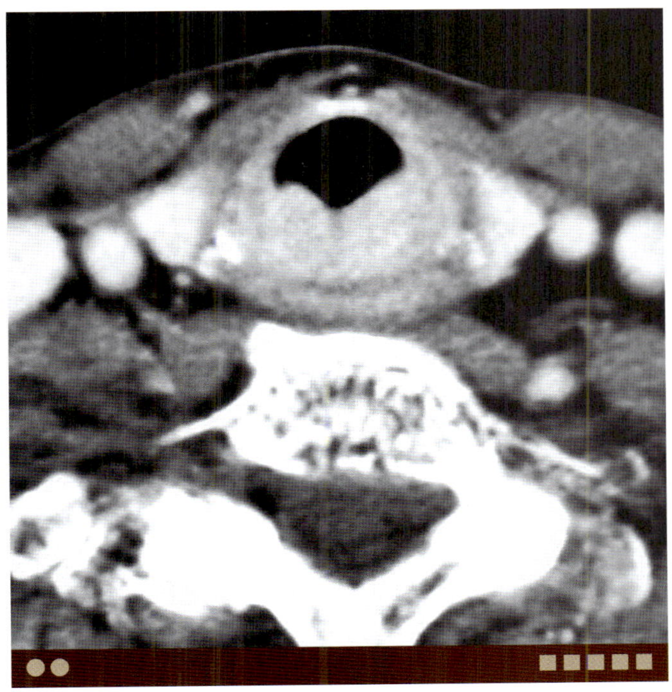

I. Plasmacytoma. Axial contrast-enhanced CT shows a homogeneously enhancing tumor in the posterior subglottis.

Case 10–16 Laryngeal Hemangioma

Akifumi Fujita, Osamu Sakai

PRESENTATION

Difficulty in breathing.

FINDINGS

MRI demonstrates a well-circumscribed, lobulated lesion in the larynx showing fairly high signal on T2W images and avid enhancement.

DIFFERENTIAL DIAGNOSIS

- Squamous cell carcinoma (SCCA): This is the most common malignant laryngeal tumor. Most SCCAs are diagnosed clinically; therefore, the role of cross-sectional imaging is to evaluate local extension of the tumor and nodal metastasis.
- Schwannoma: Laryngeal schwannoma usually grows very slowly and is often diagnosed between 50 and 60 years old with female predominance. The symptom varies depending on its location and size.
- Lymphoma: This condition usually demonstrates a submucosal, homogeneous, relatively low-signal lesion on T2W images.
- Papillomas: This condition usually occurs in children.
- Laryngocele: This condition usually contains air (laryngocele) or fluid (saccular cyst) inside the lesion. Peripheral enhancement may be seen on postcontrast images.

COMMENTS

This is a 33-year-old man with an incidentally found supraglottic mass without complaint of airway obstruction.

Laryngeal hemangioma is a benign nonepithelial or mesenchymal tumor, typically located in the glottic or subglottic region. They are more common in adults than in children, but pediatric type is more likely to occur in the subglottic area that may cause airway obstruction. Although they often regress, intervention may be necessary due to airway compromise. In adults, hemangiomas (or venous malformations) tend to be localized in the glottic and supraglottic. Extralaryngeal hemangiomas rarely extend into the larynx.

Hemangioma is seen as a well-circumscribed lobular mass on CT and MRI. Phleboliths may be seen in large lesions. Hemangiomas typically demonstrate very high signal on T2W MR images, and enhancement both on CT and MRI. These findings are very helpful to differentiate from other benign mesenchymal tumors, such as neurogenic tumor, paraganglioma, lipoma, leiomyoma, rhabdomyoma, chondroma, as well as malignant tumors, such as squamous cell carcinoma, minor salivary gland carcinoma, sarcoma especially chondrosarcoma, lymphoma, and metastasis.

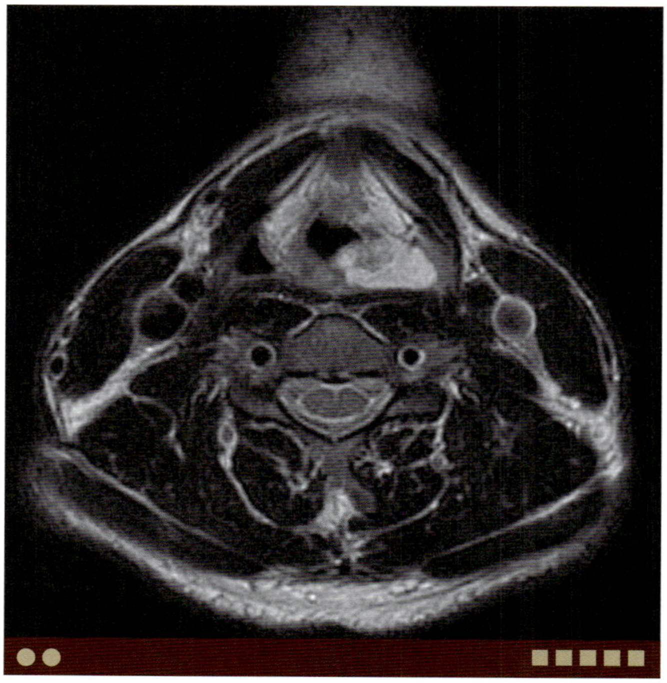

A. Laryngeal hemangioma. Axial T2W MR image demonstrates a well-circumscribed lobulated, fairly high-signal mass in the left supraglottic larynx.

PEARLS

- **Laryngeal hemangioma is more common in adults, often in the supraglottic and glottic larynx.**
- **Pediatric lesions tend to occur in the subglottic larynx and receive more attention because they often cause airway obstruction.**
- **Fairly high signal on T2W images is characteristic for hemangiomas.**

ADDITIONAL IMAGES (B-D)

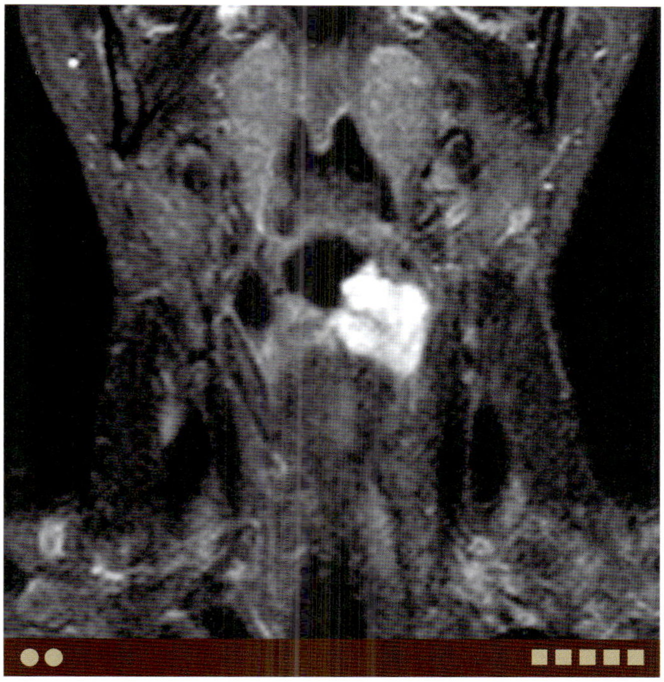

B. Laryngeal hemangioma, same patient as A. Coronal STIR image demonstrates a very high-signal mass in the left supraglottic and glottic larynx.

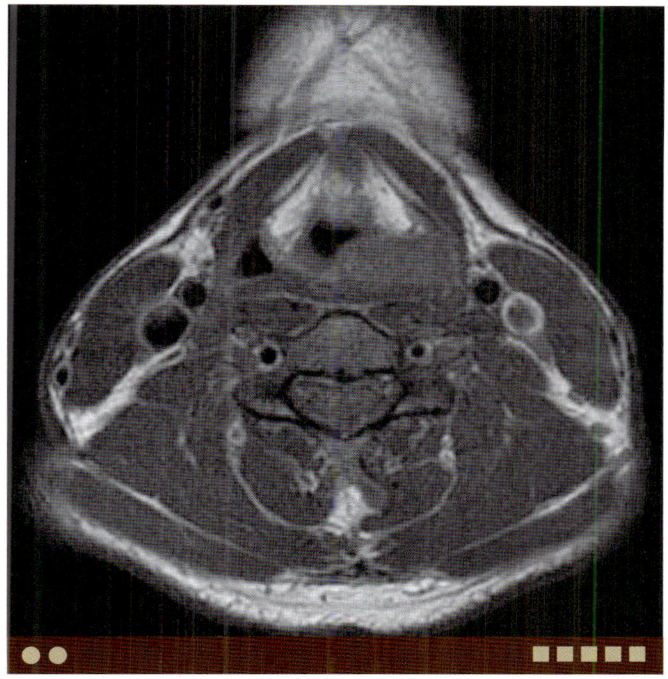

C. Laryngeal hemangioma, same patient as A. Axial T1W image demonstrates low signal of the left supraglottic lesion.

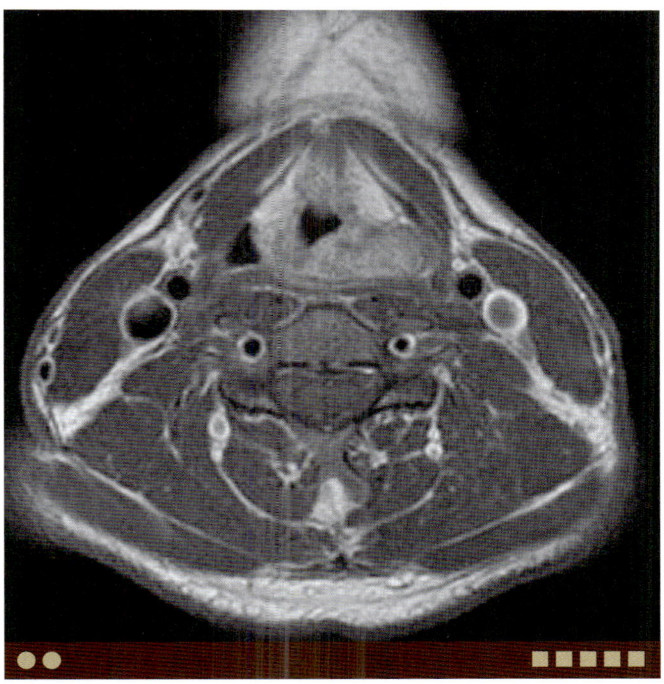

D. Laryngeal hemangioma, same patient as A. Axial postcontrast T1W image demonstrates homogeneous, avid enhancement of the lesion.

DIFFERENTIAL DIAGNOSIS IMAGES (E-I)

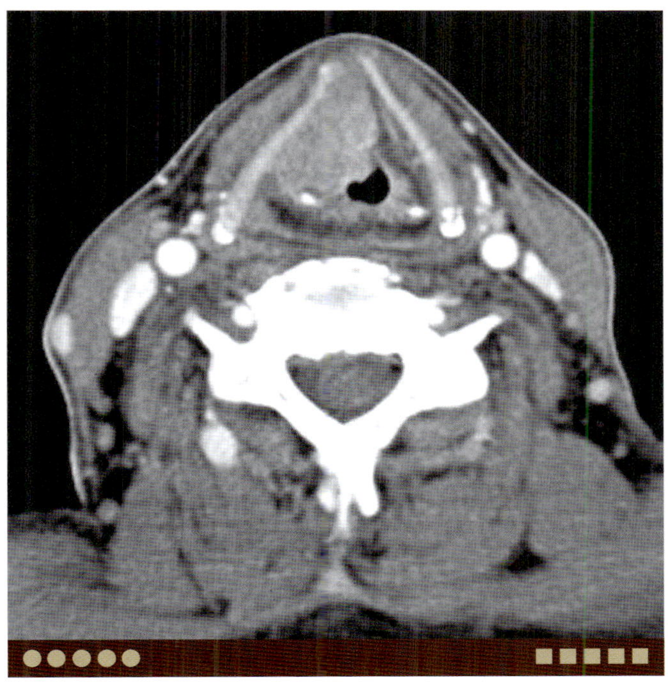

E. SCCA. Axial postcontrast CT demonstrates a heterogeneously enhancing right glottic mass extending into the paraglottic space.

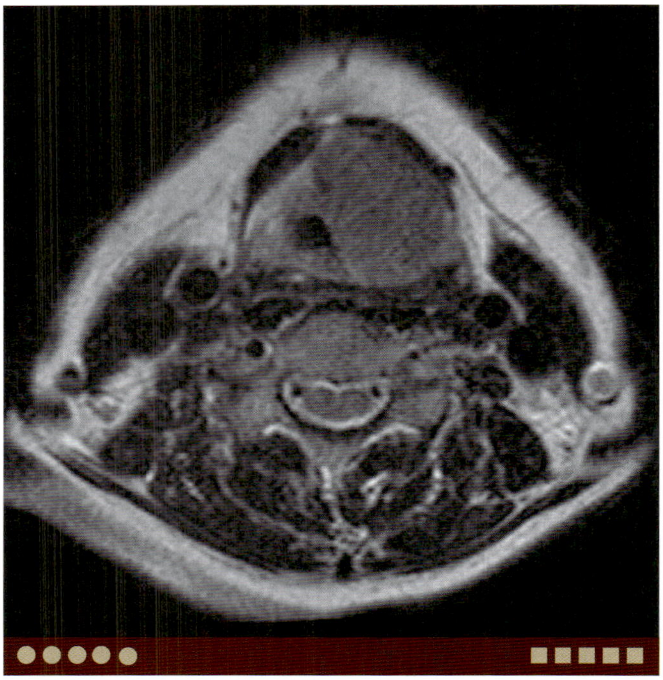

F. SCCA in a different patient. Axial T2W image demonstrates a relatively low-signal intensity mass in the left supraglottic larynx.

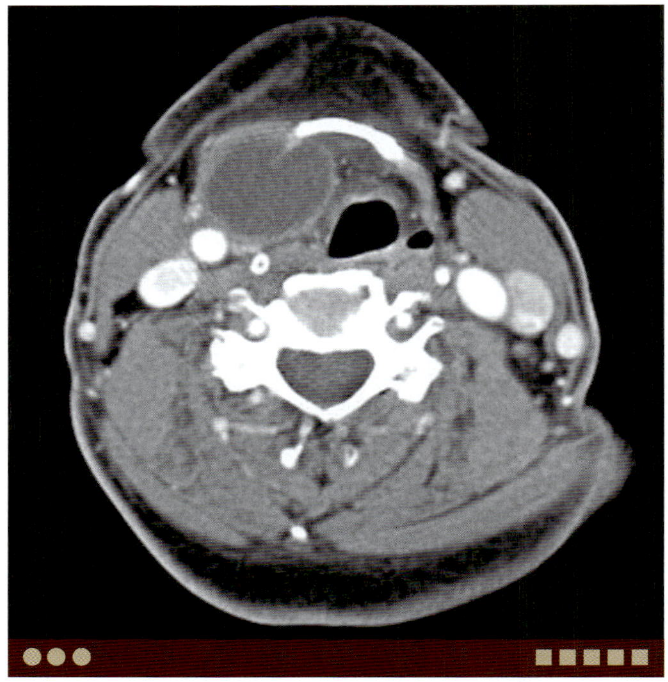

G. Saccular cyst. Axial postcontrast CT image demonstrates a cystic mass in the right paraglottic space with lateral extension.

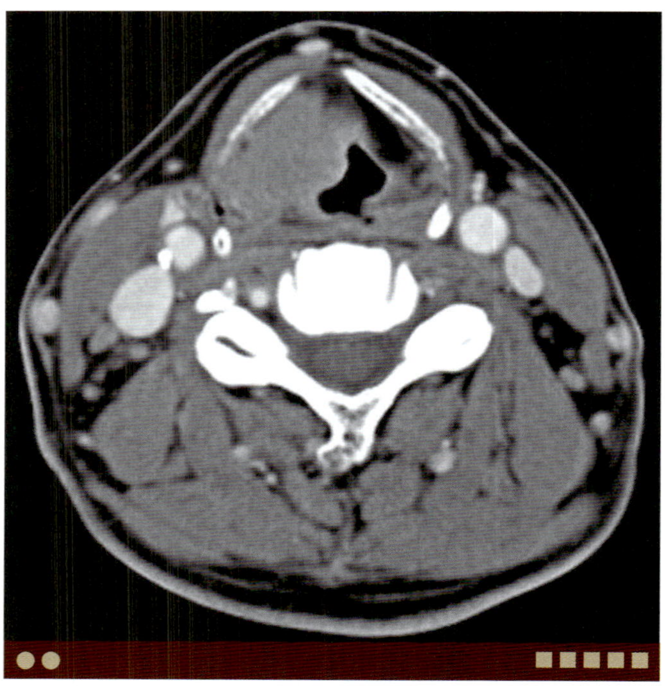

H. MALT lymphoma. Axial postcontrast CT demonstrates a well-circumscribed homogeneously enhancing submucosal mass in the right supraglottic larynx.

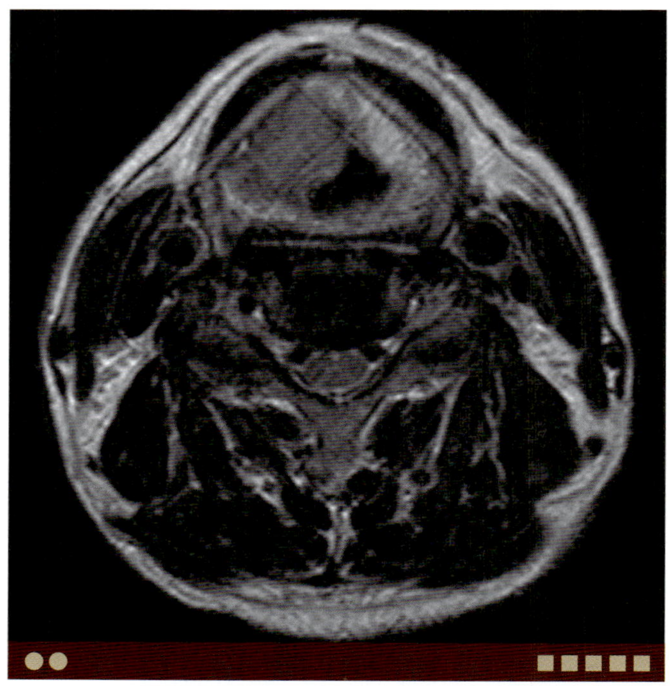

I. MALT lymphoma, same patient as H. Axial T2W image demonstrates a homogeneous relatively low-signal intensity right submucosal mass extending to the paraglottic space.

Case 10–17 Rhabdomyoma

Osamu Sakai, Jimmy Wang

PRESENTATION

Hoarseness.

FINDINGS

CT demonstrates a well-marginated, homogeneously enhancing mass in the larynx.

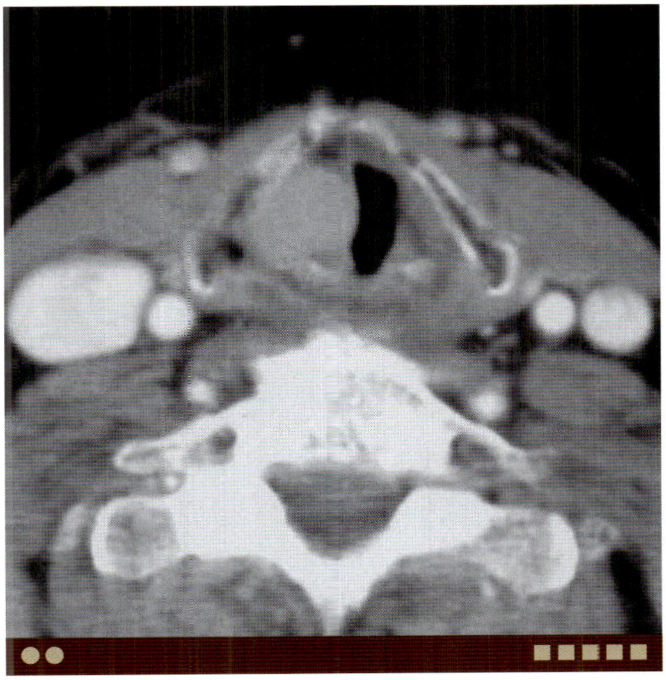

A. Rhabdomyoma. Axial postcontrast CT demonstrates a homogeneously enhancing submucosal lesion in the right vocal cord.

DIFFERENTIAL DIAGNOSIS

- Rhabdomyosarcoma: This is a rare malignant tumor in the larynx. Imaging findings are similar to those of rhabdomyoma, often with more aggressive features.
- Squamous cell carcinoma (SCCA): SCCA is the most common malignant tumor of the larynx, and occasionally presents as a submucosal mass with relatively well-defined margins.
- Lymphoma: This laryngeal presentation usually demonstrates a submucosal, homogeneous, density/signal lesion with intermediate signal on T2W images.
- Amyloidosis: This is a rare deposition disorder of abnormal amount of proteins and demonstrates nodular soft tissue thickening or a submucosal mass, often with calcification.
- Schwannoma: Laryngeal schwannoma usually is rare, and grows very slowly. It is often diagnosed between 50 and 60 years old with female predominance. It shows similar appearance to schwannomas anywhere else.
- Granular cell tumor: Also known as Abrikossoff tumor, is a rare benign, slowly growing neoplasm. They show relatively homogeneous enhancement on CT, slightly hypointense signal on T1W, heterogeneously increased signal on T2W images, and homogeneous enhancement.

COMMENTS

This is a 65-year-old man with hoarseness.

Rhabdomyoma is a rare benign tumor originating in striated muscles, most commonly in the heart. Extracardiac rhabdomyoma is considered distinct from cardiac rhabdomyoma, which is believed to be a hamartoma and not a true neoplasm. Cardiac rhabdomyoma is usually diagnosed in children and associated with tuberous sclerosis.

Laryngeal rhabdomyoma is extremely rare, although extracardiac rhabdomyomas most commonly occur in the head and neck region, usually in the upper aerodigestive tract. Clinical course of laryngeal rhabdomyoma reflects slow growth and common clinical presentation includes progressive dysphagia, hoarseness, dyspnea, or foreign-body sensation.

Radiologically, rhabdomyoma usually appears as a benign neoplasm with well-circumscribed margins, absence of invasion into surrounding soft tissues, and submucosal location, although findings mimicking malignant tumors such as indistinct borders have been reported. On CT, rhabdomyomas demonstrate homogeneous density, similar to muscle. On MRI, they are usually isointense or slightly hyperintense to muscle, and homogeneously enhance without necrosis or hemorrhage.

PEARLS

- **Laryngeal rhabdomyoma is extremely rare, although extracardiac rhabdomyomas most commonly occur in the head and neck region.**
- **Rhabdomyoma usually appears as a benign neoplasm with well-circumscribed margins, absence of invasion into surrounding soft tissues, and submucosal location.**
- **Rhabdomyomas demonstrate similar density to muscle on CT. On MRI, they are usually isointense or slightly hyperintense to muscle, and homogeneously enhance.**

The differential diagnosis includes various malignant tumors, such as squamous cell carcinoma and rhabdomyosarcoma, as well as benign lesions, such as hemangiomas, lipomas, amyloidomas, neurofibromas, granular cell tumors, and leiomyomas. Although grossly similar to rhabdomyoma, microscopically rhabdomyosarcoma can be distinguished by the presence of atypical mitotic figures, nuclear pleomorphism, and foci of invasion. Granular cell tumors, when occurring in the larynx, can be quite readily distinguished from rhabdomyomas histologically.

ADDITIONAL IMAGES (B-E)

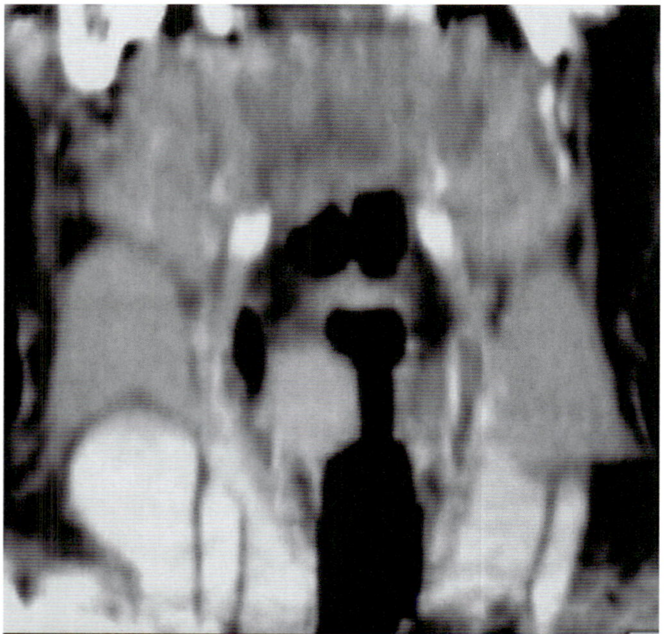

B. Rhabdomyoma, same patient as A. Coronal postcontrast CT demonstrates a homogeneously enhancing submucosal lesion in the right vocal cord.

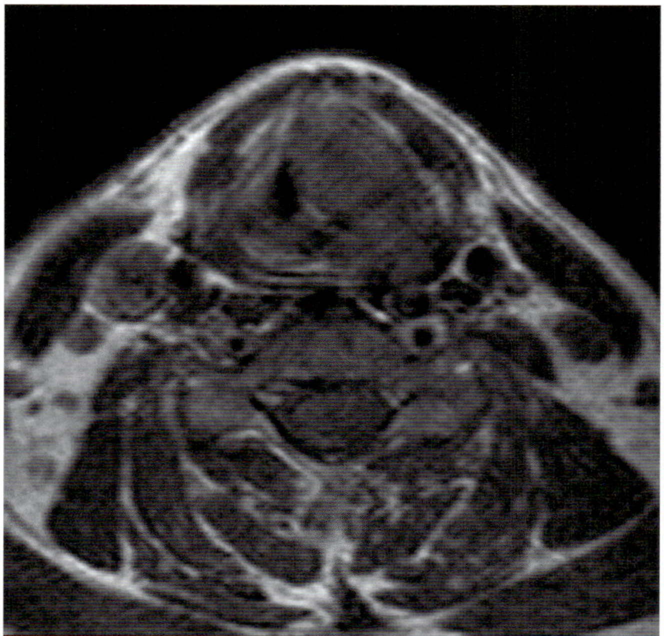

C. Rhabdomyoma in a different patient. Axial T1W image demonstrates a low-signal lesion in the left supraglottic larynx.

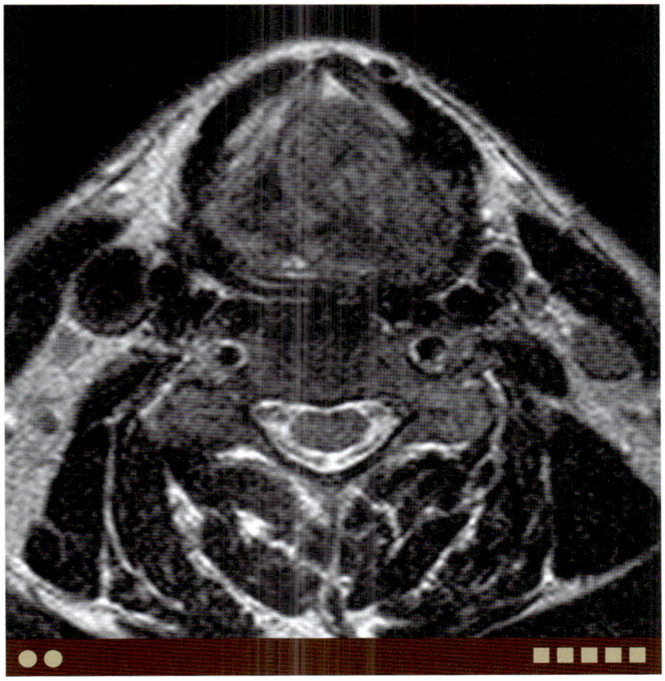

D. Rhabdomyoma, same patient as C. Axial T2W image demonstrates an intermediate-to-low signal lesion in the left supraglottic larynx.

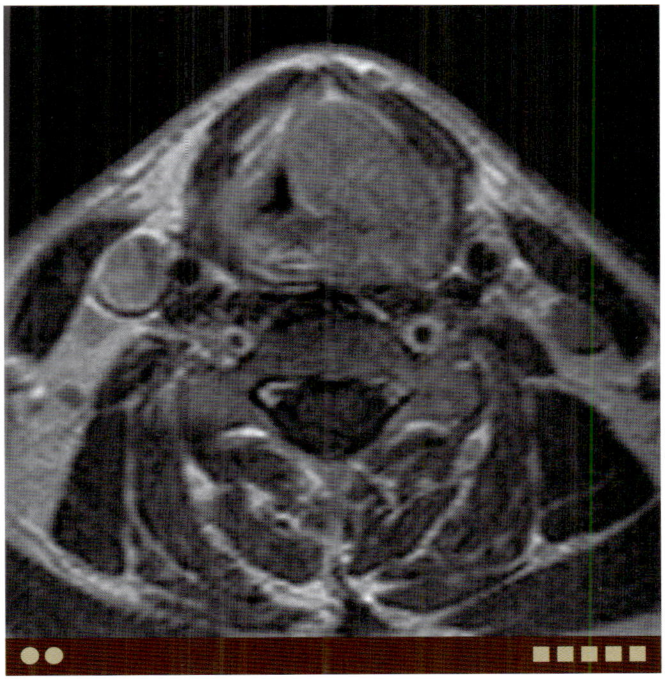

E. Rhabdomyoma, same patient as C. Axial postcontrast T1W image demonstrates mild enhancement of the lesion.

DIFFERENTIAL DIAGNOSIS IMAGES (F-J)

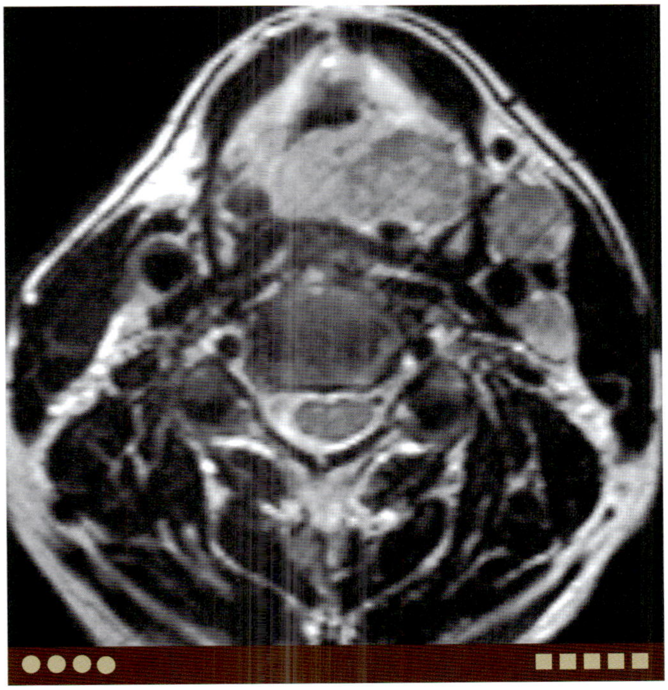

F. SCCA. Axial T2W MR image shows a heterogeneous signal lesion in the left supraglottic larynx. The metastatic nodes in the left level III demonstrate similar signal to the primary lesion.

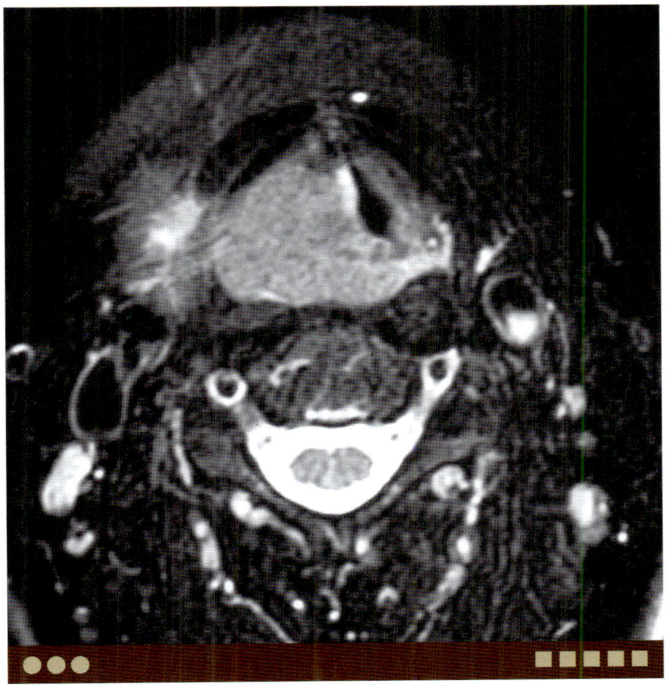

G. Lymphoma. Axial T2W MR image demonstrates homogeneous intermediate-signal lesion centered in the right paraglottic space in the supraglottis and glottis. The vocal cord is deviated to the left.

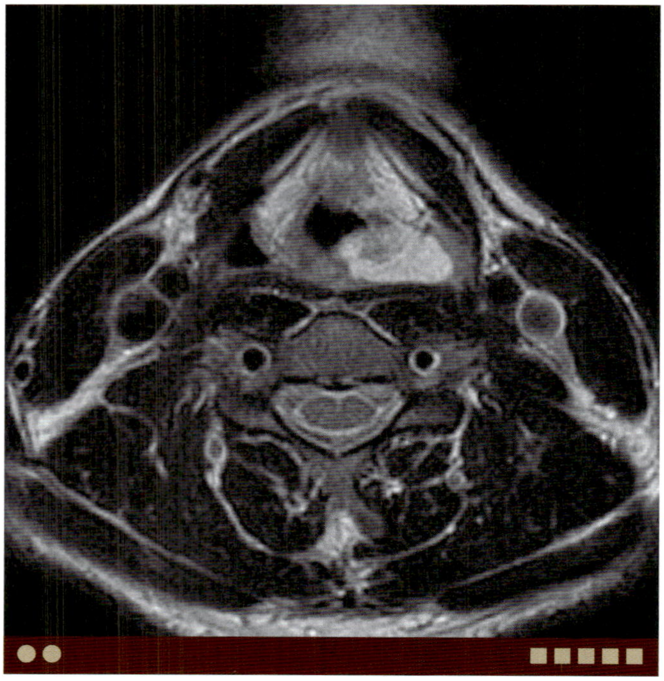

H. Hemangioma. Axial T2W MR image demonstrates a well-circumscribed, lobulated, fairly high-signal mass in the left supraglottic larynx.

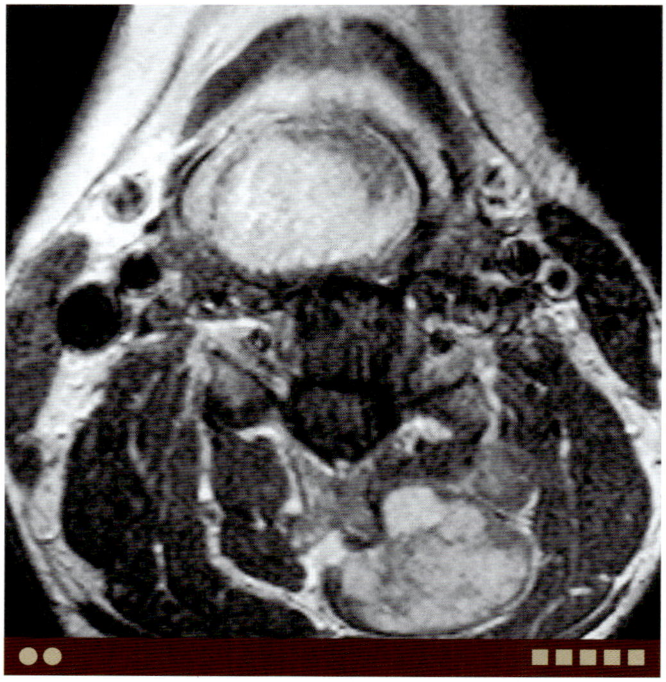

I. Schwannoma. Axial postcontrast T1W image shows a round enhancing lesion in the supraglottic larynx.

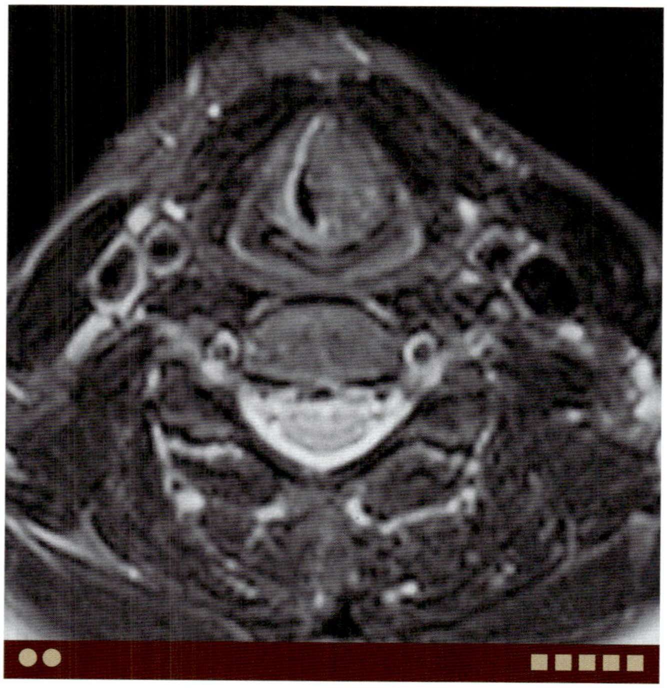

J. Granular cell tumor. Axial T2W image shows a left vocal cord lesion demonstrating slightly heterogeneous increased signal.

Case 10–18 Laryngotracheobronchitis

Osamu Sakai, Benjamin Ludwig

PRESENTATION

Inspiratory stridor and "barking" cough.

FINDINGS

Frontal soft tissue neck radiograph demonstrates narrowing of the subglottic airway, with loss of normal shoulders of the subglottic trachea.

DIFFERENTIAL DIAGNOSIS

- Epiglottitis: Emergent condition which presents with respiratory distress, fever, and posturing, with imaging findings of epiglottic and aryepiglottic fold thickening.
- Foreign body: Produces similar clinical symptoms, but radiographs may demonstrate a radio-opaque foreign body or soft tissue density within the airway, or mass effect from foreign body within esophagus.
- Subglottic stenosis: Symmetric narrowing of the subglottic airway with history of prolonged intubation. Congenital form is associated with other laryngotracheal abnormalities.
- Bacterial tracheitis: Narrowing of the subglottic airway, possibly with soft tissue density adherent to the wall of the airway, representing exudative plaque.
- Subglottic hemangioma: Typically seen within the first year of life, and then regresses, with asymmetric subglottic narrowing.

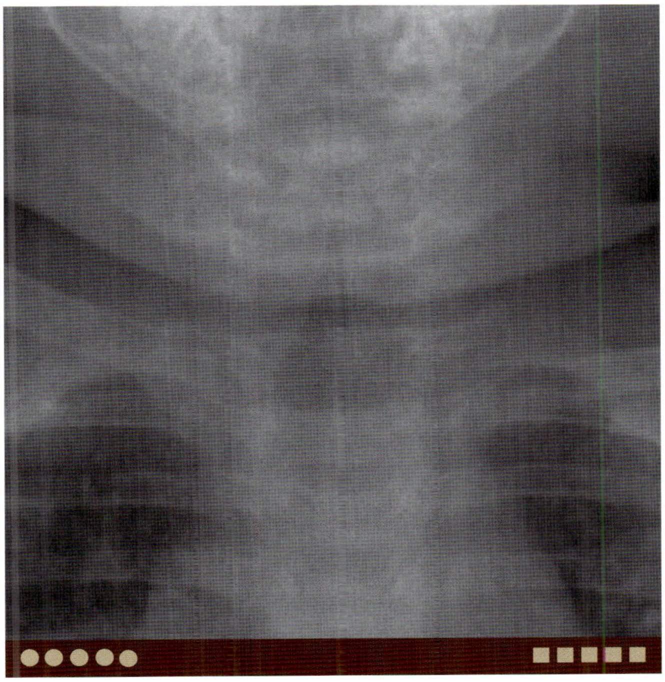

A. Laryngotracheobronchitis. Frontal radiograph demonstrates loss of normal convex shoulders of the subglottic airway, the "steeple sign."

COMMENTS

This patient is a 2-year-old girl with a fever and "barking" cough.

Laryngotracheobronchitis or croup, most commonly occurs from ages 6 months to 3 years. Viral etiologies, including human parainfluenza virus (HPIV), particularly HPIV-1 and HPIV-2, are most commonly implicated.

Patient presentation includes inspiratory stridor, hoarseness, and the classic "barking" cough, typically during the fall and winter months with preceding symptoms of a lower respiratory tract infection. Subglottic edema results in airway narrowing and inspiratory stridor, while inflammation in the larynx and vocal cords results in cough and hoarseness.

The role of imaging in croup is to evaluate other potential causes of inspiratory stridor, often when the clinical diagnosis of croup is not clear.

The frontal radiograph demonstrates straightening of the normal convex "shoulders" of the subglottic airway, termed the "steeple sign." Lateral radiographs also show narrowing of the subglottic airway, usually with overdistention of the hypopharynx. Of note, the subglottic narrowing is symmetric, and the epiglottis and aryepiglottic folds are normal.

Other emergent conditions with similar presentations include epiglottitis, upper airway foreign body, subglottic stenosis, bacterial tracheitis, and subglottic hemangioma. Clinical history, physical examination, and radiographic features distinguish croup from these other entities.

Croup is often managed on an outpatient basis with oral and inhaled corticosteroids. Inpatient management, with racemic epinephrine nebulizers, corticosteroids, and possible intubation are reserved for severe cases.

PEARLS

- **The role of imaging in suspected croup is to evaluate for emergent conditions with similar presentations, including airway foreign body and epiglottitis.**
- **Classic presentation includes inspiratory stridor and barking cough in children 6 months to 3 years of age. Consider other causes in older children.**
- **Frontal radiograph demonstrates symmetric subglottic narrowing, with straightening of the normal convexities of the subglottic airway ("steeple sign").**

ADDITIONAL IMAGE

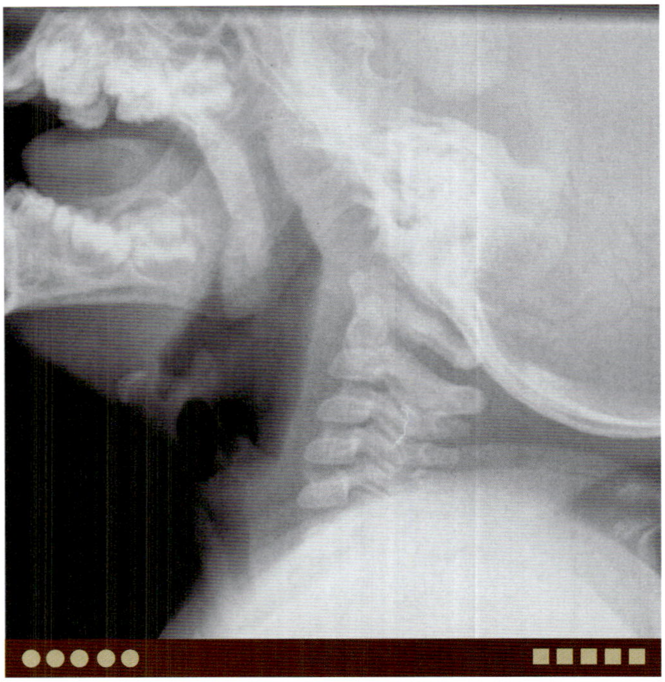

B. Laryngotracheobronchitis, same patient as A. Lateral radiograph demonstrates subglottic narrowing and overdistension of the hypopharynx.

DIFFERENTIAL DIAGNOSIS IMAGES (C-E)

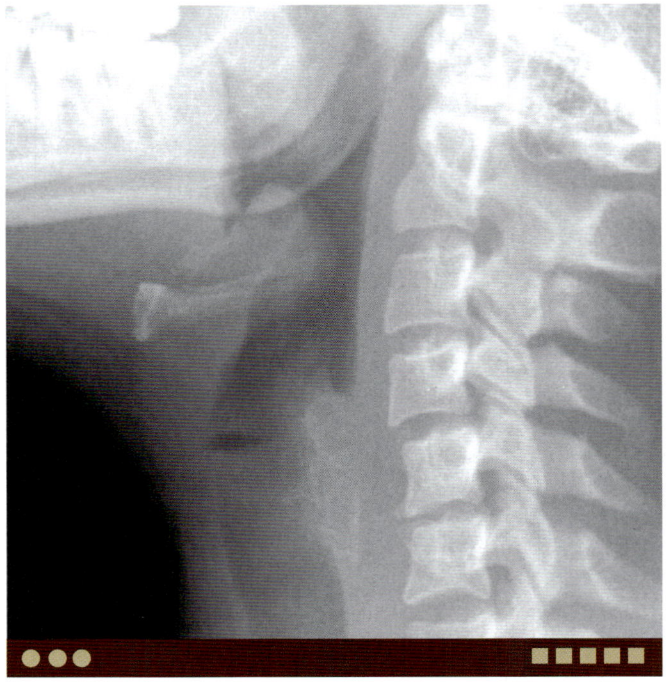

C. Epiglottitis. Lateral radiograph demonstrates a thickened, bulbous epiglottis.

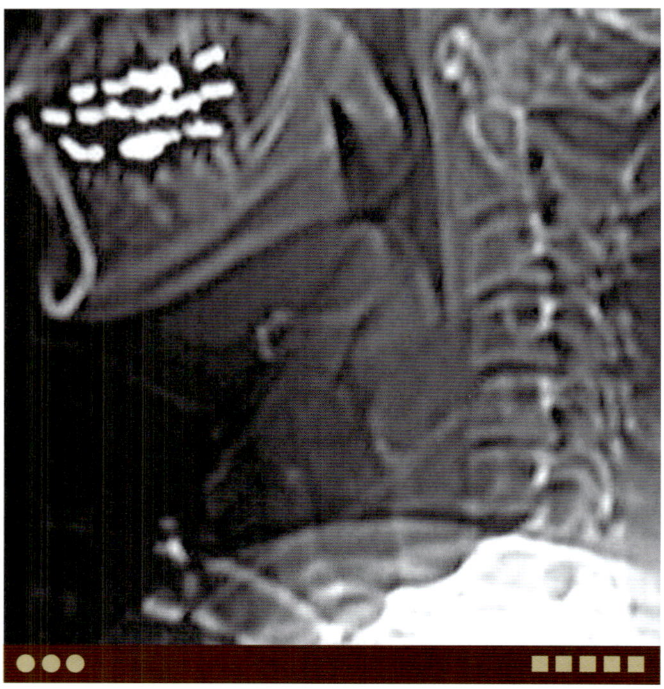

D. Epiglottitis in a different patient. Lateral scout image of CT demonstrates significantly thickened epiglottis.

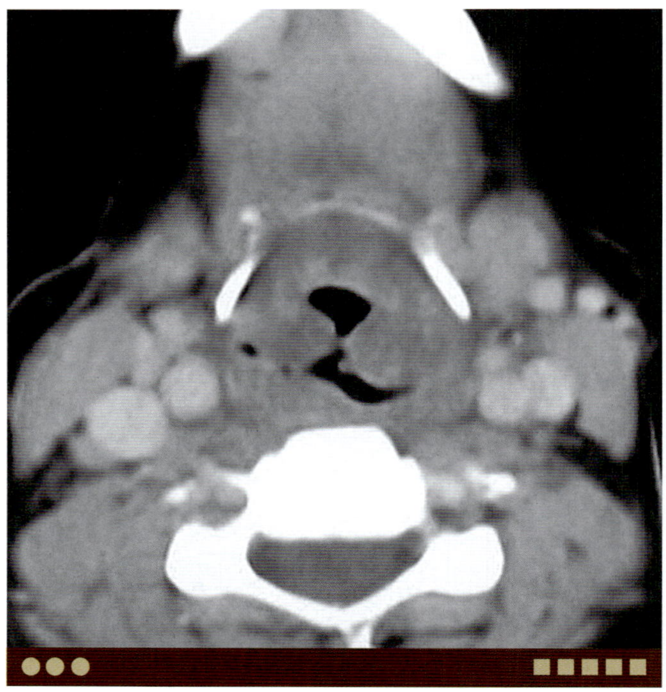

E. Epiglottitis, same patient as D. Axial contrast-enhanced CT demonstrates thickened aryepiglottic folds.

Case 10–19 Subglottic/Tracheal Stenosis

Osamu Sakai, Benjamin Ludwig

PRESENTATION

Stridor, history of intubation.

FINDINGS

Axial CT demonstrates narrowing of the subglottic or tracheal lumen, with concentric wall thickening

DIFFERENTIAL DIAGNOSIS

- Malignant tumors: The most common malignant tumors in adults include squamous cell carcinoma and adenoid cystic carcinoma, followed by carcinoid and mucoepidermoid carcinoma. Malignancy originating from chondroid may also occur in the trachea given the presence of cartilage.
- Benign tumors: Common benign tumors in the trachea include papilloma, fibroma, and hemangioma.
- Wegener's granulomatosis: A disease of unknown etiology characterized by necrotizing granulomatous vasculitis that can involve the upper and lower airways, lungs, and kidneys. Tracheal involvement is characterized by concentric tracheal wall thickening, luminal narrowing, and calcifications associated with tracheal rings.
- Amyloidosis: A systemic disease characterized by progressive deposition of amyloid in the extracellular tissues. The larynx, pharynx, and trachea are often involved. CT demonstrates nodular wall thickening and luminal narrowing, commonly with calcification.
- Relapsing polychondritis: This is a systemic, destructive autoimmune disorder involving all types of cartilaginous structures, including the trachea, nose, and ear. Imaging findings include airway narrowing and concentric wall thickening, with calcification within the tracheal rings.
- Tracheobronchopathia osteochondroplastica: A rare idiopathic disease characterized by formation of cartilaginous, osseous, or mixed nodules in the tracheal and bronchial submucosa. CT demonstrates irregular thickening of the tracheal wall with small nodules and calcifications, which classically spares the posterior tracheal wall.

COMMENTS

This is a 57-year-old man with stridor and history of endotracheal intubation.

Subglottic or tracheal stenosis may be congenital, idiopathic, or secondary to trauma (including intubation), chemical exposure, tracheostomy, neoplasm, granulomatous disease such as Wegener's granulomatosis, or depositional disease such as amyloidosis.

This condition is most commonly seen as a complication of prolonged endotracheal intubation. A hyperinflated cuff during intubation results in pressure/ischemic mucosal and cartilaginous necrosis with consequent scarring and fibrosis. This is seen as a smooth, focal subglottic/tracheal stenosis, while tracheostomy-related stenosis tends to show irregular, longer stenosis. The clinical presentation includes dyspnea, shortness of breath, stridor, and wheezing, and is often confused with asthma clinically.

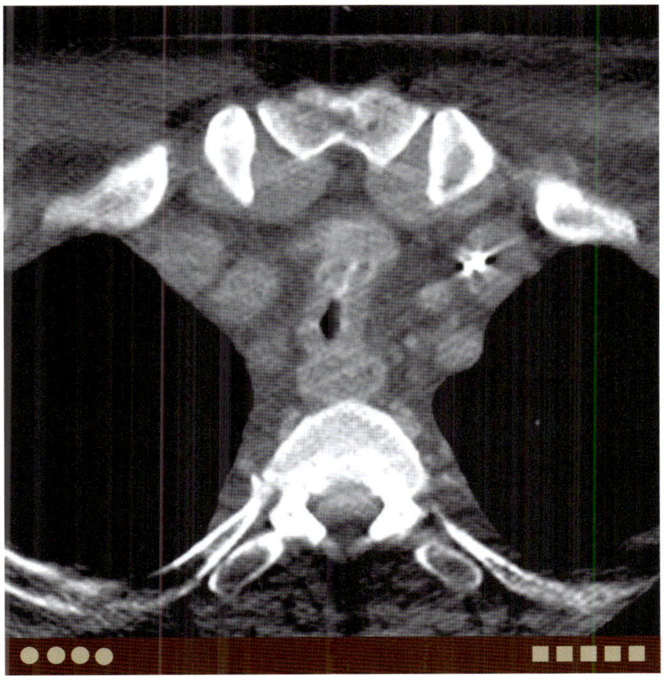

A. Tracheal stenosis. Axial CT demonstrates wall thickening and stenosis of the trachea at the level of the manubrium.

CT allows one to localize and quantify the degree of stenosis, and identify the underlying etiology. Multiplanar reconstructions as well as volume-rendered 3D images are helpful for diagnosis and surgical planning.

Treatment options include endoscopic tracheal dilatation, tracheal stent placement, and tracheal resection/reconstruction, depending on the cause, location, and length of stenosis.

PEARLS

- **Subglottic or tracheal stenosis can be secondary to multiple etiologies, the most common of which is prolonged intubation.**
- **Clinical presentations include dyspnea, shortness of breath, stridor, and wheezing, and may mimic asthma.**
- **CT is helpful to localize and characterize the degree of stenosis for surgical planning.**

ADDITIONAL IMAGES (B-E)

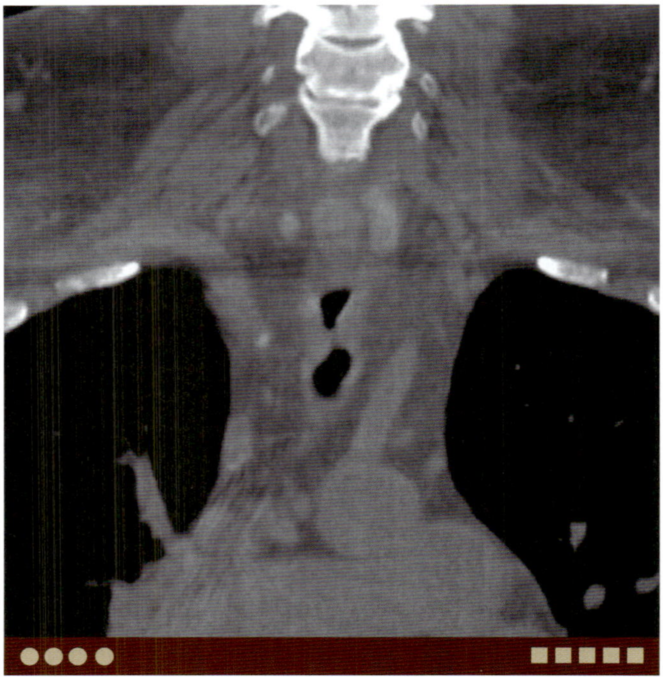

B. Tracheal stenosis, same patient as A. Coronal CT demonstrates wall thickening and focal stenosis of the trachea.

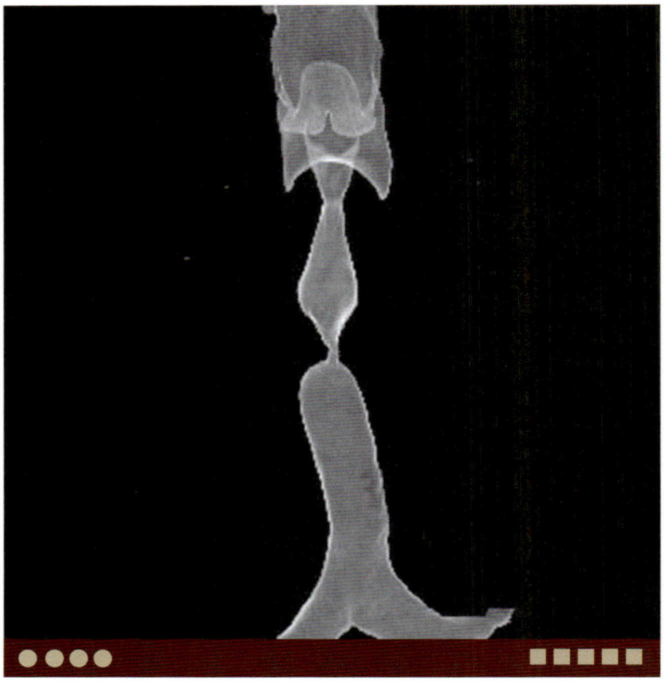

C. Tracheal stenosis, same patient as A. Frontal projection of volume-rendering 3D image demonstrates a focal stenosis of the trachea.

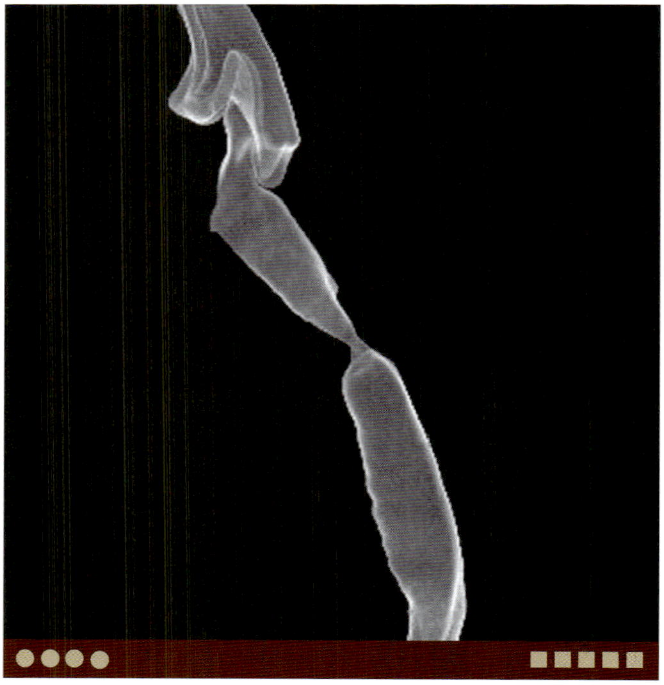

D. Tracheal stenosis, same patient as A. Lateral projection of volume-rendering 3D image demonstrates a focal stenosis of the trachea.

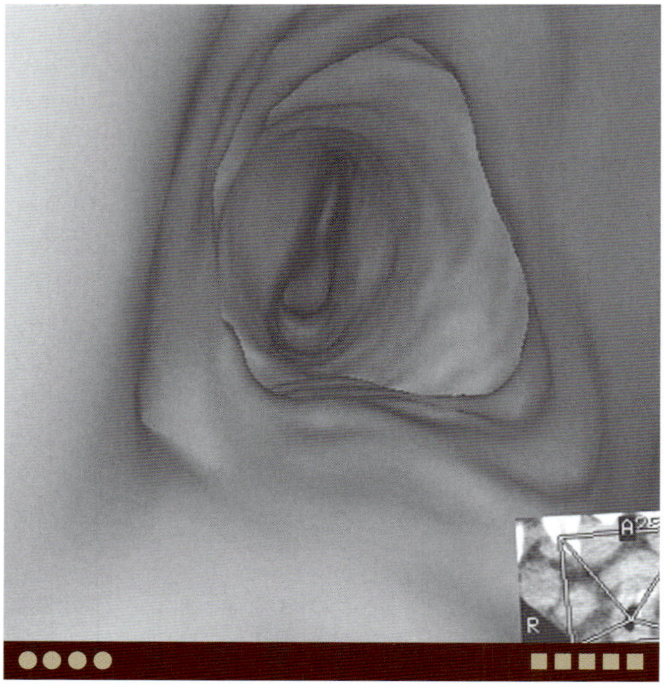

E. Tracheal stenosis, same patient as A. Virtual endoscopic image demonstrates a focal stenosis of the trachea.

DIFFERENTIAL DIAGNOSIS IMAGES (F-J)

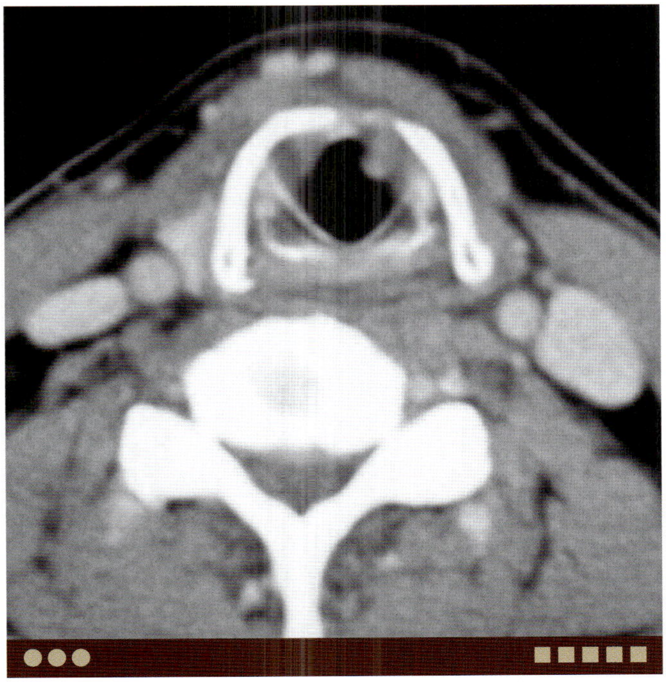

F. Laryngeal papillomatosis. Axial postcontrast CT through the subglottic larynx demonstrates a polypoid lesion arising from the left anterolateral wall of the trachea.

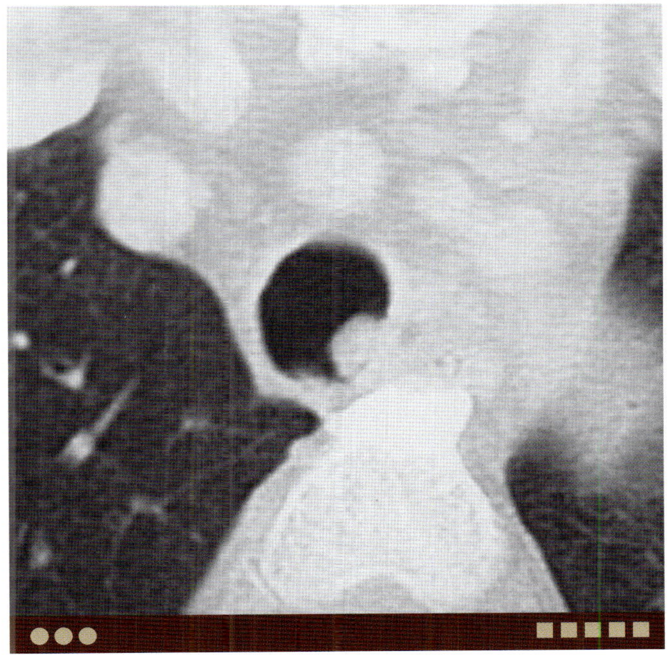

G. Laryngeal papillomatosis in a different patient. Axial CT through the trachea demonstrates a polypoid lesion arising from the left posterolateral wall of the trachea.

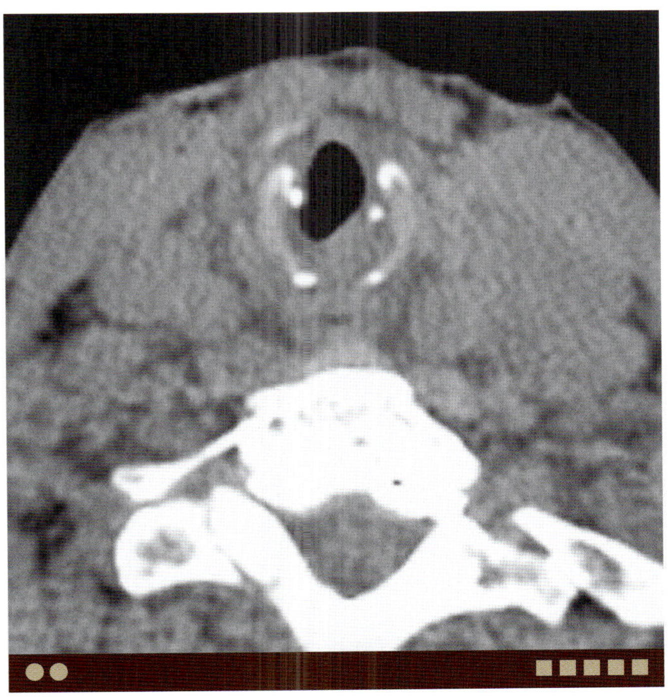

H. Amyloidosis. Axial noncontrast CT demonstrates slightly irregular concentric narrowing of the subglottic larynx. Note focal calcifications.

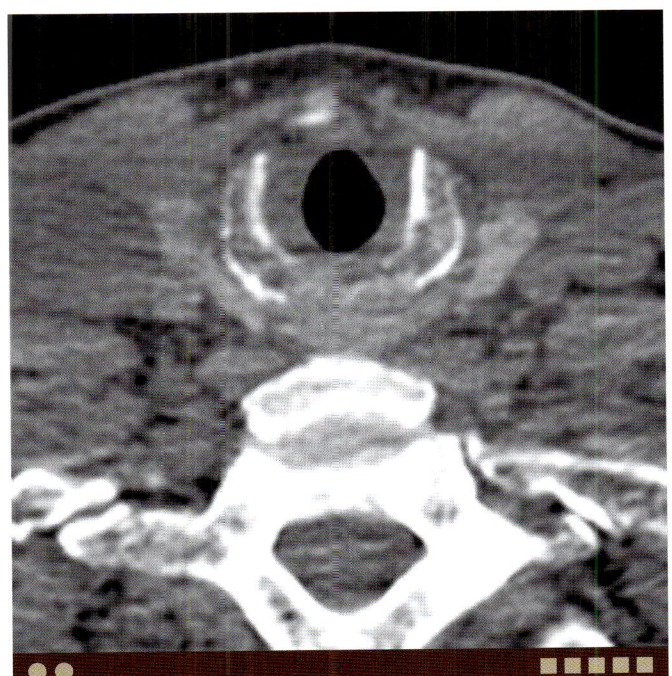

I. Wegener's granulomatosis. Axial noncontrast CT demonstrates concentric soft tissue thickening in the subglottic trachea in a patient with Wegener's granulomatosis.

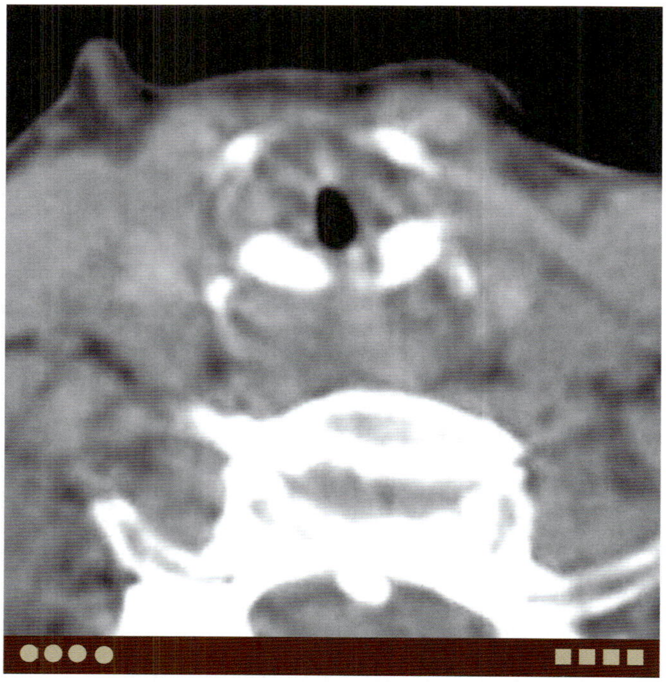

J. Tracheobronchomalacia. Axial CT demonstrates narrowing of the subglottic larynx.

Chapter 11

INFRAHYOID NECK

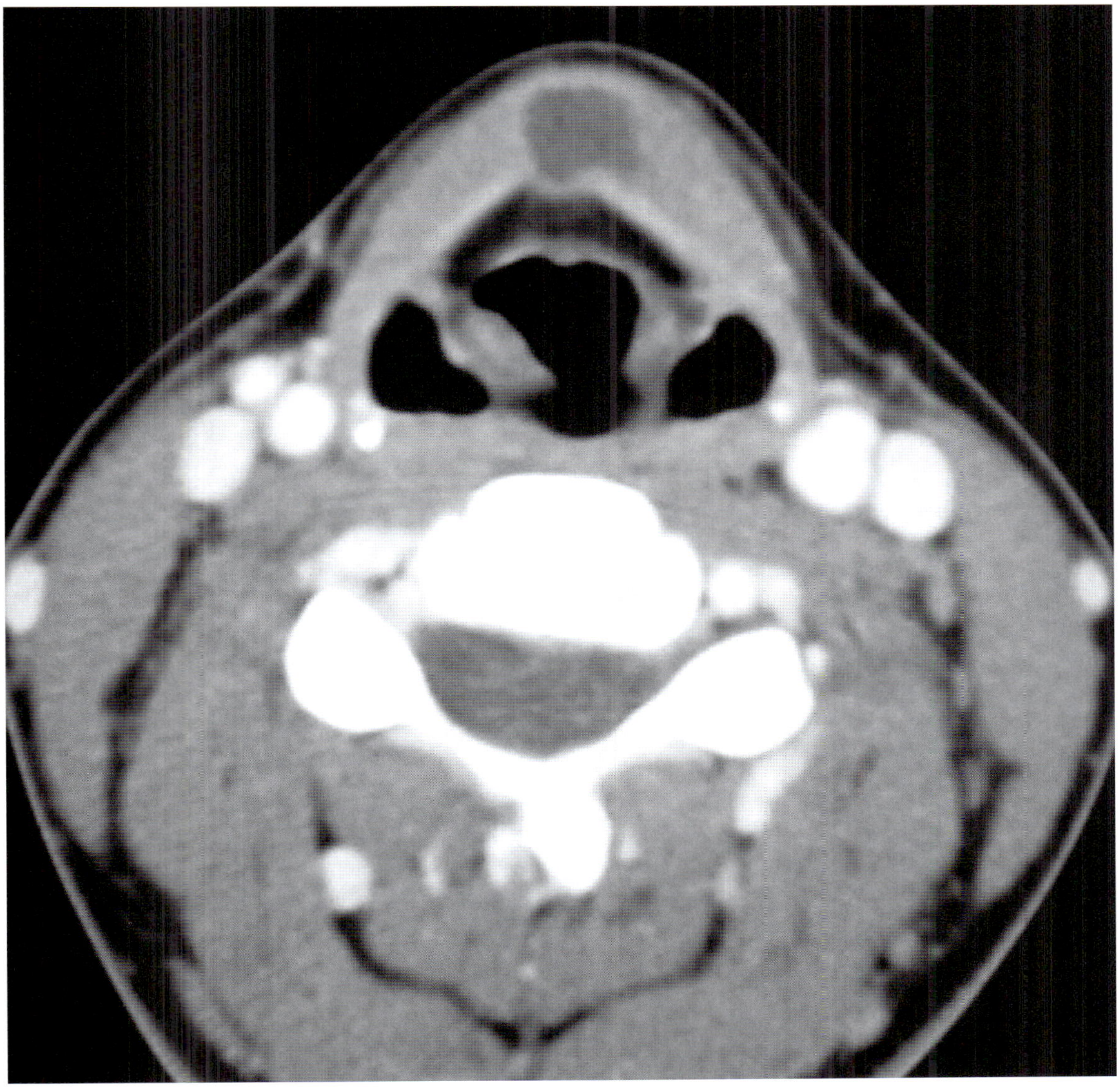

Case 11-1 Thyroglossal Duct Cyst

Osamu Sakai, June Cheng

PRESENTATION

Anterior neck mass.

FINDINGS

CT and MRI demonstrate a midline cystic lesion embedded in the strap muscle.

DIFFERENTIAL DIAGNOSIS

- Dermoid/epidermoid cyst: Dermoid and epidermoid cysts are located superficial to the strap muscle. Differentiation between dermoid and epidermoid is often difficult by imaging; however, the presence of fat strongly suggests a dermoid.
- Necrotic lymph node: Lymph nodes are located superficial to the strap muscle. Once a necrotic node is identified, a primary source should be determined.
- Branchial cleft cyst: Branchial cleft cysts are located lateral or off-midline. Second brachial cleft cyst is most common and located posterior to the submandibular gland.

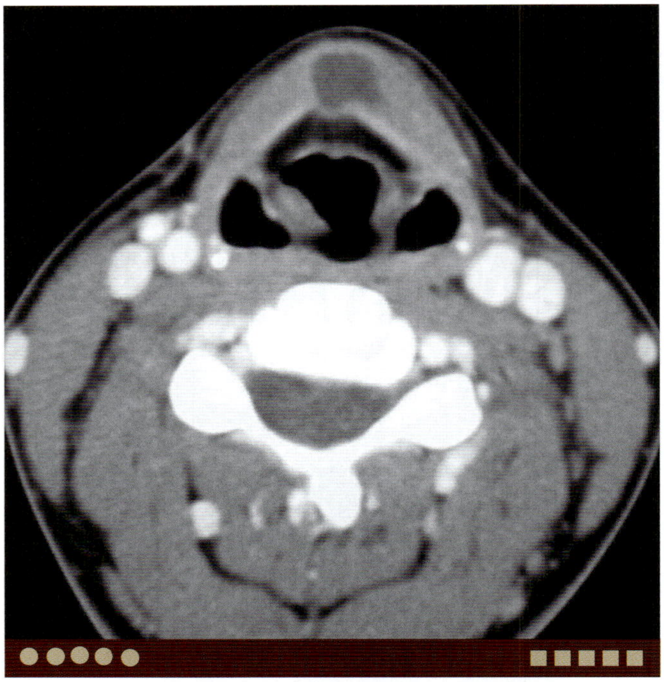

A. Thyroglossal duct cyst. Axial contrast-enhanced CT shows a cystic lesion embedded midline in the strap muscle.

COMMENTS

This is a 21-year-old woman with an anterior neck mass.

Thyroglossal duct cyst is a common congenital/developmental cystic lesion and usually located in the midline anterior neck. Patients often present in the third decade or later. It occurs along the thyroglossal duct, between the foramen cecum and thyroid, and most often seen around the level of the hyoid. About three-fourths of these lesions occur midline, and one-fourth occur off-midline. The internal density or signal is similar to that of water. However, increased density on CT or signal on T1W images may be seen with proteinaceous contents.

The differential diagnosis includes other cystic lesions, such as necrotic nodes and dermoid/epidermoid cysts. The most important distinguishing feature is that the thyroglossal duct cyst is embedded in the strap muscle, deep to the superficial surface of the muscle. However, dumbbell-shaped anterior protrusion is often seen.

Although the cyst wall is usually thin, it can irregularly thicken and enhance with infection. Residual or ectopic thyroid tissue is occasionally found as a high-density nodule within the cyst or along the course of the thyroglossal duct. The residual/ectopic thyroid tissue demonstrates signal and enhancement characteristics similar to normal thyroid tissue.

Malignancy, usually papillary carcinoma, rarely occurs from thyroglossal duct cysts. Follicular variant of papillary carcinoma, pure follicular carcinoma, anaplastic carcinoma, and squamous cell carcinoma have also been reported.

PEARLS

- **Thyroglossal duct cyst is a common congenital/developmental cystic lesion and usually seen in the midline anterior neck.**
- **It occurs anywhere along the course of the thyroglossal duct, between the foramen cecum and thyroid, and often seen around the level of the hyoid.**
- **Thyroglossal duct cyst is embedded in the strap muscle, deep to the superficial surface of the muscle.**
- **Residual thyroid tissue is occasionally seen in the cyst.**

ADDITIONAL IMAGES (B-G)

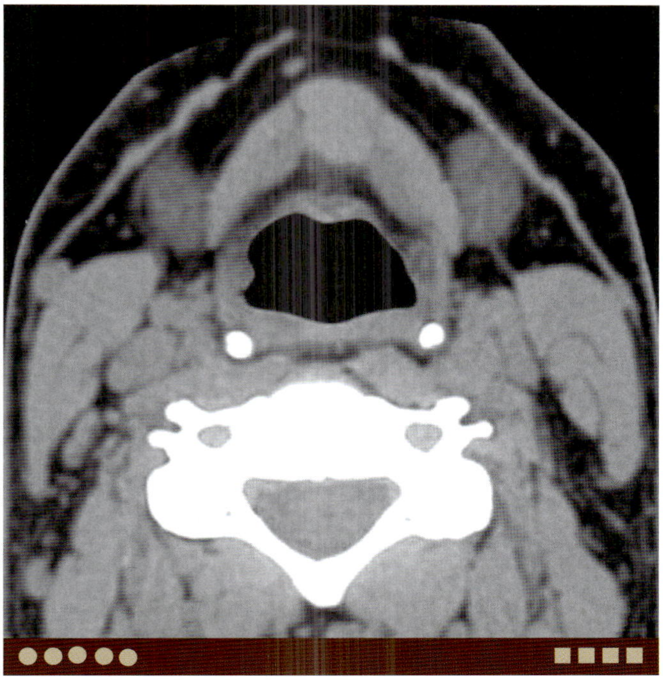

B. Thyroglossal duct cyst in a different patient. Axial noncontrast-enhanced CT shows a slightly hyperattenuating lesion embedded midline in the strap muscle, consistent with proteinaceous contents.

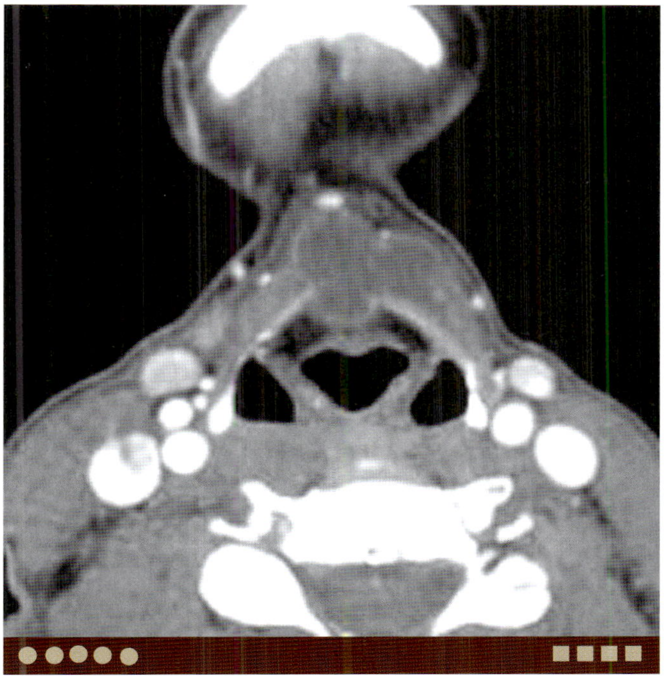

C. Thyroglossal duct cyst in a different patient. Axial contrast-enhanced CT shows a lobulated cystic lesion protruding anterior to the thyroid lamina. However, the lesion is still deep to the superficial surface of the strap muscle.

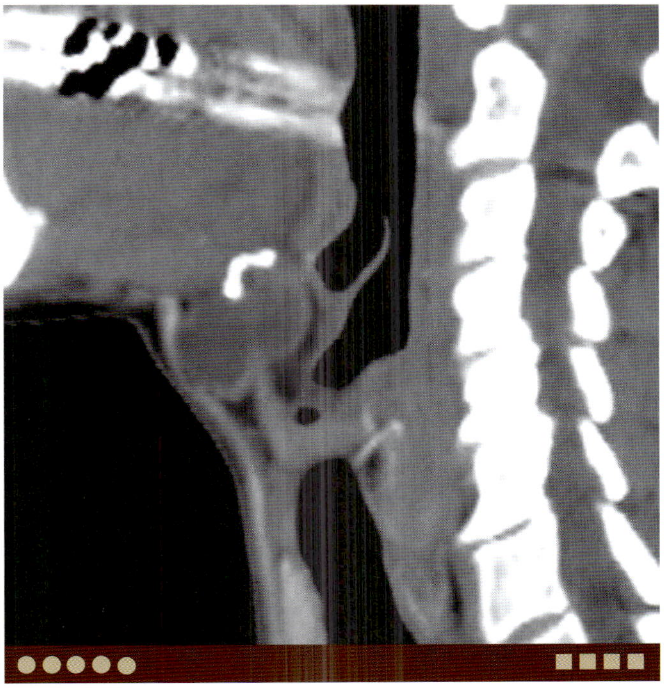

D. Thyroglossal duct cyst, same patient as C. Sagittal contrast-enhanced CT shows a lobulated cystic lesion with anterior protrusion below the hyoid.

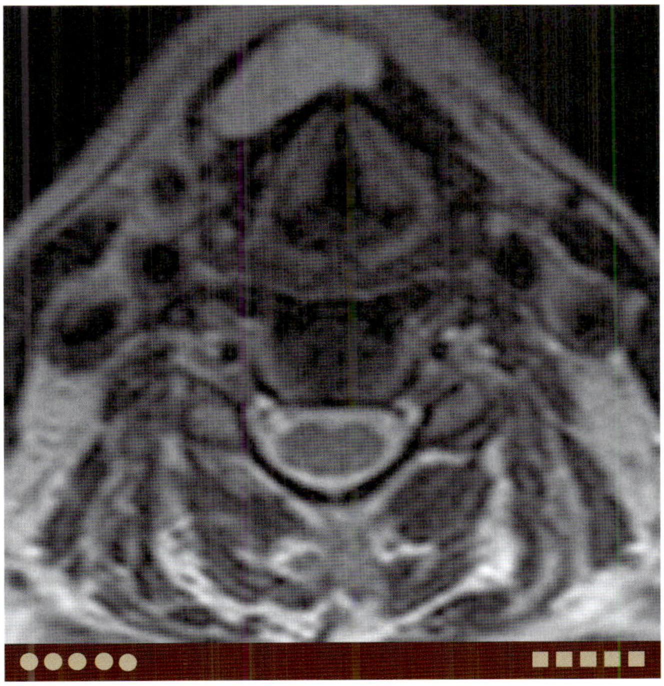

E. Thyroglossal duct cyst in a different patient. Axial T2W MR image demonstrates a high-signal cystic lesion embedded in the strap muscle.

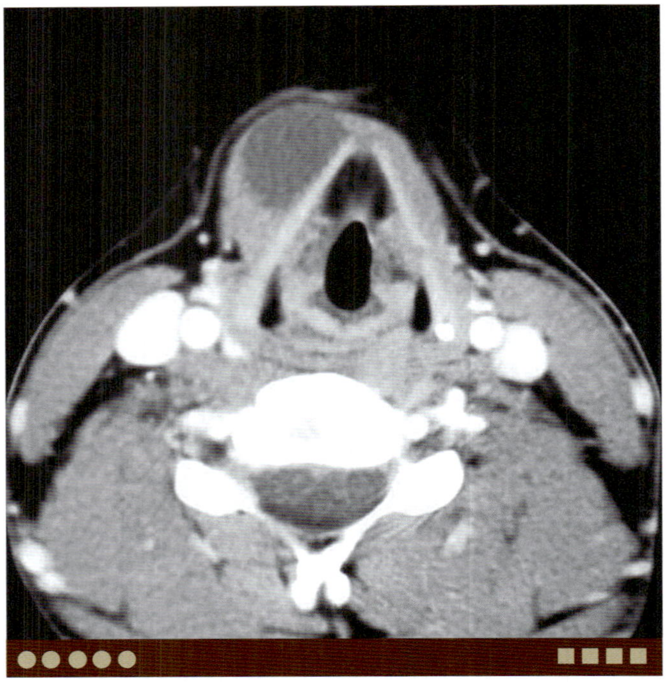

F. Thyroglossal duct cyst in a different patient. Axial contrast-enhanced CT shows a cystic lesion seen off-midline on the right. However, the lesion is still deep to the superficial surface of the strap muscle.

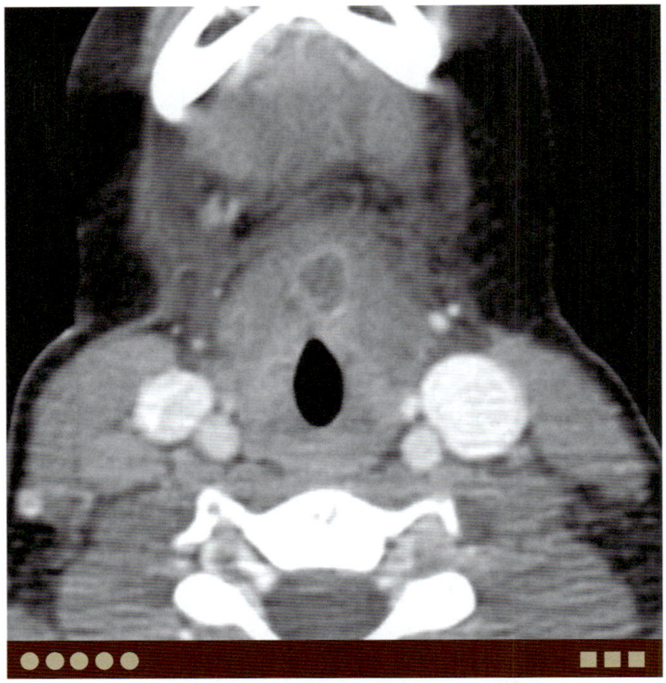

G. Infected thyroglossal duct cyst. Axial contrast-enhanced CT image demonstrates a midline cystic lesion with irregular rim enhancement embedded in the strap muscles. Note heterogeneously increased density in the surrounding fat due to inflammation.

DIFFERENTIAL DIAGNOSIS IMAGES (H-J)

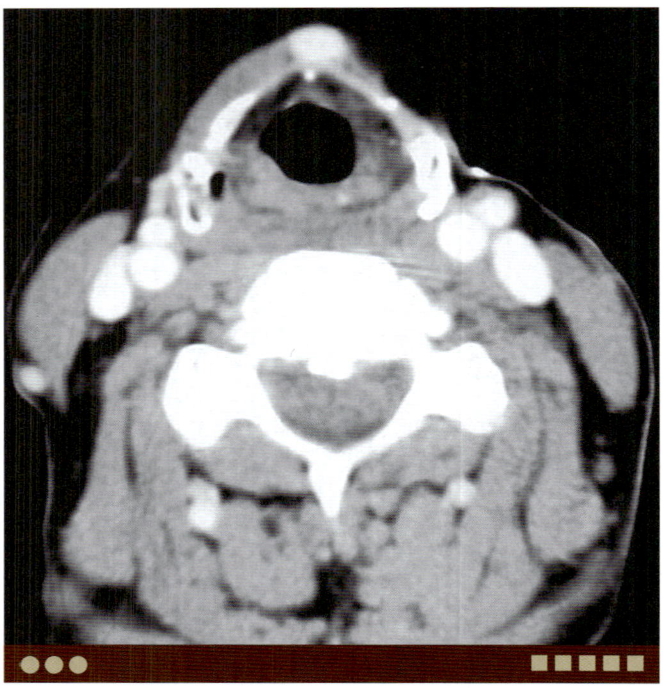

H. Residual/ectopic thyroid tissue. Axial contrast-enhanced CT shows a high-density nodular lesion in a midline location, anterior to the thyroid lamina and deep to the superficial surface of the strap muscle.

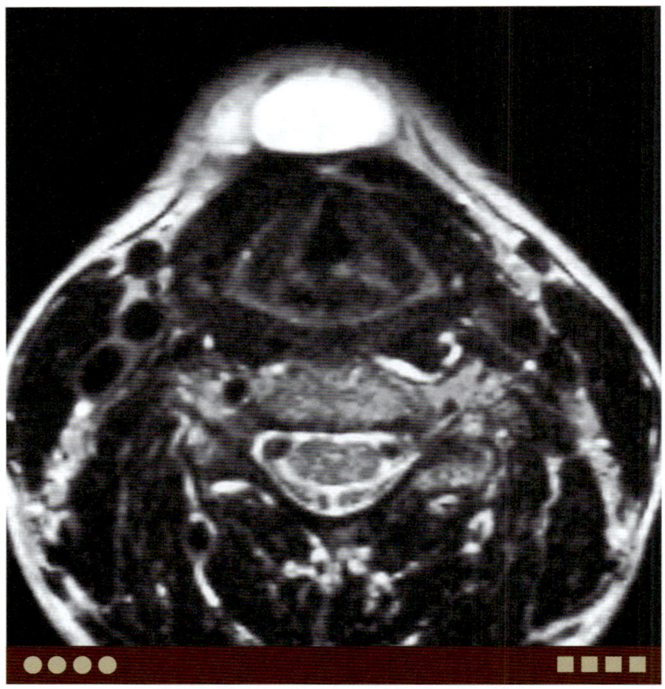

I. Dermoid cyst. Axial T2W MR image demonstrates a high-signal cystic lesion superficial to the strap muscle in midline.

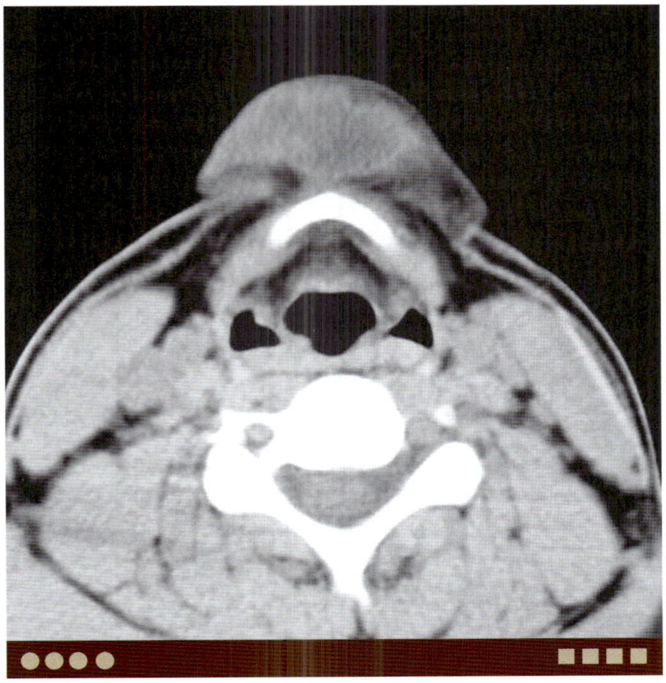

J. Ruptured dermoid cyst. Axial noncontrast-enhanced CT shows an irregularly shaped cystic lesion superficial to the strap muscle in a midline location. Note heterogeneously increased density in the surrounding fat due to inflammation.

Case 11–2 Dermoid

Osamu Sakai, Elisa Flower

PRESENTATION

Anterior neck mass.

FINDINGS

CT demonstrates a cystic lesion in the anterior neck superficial to the strap muscle.

DIFFERENTIAL DIAGNOSIS

- Thyroglossal duct cyst: This is a common developmental cyst embedded in or deep to the strap muscle.
- Necrotic lymph node: This is seen superficial to the strap muscle, often with a thick, irregular wall. Metastases from squamous cell carcinoma and papillary thyroid carcinoma as well as tuberculosis should be considered.
- Brachial cleft cyst: This is more laterally located. Second branchial cleft cyst is the most common type and seen posterior to the submandibular gland.

COMMENTS

This is a 12-year-old girl with an anterior neck mass.

Dermoids and epidermoids are congenital/developmental cystic lesions, often categorized as choristoma, and formed by migration of the ectodermal tissue. A dermoid cyst is lined with epithelium which contains tissues and cells normally present in skin layers, such as hair follicles, sebaceous and sweat glands, while an epidermoid is made of a thin layer of squamous epithelium.

A dermoid is usually diagnosed in the first or second decade of life; however, occasionally it occurs in the deeper tissues, grows gradually, and is discovered later in life. When it occurs in the anterior neck in the midline, it is important to differentiate it from thyroglossal duct cyst. Location is very important; dermoid occurs superficial to the strap muscle, close to the skin, whereas thyroglossal cyst is embedded in or deep to the strap muscle.

If fatty density or signal is identified, dermoid is easily diagnosed; however, it is not commonly seen. Necrotic node, ranula, and lymphatic malformation (lymphangioma or cystic hygroma) should be always considered as the differential diagnosis.

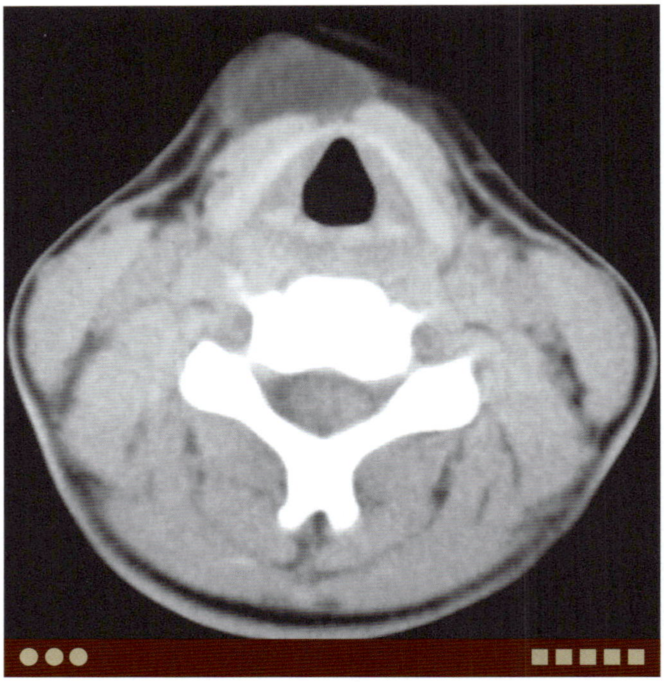

A. Dermoid. Axial noncontrast CT shows a cystic lesion superficial to the strap muscle. Note the density is slightly lower than the cerebrospinal fluid (CSF) suggesting presence of fat.

PEARLS

- **Dermoid is a common congenital/developmental cystic lesion, often seen in the anterior neck.**
- **Dermoid is located superficial to the strap muscle. This is important to differentiate it from thyroglossal duct cyst.**
- **When ruptured, inflammatory change is often seen in the surrounding soft tissue due to chemical irritation.**

ADDITIONAL IMAGES (B-F)

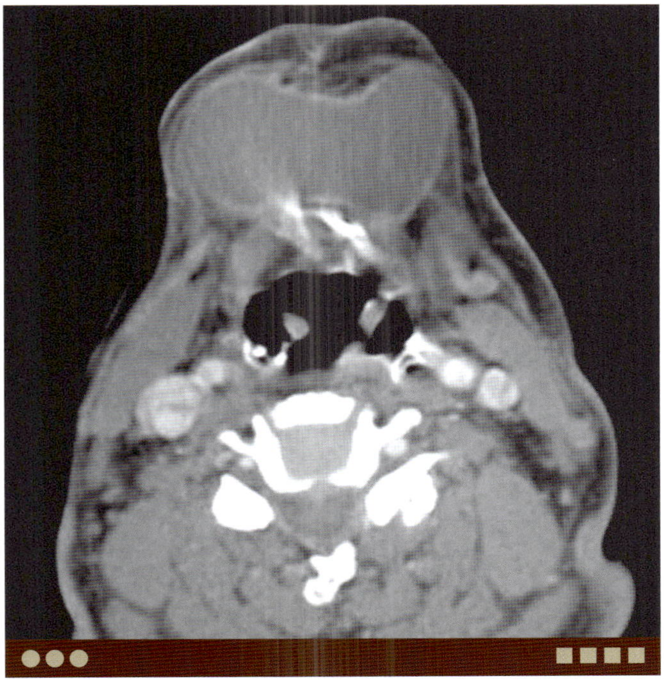

B. Dermoid in a different patient. Axial postcontrast CT shows a large cystic lesion superficial to the strap muscle.

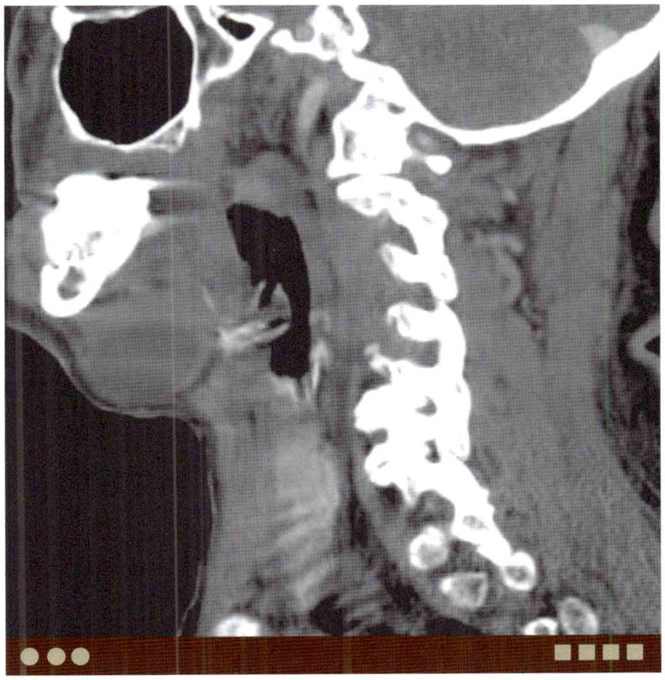

C. Dermoid, same patient as B. Sagittal postcontrast CT shows a large cystic lesion superficial to the strap muscle in the submental region.

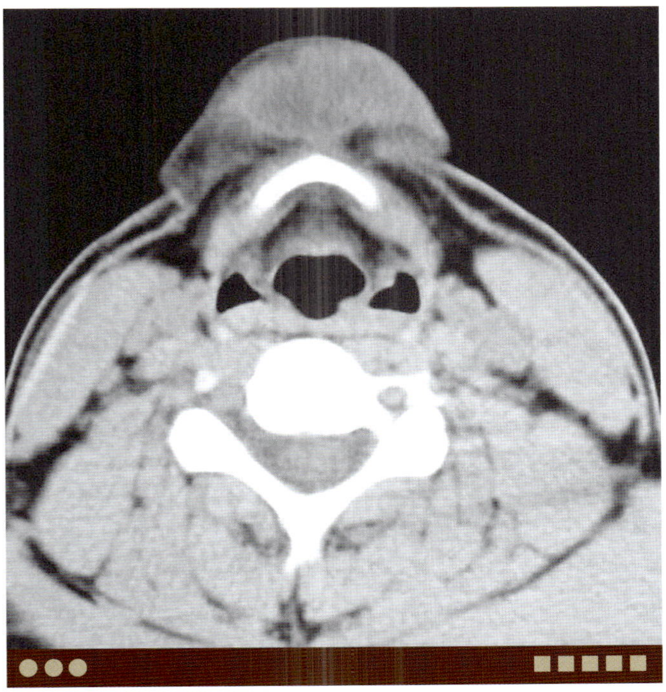

D. Ruptured dermoid. Axial noncontrast CT shows a slightly lobulated cystic lesion with surrounding inflammatory change in the anterior neck close to the skin, superficial to the strap muscle.

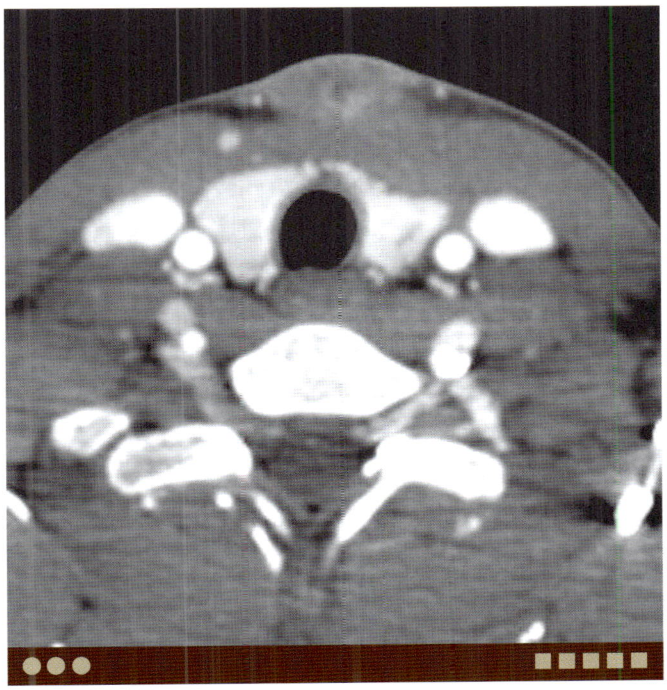

E. Ruptured dermoid in a different patient. Axial postcontrast CT shows a lesion with enhancing irregular wall in the anterior neck close to the skin, superficial to the strap muscle. Note inflammatory change around the lesion from chemical irritation.

DIFFERENTIAL DIAGNOSIS IMAGES (G-J)

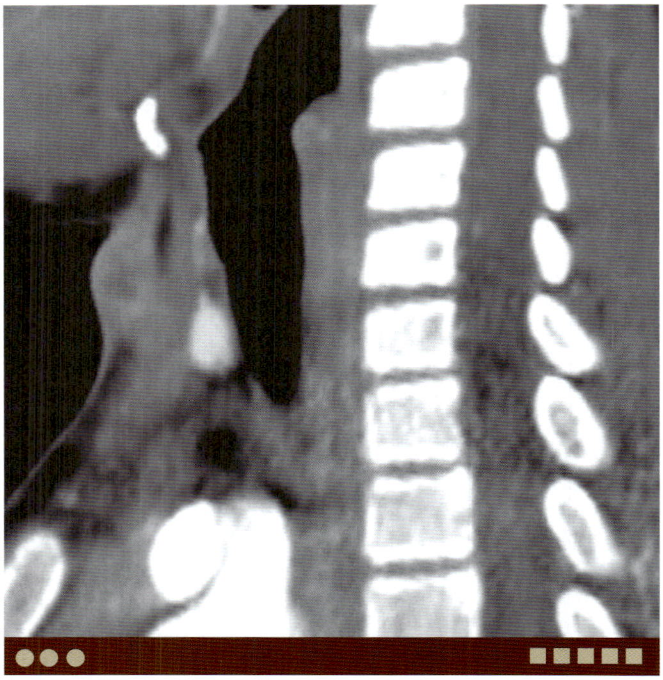

F. Ruptured dermoid, same patient as E. Sagittal postcontrast CT demonstrates the lesion with thick enhancing wall, superficial to the strap muscle.

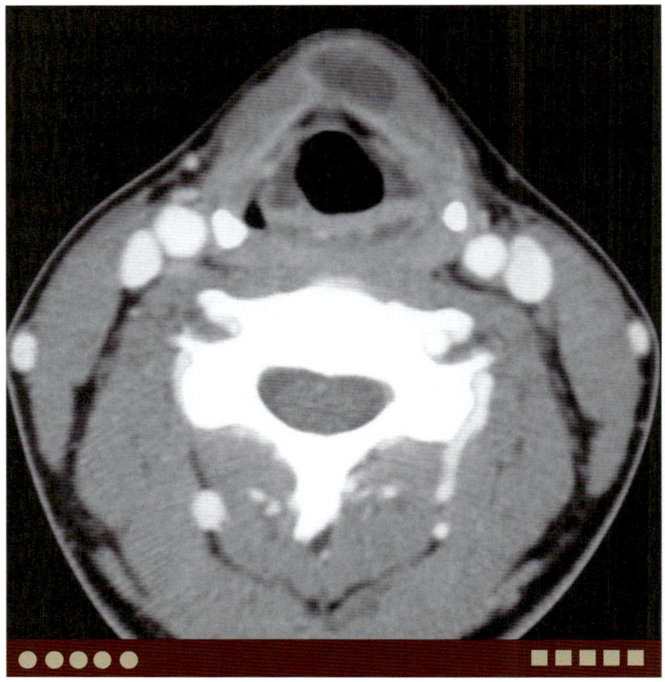

G. Thyroglossal duct cyst. Axial postcontrast CT demonstrates a cystic lesion in the anterior neck, embedded in the strap muscle.

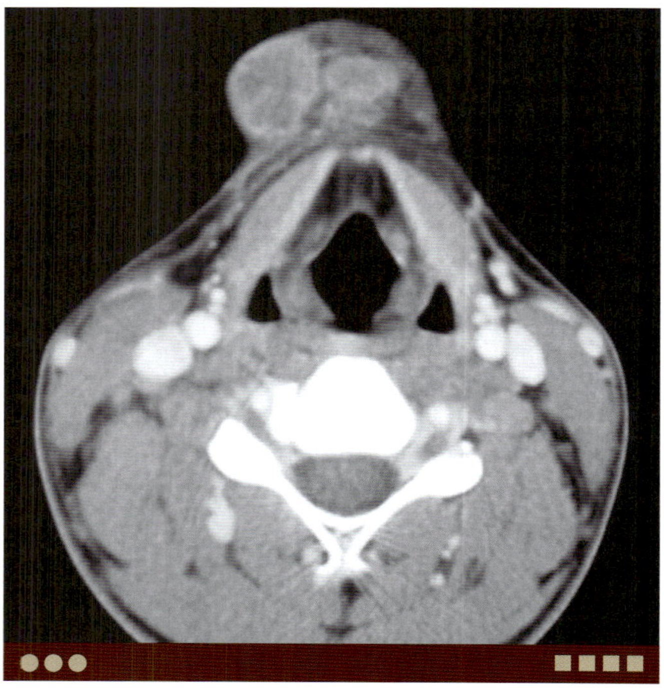

H. Necrotic node, tuberculous lymphadenitis. Axial contrast-enhanced CT demonstrates enlarged nodes with central low densities with surrounding inflammation.

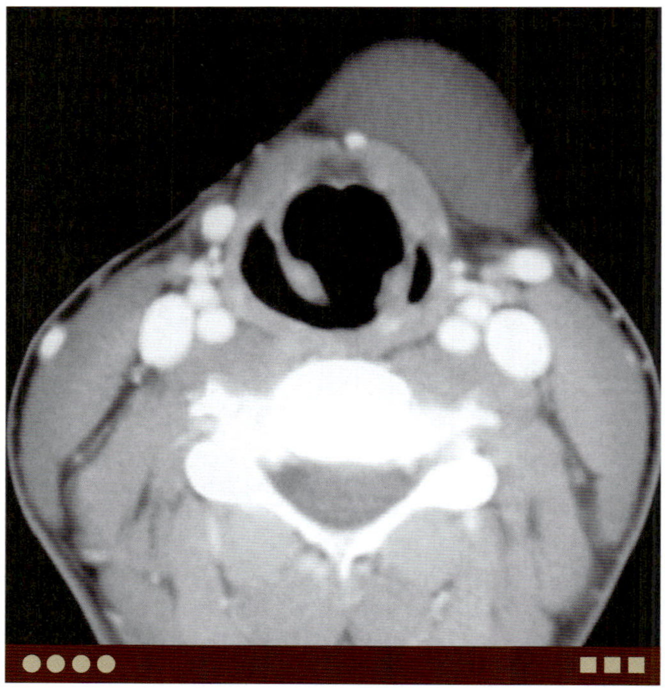

I. Diving ranula. Axial postcontrast CT demonstrates a cystic lesion in the anterior neck superficial to the strap muscle.

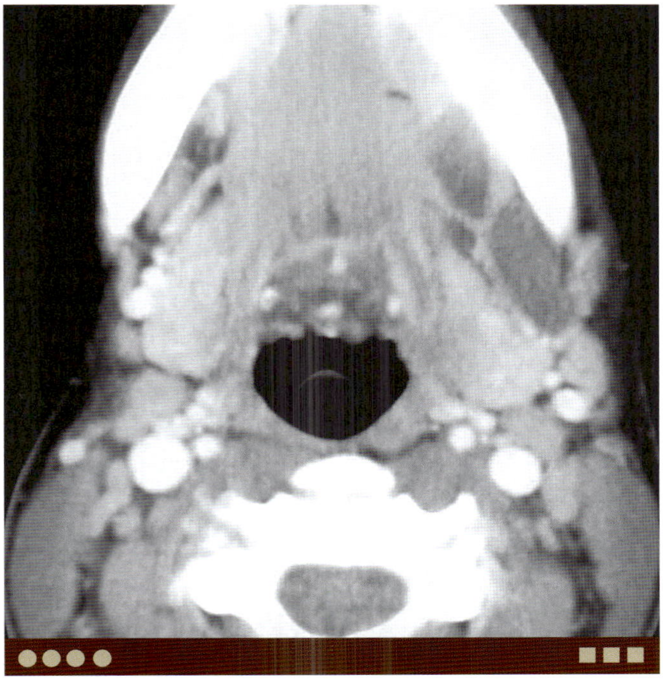

J. Diving ranula, same patient as I. Axial postcontrast CT through the sublingual and submandibular glands demonstrates a septated diving ranula on the left.

Case 11-3 Pyriform Sinus Fistula

Osamu Sakai, June Cheng

PRESENTATION

History of recurrent left neck infection and thyroiditis.

FINDINGS

CT demonstrates a rim-enhancing lesion in the left neck involving the left lobe of the thyroid.

DIFFERENTIAL DIAGNOSIS

- Hypopharyngeal cancer with necrotic metastatic lymph nodes: This may present with very similar findings to pyriform sinus fistula; however, involvement of the thyroid is rare. Patients are usually old men, not young women.
- Thyroid tumors: Thyroid tumors arising in the superior pole of the thyroid demonstrate similar findings; however, hypopharyngeal abnormality is rare.
- Branchial cleft cyst: Second branchial cleft cyst is the most common type and seen posterior to the submandibular gland and anteromedial to the sternocleidomastoid muscle. Infected branchial cleft cyst demonstrates a cystic lesion with thick, irregular enhancing wall.

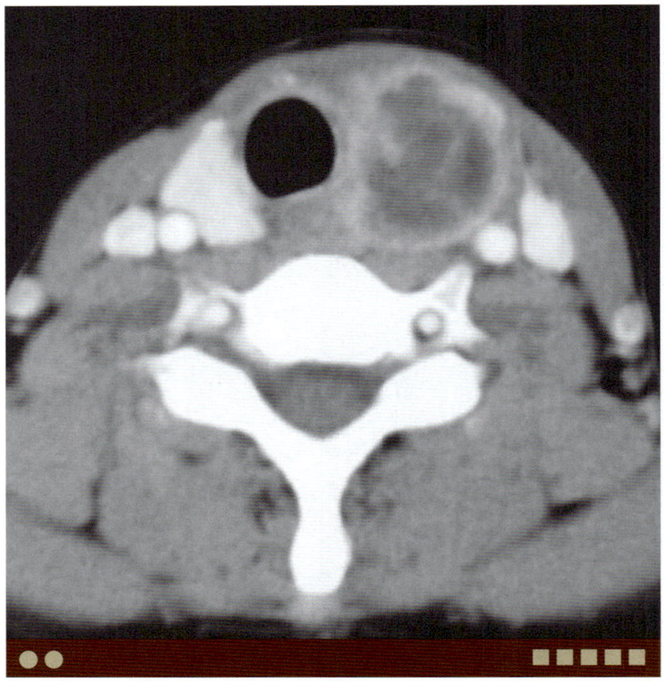

A. Pyriform sinus fistula and suppurative thyroiditis. Axial contrast-enhanced CT through the thyroid gland demonstrates an enhancing lesion involving the left lobe of the thyroid consistent with suppurative thyroiditis.

COMMENTS

This is a 30-year-old woman with a left-sided tender neck mass.

Pyriform sinus fistula usually presents as infection or inflammation in the neck, often involving the thyroid, causing recurrent suppurative thyroiditis or subcutaneous abscess. This is a developmental abnormality associated with a residual third or fourth branchial pouch. The third and fourth pharyngeal pouches form the pyriform. Persistent ducts from either of these pharyngeal pouch sinuses may drain into the pyriform sinus. It has been proposed that the third pouch fistula drains anterior to the fold made by the internal laryngeal nerve, and that the fourth pouch fistula drains posterior to this fold.

The patient is typically a young woman with a history of recurrent neck infection or thyroiditis. The first episode of neck inflammation/infection usually occurs before 10 years of age. However, the patient may present later in life. A pyriform sinus fistula usually occurs on the left side (>80%). Embryologically, the left fourth branchial arch artery forms a part of the aortic arch, while the right one forms the right subclavian artery. Normal asymmetry in the lower neck development may be associated with left-sided predominance of the fistula, which may support the fourth branchial pouch origin of this condition.

Suppurative thyroiditis is rare because of the high concentration of iodine and hypervasularity of the thyroid. Therefore, this condition should always be considered in a patient with suppurative thyroiditis.

It is usually difficult to identify the fistula directly on CT. Barium swallow is required to make a diagnosis. However, the fistula may not be demonstrated in the acute inflammatory phase due to edema from infection and inflammation. Therefore, barium swallow should be performed after 2 weeks of antibiotic therapy.

PEARLS

- **Pyriform sinus fistula is a developmental abnormality associated with a residual third or fourth branchial pouch and present with recurrent suppurative thyroiditis or subcutaneous abscess.**
- **It usually occurs in a young woman on the left side.**
- **This condition should always be considered in a patient with suppurative thyroiditis.**

ADDITIONAL IMAGES (B-H)

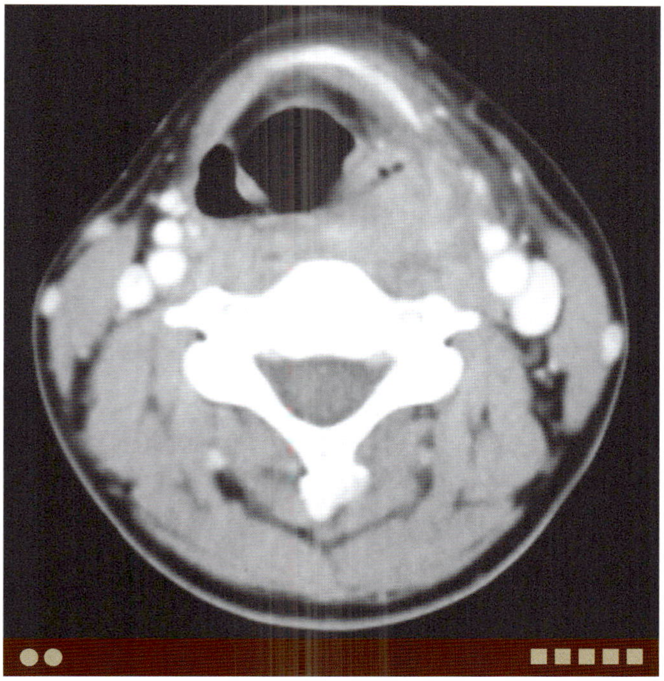

B. Pyriform sinus fistula, same patient as A. Axial contrast-enhanced CT through the hypopharynx demonstrates inflammatory change in and around the left pyriform sinus.

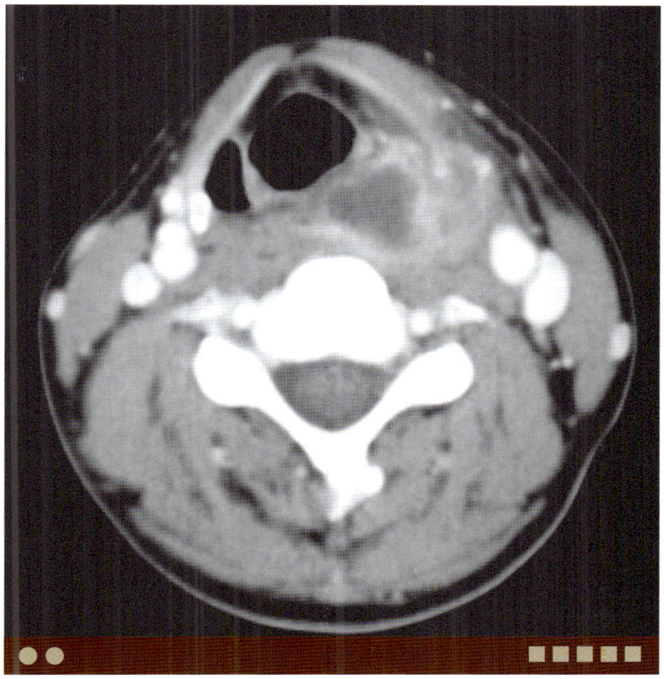

C. Pyriform sinus fistula, same patient as A. Axial contrast-enhanced CT through slightly lower level demonstrates a rim-enhancing lesion consistent with abscess.

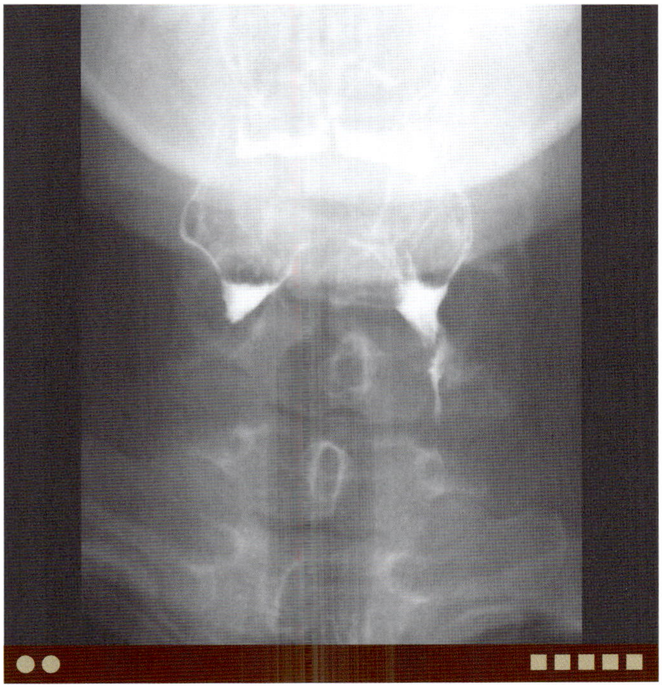

D. Pyriform sinus fistula, same patient as A. Barium swallow after 2 weeks of antibiotics therapy demonstrates fistula tract from the left pyriform sinus.

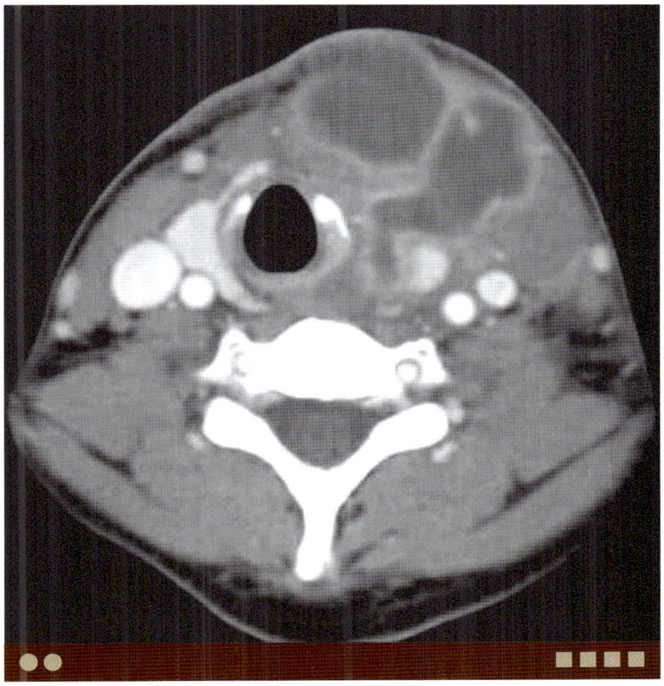

E. Pyriform sinus fistula and neck abscess in a different patient. Axial contrast-enhanced CT through the thyroid gland demonstrates lobulated rim-enhancing abscesses in the left anterior neck. Note involvement of the left lobe of the thyroid.

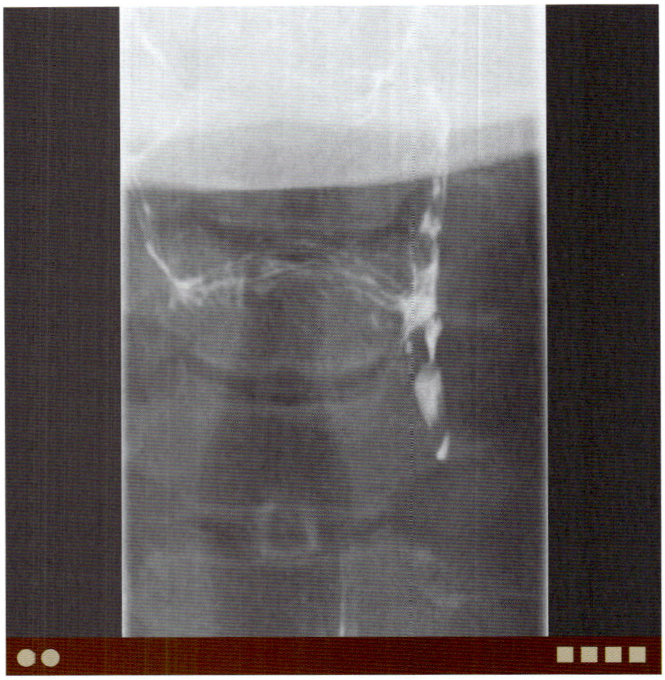

F. Pyriform sinus fistula and neck abscess, same patient as E. Barium swallow after 2 weeks of antibiotics therapy demonstrates fistula tract from the left pyriform sinus.

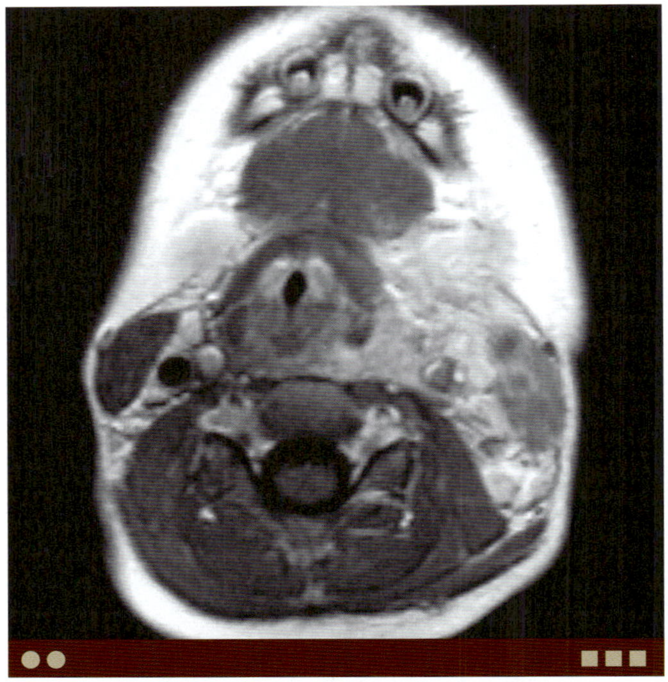

G. Pyriform sinus fistula in a 3-year-old girl. Axial postcontrast T1W image demonstrates an enhancing lesion in the left pyriform sinus with surrounding inflammatory change.

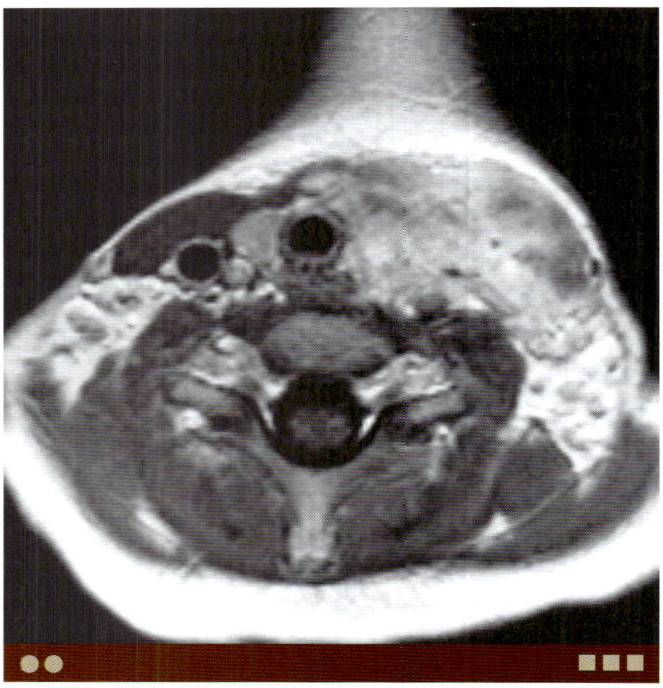

H. Pyriform sinus fistula, same patient as G. Axial postcontrast T1W image through the thyroid demonstrates extensive inflammatory changes involving the left lobe of the thyroid and surrounding tissue.

DIFFERENTIAL DIAGNOSIS IMAGES (I-J)

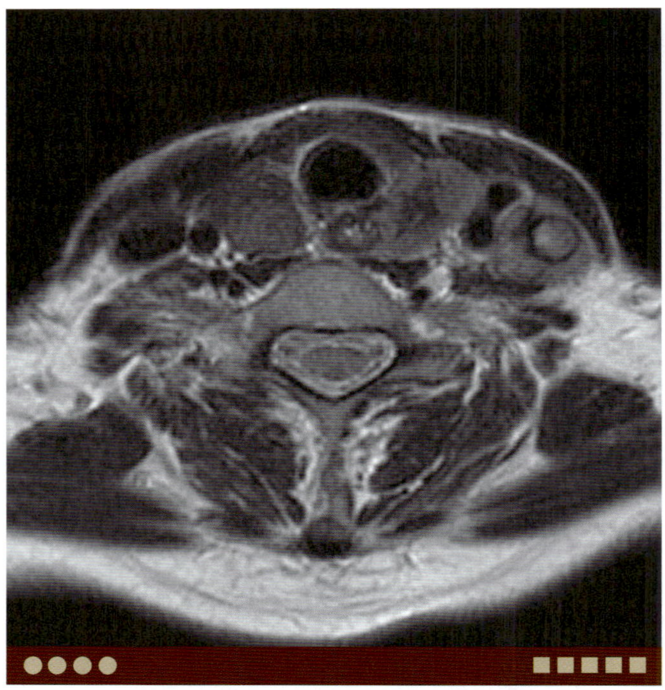

I. Papillary thyroid carcinoma. Axial T2W image demonstrates left thyroid tumor and enlarged left cervical lymph nodes. Note the extracapsular extension of the thyroid tumor and invasion into the esophagus.

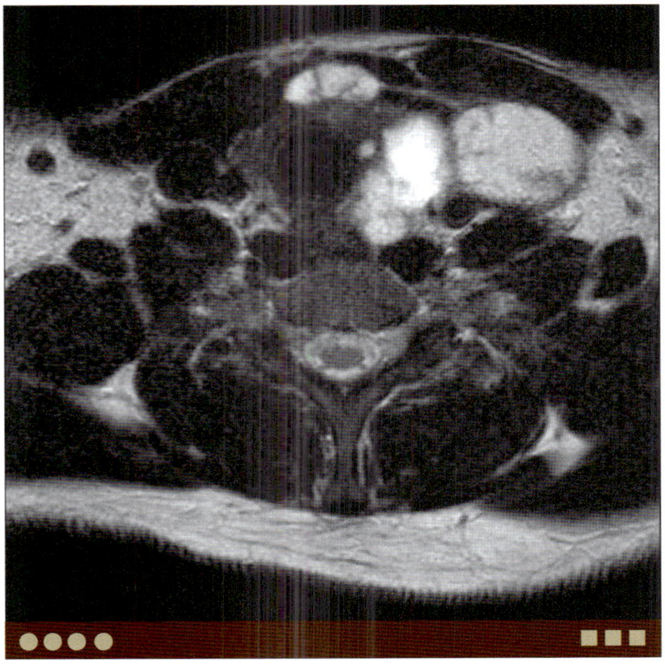

J. Papillary thyroid carcinoma with nodal metastases. Axial T2W MR image demonstrates multiple cystic lesions showing variable signal in the left neck.

Case 11–4 Secondary Hyperparathyroidism

Akifumi Fujita, Margaret Chapman, Osamu Sakai

PRESENTATION

Hypercalcemia.

FINDINGS

CT demonstrates enlarged parathyroid glands, posterior to the inferior poles of the thyroid gland.

DIFFERENTIAL DIAGNOSIS

- Thyroid tumors: Exophytic mass lesions arising from the thyroid can mimic parathyroid lesions. It is often difficult to localize the lesion internal or external to the thyroid.
- Lymph nodes: These may present with similar findings. Careful evaluation for possible primary lesions should always be performed.

COMMENTS

This is a 65-year-old man with a history of long-term hemodialysis.

Secondary hyperparathyroidism can often be seen in patients on long-term hemodialysis. The role of head and neck imaging is to identify enlarged parathyroid glands for surgical resection. Locally, ultrasound is very useful; however, ectopic parathyroid glands may be difficult to detect by ultrasound alone. CT is also useful, particularly with thin slices and multiplanar reconstruction with multidetector computed tomography (MDCT). On CT, the lesion may demonstrate similar findings to enlarged lymph nodes. Artifacts from the bones and shoulders often degrade the images and may make evaluation difficult. MRI is also reported as useful in demonstrating enlarged parathyroid glands as T1 isointense and T2 hyperintense lesions. However, images are often degraded by artifacts from motion, swallowing, susceptibility, or poor signal from the use of inappropriate coils or sequences.

Nuclear medicine studies have an important role in diagnosing parathyroid lesions. Recently, ^{99m}Tc-MIBI with early and delayed imaging is most commonly used, while ^{201}Tl-^{99m}TcO^{4-} subtraction was used in the past. Nuclear medicine studies are sensitive and useful for the detection of ectopic parathyroid glands.

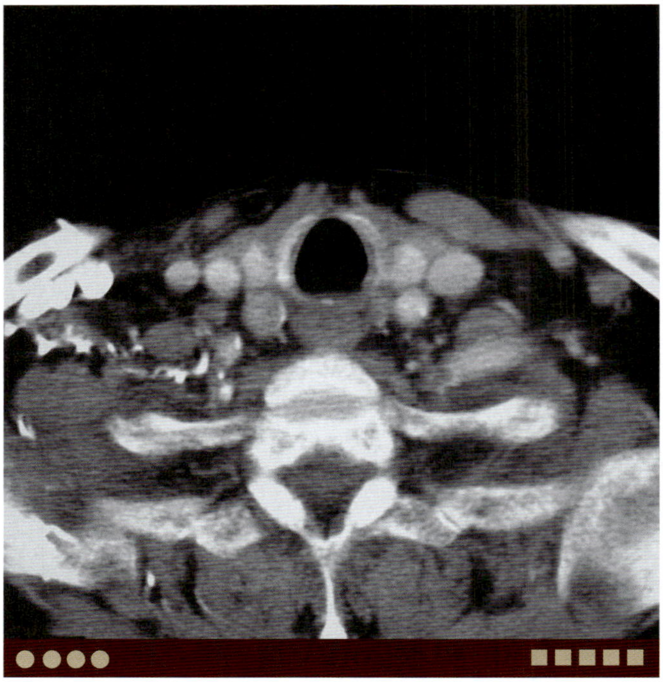

A. Parathyroid hyperplasia, secondary hyperparathyroidism. Axial postcontrast CT demonstrates enlarged parathyroid glands posterior to the inferior poles of the thyroid glands, right larger than left.

Secondary osseous changes are often seen on CT, including loss of normal trabeculation and diffuse sclerotic changes in the skull base and maxillofacial bones, known as osteitis fibrosa cystica. "Brown tumors" are not commonly seen in the head and neck, however, may result in mass effect into the adjacent structures.

PEARLS

- **Secondary hyperparathyroidism is often seen in patients on long-term hemodialysis.**
- **^{99m}Tc-MIBI with early and delayed imaging is most commonly used.**
- **Ultrasound is useful locally; however detection of ectopic parathyroid glands may be difficult.**
- **CT and MRI are also useful. These scans should cover from the hyoid to the mediastinum.**

ADDITIONAL IMAGES (B-G)

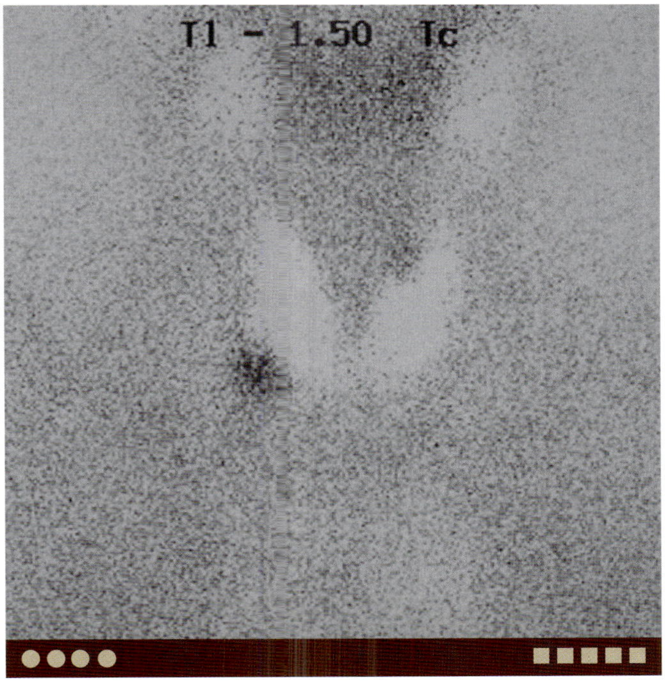

B. Parathyroid hyperplasia, secondary hyperparathyroidism, same patient as A. ^{201}Tl-$^{99m}TcO^{4-}$ subtraction study demonstrates increased uptake inferior to the lower pole of the right lobe of the thyroid. A smaller amount of increased uptake is also seen superior to the superior pole of the left lobe of the thyroid.

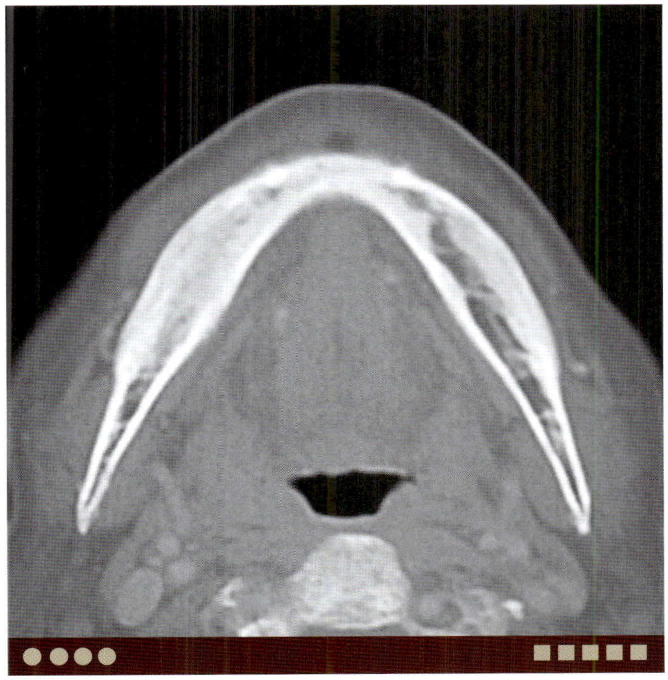

C. Parathyroid hyperplasia, secondary hyperparathyroidism, same patient as A. Bone window CT demonstrates diffuse sclerotic changes of the mandible.

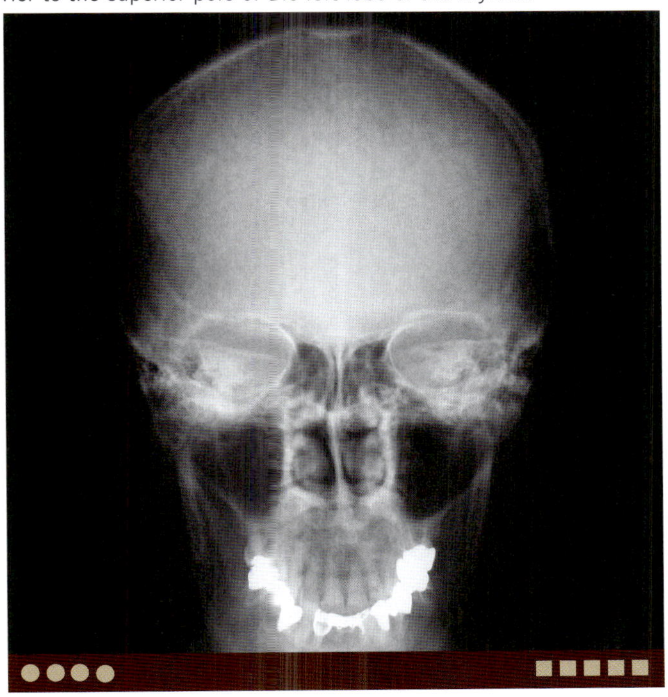

D. Parathyroid hyperplasia, secondary hyperparathyroidism, same patient as A. Skull radiograph demonstrates trabecular bone resorption of the cranial vault. Alternating areas of lucency and sclerosis produce a "salt and pepper" appearance.

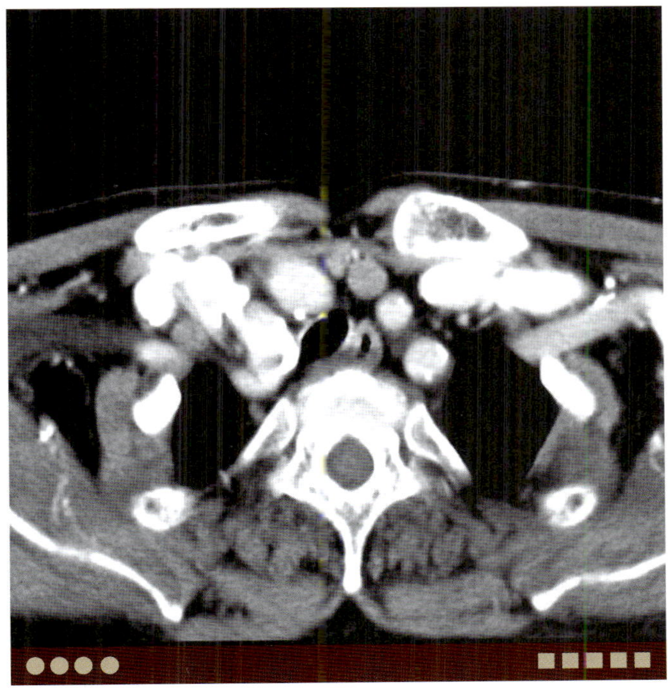

E. Parathyroid hyperplasia, secondary hyperparathyroidism in a different patient. Axial postcontrast CT demonstrates enlarged parathyroid gland caudal to the inferior pole of left thyroid gland.

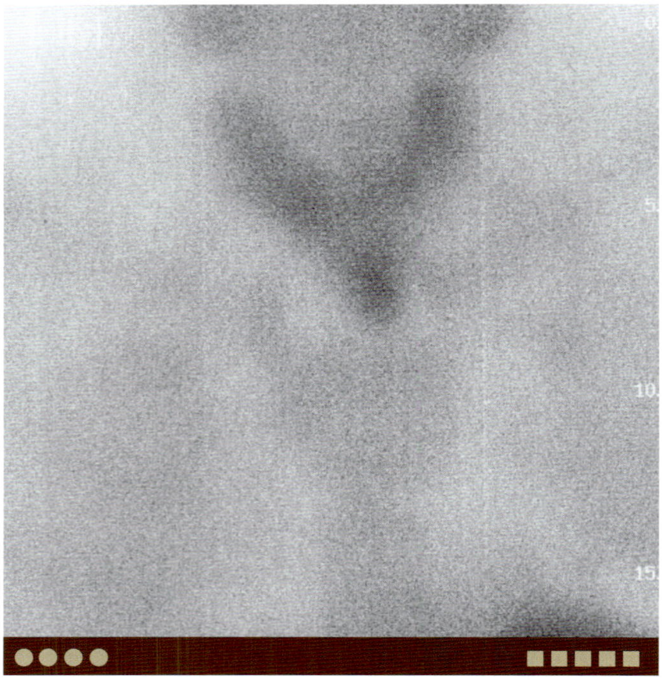

F. Parathyroid hyperplasia, secondary hyperparathyroidism, same patient as E. ^{99m}Tc-MIBI study demonstrates nodular uptake in the region inferior to left thyroid gland in this early image.

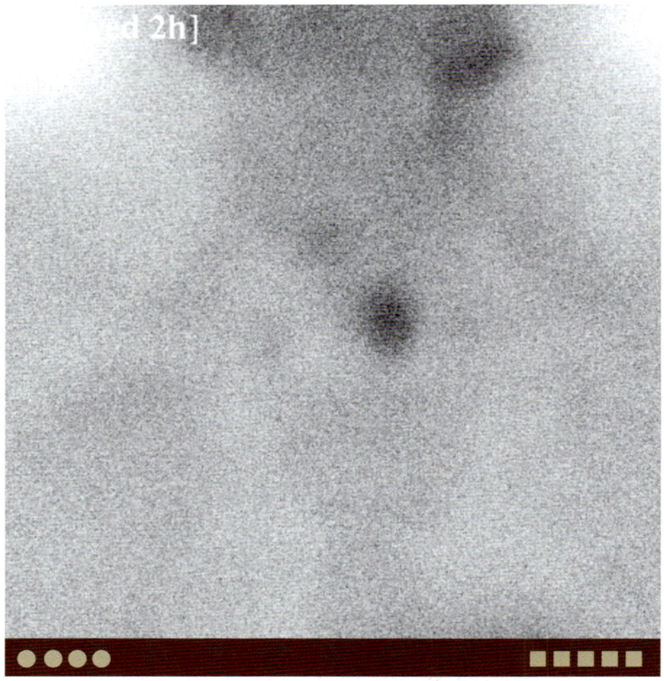

G. Parathyroid hyperplasia, secondary hyperparathyroidism, same patient as E. Delayed image of ^{99m}Tc-MIBI study demonstrates prolonged uptake of the parathyroid hyperplasia.

DIFFERENTIAL DIAGNOSIS IMAGES (H-J)

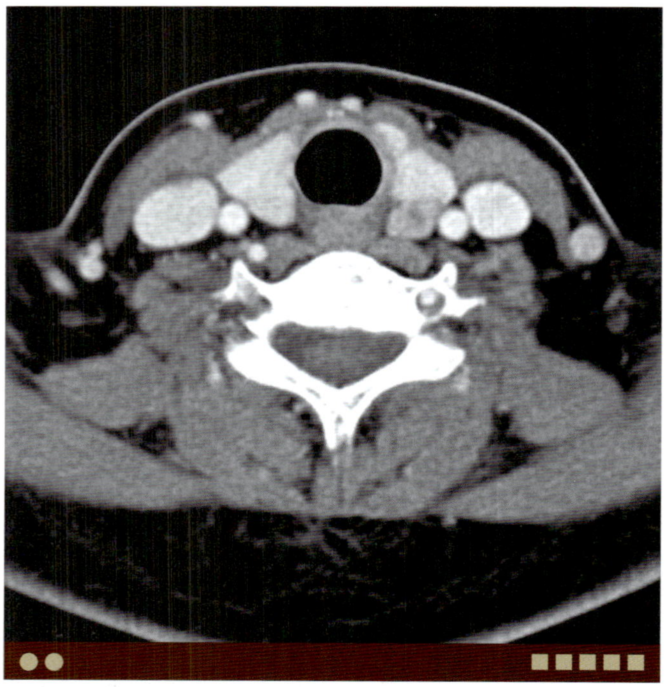

H. Parathyroid adenoma, primary hyperparathyroidism. Axial postcontrast CT shows a moderately enhancing nodular tumor posterior to the left lobe of the thyroid gland.

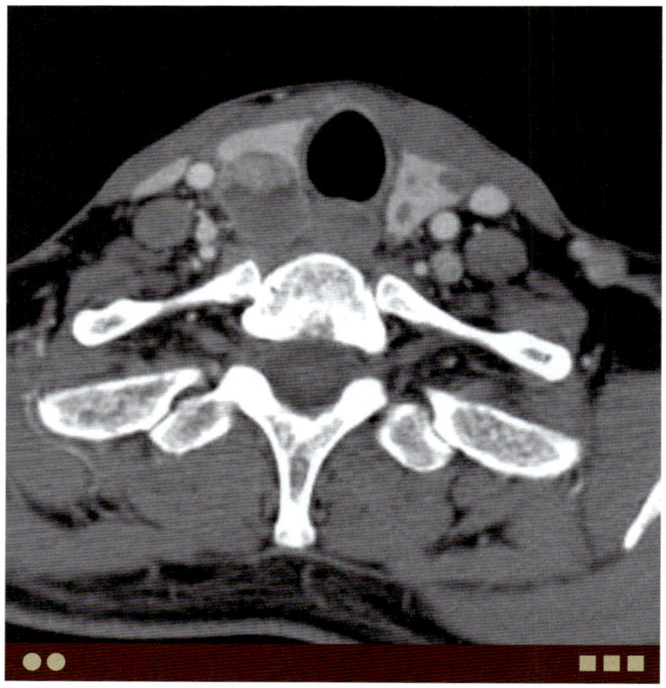

I. Parathyroid carcinoma. Axial postcontrast CT demonstrates a partially cystic lesion with a mural nodule, located in the right lower neck, posterior to the right lobe of the thyroid gland. (*Courtesy of Dr. Hiroki Kato*)

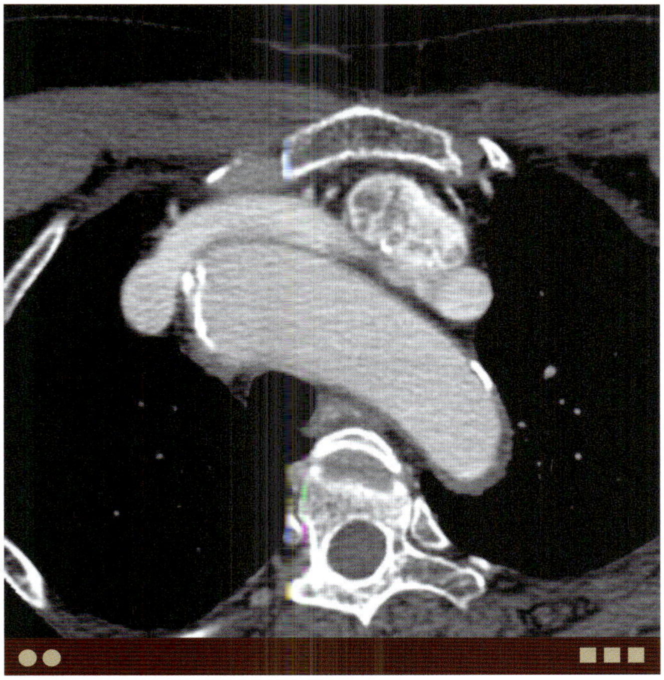

J. Goiter. Axial postcontrast CT demonstrates a heterogeneously enhancing mass posterior to the sternum.

Case 11-5 Lymphoma of the Thyroid

Akifumi Fujita, Margaret Chapman, Osamu Sakai

PRESENTATION

Enlarging anterior neck mass.

FINDINGS

CT demonstrates a markedly enlarged thyroid gland with heterogeneously decreased density.

DIFFERENTIAL DIAGNOSIS

- Goiter: This condition tends to show a heterogeneous, enlarged thyroid gland usually with some preservation of the normal high-density attenuation of the thyroid. Without appropriate clinical history or endocrinologic data, these conditions may be difficult to distinguish by imaging alone.
- Anaplastic carcinoma of the thyroid: This demonstrates similar findings but is usually more aggressive with invasion of the adjacent structures.
- Hashimoto thyroiditis: This condition also demonstrates diffuse enlargement of the thyroid gland and may be impossible to differentiate from lymphoma by imaging alone. Clinical history and examination findings may be beneficial in differentiation.

COMMENTS

This is a 68-year-old woman with a history of Hashimoto thyroiditis.

Primary lymphomas of the thyroid gland are rare. When encountered, they are usually non-Hodgkin lymphomas (NHL), with primary Hodgkin disease of the thyroid gland being extremely rare. Thyroid lymphoma constitutes about 3% of all NHLs and 5% of all thyroid tumors. It most often occurs in elderly women (M:F = 1:3). Rapid increase in thyroid size causes mass effect to the trachea and esophagus and results in dyspnea and dysphagia. Thyroid lymphoma is often associated with Hashimoto thyroiditis, a condition which is characterized by chronic thyroiditis with lymphocytic infiltration. Secondary lymphoma may occur as metastasis or direct invasion of lymphoma from adjacent nodal or extranodal origins.

Imaging findings of thyroid lymphoma are often nonspecific and may be similar to goiter and anaplastic carcinoma. Lymphomas are usually large at the time of diagnosis (5-10 cm) and often demonstrate slight heterogeneity and low density on CT and relatively low signal on both T1W and T2W images. Calcification is usually not seen, although the presence of calcification does not exclude lymphoma. Extracapsular extension and invasion to the adjacent structures are aggressive features suggestive of malignancy.

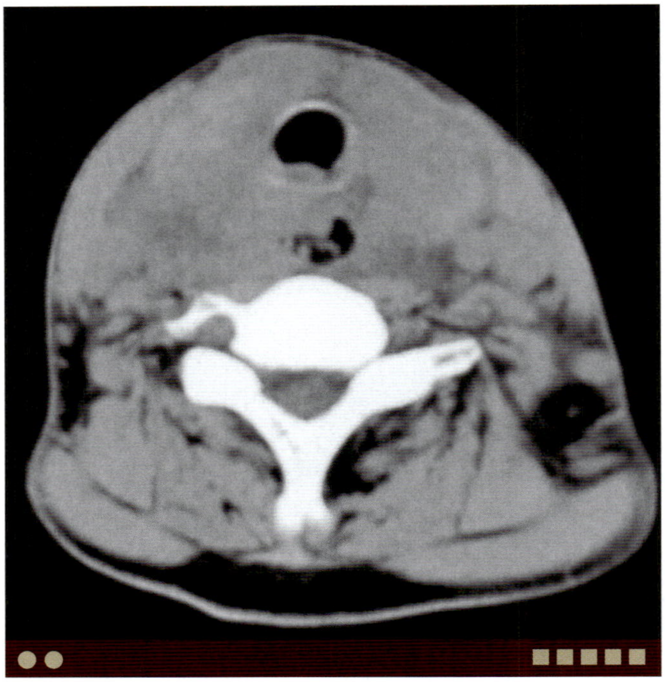

A. Lymphoma. Axial noncontrast CT demonstrates an enlarged thyroid gland displacing the trachea anteriorly.

Lymphoma is not common in the thyroid and imaging findings are similar to anaplastic carcinoma. However, as lymphoma responds to chemotherapy and radiation and is potentially curable, early diagnosis and appropriate therapy are essential for improved outcome.

PEARLS

- **Primary lymphoma of the thyroid is rare, and is often associated with Hashimoto thyroiditis.**
- **Imaging findings of lymphoma are often nonspecific and may be similar to goiter and anaplastic carcinoma. Enlarging thyroid with heterogeneously decreased density is a common finding.**
- **Thyroid lymphoma commonly occurs in elderly women.**
- **Patients with Hashimoto disease have a higher incidence of primary thyroid lymphoma.**
- **Signal characteristics include homogeneous low density on CT and relatively low signal on both T1W and T2W images.**

ADDITIONAL IMAGES (B-D)

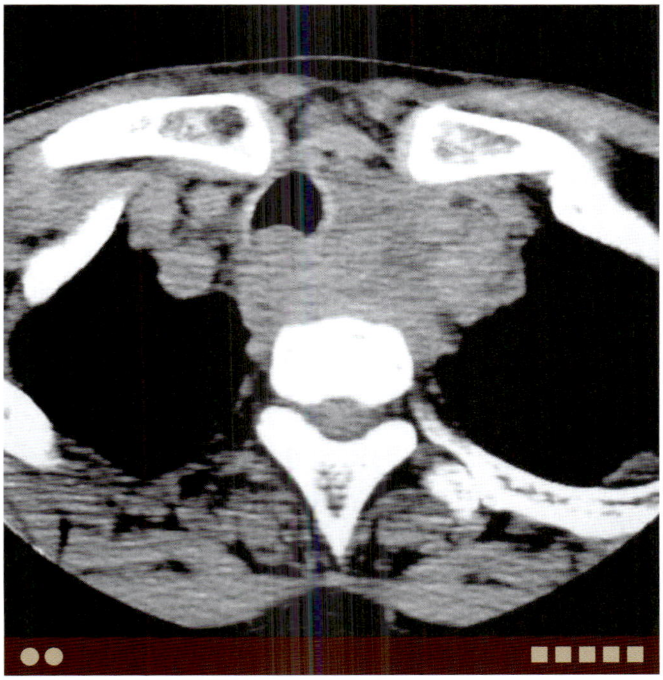

B. Lymphoma, same patient as A. Axial noncontrast CT demonstrates intrathoracic extension of the tumor obliterating the fat planes around the major branches of the aorta.

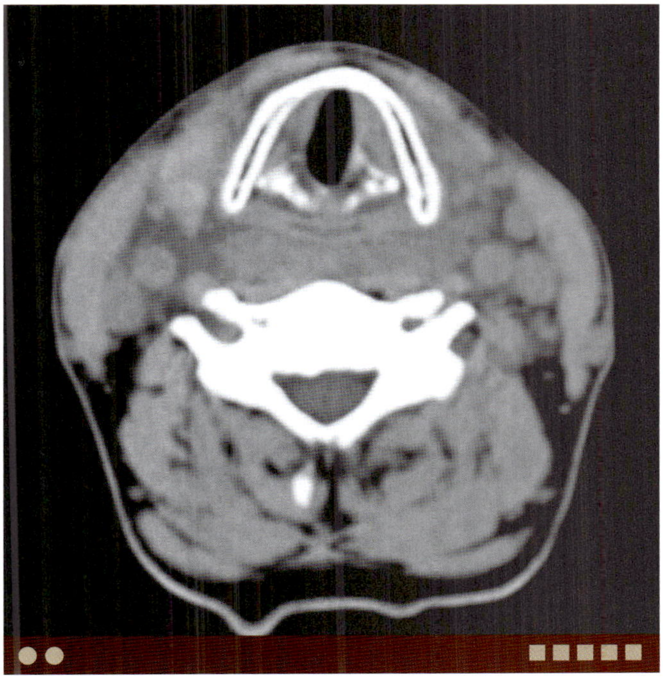

C. Lymphoma, same patient as A. Axial noncontrast CT through the level of the cricoid demonstrates retropharyngeal edema.

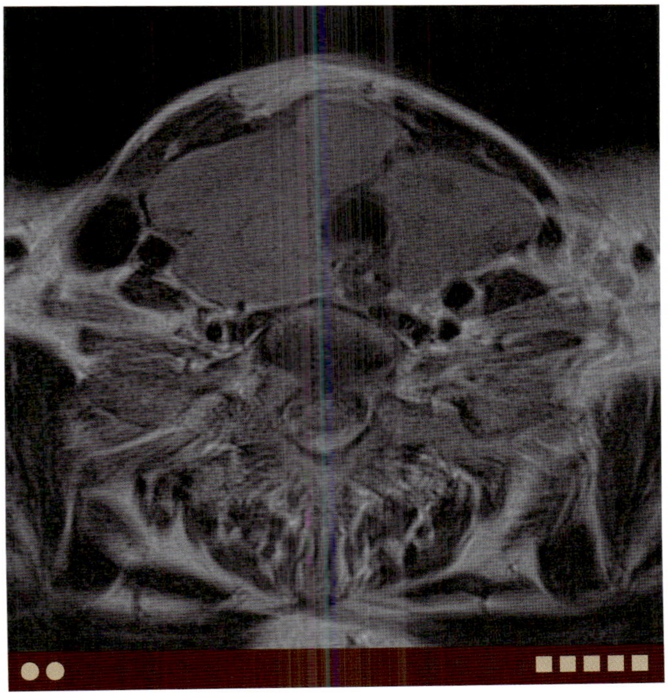

D. Lymphoma in a different patient. Axial T2W image demonstrates diffuse enlargement of the bilateral thyroid lobes with homogeneously low signal.

DIFFERENTIAL DIAGNOSIS IMAGES (E-I)

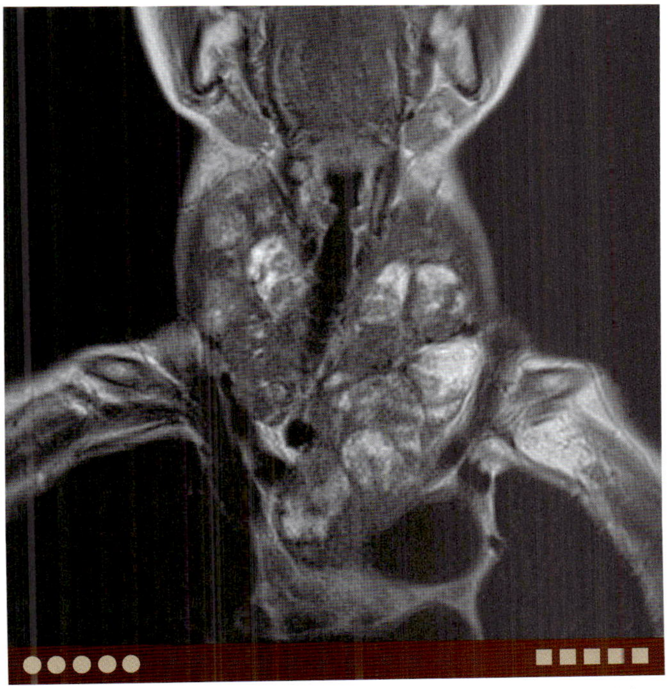

E. Adenomatous goiter. Coronal T2W image demonstrates multinodular enlargement of the bilateral thyroid glands. Note the heterogeneous signal intensity of the tumor.

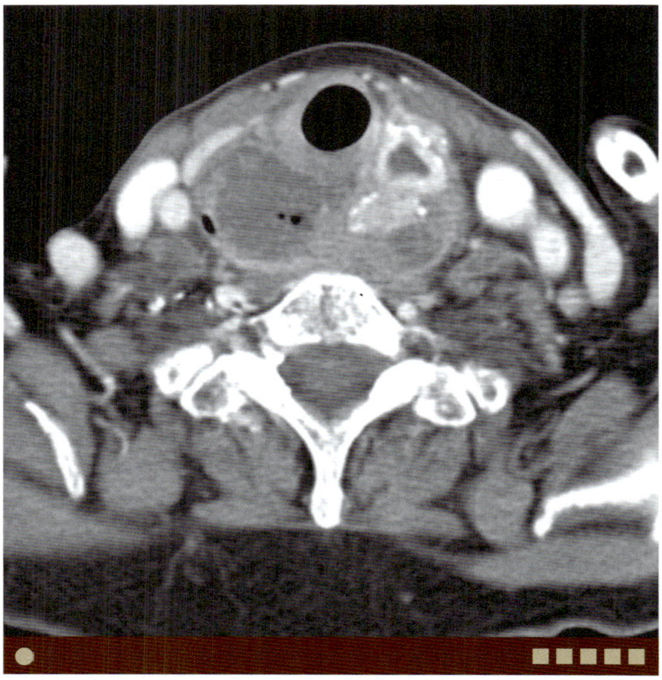

F. Anaplastic carcinoma. Axial contrast-enhanced CT demonstrates a heterogeneously enhancing thyroid tumor displacing the trachea anteriorly.

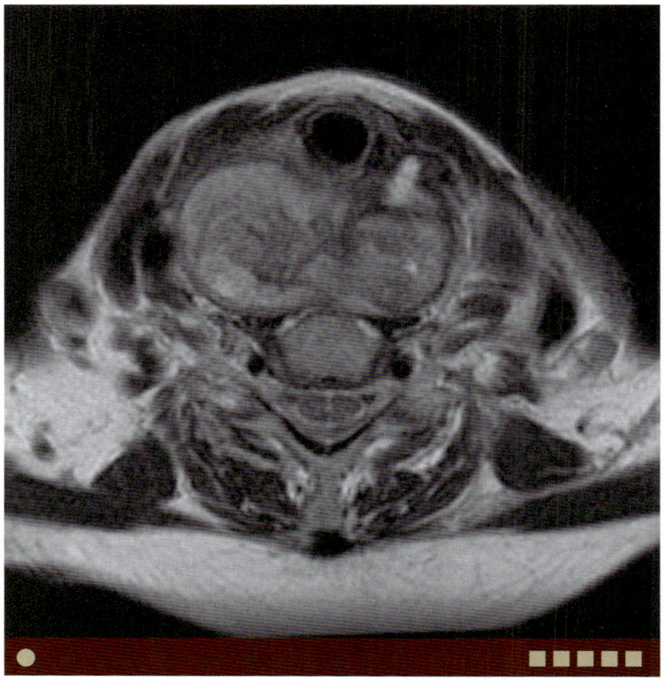

G. Anaplastic carcinoma, same patient as F. Axial T2W image demonstrates heterogeneous signal intensity of the tumor displacing the trachea anteriorly.

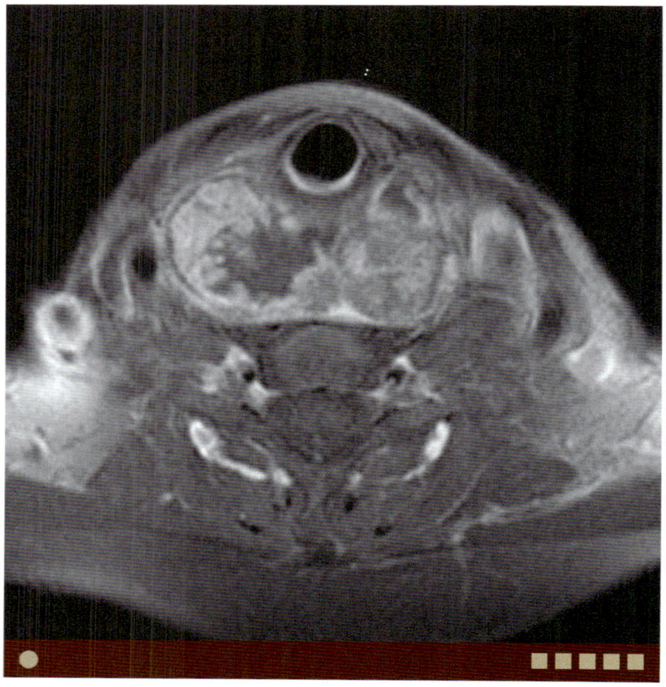

H. Anaplastic carcinoma, same patient as F. Axial postcontrast fat-suppressed T1W image demonstrates a heterogeneously enhancing tumor displacing the trachea anteriorly.

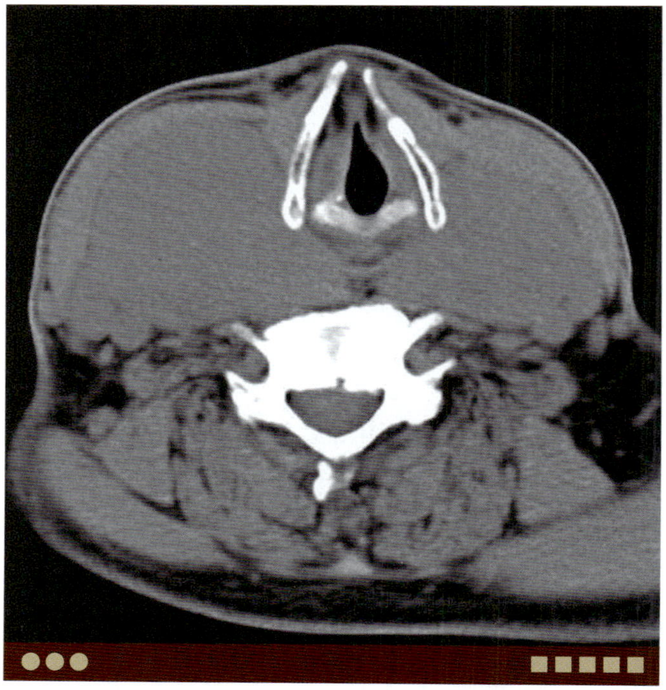

I. Hashimoto thyroiditis. Axial CT demonstrates homogeneous low-density enlargement of the thyroid gland.

Case 11–6 Papillary Thyroid Carcinoma

Akifumi Fujita, Margaret Chapman, Osamu Sakai

PRESENTATION

Hoarseness.

FINDINGS

CT and MRI show a thyroid tumor and multiple enlarged lymph nodes with variable appearance.

DIFFERENTIAL DIAGNOSIS

- Tuberculosis: This demonstrates variable appearance of lymph nodes; avid enhancement, cystic change, and calcification.
- Squamous cell carcinoma: Nodal metastasis often demonstrates intranodal necrosis. Calcification is not common.
- Kaposi's sarcoma: This condition is often associated with HIV infection and can present with enhancing metastatic nodes.
- Others: Cat scratch disease and Kikuchi-Fujimoto disease (histiocytic necrotizing lymphadenitis) may demonstrate similar findings.

COMMENTS

This is a 61-year-old woman with a history of a rapidly growing neck mass.

Papillary thyroid carcinoma is the most common carcinoma of the thyroid, representing 55% to 80% of all thyroid carcinomas. Follicular carcinoma and anaplastic carcinoma are relatively rare (5%-15% of thyroid carcinomas), and medullary carcinoma is the least common (<5%). Medullary carcinoma is often associated with multiple endocrine neoplasia (MEN).

Ultrasound is the first-line modality for evaluation and diagnosis of papillary thyroid cancer as fine-needle aspiration (FNA) can be performed immediately under ultrasound guidance. Recently, FNA has been recommended for thyroid masses over 1 cm in diameter.

The role of CT and MRI in evaluation of papillary thyroid cancers is to evaluate for invasion into the adjacent structures and/or nodal metastasis, not for localization of the lesion in the thyroid gland. A careful search for extracapsular extension, invasion into the trachea, esophagus, paraspinal muscles, carotid artery, and jugular vein should be performed. However, without apparent tumor protrusion into the lumen, it may be difficult to diagnose tumor invasion into the adjacent airway or vessels.

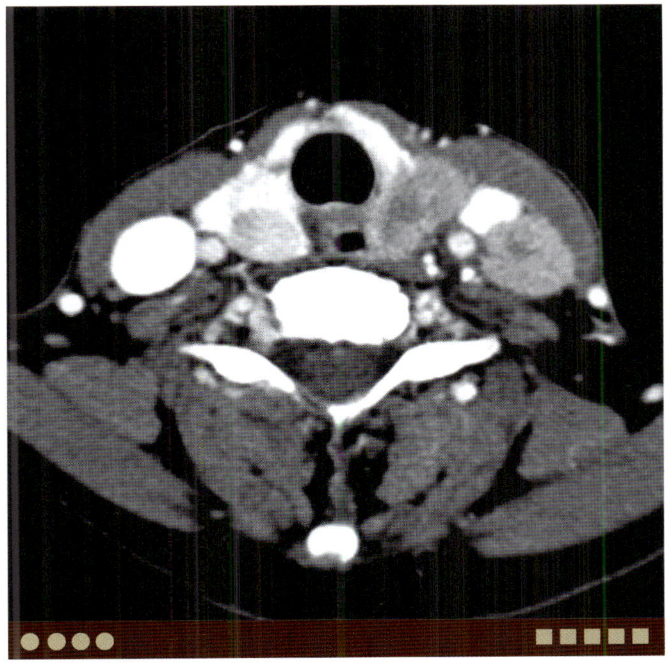

A. Papillary thyroid carcinoma. Axial contrast-enhanced CT demonstrates left thyroid tumor and left cervical lymph node swelling. Both the thyroid tumor and lymph node show avid enhancement.

Nodal metastasis from papillary carcinoma demonstrates variable findings, such as avid enhancement, cystic or necrotic appearance, calcification, or nonenhancing enlargement. The primary lesion may often be small and not well detected on CT or MRI. Therefore, whenever variable appearance of lymph nodes is seen particularly in young women, papillary thyroid carcinoma and tuberculosis should be considered. Remember papillary thyroid carcinoma can be seen in young females even in their teens and early twenties.

PEARLS

- **Ultrasound is the first-line modality for evaluation. Fine-needle aspiration (FNA) can be performed under ultrasound guidance, and is recommended for a mass over 1 cm in diameter.**
- **Papillary thyroid carcinoma is the most common thyroid carcinoma, and demonstrates variable appearance of metastatic lymph nodes.**
- **The primary lesion in the thyroid may be small and the patient may initially present with a nodal mass.**

ADDITIONAL IMAGES (B-E)

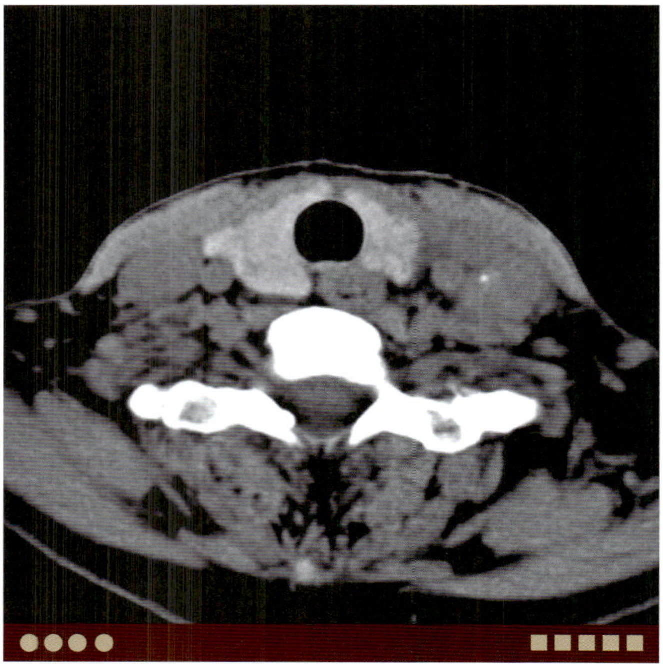

B. Papillary thyroid carcinoma, same patient as A. Axial noncontrast-enhanced CT at a level lower than A demonstrates an enlarged node with calcification.

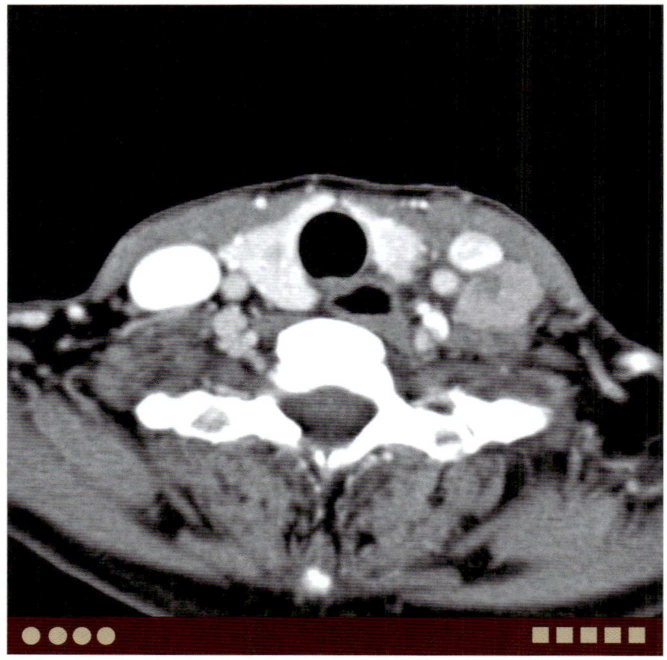

C. Papillary thyroid carcinoma, same patient as A. Axial contrast-enhanced CT at the same level as B demonstrates enhancement of the node.

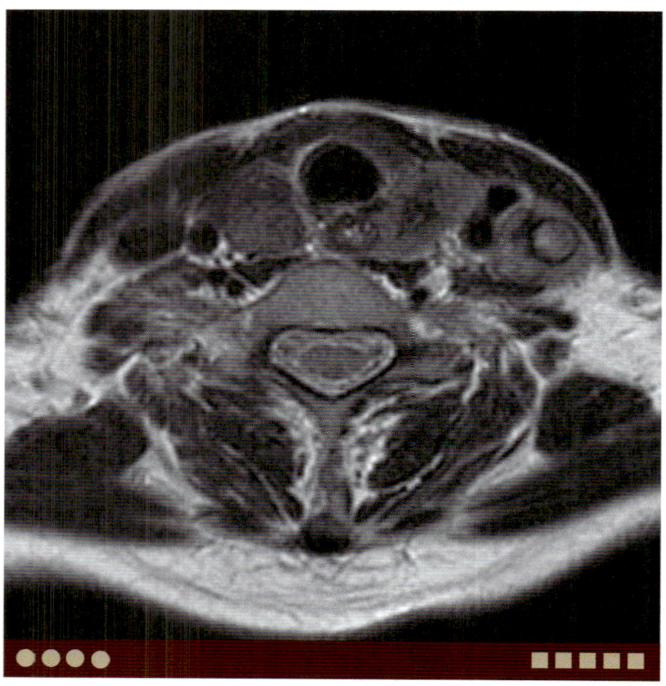

D. Papillary thyroid carcinoma, same patient as A. Axial T2W image demonstrates left thyroid tumor and enlarged left cervical lymph nodes. Note the extracapsular extension of the thyroid tumor and invasion into the esophagus.

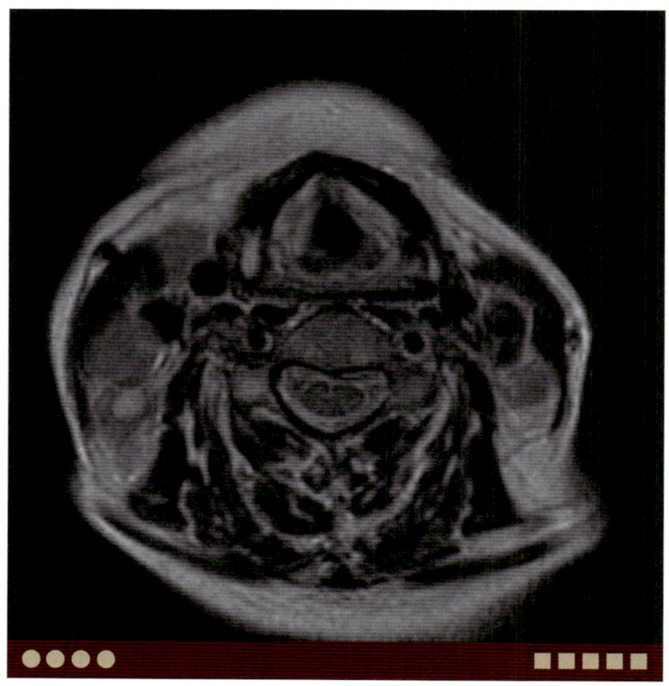

E. Papillary thyroid carcinoma in a different patient. Axial T2W image demonstrates bilateral cervical lymphadenopathy. Note the cystic change of the right node.

DIFFERENTIAL DIAGNOSIS IMAGES (F-H)

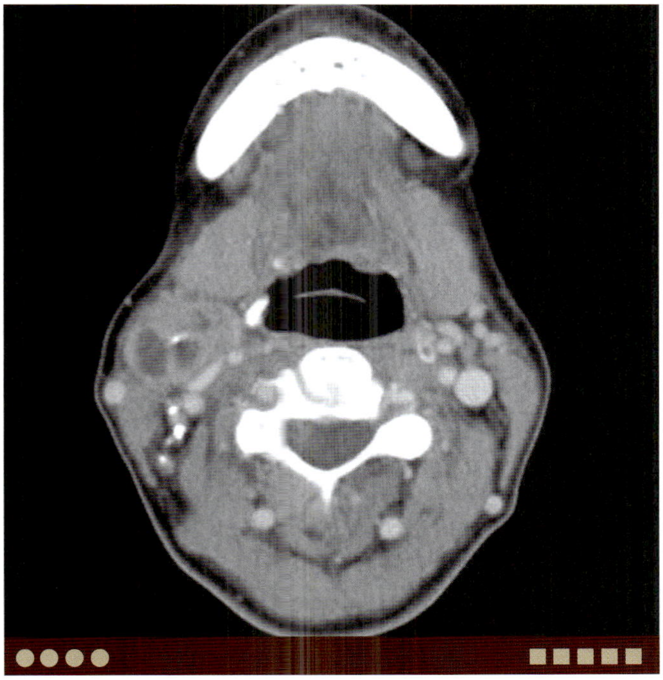

F. Tuberculosis. Axial contrast-enhanced CT demonstrates multiple enlarged lymph nodes with cystic change and calcification.

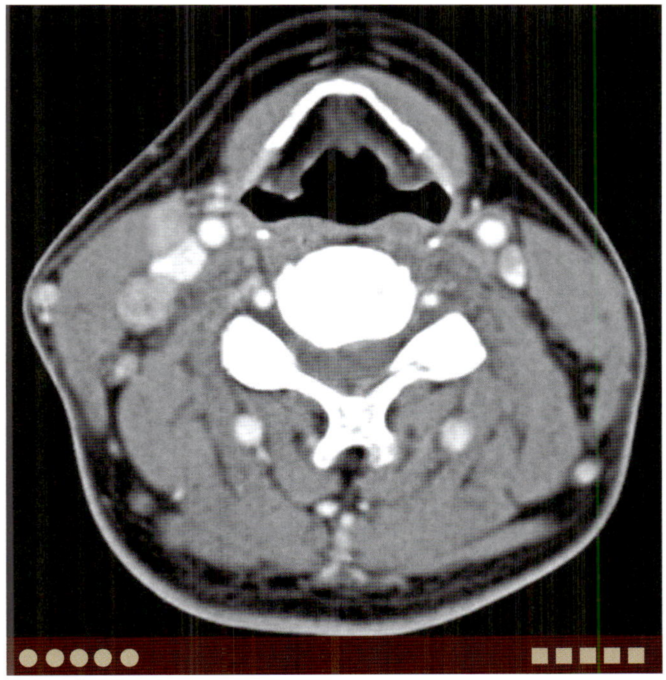

G. Squamous cell carcinoma. Axial contrast-enhanced CT demonstrates multiple heterogeneously enhancing enlarged lymph nodes with central necrosis.

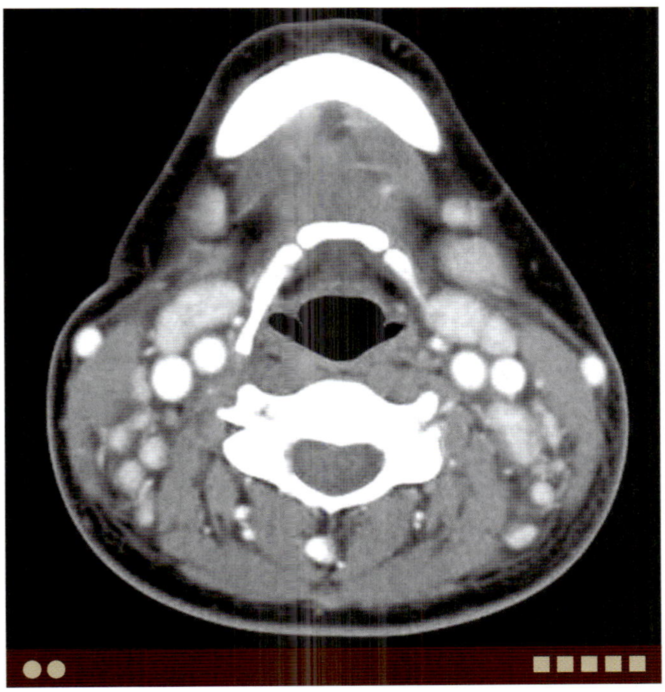

H. Kikuchi-Fujimoto disease. Axial contrast-enhanced CT demonstrates multiple swollen lymph nodes with avid enhancement. Note fat stranding around the involved nodes.

Case 11–7 Follicular Adenoma: Thyroid

Hiroki Kato, Asim Mian, Osamu Sakai

PRESENTATION

Slowly enlarging thyroid mass without pain.

FINDINGS

CT and MRI demonstrate a well-demarcated, encapsulated thyroid tumor.

DIFFERENTIAL DIAGNOSIS

- Papillary carcinoma: Imaging findings of papillary carcinoma are variable and include a dominant nodule, multifocal nodules, and diffuse infiltrative change of the gland. Papillary thyroid carcinoma may be encapsulated with well-demarcated margins mimicking benign lesions.
- Follicular carcinoma: Although follicular carcinomas are well differentiated, relative low-grade malignancy, they are either encapsulated or invasive. The appearance of minimally invasive follicular carcinoma may have some features in common with those of follicular adenoma.
- Medullary carcinoma: Medullary carcinomas have a higher mortality rate than well-differentiated papillary and follicular malignancies. They may also be either encapsulated or infiltrative.

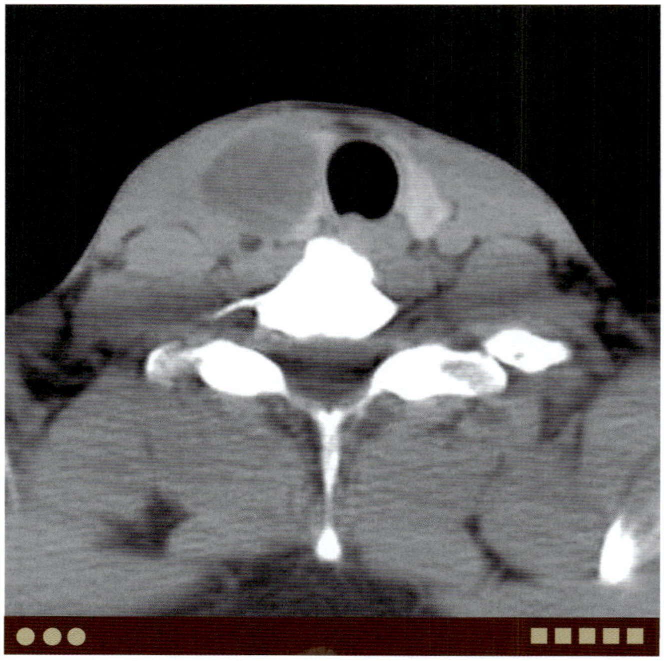

A. Follicular adenoma. Axial unenhanced CT demonstrates a homogeneously well-demarcated, hypodense lesion in the right thyroid gland.

COMMENTS

This is a 39-year-old man with slowly enlarging thyroid mass without pain.

The follicular adenoma is a common benign tumor of the thyroid gland. They present as a solitary nodule, usually as a painless, slow-growing mass. Most occur in middle-aged women that are euthyroid, as a painless thyroid nodule. It may be found during a routine physical examination. Grossly, adenomas are round to oval, with a fibrous capsule that is usually regular and thin. They typically range in size between 1 and 3 cm, not exceeding 4 cm. Histopathologically, follicular adenomas may have cystic degeneration, hemorrhage, ossification, calcification, fibrosis, and even necrosis can be seen. Sudden enlargement of a follicular adenoma is usually related to spontaneous hemorrhage within tumor.

The differential diagnosis of a follicular adenoma includes a dominant hyperplastic nodule, minimally invasive follicular carcinoma, and encapsulated variant of papillary thyroid carcinoma. The differential diagnosis between a follicular adenoma and a follicular carcinoma may be confusing. Cytology cannot distinguish between an adenoma and a carcinoma and excisional biopsy is needed. The pathologist must carefully observe the entire capsule in order to exclude capsular invasion, which is the hallmark of malignancy. Although it is difficult to distinguish follicular adenoma from follicular carcinoma, follicular adenomas are approximately five times more frequently encountered than follicular carcinomas.

Imaging findings are often nonspecific. Smooth margin is often seen in follicular adenomas on ultrasound, CT, and MRI reflecting the fibrous capsule. Calcifications and cystic degeneration may be present in the tumor.

PEARLS

- **Follicular adenoma demonstrates a well-demarcated, encapsulated mass.**
- **Follicular adenoma may include calcifications and cystic degeneration.**
- **It is difficult to distinguish follicular adenoma from follicular carcinoma by imaging alone. Further, cytology cannot distinguish between an adenoma and a carcinoma.**

DIFFERENTIAL DIAGNOSIS IMAGES (B-H)

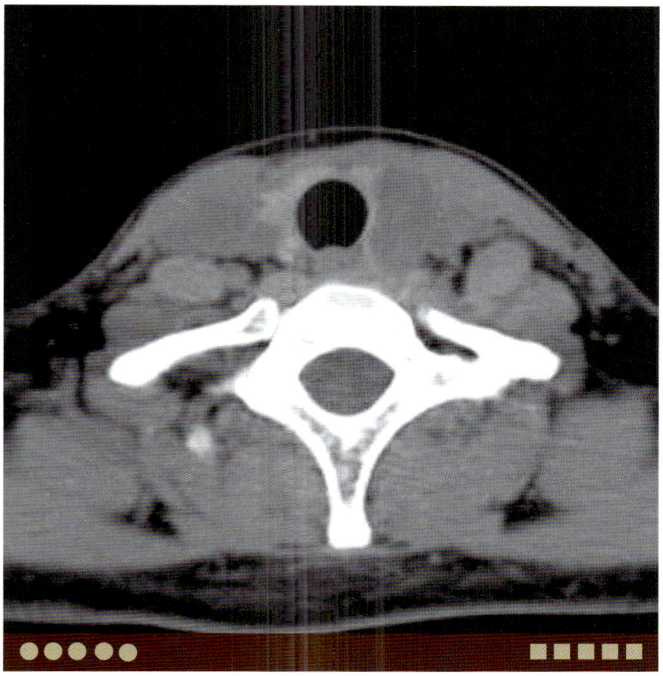

B. Thyroid papillary carcinoma. Axial unenhanced CT demonstrates homogeneously well-demarcated, hypodense tumor in the left thyroid gland.

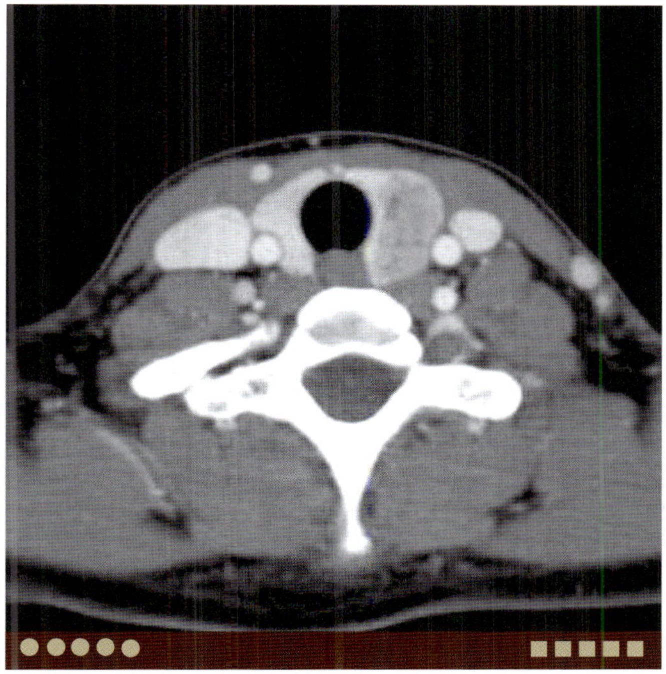

C. Thyroid papillary carcinoma, same patient as B. Axial enhanced CT demonstrates heterogeneous enhancement in the tumor.

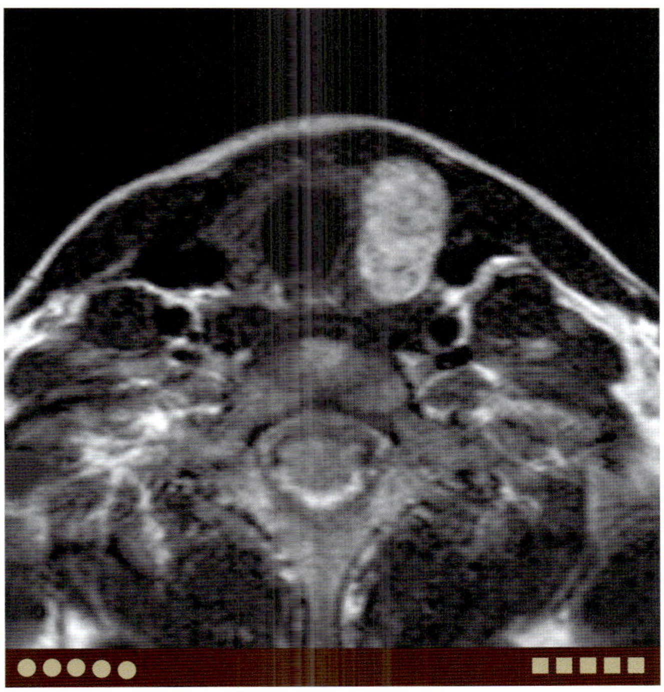

D. Thyroid papillary carcinoma, same patient as B. Axial T2W image demonstrates a heterogeneously well-demarcated, hyperintense tumor.

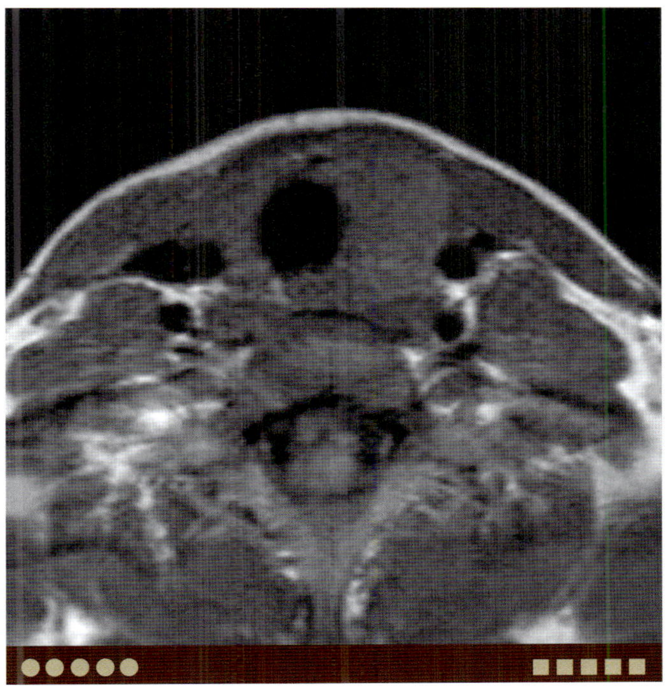

E. Thyroid papillary carcinoma, same patient as B. Axial T1W image demonstrates low-signal intensity in the tumor.

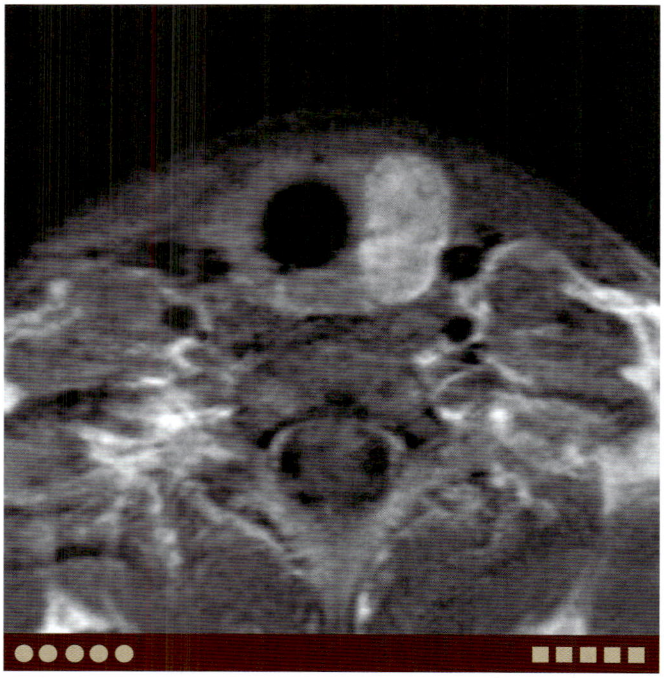

F. Thyroid papillary carcinoma, same patient as B. Axial postcontrast fat-suppressed T1W image demonstrates heterogeneous enhancement in the tumor.

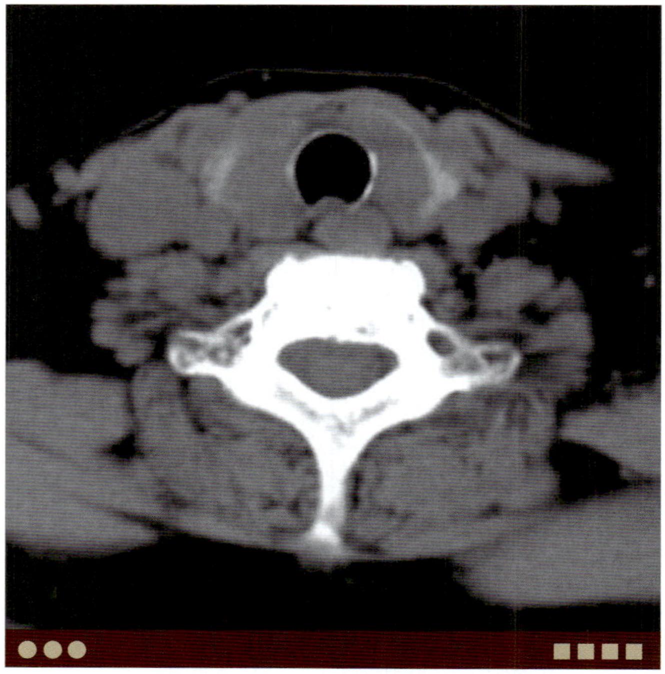

G. MALT lymphoma. Axial unenhanced CT demonstrates well-demarcated, homogeneously hypodense lesions in the bilateral thyroid gland.

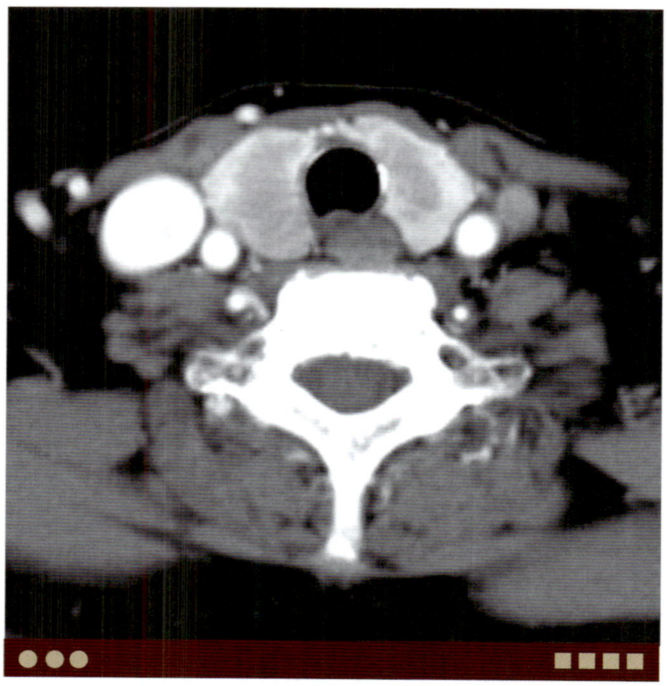

H. MALT lymphoma, same patient as G. Axial enhanced CT demonstrates homogeneous enhancement in the tumors.

Case 11–8 Primary Hyperparathyroidism

Akifumi Fujita, Margaret Chapman, Osamu Sakai

PRESENTATION

Bone pain.

FINDINGS

CT demonstrates a craniocaudally elongated, "teardrop"-shaped lesion posterior to the inferior or superior pole of the thyroid gland, showing lower density than the thyroid gland on noncontrast CT.

DIFFERENTIAL DIAGNOSIS

- Thyroid tumors: Exophytic mass lesions arising from the thyroid can mimic parathyroid lesions. It is often difficult to localize the lesion internal or external to the thyroid.
- Lymph nodes: These may present with similar findings. Careful evaluation for possible primary lesions should always be performed.

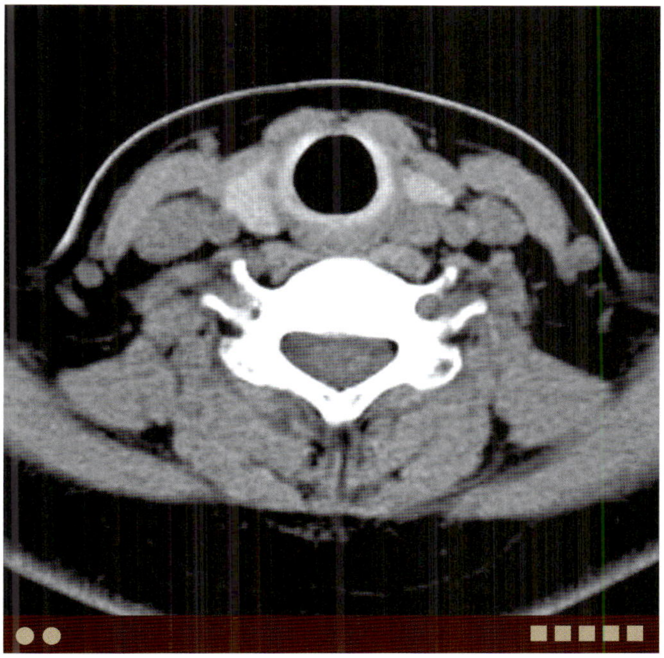

A. Parathyroid adenoma, primary hyperparathyroidism. Axial noncontrast CT demonstrates a round tumor posterior to the superior pole of the left thyroid gland.

COMMENTS

This is a 36-year-old woman with a history of multifocal bone pain.

Primary hyperparathyroidism may be asymptomatic, or may present with bone pain, renal calculi, or pancreatitis due to hypercalcemia. The role of head and neck imaging is to identify potential parathyroid adenomas for surgical resection. Locally, ultrasound is very useful; however, ectopic parathyroid glands may be difficult to detect by ultrasound alone. CT is also useful, particularly with thin slices and multiplanar reconstruction using MDCT. Parathyroid adenomas are usually seen as craniocaudally elongated, "teardrop"-shaped lesions, posterior to the thyroid glands. They show lower density than normal thyroid tissue on noncontrast CT, and enhance differently from the thyroid and lymph node, often with rapid enhancement and rapid washout. Therefore, dynamic contrast-enhanced study may be helpful. Multiplanar reconstruction is helpful to differentiate a parathyroid adenoma from an exophytic mass lesion in the thyroid gland. Artifacts from the bones and shoulders often degrade the images and may make evaluation difficult. MRI is also reported as useful in demonstrating enlarged parathyroid glands as T1 isointense and T2 hyperintense lesions. However, images are often degraded by artifacts from motion, swallowing, susceptibility, or poor signal from the use of inappropriate coils or sequences.

Nuclear medicine studies have an important role in diagnosing parathyroid lesions. Recently, ^{99m}Tc-MIBI with early and delayed imaging is most commonly used, while ^{201}Tl-^{99m}TcO^{4-} subtraction was used in the past. Nuclear medicine studies are sensitive and useful for detection of ectopic parathyroid glands, although small lesion may not be detected secondary to poor spatial resolution.

PEARLS

- **Primary hyperparathyroidism may be asymptomatic, or may present with bone pain, renal calculi, or pancreatitis.**
- **^{99m}Tc-MIBI with early and delayed imaging is most commonly used.**
- **Ultrasound is useful locally; however, detection of ectopic parathyroid glands may be difficult.**
- **CT and MRI are also useful. These scans should cover from the hyoid to the mediastinum.**
- **Parathyroid adenoma demonstrates low density on noncontrast CT and moderate enhancement after contrast administration.**

ADDITIONAL IMAGES (B-H)

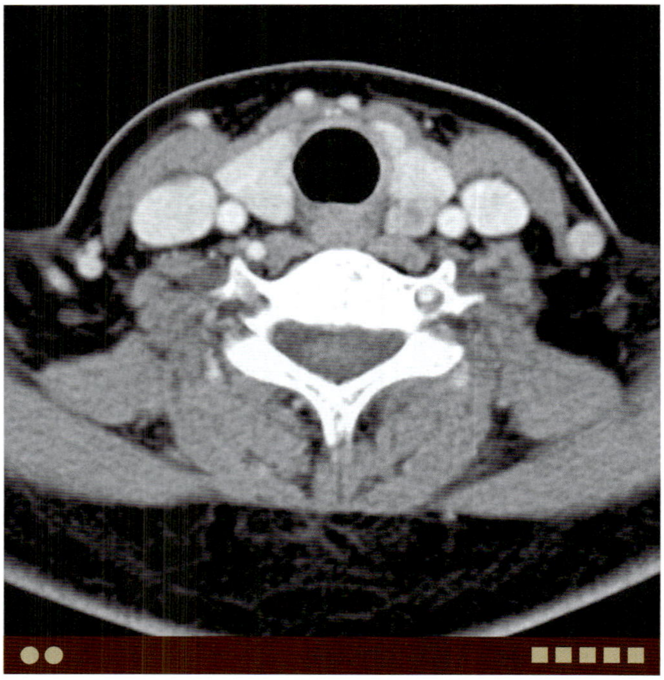

B. Parathyroid adenoma, primary hyperparathyroidism, same patient as A. Axial contrast-enhanced CT shows moderate enhancement of the adenoma.

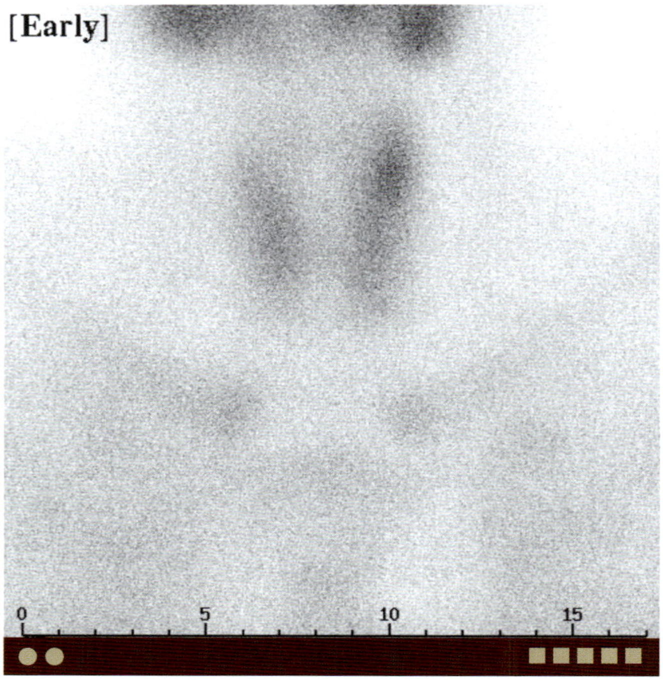

C. Parathyroid adenoma, primary hyperparathyroidism, same patient as A. Early image of ^{99m}Tc-MIBI study demonstrates nodular uptake within the posterior region of the superior pole of the left thyroid gland.

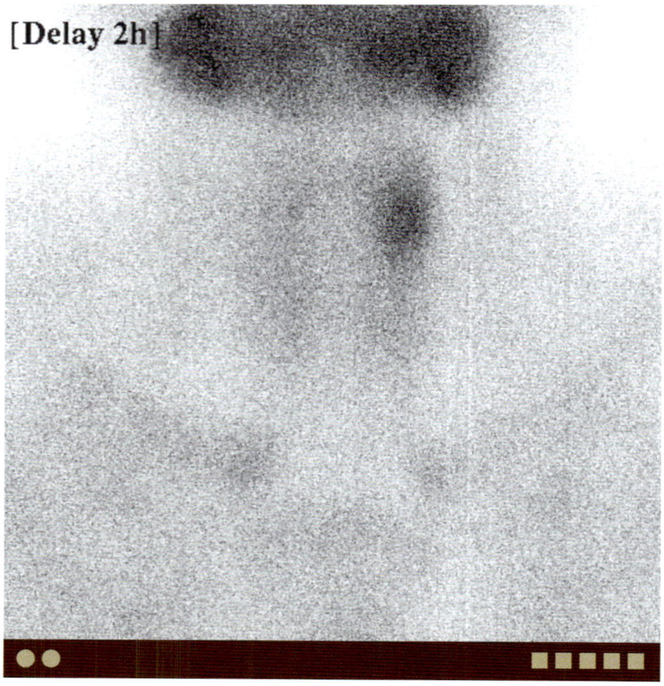

D. Parathyroid adenoma, primary hyperparathyroidism, same patient as A. Delayed image of ^{99m}Tc-MIBI study demonstrates prolonged uptake of the parathyroid adenoma.

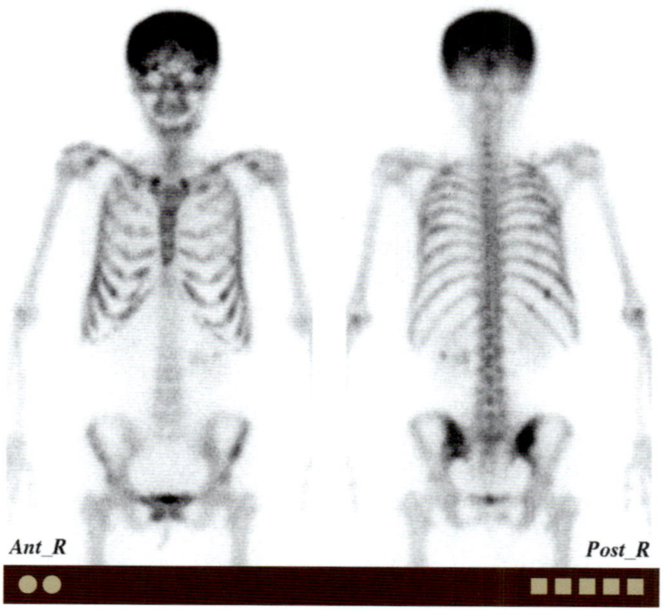

E. Parathyroid adenoma, primary hyperparathyroidism, same patient as A. ^{99m}Tc-HMDP bone scintigraphy shows diffuse uptake of the cranial vault. Note the multiple foci of nodular uptake within the ribs suggestive of pathologic fractures.

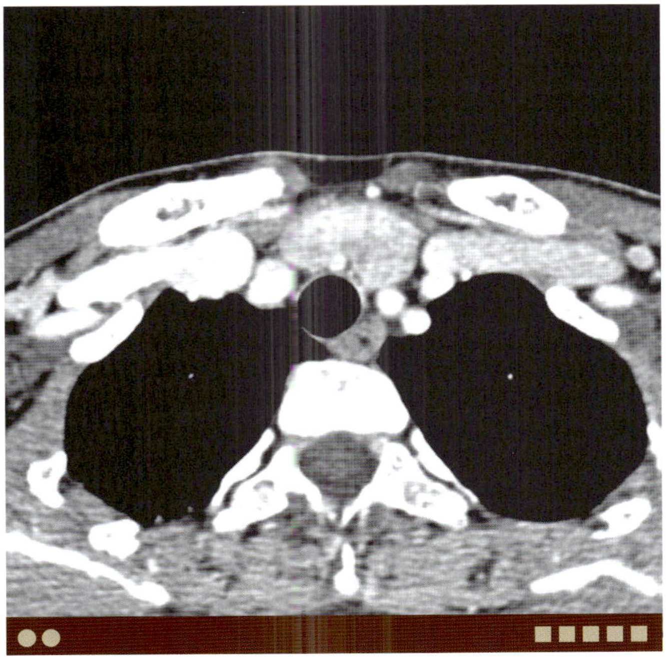

F. Parathyroid adenoma, primary hyperparathyroidism in a different patient. Axial contrast-enhanced CT demonstrates moderately enhanced lesion in the upper mediastinum. This was difficult to differentiate from a thyroid tumor because of its similar density on enhanced CT.

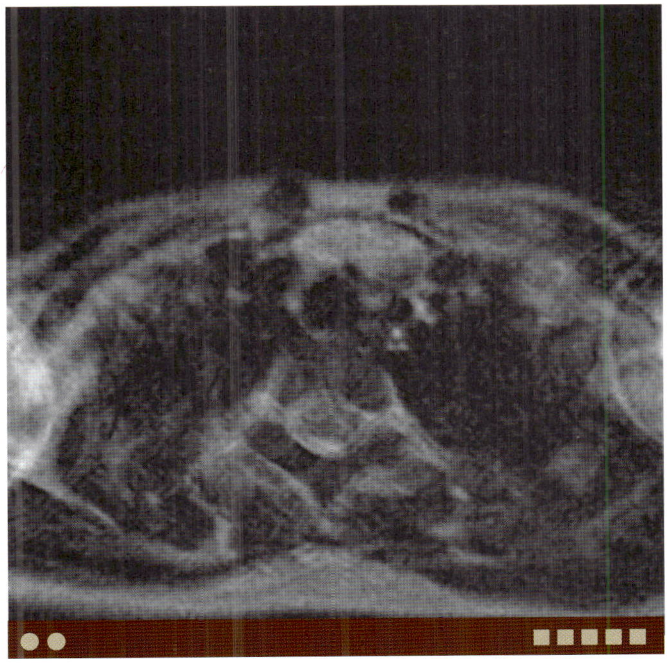

G. Parathyroid adenoma, primary hyperparathyroidism, same patient as F. Axial T2W image demonstrates hyperintense mass in the upper mediastinum.

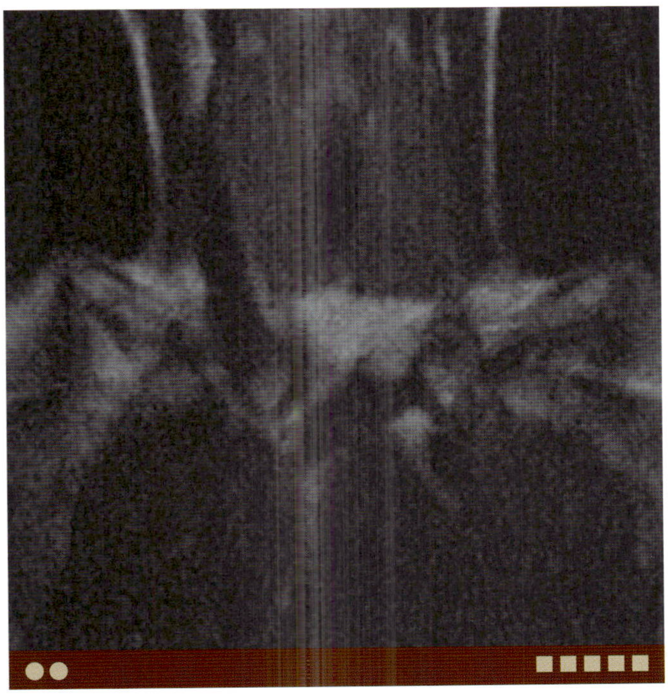

H. Parathyroid adenoma, primary hyperparathyroidism, same patient as F. Coronal T2W image demonstrates a hyperintense mass caudal to thyroid gland. MRI shows better contrast between parathyroid adenoma and thyroid gland, but motion artifact is also obvious.

DIFFERENTIAL DIAGNOSIS IMAGES (I-J)

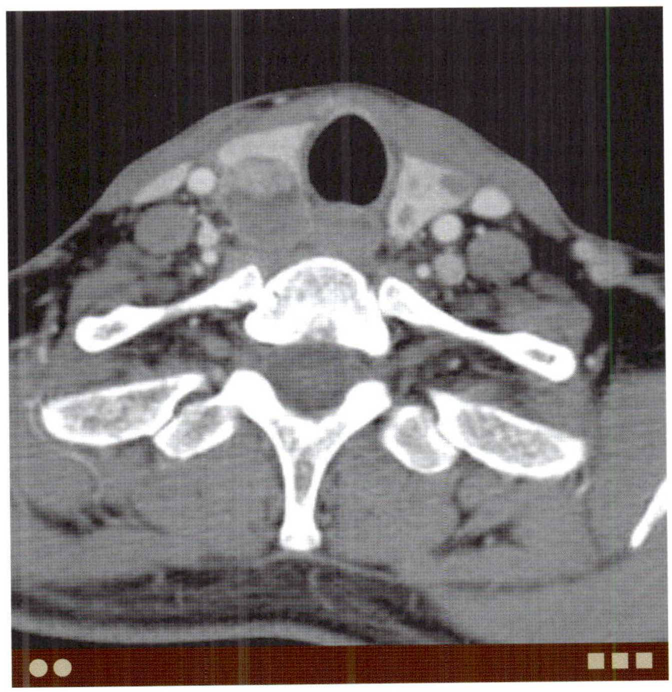

I. Parathyroid carcinoma. Axial postcontrast CT demonstrates a partially cystic lesion with a mural nodule, located in the right lower neck, posterior to the right lobe of the thyroid gland. (*Courtesy of Dr. Hiroki Kato*)

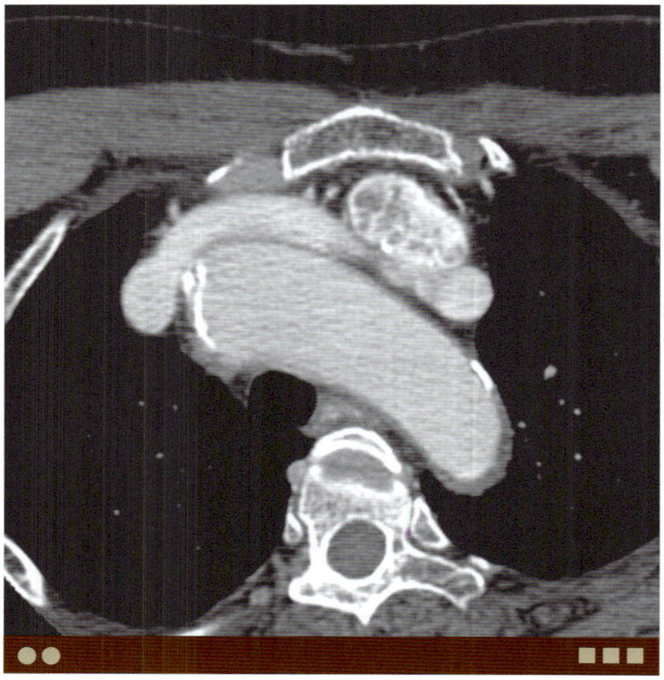

J. Goiter. Axial postcontrast CT demonstrates a heterogeneously enhancing mass posterior to the sternum.

Case 11–9 Goiter

Osamu Sakai, Akifumi Fujita, Asim Mian

PRESENTATION

Neck mass.

FINDINGS

CT and MR images demonstrate enlarged thyroid glands.

DIFFERENTIAL DIAGNOSIS

- Thyroid papillary carcinoma: This tends to be more heterogeneous and focal; however, histological diagnosis by imaging alone is difficult. Extracapsular extension, invasion to adjacent structures, and metastasis suggest malignancy.
- Anaplastic carcinoma of the thyroid: This is a rapidly growing aggressive tumor and invades the adjacent structures.
- Lymphoma: This shows enlargement of the thyroid gland with homogeneous density or signal and is often associated with Hashimoto disease.

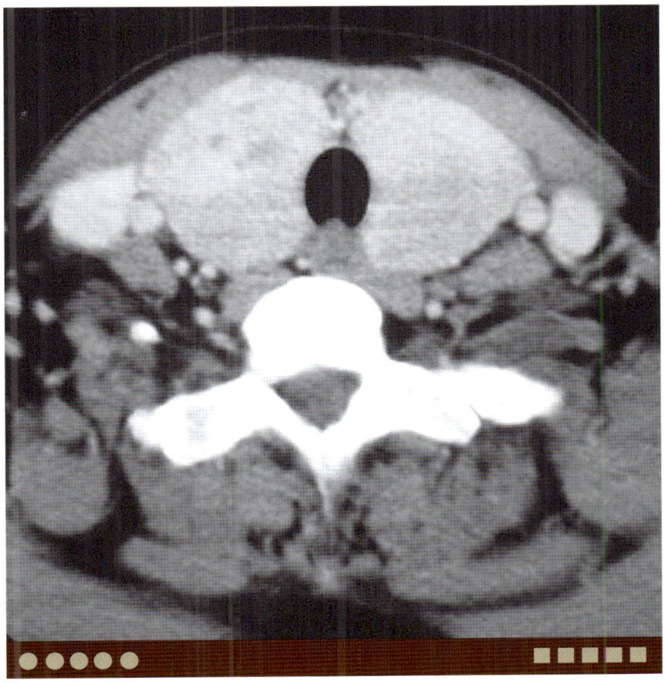

A. Goiter. Axial contrast-enhanced CT demonstrates heterogeneously enhancing enlarged thyroid glands.

COMMENTS

This is a 38-year-old woman with history of slowly growing neck mass.

Goiter is a generalized term and refers to the abnormal enlargement of the thyroid gland. Thyroid function can be normal (euthyroidism) or abnormal (hypothyroidism or hyperthyroidism). The etiology is variable, but in the United States most goiters are due to autoimmune thyroiditis such as Hashimoto disease. There is no racial predilection and the female-to-male ratio is 4:1. Enlargement of the thyroid gland can be diffuse or nodular and the thyroid may extend inferiorly into the mediastinum or the retrosternal space. Mass effect to the larynx, trachea, esophagus, laryngeal nerves, and vessels is common. Most goiters are benign. Invasion to those structures suggests malignancy.

Ultrasound is the first-line modality for diagnosis and fine-needle aspiration (FNA) can be performed under ultrasound guidance. Currently, FNA is recommended for a mass over 1 cm in diameter.

The role of CT and MRI is to evaluate for invasion to the adjacent structures and nodal metastasis, not localization of the lesion in the thyroid gland. Extracapsular extension, invasion to the trachea, paraspinal muscles, carotid artery, and jugular vein should be carefully evaluated. However, without apparent tumor protrusion into the lumen, it may be difficult to diagnose tumor invasion to the airway or vessels.

PEARLS

- **Goiter is a generalized term and refers to the abnormal enlargement of the thyroid gland, more commonly seen in women than men.**
- **Enlargement of the thyroid gland can be diffuse or nodular and the thyroid may extend inferiorly into the mediastinum or the retrosternal space.**
- **Mass effect to the adjacent structures is common. However, invasion to those structures suggests malignancy.**

ADDITIONAL IMAGES (B-H)

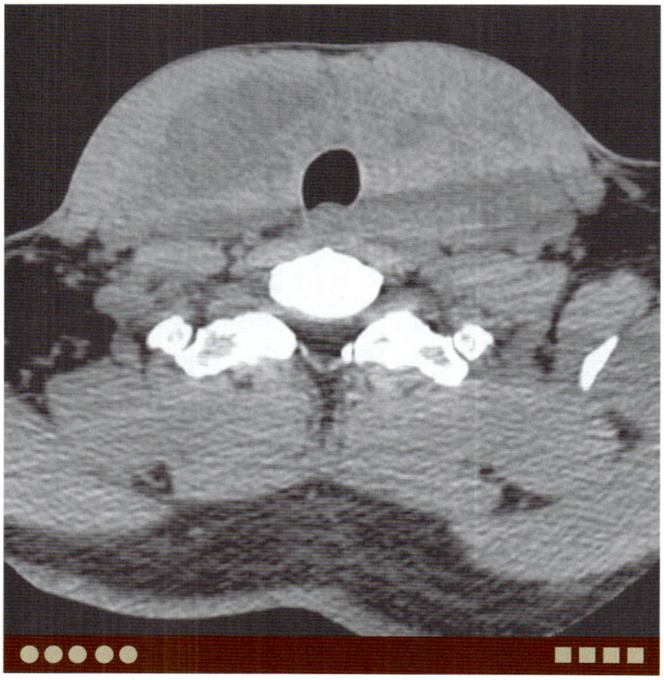

B. Goiter in a different patient. Axial noncontrast CT demonstrates enlarged bilateral thyroid glands with heterogeneous internal densities.

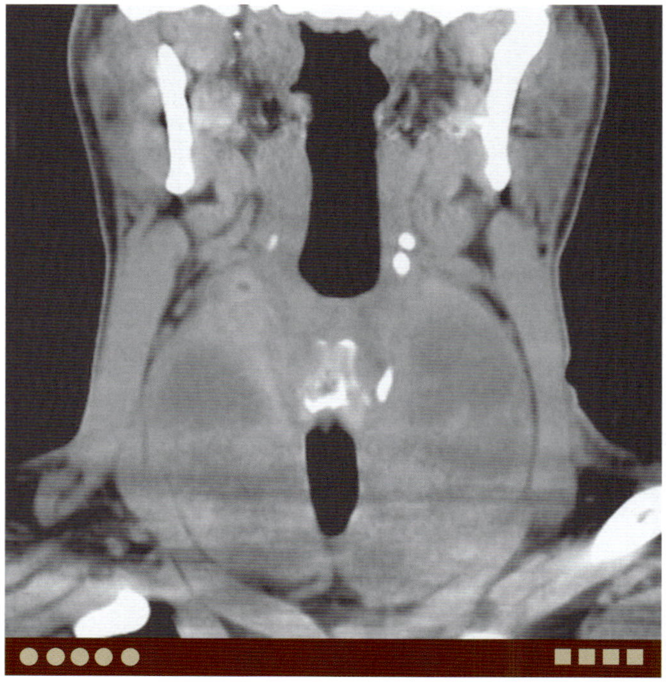

C. Goiter, same patient as B. Coronal noncontrast CT demonstrates enlarged bilateral thyroid glands extending craniocaudally. Significant mass effect to the adjacent structures is present; however, there is no evidence of invasion.

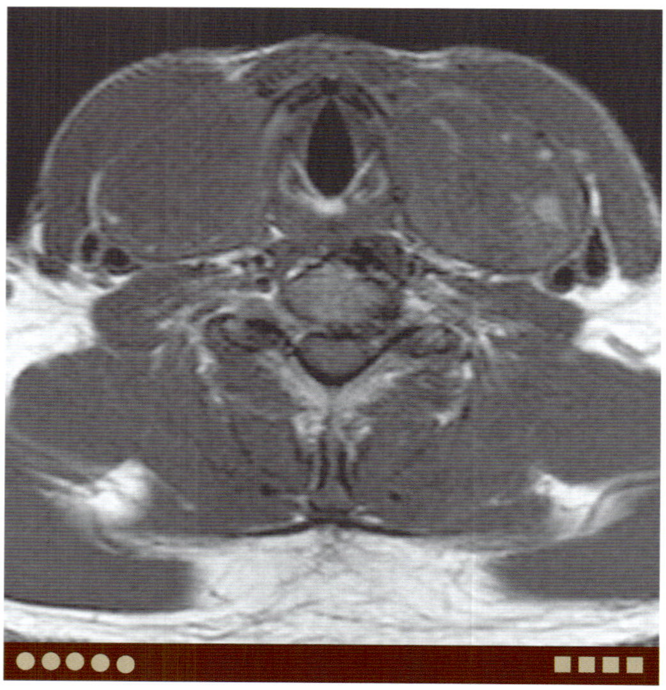

D. Goiter in a different patient. Axial T1W MR image demonstrates enlarged bilateral thyroid glands with heterogeneous internal signal displacing the carotid vessels.

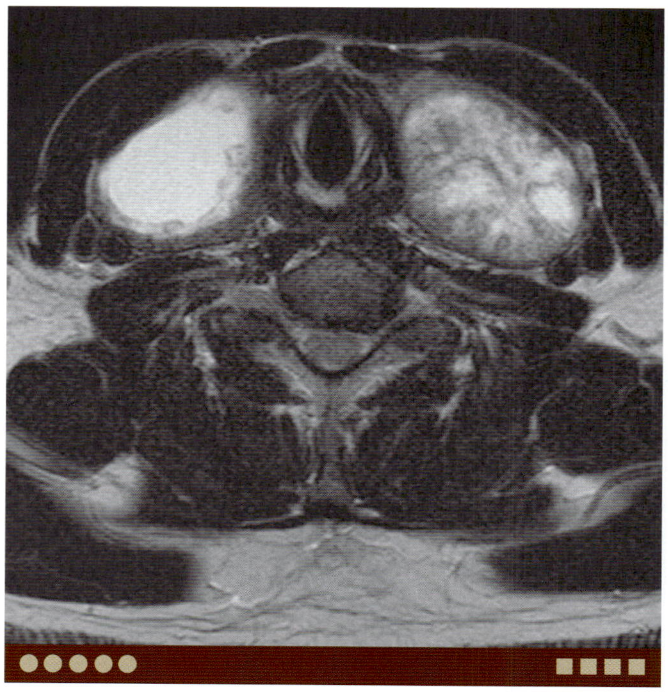

E. Goiter, same patient as D. Axial T2W MR image demonstrates more cystic degeneration in the right lobe of the thyroid gland. No invasive change is seen despite significant mass effect to the adjacent structures.

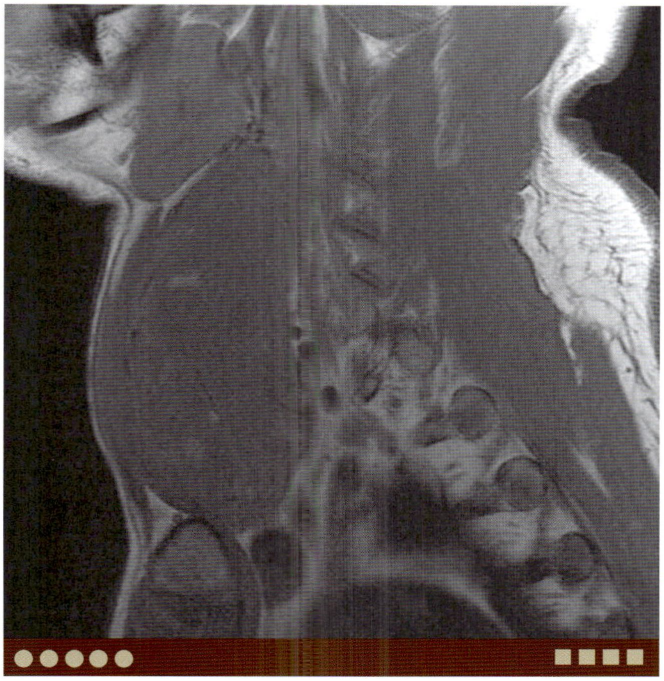

F. Goiter, same patient as D. Sagittal T1W MR image demonstrates craniocaudal extension of the goiter, from the submandibular region to the manubrium.

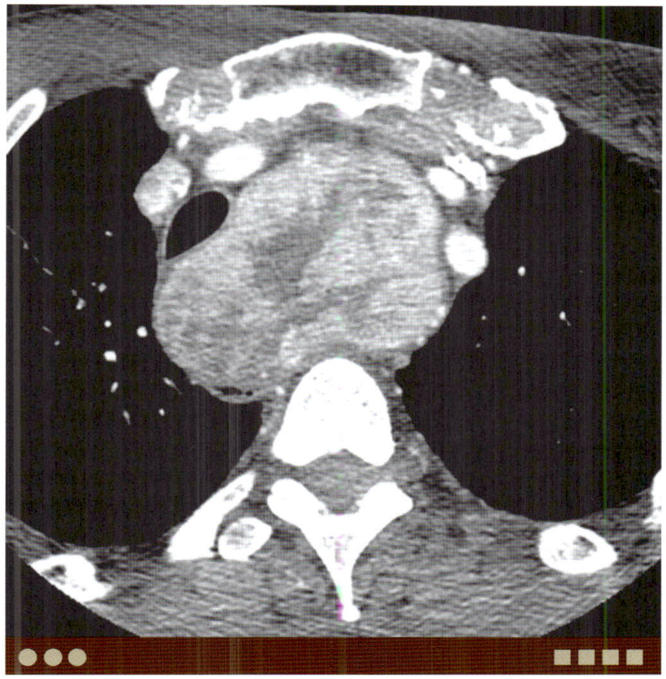

G. Goiter in a different patient. Axial contrast-enhanced CT demonstrates heterogeneously enhancing enlarged left thyroid with substernal extension, displacing the trachea and esophagus.

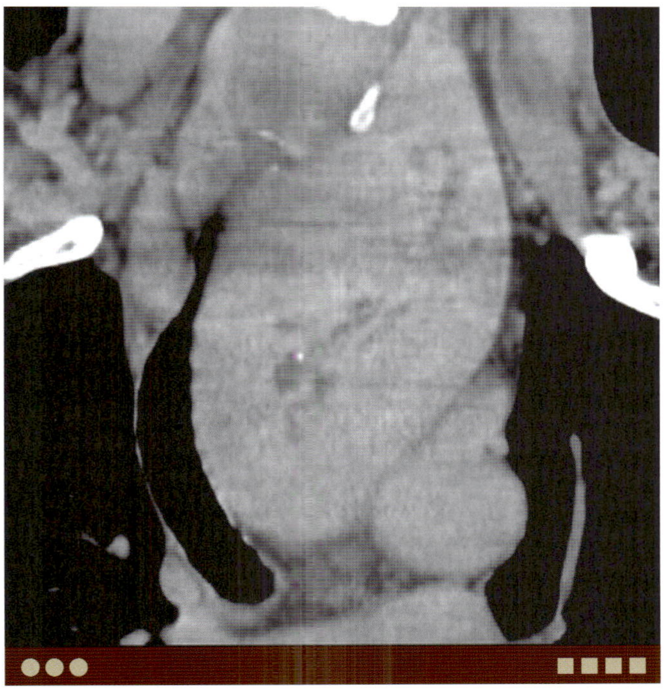

H. Goiter, same patient as G. Coronal contrast-enhanced CT demonstrates markedly enlarged left thyroid extending between the aorta and trachea. Note no invasive finding despite significant mass effect.

DIFFERENTIAL DIAGNOSIS IMAGES (I-J)

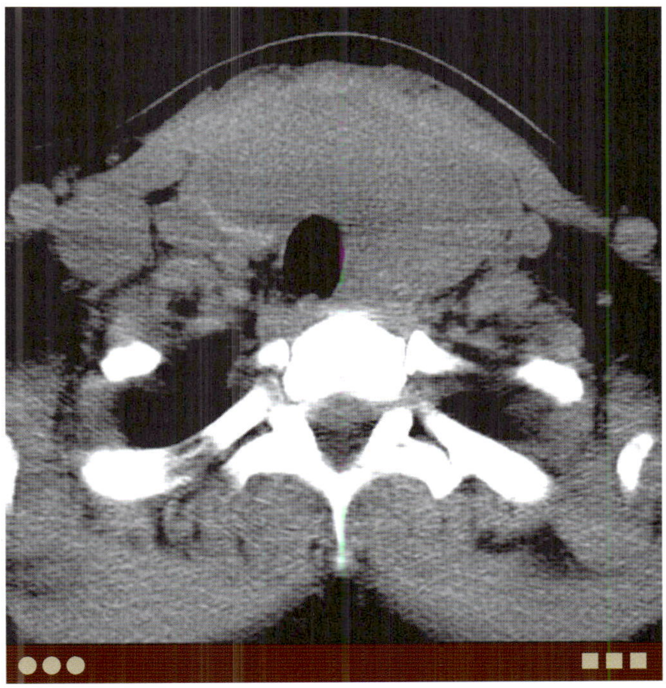

I. Poorly differentiated follicular thyroid carcinoma. Axial noncontrast CT demonstrates enlarged left thyroid causing mass effect to the adjacent structures.

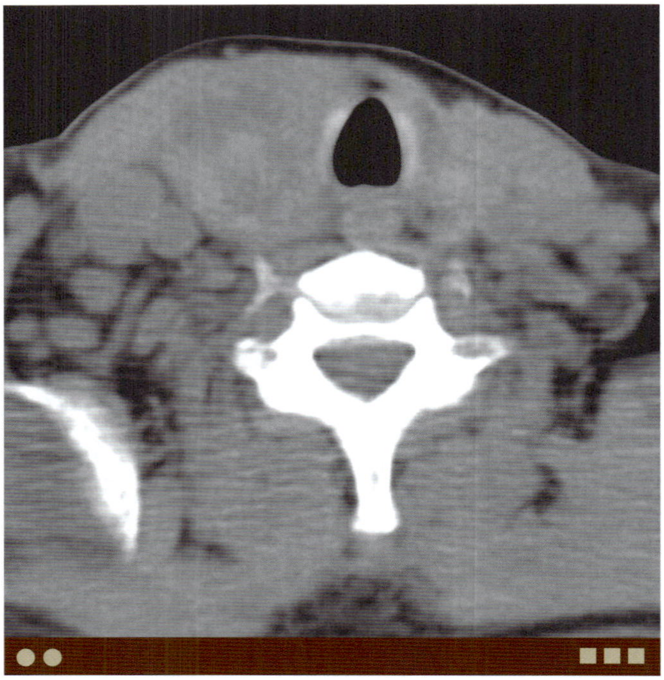

J. Lymphoma. Axial noncontrast CT demonstrates enlarged thyroid glands, right more than left. Margins are not well defined and slight increase in density of the surrounding fat is seen suggesting edema.

Case 11–10 Medullary Thyroid Carcinoma

Akifumi Fujita, Asim Mian, Osamu Sakai

PRESENTATION

Thyroid nodules.

FINDINGS

CT demonstrates a nodular lesion with punctate calcification in the thyroid. MRI shows a nonspecific nodular lesion with T2W high signal and enhancement.

DIFFERENTIAL DIAGNOSIS

- Papillary thyroid carcinoma: This is the most common thyroid cancer and mimics medullary thyroid carcinoma. It is difficult to differentiate by cross-sectional imaging.
- Multinodular goiter: This condition shows diffuse enlargement with multiple nodules. Heterogeneous density/intensity may be seen due to cystic degeneration, calcification, and fibrosis.
- Follicular adenoma: This condition is usually not invasive.
- Hashimoto thyroiditis: This condition usually demonstrates diffuse symmetrical enlargement of the thyroid glands with low density on CT.

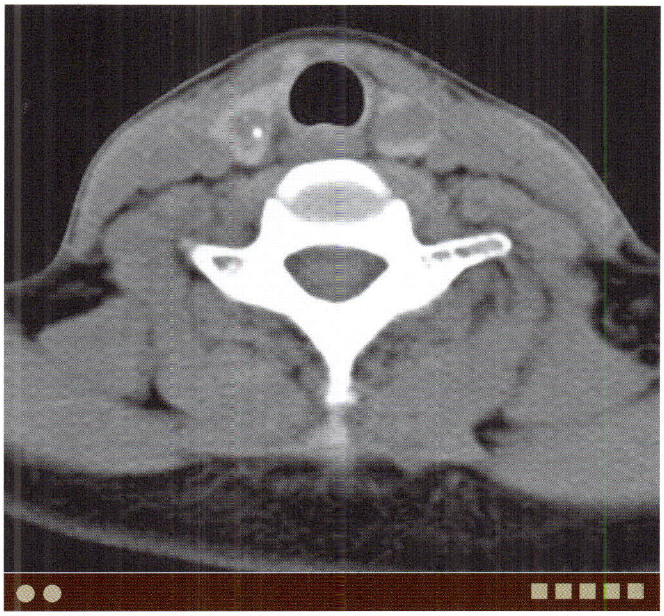

A. Medullary thyroid carcinoma. Axial noncontrast CT demonstrates bilateral low density, well-circumscribed nodules in the thyroid. Note the punctate calcification of the nodule in the right lobe.

COMMENTS

This is a 49-year-old woman with painless thyroid nodules. After diagnosis of medullary carcinoma (MTC) with fine-needle aspiration (FNA), total thyroidectomy with bilateral neck dissection was performed. She did not have multiple endocrine neoplasia (MEN) syndrome.

MTC is a rare tumor arising from calcitonin-producing C cells of the thyroid. The incidence of MTC is 2% to 8% of all thyroid cancers. MTC usually occurs sporadically, but may occur in familial form associated with MEN and familial form without MEN. MEN syndromes are inherited as autosomal dominant. MTC is associated with pheochromocytoma and parathyroid hyperplasia/adenoma as type IIA and with pheochromocytoma and mucosal neuromas as type IIB. MTC associated with MEN is more often multifocal and bilateral than sporadic MTC.

Ultrasound (US) is usually the first modality used in the diagnostic workup for a thyroid nodule. It is a handy noninvasive procedure and US-guided FNA can be performed if the lesion is more than 1 cm. CT and MRI are not always necessary for thyroid nodules, but may be preferred for assessment of large tumors, extraglandular extension, and metastatic lymph nodes.

MTC usually shows a solid low-density, well-circumscribed mass in the thyroid on CT. Fine punctate calcifications may be found in the primary tumor and in metastatic nodes. Irregular margins and extraglandular extension may be seen; however, MTC usually has well-defined margins. Unlike papillary and follicular subtypes of thyroid carcinomas, MTC does not concentrate radioiodine. But radionuclides specific for neuroendocrine tissue such as I-131 MIBG and FDG-PET may be helpful for detecting metastasis and recurrence.

PEARLS

- **MTC is usually sporadic, but may be associated with MEN syndromes.**
- **Ultrasound with FNA is the first diagnostic modality for MTC. CT and MRI are preferred to assess large tumors, extraglandular extension, and nodal metastasis.**
- **MTC is often well circumscribed on cross-sectional imaging, but irregular margins and lymph node metastasis may be seen.**

ADDITIONAL IMAGES (B-D)

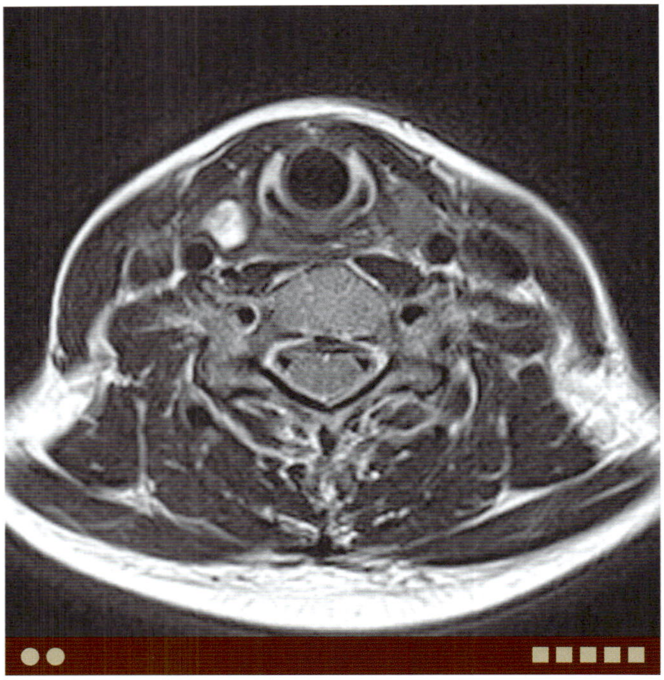

B. MTC, same patient as A. Axial T2W image demonstrates high-signal intensity of the nodule in the right lobe. There is no extraglandular extension.

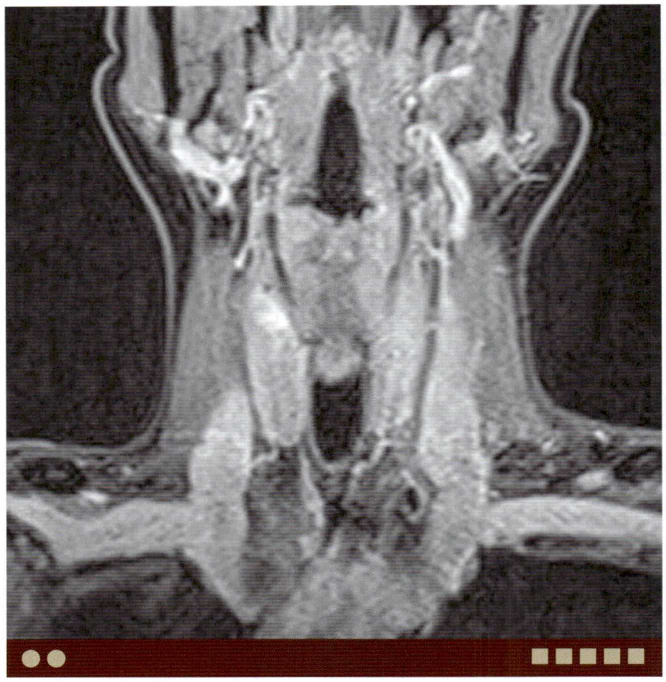

C. MTC, same patient as A. Coronal postcontrast T1W image demonstrates enhancement of the nodule in the right lobe.

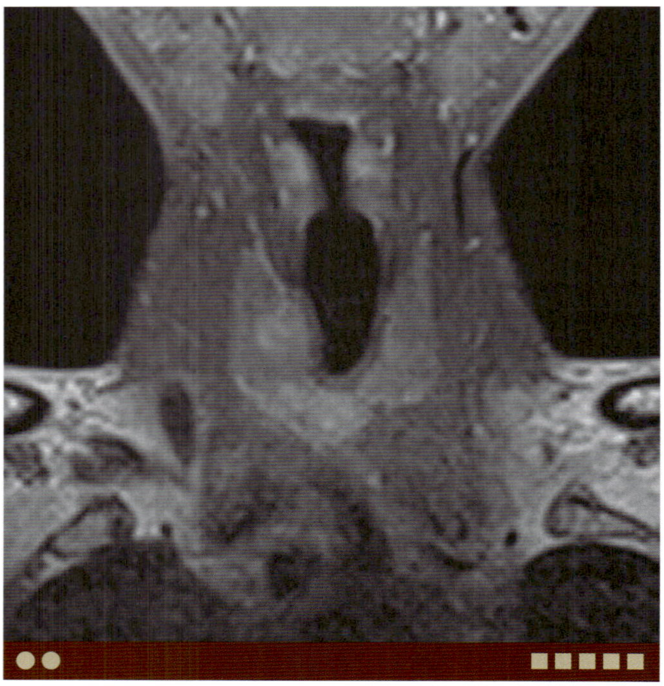

D. MTC in a different patient. Coronal postcontrast T1W image demonstrates multiple enhancing nodules in the right lobe and isthmus.

DIFFERENTIAL DIAGNOSIS IMAGES (E-I)

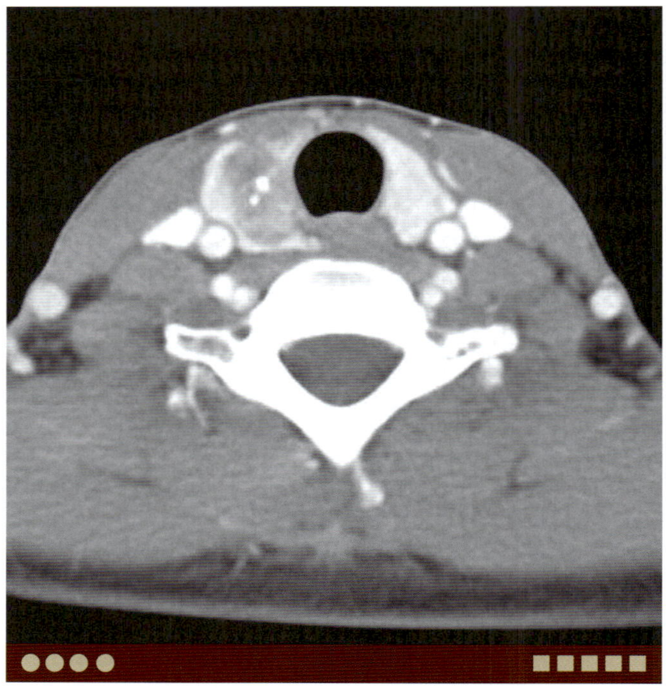

E. Papillary thyroid carcinoma. Axial postcontrast CT demonstrates solid nodule in the right lobe of the thyroid with calcification.

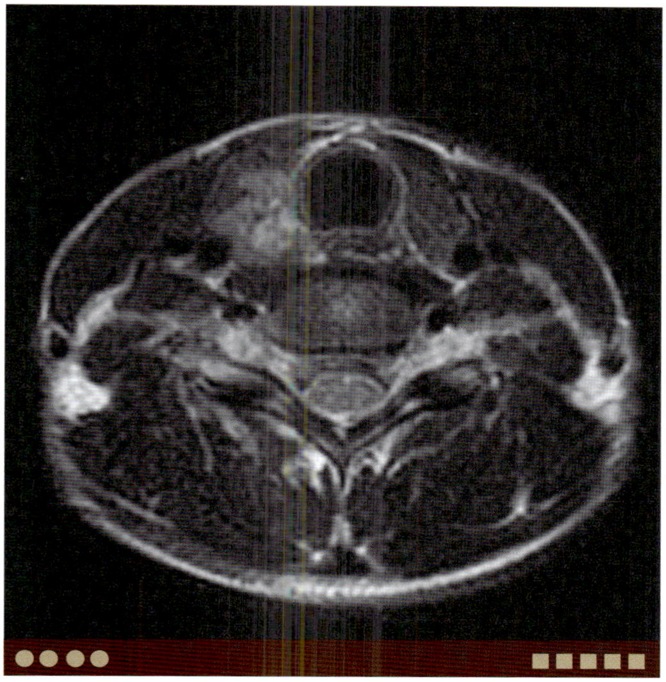

F. Papillary thyroid carcinoma, same patient as E. Axial T2W image demonstrates a high-signal nodule in the right lobe of the thyroid.

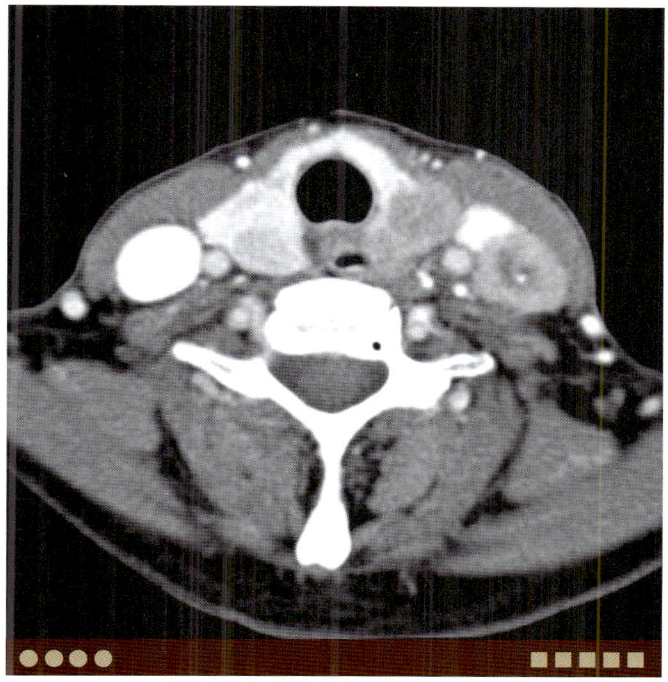

G. Papillary thyroid carcinoma in a different patient. Axial postcontrast CT demonstrates solid enhancing nodules in the thyroid bilaterally. Note nodal metastases in the left jugular chain. Total thyroidectomy proved papillary carcinoma of the left lobe with metastatic nodes and follicular adenoma in the right lobe.

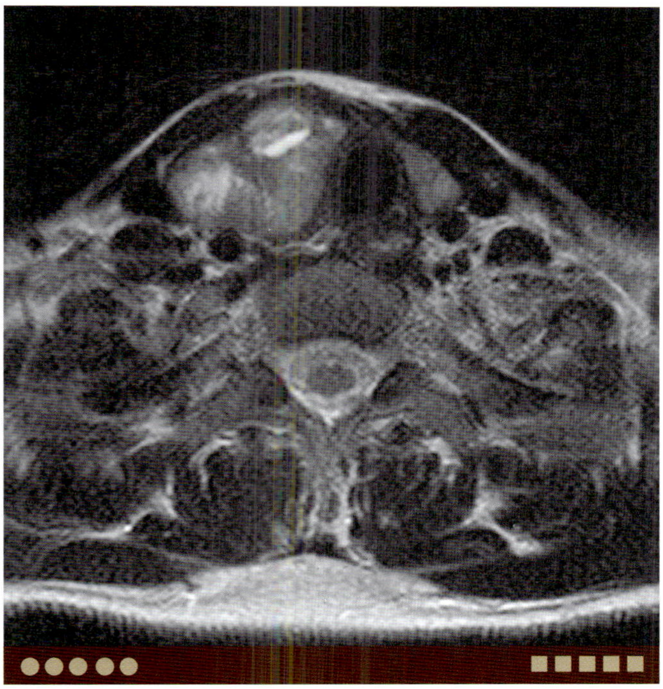

H. Multinodular goiter. Axial T2W image demonstrates a multinodular heterogeneous signal intensity mass of the right lobe. Cystic degeneration, fibrosis, and calcification were noted pathologically.

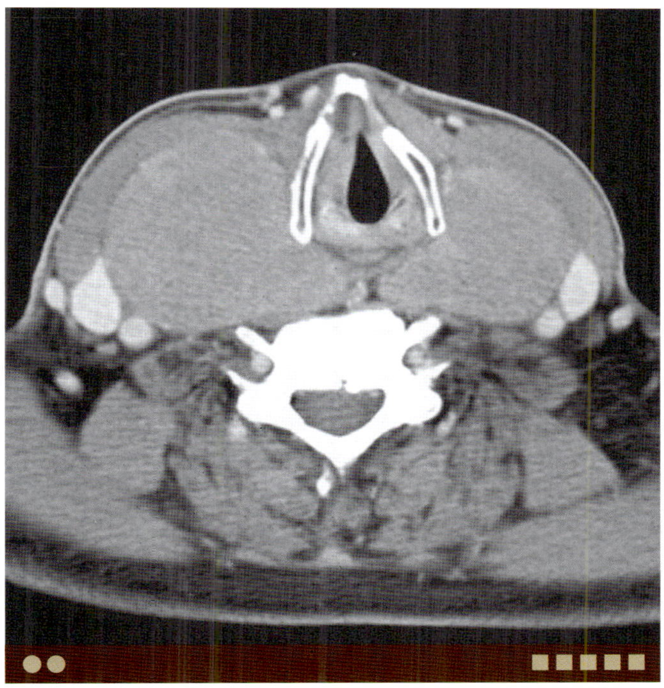

I. Hashimoto thyroiditis. Axial postcontrast CT demonstrates diffuse low-density enlargement of the bilateral thyroid. No necrosis or calcification is noted.

Case 11–11 Jugular Vein Thrombosis

Akifumi Fujita, Margaret Chapman, Osamu Sakai

PRESENTATION

Tenderness of the neck associated with fever.

FINDINGS

CT demonstrates nonopacified internal jugular vein.

DIFFERENTIAL DIAGNOSIS

- Normal asymmetric and heterogeneous enhancement of the internal jugular vein: Delayed and/or heterogeneous opacification is often seen in the jugular vein, particularly on the left without associated abnormality. This does not show surrounding inflammatory change.
- Necrotic metastatic lymph nodes and intranodal abscess: These conditions mimic jugular vein thrombosis. Lack of tubular appearance usually aids in diagnosis. However, these conditions can cause jugular vein thrombosis.

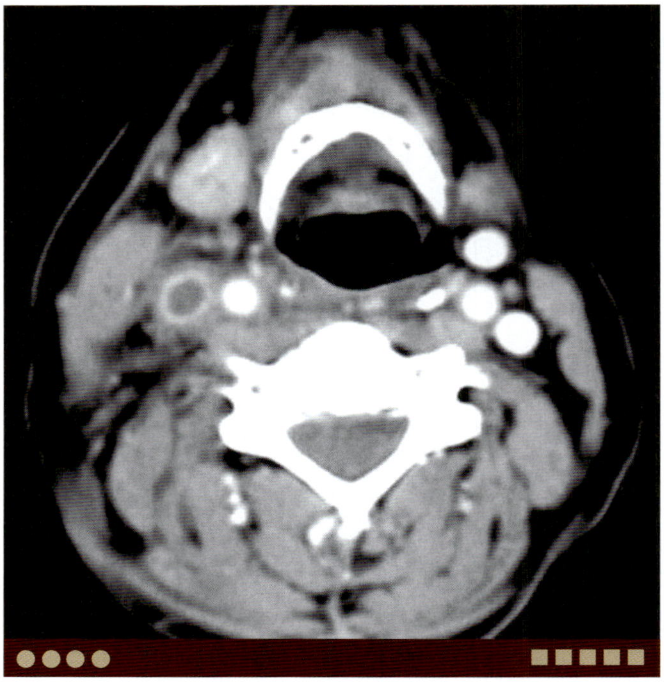

A. Jugular vein thrombosis. Axial postcontrast CT demonstrates filling defect and ringlike enhancement of the right internal jugular vein. Note increased density in the surrounding fatty tissue reflecting inflammation and mild retropharyngeal edema.

COMMENTS

This is a 40-year-old man with lung cancer status post central catheter placement through the right internal jugular vein.

Jugular vein thrombosis is often associated with central venous catheter placement, intravenous drug use, malignancy, and disorders of hypercoagulopathy. It is rare in healthy individuals. In the acute phase of venous thrombosis, inflammation and edema occur in the surrounding soft tissues and symptoms similar to infection, such as pain and masses, are often encountered. However, chronic thrombosis may present as a painless mass.

Lemierre syndrome is a condition characterized by thrombosis of the internal jugular vein that develops following an oropharyngeal infection, usually caused by *Fusobacterium necrophorum*. This condition may affect healthy young adults. Fusobacteria are normal oropharyngeal flora. Sepsis and septic metastases frequently affect the lungs, the musculoskeletal system, and occasionally the liver. Anticoagulation and surgical intervention can be helpful in advanced cases.

On contrast-enhanced CT, a filling defect and ringlike enhancement is seen in the internal jugular vein, often with increased caliber. In acute thrombosis or thrombophlebitis, irregular ringlike enhancement and increased density in the surrounding fatty tissue are seen reflecting inflammation; however, these findings may not be seen in chronic disease.

Asymmetric and heterogeneous enhancement of the internal jugular vein is often seen without abnormality, particularly on the left, most likely due to compression of the brachiocephalic vein by the aortic arch or bracheocephalic artery. This condition lacks ringlike enhancement, surrounding inflammatory change, and increase in caliber, and should be easily distinguished from real thrombosis.

PEARLS

- **Jugular vein thrombosis is often associated with central venous catheter placement, intravenous drug use, and malignancy.**
- **Filling defect, ringlike enhancement, and increased caliber accompanied with surrounding inflammation are typical findings of acute thrombosis or thrombophlebitis.**
- **Asymmetric and heterogeneous enhancement of the internal jugular vein is often seen without abnormality, particularly on the left, without ringlike enhancement, surrounding inflammatory change, or increased caliber.**

ADDITIONAL IMAGES (B-D)

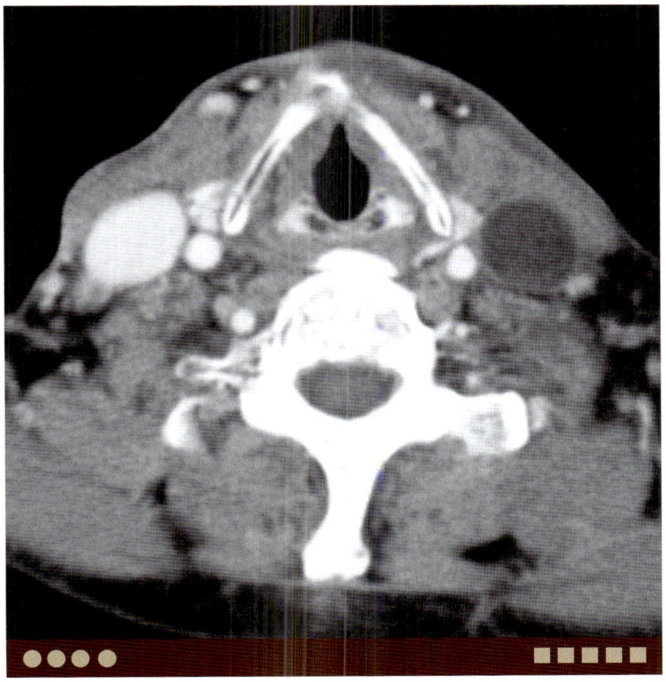

B. Jugular vein thrombosis in a different patient. Axial postcontrast CT demonstrates lack of contrast enhancement in the left jugular vein.

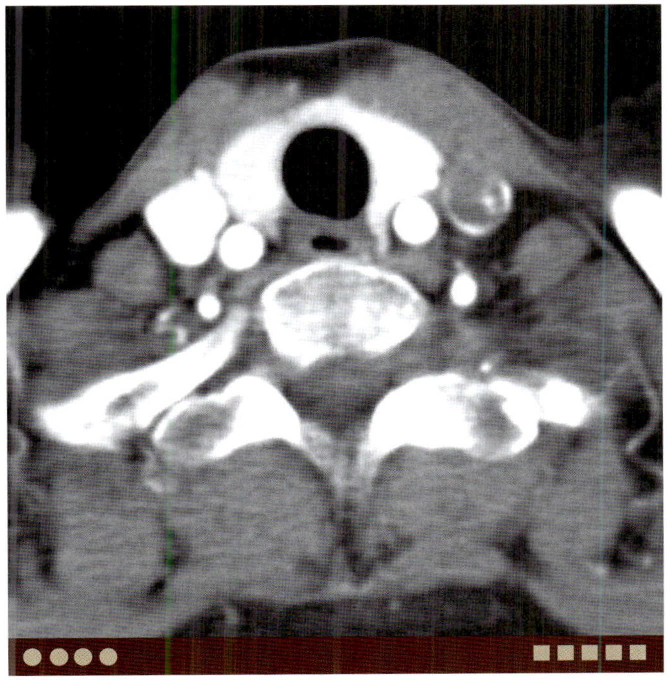

C. Jugular vein thrombosis in a different patient. Axial postcontrast CT demonstrates a low-density defect within the left internal jugular vein.

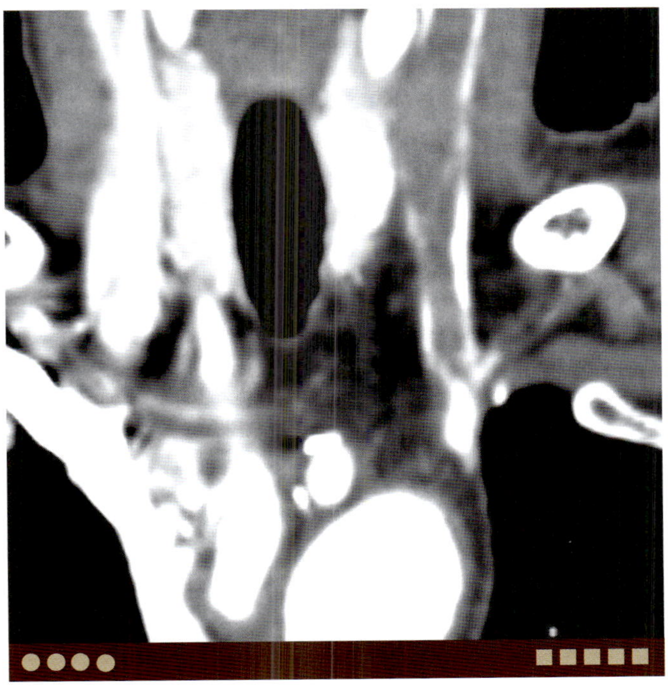

D. Jugular vein thrombosis, same patient as C. Coronal postcontrast CT demonstrates the inferior extent of the low-density defect noted within the left internal jugular vein.

DIFFERENTIAL DIAGNOSIS IMAGES (E-J)

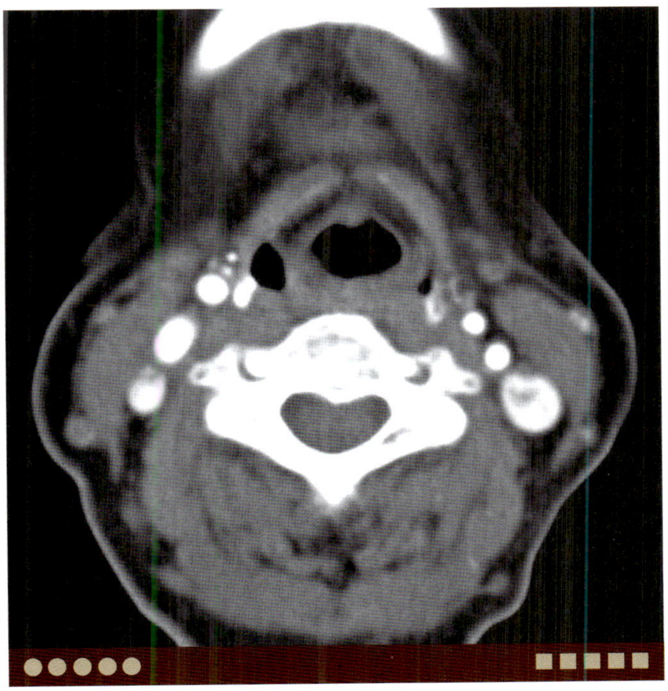

E. Normal asymmetric and heterogeneous enhancement of the internal jugular vein. Axial postcontrast CT demonstrates heterogeneous enhancement of the left internal jugular vein.

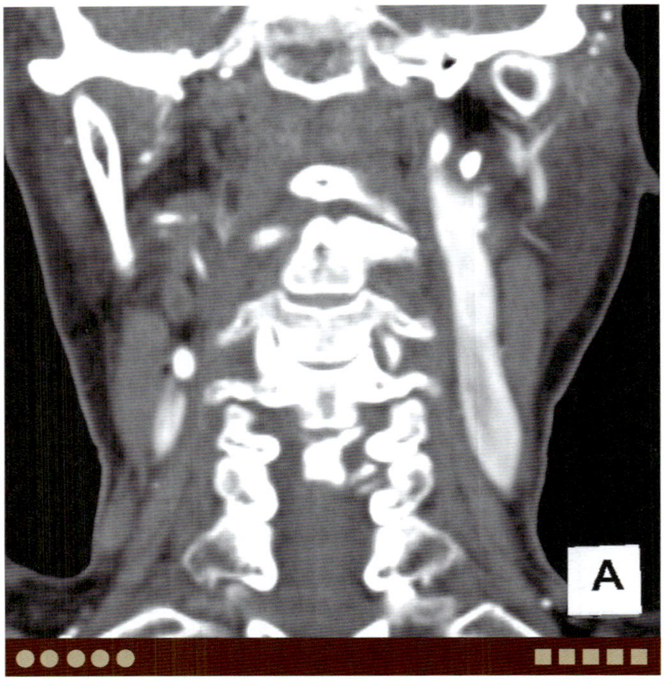

F. Normal asymmetric and heterogeneous enhancement of the internal jugular vein. Coronal postcontrast CT demonstrates heterogeneous enhancement of the left internal jugular vein.

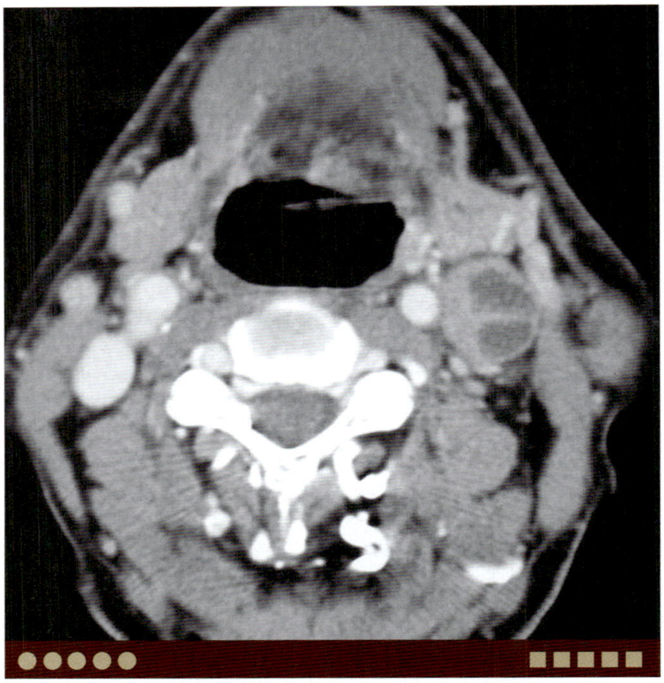

G. Necrotic metastatic lymph node. Axial postcontrast CT demonstrates a nodular lesion in the left jugular chain with central necrosis.

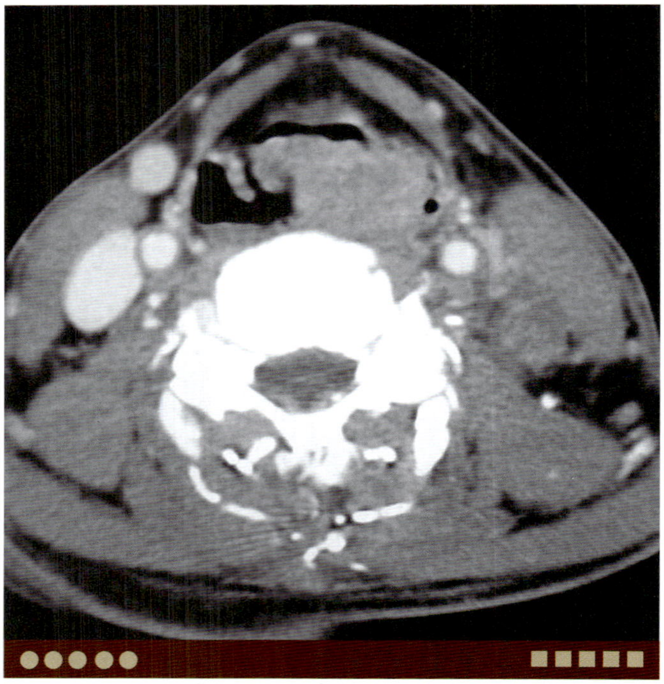

H. Necrotic metastatic lymph node, same patient as G. Axial postcontrast CT demonstrates poorly enhancing nodular lesions in the left jugular chain. Note the primary tumor within the left hypopharynx.

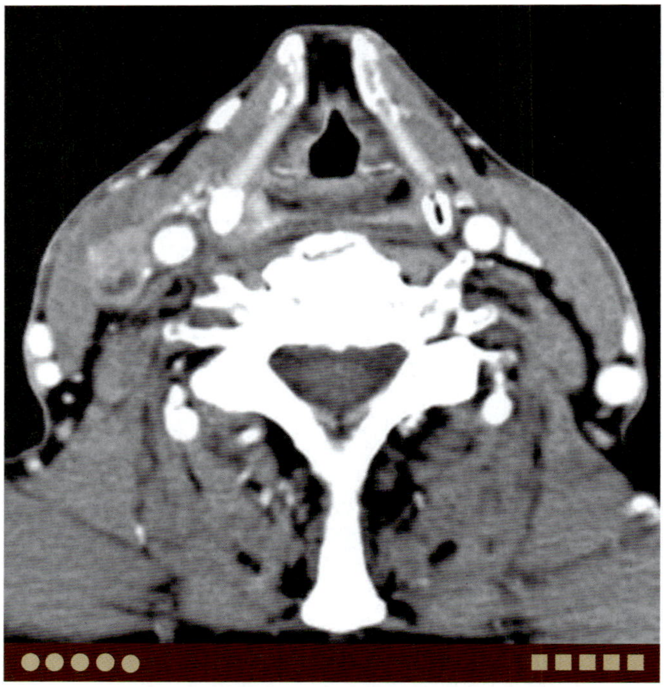

I. Necrotic metastatic lymph node in a different patient. Axial postcontrast CT demonstrates a heterogeneously enhancing nodular lesion in the right jugular chain. Note the compression of the right internal jugular vein medially.

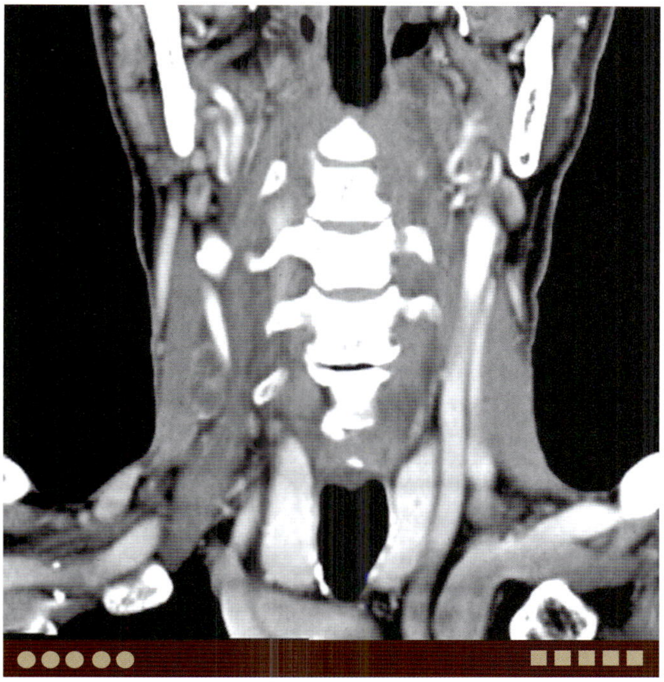

J. Necrotic metastatic lymph node, same patient as I. Coronal postcontrast CT demonstrates heterogeneously enhancing nodular lesions along the right jugular chain.

Case 11–12 Asymmetry of Internal Jugular Veins

Osamu Sakai, Elisa Flower

PRESENTATION

Right neck mass.

FINDINGS

Contrast-enhanced CT demonstrates a large right and a small left internal jugular vein.

DIFFERENTIAL DIAGNOSIS

- Jugular vein thrombosis: This is often associated with central venous catheter placement, intravenous drug use, malignancy, and hypercoagulopathy, and is rare in healthy individuals. Inflammatory change is often seen in the adjacent soft tissue.
- Branchial cleft cyst: Among branchial cleft cysts, second branchial cleft cyst is most common and usually located posterior to the submandibular gland and anteromedial to the sternocleidomastoid muscle and lacks tubular craniocaudal extension.
- Necrotic or cystic lymph node: This lacks tubular craniocaudal extension, however, can be multiple and mimic a thrombosed vein.
- Lymphatic malformation (lymphangioma): This may demonstrate internal septi and a lobulated appearance.

COMMENTS

This is a 44-year-old woman with a palpable right neck mass.

Asymmetry of the internal jugular veins (IJVs) is often seen in healthy individuals, raging from severe hypoplasia or aplasia (not identified on CT or MRI) to complete symmetry. The right internal jugular vein is usually larger than the left.

Abnormal signal on MRI and heterogeneous enhancement on CT is often seen in the left IJV, and sometimes mistaken as venous thrombosis, necrotic node, or cystic tumor. There are several causes for this phenomenon. One of the major reasons is compression of the left brachiocephalic vein by the aortic arch or brachiocephalic artery, which results in stasis of the venous blood. Moreover, reflux of contrast into the IJV, even to the transverse sinus, can be seen when the contrast is injected into the vein of the left upper extremity. Therefore, contrast should be injected into the right antecubital vein when performing a dynamic contrast-enhanced study such as CT or MR angiography to obtain better bolus of contrast.

Asymmetric and heterogeneous enhancement of the IJV is more often seen with a multidetector-row CT because of fast scanning. An additional delayed scan easily demonstrates homogeneous enhancement of the veins, although this has the drawback of additional radiation. Alternatively, ultrasound can be performed to confirm patency. However, usually this normal asymmetric enhancement can be easily differentiated from true venous thrombosis by absence of thick and irregular ringlike enhancement of the vein and surrounding inflammatory change.

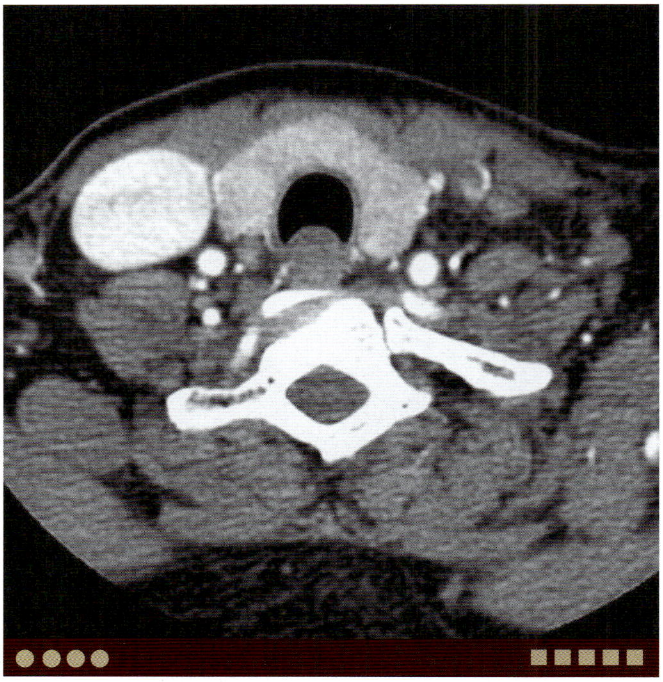

A. Normal asymmetry in the IJVs. Axial contrast-enhanced CT demonstrates large and well-opacified right IJV.

PEARLS

- **Asymmetry of the IJVs is often seen, ranging from severe hypoplasia or aplasia to complete symmetry. The right internal jugular vein is usually larger than the left.**
- **Asymmetric and heterogeneous enhancement of the IJV is often seen on the left.**
- **Asymmetric and heterogeneous enhancement of the IJV is usually differentiated from true venous thrombosis by lack of thick and irregular ringlike enhancement of the vein and surrounding inflammatory change.**

ADDITIONAL IMAGES (B-H)

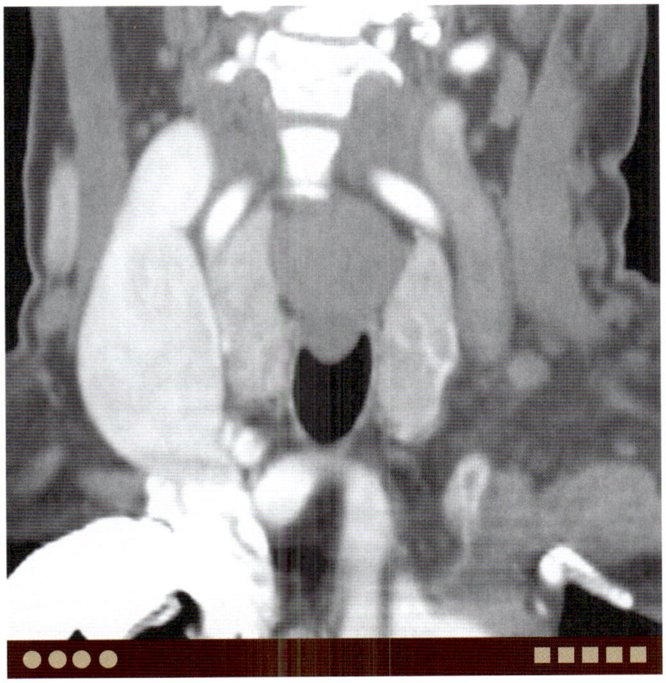

B. Normal asymmetry in the IJVs, same patient as A. Coronal CT demonstrates large right IJV. The left IJV is small and less opacified.

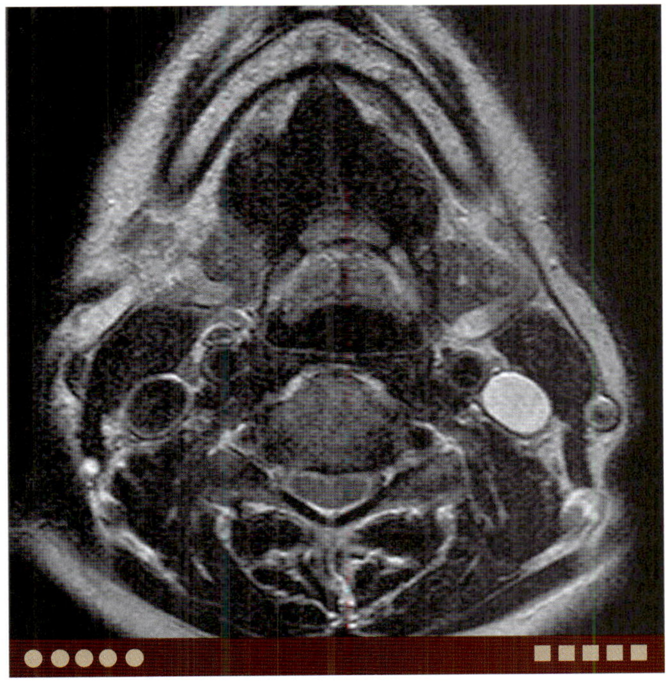

C. Normal asymmetry in signal. Axial T2W MR image demonstrates homogeneous high signal in the left IJV. The right IJV shows a signal-void.

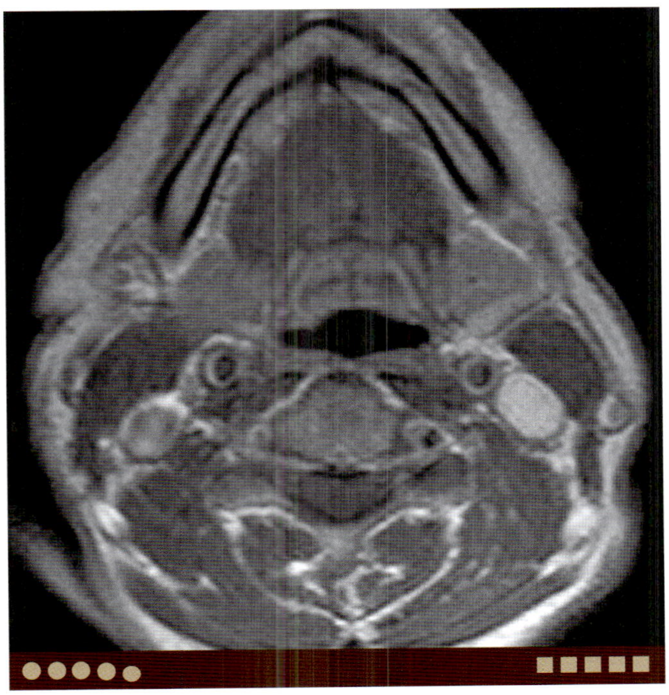

D. Normal asymmetry in signal, same patient as C. Axial postcontrast T1W MR image demonstrates enhancement in the IJVs bilaterally

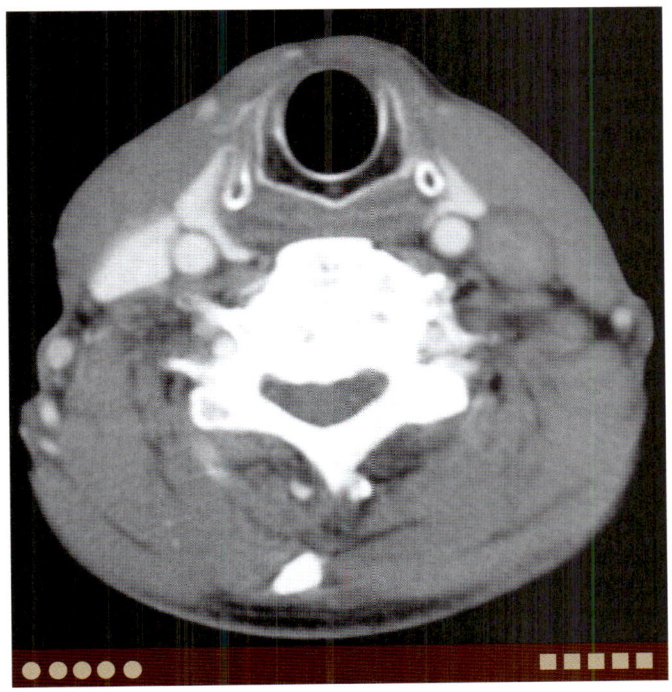

E. Normal asymmetric enhancement. Axial contrast-enhanced CT demonstrates no contrast enhancement in the left IJV.

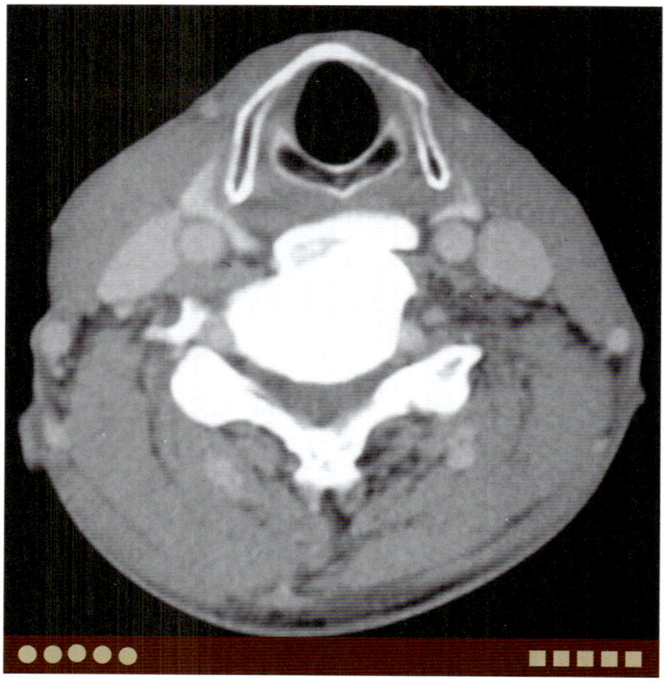

F. Normal asymmetric enhancement, same patient as E. Delayed scan demonstrates symmetric and homogeneous enhancement in the IJVs.

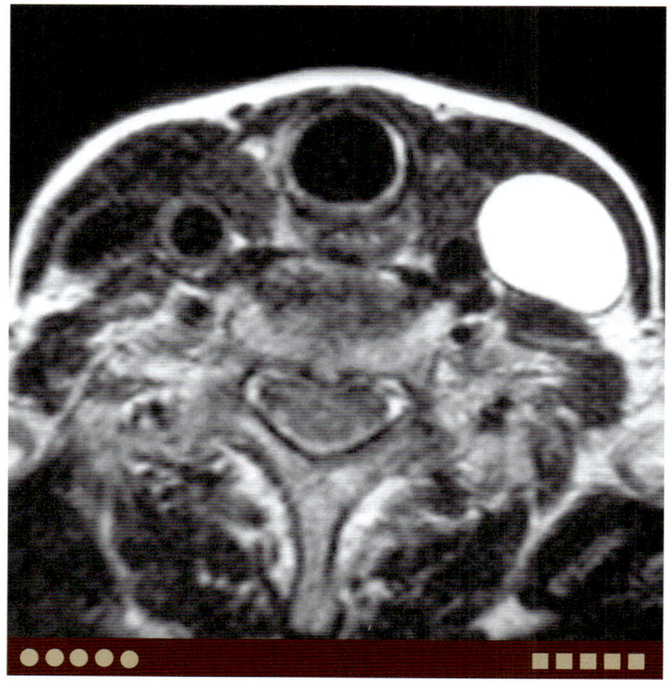

G. Normal asymmetry in size and signal. Axial T2W MR image demonstrates enlarged left IJV with high signal.

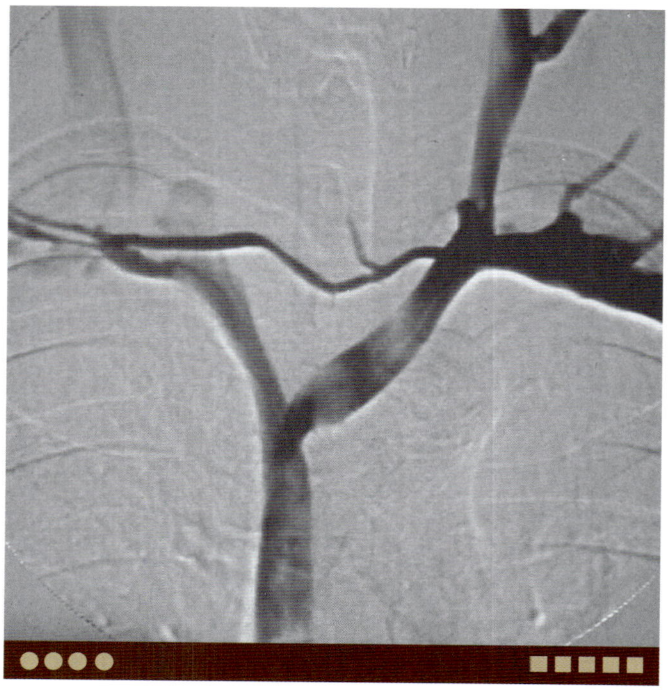

H. Normal contrast reflux into the left IJV. Digital subtraction angiography (DSA) demonstrates contrast reflux into the left IJV without an obstructive lesion in the left brachiocephalic vein or superior vena cava.

DIFFERENTIAL DIAGNOSIS IMAGES (I-J)

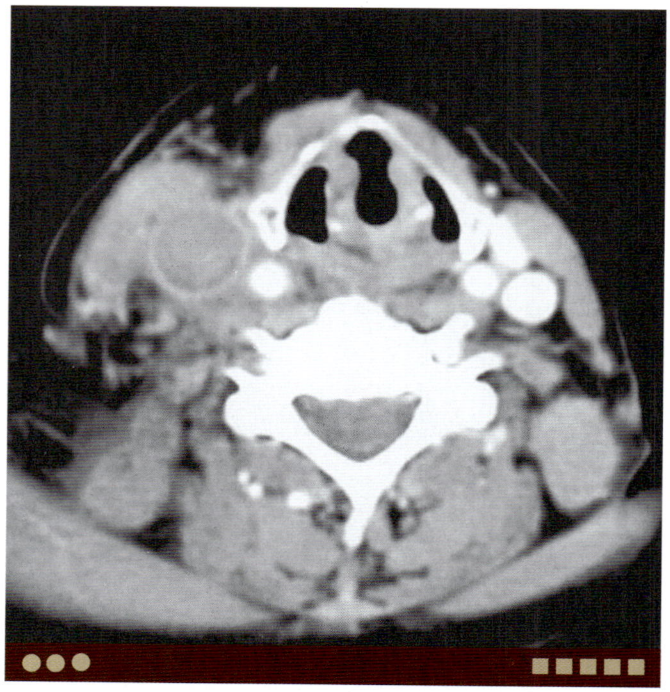

I. IJV thrombophlebitis. Axial contrast-enhanced CT demonstrates a thrombosed right IJV. Note ringlike enhancement and expansion of the vessel as well as surrounding inflammatory change.

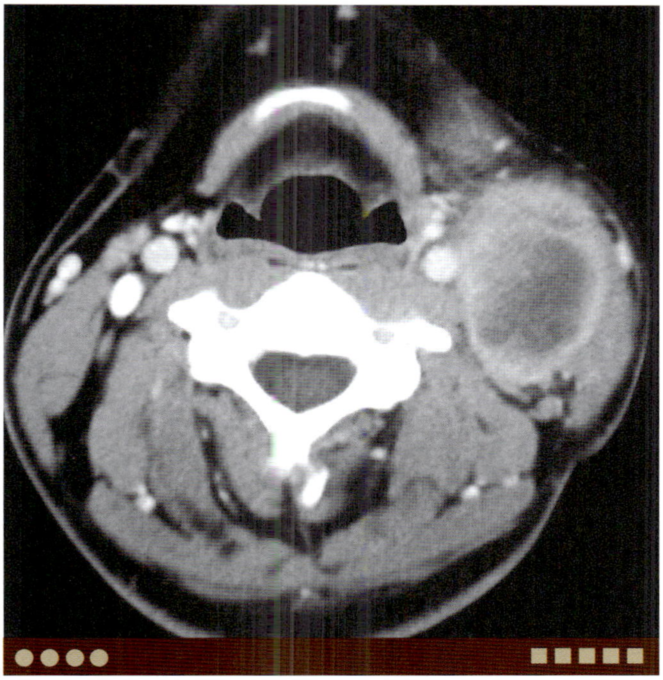

J. Necrotic metastatic node. Axial contrast-enhanced CT demonstrates a large heterogeneously enhancing lesion lateral to the left common carotid artery. The left IJV is not identified. Ill-defined boundary of the lesion suggests extracapsular tumor spread.

Case 11–13 Takayasu Arteritis

Osamu Sakai, Elisa Flower

PRESENTATION

No pulse in the upper extremities.

FINDINGS

CT and MRI demonstrate concentric wall thickening and narrowing of the common carotid artery in a young woman.

DIFFERENTIAL DIAGNOSIS

- Atherosclerotic disease: This is more often seen in elderly patients. Proximal internal carotid arteries and intracranial arteries are often involved. Calcification is common.
- Other vasculitides: By imaging alone it is difficult to differentiate it from other vasculitides.
- Moyamoya disease: This is a vascular occlusive disease which occurs in the intracranial arteries, particularly in the circle of Willis. Dilatation of the perforating arteries occurs, demonstrating a moyamoya or "puff of smoke" appearance

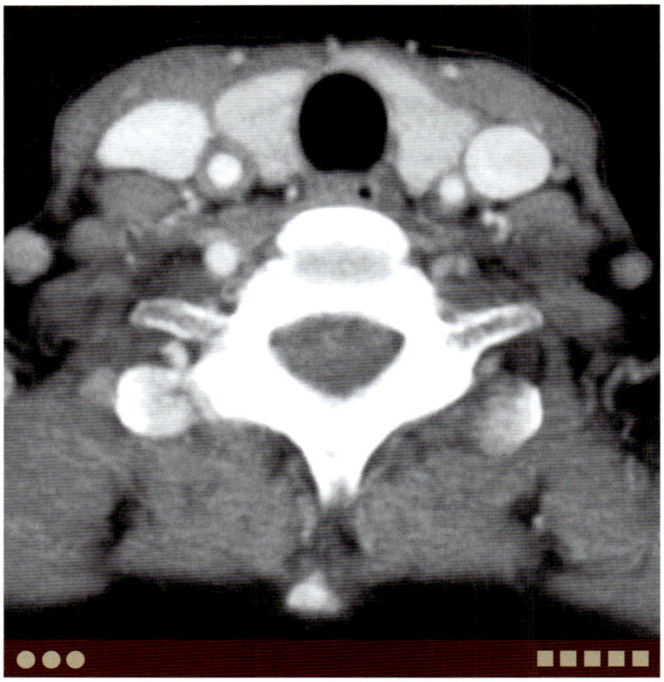

A. Takayasu arteritis. Axial contrast-enhanced CT demonstrates thickening of the wall of the common carotid artery bilaterally.

COMMENTS

This is a 57-year-old woman with pulseless upper extremities.

Takayasu arteritis is also known as aortitis syndrome or pulseless disease. This disease is a vasculitis of unknown etiology which involves mid-to-large size arteries including pulmonary arteries. Patients are often young women with a female-to-male ratio of 8:1. They are usually diagnosed by age 30. Takayasu arteritis is more frequently seen in Asia and India than in western Europe and North America, although it has a worldwide distribution.

The aorta as well as the brachiocephalic, subclavian, carotid, and vertebral arteries are often involved, and demonstrate wall thickening, stenosis, and occlusion. The aortic arch is often involved in Japanese patients while the left subclavian, superior mesenteric, and abdominal aorta are often involved in patients in the United States. Intracranial arteries are usually preserved. Rarely, cerebral aneurysms occur in patients with Takayasu arteritis, which can rupture and cause subarachnoid hemorrhage. In the active phase, enhancement of the arterial wall is commonly seen.

Historically, catheter angiogram had been performed to make the diagnosis; however, currently noninvasive imaging such as MRI/MRA and CT/CTA is performed. Dynamic contrast-enhanced MRA is very useful to evaluate patency of the vasculature, and postcontrast transverse imaging is useful to assess activity of the disease. Prominent wall enhancement is seen in the active inflammatory phase. CT/CTA also easily demonstrates concentric narrowing of the vessels and is useful to assess the patency due to high spatial resolution. However, CT/CTA is not an ideal imaging modality for follow-up due to radiation, particularly in young patients.

PEARLS

- **Takayasu arteritis or aortitis syndrome is also known as pulseless disease, which involves mid-to-large size arteries, such as branches of the aorta.**
- **Takayasu arteritis is commonly seen in young females, particularly Asian population.**
- **Intracranial arteries are usually preserved. Rarely, cerebral aneurysms occur.**

ADDITIONAL IMAGES (B-G)

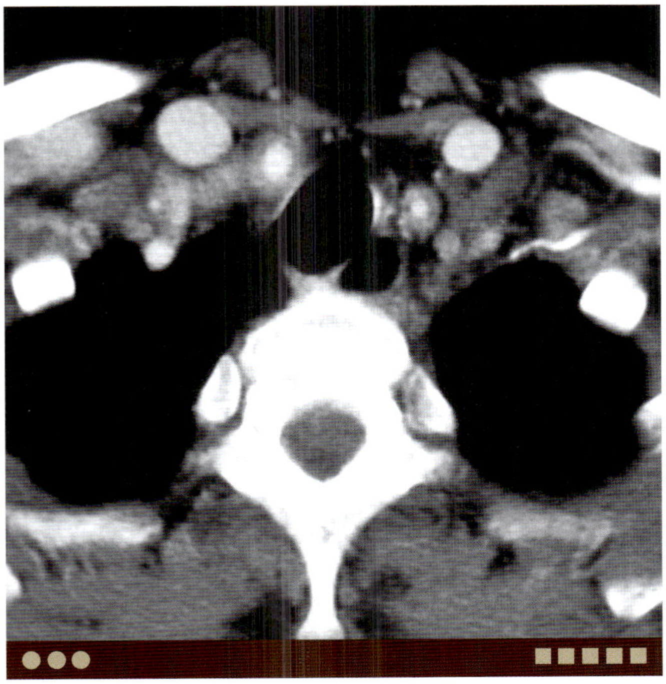

B. Takayasu arteritis, same patient as A. Axial contrast-enhanced CT through the thoracic inlet demonstrates narrowing of the left common carotid artery as well as wall thickening of the bilateral common carotid arteries.

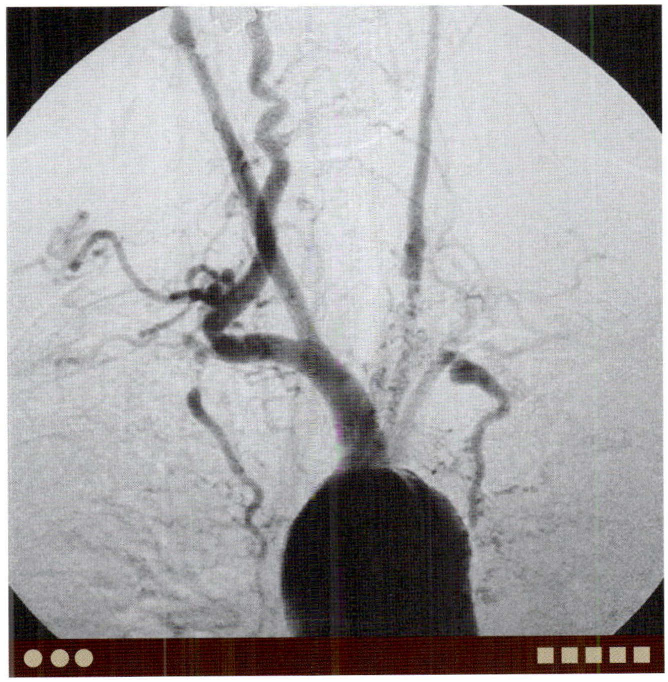

C. Takayasu arteritis, same patient as A. Digital subtraction aortogram demonstrates occlusion of the bilateral subclavian and left vertebral arteries. Long-segment narrowing is seen in the bilateral common carotid arteries, on the left much worse than on the right. Compensatory dilatation of the right vertebral artery is present.

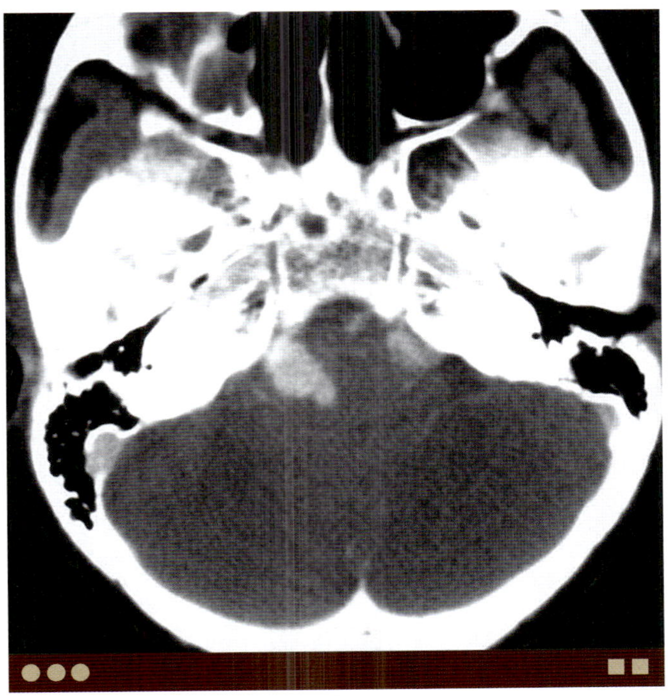

D. Takayasu arteritis, same patient as A. Axial contrast-enhanced CT through the posterior fossa demonstrates a round enhancing structure close to the right vertebral artery.

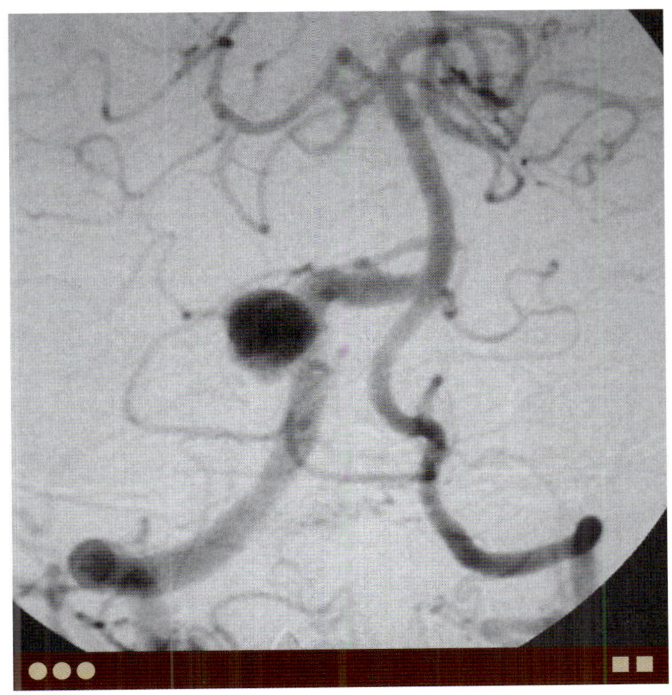

E. Takayasu arteritis, same patient as A. Digital subtraction angiogram of the posterior circulation demonstrates an aneurysm at the origin of the right posterior inferior cerebellar artery.

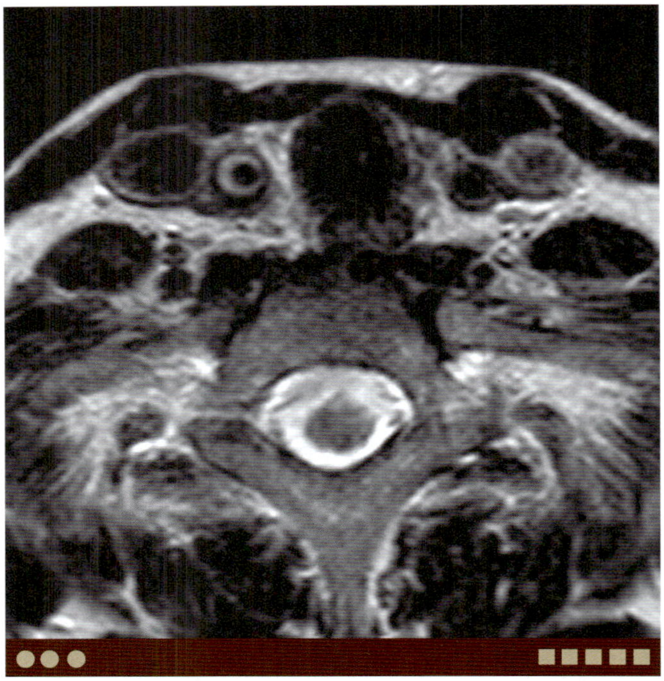

F. Takayasu's arteritis in a different patient. Axial T2W MR image demonstrates wall thickening of the right common carotid artery. Note thickened intima showing hyperintensity.

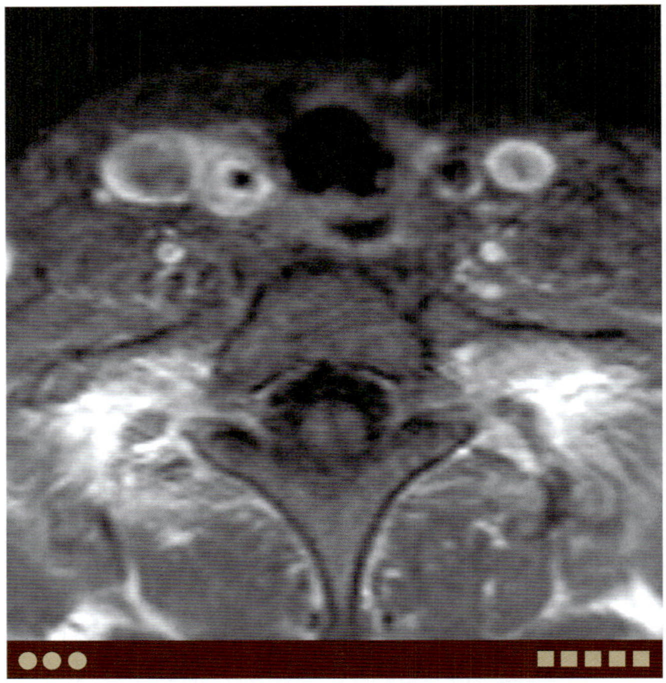

G. Takayasu arteritis, same patient as F. Axial postcontrast fat-suppressed T1W image demonstrates enhancement of the thickened wall of the right common carotid artery, suggestive of active inflammation.

DIFFERENTIAL DIAGNOSIS IMAGES (H-I)

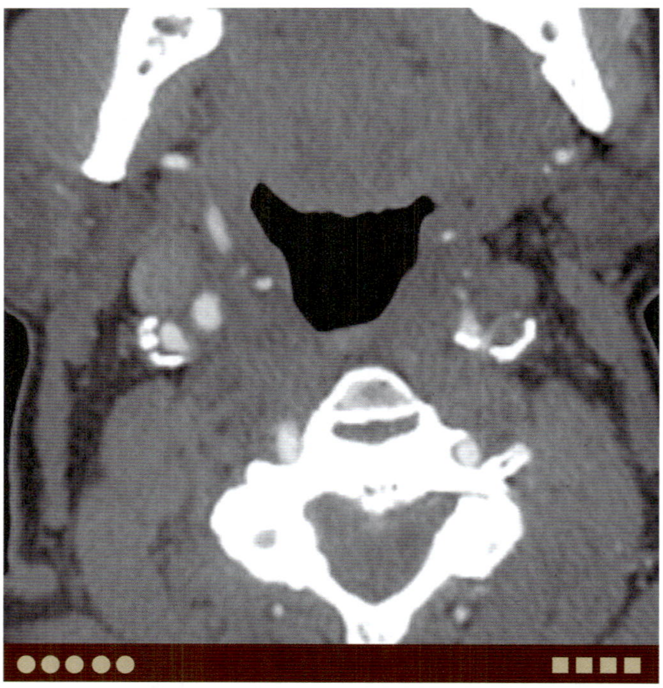

H. Atherosclerosis. Axial CTA image demonstrates severe stenosis of the internal carotid arteries, left worse than right, with calcified and noncalcified plaques.

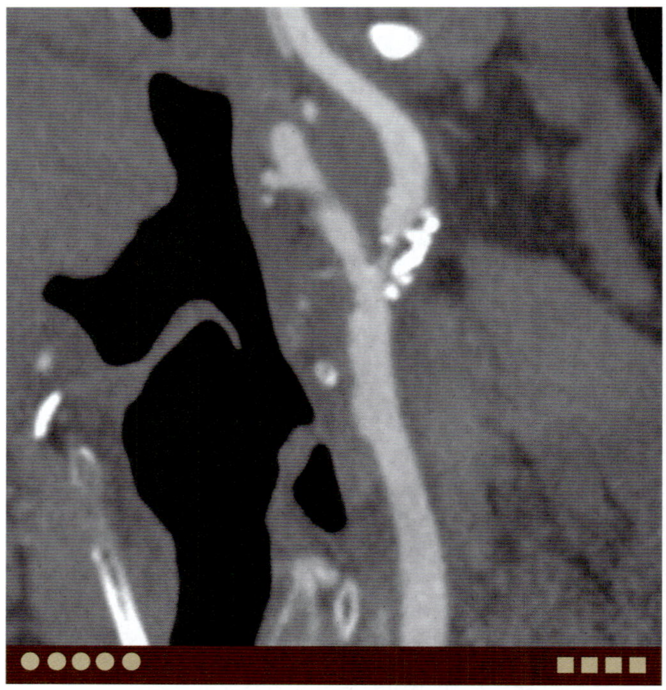

I. Atherosclerosis, same patient as H. Curved reformation from axial CTA demonstrates severe stenosis of the left internal carotid artery with calcified and noncalcified plaques.

Case 11–14 Lipoma

Osamu Sakai, Francisco Contreras

PRESENTATION

Painless mass.

FINDINGS

CT demonstrates a fat density mass in the superficial soft tissues.

DIFFERENTIAL DIAGNOSIS

- Liposarcoma: This is a common soft tissue sarcoma, often presenting with a soft tissue component in addition to a pure fatty compartment. Although well differentiated, liposarcomas are mainly composed of fat with septa or nodules. Myxoid liposarcoma is the most common type of liposarcoma, and fatty density or signal is often not seen in imaging.
- Dermoid: This is a congenital/developmental cyst. It is often impossible to be differentiated from an epidermoid by imaging. The presence of fat favors dermoid rather than epidermoid.
- Madelung disease: A rare condition of diffuse, symmetric fatty proliferation in the neck and upper trunk. Increased fat proliferation in the superficial soft tissues does not demonstrate abnormal soft tissue component or enhancement.

COMMENTS

This is a 67-year-old man with a painless mass in the neck.

Lipoma is the most common soft tissue mass. This is benign neoplasm composed entirely of mature fat contained within a thin, smooth, noninfiltrative capsule. The majority demonstrate a homogeneous fat content with little-to-no internal architecture. As they grow, they typically displace the adjacent structures. A very small percentage of these benign growths have a minor portion of nonfatty soft tissue components.

In the head and neck, it often occurs in the superficial soft tissues or muscles, which can be intra- or intermuscular. The most common sites of origin in the neck are in the posterior cervical, submandibular, anterior cervical, and within the parotid spaces. Further, lipoma may involve multiple fascia-defined spaces. It often presents as a longstanding painless soft mass, or incidentally found at a doctor's visit for other reasons. No intervention is required and often just watched clinically; however, surgery can be performed for cosmetic reasons.

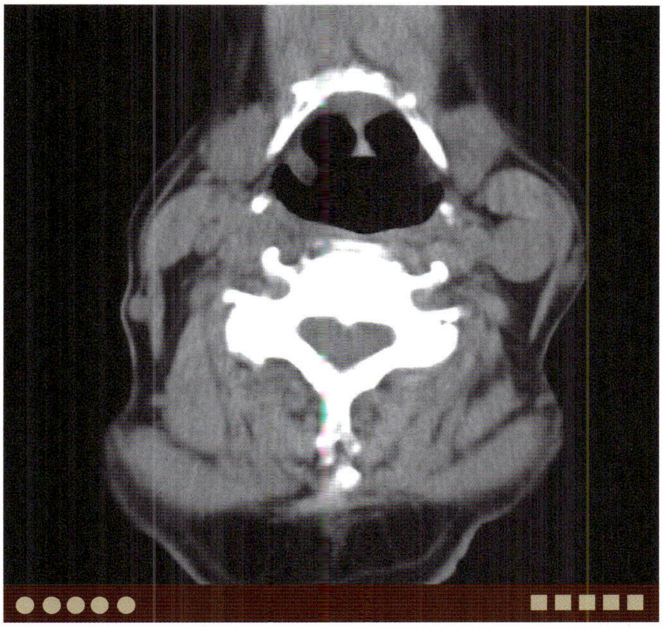

A. Lipoma. Axial noncontrast-enhanced CT shows a focal proliferation of the fat in the posterior neck in midline.

PEARLS

- **Lipoma is the most common soft tissue mass and composed of benign mature fat.**
- **Lipoma typically occurs as a painless long-standing mass that requires no intervention.**
- **Lipoma may involve multiple fascia-defined spaces.**

ADDITIONAL IMAGES (B-F)

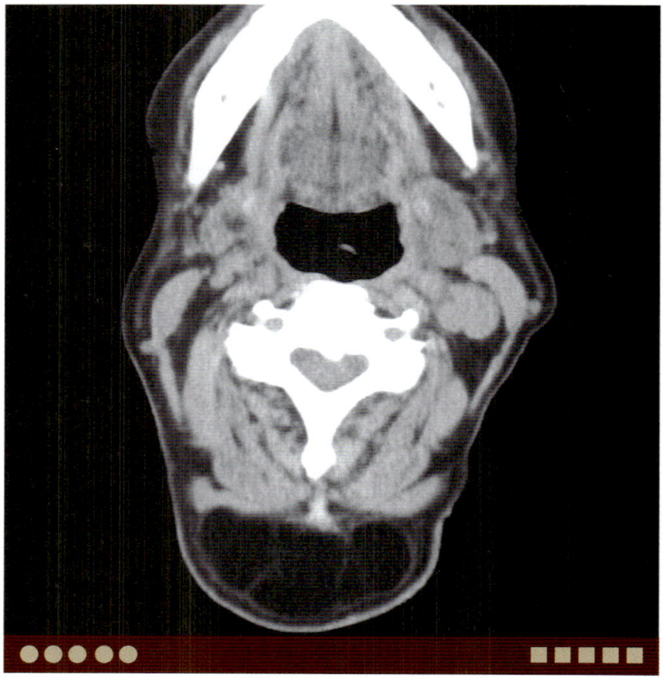

B. Lipoma, same patient as A. Axial noncontrast-enhanced CT shows a focal proliferation of the fat in the posterior neck in midline.

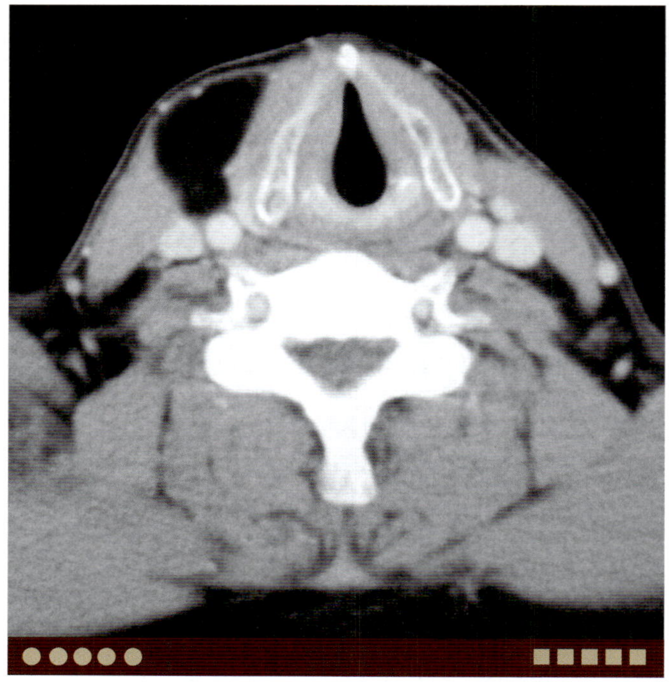

C. Lipoma in a different patient. Axial contrast-enhanced CT shows a focal proliferation of the fat in the anterior right neck.

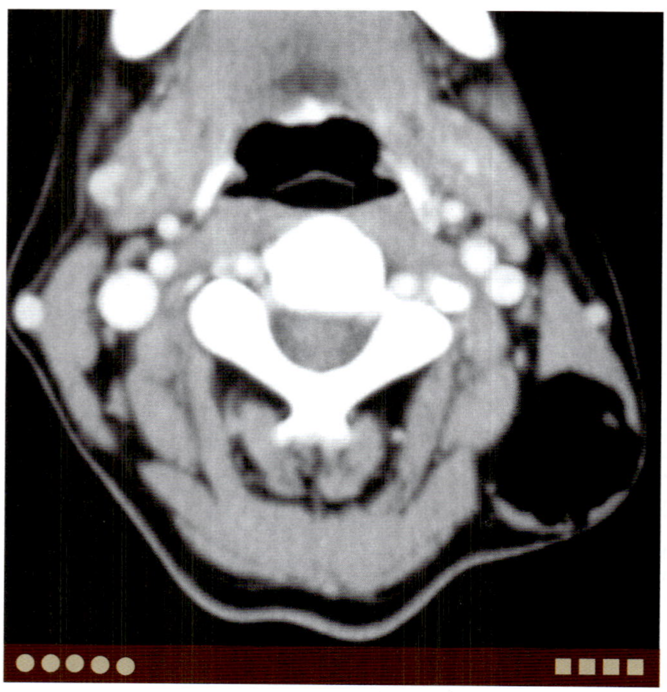

D. Lipoma in a different patient. Axial contrast-enhanced CT shows a focal intramuscular proliferation of the fat in the left sternocleidomastoid muscle.

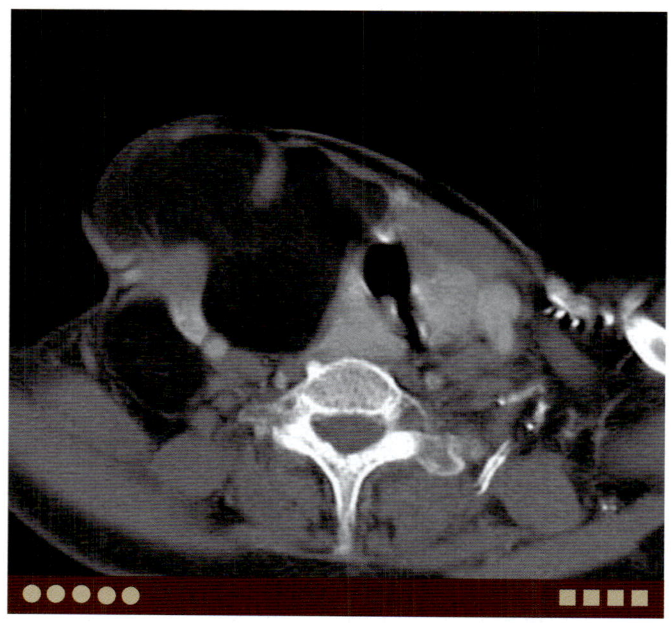

E. Lipoma in a different patient. Axial contrast-enhanced CT shows a lobulated fatty proliferation in the right anterior neck with intramuscular component involving the sternocleidomastoid muscle.

DIFFERENTIAL DIAGNOSIS IMAGES (G-H)

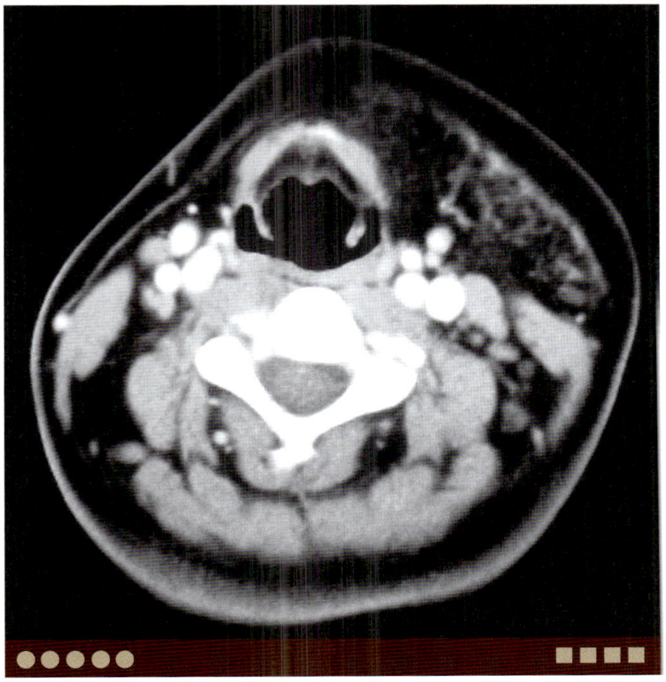

F. Lipoma in a different patient. Axial contrast-enhanced CT shows proliferation of the fat in the anterior left neck with a minor soft tissue component.

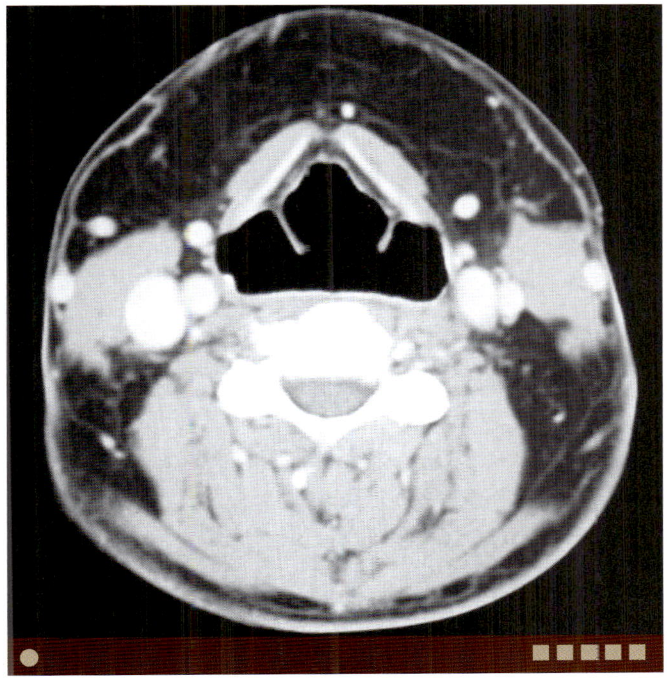

G. Madelung disease. Axial contrast-enhanced CT shows diffuse, symmetric fatty deposition beneath the platysma without areas of enhancement or focal soft tissue nodule.

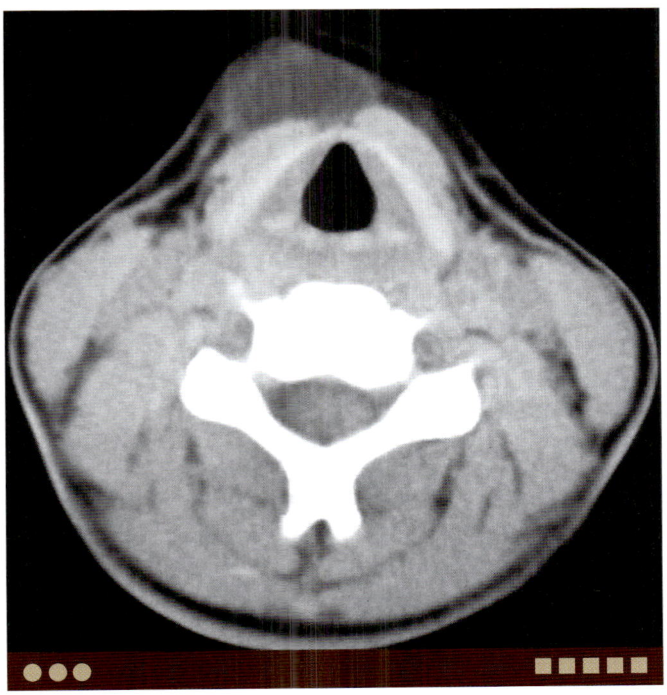

H. Dermoid. Axial noncontrast CT shows a cystic lesion superficial to the strap muscle. Note the density is slightly lower than the CSF suggesting presence of fat.

Case 11–15 Parathyroid Cyst

Hiroki Kato, Asim Mian, Osamu Sakai

PRESENTATION

Mostly asymptomatic. Rarely causes tracheal and esophageal compression, hoarseness, and pain.

FINDINGS

CT and MRI demonstrate a cystic lesion located posterior to the thyroid gland.

DIFFERENTIAL DIAGNOSIS

- Thyroid cyst: Thyroid cysts are usually filled with brownish or hemorrhagic fluid with increased thyroglobulin concentration. The differentiation from parathyroid cyst is difficult by imaging alone.
- Cervical thymic cyst: Cervical thymic cyst often occurs in association with the thymopharyngeal duct or tract. It is typically located in the anterior triangle, either superficial or deep to the sternocleidomastoid muscle, contacting the carotid sheath.
- Lymphatic malformation (cystic hygroma): Lymphatic malformation often occurs in the posterior triangle and manifests early in life.

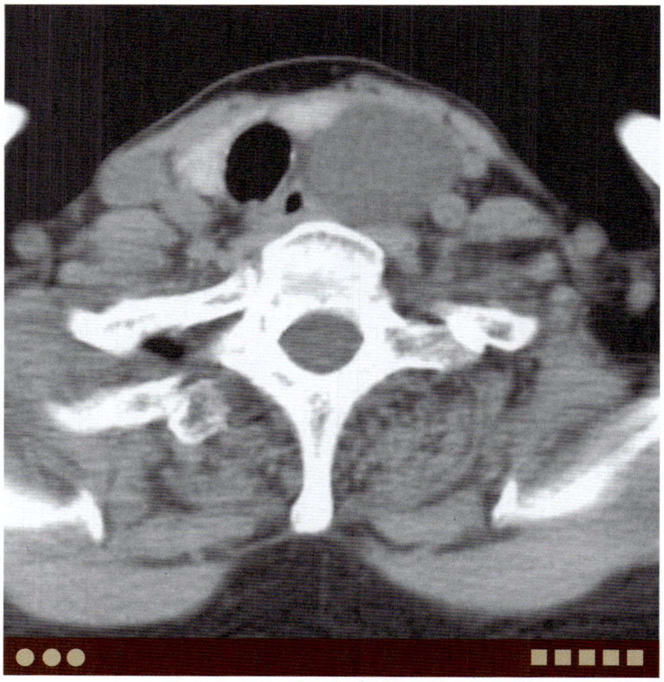

A. Parathyroid cyst. Axial unenhanced CT demonstrates a well-demarcated, homogeneously hypodense lesion, located in the left lower neck posterior to the left lower pole of the thyroid gland.

COMMENTS

This is a 69-year-old woman with discomfort from the lower neck to the upper chest.

The origin of parathyroid cyst is unclear, but parathyroid cysts are classified based on the presumptive mechanism of cyst formation: (1) congenital cyst from pharyngeal pouch remnants, (2) coalescence of parathyroid microcysts, and (3) parathyroid pseudocysts (infarction, hemorrhage, or cystic degeneration within a parathyroid adenoma). Although parathyroid microcysts are a common benign disease, large parathyroid cysts are not common. Parathyroid cysts are divided into two groups: nonfunctioning and functioning. The majority of these cysts are nonfunctional, but some (10%-15%) are functional and diagnosed due to primary hyperparathyroidism with elevated serum calcium and parathyroid hormone (PTH) levels. Regardless of being nonfunctional or functional, parathyroid cysts are usually filled with serous fluid with a high level of PTH. Confirmation of elevated PTH level in the contained fluid by aspiration may facilitate diagnosis when a parathyroid cyst is suspected.

Parathyroid cysts can occur anywhere from the angle of the mandible down to the mediastinum. Parathyroid cysts most commonly arise in the inferior parathyroid glands (65%). Especially, nonfunctional parathyroid cysts occur almost exclusively in the inferior parathyroid glands (95%). In general, a nonfunctional parathyroid cyst demonstrates a unilocular homogeneous cystic lesion with thin walls on CT and MRI. Content fluid is isodense and isointense to the cerebrospinal fluid, reflecting its serous fluid contents. However, functional parathyroid cysts have variable MRI and CT characteristics depending on their protein content.

PEARLS

- **Parathyroid cyst is located posterior to the thyroid gland.**
- **Nonfunctional parathyroid cyst is often a unilocular cystic lesion with thin walls.**
- **Differentiating parathyroid cysts from thyroid cysts is often difficult by imaging alone.**

ADDITIONAL IMAGES (B-D)

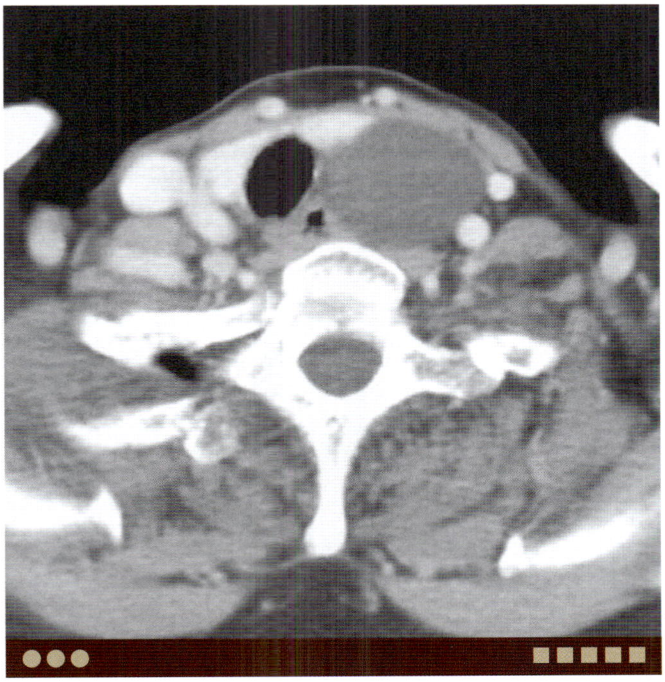

B. Parathyroid cyst, same patient as A. Axial contrast-enhanced CT demonstrates no enhancement in the lesion.

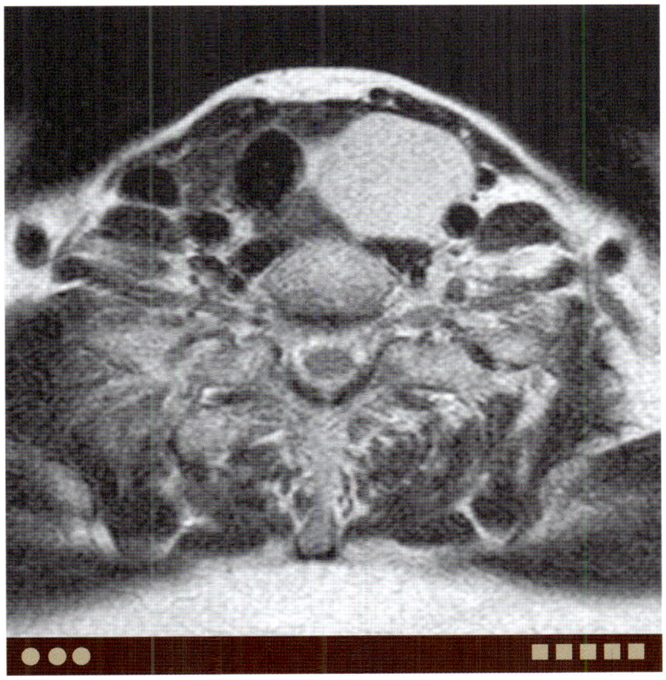

C. Parathyroid cyst, same patient as A. Axial T2W image demonstrates homogeneously high-signal intensity.

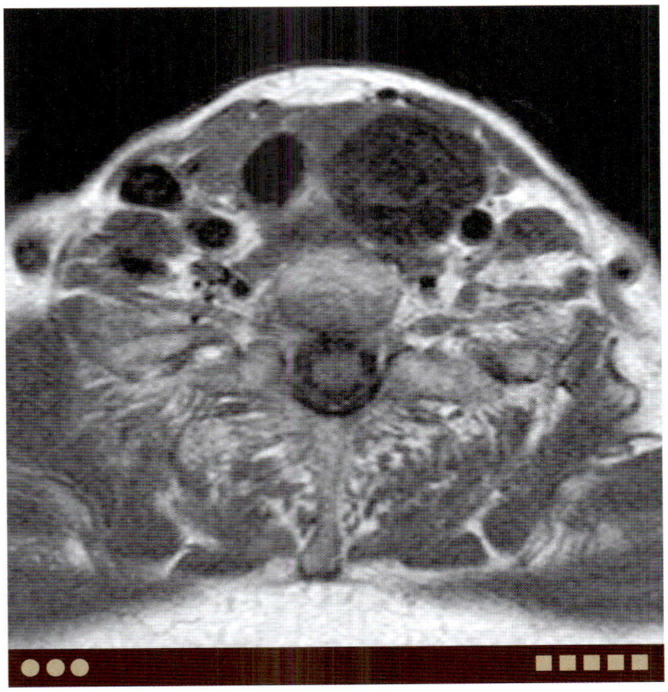

D. Parathyroid cyst, same patient as A. Axial T1W image demonstrates low-signal intensity

DIFFERENTIAL DIAGNOSIS IMAGES (E-G)

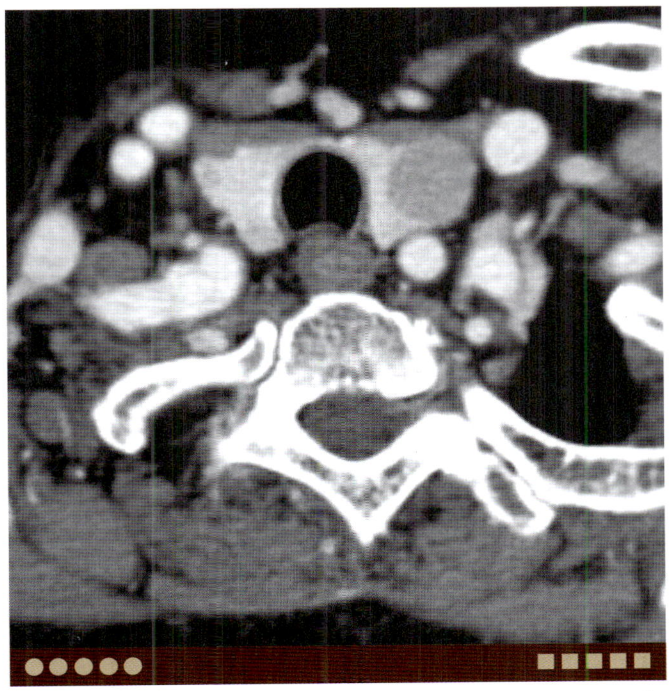

E. Thyroid cyst. Axial contrast-enhanced CT demonstrates a cystic lesion in the left lobe of the thyroid gland.

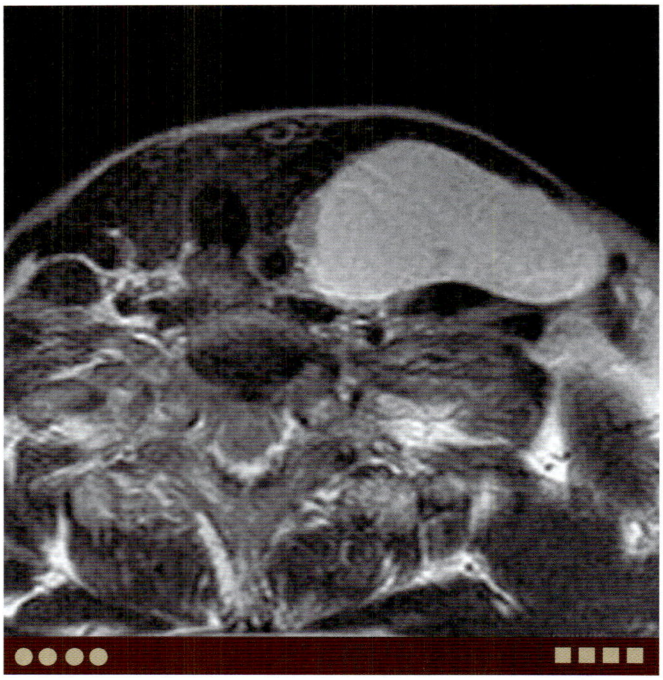

F. Lymphatic malformation. Axial T2W image demonstrates a cystic lesion displacing the thyroid and other adjacent structures in the left lower neck.

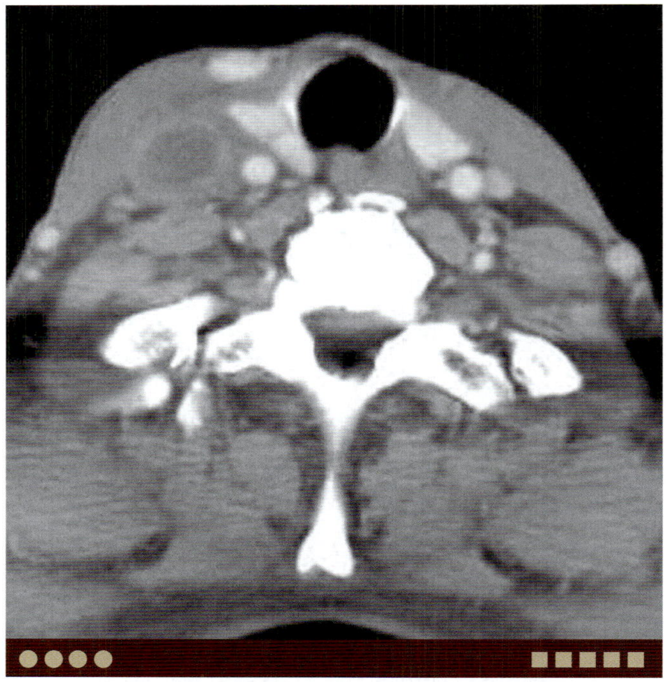

G. Internal jugular vein thrombosis. Axial contrast-enhanced CT demonstrates lack of enhancement in the lumen of the right internal jugular vein. Note expansion of the vein, thick ringlike enhancement of the wall and inflammatory change in the surrounding fat.

Case 11–16 Madelung Disease

Osamu Sakai, Francisco Contreras

PRESENTATION

Neck swelling.

FINDINGS

CT and MRI demonstrate symmetrically increased fatty tissue in the superficial neck.

DIFFERENTIAL DIAGNOSIS

- Obesity: Although diffuse fatty deposition is also seen, there is typically a more evenly distributed fat deposition throughout the entire body and not isolated to the neck and upper body.
- Lipoma: These lesions typically present as focal, localized fatty tissue proliferation.
- Liposarcoma: This is true neoplastic process and often contains soft tissue components. The well-differentiated type will demonstrate a lobulated, nonenhancing fatty mass with internal septations or nodules. The less well-differentiated types appear as heterogeneous, enhancing soft tissue masses with amorphous fatty portions within the margins of the lesion.

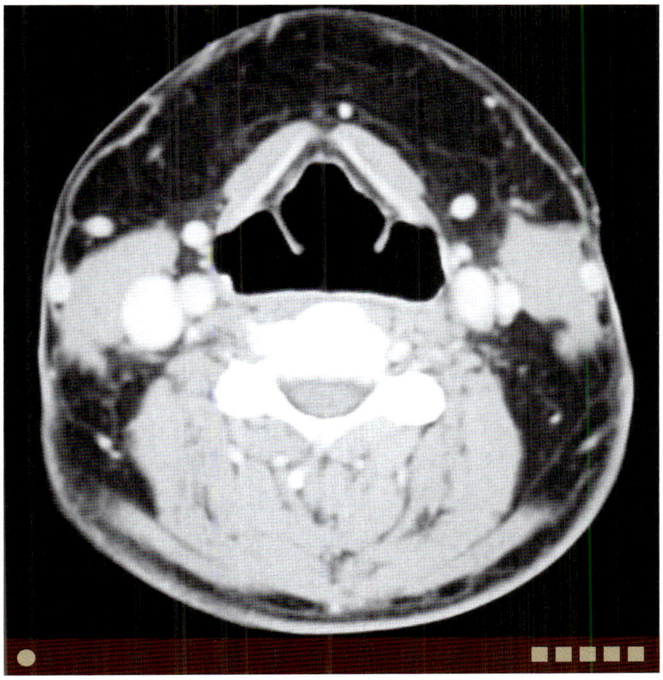

A. Madelung disease. Axial contrast-enhanced CT shows diffuse, symmetric fatty deposition beneath the platysma without areas of enhancement or focal soft tissue nodule.

COMMENTS

This is a 38-year-old man with increasing neck circumference.

Madelung disease is also known as multiple symmetrical lipomatosis, cephalothoracic lipodystrophy, and Launois-Bensaude syndrome. It is a rare condition consisting of diffuse, symmetric fat proliferation in the neck and upper trunk. The deposition of fat usually increases slowly for the first few years, but occasionally shows acceleration over a course of several months.

This disease often affects men and is most commonly reported in the Mediterranean area. Madelung disease is typically reported in middle-aged white men with a male-to-female ratio of 4:1, although both women and other races can be affected. Familial cases have been reported. It is thought to be genetic, but its exact mode of inheritance is uncertain. It is postulated to be an inherited mitochondrial DNA disease. However, most of the cases are sporadic.

Anemia, liver dysfunction, and alcohol have been thought to be associated with this condition; however, the etiology remains uncertain. Histologically, there is a proliferation of normal fatty tissue without encapsulation. Dyspnea due to mass effect upon the trachea or larynx from increased fatty tissue has been reported; however, patients usually seek medical treatment because of cosmetic concerns.

CT and MRI demonstrate symmetrically increased fat in the superficial soft tissue of the neck without abnormal soft tissue component or enhancement.

PEARLS

- **Symmetrically increased fat deposition in the superficial soft tissue of the neck without abnormal soft tissue component or enhancement.**
- **The presence of any component of enhancement should raise the suspicion of a malignant process such as a liposarcoma.**

ADDITIONAL IMAGES (B-F)

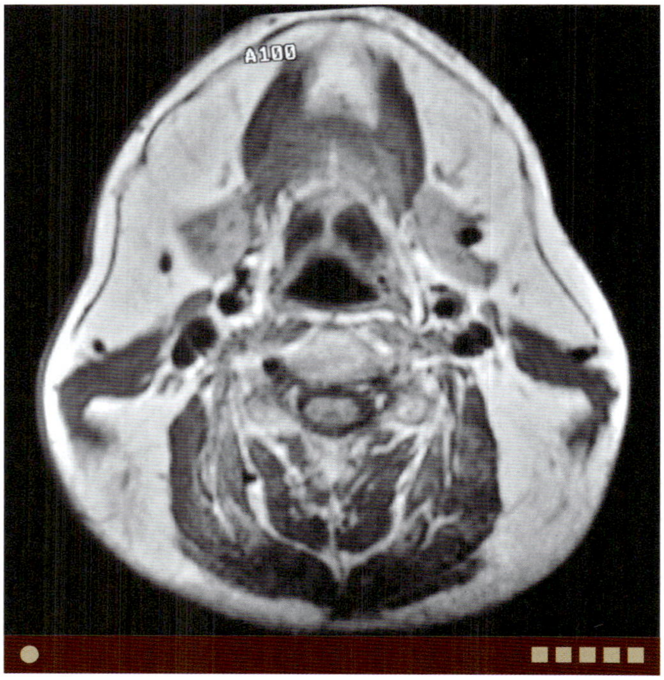

B. Madelung disease, same patient as A. Axial T1W MR image shows diffuse, symmetric fatty deposition in the anterior neck beneath the platysma as well as in the posterior triangles.

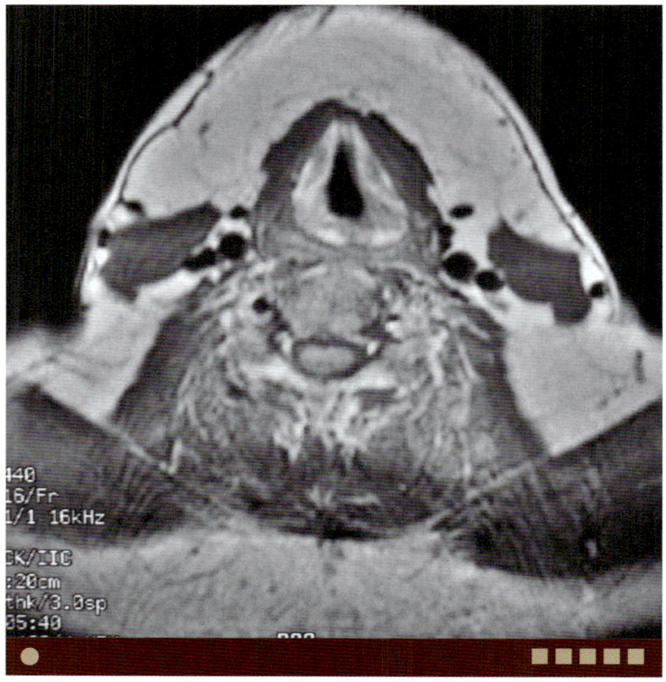

C. Madelung disease, same patient as A. Axial T1W MR image through the larynx shows prominent, symmetric fatty deposition in the anterior neck as well as in the back.

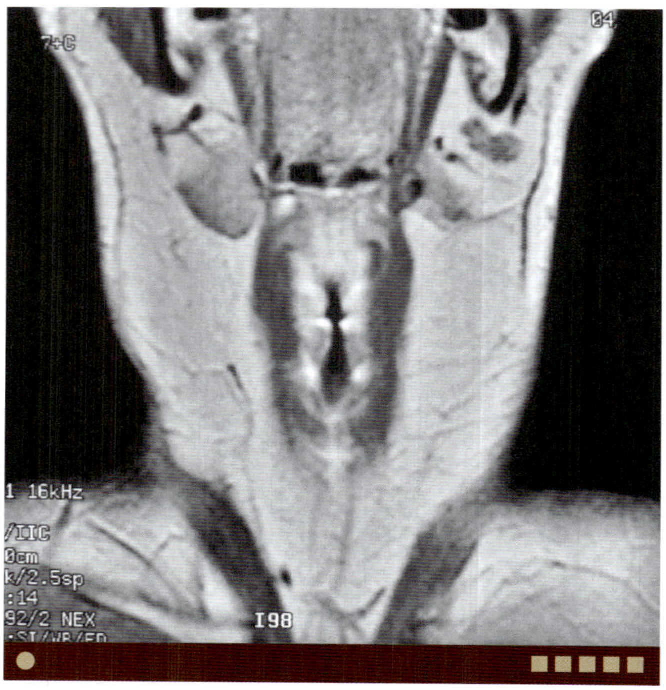

D. Madelung disease, same patient as A. Coronal T1W MR image shows symmetric fatty deposition within the subcutaneous tissues of the neck.

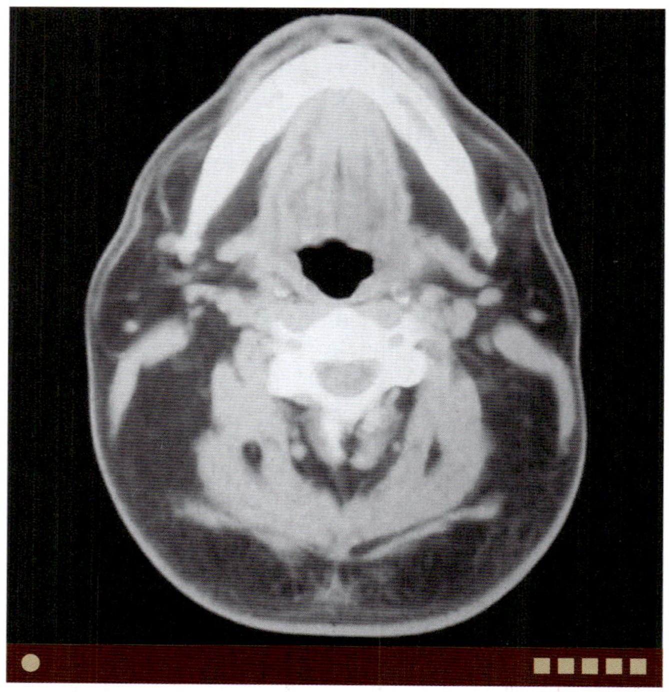

E. Madelung disease in a different patient. Axial noncontrast-enhanced CT shows diffuse, symmetric fatty deposition within the subcutaneous tissues of the neck, more prominent in the posterior triangle.

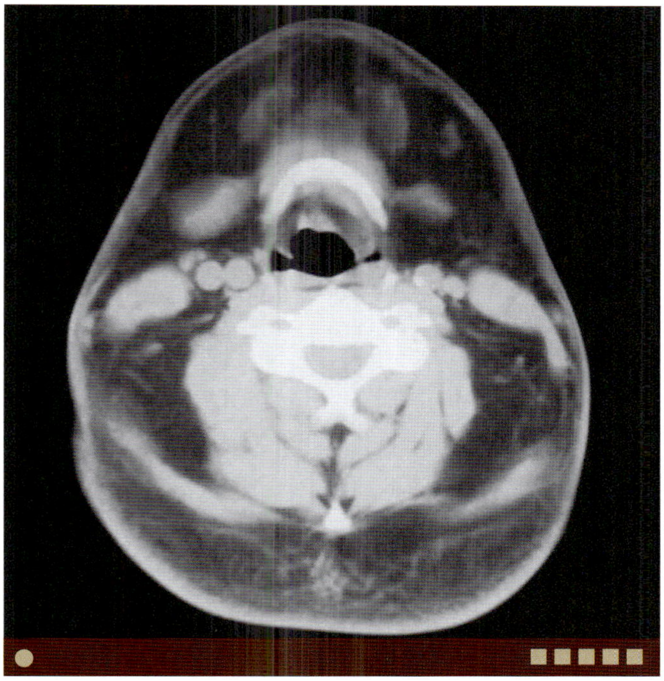

F. Madelung disease, same patient as E. Axial noncontrast-enhanced CT shows diffuse, symmetric fatty deposition in the anterior and posterior neck.

DIFFERENTIAL DIAGNOSIS IMAGES (G-H)

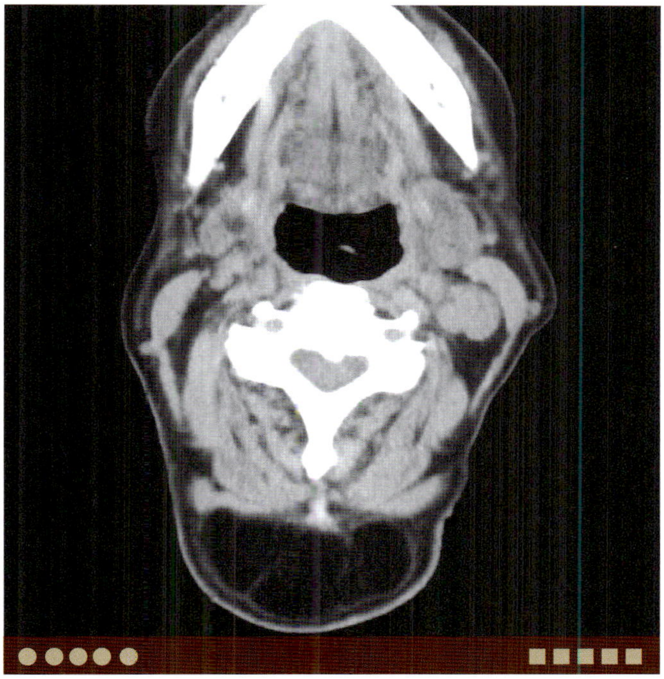

G. Lipoma. Axial noncontrast-enhanced CT shows a focal proliferation of fat in the midline posterior neck.

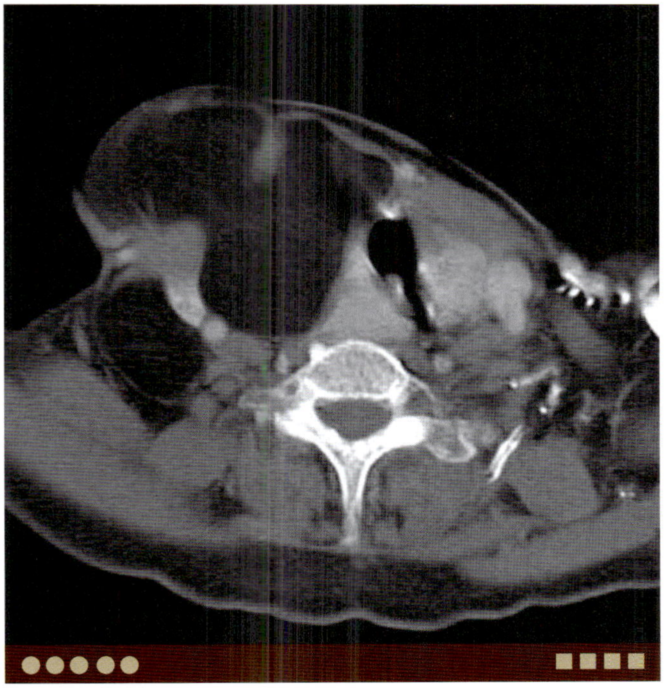

H. Lipoma in a different patient. Axial contrast-enhanced CT shows a lobulated, fatty proliferation in the right anterior neck with an intramuscular component involving the sternocleidomastoid muscle.

Case 11–17 Hashimoto Thyroiditis

Osamu Sakai, Akifumi Fujita, Asim Mian

PRESENTATION

Increasing anterior neck mass.

FINDINGS

CT demonstrates enlarged thyroid glands with heterogeneously decreased density.

DIFFERENTIAL DIAGNOSIS

- Goiter: This tends to show heterogeneously enlarged thyroid glands with normal thyroid demonstrating higher density, although it may be difficult to distinguish each other by imaging only without appropriate clinical history or endocrinological data.
- Lymphoma: This is often associated with Hashimoto thyroiditis. Rapid increase in size of the thyroid in a patient with Hashimoto thyroiditis strongly suggests lymphoma.
- Anaplastic carcinoma of the thyroid: This demonstrates similar findings but more aggressive and invades the adjacent structures.

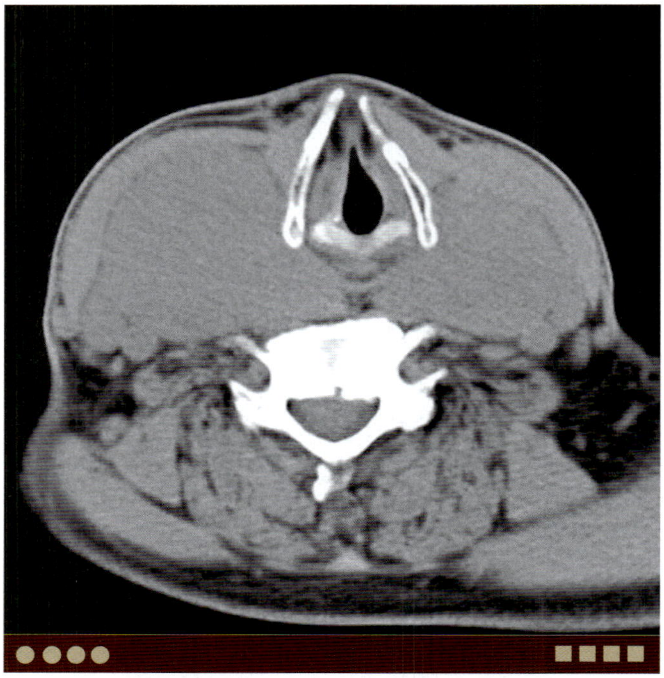

A. Hashimoto thyroiditis. Axial noncontrast CT demonstrates significantly enlarged thyroid glands with decreased density bilaterally.

COMMENTS

This is a 65-year-old man with history of chronic thyroiditis.

Hashimoto thyroiditis or chronic lymphocytic thyroiditis is a chronic thyroiditis with lymphocytic infiltration characterized by the destruction of thyroid cells by various cell- and antibody-mediated immune processes. This condition occurs more often in women than in men (F:M = 10-20:1), commonly between 45 and 65 years of age. This is the most common cause of primary hypothyroidism in North America after the age of 6.

Morbidity often results from failure to make the diagnosis and failure to institute l-thyroxine replacement therapy in adequate doses. Notably, patients with Hashimoto thyroiditis have significantly increased risk (×70-80) of lymphoma which is usually B-cell non-Hodgkin lymphoma (NHL) just like other lymphomas in the head and neck. It is believed that chronic antigenic stimulation secondary to the autoimmune disorder causes chronic proliferation of lymphoid tissue and its clonal proliferation. In addition, other malignancies, such as papillary carcinoma, Hurthle cell tumor, leukemia, and plasmacytoma may occur in patients with Hashimoto thyroiditis.

Imaging findings of Hashimoto thyroiditis are very nonspecific. Diffuse enlargement of the thyroid glands with decreased density is often seen. Calcification or necrosis is not common. Rapid increase in size of the thyroid and presence of aggressive features such as extracapsular extension and invasion to the adjacent structures in a patient with Hashimoto thyroiditis strongly suggests lymphoma.

PEARLS

- **Hashimoto thyroiditis is chronic thyroiditis with lymphocytic infiltration.**
- **Imaging findings are nonspecific. However, diffuse enlargement of the thyroid glands with decreased density is often seen.**
- **Patients with Hashimoto thyroiditis have significantly increased risk of primary thyroid lymphoma.**
- **Other malignancies, such as papillary carcinoma, Hurthle cell tumor, leukemia, and plasmacytoma may occur in patients with Hashimoto thyroiditis.**

ADDITIONAL IMAGES (B-C)

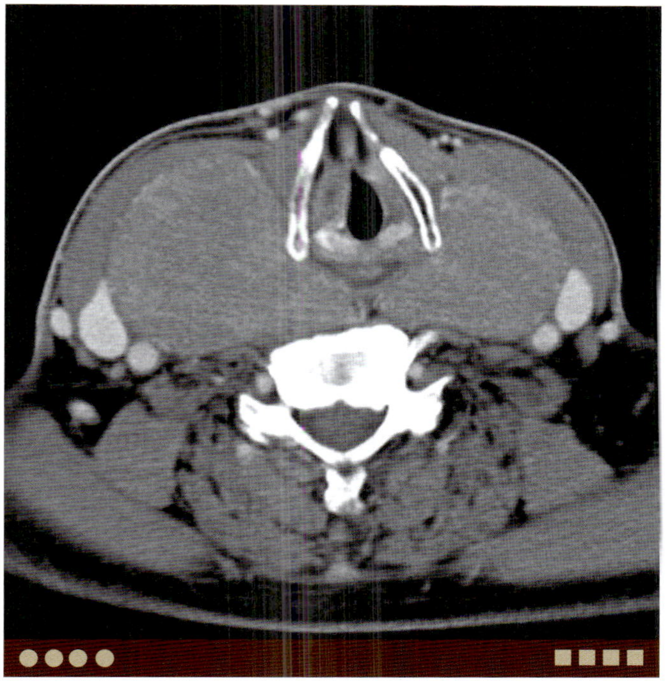

B. Hashimoto thyroiditis, same patient as A. Axial contrast-enhanced CT demonstrates minimal enhancement of the enlarged thyroid glands.

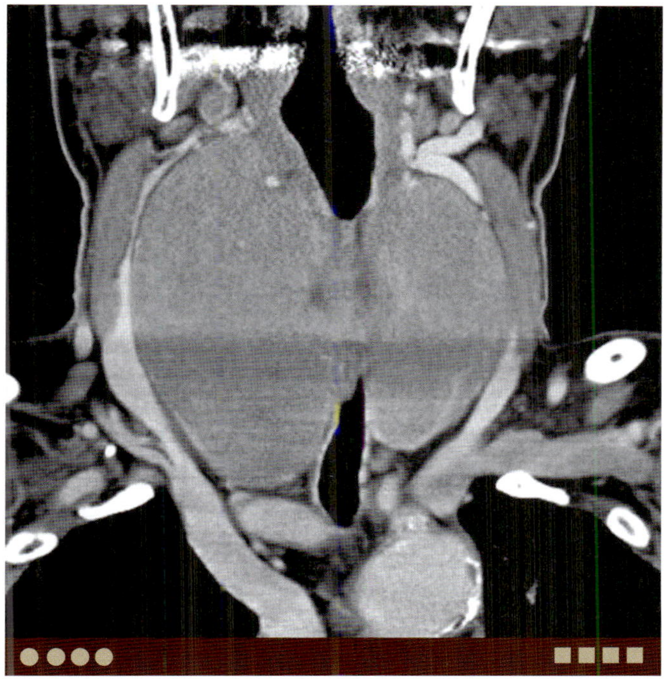

C. Hashimoto thyroiditis, same patient as A. Coronal contrast-enhanced CT demonstrates minimal enhancement of the significantly enlarged thyroid glands.

DIFFERENTIAL DIAGNOSIS IMAGES (D-G)

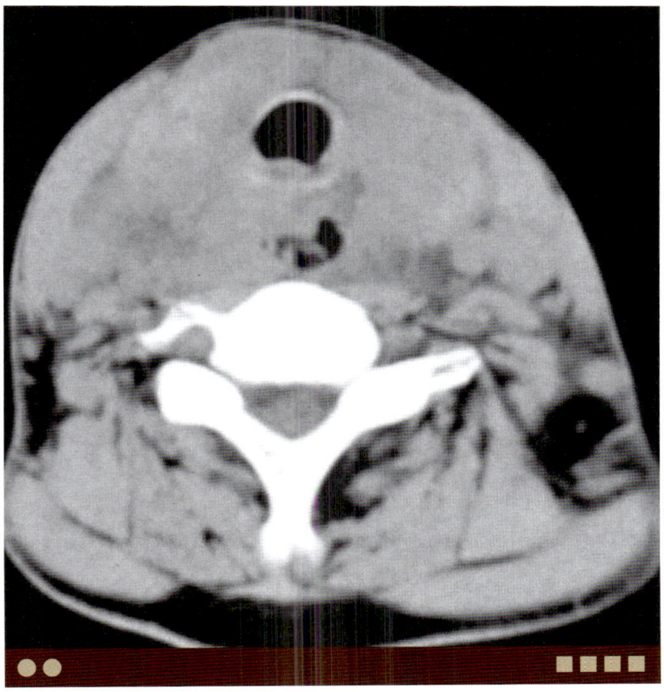

D. Lymphoma from Hashimoto thyroiditis. Axial noncontrast CT demonstrates enlarged thyroid glands displacing the trachea anteriorly and carotid vessels laterally. Note poorly defined margins of the thyroid glands.

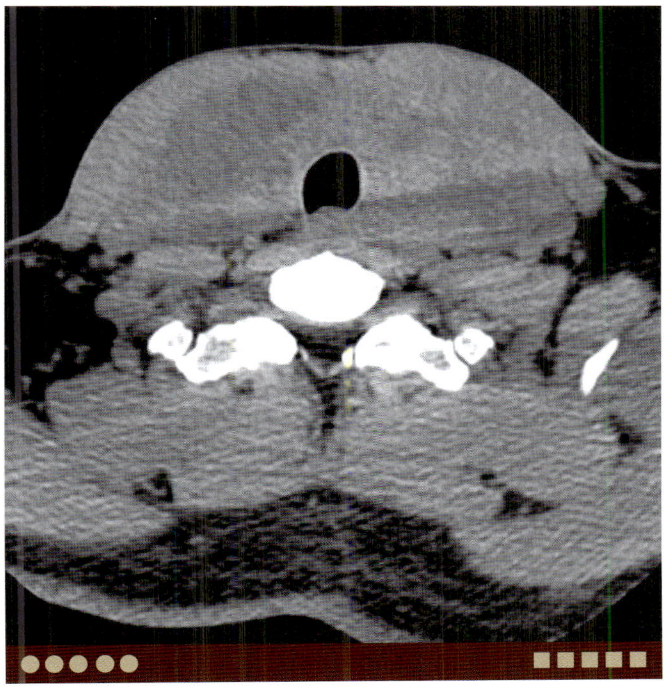

E. Goiter. Axial noncontrast CT demonstrates more cystic degeneration in the right lobe of the thyroid gland. No invasive change is seen despite significant mass effect to the adjacent structures.

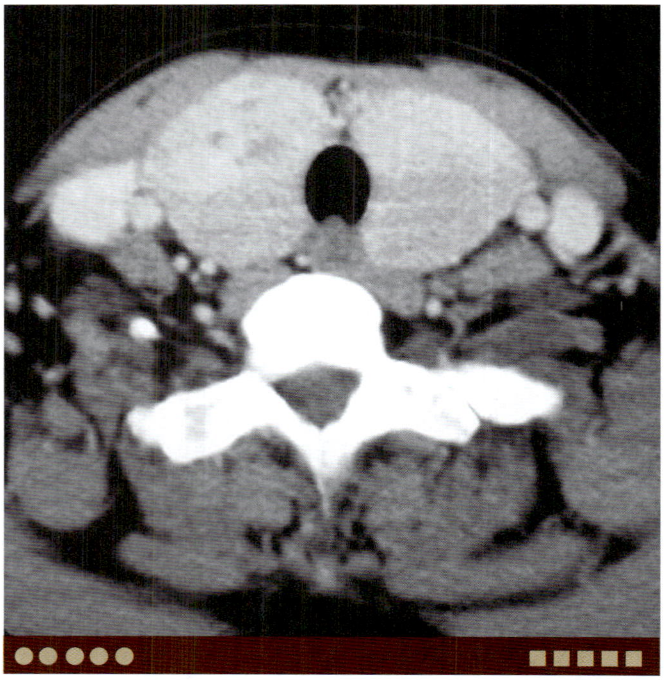

F. Goiter in a different patient. Axial contrast-enhanced CT demonstrates diffuse enhancement of the enlarged thyroid glands with slight heterogeneity.

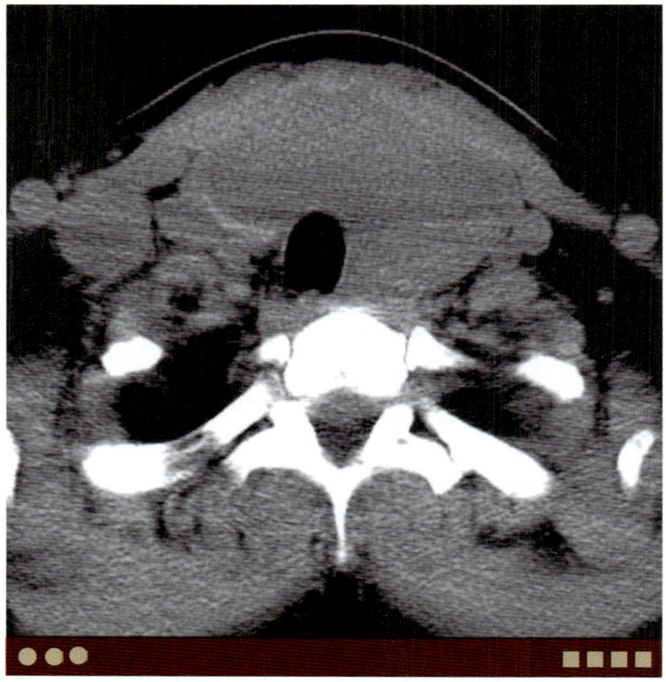

G. Poorly differentiated follicular thyroid carcinoma. Axial noncontrast CT demonstrates significantly enlarged left lobe of the thyroid.

Case 11–18 Thymic Cyst

Memi Watanabe, Hiroki Kato, Benjamin Ludwig, Osamu Sakai

PRESENTATION

Anterior lower neck mass or incidental imaging finding.

FINDINGS

CT and MRI demonstrate a cystic mass in the anterior neck extending into the mediastinum.

DIFFERENTIAL DIAGNOSIS

- Thymoma: This may present a well-circumscribed soft tissue mass in the anterior mediastinum, and may be indistinguishable from complex thymic cyst on CT. MRI may be useful in differentiating between the two. A thymoma shows signal intensity similar to that of normal thymic tissue, and contrast-enhanced MR images may demonstrate enhancing solid components.
- Teratoma: Cystic teratoma may mimic a thymic cyst; however, a teratoma includes complex components and contains soft tissue, fat, and calcification.
- Thyroid cyst: Cystic lesions in the thyroid gland are relatively common. Cysts may contain thymoglobulin and proteinaceous materials and show high attenuation on CT and increased T1 signal on MRI.
- Lymphatic malformation (lymphangioma): This is more common in the posterior neck and axilla, however, may be seen in the anterior neck and extend into the mediastinum. This can be uni- or multilocular, and CT typically demonstrates homogeneous low attenuation. Increased or heterogeneous attenuation may result from superimposed infection or hemorrhage.
- Parathyroid cyst: Parathyroid cysts can occur anywhere from the angle of the mandible down to the mediastinum, although they most commonly arise in the inferior parathyroid glands.

COMMENTS

Thymic cysts are uncommon, and may be congenital or acquired. Congenital thymic cysts arise from a persistent remnant of the thymopharyngeal duct. They may arise anywhere along the path of the duct, found immediately adjacent to the carotid sheath from the angle of the mandible to the level of diaphragm. Cysts may present as slowly enlarging, painless masses, either superficial or deep to the sternocleidomastoid muscle. They are often asymptomatic and discovered incidentally on imaging. Congenital thymic cysts are typically unilocular and contain serous fluid. CT demonstrates a well-defined, thin-walled cyst with simple fluid attenuation.

Acquired thymic cysts are associated with degeneration of the Hassall corpuscles within the thymus. Cysts may be seen in the setting of both HIV and Hodgkin lymphoma.

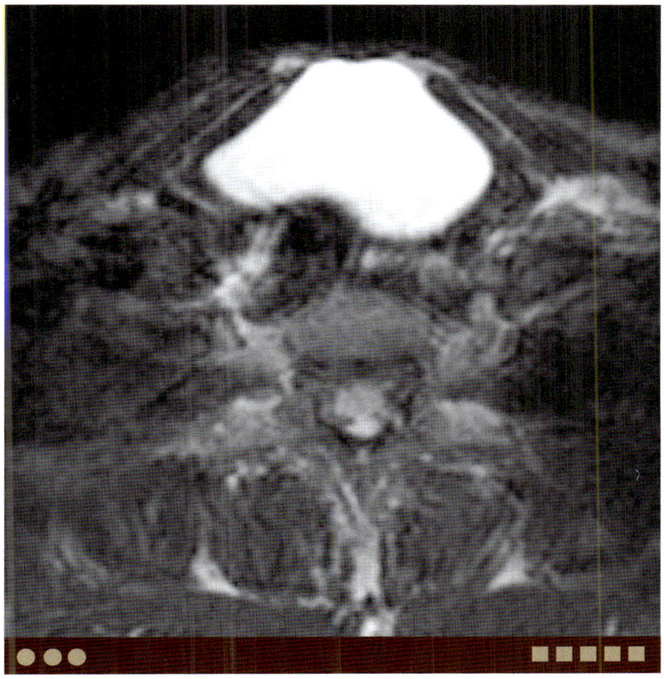

A. Thymic cyst. Axial fat-suppressed T2W image demonstrates a unilocular cystic mass with high-signal intensity at the thoracic inlet.

Acquired thymic cysts can be uni- or multilocular, and often contain hemorrhage or mucin. This results in increased attenuation/signal intensity within the cysts, and may lead to difficulty in differentiation from solid masses. Calcification of cyst wall can be seen.

MRI is useful in differentiating between complex thymic cysts and other neck masses. While MR images may demonstrate a cystic mass with fluid signal intensity, if hemorrhage or infection occurs, the cyst may demonstrate high-signal intensity on both T1W and T2W images, as well as a fluid–fluid level. Contrast-enhanced MRI typically demonstrates a thin wall in thymic cysts, whereas cystic thymomas or teratomas contain enhancing solid components.

PEARLS

- **Thymic cysts can be congenital or acquired.**
- **CT demonstrates either unilocular or multilocular cystic mass with simple fluid attenuation. However, infectious or mucin-containing thymic cyst may demonstrate high attenuation on CT, and may be indistinguishable from other cystic or solid masses, such as thymoma.**
- **MRI demonstrates a cystic mass with fluid signal intensity, or high-signal intensity on T1W images due to hemorrhage or mucinous content. Contract-enhanced MR images may aid in differentiation from cystic thymoma or other cystic masses.**

ADDITIONAL IMAGES (B-C)

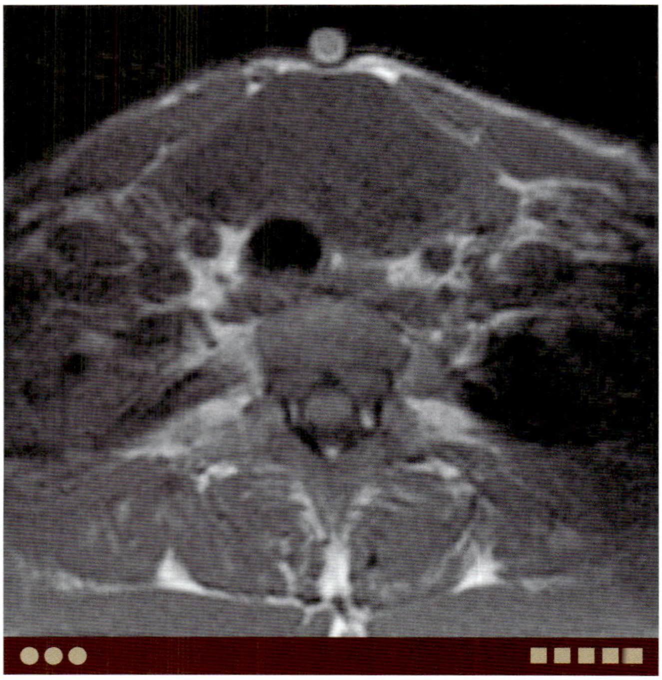

B. Thymic cyst, same patient as A. Axial T1W image demonstrates a low-signal intensity mass, which displaces the trachea.

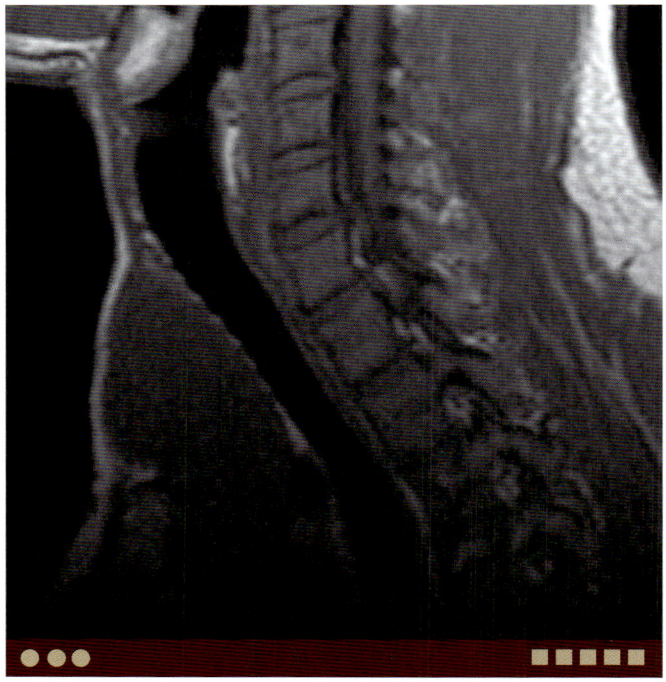

C. Thymic cyst, same patient as A. Sagittal T1W image demonstrates a lower cervical cystic mass extending to the thoracic inlet.

DIFFERENTIAL DIAGNOSIS IMAGES (D-G)

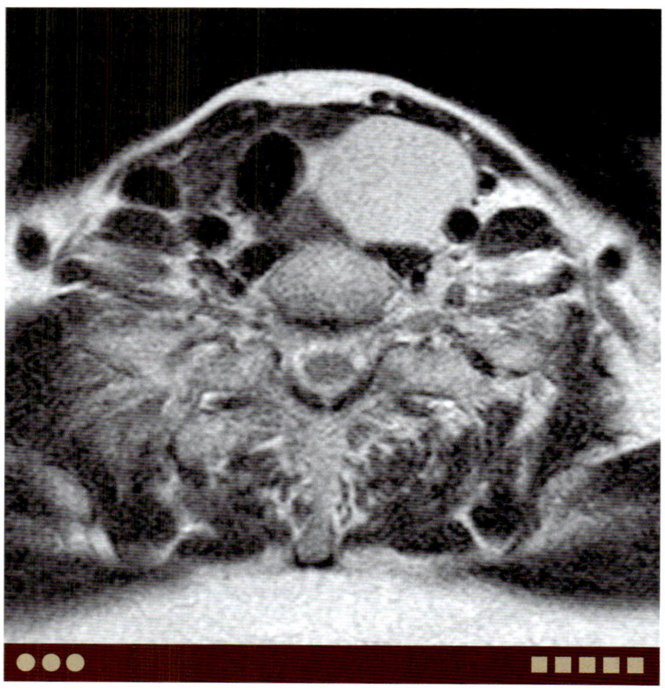

D. Parathyroid cyst. Axial T2W image demonstrates a homogeneous fluid signal intensity lesion inferior to the thyroid gland

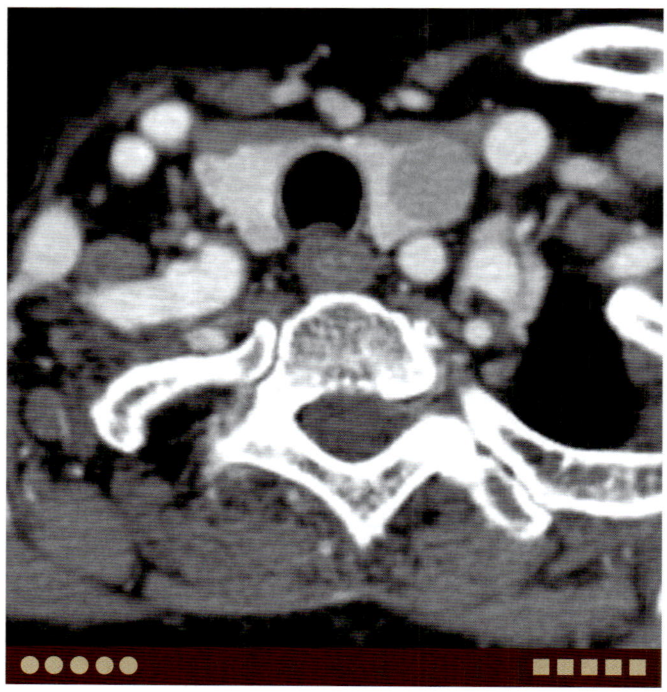

E. Thyroid cyst. Axial contrast-enhanced CT demonstrates a cystic lesion in the left lobe of the thyroid gland.

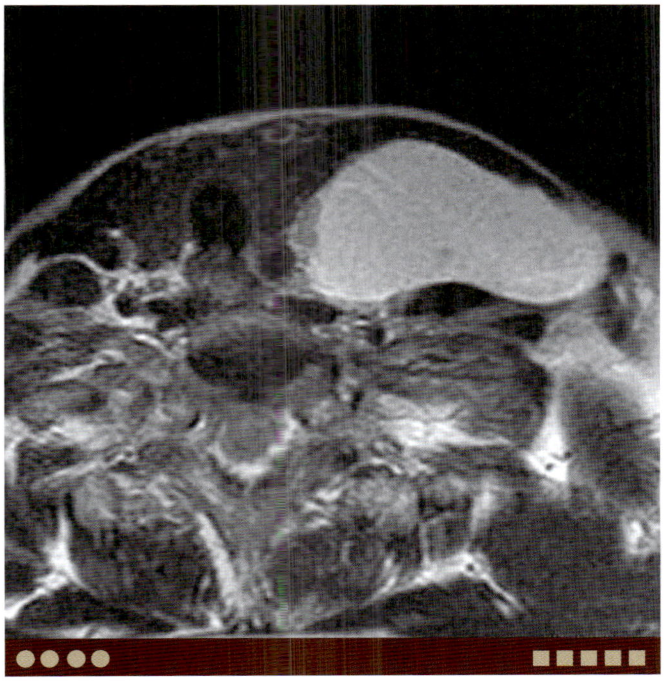

F. Lymphatic malformation. Axial T2W image demonstrates a cystic lesion displacing the thyroid and other adjacent structures in the left lower neck.

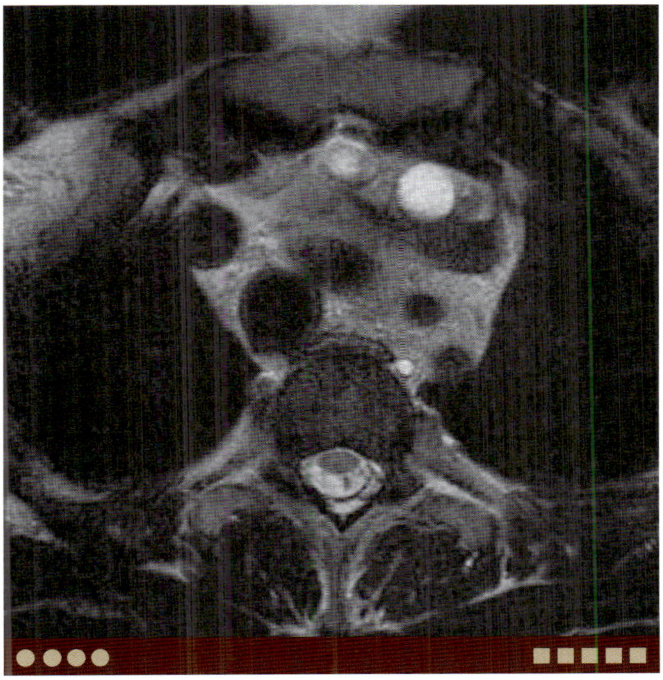

G. Cystic nodal metastasis from papillary thyroid carcinoma. Axial T2W image demonstrates a cystic lesion in the left anterior mediastinum.

Case 11–19 Schwannoma: Brachial Plexus

Hiroki Kato, Asim Mian, Osamu Sakai

PRESENTATION

Palpable neck mass with tenderness and pain radiating to the arm along the distribution of the affected nerve.

FINDINGS

MRI demonstrates an elongated, well-defined, smoothly marginated lesion along a brachial plexus nerve root.

DIFFERENTIAL DIAGNOSIS

- Neurofibroma: Neurofibroma is the second most common tumor arising from the brachial plexus. "Target sign," central low signal on T2W images is often seen; however, presence of the target sign does not differentiate neurofibroma from schwannoma completely.
- Lymphoma: Lymphoma can arise anywhere in the head and neck but often from the Waldeyer ring, orbit, nasal cavity, paranasal sinuses, thyroid gland, and salivary glands. CT and MRI demonstrate a homogeneous lesion.
- Lymph node metastasis: Nodal metastasis in the lower neck or supraclavicular fossa predominantly occurs in patients with malignancies in the lung, breast, head, and neck.
- Pancoast tumor (superior sulcus tumor): The brachial plexus is not uncommonly involved by malignant tumors of the lung apex.

COMMENTS

This is a 52-year-old man with slowly progressive pain radiating down the arm.

Neurogenic tumors arising from the brachial plexus are rare. Histological diagnoses of the primary brachial plexus neurogenic tumors include schwannoma, neurofibroma, and malignant peripheral nerve sheath tumor with schwannoma being the most common. The most common benign nonneurogenic tumor to involve the brachial plexus is aggressive fibromatosis (extra-abdominal desmoid tumor). Malignant nonneurogenic tumors involving the brachial plexus include primary soft tissue sarcomas, such as low-grade fibrosarcoma, synovial sarcoma, and radiation-induced sarcoma. Presenting signs and symptoms of the brachial plexus tumors include palpable mass, numbness/paresthesias, radiating pain, local pain, and weakness.

Radiography is usually normal unless the tumor has extended into the neural foramen, when it may cause well-defined bony remodeling/erosion and foraminal enlargement. MRI is the most useful modality for diagnoses of brachial plexus schwannoma. Typical MRI features of benign neurogenic tumors include a well-defined, ovoid-shaped mass with the long axis in line with the nerve of origin. The brachial plexus and proximal nerves run between the anterior and middle scalene muscles and axial images are useful to identify the lesion and its relationship to the nerve. CT and MRI findings of schwannomas have been described as a well-circumscribed, heterogeneous mass which can be explained by cellularity and histological features; hypocellular regions (Antoni type B), more cellular regions (Antoni type A), and cystic degeneration. Occasionally, target sign is observed depending on the distribution of Antoni types A and B areas within the tumor.

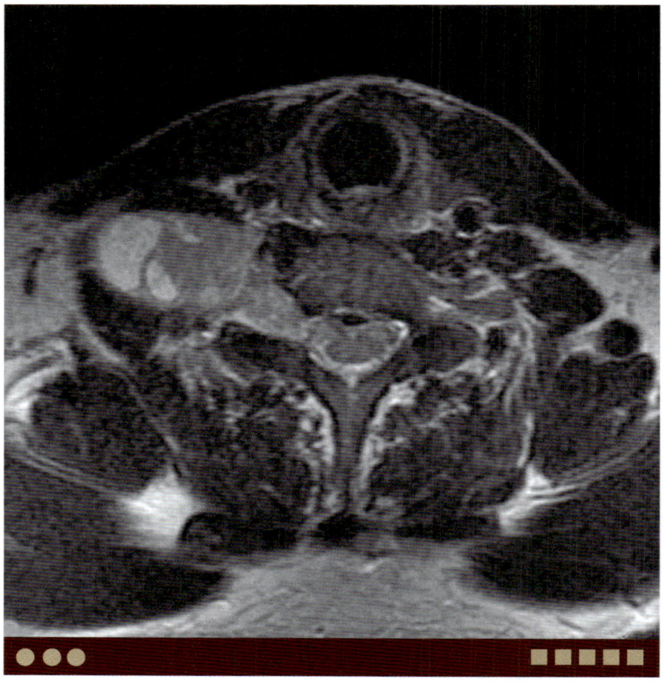

A. Brachial plexus schwannoma. Axial T2W MR image demonstrates a ovoid-shaped heterogeneous signal lesion between the anterior and middle scalene muscles. Note widening of the right neural foramen.

PEARLS

- **Schwannoma is the most common tumor associated with the brachial plexus.**
- **Brachial plexus schwannoma is located between the anterior and middle scalene muscles.**
- **The differentiation between schwannoma and neurofibroma is often difficult.**

ADDITIONAL IMAGES (B-E)

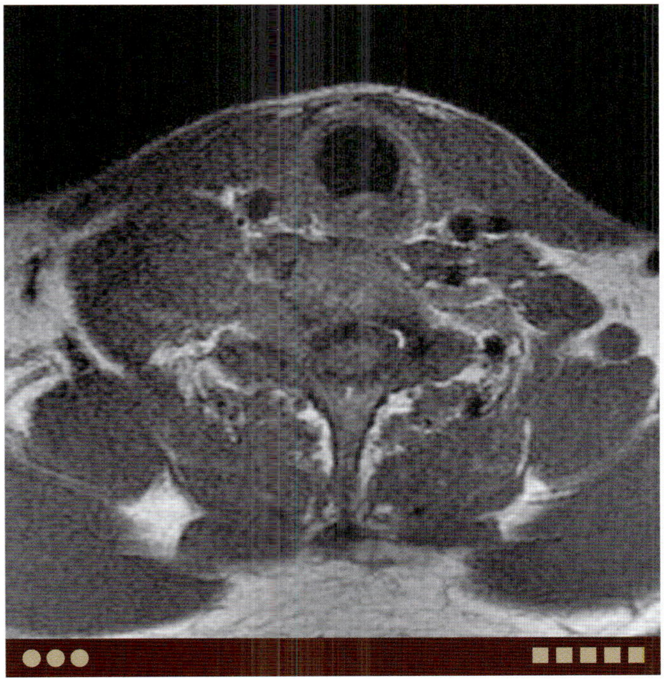

B. Brachial plexus schwannoma, same patient as A. Axial T1W MR image demonstrates low-signal intensity.

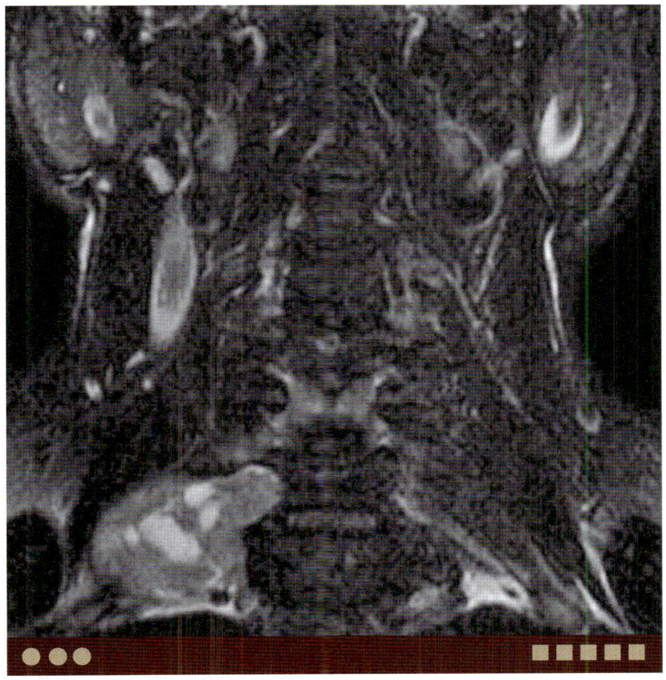

C. Brachial plexus schwannoma, same patient as A. Coronal fat-suppressed T2W image demonstrates a well-demarcated heterogeneous lesion with thickened proximal nerve.

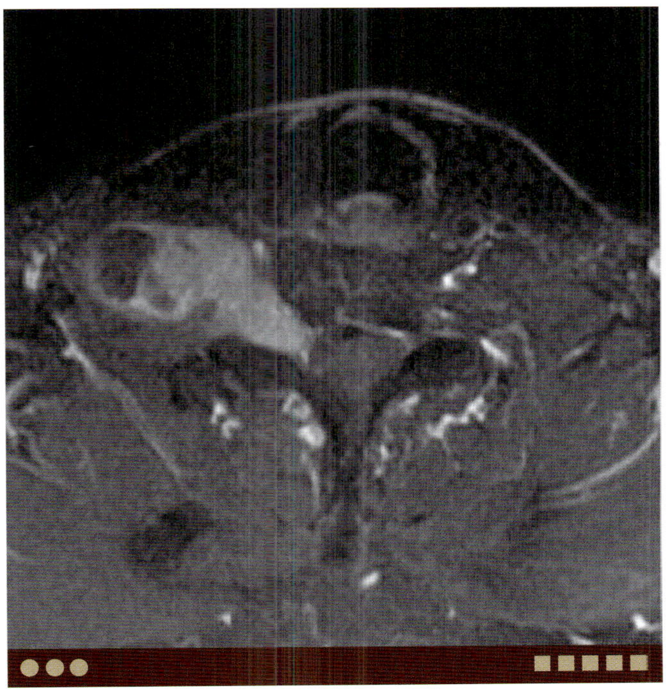

D. Brachial plexus schwannoma, same patient as A. Axial post-contrast fat-suppressed T1W image demonstrates a heterogeneously enhancing lesion with cystic degeneration.

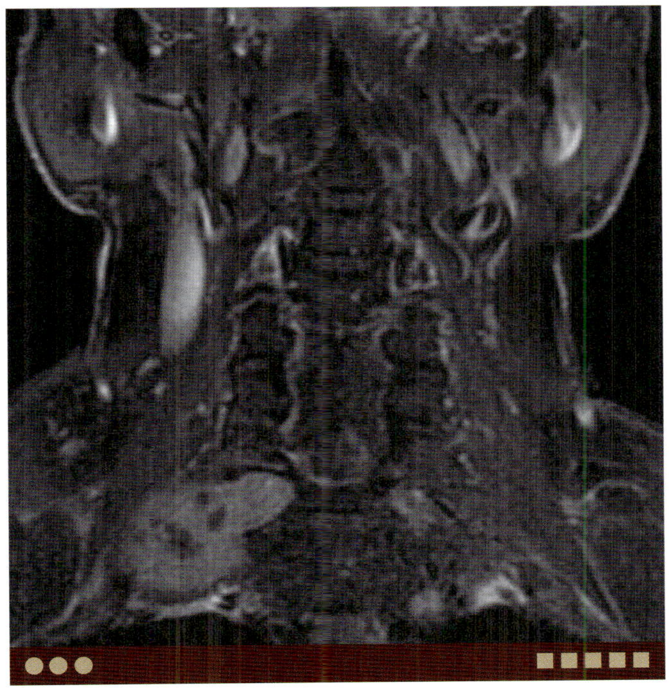

E. Brachial plexus schwannoma, same patient as A. Coronal post-contrast fat-suppressed T1W image demonstrates heterogeneously enhancing lesion with widening of the neural foramen.

DIFFERENTIAL DIAGNOSIS IMAGES (F-I)

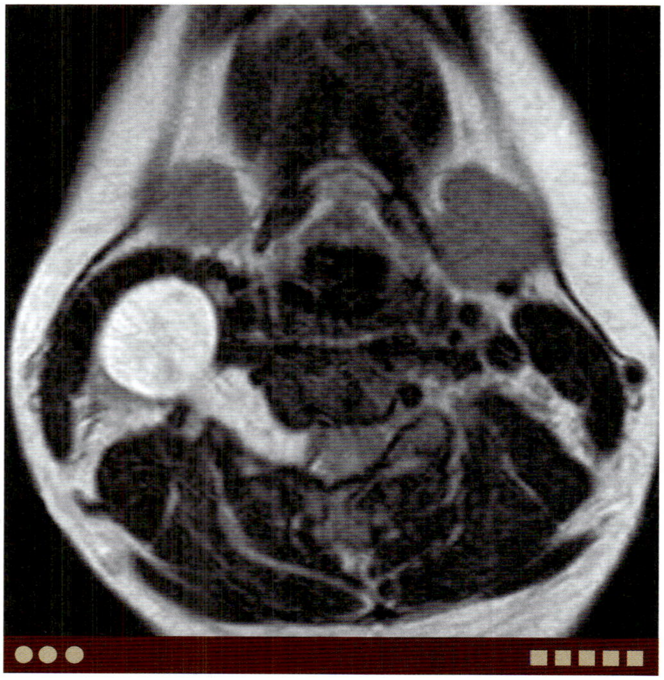

F. Brachial plexus neurofibroma. Axial T2W MR image demonstrates a well-demarcated high-signal lesion extending into the neural foramen, which is widened by the lesion.

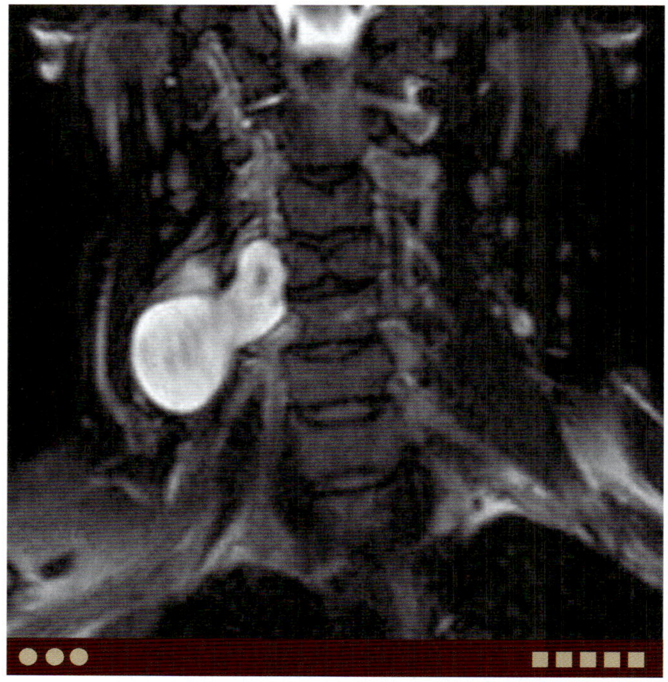

G. Brachial plexus neurofibroma, same patient as F. Coronal fat-suppressed T2W image demonstrates the "target sign," a hyperintense lesion with inhomogeneous central low signal.

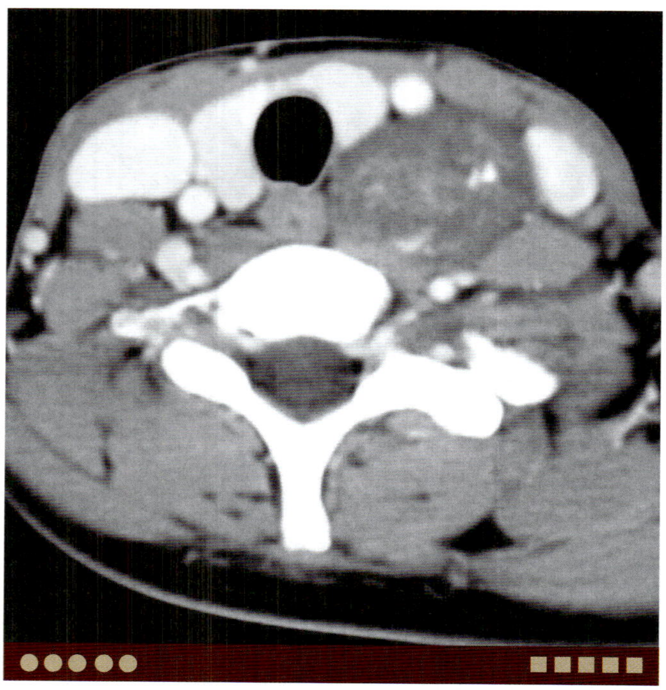

H. Schwannoma from the vagus nerve. Axial contrast-enhanced CT demonstrates a slightly heterogeneously enhancing tumor, posterolateral to the common carotid artery, medial to the internal jugular vein, and anteromedial to the anterior scalene muscle.

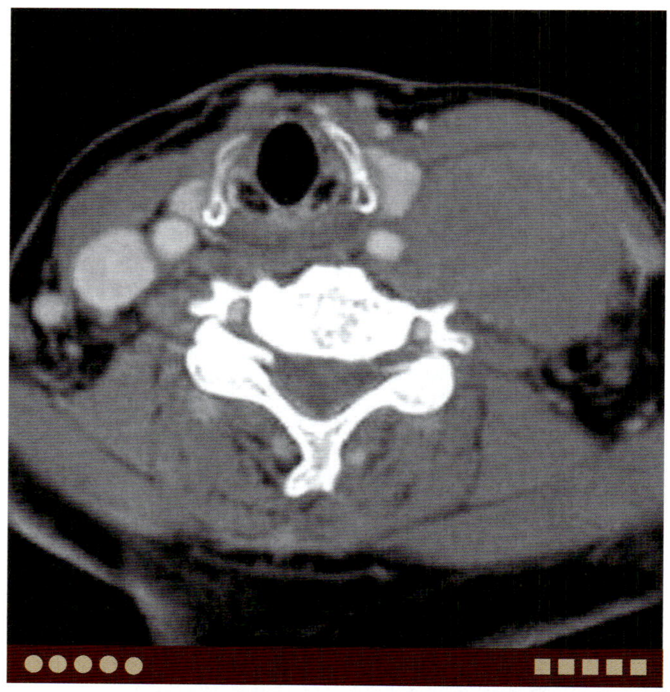

I. Diffuse large B-cell lymphoma. Axial contrast-enhanced CT demonstrates a homogeneous soft tissue mass anterior to the anterior scalene muscle.

Case 11–20 Graves Disease

Hiroki Kato, Asim Mian, Osamu Sakai

PRESENTATION

Hyperthyroidism.

FINDINGS

CT demonstrates the enlarged thyroid glands to have diffusely decreased density.

DIFFERENTIAL DIAGNOSIS

- Subacute thyroiditis: Subacute thyroiditis is a destructive thyroiditis and thyrotoxic condition. Radioiodine uptake is low, often less than 1%, reflecting thyrotoxicosis due to a discharge of preformed stores of thyroid hormone and suppressed adjacent normal thyroid tissue.
- Hashimoto thyroiditis: Hashimoto thyroiditis is characterized by autoimmune destruction of thyroid parenchyma. Thyroid scintigraphy demonstrates either increased or decreased uptake. If thyroid parenchyma is replaced by fibrous tissue, heterogeneously decreased uptake can be seen.
- Silent thyroiditis: Silent thyroiditis is initially described as a painless variant of subacute thyroiditis, however, recently considered a variant form of Hashimoto thyroiditis. This manifests as transient thyrotoxicosis followed by transient hypothyroidism. As with subacute thyroiditis, thyroid scintigraphy shows minimal uptake due to the damage of follicular cells.

COMMENTS

This is a 32-year-old woman with an enlarged thyroid gland, sweating, and palpitations.

Graves disease is the most common form of hyperthyroidism and often triggered by an infection or physical or emotional stress. This is an autoimmune disorder caused by antibodies against the thyrotropin (TSH) receptors on the cell surface of the thyroid follicle. Serum thyroid hormone levels are elevated and the pituitary TSH level is appropriately suppressed. Graves disease causes inflammation of the orbit, including extraocular muscles swelling and increase of retrobulbar fat resulting in exophthalmos and swelling of periorbital soft tissues (Graves ophthalmopathy). Rarely, patients with Graves disease develop a lumpy reddish thickening of the skin in front of the shins known as pretibial myxedema (Graves dermopathy).

Thyroid scintigraphy demonstrates diffusely enlarged thyroid and increased uptake due to both increased stimulation and function. In patients with Graves disease, the pyramidal lobe is often visualized, which is usually not seen in normal patients owing to its relatively small size. In a patient with thyrotoxicosis homogeneously increased uptake throughout the thyroid gland, especially with a visible pyramidal lobe, is highly suggestive of Graves disease.

Unenhanced CT demonstrates the enlarged thyroid glands with a lower than normal attenuation, reflecting decreased iodine concentration even though there is an overall increase in the iodine content of the gland. Even after treatment, the attenuation of the thyroid gland may not return to normal.

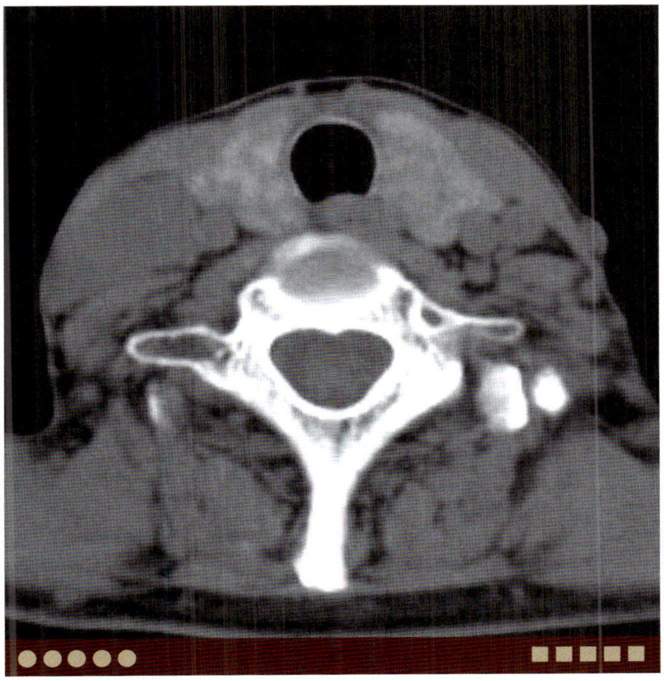

A. Graves disease. Axial unenhanced CT demonstrates diffuse swelling and decreased attenuation of the bilateral thyroid glands.

PEARLS

- **Graves disease is the most common form of hyperthyroidism and often triggered by an infection or physical or emotional stress.**
- **Thyroid scintigraphy demonstrates the enlarged thyroid glands and homogeneously increased uptake, often with a visible pyramidal lobe.**
- **CT demonstrates enlarged thyroid glands with low attenuation.**

ADDITIONAL IMAGE

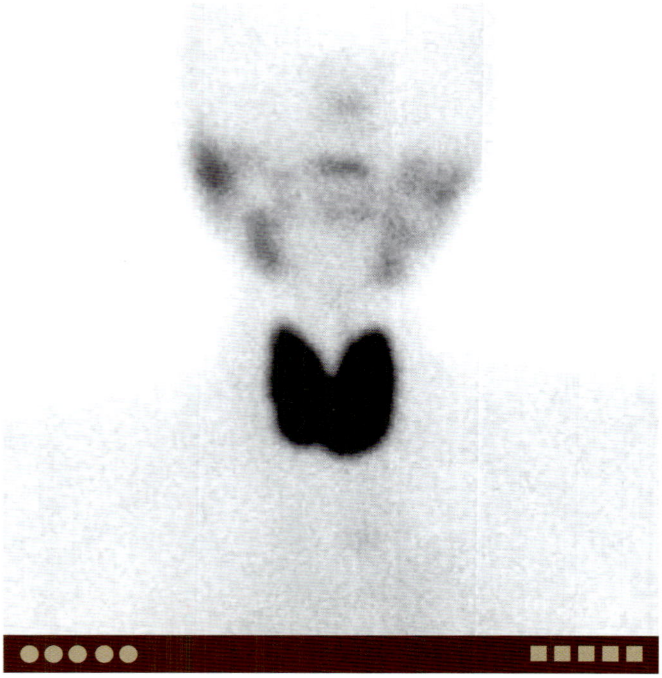

B. Graves disease, same patient as A. 99mTc-pertechnetate scintigraphy demonstrates markedly increased activity in the bilateral thyroid glands.

DIFFERENTIAL DIAGNOSIS IMAGES (C-G)

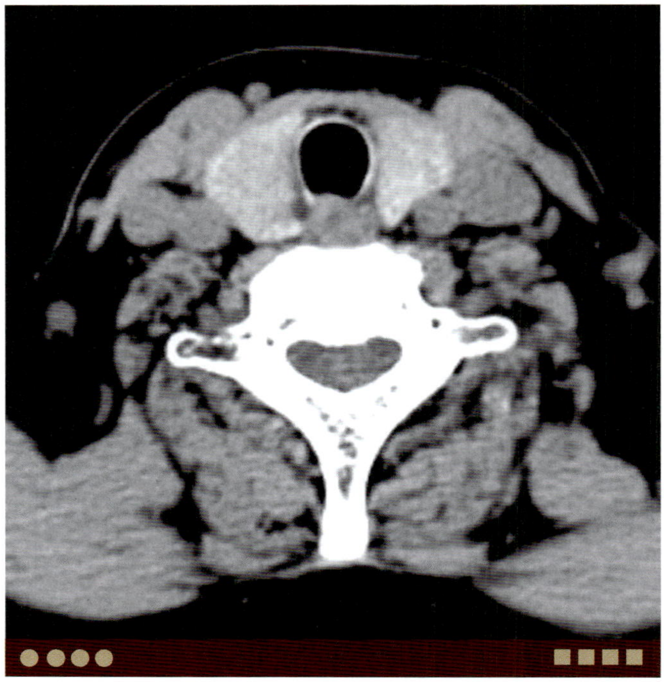

C. Hashimoto thyroiditis. Axial unenhanced CT demonstrates mild swelling and mildly decreased density of the bilateral thyroid glands.

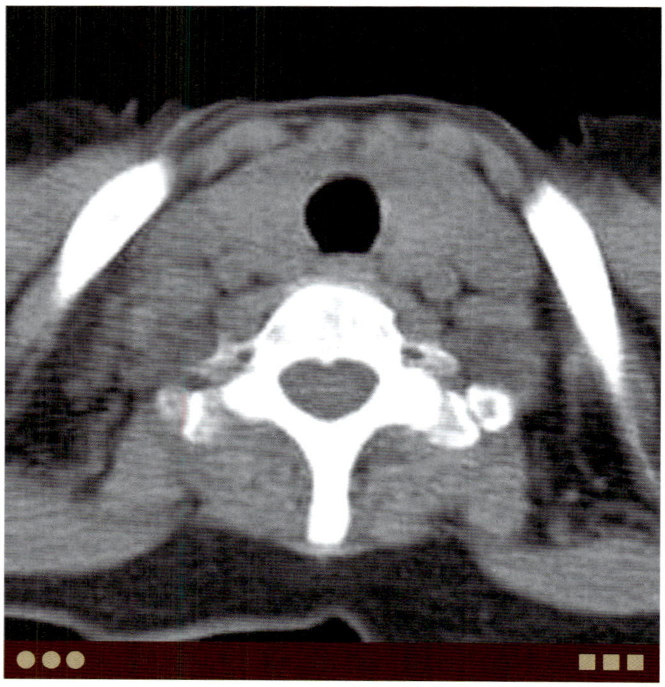

D. Silent/painless thyroiditis. Axial unenhanced CT demonstrates diffusely decreased attenuation of the bilateral thyroid glands.

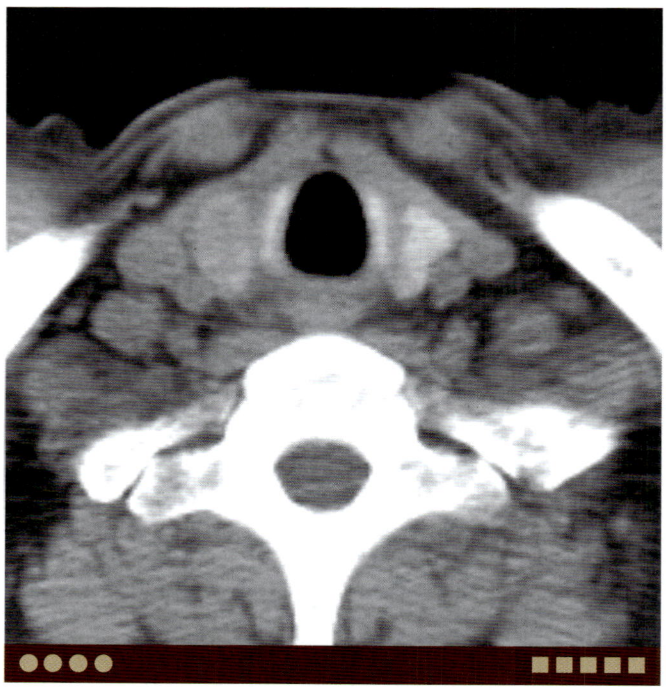

E. Subacute thyroiditis. Axial enhanced CT demonstrates a hypodense region in the right lobe of the thyroid gland.

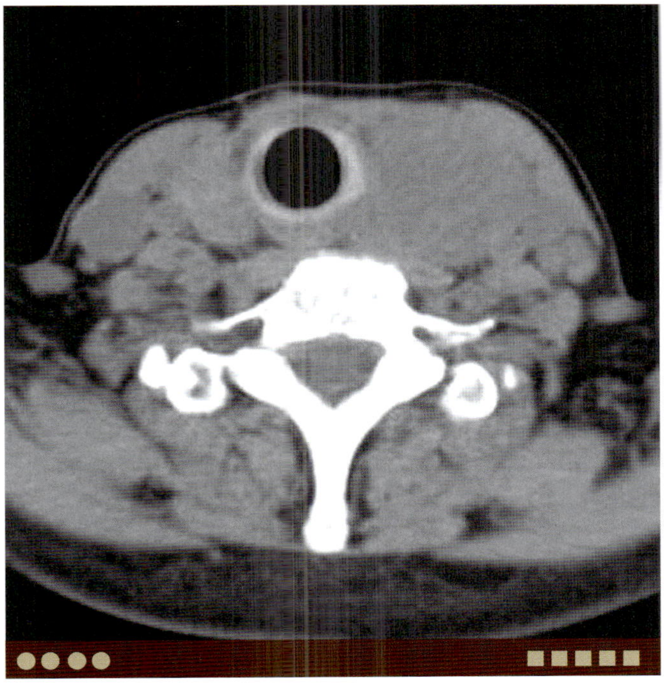

F. Diffuse large B-cell lymphoma. Axial unenhanced CT demonstrates a large hypodense lesion in the left lobe of the thyroid gland.

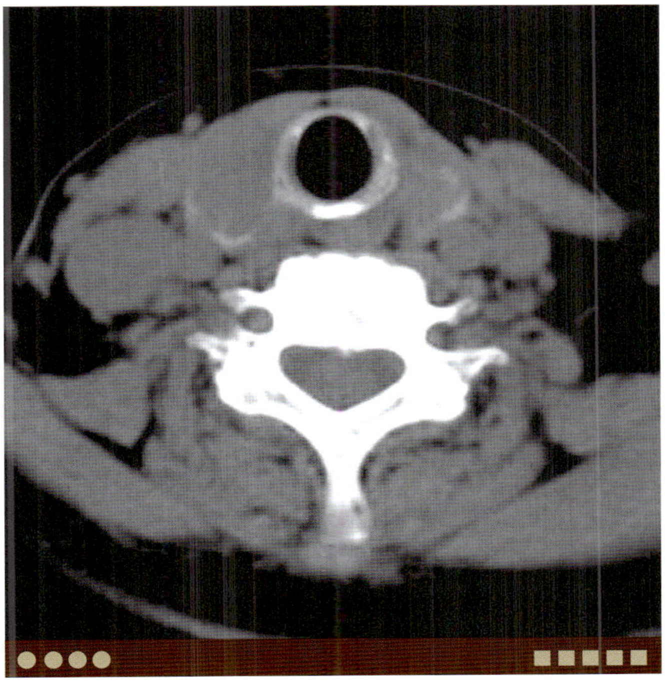

G. MALT lymphoma. Axial unenhanced CT demonstrates hypodense lesions in the bilateral thyroid glands.

Case 11-21 Parathyroid Carcinoma

Hiroki Kato, Asim Mian, Osamu Sakai

PRESENTATION

Various clinical manifestations of hyperparathyroidism with some patients being totally asymptomatic.

FINDINGS

CT and MRI demonstrate an invasive lesion located posterior to the thyroid gland.

DIFFERENTIAL DIAGNOSIS

- Parathyroid adenoma: Parathyroid adenomas show low signal on T1W and high signal on T2W images. Contrast-enhanced CT and MRI demonstrate a well-circumscribed, enhancing lesion in the characteristic location of parathyroid glands which is posterior to the thyroid gland.
- Parathyroid hyperplasia: Parathyroid hyperplasia may be associated with familial hyperparathyroidism or multiple endocrine neoplasia (MEN) syndromes. Parathyroid hyperplasia typically involves multiple parathyroid glands and is difficult to evaluate by any imaging modality due to the small size of the hyperplastic glands.
- Parathyroid cyst: Cystic lesions of the parathyroid gland can be either nonfunctioning or functioning. Functioning cystic lesions in patients with hyperparathyroidism may represent cystic degeneration within an adenoma or hyperplastic gland.

COMMENTS

This is a 38-year-old man with primary hyperparathyroidism. Serum calcium and serum parathyroid hormone (PTH) levels are elevated and serum phosphate level is decreased.

Hyperparathyroidism is diagnosed by biological tests which reveal high serum calcium or low serum phosphate levels, but direct measurement of PTH is currently performed routinely. The causes of hyperparathyroidism include a solitary parathyroid adenoma (75%-85%), parathyroid hyperplasia (10%-15%), and multiple parathyroid adenomas (2%-3%). Other rare causes include parathyroid carcinoma and parathyroid cyst. Although parathyroid carcinoma is an unusual cause of hyperparathyroidism, hyperparathyroidism accounts for clinical presentation of approximately 85% of all parathyroid carcinomas. Various clinical manifestations of hyperparathyroidism such as general malaise, urinary calculus, peptic ulceration, mental depression, and bone changes are seen in patients with parathyroid carcinomas. However, some patients may be totally asymptomatic and diagnosed on routine blood tests.

Clinical and imaging appearance of parathyroid carcinoma may be similar to adenoma. It is important to assess any invasion of adjacent structures and immobility of the abnormal gland on swallowing, which should raise the possibility of malignant nature of the lesion. Regional cervical and mediastinal nodal metastases may occur in up to one-third of patients and distant metastases (liver, lung bone) in approximately 25% of patients. In patients suspected for parathyroid carcinomas, preoperative CT or MRI is recommended for surgical planning.

99mTc-sestamibi scintigraphy may be useful to detect parathyroid carcinomas because some carcinomas may take up 99mTc-sestamibi, although it is difficult to distinguish parathyroid carcinoma from parathyroid adenoma by scintigraphy. SPECT is essential to avoid false-negative results in patients with lesions located deep in the neck or ectopic sites.

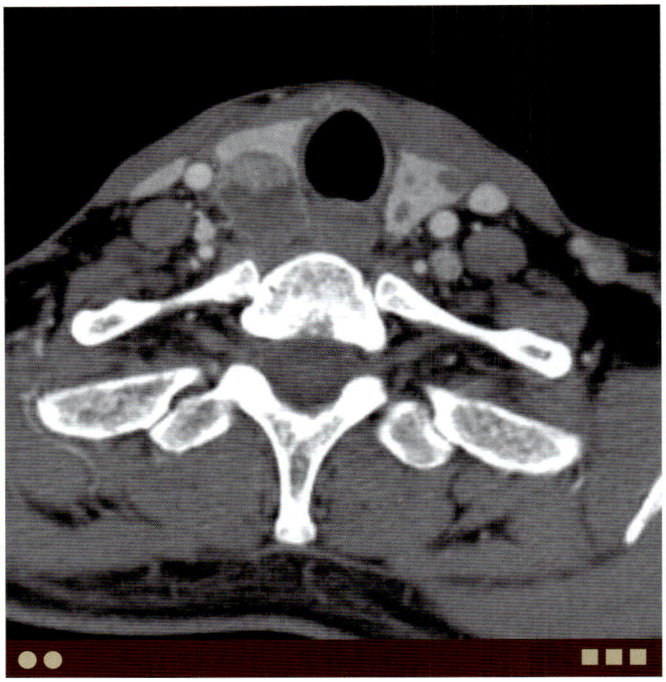

A. Parathyroid carcinoma. Axial enhanced CT demonstrates a partially cystic lesion with a mural nodule, located in the right lower neck, posterior to the right lower pole of the thyroid gland.

PEARLS

- **Imaging findings of parathyroid carcinomas are nonspecific and may be similar to parathyroid adenomas.**
- **Invasion of adjacent tissues, lymph node, or distant metastases distinguishes a parathyroid carcinoma from a parathyroid adenoma.**
- **Some parathyroid carcinomas may demonstrate uptake of 99mTc-sestamibi.**

ADDITIONAL IMAGE

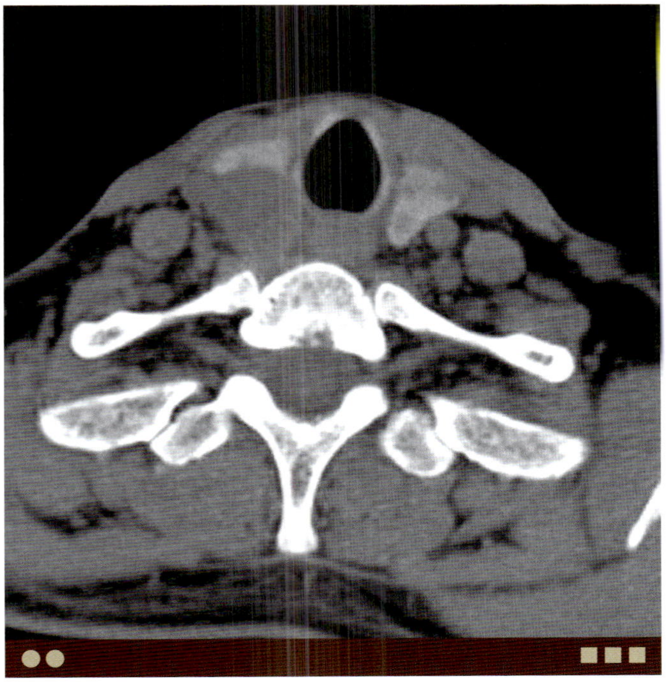

B. Parathyroid carcinoma, same patient as A. Axial unenhanced CT demonstrates a hypodense lesion.

DIFFERENTIAL DIAGNOSIS IMAGES (C-G)

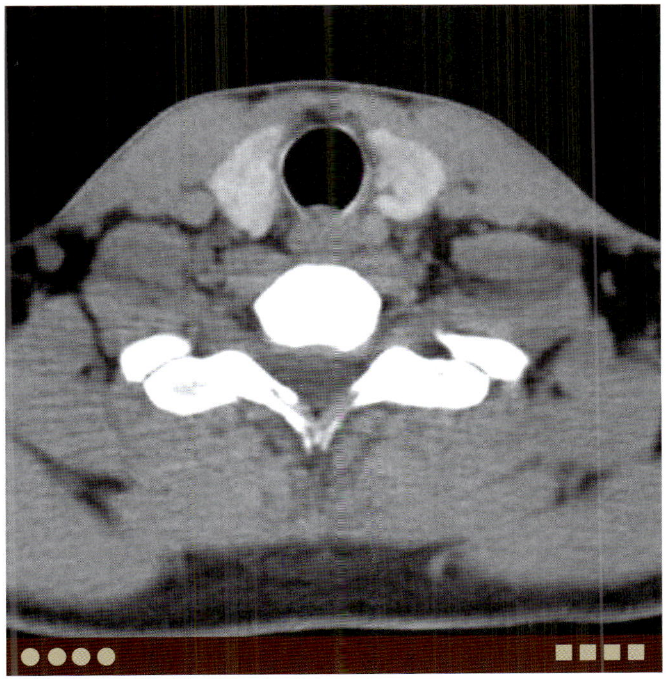

C. Parathyroid adenoma. Axial unenhanced CT demonstrates a hypodense lesion posteromedial to the left upper pole of the thyroid gland.

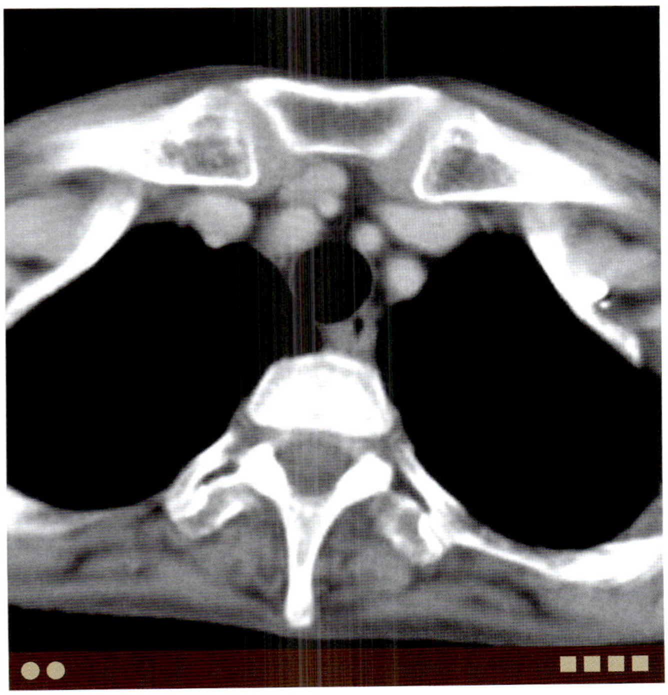

D. Ectopic parathyroid adenoma. Axial unenhanced CT demonstrates an enhanced lesion in the upper mediastinum anterior to the brachiocephalic artery.

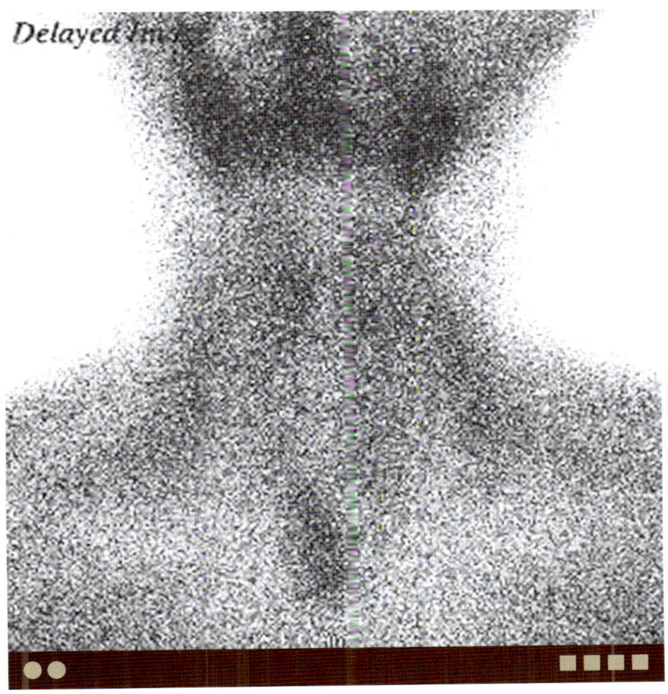

E. Ectopic parathyroid adenoma, same patient as D. 99mTc-sestamibi scintigraphy demonstrates an increased tracer uptake in the upper mediastinum.

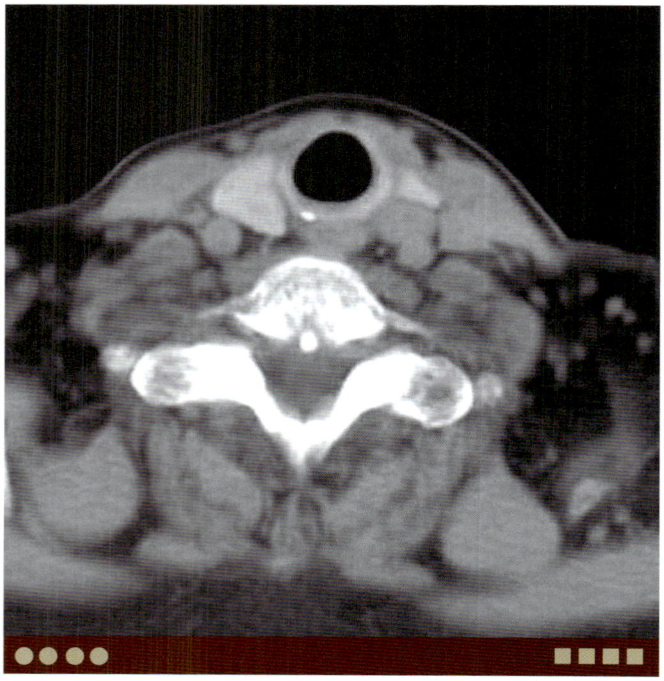

F. Parathyroid hyperplasia. Axial unenhanced CT demonstrates a hypodense lesion posterior to the left upper pole of the thyroid gland.

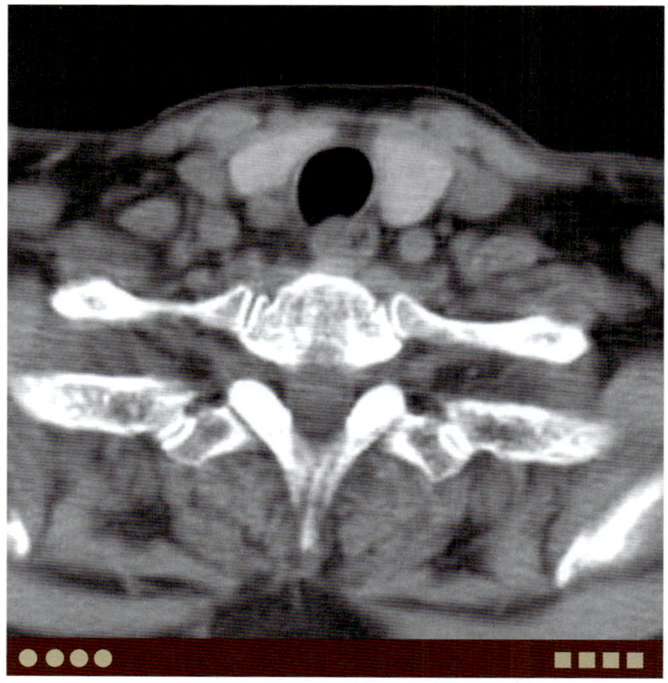

G. Parathyroid hyperplasia, same patient as F. Axial unenhanced CT demonstrates a hypodense lesion posterior to the right lower pole of the thyroid gland.

Case 11–22 Anaplastic Carcinoma: Thyroid

Hiroki Kato, Asim Mian, Osamu Sakai

PRESENTATION

Rapidly enlarging thyroid mass accompanied with symptoms related to mechanical compression, such as hoarseness, dysphagia, dyspnea, vocal cord paralysis, and cervical pain.

FINDINGS

CT and MRI demonstrate a thyroid tumor with aggressive invasion of adjacent structures.

DIFFERENTIAL DIAGNOSIS

- Lymphoma: Lymphoma predominantly occurs in women, particularly in patients with Hashimoto thyroiditis. Clinically detectable rapid growth of the tumor is most commonly seen in anaplastic thyroid carcinoma; however, lymphoma, sarcomas, and high-grade carcinomas may grow rapidly. Aggressive local invasion is also common with lymphoma and sarcomas as well as anaplastic thyroid carcinoma.
- Papillary carcinoma: Papillary carcinoma is a low-grade malignancy, and the most common primary thyroid carcinoma. Microcalcifications are found in 29% to 59% of all primary thyroid carcinomas, most commonly in papillary thyroid carcinoma.
- Adenoma: Thyroid adenomas are true benign neoplasms distinctly separated from the adjacent thyroid tissue by a fibrous capsule. Intratumoral degeneration and hemorrhage may be seen in adenomas and most thyroid cysts represent degeneration of adenoma.

COMMENTS

This is a 75-year-old man with rapidly enlarging thyroid mass and pharyngalgia.

Anaplastic thyroid carcinoma, although rare, is the most aggressive solid tumor characterized by rapid growth and extremely poor prognosis, with a 5-year survival of 5% and a mean survival of 6 months after diagnosis. Other terms of this tumor include undifferentiated, dedifferentiated, and sarcomatoid carcinoma. Local control of disease by surgery and/or external beam radiotherapy is of fundamental importance to improve survival. Ultimately, survival is limited to months and death is often caused by uncontrolled tumor, which is widely metastatic. Anaplastic thyroid carcinoma usually does not concentrate iodine or express thyroglobulin. It is essential to verify the diagnosis histologically because insular thyroid cancer, lymphomas, and medullary thyroid cancer are often similar to anaplastic thyroid carcinoma. Most of anaplastic thyroid carcinomas

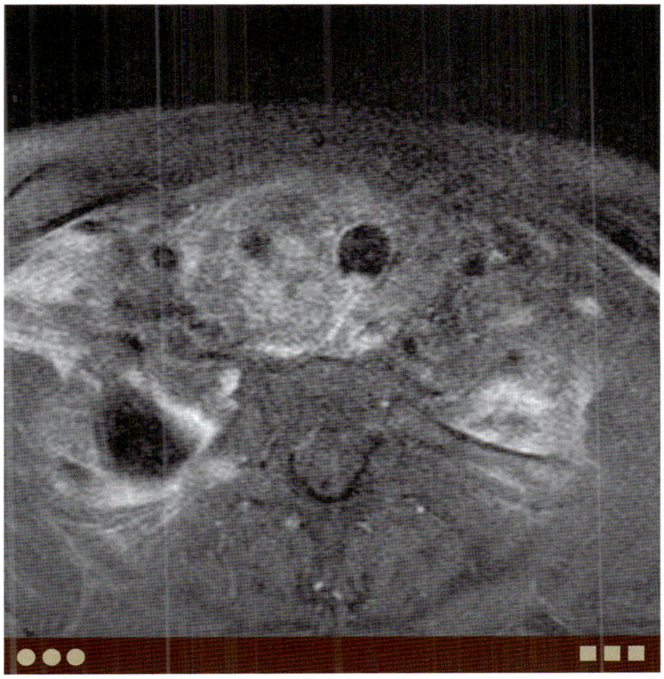

A. Anaplastic thyroid carcinoma. Axial postcontrast fat-suppressed T1W image demonstrates a right thyroid tumor with heterogeneous enhancement.

grow on a preexisting thyroid nodular goiter or on a preexisting differentiated thyroid carcinoma, especially a follicular thyroid tumor.

Anaplastic thyroid carcinoma is often larger than 5 cm. Aggressive local invasion is common, and the surrounding structures (eg, muscles, trachea, esophagus, laryngeal nerve, and larynx) are invaded at the time of diagnosis in most patients. Lymph node metastases are seen in approximately half of the patients. Distant metastases are present in 20% to 50% of cases at the time of diagnosis. The most frequent site of distant metastasis is the lung, followed by bone, skin, and brain.

On ultrasound, they are frequently hypoechoic. On CT, punctuate calcifications and necrosis are frequently present.

PEARLS

- **Anaplastic thyroid carcinoma is the most aggressive solid tumor with local invasion of the surrounding structures.**
- **Lymph node metastases and distant metastases are often seen at the time of diagnosis.**
- **Punctuate calcifications and necroses are frequently observed on CT.**

ADDITIONAL IMAGES (B-E)

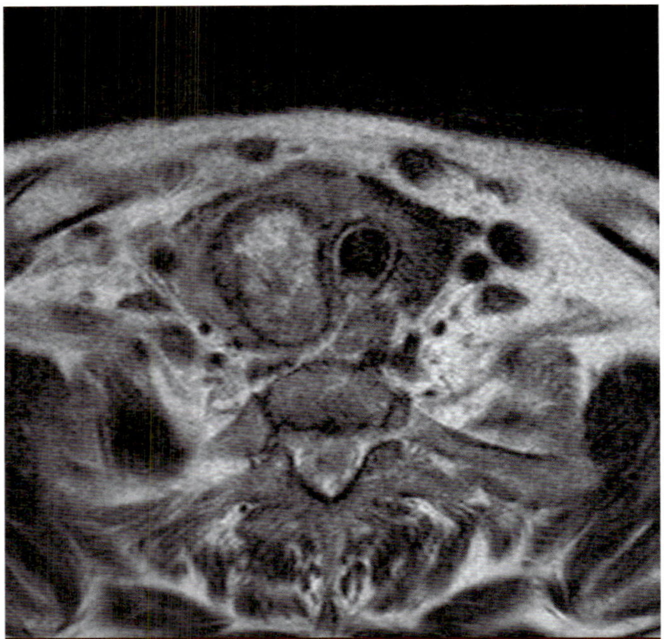

B. Anaplastic thyroid carcinoma, same patient as A. Axial T2W image demonstrates heterogeneous low to high signals within the tumor.

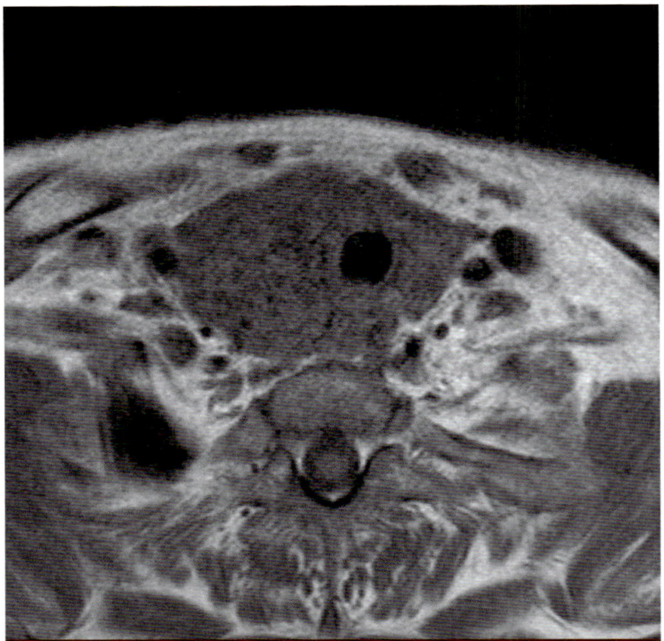

C. Anaplastic thyroid carcinoma, same patient as A. Axial T1W image demonstrates heterogeneous low-signal intensity in the tumor.

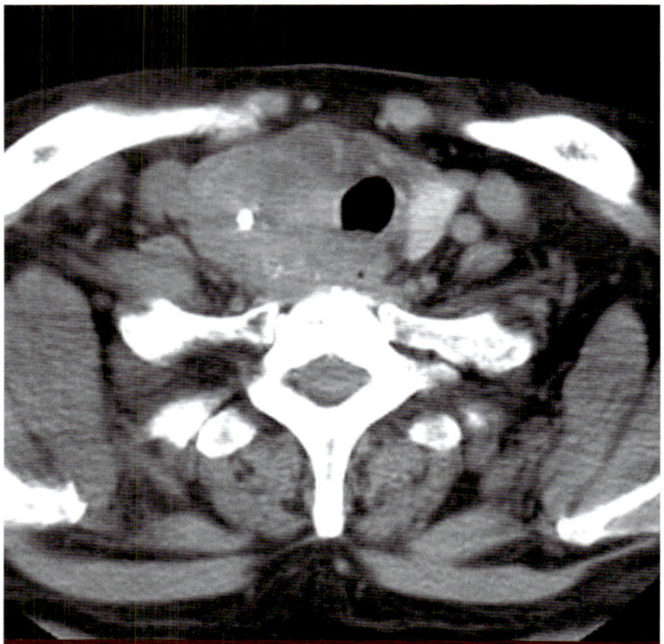

D. Anaplastic thyroid carcinoma, same patient as A. Axial unenhanced CT demonstrates a right thyroid tumor with calcification.

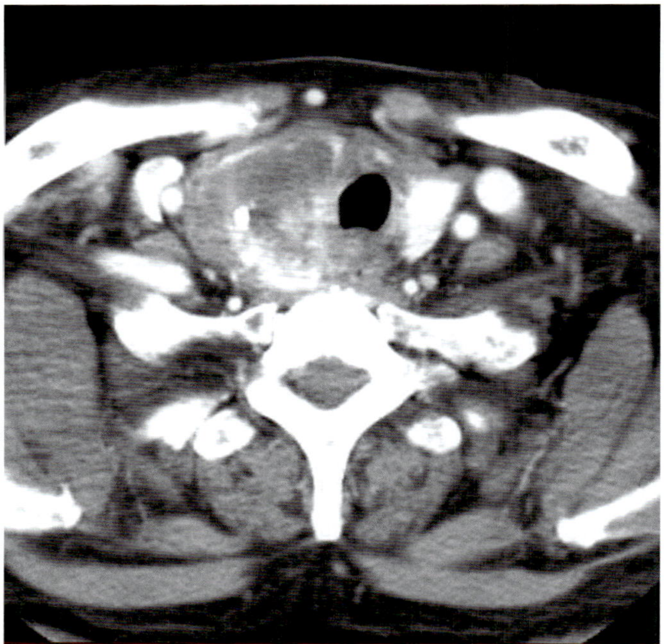

E. Anaplastic thyroid carcinoma, same patient as A. Axial contrast-enhanced CT demonstrates heterogeneous enhancement in the tumor.

DIFFERENTIAL DIAGNOSIS IMAGES (F-I)

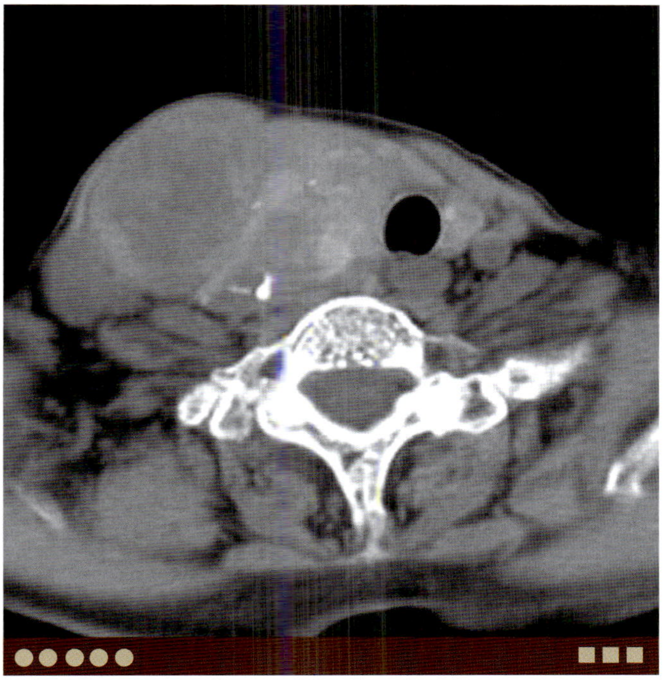

F. Thyroid adenomatous goiter. Axial unenhanced CT demonstrates a large heterogeneous density lesion arising from the thyroid gland with calcification.

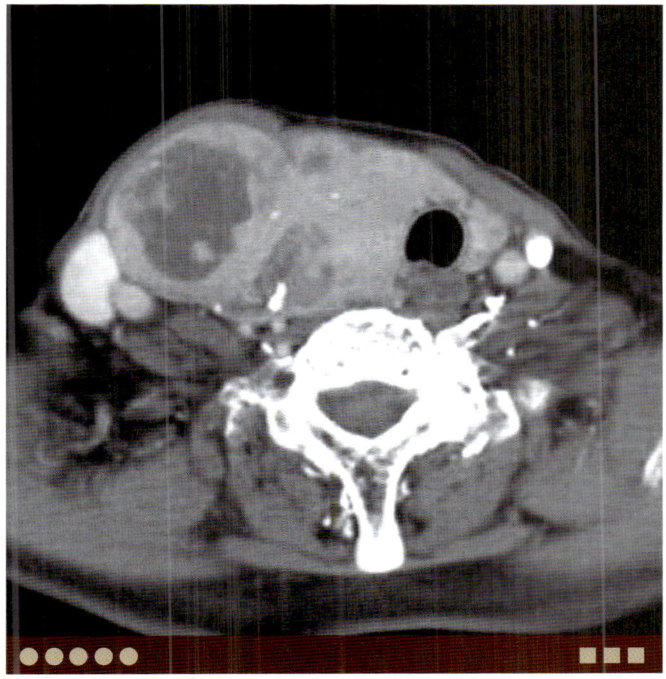

G. Thyroid adenomatous goiter, same patient as F. Axial contrast-enhanced CT demonstrates heterogeneous enhancement in the tumor.

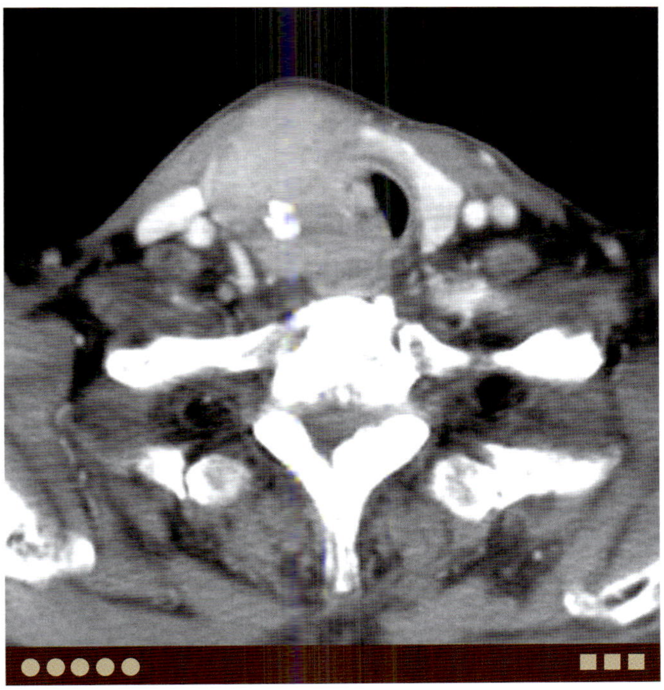

H. Thyroid papillary carcinoma. Axial contrast-enhanced CT demonstrates a right thyroid gland tumor with calcification and tracheal invasion.

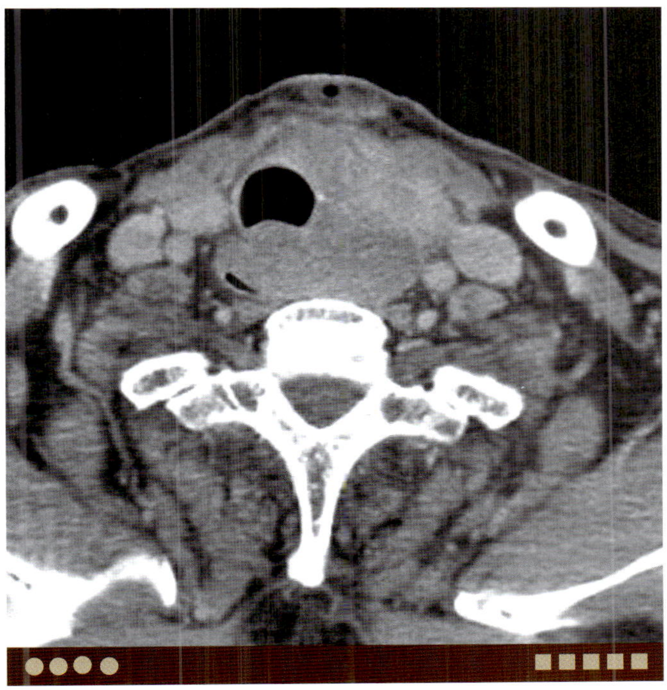

I. Diffuse large B-cell lymphoma. Axial contrast-enhanced CT demonstrates a homogeneous, hypodense lesion in the left thyroid gland.

Case 11–23 Plummer Disease (Autonomously Functioning Thyroid Nodule)

Hiroki Kato, Asim Mian, Osamu Sakai

PRESENTATION

Hyperthyroidism. Palpitations, sweating, insomnia, body weight loss, anxiety, bulging eyes, and tremors.

FINDINGS

Thyroid scintigraphy demonstrates a "hot" nodule. The accumulation cannot be suppressed with exogenous thyroid hormone.

DIFFERENTIAL DIAGNOSIS

- Nonfunctioning thyroid nodule: Nonfunctioning or "cold" thyroid nodules include both benign conditions (adenomas, cysts, and inflammation) and malignant tumors. Therefore, thyroid scintigraphy is not useful to differentiate a benign nodule from a malignant tumor. However, hot nodules are rarely malignant.
- Thyroid cancers: Although thyroid cancers usually do not show increased uptake on scintigraphy, rarely hot nodules can be malignant. Well-differentiated thyroid papillary and follicular carcinomas often concentrate iodine and 123-I imaging is useful for follow-up.
- Lymphoma: Lymphoma, usually non-Hodgkin lymphoma, is uncommon in the thyroid. It may occur as a part of generalized lymphoma or as a primary tumor, usually in the setting of Hashimoto thyroiditis. Lymphoma is typically "cold" on both 99mTc and 123-I scintigraphy.

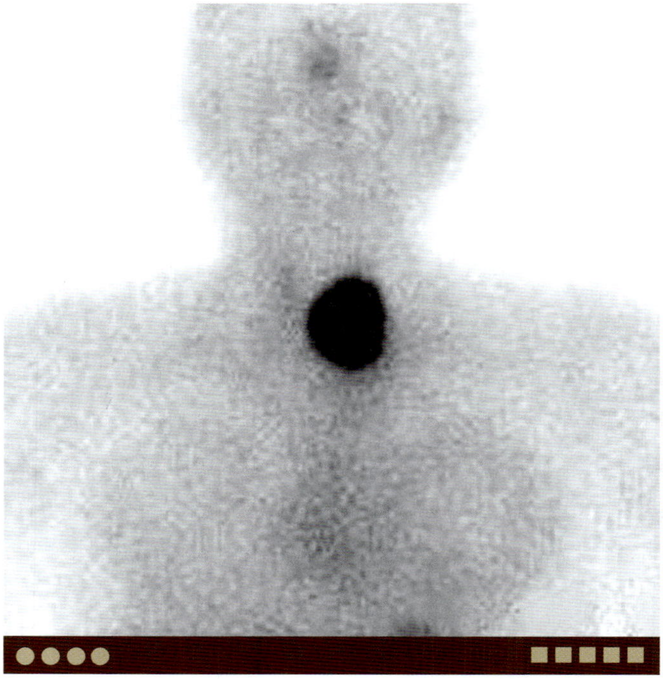

A. Plummer disease (adenoma). 99mTc-pertechnetate scintigraphy demonstrates hyperactive nodule in the left lobe and minimal activity in the remaining thyroid.

COMMENTS

This is a 47-year-old woman with symptoms of hyperthyroidism and a left thyroid nodule.

Thyroid nodules are very frequently seen and they may represent a variety of thyroid diseases. The vast majority of thyroid nodules are benign, and the most common cause of benign thyroid nodules is nodular hyperplasia. Although the main purpose of imaging is to differentiate the malignancy requiring surgical treatment from benign nodules, it is often difficult due to their nonspecific imaging findings on ultrasound, CT, and MRI.

Radionuclide scintigraphy is not used routinely to assess thyroid nodules. It is primarily of use in patients with a suppressed thyroid-stimulating hormone level, in whom it allows assessment of the functional activity of a thyroid nodule and of the whole gland. "Hot" nodules at scintigraphy reflect benign conditions in over 90% of cases, most commonly adenomas or hyperplasia. Although malignant thyroid nodules usually do not show uptake on scintigraphy, "hot nodules" rarely can be malignant. Meanwhile, although "cold" nodules are commonly thought to indicate an increased risk of malignancy, as many as 77% of cold nodules are benign (adenomas, cysts, and inflammation). Therefore, thyroid scintigraphy is also not very helpful for differentiating a benign nodule from a malignant nodule.

The term "Plummer disease" is used to indicate autonomously functioning thyroid nodules. In these conditions, although adjacent normal thyroid tissue is suppressed on scintigraphy, the autonomously functioning nodule cannot be suppressed by exogenous thyroid hormone. If a "hot" nodule is suppressed by exogenous thyroid hormone, the nodule is not considered as "Plummer disease." Most "hot" nodules suppressed by exogenous thyroid hormone are hyperplastic nodules.

PEARLS

- **The term "Plummer disease" is used to indicate an autonomously functioning thyroid nodule, and the "hot" nodule cannot be suppressed by exogenous thyroid hormone.**
- **Although most "hot" nodules are benign, they rarely can be malignant tumors.**
- **Although "cold" nodules usually indicate an increased risk of thyroid malignancy, most "cold" nodules are benign.**

ADDITIONAL IMAGE

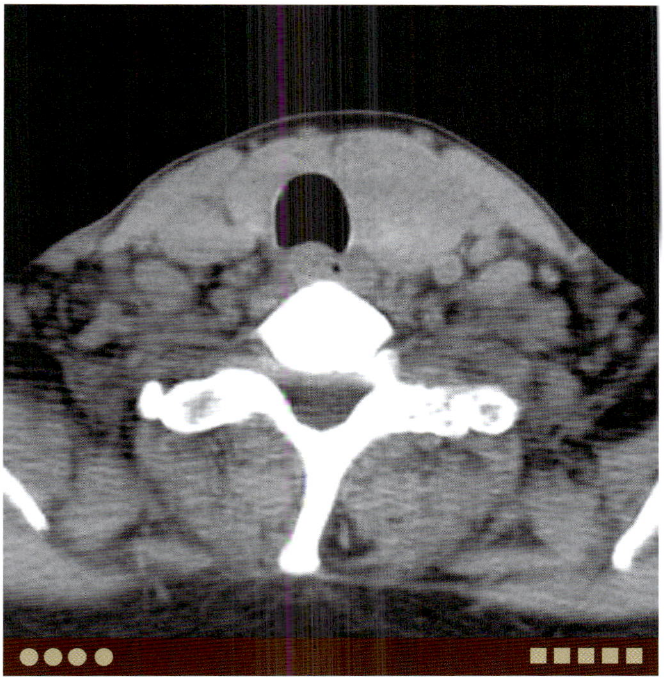

B. Plummer disease (adenoma), same patient as A. Axial unenhanced CT demonstrates a homogeneously hypodense lesion in the left lobe of the thyroid gland.

DIFFERENTIAL DIAGNOSIS IMAGES (C-H)

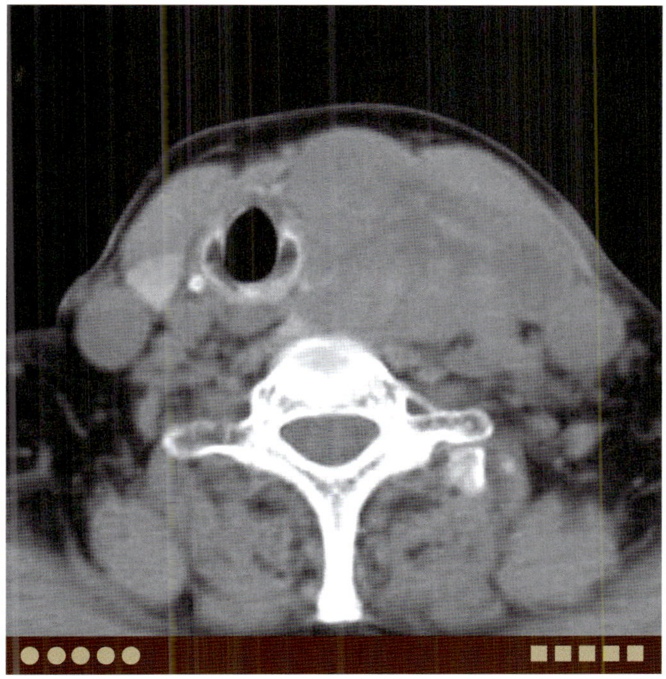

C. Nonfunctional thyroid adenomatous goiter. Axial unenhanced CT demonstrates a large hypodense lesion in the left thyroid gland.

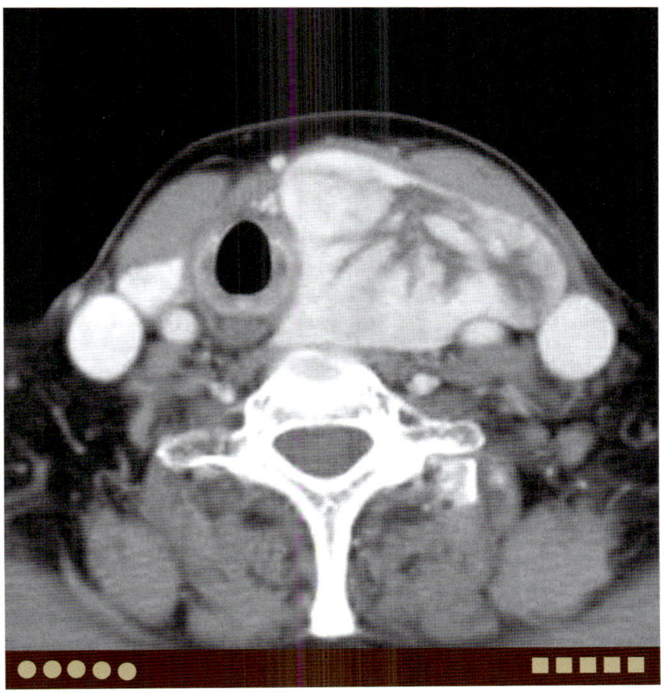

D. Nonfunctional thyroid adenomatous goiter, same patient as C. Axial contrast-enhanced CT demonstrates heterogeneous avid enhancement of the lesion.

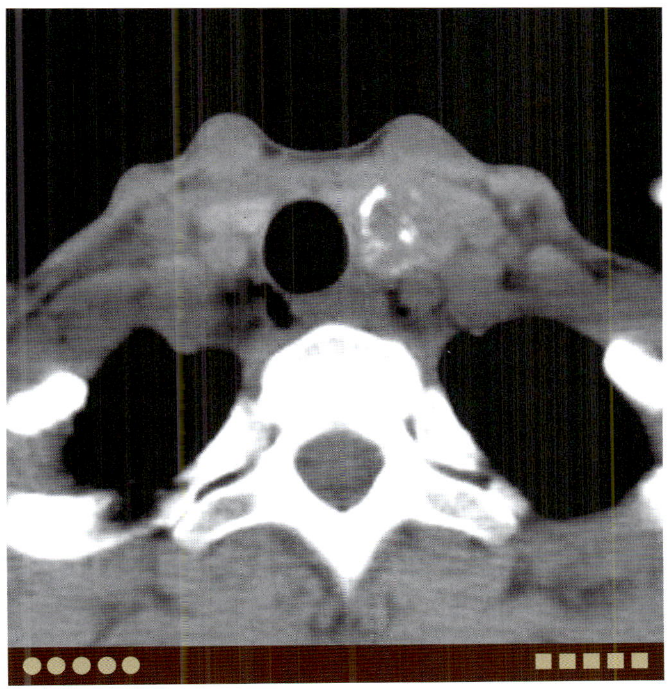

E. Thyroid papillary carcinoma. Axial unenhanced CT demonstrates a hypodense lesion with multifocal calcifications in the left lobe of the thyroid gland.

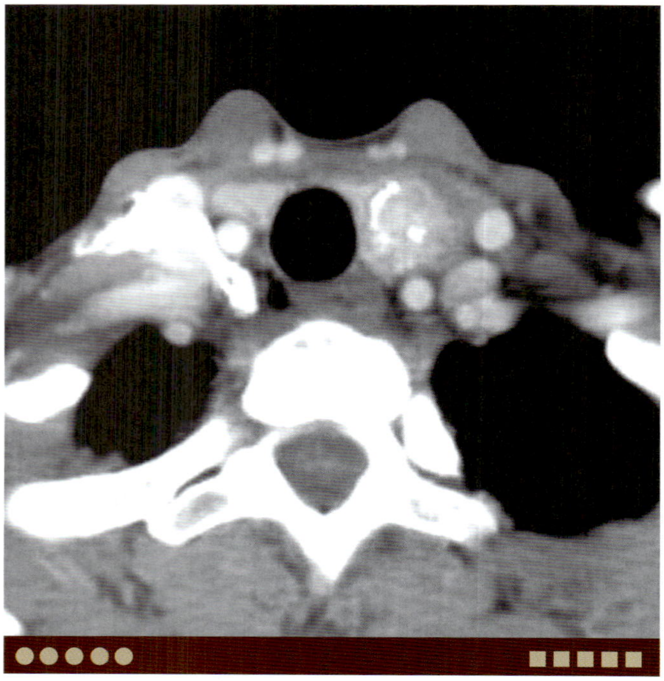

F. Thyroid papillary carcinoma, same patient as E. Axial contrast-enhanced CT demonstrates heterogeneous enhancement of the lesion.

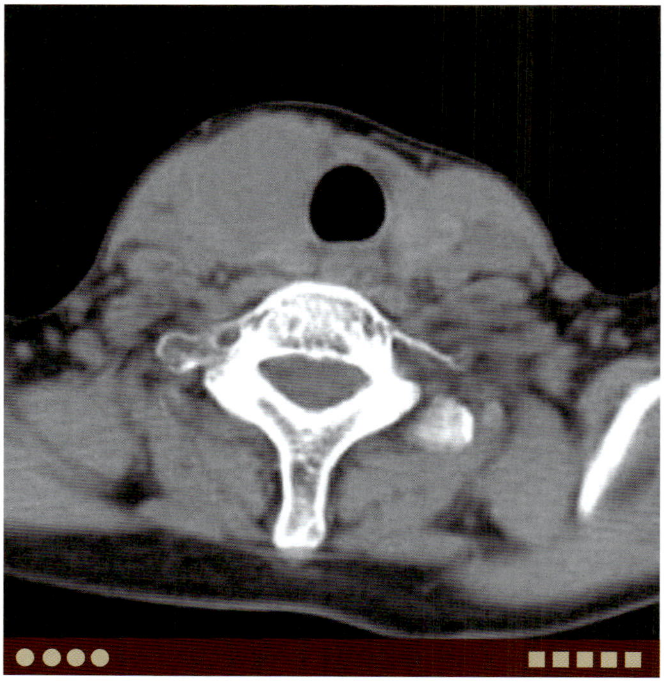

G. Diffuse large B-cell lymphoma. Axial unenhanced CT demonstrates a homogeneous, hypodense lesion in the right lobe of the thyroid gland.

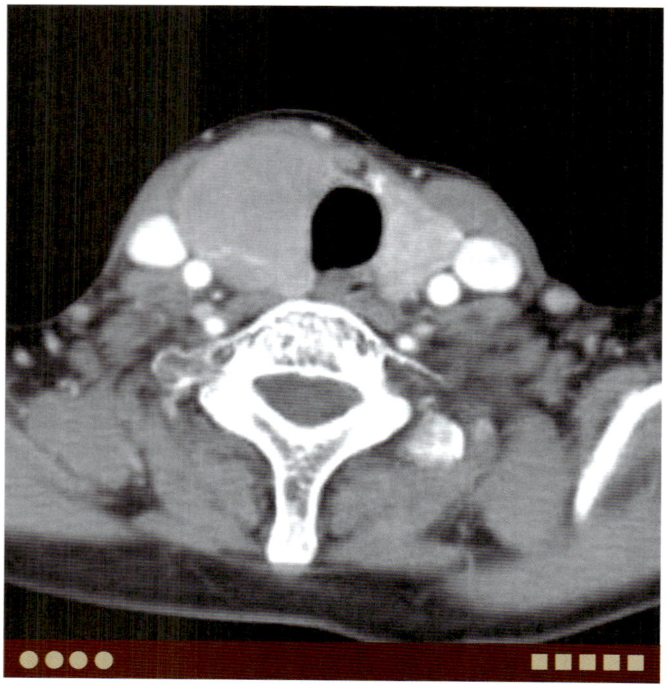

H. Diffuse large B-cell lymphoma, same patient as G. Axial contrast-enhanced CT demonstrates homogeneous enhancement of the lesion.

Case 11–24 Tracheobronchial Amyloidosis

Akira Murakami, Osamu Sakai

PRESENTATION

Shortness of breath.

FINDINGS

CT and MRI demonstrate circumferential or polypoid thickening of the trachea with calcifications.

DIFFERENTIAL DIAGNOSIS

- Wegener's granulomatosis: This condition can involve any portion of the aerodigestive tract and causes concentric narrowing of the lumen or nodular masses.
- Tracheopathia osteochondroplastica: This is an idiopathic disorder of multiple osteocartilaginous masses adjacent to the tracheal rings. Unlike amyloidosis, this tends to spare the posterior membranous portion of the trachea.
- Tracheobronchial papillomatosis: This is caused by human papillomavirus, most often acquired at birth from maternal infection, manifesting as multiple soft tissue nodules projecting into the airway.
- Relapsing polychondritis: Autoimmune connective tissue disease resulting in stricture and mural thickening, often with calcification.

COMMENTS

This is a 66-year-old woman with amyloidosis.

Amyloidosis is a family of protein-folding disorders which result in the formation and deposition of insoluble fibrillar proteins in the extracellular space. These fibrils are arranged in a beta-pleated sheet conformation which produces the classic apple-green birefringence under polarized light microscopy.

There are many different types of amyloidosis and the classification system is based on the precursor protein of the fibril. In the majority of head and neck amyloidosis, this precursor protein is produced and deposited locally by a clone of plasma cells that are confined to that location. If such plasma cells are located and proliferating in the bone marrow, the amyloidogenic light chain precursors can cause systemic amyloid deposition in virtually any organ system in the body.

Tracheobronchial amyloidomas are found in 9% of head and neck amyloidosis. They can manifest as a polypoid mass-like lesions or diffuse concentric soft tissue thickening. The deposits are homogeneous, submucosal, and soft tissue attenuating on CT, often with calcifications. There is generally little-to-no enhancement.

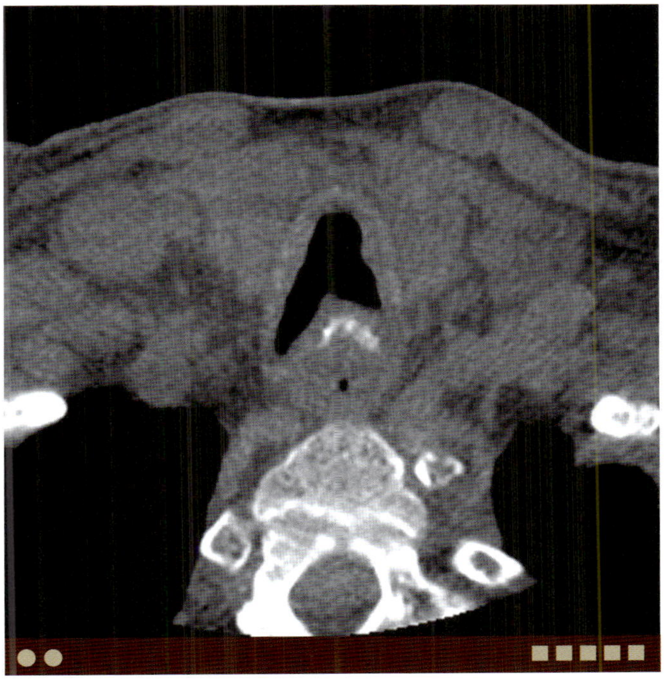

A. Amyloidosis. Axial CT demonstrates circumferential thickening of the trachea at the thoracic inlet level.

PEARLS

- **Amyloidosis is a rare lesion that can occur anywhere in the entire aerodigestive tract.**
- **Amyloid deposit is soft tissue density, which may be nodular or circumferential, and calcification is common.**
- **On MRI, amyloidomas show low signal on T1W, and low-to-intermediate signal on T2W images, with little-to-no enhancement. Calcifications are common.**
- **Although the localized form is most common in the head and neck, patients must be evaluated clinically to rule out the presence of systemic disease.**

ADDITIONAL IMAGES (B-F)

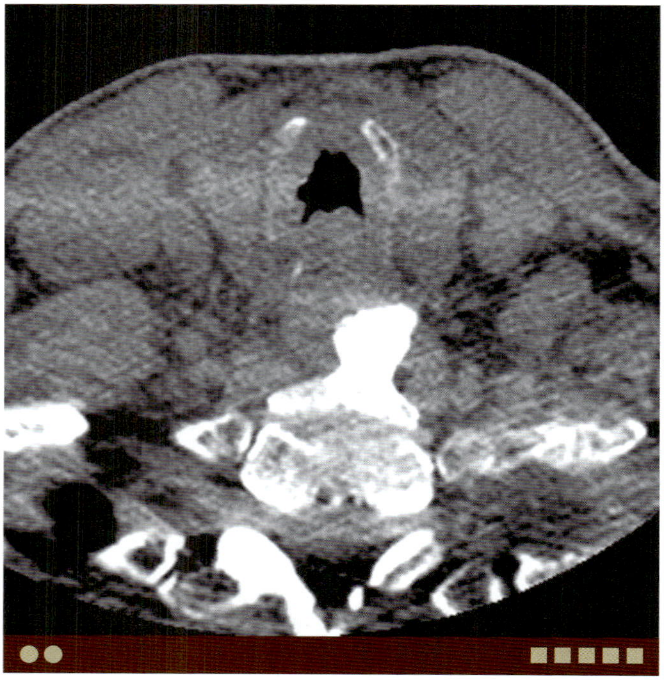

B. Amyloidosis in a different patient. Axial CT demonstrates slightly irregular circumferential thickening of the tracheal wall.

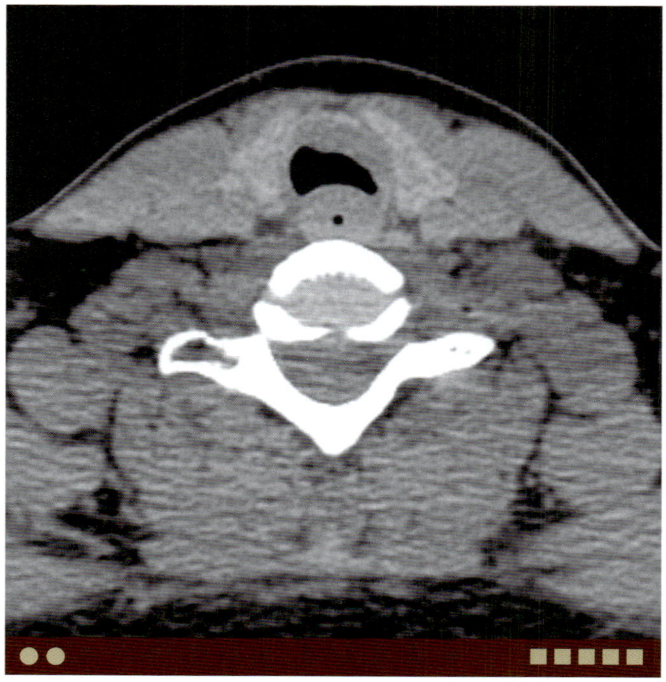

C. Amyloidosis, same patient as B. Axial CT demonstrates slightly eccentric circumferential thickening of the tracheal wall.

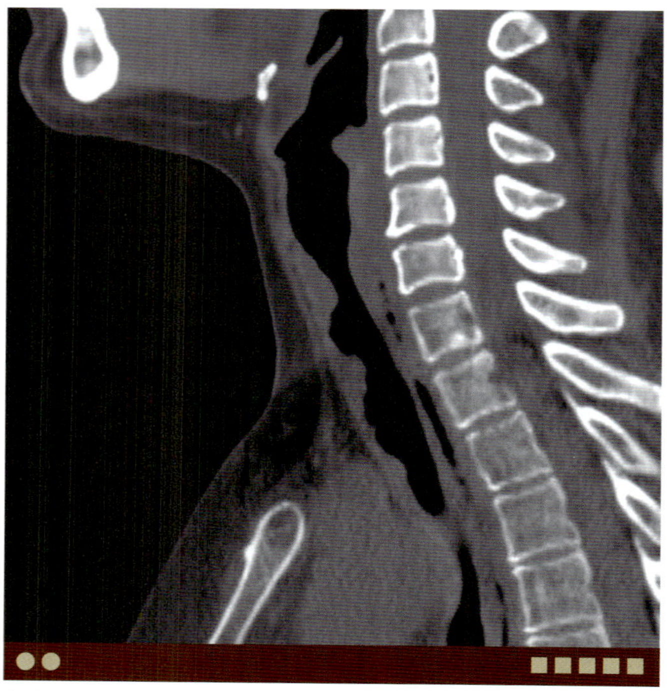

D. Amyloidosis, same patient as B. Sagittal CT demonstrates multifocal circumferential thickening of the tracheal wall.

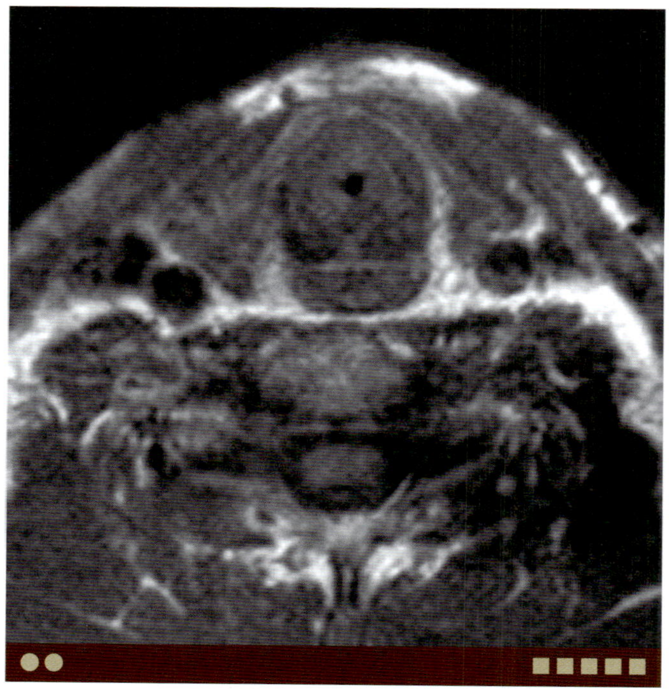

E. Amyloidosis in a different patient. Axial T1W MR image shows circumferential narrowing of the subglottis due to submucosal amyloid deposit.

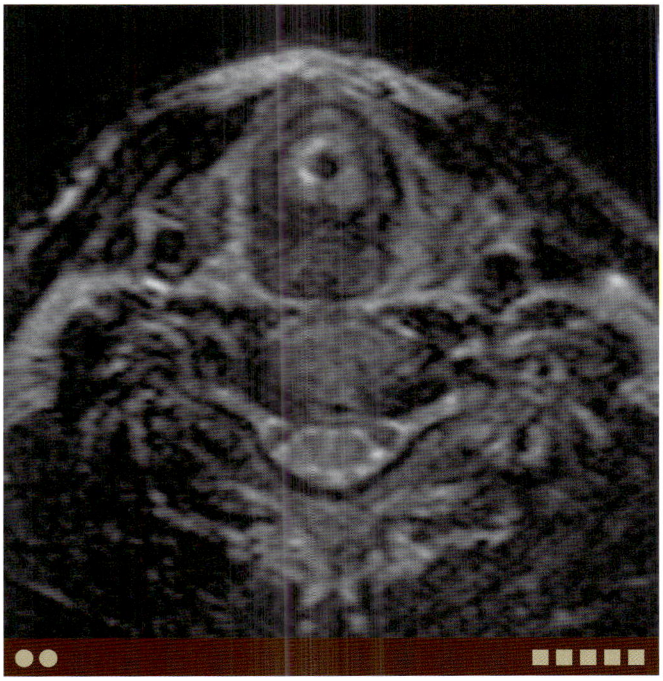

F. Amyloidosis, same patient as E. Axial T2W MR image shows circumferential narrowing of the subglottis due to submucosal amyloid deposit. Note iso-to-low signal of the lesion.

DIFFERENTIAL DIAGNOSIS IMAGES (G-I)

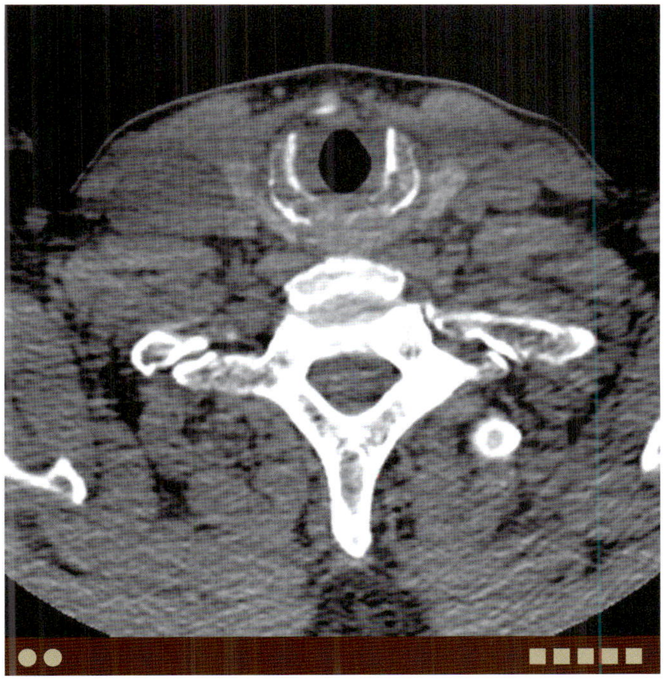

G. Wegener's granulomatosis. Axial CT demonstrates circumferential soft tissue thickening of the tracheal wall.

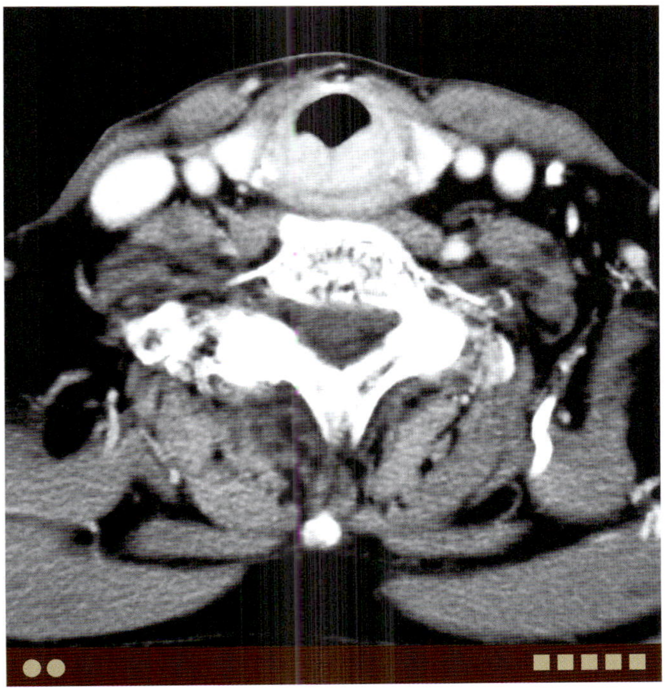

H. Plasmacytoma. Axial postcontrast CT shows a homogeneously enhancing tumor in the posterior trachea.

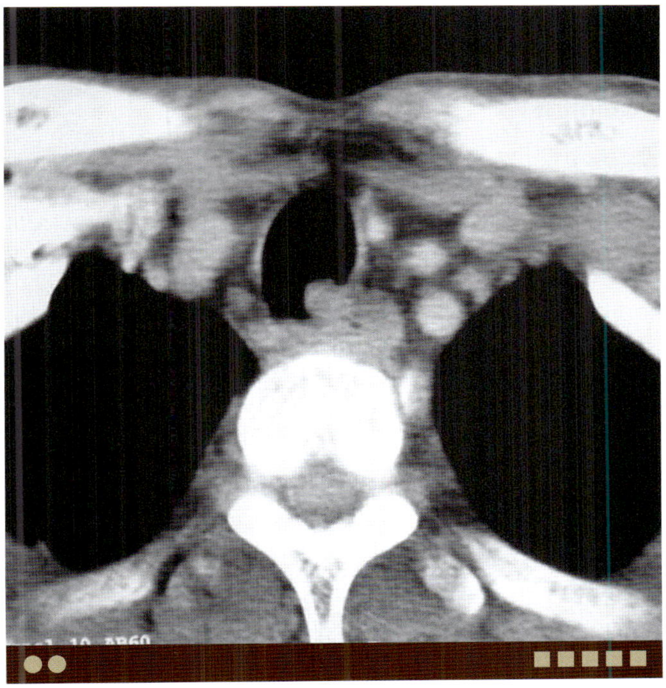

I. Papilloma. Axial postcontrast CT shows a nodular, polypoid soft tissue density in the posterior trachea.

Case 11–25 Relapsing Polychondritis

Hiroki Kato, Asim Mian, Osamu Sakai

PRESENTATION

Recurrent pain and swelling of the external ear.

FINDINGS

CT demonstrates increased attenuation and thickening of the auricles and laryngeal and tracheal walls.

DIFFERENTIAL DIAGNOSIS

- Tracheobronchopathia osteochondroplastica: This is a rare idiopathic disease characterized by formation of cartilaginous, osseous, or mixed nodules in the tracheal and bronchial submucosa. CT demonstrates irregular thickening of the tracheal wall with small nodules and calcifications/ossifications.
- Wegener's granulomatosis: This is a disease of unknown etiology characterized by necrotizing granulomatous vasculitis that may often involve the upper and lower airways, lungs, and kidneys. Paranasal sinuses and trachea are often involved.
- Amyloidosis: This condition is characterized by progressive deposition of amyloid in the extracellular tissues. The larynx, pharynx, and trachea are often involved. CT demonstrates nodular wall thickening and luminal narrowing of the airway. Calcification is commonly seen.

COMMENTS

This is a 40-year-old woman with pain, redness, swelling, and tenderness in the bilateral ears.

Relapsing polychondritis is characterized by recurrent episodes of painful inflammation, such as auricular chondritis, polyarthritis, nasal chondritis, ocular inflammation, and respiratory tract involvement. Attacks tend to vary in severity and duration usually lasting for days to weeks before resolving spontaneously. This is a systemic, widespread, and destructive inflammatory disorder involving all types of cartilaginous structures, such as elastic cartilages of the ears and nose, hyaline cartilages of peripheral joints, fibrocartilages in the axial sites, as well as cartilages in the tracheobronchial tree. Further, relapsing polychondritis also involves other proteoglycan-rich structures, such as the eye, heart, blood vessels, and inner ear.

Relapsing polychondritis must be diagnosed based on clinical findings because there is no specific laboratory test. About 25% of cases have coexistent diseases, and relapsing polychondritis appears to be closely associated with autoimmune diseases. Systemic vasculitis (polyarteritis nodosa, Takayasu arteritis, giant cell arteritis, Wegener's granulomatosis), rheumatoid arthritis, Sjögren's syndrome, systemic lupus erythematosus, progressive systemic sclerosis, Reiter syndrome, Behcet disease, thyroid disease, ulcerative colitis, and paraneoplastic syndrome have been reported with relapsing polychondritis.

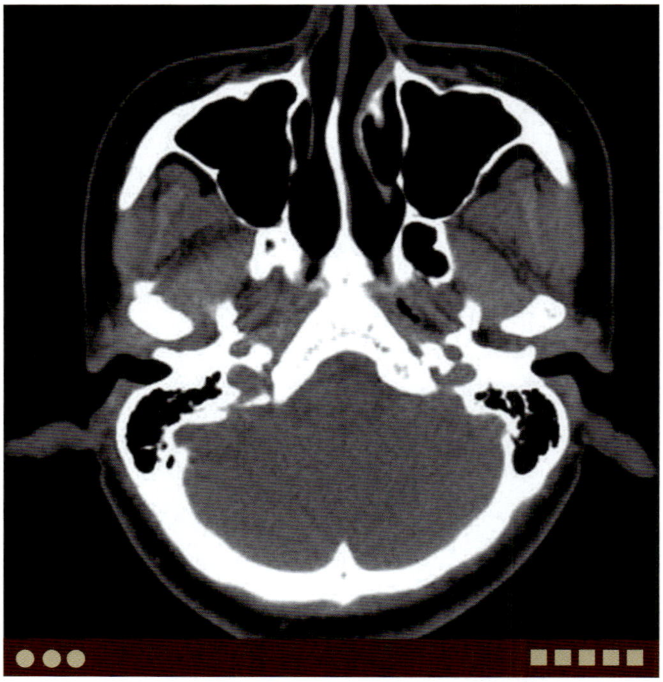

A. Relapsing polychondritis. Axial unenhanced CT demonstrates diffuse thickening of bilateral auricles.

Increased attenuation and smooth thickening of the auricles and airway walls are common findings of relapsing polychondritis. The diffuse thickening of auricles is a very specific finding for this condition. Other CT findings of this disease include calcifications of the auricles, nasal cartilage collapse, subglottic and tracheobronchial luminal narrowing, often with calcification.

PEARLS

- **Relapsing polychondritis is an uncommon, systemic disorder, which involves all types of cartilage.**
- **The diagnosis of relapsing polychondritis is made by clinical findings because there is no specific laboratory test.**
- **Increased attenuation and smooth thickening of the auricles and the airway walls are common CT findings of relapsing polychondritis.**

ADDITIONAL IMAGES (B-C)

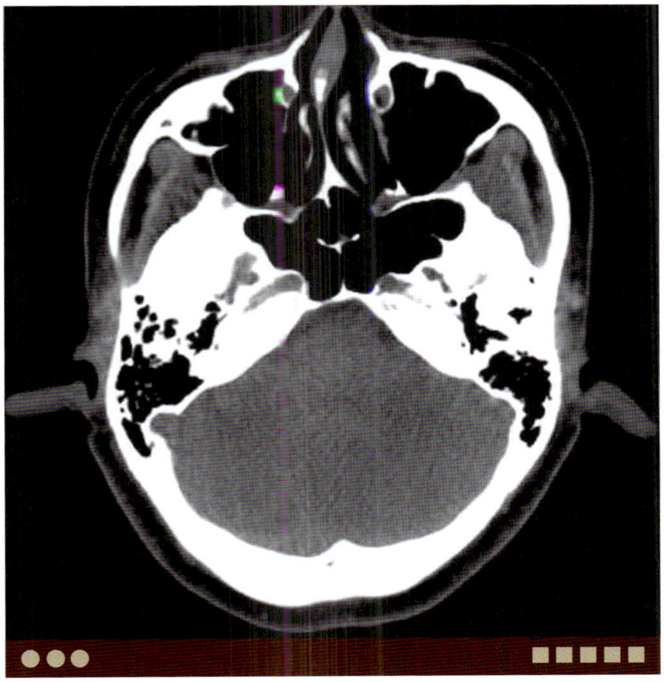

B. Relapsing polychondritis, same patient as A. Axial unenhanced CT demonstrates diffuse thickening of bilateral auricles (higher level than A).

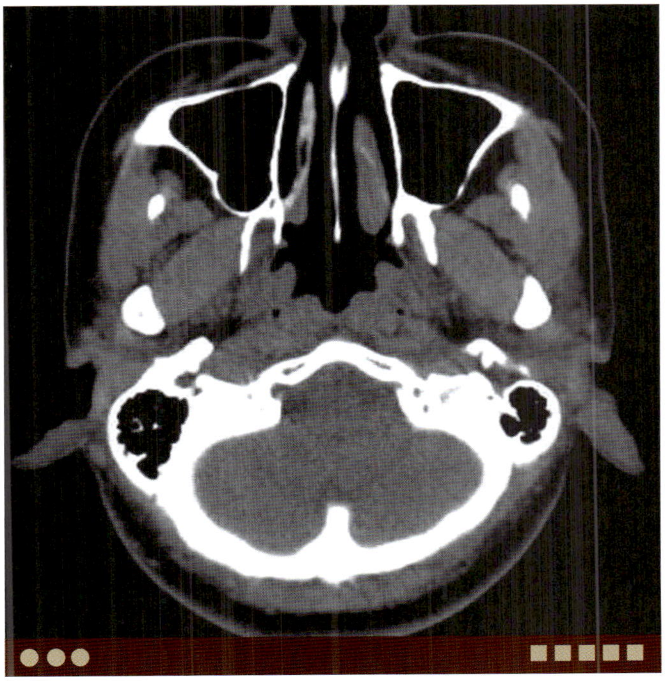

C. Relapsing polychondritis, same patient as A. Axial unenhanced CT demonstrates diffuse thickening of bilateral auricles (lower level than A).

DIFFERENTIAL DIAGNOSIS IMAGES (D-I)

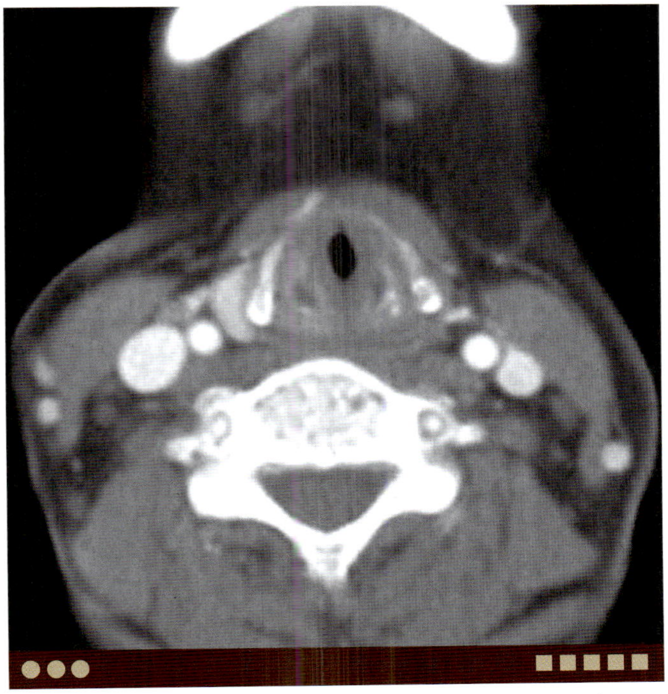

D. Amyloidosis. Axial contrast-enhanced CT demonstrates circumferential wall thickening of the subglottic larynx.

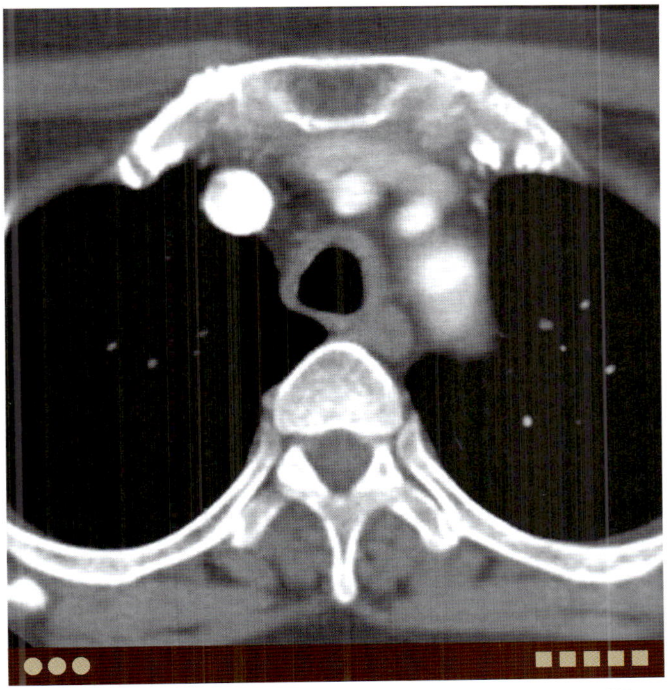

E. Amyloidosis, same patient as D. Axial contrast-enhanced CT demonstrates circumferential wall thickening of the trachea.

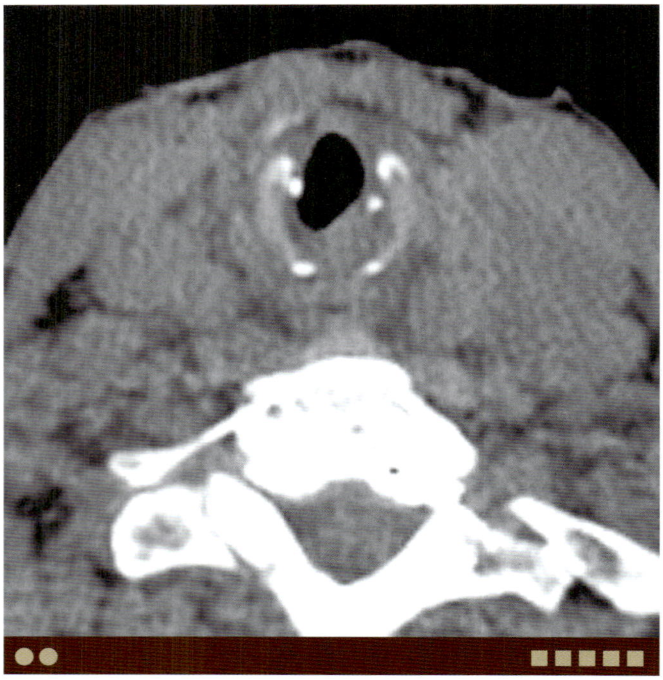

F. Amyloidosis in a different patient. Axial CT demonstrates slightly irregular concentric narrowing of the subglottic larynx. Note focal calcifications.

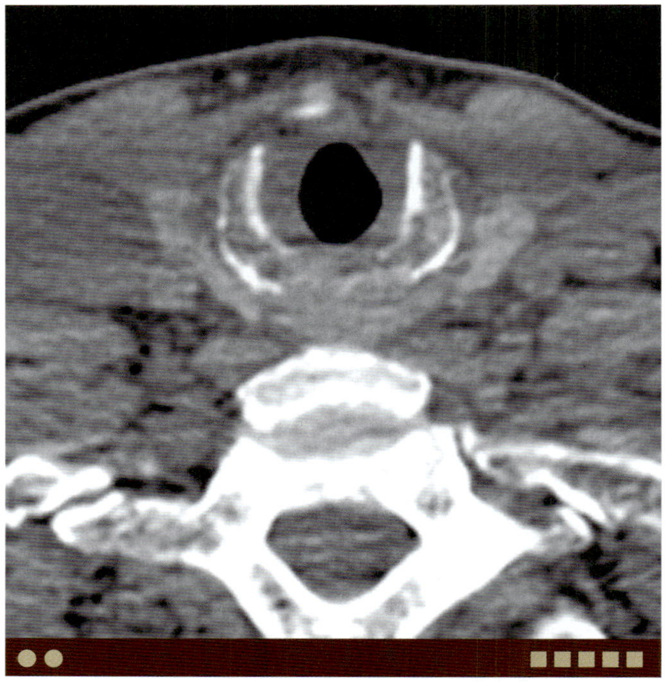

G. Wegener's granulomatosis. Axial CT demonstrates concentric soft tissue thickening in the subglottis.

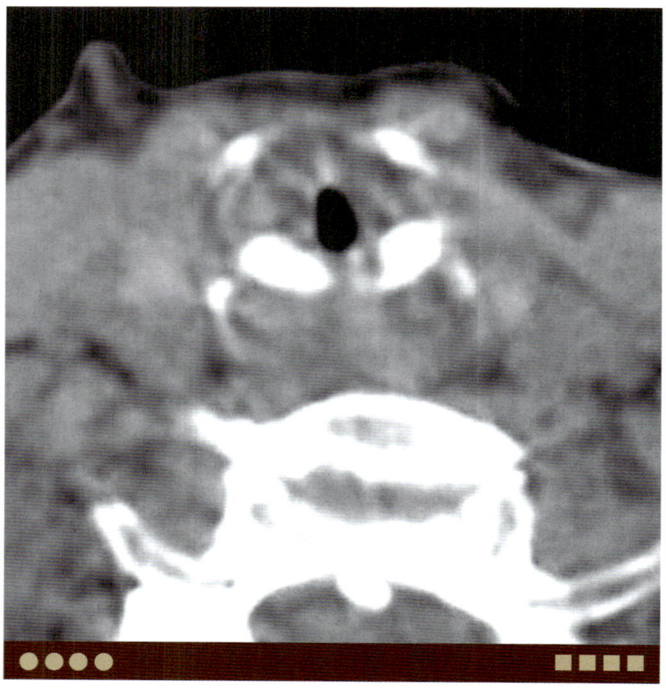

H. Tracheobronchomalacia. Axial CT demonstrates narrowing of the subglottic larynx.

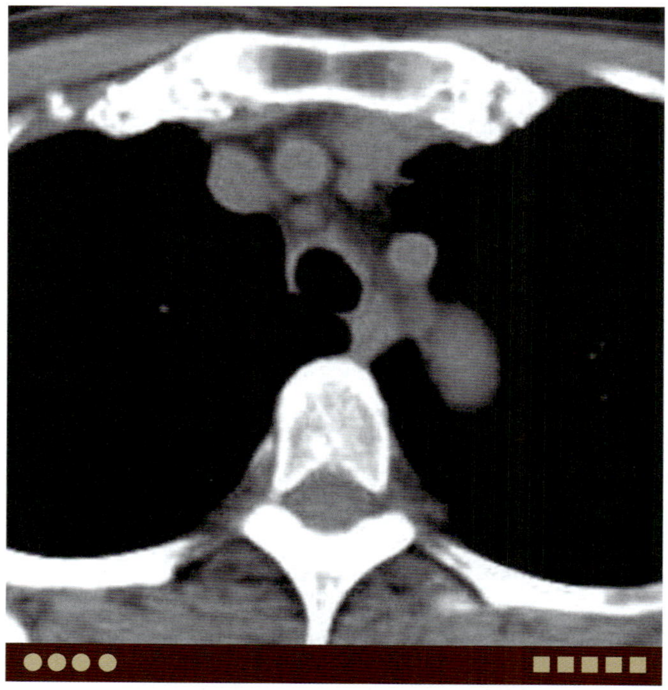

I. Tracheobronchomalacia in a different patient**.** Axial CT demonstrates wall thickening of the cartilaginous segment of the trachea.

Case 11–26 Subacute Thyroiditis

Hiroki Kato, Asim Mian, Osamu Sakai

PRESENTATION

Anterior neck pain and tenderness.

FINDINGS

CT demonstrates the thyroid gland to have diffusely decreased density.

DIFFERENTIAL DIAGNOSIS

- Graves disease: Graves disease is an autoimmune disorder caused by antibodies against the thyroid-stimulating hormone (TSH) receptors on the cell surface of the thyroid follicle. Imaging studies often demonstrate diffusely enlarged thyroid gland. On thyroid scan, increased activity through the thyroid is noted due to both increased stimulation and function of the gland.
- Hashimoto thyroiditis: This is also known as chronic autoimmune thyroiditis and is a condition characterized by autoimmune destruction due to autoimmunity to thyroid antigens and lymphocyte infiltration. Thyroid scan demonstrates areas of either increased activity (follicles responding to TSH) or decreased activity (follicles not responding to TSH).
- Thyroid tumor: Most thyroid tumors are nonfunctional. However, toxic hyperthyroidism is rarely caused by hyperfunctioning thyroid nodules, including toxic autonomous nodule and toxic multinodular goiter.

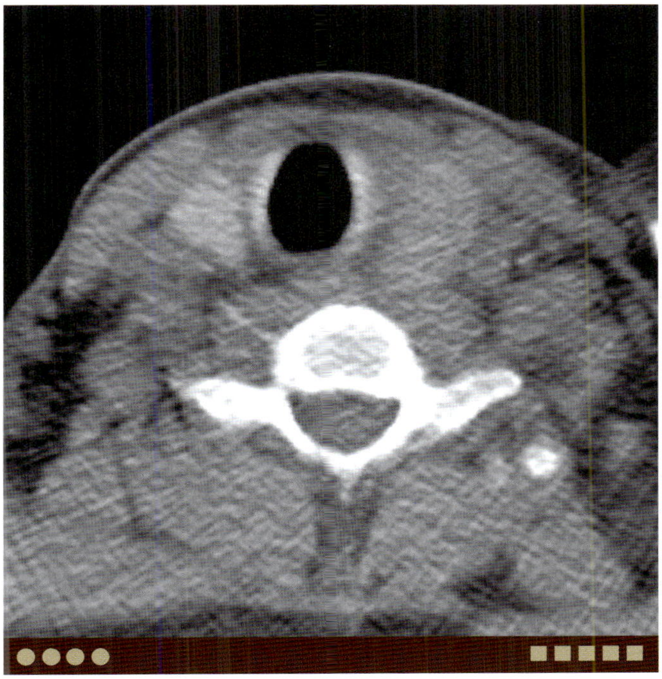

A. Subacute thyroiditis. Axial unenhanced CT demonstrates swelling and decreased attenuation of the left lobe of the thyroid gland.

COMMENTS

This is a 27-year-old woman with painful enlargement of the left thyroid gland for a few weeks.

Subacute thyroiditis is a destructive thyroiditis and thyrotoxic condition, and also known as subacute granulomatous thyroiditis, giant cell thyroiditis, or de Quervain thyroiditis. Subacute thyroiditis is presumed to be caused by a self-limited inflammatory process and usually occurs following upper respiratory tract infection caused by Coxsackie virus and mumps. Postviral inflammatory response leads to giant cell infiltration into the thyroid follicles, ultimately resulting in follicular swelling and disruption with release of stored thyroid hormone into the circulation. Swelling of the thyroid follicles results in stretching of the thyroid capsule with subsequent pain and tenderness, while the release of excess thyroid hormone results in thyrotoxic signs and symptoms. Neck pain frequently radiates to the ears and increases during swallowing.

Thyroid scintigraphy shows a variable pattern that usually reverts to normal as the patient returns to the euthyroid state. However, in the initial stage, subacute thyroiditis usually shows no or minimal uptake on thyroid scan, probably because of follicular cell destruction and suppressed adjacent normal thyroid tissue.

Unenhanced CT demonstrates the enlarged thyroid glands with a lower than normal attenuation. On MRI, mild hyperintensity on T1W and more pronounced hyperintensity on T2W images compared with the muscle are seen. Postcontrast studies demonstrate moderate enhancement with some heterogeneity reflecting inflammatory nature of the disease process.

PEARLS

- **Subacute thyroiditis is a self-limited inflammatory disease and often occurs secondary to viral upper respiratory tract infection.**
- **In the acute stage of subacute thyroiditis, thyroid scintigraphy usually shows no or minimal uptake.**
- **CT demonstrates enlarged thyroid glands with low attenuation. MRI demonstrates mild hyperintensity on T1W and more pronounced hyperintensity on T2W images. Postcontrast studies demonstrate moderate enhancement with some heterogeneity.**

ADDITIONAL IMAGE

B. Subacute thyroiditis, same patient as A. 99mTc-pertechnetate scintigraphy demonstrates very minimal activity in the thyroid gland.

DIFFERENTIAL DIAGNOSIS IMAGES (C-G)

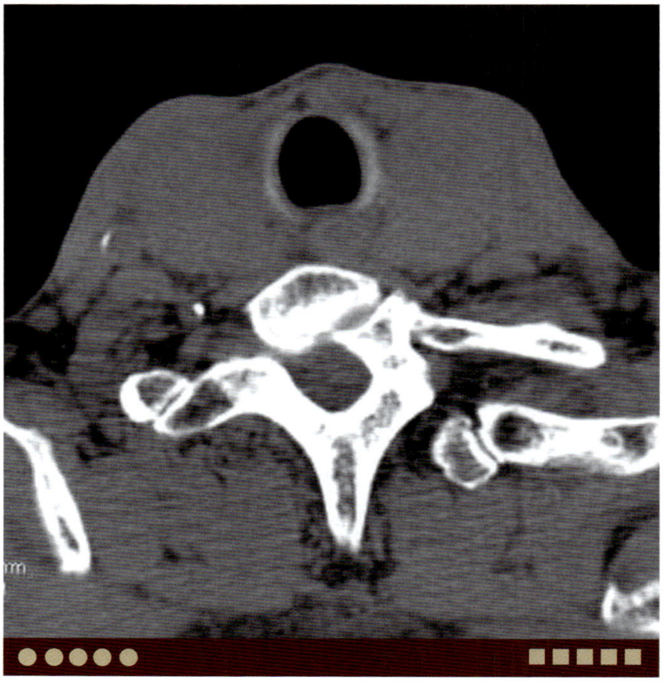

C. Graves disease. Axial unenhanced CT demonstrates diffuse swelling and decreased density of the bilateral thyroid glands.

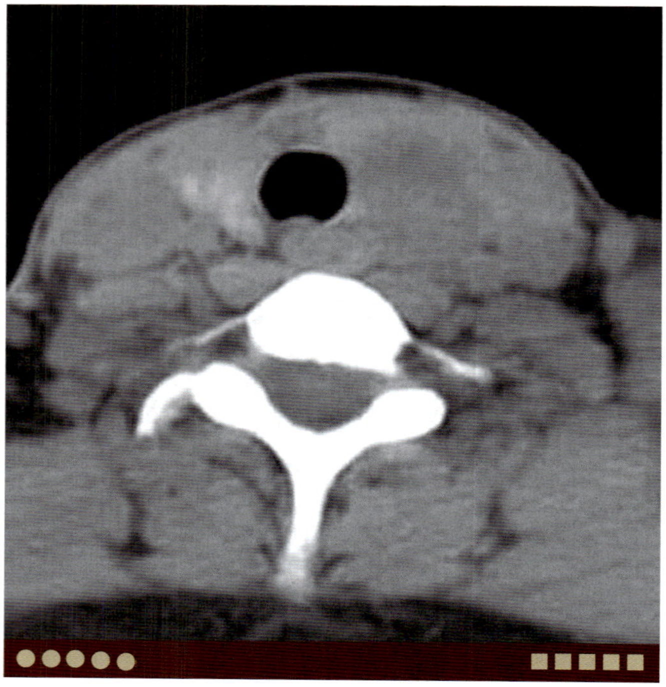

D. Adenomatous goiter. Axial unenhanced CT demonstrates an ill-defined hypodense lesion in the left lobe of the thyroid gland.

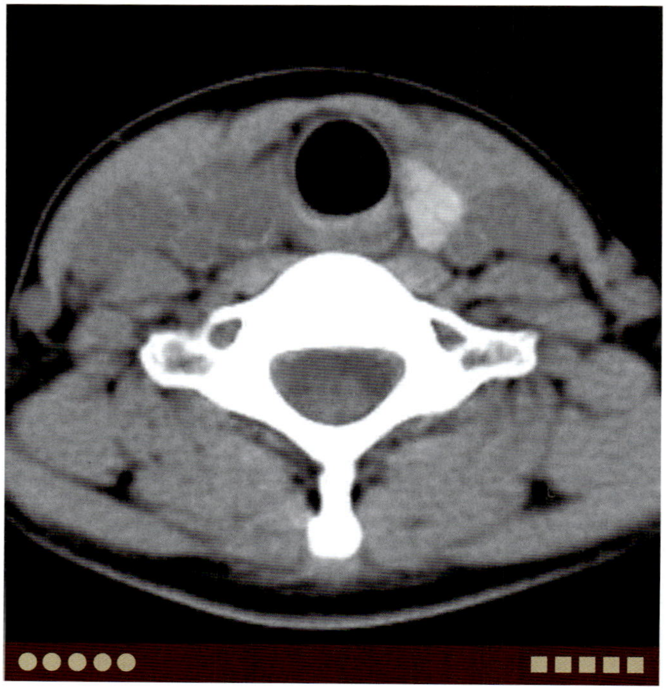

E. Papillary carcinoma. Axial unenhanced CT demonstrates a hypodense lesion in the right lobe of the thyroid gland.

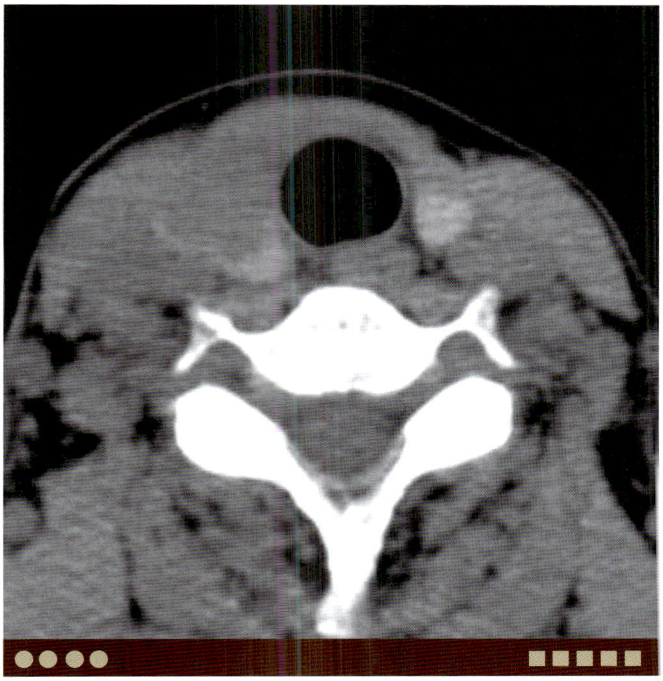

F. MALT lymphoma. Axial unenhanced CT demonstrates a hypodense lesion in the right lobe of the thyroid gland.

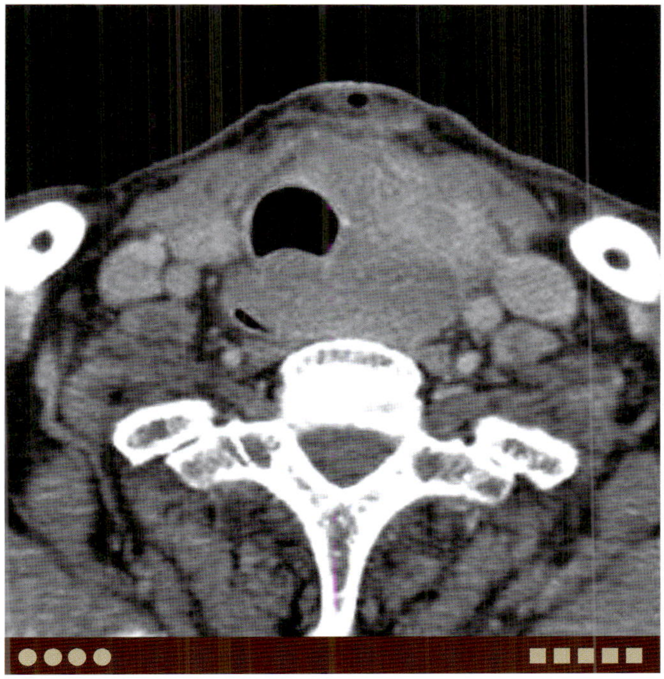

G. Diffuse large B-cell lymphoma. Axial enhanced CT demonstrates a homogeneous, hypodense lesion in the left lobe of the thyroid gland.

Case 11–27 Fibromatosis Colli

Benjamin Ludwig, Osamu Sakai

PRESENTATION

Three-week-old infant with neck mass and torticollis.

FINDINGS

Grayscale ultrasound demonstrates a circumscribed lesion within the caudal aspect of the sternocleidomastoid muscle.

DIFFERENTIAL DIAGNOSIS

- Cervical lymphadenopathy/lymphoma: Enlarged nodes may present as palpable neck masses in infants, but are not intramuscular in location.
- Rhabdomyosarcoma: This entity may be seen in neonates, and presents with an intramuscular, rapidly enlarging neck mass. Imaging findings are typically aggressive, with muscular and soft tissue infiltration, enhancement/hypervascularity, and rapid progression.
- Congenital cystic neck lesions: Entities such as branchial pouch remnants, dermoid/epidermoid, and lymphatic malformations (lymphangiomas) may present as neck masses, but are extramuscular and demonstrate cystic characteristics on imaging.
- Hematoma: Intramuscular hematoma secondary to birth trauma may present with a palpable neck mass. Imaging features depend on the age of the hemorrhage, and enhancement can be seen in organizing hematomas. A history of birth trauma may aid in diagnosis.

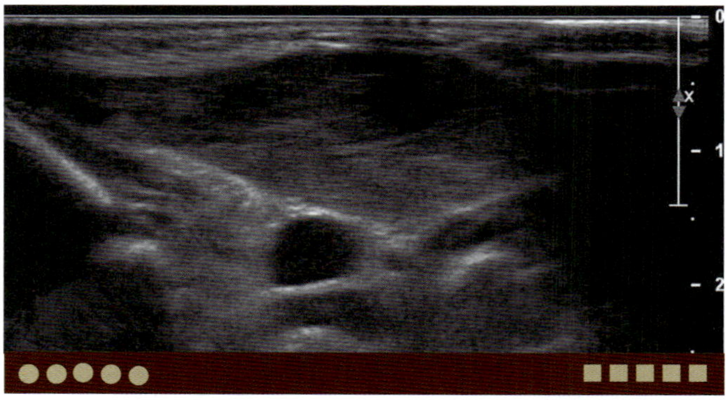

A. Fibromatosis colli. Sagittal grayscale ultrasound of the right sternocleidomastoid muscle shows fusiform enlargement of the inferior sternocleidomastoid, without evidence of focal lesion.

COMMENTS

This is a 3-week-old infant with a palpable neck mass and torticollis.

Fibromatosis colli, or pseudotumor of the sternocleidomastoid, presents as a palpable neck mass in 2- to 4-week-old infants, and may be associated with torticollis. It is believed to be secondary to fibrocollagenous infiltration of the muscle. The condition is most commonly seen after breech or forceps deliveries, and typically affects the mid to lower third of the sternocleidomastoid muscle.

Ultrasound findings include focal or diffuse muscular enlargement, with variable echogenicity of the abnormality. In cases in which the ultrasound findings are atypical, MRI can be obtained. MRI findings similarly include focal or diffuse muscular enlargement, which is T1 isointense and slightly T2 hyperintense relative to normal muscle. Enhancement can also be seen after contrast administration, which can simulate a more aggressive lesion.

Fibromatosis colli is a benign, self-limiting process, which usually undergoes complete resolution within the first year of life. The recognition of age of onset, obstetrical history, and imaging findings allow for the diagnosis, and prevention of unnecessary biopsies or surgical intervention.

PEARLS

- **Fibromatosis colli is a benign, self-limiting condition that affects infants, and typically resolves within the first year of life.**
- **Imaging features on ultrasound and MRI, combined with clinical history and patient age, can lead to the diagnosis.**
- **Location within the mid to lower third of the sternocleidomastoid is characteristic.**

ADDITIONAL IMAGES (B-G)

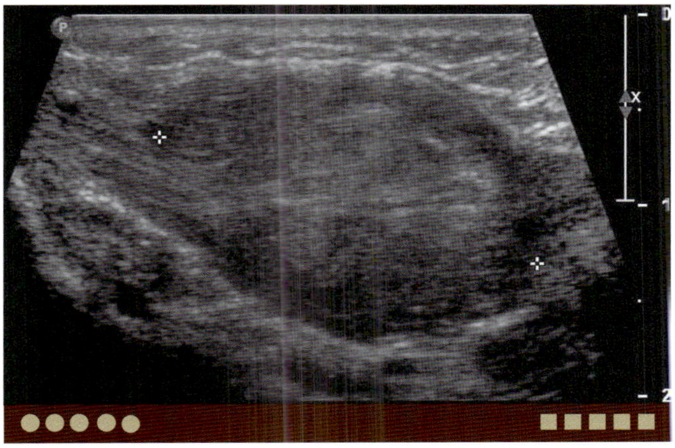

B. Fibromatosis colli, same patient as A. Transverse grayscale ultrasound of the right sternocleidomastoid shows focal enlargement of the inferior sternocleidomastoid muscle.

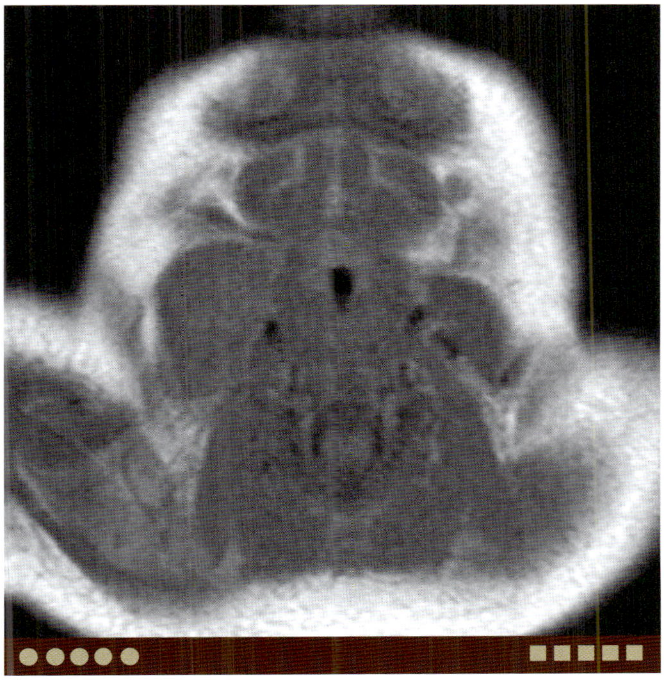

C. Fibromatosis colli in a different patient. Axial T1W MR image demonstrates focal enlargement of the right sternocleidomastoid muscle relative to the left.

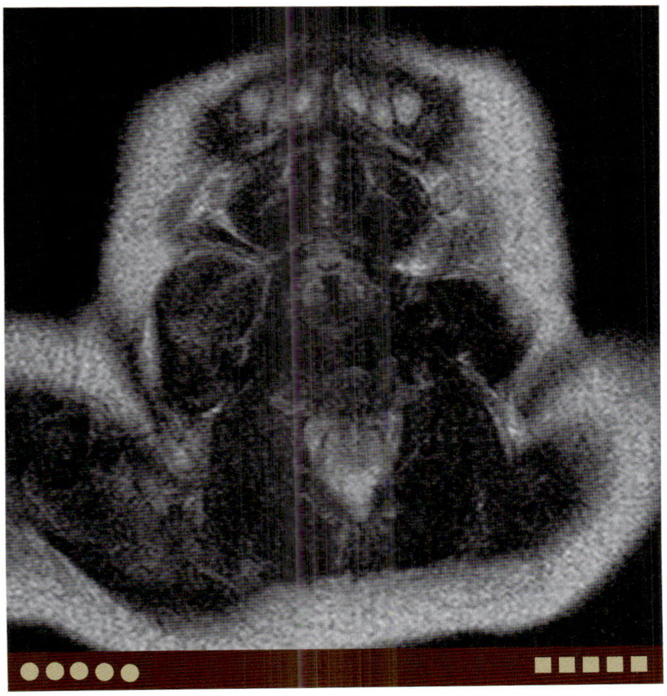

D. Fibromatosis colli, same patient as C. Axial T2W MR image shows mild T2 hyperintensity associated with focal enlargement of the right sternocleidomastoid muscle.

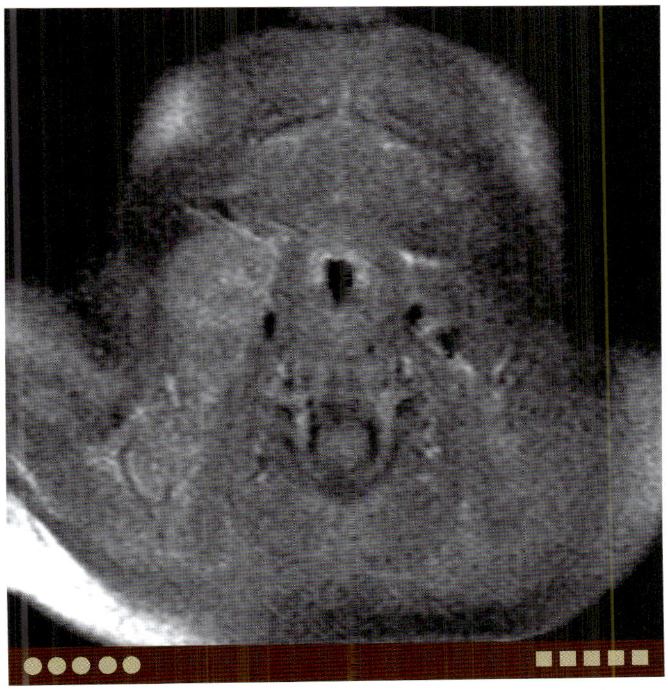

E. Fibromatosis colli, same patient as C. Axial postcontrast fat-suppressed T1W images show homogeneous enhancement within the focally expanded inferior sternocleidomastoid.

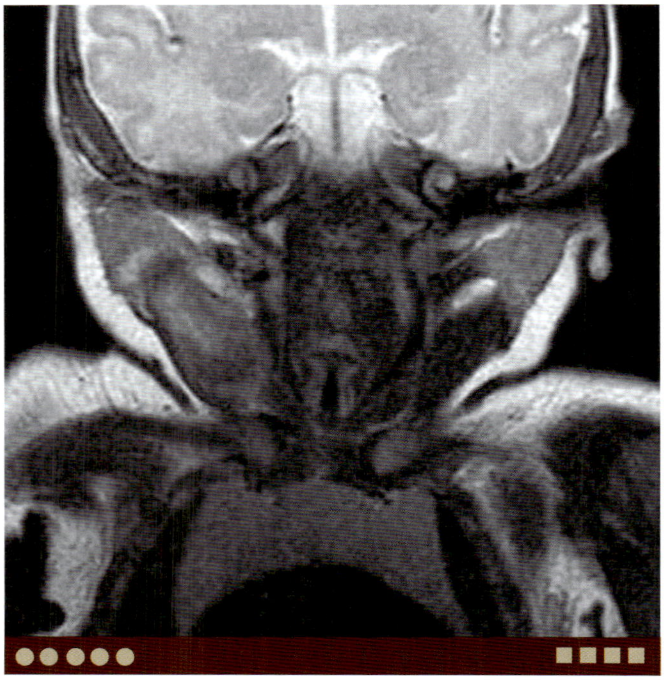

F. Fibromatosis colli, same patient as C. Coronal T2W MR image shows mild T2 hyperintensity associated with fusiform enlargement of the right sternocleidomastoid muscle.

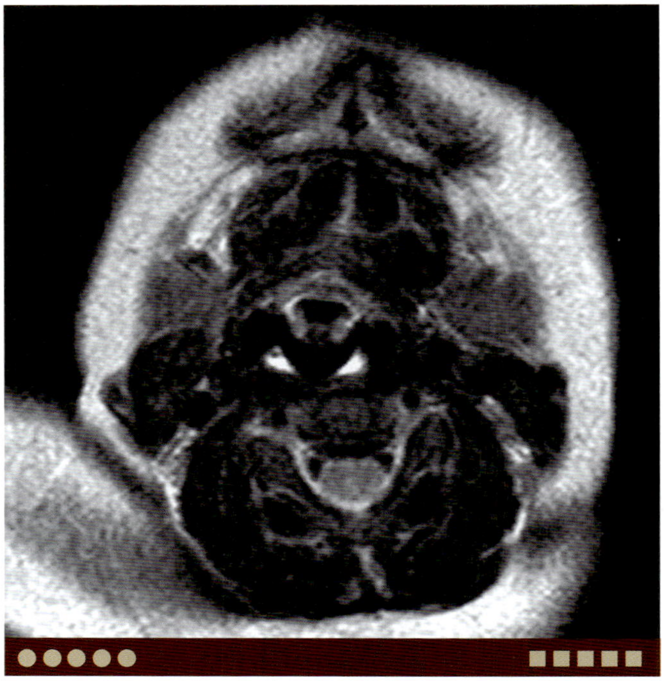

G. Fibromatosis colli, same patient as C, 3 months after diagnosis. Axial T2W MR image demonstrates near complete resolution of focal right sternocleidomastoid enlargement. Resolution is consistent with the natural history of the process.

DIFFERENTIAL DIAGNOSIS IMAGES (H-I)

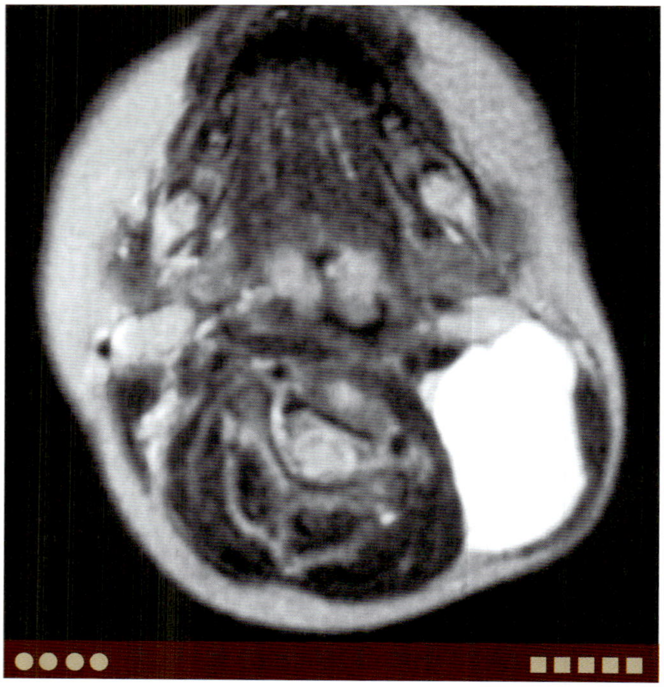

H. Lymphatic malformation. Axial T2W image shows a unilocular lesion to have homogeneous high signal in the left posterior triangle.

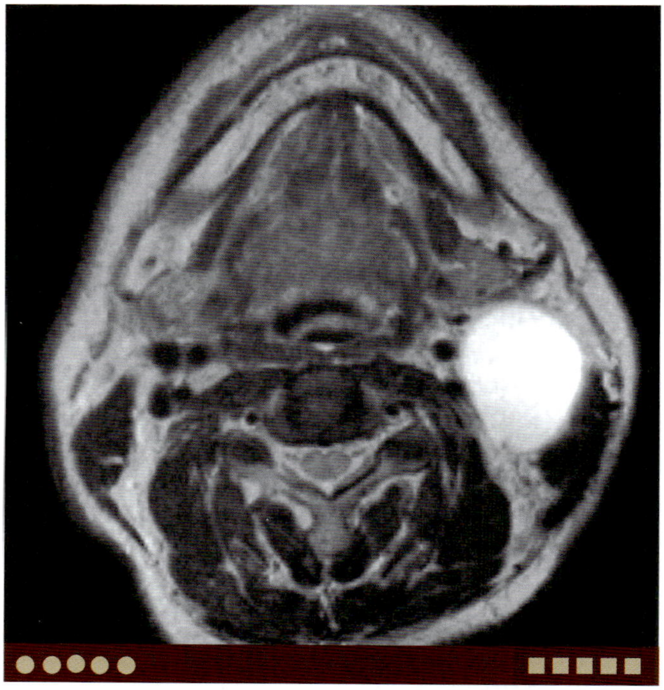

I. Second branchial cleft cyst. Axial T2W MR image shows a cystic lesion anteromedial to the left sternocleidomastoid muscle.

Case 11–28 Upper Esophageal Sphincter

Susan Langmore

PRESENTATION

Upper esophageal stricture (UES) versus hypertonic cricopharyngeus (CP) muscle.

FINDINGS

Fluoroscopy image shows restricted UES opening when swallowing a 5 mL of liquid. Normal maximum distension is 0.50 cm.

DIFFERENTIAL DIAGNOSIS

- Hypercontracted CP muscle: Neurogenic etiology with resting tone of the CP muscle high and/or which does not relax adequately, making it difficult for it to open.
- Stricture postradiotherapy: Formation of scar tissue at the region of the upper esophageal sphincter causing it to be restricted in opening diameter or even be completely closed.
- Reduced hypolaryngeal excursion: Reducing the mechanical pull on the UES to open it, even when it is relaxed.

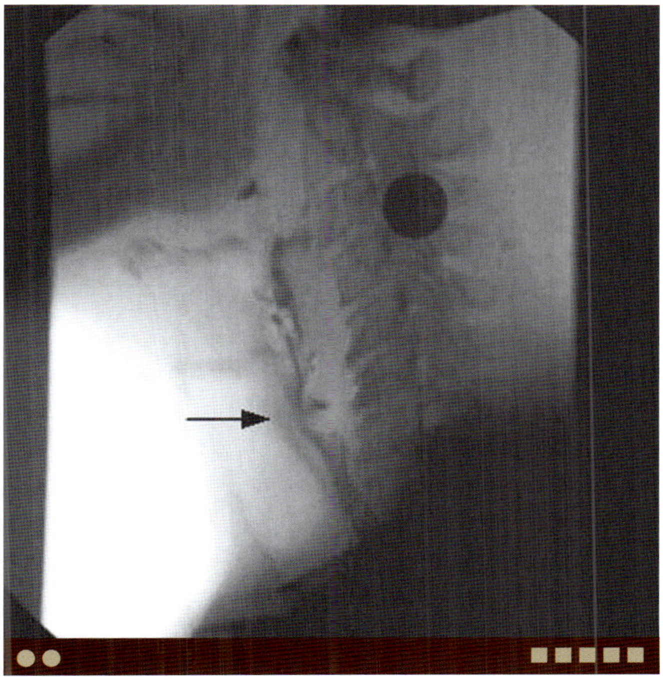

A. UES. Fluoroscopy image with a small bolus shows restricted UES opening of 0.166 cm when swallowing a 5 mL of liquid. Normal maximum distension is 0.50 cm.

COMMENTS

This is 68-year-old man with difficulty in swallowing. His dysphagia has worsened over the year despite swallow therapy. He complains that food sticks in his throat and he needs to chase it down with liquid. Medical history includes chemotherapy and radiotherapy for pharyngeal cancer completed 1 year ago and a long-standing history of gastroesophageal reflux disease (GERD) supported by the presence of a hiatal hernia, and sleep apnea.

Upper esophageal strictures are commonly reported after radiotherapy for head and neck cancer due to fibrosis of the cricopharyngeus and inferior constrictor muscles at the esophageal inlet. However, a history of gastroesophageal reflux is also associated with an increased incidence of "tight" cricopharyngeus muscle. The radiographic term for this picture is a "prominent CP bar." Our patient had both of these problems as a potential etiology.

PEARLS

- **It is only when a larger bolus was given that the true profile is revealed. A large bolus highlights the relatively patulous hypopharynx above a hypercontracted UES and forces the bolus through the tight but compliant UES. If this were a stricture, a large bolus would not increase the diameter of the UES opening.**
- **Giving the patient a large bolus is sometimes risky because many of these patients will aspirate with a larger bolus. However, it is the best way to differentiate a muscular dysfunction from a fibrotic stricture.**
- **One major difficulty is sorting out a narrowed CP segment due to a primary problem with the UES versus reduced UES opening secondary to a primary problem of reduced traction on the UES from the laryngeal structures as they are lifting superiorly and pulling anteriorly. There are two components of UES opening to keep in mind. The first stage is UES relaxation, secondary to inhibition of its tonic contractile resting state. The second stage occurs as the UES is pulled open from laryngeal structures as they lift during the swallow. If this distinction is not made, the UES can look to be the guilty structure when, in fact, it is simply not being pulled open. The large bolus will help to sort this out.**

ADDITIONAL IMAGE

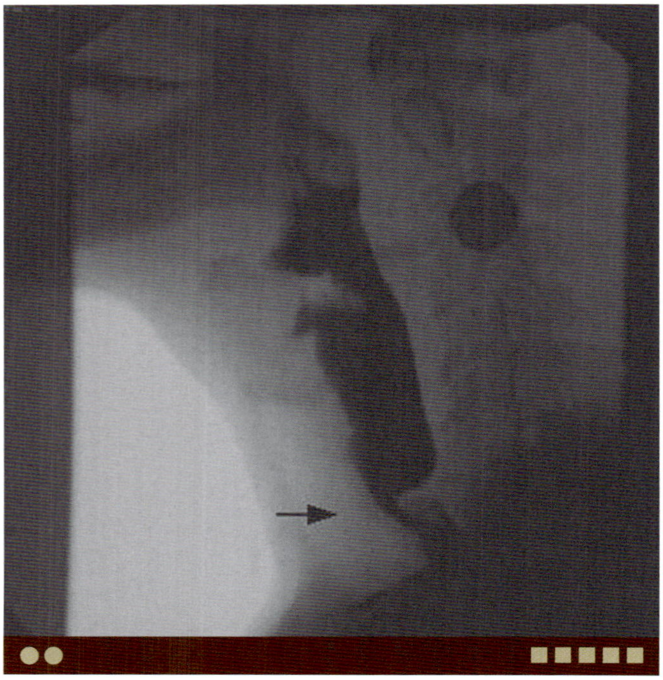

B. UES, same patient as A. Fluoroscopy image shows more apparent reduced UES opening with a large bolus. The UES opens slightly more, to a diameter of 0.297, with a patulous pharynx and widely open esophagus bordering it. This is more than 2 standard deviation (SD) below the normal maximum opening diameter of the UES for a large bolus (0.40 cm minimum).

DIFFERENTIAL DIAGNOSIS IMAGES (C-D)

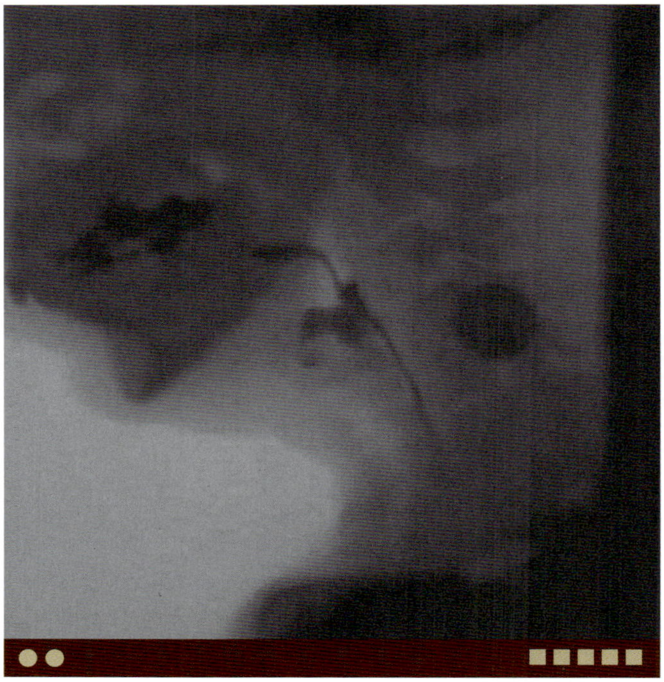

C. Stricture postradiotherapy. This 55-year-old woman has complaints of swallowing following two courses of radiotherapy and surgery for head and neck cancer and lymphoma: one recent and the other course delivered 40 years ago. She complains that food and pills stick in her throat; she also chokes on liquids. The first fluoroscopy image shows an extremely narrowed CP segment, measuring only 0.189 cm at its most narrow portion. The very narrow UES region extends more than 3 cm from the pharynx superiorly and the esophagus inferiorly from about C4 to C6.

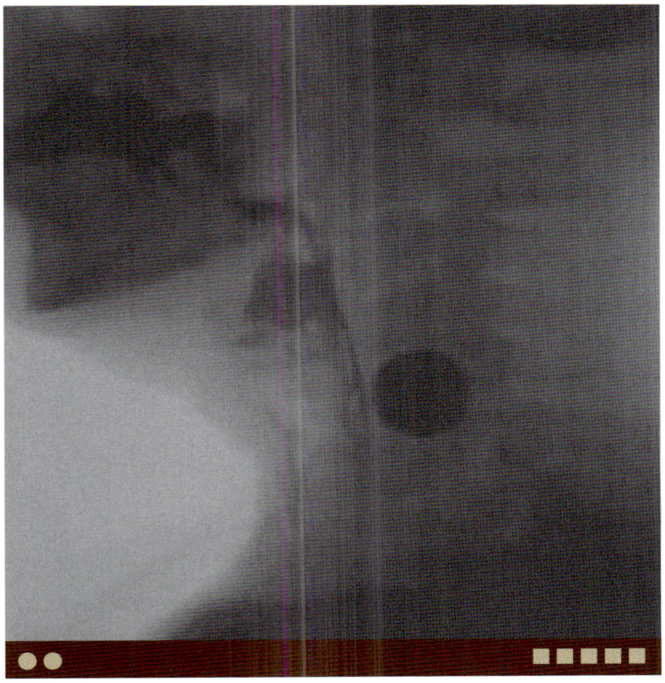

D. Stricture postradiotherapy, same patient as C. Large bolus fluoroscopy image shows the UES region does not open any more than on the small bolus. It does show the wider pharyngeal area, however. Because the patient could not clear the bolus through the UES, this bolus overflowed the laryngeal vestibule shortly thereafter and was aspirated.

Case 11–29 Reduced Bolus Clearance at the Level of the Valleculae

Susan Langmore

PRESENTATION

Residue of a 5-cc bolus of liquid in the valleculae after the swallow.

FINDINGS

Fluoroscopy image after swallowing a level teaspoon of liquid barium shows that the bolus did not clear the vallecular space and surrounding area.

DIFFERENTIAL DIAGNOSIS

- Radiotherapy: The epiglottis is a cartilage and its pliability can be damaged by radiotherapy.
- Connective tissue disease: Reduces the pliability of the epiglottis.
- Anatomic/obstruction: Osteophyte or other obstruction, pushing forward on the posterior pharyngeal wall and preventing the epiglottis from moving completely.
- Physiologic: (1) Reduced base of tongue contact against the posterior pharyngeal wall and retractive force against the epiglottis to facilitate its first bend to about 90 degrees, and (2) reduced hyoid excursion which causes the epiglottis to complete the retroflexion to about 180 degrees.

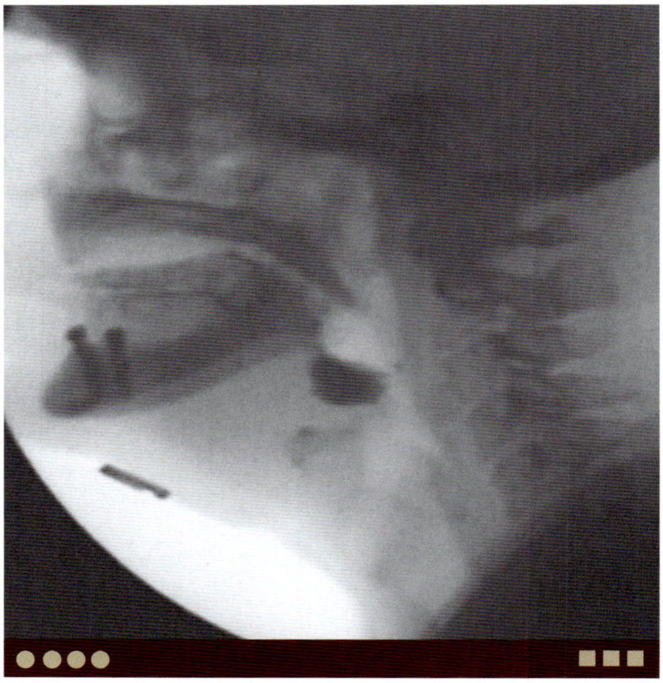

A. Reduced bolus clearance. Fluoroscopy after swallowing a level teaspoon of liquid barium showed that the bolus did not clear the vallecular space and surrounding area.

COMMENTS

This is a 65-year-old man status post chemoradiation therapy for head and neck cancer 2 years ago. He has never regained a level of swallowing that would allow him to discard his feeding tube. The small bolus of liquid shown in this still frame did not clear the vallecular space; food presented him with even a greater challenge.

During a normal swallow, the tissues within the hypopharynx completely close against each other, squeezing the bolus through and obliterating the airspace. If residue is left at the level of the valleculae, it indicates that the epiglottis did not retroflex, trapping the bolus in the valleculae. However, since the epiglottis is not a muscle, with active contractile force, the etiology is more convoluted. Either the tongue did not squeeze against the epiglottis sufficiently, or the hyoid did not lift and "torque" the epiglottis to its full retroflexed position.

Using fluoroscopy, airspace and residual contrast volume can be measured.

PEARLS

- **Location of residue has been shown to be the best indicator of the source of the problem in several studies. However, as seen by these examples, inspection of structural movement and anatomy provide further insight into the nature of the impairment.**

ADDITIONAL IMAGES (B-G)

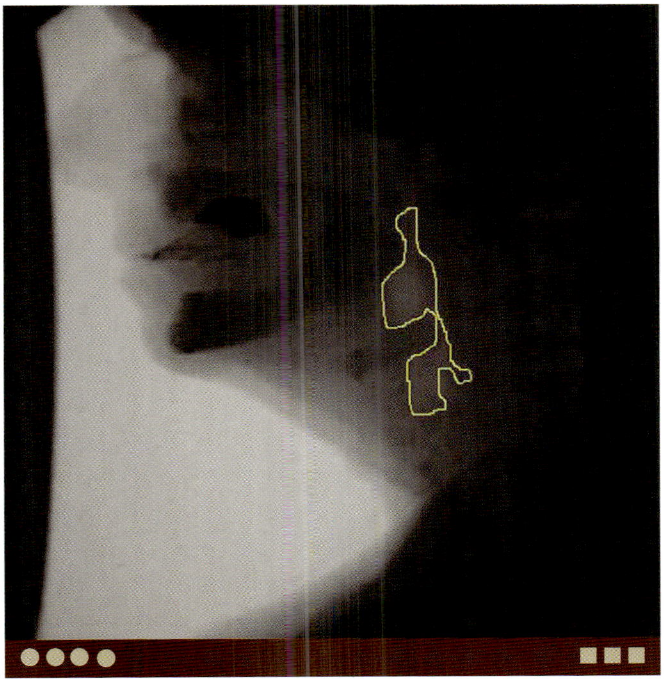

B. Reduced bolus clearance, same patient as A. Fluoroscopy shows that the area occupied by air *when the pharynx was at rest* was 5559 pixels.

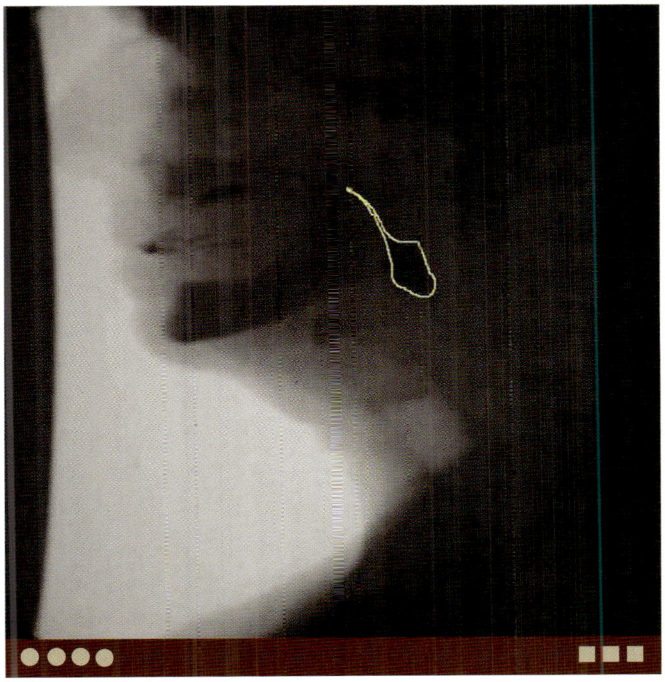

C. Reduced bolus clearance, same patient as A. Fluoroscopy shows that the area within the pharynx *at maximum pharyngeal contraction* (during the height of the swallow), where the airspace was maximally closed, was 1108 pixels; there was no airspace visible, but the bolus remained in the space left open. The ratio of 1108/5559 or 0.199, indicated that 20% of the airspace was still open (ie, not closed) at maximum pharyngeal contraction. Normal ratio = 0.02 to 0.06.

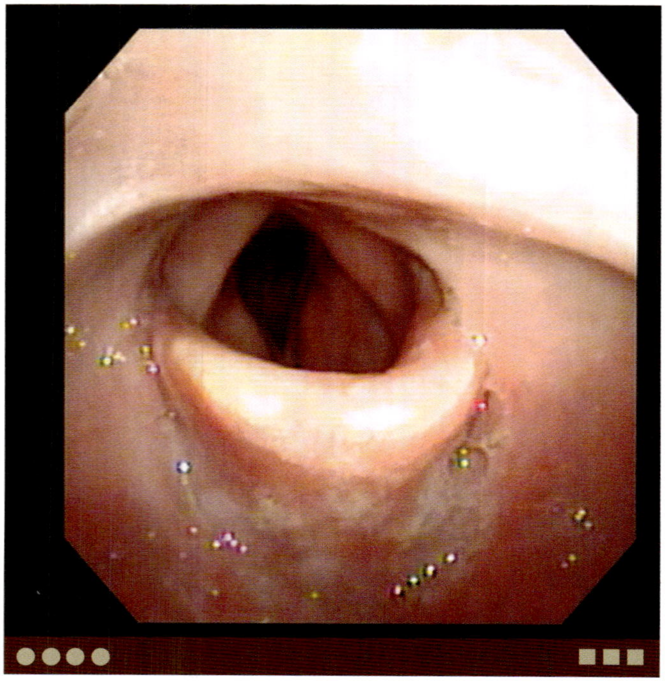

D. Reduced bolus clearance, same patient as A. Flexible laryngoscopy shows the extent of the fibrotic changes and the restricted space around the epiglottis for the bolus to flow out of the valleculae. Webbing and thickening of the tissues within the oropharynx and hypopharynx are typical after radiation therapy.

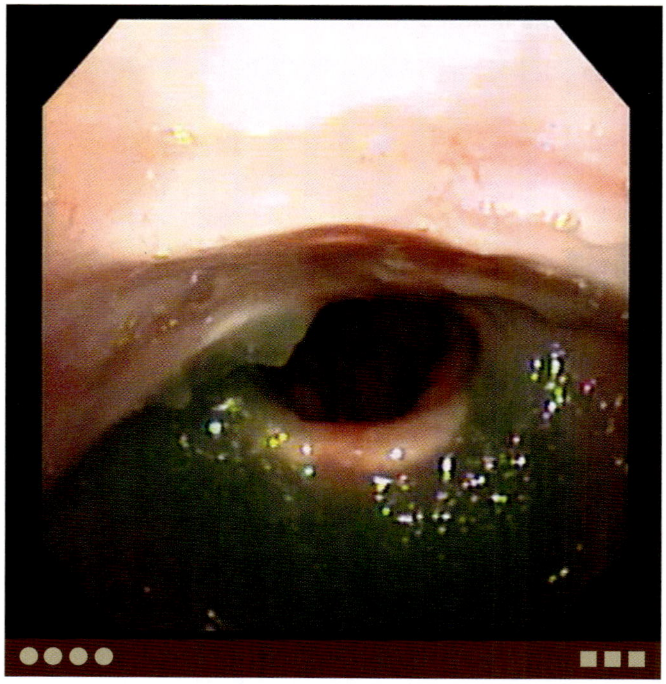

E. Reduced bolus clearance, same patient as A. Flexible laryngoscopy shows applesauce in the vallecular space and illustrate the residue in the valleculae nicely.

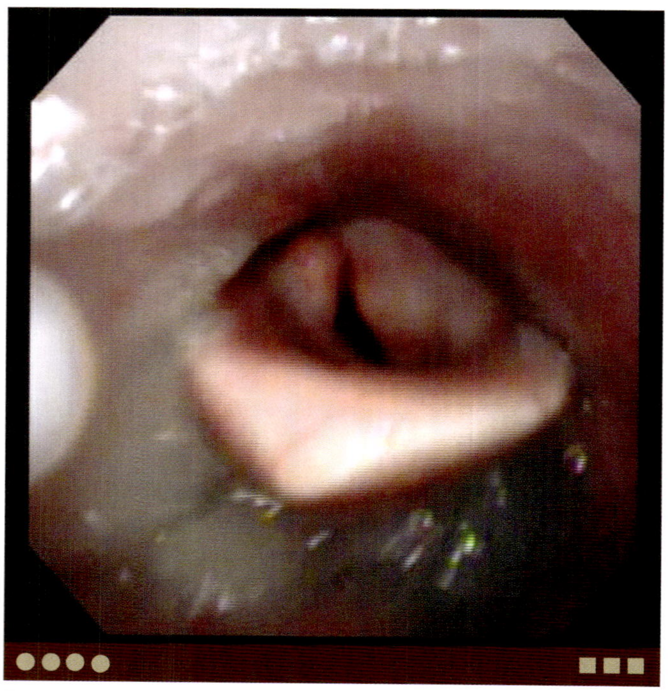

F. Reduced bolus clearance, postradiation therapy in a different patient. Flexible laryngoscopy shows similar swallowing problem, fruit cocktail not able to clear the valleculae.

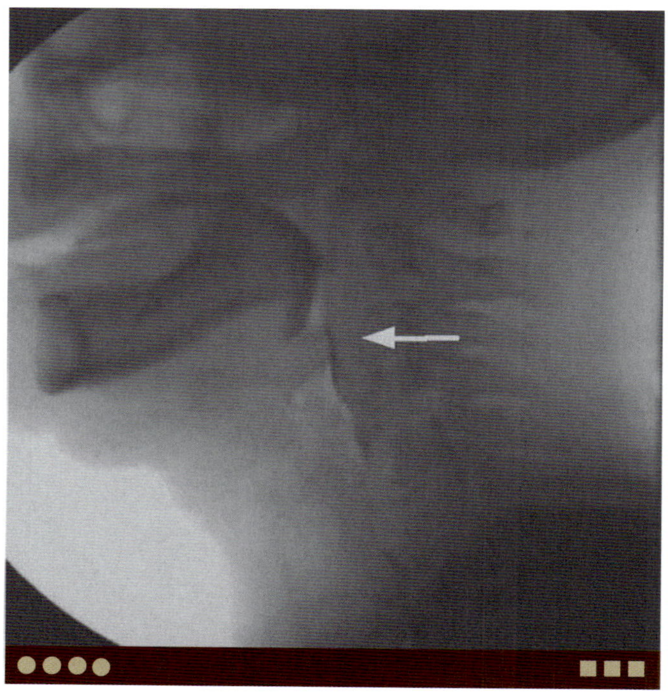

G. Reduced bolus clearance, postradiation therapy in a different patient. Fluoroscopy shows thick epiglottis and hang up in valleculae. The epiglottis is abutting the posterior pharyngeal wall in a partly retroflexed state. After radiotherapy, the epiglottis can become very stiff.

DIFFERENTIAL DIAGNOSIS IMAGES (H-I)

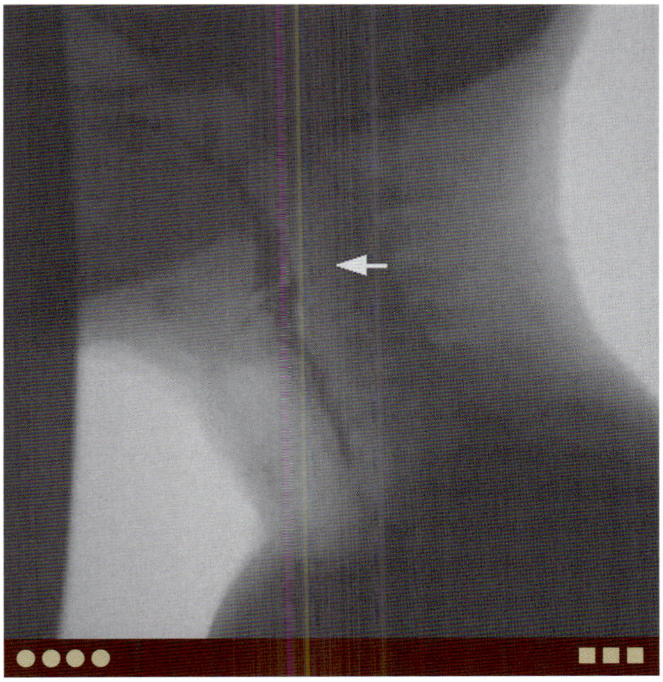

H. Residue throughout the hypopharynx. Fluoroscopy shows minimal retroflexion of the epiglottis and reduced bolus clearance. However, the residue is not concentrated in the valleculae but rather is dispersed throughout the hypopharynx. The medical etiology of this was amyloidosis, causing very stiff and limited movement of all structures.

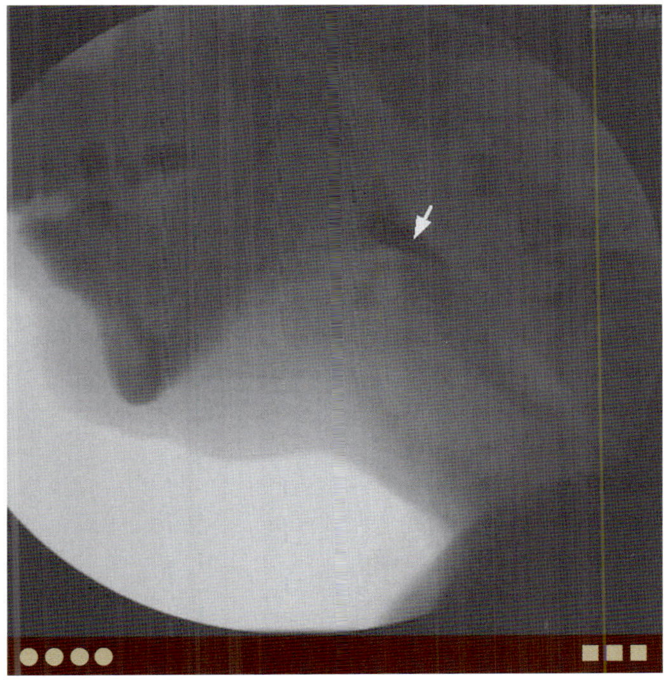

I. Residue at the valleculae in the presence of *complete* epiglottic retroflexion. Fluoroscopy shows both epiglottic retroflexion and hyoid excursion was judged to be good but residue still remained in the valleculae. The etiology of residue localized to the valleculae was attributed to reduced base of tongue retraction. In fact, after swallowing a dry cracker, the residue along the base of tongue was well visualized, in addition to the residue in the valleculae.

Chapter 12

LYMPH NODES

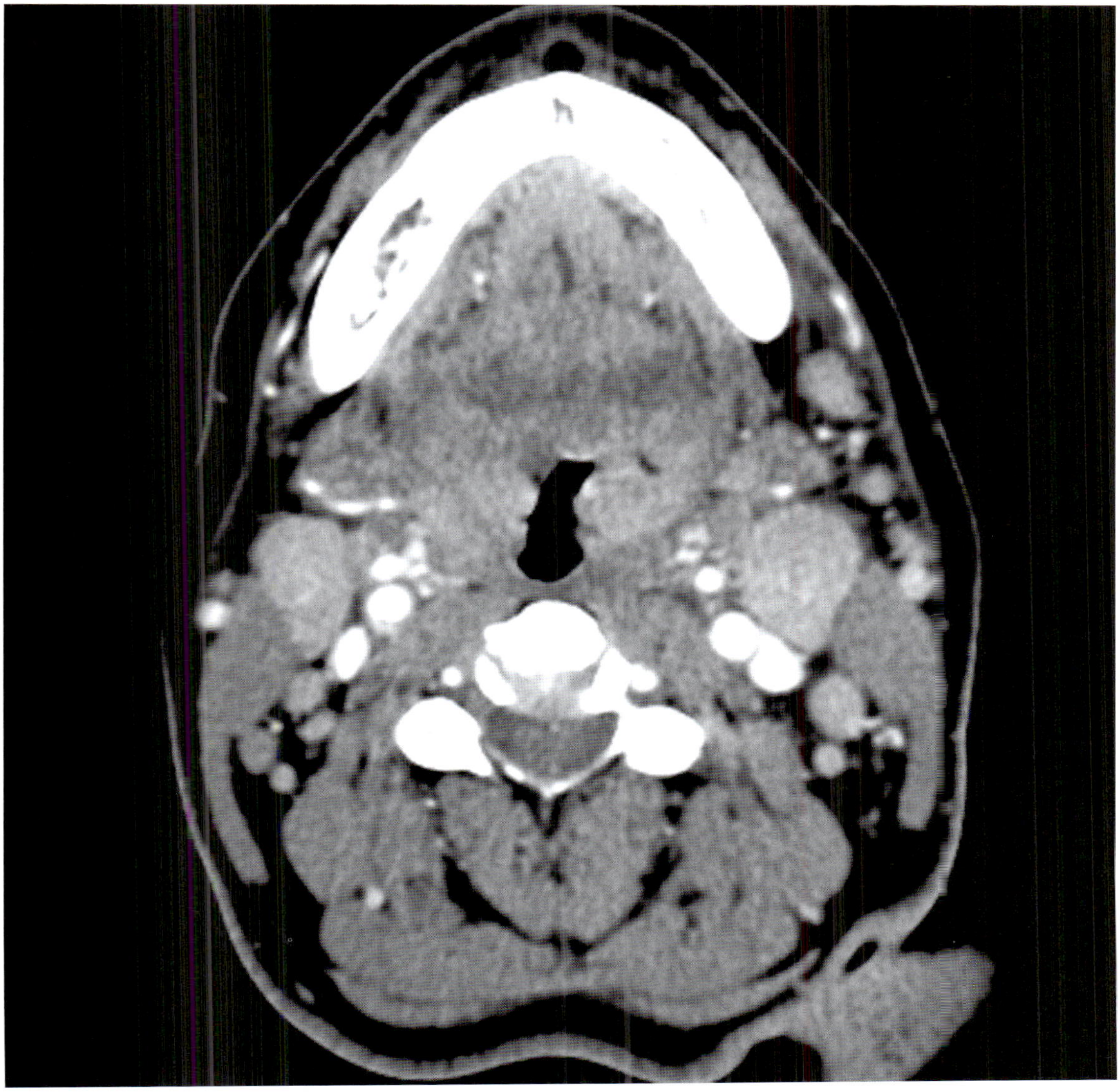

Case 12–1 Reactive Cervical Lymphadenopathy

Benjamin Ludwig, Osamu Sakai

PRESENTATION

Recent upper respiratory infection, painful cervical lymphadenopathy.

FINDINGS

Contrast-enhanced CT of the neck demonstrates multiple, enlarged, homogeneously enhancing lymph nodes.

DIFFERENTIAL DIAGNOSIS

- Suppurative lymphadenopathy: Secondary to bacterial infection, nodes typically demonstrate central hypodensity, peripheral rim enhancement, and inflammatory changes in the adjacent soft tissues or muscles.
- Metastatic lymph nodes: Imaging findings range from normal to enlarged nodes, with possible central hypodensity and peripheral enhancement in the setting of nodal necrosis. Perinodal inflammatory changes are usually absent, but loss of fat planes with adjacent tissues suggests extracapsular tumor spread.
- Nodal lipoid metaplasia: Peripheral nodal hypoattenuation, measuring fat density, which is responsible for the typical "lima-bean" shape of nodes.

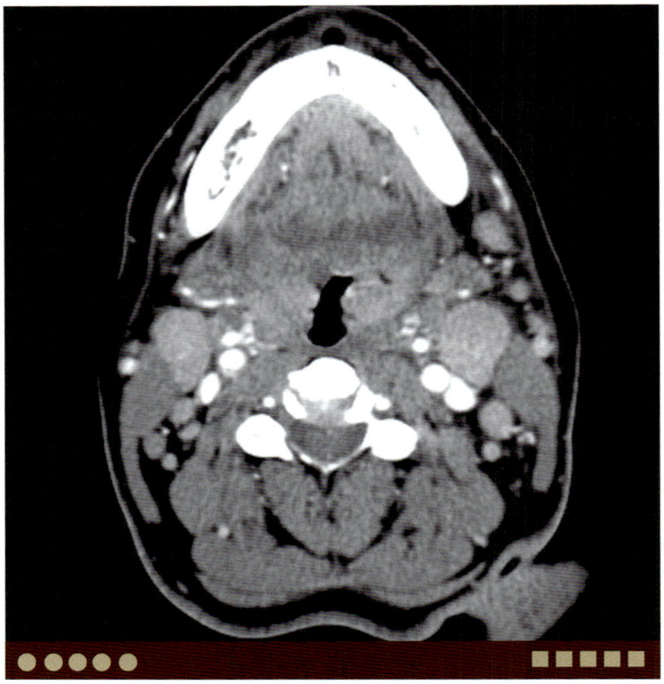

A. Reactive lymphadenopathy. Axial contrast-enhanced CT demonstrates enlarged, mildly enhancing bilateral level II lymph nodes, without central necrosis.

COMMENTS

This patient is a 57-year-old woman with sore throat and neck pain.

Reactive cervical lymphadenopathy may be due to infectious, inflammatory, lymphoproliferative, or neoplastic etiologies.

Normal lymph nodes are classified as <10 mm in long axis, with the exception of level IB and level II nodes, which may be up to 15 mm. Normal nodes are described as iso or hypoattenuating to muscle on CT, and ovoid in shape. On MRI, nodes have low-to-intermediate T1 signal intensity, and are hyperintense on T2W images. Ultrasound findings include homogenous, hypoechogenicity relative to muscle. Fat within the lymph node hilum is characteristic of normal lymph nodes.

Imaging based characterization of nodes must be correlated with the patient's age, presentation, and physical examination findings. Although some diseases or conditions may show characteristic imaging findings, diagnosis of causative agent is often difficult by imaging alone. Imaging features including size, location, attenuation, and associated head and neck findings may narrow the differential.

Benign lymph nodes are typically normal in size to slightly enlarged, and may enhance. Viral etiologies produce diffuse lymph node involvement with little surrounding inflammation.

Common viral etiologies include human immunodeficiency virus, cytomegalovirus, and infectious mononucleosis.

Bacterial etiologies tend to produce more enlarged nodes, with perinodal inflammatory change, and can progress to suppurative nodes and intranodal abscesses. Common bacterial etiologies include *Staphylococcus aureus,* Group A *streptococcus,* tuberculous and nontuberculous mycobacteria, and cat scratch disease.

PEARLS

- **While findings are often nonspecific, imaging characteristics including nodal size, attenuation and enhancement, location, associated head and neck findings, and correlation with patient history and physical examination, may aid in establishing a diagnosis.**
- **Reactive lymph nodes may result from infectious, inflammatory, lymphoproliferative, and neoplastic etiologies.**
- **Nodes with central necrosis may be related to infection or metastatic involvement. Secondary inflammatory findings, history, and clinical examination should aid in diagnosis.**

Idiopathic etiologies include Kawasaki, Kimura, Kikuchi-Fujimoto, and Castleman diseases, sarcoidosis, and post-transplant lymphoproliferative disorder. Location, enhancement characteristics, and associated head and neck findings aid in diagnosis of these entities.

Suppurative lymph nodes result from bacterial infection with pus formation within nodes, most commonly due to *S. aureus* and Group A *Streptococcus*. Nodes demonstrate central hypoattenuation with rim enhancement and inflammatory change in adjacent structures on CT. MRI findings include central T2 hyperintensity with T1 hypointensity and peripheral enhancement after gadolinium. Ultrasound findings include intranodal cyst formation with peripheral Doppler hypervascularity. Such imaging findings can also be seen in the setting of metastatic disease.

Neoplastic involvement may result from lymphoma, leukemia, or metastatic disease. Nodes may range from normal in size to enlarged, and may also demonstrate nodal necrosis. Nodes often have an ill-defined border, with loss of fat planes between and/or invasion of adjacent structures, consistent with extracapsular tumor spread. It is important to include postcontrast fat-suppressed T1W sequences in order to evaluate for the nonenhancing region of central necrosis as well as extracapsular tumor spread.

ADDITIONAL IMAGES (B–G)

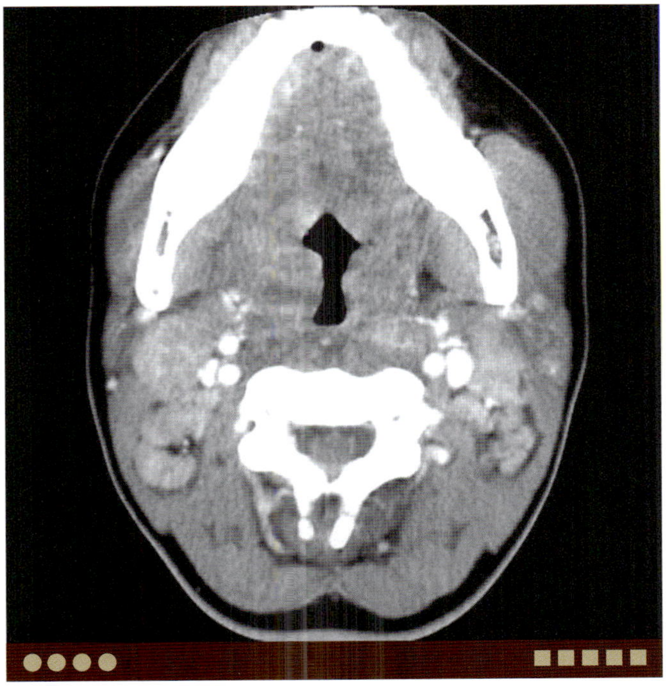

B. Mononucleosis. Axial postcontrast CT demonstrates multiple, heterogeneously enhancing, enlarged bilateral level II lymph nodes. Note enlarged, edematous palatine tonsils.

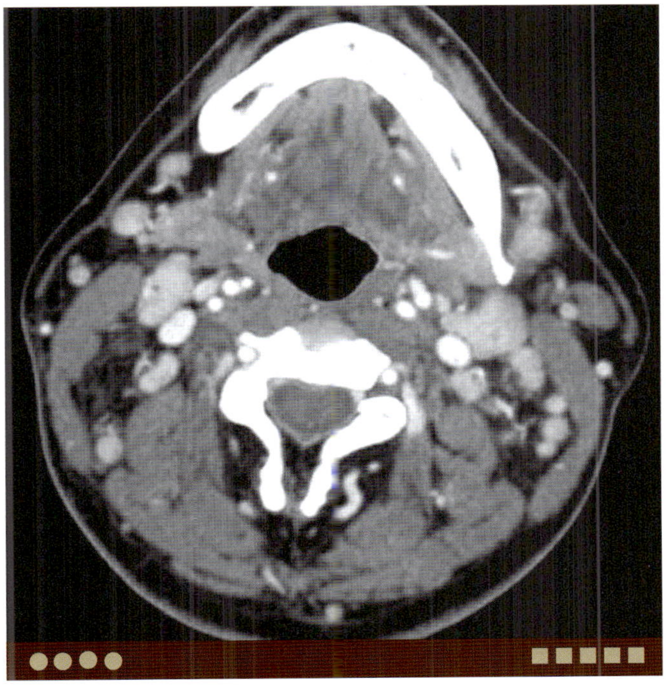

C. Lymphadenopathy associated with HIV infection. Axial postcontrast CT demonstrates multiple bilateral, homogeneously enhancing level I and II lymph nodes.

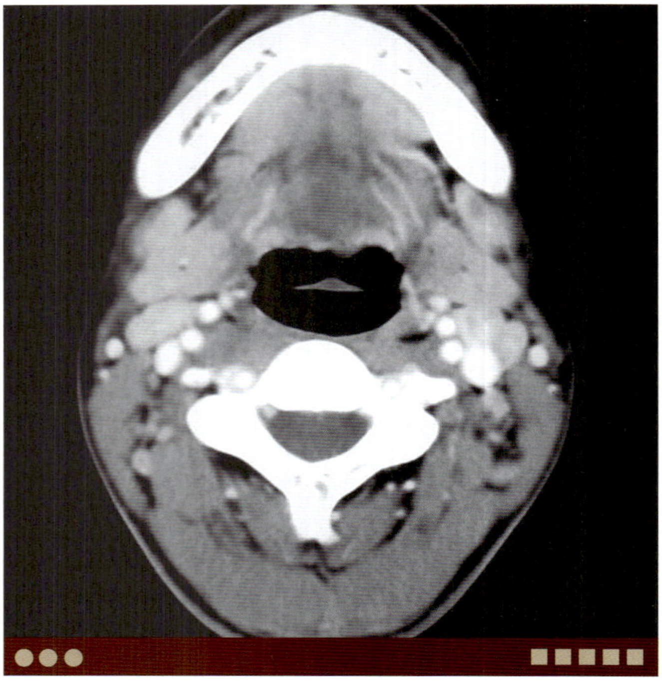

D. Sarcoidosis. Axial postcontrast CT demonstrates multiple, enhancing, enlarged bilateral level I and II lymph nodes.

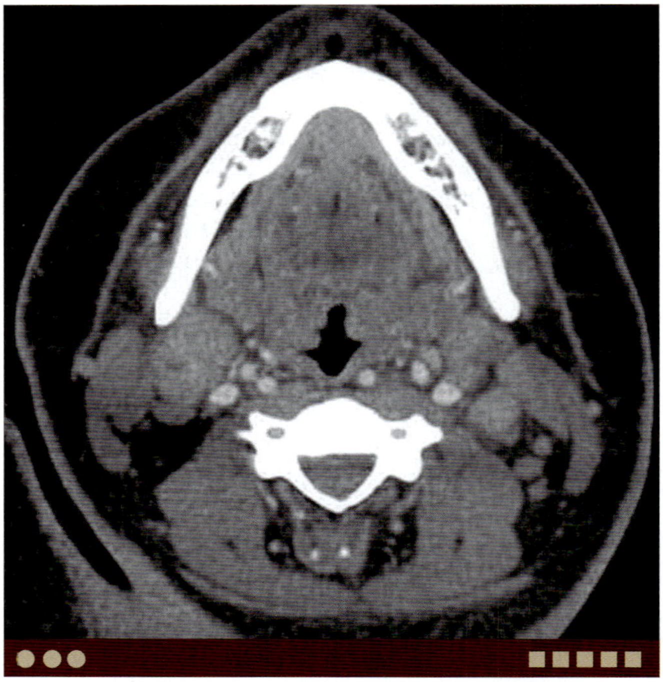

E. Cat scratch disease. Axial postcontrast CT demonstrates multiple, enhancing, enlarged bilateral level II lymph nodes. Some nodes demonstrate central hypodensity and perinodal inflammatory changes.

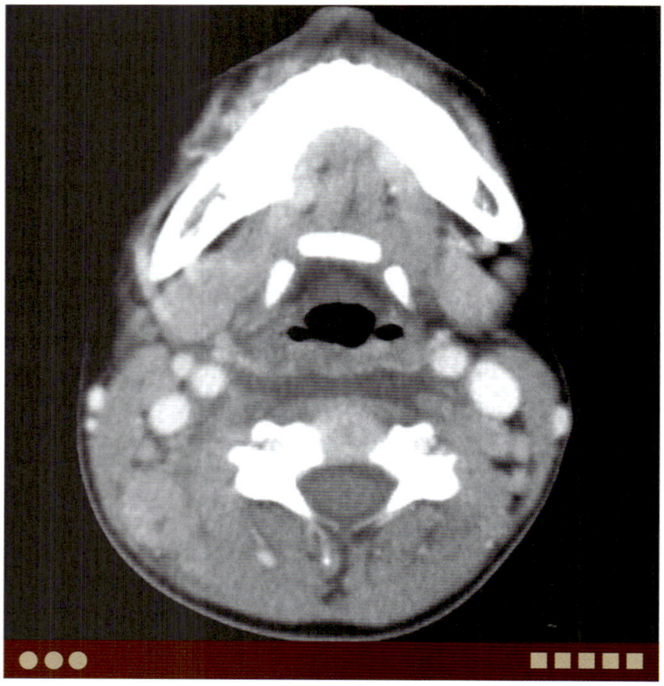

F. Kawasaki disease. Axial postcontrast CT demonstrates multiple, enhancing bilateral level II and V lymph nodes. Note associated retropharyngeal edema.

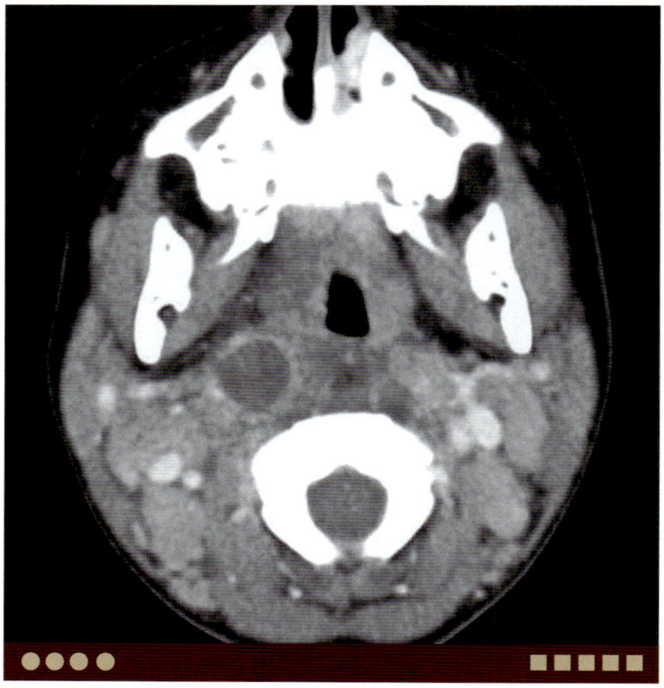

G. Lateral retropharyngeal intranodal abscess. Axial CT postcontrast demonstrates an enlarged, rim-enhancing right lateral retropharyngeal node (node of Rouvière) with adjacent phlegmon.

DIFFERENTIAL DIAGNOSIS IMAGES (H-J)

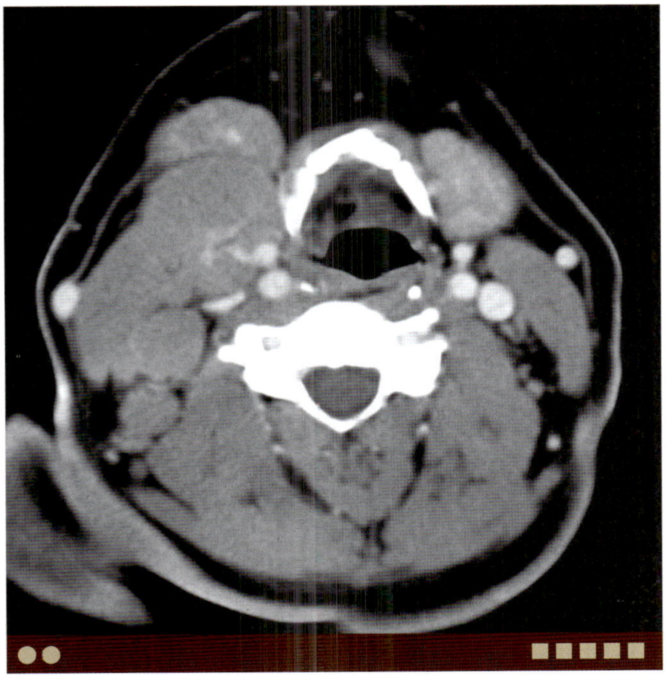

H. Lymphoma. Axial postcontrast CT demonstrates multiple, enlarged, minimally enhancing, homogeneous right level II and V lymph nodes.

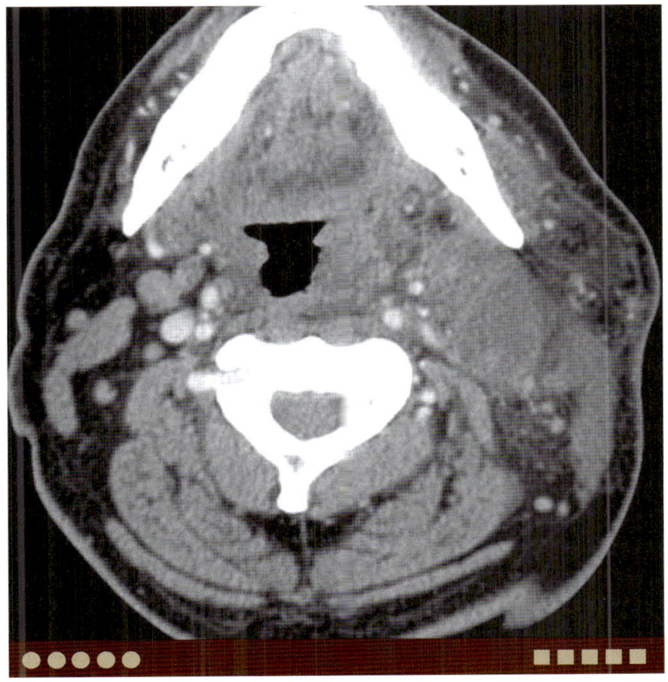

I. Metastasis from tonsillar squamous cell carcinoma. Axial postcontrast CT through the palatine tonsils demonstrates minimally enlarged left tonsil, the site of the primary neoplasm. An enlarged left level IIA node with loss of adjacent fat planes and infiltrative changes is consistent with nodal metastasis with extracapsular tumor spread.

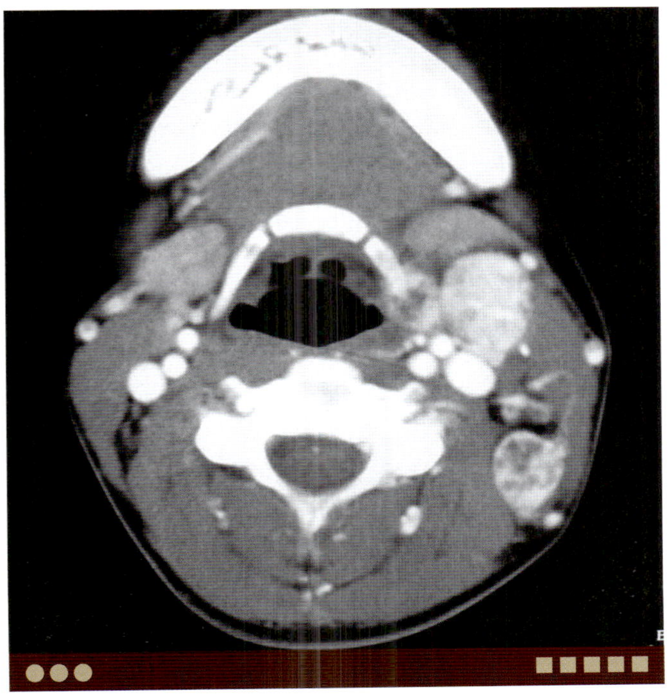

J. Metastasis from papillary thyroid carcinoma. Axial postcontrast CT demonstrates multiple, heterogeneous, avidly enhancing, enlarged left level II and V lymph nodes.

Case 12–2 Metastatic Lymphadenopathy: Necrotic Node

Osamu Sakai, Rohini Nadgir

PRESENTATION

Neck mass.

FINDINGS

CT shows a rim-enhancing nodal mass in the neck.

DIFFERENTIAL DIAGNOSIS

- Tuberculous adenitis: Involved lymph nodes demonstrate variable appearance; including avid enhancement, cystic change, and calcification. Because tuberculosis is a low-grade infection and inflammatory change around the affected node may be subtle, the finding may be similar to metastasis from squamous cell carcinoma or papillary thyroid carcinoma.
- Intranodal necrosis or abscess from bacterial infection: This often demonstrates profound inflammatory process in the adjacent soft tissue. However, inflammatory change is often seen associated with metastasis from squamous cell carcinoma.
- Infected branchial cleft cyst: This is seen as a rim-enhancing cystic lesion.

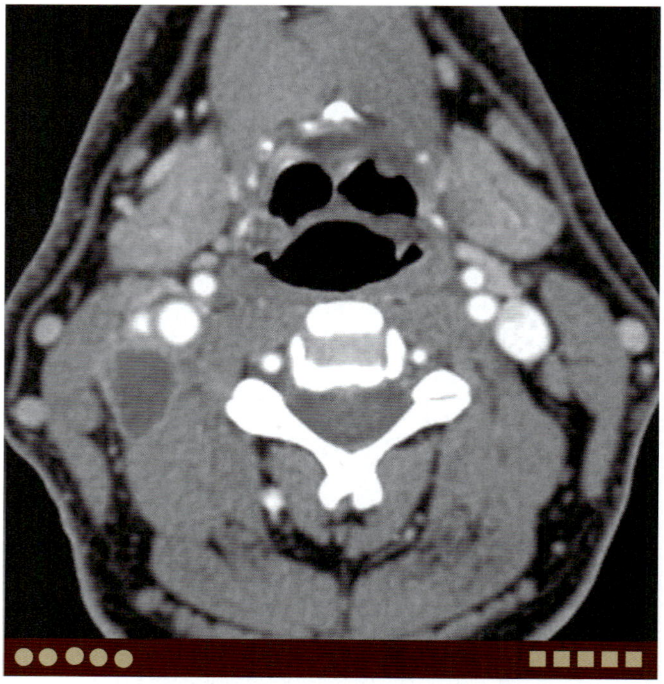

A. Metastasis from tonsillar SCCA. Axial postcontrast CT demonstrates an enlarged lymph node with central low density in the right level IIB.

COMMENTS

This is a 50-year-old man with squamous cell carcinoma (SCCA) in the right tonsil.

To evaluate lymph node for possible metastatic lesion, a classic size criterion is still widely used, even with recent advance in imaging modalities, such as MDCT and MRI, and more recently PET-CT. If the lymph node exceeds 1.5 cm in the level II, or 1 cm in anywhere else in the neck, metastasis from malignancy should be considered. Note in the head and neck, the long axis (not short axis) in the axial plane is usually measured to increase the sensitivity and to match the clinical measurement. Other findings which can suggest nodal metastasis are round shape rather than lima-bean shape, loss of fatty hilum, and conglomerate lymph nodes.

More important finding to suggest metastasis is central low density, which is often termed as central "necrosis." If there is central low density, the node is always abnormal regardless of its size; differential considerations include tumor necrosis versus intranodal abscess from infection. This is a definite finding of abnormality, whereas size criteria always have considerable overlap between normal and abnormal, and benign and malignant etiologies.

CT can detect intranodal necrosis larger than 3 mm in diameter. The differential diagnosis always should include metastasis from SCCA, papillary thyroid carcinoma, and tuberculosis. Larger nodal metastasis has a higher incidence of necrosis. On the contrary, if there is no necrosis in an enlarged lymph node larger than 3 cm, metastasis from SCCA is less likely. Other etiologies such as lymphoma should be considered in these cases.

PEARLS

- **Central low density in the lymph node is always abnormal regardless of the size of the node.**
- **Nodal metastases from SCCA and papillary thyroid carcinoma often present with intranodal tumor necrosis.**
- **Tuberculosis can mimic necrotic nodal metastasis.**

ADDITIONAL IMAGES (B-D)

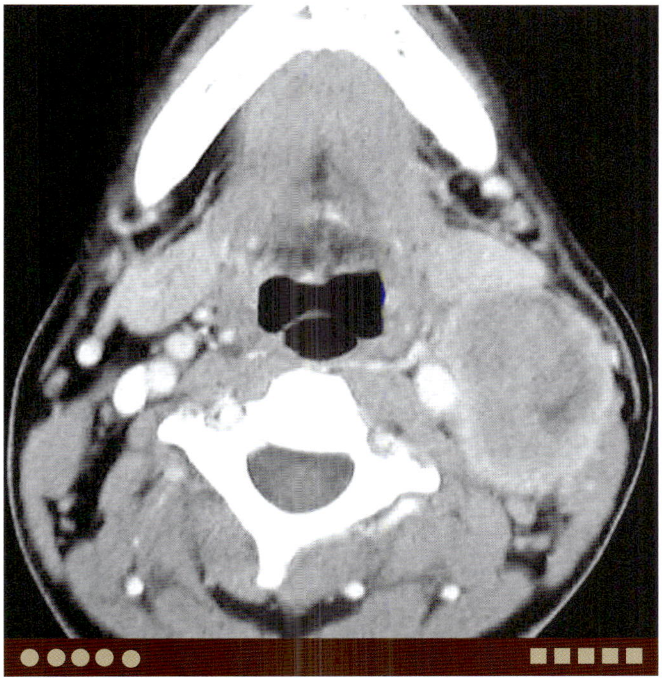

B. Metastasis from tongue SCCA. Axial postcontrast CT demonstrates an enlarged, heterogeneously enhancing node with central low density in the left level IIA.

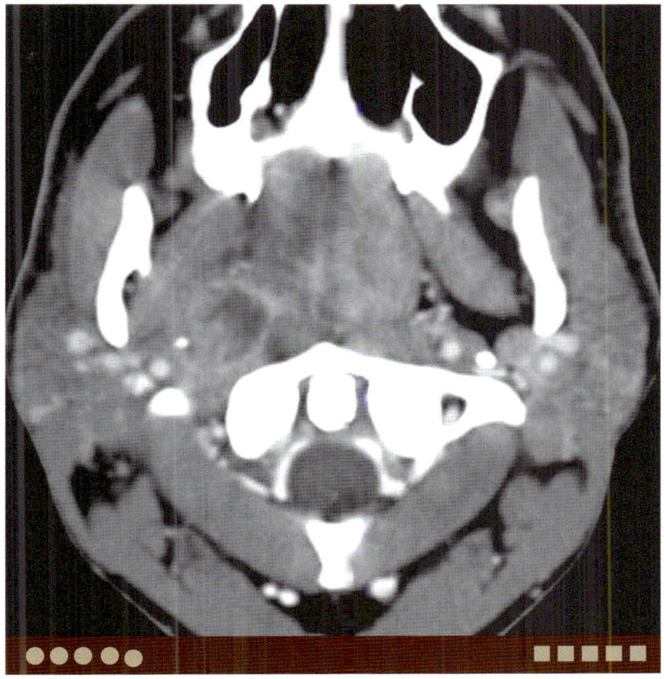

C. Metastasis from nasopharyngeal carcinoma. Axial postcontrast CT demonstrates a large necrotic right retropharyngeal node.

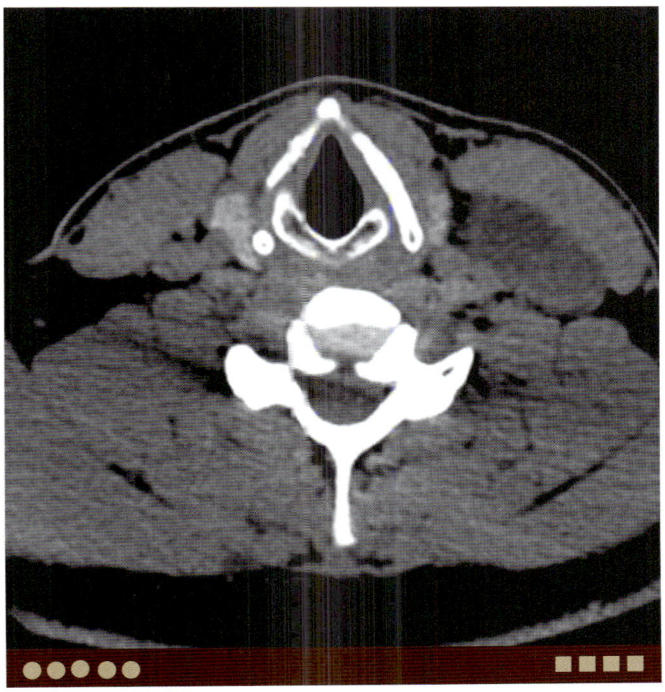

D. Metastasis from papillary thyroid cancer. Axial noncontrast CT demonstrates completely cystic node in the left level III/IV.

DIFFERENTIAL DIAGNOSIS IMAGES (E-I)

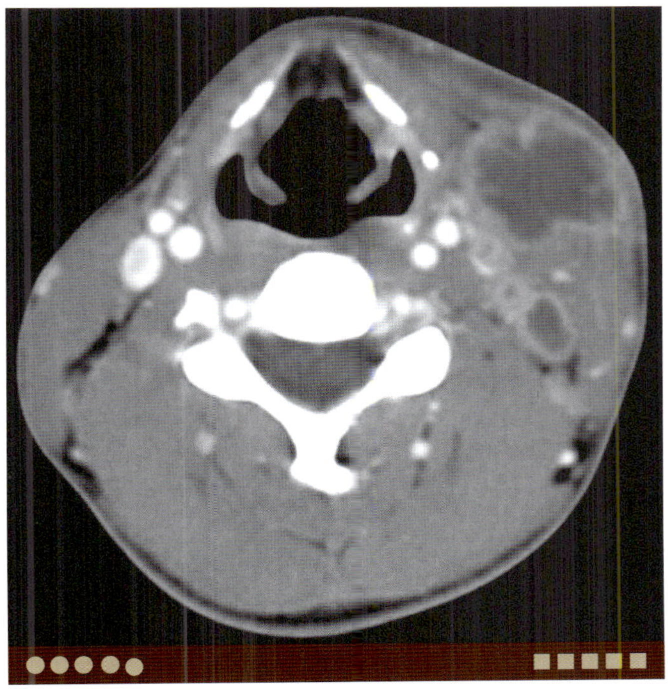

E. Tuberculosis. Axial postcontrast CT demonstrates a large necrotic node with perinodal inflammatory change and multiple smaller necrotic nodes in the left level III.

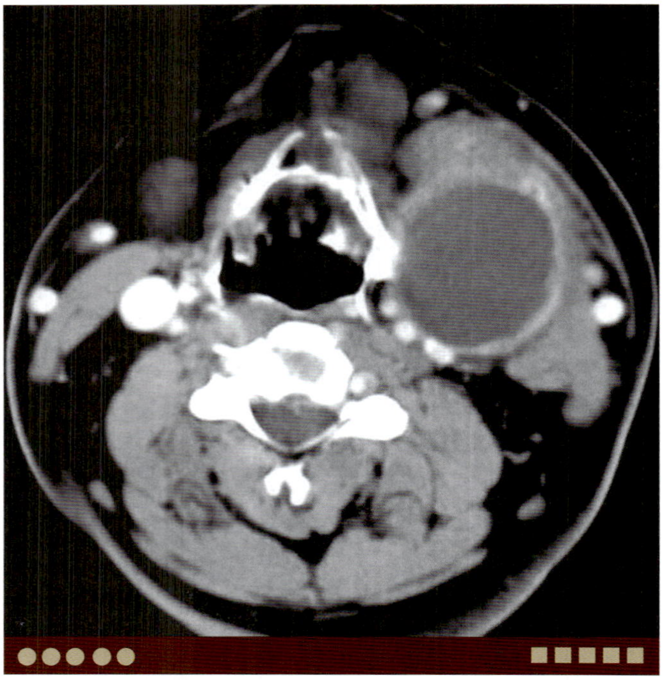

F. Infected branchial cleft cyst. Axial postcontrast CT demonstrates a large cystic lesion with thickened enhancing wall, anterolateral to the left carotid vessels, anteromedial to the sternocleidomastoid muscle, a typical location of second branchial cleft cyst.

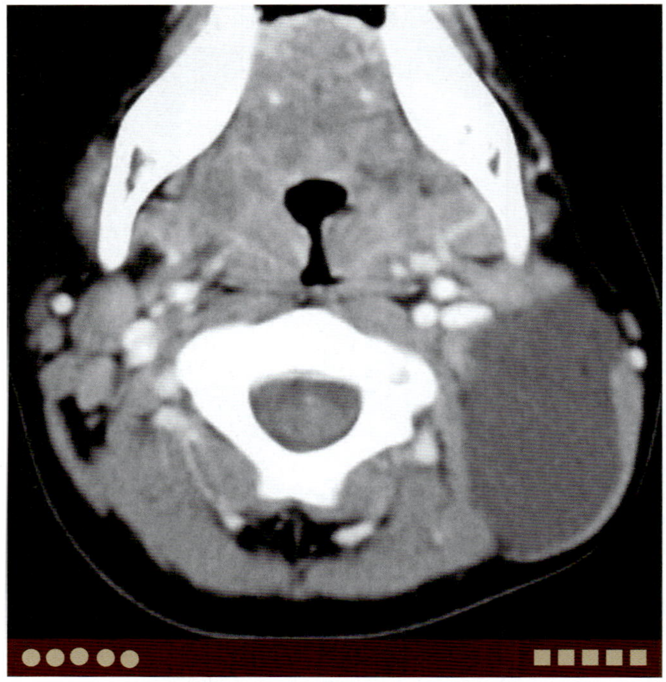

G. Lymphatic malformation. Axial postcontrast CT demonstrates a large cystic lesion in the left posterior triangle.

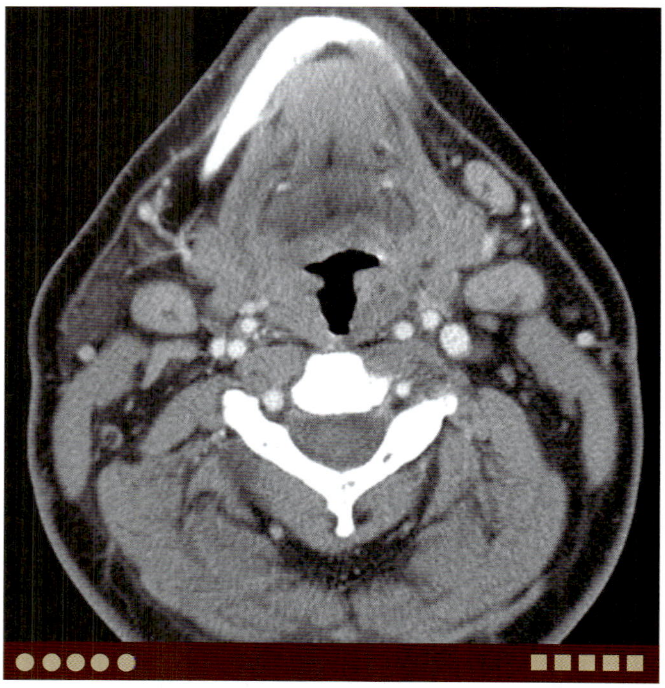

H. Reactive hyperplastic node. Axial postcontrast CT demonstrates multiple enlarged nodes with fatty hila in the bilateral levels I and II.

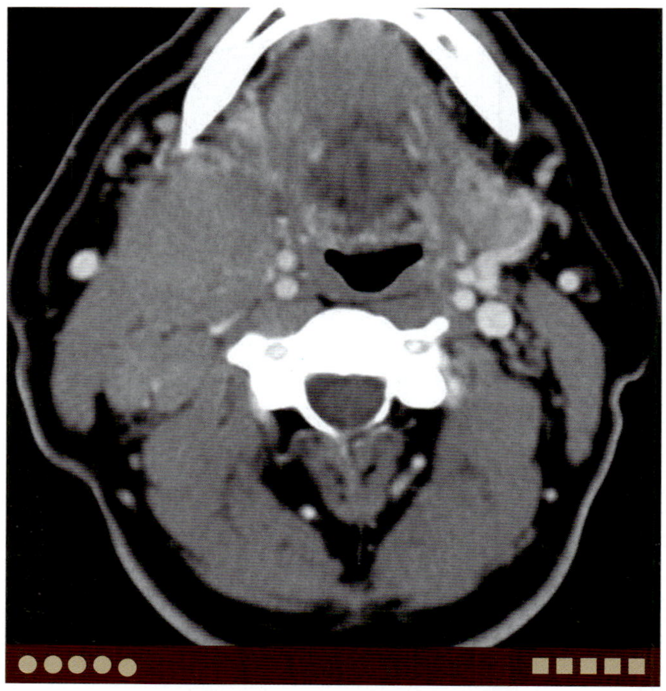

I. Lymphoma. Axial postcontrast CT demonstrates very large non-necrotic nodes in the right level II.

Case 12–3 Metastatic Lymphadenopathy: Extracapsular Tumor Spread

Osamu Sakai, Rohini Nadgir

PRESENTATION

Neck mass.

FINDINGS

CT shows a rim-enhancing lymph node with poorly defined border.

DIFFERENTIAL DIAGNOSIS

- Tuberculous adenitis: Involved lymph nodes demonstrate variable appearance; including avid enhancement, cystic change, and calcification. Because tuberculosis is a low-grade infection and inflammatory change around the affected node may be subtle, the finding may be similar to metastasis from squamous cell carcinoma (SCCA) or papillary thyroid carcinoma.
- Intranodal necrosis or abscess from bacterial infection: This often demonstrates profound inflammatory process in the adjacent soft tissue. However, inflammatory change is often seen associated with metastasis from squamous cell carcinoma.
- Infected branchial cleft cyst: This is seen as a rim-enhancing cystic lesion.

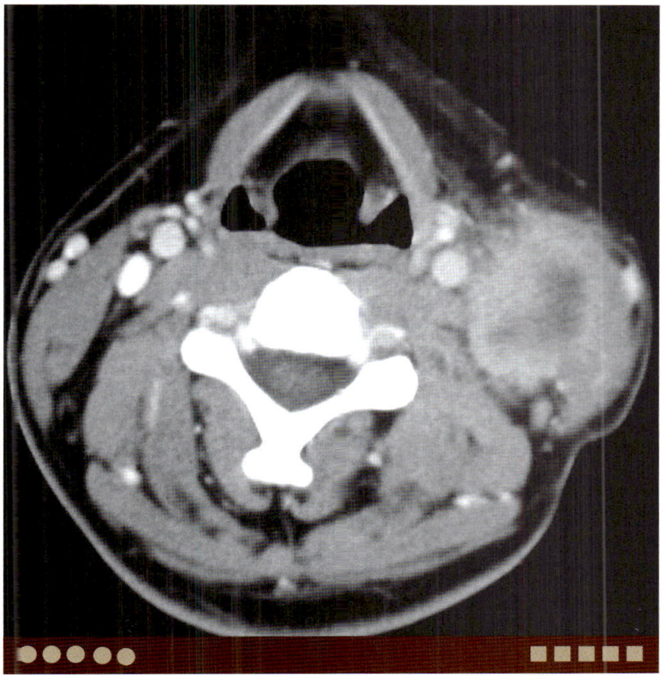

A Extranodal tumor extension, metastasis from tongue SCCA. Axial postcontrast CT demonstrates an enlarged lymph node with central low density and infiltrative margins in the left level II.

COMMENTS

This is a 21-year-old man with tongue cancer.

Tumors metastasizing to lymph nodes can extend beyond the capsule of the node, which is called extracapsular tumor spread. This condition will cut down the 5-year survival rate about 50%. This is often seen in larger nodes, however, small nodes can present extranodal tumor spread as well. Histologically, extracapsular tumor extension is found in about 25% of lymph nodes 1 cm in greatest diameter, in about 40% of lymph nodes less than 2 cm, in about 50% of nodes 2 to 3 cm, and in about 75% of nodes larger than 3 cm in diameter. Once extracapsular extension has occurred, the tumor can extend further and invade adjacent critical structures, such as the carotid artery, cranial nerves IX to XII, and the skull base. If macroscopic extracapsular tumor extension is present, the patient has about 10 times greater risk of a neck recurrence when compared with patients without such macroscopic tumor, and requires postoperative radiation.

Macroscopic extranodal tumor extension is seen on contrast-enhanced CT as an enhancing nodal rim, which is irregular and thick with infiltration of the adjacent fat planes. These criteria can be applied only if the patient has not recently had surgery, irradiation, or active infection or inflammation in the region because these conditions can cause similar imaging appearances.

PEARLS

- **Irregular and thick rim enhancement of metastatic nodes with infiltration into the adjacent fat planes suggests macroscopic extracapsular tumor spread.**
- **The patient with macroscopic extracapsular tumor has about 10 times greater risk of a neck recurrence when compared with patients without such macroscopic tumor.**
- **Histologically, extracapsular tumor extension is found in 40% of lymph nodes less than 2 cm in diameter.**

ADDITIONAL IMAGES (B-G)

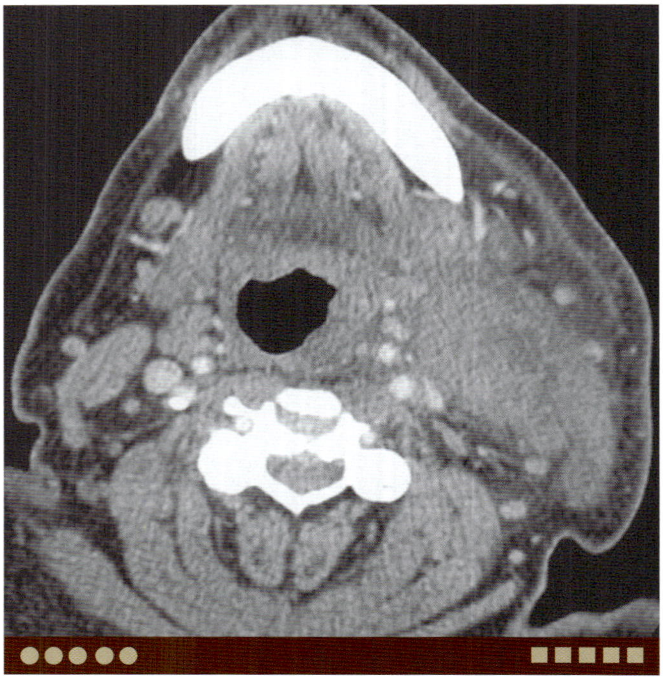

B. Metastasis from tonsillar SCCA. Axial postcontrast CT demonstrates an enlarged, heterogeneously enhancing node with central low density and poorly defined margins in the left level II. Note obscured boundaries between the node and sternocleidomastoid muscle to suggest invasion.

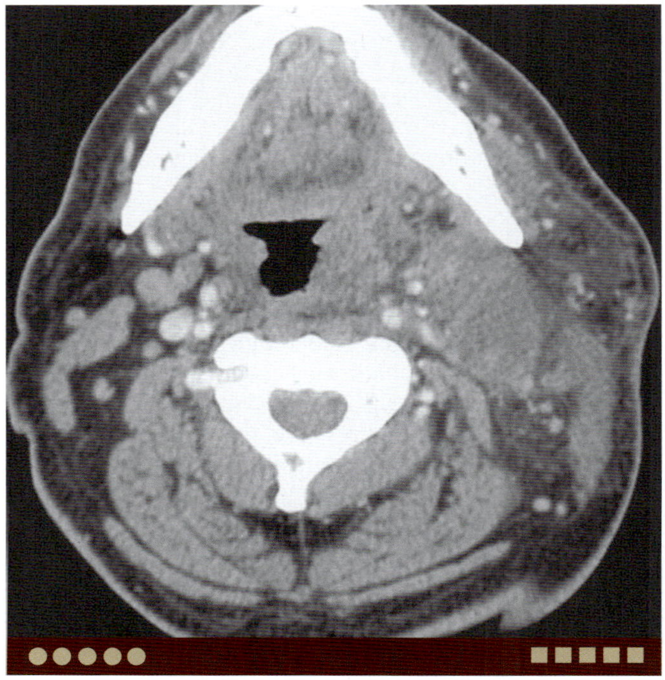

C. Metastasis from tonsillar SCCA, same patient as B. Axial postcontrast CT through the palatine tonsils demonstrates minimally enlarged left tonsil, the primary site. Again, infiltrative margins of the metastatic node are seen.

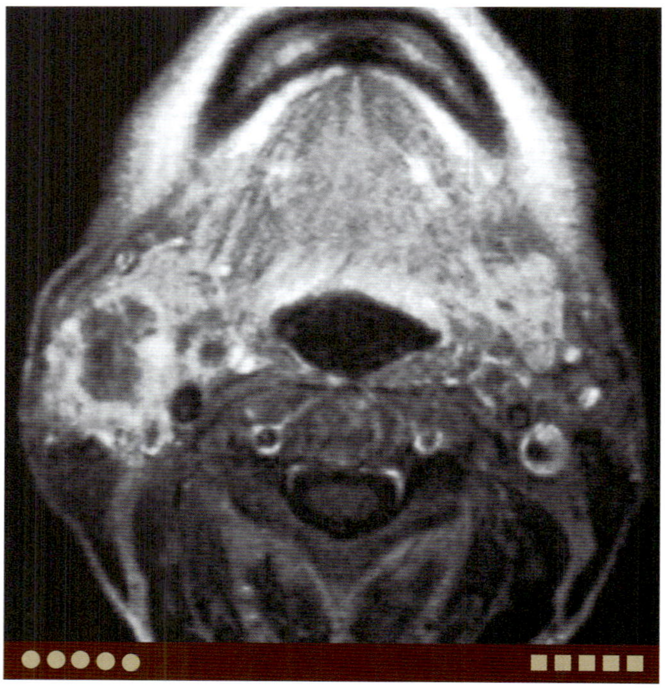

D. Metastasis from tonsillar SCCA in a different patient. Axial postcontrast fat-suppressed T1W image demonstrates a rim-enhancing lymph node with poorly defined borders in the right level II.

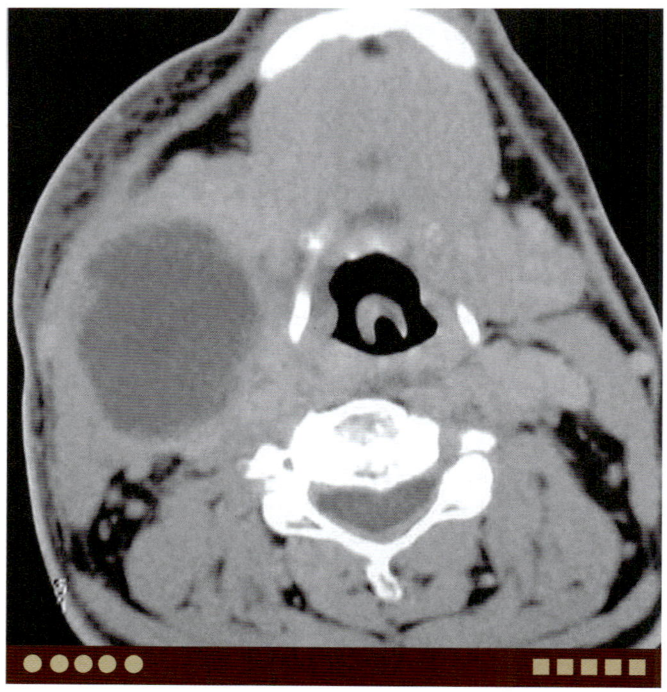

E. Metastasis from hypopharyngeal SCCA. Axial postcontrast CT demonstrates a large cystic-appearing lesion with poorly defined margins in the right level II. Fat planes around the node are obscured.

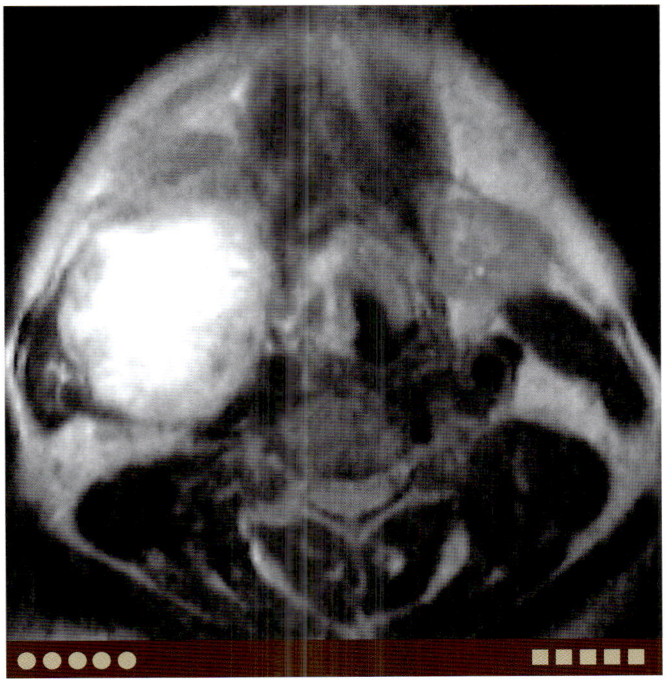

F. Metastasis from hypopharyngeal SCCA, same patient as E. Axial T2W MR image demonstrates a large cystic-appearing lesion with thick irregular margins in the right level II.

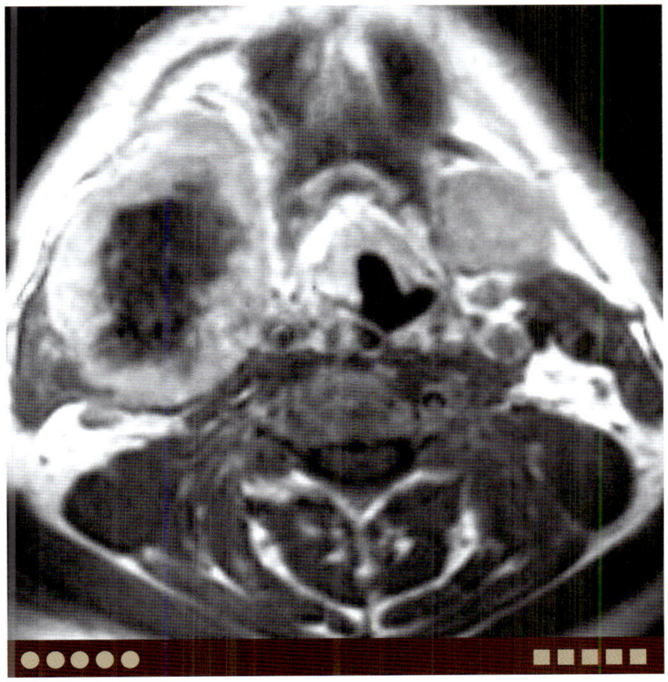

G. Metastasis from hypopharyngeal SCCA, same patient as E. Axial postcontrast T1W image demonstrates thick and irregular rim-enhancement of the lesion.

DIFFERENTIAL DIAGNOSIS IMAGES (H-J)

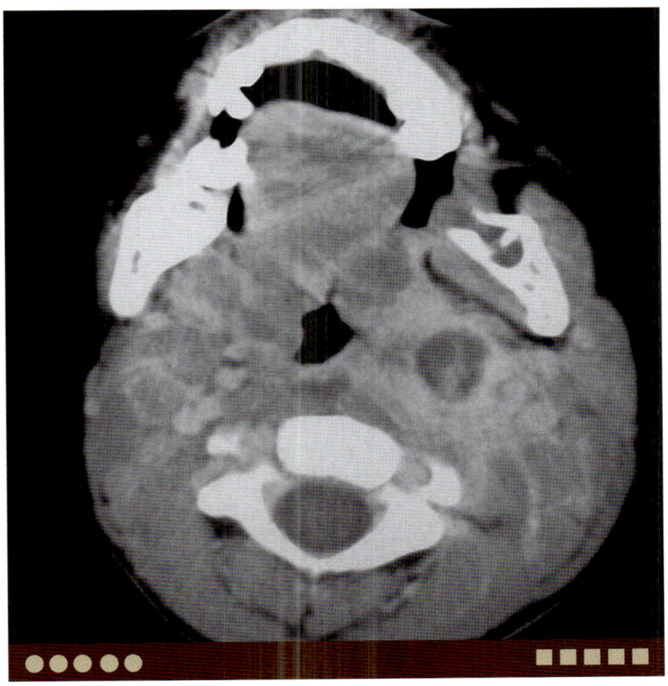

H. Intranodal abscess secondary to tonsillitis. Axial postcontrast CT demonstrates an avidly enhancing enlarged node with intranodal abscess. The fat planes around the node are completely obscured.

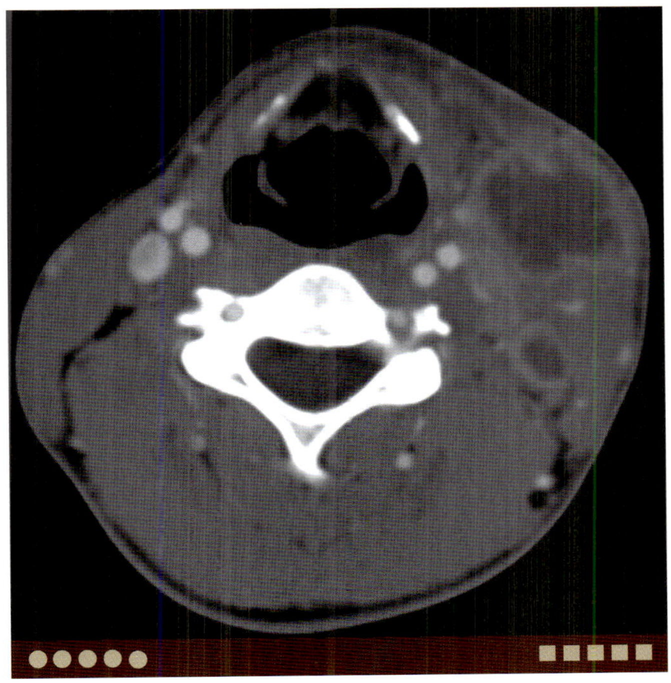

I. Tuberculosis. Axial postcontrast CT demonstrates a large necrotic node with perinodal inflammatory change and multiple smaller necrotic nodes in the left level III.

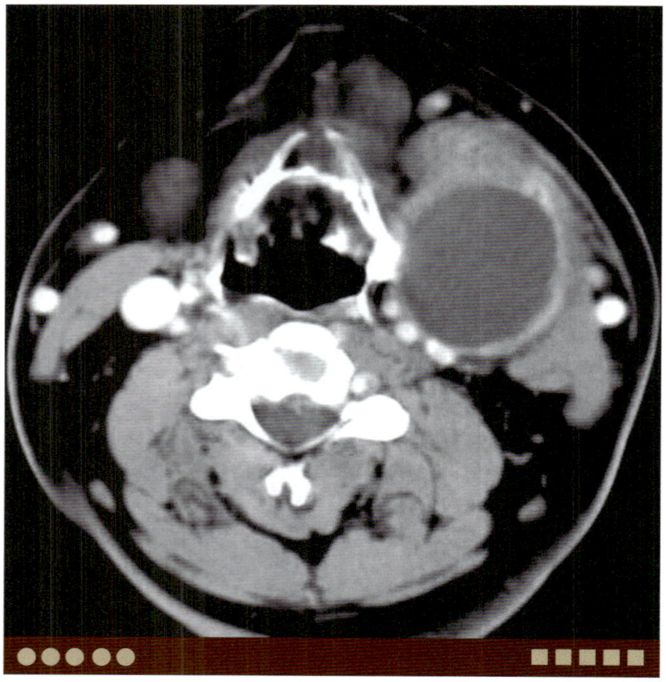

J. Infected branchial cleft cyst. Axial postcontrast CT demonstrates a large cystic lesion with thickened enhancing wall, anterolateral to the left carotid vessels, anteromedial to the sternocleidomastoid muscle, typical location for a second branchial cleft cyst.

Case 12-4 Lymphoma

Osamu Sakai, Rohini Nadgir

PRESENTATION

Enlarging neck mass.

FINDINGS

CT and MRI show enlarged lymph nodes with homogeneous density/signal without necrosis.

DIFFERENTIAL DIAGNOSIS

- Squamous cell carcinoma: This is by far the most common malignancy in the head and neck. Nodal metastasis tends to have intranodal necrosis, particularly with increase in size.
- Reactive hyperplastic nodes: This condition shows enlarged, clearly demarcated nodes with homogeneous density/intensity. Clinical picture of infection or inflammation is often present.
- Infectious mononucleosis: This condition often demonstrates multiple homogeneously enhancing nodes in the bilateral neck, often with edematous enlarged tonsils.
- Tuberculosis: Clinical symptoms of tuberculosis may be similar to that of lymphoma. However, heterogeneous enhancement, intranodal abscess, and calcification are often seen in tuberculous nodes.

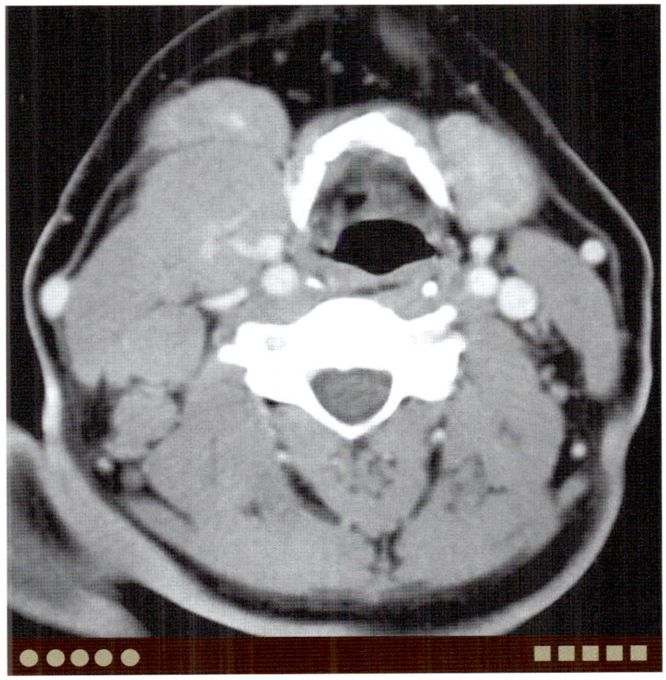

A. Lymphoma. Axial contrast-enhanced CT demonstrates significantly enlarged nodes without necrosis in the right levels II and V. Note vessels are running through the level II lesion.

COMMENTS

This is a 44-year-old man with an enlarging right neck mass.

In the head and neck, both Hodgkin disease and non-Hodgkin lymphoma occur. A distribution limited to the nodal system is characteristic for Hodgkin disease, while extranodal lesions are commonly secondary to non-Hodgkin lymphoma.

Lymphoma often presents with homogeneous, clearly demarcated nodes, similar to reactive hyperplastic lymph nodes. Imaging findings of lymphoma may be nonspecific; however, a thin nodal capsule with a central homogeneous region of slightly lower density than the muscle is a highly suggestive imaging appearance on CT for lymphomatous nodes. Large cell lymphoma may present with significantly enlarged nodes that may be nonnecrotic. Because squamous cell carcinoma usually causes necrosis in nodes larger than 3 cm in greatest diameter, a large nonnecrotic node suggests a differential diagnosis other than squamous cell carcinoma. Not only treated lymphoma, but also pretreatment lymphoma nodes may be necrotic, mimicking metastasis from squamous cell carcinomas. Therefore, presence of intranodal necrosis does not rule out lymphoma. Lymphomatous nodes also may have significant enhancement.

In patients with both squamous cell carcinoma and malignant lymphoma, local pain is usually minimal or absent.

PEARLS

- **Both Hodgkin disease and non-Hodgkin lymphoma occur in the head and neck.**
- **Enlarged nodes with homogeneous density or signal, without calcification are suggestive of lymphoma.**
- **If the lymph node exceeds 3 cm in diameter without necrosis, it will be less likely to be squamous cell carcinoma, and more likely to be lymphoma.**

ADDITIONAL IMAGES (B-G)

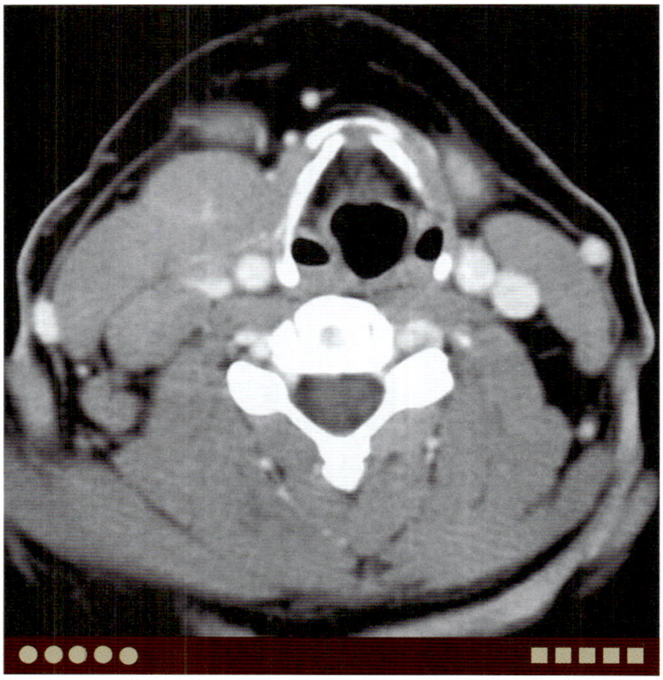

B. Lymphoma, same patient as A. Axial contrast-enhanced CT demonstrates multiple enlarged nodes without necrosis in the right levels III and V.

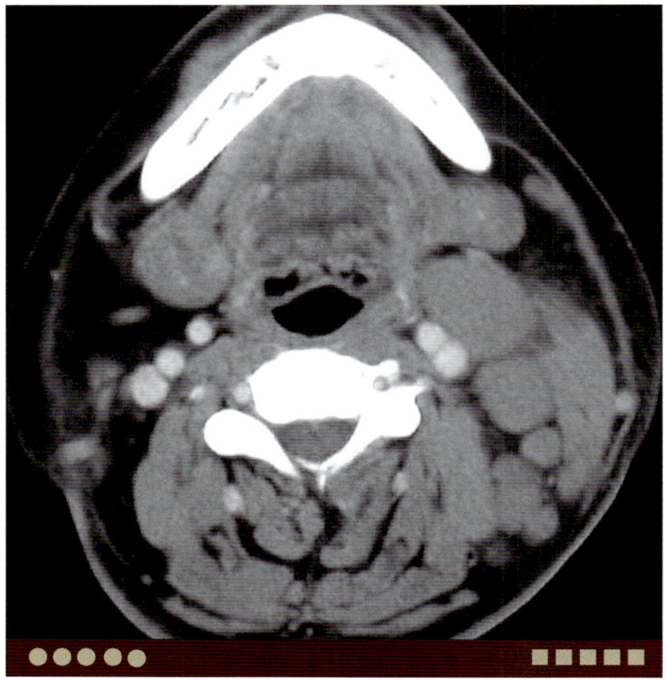

C. Lymphoma in a different patient. Axial contrast-enhanced CT demonstrates multiple enlarged nodes without necrosis in the left levels II and V.

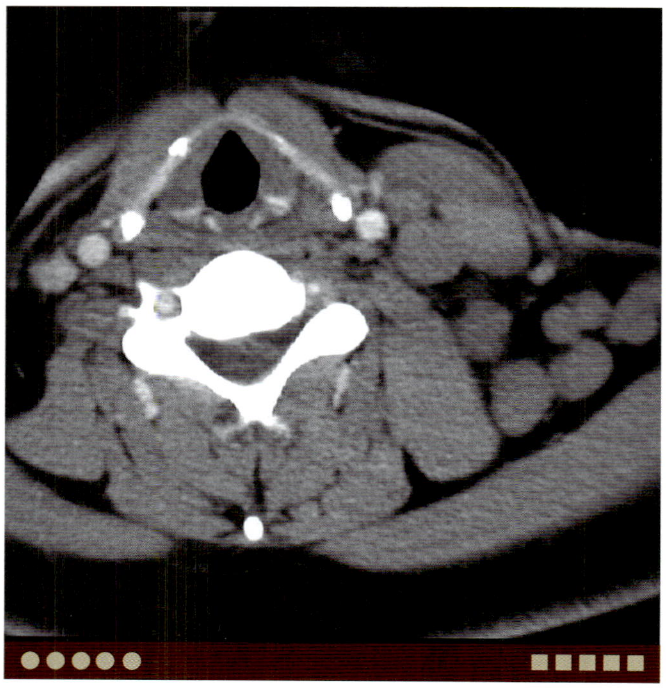

D. Lymphoma, same patient as C. Axial contrast-enhanced CT demonstrates multiple enlarged nodes without necrosis in the left levels III and V.

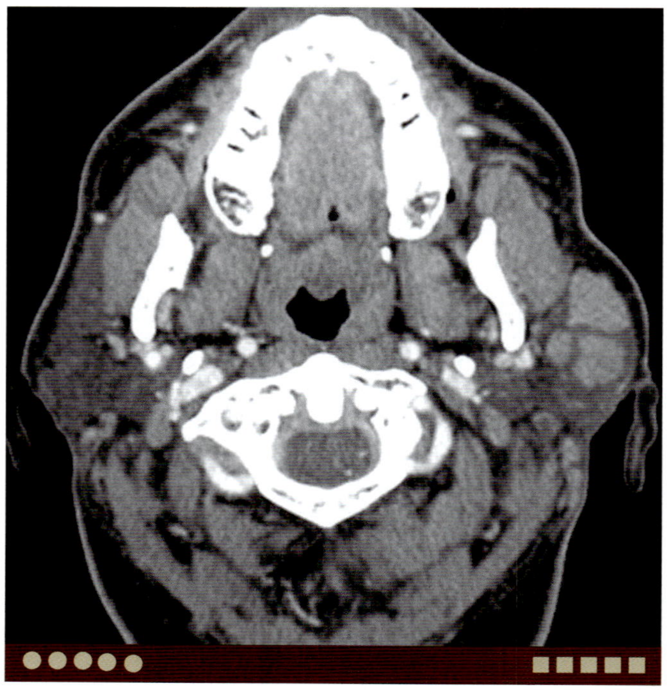

E. Lymphoma in a different patient. Axial contrast-enhanced CT demonstrates enlarged left intraparotid nodes without necrosis.

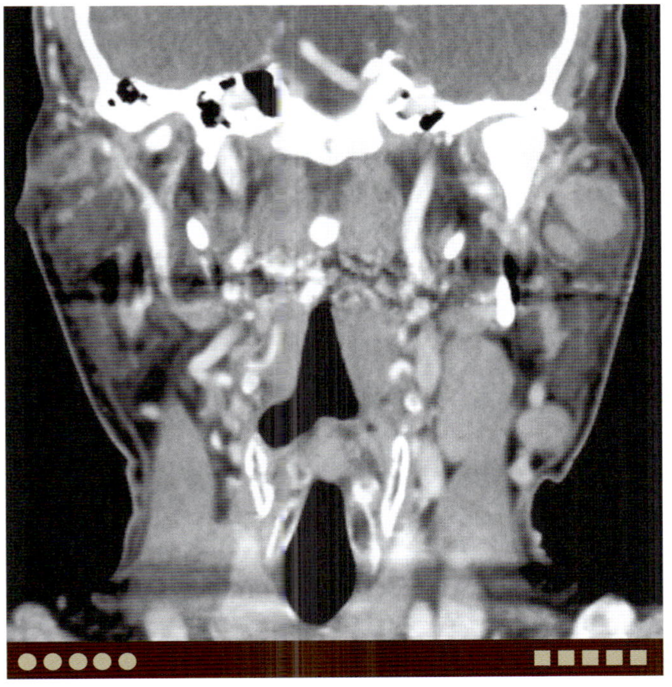

F. Lymphoma, same patient as E. Coronal contrast-enhanced CT demonstrates enlarged nonnecrotic nodes in the left parotid gland and level III.

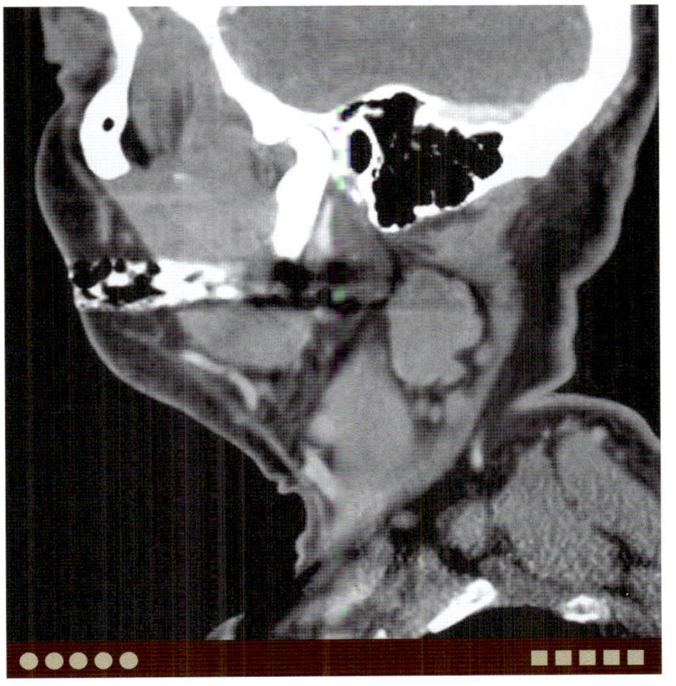

G. Lymphoma, same patient as E. Sagittal contrast-enhanced CT demonstrates an enlarged nonnecrotic node in the left level IIB.

DIFFERENTIAL DIAGNOSIS IMAGES (H-J)

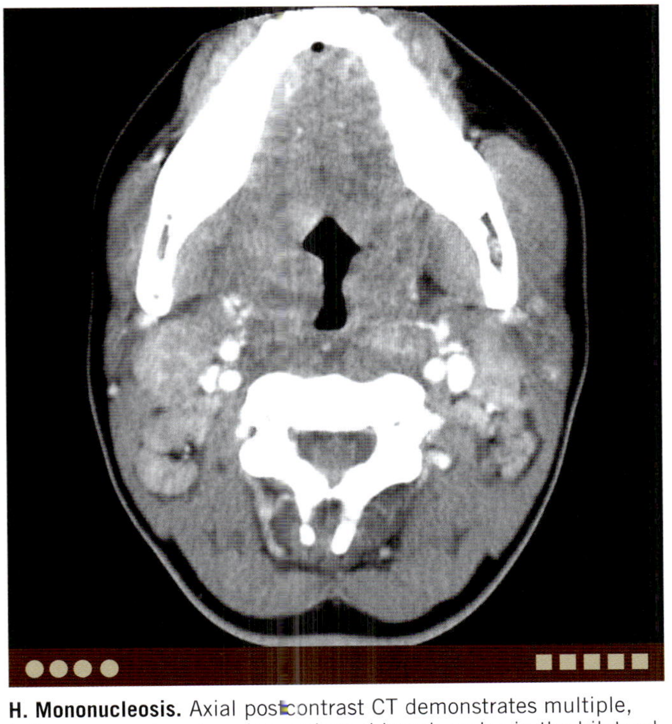

H. Mononucleosis. Axial postcontrast CT demonstrates multiple, heterogeneously enhancing, enlarged lymph nodes in the bilateral level II. Note enlarged, edematous bilateral palatine tonsils.

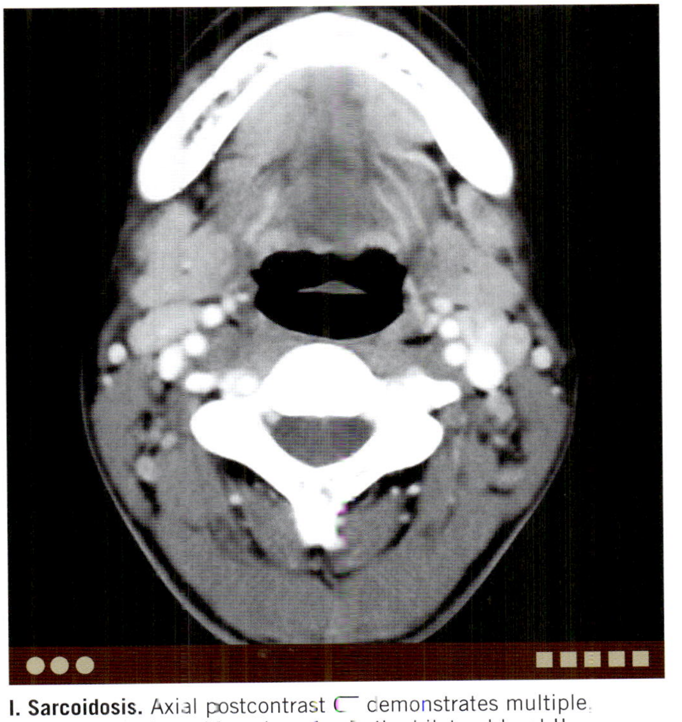

I. Sarcoidosis. Axial postcontrast CT demonstrates multiple enhancing, enlarged lymph nodes in the bilateral level II.

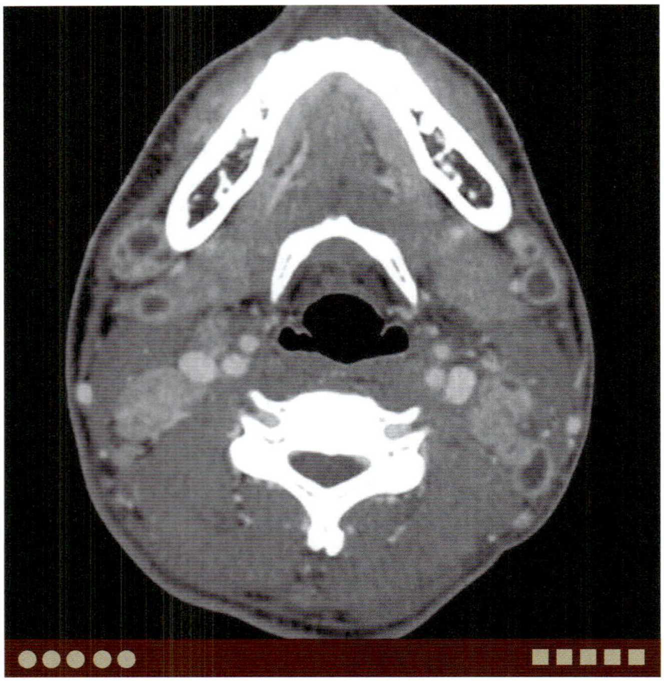

J. Tuberculosis. Axial postcontrast CT demonstrates multiple heterogeneously enhancing nodes with central low density in the bilateral levels I, II, and V.

Case 12–5 Tuberculous Lymphadenitis

Osamu Sakai, Rohini Nadgir, Benjamin Ludwig

PRESENTATION

Neck mass.

FINDINGS

CT shows multiple rim-enhancing masses in the bilateral neck, particularly in the posterior triangles.

DIFFERENTIAL DIAGNOSIS

- Intranodal necrosis or abscess from bacterial infection: This usually demonstrates profound inflammatory process in the adjacent soft tissue. However, inflammatory change may be mild if the patient is treated by antibiotics.
- Necrotic metastasis: This may present similar findings to tuberculous lymphadenitis, most often from squamous cell carcinoma (SCCA) in older patients and papillary thyroid carcinoma in younger patients.
- Infected branchial cleft cyst: This is seen as a rim-enhancing cystic lesion.

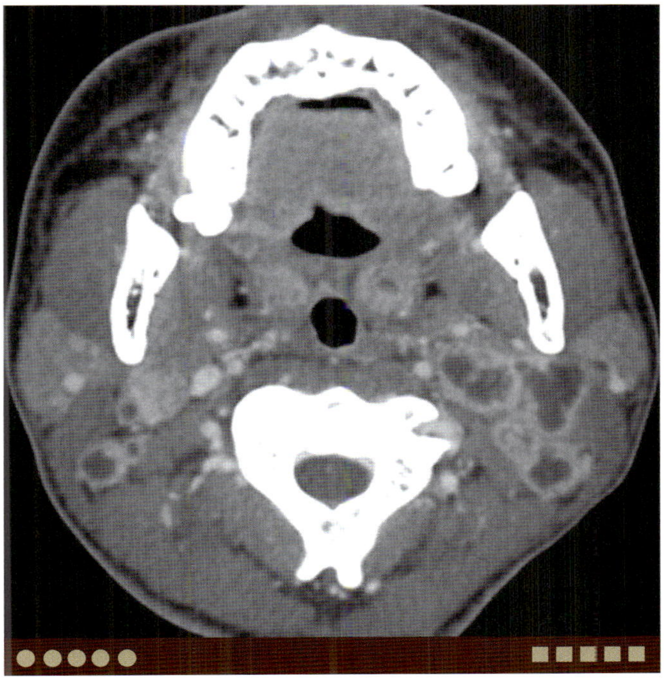

A. Tuberculosis. Axial postcontrast CT demonstrates multiple heterogeneously enhancing nodes with central low density in the bilateral level II.

COMMENTS

This is a 40-year-old man with HIV.

Tuberculous lymphadenitis shows less associated inflammatory change compared to bacterial infection or suppurative lymphadenitis, and often presents as a painless neck mass. It is important to try to differentiate this condition from nodal metastasis of unknown origin. With increasing numbers of HIV infected patients, tuberculosis is more often seen in our practice. Tuberculosis and metastasis should always be in the differential diagnosis of central low-density nodes or rim-enhancing cystic lesions. Particularly, in young female patients with variable nodal appearance, tuberculosis and papillary thyroid carcinoma should be considered.

Purified protein derivative skin test for tuberculosis can be negative in HIV infected patients with tuberculosis. Therefore, imaging can play an important role in diagnosis and appropriate treatment.

Lymph nodes with tuberculous involvement demonstrate variable imaging appearances including avid enhancement, cystic change, and calcification. Nodal calcification from tuberculosis is rare in the neck although it is very common in the mediastinum. Typically, the involved nodes demonstrate central low density with thick, irregular enhancing rim, although in the early stage the nodes can demonstrate avid enhancement without central necrosis. Inflammatory change is often seen in the surrounding fat planes and soft tissue, however, it is milder compared to intranodal abscess from bacterial infection. Necrotic nodes can coalesce and form a larger abscess (cold abscess), which is typical for tuberculosis.

All nodal chains can be involved including the jugular chains (levels II, III, and IV), but posterior triangle nodes (level V) are more often involved.

PEARLS

- **Tuberculous adenitis demonstrates variable nodal appearance; avid enhancement, cystic change, and calcification.**
- **Nodal calcification from tuberculosis is not common in the neck although it is very common in the mediastinum.**
- **Always consider metastasis as a differential diagnosis, even in young patients.**

ADDITIONAL IMAGES (B-G)

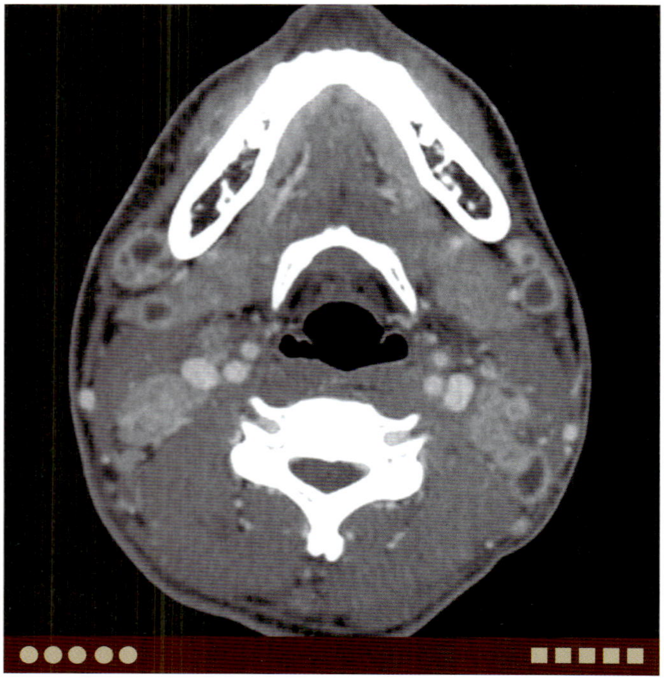

B. Tuberculosis, same patient as A. Axial postcontrast CT demonstrates multiple heterogeneously enhancing nodes with central low density in the bilateral levels I, II, and V.

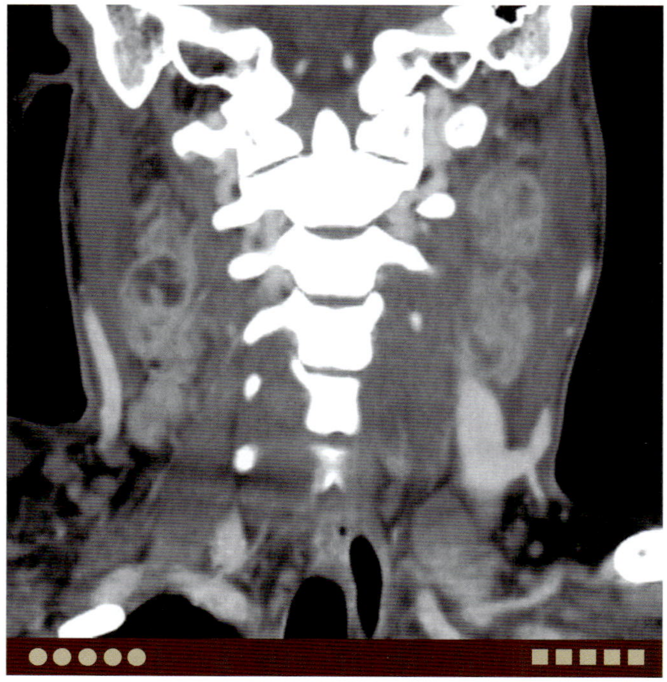

C. Tuberculosis, same patient as A. Coronal postcontrast CT demonstrates multiple heterogeneously enhancing nodes with central low density in the bilateral level II through IV.

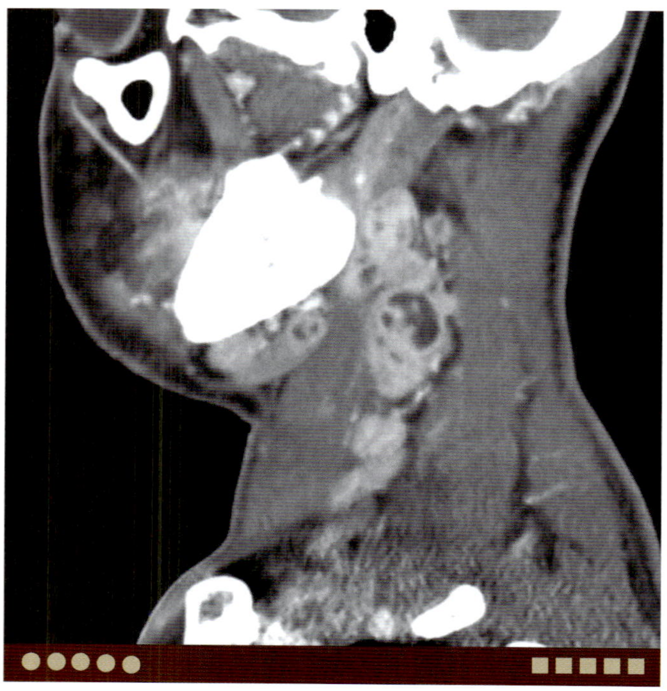

D. Tuberculosis, same patient as A. Sagittal postcontrast CT demonstrates multiple heterogeneously enhancing nodes with central low density in the level I through IV.

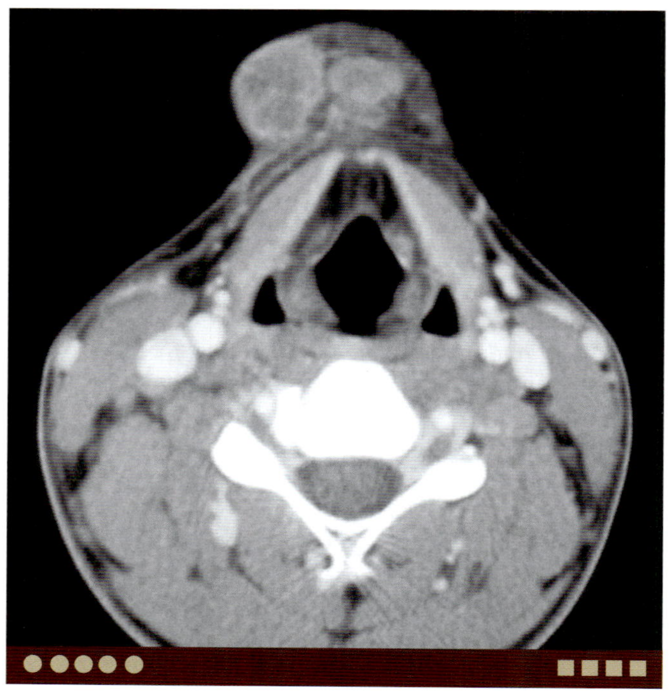

E. Tuberculosis in a different patient. Axial postcontrast CT demonstrates isolated heterogeneously enhancing nodes with central low density in the level I.

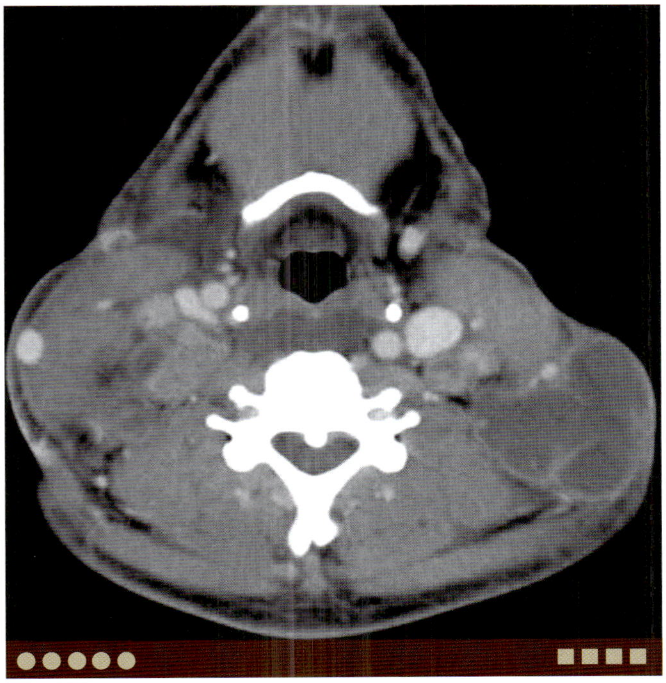

F. Tuberculosis in a different patient. Axial postcontrast CT demonstrates cystic-appearing, septated lesions in the bilateral levels II and V. Note retropharyngeal edema.

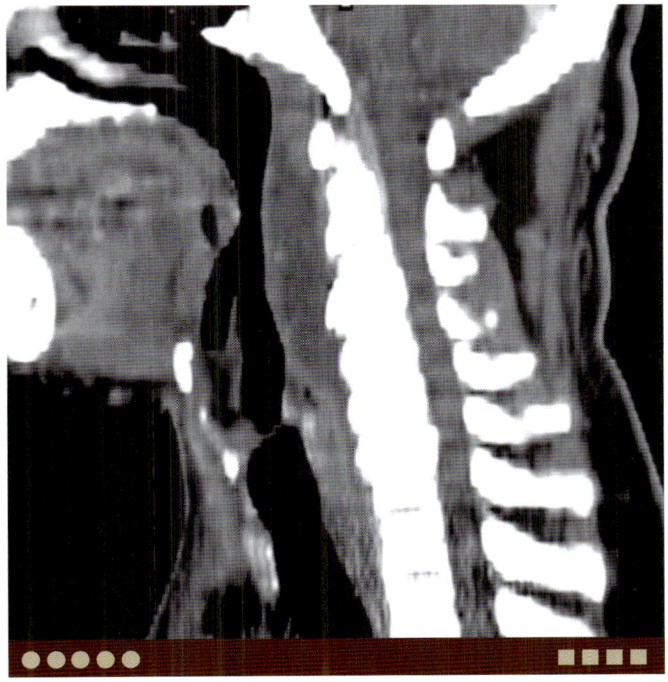

G. Tuberculosis, same patient as F. Sagittal postcontrast CT demonstrates retropharyngeal edema, without rim enhancement to suggest abscess.

DIFFERENTIAL DIAGNOSIS IMAGES (H-J)

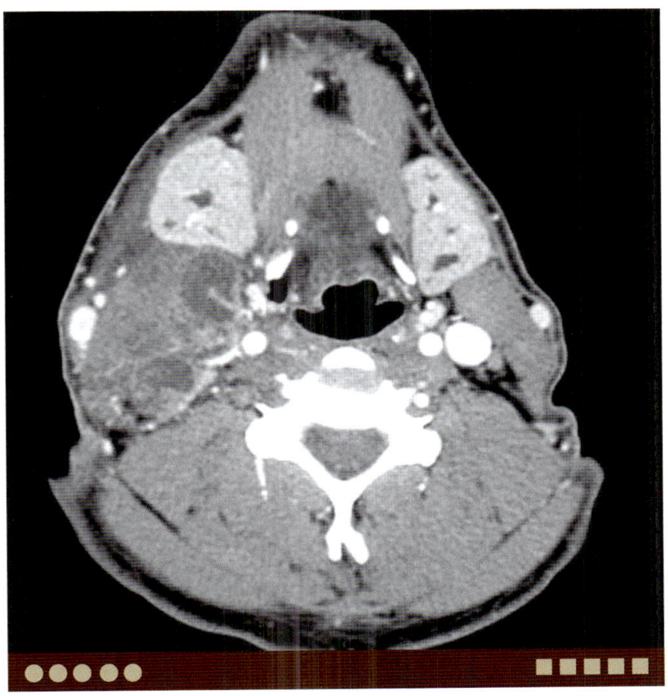

H. Metastasis from tonsillar SCCA. Axial postcontrast CT demonstrates poorly defined heterogeneously enhancing metastatic nodes in the right level II. Ill-defined borders suggest extracapsular tumor spread.

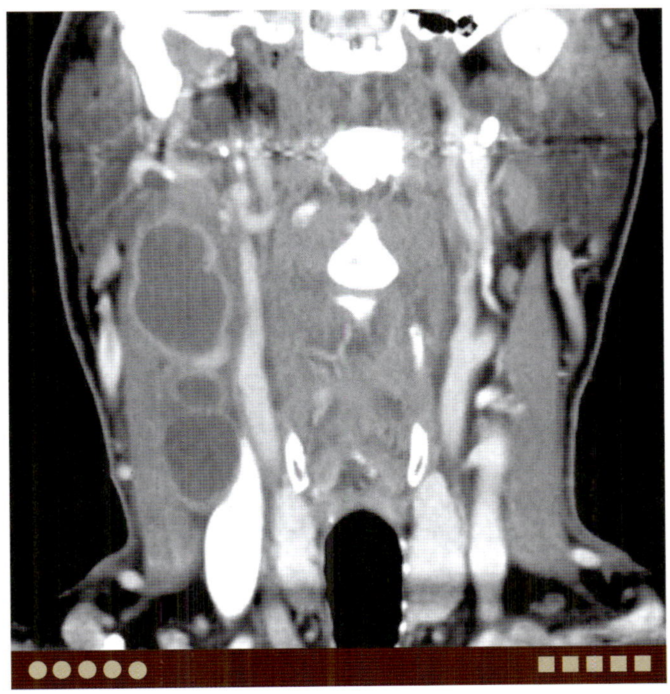

I. Metastasis from base of tongue SCCA. Coronal postcontrast CT demonstrates multiple, cystic-appearing, rim-enhancing metastatic nodes in the right levels II and III.

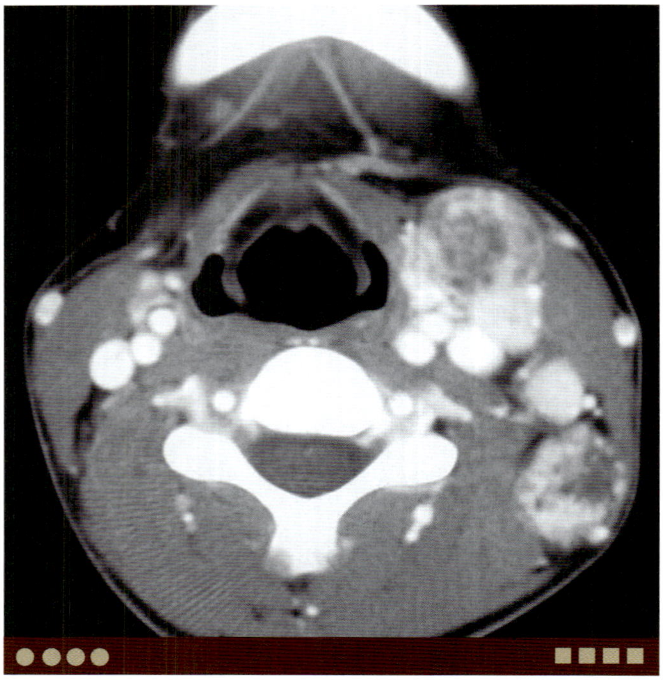

J. Metastasis from papillary thyroid carcinoma. Axial postcontrast CT demonstrates multiple heterogeneously enhancing nodes with intranodal low densities in the left levels II and V.

Case 12–6 Sarcoidosis: Lymph Node

Naoko Saito, Jimmy Wang, Osamu Sakai

PRESENTATION

Bilateral lymph nodes swelling.

FINDINGS

CT demonstrates multiple bilateral, homogeneously enhancing cervical lymph nodes.

DIFFERENTIAL DIAGNOSIS

- Lymphoma: Multiple homogeneously enhancing lymph nodes are typically seen. Cystic or necrotic change, or calcification is rare without treatment.
- Human immunodeficiency virus (HIV) infection: Cervical lymphadenopathy, nasopharyngeal lymphoid enlargement, and lymphoepithelial lesions of the parotid gland are the three major head and neck imaging findings for HIV infection.
- Kikuchi-Fujimoto disease: This is a histiocytic necrotizing lymphadenitis, and most commonly seen in Japanese women younger than 30 years of age. Multiple homogeneously enhancing lymph nodes with perinodal infiltration are frequently seen.
- Amyloidosis: This is a disease in which an abnormal protein (amyloid) builds up in organs and tissues, impairing their function. Multiple enlarged nodes with nodal calcification are often seen.

COMMENTS

This is a 55-year-old woman with bilateral lymph nodes swelling and difficulty of swallowing.

Sarcoidosis is a systemic disease characterized by noncaseating granulomas, and can affect any organ. In the head and neck, sarcoidosis involves cervical lymph nodes, eyes, parotid glands, lacrimal glands, and the upper respiratory tract. It is often seen between 20 and 40 years of age with a slightly higher prevalence in women. Patients present with nonspecific symptoms such as fever, malaise, weight loss, and erythema nodosum.

About one third of the patients with sarcoidosis present with cervical lymphadenopathy. Intraparotid lymph nodes are often involved. In cases of cervical lymphadenopathy with intraparotid lymph nodes swelling, the most likely diagnosis is either sarcoidosis or lymphoma. Enlarged mediastinal lymph nodes are also seen, which help to differentiate from other disease.

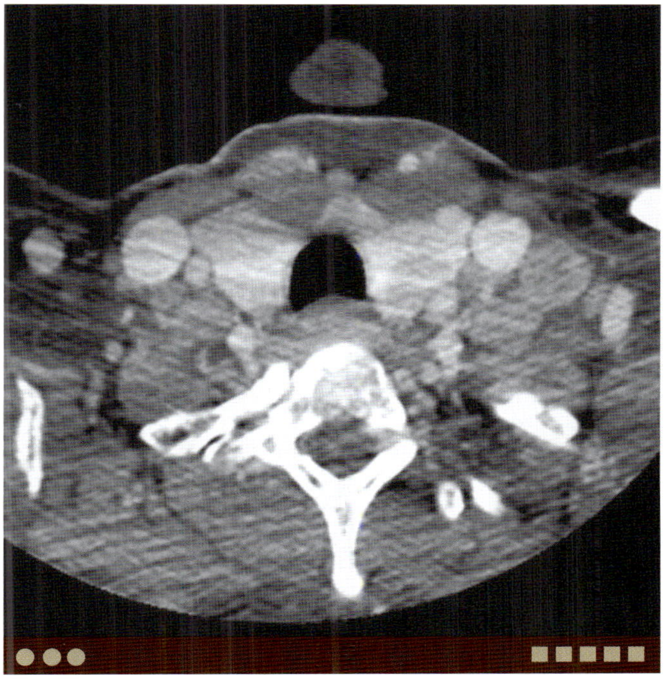

A. Sarcoidosis. Axial contrast-enhanced CT demonstrates multiple bilateral, enlarged lymph nodes. The lymph nodes are homogeneously enhanced.

On imaging, sarcoidosis demonstrates multiple enlarged lymph nodes. The lymph nodes are usually homogeneous and have sharp margins. These nodes are often larger than 2 cm in size. Nodal calcification, especially eggshell type, can be seen. Eggshell calcification may also be seen in patients with fungal infection, silicosis, pneumoconiosis, amyloidosis, tuberculosis, and so on.

PEARLS

- **About one third of the patients with sarcoidosis present with cervical lymphadenopathy.**
- **Intraparotid lymph nodes are often involved.**
- **Sarcoidosis demonstrates multiple enlarged, homogeneous lymph nodes with sharp margins.**

ADDITIONAL IMAGES (B-G)

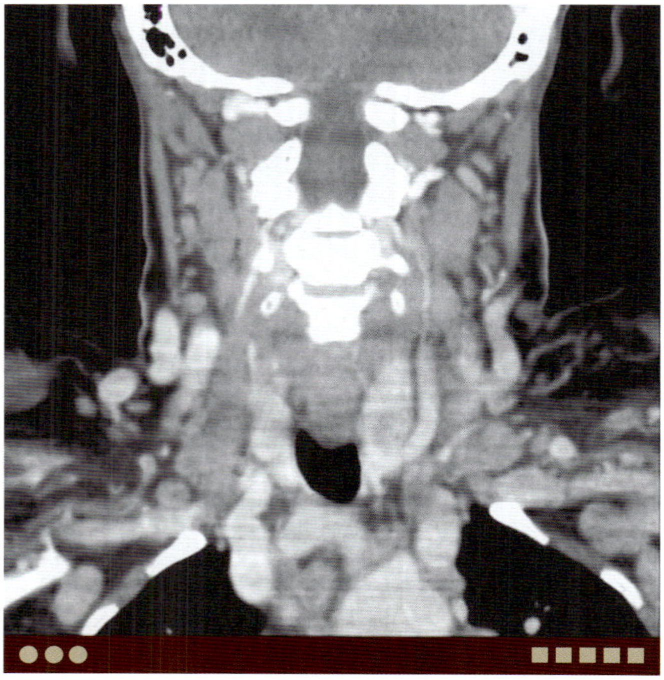

B. Sarcoidosis, same patient as A. Coronal contrast-enhanced CT demonstrates multiple enlarged cervical and supraclavicular lymph nodes bilaterally. Multiple mediastinal lymph nodes are also noted.

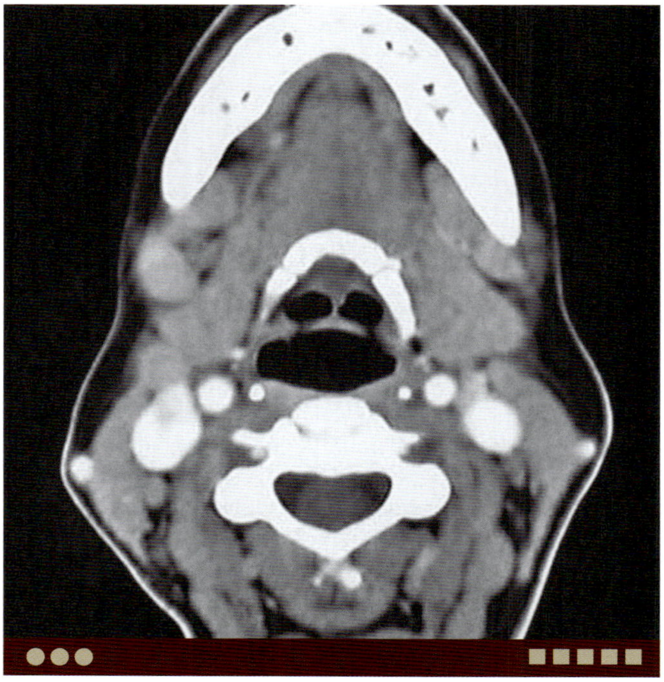

C. Sarcoidosis in a different patient. Axial contrast-enhanced CT demonstrates multiple bilateral, homogeneously enhancing lymph nodes.

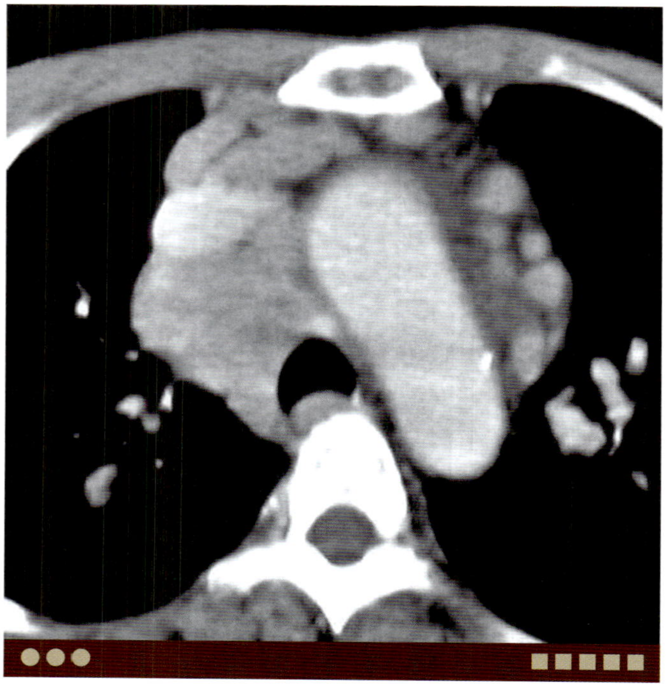

D. Sarcoidosis, same patient as C. Axial contrast-enhanced CT demonstrates multiple enlarged mediastinal lymph nodes, most prominently in the right paratracheal region.

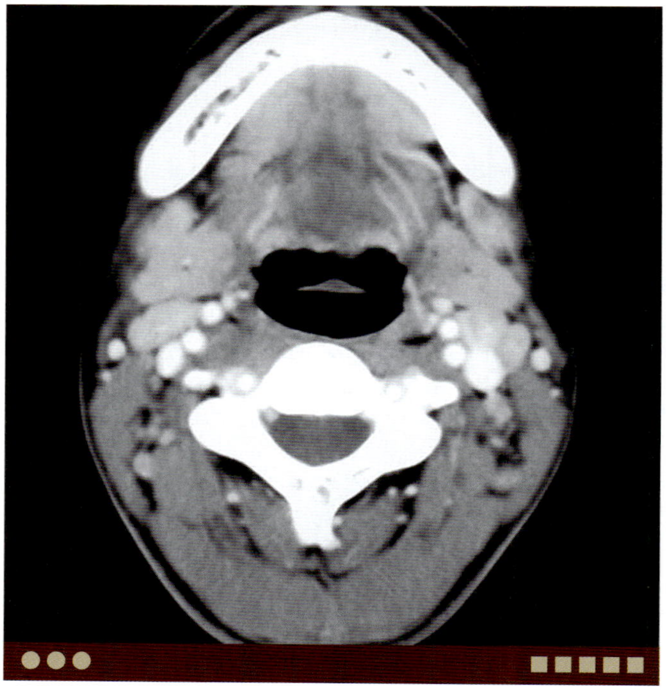

E. Sarcoidosis in a different patient. Axial contrast-enhanced CT demonstrates multiple homogeneously enhancing lymph nodes in the levels I and II bilaterally.

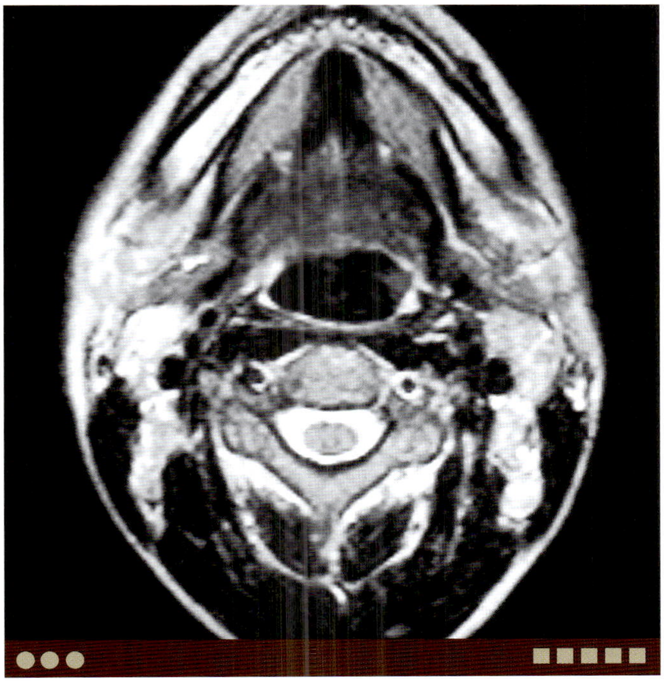

F. Sarcoidosis, same patient as E. Axial T2W MR image demonstrates high signal in the enlarged bilateral levels I and II nodes.

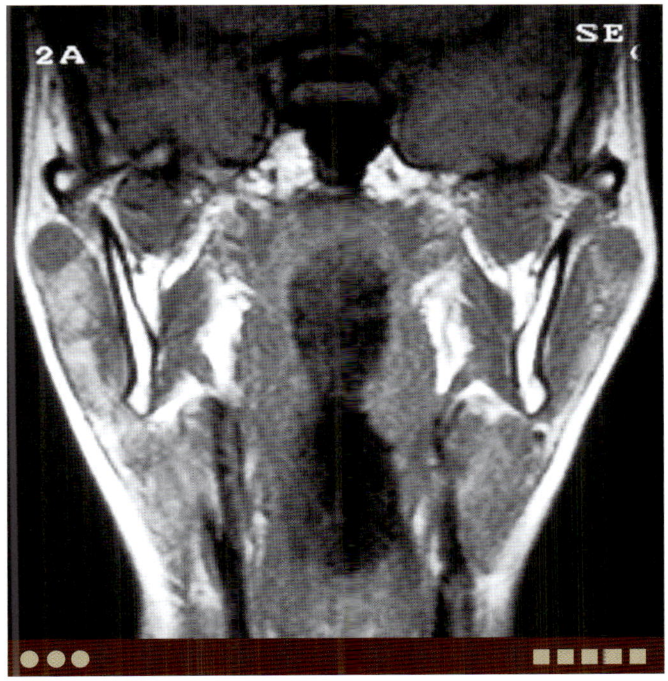

G. Sarcoidosis, same patient as E. Coronal T2W MR image demonstrates enlarged intraparotid nodes bilaterally.

DIFFERENTIAL DIAGNOSIS IMAGES (H-J)

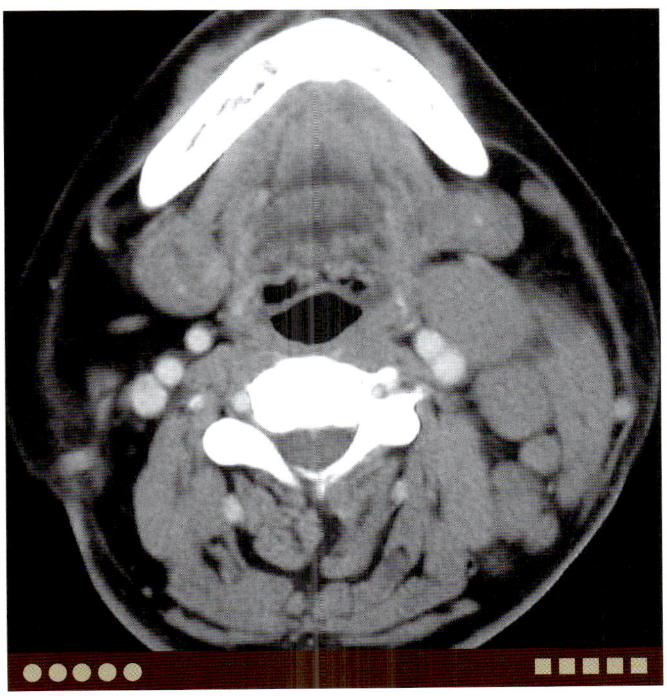

H. Lymphoma. Axial contrast-enhanced CT demonstrates multiple enlarged lymph nodes in the left levels II and V without necrosis or calcification.

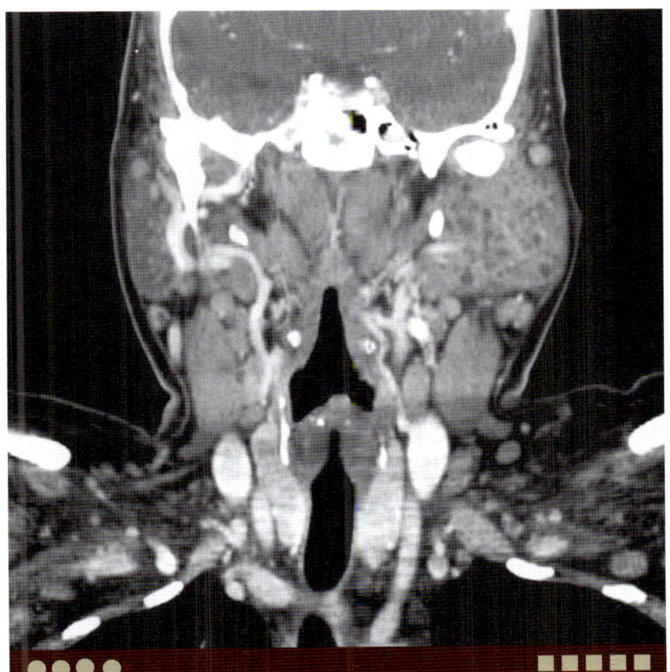

I. HIV infection. Coronal contrast-enhanced CT demonstrates multiple bilateral, enhancing lymph nodes. Multiple cystic lesions in bilateral parotid glands are also noted, which is a characteristic finding of lymphoepithelial lesions associated with HIV infection.

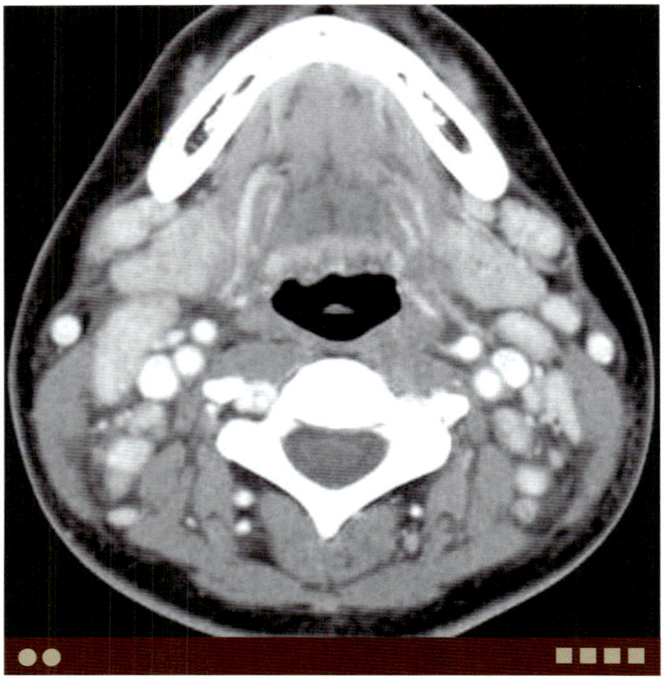

J. Kikuchi-Fujimoto disease. Axial contrast-enhanced CT demonstrates multiple bilateral, enhancing lymph nodes. Note infiltration of adjacent fat tissues.

Case 12–7 Kikuchi-Fujimoto Disease

Atsuko Sakamoto, Akifumi Fujita, Jimmy Wang, Osamu Sakai

PRESENTATION

Cervical lymphadenopathy with tenderness.

FINDINGS

CT shows multiple enhancing cervical lymph nodes with or without central low density.

DIFFERENTIAL DIAGNOSIS

- Infectious mononucleosis: This is a condition related to Epstein-Barr virus (EBV) infection and commonly seen in children and young adults, "kissing disease," often bilateral.
- Tuberculous adenitis: This condition shows variable appearance of affected lymph node; homogeneous enhancement, heterogeneous enhancement, intranodal abscess/necrosis, and occasionally calcification.
- Lymphoma: Lymphoma demonstrates unilateral or bilateral lymphadenopathy usually with homogeneous density and mild enhancement, but it may be variable in appearance.
- Suppurative adenopathy: This condition is intranodal abscess formation. Heterogeneously enhancing nodes with central low densities are seen.
- Metastatic nodal disease: Metastasis causes heterogeneous enhancement of nodes. Squamous cell carcinoma is the most common malignancy in the neck, however, thyroid cancer should also be considered, particularly in young women.

COMMENTS

This is a 38-year-old woman with mildly enlarged lymph nodes on both sides of the neck.

Kikuchi-Fujimoto disease or histiocytic necrotizing lymphadenopathy is a rare lymphadenitis of unknown etiology which suggests an immune response of T cell and histiocytes to a viral infectious agent. This disease is mainly seen in Japan but isolated cases are reported in the United States and Europe. This disease affects mainly young adults with slight female preponderance. Most patients are less than 40 years of age.

Course of the disease is generally benign and self-limiting. Lymphadenopathy spontaneously improves or resolves completely within several weeks to 8 months. Common symptoms are fever and cervical lymphadenopathy. Some patients show leukopenia. Excisional lymph node biopsy is useful for diagnosis.

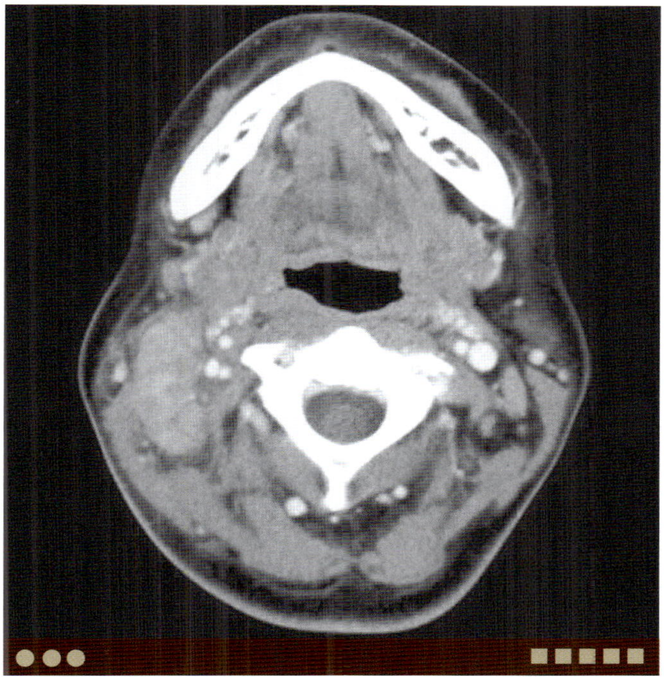

A. Kikuchi-Fujimoto disease. Axial postcontrast CT image demonstrates heterogeneously enhancing enlarged right level II node with perinodal infiltration.

CT shows multiple, mildly enlarged lymph nodes with homogeneous enhancement and perinodal infiltration. Sometime intranodal necrosis is seen. Lymphadenopathy can develop anywhere else, but the most common sites are unilateral cervical regions, frequently in the level II to V.

The differential diagnosis includes systemic lupus erythematodes, tuberculous adenitis, sarcoidosis, viral lymphadenitis, lymphoma, and metastasis. Nodal metastasis from papillary thyroid cancer may demonstrate similar findings and often affects young women, similar population to Kikuchi-Fujimoto disease.

PEARLS

- **Kikuchi-Fujimoto disease affects cervical lymph nodes, frequently in the level II to V, often bilateral.**
- **CT shows multiple, mildly enlarged lymph nodes with homogeneous enhancement and perinodal infiltration. Intranodal necrosis may be seen.**

ADDITIONAL IMAGES (B-C)

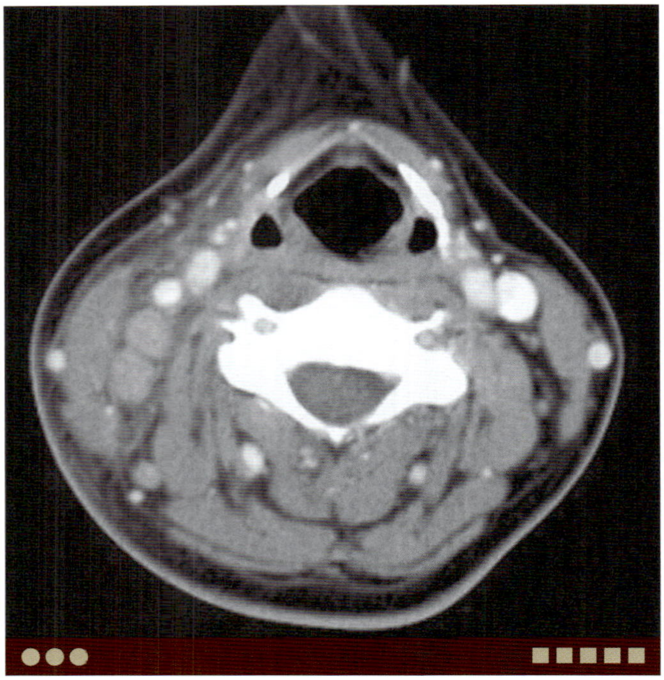

B. Kikuchi-Fujimoto disease, same patient as A. Axial postcontrast CT demonstrates multiple heterogeneously enhancing nodes with perinodal infiltration in the right level III.

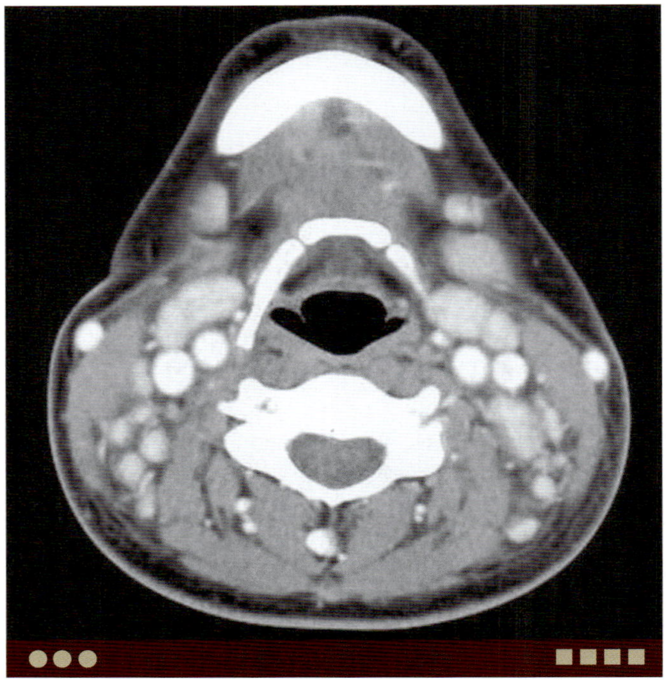

C. Kikuchi-Fujimoto disease in a different patient. Axial postcontrast CT demonstrates avidly enhancing multiple enlarged nodes with perinodal infiltration in the bilateral level II.

DIFFERENTIAL DIAGNOSIS IMAGES (D-G)

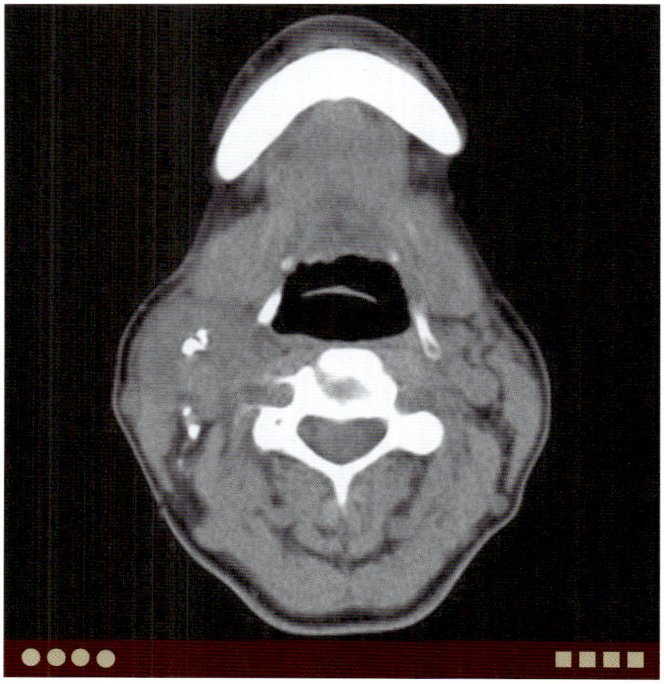

D. Tuberculous adenitis. Axial noncontrast CT demonstrates enlarged right level II nodes with mild perinodal infiltration and calcification.

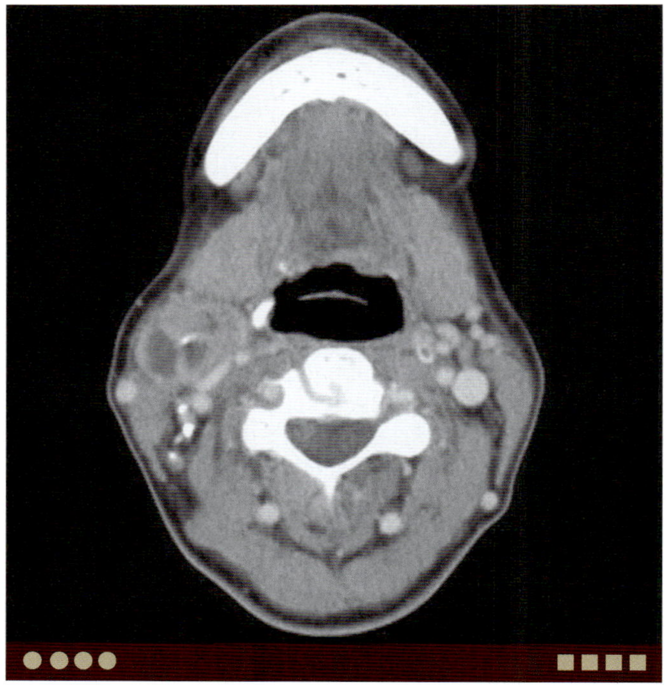

E. Tuberculous adenitis, same patient as D. Axial postcontrast CT demonstrates heterogeneous enhancement in the affected nodes.

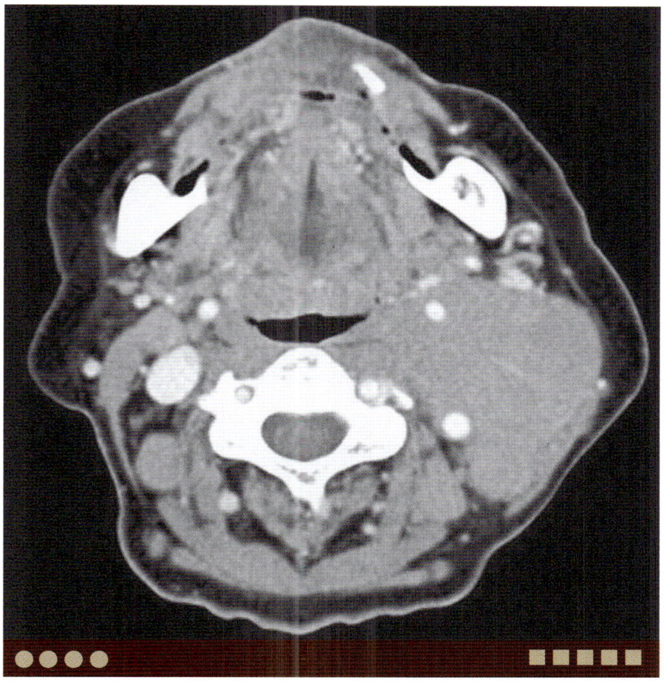

F. Lymphoma. Axial postcontrast CT demonstrates a very large, mildly enhancing, homogenous density mass in the left level II.

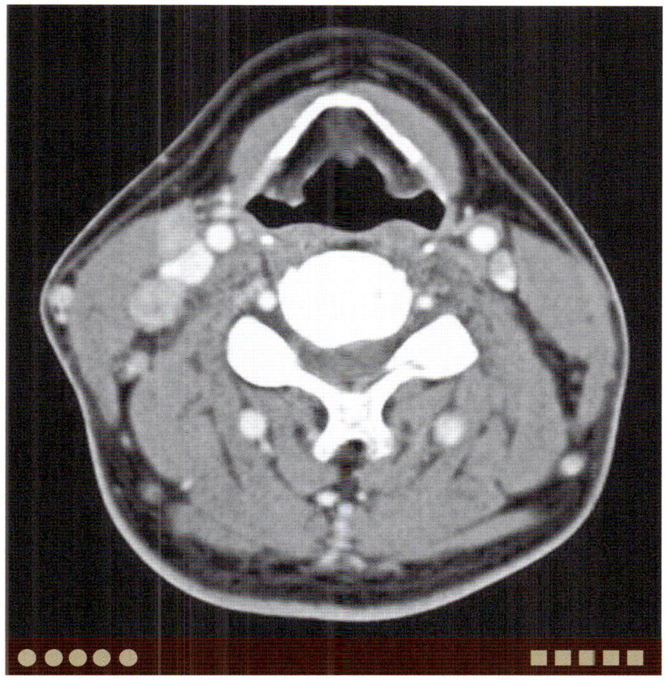

G. Metastasis from squamous cell carcinoma. Axial postcontrast CT demonstrates heterogeneously enhancing right level III nodes.

Case 12–8 Kawasaki Disease

Yukio Kimura, Akifumi Fujita, Osamu Sakai

PRESENTATION

Fever, sore throat, and bilateral cervical lymphadenopathy.

FINDINGS

CT shows mildly enhancing, enlarged cervical lymph nodes bilaterally with fluid density in the retropharyngeal space (RPS).

DIFFERENTIAL DIAGNOSIS

- Infectious mononucleosis: This condition is related to Epstein-Barr virus (EBV) infection and commonly seen in children and young adults, "kissing disease." Sore throat with cervical lymphadenopathy is a common presentation. Splenomegaly is also seen. Clinical and imaging findings may be very similar to Kawasaki disease.
- Suppurative adenopathy: This condition is related to intranodal abscess formation. Heterogeneously enhancing nodes with central low densities are seen. If the RPS is involved, commonly this is seen in the lateral retropharyngeal node, just medial to the internal carotid artery. Rarely medial retropharyngeal node involvement may be seen.
- Retropharyngeal abscess: This usually demonstrates a rim-enhancing fluid collection, typically bow-tie appearance, in the RPS. Early abscess may not have rim enhancement and is thus difficult to differentiate from edema.

COMMENTS

This is a 6-year-old girl with 3-day history of fever and sore throat, and 1-day history of bilateral cervical lymphadenopathy. She was initially diagnosed as retropharyngeal abscess, but a few days later, other symptoms of conjunctivitis, strawberry tongue, and rash became obvious.

Kawasaki disease (KD), also known as acute febrile mucocutaneous lymph node syndrome, is a systemic vasculitis of unknown etiology affecting infants and young children. KD is defined by the presence of at least 4 of the following 5 clinical signs: fever, bilateral nonexudative conjunctivitis, changes of the oropharyngeal mucosa, changes in the peripheral extremities, skin rash, and cervical lymphadenopathy. Further, KD is associated with coronary aneurysms. Patients whose illness does not meet the above definition but who have fever and coronary artery abnormalities are classified as having atypical or incomplete KD. No definitive diagnostic test exists in KD.

CT demonstrates enhancing enlarged cervical lymph nodes as one of the major radiological findings, and fluid density without rim enhancement in the RPS. The most important differential diagnosis is retropharyngeal abscess, which is a life-threatening condition and may require immediate surgical drainage. Retropharyngeal abscess usually demonstrates retropharyngeal fluid collection, typically bow-tie shaped, with rim enhancement on postcontrast CT. However, early abscess may not demonstrate apparent rim enhancement. Intranodal abscess of the lateral retropharyngeal node is seen just medial to the internal carotid artery, not crossing midline.

In KD, surgical exploration of the parapharyngeal space or RPS is not recommended, as drainage is not therapeutic, biopsy is not diagnostic except for nonspecific vasculitis, and there is an anesthetic risk associated with possible cardiac complications in patients with KD.

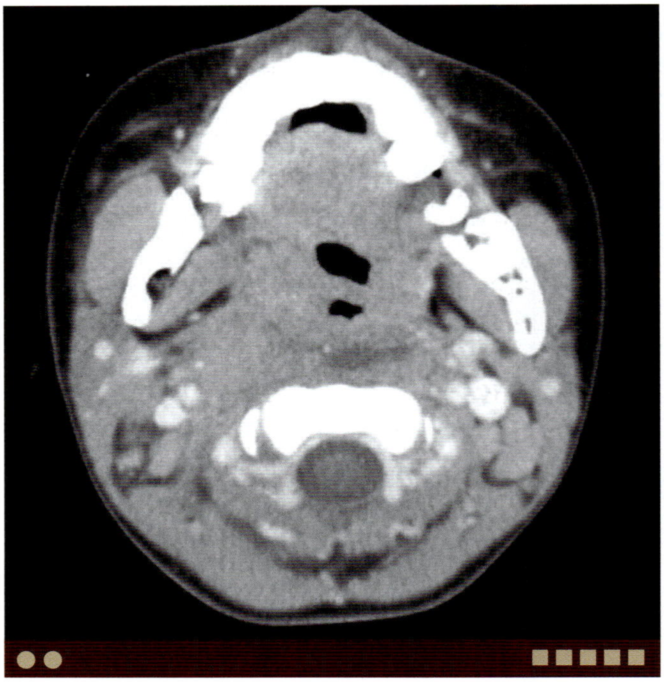

A. Kawasaki disease. Axial postcontrast CT image demonstrates enlarged right lateral retropharyngeal lymph node and fluid density in the RPS without peripheral rim enhancement. Enlarged lymph nodes are also seen in the bilateral level II.

PEARLS

- **Clinical and imaging findings of KD may be similar to infectious mononucleosis. Thorough clinical evaluation is critical.**
- **CT demonstrates enlarged cervical nodes with fluid density in the RPS without rim enhancement.**
- **Rim-enhancing fluid collection in the RPS suggests abscess, which often requires surgical intervention.**

ADDITIONAL IMAGES (B-C)

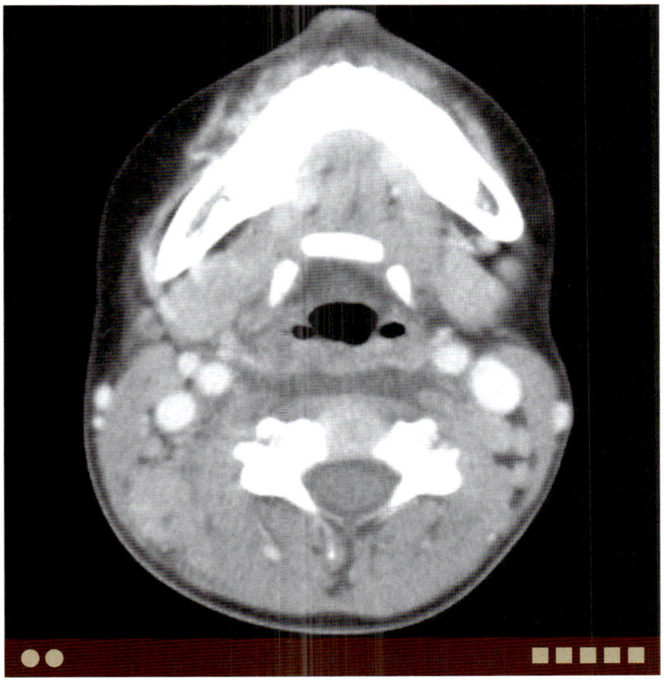

B. Kawasaki disease, same patient as A. Axial postcontrast CT through the hyoid demonstrates the fluid density in the RPS and bilateral cervical lymphadenopathy.

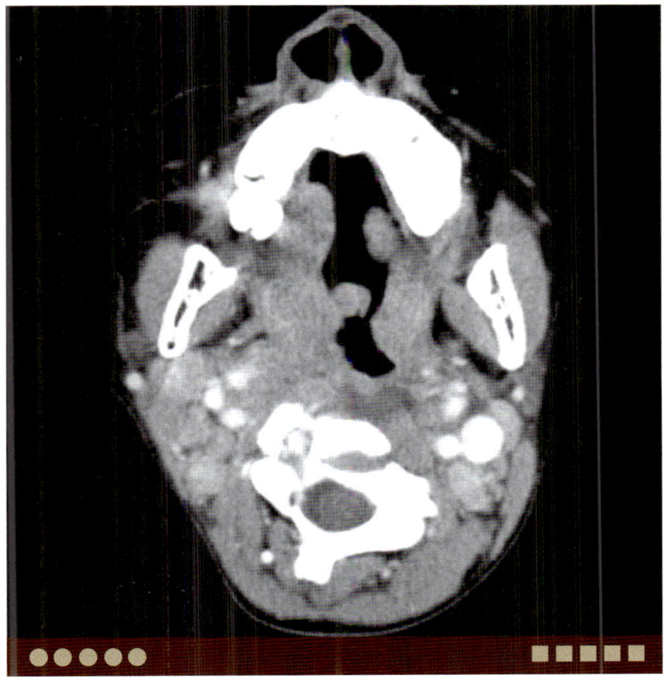

C. Kawasaki disease in a different patient. Axial postcontrast CT shows fluid density in the RPS without rim enhancement and bilateral lymphadenopathy. This is an 8-year-old girl with fever and sore throat as initial presentation.

DIFFERENTIAL DIAGNOSIS IMAGES (D-G)

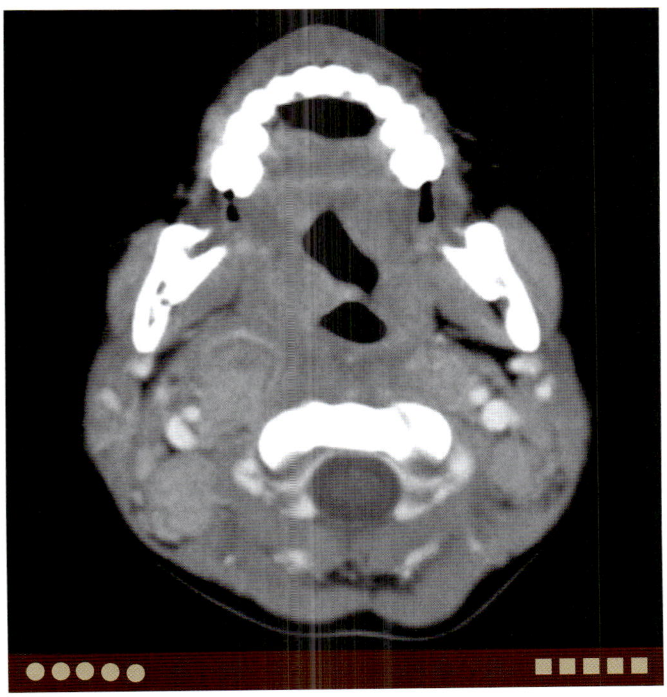

D. Suppurative adenopathy. Axial postcontrast CT shows heterogeneously enhancing enlarged bilateral lateral retropharyngeal and level IIB lymph nodes with RPS edema.

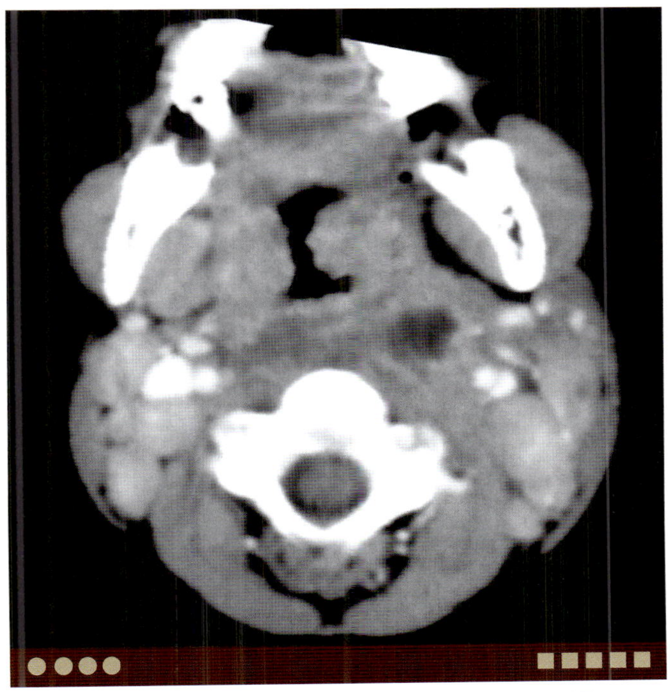

E. Retropharyngeal intranodal abscess. Axial postcontrast CT demonstrates rim-enhancing low density in the enlarged left lateral retropharyngeal node and edema in the RPS.

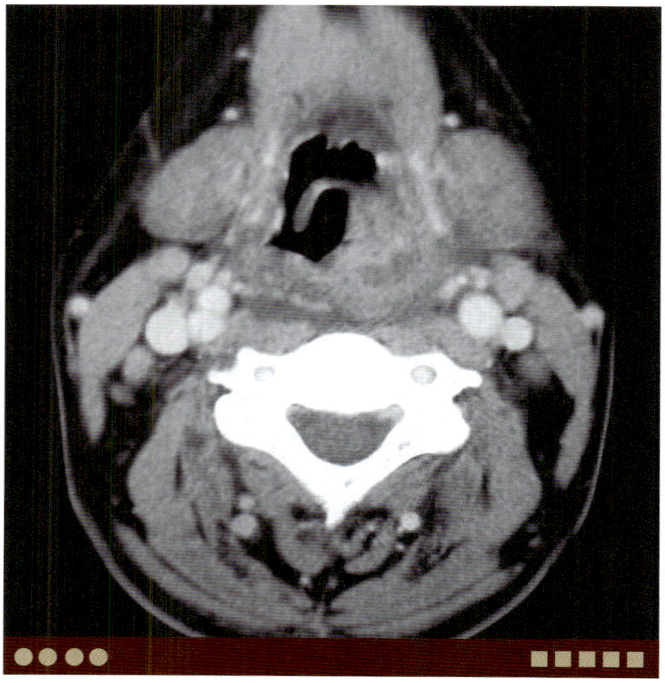

F. Retropharyngeal abscess. Axial postcontrast CT demonstrates rim-enhancing fluid collection centered in the left hypopharynx as well as fluid collection with mild rim enhancement in the RPS.

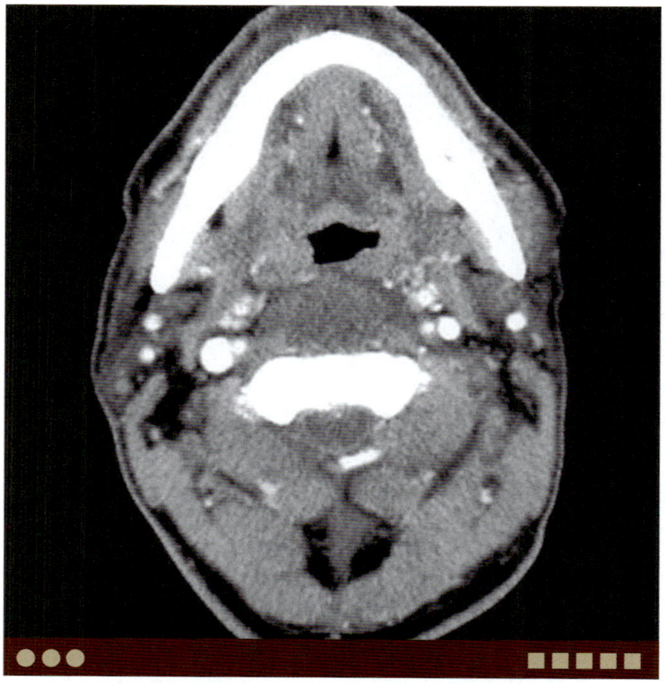

G. Prevertebral hematoma. Axial postcontrast CT demonstrates high-density collection in the prevertebral space. Trace fat density in the RPS is preserved on the right, however, RPS edema is seen on the left.

Case 12–9 Castleman Disease

Osamu Sakai, Rohini Nadgir

PRESENTATION

Neck mass.

FINDINGS

CT demonstrates an avidly enhancing, enlarged lymph node in the neck.

DIFFERENTIAL DIAGNOSIS

- Paraganglioma: This usually demonstrates abnormal flow-voids and "salt-and-pepper" appearance and is commonly seen in the carotid bifurcation (carotid body tumor), skull base (glomus jugulare and glomus vagale), or tympanic cavity (glomus tympanicum, glomus jugulotympanicum).
- Schwannoma: Schwannoma is usually not very hypervascular; however, up to 10% of Castleman disease is not hypervascular and may mimic schwannoma.
- Metastatic lymph node: Metastasis from hypervascular primary tumors such as melanoma and thyroid cancer can demonstrate enhancing nodes. Metastatic nodes are usually multiple.
- Lymphoma: Lymphoma usually shows homogeneous density/signal within multiple enlarged nodes with minimal-to-mild, (not avid) enhancement.

COMMENTS

This is a 45-year-old man with a painless mass in the left neck.

Castleman disease is one of the benign lymphoproliferative disorders and is also known as giant lymph node hyperplasia and angiomatous lymphoid hamartoma. The etiology is unknown, however, it is speculated to occur secondary to hamartomatous, infectious, and inflammatory processes. Histologically, it can be divided into two types; hyaline-vascular type and plasmacytic type. Most of localized unicentric Castleman disease is hyaline-vascular type, and this is the more common type seen in the head and neck. The patient is usually asymptomatic and presents with a painless mass, curable by surgical resection. Plasmacytic type is often seen in the mesentery and retroperitoneum, and is accompanied with lymphoma-like symptoms, such as fever, anemia, weight loss, increased IgG, elevated erythrocyte sedimentation rate, hypergammoglobulinemia and hypoalbunemia. Close follow-up is necessary after resection and often chemotherapy is required.

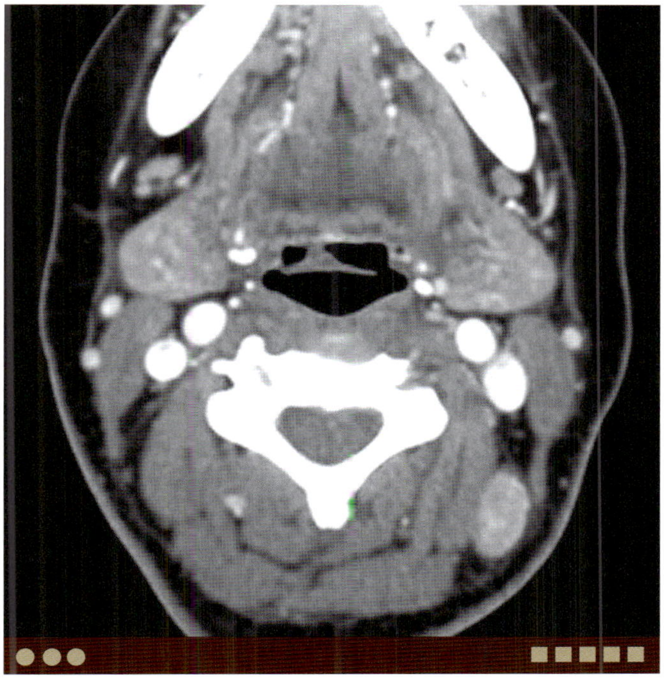

A. Castleman disease. Axial contrast enhanced CT demonstrates an avidly enhancing enlarged node in the left level V.

Castleman disease is often seen as an enlarged, avidly enhancing solitary lymph node (hyaline-vascular type), however, up to 10% may not show prominent enhancement. Calcification is often seen. On MRI, it demonstrates homogeneous low signal on T1W and relatively high signal on T2W images. On T2W images, central low-signal reflecting fibrosis is occasionally noted. Relatively homogeneous avid enhancement is usually seen after intravenous contrast administration.

PEARLS

- **Castleman disease is usually seen as an enlarged, avidly enhancing solitary lymph node in the head and neck.**
- **Up to 10% of Castleman disease is not hypervascular.**
- **Plasmacytic type is often multiple and associated with systemic lymphoma-like symptoms.**

ADDITIONAL IMAGES (B-G)

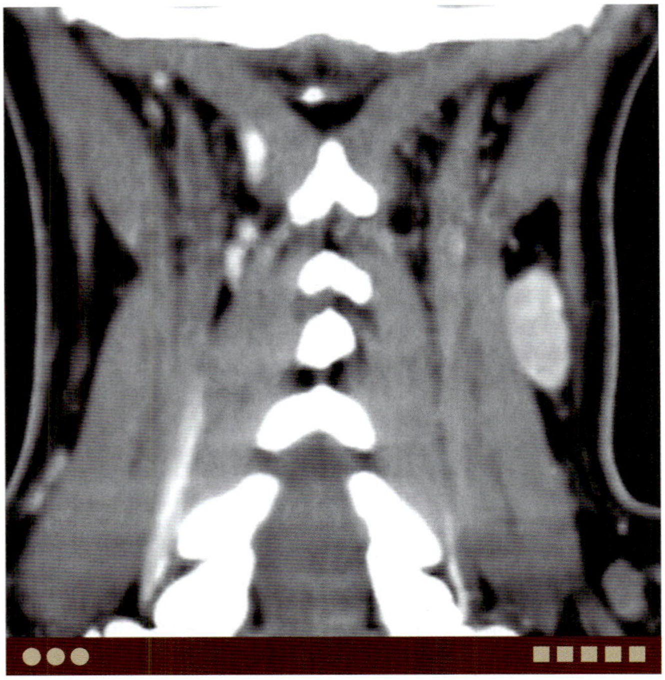

B. Castleman disease, same patient as A. Coronal contrast-enhanced CT demonstrates an avidly enhancing, enlarged node in the left level V.

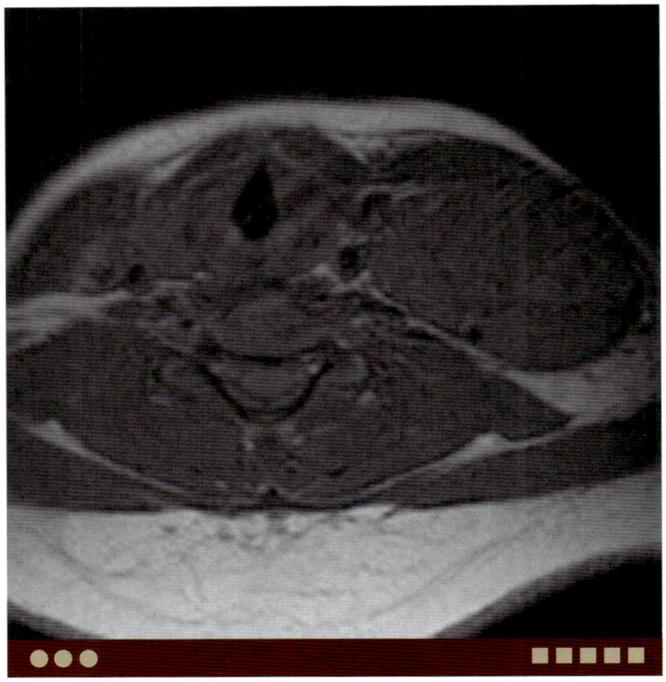

C. Castleman disease in a different patient. Axial T1W MR image demonstrates a large, homogeneous low-signal lesion posteromedial to the left sternocleidomastoid muscle (level IIIB).

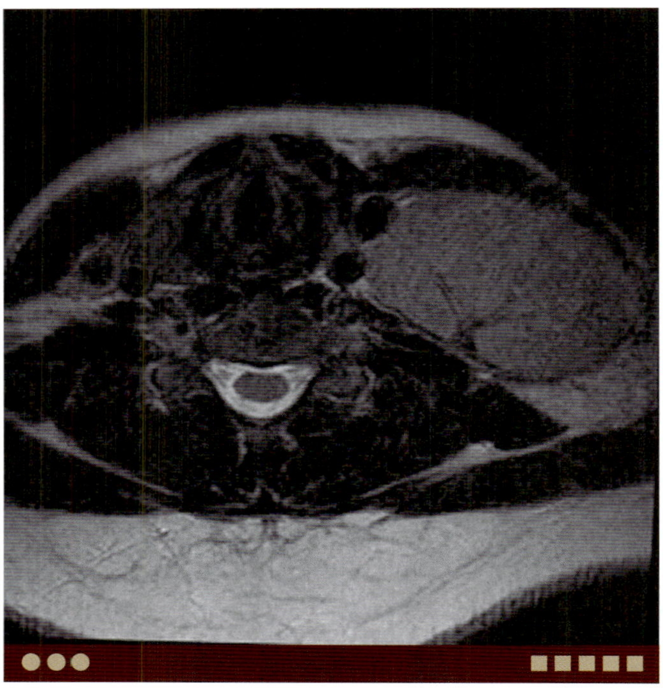

D. Castleman disease, same patient as C. Axial T2W MR image demonstrates the lesion showing homogeneous high signal.

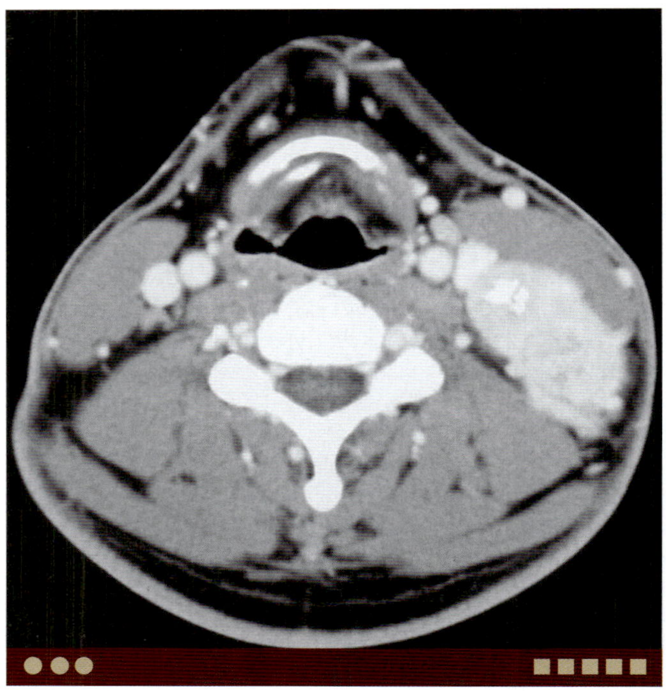

E. Castleman disease in a different patient. Axial contrast-enhanced CT demonstrates avidly enhancing lesion posteromedial to the left sternocleidomastoid muscle (level II/III). A focal calcification is noted in the anteromedial portion of the lesion.

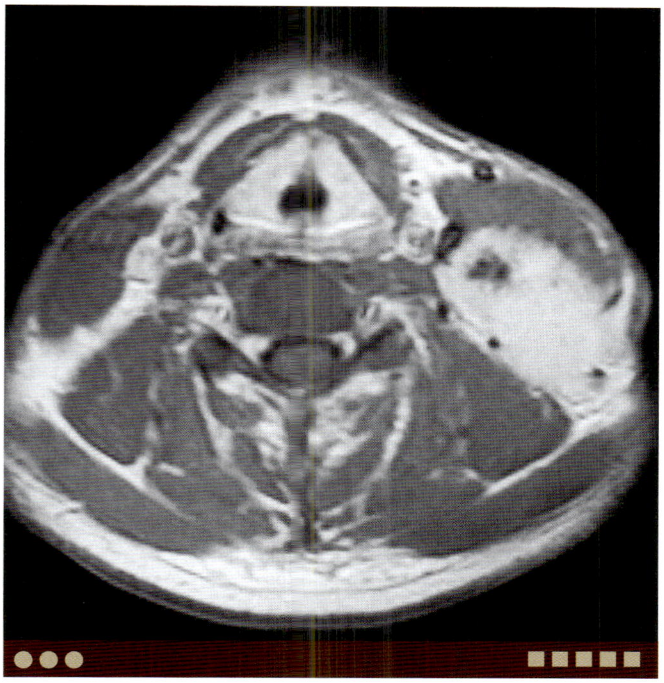

F. Castleman disease, same patient as E. Axial postcontrast T1W MR image demonstrates avid enhancement of the lesion. Signal-voids due to calcification are noted in the anteromedial portion of the lesion.

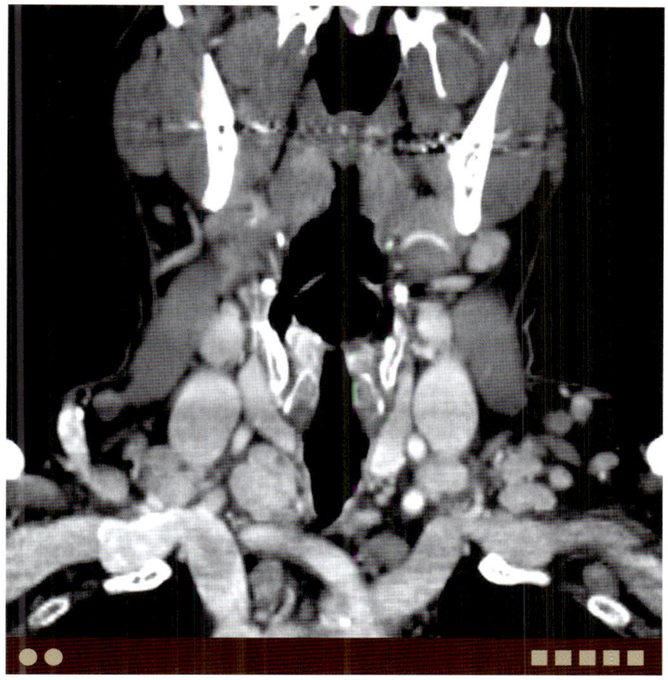

G. Castleman disease, plasmacytic type. Coronal contrast-enhanced CT demonstrates multiple homogeneously enhancing nodes bilaterally.

DIFFERENTIAL DIAGNOSIS IMAGES (H-J)

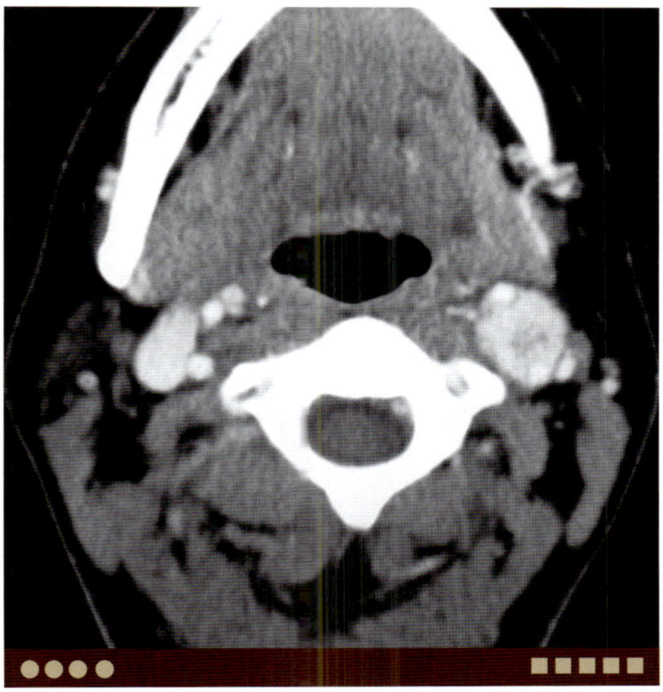

H. Paraganglioma. Axial contrast-enhanced CT demonstrates an avidly enhancing lesion at the left carotid bifurcation, splaying the internal and external carotid arteries, a typical appearance of carotid body tumor.

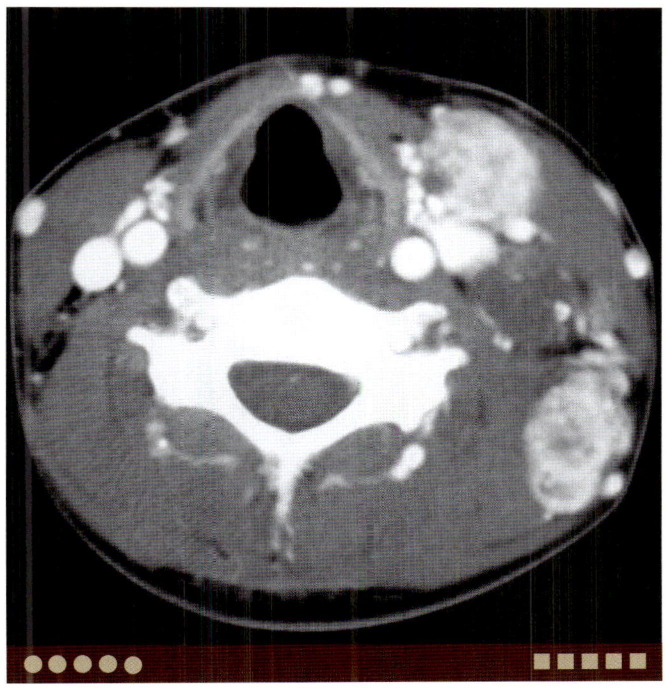

I. Metastasis from papillary thyroid carcinoma. Axial contrast-enhanced CT demonstrates multiple avidly enhancing nodes in the left levels III and V as well as a nonenhancing node in the left level III.

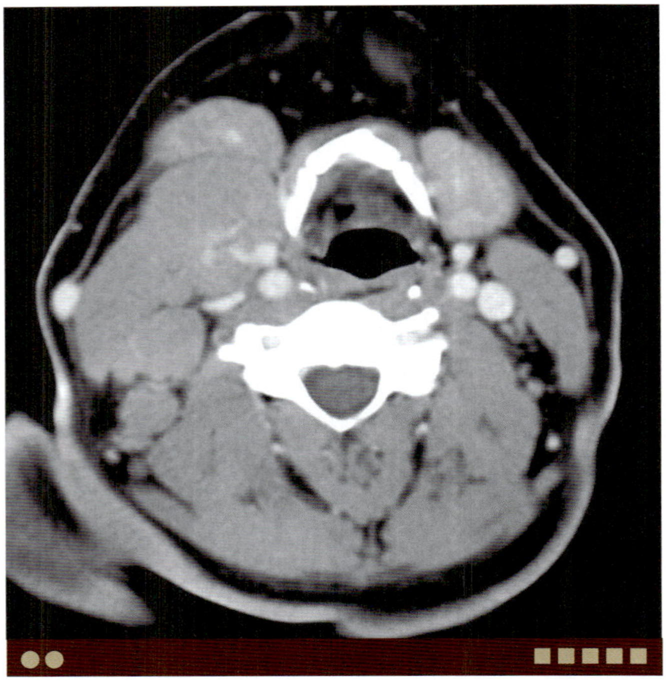

J. Lymphoma. Axial contrast-enhanced CT demonstrates multiple, enlarged, minimally enhancing, homogeneous density nodes in the right levels II and V.

Case 12–10 Cat Scratch Disease

Naoko Saito, Jimmy Wang, Osamu Sakai

PRESENTATION

Neck mass.

FINDINGS

CT demonstrates enhancing enlarged lymph nodes with surrounding edema. Some nodes show intranodal necrosis.

DIFFERENTIAL DIAGNOSIS

- Tuberculous lymphadenitis: This condition shows a wide variety of imaging findings, but enlarged nodes with central necrosis are the most common characteristic. Nodal calcification can be seen, however, it is relatively rare.
- Sarcoidosis: This is a systemic disease characterized by noncaseating granulomas. Multiple homogeneously enhancing lymph nodes are seen, often with sites of extranodal involvement in the parotid gland, orbit, and upper respiratory tract.
- Human immunodeficiency virus (HIV) infection: Cervical lymphadenopathy, nasopharyngeal lymphoid enlargement, and lymphoepithelial lesions of the parotid gland are the three major head and neck imaging findings for HIV infection.
- Kikuchi-Fujimoto disease: This is a histiocytic necrotizing lymphadenitis, and most commonly seen in Japanese women younger than 30 years of age. Multiple homogeneously enhancing lymph nodes with perinodal infiltration are frequently seen. Central necrosis is also seen.
- Lymphoma: Enlarged lymph nodes with homogeneous density/signal and mild enhancement are typical findings for lymphoma. Cystic or necrotic change, or calcification is rare without treatment.

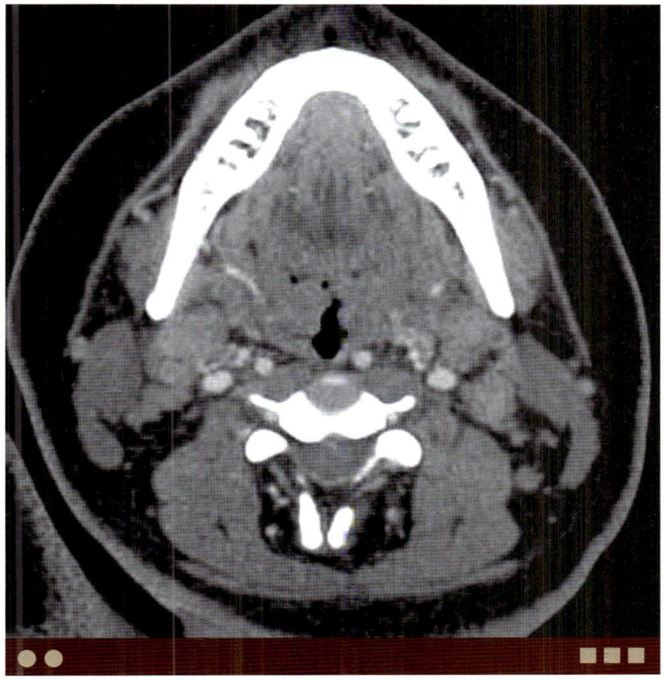

A. Cat scratch disease. Axial contrast-enhanced CT demonstrates multiple enlarged lymph nodes in the level II bilaterally.

COMMENTS

This is a 23-year-old man with bilateral neck masses.

Cat scratch disease is a zoonotic disease caused by *Bartonella henselae* and characterized by necrotizing granulomatous regional lymphadenitis. The bacteria are introduced at a skin site by a scratch of a cat. The exposure to dogs has also been reported to cause the disease, however, it is rare. Cat scratch disease is seen worldwide, and often seen in children and young adults.

Three to 10 days after being scratched or bitten by a cat, the primary site develops a granulomatous skin lesion. The inoculation sites are usually on the hands, arms, or chest. This skin lesion resolves spontaneously within 1 to 3 weeks. Then, painful regional lymphadenopathy appears within weeks after the primary skin lesion. The cervical and axillary lymph nodes are the most commonly affected. This lymphadenopathy usually resolves within 2 to 4 months.

Cat scratch disease usually demonstrates markedly enlarged lymph nodes with extensive surrounding edema. On contrast-enhanced CT, central low density with peripheral enhancement representing intranodal necrosis can sometimes be observed.

Typically cat scratch disease is benign and self-limiting, however, 1% to 2 % of the patients progress to severe systemic infections including encephalitis, osteomyelitis, hepatitis, and pleuritis.

PEARLS

- **Cat scratch disease is characterized by necrotizing granulomatous, regional lymphadenitis.**
- **Painful regional lymphadenopathy appears within weeks after the primary skin lesion.**
- **Contrast-enhanced CT sometimes demonstrates central low density with peripheral enhancement representing intranodal necrosis.**

ADDITIONAL IMAGES (B-C)

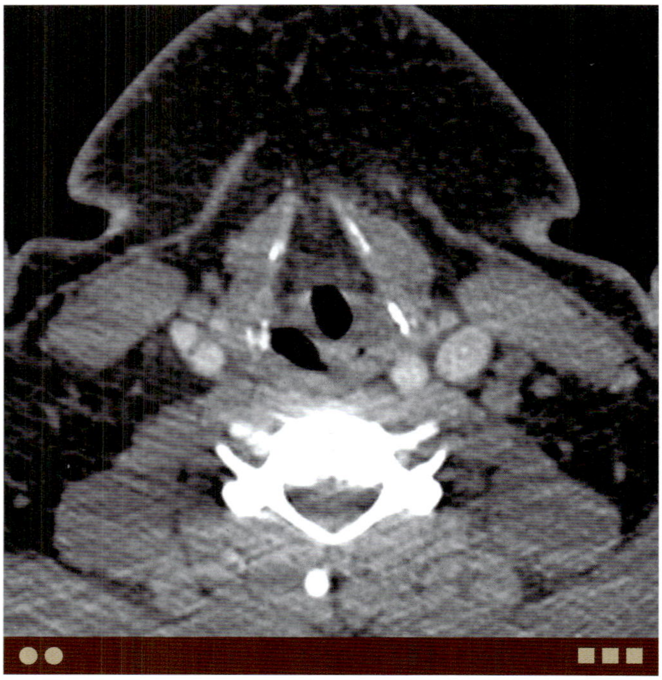

B. Cat scratch disease, same patient as A. Axial contrast-enhanced CT at the lower level demonstrates enhancing several left level III lymph nodes with central low-density area representing central necrosis.

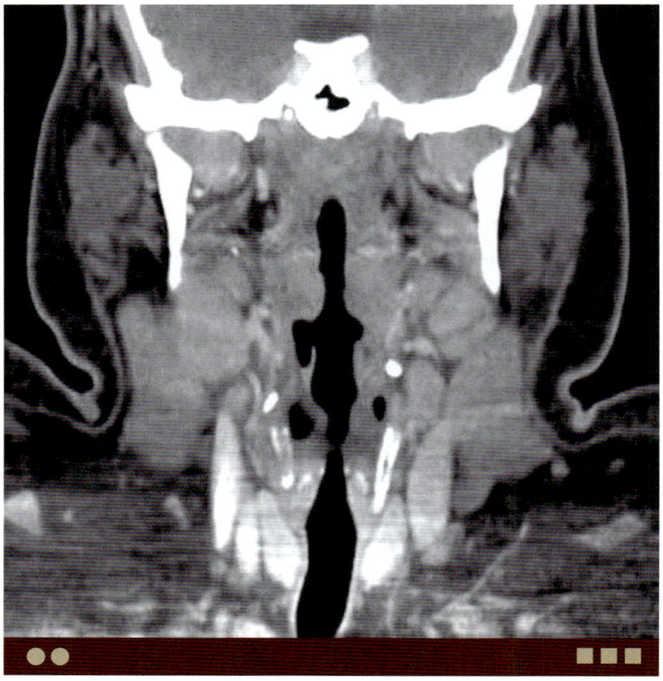

C. Cat scratch disease, same patient as A. Coronal contrast-enhanced CT demonstrates multiple bilateral enlarged, homogeneously enhancing lymph nodes.

DIFFERENTIAL DIAGNOSIS IMAGES (D-G)

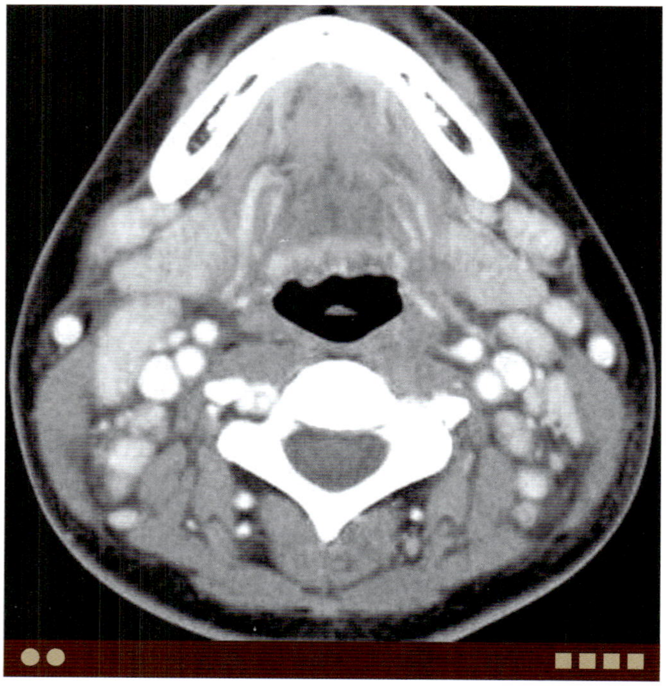

D. Kikuchi-Fujimoto disease. Axial contrast-enhanced CT demonstrates multiple bilateral, enhancing lymph nodes. Note infiltration of adjacent fat tissues.

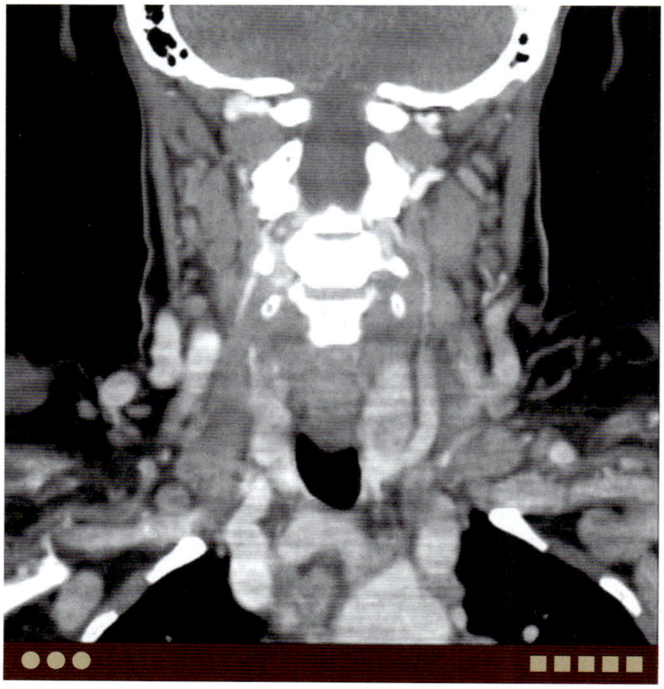

E. Sarcoidosis. Coronal contrast-enhanced CT demonstrates multiple bilateral, enlarged cervical, supraclavicular, and mediastinal lymph nodes.

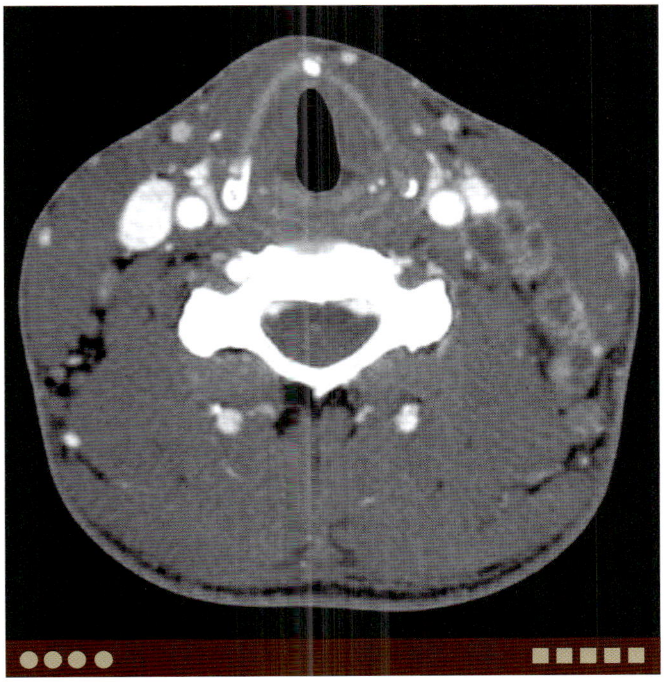

F. Tuberculous lymphadenitis. Axial contrast-enhanced CT demonstrates multiple left levels II and V lymph nodes with central necrosis.

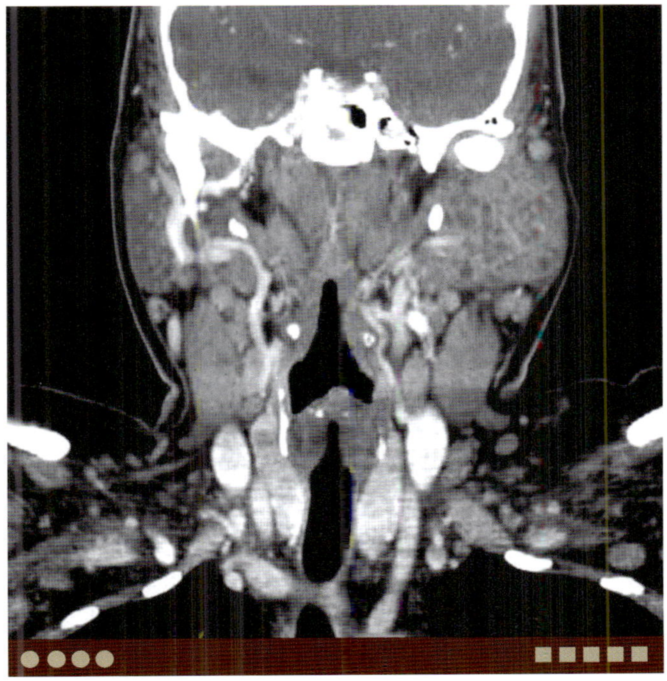

G. HIV infection. Coronal contrast-enhanced CT demonstrates multiple bilateral, enhancing lymph nodes. Multiple cystic lesions in bilateral parotid glands are also noted, which is a characteristic finding of lymphoepithelial lesions associated with HIV infection.

Case 12–11 Mononucleosis

Asim Mian, Osamu Sakai

PRESENTATION

Bilateral cervical lymphadenopathy with sore throat, difficulty swallowing, and low-grade fevers.

FINDINGS

CT demonstrates bilateral enlarged, enhancing cervical lymph nodes with marked enlargement of the nasopharyngeal and palatine tonsils.

DIFFERENTIAL DIAGNOSIS

- Suppurative adenopathy: This condition is intranodal abscess formation. Heterogeneously enhancing nodes with central low densities are seen.
- Tuberculous adenitis: This condition shows variable appearance of affected lymph node; homogeneous enhancement, heterogeneous enhancement, intranodal abscess/necrosis, and occasionally calcification.
- Kawasaki disease: It is also known as acute febrile mucocutaneous lymph node syndrome which is a systemic vasculitis of unknown etiology affecting infants and young children.
- Kikuchi-Fujimoto disease: This is also known as histiocytic necrotizing lymphadenopathy, and is a rare lymphadenitis of unknown etiology. This disease is mainly seen in Japan but cases are reported in the United States and Europe.
- Metastatic nodal disease: Metastasis causes heterogeneous enhancement of nodes. Squamous cell carcinoma is the most common malignancy in the neck, however, thyroid cancer should also be considered, particularly in young women.
- Lymphoma: Lymphoma demonstrates unilateral or bilateral lymphadenopathy usually with homogeneous density and mild enhancement, but it may be variable in appearance.

COMMENTS

This is a 16-year-old girl with sore throat and bilateral cervical lymphadenopathy.

Mononucleosis is a viral infection caused by Epstein-Barr virus (EBV). It typically presents with fevers, sore throat, markedly enlarged tonsils, and lymphadenopathy. It is usually spread by saliva and close contact. Although it can occur at any age, it usually occurs in adolescents and called the "kissing disease." There are many constitutional symptoms and complications including, but not limited to, generalized fatigue (weeks to months), rash, splenomegaly, hepatitis and jaundice, Guillain-Barre syndrome, and seizures.

CT usually demonstrates extensive, multiple enhancing nodes throughout the neck bilaterally. Markedly enlarged, heterogeneously enhancing tonsils (adenoid, palatine, lingual) are seen without peripherally enhancing collection as is seen with tonsillar abscess. Inflammatory changes from this process can extend into the retropharyngeal space resulting in edema without abscess.

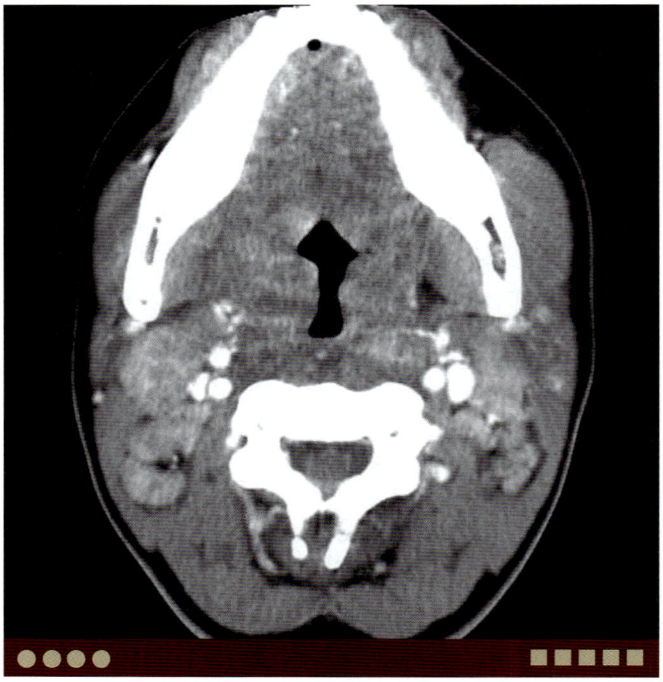

A. Mononucleosis. Axial postcontrast CT demonstrates multiple, heterogeneously enhancing, enlarged lymph nodes in the bilateral level II. Note enlarged, edematous bilateral palatine tonsils.

PEARLS

- **Mononucleosis is a viral infection caused by EBV, commonly seen in children and young adults.**
- **Mononucleosis demonstrates multiple enhancing cervical nodes and markedly enlarged tonsils with heterogeneous enhancement.**

ADDITIONAL IMAGE

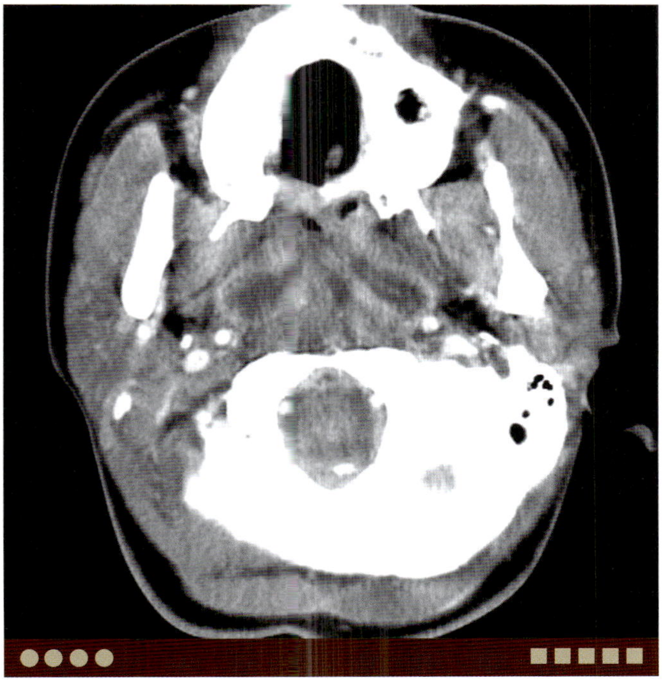

B. Mononucleosis, same patient as A. Axial postcontrast CT demonstrates significantly enlarged, heterogeneously enhancing nasopharyngeal tonsils, obliterating the nasopharyngeal lumen.

DIFFERENTIAL DIAGNOSIS IMAGES (C-F)

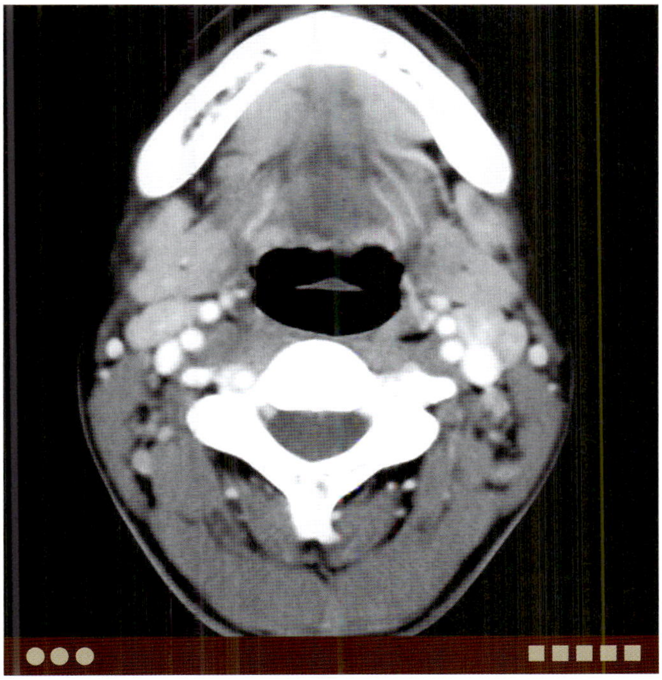

C. Sarcoidosis. Axial postcontrast CT demonstrates multiple, enhancing, enlarged lymph nodes in the bilateral level II.

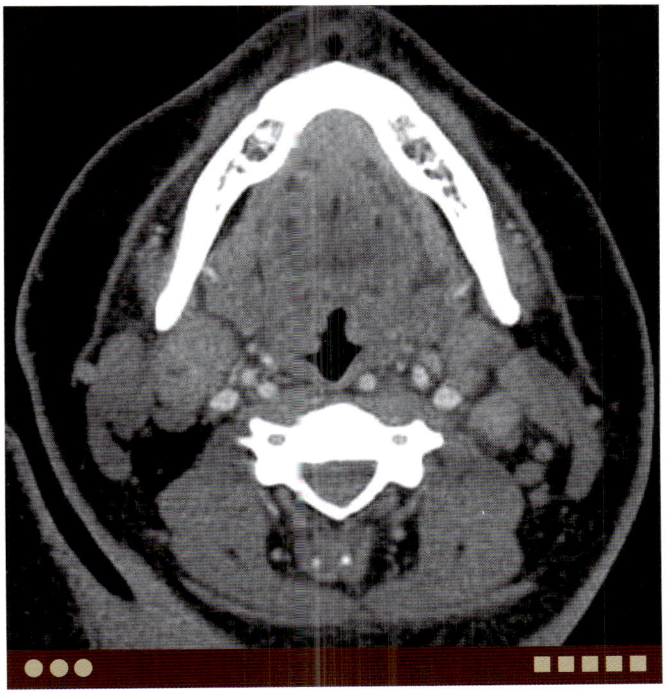

D. Cat scratch disease. Axial postcontrast CT demonstrates multiple, enhancing, enlarged lymph nodes in the bilateral level II. Some nodes have central low densities and perinodal infiltrative changes.

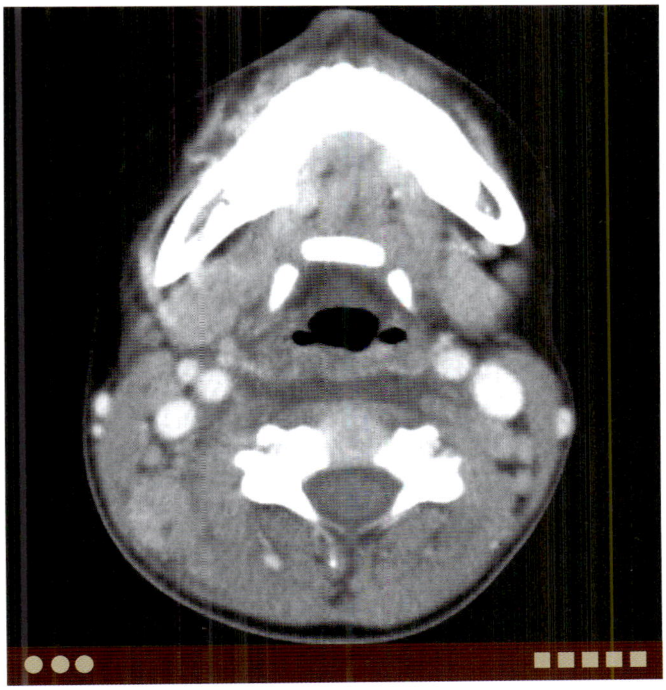

E. Kawasaki disease. Axial postcontrast CT demonstrates multiple, enhancing lymph nodes in bilateral levels II and V. Note retropharyngeal edema.

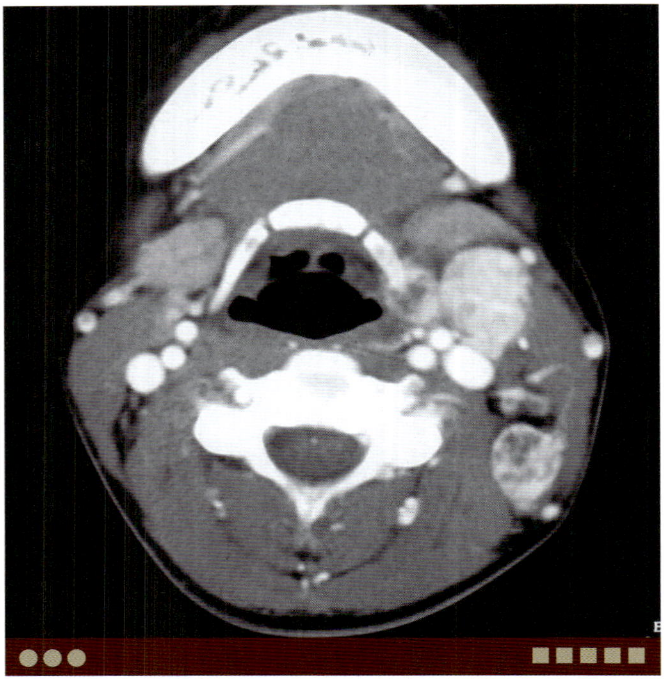

F. Metastasis from papillary thyroid carcinoma. Axial postcontrast CT demonstrates multiple, heterogeneous, avidly enhancing, enlarged lymph nodes in the left levels II and V.

Case 12–12 Nodal Metastasis from Papillary Thyroid Carcinoma

Osamu Sakai, Rohini Nadgir

PRESENTATION

Neck mass.

FINDINGS

CT and MRI show various appearance of cervical lymph nodes; homogeneous and heterogeneous enhancement, cystic change, necrosis, and calcification.

DIFFERENTIAL DIAGNOSIS

- Tuberculosis: Involves lymph nodes that demonstrate variable appearance including avid enhancement, cystic change, and calcification.
- Squamous cell carcinoma: Nodal metastasis often demonstrates intranodal necrosis. Calcification is not common.
- Kaposi's sarcoma: This is often associated with HIV infection and can present with enhancing metastatic nodes.
- Other inflammatory conditions: Cat scratch disease and Kikuchi-Fujimoto disease (histiocytic necrotizing lymphadenitis) may demonstrate similar findings.
- Lymphoma: Lymphoma usually demonstrates large, homogeneous density nodes which mildly enhance. Necrosis is unusual but can be seen without treatment.

COMMENTS

This is a 26-year-old woman with a rapidly growing left neck mass.

Papillary thyroid carcinoma is most common among carcinomas of the thyroid and represents the majority of all thyroid carcinomas (55% to 80%). Primary tumor in the thyroid may not be apparent, and the patient may present with a painless neck mass.

On CT, metastatic nodes from papillary thyroid cancer demonstrate various appearances; homogeneous enhancement simulating hyperplastic lymph nodes, avid enhancement, almost no enhancement, intranodal necrosis, completely cystic appearance or calcification. Imaging finding may be very similar to that of tuberculosis. However, perinodal inflammatory change is usually not seen with metastasis from thyroid cancer. Metastasis from papillary thyroid carcinoma should be considered in the differential diagnosis as well as tuberculosis, whenever variable appearance of lymph nodes is seen, particularly in young women, even in teenagers.

On MRI, the central low density on CT may show increased signal on both T1W and T2W images due to increased protein concentration from thyroglobulin accumulation, tumor necrosis, and hemorrhage.

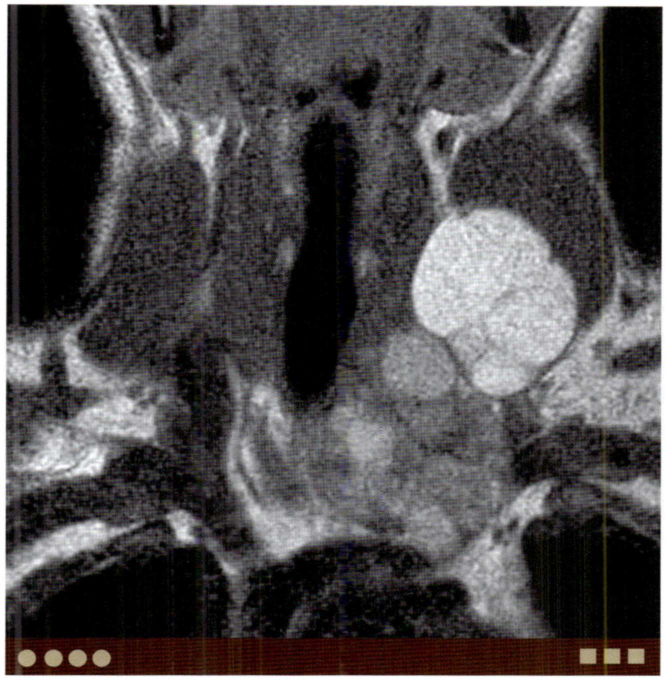

A. Nodal metastasis from papillary thyroid carcinoma. Coronal T1W MR image demonstrates mult cystic lesions showing variable signal in the left lower neck.

PEARLS

- **Papillary thyroid carcinoma demonstrates variable appearance of metastatic lymph nodes.**
- **Papillary thyroid carcinoma can be seen in young patients, even in teenagers.**
- **The primary lesion in the thyroid may be small and not clearly identified on CT or MR.**

ADDITIONAL IMAGES (B-G)

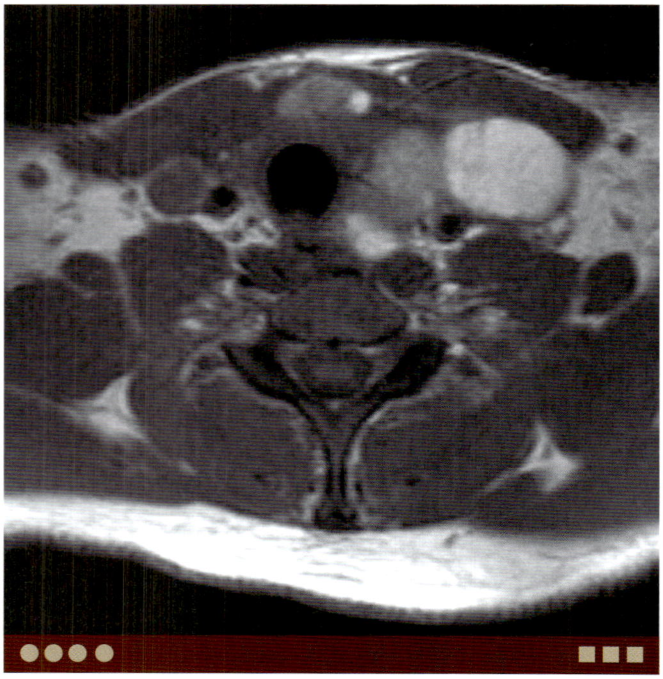

B. Metastasis from papillary thyroid carcinoma, same patient as A. Axial T1W MR image demonstrates multiple cystic lesions showing variable signal in the left neck.

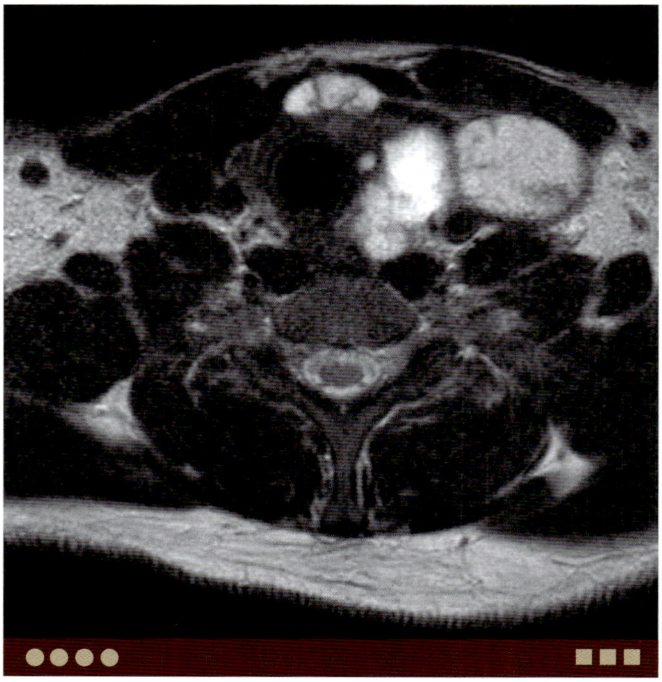

C. Metastasis from papillary thyroid carcinoma, same patient as A. Axial T2W MR image demonstrates multiple cystic lesions showing variable signal in the left neck.

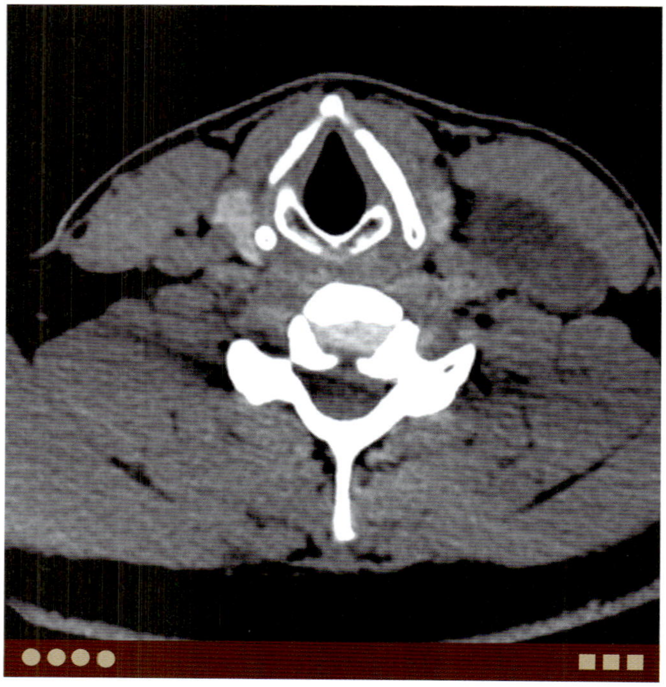

D. Metastasis from papillary thyroid carcinoma, same patient as A. Axial noncontrast CT demonstrates cystic node in the left level III/IV.

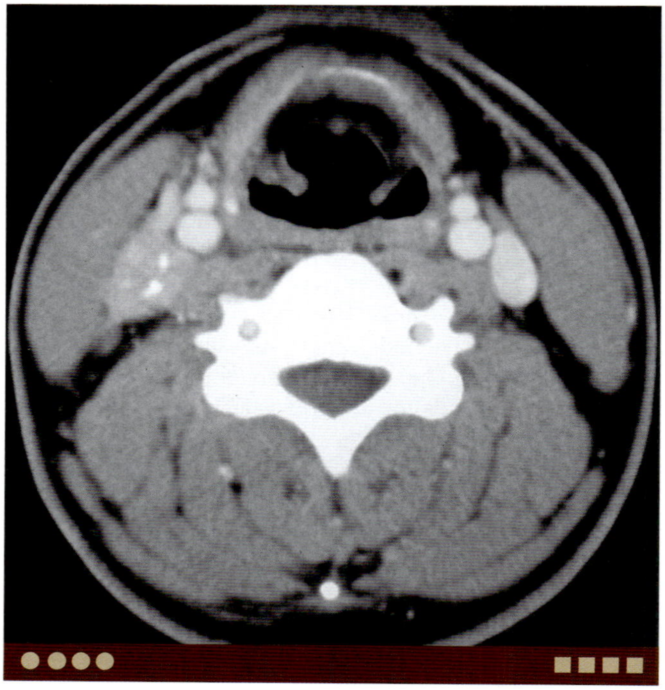

E. Metastasis from papillary thyroid carcinoma in a different patient. Axial postcontrast CT demonstrates a moderately enhancing, enlarged node with punctate calcifications in the right level III.

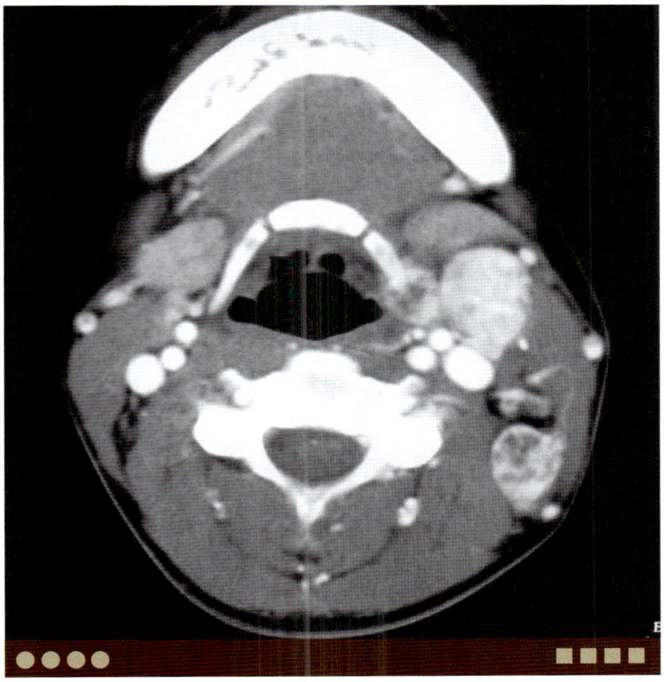

F. Metastasis from papillary thyroid carcinoma in a different patient. Axial postcontrast CT demonstrates multiple heterogeneously enhancing nodes in the left levels II and V.

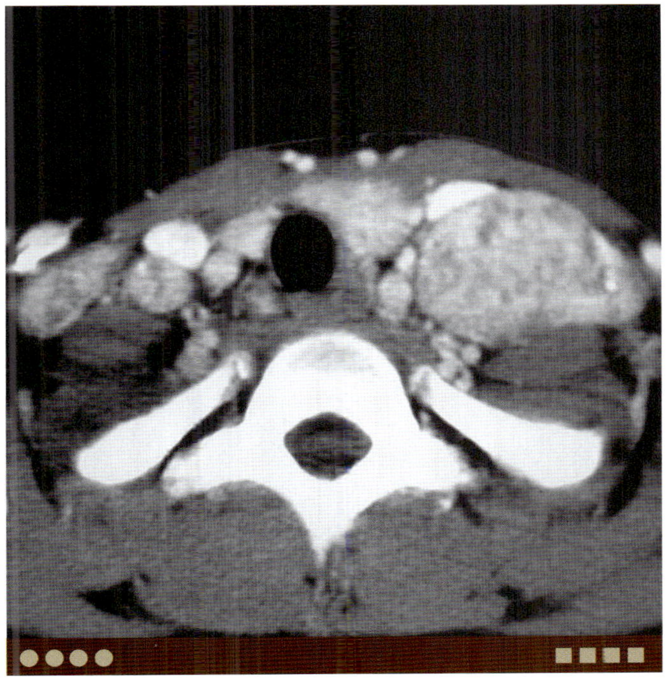

G. Metastasis from papillary thyroid carcinoma, same patient as F. Axial postcontrast CT demonstrates multiple heterogeneously enhancing nodes in the bilateral levels IV and VI and supraclavicular fossae.

DIFFERENTIAL DIAGNOSIS IMAGES (H-J)

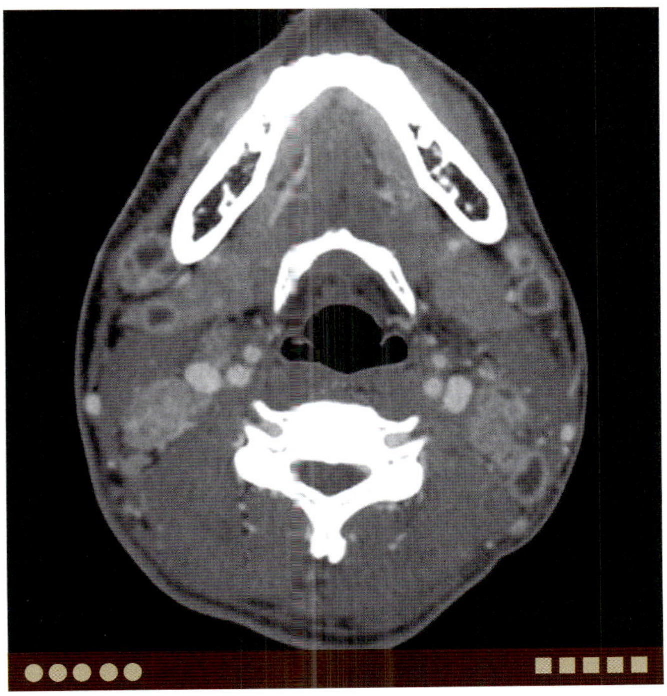

H. Tuberculosis. Axial postcontrast CT demonstrates multiple heterogeneously enhancing nodes with central low density in the bilateral levels I, II, and V.

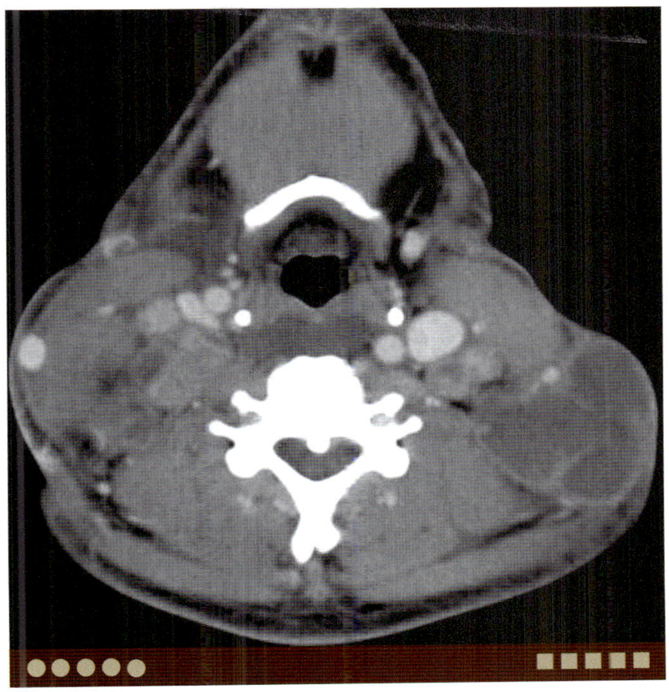

I. Tuberculosis in a different patient. Axial postcontrast CT demonstrates multiple, predominantly cystic lesions in the bilateral neck. Edema is noted in the retropharyngeal space.

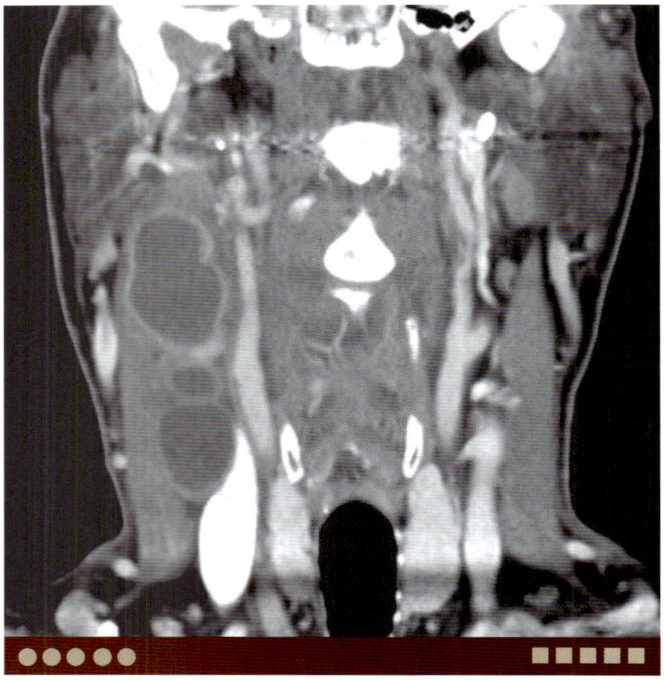

J. Metastasis from base of tongue squamous cell carcinoma. Coronal postcontrast CT demonstrates multiple, cystic-appearing, rim-enhancing metastatic nodes in the right levels II and III.

Case 12–13 Leukemia

Hiroki Kato, Jimmy Wang, Osamu Sakai

PRESENTATION

Cervical lymphadenopathy.

FINDINGS

CT and MRI demonstrate bilateral cervical lymphadenopathy.

DIFFERENTIAL DIAGNOSIS

- Reactive hyperplastic nodes: Enlarged nodes are often seen in non-neoplastic conditions. These nodes preserve kidney-bean shape and fatty hilum without intranodal necrosis.
- Lymphoma: Non-Hodgkin lymphoma generally presents with widespread lymphadenopathy, while Hodgkin lymphoma is characterized by its localized presentation and spreads to contiguous nodal regions orderly.
- Nodal metastasis: Lymph node size is one of the most frequently used criteria for discriminating metastatic from nonmetastatic (benign reactive) nodes, >1.5 to 2.0 cm in level II and >1 cm in other locations. Furthermore, central necrosis/low density is abnormal in any size and suggestive of metastatic disease.
- Lymphadenitis: Bacterial infection in the head and neck as well as viral infection such as cytomegalovirus and adenovirus causes lymphadenitis. Tuberculous lymphadenitis is also commonly seen in people from epidemic areas and immunocompromised patients.

COMMENTS

This is a 65-year-old woman with slowly progressive bilateral cervical lymphadenopathy.

Acute lymphoblastic leukemia (ALL) is predominantly seen in children, while acute myelogenous leukemia (AML) typically affects older individuals. Patients with acute leukemia generally present with fatigue, fever, and bleeding. Physical examination reveals a pale appearance with purpura and petechiae, lymphadenopathy, and splenomegaly. In ALL lymphadenopathy and splenomegaly are more common, while lymphadenopathy is unusual in adult AML.

Chronic lymphoblastic leukemia (CLL) predominantly affects older individuals. Most patients with CLL are asymptomatic at presentation, while those who are symptomatic present with fatigue or lymphadenopathy. Chronic myelogenous leukemia (CML) typically presents in the middle ages with fatigue, night sweats, and low-grade fever. Some patients present symptoms related to marked splenomegaly with left upper quadrant pain. Lymphadenopathy is seen as the disease accelerates. In patients with leukemia, peripheral lymphadenopathy is more commonly seen in patients with lymphoblastic leukemia rather than the myelogenous leukemia.

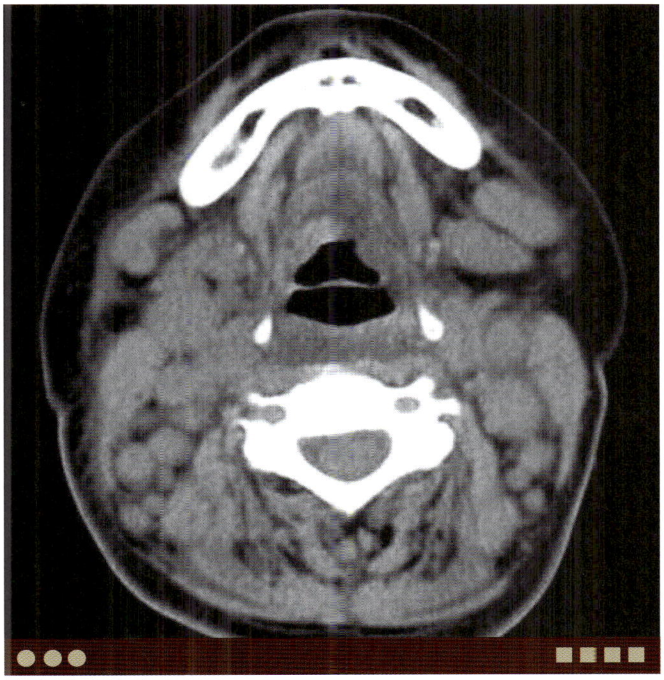

A. Adult T-cell leukemia. Axial unenhanced CT demonstrates bilateral upper cervical (levels I and II) lymphadenopathy without central necrosis. Note retropharyngeal edema.

More than 25% of malignant tumors in children occur in the head and neck, and the cervical lymph nodes are the most common site. During the first 6 years of life, neuroblastoma and leukemia are the most common malignancy associated with cervical lymphadenopathy, followed by rhabdomyosarcoma and non-Hodgkin lymphoma. Viral infection, malignancies such as leukemia or lymphoma, and collagen vascular diseases such as juvenile rheumatoid arthritis or systemic lupus erythematosus are more commonly associated with generalized lymphadenopathy. Supraclavicular or posterior cervical lymphadenopathy is more often associated with malignancy compared with anterior cervical lymphadenopathy.

PEARLS

- **ALL predominantly affects children, and lymphadenopathy and splenomegaly are commonly seen.**
- **Peripheral lymphadenopathy is more commonly seen in patients with lymphoblastic leukemia rather than myelogenous leukemia.**
- **During the first 6 years of life, neuroblastoma and leukemia are the most common malignancy associated with cervical lymphadenopathy.**

ADDITIONAL IMAGES (B-C)

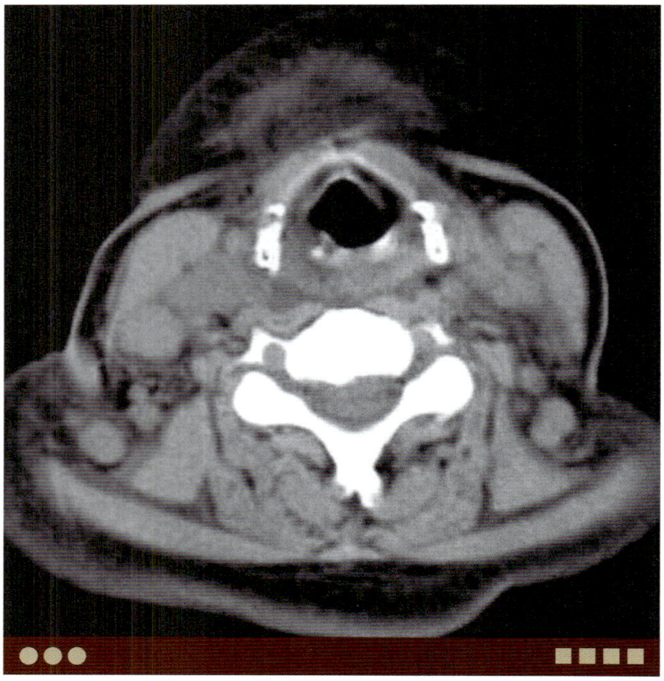

B. Adult T-cell leukemia, same patient as A. Axial unenhanced CT demonstrates bilateral mid cervical (levels III and V) lymphadenopathy without central necrosis.

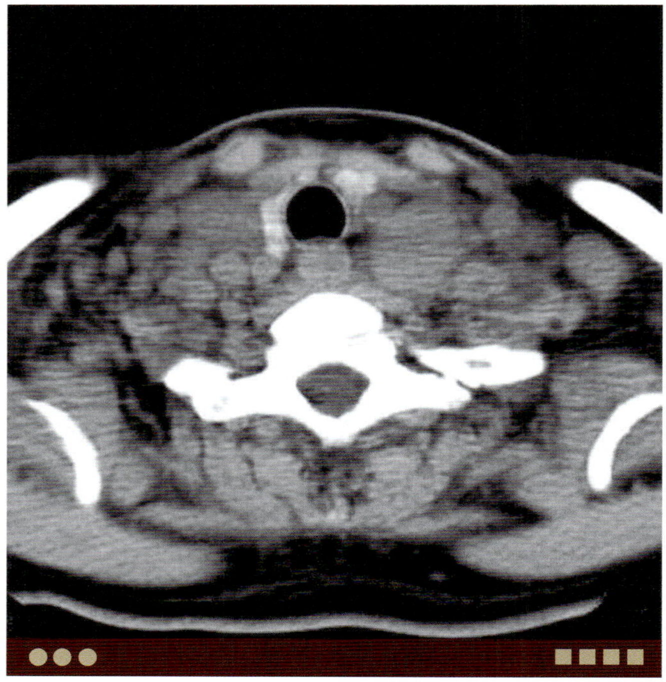

C. Adult T-cell leukemia, same patient as A. Axial unenhanced CT demonstrates bilateral lower cervical (level IV and supraclavicular) lymphadenopathy without central necrosis.

DIFFERENTIAL DIAGNOSIS IMAGES (D-H)

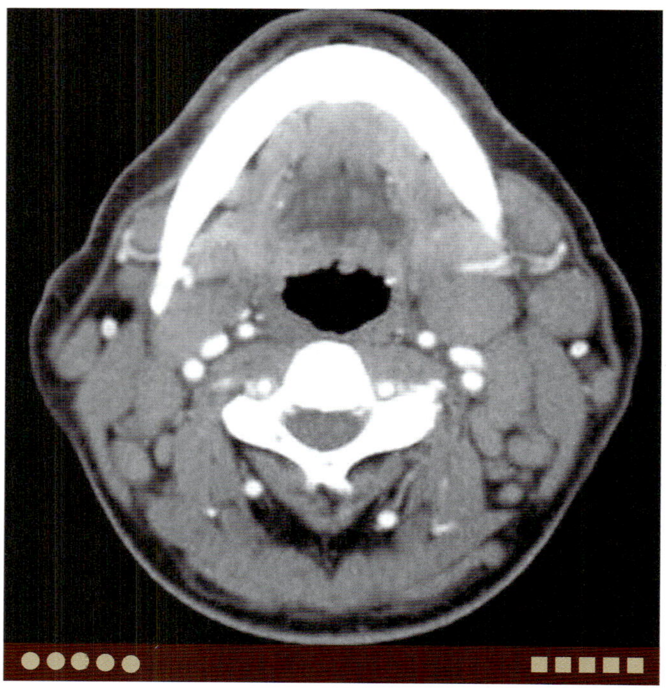

D. Diffuse large B-cell lymphoma. Axial contrast-enhanced CT demonstrates bilateral upper cervical (level II) lymphadenopathy without necrosis.

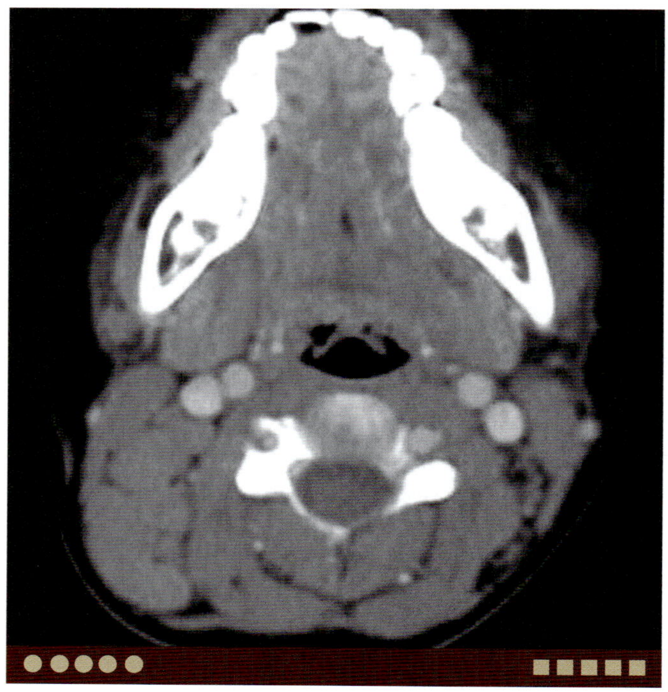

E. Hodgkin disease. Axial contrast-enhanced CT demonstrates right levels IIB and V lymphadenopathy without necrosis.

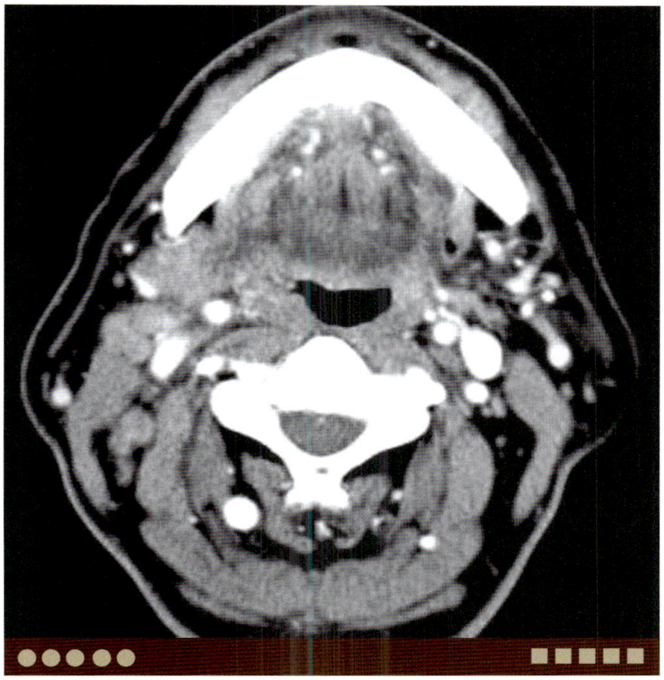

F. Nodal metastasis from oropharyngeal squamous cell carcinoma. Axial contrast-enhanced CT demonstrates heterogeneously enhancing right level II nodes.

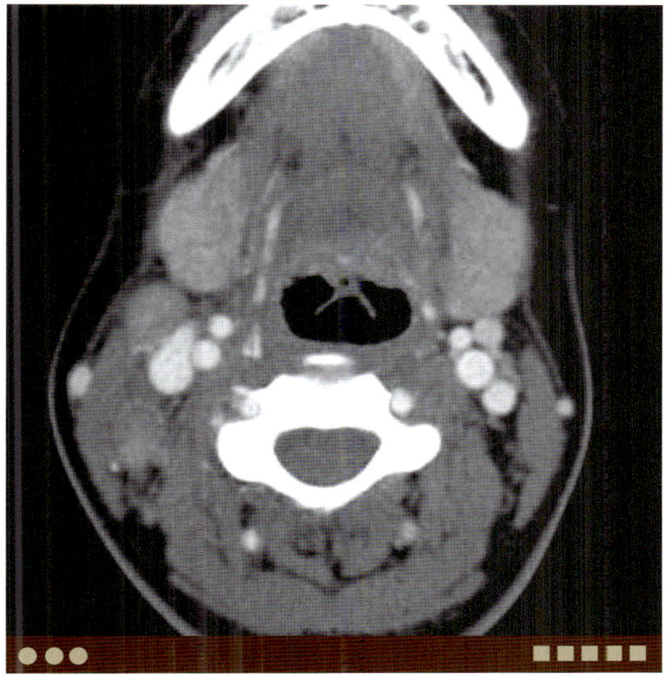

G. Kikuchi-Fujimoto disease (histiocytic necrotizing lymphadenitis). Axial contrast-enhanced CT demonstrates heterogeneously enhancing right level II nodes with surrounding inflammatory change.

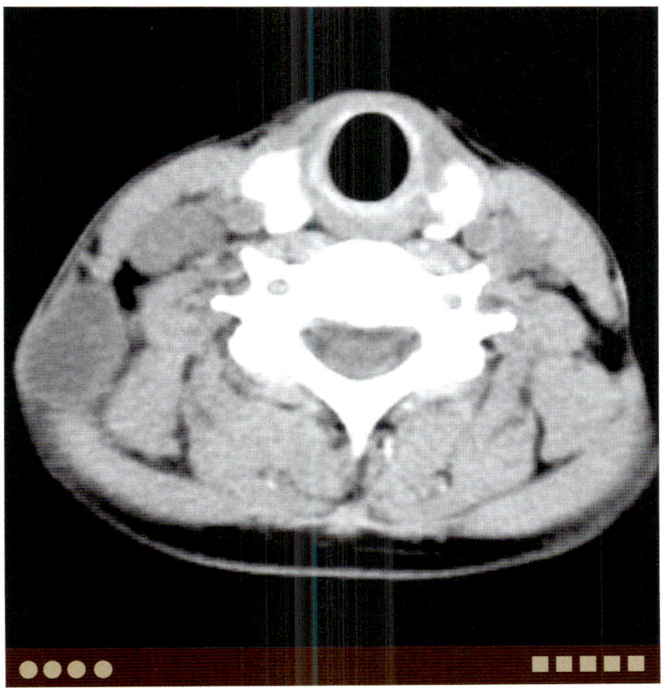

H. Tuberculosis lymphadenitis. Axial unenhanced CT demonstrates an enlarged right level V node with central necrosis.

Case 12–14 Lymphadenopathy Associated with HIV Infection

Naoko Saito, Jimmy Wang, Osamu Sakai

PRESENTATION

Multiple cervical lymph nodes swelling.

FINDINGS

CT demonstrates multiple bilateral, homogeneously enhancing lymph nodes.

DIFFERENTIAL DIAGNOSIS

- Sarcoidosis: This is a systemic disease characterized by noncaseating granulomas. Multiple homogeneously enhancing lymph nodes are seen with extranodal sites of involvement including parotid glands, orbit, and upper respiratory tract.
- Lymphoma: Multiple homogeneously enhancing lymph nodes are seen. Cystic change is rare without treatment.
- Tuberculous adenitis: This condition shows variable appearance of affected lymph node; homogeneous enhancement, heterogeneous enhancement, intranodal abscess/necrosis, and occasionally calcification.
- Metastatic nodal disease: Metastasis causes heterogeneous enhancement of nodes. Squamous cell carcinoma is the most common malignancy in the neck, however, thyroid cancer should also be considered, particularly in young women.
- Kikuchi-Fujimoto disease: This is a histiocytic necrotizing lymphadenitis, and most commonly seen in patients younger than 30 years of age. This disease is more commonly seen in Japan. Multiple enhancing lymph nodes with perinodal infiltration are frequently seen.

COMMENTS

This is a 54-year-old human immunodeficiency virus (HIV) positive man with cervical lymphadenopathy.

HIV is a retrovirus that infects cells of the immune system and destroys or disrupts their function. In the more advanced stages of HIV infection, acquired immunodeficiency syndrome (AIDS) develops.

About 70 % of the patients with HIV develop persistent, generalized lymphadenopathy within the first 3 months after primary infection. Cervical reactive lymphadenopathy without associated infection is seen in up to 50% of the patients. Secondary infection may also cause lymphadenopathy. Tuberculosis is seen, particularly in patients with a CD4 count below 400.

On imaging, HIV infection demonstrates nonspecific multiple, bilateral, homogeneous cervical lymphadenopathy.

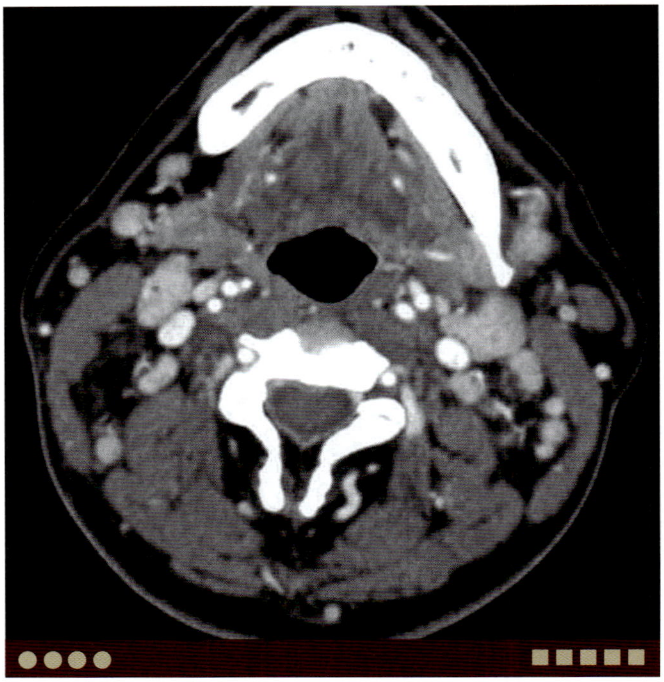

A. Lymphadenopathy associated with HIV infection. Axial contrast-enhanced CT demonstrates multiple bilateral, homogeneously enhancing lymph nodes.

It is suggested that increasing lymph node size correlates with decreasing CD4 levels. Cervical lymphadenopathy is often accompanied with lymphoepithelial lesions of the parotid gland and nasopharyngeal lymphoid enlargement. They are the three major imaging findings in head and neck for HIV infection.

Non-Hodgkin lymphoma is the second most common neoplasm arising in patients with HIV infection and AIDS after Kaposi's sarcoma. The risk of non-Hodgkin lymphoma in patients with AIDS is about 60 times higher than normal population.

PEARLS

- **Cervical lymphadenopathy is seen in up to 50% of the patients with HIV infection.**
- **In head and neck, cervical lymphadenopathy, nasopharyngeal lymphoid enlargement, and lymphoepithelial lesions of the parotid gland are the three major imaging findings for HIV infection.**
- **The risk of non-Hodgkin lymphoma in patients with AIDS is about 60 times higher than normal population.**

ADDITIONAL IMAGES (B–F)

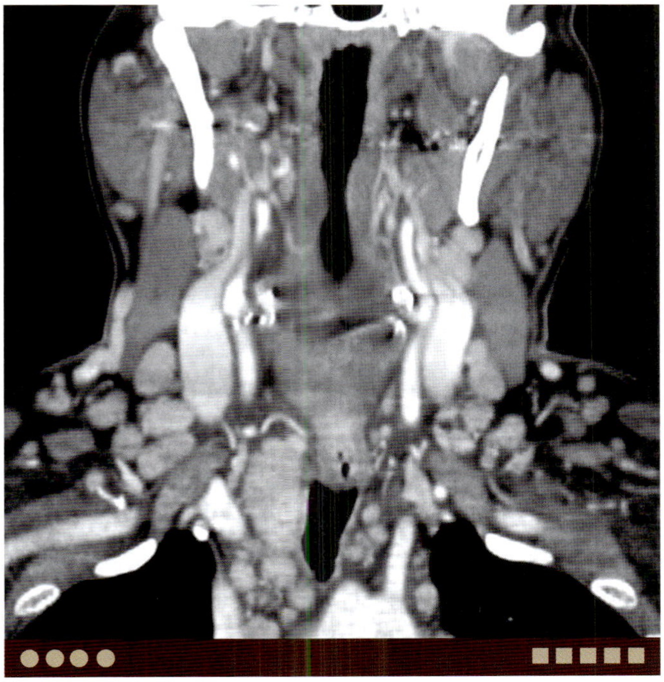

B. Lymphadenopathy associated with HIV infection, same patient as A. Coronal contrast-enhanced CT demonstrates multiple cervical, supraclavicular, and mediastinal lymph nodes.

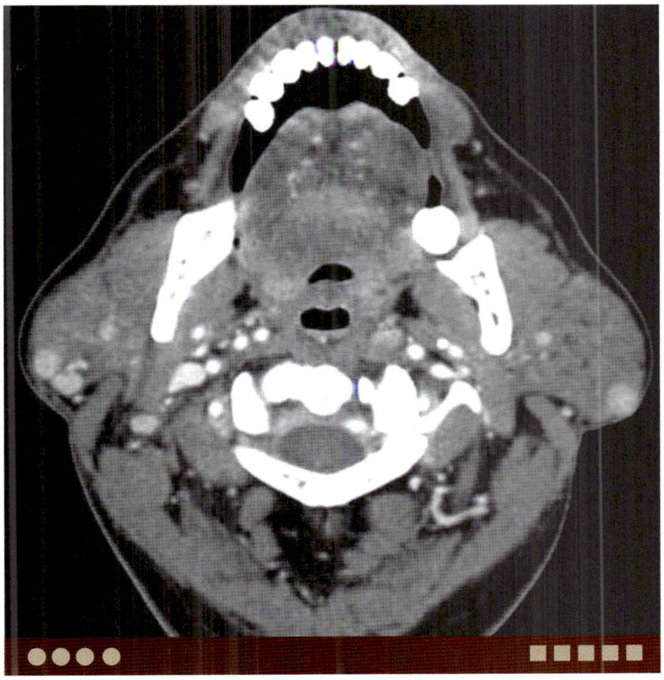

C. Lymphadenopathy associated with HIV infection, same patient as A. Axial contrast-enhanced CT demonstrates small cystic lesions in bilateral parotid glands as well as enhancing intraparotid lymph nodes.

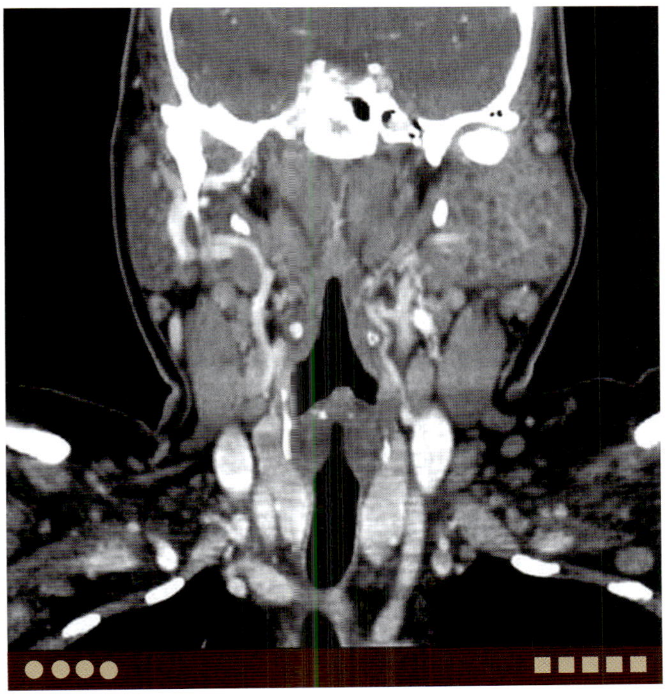

D. Lymphadenopathy associated with HIV infection in a different patient. Coronal contrast-enhanced CT demonstrates multiple lymphadenopathy and lymphoepithelial cysts in bilateral parotid glands. Note the nasopharyngeal lymphoid enlargement.

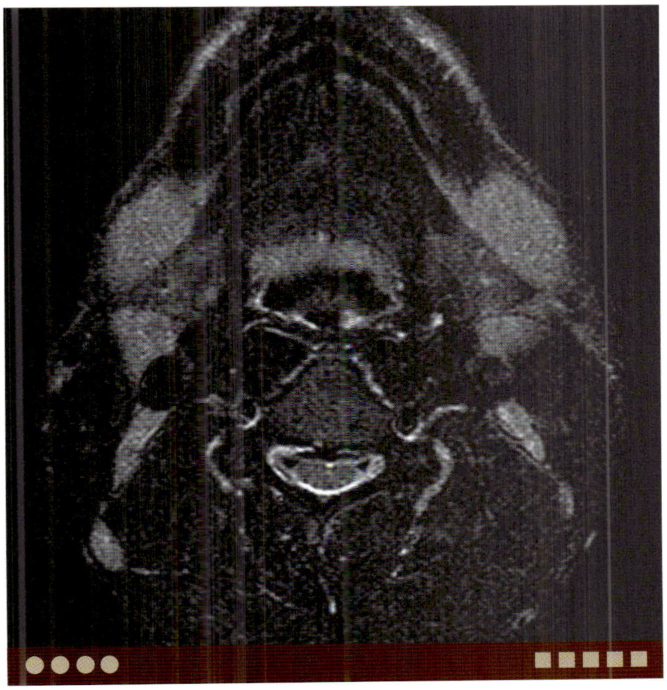

E. Lymphadenopathy associated with HIV infection in a different patient. Axial STIR image demonstrates multiple bilateral, homogeneous high-signal lymph nodes.

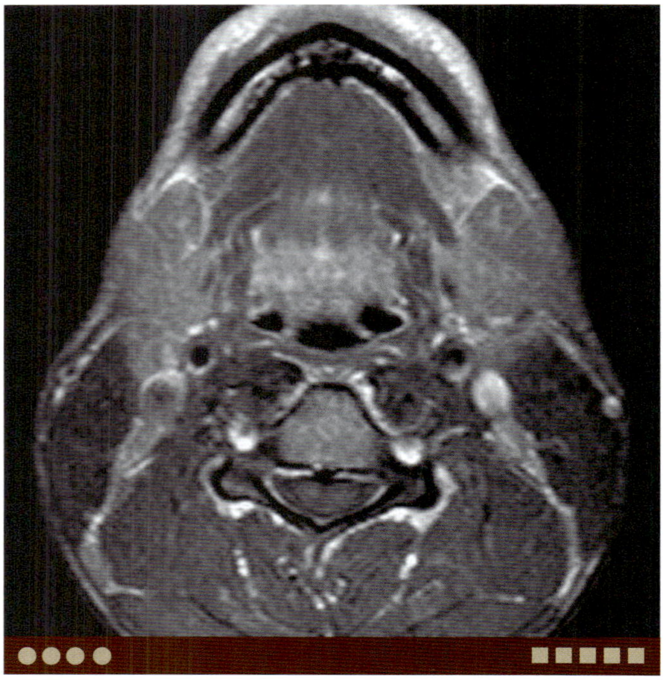

F. Lymphadenopathy associated with HIV infection, same patient as E. Axial postcontrast T1W image demonstrates homogeneously enhancing lymph nodes.

DIFFERENTIAL DIAGNOSIS IMAGES (G-I)

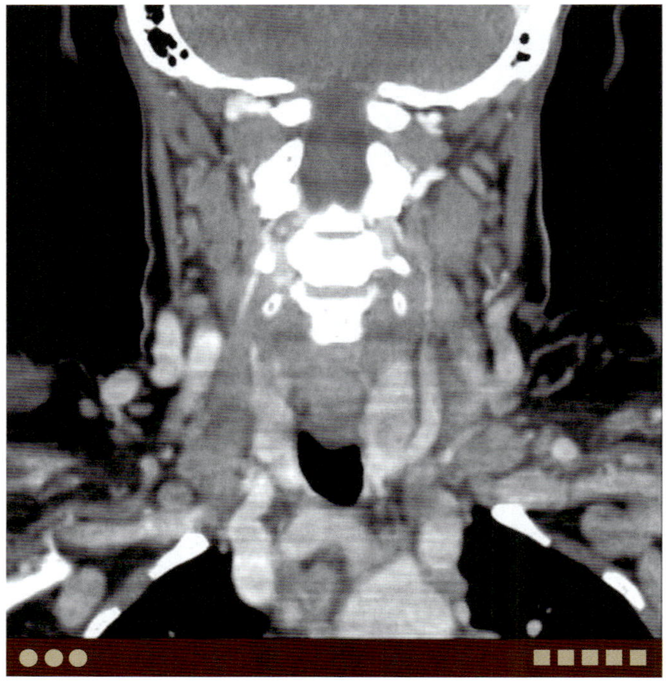

G. Sarcoidosis. Coronal contrast-enhanced CT demonstrates multiple enhancing cervical, supraclavicular, and mediastinal lymph nodes.

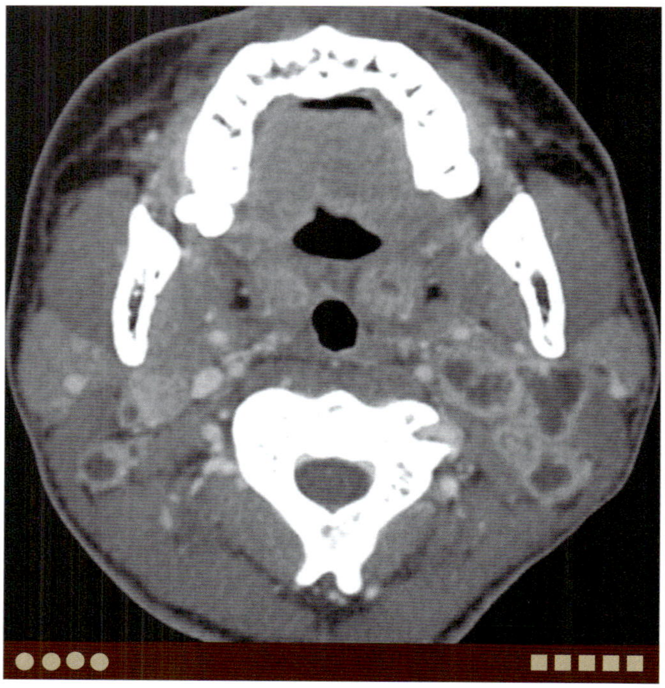

H. Tuberculosis in a patient with HIV infection. Axial contrast-enhanced CT demonstrates multiple, enhancing lymph nodes with central necrosis bilaterally.

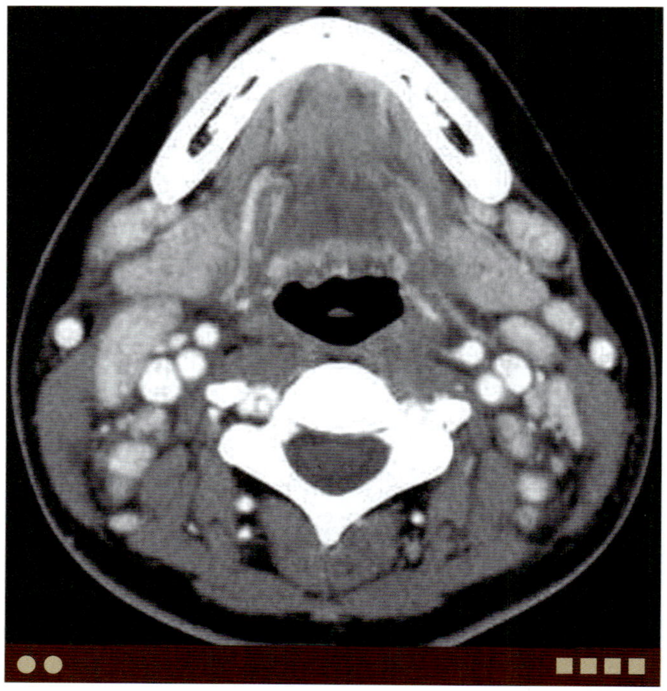

I. Kikuchi-Fujimoto disease. Axial contrast-enhanced CT demonstrates multiple enhancing lymph nodes bilaterally. Note infiltration in the adjacent fat planes.

Case 12–15 Syphilis

Hiroki Kato, Jimmy Wang, Osamu Sakai

PRESENTATION

Cervical lymphadenopathy.

FINDINGS

CT and MRI demonstrate multiple enlarged lymph nodes in the neck with or without central necrosis.

DIFFERENTIAL DIAGNOSIS

- Tuberculosis: Tuberculous lymphadenitis may be unilateral or bilateral, and found anywhere in the neck, but more common in the spinal accessory chain (level V). Homogeneously nonnecrotic nodes are seen in the early phase of infection. As the disease progresses, necrotic nodes with thick rim enhancement are demonstrated. Calcification is common in the mediastinum, however, rare in the neck.
- Pyogenic lymphadenitis: This condition demonstrates intranodal abscess, central low density and rim enhancement in affected nodes. *Staphylococcus aureus* and Group A beta-hemolytic streptococci are common pathogens for pyogenic lymphadenitis.
- Metastatic node: Nodal metastasis should always be included in the differential diagnosis of lymph nodes with central low density. Squamous cell carcinoma as well as papillary thyroid carcinoma should be considered.

COMMENTS

This is a 62-year-old man with pain, swelling, and tenderness in the right neck.

Syphilis is a sexually transmitted disease (STD) caused by *Treponema pallidum*. The route of transmission of syphilis is almost always through sexual contact, however, much less often, through blood transfusion or fetal transmission from mother to fetus in the uterus. The natural course of this disease is divided into three stages; primary (chancre of the genitals, rectum or mouth), secondary (generalized macular/popular rash, fever, sore throat, malaise, weight loss, headache, and enlarged lymph nodes throughout the body), and tertiary (cardiovascular syphilis, neurosyphilis, and syphilitic gummas). Although the genitals are the most common site of chancre formation in primary syphilis, any mucous membrane can be involved. In the head and neck, it is most commonly seen in the lips, tongue, and tonsils.

Regional lymphadenopathy is one of the clinical manifestations of primary syphilis, and generalized lymphadenopathy often occurs during the second stage. Lymphadenopathy may also be associated with latent or early tertiary syphilis.

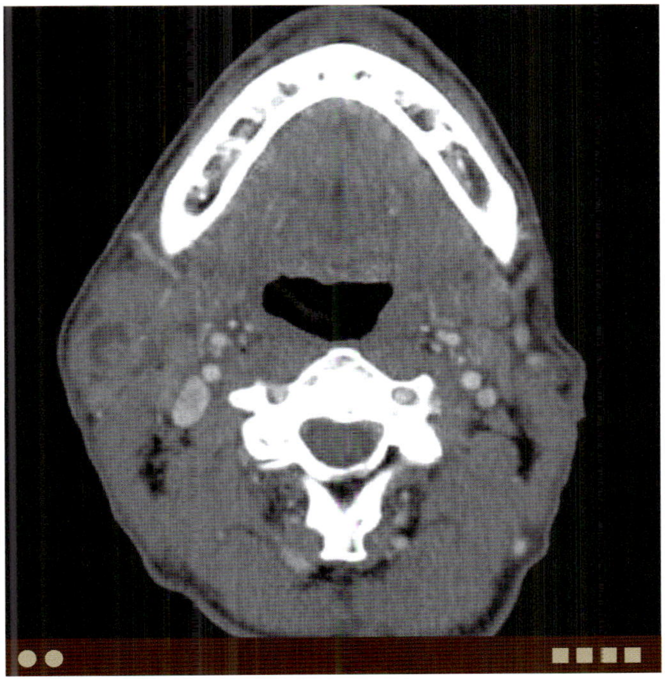

A. Syphilis. Axial contrast-enhanced CT demonstrates enlarged lymph nodes with central necrosis and surrounding inflammatory change in the right level II.

Although any nodes in the neck may be involved, the preauricular nodes are often involved.

CT and MR imaging appearance of syphilitic lymphadenitis may be variable and nonspecific, however, it often shows multiple enlarged nodes with or without central necrosis. Necrosis or cystic change may also be demonstrated after antibiotic therapy for syphilis.

Although syphilis is not a common cause of cervical lymphadenopathy, it should be in the differential diagnosis of unexplained lymphadenopathy even without a history of primary syphilis, or obvious risk factor for STD, because this is a curative but potentially life-threatening disease.

PEARLS

- **Lymphadenopathy is one of the clinical manifestations of syphilis in all stages.**
- **CT and MR imaging appearance of syphilitic lymphadenitis may be variable and nonspecific; however, it often shows multiple enlarged nodes with or without central necrosis.**
- **Syphilitic cervical lymphadenitis is rare, however, it should be in the differential diagnosis of unexplained lymphadenopathy.**

ADDITIONAL IMAGE

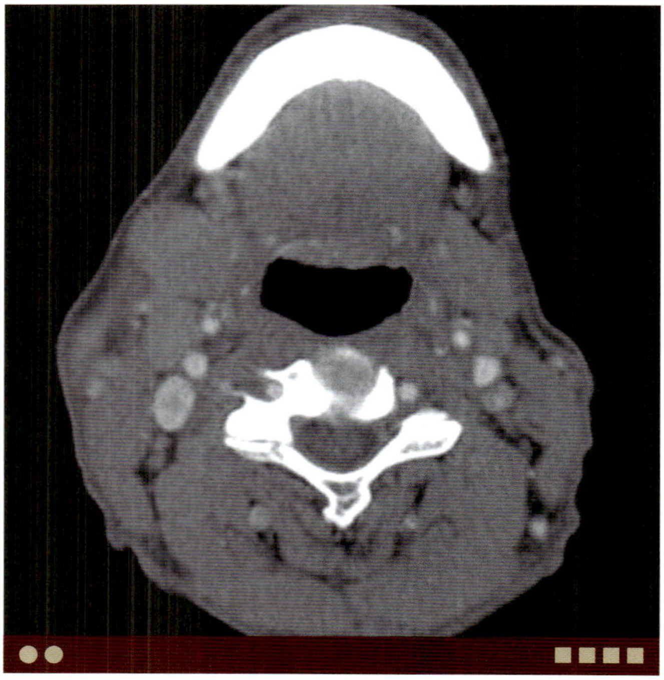

B. Syphilis, same patient as A. Axial contrast-enhanced CT demonstrates enlarged right jugulodigastric node without central necrosis.

DIFFERENTIAL DIAGNOSIS IMAGES (C-H)

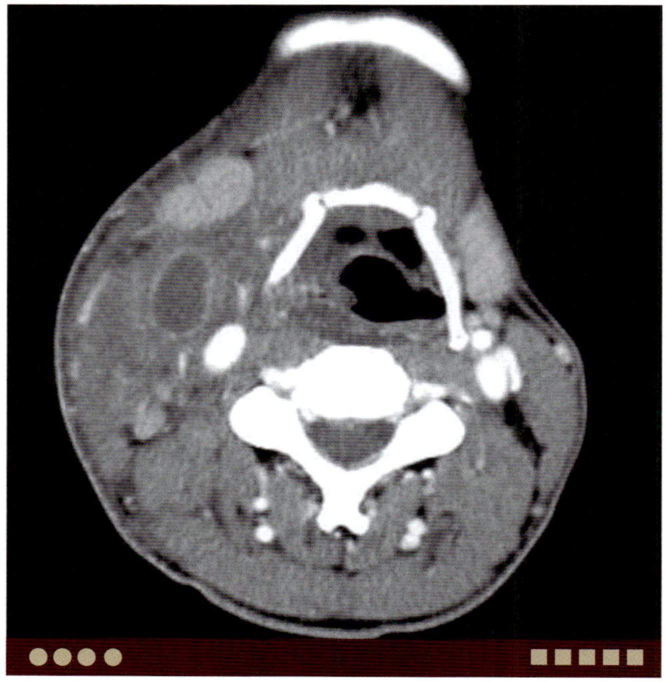

C. Pyogenic lymphadenitis. Axial contrast-enhanced CT demonstrates right upper cervical lymphadenopathy with central necrosis. Note significant inflammatory change in the fat adjacent to the affected node.

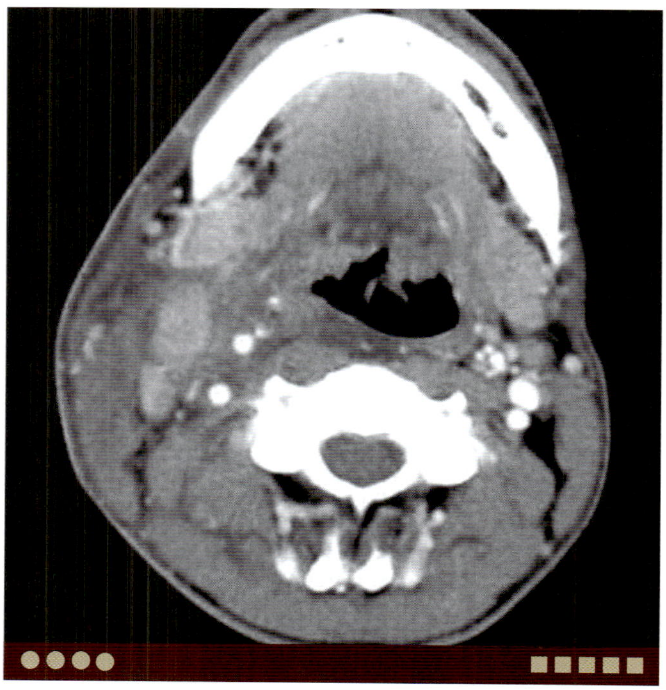

D. Pyogenic lymphadenitis, same patient as C. Axial contrast-enhanced CT demonstrates right upper cervical lymphadenopathy without central necrosis.

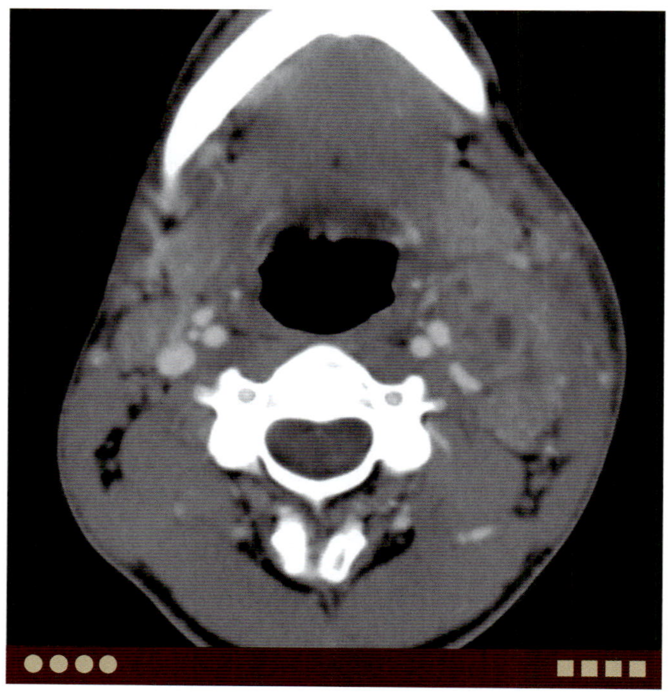

E. Tuberculosis. Axial contrast-enhanced CT demonstrates heterogeneously enhancing level II nodes bilaterally. Note intranodal abscesses in the left jugulodigastric node.

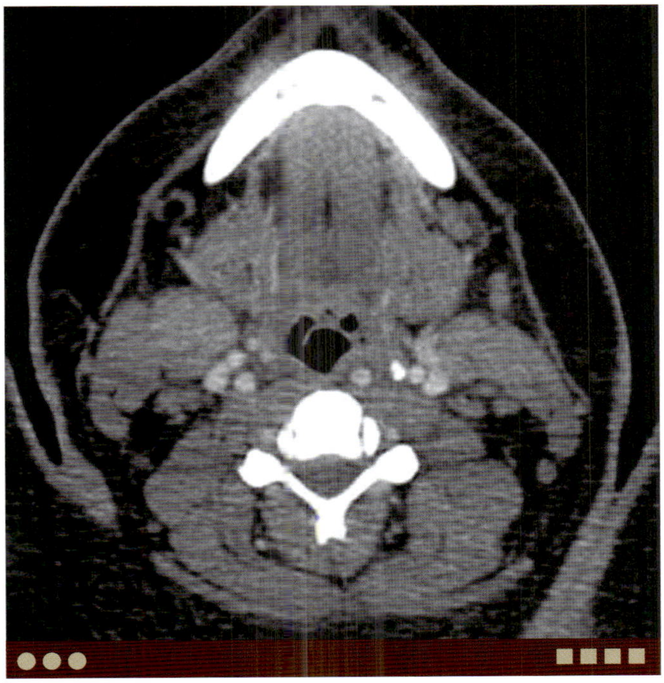

F. Cat scratch disease. Axial contrast-enhanced CT demonstrates enhancing, enlarged bilateral level II nodes, right greater than left.

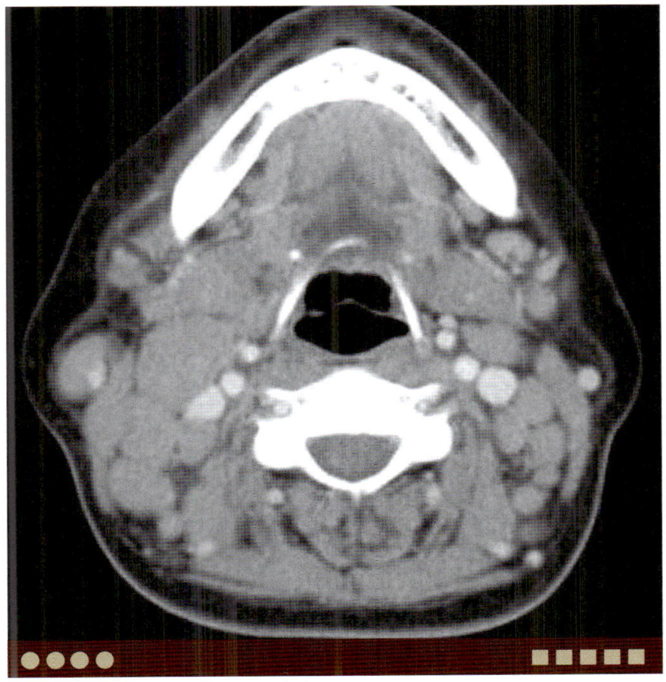

G. Diffuse large B-cell lymphoma. Axial contrast-enhanced CT demonstrates homogeneously enhancing level II nodes bilaterally, right more than left, without central necrosis.

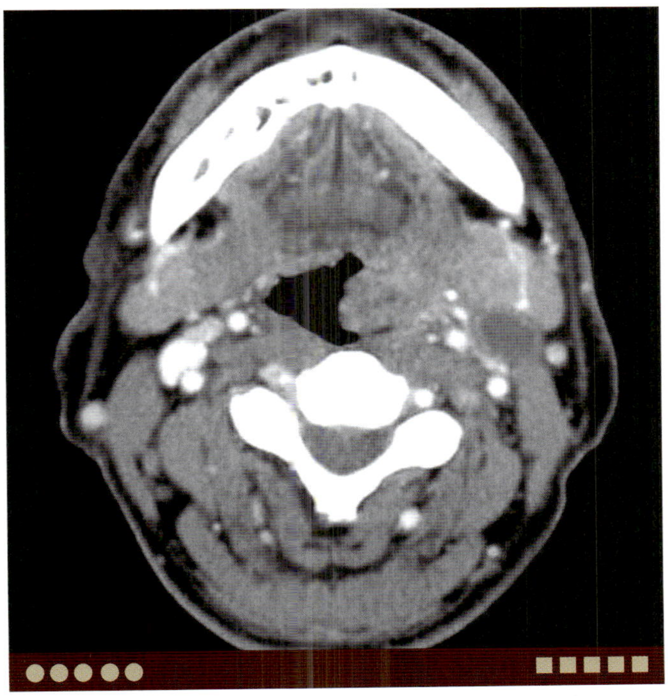

H. Nodal metastasis from oropharyngeal squamous cell carcinoma. Axial contrast-enhanced CT demonstrates left tonsillar cancer with necrotic left level II lymph node.

Case 12–16 Kimura Disease

Osamu Sakai, Akifumi Fujita

PRESENTATION

Submental mass.

FINDINGS

CT and MRI demonstrate multiple enlarged cervical lymph nodes, including parotid regions, without necrosis.

DIFFERENTIAL DIAGNOSIS

- Tuberculous lymphadenitis: This condition shows a wide variety of imaging findings, but enlarged nodes with central necrosis are the most common characteristic. Nodal calcification can be seen, however, it is relatively rare in the neck.
- Kikuchi-Fujimoto disease: This is a histiocytic necrotizing lymphadenitis, and most commonly seen in Japanese women younger than 30 years of age. Multiple homogeneously enhancing lymph nodes with perinodal infiltration are frequently seen. Central necrosis is also seen.
- Sarcoidosis: This is a systemic disease characterized by noncaseating granulomas. Multiple homogeneously enhancing lymph nodes are seen, often with sites of extranodal involvement in the parotid gland, orbit, and upper respiratory tract.
- Papillary thyroid cancer nodal metastasis: Metastatic nodes from papillary thyroid cancers demonstrate various appearances; homogeneous enhancement simulating hyperplastic lymph nodes, avid enhancement, almost no enhancement, intranodal necrosis, completely cystic appearance, or calcification.
- Lymphoma: Both Hodgkin and non-Hodgkin lymphomas involve lymph nodes in the neck and usually show homogeneous density.

COMMENTS

This is a 40-year-old man with a submental mass.

Kimura disease is a benign chronic granulomatous disease of unknown etiology, which occurs most commonly in the head and neck. This disease is characterized histopathologically by eosinophilic lymphfolliculoid granuloma, often with concomitant peripheral blood eosinophilia and elevated serum IgE. Kimura disease is more commonly seen in Japan and other Asian countries, and affects mostly males from second to fourth decade, affects salivary glands as well as lymph nodes. Beyond head and neck regions, this disease often affects axillary and inguinal lymph nodes and cubital subcutaneous soft tissues. Typical clinical presentation includes asymmetrical lymphadenopathy and subcutaneous soft tissue masses in the head and neck region. These lesions are usually painless, sometimes with itching of the surrounding skin, and slowly progressive for years.

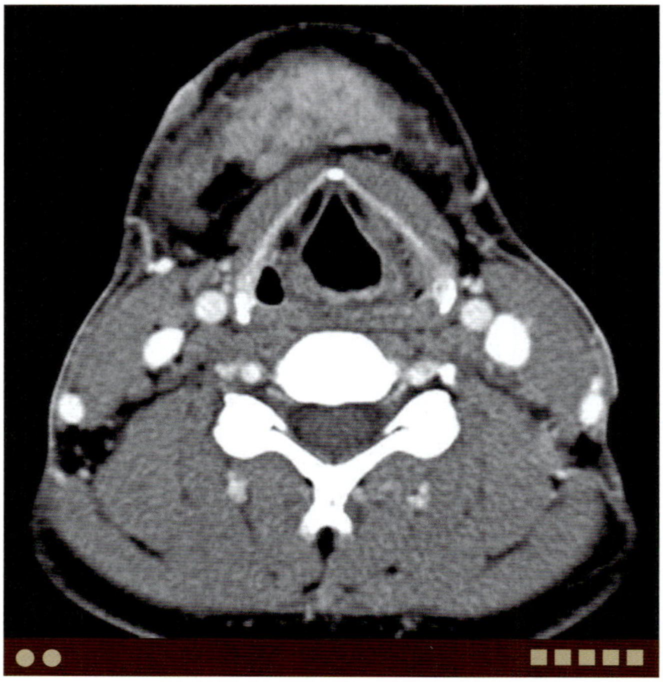

A. Kimura disease. Axial postcontrast CT demonstrates an ill-defined enhancing submental soft tissue mass.

The differential diagnosis of Kimura disease includes angiolymphoid hyperplasia with eosinophilia, Hodgkin disease, angioimmunoblastic T-cell lymphoma, Langerhans cell histiocytosis, florid follicular hyperplasia, Castleman disease, dermatopathic lymphadenopathy, Churg-Strauss syndrome, drug reaction, and parasitic lymphadenitis.

PEARLS

- **Kimura disease commonly affects salivary glands and cervical lymph nodes without necrosis.**
- **Avid enhancement of the lesion and affected nodes is usually seen on postcontrast images.**
- **Kimura disease is important for the differential diagnosis of avidly enhancing lymph nodes, although it is difficult to be differentiated from other etiologies by imaging alone.**

Enlarged lymph nodes are often oval shape without central necrosis. A salivary gland lesion tends to be ill-defined, and often infiltrates beyond the capsule invading adjacent structures. On MRI, it shows various signals on T2W images depending on the degree of fibrosis. In the incipient period with less fibrosis it shows high signal, however, with advanced fibrosis it shows low signal. Postcontrast images demonstrate avid enhancement, but with advanced fibrosis, it shows less enhancement. Avid enhancement is also seen in affected lymph nodes with postcontrast images.

ADDITIONAL IMAGES (B-G)

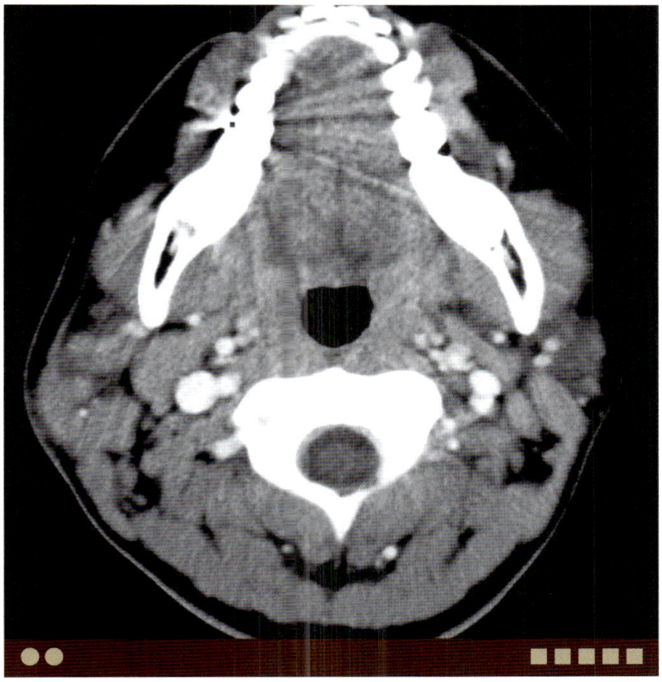

B. Kimura disease in a different patient. Axial contrast-enhanced CT demonstrates multiple enlarged right level II and periparotid nodes.

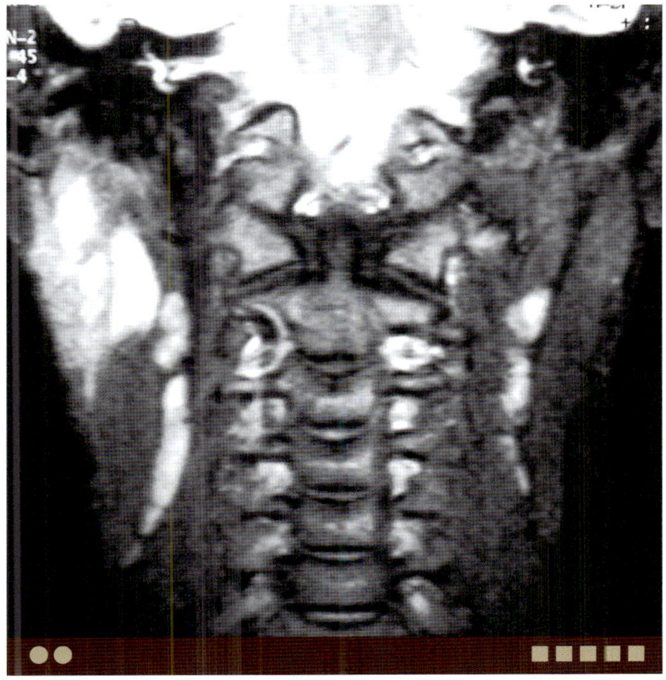

C. Kimura disease, same patient as B. Coronal STIR image demonstrates high-signal, enlarged right intra-/peri-parotid nodes.

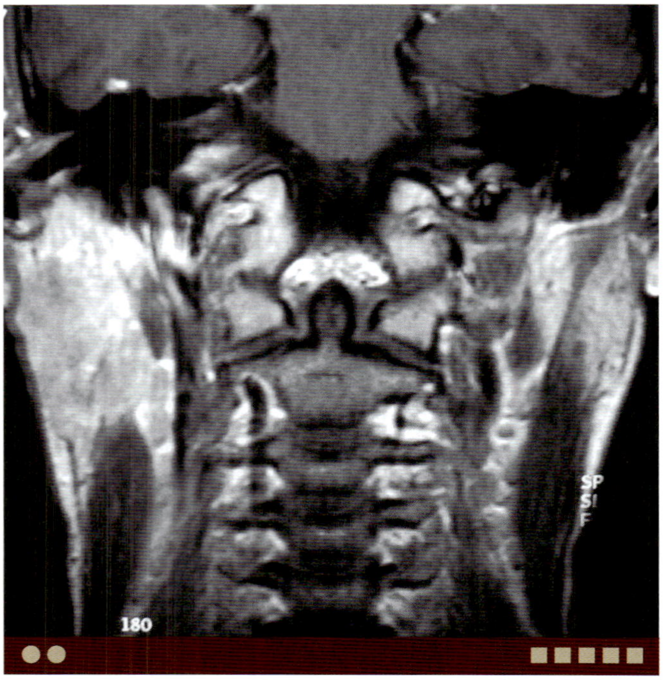

D. Kimura disease, same patient as B. Coronal postcontrast T1W image demonstrates homogeneous enhancement of the enlarged nodes.

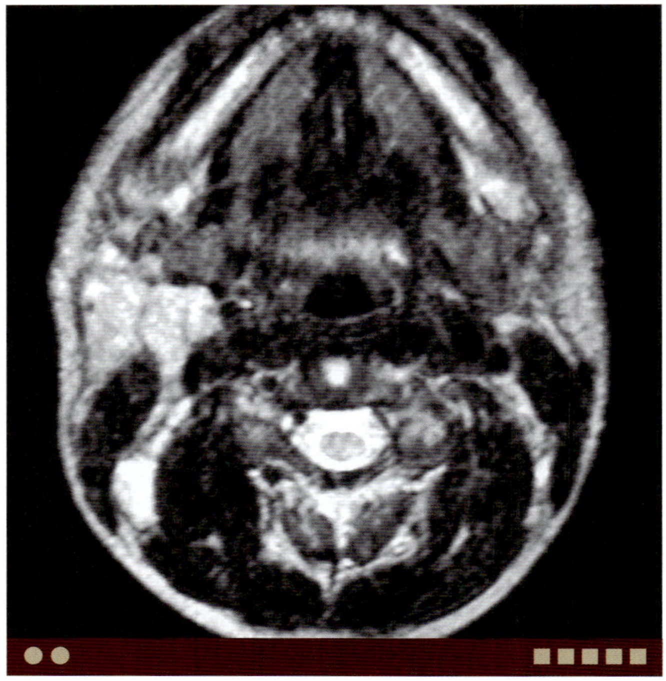

E. Kimura disease, same patient as B. Axial T2W MR image demonstrates multiple enlarged high-signal nodes in the right level II.

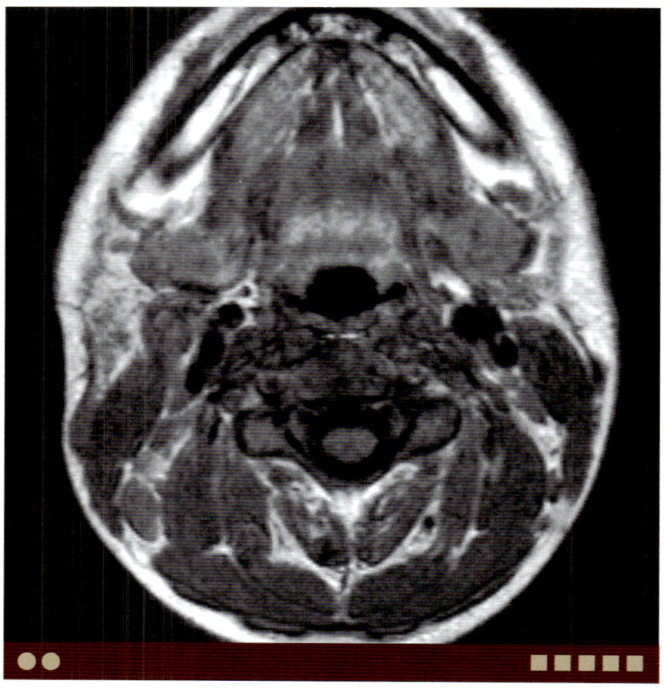

F. Kimura disease, same patient as B. Axial T1W MR image demonstrates low signal of the enlarged right level II nodes.

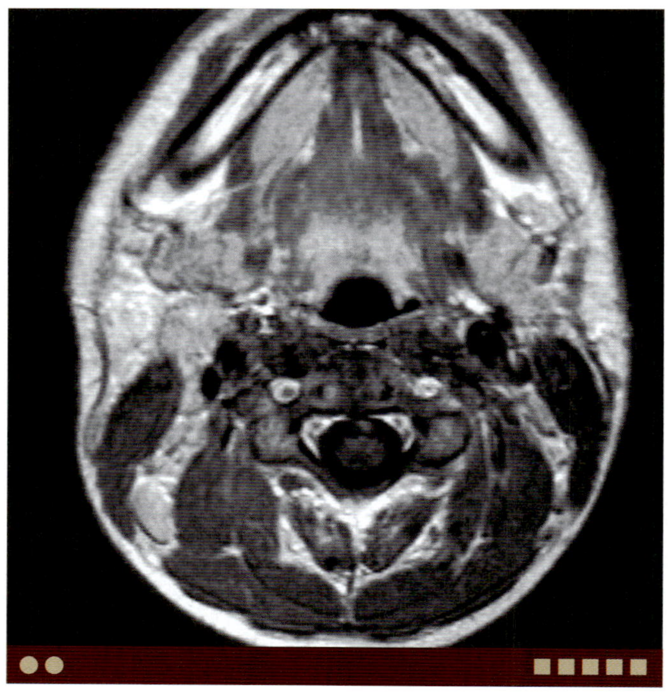

G. Kimura disease, same patient as B. Axial contrast-enhanced T1W MR image demonstrates homogeneous enhancement of the enlarged right level II nodes.

DIFFERENTIAL DIAGNOSIS IMAGES (H-J)

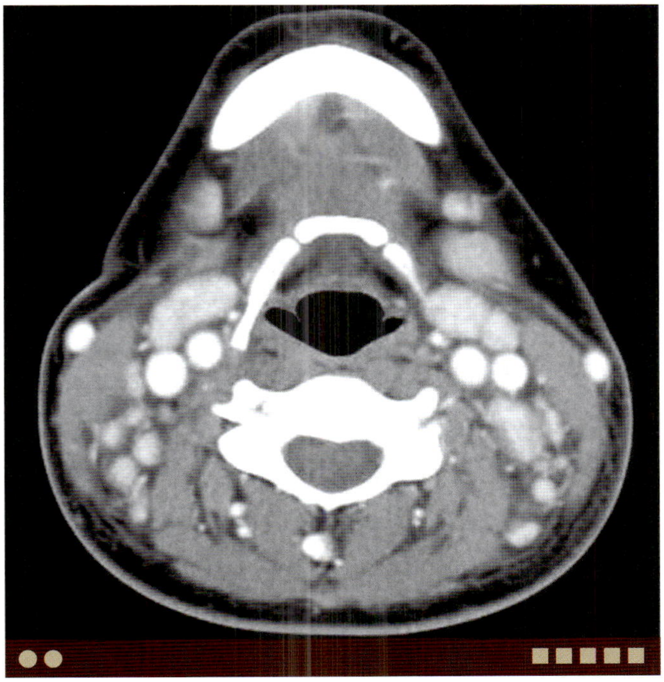

H. Kikuchi-Fujimoto disease. Axial contrast-enhanced CT demonstrates multiple, avidly enhancing nodes with perinodal infiltrative inflammatory changes.

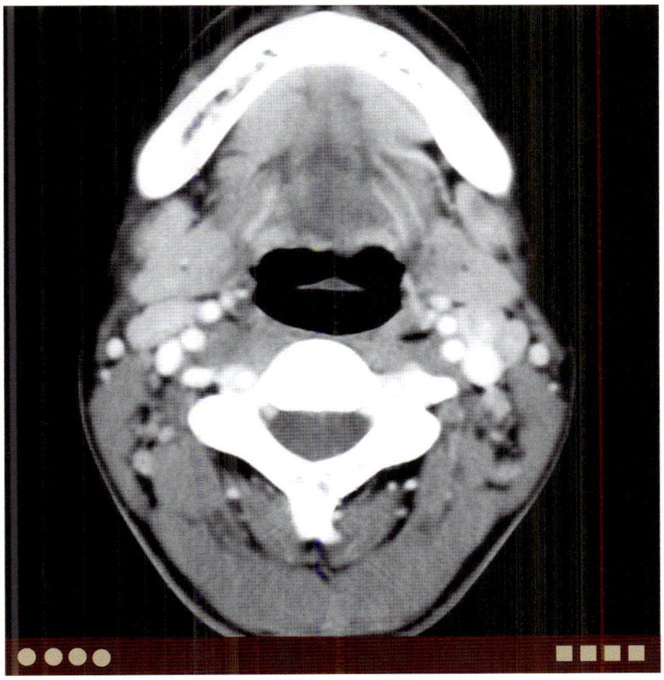

I. Sarcoidosis. Axial contrast-enhanced CT demonstrates multiple, enlarged enhancing nodes without perinodal infiltrative inflammatory changes.

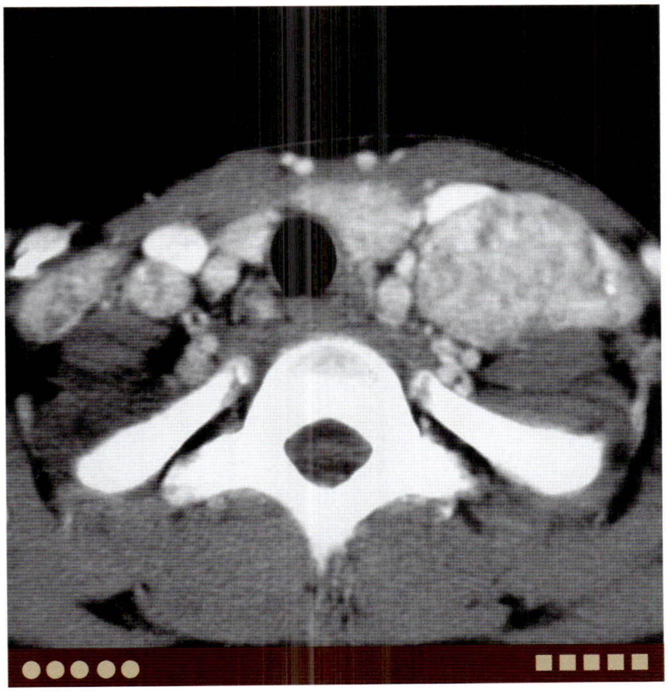

J. Metastasis from papillary thyroid carcinoma. Axial contrast-enhanced CT demonstrates avidly enhancing nodes in the bilateral level IV and supraclavicular fossa. Note ill-defined primary lesion in the left lobe of the thyroid gland.

Chapter 13

PET/CT

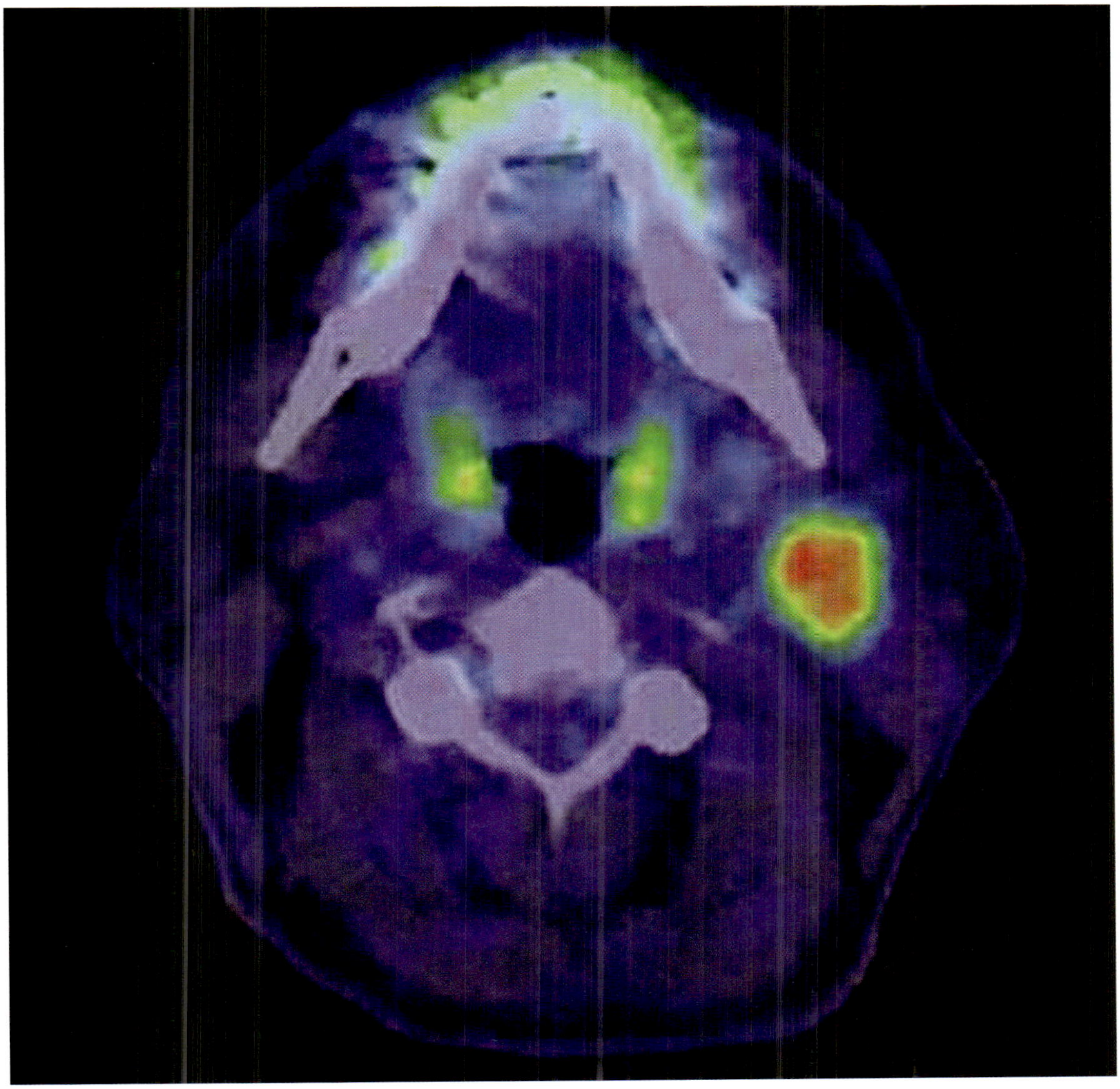

Case 13–1 Unknown Primary Squamous Cell Carcinoma

Ari Sacks, Shilpa Surasi, Rathan Subramaniam

PRESENTATION

Neck mass in patients without known primary tumors.

FINDINGS

Positron emission tomography/computed tomography (PET/CT) demonstrates intense 2-[^{18}F] fluoro-2-deoxy-D-glucose (FDG) hypermetabolic activity within the left palatine tonsil, which is the primary site.

DIFFERENTIAL DIAGNOSIS

- Lymphoma: Lymphomas show very similar imaging findings to nasopharyngeal carcinoma (NPC), particularly WHO type III, and is very difficult to differentiate from NPC. Lymphoma may show more homogeneous signal and infiltrative invasion rather than destruction.
- Inflammation of the tonsils: Infection and inflammation of the tonsils demonstrate increased FDG uptake, usually bilaterally.
- Physiological uptake: Palatine tonsils can demonstrate intense physiological FDG uptake which is symmetrical. Asymmetric uptake in the palatine tonsils raises a possibility of neoplastic process.

COMMENTS

This is a 65-year-old man with left-sided neck mass without known primary tumors.

Head and neck cancers (HNCs) are the fifth most common cancer worldwide and are increasing in incidence. Primary risk factors for squamous cell carcinoma (SCCA) of the head and neck include alcohol and tobacco use. About 5% to 10% of HNCs present as a neck nodal mass with unknown site of primary, as seen in this case. Conventional investigations to find the primary lesion and stage the cancer include clinical examination, panendoscopy, and either CT or MRI. Failure to identify the primary tumor impedes treatment planning and may negatively influence patient prognosis. Common primary sites of "unknown primary" cancers are nasopharynx, tonsils, base of tongue, and pyriform sinuses.

PET/CT plays an increasing role in the diagnosis, staging, and prognosis of HNC. SCCAs in the head and neck typically have high glycolytic activity and thus high FDG uptake. This permits FDG-PET/CT scans to identify metabolically active, small or superficial lesions that are not well seen on CT or MRI. Studies show FDG-PET alone in HNC has an overall sensitivity, specificity, and accuracy rate in detecting unknown primary tumors of 88.3%, 74.9%, and 78.8%, respectively. Furthermore, FDG-PET detected 24.5% of tumors that were not apparent after conventional work-up. In comparison studies, FDG-PET has been found to be the most reliable imaging procedure in the detection of primary tumors and recurrent carcinomas localized in the head and neck region.

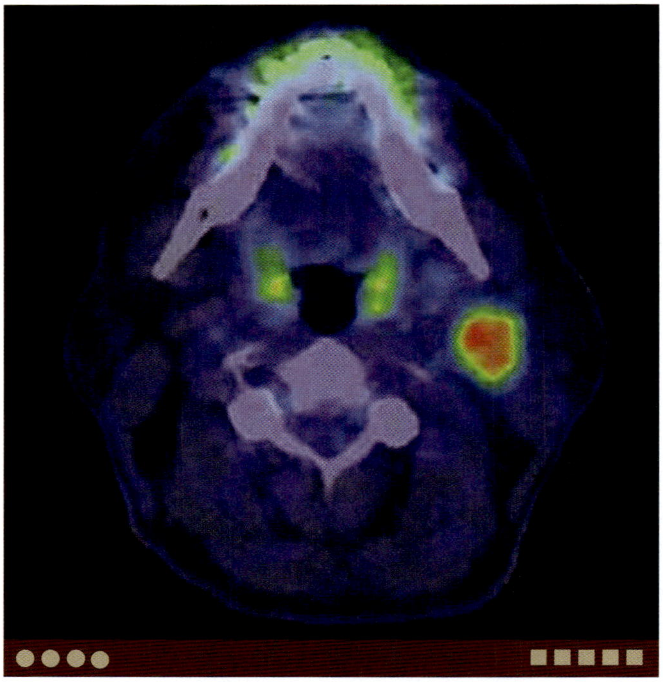

A. Unknown primary cancer. Axial fused FDG-PET/CT image demonstrates intense FDG hypermetabolism in the left level IIA lymph node.

PEARLS

- **About 5% to 10% of head and neck squamous cell carcinomas present with cervical node involvement with an unknown primary.**
- **FDG-PET/CT detects about one third of primary tumors that were undetected by other modalities in the head and neck.**
- **Detection of an unknown primary changes the management such as the radiation therapy field.**
- **Common primary sites of "unknown primary" cancers are nasopharynx, tonsils, base of tongue, and pyriform sinuses.**

ADDITIONAL IMAGE

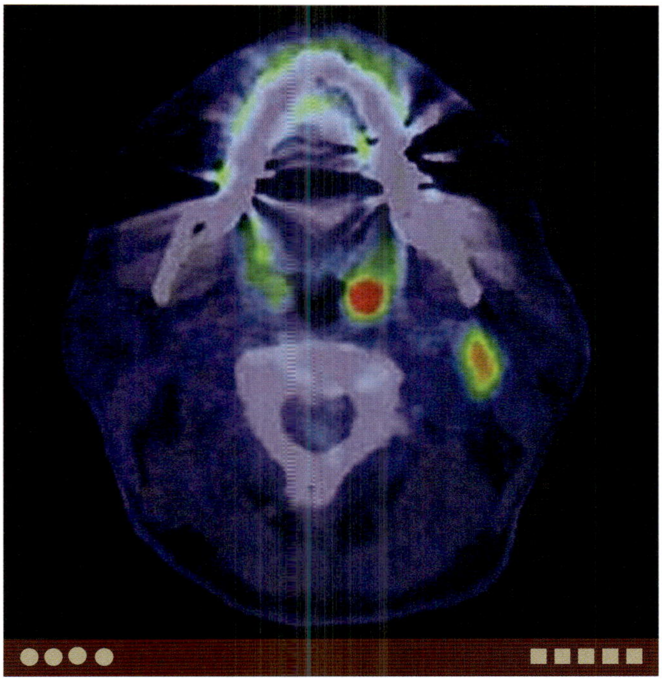

B. Unknown primary cancer, same patient as A. Axial fused FDG-PET/CT image demonstrates asymmetric, increased FDG uptake noted in the left palatine tonsil, the primary site, proven by tissue diagnosis.

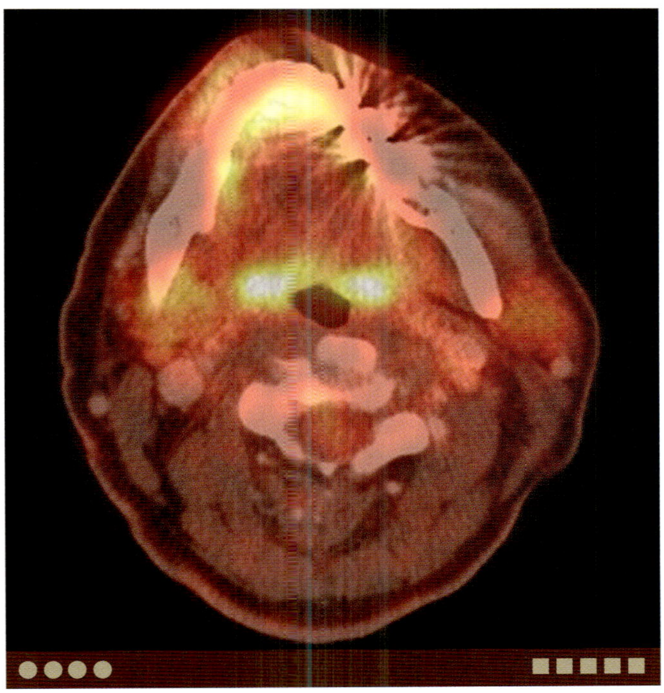

D. Physiological uptake, same patient as C. Axial fused FDG-PET/CT image demonstrates intense, symmetric FDG hypermetabolism in the palatine tonsils.

DIFFERENTIAL DIAGNOSIS IMAGES (C-D)

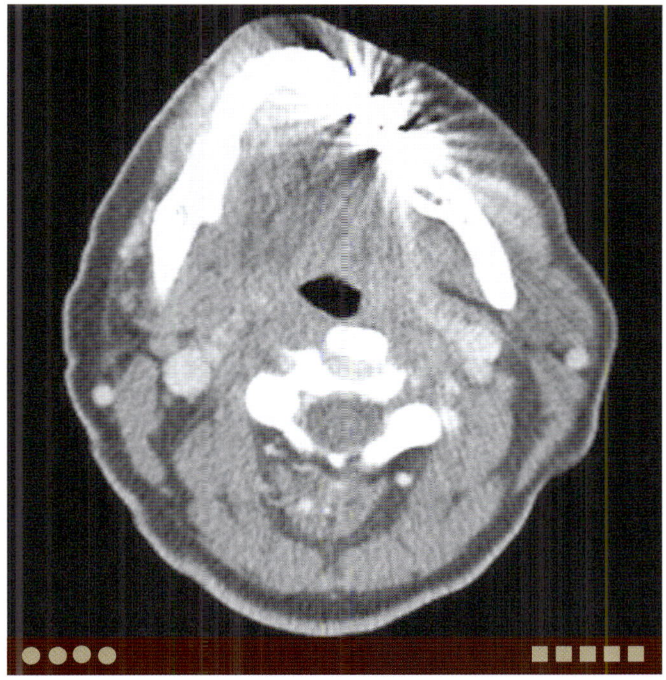

C. Physiological uptake. Axial postcontrast CT demonstrates symmetric unremarkable palatine tonsils.

Case 13–2 Floor of Mouth Squamous Cell Carcinoma

Jessica Davison, Shilpa Surasi, Rathan Subramaniam

PRESENTATION

Mouth ulcer under the tongue.

FINDINGS

PET/CT demonstrates an area of FDG hypermetabolism in the floor of mouth.

DIFFERENTIAL DIAGNOSIS

- Verrucous carcinoma: A diffuse, papillary, nonmetastasizing, well-differentiated, malignant neoplasm of the epidermis of oral epithelium. It demonstrates intense FDG hypermetabolism.
- Physiological uptake: Normal sublingual salivary glands demonstrate moderate FDG hypermetabolism. However, this would be symmetrical.

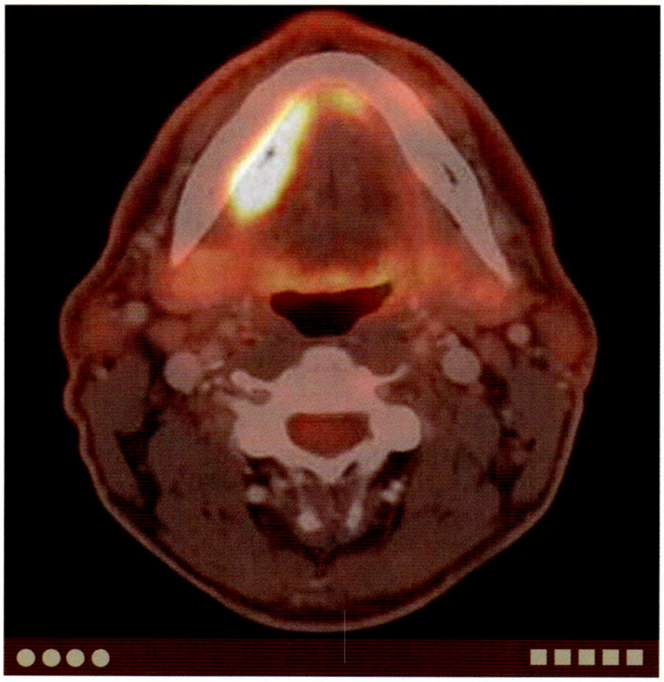

A. SCCA of FOM. Axial fused FDG-PET/CT image demonstrates an intense FDG hypermetabolic activity in the right FOM with a SUVmax of 16.

COMMENTS

This is a 54-year-old man with a mouth ulcer under his tongue for 2 months prior to presentation. Pain was exacerbated by hot and spicy food.

Oral squamous cell carcinoma (SCCA) affects approximately 30,000 Americans each year. In the United States, 3% of cancers in men and 2% in women are oral SCCAs and often occur in patients over the age of 50. The chief risk factors are smoking, especially >2 packs/day, and alcohol use. Chronic irritations such as dental caries, overuse of mouthwash, chewing tobacco, and the use of betel quid are also associated with an increased risk. Recent studies show that about 25% of mouth and 35% of throat cancers are caused by oral human papilloma virus (HPV). However, oral SCCA may arise in patients with no identifiable risk factors. Symptoms may include a poorly healing mouth ulcer, a hoarse voice, or other persistent problems in the area. Early curable lesions are often asymptomatic, and thus, screening is essential for early detection.

Approximately 40% of intraoral SCCA begin on the floor of the mouth (FOM) or on the lateral and ventral surfaces of the tongue, while 38% occur on the lower lip and are usually consequent to solar exposure. The remaining 11% begin in the palate and tonsillar area. Definitive diagnosis is made via biopsy of the lesion.

For localized SCCA of the FOM, 5-year survival is 65%. Lymph node metastasis decreases survival rate by about 50%. The 5-year disease-free survival rate for HPV positive cancer is significantly higher when appropriately treated with surgery, radiation, and chemotherapy as compared to non-HPV positive cancer, substantiated by multiple studies. In one study, multivariate analysis confirms that increasing tumor thickness, rather than tumor stage, had the best correlation with treatment failure and survival.

Metastases reach the regional lymph nodes first and later the lungs. Treatment is usually with surgery and radiotherapy. FDG-PET/CT is very useful in staging, therapy assessment and surveillance of SCCA of the FOM.

PEARLS

- **SCCA and verrucous carcinoma usually demonstrate intense FDG hypermetabolism. Physiological sublingual salivary gland FDG uptake would be symmetrical.**
- **Superficial lesions (T1) are difficult to diagnose by imaging.**
- **For localized carcinoma of the FOM, 5-year survival is 65%. Lymph node metastasis decreases the survival rate by 50%.**

ADDITIONAL IMAGES (B-C)

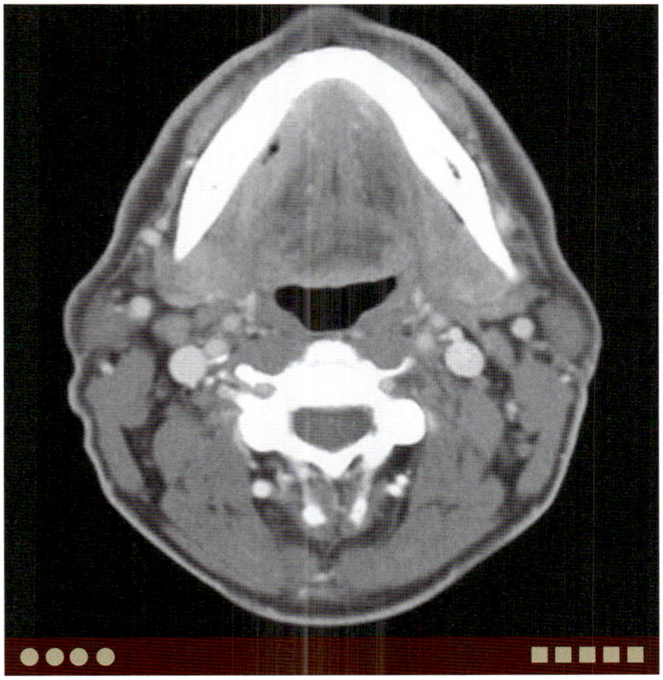

B. SCCA of FOM, same patient as A. Axial soft tissue window CT demonstrates an enhancing soft tissue mass in the right FOM.

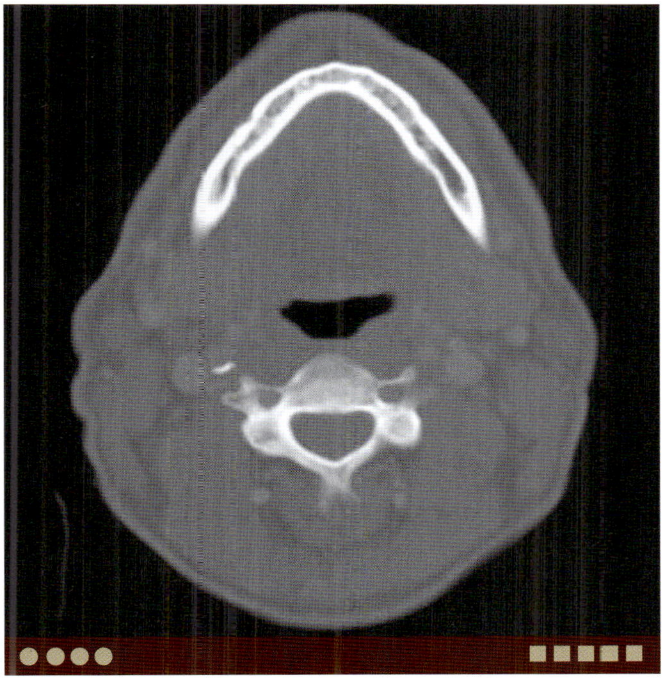

C. SCCA of FOM, same patient as A. Axial bone window CT demonstrates no involvement of the cortical bone of the mandible.

DIFFERENTIAL DIAGNOSIS IMAGES (D-E)

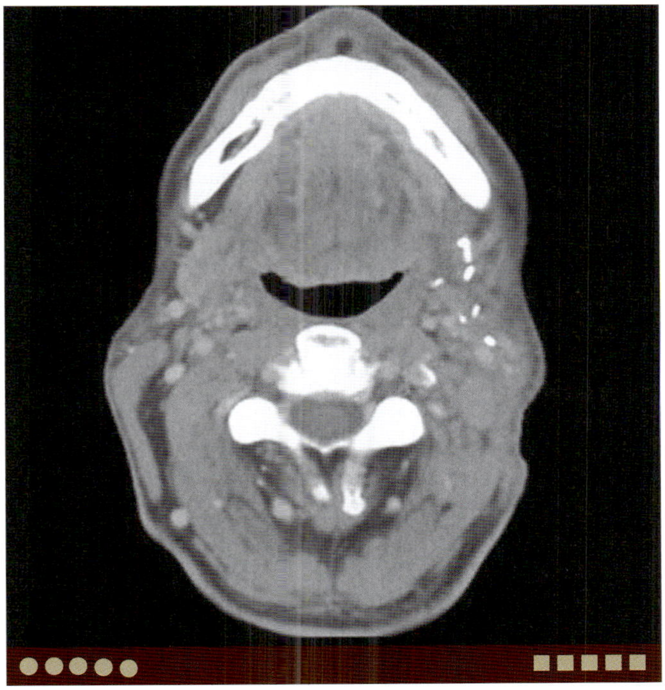

D. Physiological uptake. Axial postcontrast soft tissue window CT demonstrates unremarkable sublingual glands bilaterally.

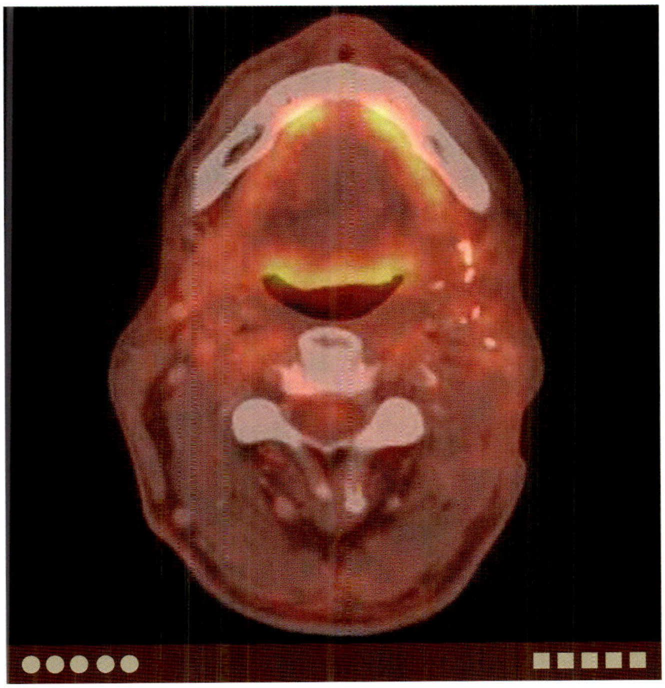

E. Physiological uptake, same patient as D. Axial fused FDG-PET/CT image demonstrates symmetric physiological FDG uptake in the sublingual glands.

Case 13–3 Base of Tongue Squamous Cell Carcinoma

Ankit Agarwal, Amol Mehta, Shilpa Surasi, Rathan Subramaniam

PRESENTATION

Throat pain, neck mass, dysphagia.

FINDINGS

FDG-PET/CT demonstrates FDG hypermetabolism in the posterior third of the tongue.

DIFFERENTIAL DIAGNOSIS

- Benign uptake in the tongue base: This can occur due to movement of the tongue muscles after injection with the radiotracer which leads to FDG uptake in that area.
- Lingual tonsillar lymphoma: Demonstrates intense FDG hypermetabolism similar to tongue-base squamous cell carcinoma.

COMMENTS

This is a 54-year-old woman with dysphagia, odynophagia, and a neck mass.

Base of tongue (BOT) squamous cell carcinoma (SCCA) is a relatively rare form of head and neck cancer. It has an estimated incidence of between 1 and 2 people per 100,000 per year. BOT SCCA is relatively asymptomatic and is usually biologically aggressive by the time it is detected in patients. Thus, survival rates for BOT SCCA can be as low as 20%, but the survival rate improves significantly 50% to 70% if it is detected and treated while still localized to the tongue area. In later stages, BOT SCCA can manifest through symptoms such as pain, difficulty in swallowing, and changes in voice.

PET/CT is useful in both detecting BOT SCCAs and surgical planning for BOT SCCAs. Studies show that PET/CT is useful in identifying the unknown primary tumor in BOT SCCA cases in approximately one third of patients. FDG PET is also more sensitive to the nodal metastasis on a level-by-level basis than CT or MRI.

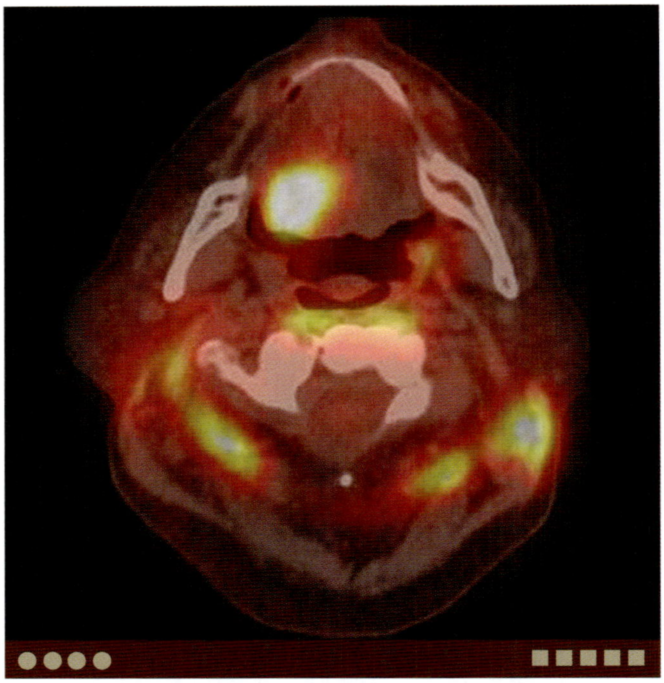

A. BOT SCCA. Axial fused FDG-PET/CT image demonstrates a mass in the right posterior third of the tongue with a SUVmax of 11.There is physiological brown fat uptake in the posterior cervical space.

PEARLS

- **BOT SCCA remains asymptomatic until the disease is relatively advanced, leading to many patients with late stage disease and widespread metastases at initial presentation.**
- **Therefore a sensitive and specific biomarker for the early detection, diagnosis, and treatment of BOT SCCA is critical.**

ADDITIONAL IMAGE

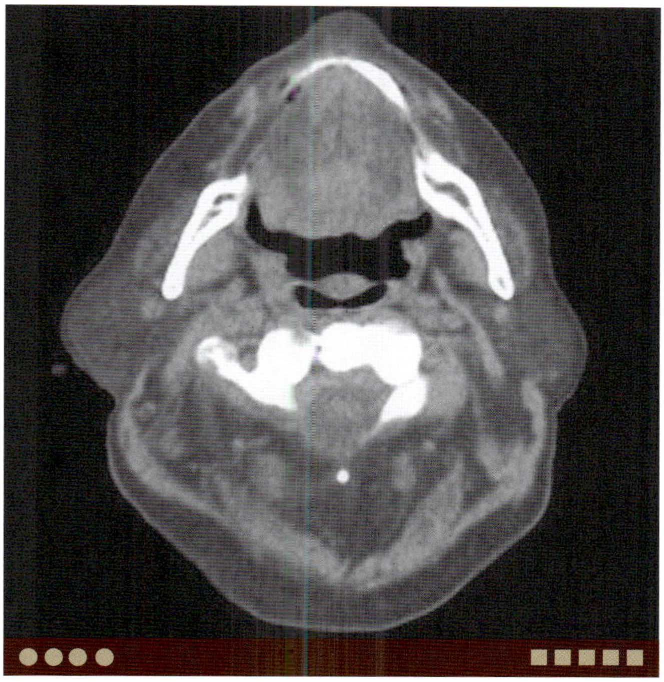

B. BOT SCCA, same patient as A. Axial soft tissue window CT hardly demonstrates the tumor in the right BOT. Note normal fat density in the bilateral posterior cervical space.

DIFFERENTIAL DIAGNOSIS IMAGES (C-D)

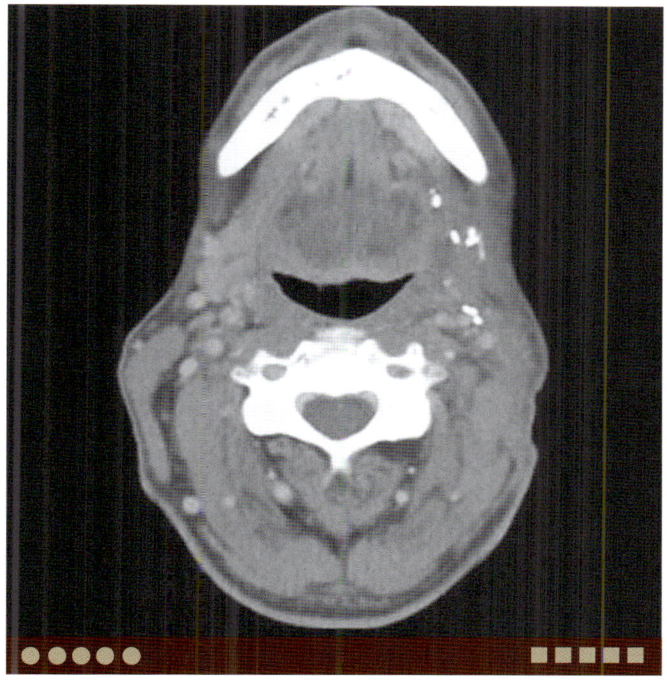

C. Physiological uptake. Axial soft tissue window CT demonstrates unremarkable BOT.

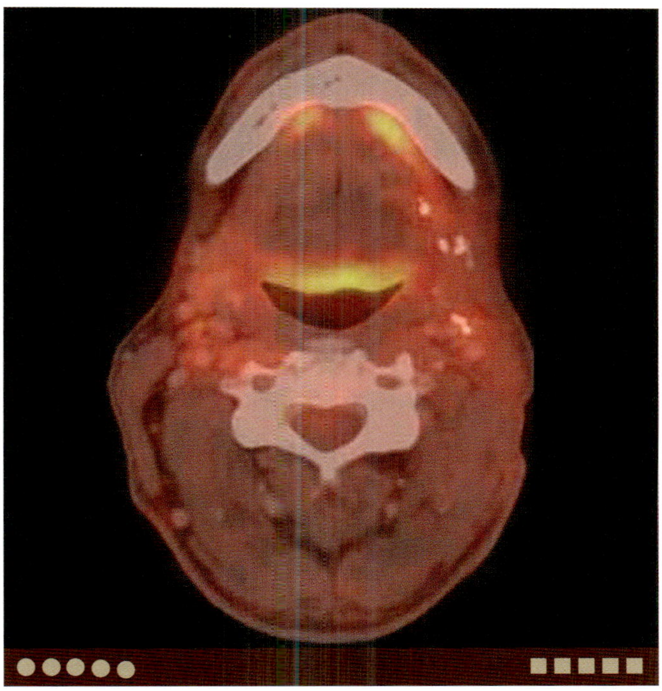

D. Physiological uptake, same patient as C. Axial fused FDG-PET/CT image demonstrates symmetric physiological FDG uptake in the BOT.

Case 13-4 Tonsillar Squamous Cell Carcinoma

Jessica Davison, Tim Ryan, Shilpa Surasi, Rathan Subramaniam

PRESENTATION

Persistent neck and throat pain.

FINDINGS

FDG-PET/CT demonstrates intense FDG uptake in the palatine tonsils.

DIFFERENTIAL DIAGNOSIS

- Tonsillar lymphoma: Usually demonstrates intense FDG hypermetabolism similar to tonsillar squamous cell carcinoma (SCCA).
- Physiological uptake: Usually symmetrical moderate to intense FDG uptake.

COMMENTS

This is a 62-year-old man with persistent left neck and throat soreness for 1 year.

Tonsillar SCCA is second in frequency only to laryngeal cancer among head and neck cancers. Of oropharyngeal cancers, most (>90%) are SCCAs. The majority of oropharyngeal SCCAs are advanced (60%) when first detected. Major risk factors for developing oropharyngeal SCCA include age above 50, tobacco and alcohol use, especially when used concurrently (relative risk 40).

The incidence of oropharyngeal cancers appears to be increasing in Western societies, especially among young men who do not have the usual risk factors, including smoking. In these cases, sexually transmitted human papilloma virus (HPV) type 16 is frequently associated (>50% of cases) with carcinomas of the palatine tonsil and base of tongue. HPV-positive tonsillar SCCAs have a better prognosis (lower risk of recurrence, longer survival) than patients with HPV-negative SCCAs. An association between tonsillar and base of tongue SCCAs and the oncogenic Epstein-Barr virus (EBV) has also been demonstrated.

Non-Hodgkin lymphoma is the second most common head and neck malignancy. Most of these are B-cell lymphomas. Moreover, the most common site of pathology is the tonsil. It is difficult to differentiate a high-grade lymphoma and SCCA by FDG uptake alone.

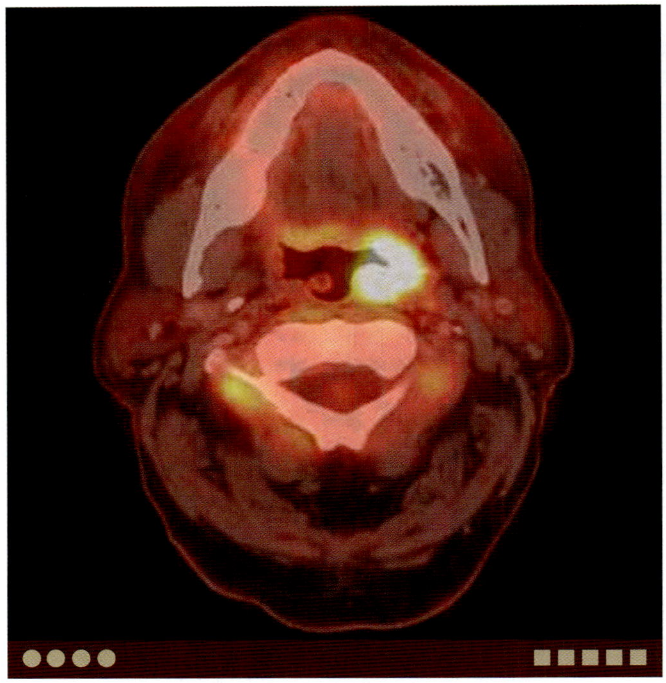

A. Tonsillar SCCA. Axial fused FDG-PET/CT image demonstrates a hypermetabolic left tonsillar mass with a SUVmax of 17.

PEARLS

- **Tonsillar SCCAs represent approximately 15% to 20% of all intraoral and oropharyngeal SCCAs in the United States.**
- **Tobacco and alcohol are the leading causes of oral cancer.**
- **HPV (type 16 especially) is associated with tonsillar and tongue-base SCCA, especially in young men without the risk factors of smoking or alcohol. HPV-16 associated oropharyngeal SCCA has better prognosis.**
- **Both tonsillar SCCA and lymphoma can present with intense FDG uptake.**

ADDITIONAL IMAGE

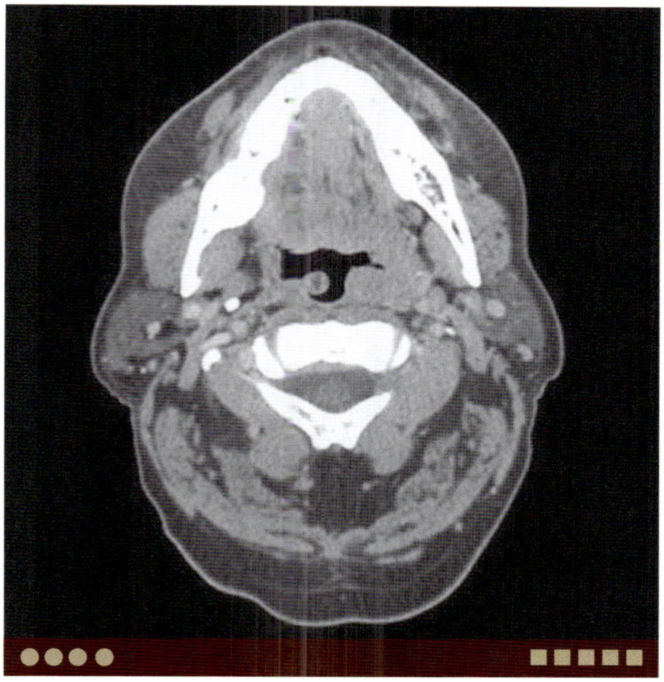

B. Tonsillar SCCA, same patient as A. Axial soft tissue window CT hardly demonstrates a soft tissue mass in the left tonsillar fossa.

DIFFERENTIAL DIAGNOSIS IMAGES (C-D)

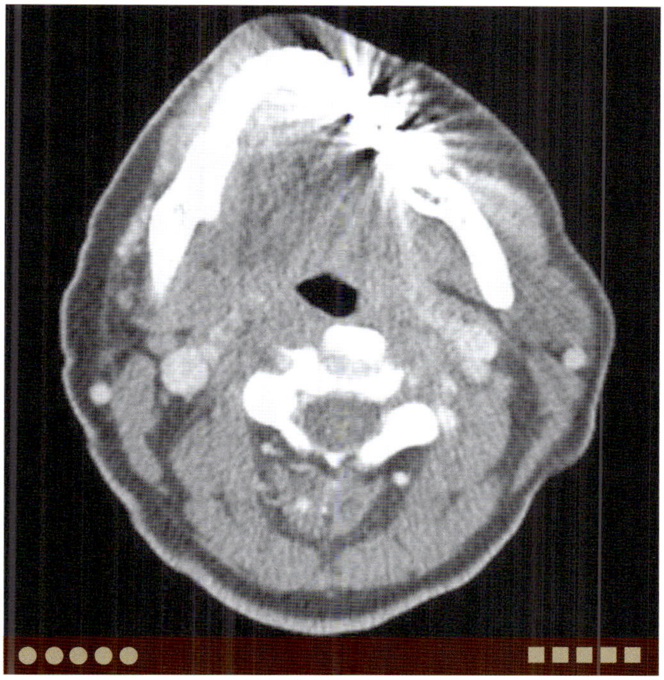

C. Physiological uptake. Axial soft tissue window CT demonstrates unremarkable palatine tonsils.

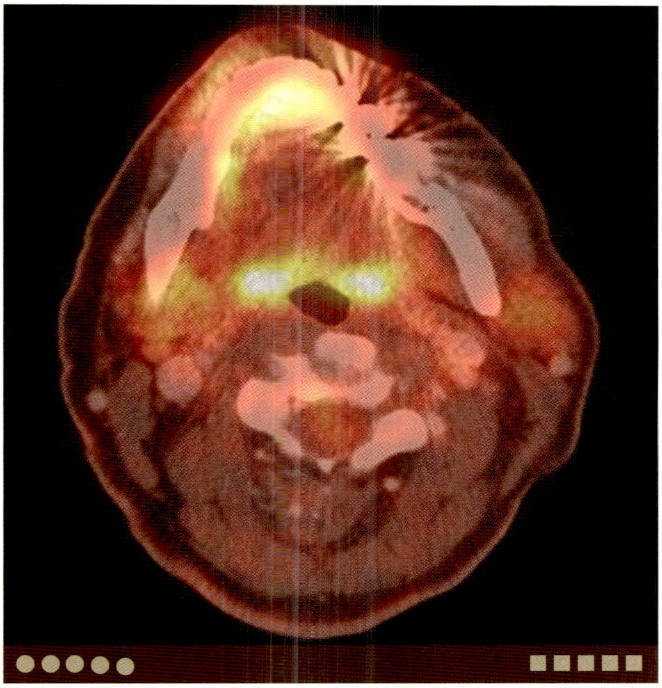

D. Physiological uptake, same patient as C. Axial fused FDG-PET/CT image demonstrates symmetric physiological FDG uptake in the palatine tonsils.

Case 13-5 Laryngeal Squamous Cell Carcinoma

Ankit Agarwal, Amol Mehta, Shilpa Surasi, Rathan Subramaniam

PRESENTATION

Increasing hoarseness of voice.

FINDINGS

FDG-PET/CT demonstrates intense FDG uptake in a laryngeal lesion.

DIFFERENTIAL DIAGNOSIS

- Physiological uptake or phonation artifact: Mild-to-moderate FDG hypermetabolism may be observed in vocal cords with physiological uptake or phonation artifact.
- Vocal cord Teflon granuloma: Teflon injection is used to improve phonation of a paralyzed vocal cord and the chronic inflammation induced by Teflon is intensely FDG-avid.

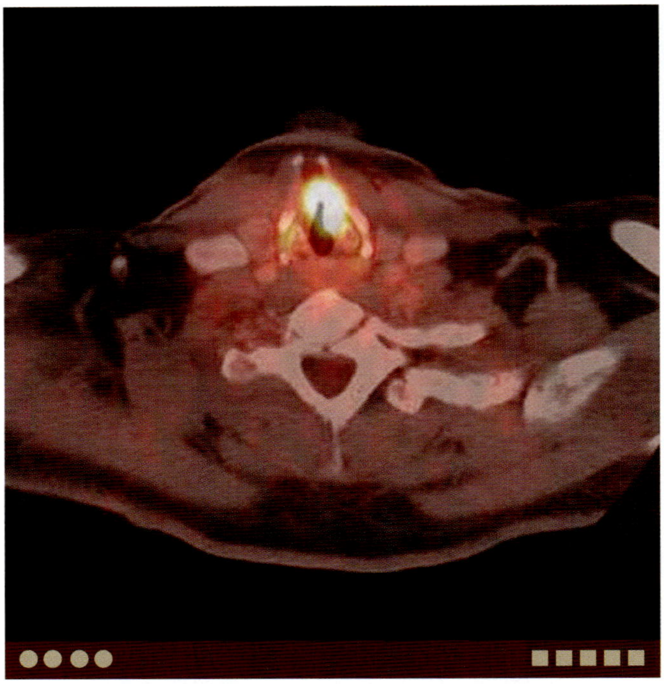

A. Laryngeal SCCA. Axial fused FDG-PET/CT image demonstrates hypermetabolic activity with a SUVmax of 19 involving the left vocal cord crossing the anterior commissure and involving the anterior part of the right vocal cord.

COMMENTS

This is a 75-year-old man with increasing hoarseness of voice, a laryngeal mass and ulcerative lesions involving both vocal cords.

Laryngeal squamous cell carcinomas (SCCAs) account for about 2% of all human cancers. They are most frequently found in men over 60 years old. HPV infections and carcinogens inhaled by heavy smokers increase the likelihood of developing this condition. Laryngeal SCCAs can be subdivided into three main categories based on their anatomical location and in order of decreasing frequency: glottic, supraglottic, and subglottic carcinomas. Carcinomas of the supraglottic and subglottic area have a tendency to be larger at time of diagnosis and metastasize early in 20% to 40% of cases.

Most laryngeal SCCAs present with symptoms similar to chronic laryngitis. Patients usually report hoarseness of voice, a persistent sore throat, and a persistent cough. Lumps on the vocal cords can also be clinically seen. However, due to the clinical similarities with noncancerous conditions, biopsy is warranted in the diagnosis of potential vocal cord cancer cases.

Studies have shown significantly higher FDG uptake and SUVmax in laryngeal SCCAs than in benign lesions or physiological uptake due to phonation artifact. Teflon injections performed to improve phonation of a paralyzed vocal cord can induce chronic inflammation and demonstrates intense FDG uptake simulating malignancy. However, the CT images would demonstrate high-density Teflon in the vocal cords.

PEARLS

- **Laryngeal cancer can present with symptoms similar to chronic laryngitis.**
- **Laryngeal SCCA presents with intense, focal FDG uptake. However, small T1 lesions may not be detected by PET/CT.**
- **Intense FDG uptake from Teflon granuloma or moderate-to-intense FDG uptake from phonation artifact can mimic SCCA uptake.**
- **Supraglottic and subglottic SCCAs tend to be larger at time of diagnosis with metastasis in 20% to 40% of cases.**

ADDITIONAL IMAGE

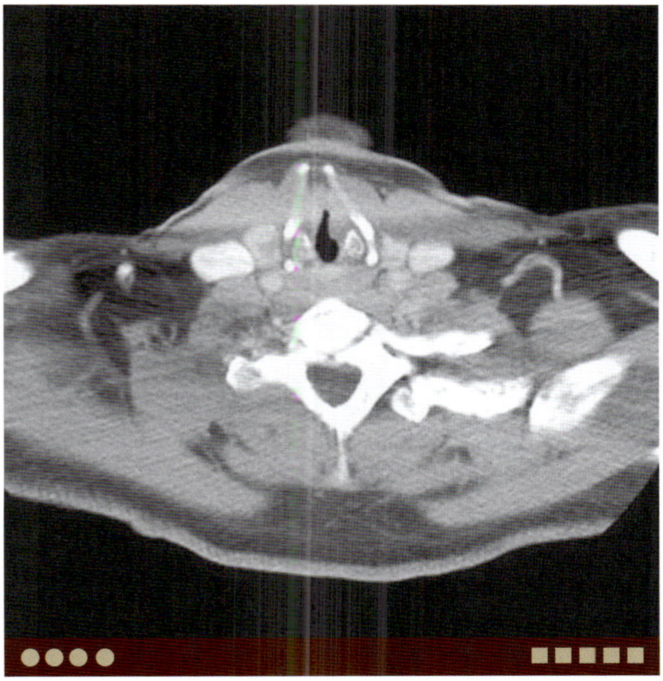

B. Laryngeal SCCA, same patient as A. Axial soft tissue window CT demonstrates a soft tissue mass involving the left vocal cord and crossing the anterior commissure to involve the anterior part of the right vocal cord.

DIFFERENTIAL DIAGNOSIS IMAGES (C-E)

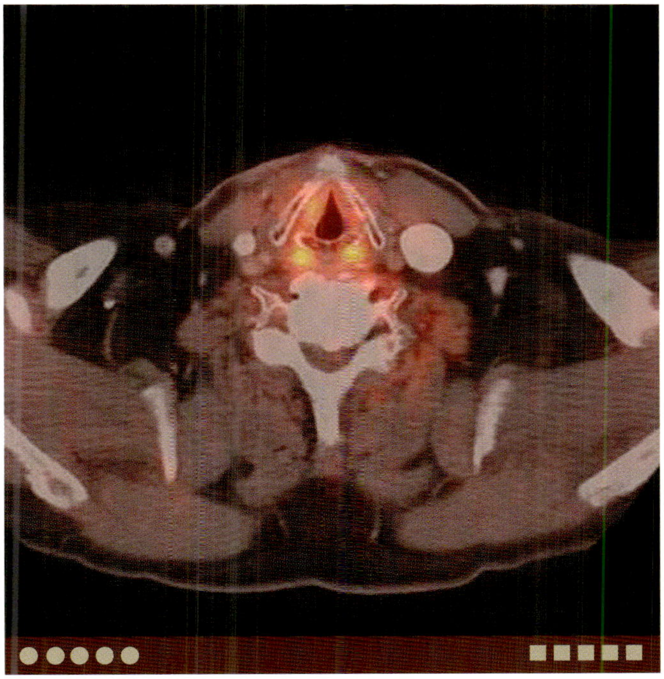

C. Physiological uptake. Axial fused FDG-PET/CT image demonstrates physiological FDG uptake in the right vocal cord and in the postcricoid soft tissues.

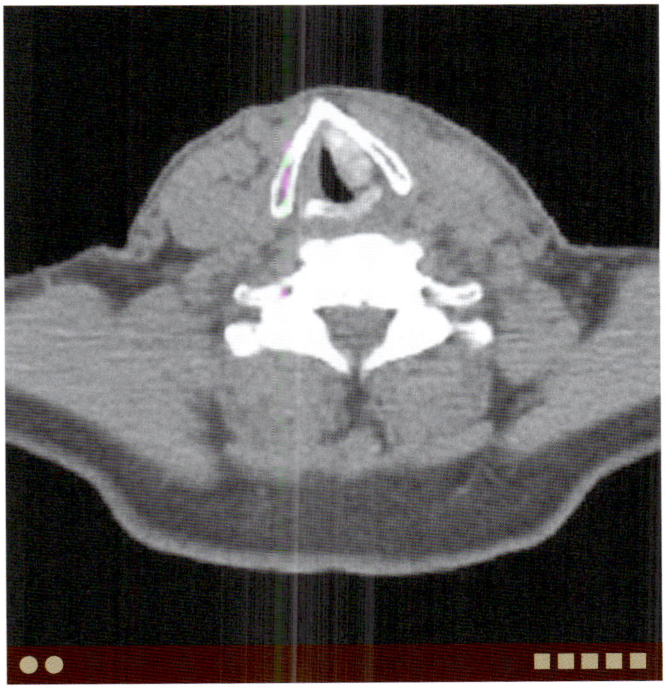

D. Teflon injection. Axial CT demonstrates high-density material in the left vocal cord due to the Teflon injection.

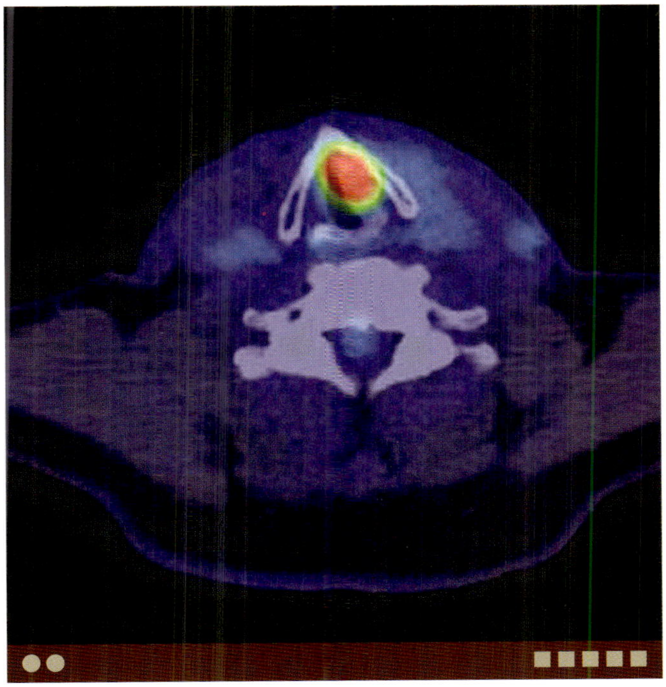

E. Teflon injection, same patient as D. Axial fused FDG-PET/CT image demonstrates intense FDG uptake in the left vocal cord due to chronic inflammation which can last for many years.

Case 13–6 Mucoepidermoid Carcinoma

Jessica Davison, Dan Filitis, Shilpa Surasi, Rathan Subramaniam

PRESENTATION

Parotid mass.

FINDINGS

PET/CT demonstrated an FDG hypermetabolic cystic and solid parotid gland mass.

DIFFERENTIAL DIAGNOSIS

- Squamous cell carcinoma (SCCA): Primary or metastatic SCCA usually demonstrates intense FDG hypermetabolism and can consist of necrotic areas.
- Lymphoma: High-grade lymphoma is usually intensely FDG-avid but necrotic areas are rare.
- Warthin tumor: Though benign, Warthin tumor demonstrates moderate-to-intense FDG hypermetabolism.

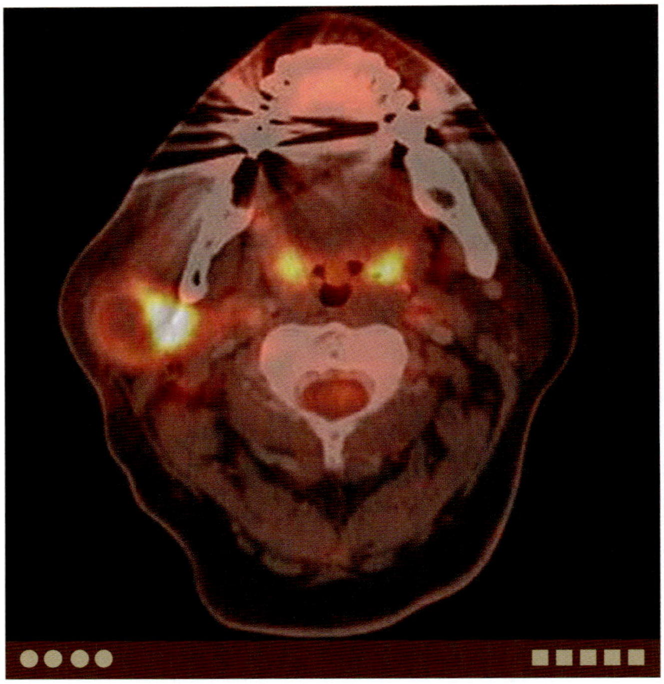

A. Parotid mucoepidermoid carcinoma. Axial fused FDG-PET/CT image demonstrates hypermetabolic activity with a SUVmax of 15 corresponding to a mixed cystic and solid lesion replacing the entire parenchyma of the right parotid gland. Bilateral physiological tonsillar uptake is noted.

COMMENTS

This is a 45-year-old man with 2-month history of pain and swelling in the right preauricular region.

Salivary gland tumors represent 2% to 4% of all head and neck neoplasms. Most salivary gland tumors originate in the parotid gland, from which 10% to 15% are found to be malignant. Mucoepidermoid carcinoma (MEC) is the most common malignant tumor of the parotid gland and constitutes approximately 30% of all salivary gland malignancies. MEC is composed of three cell types, which occur in varying amounts: mucus-secreting cells, epidermoid cells, and intermediate cells. The composition of these cells determines the grade; I to III. Grade I is considered low grade and has a very low recurrence rate. Grades II and III are considered high grade and do considerably worse. If a tumor is low grade the 5-year disease-free survival rate is 97.0%, while if it is high grade it is only 22.5%. High-grade MEC of the parotid gland is an aggressive disease that frequently presents at advanced stage. High-grade tumors at presentation have increased tumor size, higher tumor, node, metastasis (TNM) stage, increased lymph node spread, and recurrence. In contrast to SCCA, the histologic grade for MEC may be at least as important as TNM stage as a prognostic tool. Presence of anaplasia, necrosis, cystic formation, and neural or vascular involvement are statistically significant independent predictors of outcome. Most patients with a parotid tumor present with an enlarging, asymptomatic, unilateral parotid mass. Facial nerve paralysis or paresis, pain, and a firm-fixed position with a parotid mass are highly indicative of a malignant tumor.

PEARLS

- **The FDG avidity of the MEC varies with histological grade. The high-grade MEC is intensely FDG-avid and the low-grade MEC is mild-to-moderate FDG-avid.**
- **The histological grade and FDG avidity of MEC predicts prognosis.**
- **High-grade MEC may demonstrate perineural spread which is best imaged by MRI than PET/CT due to low volume disease and lower spatial resolution of PET.**

ADDITIONAL IMAGES (B-C)

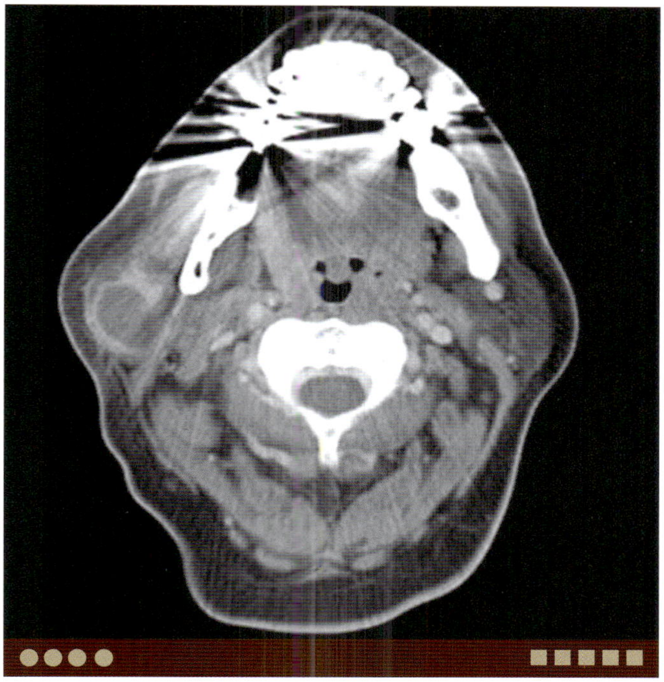

B. Parotid MEC, same patient as A. Axial soft tissue window CT demonstrates enlarged right parotid gland with central hypodensity suggesting necrosis.

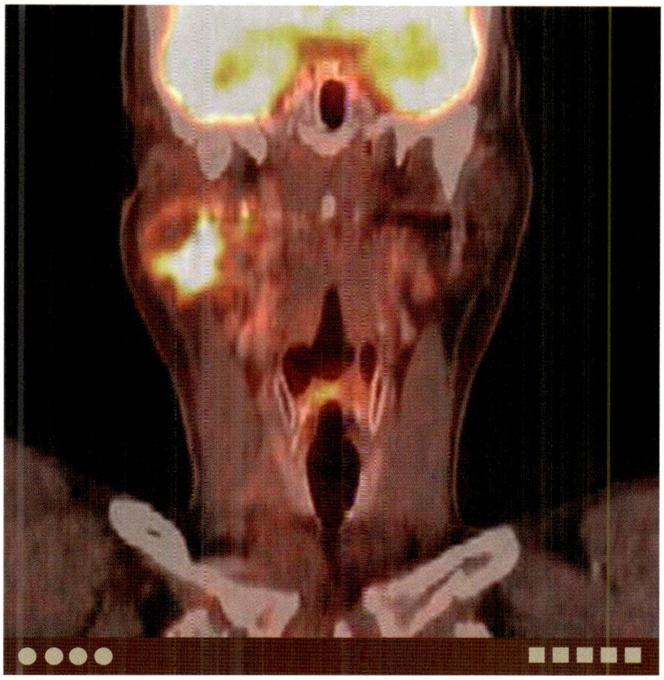

C. Parotid MEC, same patient as A. Coronal fused FDG-PET/CT image demonstrates the right parotid tumor. The cystic areas demonstrate FDG hypometabolism consistent with necrosis and the solid areas demonstrate intense FDG hypermetabolism consistent with high-grade mucoepidermoid carcinoma.

DIFFERENTIAL DIAGNOSIS IMAGES (D-H)

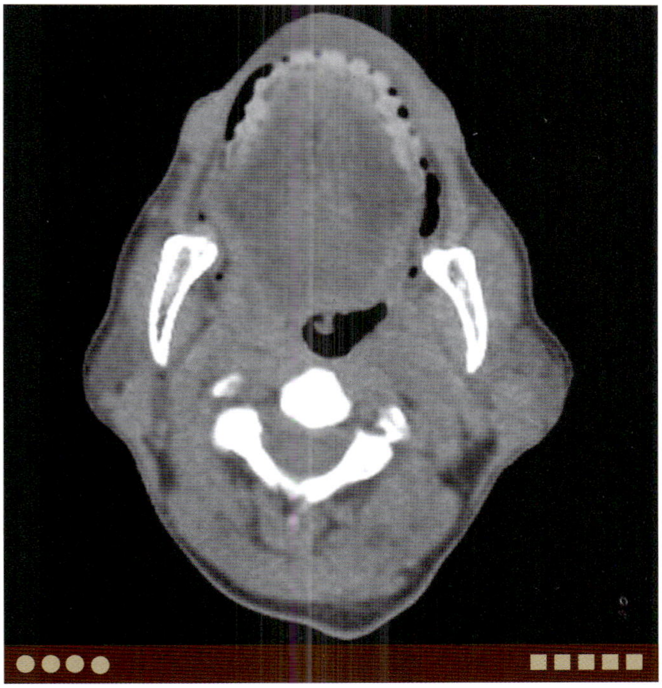

D. Lymphoma. Axial CT demonstrates a soft tissue density mass in the left parotid gland.

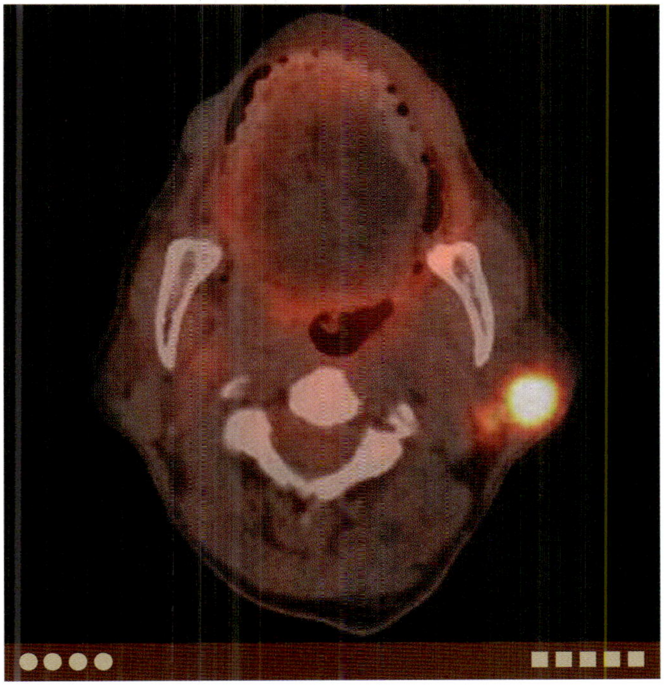

E. Lymphoma, same patient as D. Axial fused FDG-PET/CT image demonstrates intense FDG hypermetabolism in the left parotid tumor.

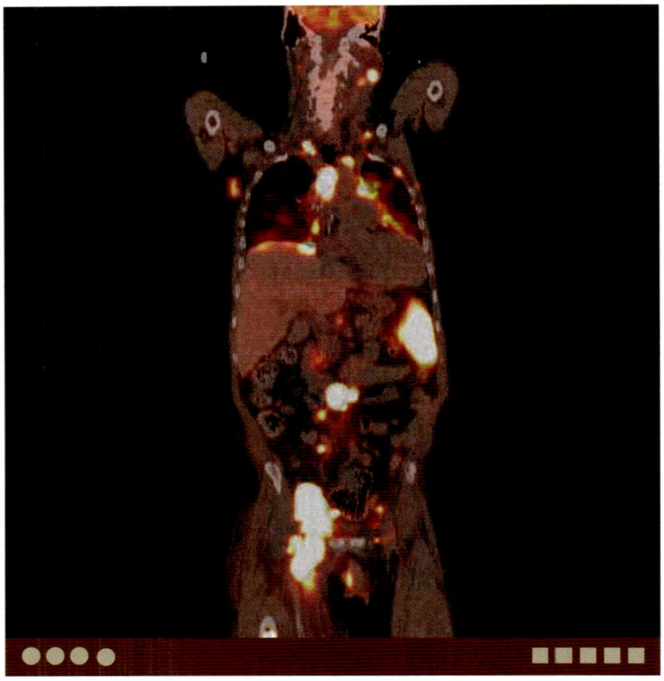

F. Lymphoma, same patient as D. Coronal fused FDG-PET/CT image demonstrates many other FDG hypermetabolic foci in the body consistent with biopsy-proven diffuse large cell lymphoma.

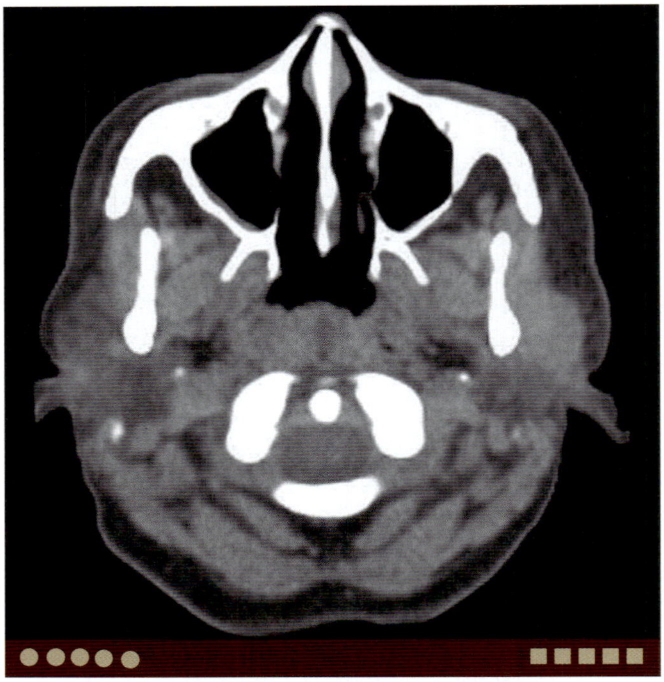

G. Warthin tumor. Axial CT demonstrates a soft tissue density mass in the left parotid gland.

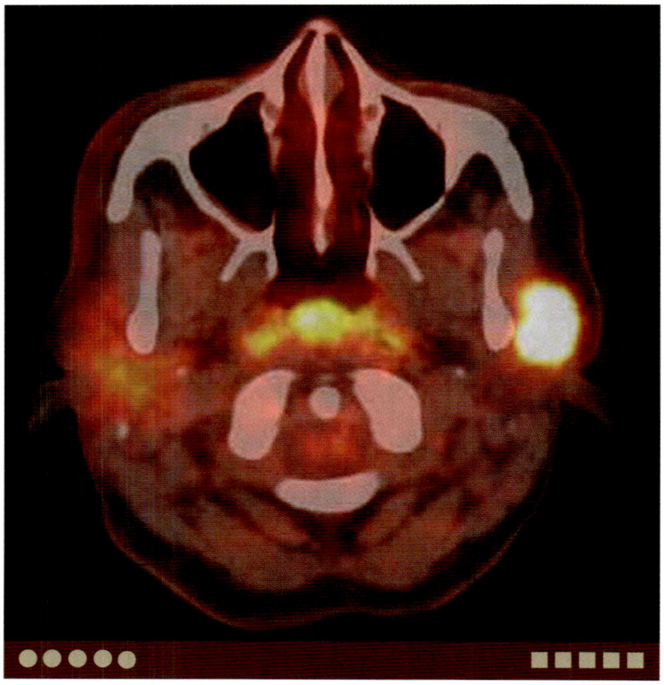

H. Warthin tumor, same patient as G. Axial fused FDG-PET/CT image demonstrates intense FDG hypermetabolism in the left parotid tumor consistent with biopsy-proven Warthin tumor.

Case 13–7 Esthesioneuroblastoma

Shilpa Surasi, Ankit Agarwal, Amol Mehta, Rathan Subramaniam

PRESENTATION

Mass in the superior nasal cavity.

FINDINGS

FDG-PET/CT scan demonstrates a FDG hypermetabolic mass in the superior nasal cavity.

DIFFERENTIAL DIAGNOSIS

- Lymphoma: Sinonasal lymphomas are usually non-Hodgkin type and most of these in the United States are of B-cell origin. It is usually FDG-avid and cannot be differentiated from esthesioneuroblastoma based on FDG avidity only.
- Squamous cell carcinoma (SCCA): SCCA comprises 80% to 90% of all primary sinonasal malignancies. Most of them occur in the maxillary antrum, followed by the nasal cavity. It is usually FDG-avid and cannot be differentiated from esthesioneuroblastoma based on FDG avidity only.
- Sinonasal undifferentiated carcinoma (SNUC): SNUC demonstrates intense FDG avidity.
- Metastasis: Nasal cavity and ethmoids are common sites for metastasis of a variety of highly vascular tumors with renal cell carcinoma being the most common. Carcinomas of breast, lung, testis, and thyroid follow in the decreasing order of frequency. The FDG avidity is variable depending on the primary tumor.

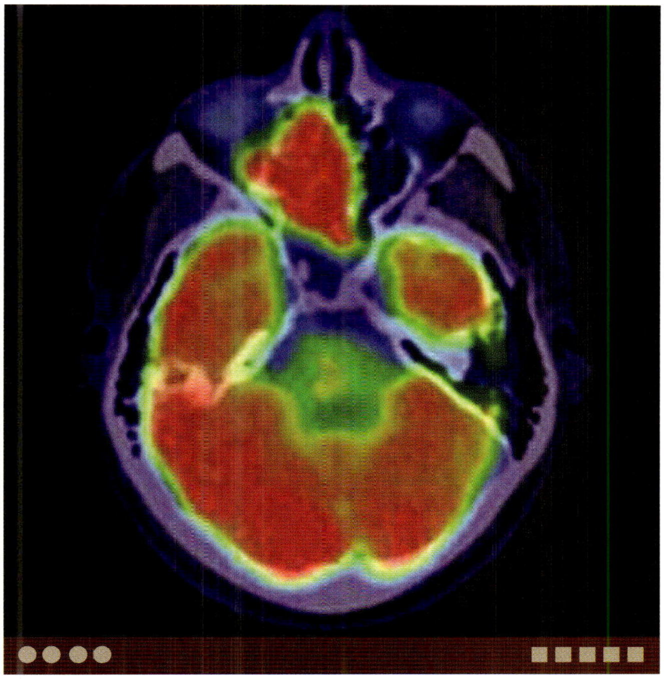

A. Esthesioneuroblastoma. Axial fused FDG-PET/CT image demonstrates a FDG hypermetabolic mass in the right nasal cavity.

COMMENTS

Esthesioneuroblastoma or olfactory neuroblastoma is a rare, locally aggressive sinonasal tumor. The most common site of origin is high in the nasal vault from the olfactory epithelium, most of which is located at the cribriform plate. Esthesioneuroblastoma has two peaks of incidence: the first in young men and the second between the ages of 50 and 60 years. Symptoms and signs include nasal pressure, headache, nasal discharge, and inability to breathe through the nose or smell.

Esthesioneuroblastomas vary in biological aggressiveness. They can either be small, slow developing, or rapidly growing tumors. Patient survival is estimated to vary from a few months to 20 years or more depending on the size and rate of growth of the tumor.

PET/CT imaging has been used to anatomically and functionally stage esthesioneuroblastomas and is a more accurate diagnostic technique than either CT or MRI. Later stage tumors such as regional or distant metastases of esthesioneuroblastoma can be identified by PET/CT. FDG-PET/CT also provides prognostic information prior to surgery and useful in posttherapy assessment.

PEARLS

- **Esthesioneuroblastoma is a neural crest derived neoplasm arising from the olfactory mucosa in the superior nasal fossa.**
- **Locoregional and distant metastasis occurs in up to 38% of patients. Late recurrences or metastatic disease can occur up to two decades after initial presentation.**
- **PET/CT is useful in the staging, prognosis, and therapy assessment of esthesioneuroblastomas.**

DIFFERENTIAL DIAGNOSIS IMAGES (B-C)

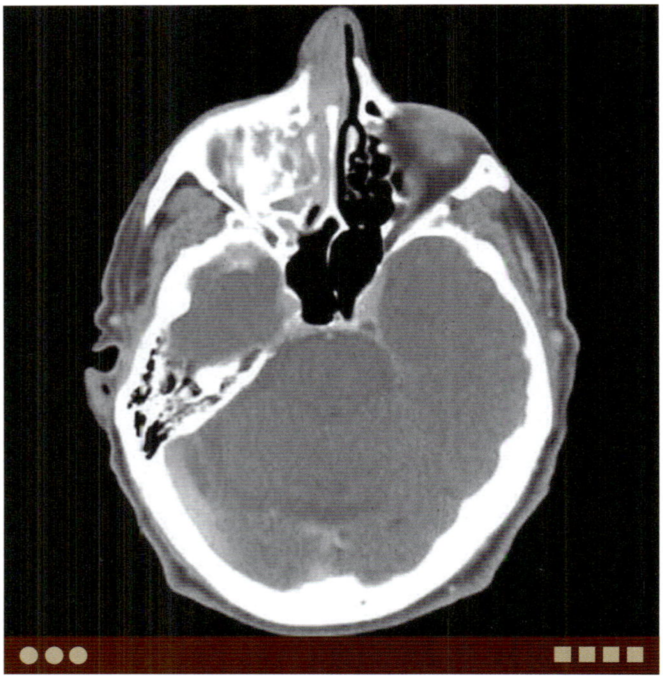

B. SNUC. Axial CT demonstrates a soft tissue density mass in the right nasal cavity.

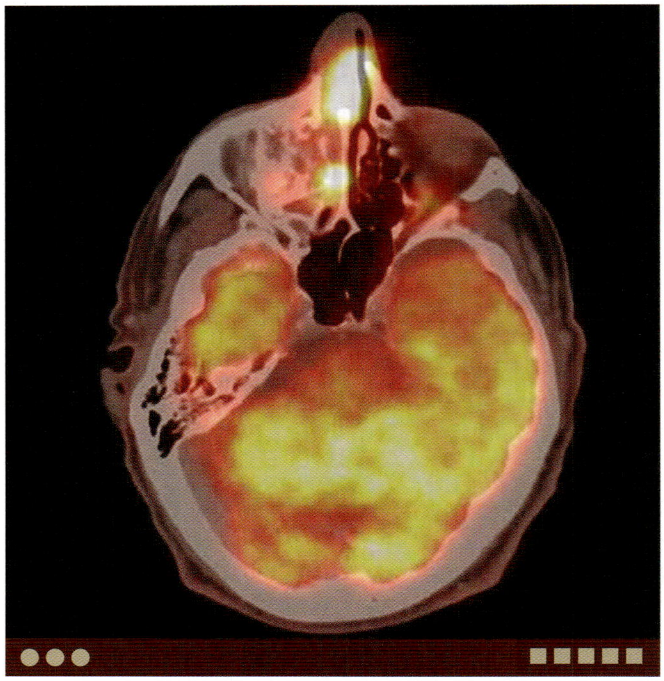

C. SNUC, same patient as B. Axial fused FDG-PET/CT image demonstrates a FDG hypermetabolism in the right nasal cavity mass.

Case 13–8 Thyroid Carcinoma

Jessica Davison, Shilpa Surasi, Rathan Subramaniam

PRESENTATION

Incidental, painless and palpable solitary thyroid nodule or mass.

FINDINGS

PET/CT demonstrates a hypermetabolic thyroid mass.

DIFFERENTIAL DIAGNOSIS

- Benign follicular neoplasm: This condition demonstrates hyperplastic follicular cell growth. Clinical presentation may be similar to follicular carcinoma. This may demonstrate intense, focal FDG hypermetabolism.
- Thyroiditis: This is an autoimmune condition that displays inflammation of the thyroid tissue. Patients usually presents with fatigue and vague pain. It demonstrates diffuse FDG uptake throughout the thyroid gland than focal FDG uptake.

COMMENTS

This is a 57-year-old man with rapidly enlarging left thyroid mass.

Palpable thyroid nodules exist in 4% to 7% of the US adult population. They are more frequently found in women and associated with both aging and a decrease in iodine intake. Of these nodules, only 5% are manifestations of thyroid cancer, with an incidence of 2 to 4 per 100,000 people per year, constituting 1% of all cancers and 0.5% of all cancer deaths. Thyroid cancer can be classified into four commonly observed cell types in the order of decreasing frequency: papillary, follicular, medullary, and anaplastic. There are also rare incidences of primary thyroid lymphoma and sarcoma.

Most thyroid nodules cause no symptoms and are incidentally discovered through self-observation, observation by others, or physical examinations by physicians. Occasionally, pain, hoarseness, or dysphagia can manifest symptoms. Though clinically palpable, clinical examination has low sensitivity and specificity for detecting thyroid nodules. Therefore, laboratory evaluation of serum thyrotropin is warranted and imaging procedures can greatly aid in the diagnosis of potential thyroid cancer cases.

Ultrasonography is useful in distinguishing cystic nodules from solid nodules and in guiding diagnostic fine-needle aspiration biopsies. However, it is not reliable in diagnosing malignant lesions. CT and MRI are also unreliable in differentiating between malignant and benign nodules and rarely indicated in the evaluation of thyroid nodule. Radionuclide scanning is helpful in determining if the nodule is functioning. Nonfunctioning or cold nodules would increase the likelihood of thyroid cancer (15%-25%).

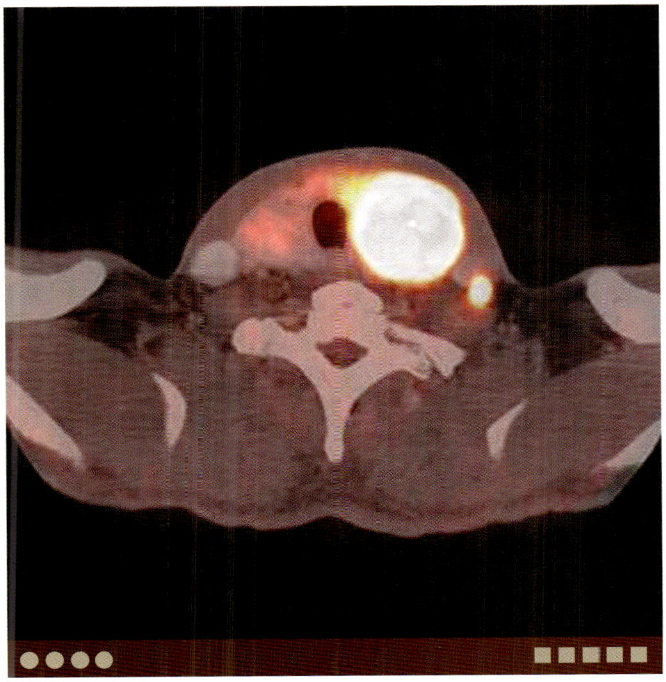

A. Anaplastic thyroid carcinoma. Axial fused FDG-PET/CT image demonstrates a large FDG hypermetabolic lesion in the left lobe of the thyroid gland with a SUVmax of 17 and a hypermetabolic lymph node in the left level IV consistent with metastasis.

Studies have shown that the use of PET/CT shows significantly higher SUVmax in thyroid cancer than in benign lesions. High glucose metabolism signifies poorly differentiated tumors and greater malignant potential and vice versa. An incidentally identified FDG-avid focal nodule has 30% to 40% chance of being malignant. For differentiated thyroid cancers, PET/CT is advocated in the follow-up of patients who have elevated serum thyroglobulin but negative radioiodine whole body scans. For medullary and anaplastic thyroid cancers, PET/CT has a significant role in staging, assessing treatment response, monitoring tumor recurrence or metastasis, and predicting prognosis based on FDG uptake.

PEARLS

- **Incidentally identified FDG-avid focal nodule has 30% to 40% chance of being malignant.**
- **PET/CT is useful in identifying the metastases and prognosis of patients with differentiated thyroid cancer who has rising thyroglobulin levels and a negative radioactive iodine scan.**
- **PET/CT is very valuable in staging, therapy response, and prognosis of patients with medullary and anaplastic thyroid cancers.**

ADDITIONAL IMAGES (B-D)

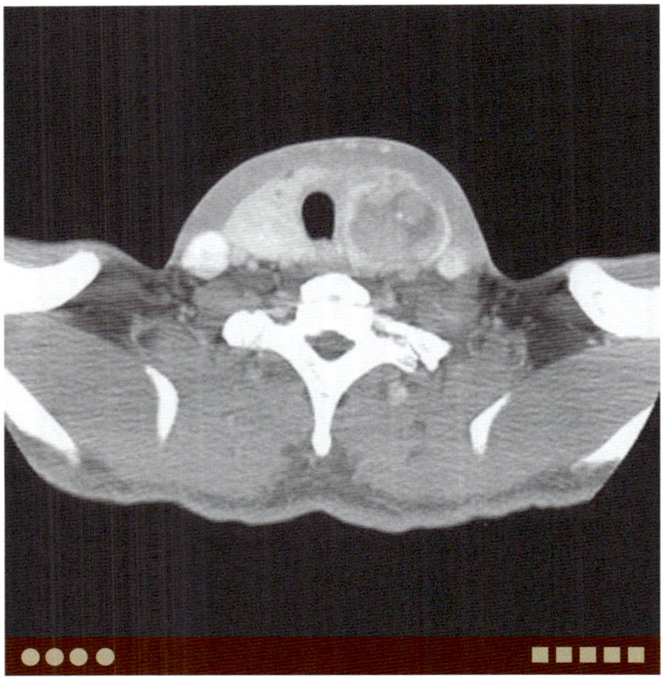

B. Anaplastic thyroid carcinoma, same patient as A. Axial soft tissue algorithm CT demonstrates a large, heterogeneous density lesion in the left lobe of the thyroid with low-density areas likely representing necrosis. Note the metastatic node posterolateral to the left internal jugular vein.

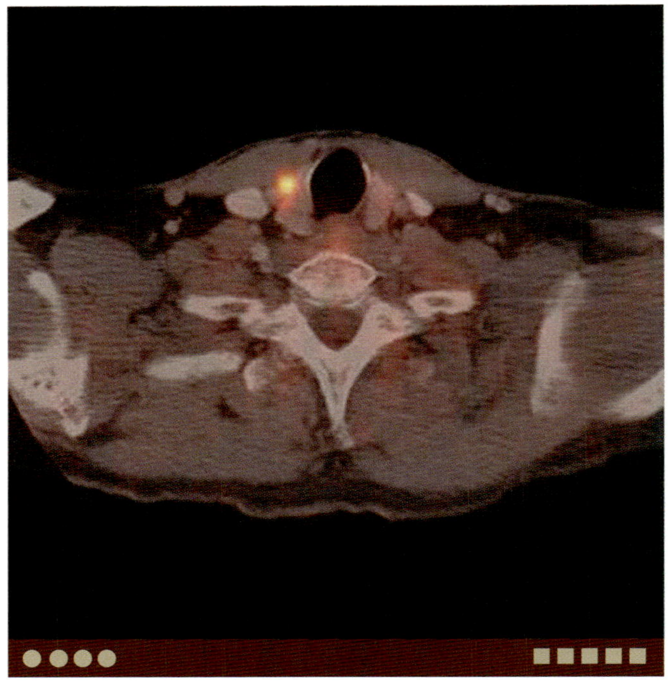

C. Papillary thyroid carcinoma in a 53-year-old man with AIDS and Kaposi sarcoma. Axial fused FDG-PET/CT image demonstrates an intense focal hypermetabolism with a SUVmax of 8 in the right lobe of the thyroid.

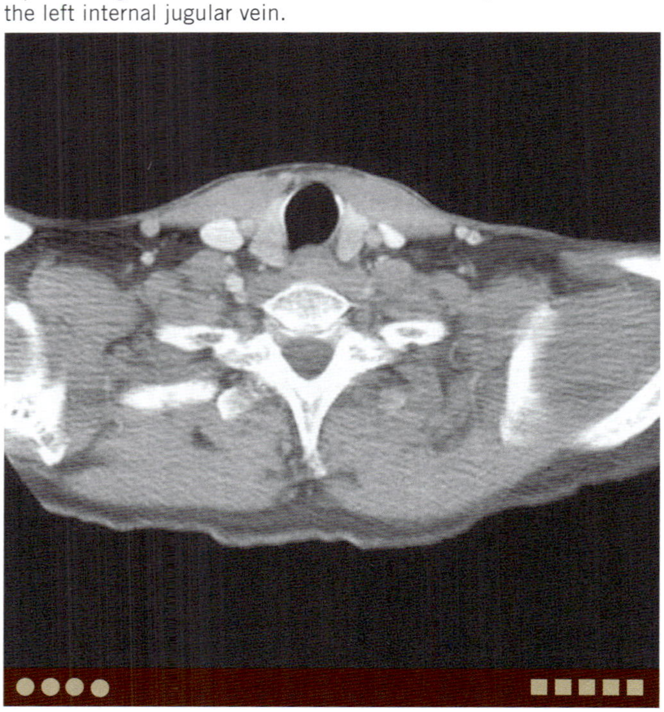

D. Papillary thyroid carcinoma, same patient as C. Axial soft tissue algorithm CT hardly demonstrates a low-density focal nodule in the right lobe of the thyroid gland.

Case 13–9 Treatment Assessment in Head and Neck Squamous Cell Carcinoma

Shilpa Surasi, Jessica Davison, Rathan Subramaniam

PRESENTATION

Neck mass.

FINDINGS

Restaging FDG-PET/CT scan in a patient with treated head and neck squamous cell carcinoma (SCCA) demonstrates no hypermetabolic uptake consistent with complete metabolic response at the primary site.

DIFFERENTIAL DIAGNOSIS

- Posttreatment inflammation: Chemo and radiotherapy can cause metabolic flare attributed to the activation of macrophages making it difficult to distinguish between benign inflammation and residual or recurrent malignancy.
- Recurrence of the tumor: Patients who have received potentially curative treatment for head and neck cancer are still at risk of recurrences and second (metachronous) primary tumors.

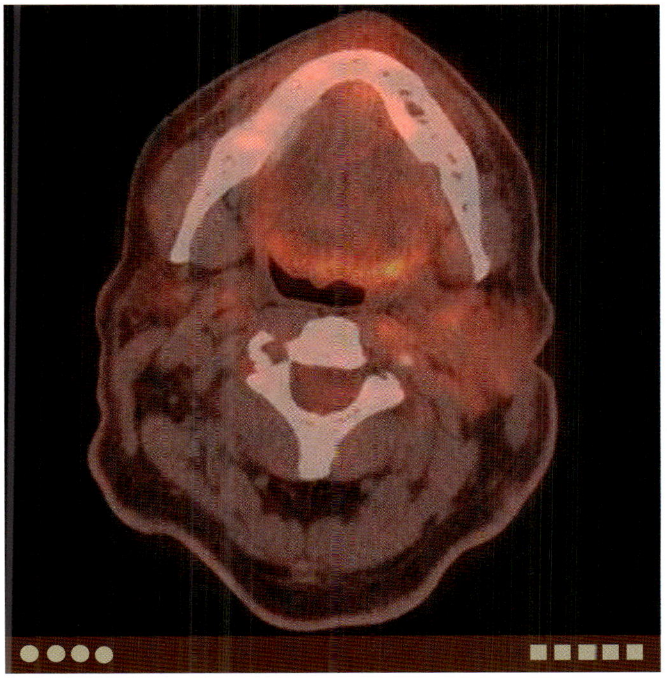

A. Complete metabolic response of tonsillar/base of tongue SCCA with level II nodal metastasis. Axial fused FDG-PET/CT done 3 months after chemotherapy demonstrates no FDG uptake consistent with a complete metabolic response.

COMMENTS

This is a 49-year-old man with a mass in the left neck.

Head and neck SCCA is the fifth most common cancer worldwide. Patients who have undergone potentially curative treatments require routine follow-up to detect and instigate early treatment of recurrences, so that there is a better chance of cure. Posttreatment surveillance also helps in the evaluation of disease control, rehabilitation of functional loss, and pain management thus impacting on the emotional and psychological well being of the patient.

The imaging modalities used to assess therapy response include CT, MRI, and PET/CT. The differentiation between residual or recurrent tumor, fibrosis, osteoradionecrosis, inflammation, and scars is difficult in both CT and MRI. FDG uptake is helpful in differentiating residual or recurrent tumor from scar tissue and is the best imaging modality to establish posttherapy assessment. PET/CT being a whole body study from the vertex to the mid-thigh helps in detecting distant metastases, unlike the other anatomic imaging techniques.

Despite high diagnostic accuracy, FDG-PET/CT scan has its own limitations. FDG, being a glucose analog is affected by conditions such as inflammation, high glucose levels, and altered permeability or vascularity. Recent studies have shown increased specificity of [F-18] fluorothymidine ([F-18] FLT) which is a novel radiotracer measuring thymidine kinase 1 (TK1) activity, an enzyme that is closely related to cellular proliferation. It is reported to be stable in vitro and accumulates in the proliferating tissues and malignant tumors. FDG is usually done 8 to 12 weeks post-chemoradiation to minimize the inflammatory effect. On the other hand, FLT-PET/CT as a proliferative marker is less prone for inflammatory uptake and can be done as early as 1 week after the start of therapy.

PEARLS

- **FDG-PET/CT posttreatment surveillance of head and neck SCCA patients plays an important role in detecting recurrences and an early diagnosis increases the chances of cure.**
- **PET/CT imaging has a better accuracy than other imaging modalities for therapy assessment.**
- **A posttherapy FDG-PET/CT is done about 8-12 weeks after the completion of radiation therapy to minimize the effects of radiation-induced inflammation.**
- **[F-18] FLT-PET/CT is a proliferative marker and may be used to image at early stages of therapy to assess the success or failure of therapy.**

ADDITIONAL IMAGES (B-D)

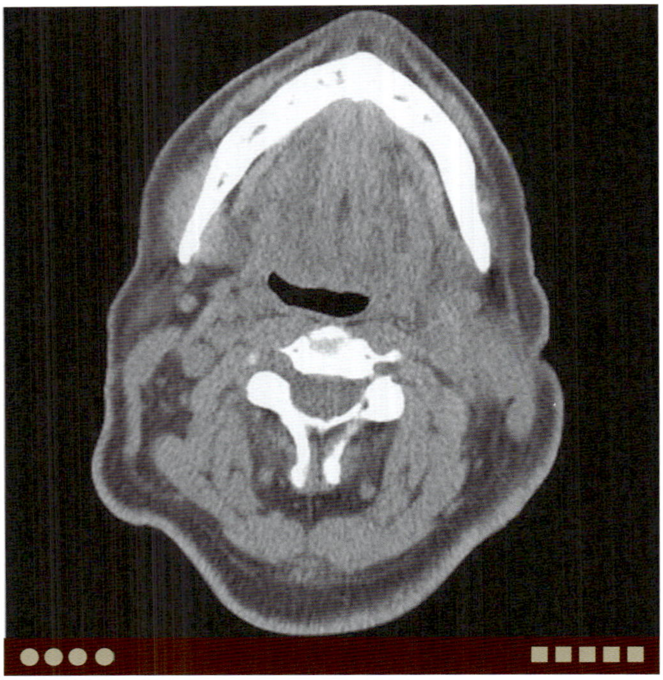

B. Complete metabolic response of SCCA, same patient as A. Axial soft tissue algorithm CT demonstrates a residual mass, although smaller than pretreatment CT, in the left level II.

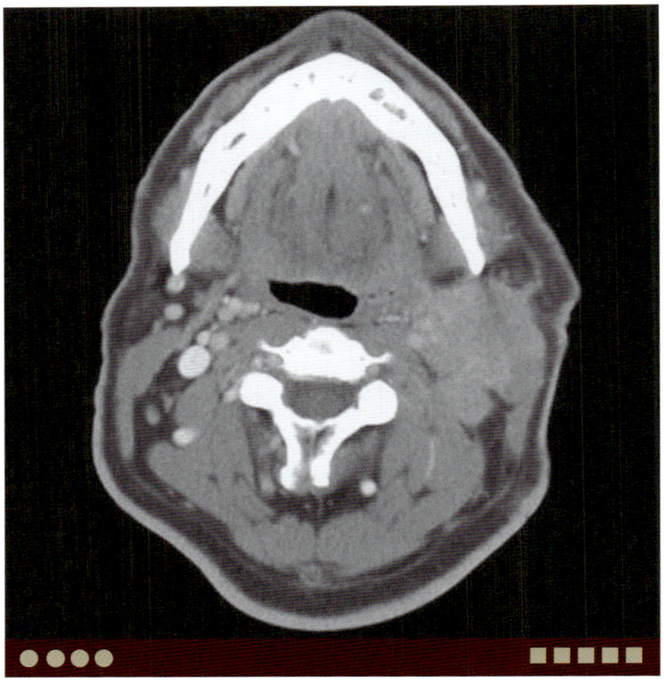

C. Pretreatment CT, same patient as A. Axial soft tissue algorithm CT demonstrates an enhancing soft tissue mass in the left level II with involvement of the carotid vessels.

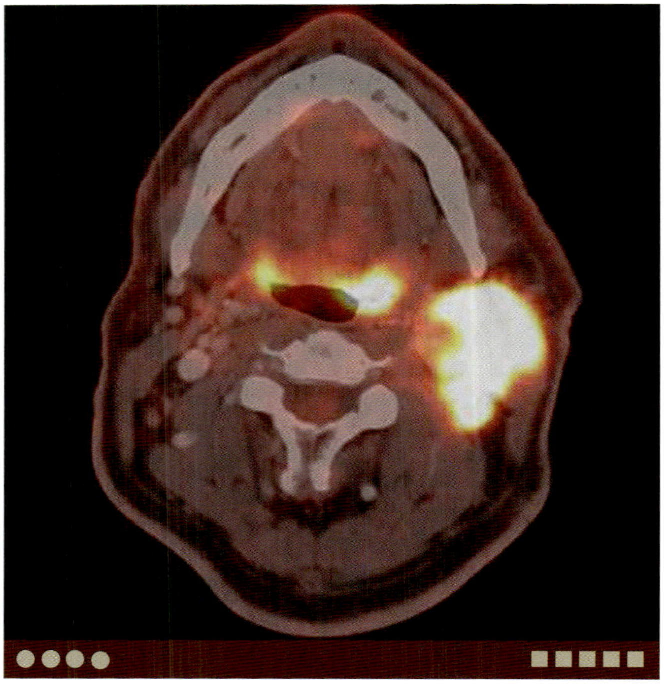

D. Pretreatment CT, same patient as A. Axial fused FDG-PET/CT prior to treatment demonstrates a hypermetabolic confluent left neck mass with a SUVmax of 16. Increased hypermetabolic activity is also seen in the left tonsillar pillar and BOT.

Chapter 14

INTERVENTIONAL HEAD AND NECK RADIOLOGY

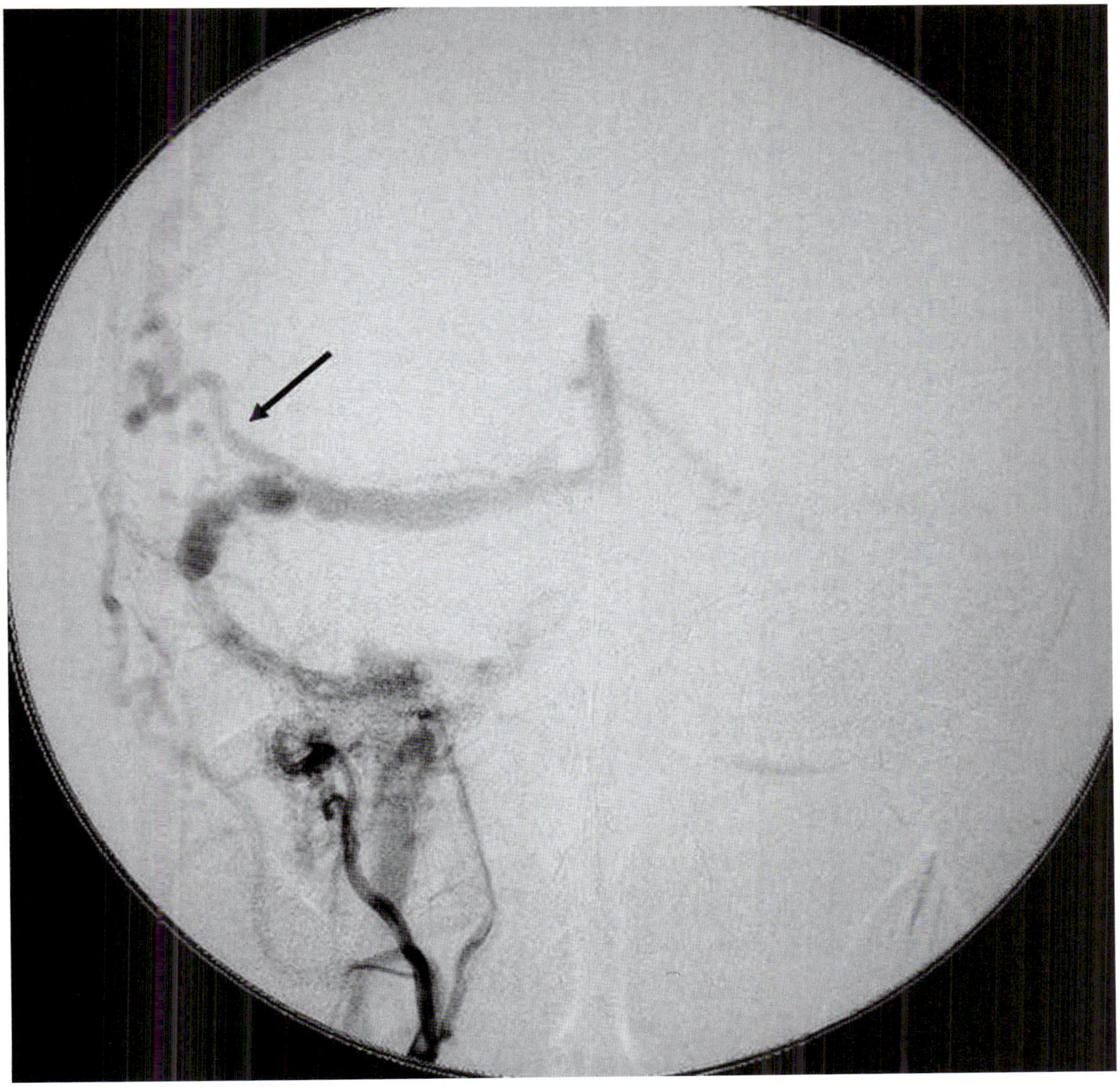

Case 14–1 Dural Arteriovenous Fistula of the Sigmoid Sinus

Morio Nagahata, Yoshinao Abe

PRESENTATION

Pulsatile tinnitus disruptive to sleep.

FINDINGS

External carotid angiogram demonstrates an early visualization of the sigmoid sinus supplied by the branches of occipital artery and posterior auricular artery. The shunting flow drains into both the internal jugular vein and the transverse sinus with marked reflux into the vein of Labbe.

DIFFRENTIAL DIAGNOSIS

- Dural arteriovenous fistula (AVF) of the transverse/sigmoid sinus without cortical venous drainage: Patients with this dural AVF without cortical venous drainage usually complain of tinnitus only, or have no symptom. This condition does not need aggressive therapy. It is important to observe the course by MRI/MRA paying attention to the change of the venous draining routes.

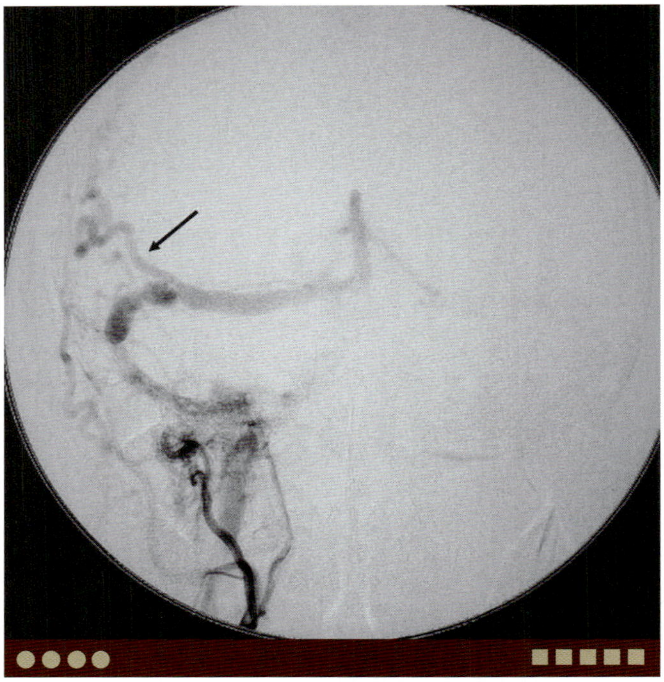

A. Right external carotid arteriogram (frontal projection) shows early opacification of the right internal jugular vein and sigmoid/transverse sinus with marked reflux into the right vein of Labbe (arrow).

COMMENTS

This is a 78-year-old woman with right-sided pulsatile tinnitus disruptive to sleep.

CT can hardly reveal the dural AVF. MRI, especially MR angiography (MRA), is helpful to identify this disease. Cerebral angiography is necessary, however, for accurate diagnosis, because evaluation of the draining pattern is important to manage patients. The symptoms of the dural AVF of this region varied from tinnitus to visual symptoms, altered mental status, and neurological deficits. The severity of the symptoms and the potential risk of hemorrhage depend on the venous draining pattern.

The patients with cortical venous drainage should be treated. Transarterial embolization (TAE) via the branches of the external carotid artery usually results in a palliative reduction in flow. Dural AVF is not usually cured by TAE alone. Transvenous coil embolization of the involved sinus can cure some patients with this disease. Transvenous sinus packing is effective for the involved sinus with the retrograde flow. This procedure is not suitable, however, for an involved sinus with antegrade flow. The involved sinus with antegrade flow is sometimes difficult to treat by transvenous embolization (TVE), because the sinus should be preserved for normal intracranial venous outflow. Superselective TVE of the affected compartment within the sinus may successfully occlude the AVF preserving the patency of sinus in such cases. Dural AVF with occluded sinus, draining into the enlarged cortical veins only, is also difficult to treat by TVE. Surgical isolation of the sinus or palliative TAE is preferable.

PEARLS

- **It is important to evaluate the presence or absence of cortical venous drainage and to evaluate the venous flow direction (antegrade or retrograde) of the affected sinus.**
- **Clinical symptoms and the venous draining pattern should be considered to make a therapeutic decision.**
- **Never obstruct the antegrade flow of the vein of Labbe, and never obstruct the torcular Herophili by coils.**

ADDITIONAL IMAGES (B-I)

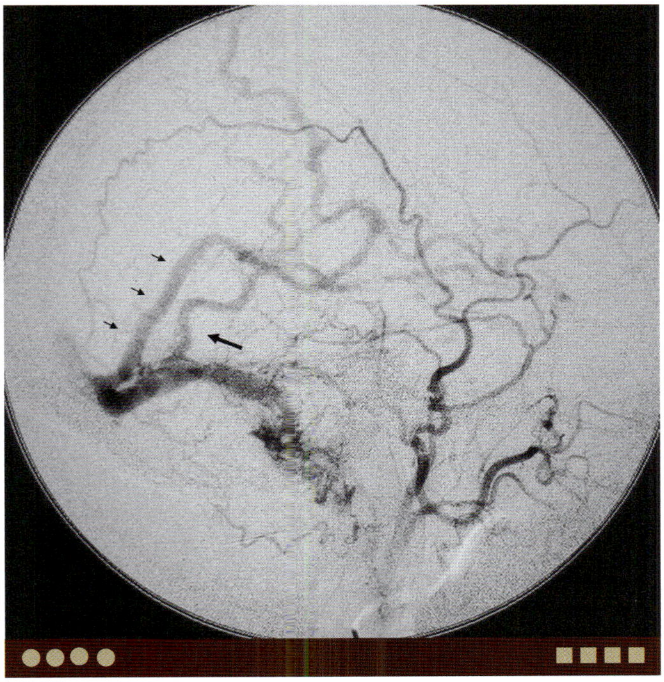

B. Right external carotid arteriogram (lateral projection) clearly demonstrates the marked cortical venous drainage into the vein of Labbe (arrow). Reflux into the straight sinus (small arrows) is also seen in this case.

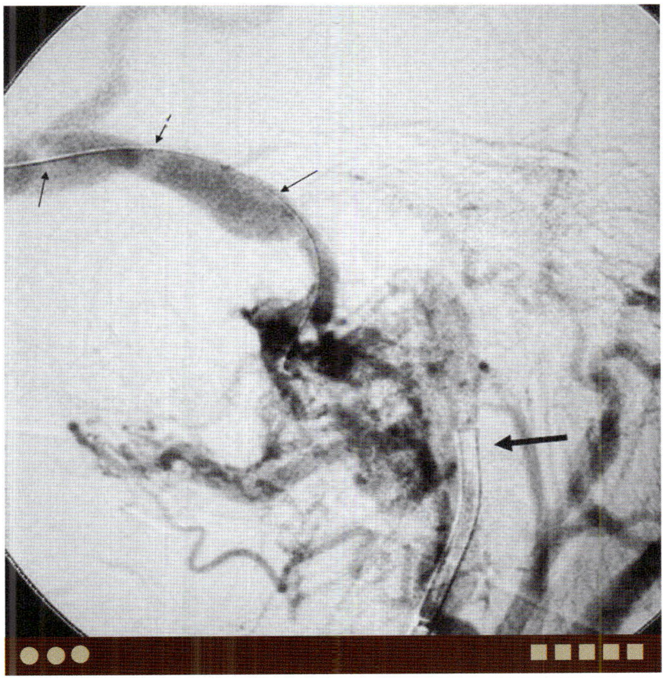

C. Magnified lateral projection demonstrates a dural AVF around the sigmoid sinus. Arrow indicates a guiding catheter tip at the right jugular bulb. Small arrows indicate the micro guide-wire reaching to the normal transverse sinus.

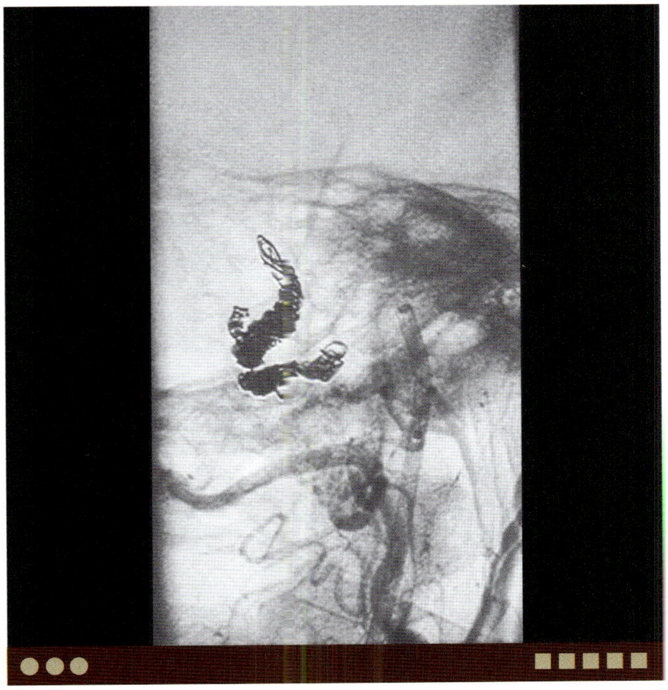

D. Magnified lateral projection demonstrates the delivered detachable coils in the right sigmoid sinus.

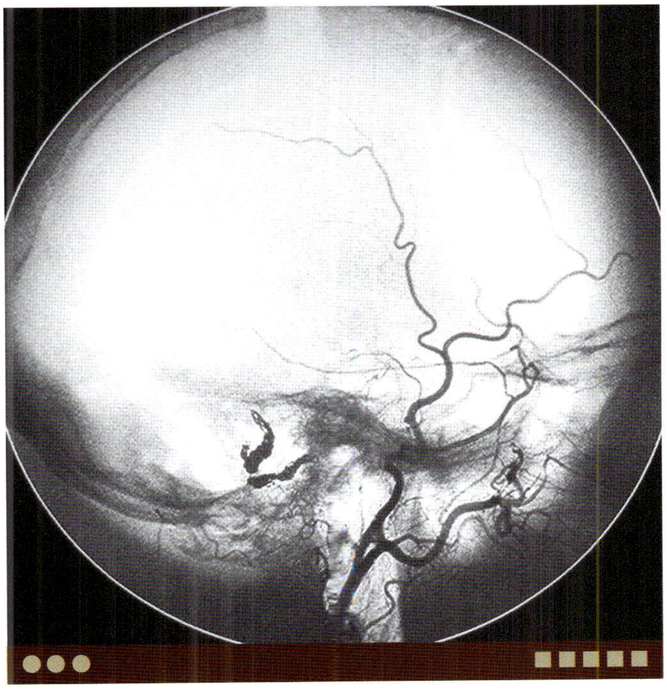

E. Right external carotid arteriogram (lateral projection) obtained 2 weeks after the TVE confirms a disappearance of the dural AVF.

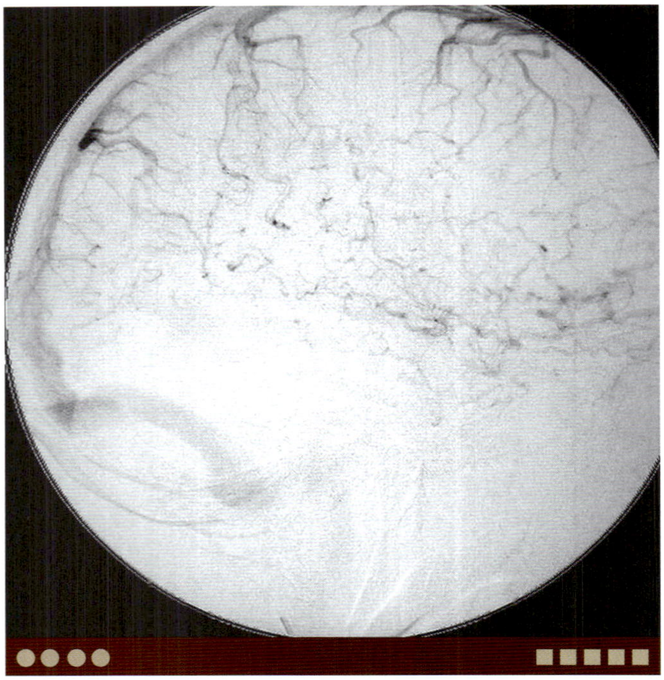

F. Preprocedural right internal carotid arteriogram demonstrates congested and tortuous cortical veins in the venous phase.

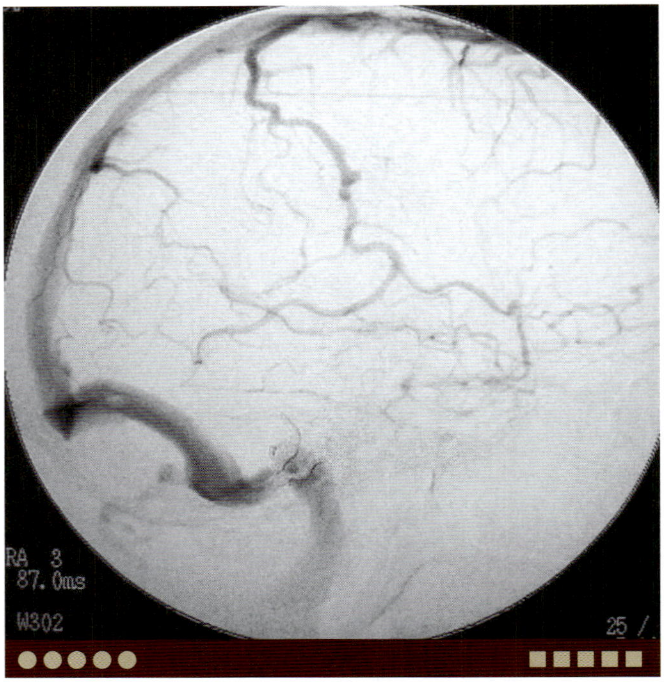

G. Right internal carotid arteriogram obtained 2 weeks after the TVE demonstrates normalized opacification of the cortical veins in the venous phase.

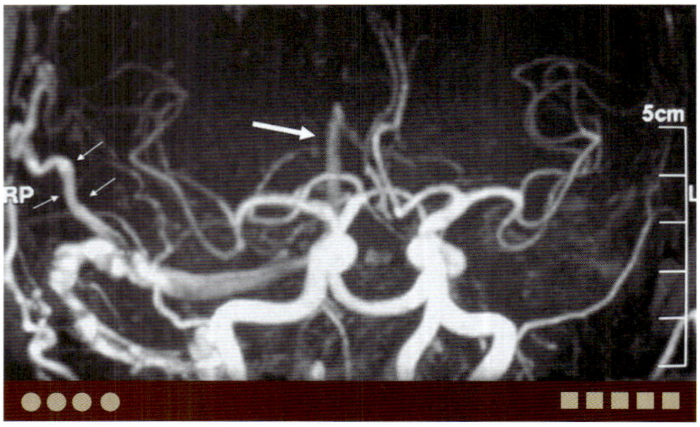

H. Right anterior oblique projection of MR angiography demonstrates a visualization of the right transverse/sigmoid sinus, straight sinus (arrow), and the vein of Labbe (small arrows).

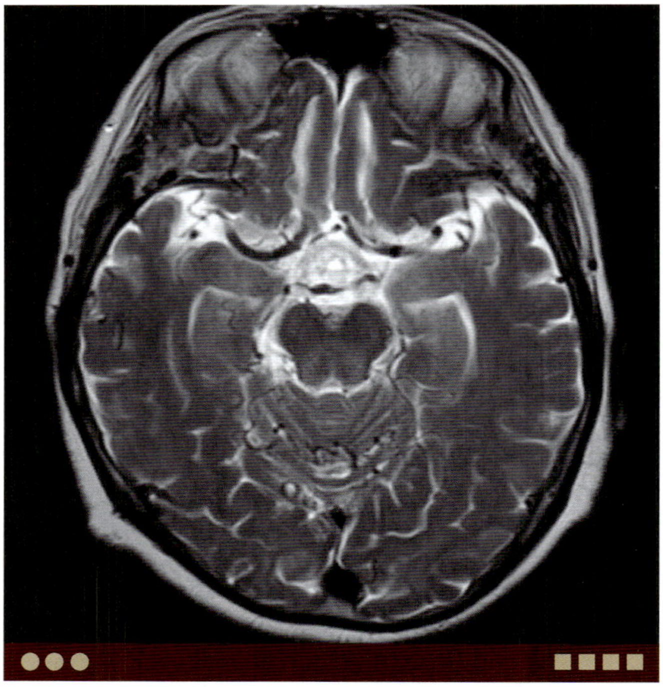

I. Axial T2W image demonstrates prominent flow-voids on the superior surface of the cerebellum, which suggest the dilated and tortuous cortical veins.

DIFFERENTIAL DIAGNOSIS IMAGE

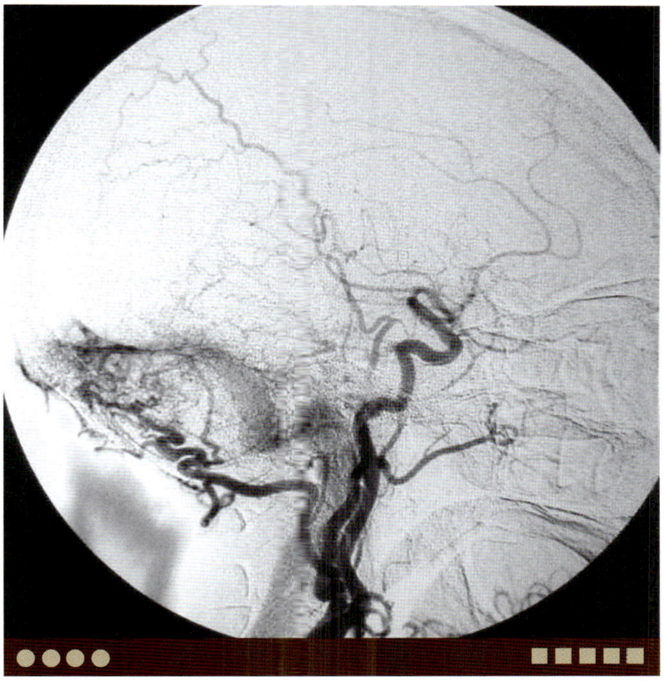

J. Dural AVF of the transverse sinus without cortical venous drainage (74F). Right external carotid arteriogram (lateral projection) demonstrates a dural AVF of the transverse sinus draining into the right internal jugular vein. Note the nonvisualization of the vein of Labbe or other cortical veins.

Case 14–2 Orbital Arteriovenous Fistula

Thanh Nguyen, Mostafa Mahmoud, Daniel Roy, Francois Guilbert, Jean Raymond, Alain Weill

PRESENTATION

Progressive diplopia, exophthalmos, chemosis, and proptosis.

FINDINGS

CT reveals a hypervascular mass in the inferior orbital fissure and angiography shows an intraorbital arteriovenous fistula.

DIFFERENTIAL DIAGNOSIS

- The differential for hypervascular masses in the orbit includes carotid cavernous fistula, either direct or indirect physiology with secondary orbital venous hypertension. Less commonly indirect orbital vein fistula may be encountered, as was confirmed with this case.

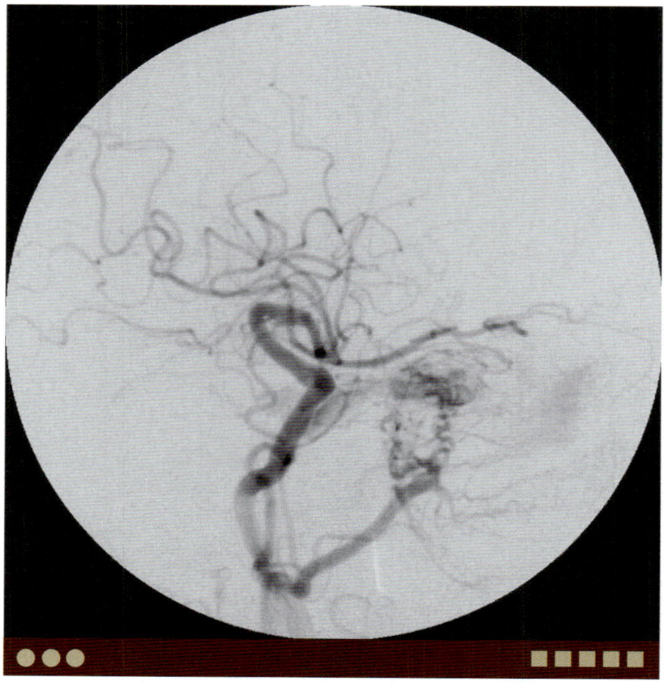

A. Arteriovenous fistula (AVF). Late arterial phase of common carotid artery (CCA) injection shows supply by the right internal maxillary artery and distal ophthalmic artery to a vascular network draining through an enlarged inferior ophthalmic vein.

COMMENTS

A 53-year-old man presented with 2 months of progressive diplopia, right eye exophthalmos, chemosis, and proptosis.

Orbital arteriovenous fistulas are anomalous communications between an artery and vein at the level of the orbit. Isolated orbital dural arteriovenous fistula (DAVF) are rare, and have been described at the level of the optic nerve sheath dura, which are known to possess arachnoid cells. Dura may also be present in the periorbital region which is composed of fibrous tissue. Patients with intraorbital dural fistula present with proptosis and chemosis, which mimics the symptoms of a carotid-cavernous fistula.

Transarterial embolization of the arteriovenous orbital fistula could be challenging in curing the disease, whereas surgical exposure has been reported with high hemorrhagic risk. When undertaking a transvenous approach, it is important to approach as close as possible to the fistula site to prevent alternate venous drainage and venous hypertension.

Treatment options of arteriovenous orbital fistula are (1) transvenous embolization with or without preceding transarterial reduction, (2) arterial embolization——reflux embolization through the central retinal artery is an important concern, (3) surgery——safe and adequate surgical exposure of the orbit is challenging and such procedures have been reported with high risk of hemorrhage, and (4) observation.

Intervention: Under general anesthesia, 5F and 7F sheaths were placed in the left femoral artery and right femoral vein, respectively. To enhance catheter navigation stability, a triaxial catheter system was mounted with a 7F guide catheter placed at the right inferior petrosal sinus, over a Tracker 38 catheter (Boston Scientific, Natick MA) at the right cavernous sinus, over a microcatheter navigated to the fistula site at the inferior ophthalmic vein (G). The venous pouch was embolized with four GDC coils, after which angiographic cure was achieved (H and I). At 1-month follow-up, there was complete resolution of the patient's exophthalmos, chemosis, and diplopia.

ADDITIONAL IMAGES (B-J)

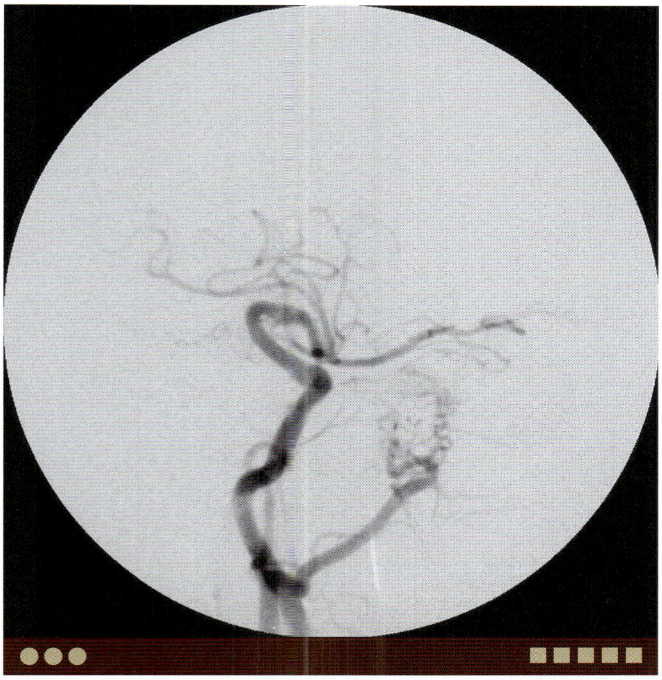

B. AVF, same patient as A. Late arterial phase of CCA injection shows supply by the right internal maxillary artery and distal ophthalmic artery to the vascular network.

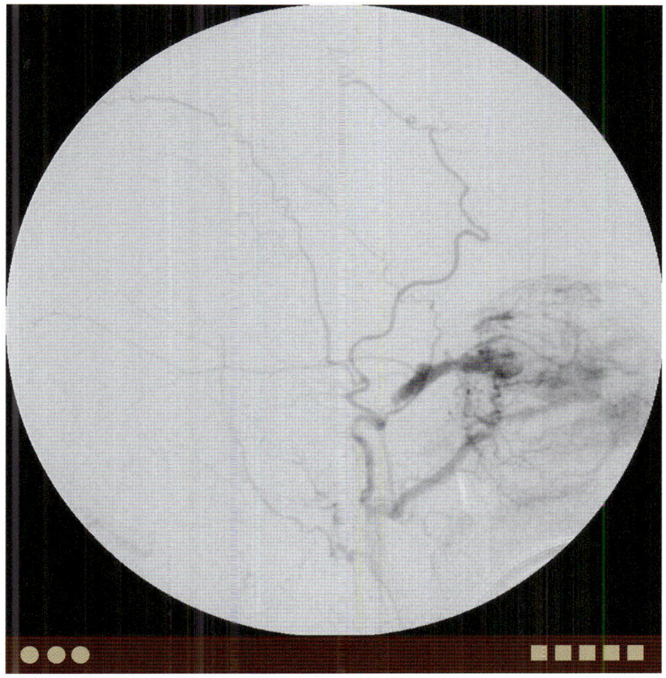

C. AVF, same patient as A. Late phase of external carotid artery (ECA) injection shows supply by the right internal maxillary artery and distal ophthalmic artery to a vascular network draining through an enlarged inferior ophthalmic vein.

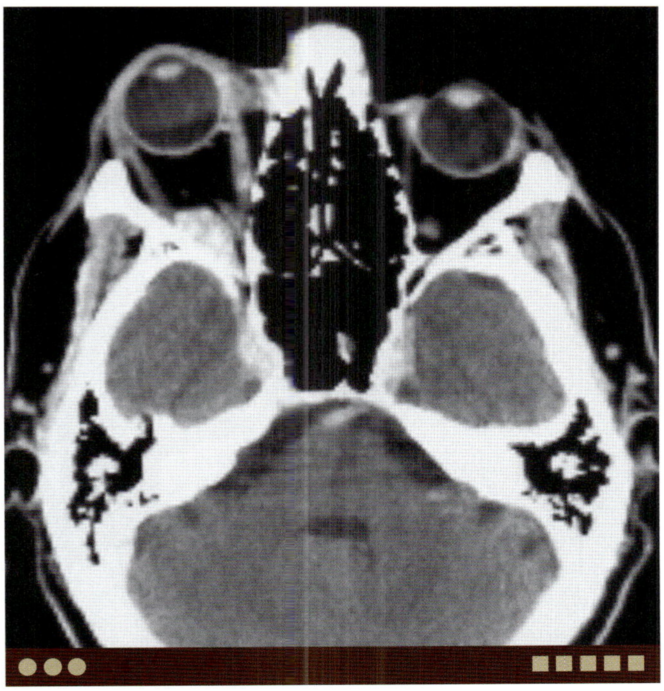

D. AVF, same patient as A. Axial postcontrast CT shows an enhancing mass at the right orbital apex and proptosis of the right eye.

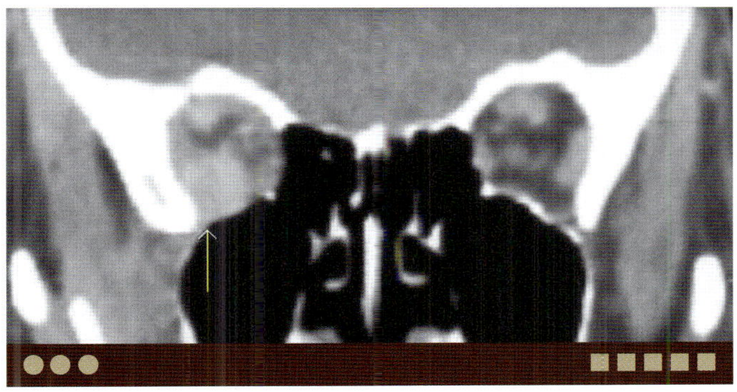

E. AVF, same patient as A. Coronal postcontrast CT shows enlarged right inferior ophthalmic vein (arrow).

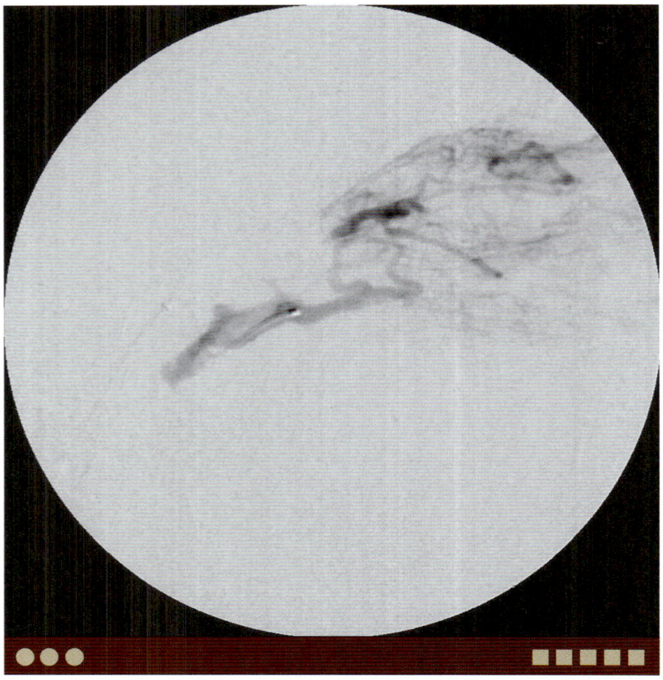

F. Microcatheter injection via the inferior ophthalmic vein (lateral view) shows opacification of the orbit.

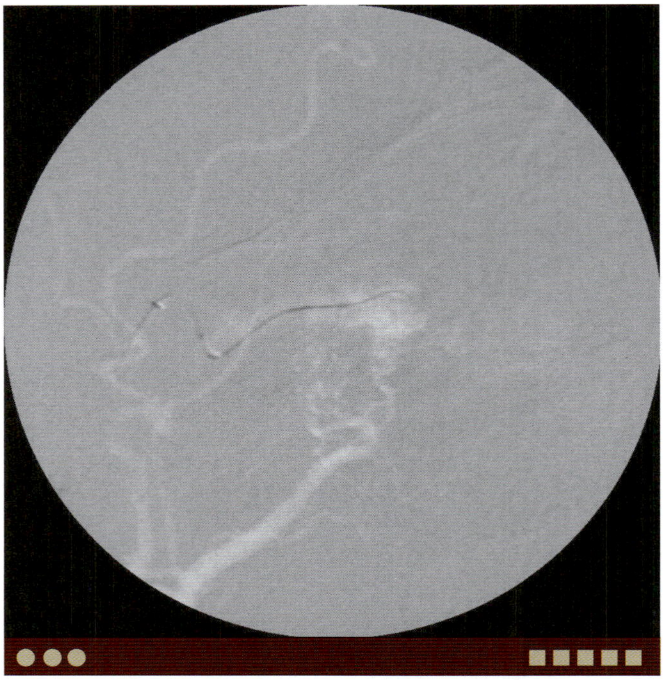

G. AVF, same patient as A. Right ECA roadmap shows placement of a microguidewire at the fistula site through the inferior ophthalmic vein.

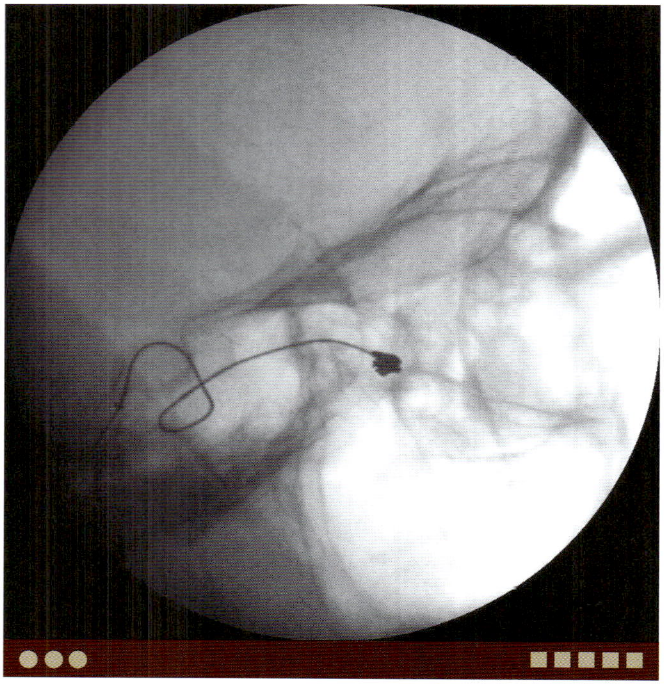

H. AVF, same patient as A. Lateral unsubtracted view shows partial coiling of the inferior ophthalmic vein.

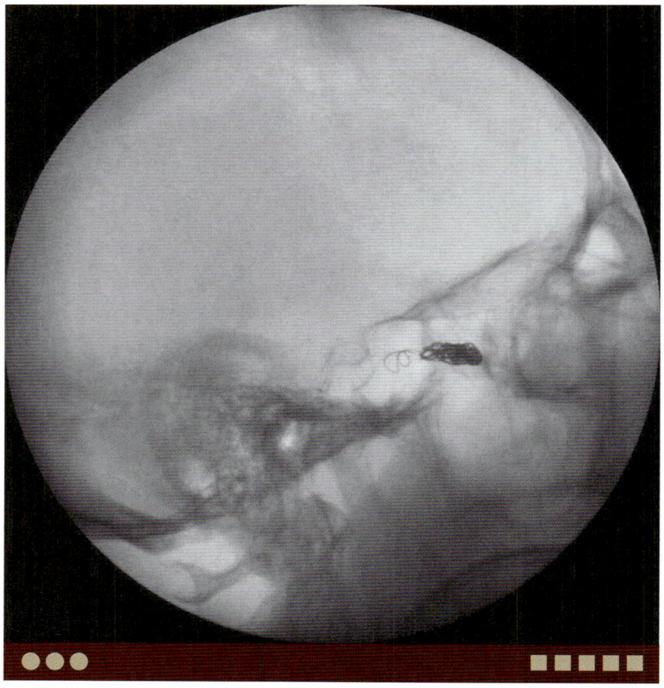

I. AVF, same patient as A. Lateral unsubtracted view shows complete coiling of the inferior ophthalmic vein.

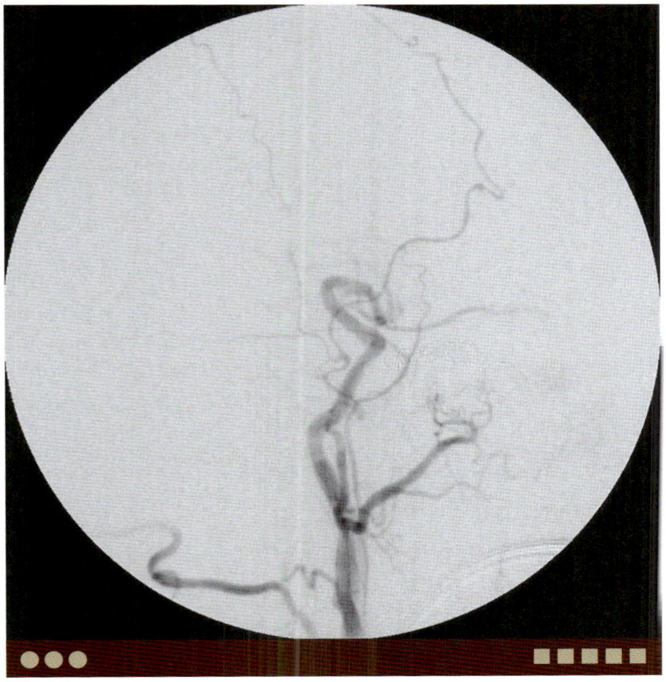

J. AVF, same patient as A. Control angiography via the right CCA shows absence of shunt, confirming fistula cure.

Case 14-3 Epistaxis

Junaid Kalia, Osama O. Zaidat

PRESENTATION

Intractable nose bleed.

FINDINGS

Characteristic nasal blush and hyperemia of the nasal septum is noticed on angiograms. Most often the nasal septum is supplied by the internal maxillary and facial branches of the external carotid artery (ECA), and superselective injection is required to distinguish the major arterial supply.

DIFFRENTIAL DIAGNOSIS

- Traumatic, infectious etiology, allergic rhinitis, neoplasm such as juvenile angiofibroma, hereditary telangiectasias, and idiopathic conditions may cause epistaxis.

COMMENTS

A 53-year-old woman who presented with left nasal epistaxis via anterior and posterior nasal septum was treated by endovascular embolization of bilateral internal maxillary branches of the ECA using polyvinyl alcohol (PVA) and pushable coils.

Epistaxis is highly prevalent and afflicts 60% of the population while only 6% requires medical attention. Anterior epistaxis is amenable to anterior packing and rarely requires intervention. Epistaxis originating from the posterior nasal septum is more challenging; requiring posterior packing and endoscopic cauterization with moderate success rate and potential complication such as pressure necrosis and patient discomfort. Arterial embolization is indicated for epistaxis refractory to the above measures.

The epistaxis differential diagnosis includes traumatic, infectious etiology, allergic rhinitis, neoplasm such as juvenile angiofibroma, hereditary telangiectasias, and idiopathic.

After the initial treatment of epistaxis fails, the patient is usually referred for endovascular embolization. The intraprocedure baseline digital subtraction angiography should include careful evaluation and assessment of the arteries supplying the nasal cavity and their collaterals. This is crucial to decide on the treatment plan and in avoiding reflux of embolic materials into vital collaterals. In particular, evaluation of the proximal intracranial internal carotid artery, ethmoidal branches of the ophthalmic artery, internal maxillary and facial artery branches is of paramount significance in endovascular treatment planning.

The embolic agents of choice are PVA particles and Gelfoam. Liquid embolic materials such as Onyx (ethylene vinyl alcohol copolymer) and NBCA (*N*-butyl 2-cyanoacrylate) are rarely used to achieve fast hemostasis. Pushable coils may be used for proximal control in refractory epistaxis.

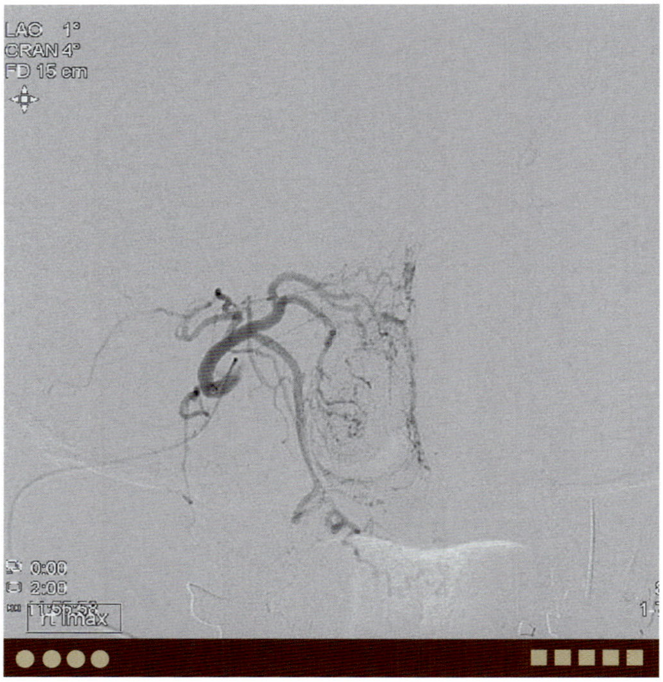

A. Epistaxis. Preembolization superselective distal right internal maxillary arteriogram (frontal projection) demonstrates hyperemia and characteristic nasal blush via sphenopalatine branches which are the major supplier of the nasal cavity.

PEARLS

- **Recurrent or multiple episodes of epistaxis with family history favor diagnosis Rendu-Osler-Weber syndrome or hereditary hemorrhagic telangiectasia (HHT).**
- **Most of the angiographic evaluation is performed while the patient is packed and extravasation may not be seen.**
- **Sphenopalatine branches of the internal maxillary artery are major arterial supply to the nasal fossa, and bilateral embolization may be required.**
- **Facial artery supply to the nasal cavity and collateral to the sphenopalatine arteries may necessitate additional embolization of the nasal branches of the facial artery. Careful facial artery embolization to avoid alar necrosis is necessary.**
- **Ethmoidal branches of ophthalmic artery may contribute to the epistaxis; however, embolization is not routinely performed as loss of vision is a possible complication.**

Distal internal maxillary sphenopalatine arteries are usually the main target for embolization as well as the superior labial branch of the facial artery. Ethmoidal arteries embolization is particularly risky as loss of vision may occur and hence not routinely recommended.

It is recommended to unpack the nasal cavity 24 to 48 hours after embolization rather than immediately. If bleeding persists, follow-up angiography is recommended with intraprocedure unpacking for further assessment for any potential additional embolization. If no additional nasal branches can be safely embolized, surgical ligation of the ethmoidal arteries is recommended.

ADDITIONAL IMAGES (B-H)

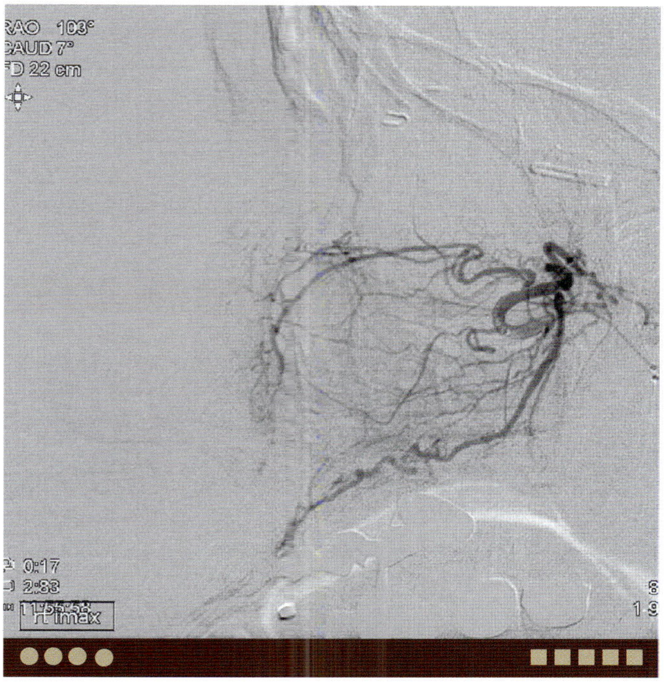

B. Epistaxis, same patient as A. Preembolization superselective right internal maxillary artery injection (lateral projection) shows blood flow to the nasal cavity via the sphenopalatine arteries.

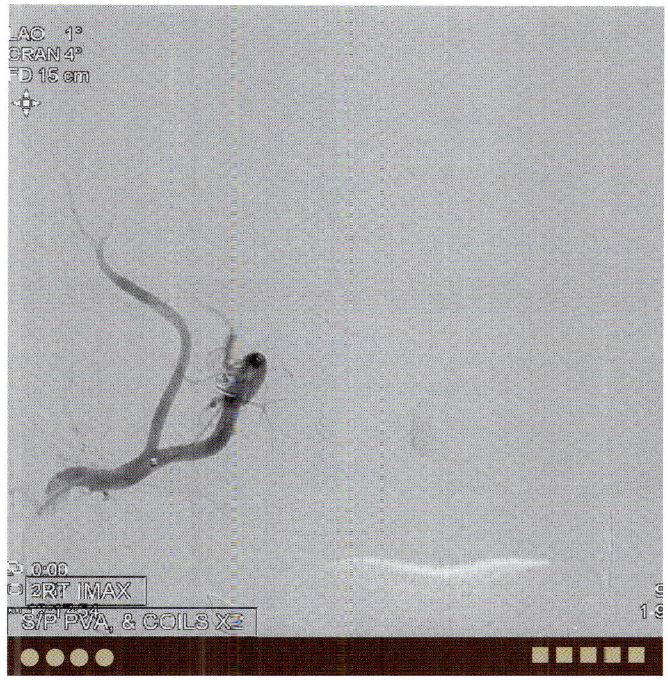

C. Epistaxis, same patient as A. Postembolization superselective right internal maxillary artery injection (frontal projection). Embolization was performed via microcatheter injection of PVA microparticles (45-150 μm and then 150-250 μm); further stagnation of flow was achieved via deployment of two pushable coils at the distal internal maxillary artery measuring 2 mm × 1 cm each.

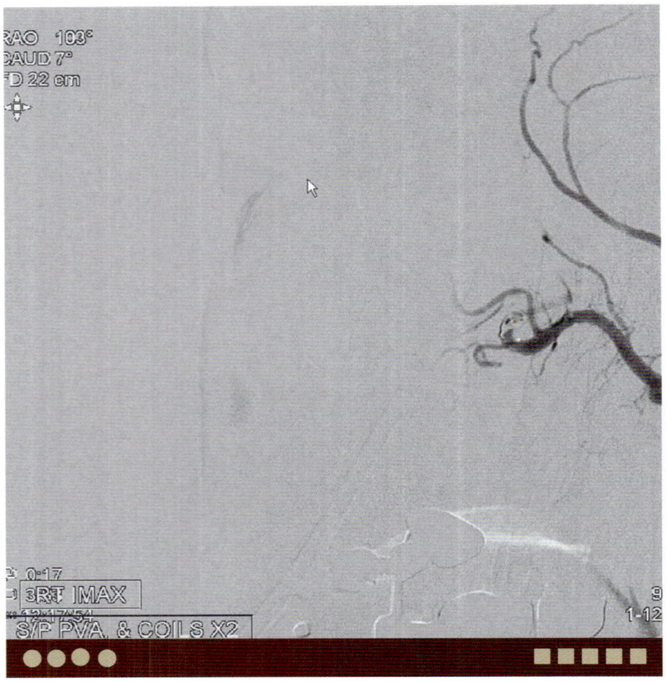

D. Epistaxis, same patient as A. Postembolization superselective right internal maxillary artery injection (lateral projection) shows no significant flow via the sphenopalatine artery into the nasal cavity.

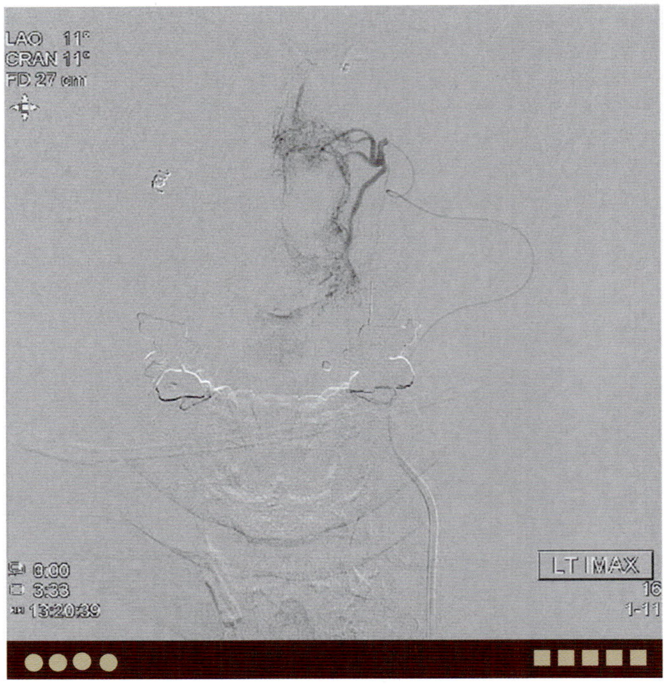

E. Epistaxis, same patient as A. Preembolization superselective left internal maxillary artery injection (frontal projection) confirms the dominant arterial supply to the nasal septum from the left internal maxillary artery.

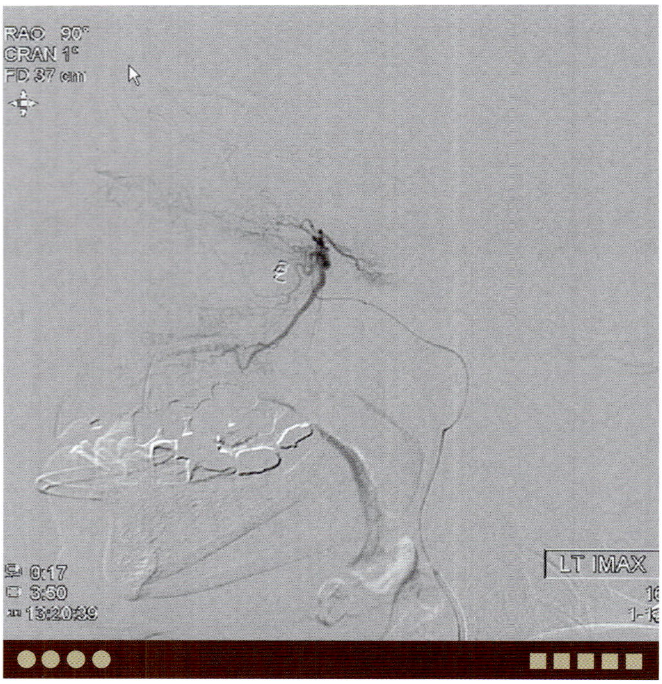

F. Epistaxis, same patient as A. Preembolization superselective left internal maxillary artery injection (lateral projection) shows blood flow to the nasal cavity via the sphenopalatine arteries.

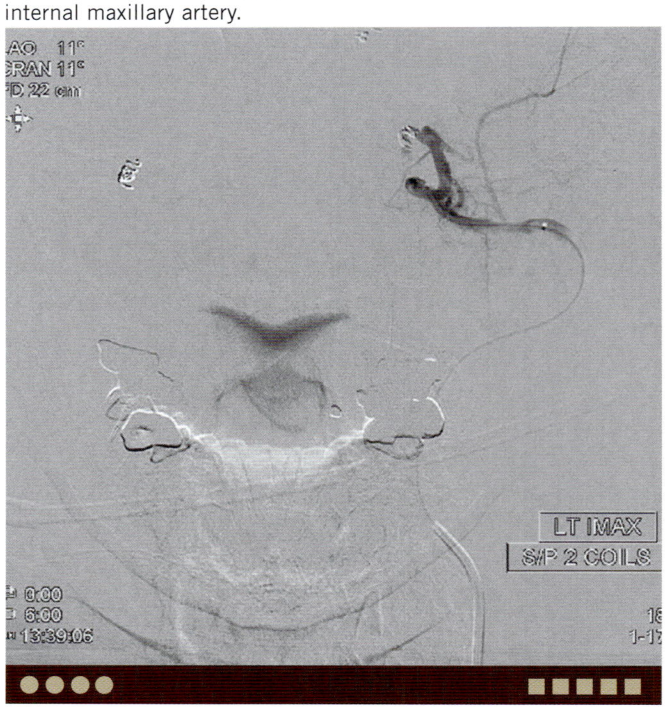

G. Epistaxis, same patient as A. Postembolization superselective left internal maxillary artery injection (frontal projection). Embolization was performed via microcatheter injection of PVA microparticles (45-150 µm and then 150-250 µm) further stagnation of flow was achieved via deployment of two pushable coils at the distal internal maxillary artery measuring 2 mm × 1 cm each.

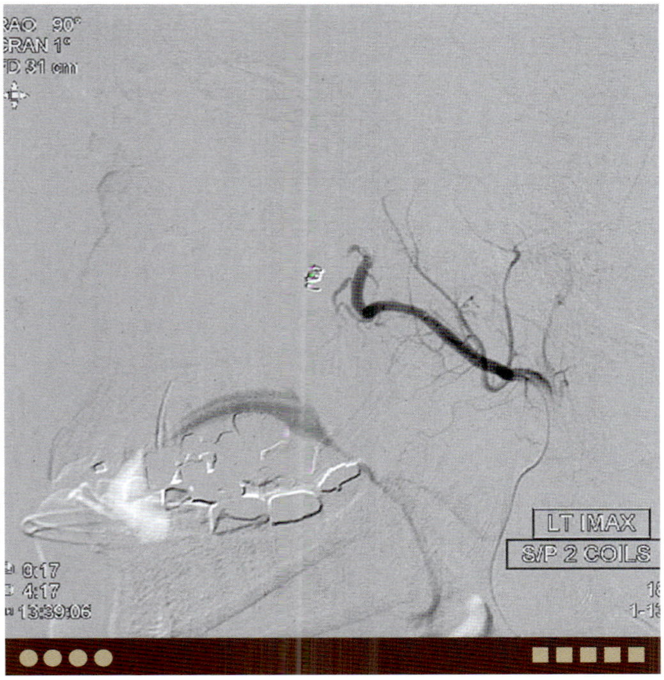

H. Epistaxis, same patient as A. Postembolization superselective left internal maxillary artery injection (lateral projection) shows no significant flow into the nasal cavity.

Case 14-4 Carotid Body Tumor

Junaid Kalia, Osama O. Zaidat

PRESENTATION

Gradually increasing painless pulsatile neck mass, cranial nerve impingement symptoms.

FINDINGS

Paragangliomas share common imaging findings and differ in location. Carotid body tumor has typical angiographic appearance located at the bifurcation of carotid artery as a with "tumor blush" rounded vascular mass. Contrast accumulates and produces a dense attenuation and puddling effect with prolonged intense blush. There may be splaying of the proximal internal carotid artery (ICA) and external carotid artery (ECA). The typical T2W MR finding is a "salt-and-pepper" hyperintense mass.

DIFFRENTIAL DIAGNOSIS

- Other paragangliomas: Paragangliomas (glomus jugulare, glomus vagale, and carotid body tumor) all have similar characteristics on angiography and MRI. The location is the differentiating factor for each subtype.

COMMENTS

This is a 42-year-old man who presented with a pulsatile right submandibular mass that was consistent with carotid body tumor on noninvasive imaging and treated with presurgical endovascular embolization.

Carotid body tumors are rare, benign tumors arising from glomus cells, originating from the embryonic neuroepithelium, which are chemoreceptors along blood vessels. Carotid body tumor accounts for 60% to 70% of head and neck paragangliomas. Paragangliomas are rare disorders that often affect women in there fifties and sixties presenting with a neck or oropharyngeal vascular mass and may cause cranial nerve symptoms.

Surgical excision is the treatment of choice for an enlarging symptomatic mass with preoperative embolization. Presurgical arteriography serves critical function in carotid body tumor evaluation including its exact location, extension, and its arterial feeders to different compartments of the tumor. It is vital during angiography to test the feasibility of temporarily occluding carotid artery that may be necessary intraoperatively to control bleeding. Arterial embolization is recommended in all carotid body tumors since by definition they are hypervascular. Superselective arteriography is recommended to identify dangerous anastomosis with ICA or vertebral artery as reflux of embolization material may lead to major neurological complications. Preferred embolization material is polyvinyl alcohol (PVA); size ranging from 45 to 510 μm in diameter as it has been shown to be safe and effective in reducing intraoperative hemorrhage.

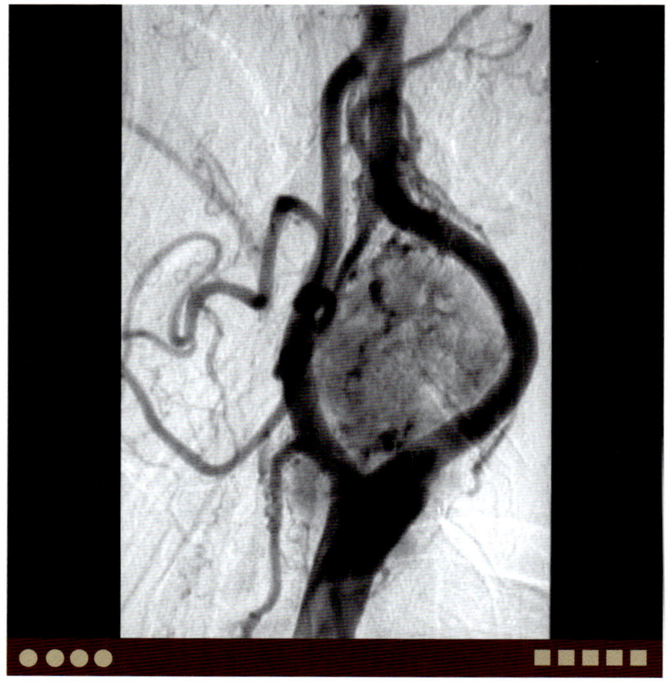

A. Carotid body tumor. Right common carotid arteriogram (lateral projection) at baseline shows a typical well-outlined dense vascular mass. A characteristic tumor blush at carotid bifurcation is appreciated consistent with diagnosis of carotid body tumor. Splaying of ICA and ECA is also seen.

PEARLS

- **Neither biopsy nor fine-needle aspiration is recommended due to high vascularity of the tumor.**
- **Preoperative angiography is mandatory for preoperative tumor evaluation including compartments, arterial feeders, dangerous anastomosis, and nerve impingement if any.**
- **Determination of the safety of temporarily occluding the carotid artery during open surgery should always be evaluated during preoperative angiography with balloon test occlusion.**
- **Preoperative embolization is recommended in all surgical cases to reduce intraoperative risk of major blood loss.**
- **Embolization is usually performed using particle of PVA from 45 to 510 μm in diameter.**
- **Surgical excision is recommended within a week to ensure no dissolution of the PVA particles in the interim.**

ADDITIONAL IMAGES (B-F)

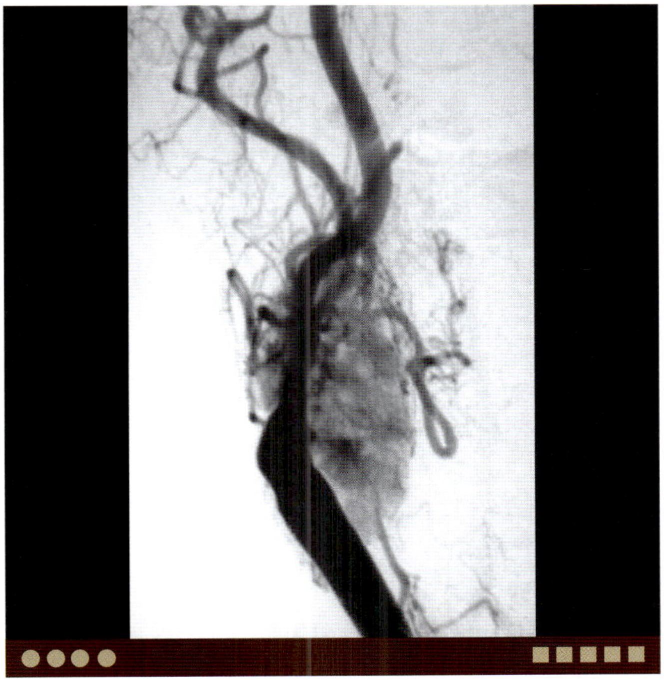

B. Carotid body tumor, same patient as A. Right common carotid arteriogram (frontal projection) at baseline shows characteristic tumor blush at carotid bifurcation. Overlapping of ICA and ECA is noted on the frontal projection.

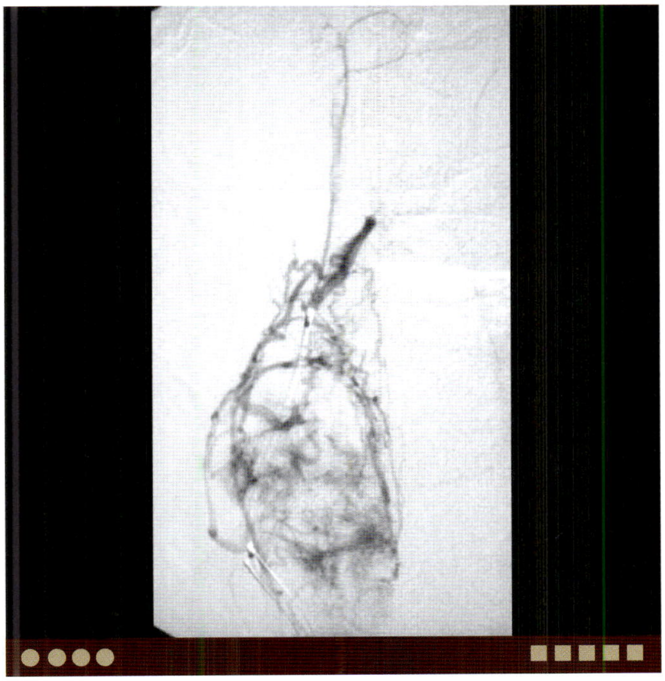

C. Carotid body tumor, same patient as A. Right ascending-pharyngeal superselective arteriogram (lateral projection) is performed to visualize anastomosis or collaterals and to identify major feeders.

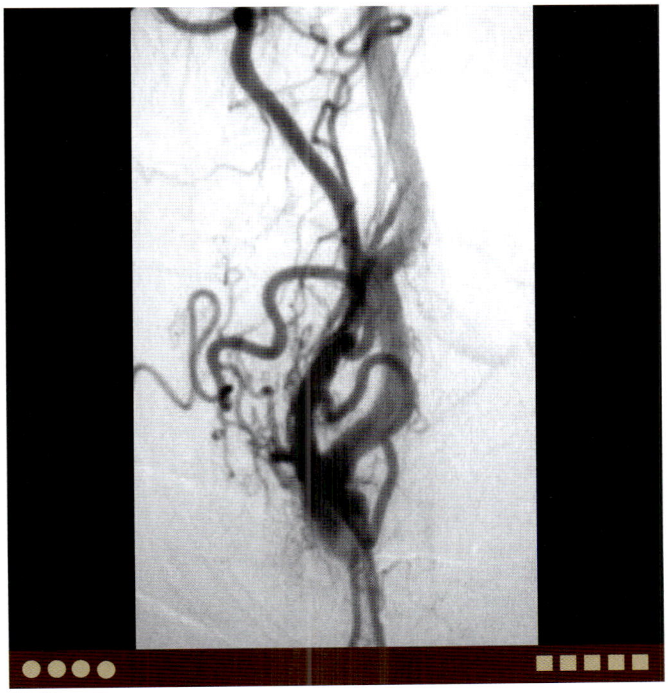

D. Carotid body tumor, same patient as A. Right common carotid arteriogram (frontal projection) postembolization with PVA particles shows near complete devascularization of the tumor.

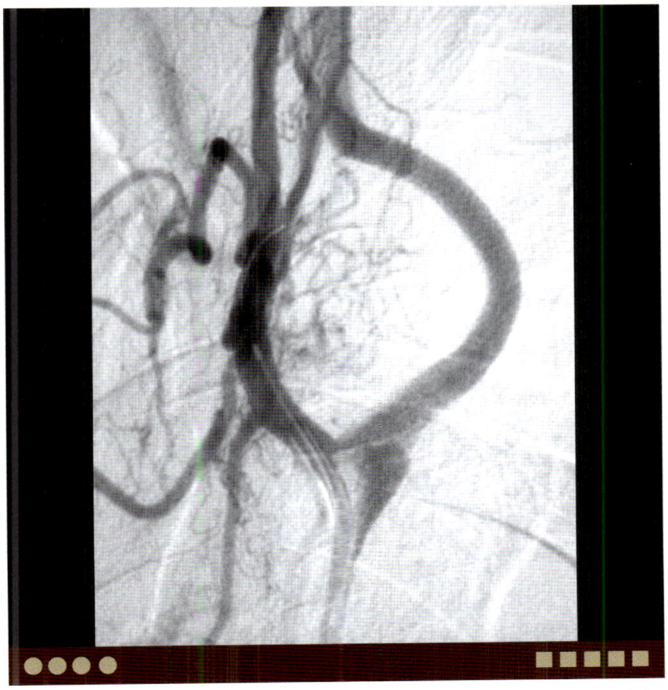

E. Carotid body tumor, same patient as A. Right common carotid arteriogram (lateral projection) postembolization with PVA particles shows near complete obliteration of the tumor blush.

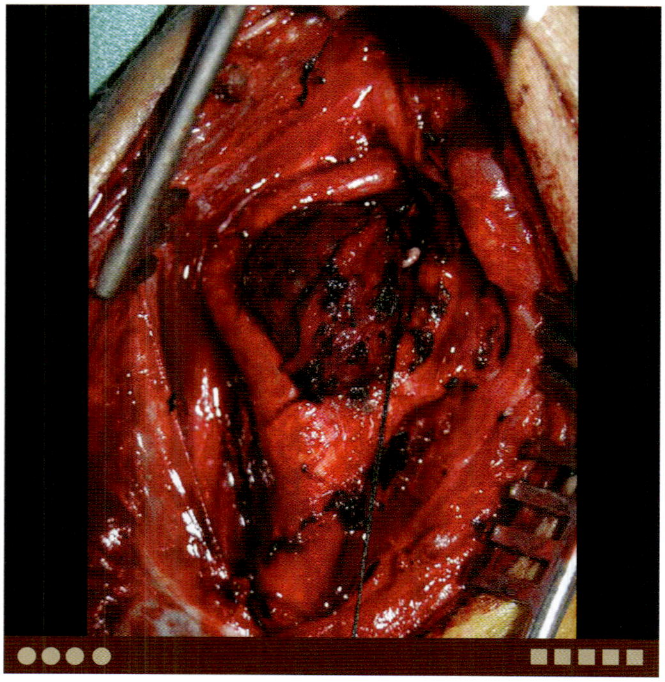

F. Carotid body tumor, same patient as A. Right common carotid bifurcation open surgical view shows splaying of carotid bifurcation and necrosis of the tumor from the embolization.

Case 14–5 Meningioma

Junaid Kalia, Osama O. Zaidat

PRESENTATION

Incidental extra-axial mass, seizures, neurological symptoms depending on location.

FINDINGS

Digital subtraction angiography reveals tumor vascular blush that takes the "spoke-wheel" appearance; where the main feeding meningeal artery is the center of the wheel and the intratumor capillary blush as the spoke. Tumor blush is appreciated according to the vascularity and size of the tumor characteristically comes early and leaves late. Intratumor arteriovenous shunting may also be seen. Mass effect with displacement of the intracranial arteries or occlusion of the venous sinuses may also be seen.

DIFFRENTIAL DIAGNOSIS

- Hemangiopericytoma: They are neoplasms of pericytes that originate in the meninges. Imaging findings of hemangiopericytoma may be similar to meningioma, but it is very vascular and locally aggressive, without bone thickening or intratumoral calcification.
- Metastasis: Dural metastases are seen as extra-axial masses. They tend to be multiples and less enhancing, although imaging findings can be very similar to meningioma.

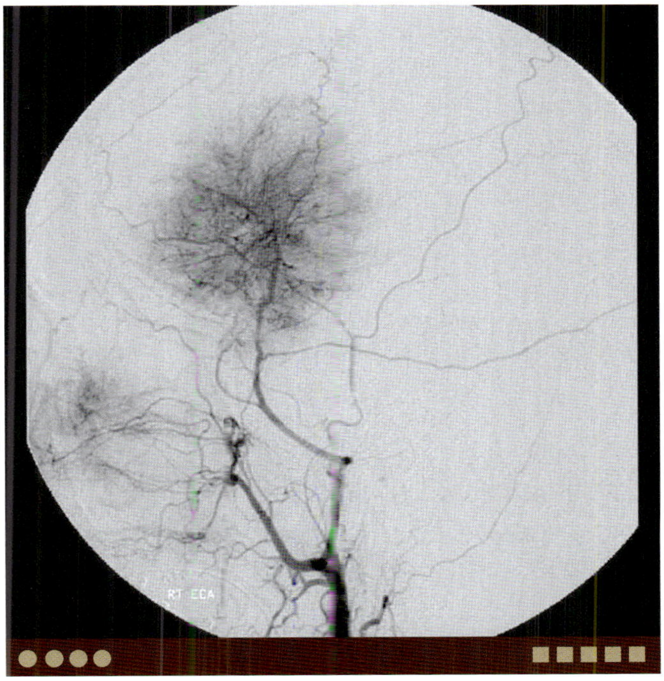

A. Meningioma. Right external carotid arteriogram (lateral projection) demonstrates hypervascular mass with typical "spoke-wheel" appearance tumor blush, consistent with meningioma. The main arterial feeder is via the frontoparietal branches of the right middle meningeal artery. A prominent nasal blush is also appreciated and should not be mistaken for meningioma.

COMMENTS

This is a 59-year-old woman presented with mental status change. MRI revealed an enhancing extra-axial mass along the right frontal lobe convexity with dural tail consistent with meningioma.

Meningiomas account for 15% of all intracranial tumors; present more commonly in adults (40-60 years) and in women (3:1). Meningiomas arise in intracranial convexities; parasagittal convexity (46%) being the most common. Most meningiomas do not require aggressive therapy. Asymptomatic incidental meningioma should be followed up with serial imaging for increase in size as roughly 7% of patients become symptomatic.

Angiographic evaluation is recommended in all meningioma cases preoperatively for surgical planning and possible preoperative embolization to reduce intraoperative blood loss, delineate the relationship to the adjacent venous and arterial structures to avoid venous or arterial infarcts, and for potentially easier resection of the necrotic tumor tissue after embolization. Vascular supply of meningiomas is usually via dural arteries. Highly vascular or large

PEARLS

- **Preoperative embolization of large and highly vascular tumors is recommended.**
- **It is essential to evaluate anastomosis and collaterals before embolization, particularly meningo-ophthalmic and ICA/ECA collateral that may lead to inadvertent intracranial particles migration and strokes.**
- **Embolization should be performed slowly to avoid particle reflux into proximal vessels, and using the largest inner-diameter microcatheter possible to avoid microcatheter occlusion.**
- **Combination of technique and material can be used depending on tumor location and feeders. Most commonly used material for preoperative tumor embolization is polyvinyl alcohol particles.**

tumors are recommended for preoperative embolization. Complete angiographic survey of all anastomosis and collateral circulation should be done prior to embolization. Major complications arise when material for embolization pass through collaterals into the intracranial circulation causing neurological deficits and stroke; especially when liquid agents are used. Particulate (polyvinyl alcohol [PVA], Gelfoam, etc.) or microspheres (gelatin, dextran, etc.) embolization should be performed as close as possible to the tumor bed and slowly to avoid reflux of particles into normal proximal vessels. Size of particle for embolization should be carefully chosen as smaller particles are preferred because of better tumor-bed penetration but may increase complication rates when injected proximally, since they may end up in more vital branches that are supplying cranial nerves. Using the largest inner-diameter microcatheter possible is recommended since it less likely to be prone to occlusion; as the particles tend to clog the smaller diameter microcatheters. There is currently no agreement on any one standardized technique or embolization material. The choice of technique and material is based on experience, vasculature, location, and accessibility. In general, expensive liquid agents are not preferred in preoperative tumor embolization.

ADDITIONAL IMAGES (B-J)

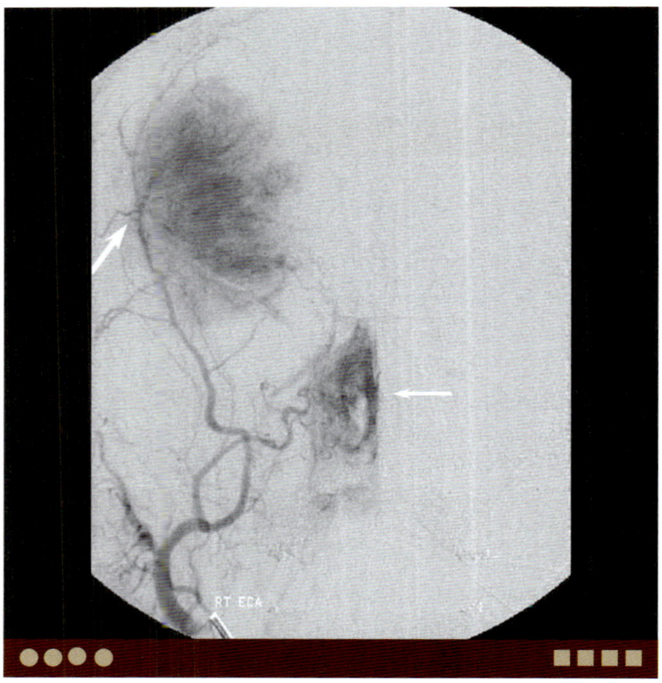

B. Meningioma, same patient as A. Right external carotid arteriogram (frontal projection) demonstrates a hypervascular mass consistent with meningioma. The main arterial feeder is via the frontoparietal branches of the right middle meningeal artery (arrow). A prominent nasal blush is also appreciated and should not be mistaken for meningioma (small arrow).

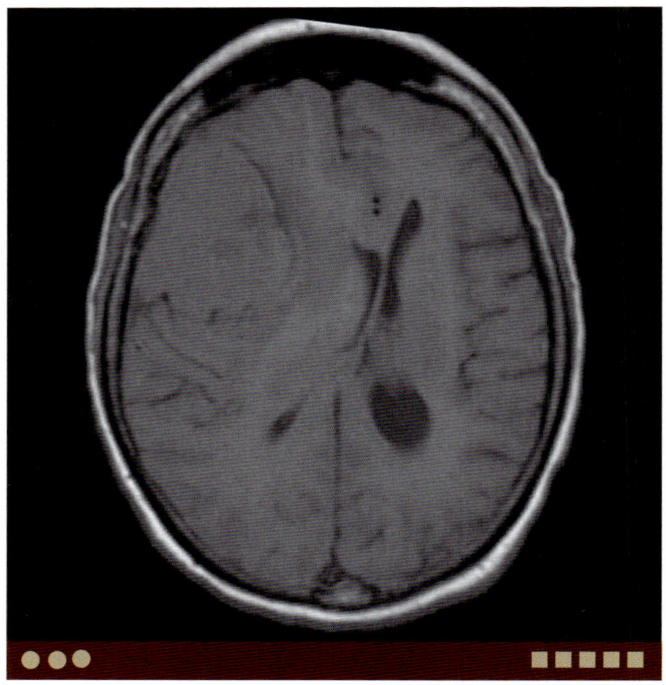

C. Meningioma, same patient as A. Axial precontrast T1W MR image shows a large extra-axial frontal mass with significant amount of surrounding vasogenic edema and causing mass effect.

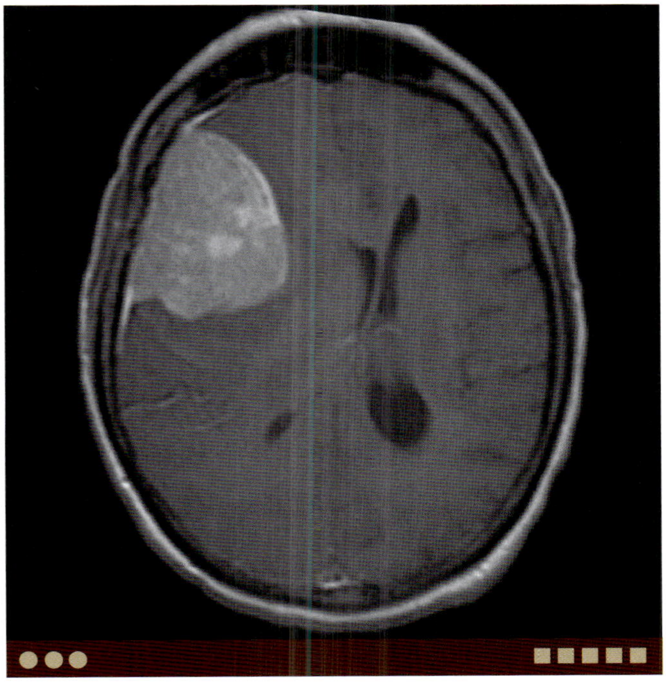

D. Meningioma, same patient as A. Axial postcontrast T1W image shows homogenous enhancement of the lesion with dural tail sign consistent with meningioma.

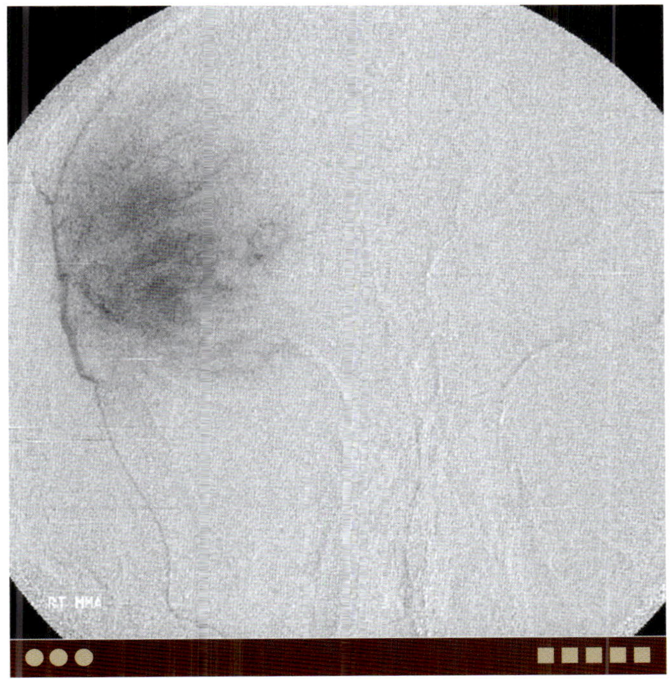

E. Meningioma, same patient as A. Superselective right middle meningeal artery injection (frontal projection) confirms the dominant arterial supply to the tumor from the right middle meningeal artery without collateral or anastomosis with the intracranial circulation.

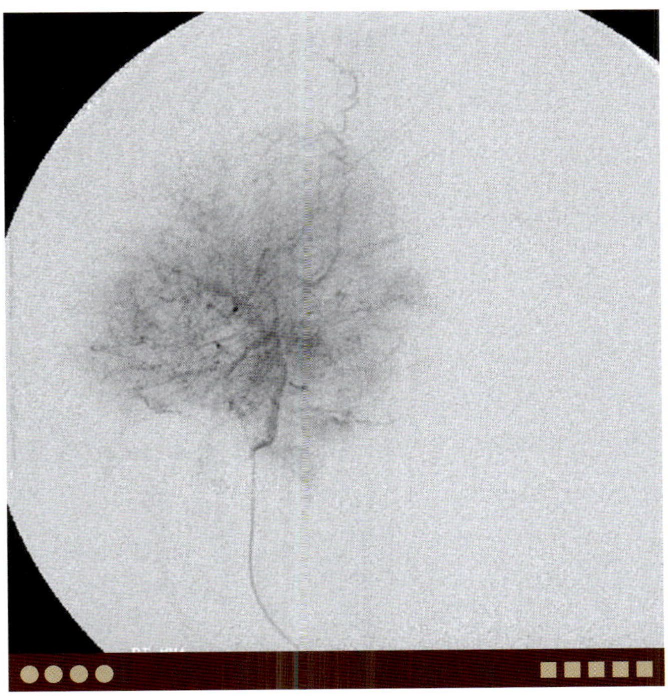

F. Meningioma, same patient as A. Superselective right middle meningeal artery injection (lateral projection) confirms the dominant arterial supply to the tumor from the right middle meningeal artery without collateral or anastomosis with the intracranial circulation.

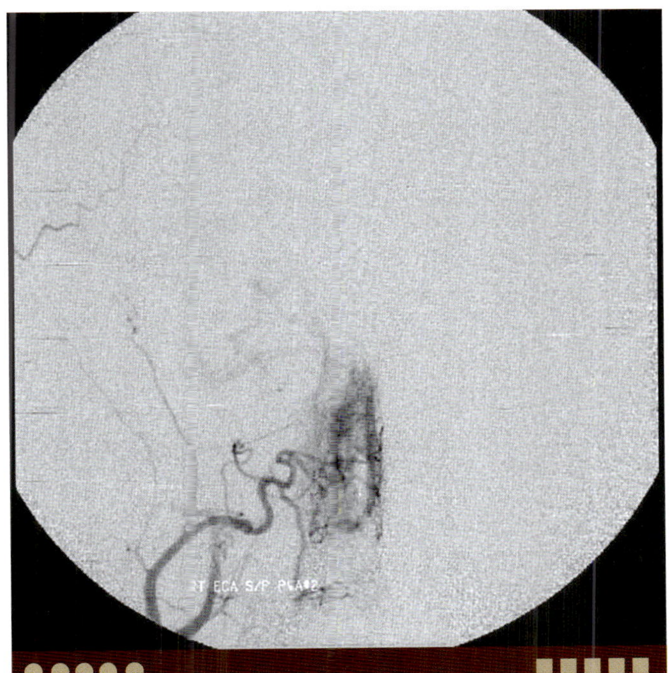

G. Meningioma, same patient as A. Embolization was performed via microcatheter injection of PVA microparticles (45-150 μm, 150-250 μm). Postembolization right external carotid arteriogram (frontal projection) shows negligible residual tumor blush.

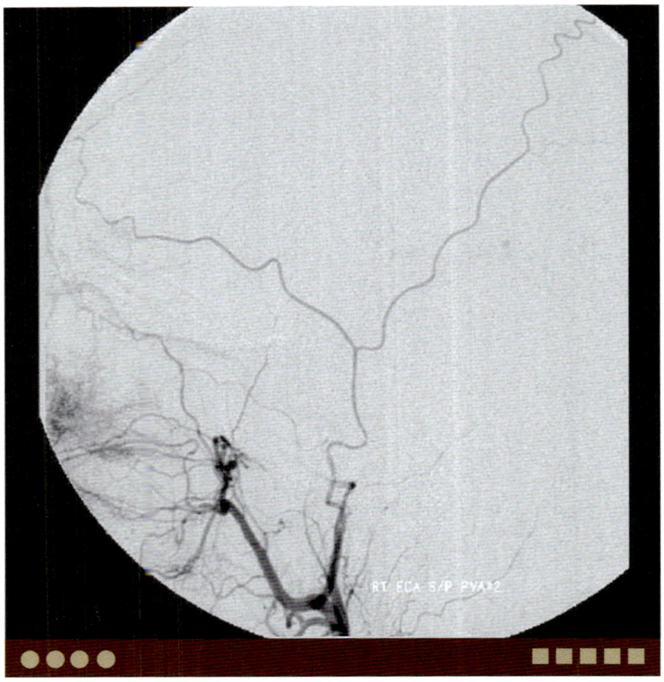

H. Meningioma, same patient as A. Postembolization right external carotid arteriogram (lateral projection) shows negligible residual tumor blush.

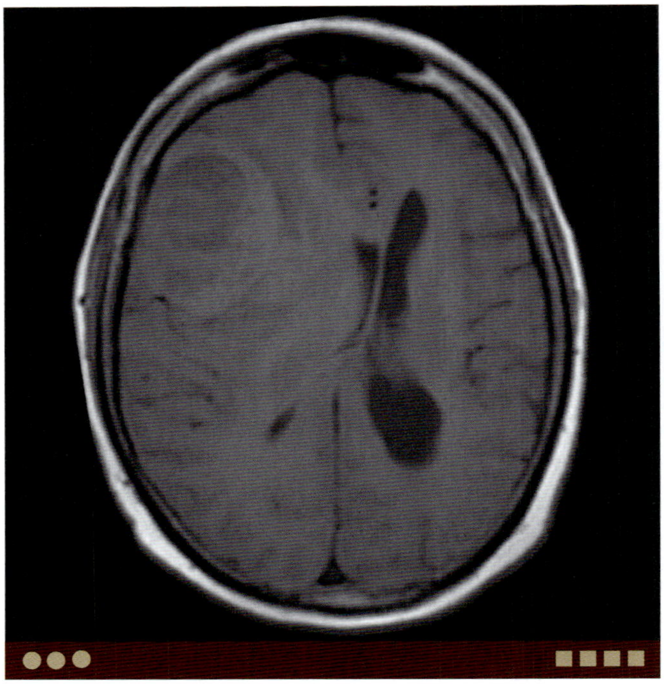

I. Meningioma, same patient as A. Postembolization axial T1W image shows a new low-signal area within the tumor.

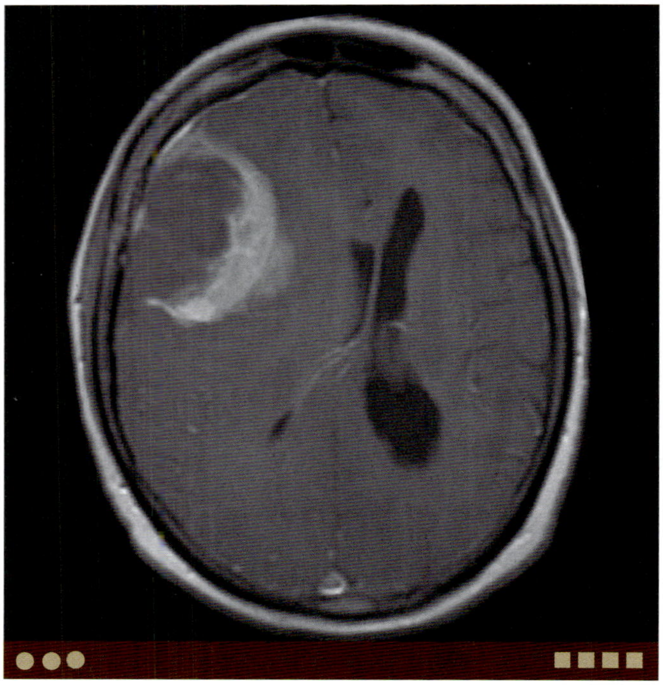

J. Meningioma, same patient as A. Postembolization axial postcontrast T1W image shows a nonenhancing area within the tumor consistent with devascularization by embolization.

Case 14–6 Meningioma

Thanh Nguyen, Daniel Roy, Francois Guilbert

PRESENTATION

Four months of progressive headache.

FINDINGS

MRI demonstrates an avidly enhancing extra-axial mass with dural tail and often with hyperostosis of the adjacent skull. Angiography reveals a hypervascular tumoral blush supplied by branches of the middle meningeal artery. The staining appears early, and persists into the venous phase.

DIFFRENTIAL DIAGNOSIS

- Hemangiopericytoma: They are neoplasms of pericytes that originate in the meninges. Imaging findings of hemangiopericytoma may be similar to meningioma, but it is very vascular and locally aggressive, without bone thickening or intratumoral calcification.
- Metastasis: Dural metastases are seen as extra-axial masses. They tend to be multiples and less enhancing, although imaging findings can be very similar to meningioma.

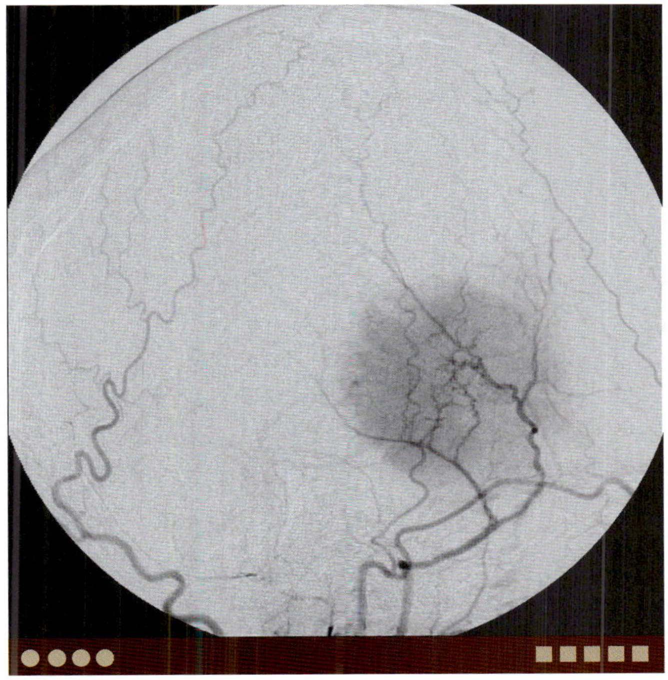

A. Meningioma. Right external carotid arteriogram (lateral projection) demonstrates a hypervascular tumoral blush supplied by two branches of the middle meningeal artery.

COMMENTS

A 43-year-old woman presented with 4 months of progressive headache.

Meningiomas are commonly located at the surface of the brain, at the skull base or its convexity. They arise from arachnoidal cap cells, which is located in the arachnoid layer covering the surface of the brain. Preoperative angiographic evaluation of meningioma is helpful to plan for the surgical resection of the tumor.

Angiographic findings of meningioma are hypervascular tumoral blush, with centrifugal or radial pattern, and prolonged blush, which appears early in the arterial phase and persists to late venous phase. Frequent supplies are middle meningeal artery (MMA), accessory meningeal, ascending pharyngeal, tentorial and inferolateral trunk. Infrequently, pial supply may occur secondarily via anterior cerebral artery, middle cerebral artery, and posterior cerebral artery. Retinal choroid blush and retinal supply should be identified prior to embolization. Further, venous sinus involvement should be identified for surgical planning

Preoperative embolization is helpful in reducing intraoperative blood loss, and is usually performed within a week of the operation. Identification of dangerous anastomosis and peripheral nerve supply is important. MMA anastomosis to the orbit, via the recurrent meningeal artery through the superior orbital fissure and MMA supplies the lacrimal gland, via the meningolacrimal branch through Hyrtl canal. Maxillary artery and cavernous internal carotid artery (ICA) anastomosis via inferolateral trunk through foramen of rotundum. In addition, neuromeningeal trunk of the ascending pharyngeal artery and supply to cranial nerves 9,10, and 11.

Intervention: Microcatheterization of the MMA showed the tumoral blush and absence of orbital anastomoses. Embolization of two branches of the MMA with 355 to 500 µm particles (Boston Scientific, Natick, MA). After embolization through the distal MMA branch, microcatheter injection showed reflux opacification to the ophthalmic artery and orbit. The more proximal MMA branch was then embolized with careful attention not to reflux to the opthalmic artery anastomosis. Postembolization angiogram showed good devascularization of the tumor.

Clinical course: The patient did well, without visual sequelae.

PEARLS

- **Dangerous anastomoses are always present, even if not angiographically visible. The preferential flow to the tumor may mask these anastomoses prior to embolization. These anastomoses may open or become apparent after embolization due to flow redirection.**
- **Larger particle injection may be less vulnerable to embolization to the most distal end organs (ie, retina).**

ADDITIONAL IMAGES (B-H)

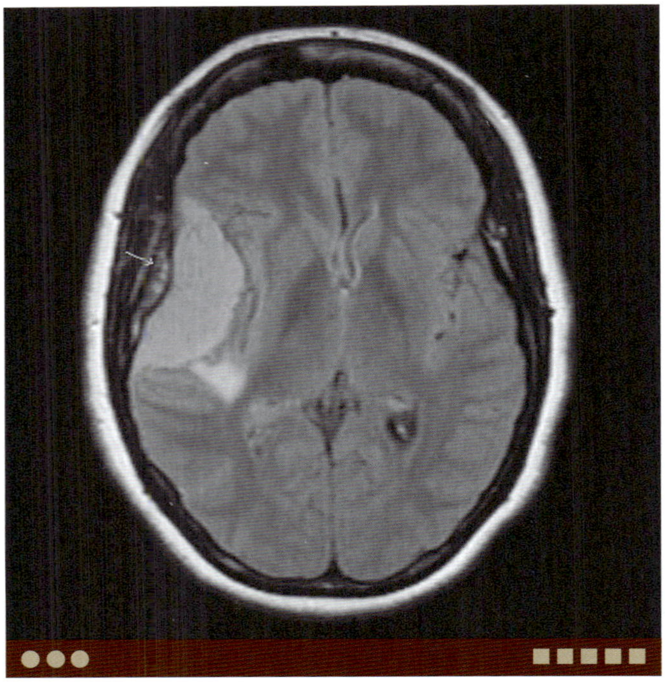

B. Meningioma, same patient as A. Axial FLAIR MR image shows a hyperintense right frontal extra-axial mass. Note hyperostosis of the adjacent skull (arrow).

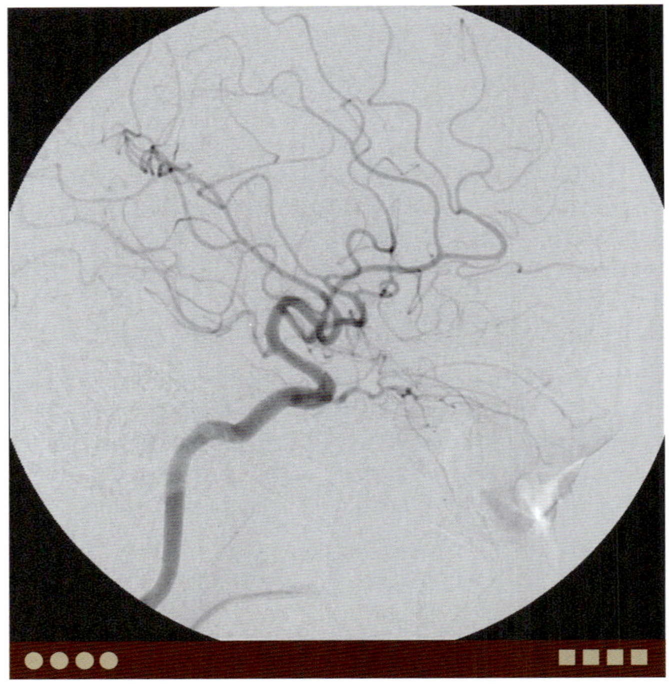

C. Meningioma, same patient as A. Right ICA injection (lateral projection) demonstrates a low ophthalmic artery origin and its supply to the orbit and retina.

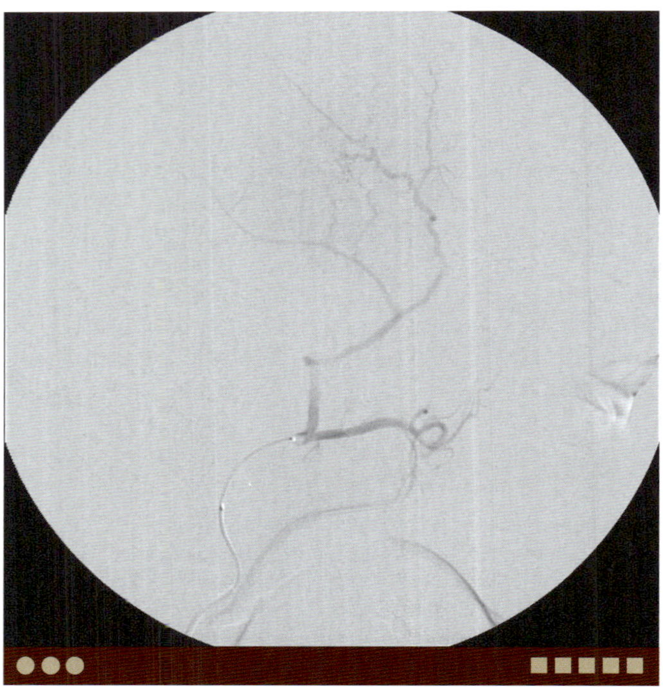

D. Meningioma, same patient as A. Preembolization microcatheter selective MMA injection (lateral projection) demonstrates no orbital anastomosis.

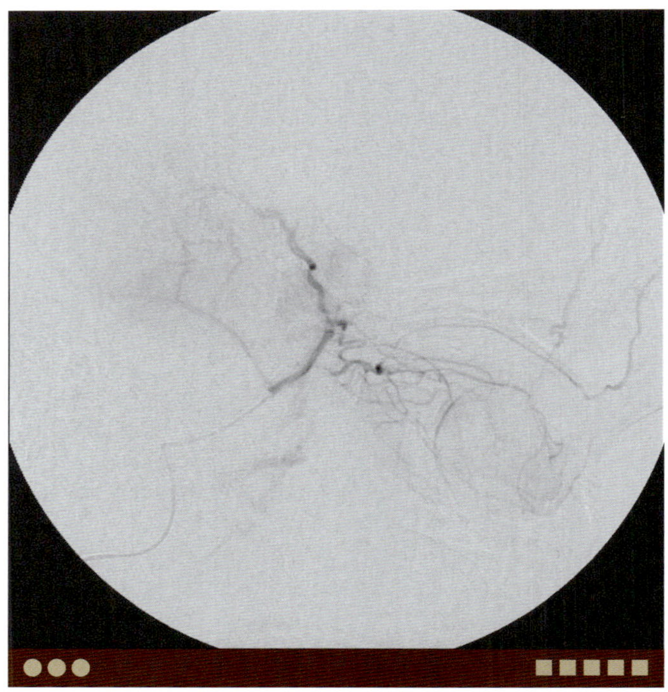

E. Meningioma, same patient as A. After embolization of a distal branch of the MMA, microcatheter injection (lateral projection) shows reflux opacification to an ophthalmic artery anastomosis (arrow).

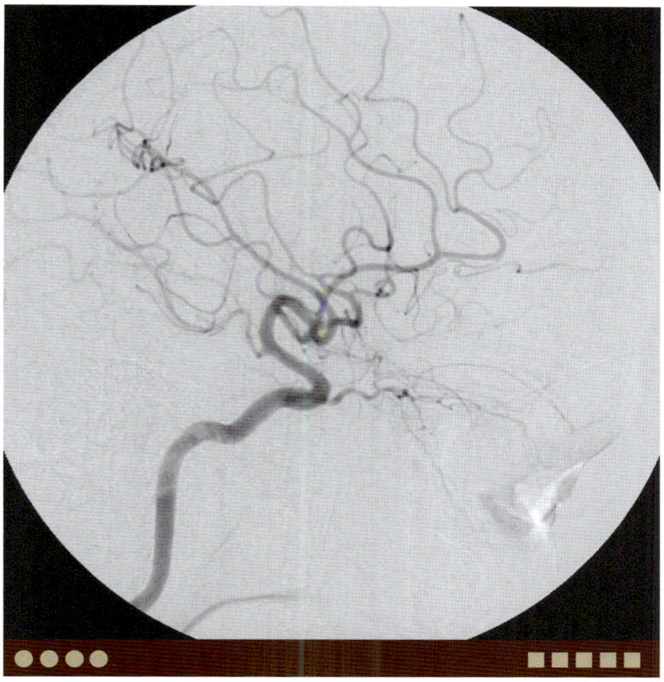

F. Meningioma, same patient as A. Comparison view of right ICA injection (lateral projection) shows the ophthalmic artery anastomosis to MMA.

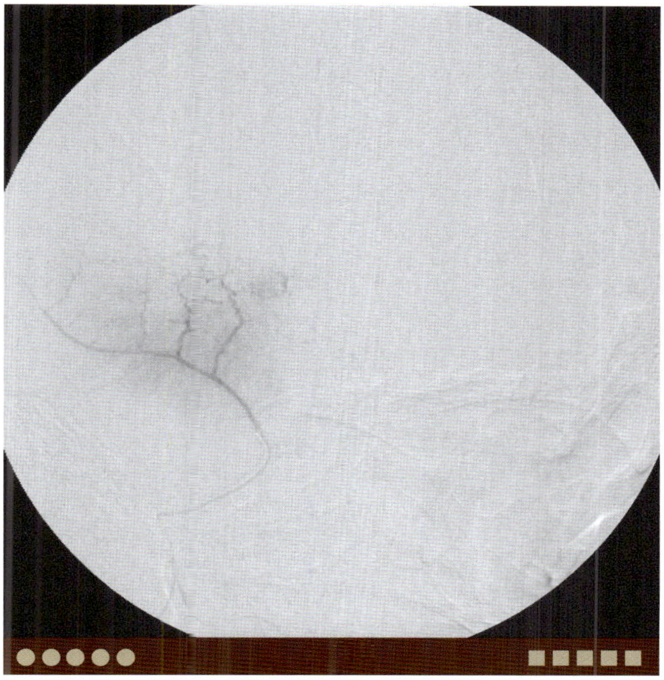

G. Meningioma, same patient as A. Selection of a proximal MMA branch (lateral projection) and embolization with 355 to 500 μm particles.

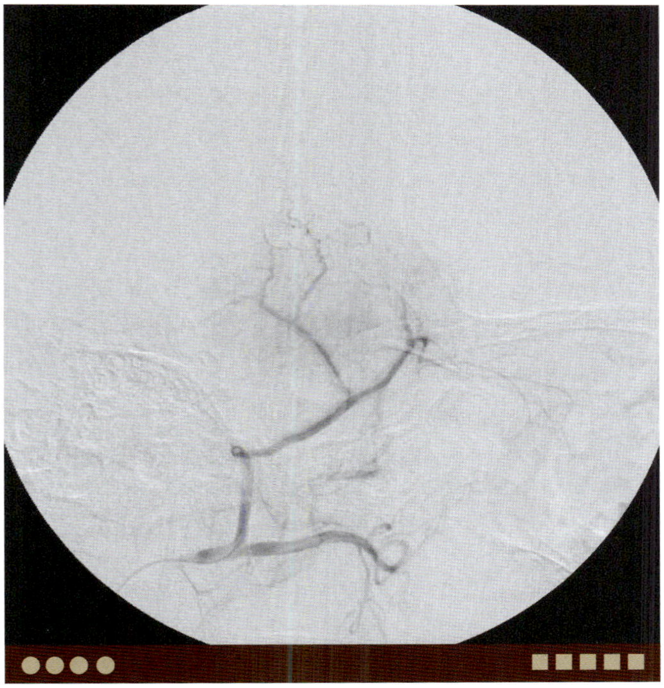

H. Meningioma, same patient as A. Control angiography postembolization (lateral projection) shows good devascularization of the tumor.

Case 14–7 Juvenile Angiofibroma

Thanh Nguyen, Alexander Norbash

PRESENTATION

Nasal obstruction, epistaxis, and headache.

FINDINGS

MRI revealed a large hypervascular nasopharyngeal lesion, centered on the pterygopalatine fossa and extending both medially into the nasopharynx, and laterally into the masticator space through the pterygomaxillary fissure.

DIFFERENTIAL DIAGNOSIS

- In the differential, other causes of nasal obstruction could be considered: nasal polyps, antrochoanal polyp, teratoma, encephalocele, dermoids, inverted papilloma, rhabdomyosarcoma, and squamous cell carcinoma. The combination of hypervascular enhancement and flow-voids, when considered with the anatomic lesion centering in the sphenopalatine foramen, is rather specific.

COMMENTS

A 20-year-old man presented with nasal congestion over a year, and one episode of epistaxis. He also complained of loss of sense of smell and taste.

Juvenile angiofibromas are benign and often bulky tumors of the sinonasal cavity and nasopharynx which are highly vascular with dense enhancement and flow-voids. The typical presentation is recurrent epistaxis in young males, often associated with nasal obstruction.

Frequent blood vessel supply includes the internal maxillary artery branches, and often the ascending pharyngeal artery in addition to other surrounding distal territorial branch vessels. These tumors frequently recur after surgery (up to 60% of the time).

Selective microcatheter catheterization with presurgical particulate suspension embolization using 250 to 350 μm particles was performed. Postembolization angiography showed near-complete devascularization of the tumor.

The patient underwent postembolic surgical resection of the juvenile angiofibroma, resulting in 300 cc of blood loss and improvement of his symptoms.

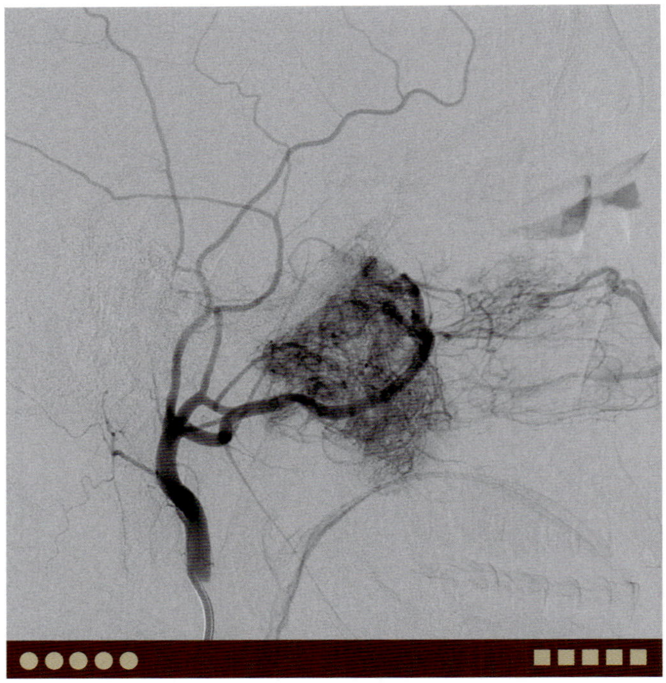

A. Juvenile angiofibroma. Selective external carotid artery injection (lateral view) shows a hypervascular blush with feeding primarily from a prominent internal maxillary artery.

PEARLS

- **Juvenile angiofibromas occur almost exclusively in young males.**
- **The tumor usually is centered behind the maxillary sinus within the sphenopalatine foramen, and bows the posterior wall of the maxillary sinus forward, often extending medially to the nasal cavity, laterally to the masticator space, inferiorly to the palate, and superiorly to the inferior orbital fissure and often the orbit.**
- **Avid enhancement on CT and dense enhancement with multiple flow-voids on MRI are characteristic findings.**

ADDITIONAL IMAGES (B-G)

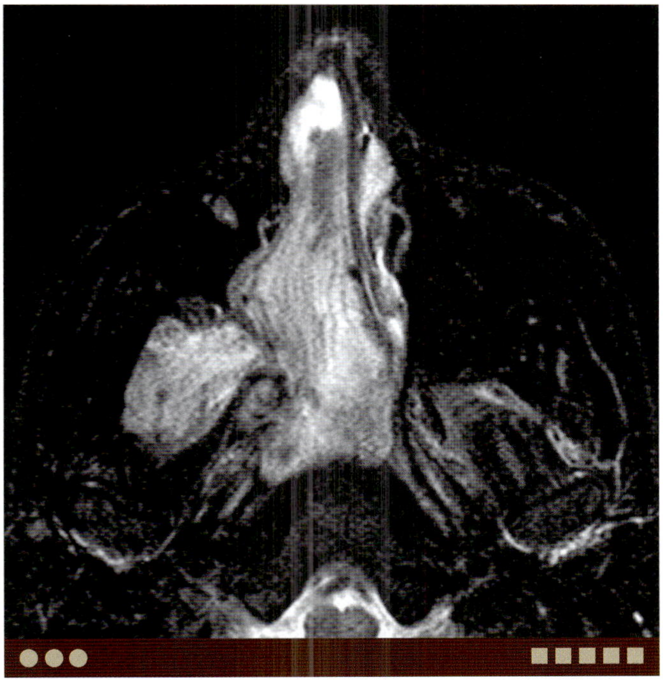

B. Juvenile angiofibroma, same patient as A. Axial fat-suppressed T2W image demonstrates the hyperintense tumor occupying and expanding the right pterygopalatine fossa with medial extension through the sphenopalatine foramen into the nasal cavity, and lateral extension to the pterygomaxillary fissure, and secondarily to the masticator space. Note flow-voids within the lesion.

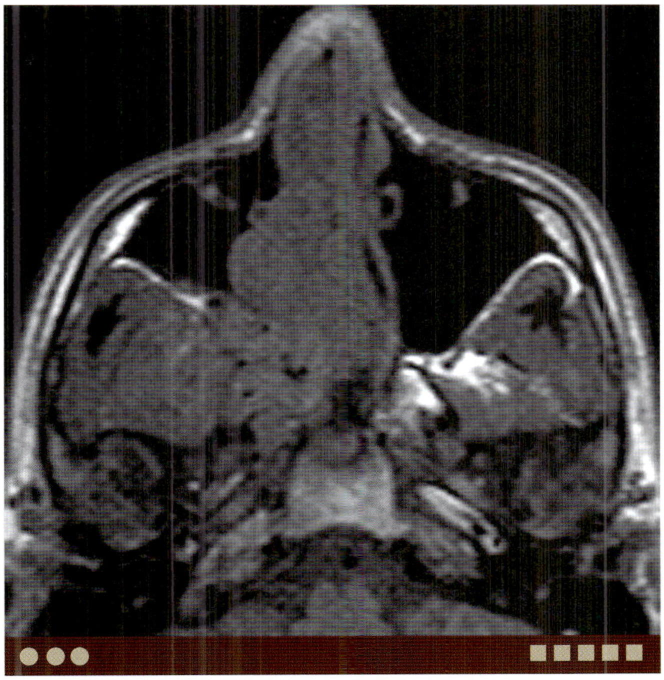

C. Juvenile angiofibroma, same patient as A. Axial T1W images demonstrate a low-signal lesion with internal flow-voids extending into the pterygopalatine fossa.

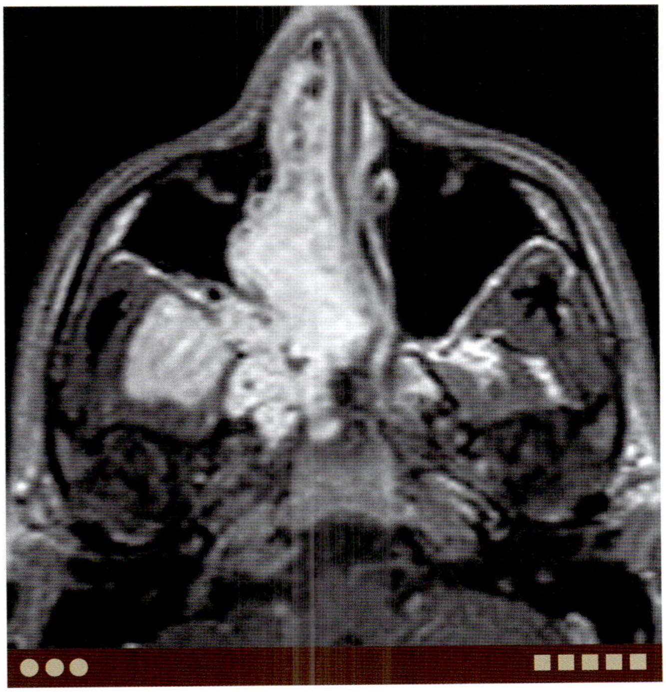

D. Juvenile angiofibroma, same patient as A. Axial postcontrast T1W images demonstrate avid enhancement of the hypervascular tumor. Flow-voids are again noted.

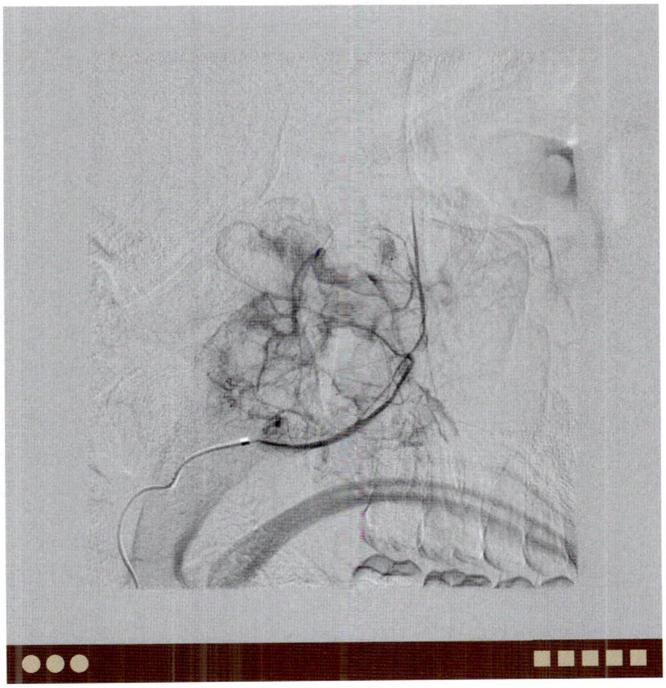

E. Juvenile angiofibroma, same patient as A. Preembolization superselective distal right internal maxillary artery injection (lateral view) confirms the hypervascular blush with less overlying external carotid artery branches shown in image "A."

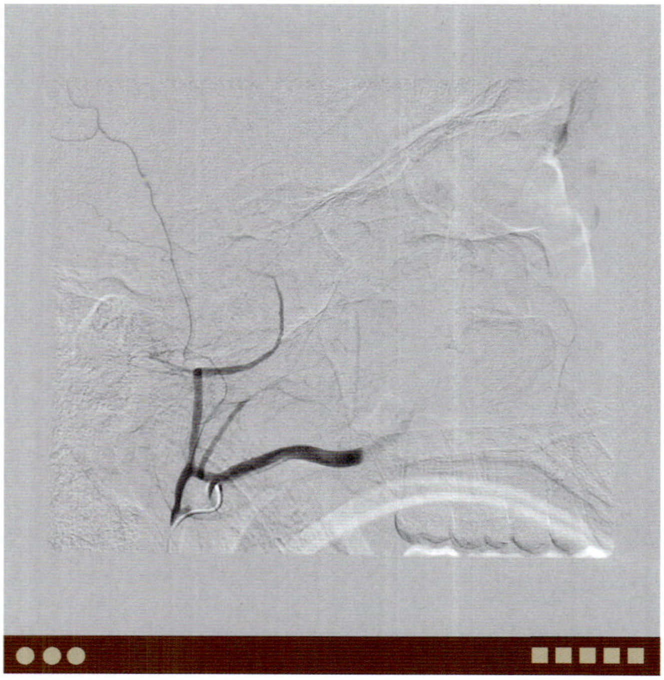

F. Juvenile angiofibroma, same patient A. Superselective distal right internal maxillary artery injection (lateral view) after particulate suspension embolization shows devascularization of the previously hypervascular tumor.

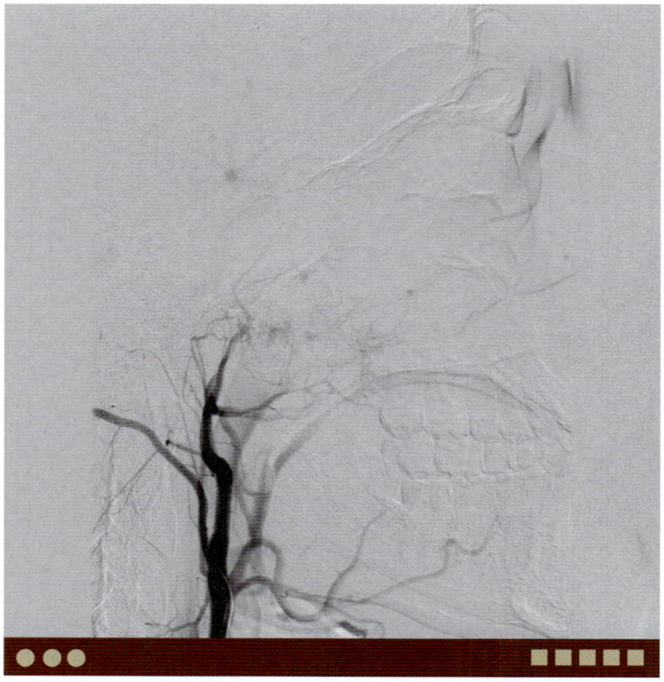

G. Juvenile angiofibroma, same patient A. Selective external carotid artery injection (lateral view) following particle embolization, compared with image "A," shows near-complete devascularization of the tumor.

Case 14–8 Arteriovenous Malformation

Hideki Hyodoh

PRESENTATION

Cheek swelling.

FINDINGS

Angiographic images demonstrate meandering arteries and draining veins

COMMENTS

This is a 56-year-old man with swelling of the right cheek.

Vascular malformation can be classified according to blood flow rate. High-flow malformations have many arterial components, whereas low-flow malformations have capillary, venous, lymphatic, or a combination of these components. This classification is accepted as the International Society for the Study of Vascular Anomalies (ISSVA) classification.

Arteriovenous malformation (AVM) is a benign, however, locally aggressive condition. AVMs can occur anywhere in the body, however, often arise in the head and neck.

On MRI, AVM demonstrates multiple meandering flow-voids, better seen on T2W image, and heterogeneous enhancement on postcontrast T1W images. MR fluoroscopy demonstrates the vascular circulation and blood flow. MR imaging is very helpful for therapeutic planning as well as to evaluate the therapeutic effect.

Complete destruction of the nidus is the only potential cure. Decreasing the clinical symptoms is another goal in treating problematic arteriovenous malformations. Nidus sclerotherapy is currently considered the best treatment. Surgical resection, medical therapy, and transarterial embolization have shown limited success but are associated with a high rate of recurrence and exacerbation.

Nidus ablation (occlusion) is the key to success. Nidus ablation with sclerotherapy is recommended, and proximal (or distal) embolization must be avoided. General anesthesia or nerve block is recommended during sclerotherapy except polidocanol sclerotherapy. The following sclerosants are used; 1) absolute ethanol: the most effective material, only well-trained hand can use, high rate of complication (skin necrosis, nerve damage), maximum dose 1.0 mL/kg, 2) ethanolamine oleate (EO): the second most effective material, mixed with nonionized contrast, flow control technique (balloon, tourniquet) must be used, risk for complications (hemolysis, skin necrosis), maximum dose 5% EO 0.4 mL/kg (0.02 g/kg, and 3) polidocanol: mixed with contrast (1-2 mL) or air (4 mL), risk for complications (skin necrosis, bradycardia), maximum dose 2 mg/kg.

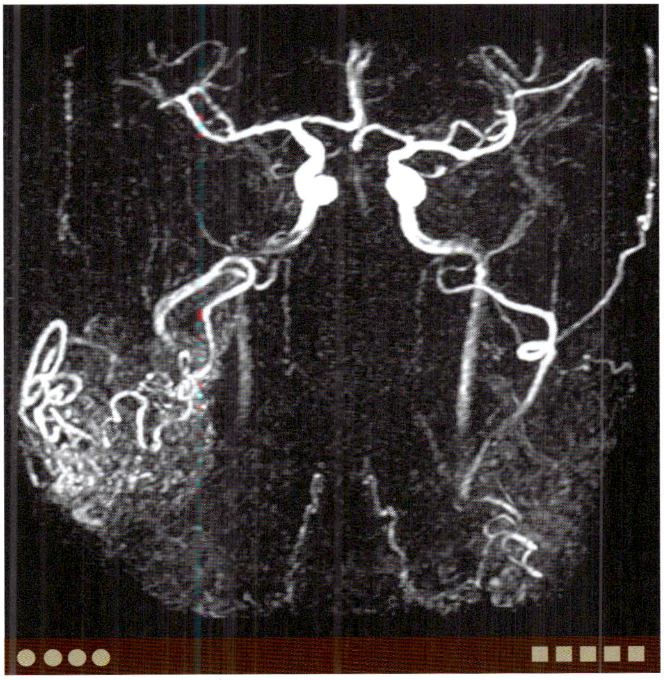

A. AVM. Contrast-enhanced MR angiography using the 3D time-resolved imaging of contrast kinetics technique (3D-TRICKS) demonstrates a large vascular mass with meandering arteries and draining veins in the right cheek.

PEARLS

- **AVM is the anomalous connection between the artery and vein without normal capillary bed.**
- **Conventional catheter angiogram is the gold standard. But contrast-enhanced MRA is very helpful for treatment planning and follow-up.**
- **Nidus sclerotherapy is the key to the success of the interventional radiology procedure.**

ADDITIONAL IMAGES (B-F)

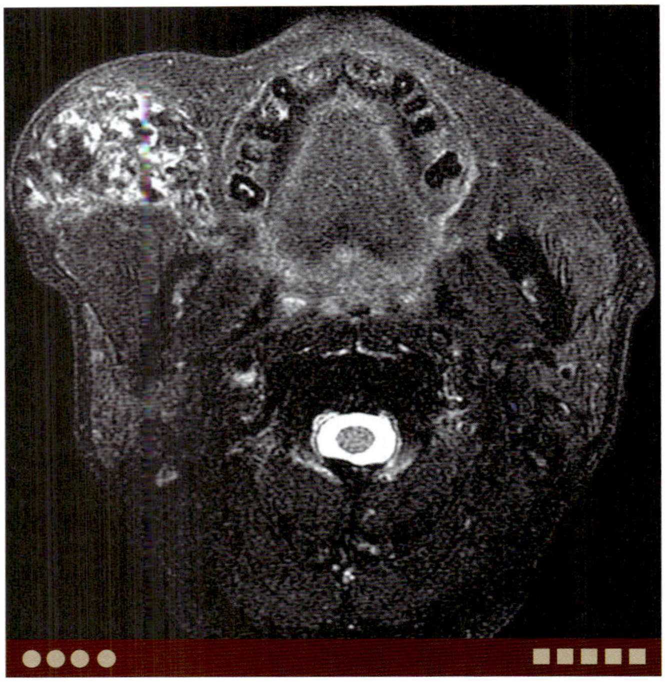

B. AVM. Axial fat-suppressed T2W image with demonstrates an ill-defined high-signal intensity mass with multiple flow-voids.

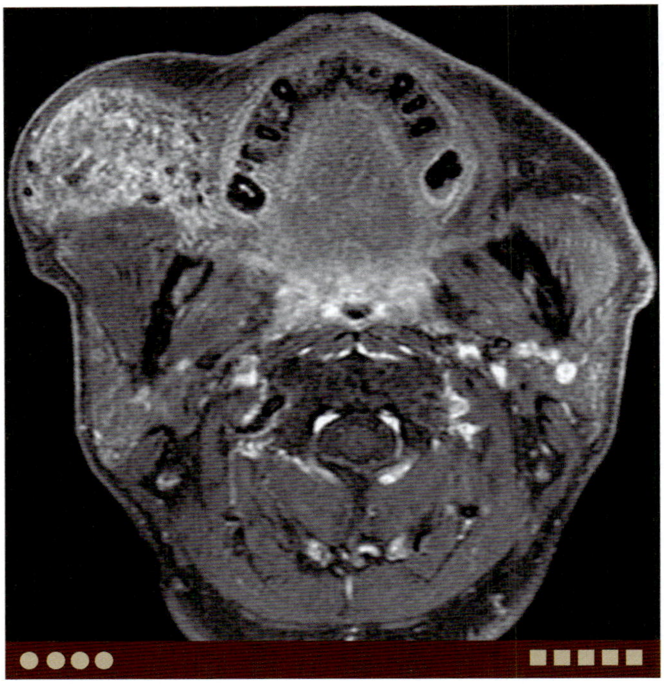

C. AVM. Axial postcontrast fat-suppressed T1W image demonstrates heterogeneous enhancement of the lesion with numerous flow-voids, extending from the buccal space to the masticator space.

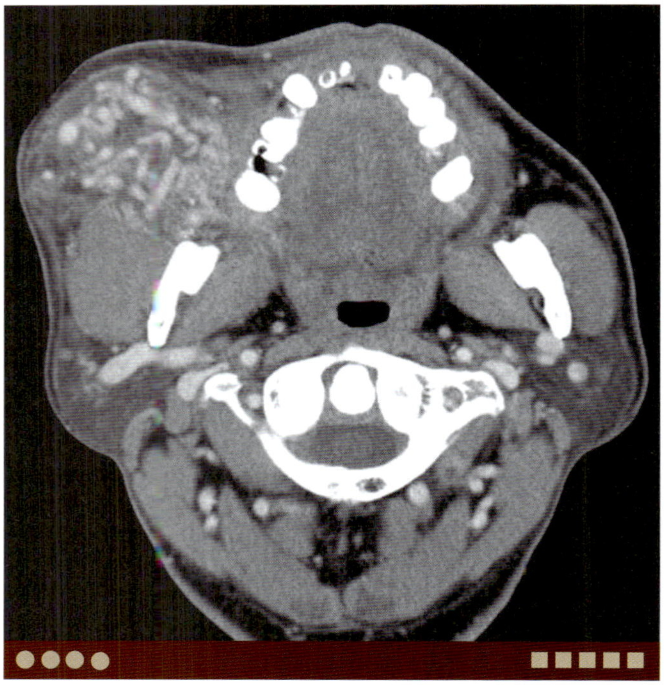

D. AVM. Axial contrast-enhanced CT demonstrates dilated vasculature within the lesion.

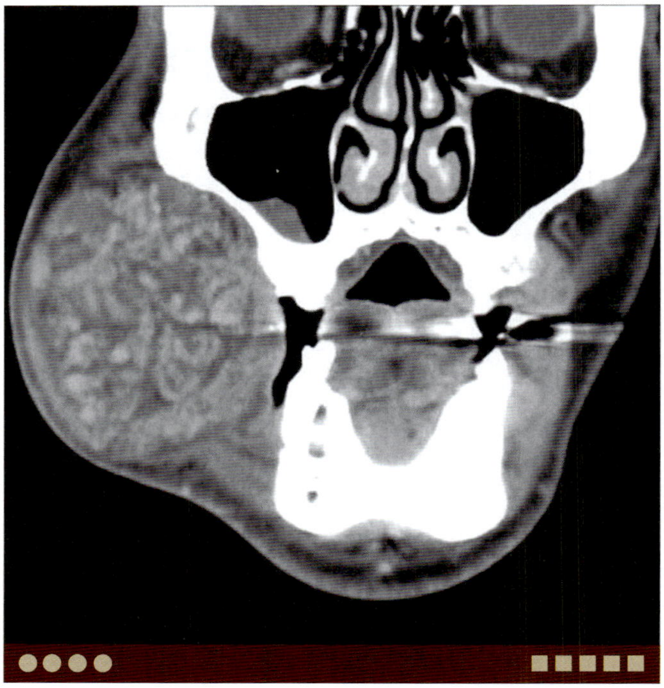

E. AVM. Coronal contrast-enhanced CT demonstrates a large heterogeneously enhancing lesion with numerous meandered vasculatures in the right cheek.

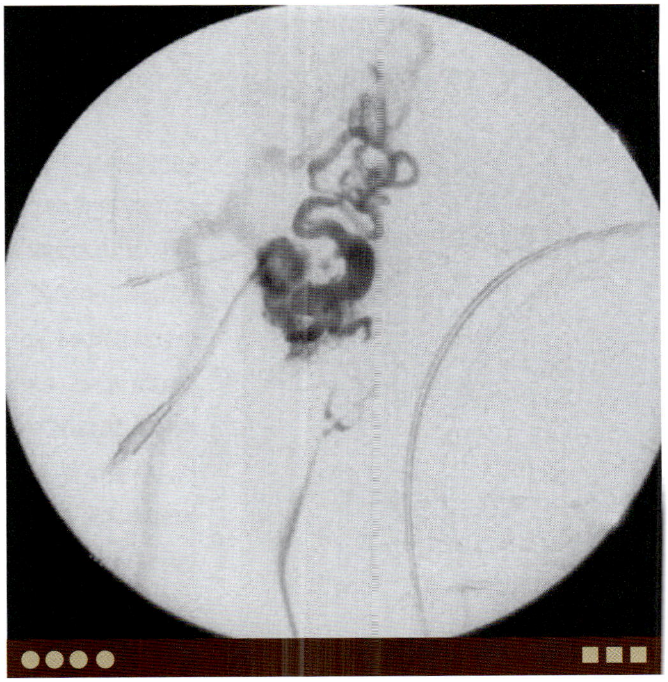

F. **AVM.** Direct puncture digital subtraction angiography (DSA) shows an ill-defined, meandered vasculature. Occlusion balloon catheter is placed in the right external carotid artery.

DIFFERENTIAL DIAGNOSIS IMAGE (G)

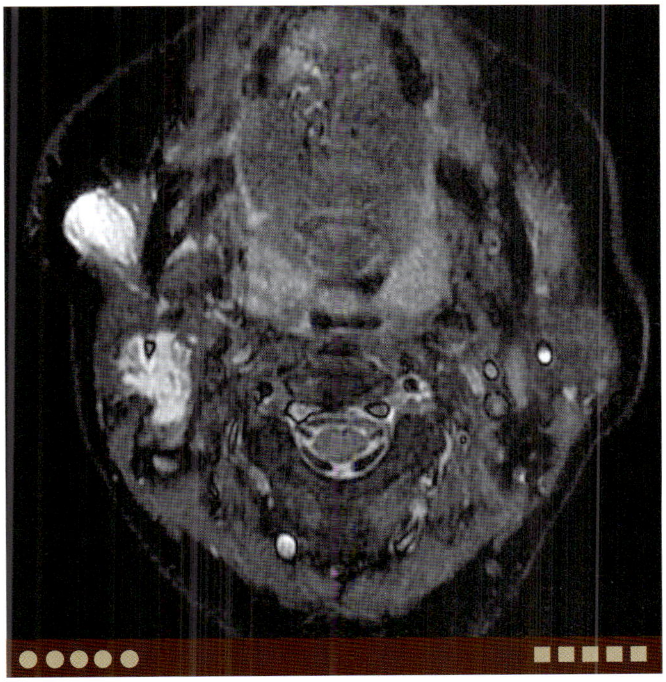

G. Venous malformation in a 58-year-old woman. Axial fat-suppressed T2W MR image demonstrates high-signal intensity lesions without flow-voids in the right masticator, buccal and parotid spaces.

Chapter 15

RADIOTHERAPY

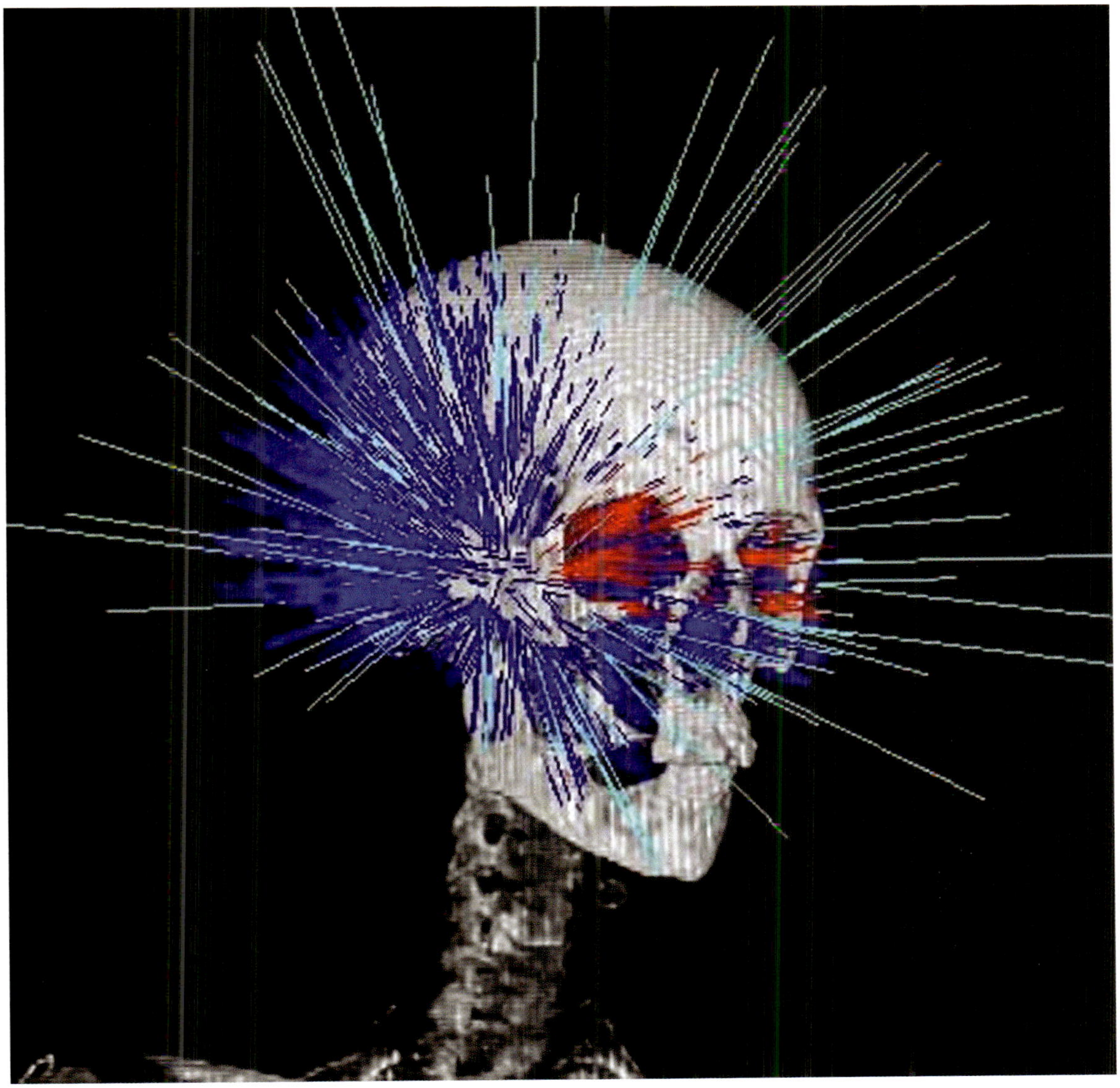

Case 15-1 Nasopharyngeal Carcinoma

Danielle Margalit, Osamu Sakai, Minh Tam Truong

PRESENTATION

Neck mass, hearing loss, otalgia, otitis media secondary to obstruction of the eustachian tube, nasal bleeding or obstruction, cranial nerve deficits, or trismus.

FINDINGS

CT and MRI show a mass involving the fossa of Rosenmüller with opacified mastoid air cells.

DIFFERENTIAL DIAGNOSIS

- Lymphoma: Lymphomas show very similar imaging findings to nasopharyngeal carcinoma (NPC), particularly WHO type III, and is very difficult to be differentiated from NPC. Lymphoma may show more homogeneous signal and infiltrative invasion rather than destruction.
- Enlarged adenoids: Proliferation of lymphoid tissue without involvement of the prevertebral muscles or clivus.
- Minor salivary gland tumors: More focal or localized, mass formation initially.

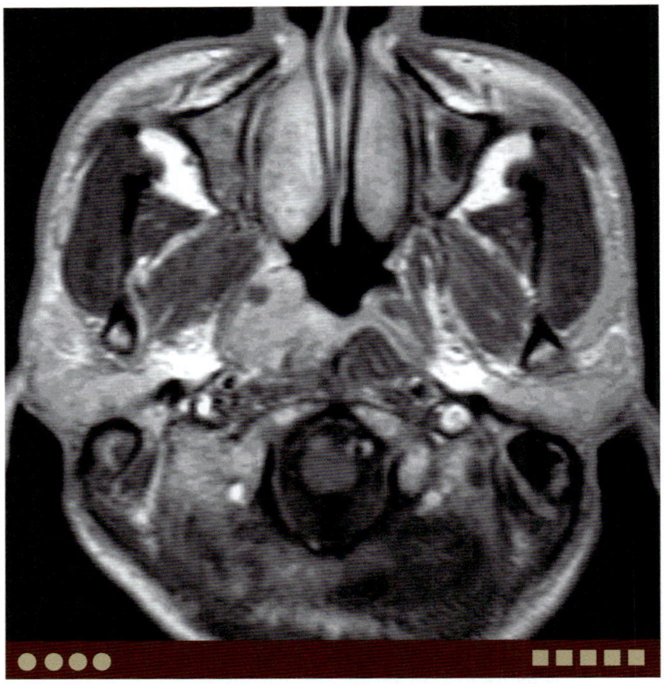

A. Nasopharyngeal carcinoma. Axial Postcontrast T1W image demonstrates an enhancing mass in the right nasopharynx obliterating the fossa of Rosenmüller with infiltration into the right longus colli muscle.

COMMENTS

This is a 44-year-old Asian man who presented with progressive right hearing loss, right otalgia, and a right middle ear effusion. Flexible nasolaryngoscopy revealed a mass based in the right fossa of Rosenmüller compressing the eustachian tube orifice. CT and MRI of the neck revealed a heterogeneously enhancing mass in the right nasopharynx obliterating the fossa of Rosenmüller and invasion of the right longus colli muscles and sphenoid sinus. There was abnormal soft tissue in the right pterygopalatine fossa and widening of the Vidian canal. There was an enlarged right level IIB lymph node. Biopsy revealed invasive nasopharyngeal carcinoma, undifferentiated nonkeratinizing type, World Health Organization (WHO) type III. The polymerase chain reaction (PCR) assay for Epstein-Barr virus (EBV) demonstrated EBV DNA was present. The clinical stage was T4N1M0, stage IV. The patient received concurrent chemoradiation therapy using cisplatin and a total dose of 70 Gy to the primary tumor and involved lymph node and 56 Gy to the uninvolved bilateral neck. Intensity-modulated radiation therapy was used to minimize dose to the temporal lobes, brain, brain stem, spinal cord, parotid glands, larynx, and esophagus.

Primary radiotherapy is the standard of care for early- and advanced-stage nasopharyngeal carcinoma. The Intergroup 0099 randomized control trial demonstrated an overall survival and progression-free survival benefit with the addition of concurrent cisplatin to radiation therapy in patients with locally advanced nonmetastatic nasopharyngeal carcinoma. Subsequent meta-analysis confirmed the benefit of adding cisplatin based chemotherapy to radiation therapy.

PEARLS

- **There are three histologic types of nasopharyngeal carcinoma: WHO type I (keratinizing squamous cell carcinoma), WHO type II (differentiated nonkeratinizing carcinoma), and WHO type III (undifferentiated carcinoma.). WHO type III is most prevalent in Southeast Asia where the incidence is 25 to 50 per 100,000.**
- **Primary radiation (+/– chemotherapy) is the standard treatment for nasopharyngeal cancer encompassing the primary tumor and bilateral elective regional neck nodes.**
- **Skull-base involvement can lead to cranial nerve neuropathies.**

While nasopharyngeal cancer is uncommon in the United States, it is prevalent in Southeast Asia, North Africa, and among the Inuit of Alaska. Environmental, viral, and genetic factors play more of a role than alcohol and tobacco which are typically risk factors for the sporadic WHO type I form. Epstein-Barr virus has been shown to be a potential etiologic factor. Response to treatment correlates with decreasing serum EBV titers in patients with EBV-positive NPC. Additional risk factors include smoking, and a diet high in salt-cured fish. There is a high incidence of lymphadenopathy at presentation and 50% of patients present with bilateral neck disease. The most commonly involved lymph nodes are the retropharyngeal nodes. A common pathway of early skull-base invasion is via the foramen lacerum and the petroclinoid fissure. Approximately 20% of patients present with cranial nerve involvement of which cranial nerves V2, V3, and V1 are most commonly involved.

TREATMENT

Radiation therapy alone for early T stage, lymph node–negative disease. Radiation therapy with concurrent cisplatin based chemotherapy for locally advanced disease (stage T2 and higher) followed by adjuvant chemotherapy is recommended based on the Intergroup study.

ADDITIONAL IMAGES (B-G)

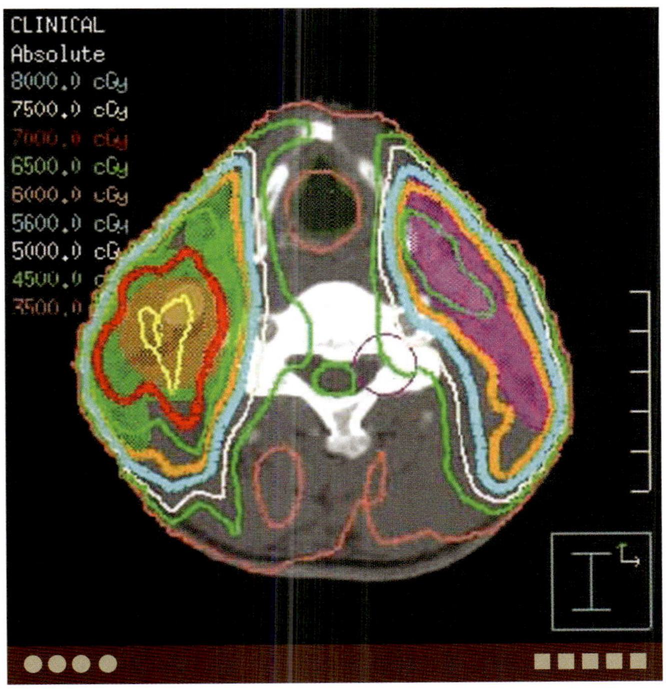

B. NPC, same patient as A. Axial radiation treatment plan using intensity-modulated radiation therapy (IMRT). Red line represents 70-Gy line encompassing primary tumor and involved nodes. Orange line represents 60-Gy line encompassing upper neck. Light blue line represents 56-Gy line encompassing lower neck.

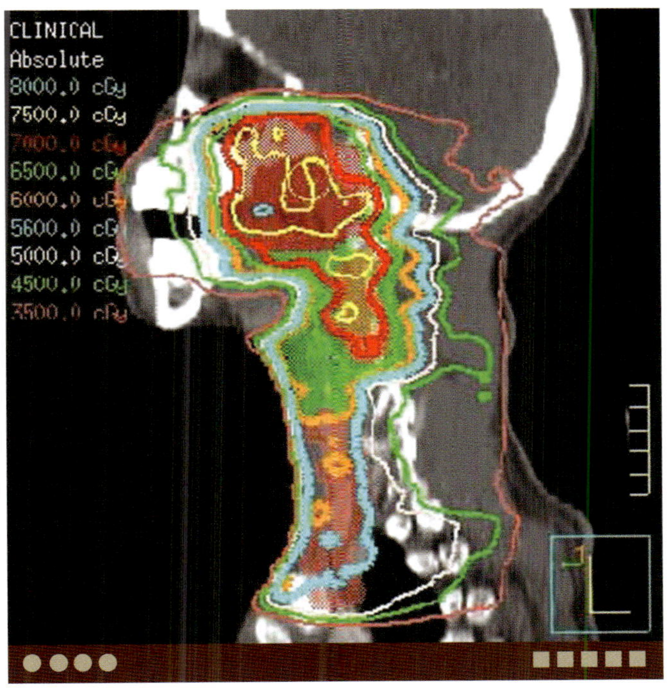

C. NPC, same patient as A. Sagittal radiation treatment plan using IMRT. Bilateral parotid glands, oral cavity, larynx, postcricoid area, and spinal cord are spared to minimize toxicity.

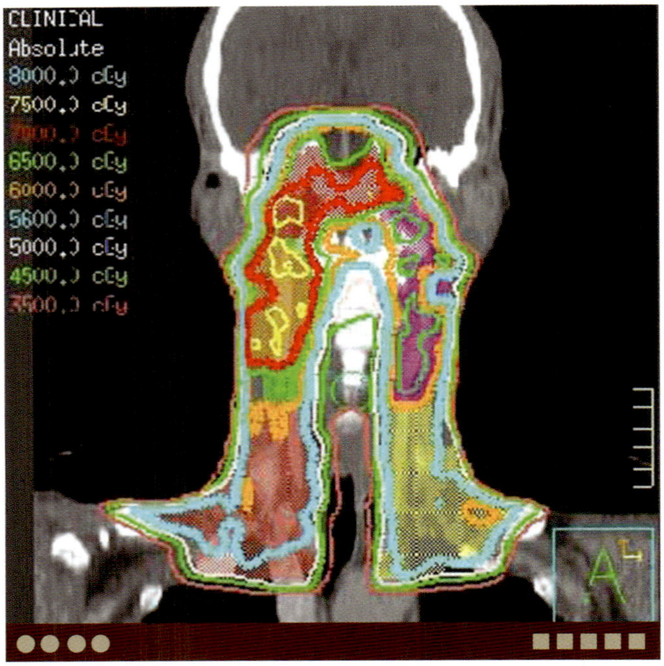

D. NPC, same patient as A. Coronal radiation treatment plan using IMRT. Bilateral parotid glands, oral cavity, larynx, postcricoid area, and spinal cord are spared to minimize toxicity.

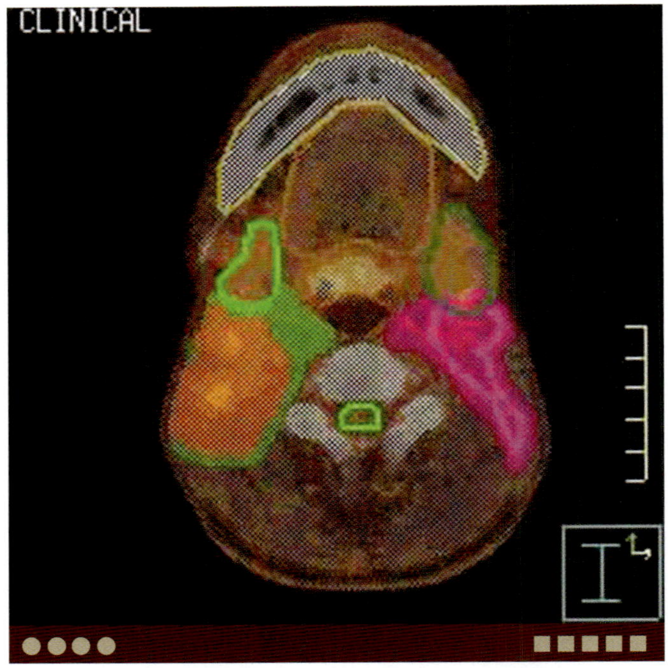

E. NPC, same patient as A. Axial PET/CT fusion for radiation planning. Bilateral submandibular glands, oral tongue, spinal cord, and involved and elective nodal volumes are contoured. The red colorwash represents the primary tumor, orange colorwash represents involved nodes, green and purple colorwash represent upper nodal volumes, orange and yellow colorwash represent lower elective nodal volumes.

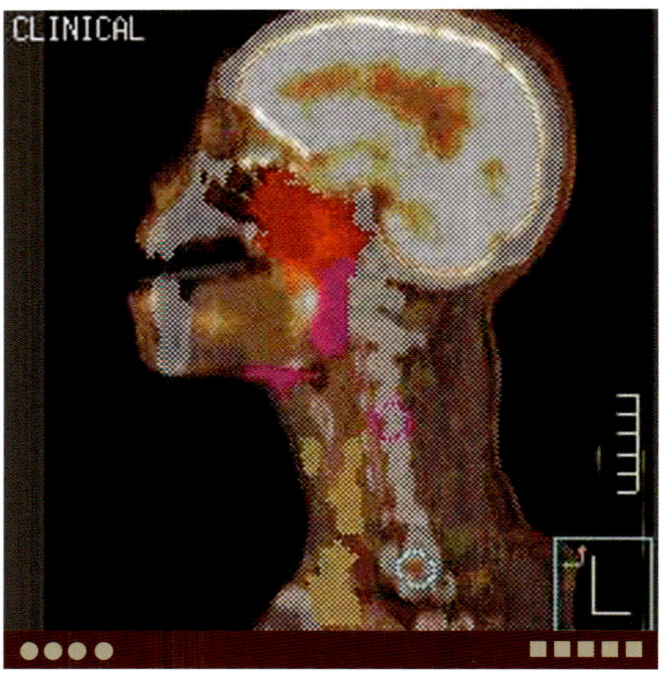

F. NPC, same patient as A. Sagittal PET/CT fusion for radiation planning. The red colorwash represents the primary tumor, orange colorwash represents involved nodes, green and purple colorwash represent upper nodal volumes, orange and yellow colorwash represent lower elective nodal volumes.

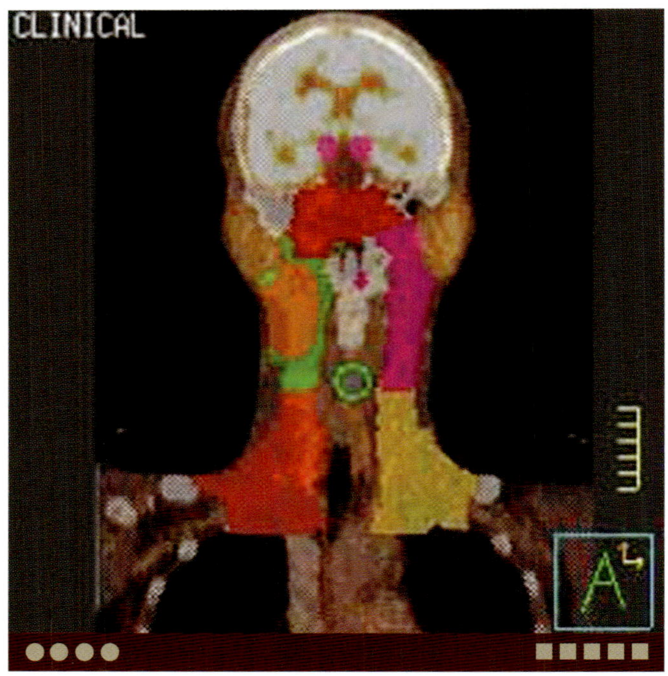

G. NPC, same patient as A. Coronal PET/CT fusion for radiation planning. The red colorwash represents the primary tumor, orange colorwash represents involved nodes, green and purple colorwash represent upper nodal volumes, orange and yellow colorwash represent lower elective nodal volumes.

DIFFERENTIAL DIAGNOSIS IMAGES (H-I)

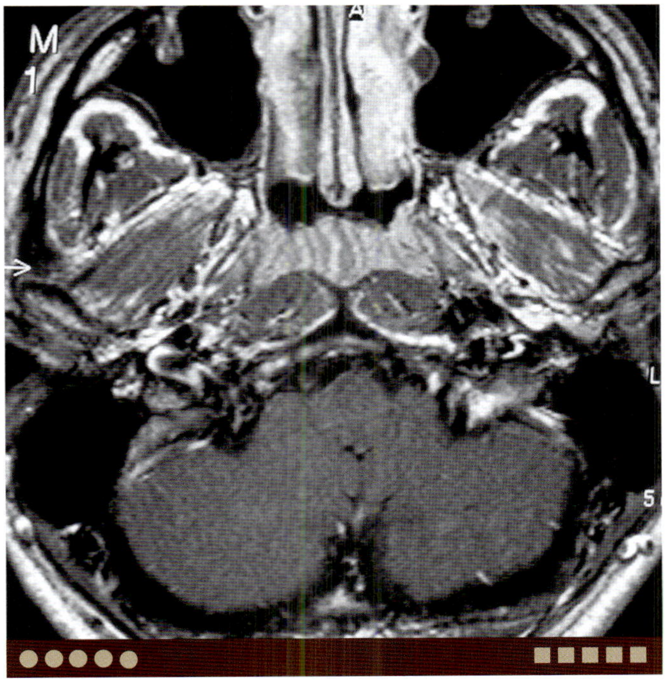

H. Adenoid hypertrophy. Axial postcontrast T1W MR image demonstrates enlarged adenoids with preserved striation.

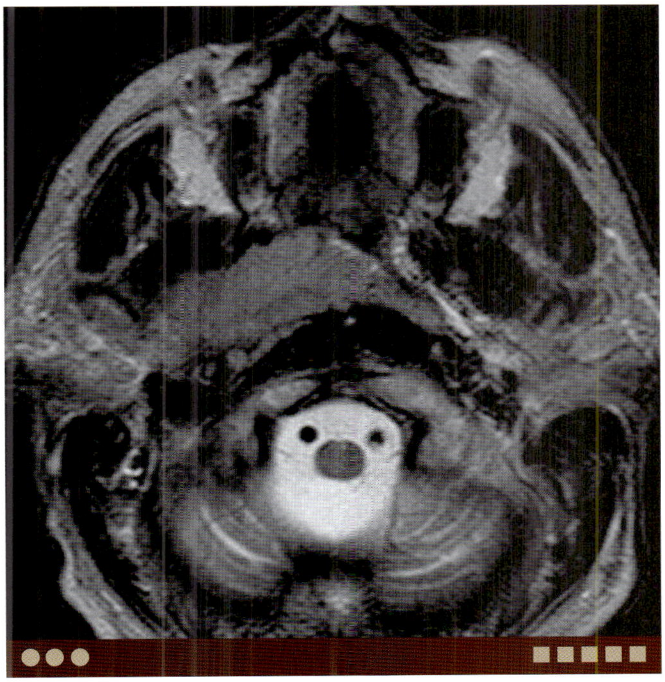

I. Lymphoma. Axial T2W MR image demonstrates an intermediate homogeneous signal lesion centered in the right fossa of Rosenmüller. Note involvement of the right parapharyngeal and masticator spaces as well as prevertebral space.

Case 15–2 Tonsillar Squamous Cell Carcinoma

Minh Tam Truong, Danielle Margalit, Paramjit Singh, Osamu Sakai

PRESENTATION

Unilateral otalgia, sore throat, dysphagia, trismus, asymptomatic neck mass.

FINDINGS

CT demonstrates a large neck mass.

DIFFERENTIAL DIAGNOSIS

- Lymphoid hyperplasia of the tonsils: Tonsillar prominence is common in children and young adults; typically bilateral and symmetric and often associated with prominent adenoids and cervical lymphadenopathy. Enhancing septa are seen on contrast-enhanced CT and MR.
- Lymphoma: Second most common malignancy in the palatine tonsils. Lymphoma usually shows homogeneous density/signal with enlarged, nonnecrotic lymph nodes.
- Peritonsillar abscess: Commonly seen in young adults, although it occurs at any age. It usually begins with acute tonsillitis manifested by tonsillar edema superficially and progresses into the deep soft tissues.
- Benign mixed tumor: Typically a well-circumscribed mass arising from the minor salivary glands in the pharyngeal mucosa.

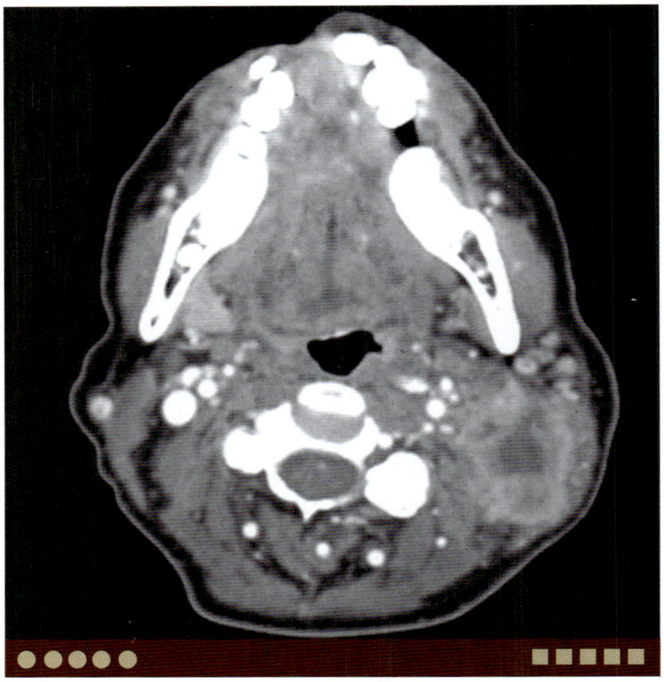

A. Tonsillar SCCA. Axial contrast-enhanced CT demonstrates a large necrotic node with extracapsular tumor spread in the left level IIB. Note a small enhancing primary lesion in the left palatine tonsil.

COMMENTS

This 48-year-old woman presented with sore throat, left otalgia, and a fixed left neck mass. An examination showed an ulcerative lesion of the left palatine tonsil. Biopsy of the left tonsil showed moderately to poorly differentiated invasive squamous cell carcinoma (SCCA). A PET/CT also detected bilateral 2-[^{18}F] fluoro-2-deoxy-D-glucose (FDG)-avid level II, III, and IV lymphadenopathy. The clinical stage was T2N2b tonsillar carcinoma.

The patient was treated with definitive chemoradiation therapy to the primary tumor and bilateral neck to a total dose of 70 Gy to the gross disease, with concurrent cisplatin and achieved a complete response by PET/CT scan at 8 weeks.

Alcohol and tobacco are traditional risk factors for tonsillar carcinoma. The human papilloma virus (HPV) is now recognized to play a role in carcinogenesis with HPV-16 being the most commonly implicated. Patients with HPV-related oropharyngeal cancer have an improved prognosis than HPV-negative cancers. The oropharynx is composed of four different sites: the soft palate, tonsillar region, base of tongue, and pharyngeal wall. The primary lymphatic drainage is to the upper deep jugular chain and the retropharyngeal lymph nodes. Advanced tumors of the tonsillar fossa may invade the medial pterygoid muscle and cause trismus.

TREATMENT

Single modality therapy is preferred for early-stage tonsillar carcinoma with either radiation therapy or surgery. Functional outcomes are typically better for radiation therapy. Chemotherapy is combined with radiation therapy for more advanced lesions. Neck dissection is recommended for residual nodal disease after chemoradiation.

PEARLS

- **Chemoradiotherapy is the treatment of choice for locally advanced tonsillar carcinoma.**
- **The bilateral lymph nodes are electively treated for locally advanced disease.**
- **Persistent neck disease after chemoradiotherapy can be salvaged by neck dissection.**

ADDITIONAL IMAGES (B-F)

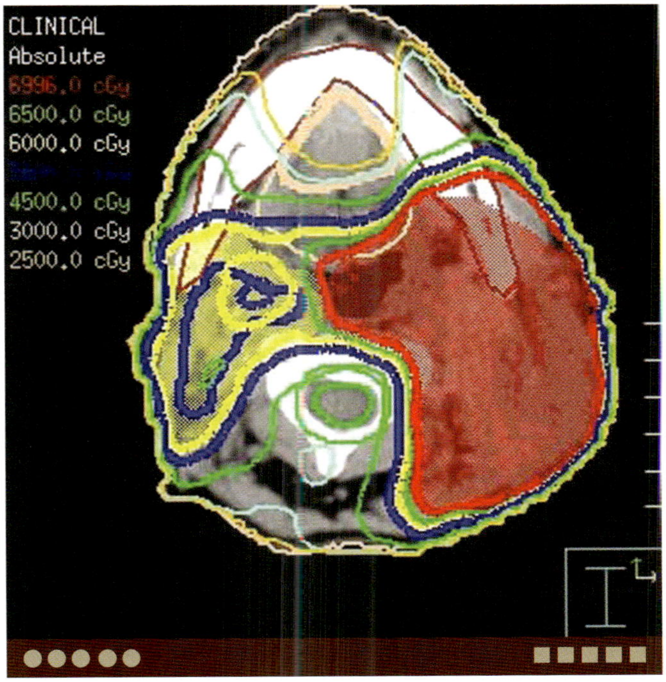

B. Tonsillar SCCA, same patient as A. Axial radiation treatment plan using intensity-modulated radiation therapy (IMRT).

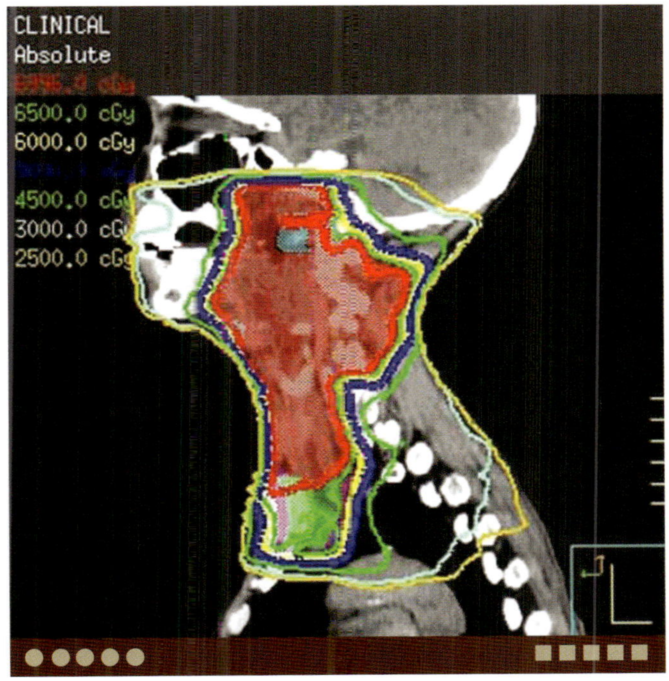

C. Tonsillar SCCA, same patient as A. Sagittal radiation treatment plan using IMRT.

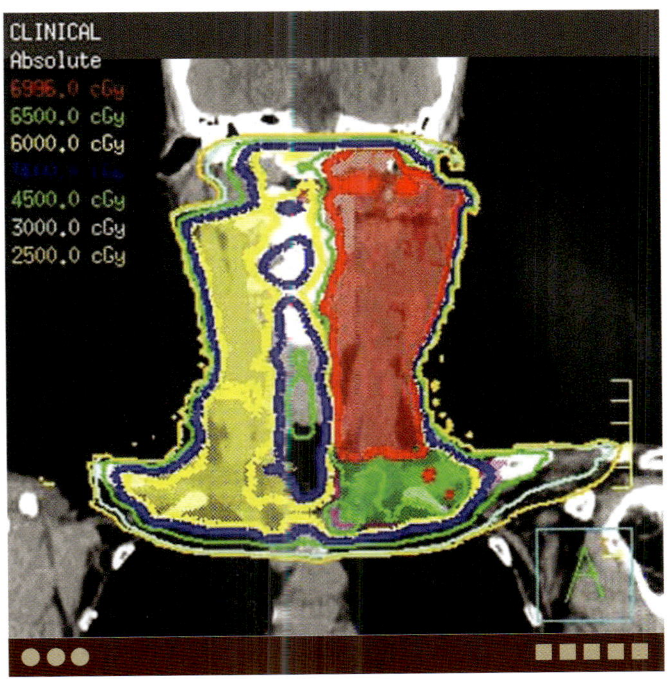

D. Tonsillar SCCA, same patient as A. Coronal radiation treatment plan using IMRT.

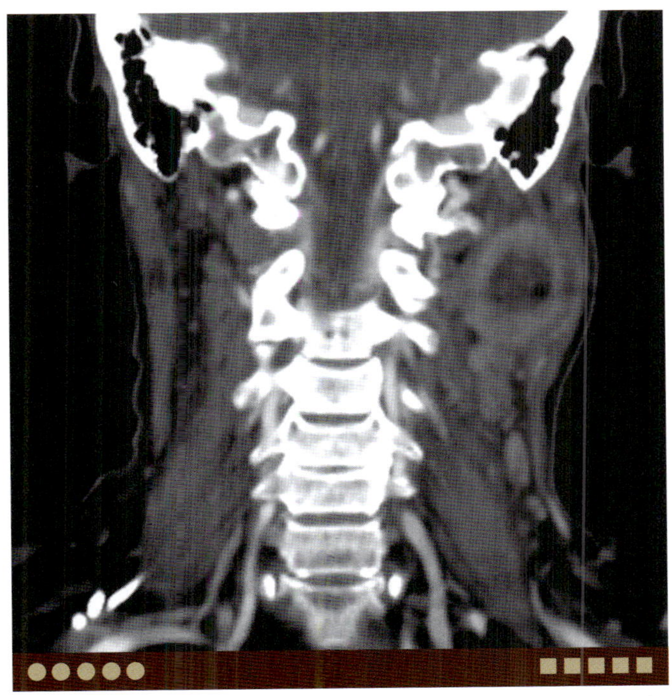

E. Tonsillar SCCA, same patient as A. Coronal contrast-enhanced CT demonstrates a large necrotic node with extracapsular tumor spread in the left level II. Smaller metastatic nodes are also seen in the left level III and IV.

DIFFERENTIAL DIAGNOSIS IMAGES (G-I)

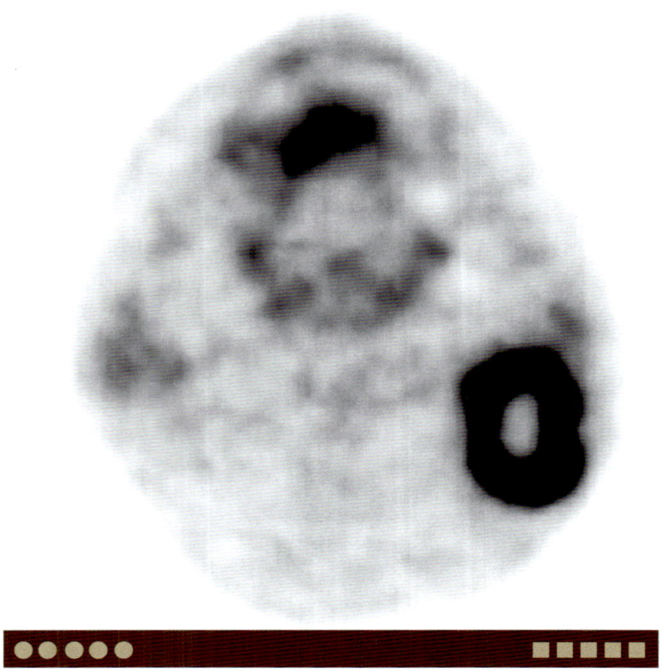

F. Tonsillar SCCA, same patient as A. Axial PET image demonstrates increased uptake in the necrotic left level IIB node.

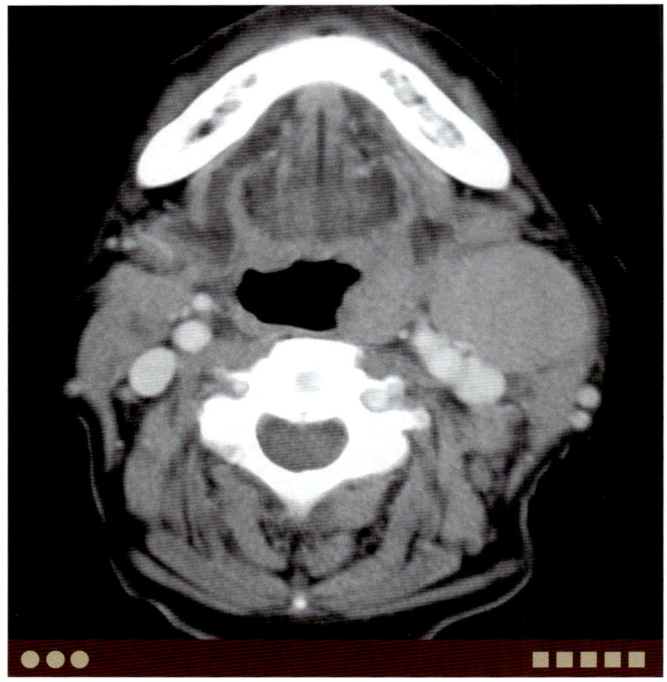

G. Lymphoma. Axial contrast-enhanced CT demonstrates a mildly enhancing lesion arising from the left palatine tonsil. Note large, mildly enhancing, nonnecrotic left level II node.

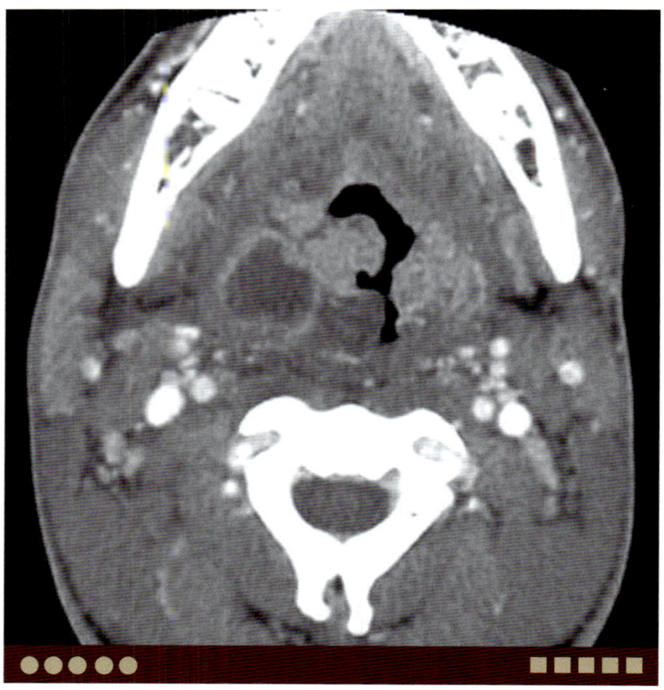

H. Peritonsillar abscess. Axial postcontrast CT demonstrates a rim-enhancing fluid collection in the right peritonsillar region. The right palatine tonsil is displaced medially and there is narrowing of the oropharyngeal lumen.

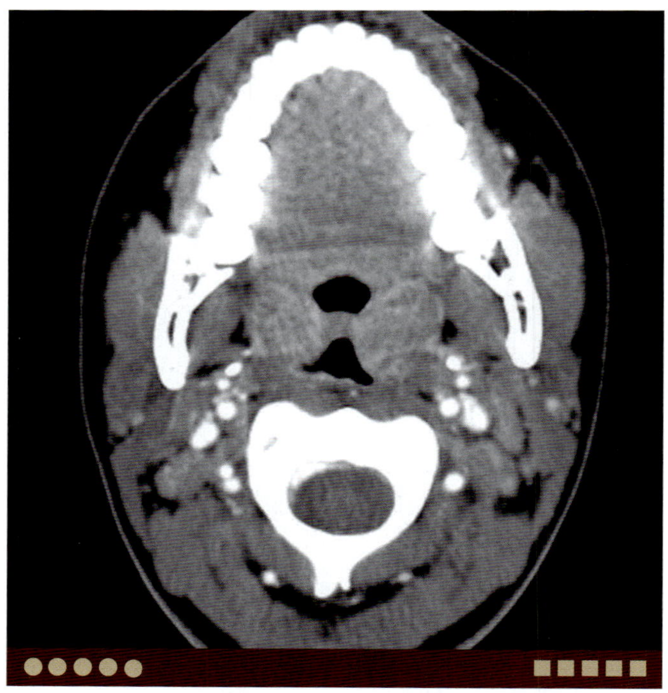

I. Tonsillitis. Axial postcontrast CT demonstrates enlarged, enhancing tonsils bilaterally. Striation is seen, however, no apparent mass is noted in the tonsils.

Case 15–3 Oral Tongue Carcinoma

Paul Romesser, Osamu Sakai, Minh Tam Truong

PRESENTATION

Tongue mass, pain, otalgia, odynophagia.

FINDINGS

CT demonstrates a heterogeneously enhancing lesion in the lateral tongue.

DIFFERENTIAL DIAGNOSIS

- Adenoid cystic carcinoma: Salivary gland tumor that often occurs in the sublingual gland and may involve the tongue. Perineural tumor spread is common.
- Mucoepidermoid carcinoma: Also a salivary gland tumor that often occurs in the sublingual gland and may involve the tongue. High-grade tumors tend to be solid and infiltrative.

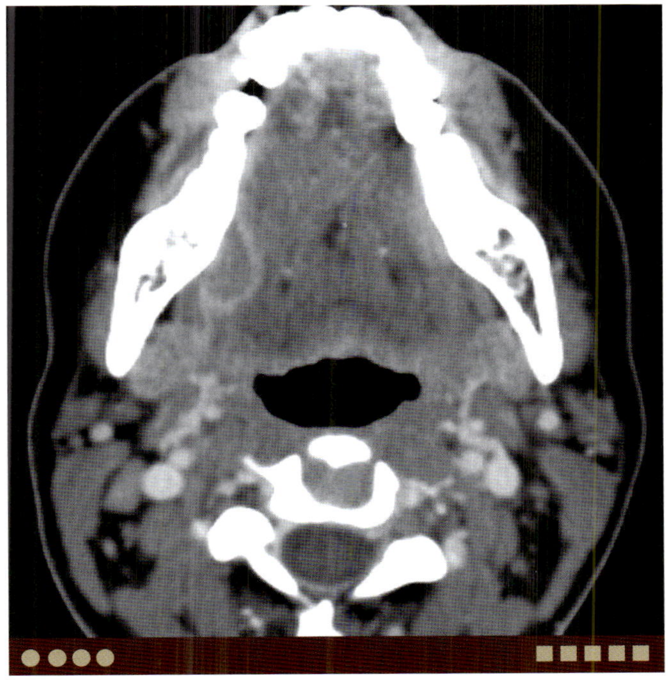

A. SCCA of the oral tongue. Axial postcontrast CT demonstrates a peripherally enhancing tumor in the right lateral tongue.

COMMENTS

This 36-year-old woman developed a painful mass on her right lateral tongue. Over a 3-month interval she developed worsening pain, right otalgia, odynophagia, and occasional bleeding. A biopsy of this lesion revealed moderately differentiated squamous cell carcinoma (SCCA). A PET/CT showed a focus of intense hypermetabolic activity in the right lateral tongue with a maximum SUV of 11.7, corresponding to an ovoid lesion measuring 9 × 15 mm in size on CT without nodal metastasis. She underwent a partial right glossectomy and a right neck dissection. Pathology revealed a 2.5 cm SCCA of the right lateral tongue with a depth of invasion of 9 mm. One of 11 nodes was positive in right level II with extracapsular tumor extension. The tumor stage was American Joint Committee on Cancer Staging system (AJCC) pT2N1M0 (stage III).

The mobile anterior two-third of the tongue is considered as a part of the oral cavity. The oral tongue is bound posteriorly by the circumvallate papillae, inferiorly by the floor of the mouth. Six muscles comprise the bulk of the tongue, three intrinsic muscles including lingual, vertical, and transversus muscles and three extrinsic muscles including genioglossus, hyoglossus and styloglossus. Risk factors for tongue carcinomas include tobacco, alcohol, human papilloma virus (HPV), herpes simplex virus, and oral leukoplakia. Increasing incidence of oral cavity cancers in nonsmokers and younger patients are attributed to increased HPV infection. Tumor invasion of the primary lesion greater than 4 mm is seen on pathology necessitates addressing the regional nodes either with elective neck dissection or elective nodal irradiation. The lymphatic drainage of the tongue involves levels IA, IB, II, III, and IV. The large majority of cancers identified in the oral cavity are SCCA.

Treatment often involves initial surgical management (wide excision with or without elective neck dissection) followed by postoperative radiation with or without chemotherapy, depending on adverse pathological features including advanced T stage, positive nodes, microscopic positive margins, extracapsular nodal extension, lymphovascular invasion, and perineural invasion.

PEARLS

- **Early oral tongue SCCA can be detected from careful physical of the oral cavity. Initial surgical management is preferred for oral cavity cancers.**
- **Postoperative radiation is added depending on pathological features.**
- **Chemoradiation therapy is used for locally advanced or unresectable oral cavity cancers.**
- **Subclinical cervical nodal metastases in patients presenting with oral tongue carcinoma and can be predicted by the depth of invasion of the primary lesion.**

ADDITIONAL IMAGES (B-G)

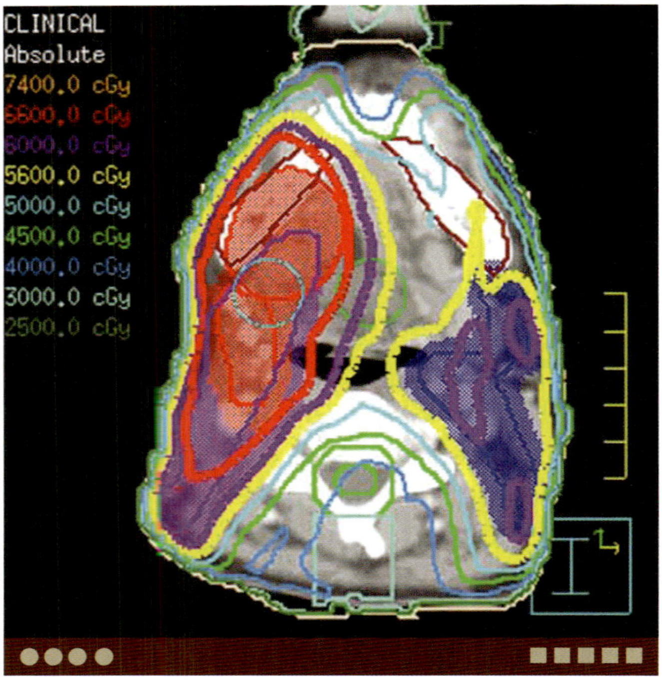

B. SCCA of the oral tongue, same patient as A. Axial intensity-modulated radiation therapy (IMRT) radiation treatment plan encompassing surgical bed and bilateral neck.

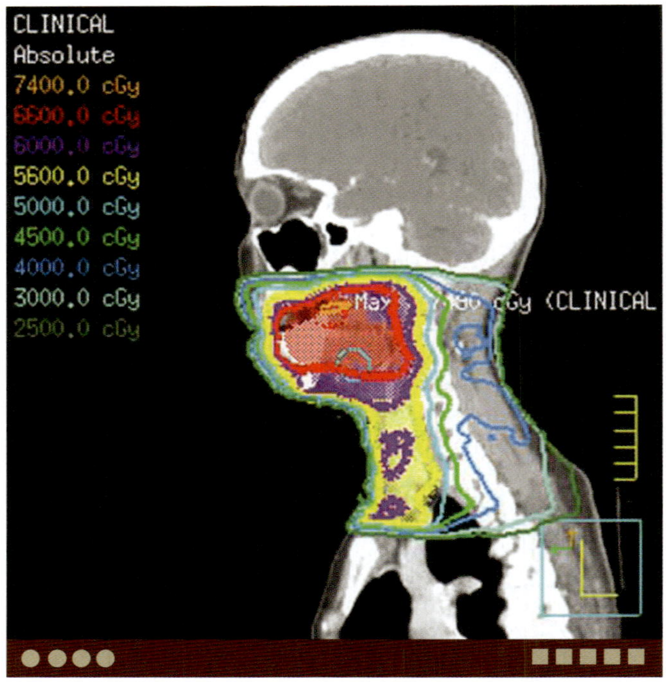

C. SCCA of the oral tongue, same patient as A. Sagittal IMRT radiation treatment plan of surgical bed and bilateral neck.

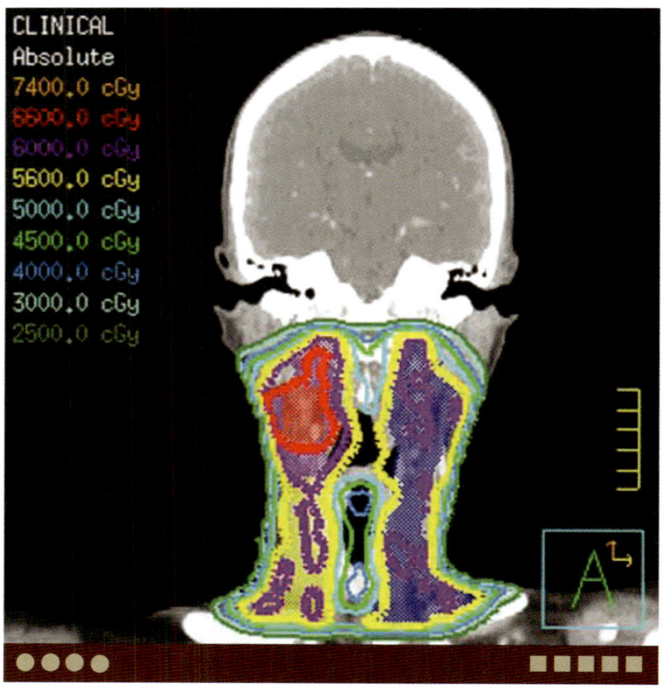

D. SCCA of the oral tongue, same patient as A. Coronal IMRT radiation treatment plan of surgical bed and bilateral neck.

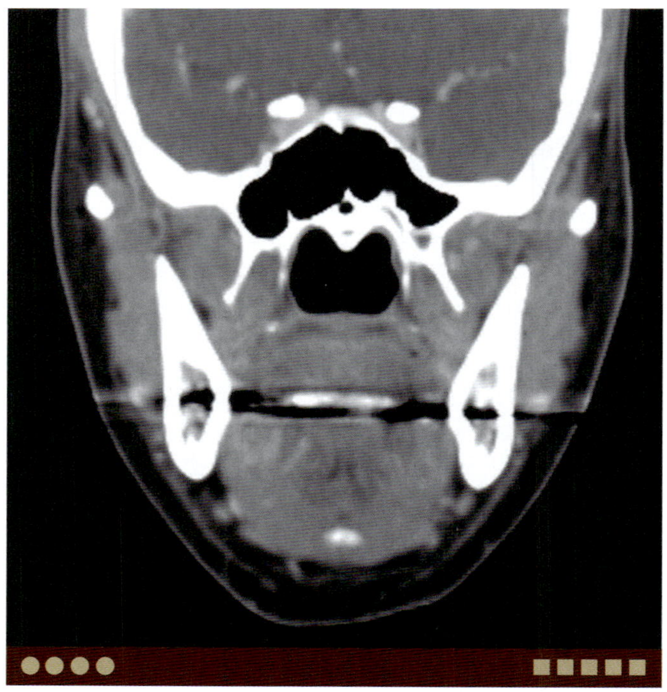

E. SCCA of the oral tongue, same patient as A. Coronal postcontrast CT demonstrates a peripherally enhancing tumor in the right lateral tongue.

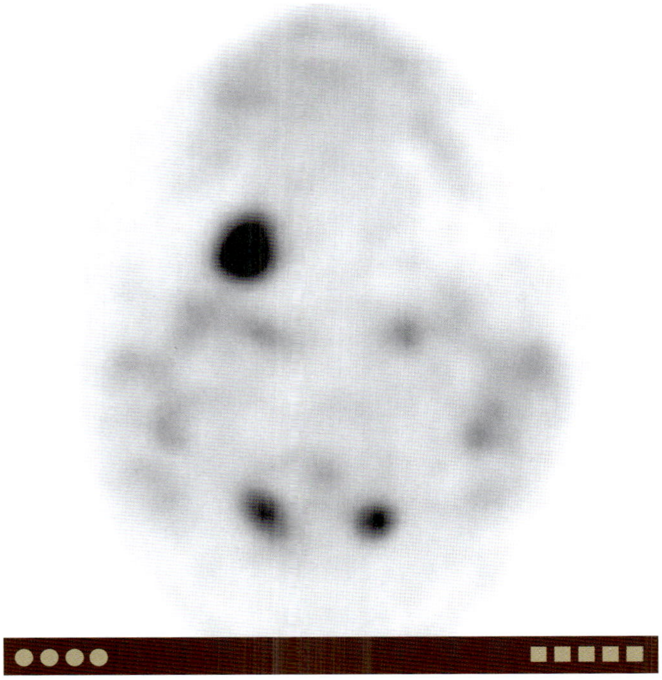

F. SCCA of the oral tongue, same patient as A. Axial PET image demonstrates a focal FDG uptake in the right lateral tongue.

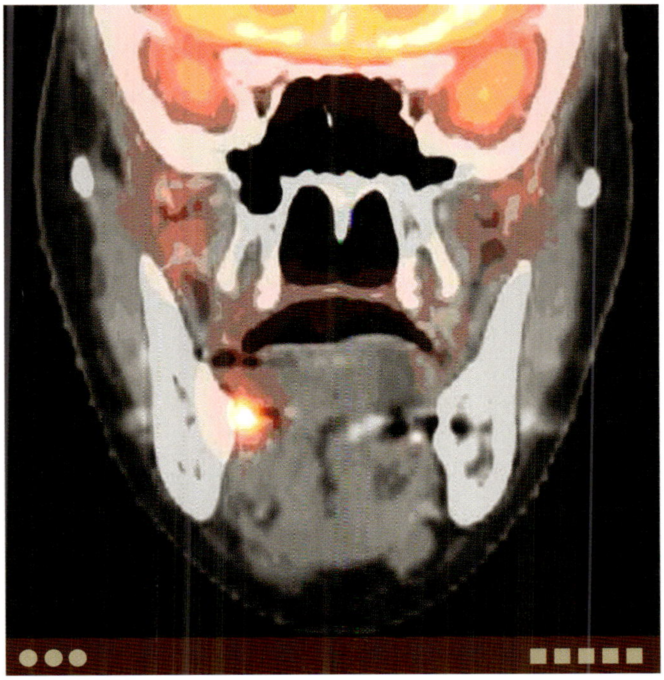

G. SCCA of the oral tongue, same patient as A. Coronal PET/CT image demonstrates a hypermetabolic tumor in the right lateral tongue.

DIFFERENTIAL DIAGNOSIS IMAGES (H-J)

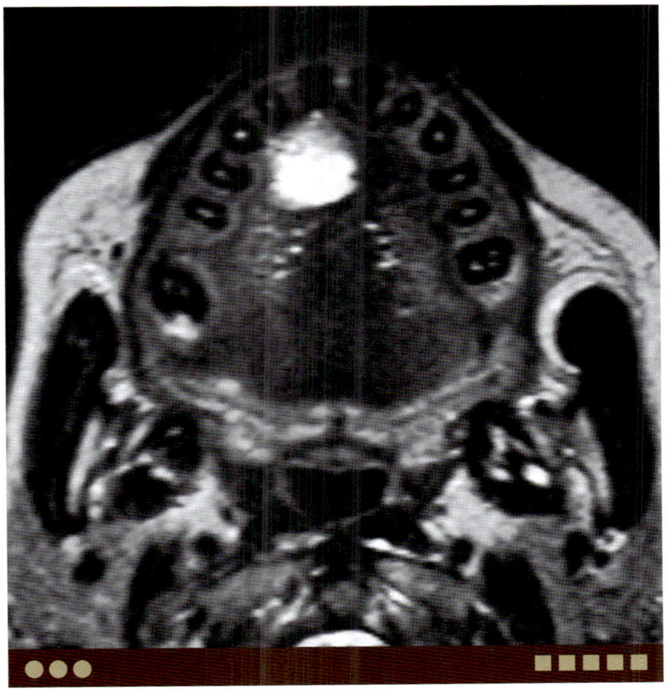

H. Hemangioma. Axial T2W image demonstrates a well-demarcated, very high-signal lesion in the anterior right tongue.

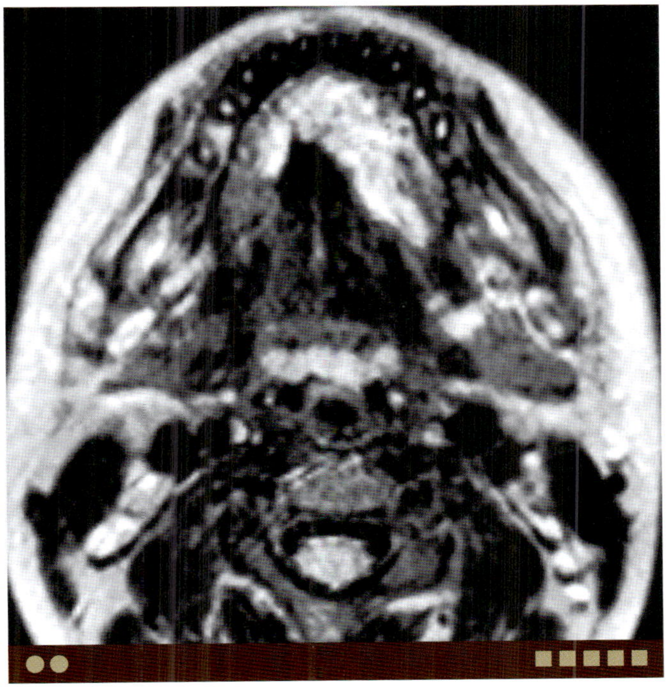

I. Neurofibroma. Axial T2W image demonstrates a slightly lobulated, high-signal lesion centered in the anterior left tongue crossing midline.

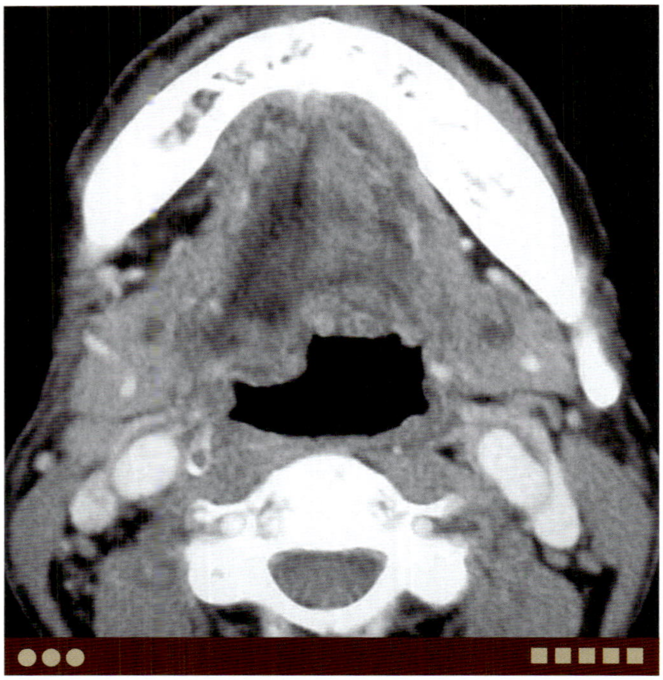

J. Denervation myositis. Axial postcontrast CT in a patient with nasopharyngeal carcinoma demonstrates decreased density and posterior protrusion of the right tongue consistent with subacute to chronic denervation myositic change due to hypoglossal nerve invasion.

Case 15–4 Base of Tongue Squamous Cell Carcinoma

Minh Tam Truong, Danielle Margalit, Paramjit Singh, Osamu Sakai

PRESENTATION

Otalgia, dysphagia, odynophagia, and dysarthria.

FINDINGS

MRI and CT demonstrate a heterogeneously enhancing lesion at the base of tongue (BOT) and filling the valleculae.

DIFFERENTIAL DIAGNOSIS

- Lymphoid hypertrophy: Normal or nonneoplastic enlarged lingual tonsils located at the BOT may enhance on CT and MRI and increased FDG uptake on PET. This should not be confused with tumor.
- Lymphoma: Lymphomas occur in the Waldeyer ring including base of tongue although it is not very common (tonsil > nasopharynx > BOT).
- Minor salivary gland tumors: Mucoepidermoid carcinoma and adenoid cystic carcinoma can occur at the BOT.

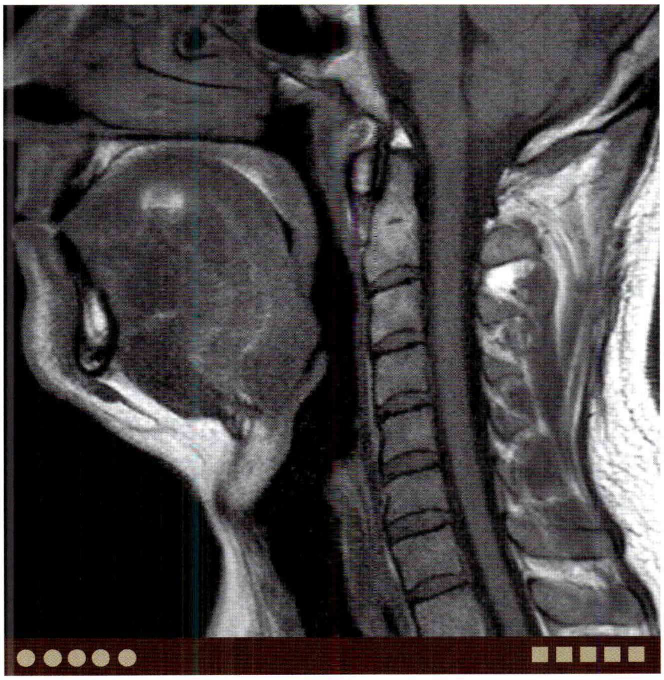

A. BOT SCCA. Sagittal T1W MRI image shows an abnormal mass at the base of tongue. There is no apparent invasion of the intrinsic tongue musculature which is the criteria for T4 classification per AJCC staging.

COMMENTS

This 46-year-old man presented with a right neck mass. An examination revealed right cervical and submandibular lymphadenopathy. MRI and CT demonstrated a heterogeneously enhancing lesion at the BOT and right level II, III, and IV lymphadenopathy. Endoscopy revealed an ulcerated lesion of the BOT extending to the lingual surface of the epiglottis. Fine-needle aspiration (FNA) of the mass revealed invasive squamous cell carcinoma (SCCA). PET/CT showed a right BOT lesion with lymphadenopathy in levels II to IV and left level II lymphadenopathy. The clinical stage was T1N2c SCCA of the BOT. The patient received definitive radiation therapy with concurrent cisplatin.

The BOT includes the posterior one-third of tongue and valleculae, is bounded anteriorly by the circumvallate papillae, laterally by the glossopharyngeal sulci, and posteriorly by the junction between the valleculae and base of the epiglottis. Tumors that involve the valleculae can spread to the lingual surface of the epiglottis and can also extend to the preepiglottic space submucosally. Lateral BOT tumors can extend to the glossotonsillar sulcus. BOT tumors may spread anteriorly to involve the floor of mouth and oral tongue. Palpation of the BOT and oral tongue is important to detect submucosal spread. BOT carcinomas have a high rate of lymph node spread. Approximately 75% of patients have clinically positive lymph nodes at presentation.

Definitive radiation therapy is performed for early-stage T1 and T2 lesions. T3 or T4 lesions and more advanced carcinoma of the BOT are treated with radiation therapy and concurrent chemotherapy. Occasionally, interstitial brachytherapy is used to supplement dose to residual primary tumor. Lymph nodes on both sides of the neck are irradiated due to high incidence of bilateral regional nodal spread.

PEARLS

- **Lymph node metastases are frequently bilateral due to the midline position of most tumors and the rich capillary lymphatic networks.**
- **There is a high rate of subclinical cervical lymph nodes metastases in patients presenting with base of tongue carcinoma.**
- **The normal lingual tonsils located at the tongue base may enhance on CT and MRI and show increased FDG uptake on PET. This should not be confused with tumor.**

ADDITIONAL IMAGES (B-G)

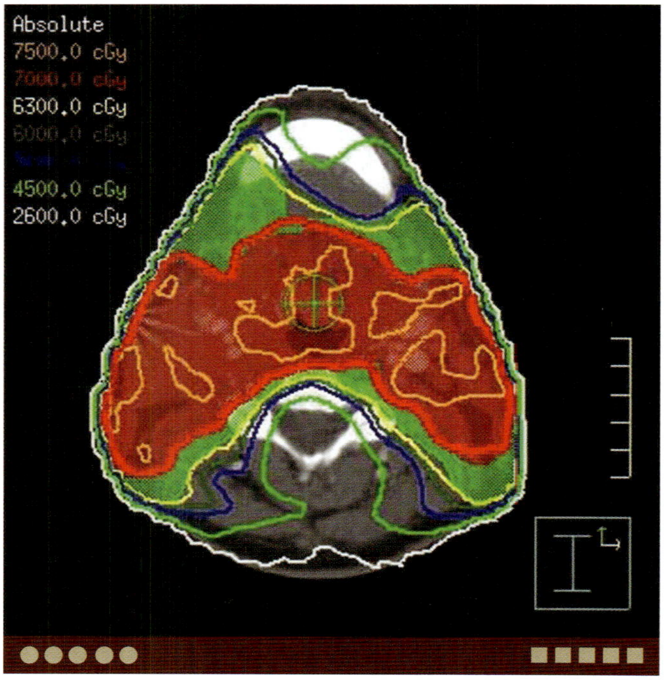

B. BOT SCCA, same patient as A. Axial radiation treatment plan using intensity-modulated radiation therapy (IMRT).

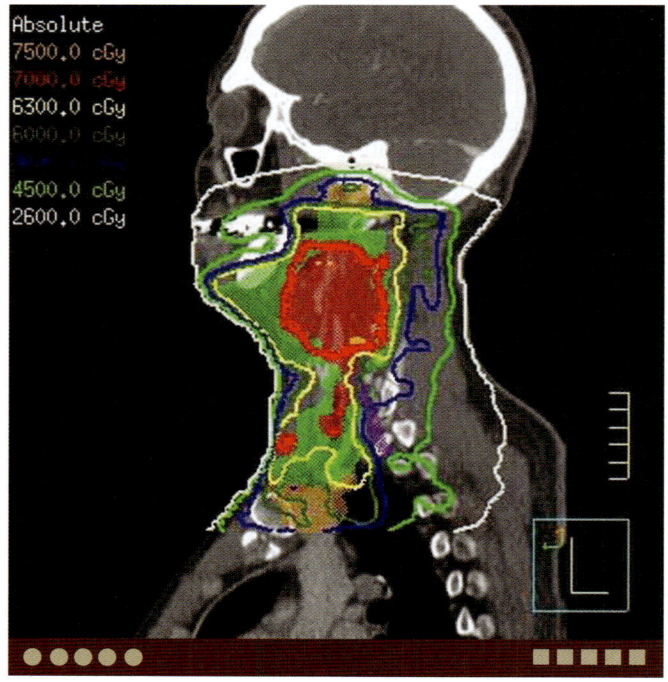

C. BOT SCCA, same patient as A. Sagittal radiation treatment plan using IMRT.

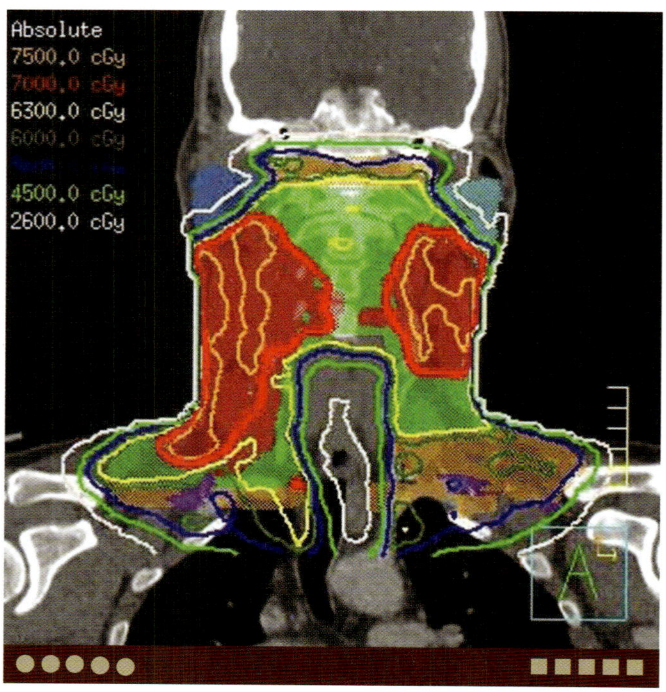

D. BOT SCCA, same patient as A. Coronal radiation treatment plan using IMRT.

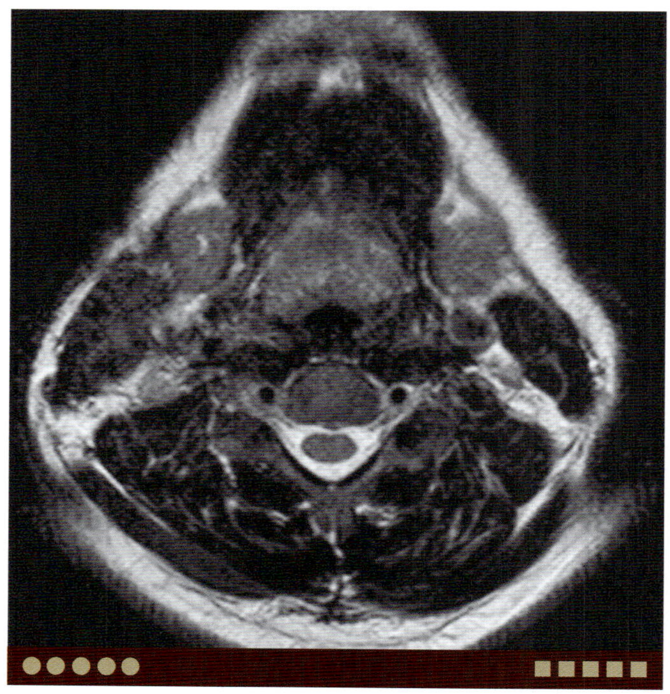

E. BOT SCCA, same patient as A. Axial T2W image demonstrates a mildly hyperintense lesion in the BOT filling the valleculae. Note metastatic nodes in the right level II.

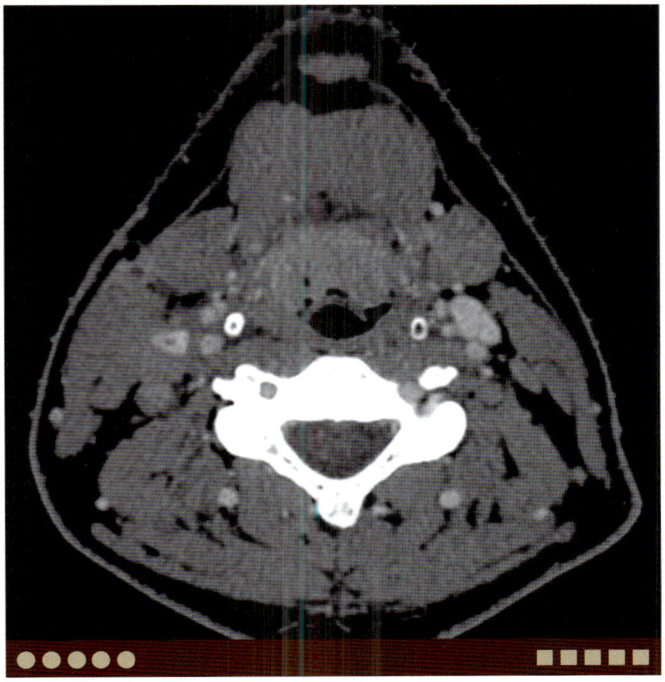

F. BOT SCCA, same patient as A. Axial contrast-enhanced CT demonstrates a mildly enhancing tumor in the BOT filling the valleculae. Note metastatic nodes in the right level II.

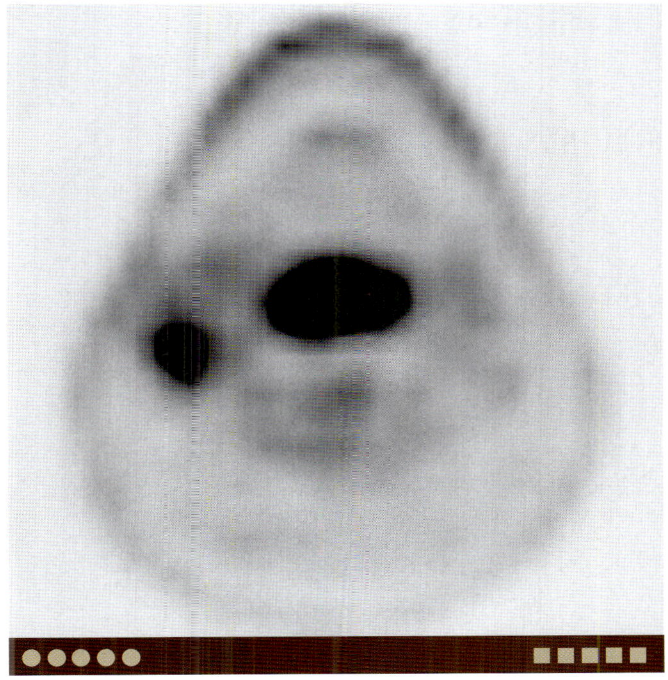

G. BOT SCCA, same patient as A. Axial PET image demonstrates an avid FDG uptake in the primary lesion as well as in the right level II metastatic node.

DIFFERENTIAL DIAGNOSIS IMAGES (H-I)

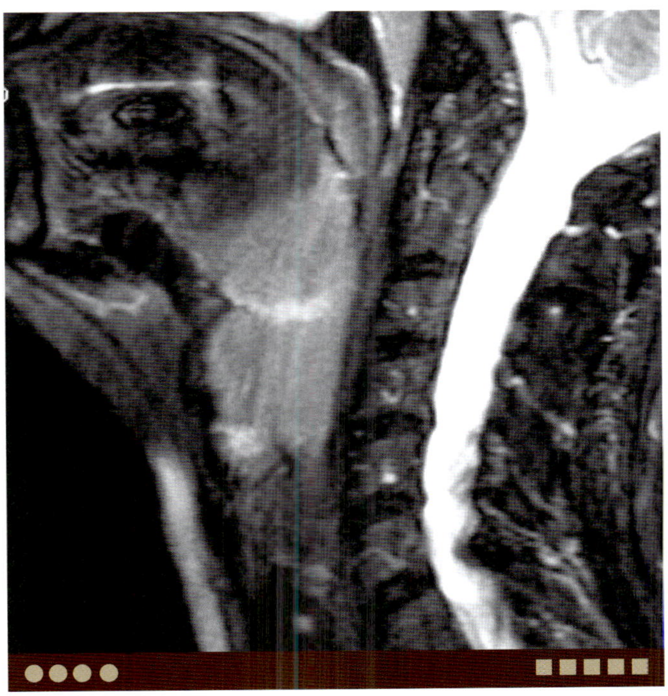

H. Lymphoma. Sagittal STIR image shows a homogeneous intermediate-signal lesion involving the base of tongue and hypopharynx.

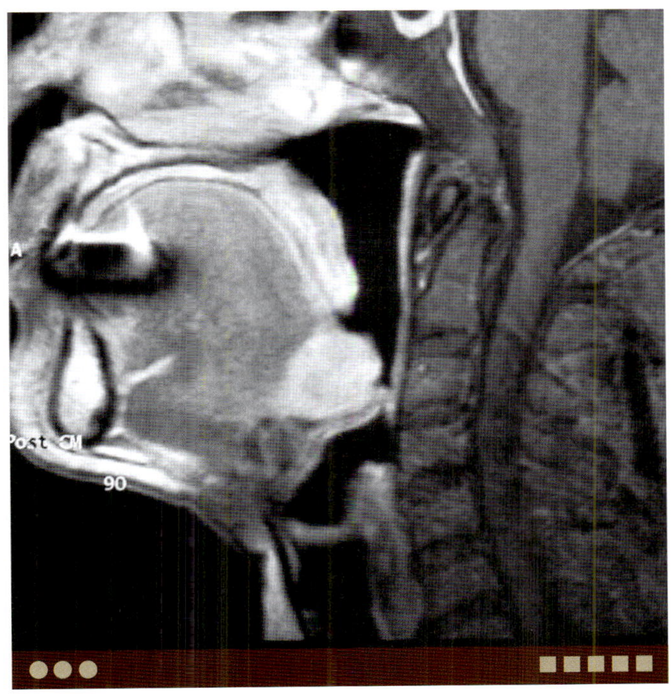

I. Mucoepidermoid carcinoma. Sagittal postcontrast T1W image demonstrates an enhancing tumor at the base of tongue.

Case 15–5 Hypopharyngeal Squamous Cell Carcinoma

Danielle Margalit, Osamu Sakai, Minh Tam Truong

PRESENTATION

Dysphagia with solids, weight loss, otalgia.

FINDINGS

CT and MRI demonstrate a soft tissue mass within the pyriform sinus and involving the aryepiglottic fold.

DIFFERENTIAL DIAGNOSIS

- Lymphoma: This usually demonstrates more homogeneous density or signal compared with squamous cell carcinoma (SCCA).
- Adenoid cystic carcinoma: This is a relatively rare tumor. Imaging findings can be similar to SCCA and indistinguishable.
- Amyloidosis: This demonstrates nodular mucosal thickening or submucosal mass often with calcification.

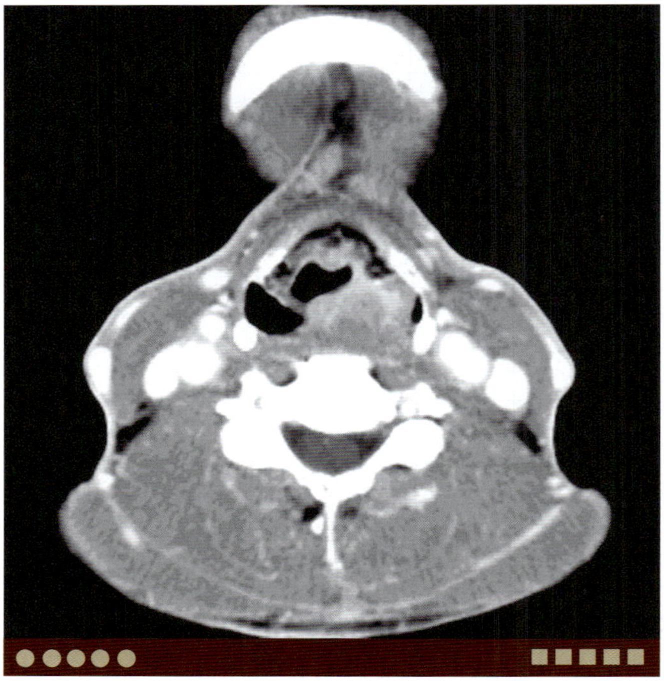

A. HPC. Axial contrast-enhanced CT demonstrates a soft tissue mass within the left pyriform sinus involving the left aryepiglottic fold.

COMMENTS

This 61-year-old man developed a sensation of a "lump" in his throat, dysphagia with solids, left otalgia, unintentional weight loss, and hoarseness.

Flexible laryngoscopy performed showed a mass involving the medial left pyriform sinus extending to the pharyngoepiglottic fold and involving the left arytenoid with pooling of secretions in the left pyriform sinus. The left false vocal cord was fixed. The mass appeared to invade the left false vocal cord as evidenced by fat effacement on CT. CT and MRI showed no invasion of the thyroid or cricoid cartilage, hyoid bone, thyroid gland, or esophagus, or nodal metastasis. An examination under anesthesia also confirmed the pyriform sinus mass extending to the postcricoid region. A biopsy confirmed squamous cell carcinoma. The patient was staged as AJCC T3N0M0 based on fixation of the ipsilateral hemilarynx.

The three major subsites of the hypopharynx include the pyriform sinuses, posterior and lateral hypopharyngeal walls, and the postcricoid area. The pyriform sinus is the most common site of hypopharyngeal SCCA (HPC). Submucosal spread is a characteristic feature of HPC. Due to the rich lymphatic supply, lymph node involvement is common with 75% of patients having clinically positive neck lymph nodes at presentation. The typical lymph node drainage from the hypopharynx includes levels II to V, and the retropharyngeal lymph nodes. Tumors that involve the lower hypopharynx and postcricoid area may result in lymph node drainage to paratracheal and paraesophageal lymph nodes. External auditory canal pain may be referred via the superior laryngeal nerve through the auricular nerve of Arnold (CN X). The initial office-based history and examination and subsequent radiologic imaging is directed toward determining the extent of the primary tumor and involved lymph nodes excluding distant metastatic disease.

Select T3 lesions are appropriate for irradiation and concurrent chemotherapy. Traditionally, the standard of care for T3-4 HPC is surgery involving a total laryngectomy and partial pharyngectomy and bilateral lymph node dissections. However, an organ preservation approach has been shown to be equivalent to surgery based on a European study randomizing patients to surgery versus induction chemotherapy and radiation therapy. Often concurrent chemoradiation therapy is used for HPC based on extrapolated data from

PEARLS

- **Locally advanced HPCs have a high risk of lymph node metastases, necessitating elective nodal irradiation to the bilateral neck and including the retropharyngeal lymph nodes in addition to the jugular lymph node chain.**
- **Chemoradiation therapy is an organ preservation approach equivalent to definitive surgery.**

larynx cancer showing improved laryngeal preservation rates with concurrent chemoradiation therapy when compared to induction chemotherapy followed by radiation alone.

The patient received definitive radiation therapy and concurrent cisplatin-based chemotherapy. He received 70 Gy to the primary lesion and 56 Gy to the nodal regions of lower risk of microscopic spread using intensity-modulated radiation therapy. The patient has achieved a complete clinical and radiological response by PET/CT and is without evidence of disease at 1-year follow-up.

ADDITIONAL IMAGES (B-F)

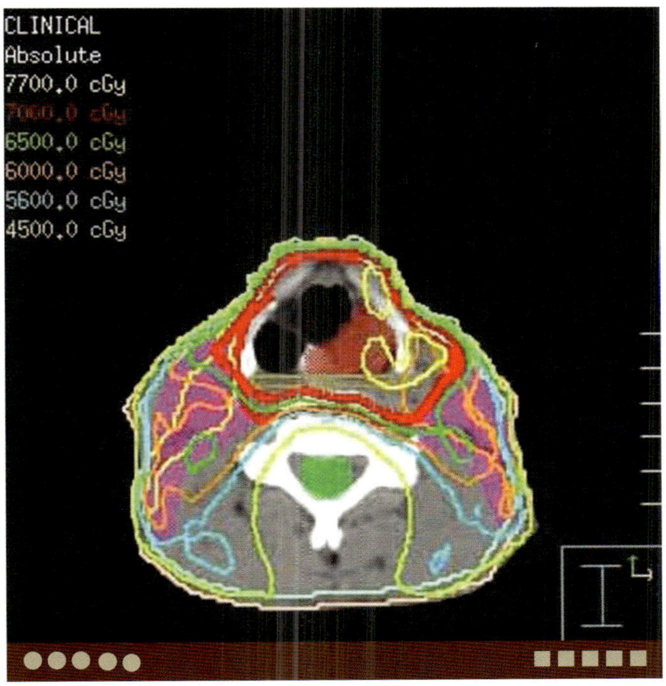

B. HPC, same patient as A. Axial radiation treatment plan using intensity-modulated radiation therapy (IMRT).

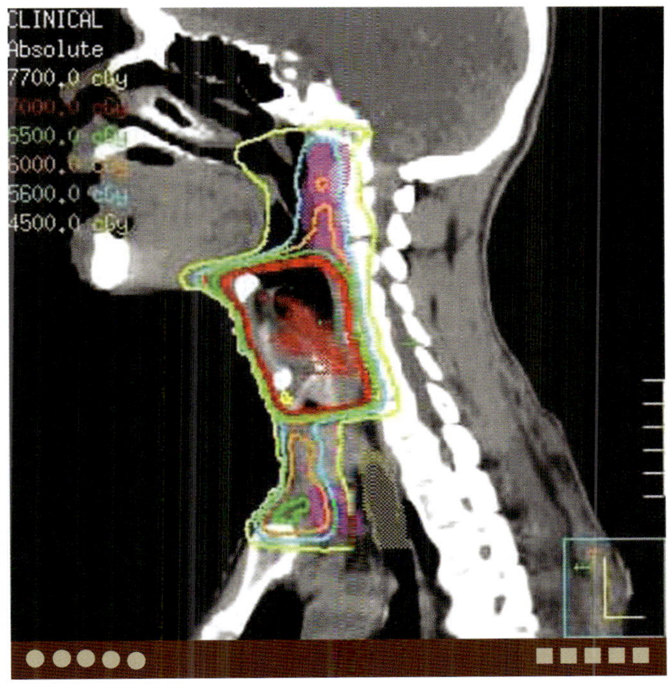

C. HPC, same patient as A. Sagittal radiation treatment plan using IMRT.

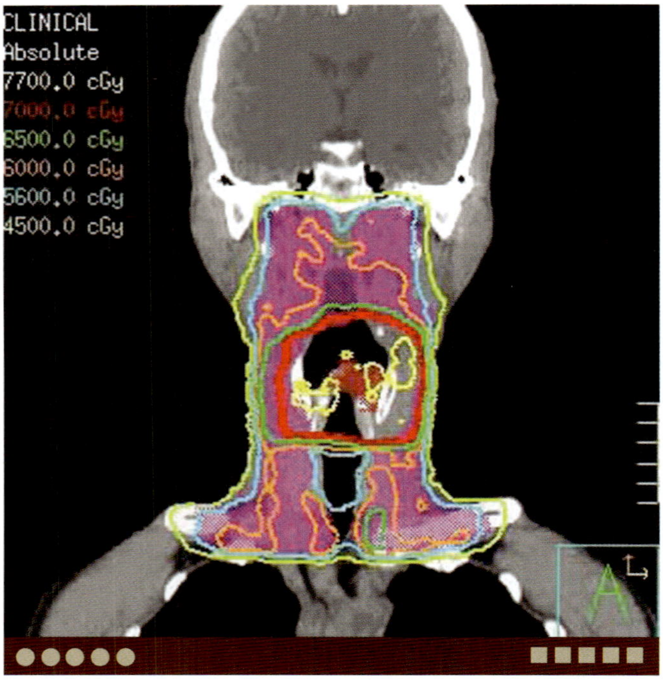

D. HPC, same patient as A. Coronal radiation treatment plan using IMRT.

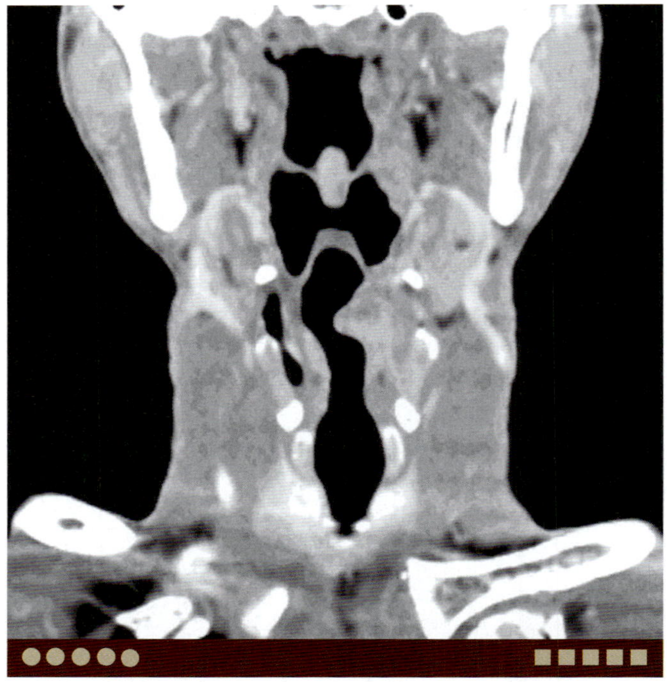

E. HPC, same patient as A. Coronal contrast-enhanced CT demonstrates a tumor in the left hypopharynx obliterating the paraglottic fat.

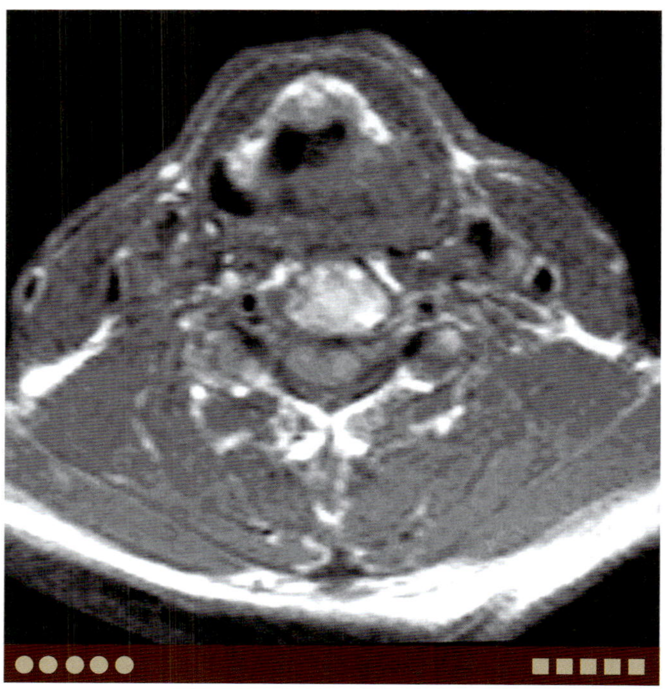

F. HPC, same patient as A. Axial T1W image demonstrates a tumor involving the left aryepiglottic fold and obliterating the paraglottic fat.

DIFFERENTIAL DIAGNOSIS IMAGES (G-H)

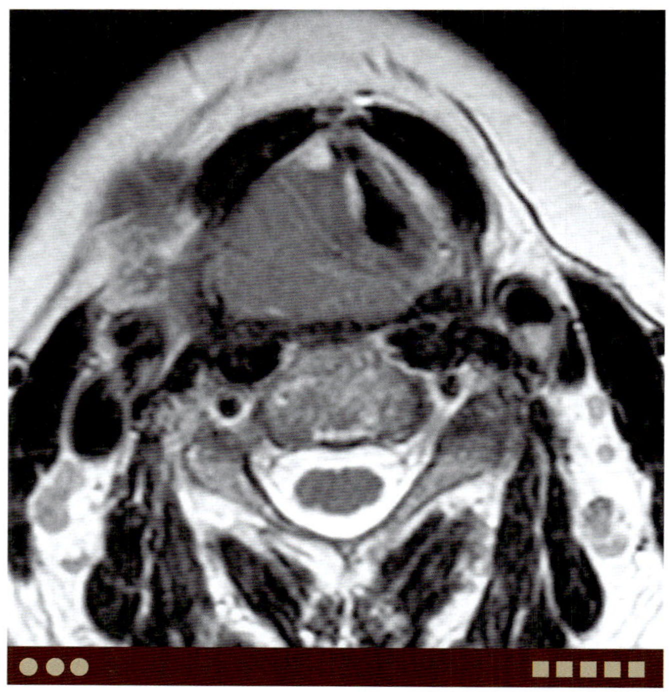

G. Lymphoma. Axial T2W image shows a homogeneous, intermediate-signal lesion involving the right paraglottic space and displacing the cord medially.

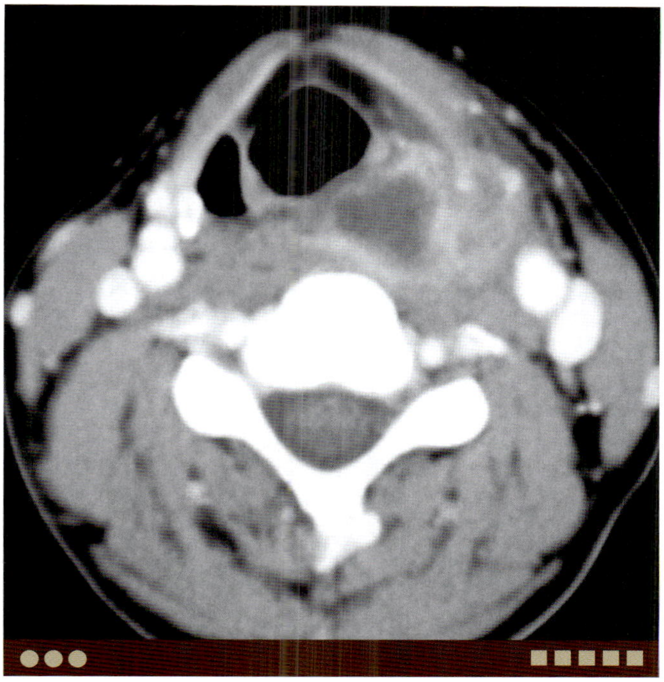

H. Pyriform sinus fistula, developmental anomaly. Axial postcontrast CT demonstrates a heterogeneous rim-enhancing lesion centered in the left pyriform sinus. Lower slices demonstrate abscess in the left lobe of the thyroid (not shown).

Case 15-6 Laryngeal Carcinoma

David Kozono, Danielle Margalit, Osamu Sakai, Minh Tam Truong

PRESENTATION

Glottic cancers may present initially with hoarseness; more advanced lesions may cause airway obstruction, pain, dysphagia, and referred otalgia. Subglottic cancers may present with stridor or dyspnea on exertion. Supraglottic cancers may present with pain on swallowing, change in voice quality (hot potato voice), and referred otalgia.

FINDINGS

CT demonstrates asymmetric thickening or a mass in the larynx.

DIFFERENTIAL DIAGNOSIS

- Lymphoma: This usually demonstrates homogeneous density/signal and mild enhancement.
- Rhabdomyoma and rhabdomyosarcoma: These are rare submucosal tumors. Rhabdomyosarcoma tends to demonstrate more aggressive features.
- Adenoid cystic carcinoma: This is rare. The imaging findings are similar to squamous cell carcinoma (SCCA) and often indistinguishable.
- Schwannoma: This is a rare tumor, however, important for the differential diagnosis of submucosal tumors in the larynx. This often arises in the supraglottic larynx.

COMMENTS

This is a 55-year-old woman who presented with progressive hoarseness. Flexible nasolaryngoscopy revealed nodularity of the epiglottis with thickening of the aryepiglottic folds bilaterally and decreased mobility of the vocal folds bilaterally. Examination under anesthesia confirmed the abnormality of the epiglottis extending to the false vocal cords bilaterally. Biopsy showed moderately differentiated invasive SCCA. CT revealed an ill-defined, heterogeneously enhancing lesion of the epiglottis with infiltration of the preepiglottic fat. There was thickening and nodularity of the bilateral aryepiglottic folds and left pyriform sinus. There were no pathologically enlarged lymph nodes of the neck. The patient was staged as T3N0 carcinoma of the supraglottic larynx arising from the epiglottis.

The patient elected to receive a voice-preserving treatment approach with definitive radiation therapy and concurrent cisplatin. The patient is clinically free of disease at 2 years of follow-up.

The landmark VA larynx study was a randomized study that compared induction chemotherapy followed by radiation versus total laryngectomy and postoperative radiation. This study showed that patients who received chemotherapy followed by radiation had a 64% larynx preservation rate at 2 years with no significant difference in 2-year survival compared with the surgical group. A subsequent large

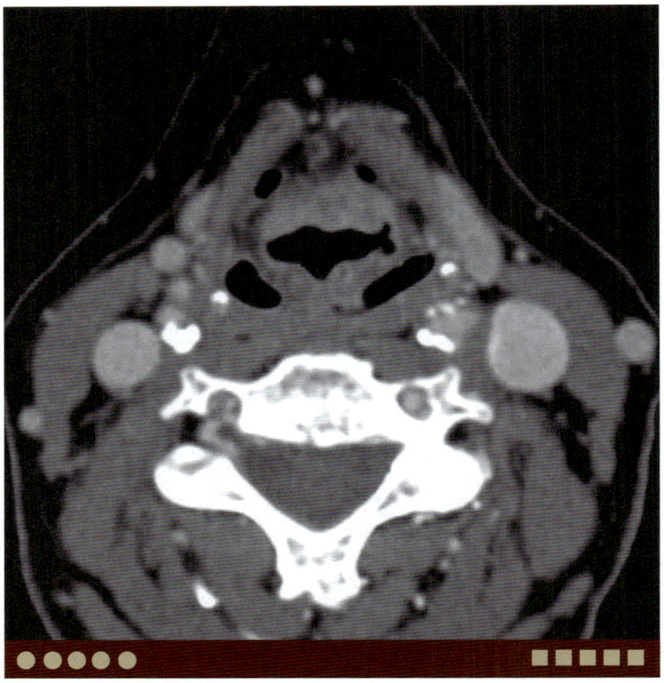

A. Supraglottic SCCA. Axial postcontrast CT demonstrates irregularity and heterogeneous enhancement of the epiglottis and aryepiglottic folds, left more then right.

PEARLS

- **Laryngeal cancer is the most common head and neck cancer, and SCCA is the most common histology.**
- **The larynx is divided into three anatomic regions: supraglottic larynx, glottic larynx, and subglottic larynx. Carcinomas have a distinctive pattern of spread and incidence of lymph node involvement depending on the laryngeal subsite involved.**
- **Advanced-stage laryngeal carcinoma was traditionally treated with total laryngectomy with postoperative radiation therapy. Randomized control trials have shown that combined modality therapy with chemotherapy and radiation therapy offer the chance for organ preservation without compromising survival.**

randomized study, RTOG 91-11, subsequently showed improved larynx preservation rates using concurrent chemoradiation compared to radiation alone or induction chemotherapy followed by radiation.

TREATMENT

Early lesions (T1 and T2) can typically be treated with a single modality such as voice-preserving surgery or radiation therapy. Locally advanced T3 and nonbulky T4 lesions are treated with radiation with concomitant chemotherapy as a method of larynx/voice preservation. For bulky T4 lesions, total laryngectomy followed by adjuvant radiotherapy with or without concomitant chemotherapy is the standard treatment. Indications for postoperative radiation therapy with concurrent chemotherapy include extracapsular extension and positive surgical margins. The bilateral jugular nodal chains are addressed electively either surgically or by radiation therapy for T3 and T4 glottic lesions. For T1-4 supraglottic cancer, elective nodal irradiation or neck dissection is performed as the risk of occult lymphatic spread is high even for T1 lesions.

ADDITIONAL IMAGES (B-F)

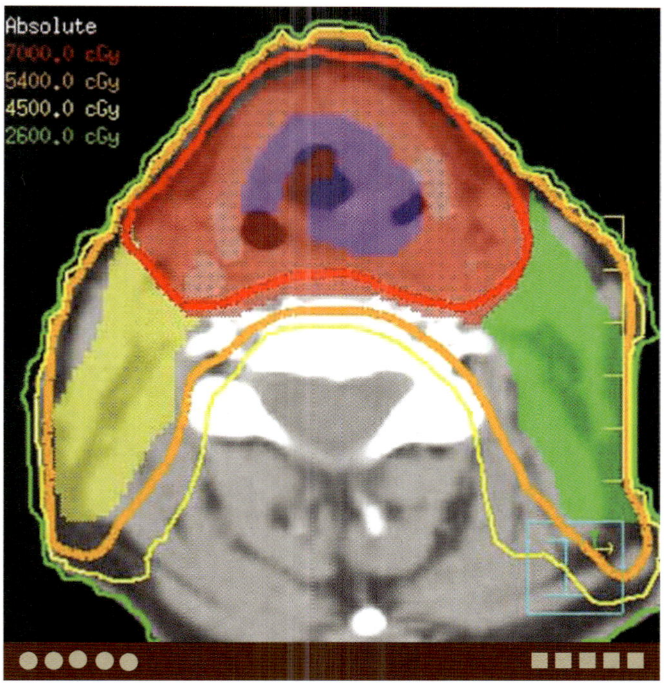

B. Supraglottic SCCA, same patient as A. Axial radiation treatment plan using intensity-modulated radiation therapy (IMRT). The primary gross tumor volume (GTV) is shaded in violet. The primary planning target volume (PTV) containing the GTV plus clinical and setup margins is shaded in red and prescribed to 70 Gy. The right and left neck elective nodal PTVs are shaded in yellow and green, respectively, and prescribed to 54 Gy. The primary and bilateral neck PTVs are simultaneously treated in 33 daily fractions with dose painting. Isodose lines colored red (70 Gy), orange (54 Gy), yellow (45 Gy), and green (26 Gy) show excellent coverage of the PTVs with good sparing of the esophagus, spinal cord, parotids, and other critical structures.

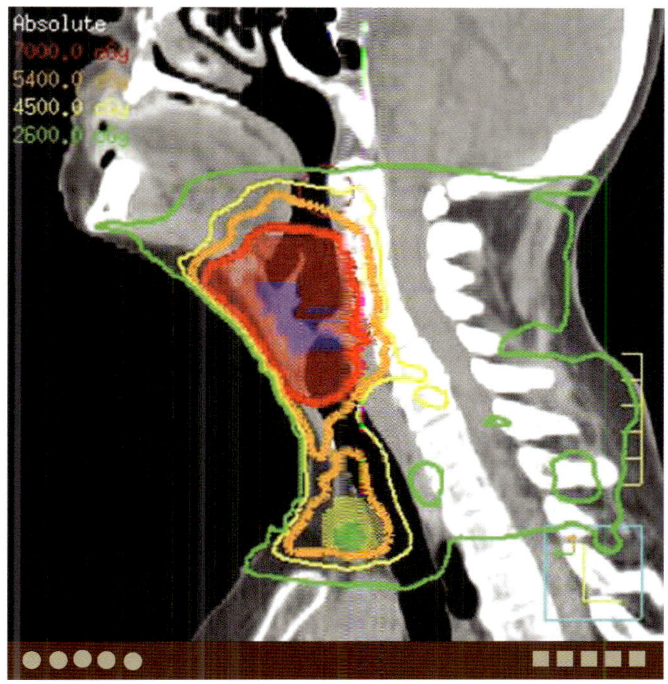

C. Supraglottic SCCA, same patient as A. Sagittal radiation treatment plan using IMRT.

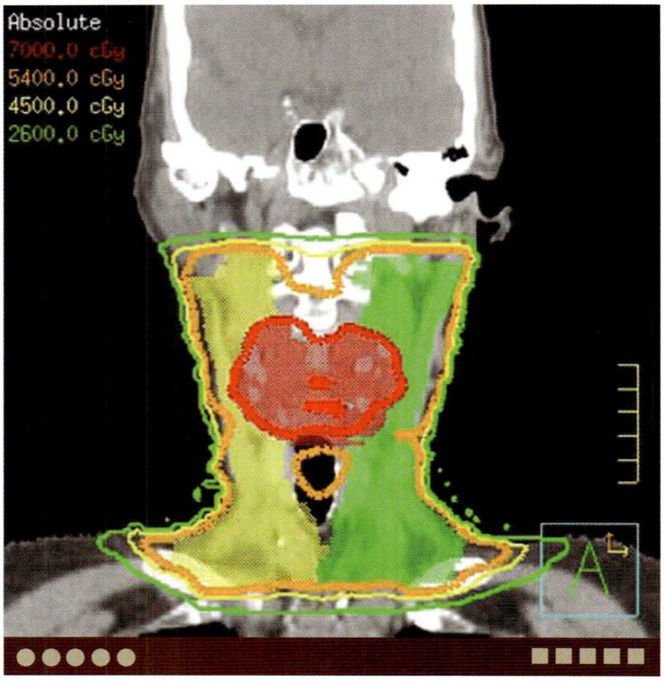

D. Supraglottic SCCA, same patient as A. Coronal radiation treatment plan using IMRT.

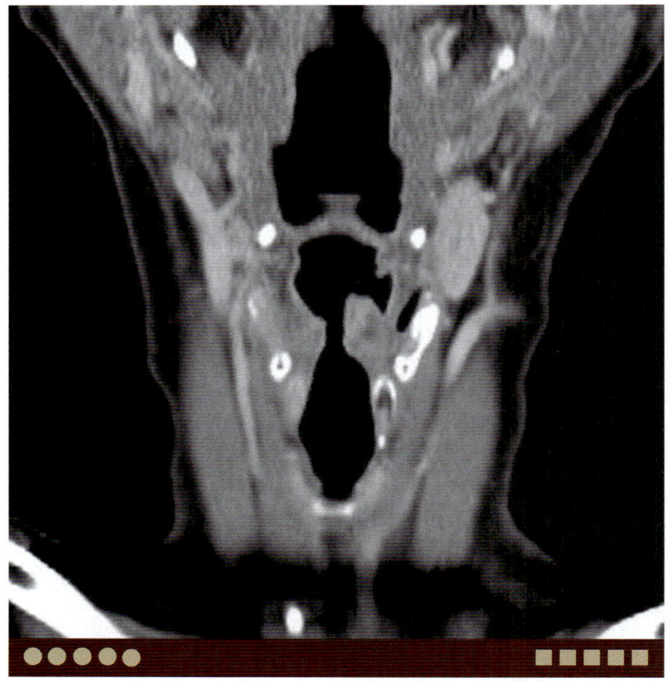

E. Supraglottic SCCA, same patient as A. Coronal postcontrast CT demonstrates irregularity and thickening of aryepiglottic folds, left more then right.

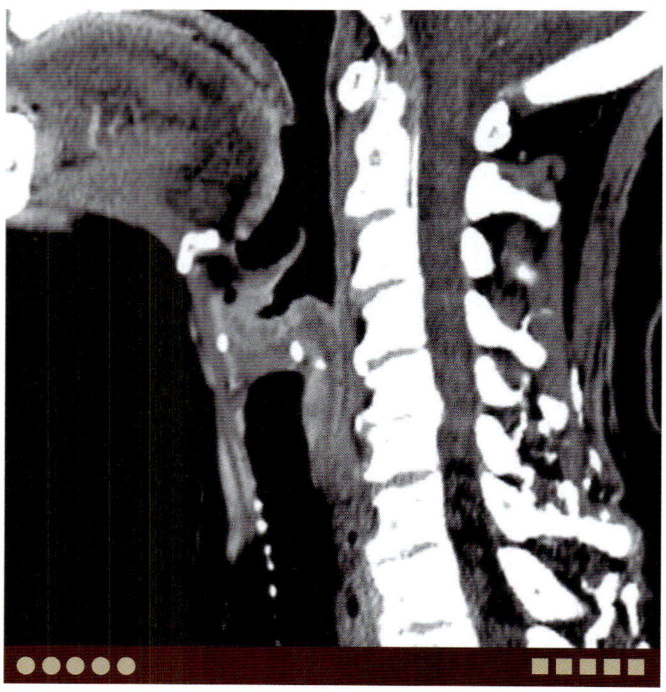

F. Supraglottic SCCA, same patient as A. Sagittal postcontrast CT demonstrates heterogeneously enhancing tumor involving the aryepiglottic fold.

DIFFERENTIAL DIAGNOSIS IMAGES (G-I)

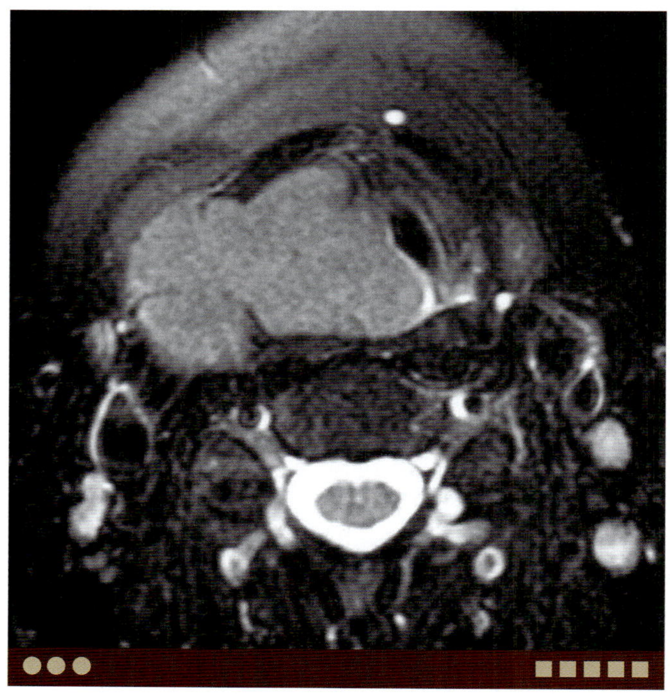

G. Lymphoma. Axial T2W image shows an intermediate-signal lesion involving the right aryepiglottic fold with lateral extension. Note homogeneous signal of the lesion without necrosis.

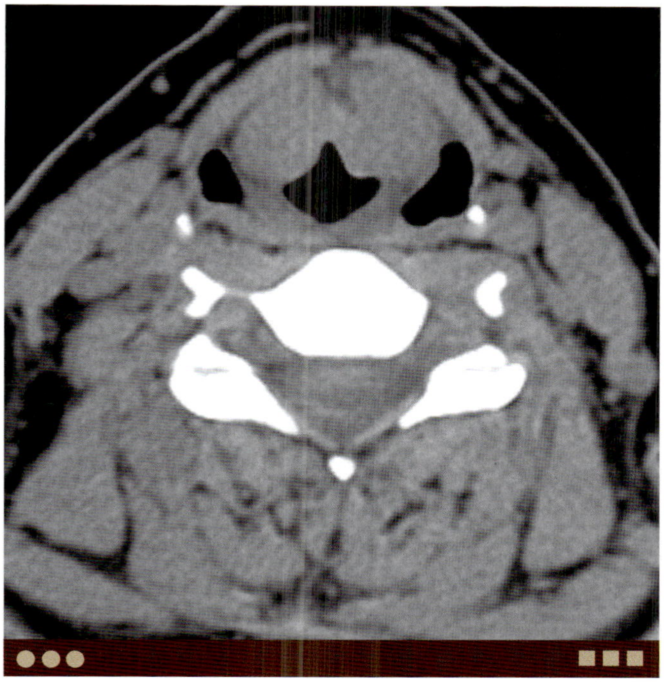

H. Amyloidosis. Axial noncontrast CT demonstrates homogeneous density lesions involving the aryepiglottic folds.

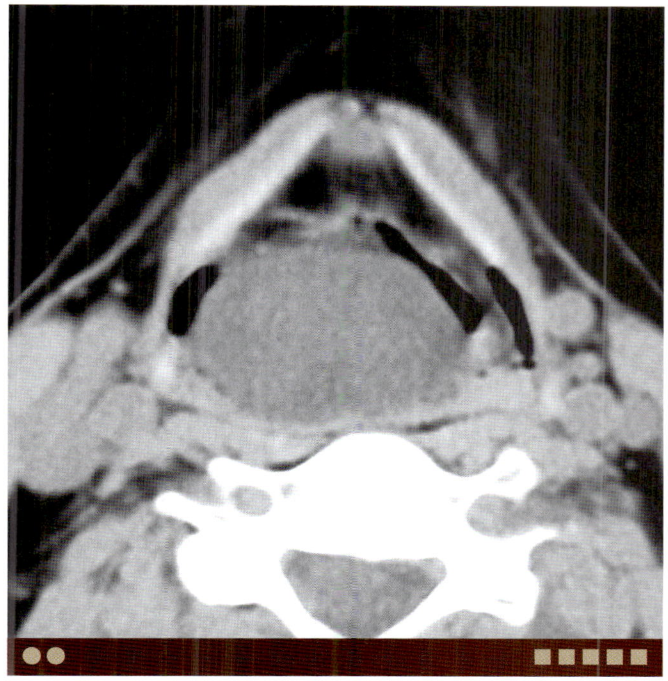

I. Schwannoma. Axial noncontrast CT demonstrates a homogeneous low-density lesion in the supraglottic larynx.

Case 15-7 Paranasal Sinus Malignancies

Paul Romesser, Osamu Sakai, Minh Tam Truong

PRESENTATION

Nasal congestion, facial swelling, cranial neuropathy, and epistaxis.

FINDINGS

CT and MRI demonstrate a soft tissue mass within the maxillary sinus with bone destruction and extension to the outside of the sinus.

DIFFERENTIAL DIAGNOSIS

- Squamous cell carcinoma (SCCA): Most common sinonasal malignant tumor, most commonly occurs in the maxillary sinus.
- Lymphoma: Large, nonnecrotic mass is a common finding. Among extranodal lymphoma in the head and neck, 40% to 50% occurs in the sinonasal cavity, commonly in the nasal cavity and maxillary sinus.
- Adenoid cystic carcinoma, mucoepidermoid carcinoma, and adenocarcinoma: Malignant tumors which arise from the minor salivary gland. Perineural tumor spread is commonly seen with adenoid cystic carcinomas.
- Neuroendocrine carcinoma and esthesioneuroblastoma: These tumors often arise in the upper nasal cavity and imaging findings of these tumors are identical and difficult to differentiate, although histologically, they can be differentiated by epithelial markers.

COMMENTS

This is an 80-year-old man with 40-pack-year smoking history who presented with 2 months of facial swelling and periorbital slight numbness. CT demonstrated a heterogeneous density tumor in the left maxillary sinus and left nasal cavity, with destruction of the anterior and posterolateral walls of the left maxillary sinus, involving the retroantral fat pad and pterygopalatine fossa with slight extension into the Vidian canal. PET/CT demonstrated a single 12 mm left level IB nodal metastasis. MRI showed involvement of the infraorbital nerve, pterygopalatine fossa, Vidian canal, and foramen rotundum. Biopsy revealed small cell type, neuroendocrine carcinoma. Due to tumor extension into the orbit and skull base, the patient underwent definitive chemoradiation.

Paranasal sinus malignancies are relatively rare head and neck malignancies, with an incidence of approximately 0.75 cases per 100,000. They present in a variety of anatomic sites and histopathologic types and are often diagnosed at an advanced-stage disease. Surgical resection

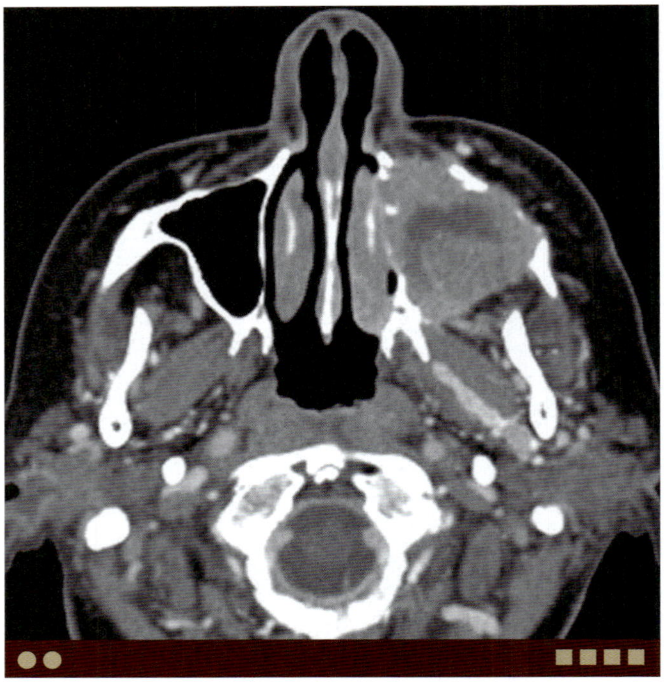

A. Maxillary sinus neuroendocrine carcinoma. Axial postcontrast CT demonstrates a solid enhancing tumor with central necrosis, occupying the left maxillary sinus with evidence of destruction.

of the primary tumor, in combination with radiation therapy, is often the mainstay of treatment. The maxillary sinus is the most common site of presentation for paranasal sinus malignancies. Ohngren line is a plane dividing the maxillary sinus into superior and inferior structures. Tumors superior to Ohngren line have a worse prognosis and commonly extend into the nasal cavity, ethmoid air cells, orbit, pterygopalatine fossa, infratemporal fossa, and base of skull. The tumors inferior to Ohngren line have a better prognosis and often infiltrate the palate, alveolar process,

PEARLS

- **Malignancies of the maxillary sinus often present at a locally advanced stage.**
- **Initial surgical resection is the mainstay of treatment followed by adjuvant radiotherapy with or without chemotherapy.**
- **Incidence of lymph node metastases and nodal recurrence depends on site and histological type and elective treatment of the regional nodes should be based upon the site and extent of primary tumor spread and also histology.**

gingivobuccal sulcus, soft tissues of the check, nasal cavity, and pterygoid fossa. The maxillary sinuses have a poor lymphatic supply and consequently nodal involvement at presentation is thought to be relatively uncommon with reported incidences at presentation ranging from 2.3% to 14%. This is in contrast to the nodal relapse rates which range between 3.8% and 38% depending on the primary site and histology. Nodal recurrences are more frequent for SCCA, neuroendocrine carcinomas, and rhabdomyosarcomas of the paranasal sinus and often elective nodal radiotherapy is considered for these histological types. For adenoid cystic carcinomas, perineural spread along cranial nerves to the skull base constitute the main pattern of spread, while lymph node metastases are uncommon.

TREATMENT

Maxillary sinus malignancies are the most common paranasal sinus malignancies which often present as locally advanced tumors and are typically managed with initial surgical resection followed by postoperative radiation with or without chemotherapy. Chemoradiotherapy can be used for unresectable tumors or advanced tumors invading into the skull base or orbit.

ADDITIONAL IMAGES (B-G)

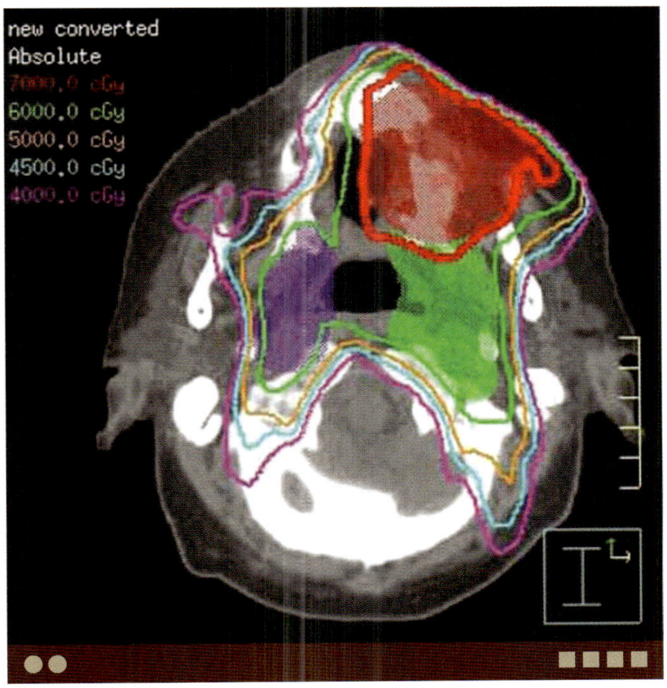

B. Maxillary sinus neuroendocrine carcinoma, same patient as A. Axial radiation treatment plan using intensity-modulated radiation therapy (IMRT). Red line represents the 70-Gy isodose line and planning target volume including the primary tumor (red colorwash) and involved node (purple colorwash). The bilateral elective regional nodes were treated to 60 Gy in the upper bilateral neck (green colorwash) and 50 Gy in the lower neck.

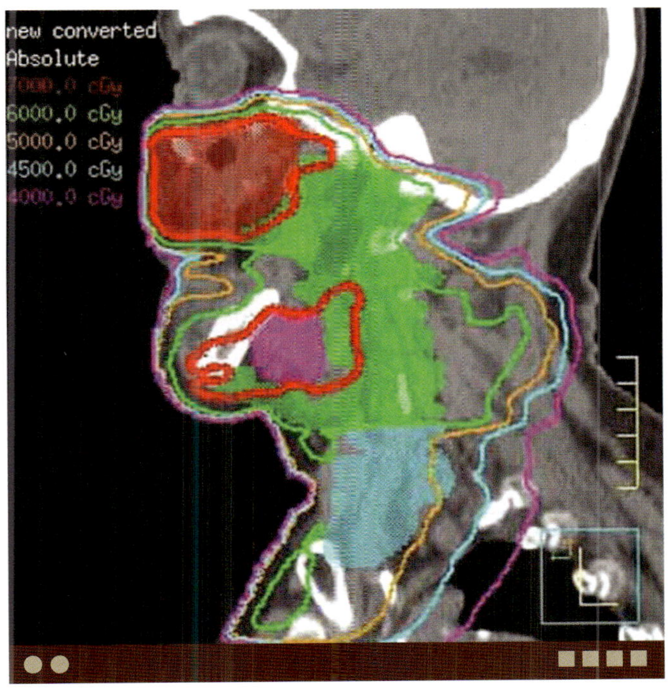

C. Maxillary sinus neuroendocrine carcinoma, same patient as A. Sagittal radiation treatment plan using IMRT.

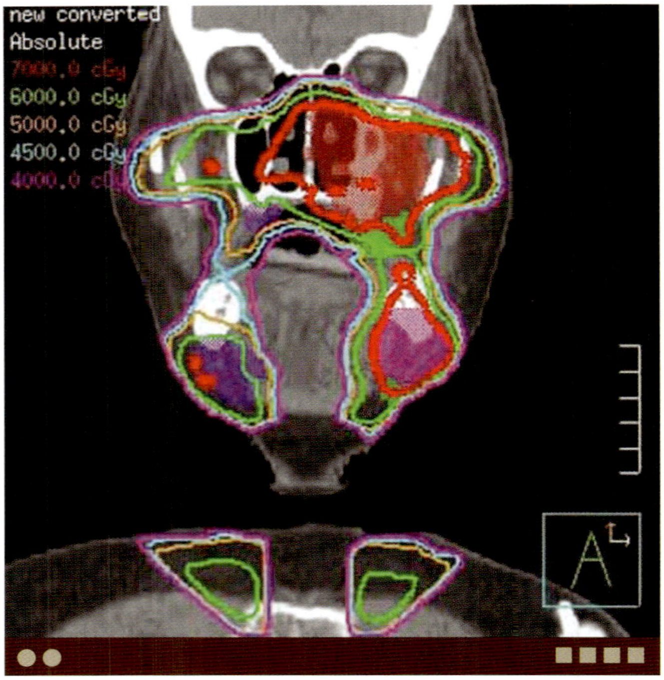

D. Maxillary sinus neuroendocrine carcinoma, same patient as A. Coronal radiation treatment plan using IMRT.

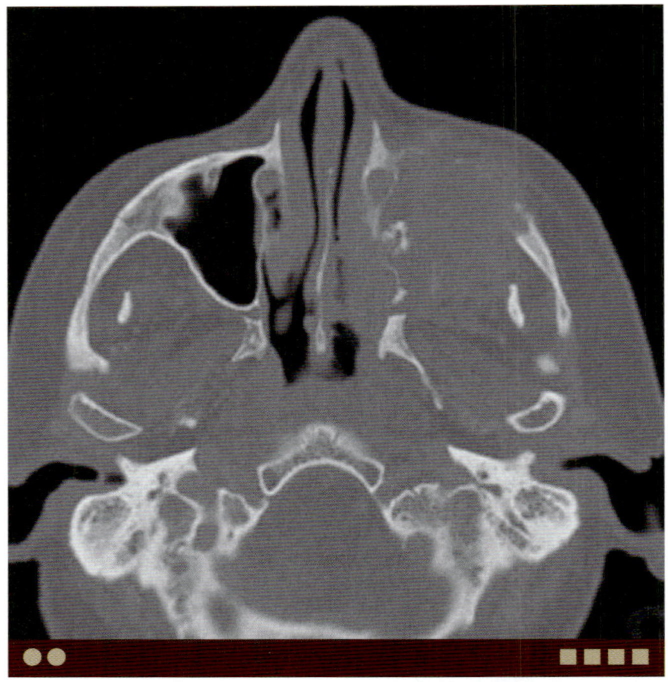

E. Maxillary sinus neuroendocrine carcinoma, same patient as A. Axial CT in bone window better demonstrates bone destruction by the tumor.

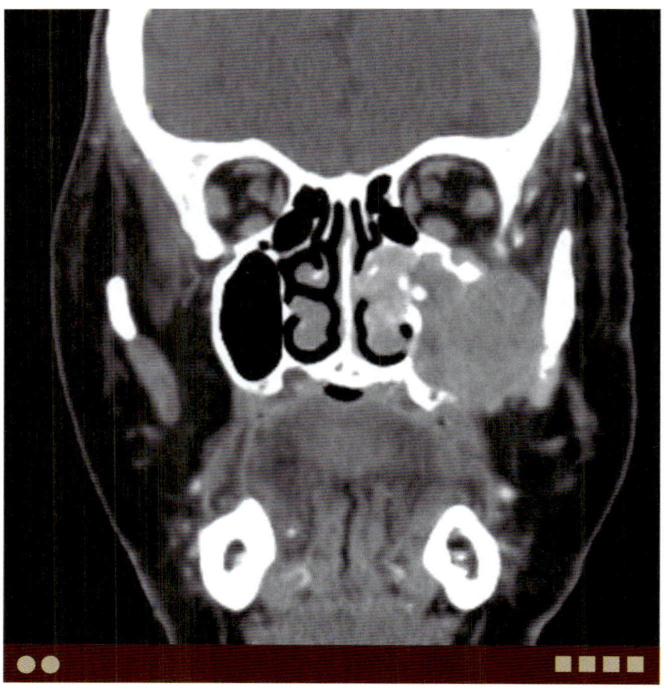

F. Maxillary sinus neuroendocrine carcinoma, same patient as A. Coronal postcontrast CT demonstrates the tumor invading the buccal space and inferior orbital fissure with destruction of the lateral wall of the left maxillary sinus. Thickening of the infraorbital nerve suggests perineural tumor spread.

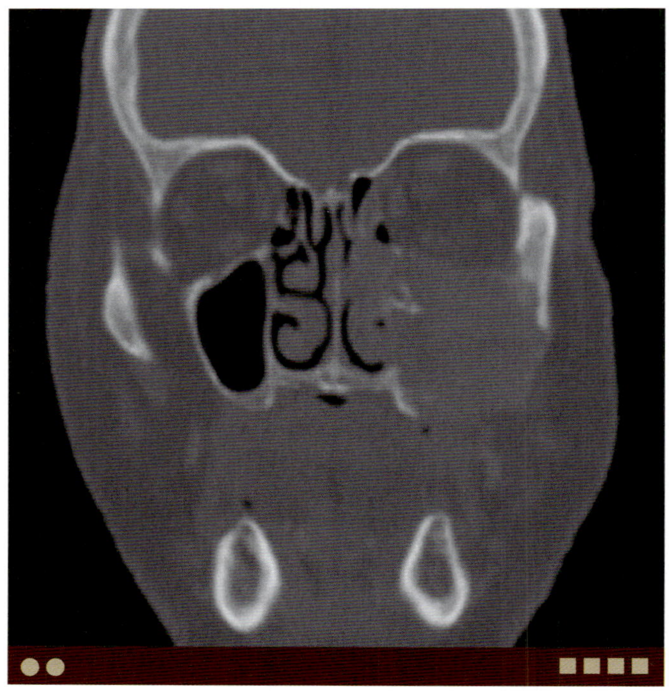

G. Maxillary sinus neuroendocrine carcinoma, same patient as A. Axial CT in bone window better demonstrates bone destruction by the tumor.

DIFFERENTIAL DIAGNOSIS IMAGES (H-I)

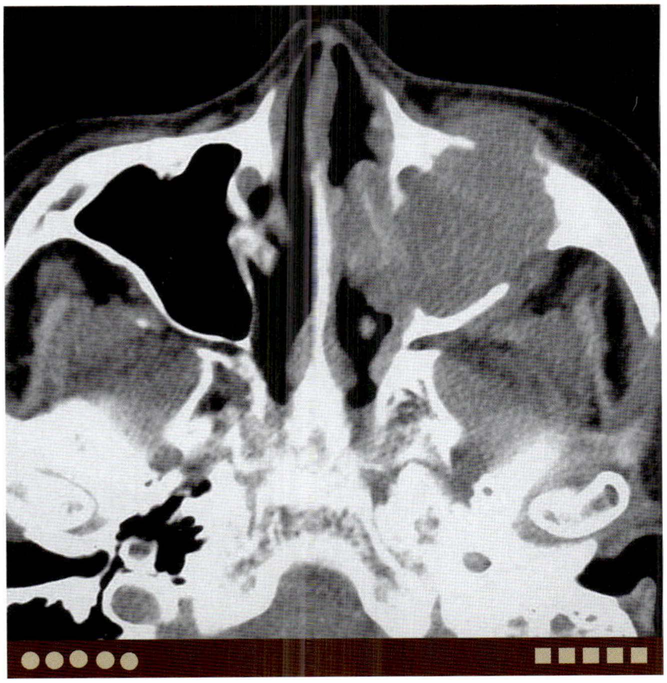

H. SCCA. Axial CT demonstrates a solid tumor occupying the left maxillary sinus, with destruction of the anterior wall and extension to the superficial soft tissue.

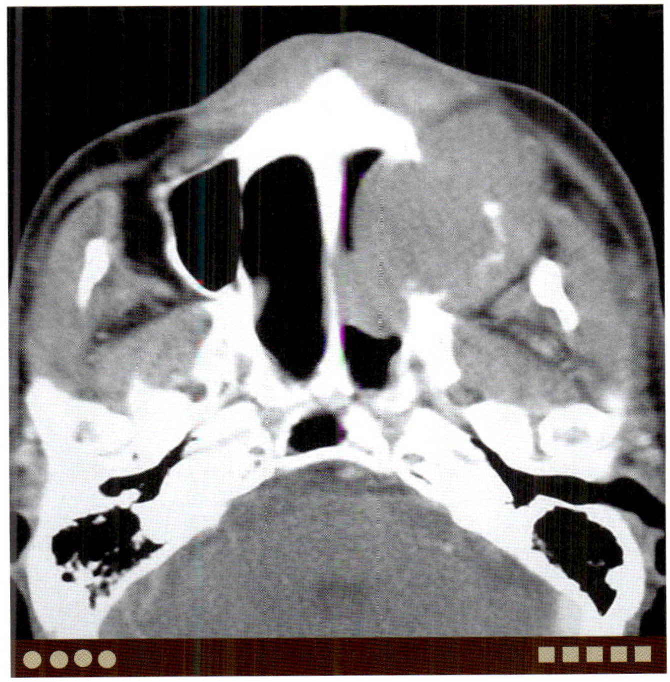

I. Lymphoma. Axial postcontrast CT demonstrates a solid tumor occupying the left maxillary sinus, with destruction of the anterior wall and extension to the superficial soft tissue.

Case 15-8 Adenoid Cystic Carcinoma of the Parotid Gland

Minh Tam Truong, Paul Romesser, Osamu Sakai

PRESENTATION

Atypical facial pain, otalgia, swelling of the parotid gland, and facial nerve paralysis.

FINDINGS

MRI demonstrates a T1 and T2 hypointense, mildly enhancing lesion in the parotid gland.

DIFFERENTIAL DIAGNOSIS

- Mucoepidermoid carcinoma: This is the most common malignant parotid gland tumor. Regional nodal metastasis is commonly seen.
- Acinic cell carcinoma: This is a rare parotid gland tumor and can be multiple and bilateral. Hemorrhage, fibrosis, and calcification are occasionally seen.
- Adenocarcinoma: This is a rare aggressive tumor with rapid growth. Imaging findings are nonspecific. Adenocarcinoma may arise from preexisting pleomorphic adenoma (carcinoma ex pleomorphic adenoma).

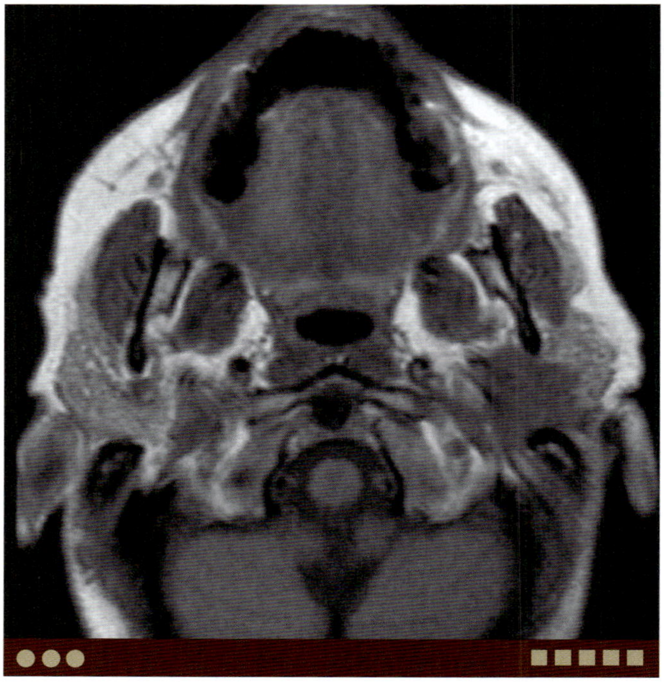

A. ACC. Axial T1W image demonstrates a low-signal infiltrative lesion involving the entire deep lobe and part of the superficial lobe of the left parotid to the stylomastoid foramen.

COMMENTS

This is a 62-year-old woman with a 3-month history of atypical facial pain, left otalgia, left parotid swelling, and acute onset of facial nerve paresis. MRI revealed signal abnormality in the deep lobe of the left parotid gland, involving the stylomastoid foramen. Fine-needle aspiration (FNA) of the lesion did not reveal malignancy. Due to sudden onset of facial nerve paralysis, open incisional biopsy was performed, and pathology revealed adenoid cystic carcinoma (ACC). Total parotidectomy with facial nerve sacrifice and selective left neck dissection was performed. Findings at operation revealed a poorly circumscribed tumor in the deep and superficial lobes of the parotid gland and tail of the gland, encasing the left external carotid artery and invading the facial nerve. Pathology revealed extensive perineural tumor spread along the facial nerve, and positive margins, without nodal metastasis. Postoperative MRI suggested a residual disease at the stylomastoid foramen.

It is important in the work-up of a parotid mass, that clinical examination finding of facial nerve paralysis is highly suggestive of malignancy. Other features suggestive of a malignant parotid tumor include pain, rapid growth, skin involvement, and cervical lymphadenopathy. A negative FNA does not exclude the possibility of malignancy and pursuing additional open biopsies or proceeding to a parotidectomy may be indicated. ACC has a high recurrence rate and postoperative irradiation is usually indicated.

Perineural spread is common in ACCs. If the facial nerve is involved, then radiation therapy should target the nerve back to the skull base to cover the facial canal and geniculate ganglion. Intensity-modulated radiation therapy (IMRT) allows highly conformal dose distributions and rapid dose fall off to spare adjacent critical structures including the spinal cord, brainstem, brain, and oral cavity.

PEARLS

- **Hallmark of parotid malignancies include rapidly enlarging parotid mass associated with facial pain and facial nerve paralysis.**
- **Indications for postoperative radiation therapy for parotid malignancies include ACC histology, high grade, facial nerve involvement, perineural invasion, and positive margins.**
- **When the facial nerve is involved by tumor, the radiation field should encompass the nerve traced back to the skull base.**

TREATMENT

Indications for postoperative radiation therapy for parotid cancer include ACC histology, positive margins, tumor adherence or invasion to the facial nerve, and perineural tumor spread. The patient underwent IMRT to the parotid bed and skull base with coverage of the stylomastoid foramen, facial canal, geniculate ganglion, and ipsilateral elective nodal irradiation. A total dose of 70 Gy in 33 fractions was delivered to the tumor bed and areas of gross residual disease seen on postoperative MRI. For high-risk subclinical disease, or microscopic positive margins a total dose of 66 Gy was delivered.

ADDITIONAL IMAGES (B-G)

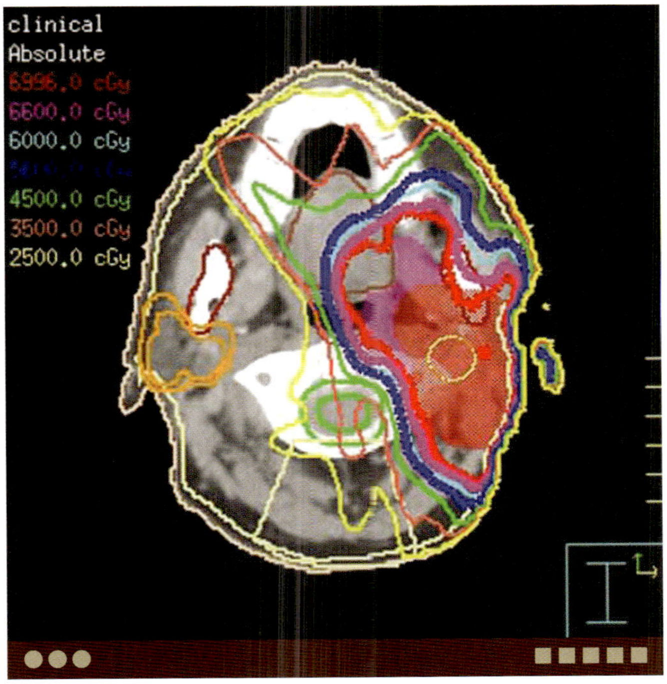

B. ACC, same patient as A. Axial radiation treatment plan using IMRT. Clinical target volume (CTV) is contoured using surgical information, pathology report, and pre- and postoperative imaging. Treatment delivered with IMRT with isodoses demonstrating conformal coverage of clinical target and sparing adjacent brain, brainstem, and oral cavity.

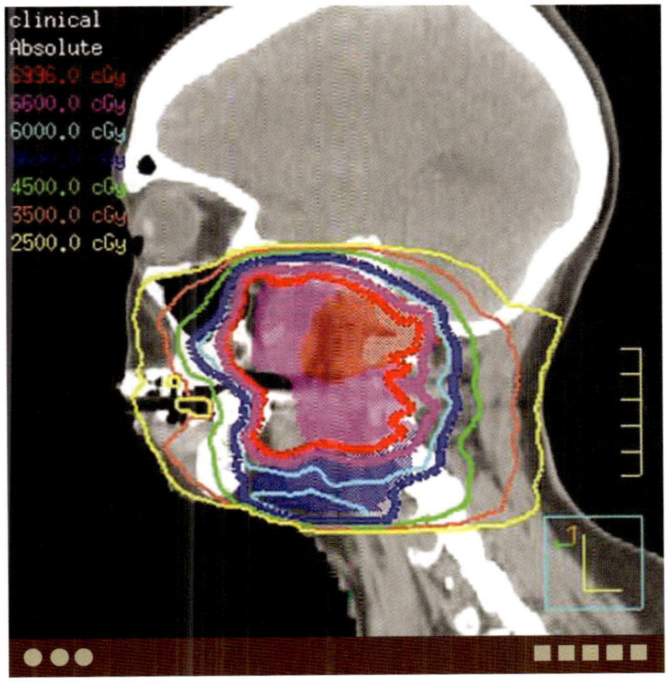

C. ACC, same patient as A. Sagittal radiation treatment plan using IMRT. CTV is contoured using surgical information, pathology report, and pre- and postoperative imaging. Treatment delivered with IMRT with isodoses demonstrating conformal coverage of clinical target and sparing adjacent brain, brainstem, and oral cavity.

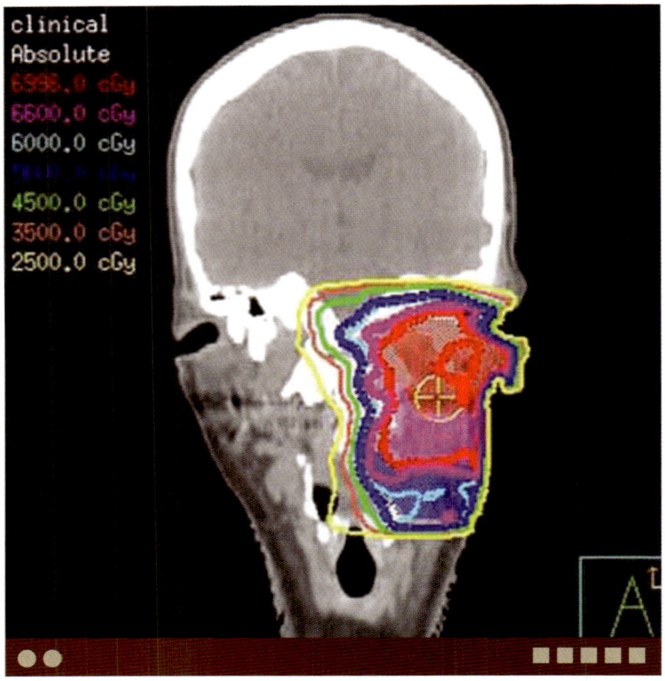

D. ACC, same patient as A. Coronal radiation treatment plan using IMRT. CTV is contoured using surgical information, pathology report, and pre- and postoperative imaging. Treatment delivered with IMRT with isodoses demonstrating conformal coverage of clinical target and sparing adjacent brain, brainstem, and oral cavity.

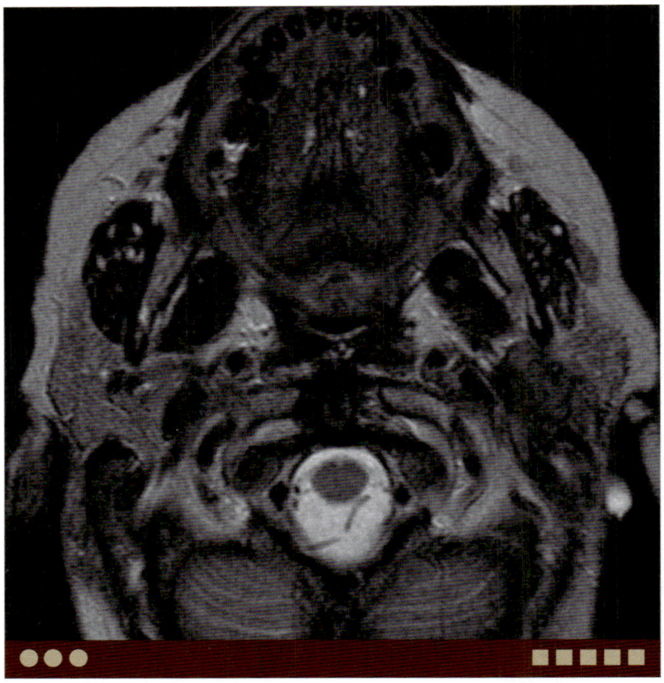

E. ACC, same patient as A. Axial T2W image demonstrates a low-signal infiltrative lesion involving the deep lobe of the left parotid extending to the stylomastoid foramen.

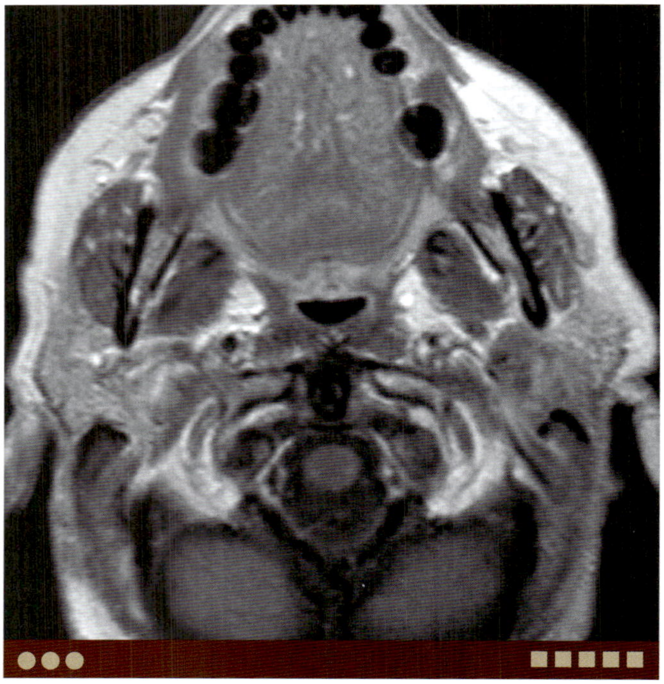

F. ACC, same patient as A. Axial postcontrast T1W image demonstrates mild, heterogeneous enhancement of the lesion.

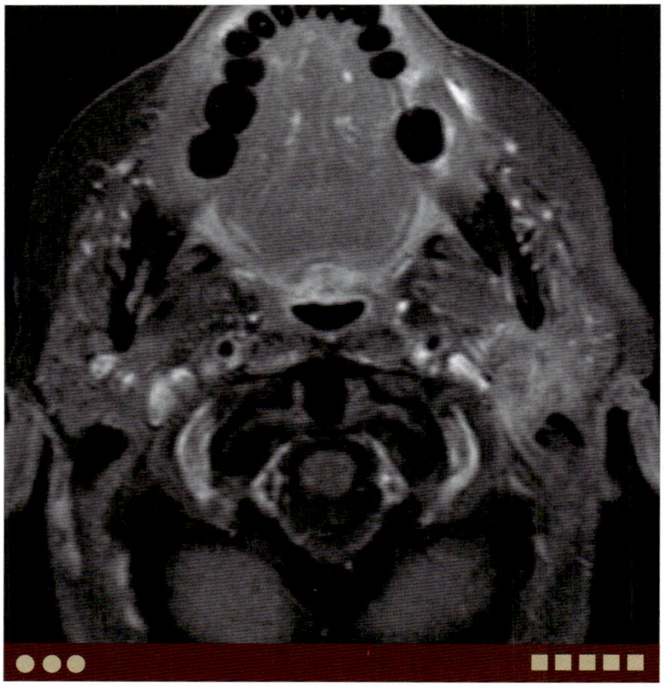

G. ACC, same patient as A. Axial postcontrast fat-suppressed T1W image demonstrates mild, heterogeneous enhancement of the lesion.

DIFFERENTIAL DIAGNOSIS IMAGES (H-J)

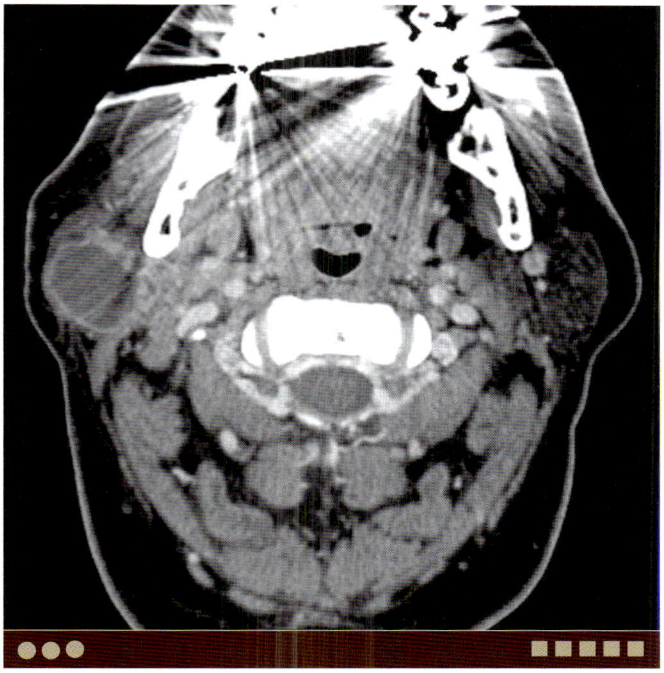

H. Mucoepidermoid carcinoma (high grade). Axial contrast-enhanced CT demonstrates a cystic appearing tumor with rim enhancement and infiltrative margins in the right parotid gland.

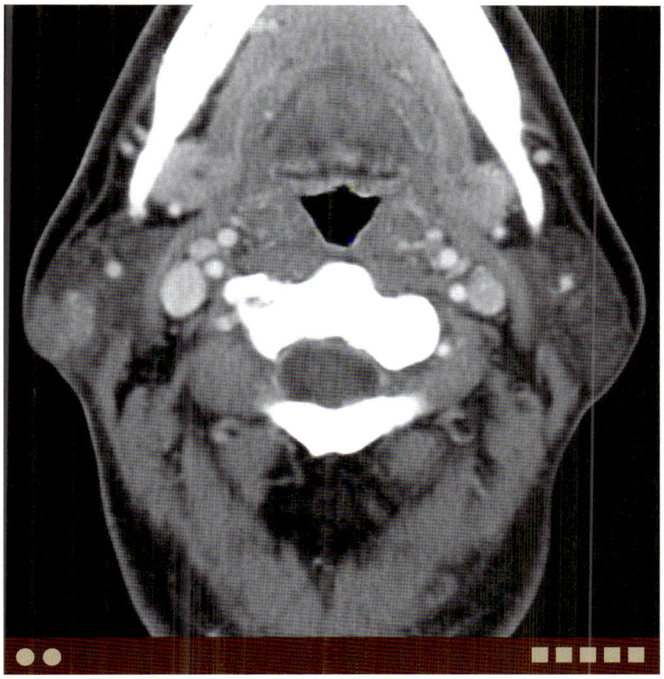

I. Acinic cell carcinoma. Axial contrast-enhanced CT demonstrates a lobulated mass in the superficial lobe of the right parotid gland. There is tumor invasion into the subcutaneous fat and skin.

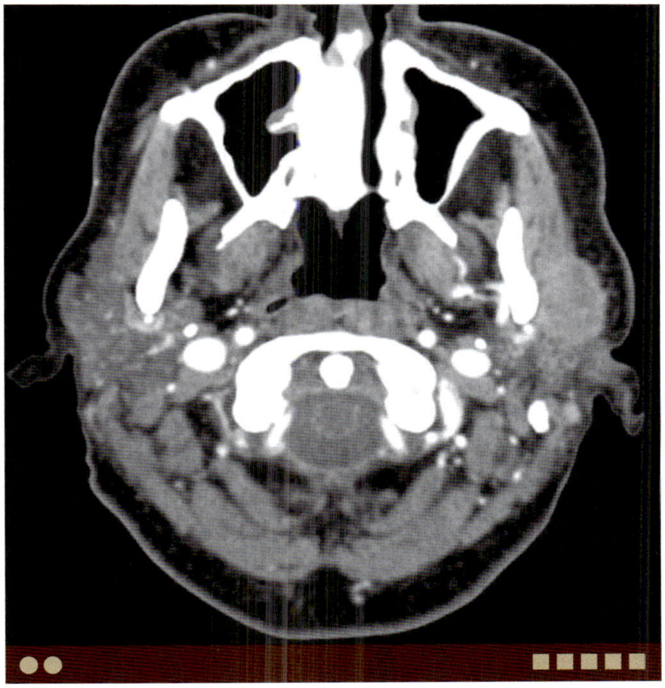

J. Adenocarcinoma. Axial contrast-enhanced CT demonstrates a heterogeneously enhancing tumor with irregular margins in the superficial lobe of the left parotid gland.

Case 15-9 Vestibular Schwannoma

Mayur Jayarao, Paramjit Singh, Minh Tam Truong, Kurtis G. Birch, Lawrence Chin

PRESENTATION

Sensorineural hearing loss, tinnitus, headaches, orofacial pain, and vestibular problems.

FINDINGS

CT and MRI demonstrate a homogeneously enhancing, extra-axial, cerebellopontine angle mass which extends through the porus acousticus and into the internal auditory canal.

DIFFERENTIAL DIAGNOSIS

- Meningioma: Constituting approximately 20% of cerebellopontine angle lesions, these well-circumscribed tumors can arise from the tentorial edge, occupy the cerebellopontine angle, and on MRI demonstrate homogeneous avid enhancement. Total surgical resection remains the treatment of choice, with radiosurgery being considered for postoperative tumor control. Small tumors may be treated with radiosurgery primarily.
- Metastasis: Metastases are usually found in the brain parenchyma, although they can rarely be found in the cerebellopontine angle as well. When present, they demonstrate avid enhancement on MRI and can cause significant mass effect which may require surgical decompression. Lesions without significant mass effect and up to 3 cm can be alternatively treated by stereotactic radiosurgery.
- Epidermoid cyst: These tumors arise from ectopic ectodermal cells that are retained within the neural groove at the time of closure. If extradural, they most frequently occur at the cerebellopontine angle. MRI is the imaging modality of choice, and surgical resection is the only treatment modality for symptomatic patients.
- Nonvestibular nerve schwannomas: Cranial nerves V, IX, and X are commonly affected, with total surgical resection being the primary treatment option for symptomatic patients. Stereotactic radiosurgery is useful for postoperative residual tumors and recurrent tumors. Small schwannomas may be treated primarily with radiosurgery particularly when incidentally found.
- Arachnoid cyst: They are usually asymptomatic but can cause symptoms secondary to mass effect. CT and MRI demonstrate water density/signal similar to the cerebrospinal fluid (CSF). When indicated, treatment consists of cyst fenestration with cystoperitoneal shunting reserved for persistent cysts.

COMMENTS

A 48-year-old woman with normal right-sided hearing, and left-sided conductive hearing loss with tinnitus of unknown etiology was referred for management of a right-sided cerebellopontine angle mass. MRI demonstrated a 1.5 cm mass at the right cerebellopontine angle adjacent to the

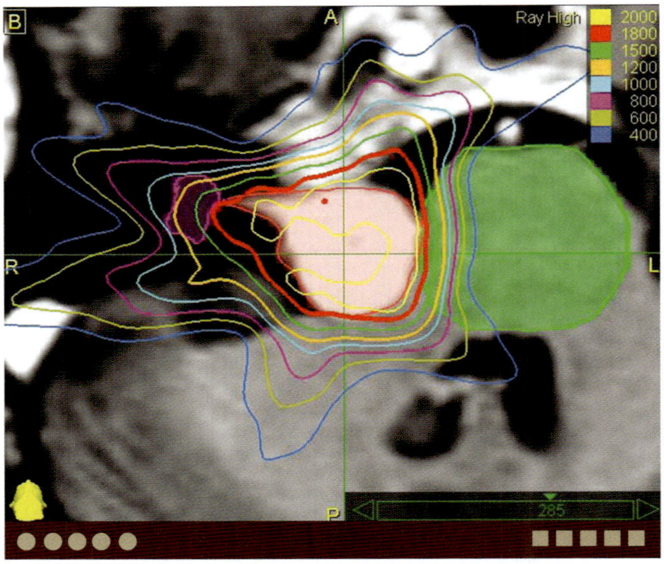

A. Vestibular schwannoma, axial CyberKnife® treatment plan. The red lines indicate the prescription isodose lines, and represent 80% of the central dose. The patient received a total of 18 Gy delivered in a dose fractionation scheme of 6 Gy × 3. Hundred percent of the tumor was covered with the rapid fall-off of the radiation isodose lines seen on the brainstem (shaded green) and right cochlea (shaded pink) sides.

PEARLS

- **Acoustic neuromas arise from Schwann cells that invest the VIII cranial nerve and are located at the cerebellopontine angle. They can extend into the internal auditory canal, with patients commonly presenting with unilateral hearing loss.**
- **Contrast-enhanced T1W MR imaging is the imaging modality of choice and demonstrates avid enhancement of the tumor.**
- **Total surgical resection can lead to a cure, with postoperative radiosurgery being utilized for residual tumor control.**
- **Stereotactic radiosurgery can be used as the definitive treatment modality for tumors less than 3 cm and in patients who do not want to undergo surgery with comparable rates of local control.**

brainstem and VII/VIII cranial nerve complex. Due to the small size of the lesion, preexisting left-sided hearing loss and the risk of right-sided hearing loss secondary to surgical resection, the patient elected to undergo CyberKnife® robotic radiosurgery. A dose of 18 Gy fractionated over three treatments was prescribed to the 80% isodose line encompassing the target volume. Radiation dose to the adjacent brainstem and right VII/VIII cranial nerve complex was minimized. The patient had no treatment-related sequelae and preservation of her hearing.

Acoustic neuromas are intracranial, extra-axial tumors that arise from the Schwann cells surrounding the vestibular or cochlear portion of the VIII cranial nerve, although 95% arise exclusively from the vestibular portion. Bilateral acoustic neuromas are a diagnostic hallmark of neurofibromatosis type II (chromosome 22q12.2). The most common presenting symptom is unilateral hearing loss secondary to either mass effect on the VIII cranial nerve and/or disruption of the cochlear blood supply. Other symptoms include headache, tinnitus, facial numbness, vertigo, and disequilibrium.

Avid homogeneous enhancement of the acoustic neuroma can be appreciated on postcontrast T1W MR images demonstrating the classic "ice cream–cone" appearance of an acoustic neuroma that has both intracanalicular and cisternal components. CT-cisternography may be utilized for patients in whom MRI is contraindicated.

Treatment options for acoustic neuromas include observation with serial imaging, surgical resection, stereotactic radiosurgery (in one to three fractions) and conventionally fractionated stereotactic radiotherapy over 5 weeks. While surgical resection remains the treatment of choice, radiosurgery can be considered instead for tumors less than 3 cm, although it cannot relieve ongoing brainstem compression. Local control rates with stereotactic radiosurgery using a single dose of 12 Gy and radiotherapy are greater than 95% with high rates of preservation of serviceable hearing of approximately 70%. An alternative fractionation schedule of 18 Gy divided into three fractions of 6 Gy each provide similar results using CyberKnife® radiosurgery. Additionally, stereotactic radiosurgery can be used postoperatively for residual tumor control. Fractionated stereotactic radiotherapy over 5 weeks using conventional fractionation is also a treatment option for acoustic neuromas of all sizes with comparable local control rates to single dose stereotactic radiosurgery, although for large tumors (greater than 3 cm), radiation does not reduce the mass effect of the tumor mass.

ADDITIONAL IMAGES (B-F)

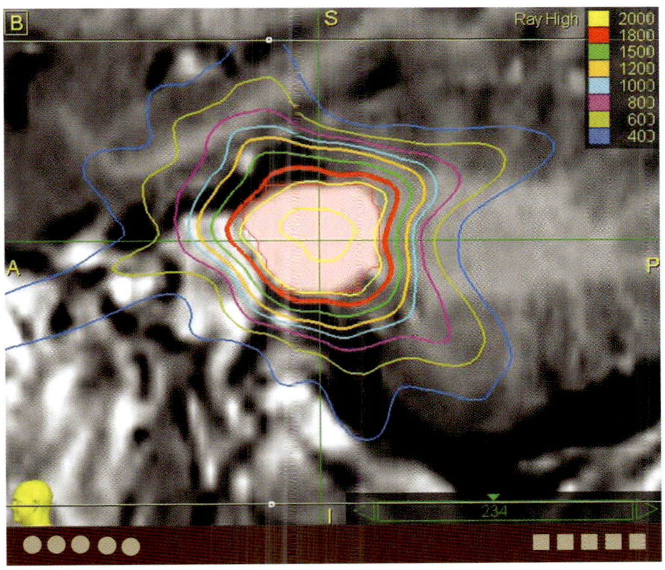

B. Vestibular schwannoma, sagittal CyberKnife® treatment plan. The red lines indicate the prescription isodose lines, and represent 80% of the central dose. The conformity index was 1.6.

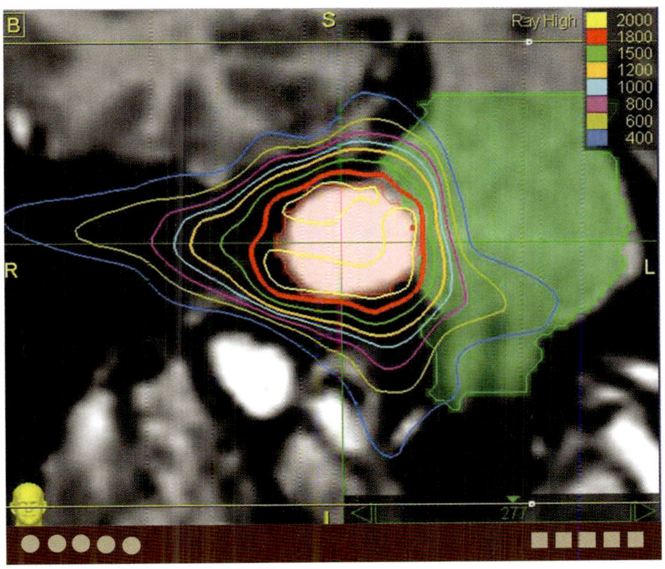

C. Vestibular schwannoma, coronal CyberKnife® treatment plan. The red line indicates the prescription isodose line, with the maximal dosing being localized over the tumor. Rapid fall-off of the isodose lines can be seen on the brainstem side (shaded green).

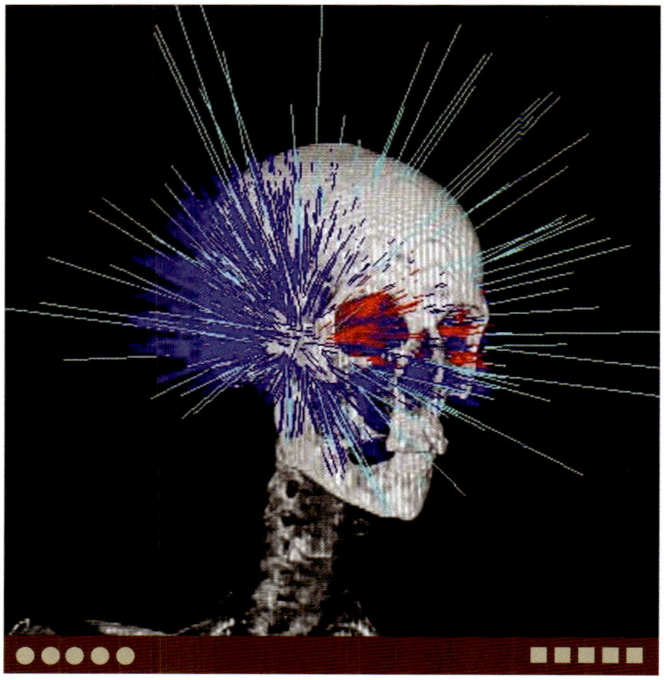

D. Vestibular schwannoma, three-dimensional x-ray beam projections CyberKnife® treatment plan. In all, 71 nodes and 99 beams were used to deliver the 18 Gy delivered in a dose fractionation scheme of 6 Gy × 3.

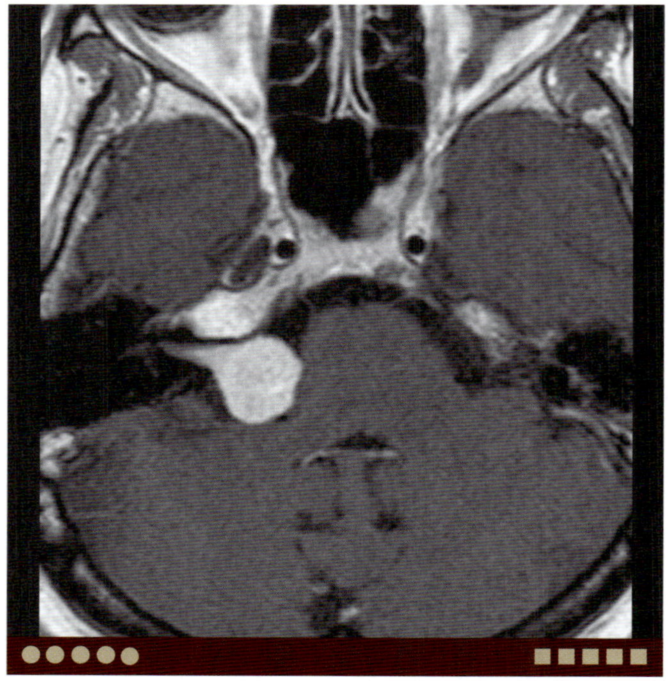

E. Vestibular schwannoma, same patient as A. Axial postcontrast T1W image demonstrates a homogeneously enhancing right cerebellopontine angle tumor extending through the porus acousticus into the right internal auditory canal. Note the resulting mass effect on the cerebellopontine angle.

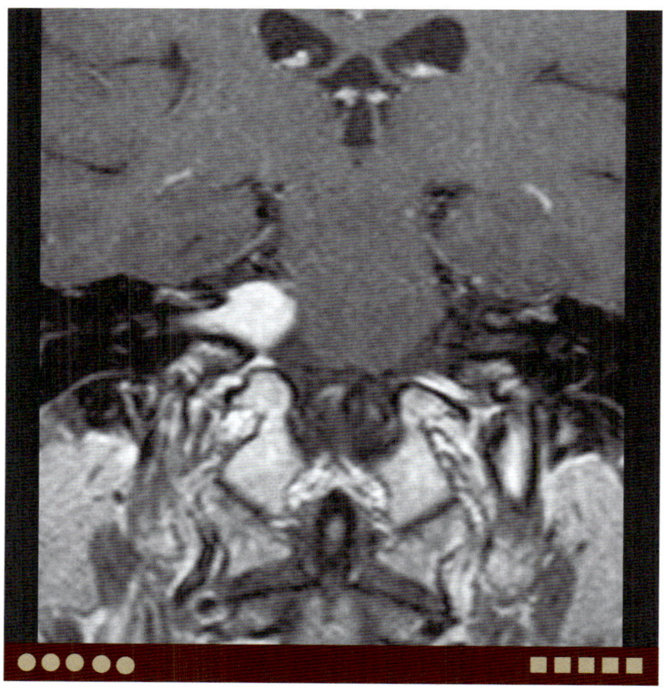

F. Vestibular schwannoma, same patient as A. Coronal postcontrast T1W image demonstrates a homogeneously enhancing right cerebellopontine angle mass extending through the porus acousticus into the right internal auditory canal.

DIFFERENTIAL DIAGNOSIS IMAGES (G-I)

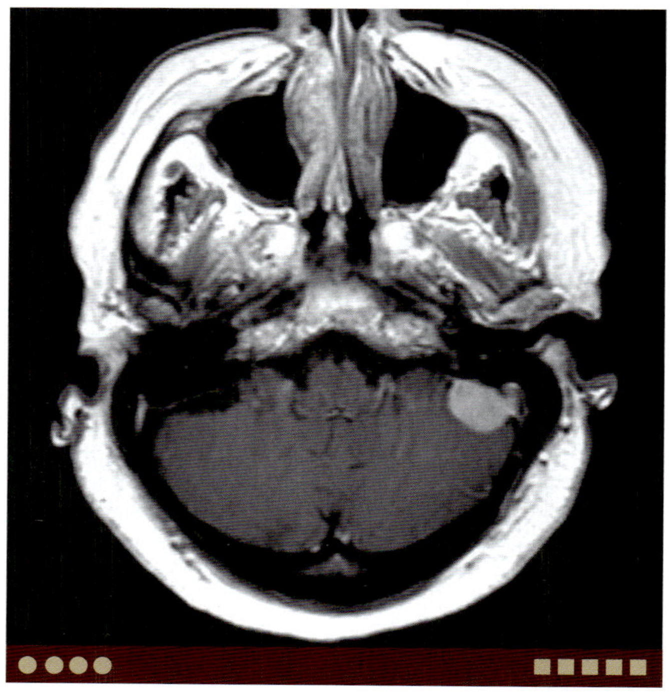

G. Meningioma. Axial postcontrast T1W image demonstrates a homogeneously enhancing dural-based mass immediately adjacent to the left sigmoid sinus and left cerebellar hemisphere.

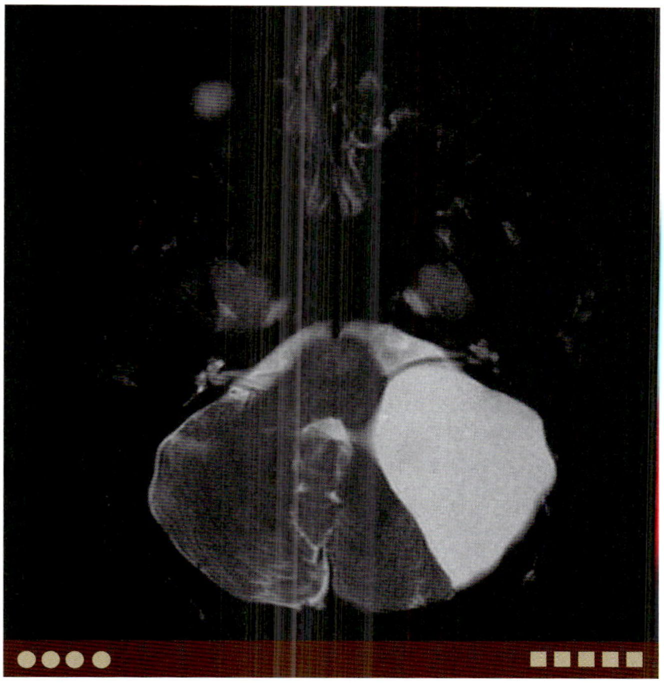

H. Arachnoid cyst. Axial T2W image demonstrates a large cystic lesion in the left cerebellopontine angle with resulting mass effect upon the pons, left cerebellum and left VII/VIII cranial nerve complex.

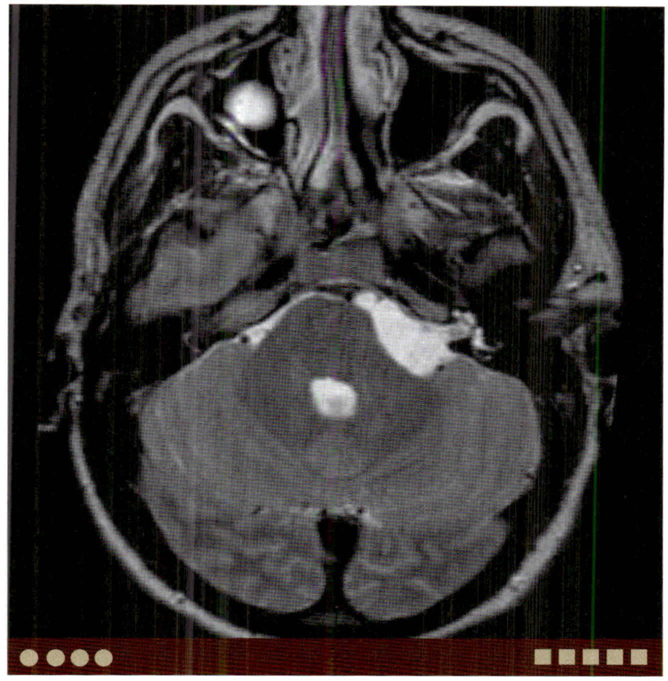

I. Epidermoid cyst. Axial T2W image demonstrates a hyperintense lesion in the left cerebellopontine angle with resulting mass effect on the adjacent pons.

Case 15–10 Meningioma: Cerebellopontine Angle

Mayur Jayarao, Minh Tam Truong, Kurtis G. Birch, Lawrence Chin

PRESENTATION

Headaches, hearing loss.

FINDINGS

CT and MRI demonstrate an extra-axial, well-circumscribed avidly enhancing mass in the petrous region posterior to the cerebellopontine angle and adjacent to the sigmoid sinus with dural-based attachment and a "meningeal tail."

DIFFERENTIAL DIAGNOSIS

- Acoustic neuroma: These extra-axial tumors arise from the Schwann cells that invest the VIII cranial nerve and are usually found in the cerebellopontine angle with extension into the internal auditory canal. They enhance homogeneously on MRI and can be cured with total surgical resection. Stereotactic radiosurgery is best reserved for lesions less than 3 cm to achieve tumor stabilization and control.
- Metastasis: Metastases are more frequently found in the brain parenchyma, and enhance on MRI. In general, up to three metastatic lesions with maximal diameters of 3 cm can be simultaneously and effectively treated with stereotactic radiosurgery, but there is no universally accepted limit to either number or size.
- Hemangioblastoma: These are benign tumors that on MRI can characteristically demonstrate a cyst with an enhancing mural nodule. Angiography is useful in preoperative localization of feeding vessels and embolization. Treatment options include total surgical resection (curative) with postoperative radiotherapy for tumor control, and stereotactic radiosurgery for tumors less than 3 cm in size and those in eloquent locations.
- Epidermoid cyst: These tumors arise from ectopic ectodermal neural cells and are commonly found in the cerebellopontine angle. MRI characteristics are variable and depend upon the fat and protein content of the cyst. Surgical resection is the only treatment option for symptomatic patients.

COMMENTS

A 72-year-old woman presented with recurrent headaches and a normal physical examination. MRI revealed a homogeneously enhancing 2-cm meningeal-based extra-axial lesion in the left petrous region posterior to the cerebellopontine angle and adjacent to the sigmoid sinus. The headaches subsequently resolved spontaneously and upon follow-up the patient expressed a desire to receive treatment for the lesion. Based on the tumor location and size, she was offered the option of surgical resection versus stereotactic radiosurgery, and elected to undergo the latter. She underwent CyberKnife® robotic radiosurgery and

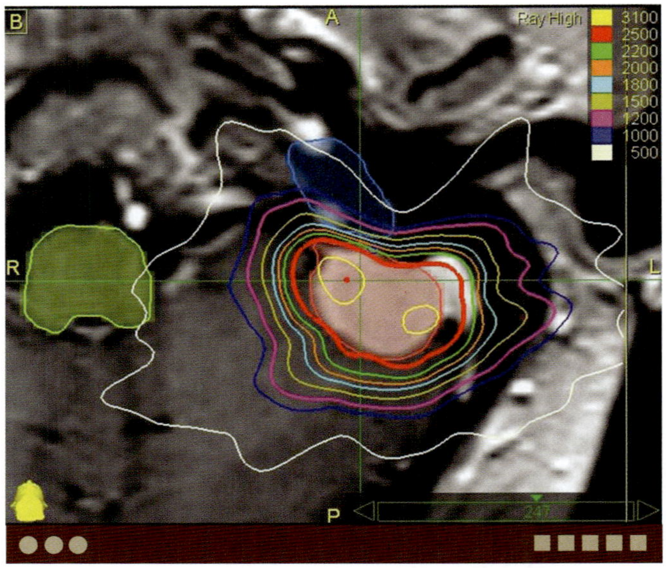

A. Meningioma, axial CyberKnife® treatment plan. The red lines indicate the prescription isodose lines, and represent 75% of the central dose. The patient received a total of 25 Gy delivered in a dose fractionation scheme of 5 Gy × 5. Over 99% of the tumor was covered with the rapid fall-off of the radiation isodose lines seen at the left cochlea (shaded blue). The brainstem is shaded green.

PEARLS

- **Meningiomas are slow growing, benign tumors that arise from arachnoid cap cells in the meninges.**
- **CT and MRI demonstrate avidly enhancing, well-circumscribed tumors that may have a characteristic "meningeal tail."**
- **Total surgical resection can afford a cure with radiotherapy reserved for residual tumor control.**
- **Stereotactic radiosurgery is most effective for tumors less than 3 cm and/or for tumors in surgically inaccessible locations.**

received a dose of 25 Gy in a dose fractionation scheme of 5 Gy × 5 to the 75% prescription isodose line.

Meningiomas arise from arachnoid cap cells and are benign, slow growing, well-circumscribed solid tumors that occasionally contain a necrotic, cystic, or calcified component. Meningiomas are almost always found on the surface of the brain and about 90% occur in the supratentorial compartment. Symptoms at initial presentation vary widely, and are reflective of tumor location and the adjacent structures. These tumors are usually noninfiltrative, cause adjacent bony erosion or hyperostosis, and very rarely can undergo malignant transformation.

On CT and MRI, meningiomas appear as well-circumscribed, avidly enhancing tumors which if large can cause substantial perilesional vasogenic edema. Postcontrast MRI may also reveal an associated "meningeal tail." Angiography may be useful for preoperative planning and embolization.

Treatment options for meningioma include observation, surgical resection, stereotactic radiosurgery, or fractionated external beam radiotherapy.

Being benign, meningiomas can be cured by total surgical resection. Radiotherapy is mainly used as an adjuvant for tumor control of residual postoperative tumors. Stereotactic radiosurgery may be considered as the initial and definitive form of tumor control for tumors less than 3 cm, or if the tumor is in an inaccessible location, or if the surgery carries a high risk of morbidity. Stereotactic radiosurgery can be delivered in a single dose of 14 Gy or with frameless systems, a hypofractionated course of 5 Gy × 5 fractions provides similar high rates of local control. For conventionally fractionated external beam radiotherapy in the definitive or postoperative setting, treatment is delivered daily over 5 weeks to doses of 50.4 Gy for benign meningiomas, 54 Gy for atypical, and 59.4 to 60 Gy for malignant meningiomas. For small meningiomas which do not demonstrate any serial interval change in size and are asymptomatic, observation is a reasonable management option.

ADDITIONAL IMAGES (B–F)

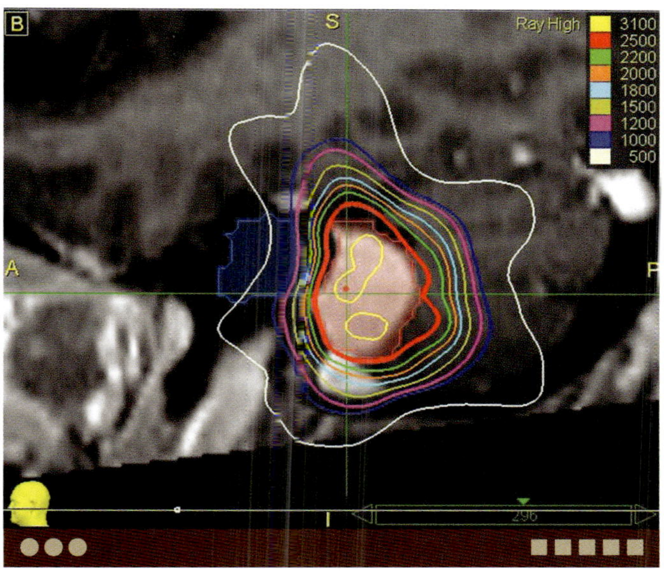

B. Meningioma, sagittal CyberKnife® treatment plan. The red lines indicate the prescription isodose lines, and represent 75% of the central dose. Rapid fall-off of the radiation isodose lines is seen at the left cochlea (shaded blue).

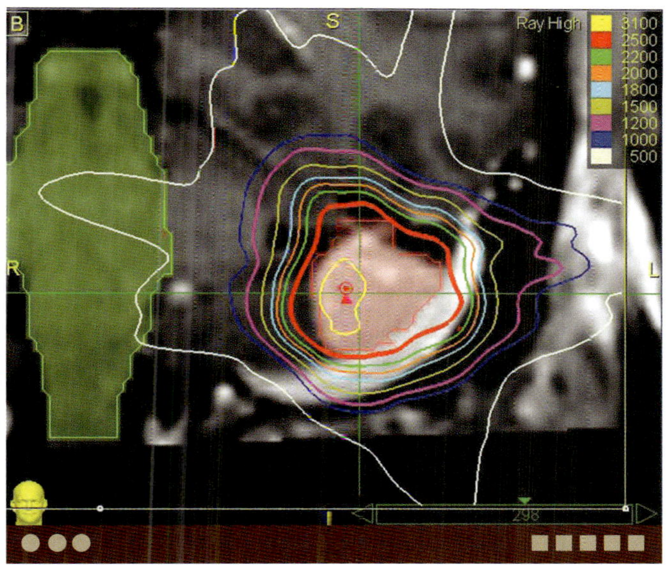

C. Meningioma, coronal CyberKnife® treatment plan. The red line indicates the prescription isodose line, with the maximal dosing being localized over the tumor (shaded red). The conformity index was 1.5, and the brainstem is shaded green demonstrating the rapid fall-off of the isodose lines before reaching the brainstem region.

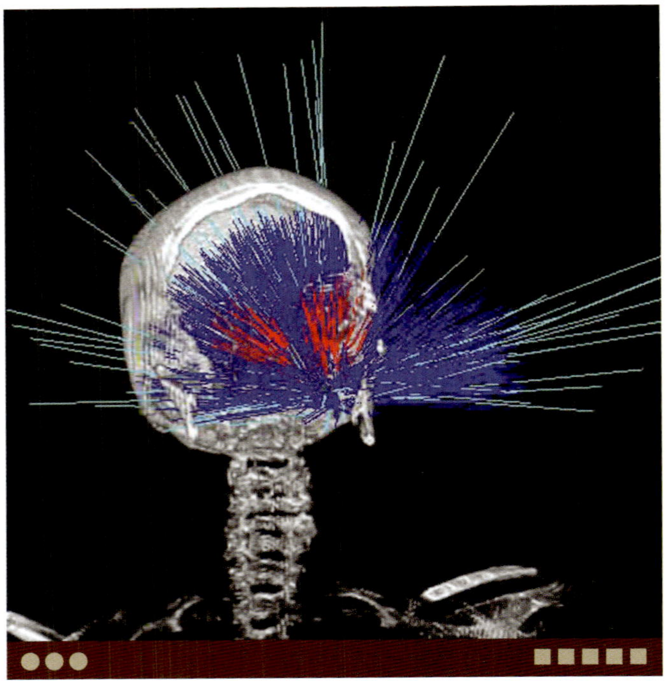

D. Meningioma, three-dimensional x-ray beam projections CyberKnife® treatment plan. In all, 52 nodes and 89 beams were used to deliver the 25 Gy in a dose fractionation scheme of 5 Gy × 5.

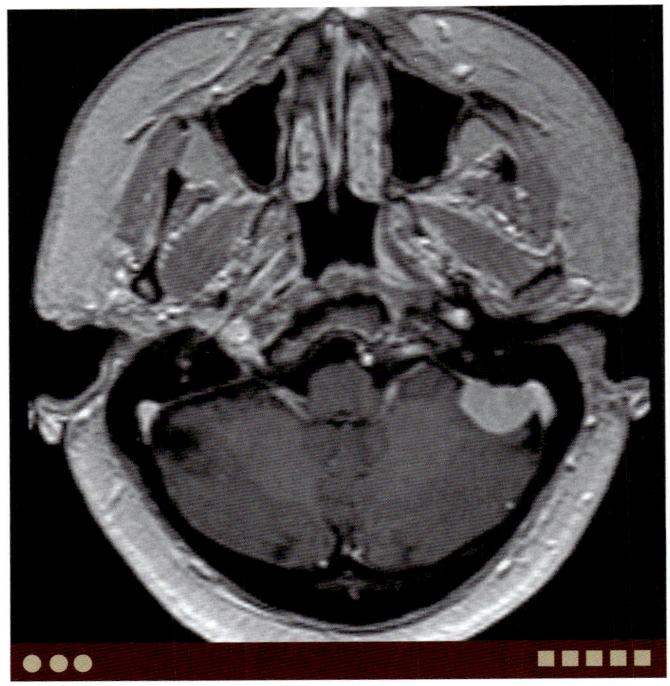

E. Meningioma, same patient as A. Axial postcontrast T1W image demonstrates an extra-axial, well-circumscribed avidly enhancing mass in the left petrous region posterior to the left cerebellopontine angle and adjacent to the left sigmoid sinus with dural-based attachment and a "meningeal tail."

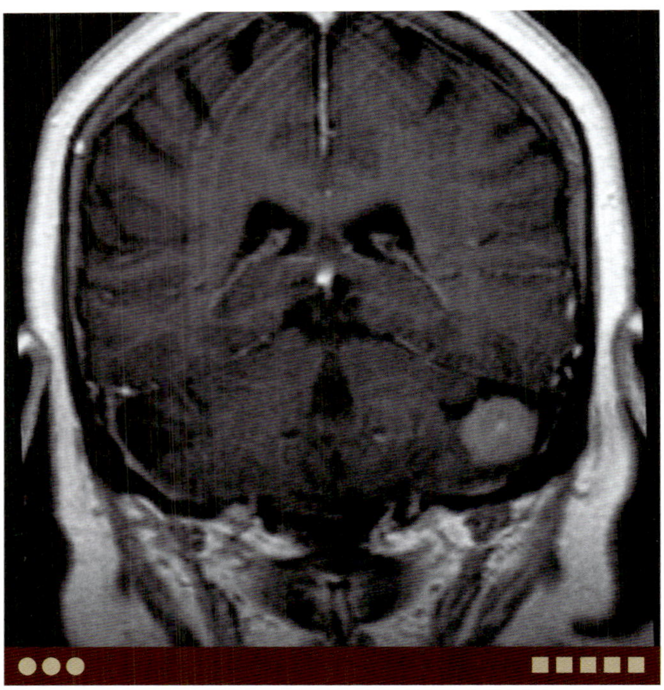

F. Meningioma, same patient as A. Coronal postcontrast T1W image demonstrates a homogeneously enhancing extra-axial left posterior fossa mass with resulting displacement of the left cerebellar hemisphere.

DIFFERENTIAL DIAGNOSIS IMAGES (G-I)

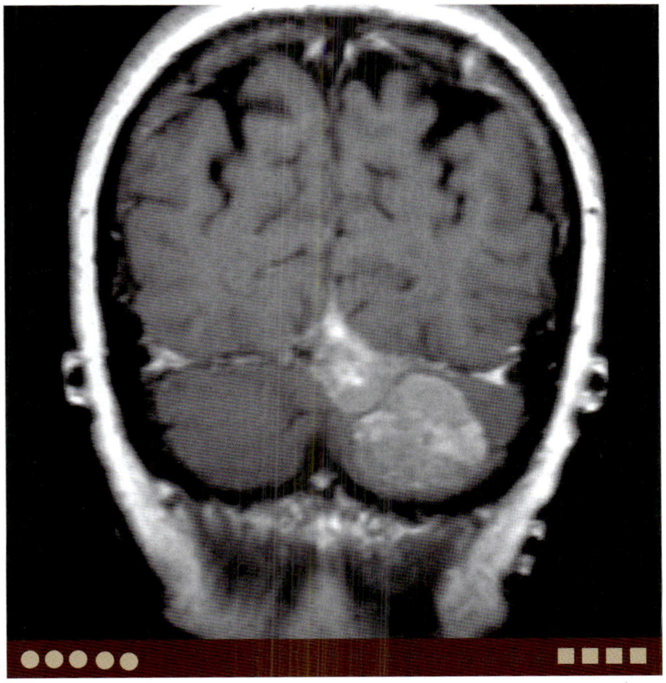

G. Metastasis. Coronal postcontrast T1W image demonstrates a larger intra-axial heterogeneously enhancing left cerebellar hemisphere mass. A smaller, extra-axial, heterogeneously enhancing mass is also seen at the left inferolateral margin of the torcular herophili with meningeal attachment and possible invasion of the sinus.

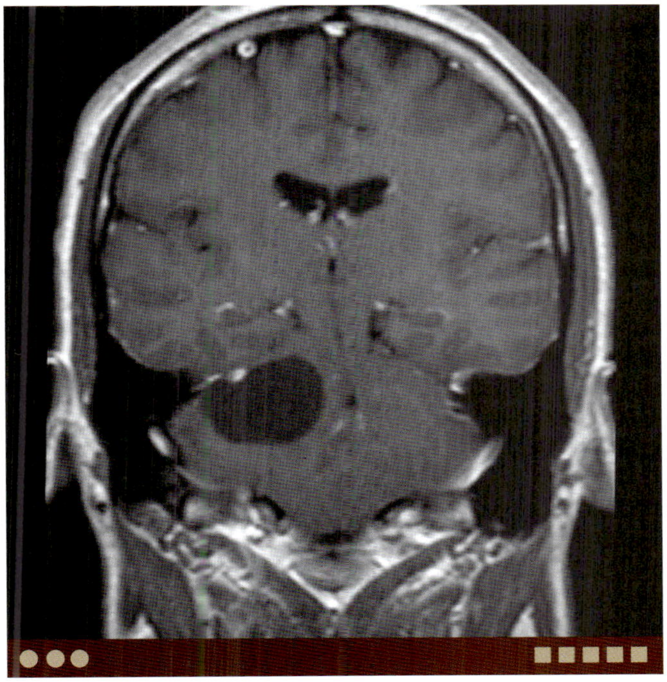

H. Hemangioblastoma. Coronal postcontrast T1W image demonstrates a cystic lesion with a small enhancing mural nodule in the right cerebellar hemisphere.

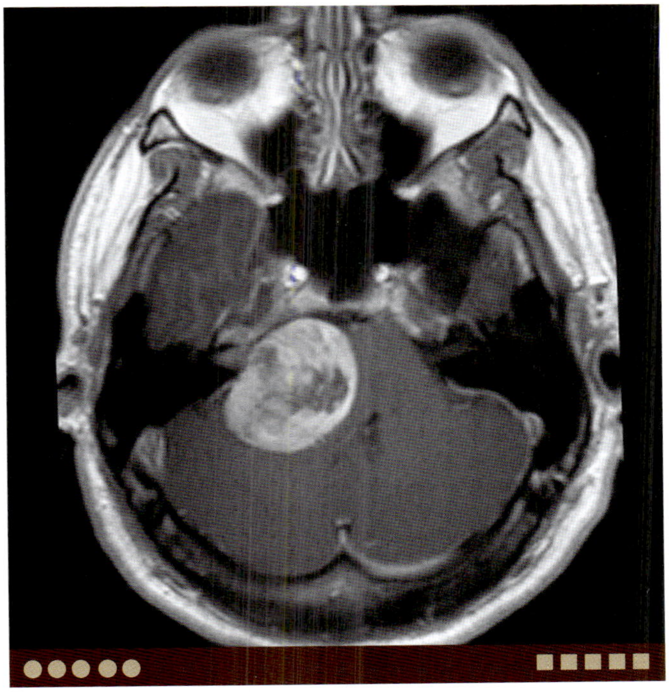

I. Vestibular schwannoma. Axial postcontrast T1W image demonstrates a large heterogeneously enhancing tumor at the right cerebellopontine angle.

Case 15–11 Meningioma: Paracavernous Region

Minh Tam Truong, Paramjit Singh, Osamu Sakai

PRESENTATION

Headaches, cranial neuropathies, focal seizures, slowly progressive neurologic deficits.

FINDINGS

CT and MRI scans demonstrated an enhancing lesion in the cavernous sinus.

DIFFERENTIAL DIAGNOSIS

- Pituitary adenoma: With macroadenomas, patients often present with visual field loss, commonly bitemporal hemianopia, by compression of the optic chiasm, and require decompression surgery. Tumors can also invade into the cavernous sinus resulting in cranial neuropathies of the third, fourth, fifth, and sixth cranial nerves.
- Schwannoma: Schwannoma can arise from the trigeminal nerve and is seen as a spindle or dumbbell-shaped mass; low signal on T1W and intermediate-to-high signal on T2W lesion which demonstrates homogeneous avid enhancement without meningeal tail sign after contrast.
- Metastasis: Metastases seen in the paracavernous region may be metastasis to the pituitary gland, bone metastasis to the clinoid or clivus, or perineural tumor extension most often along the trigeminal nerve.

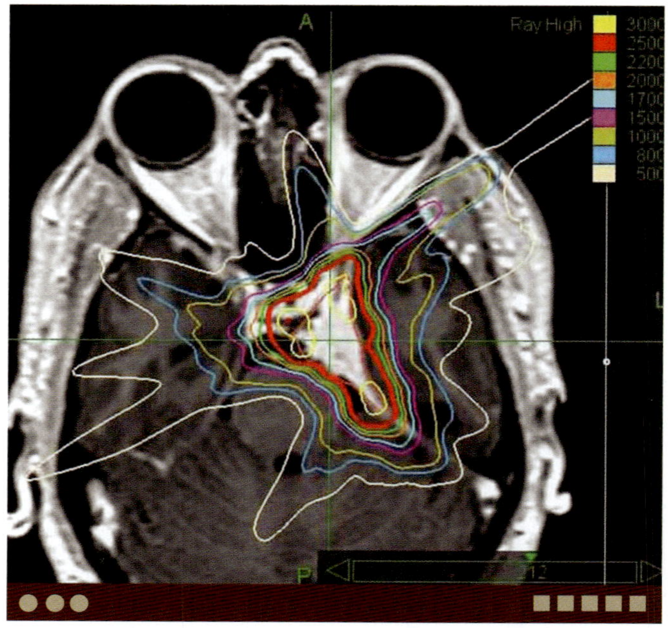

A. Paracavernous meningioma, axial CyberKnife® treatment plan. The red lines indicate the prescription isodose lines, and represent 75% of the central dose. The patient received a total of 25 Gy delivered in a dose fractionation scheme of 5 Gy × 5. Over 99% of the tumor was covered with the rapid fall-off of the radiation isodose lines.

COMMENTS

A 49-year-old woman initially presented with severe bitemporal headaches and left-sided facial numbness. Imaging findings were consistent with a cavernous sinus meningioma. Due to the location of the tumor, in close proximity to the internal carotid artery and cranial nerves traversing the cavernous sinus, and optic apparatus, surgery was not recommended. The patient was treated using hypofractionated stereotactic radiotherapy using the CyberKnife® to a total dose of 25 Gy in five fractions.

Meningiomas account for roughly 15% of all primary intracranial tumors. Meningiomas arise from arachnoid cap cells and are benign, slow growing, well-circumscribed solid tumors that occasionally contain a necrotic, cystic, or calcified component. Cavernous sinus meningiomas pose a unique therapeutic challenge due to the location and often making complete surgically extirpation difficult due to intimate proximity to cranial nerves and blood vessels.

On CT and MRI, meningiomas appear as well-circumscribed, avidly enhancing tumors which if large can cause substantial perilesional vasogenic edema. Postcontrast MRI may also

PEARLS

- **Meningiomas are slow growing, benign tumors that arise from arachnoid cap cells in the meninges.**
- **CT and MRI demonstrate avidly enhancing, well-circumscribed tumors that may have a characteristic "meningeal tail."**
- **Stereotactic radiosurgery and fractionated radiotherapy offers comparable local control rates with radiosurgery most effective for tumors less than 3 cm and/or for tumors in surgically inaccessible locations and fractionated radiotherapy for large tumors or patients with residual tumor after surgery.**
- **Cavernous sinus meningiomas may cause cranial nerve deficits, since cranial nerves III, IV, V, and VI traverse the cavernous sinus and are often difficult to achieve a complete resection.**
- **Treatment with stereotactic radiosurgery or fractionated stereotactic radiotherapy offers high rates of local control to these tumors while sparing adjacent critical normal tissue.**

reveal an associated "meningeal tail." Angiography may be useful for preoperative planning and embolization.

Treatment options for meningioma include observation, surgical resection, stereotactic radiosurgery, or fractionated radiotherapy. Surgical access to the cavernous sinus is often difficult due to the proximity of cranial nerves and carotid artery, optic structures. Fractionated stereotactic radiotherapy can deliver highly conformal treatment while sparing adjacent normal tissue. This may be done over 5 weeks to doses of 50.4 Gy in 28 fractions. Stereotactic radiosurgery may be considered as the initial and definitive form of tumor control for tumors less than 3 cm, or if the tumor is in an inaccessible location, or if the surgery carries a high risk of morbidity. Hypofractionated CyberKnife® radiosurgery may be used in 3-5 fractions offering similar local control rates and sparing of adjacent critical structures.

ADDITIONAL IMAGES (B-G)

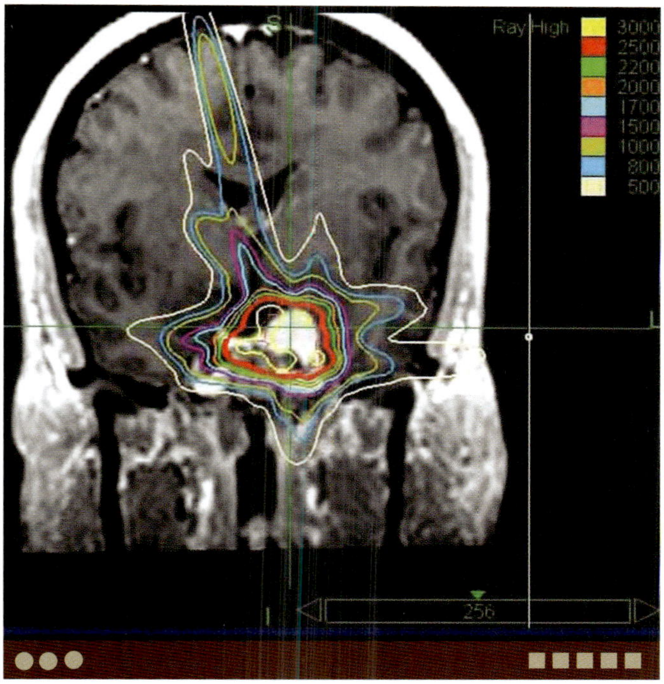

B. Paracavernous meningioma, coronal CyberKnife® treatment plan. The red lines indicate the prescription isodose lines, and represent 75% of the central dose. Rapid fall-off of the radiation isodose lines is seen.

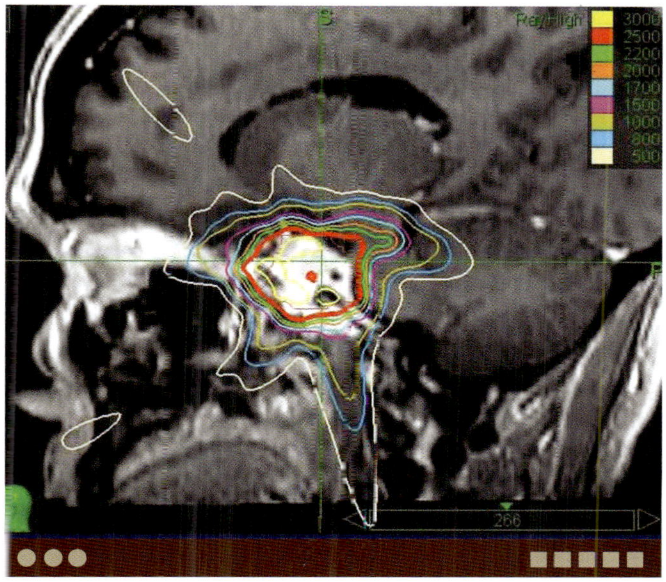

C. Paracavernous meningioma, sagittal CyberKnife® treatment plan. The red line indicates the prescription isodose line, with the maximal dosing being localized over the tumor (shaded red). The conformity index was 1.5.

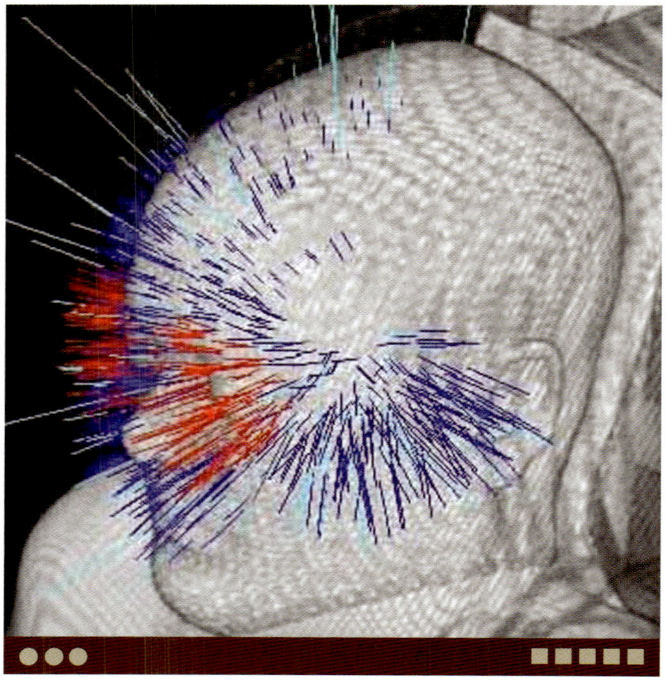

D. Paracavernous meningioma, three-dimensional x-ray beam projections CyberKnife® treatment plan. In all, 52 nodes and 89 beams were used to deliver the 25 Gy in a dose fractionation scheme of 5 Gy × 5.

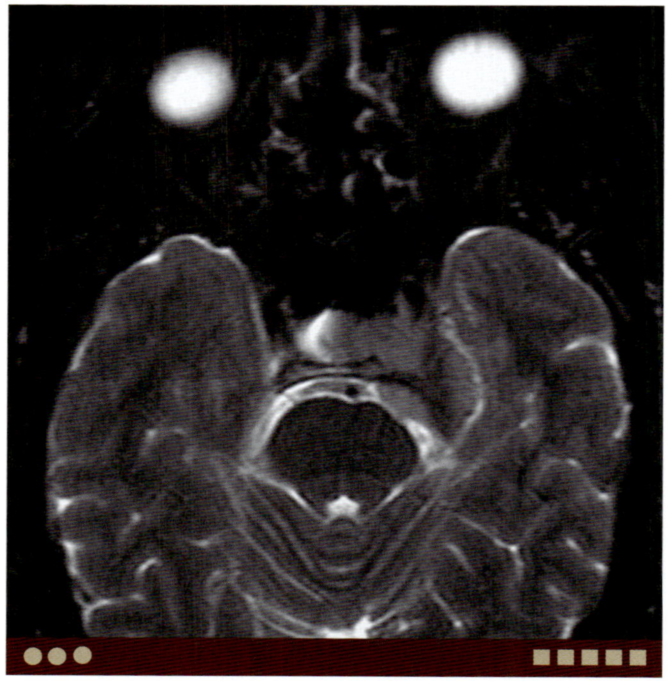

E. Paracavernous meningioma, same patient as A. Axial T2W image demonstrates a dural-based intermediate-signal lesion in the left paracavernous region.

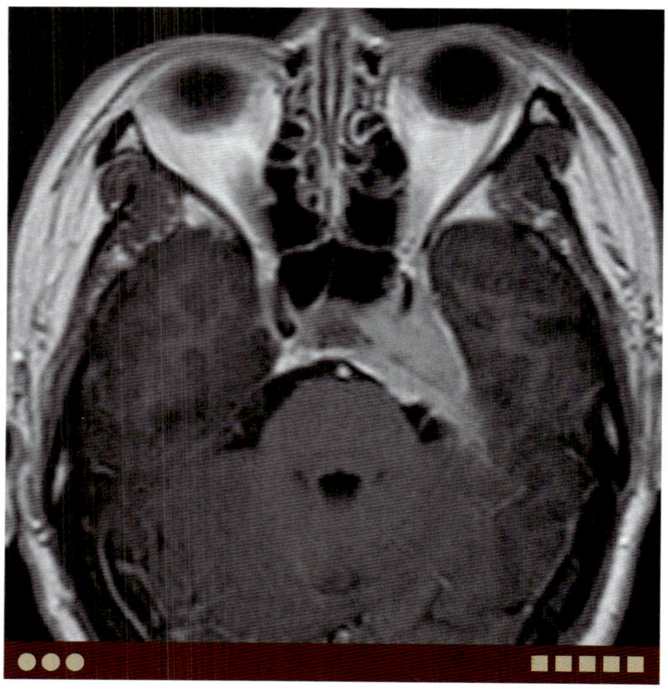

F. Paracavernous meningioma, same patient as A. Axial postcontrast T1W image demonstrates avid, homogeneous enhancement of the lesion along the dura and cerebellar tentorium.

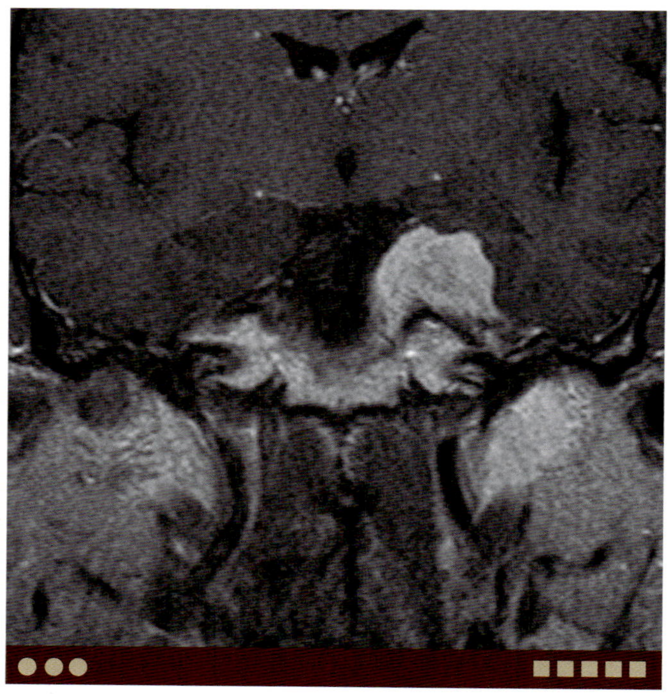

G. Paracavernous meningioma, same patient as A. Coronal postcontrast T1W image demonstrates avid, homogeneous enhancement of the lesion along the dura and cerebellar tentorium.

DIFFERENTIAL DIAGNOSIS IMAGES (H-J)

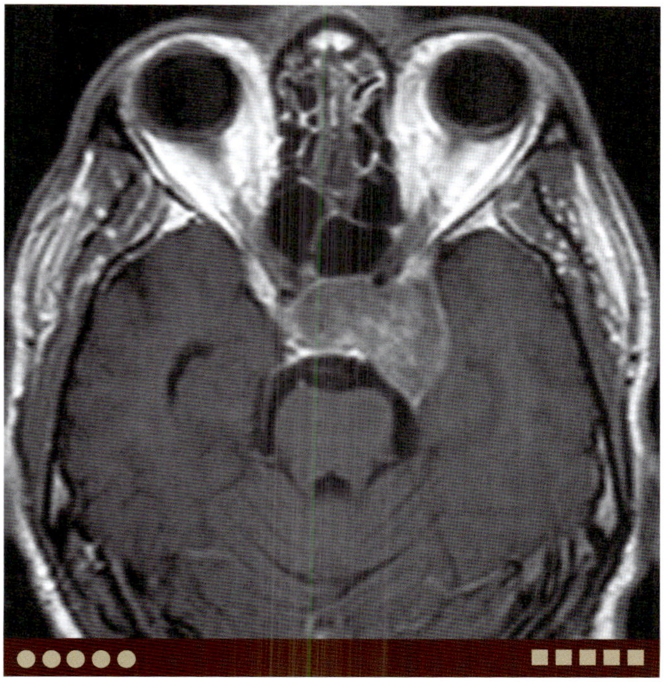

H. Pituitary adenoma. Axial postcontrast T1W image demonstrates a mildly enhancing lesion centered in the sella extending to the left paracavernous region, displacing the left internal carotid artery anteriorly.

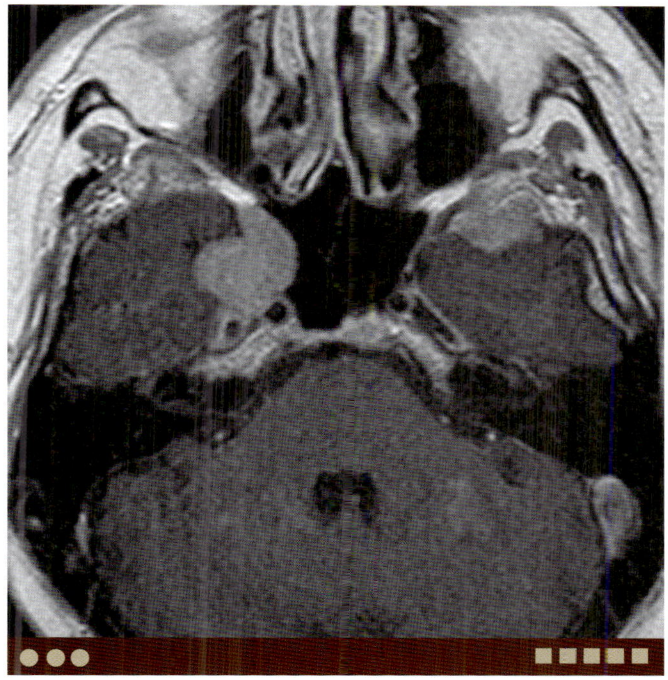

I. Trigeminal schwannoma. Axial postcontrast T1W image demonstrates a homogeneously enhancing lobulated lesion in the right paracavernous region without meningeal tail sign.

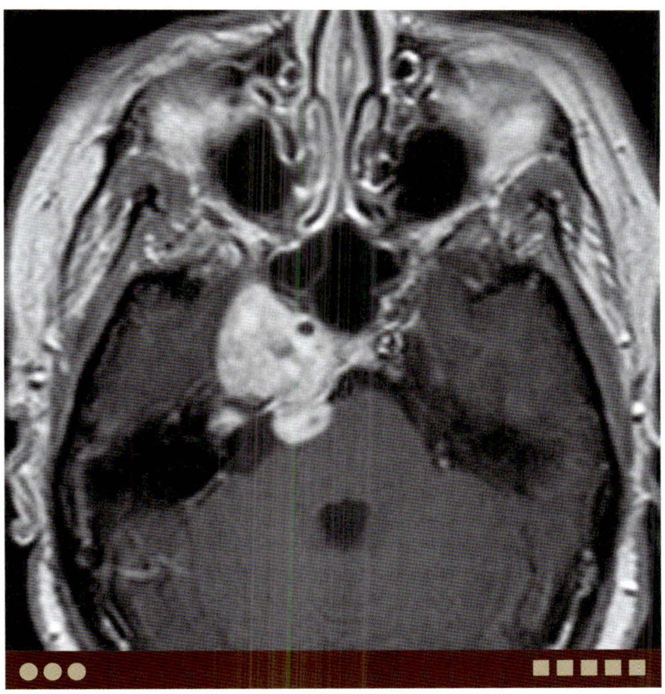

J. Perineural tumor spread, adenoid cystic carcinoma of the parotid gland. Axial postcontrast T1W image demonstrates a heterogeneously enhancing lobulated lesion in the right paracavernous region along the course of the trigeminal nerve, invading the right cavernous sinus.

Case 15–12 Arteriovenous Malformation

Mayur Jayarao, Minh Tam Truong, Kurtis G. Birch, Lawrence Chin

PRESENTATION

Facial and retromandibular pain associated with orofacial dyskinesias (Meige syndrome).

FINDINGS

MRI/MRA of the head demonstrates a tangle of tortuous abnormal vessels in the cerebellum.

DIFFERENTIAL DIAGNOSIS

- Cavernous malformation: Consists of enlarged capillaries and are generally not associated with enlarged feeding arteries or veins. Their hallmark on MRI is the presence of blood products of various ages from prior microhemorrhages. Cerebral angiograms demonstrate no abnormalities and surgical resection is the treatment of choice for symptomatic patients.
- Developmental venous anomaly: This is the commonest intracranial vascular anomaly that consists of an enlarged collection of veins and may be found associated with a cavernous malformation. The veins appear as a radial arrangement that converge on a central venous trunk, which gives them the pathognomic "hydra" or caput medusae appearance. Surgical management is considered only for lesions that have ruptured.
- Capillary telangiectasia: These are characterized by the presence of capillary vessels with saccular or fusiform dilations. They are almost always clinically silent. Faint enhancement is seen on MRI without other signal abnormality, although very subtle signal change may be seen on T2W images.
- Cerebral aneurysm: Aneurysms are classified as saccular, fusiform, or dissecting aneurysms. CTA and MRA can demonstrate the aneurysm, but angiography is the gold standard. Treatment options vary from serial monitoring of very small incidentally found aneurysms to endovascular coiling and surgical clipping for larger aneurysms. The choice between coiling and clipping depends upon patient's age and preference, aneurysm location, size, and its angiographic characteristics.

COMMENTS

A 33-year-old right-handed male with a history of a left cerebellar arteriovenous malformation (AVM) presented with facial and retromandibular pain associated with orofacial dyskinesias (Meige syndrome). Physical examination was noncontributory. MRA demonstrated a tangle of tortuous abnormal vessels in the left cerebellar hemisphere. Cerebral angiography revealed a left posteromedial cerebellar hemisphere AVM (Spetzler-Martin grade III) with a 2.5 cm compact nidus. The patient was offered management by surgical resection, radiosurgery, endovascular embolization. The patient elected to undergo CyberKnife® robotic radiosurgery and received 20 Gy in a single treatment dose.

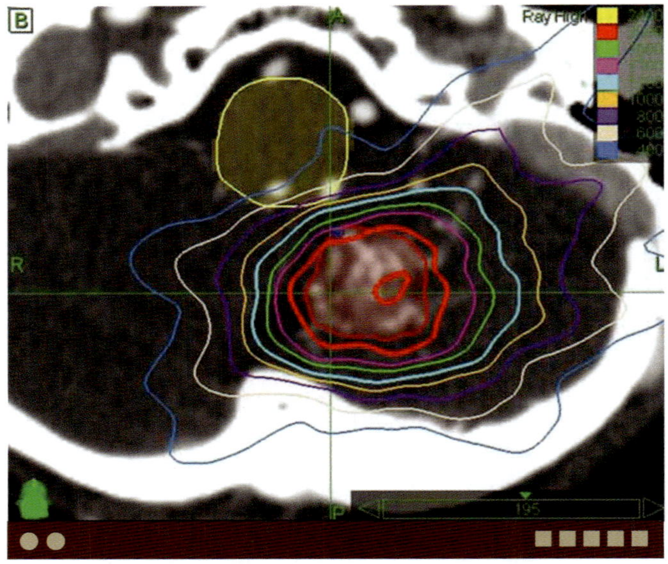

A. AVM, axial CyberKnife® treatment plan. The red lines indicate the prescription isodose lines, and represent 73% of the central dose. The patient received a total of 20 Gy delivered in a single dose. Over 98% of the tumor was covered with the rapid fall-off of the radiation isodose lines seen on the brainstem side (shaded yellow).

PEARLS

- **AVMs are congenital vascular lesions of arteries and veins that conglomerate at their nidus.**
- **CT and MRI provide information regarding AVM location and size, but catheter angiogram is the gold standard.**
- **Treatment options for AVMs include total surgical resection, endovascular embolization, and stereotactic radiosurgery.**
- **All treatment options can lead to curative outcomes, but stereotactic radiosurgery is best reserved for AVMs less than 3 cm with a compact nidus and in areas of eloquence.**

AVMs are congenital vascular lesions that result in an aberrant complex mass of tangled arteries and veins connected by one or more fistulas. The conglomerate of vessels is called the nidus, where feeding arteries drain directly into veins at a high velocity, thereby causing the veins to dilate. AVMs cause neurological dysfunction through hemorrhage, seizures, or the "steal phenomenon." Symptoms vary based on location, and approximately 12% of patients with AVMs become symptomatic, with hemorrhage being the commonest presentation. The overall risk for hemorrhage in patients with AVMs is 2% to 4% per year.

AVMs are graded using the Spetzler-Martin grade, and may be treated by surgical resection, endovascular embolization, or stereotactic radiosurgery. While these options may be considered individually for treatment, frequently a combined treatment approach is used for large lesions. Total surgical resection is most effective for small, easily accessible AVMs with low procedural risk, and can lead to a cure. Likewise, the goal of endovascular embolization is complete AVM occlusion, although for large AVMs, embolization may not be completely successful. Embolization can serve as a palliative treatment option for AVMs too large for either surgery or stereotactic radiosurgery. Embolization is also effective for reducing the size and flow through the AVM nidus, thus making surgical resection safer. Stereotactic radiosurgery is best reserved for AVMs less than 3 cm with a compact nidus and in an eloquent region of the brain where surgery cannot be safely performed. The drawback of stereotactic radiosurgery in the treatment of AVMs is the long latency (1-3 years) required to obtain complete luminal obliteration, during which period the patient is at risk for hemorrhage. Complication rates from stereotactic radiosurgery are proportionate to dose and volume, larger AVMs may require staged radiosurgery procedure or may be combined with embolization to reduce the risk of radiation-induced edema or complications. Some recent data indicate that the risk of hemorrhage is reduced during this latent period. Stereotactic radiosurgery using doses of at least 20 Gy for AVMs offers greater than 80% obliteration rate of the AVM at 3 years.

ADDITIONAL IMAGES (B-H)

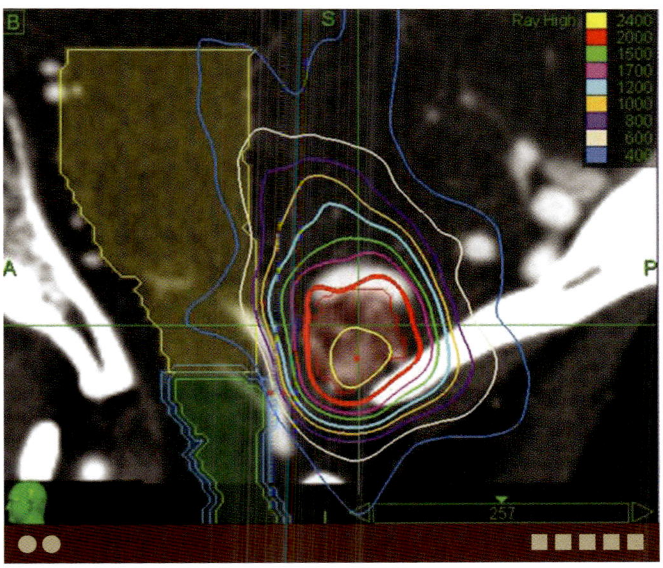

B. AVM, sagittal CyberKnife® treatment plan. The red lines indicate the prescription isodose lines, and represent 73% of the central dose. Rapid fall-off of the isodose lines can be seen at the brainstem (shaded yellow) and cervical spinal cord (shaded green).

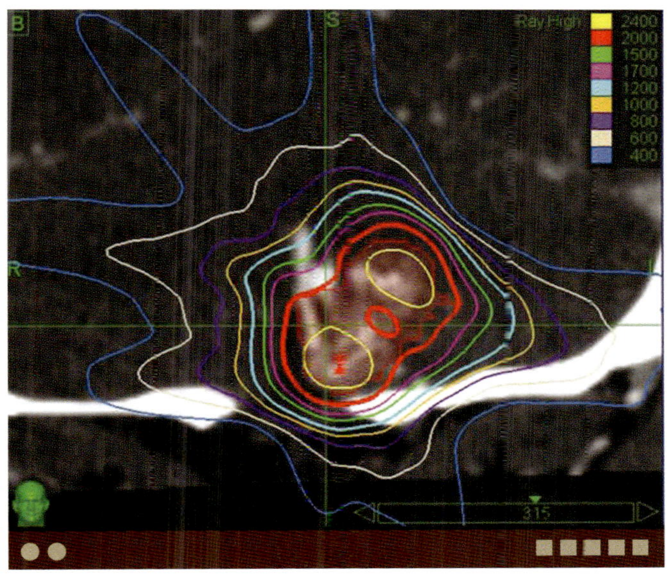

C. AVM, coronal CyberKnife® treatment plan. The red line indicates the prescription isodose line with the maximal dosing being localized over the nidus. The conformity index was 1.53.

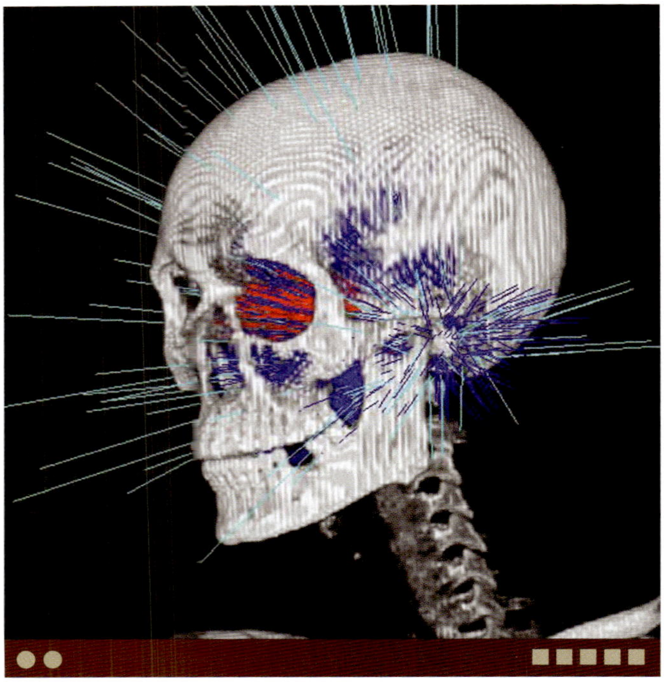

D. AVM, three-dimensional x-ray beam projections, CyberKnife® treatment plan. In all, 78 nodes and 133 beams were used to deliver the 20-Gy dose in a single treatment.

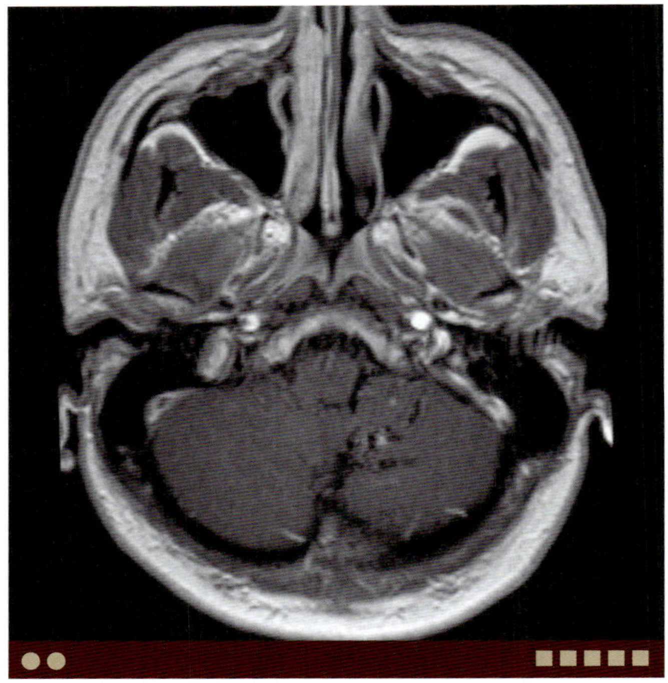

E. AVM, same patient as A. Axial postcontrast T1W image demonstrates a tangle of tortuous abnormal vessels in the inferomedial portion of the left cerebellar hemisphere.

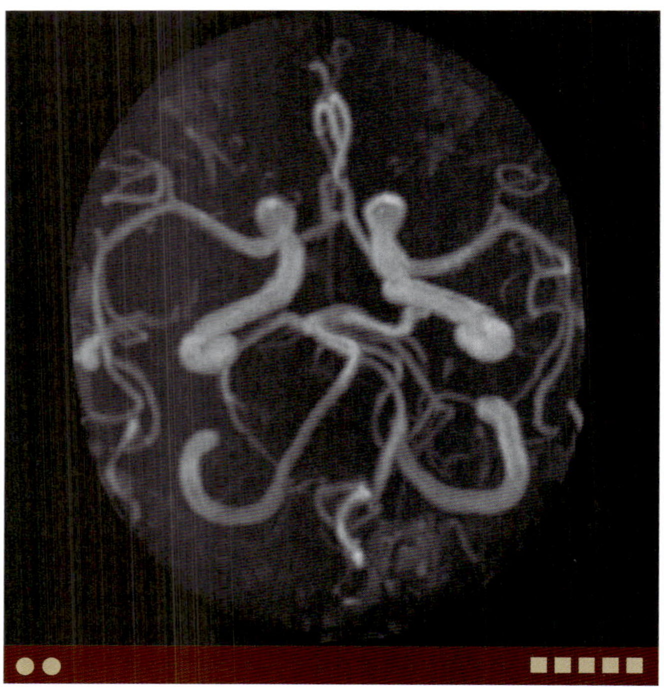

F. AVM, same patient as A. 3D-TOF MRA MIP image demonstrates the AVM with its nidus. The nidus can be seen being fed by the distal feeders of the left posterior inferior cerebellar artery.

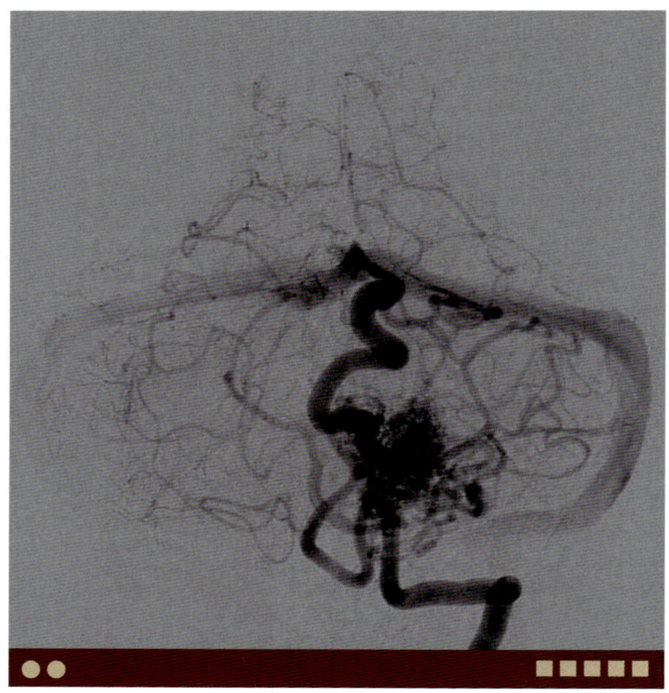

G. AVM, same patient as A. Frontal projection of left vertebral angiogram reveals the nidus of the AVM and its arterial feeders. There is preferential drainage to the left transverse sinus. The Spetzler-Martin grade is III.

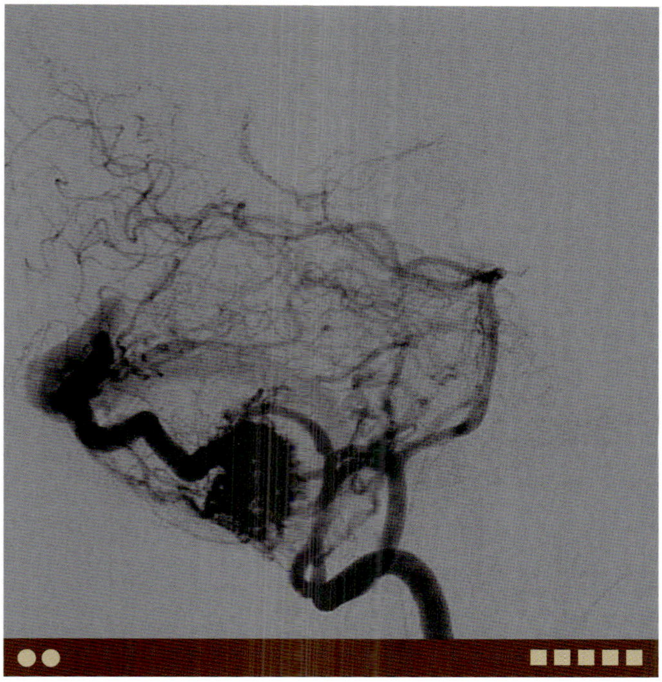

H. AVM, same patient as A. Lateral projection of left vertebral artery angiogram reveals the AVM being fed by the left posterior inferior cerebellar artery. Venous drainage of the AVM is well appreciated with a large cerebellar superficial draining vein into the torcular heterophili.

DIFFERENTIAL DIAGNOSIS IMAGES (I-J)

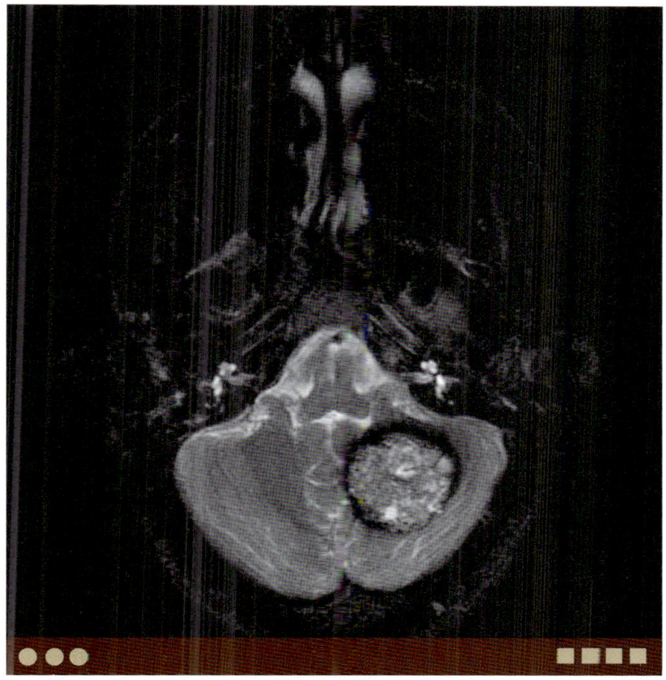

I. Cavernous malformation. Axial T2W MR image demonstrates a mass with hemosiderin rim in the left cerebellar hemisphere. Areas of high T2 signal within the lesion are suggestive of more recent blood products.

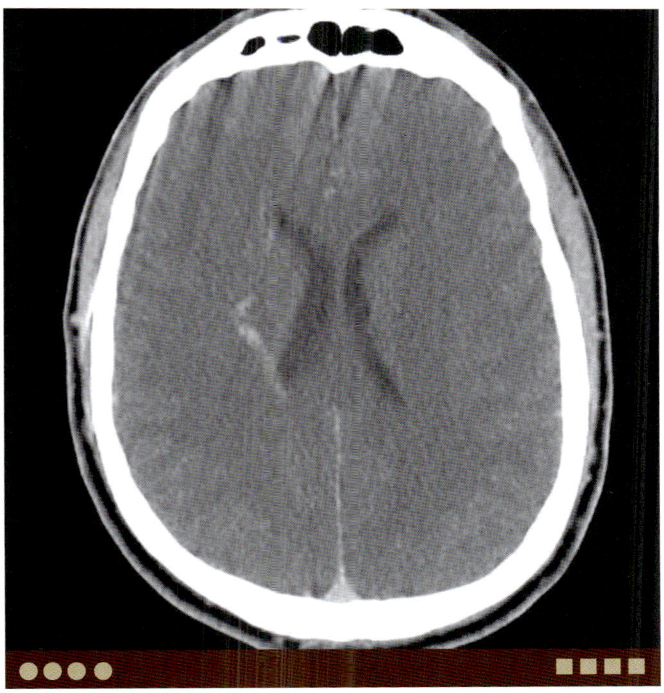

J. Developmental venous anomaly. Axial contrast-enhanced CT demonstrates liner hyperdensity that appears to be draining laterally in the right frontoparietal region.

Case 15–13 Hemangioblastoma

Mayur Jayarao, Minh Tam Truong, Kurtis G. Birch, Lawrence Chin

PRESENTATION

Worsening headache and unsteady gait for 2 weeks.

FINDINGS

CT and MRI demonstrate an avidly enhancing tumor in the cerebellum, often with a large cystic component.

DIFFERENTIAL DIAGNOSIS

- Metastasis: Metastases are the most common intracranial tumors. Lesions are often seen at the gray-white matter junction, however, they can occur anywhere in the brain, including the pia and dura. In general, up to three lesions, each with a maximal diameter of 3 cm are effectively treated by stereotactic radiosurgery, but there are no absolute guidelines regarding size and number.
- Meningioma: This is the most common benign, intracranial, extra-axial tumor. A well-circumscribed and noninfiltrative extra-axial tumor with homogeneous avid enhancement and "meningeal tail" is a characteristic fining. Total surgical resection offers the best chance for a cure with radiosurgery being performed primarily to control tumor growth either pre- or postoperatively. In some patients, radiosurgery can serve as the primary treatment for a meningioma in lieu of surgery.
- Medulloblastoma: This malignant tumor usually arises from the roof of the fourth ventricle, and often demonstrates heterogeneous enhancement on MRI. Calcification is rarely seen. CSF dissemination, "drop metastasis" commonly occurs. Treatment options include surgery, chemotherapy, and radiation, with craniospinal irradiation and posterior cranial fossa boost.
- Ependymoma: When intracranial, these generally arise within the fourth ventricle and in ~50%, demonstrate signal heterogeneity, which may indicate calcification, necrosis, blood products or tumor vascularity. Total surgical resection offers the best chance of a cure with postoperative radiation being primarily reserved for patients with WHO grade II or higher ependymomas.

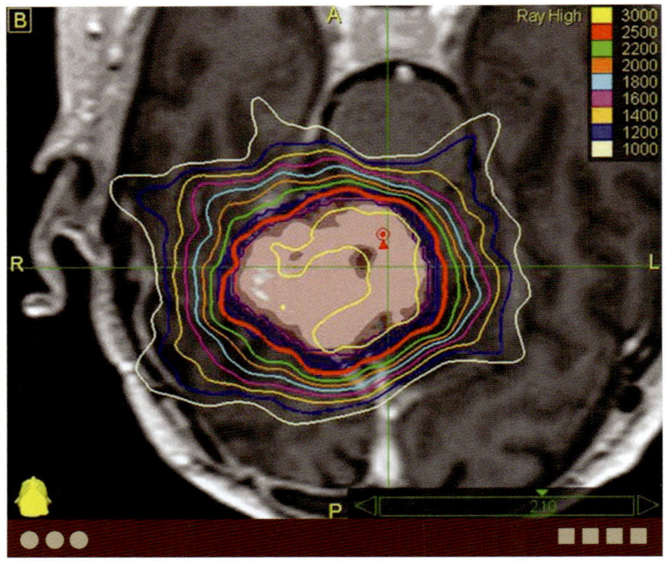

A. Hemangioblastoma, axial CyberKnife® treatment plan. The red line indicates the prescription isodose line, which represents 73% of the central dose. The patient received a total of 25 Gy delivered in a dose fractionation scheme of 5 Gy × 5. Over 99% of the tumor was covered by a dose of 25 Gy with the rapid fall-off of the radiation isodose lines seen on the brainstem side.

COMMENTS

A 53-year-old woman presented with worsening headaches and difficulty ambulating for 2 weeks. Her physical examination was significant for right upper extremity coarse tremor and gait ataxia. She underwent preoperative angiography with embolization and subsequent staged surgical debulking of the mass. Postoperatively, she received CyberKnife® robotic radiosurgery to the residual tumor with a dose of 25 Gy (in a dose fractionation scheme of 5 Gy × 5) at the 73% prescription isodose line.

Hemangioblastomas are benign tumors most commonly found in the posterior cranial fossa. The usual age at

PEARLS

- **Hemangioblastomas are commonly seen in the posterior cranial fossa in adults.**
- **A cystic lesion with an avidly enhancing mural nodule surrounded by flow-voids is characteristic of a hemangioblastoma.**
- **Total resection is the treatment of the choice in most cases, with residual tumor control achieved by postoperative radiosurgery.**
- **Stereotactic radiosurgery can be the initial and definitive treatment choice if the tumor is less than 3 cm in diameter and if the location makes surgical resection difficult. Care must be taken during dose planning in order to avoid or minimize damage to the adjacent brainstem.**

diagnosis is between the third and fifth decades. In about 25% of cases they are associated with von Hippel-Lindau (VHL) disease; the genetic hallmark of which is the loss of function of the VHL tumor suppressor gene on chromosome 3p25-26. Pathological gross examination usually reveals a tumor that does not have a capsule, is cherry red in color, and may include a cyst that contains clear or xanthochromic fluid.

Hemangioblastoma is seen as a well-circumscribed, solid, or cystic mass, with an avidly enhancing mural nodule. MRI may demonstrate serpentine signal voids, which represent dilated vessels. A cystic lesion with an enhancing mural nodule surrounded by flow-voids is characteristic of a hemangioblastoma.

Preoperative angiography remains important for defining feeding vessels and embolization. Hemangioblastoma patients can be cured by total excision and therefore surgery should be considered in all patients except in whom the risks outweigh the benefits. In these patients, radiosurgery can be considered, especially in those with tumors less than 3 cm in diameter and if the tumor is in a location that precludes surgical resection. Adjusting the dose in order to minimize radiation to the critical structures of the posterior fossa such as the brainstem must be taken into account during planning of stereotactic radiosurgery. For patients with tumors greater than 3 cm, who are not operable candidates, conventionally fractionated radiotherapy over 5 weeks is recommended.

ADDITIONAL IMAGES (B-G)

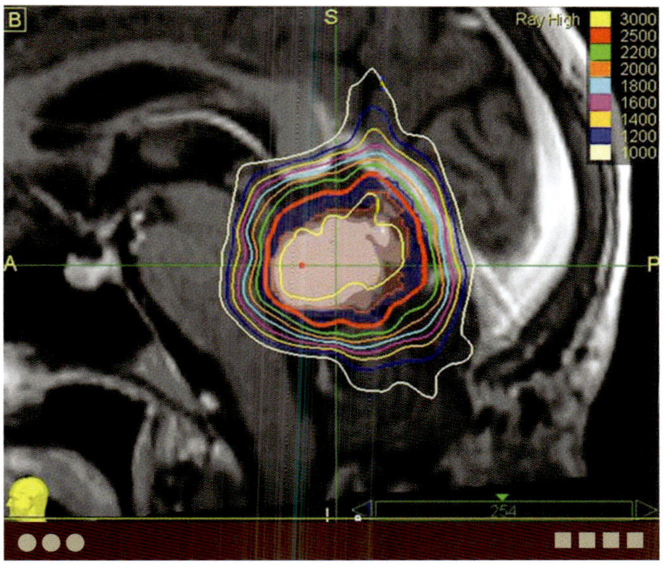

B. Hemangioblastoma, sagittal CyberKnife® treatment plan. The red line indicates the prescription isodose line, which represents 73% of the central dose. Rapid fall-off of the radiation isodose lines can be appreciated on the brainstem side.

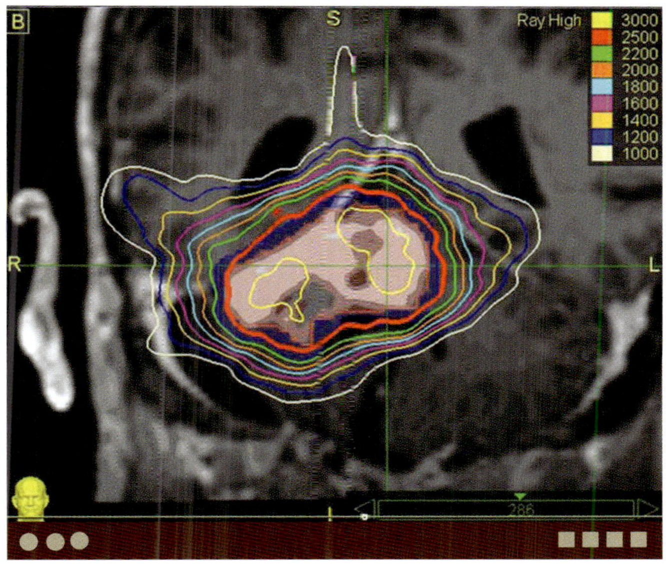

C. Hemangioblastoma, coronal CyberKnife® treatment plan. The red line indicates the 73% prescription isodose line, and the conformity index was 1.5. Rapid fall-off of the radiation isodose lines can be appreciated both supra- and infratentorially.

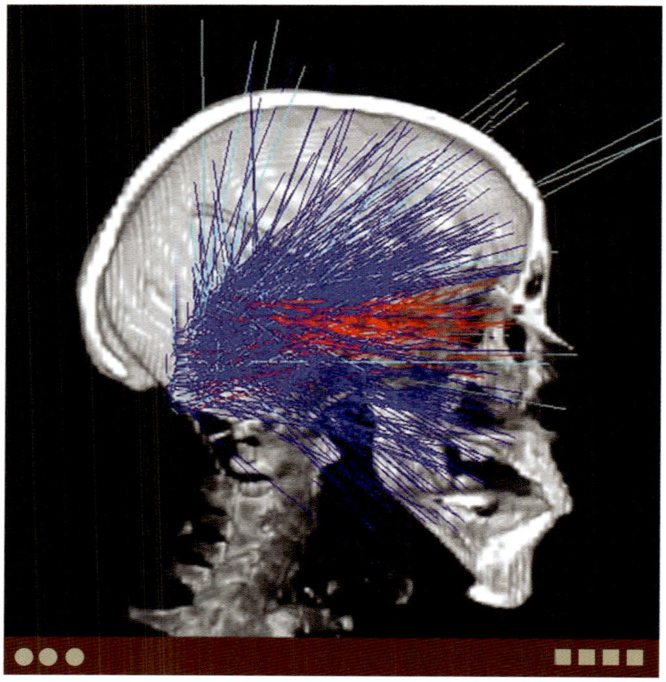

D. Hemangioblastoma, three-dimensional x-ray beam projections CyberKnife® treatment plan. In all, 74 nodes and 125 beams were used to deliver the 25-Gy dose in a dose fractionation scheme of 5 Gy × 5.

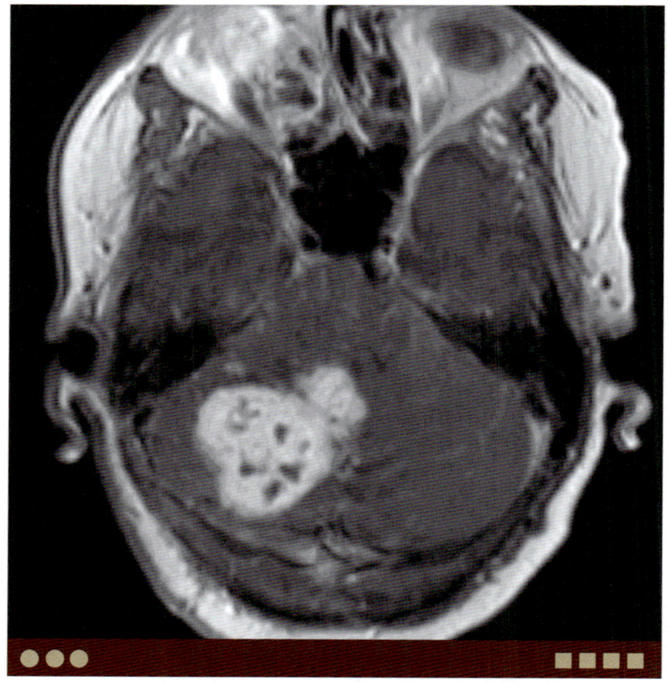

E. Hemangioblastoma, same patient as A. Axial postcontrast T1W image demonstrates a large heterogeneously enhancing tumor in the right cerebellum. Multifocal areas of fluid signal within the tumor are suggestive of cystic degeneration and/or necrosis. Associated signal voids within the lesion represent dilated afferent and/or efferent vessels.

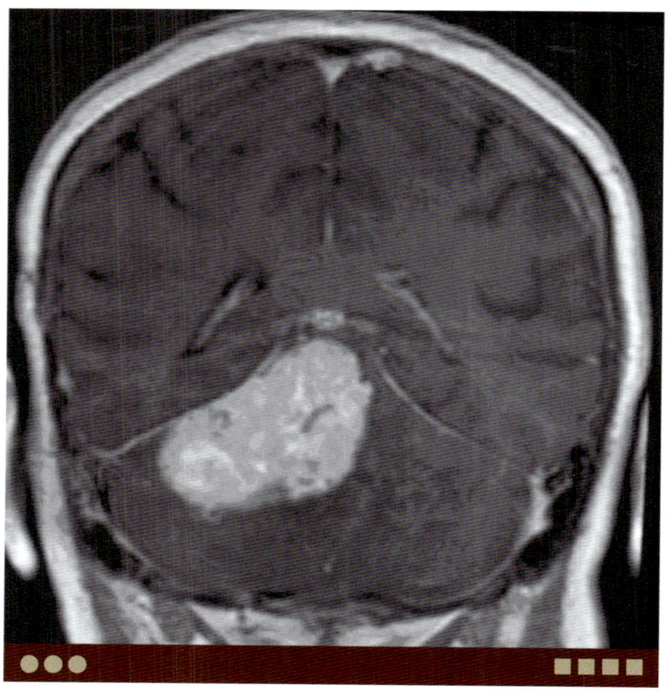

F. Hemangioblastoma, same patient as A. Coronal postcontrast T1W image demonstrates a large heterogeneously enhancing tumor in the right cerebellum. Note the upward displacement of the tentorium secondary to mass effect.

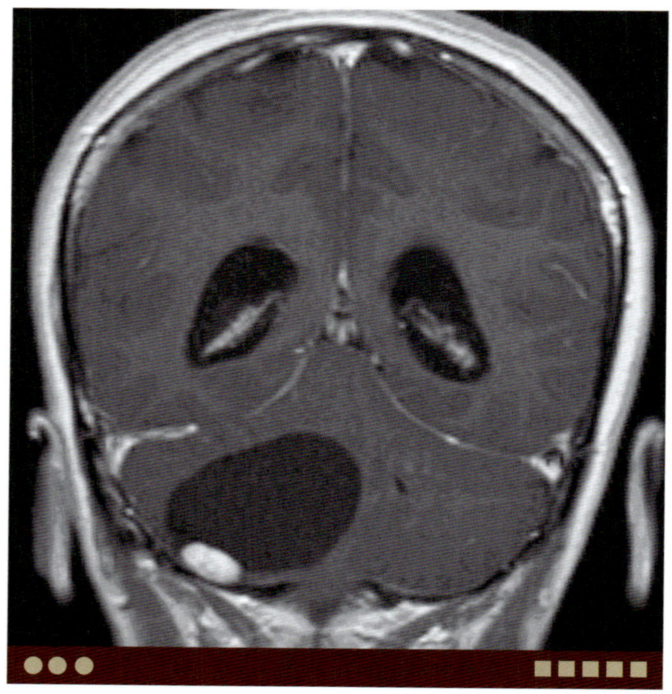

G. Hemangioblastoma in a different patient. Coronal postcontrast T1W image demonstrates a large cystic lesion with an avidly enhancing mural nodule in the right cerebellum.

DIFFERENTIAL DIAGNOSIS IMAGES (H-I)

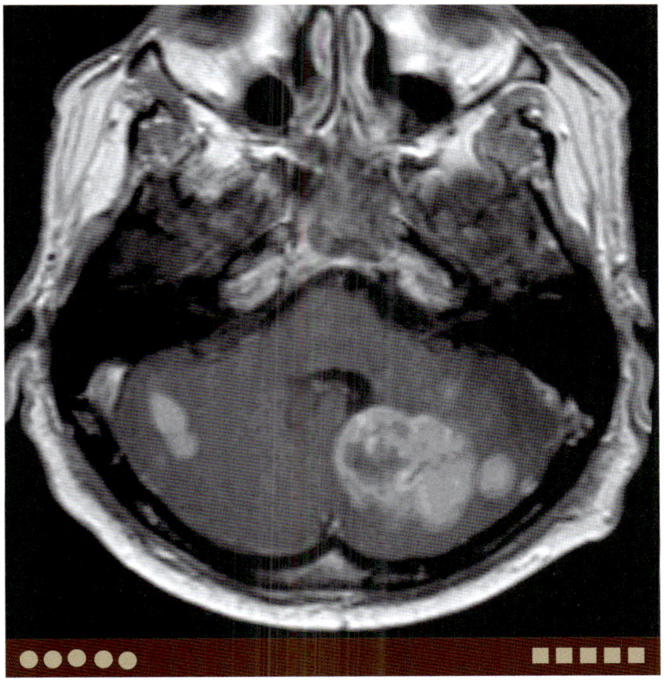

H. Metastasis. Axial postcontrast T1W image demonstrates a large heterogeneously enhancing left cerebellar lesion with multiple smaller lesions in the bilateral cerebellar hemispheres.

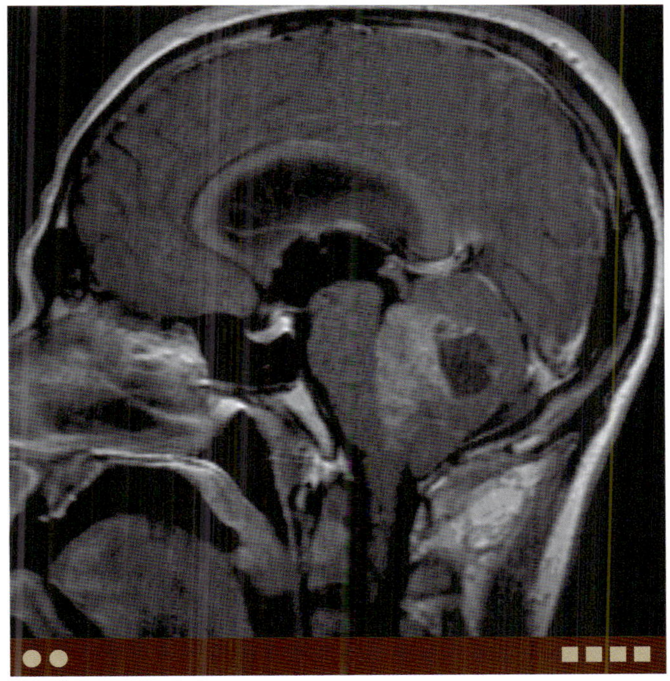

I. Medulloblastoma. Sagittal postcontrast T1W image demonstrates a large heterogeneously enhancing, solid and cystic mass which occupies and obstructs the IV ventricle, resulting obstructive hydrocephalus. Note the downward displacement of the cerebellar tonsils secondary to mass effect.

INDEX

O

R